Health Promotion Guide Charts

For a comprehensive list of additional Charts, Research Applicatio[…] Pathways, and Client Care Plans, see pp xviii–xxvi.

Universal Precautions

Universal precautions are intended to prevent parenteral, mucous membrane, and nonintact skin exposures of health care workers to blood-borne pathogens. Universal precautions apply to blood and to other body fluids containing visible blood, semen, vaginal secretions, cerebrospinal fluid, synovial fluid, pleural fluid, peritoneal fluid, pericardial fluid, and amniotic fluid. Universal precautions do not apply to feces, nasal secretions, sputum, sweat, tears, urine, and vomitus unless they contain visible blood.

Barrier Guidelines

1. Disposable gloves (vinyl, latex) should be worn when in contact or when there is potential for contact with blood, body fluids, or other fluids that may contain human immunodeficiency virus (HIV). Gloves should be removed after each client contact. Rubber gloves can be used for equipment cleaning.
2. Hands should be washed between clients, after any exposure, and after removal of gloves.
3. Protective eyewear, face shields, and/or masks should be worn during procedures that may aerosolize blood.
4. Impervious gowns should be worn when there is potential for exposure to large quantities of blood, such as in the labor and delivery area or emergency room.

Needle Precautions

1. Needles should never be recapped after use; keep in mind that most needlesticks are the result of missed needle recapping.
2. Do not cut, break, or bend needles after use; this may release aerosolized blood from the needle shaft.
3. Do not leave used needles lying around.
4. Do not dispose of needles in ordinary receptacles; instead, use appropriately labeled, impermeable needle containers.

Adapted from the Centers for Disease Control (1988). Update: Universal precautions for prevention of transmission of human immunodeficiency virus, hepatitis B virus, and other bloodborne pathogens in health-care setting. *Morbidity and Mortality Weekly Report,* 37(3), 377–388.

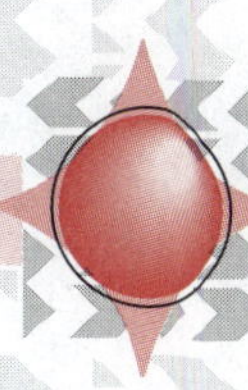

2nd Edition

MEDICAL-SURGICAL NURSING:

A NURSING PROCESS APPROACH

- Donna D. Ignatavicius, MS, RNC
- M. Linda Workman, PhD, RN, FAAN, OCN
- Mary A. Mishler, MSN, RNCS, CNN

Volume 1

W.B. SAUNDERS COMPANY

A Division of Harcourt Brace & Company

Philadelphia • London • Toronto • Montreal • Sydney • Tokyo

W.B. SAUNDERS COMPANY
A Division of Harcourt Brace & Company

The Curtis Center
Independence Square West
Philadelphia, Pennsylvania 19106

Library of Congress Cataloging-in-Publication Data

Ignatavicius, Donna D.
Medical-surgical nursing: a nursing process approach / Donna D. Ignatavicius, M. Linda Workman, Mary A. Mishler.—2nd ed.
p. cm.
Includes bibliographical references and index.
ISBN 0-7216-4863-0
1. Nursing. 2. Surgical nursing. I. Workman, M. Linda. II. Mishler, Mary A. III. Title.
[DNLM: 1. Surgical Nursing. 2. Nursing Process. WY 161 I24m 1991]
RT41.I36 1995
610.73—dc20
DNLM/DLC 94-14942

Cover Art: Georgia O'Keeffe, *Oriental Poppies,* 1928, Courtesy of the Collection Frederick R. Weisman Art Museum at the University of Minnesota, Minneapolis

Medical-Surgical Nursing:
A Nursing Process Approach, 2/e.

Single Volume ISBN 0-7216-4863-0
Volume 1 ISBN 0-7216-5909-8
Volume 2 ISBN 0-7216-5910-1
2 Volume Set ISBN 0-7216-5908-X

Printed in the United States of America.

Last digit is the print number: 9 8 7 6 5 4 3 2

To Charles and Stephanie, for their unending love, support, and patience; and to Michael J. Brown, for giving me the opportunity to have an impact on the lives of many nursing students and practitioners.

DDI

To John, David, and Gregory. Their loving support and well-developed sense of humor helped move me through the difficult times and made the good times even better.

MLW

To my now 15-year-old twins, Laura and Aaron Vogel, who are the most special people in my life; to my mother and brother, Jean and Rodney Mishler; and to Temple University, for giving me my start in nursing.

MAM

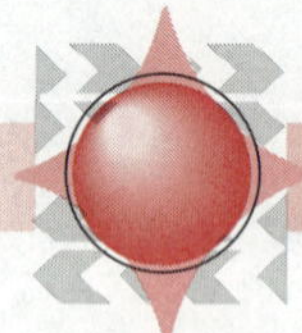

About the Authors

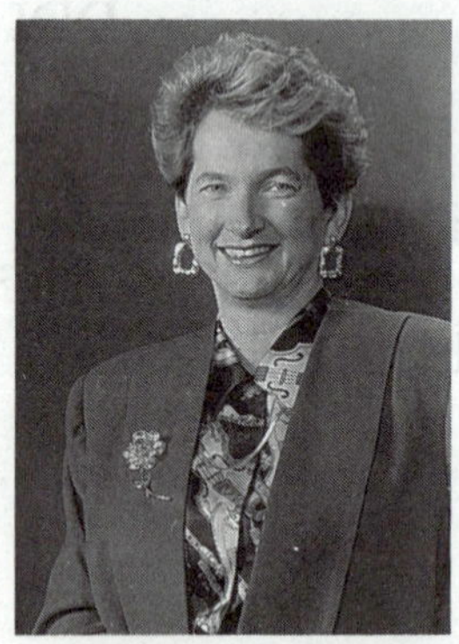

Donna D. Ignatavicius received her diploma in nursing from the Peninsula General Hospital School of Nursing in Salisbury, Maryland, in 1969. After working as a staff and charge nurse in medical-surgical nursing, she became Instructor in Staff Development at the University of Maryland Medical Center. In 1976 she received her BSN from the University of Maryland School of Nursing. For 5 years, she taught in several schools of nursing while working toward her MS in nursing, which she received in 1981. Mrs. Ignatavicius then taught in the baccalaureate program at the University of Maryland School of Nursing for six years, after which she pursued her interest in gerontology by becoming Director of Nursing at a skilled nursing facility. She has been a certified gerontological nurse since 1989. For the past 3 years, Mrs. Ignatavicius has taught at the MacQueen Gibbs Willis School of Nursing in Easton, Maryland, and has presented continuing education seminars throughout the United States.

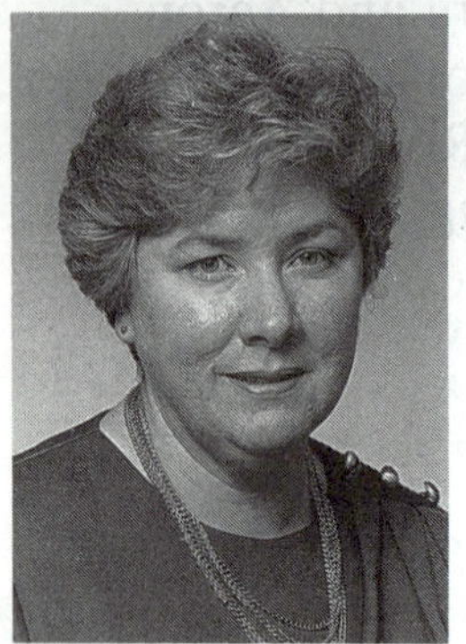

M. Linda Workman received her BSN from the University of Cincinnati College of Nursing and Health. After serving in the United States Army Nurse Corps and working as Assistant Head Nurse and Head Nurse in civilian hospitals, Ms. Workman, a native of Canada, earned her MSN from the University of Cincinnati College of Nursing and Health. She then earned a PhD in developmental biology from the College of Arts and Sciences at the University of Cincinnati. Dr. Workman's 15 years of academic experience include teaching at the diploma, associate degree, baccalaureate, and master's levels. Her areas of teaching expertise include physiology, pathophysiology, genetics, oncology, and immunology. Dr. Workman is an American Cancer Society (Ohio Division) Professor of Oncology Nursing and an Associate Professor of Nursing at the Frances Payne Bolton School of Nursing at Case Western Reserve University, Cleveland, Ohio. A special talent that Dr. Workman brings to nursing education is her ability to teach complex physiologic mechanisms and processes in a manner that is both understandable and applicable to clinical nursing practice.

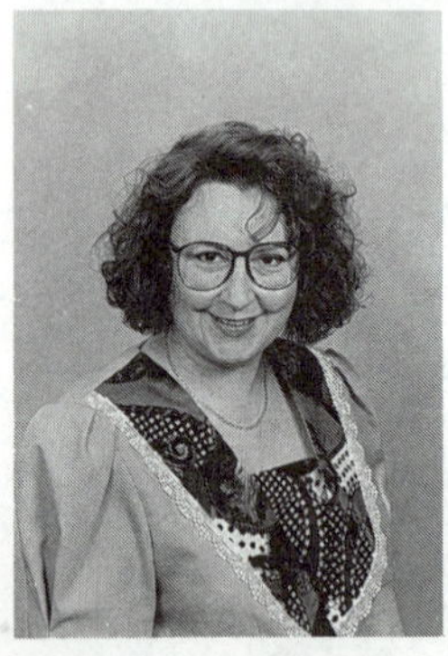

Mary A. Mishler has practiced medical-surgical nursing for her entire nursing career. She has worked as a staff nurse, staff development coordinator, nursing supervisor, and assistant director of nursing, and as a consultant. She has also served as senior-level course coordinator at a school of nursing. A 1971 graduate of Temple University Hospital School of Nursing in Philadelphia, Ms. Mishler received her BSN and MSN from the University of Pennsylvania in 1973 and 1977, respectively. A member of Sigma Theta Tau, Ms. Mishler serves as a Clinical Nurse Specialist at Our Lady of Lourdes Medical Center in Camden, New Jersey. She is certified both as a Clinical Specialist in Medical-Surgical Nursing and as a Nephrology Nurse. In 1993, she received a Certificate for Excellence in Nursing from the New Jersey State Department of Health. She has served as a member of the Standard Setting Panel for the NCLEX-RN examination and currently serves on the Editorial/Advisory Board of *Nursing Spectrum.* She also teaches continuing education seminars throughout the United States.

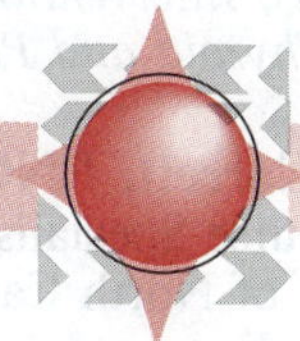

Contributors

Barbara Diebold Ahlheit, MSN, RNCS
Adjunct Instructor, Vanderbilt University. Pulmonary Clinical Nurse Specialist, Veterans Affairs Medical Center, Nashville, Tennessee.
Interventions for Clients with Lower Airway Problems

Madalon O'Rawe Amenta, RN, MN, DrPH
Executive Director, Hospice Nurses Association, Pittsburgh, Pennsylvania.
Loss, Death, and Dying

Shannon McDowell Bailey, RNCS, MS
Clinical Nurse Specialist/Consultant, St. Joseph's Hospital, Tampa, and St. Anthony's Hospital, St. Petersburg, Florida.
Assessment of the Respiratory System

Roxanne Aubol Batterden, RN, MS, CCRN
Nurse Educator, Critical Care and Medical Nursing, The Johns Hopkins Hospital, Baltimore, Maryland.
Interventions for Clients with Liver Problems; Interventions for Clients with Problems of the Gallbladder and Pancreas

Suzanne C. Beyea, RNCS, PhD
Assistant Professor, Saint Anselm College, Manchester, New Hampshire. Nurse Research Consultant, Lakes Region General Hospital, Laconia, New Hampshire.
Interventions for Clients with Stomach Disorders; Interventions for Clients with Noninflammatory Intestinal Disorders; Interventions for Clients with Inflammatory Intestinal Disorders

Marcia Sue DeWolf Bosek, DNSc, RN
Assistant Professor, Rush University. Ethics Consultant, Rush-Presbyterian–St. Luke's Medical Center, Chicago, Illinois.
Ethics

Anna M. Brock, PhD, RN, MPEd, MSN
Director, School of Nursing, and Professor, University of Southern Mississippi, Hattiesburg, Mississippi.
Adult Development

Lynne Russell Brophy, RN, MSN, OCN
Clinical Instructor, University of North Carolina at Chapel Hill, Chapel Hill, North Carolina. Clinical Nurse Specialist, Oncology, Rex Hospital, Raleigh, North Carolina.
Interventions for Clients with Breast Disorders

Jeanette K. Chambers, PhD, RNCS
Adjunct Assistant Professor, The Ohio State University. Renal Clinical Nurse Specialist and Education Specialist, Riverside Methodist Hospitals, Columbus, Ohio.
Assessment of the Renal/Urinary System; Interventions for Clients with Renal Disorders; Interventions for Clients with Chronic and Acute Renal Failure

Janice Z. Cuzzell, RN, MA
Director of Nursing, Charles R. Baxter Wound Center, Dallas, Texas.
Assessment of the Skin, Hair, and Nails; Interventions for Clients with Problems of the Skin and Nails

Lucille Sanzero Eller, RN, PhD
Postdoctoral Fellow (NINR), Rush University, Chicago, Illinois.
Interventions for Clients with Immunologic Disorders

Carol Diane Epstein, MSN, RN, CCRN
Clinical Instructor, Case Western Reserve University. Clinical Nurse, Surgical Intensive Care Unit, MetroHealth Medical Center, Cleveland, Ohio.
Research Applications for Nursing Boxes

Catherine D. Garofano BS, RN, CDE
Senior Instructor in Medicine, Hahnemann University. Nurse Specialist, Endocrinology and Diabetes, Hahnemann University Hospital, Philadelphia, Pennsylvania.
Assessment of the Endocrine System; Interventions for Clients with Pituitary and Adrenal Gland Problems; Interventions for Clients with Problems of the Thyroid and Parathyroid Glands

Cynthia Garrett, RNC, MSN
Clinical Nurse Specialist, Women's Health, University of North Carolina Hospitals, Chapel Hill, North Carolina
Interventions for Clients with Sexually Transmitted Diseases

Elizabeth F. Gloss RN, EdD
Assistant Professor, Undergraduate and Graduate Programs, SUNY Health Science Center, Brooklyn, New York.
Sensory Deprivation and Sensory Overload

Karin A. Hancher, RNCS, MSN
Formerly, Clinical Nurse Specialist, University of Virginia Medical Center, Charlottesville, Virginia.
Interventions for Clients with Oral Cavity Problems

Kathy A. Hausman, RN, MS, CNRN
Instructor, University of Maryland. Director of Organizational Development, Harbor Hospital Center, Baltimore, Maryland.
Assessment of the Nervous System; Interventions for Clients with Problems of the Central Nervous System: The Brain; Interventions for Clients with Problems of the Central Nervous System: The Spinal Cord; Interventions for Clients with Problems of the Peripheral Nervous System; Interventions for Critically Ill Clients with Neurologic Problems

Marcia J. Hill, RN, MSN
Assistant Clinical Professor, Department of Dermatology, Baylor College of Medicine. Manager, Nursing, Methodist Medical Center, Houston, Texas.
Assessment of the Skin, Hair, and Nails; Interventions for Clients with Problems of the Skin and Nails

Sue Baird Holmes, MS, RN, ONC
Courtesy Faculty Appointment, Marquette University. Clinical Nurse Specialist, St. Joseph's Hospital, Milwaukee, Wisconsin.
Body Image

Raymond H. Hull, PhD
Professor, Department of Communicative Disorders and Sciences, Audiology, The Wichita State University, Wichita, Kansas.
Assessment of the Ear and Hearing

Donna D. Ignatavicius, MS, RNC
Concepts of Health and Illness; The Nursing Profession and the Role of the Medical-Surgical Nurse; The Nursing Process; Health Care of Older Adults; Pain; Chronic and Disabling Conditions; Interventions for Clients with Connective Tissue Disease; Interventions for Clients with Infection; Assessment of the Musculoskeletal System; Interventions for Clients with Musculoskeletal Problems; Interventions for Clients with Musculoskeletal Trauma; Interventions for Clients with Other Nutritional Problems

Kathleen J. Jones, RN, MS, ANP
Clinical Nurse Specialist, Oncology, Walter Reed Army Medical Center, Washington, DC.
Interventions for Male Clients with Reproductive Problems

Mary K. Kazanowski, MS, RNC, CCRN, OCN, ARNP
Assistant Professor, Saint Anselm College, Manchester, New Hampshire.
Interventions for Clients with Vascular Problems; Interventions for Clients with Noninflammatory Intestinal Disorders; Interventions for Clients with Inflammatory Intestinal Disorders

Mary Beth Kingston, RN, MSN
Formerly, Head Nurse, Emergency Department, Hospital of the University of Pennsylvania, Philadelphia, Pennsylvania.
Assessment of the Endocrine System; Interventions for Clients with Pituitary and Adrenal Gland Problems; Interventions for Clients with Problems of the Thyroid and Parathyroid Glands

Deitra Leonard Lowdermilk, RNC, PhD
Clinical Professor, Health of Women and Children, University of North Carolina at Chapel Hill, Chapel Hill, North Carolina.
Assessment of the Reproductive System; Interventions for Clients with Gynecologic Problems

Judy Malkiewicz, RN, PhD
Associate Professor of Nursing, University of Northern Colorado, Greeley, Colorado.
Assessment of the Ear and Hearing

Jan L. Martin, RN, GNP, PhD
Associate Professor, University of Northern Colorado, Greeley, Colorado.
Interventions for Clients with Ear and Hearing Problems

Margaret Elaine McLeod, MSN, RNCS, CDE
Clinical Nurse Specialist, Veterans Administration Medical Center, Nashville, Tennessee.
Interventions for Clients with Diabetes Mellitus

Mary A. Mishler, MSN, RNCS, CNN
Interventions for Preoperative Clients; Interventions for Intraoperative Clients; Interventions for Postoperative Clients; Interventions for Critically Ill Clients with Respiratory Problems; Interventions for Clients with Diabetes Mellitus

Anne Griswold Peirce, RN, PhD
Director of Doctoral Studies, Columbia University, New York, New York.
Stress, Coping, and Adaptation

Kathleen Ouimet Perrin, MS, RN, CCRN
Associate Professor of Nursing, St. Anselm College, Manchester, New Hampshire.
Assessment of the Cardiovascular System; Interventions for Clients with Cardiac Problems; Interventions for Critically Ill Clients with Coronary Artery Disease

Carmen J. Petrin, BS, RN
Critical Care Educator, Catholic Medical Center, Manchester, New Hampshire.
Interventions for Clients with Dysrhythmias

Charon A. Pierson, RN, GNP, MSN
Instructor, Family Nurse Practitioner Program, University of Hawaii, Manoa. Geriatric Nurse Practitioner, Kaiser Permanente Medical Group, Honolulu, Hawaii.
Interventions for Clients with Urinary Problems

Rosemary C. Polomano, MSN, RN
Clinical Nurse Specialist, Pain, Hospital of the University of Pennsylvania, Philadelphia, Pennsylvania.
Pain

Lynn Rew, EdD, RNC, FAAN
Associate Professor and Assistant Dean for Student Affairs, School of Nursing, The University of Texas, Austin, Texas.
Human Sexuality

Denise A. Sadowski, RN, MSN
Independent Nurse Consultant, Burns and Critical Care, Cincinnati, Ohio.
Interventions for Clients with Burns

Judith K. Sands, RN, EdD
Associate Professor and Director of Undergraduate Studies, University of Virginia School of Nursing, Charlottesville, Virginia.
Interventions for Clients with Esophageal Problems

Karen S. Santmyer, MS, RNCS
Psychiatric Consultation Liaison Nurse, Medical University of South Carolina, Charleston, South Carolina.
Interventions for Clients with Anorexia Nervosa and Bulimia Nervosa

Teresa A. Savage, MS, RN
Practitioner-Teacher, Rush University. Practitioner-Teacher, Rush-Presbyterian–St. Luke's Medical Center, Chicago, Illinois.
Ethics

Susan Moeller Schneider, MS, RNCS, OCN
Instructor in Oncology Nursing, Case Western Reserve University. PRN Nurse, Bone Marrow Transplant Unit, University Hospitals of Cleveland, Cleveland, Ohio.
Interventions for Clients with Hematologic Problems

Pamela S. Schremp, RN, MSN, CRNO
Clinical Instructor, Case Western Reserve University. Director, Risk Management, University Hospitals of Cleveland, Cleveland, Ohio.
Assessment of the Eye and Vision; Interventions for Clients with Eye and Visual Problems

Susan Shelton, RD, LD, BS
Dietitian, Ginger Cove Life Care Center, Annapolis, Maryland.
Interventions for Clients with Other Nutritional Problems

Ann E. Furiel Sievers, RN, MA, CORLN
Assistant Adjunct Professor, University of California at San Francisco, San Francisco, California. Clinical Nurse Specialist, Otolaryngology, University of California at Davis Medical Center, Sacramento, California.
Interventions for Clients with Upper Airway Problems

Kathleen A. Singleton, MSN, RN, CNS
Instructor of Nursing, Case Western Reserve University. Clinical Nurse Specialist, Medical-Surgical Nursing, Fairview General Hospital, Cleveland, Ohio.
Interventions for Clients in Shock

Georgeanne V. Stilley, RN, MSN, OCN
Clinical Nurse Specialist, Oncology, Acute Pain Management Service, Our Lady of Lourdes Medical Center, Camden, New Jersey.
Interventions for Critically Ill Clients with Respiratory Problems

Kathleen M. White, RN, MS
Instructor, University of Maryland, Baltimore, Maryland.
Assessment of the Gastrointestinal System

M. Linda Workman, PhD, RN, FAAN, OCN
Fluid and Electrolyte Balance; Interventions for Clients with Fluid Imbalances; Interventions for Clients with Electrolyte Imbalances; Acid-Base Balance; Interventions for Clients with Acid-Base Imbalances; Inflammation and the Immune Response; Altered Cell Development and Growth; Interventions for Clients with Cancer; Interventions for Clients in Shock; Assessment of the Hematologic System

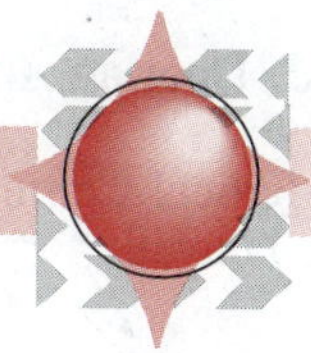

Reviewers

MaryLou Altman, RN, MSN
South Hills Health System
Pittsburgh, Pennsylvania

Sarah E. Angermuller, RN, MEd, MSN, CCRN, CNRN
Columbus College
Columbus, Georgia

Pamela A. Bachmeyer, PhD, CPNP, RN
Chicago State University
Chicago, Illinois

Roberta P. Bartee, MS, RN
Tulane University Medical Center
New Orleans, Louisiana

Janice E. Beeken, RN, PhD
University of Wyoming
Laramie, Wyoming

Margaret W. Bellak, RN, MN
Indiana University of Pennsylvania
Indiana, Pennsylvania

Nancy Berger, RNC, MSN
Charles E. Gregory School of Nursing
Perth Amboy, New Jersey

Kathleen M. Blade, RN, MS
St. Joseph Hospital School of Nursing
North Providence, Rhode Island

Nancy L. Bradley, RN, BSN, MEd
Kent State University
Kent, Ohio

Louise K. Brentin, RN, MSN
Delta College
University Center, Michigan

Barbara Brillhart, RN, PhD, CRRN
University of Colorado Health Sciences Center
Denver, Colorado

Carolyn R. Pierce Buckelew, RNCS, MA, NCC
Charles E. Gregory School of Nursing
Perth Amboy, New Jersey

Roberta Bumann, RN, MSN
Winona State University
Winona, Minnesota

Janet E. Burton, RN, MSN
St. Francis Hospital
Greenville, South Carolina

Linda Dennis Busl, RN, MEd
Good Samaritan Hospital
School of Nursing
Cincinnati, Ohio

Monica M. Capp, RN, MSN, CCRN
North Carolina Central University
Durham, North Carolina

Patricia A. Castaldi, MSN, RN
Elizabeth General Medical Center School of Nursing
Elizabeth, New Jersey

Marcia Chorba, RN, MSN
Mercy Hospital School of Nursing
Pittsburgh, Pennsylvania

Elizabeth Ann Coleman, RNP, PhD
University of Arkansas for Medical Sciences
Little Rock, Arkansas

Dianne G. Copenhaver, RN, PhD, CANP
Coppin State College
Baltimore, Maryland

Gretchen Reising Cornell, RN, PhD
Northeast Missouri State University
Kirksville, Missouri

Julie A. Coy, MS, RNC
University of Colorado Health Sciences Center
Denver, Colorado

Bridget Culhane, RN, MN, OCN
Oncology Nursing Society
Pittsburgh, Pennsylvania

Donita D'Amico, RN, EdM
William Paterson College
Wayne, New Jersey

Linda David, RN, CPAN
Yale New Haven Hospital
New Haven, Connecticut

Judy K. Davidson, MN, RNCS
Columbus College
Columbus, Georgia

Paula A. Dawson, RN, BSN, MEd, CHES
Forbes Regional Hospital
Monroeville, Pennsylvania

Ann S. Dellaira, PhD, RNC
Thomas Jefferson University
Philadelphia, Pennsylvania

Kathryn E. Dexheimer, RN, MSN
Avila College
Kansas City, Missouri

Kathleen J. Doering, RN, MN, CETN
Queens' Medical Center
Honolulu, Hawaii

Ellen Stoetzner Duke, RN, MSN, CCRN
Stephen F. Austin State University
Nacogdoches, Texas

Stella M. Dyck, RN, BScN, MContEd
University of Saskatchewan
Saskatoon, Saskatchewan

Mary E. Edwards, PhD, RNC
University of Texas at Galveston
Galveston, Texas

Lillian Elias, RN, MSN
Stanley Kaplan Organization
Jacksonville, Florida

Jan M. Ellerhorst-Ryan, RNCS, MSN
Abbey Infusion Services
Cincinnati, Ohio

Nancy L. Evans, RN, MS
St. Joseph Hospital School of Nursing
North Providence, Rhode Island

Linda J. Fahey, ANP-C, MSN
California State University, Los Angeles
Los Angeles, California

Joyce A. Feldman, RN, MSN
Visiting Nurse Association of Morris County
Morristown, New Jersey

Vickie K. Fieler, RN, MS, OCN
University of Rochester
Rochester, New York

Patricia Finder-Stone, RN, MS
Northeast Wisconsin Technical College
Green Bay, Wisconsin

Lisa M. Fiorentino, RN, MS, CRNP
University of Pittsburgh at Bradford
Bradford, Pennsylvania

Lisa Sue Flood, MSN, RNCS
Northern Michigan University
Marquette, Michigan

S. E. Fowler-Kerry, RN, PhD
University of Saskatchewan
Saskatoon, Saskatchewan

Ola Houston Fox, RNC, MSN
University of South Alabama
Mobile, Alabama

Michele A. Gerwick, MSN, RN
Indiana University of Pennsylvania
Indiana, Pennsylvania

Joyce Grant-Scott, RN, MSN
Jefferson School of Nursing
Pine Bluff, Arkansas

Milly Gutkoski, MN, RN
Formerly, Montana State University
Bozeman, Montana

Sharon E. Hannah, RNC, MPH
Hawaii Community College
University of Hawaii
Hilo, Hawaii

Nancy Hutton Haynes, RN, MN, CCRN, TNCCP
Saint Luke's College
Kansas City, Missouri

Doris J. Heaman, DSN, RN
The University of Alabama in Huntsville
Huntsville, Alabama

Adria H. Heath, RN, MSN, CNS
St. Mary's Hospital
Galveston, Texas

Lori Hendrickx, MSN, RN, CCRN
Montana State University
Missoula, Montana

Doris Hoerdeman, RN, MSN
Methodist Medical Center of Illinois School of Nursing
Peoria, Illinois

Sharon Leech Hofland, RN, MS, MN, PhD
South Dakota State University
Brookings, South Dakota

Patricia J. Hughes, EdD, RN
Pacific Lutheran University
Tacoma, Washington

Bette A. Ide, PhD, RN
University of Wyoming
Laramie, Wyoming

Charlotte L. Ingram, RNCS, MS
Columbus College
Columbus, Georgia

Patricia W. Iyer, MSN, RN
Med League Support Services
Stockton, New Jersey

Cheryl D. Johnson, RN, MSN
University of Tennessee, Memphis
Memphis, Tennessee

Joyce M. Johnson, MN, RN, FNP
South Carolina State University
Orangeburg, South Carolina

Gwendolyn C. Jones, RN, MSN
North Carolina Central University
Durham, North Carolina

Marcelle Kaplan, RN, MS, OCN
The Louis Venet, MD, Comprehensive Breast Service
Beth Israel Medical Center
New York, New York

Janet K. Kuhn, EdD, RN
Villanova University
Villanova, Pennsylvania

Nancy Kupper, RN, MSN
Tarrant County Junior College
Fort Worth, Texas

Janice G. Lanham, RN, MSN
Tri-County Technical College
Pendleton, South Carolina

Connie Leek, MSN, RNC, OCN
City of Hope National Medical Center
Duarte, California

Kay L. Luft, MN, RN, CCRN, CEN
Saint Luke's College
Kansas City, Missouri

Celeste S. Makrevis, RN, MSN, CCRN
Critical Care Concepts
Lewisburg, West Virginia

Doris M. Marshalek, RN, MSN, CCRN
Community College of Allegheny County
Pittsburgh, Pennsylvania

Donna Massey, RN, MSN, CCRN, TNS
Good Samaritan Hospital
Downers Grove, Illinois

Cindi McCarley, RN, MSN
Stephen F. Austin State University
Nacogdoches, Texas

Diana G. McLaughlin, MS, RN
Idaho State University
Pocatello, Idaho

Mary Ellen McMorrow, RN, EdD, CCRN
College of Staten Island
New York, New York

Donna V. McNelly, RN, MS
University of New England
Biddeford, Maine

Mary E. Mehok, RN, MSN, CCRN
Mercy Hospital
Pittsburgh, Pennsylvania

Dorothy Dark Mixon, RN, MSN
Coosa Valley Medical Center School of Nursing
Sylacauga, Alabama

Jean Burley Moore, PhD, RN
George Mason University
Fairfax, Virginia

Carol Nelson, RN, MSN
Spokane Community College
Spokane, Washington

Sylvia E. Nissila, PhD, RN
College of St. Catherine
Minneapolis, Minnesota

Netha O'Meara, MSN, RN
Stephen F. Austin State University
Nacogdoches, Texas

Nancy Otterness, RN, MS
Boise State University
Boise, Idaho

Brenda H. Owens, PhD, RN
Louisiana State University Medical Center School of Nursing
New Orleans, Louisiana

Doris J. Pasternak, RNC, MSN
Conemaugh School of Nursing
Johnstown, Pennsylvania

Elisabeth A. Pennington, EdD, RN
University of Massachusetts, Dartmouth
Dartmouth, Massachusetts

Sharon Ann Perrilliat-Stanley, RN, MSN
Formerly, Thomas Jefferson University
Philadelphia, Pennsylvania

Joann F. Petty, RN, MSN, OCN
La Grange Memorial Hospital
La Grange, Illinois

Barbara Ann Preib, RNC, MSN
University of Illinois
Chicago, Illinois

Janice S. Pyle, RN, MS, MSN
Jefferson State Community College
Birmingham, Alabama

Patti D. Quenzer, RN, MSN
Southern West Virginia Community College
Williamson, West Virginia

Christina Whitney Rainbolt, MSN, RN
Montana State University
Missoula, Montana

Anita C. Reinhardt, MSN, RN, CCRN
Pacific Lutheran University
Tacoma, Washington

Margueritte M. Rydlewski, MSN, RN
Richmond Memorial Hospital School of Nursing
Richmond, Virginia

Mary E. Sampel, MSN, RN
St. Louis University
St. Louis, Missouri

Linda Sarasin, MSN, RNCS
Marquette General Hospital
Marquette, Michigan

Wanda Sebastian, RN, BSN, OCN
City of Hope National Medical Center
Duarte, California

Lucinda Seidl, RN, MSN
University of Nebraska
Lincoln, Nebraska

Nance A. Seiple, CRNA, MEd
Medical Communications
Park Ridge, Illinois

Lisa K. Anderson Shaw, RNC, MSN, MA
University of Illinois at Chicago
Chicago, Illinois

Joyce A. Shireman, RN, MS, PhD
Coe College
Cedar Rapids, Iowa

Lois Fieser Short, RN, MN, ARNP
Wichita State University
Wichita, Kansas

Linda S. Sikora, RN, MSN, CCRN
Wayne State University
Detroit, Michigan

Teresa E. Kelly Snyder, MN, RNCS
Montana State University
Missoula, Montana

Mary E. Soja, MSN, MA, RN
Indiana University
Indianapolis, Indiana

Mary Ellen Stone, BSN, RN
Edustaff
Stanhope, New Jersey

Catherine Bush Strength, MN, RNC
Charity Delgado School of Nursing
New Orleans, Louisiana

Rita D. Strickland, EdD, RN, CCRN
SUNY Health Science Center at Brooklyn
Brooklyn, New York

Liz Sullivan, RN, MN, OCN, NP
City of Hope National Medical Center
Duarte, California

Patricia R. Teasley, MSN, RNCS
Columbus College
Columbus, Georgia

Paula Timmerman, RN, MSN, OCN
Good Samaritan Hospital
Downers Grove, Illinois

Kathleen C. Tully, MSN, RNCS, CCRN
Our Lady of Lourdes Medical Center
Camden, New Jersey

Janice I. Vanderlaan, RN, MSN
Stephen F. Austin State University
Nacogdoches, Texas

Marilyn J. Vontz, RN, PhD (Cand)
Bryan Memorial Hospital School of Nursing
Lincoln, Nebraska

Carole J. Petrosky Vozel, RNC, PhD
Western Pennsylvania Hospital School of Nursing
Pittsburgh, Pennsylvania

Penny Vukov-Zmora, RNCS, MS
Good Samaritan Hospital
Downers Grove, Illinois

Mary A. Ware, MEd, MSN, RN
William Carey College
New Orleans, Louisiana

Stuart L. Whitney, MS, RNCS
University of Vermont
Burlington, Vermont

Susan Karm Wieczorek, RN, MSN, CNS
St. Francis Hospital
Columbus, Georgia

Deborah F. Wilson, PhDc, RN
University of Wyoming
Laramie, Wyoming

Judith G. Winterhalter, DNSc, RNCS
Gwynedd Mercy College
Gwynedd Valley, Pennsylvania

Charlene Winters, MS, RN, CCRN
Montana State University
Missoula, Montana

Barbara J. Wirick, RN, MSc, CEN
Weber State University
Ogden, Utah

Kathy M. Witta, MSN, RN, CCRN
Pulmonary Associates
Wilmington, Delaware
Hospital of the University of Pennsylvania
Philadelphia, Pennsylvania

Carolyn Yucha, RN, PhD
University of Colorado
Denver, Colorado

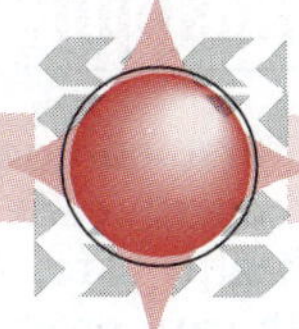

Preface

The first edition of *Medical-Surgical Nursing: A Nursing Process Approach* met with widespread acclaim as the medical-surgical nursing text of the '90s.

In the 4 years since we published that landmark first edition, changes in health care have accelerated. Hospital stays have become shorter than ever before. In the United States, health care providers, leaders in government and industry, and citizens across the land have begun to look to health care delivery in Canada and other nations as models on which to rebuild a uniquely American system of health care delivery. The health care reform movement in the United States has become a major force behind the advocacy of collaborative care—an approach that was and is foundational to this textbook.

The population of nursing students has also experienced major changes since the publication of the first edition. The "nontraditional" student has become the norm. These students balance family and work responsibilities while attending school, and time is an especially precious commodity for them.

To address the accelerating changes in health care and the changes in the student population preparing to provide it, we have undertaken an exhaustive revision of *Medical-Surgical Nursing: A Nursing Process Approach.* We have read, re-read, and revised virtually every line of the first edition. Our goal has been to ensure that the book you hold today is as current and as accessible as we can provide to help students deliver state-of-the-art health care in tomorrow's global economy.

Clinical Currency and Comprehensiveness

To ensure the book's currency and comprehensiveness, we first listened to what our readers had to tell us about their experience with the first edition. We then commissioned in-depth reviews of the first edition by experts in each subject area, many of them users of the first edition. We evaluated that feedback and formulated our revision plans. We then reassembled a team of contributors expert in each subject area to revise, rewrite, and, in some cases, draft entirely new chapters. We then commissioned nearly 500 reviews of the book's 77 chapters by instructors and clinicians from across the United States and from Canada, and we revised the chapters into their final form.

The results are a book with a strong, consistent focus on pathophysiology, collaborative care, and discharge planning, a foundation of current nursing research, and a focus on the critical "need to know" information that is a prerequisite to safe, effective care in the 1990s and beyond.

Ease of Access

To make the second edition as easy to use as possible, we broke the book into smaller chapters of more uniform length. In the first edition there were 67 chapters; in this edition there are 77. Among the subject areas now covered in their own chapters are ethics, care of the elderly, and nutritional health problems.

We also reordered the book's units, so that vital body systems, such as cardiovascular, respiratory, and neurologic, appear earlier. In those three units, we also pulled critical care content into separate chapters on management of critically ill clients with respiratory problems, coronary artery disease, and neurologic problems.

Within each chapter, we took great pains to ensure consistent readability for junior-level to senior-level students. Knowing how hard it is to focus on page after page of text after a hard day's work, we broke up blocks of text with generous use of headings, bulleted lists, tables, figures, and Charts. We concluded each chapter with a current Selected Bibliography (classic sources are noted with an asterisk—*) and Suggested Readings. The second edition also uses a fresh, new design that should help readers easily distinguish the hierarchy of headings.

Our Philosophy

As in the first edition, we take a collaborative approach to client care. We believe that in the real world of health care, nurses, clients, physicians, and other health care providers jointly *share* responsibility for the management of client problems.

We therefore discuss client care through a Collaborative Management framework. In this framework, we draw no artificial distinctions between medical treatment and nursing care. Instead, we discuss together the whole range of approaches that health care providers and their clients bring to bear to combat health problems.

However, because this is first and foremost a *nursing* text, we discuss client problems and their management from the perspective of the *nursing process.*

Integral to such a collaborative approach is to make clear, whenever appropriate, just who is responsible for what. In this second edition we have done just that. When a responsibility is primarily the nurse's, we say so. When a decision must be made jointly with a client, physician, nurse, and physical therapist, we say so. When the same care might be provided by different health care providers in different settings, we say that too.

Multinational, Multicultural, Multigenerational Focus

Ours is an era of diversity. *Medical-Surgical Nursing,* Second Edition, reflects that diversity.

To address the needs of both American and Canadian readers, we have included examples of the trade names of drugs available in the United States and of those available in Canada. (We have indicated examples of Canadian trade names with a small maple leaf next to the drug name.)

Increasingly, North American nurses are caring for clients whose race, culture, or ethnic background differs from their own. More and more, nurses must understand the differences that make us unique in order to provide the quality health care that we need. To help nurses provide quality care to clients of different races, cultures, and ethnic backgrounds, the second edition of *Medical-Surgical Nursing* highlights **Transcultural Considerations** throughout the book.

As new advances in medicine and nutrition extend our life expectancy, our populations are becoming increasingly older. Moreover, today's trend of hospitalizing only the most seriously ill clients has led to a disproportionate number of elderly clients in hospitals. To help prepare nurses to care for this elderly population, the second edition provides increased coverage of the care of the elderly. This edition includes a greater number of **Nursing Focus on the Elderly** Charts, and it highlights **laboratory values** and **drug dosages typical for elderly clients.**

Organization

The second edition of *Medical-Surgical Nursing: A Nursing Process Approach* is divided into 16 units. Unit 1, Health Promotion and Illness, lays the foundation for the health concepts incorporated throughout the book. Unit 2 includes chapters on specific biopsychosocial concepts, such as pain, altered body image, and stress. Unit 3 consists of five clear, concise chapters on fluids and electrolytes, acid-base balance, and intravenous therapy.

Unit 4 presents the perioperative nursing content that medical-surgical nurses need to know. This unit includes a great number of photographs and other learning aids to help make the perioperative environment come alive for readers. A solid grounding in these chapters should enable students to better understand the surgical content covered in the remainder of the book, where we discuss specific surgical procedures in detail.

Unit 5 includes core content on health problems related to the immune system. These chapters cover normal inflammation and the immune response, altered cell development and growth, and interventions for clients with connective tissue disease, cancer, infection, and other immunologic disorders.

The remaining 11 units present medical-surgical nursing content by body system. Each unit begins with a chapter on assessment, followed by chapters on interventions for clients with specific health problems.

Student Learning Aids

We all need structure and consistency to help us learn. Like the first edition, this edition uses consistent headings in all of its Assessment and Interventions chapters.

This edition also includes ten types of learning aids that we developed to help students quickly identify the most important information and to help them study:

- **Nursing Care Highlight** Charts draw attention to some of the most important "hands-on" nursing care covered in the book.
- **Nursing Focus on the Elderly** Charts identify the normal changes of aging that readers can expect to encounter (and the related nursing care that they can expect to provide). Additional Nursing Focus on the Elderly Charts highlight the individualized

care that elderly clients with specific conditions or undergoing specific procedures will need.

- **Education Guide** Charts demonstrate—in client-oriented language—the kinds of instructions readers must learn to provide to help clients and their families cope with life changes brought about by illness.
- **Health Promotion Guide** Charts demonstrate—again, in client-oriented language—the sorts of instructions nurses can provide to help people prevent illness and promote optimal health.
- **Lab Profile** Charts summarize important information about the laboratory tests commonly used for health problems in specific body systems. These Charts typically summarize normal ranges of laboratory values (including differences for the elderly, when appropriate) and the significance of abnormal findings.
- **Drug Therapy** Charts summarize important information about drugs commonly used for a specific illness or group of illnesses. These Charts include United States and Canadian trade names, usual dosages (including dosages for the elderly, where appropriate), nursing interventions, and rationales for these interventions.
- **Key Features** Charts highlight the clinical manifestations of important diseases and disorders.
- **Research Applications for Nursing** boxes, occurring in nearly every chapter, summarize current nursing research articles and other scientific articles applicable to nursing. Each box provides a summary of the article, a brief critique, and possible implications for nursing practice. This information should help the reader identify the strengths and weaknesses of the research and how research conclusions can translate into changes in daily practice.
- **Client Care Plans** provide examples of detailed plans of care for very specific client problems.
- **Clinical Pathways** provide examples, from across the United States, of how some hospitals are implementing a collaborative approach to care.

A Complete Teaching and Learning Package

Six companion publications complement the second edition of *Medical-Surgical Nursing* to create a complete teaching and learning package.

For Students

- Student Study Guide
- Pocket Companion

The *Student Study Guide* presents questions in a variety of formats to help students learn the content of the textbook. For this edition, questions aimed at stimulating critical thinking skills are highlighted with a special symbol. Among the Critical Thinking Exercises are Case Studies that students can complete and submit to their instructors.

The *Pocket Companion for Medical-Surgical Nursing* retains the popular alphabetical format of the first edition and now includes extensive cross-referencing to speed reader access to vital information on clinical days. The *Pocket Companion* also includes five helpful appendices, including a quick-reference to ECG interpretation.

For Instructors

- Instructor's Manual
- ExaMaster
- Test Manual
- Transparencies and Slides

The *Instructor's Manual* provides instructors with annotated learning objectives that summarize and amplify key content from the textbook. It also suggests, for each unit, fresh new ideas (including "Strategies to Promote Critical Thinking") to help clarify material for students. For each unit, the *Instructor's Manual* also includes those questions from the *Student Study Guide* that are aimed at promoting critical thinking skills, and it lists the Case Studies that appear in corresponding chapters of the *Student Study Guide.*

The computerized *ExaMaster* test bank and the printed *Test Manual* provide instructors with approximately 2000 test questions coded for correct answer, rationale, cognitive type, and objective (corresponding to a step of the nursing process). The ExaMaster program, provided free to programs adopting the text, is a comprehensive test-generation tool. It uses instructor criteria to select from the questions provided, from questions that instructors adapt to suit their own needs, and from questions that instructors themselves write.

A set of *Transparencies and Slides,* also provided free to adopters, includes 100 two-color acetates, 200 one-color transparency masters, and 125 color slides to complement lectures. Of the 125 color slides, 77 duplicate those found in the book's full-color insert, and 48 have been selected by a leading wound care expert for special relevance to the medical-surgical nurse.

All in all, the second edition of *Medical-Surgical Nursing: A Nursing Process Approach* is the comprehensive, clinically current, culturally sensitive, and reader-friendly core of a complete teaching and learning package. We hope that it will prepare students to provide quality nursing care into the 21st century.

DONNA D. IGNATAVICIUS
M. LINDA WORKMAN
MARY A. MISHLER

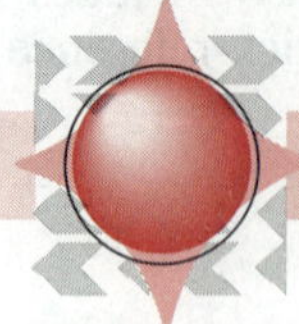

Acknowledgments

A book of this scope and depth results from the efforts of many people. Our contributors have been a pleasure to work with. They met their deadlines while producing top-quality chapters. Our reviewers, from all across the United States and from Canada, provided us with encouragement and ideas throughout the book's development.

The staff of W. B. Saunders Company worked with us throughout the planning, writing, development, and production of the second edition to help us transform our conceptual and clinical content into the teaching and learning tool that it has become. Senior Developmental Editor Lee Henderson, working with Karen Bierstedt, Hope Steele, and Terri Wood, helped us format the text and its features, paying attention to every detail. Senior Editor Barbara Nelson Cullen, who joined the project later in its development, encouraged and supported us in meeting multiple deadlines. Eileen Mann single-handedly coordinated all of the reviews that are an essential part of the development of an undergraduate textbook.

Special thanks to our copy editors, Carol Robins, Terry Russell, and Rose Marie Klimowicz, who had the enormous task of checking all of the book's editorial details while maintaining consistency throughout. Other Saunders staff who did an outstanding job are Production Manager Peter Faber, Illustration Specialist Cecelia Roberts, Designer Joan Wendt, Illustrator Sharon Iwanczuk, and Marketing Manager Maura Connor.

As we prepared the manuscript, many of our colleagues helped us: Dave Rodden, CRNA; Tom Turco, PharmD; Nazir Memon, MD, FCCP; Rod Mishler; Georgeanne Stilley, RN; Sue Zamitis, RN; and the Operating Department nursing staff of Our Lady of Lourdes Medical Center, Camden, New Jersey. The staff of our hospital and school libraries, including Lois Sanger and Fred Kafes, have been especially helpful.

Revisions in this edition have built on the work of contributors to the first edition, whose contributions the authors and publisher gratefully acknowledge:

Sally Ballenger, MS, RN
DePaul University
Chicago, Illinois
Assessment of the Nervous System

Lindy M. Beaver, MN, RNCS
Richland Memorial Hospital
Columbia, South Carolina
Interventions for Clients with Vascular Disorders

Ellen K. DeLuca, RNCS, MSN
Georgetown University
Washington, District of Columbia
Interventions for Clients with Lower Respiratory Tract Disorders

Barbara A. Given, PhD, RN, FAAN
Michigan State University
East Lansing, Michigan
Interventions for Clients with Disorders of the Stomach

Susan E. Goad, EdD, RN
Texas Woman's University
Dallas, Texas
Assessment of Clients with Disabling or Chronic Conditions

Christine Grady, RN, PhD
National Institutes of Health
Bethesda, Maryland
Interventions for Clients with Immunologic Disorders

Sally K. Graham, RN, MSN, ANP-C
Grady Hospital
Atlanta, Georgia
Interventions for Clients with Disorders of the Breast

Maureen Gröer, RN, PhD
MGH Institute of Health Professions
Boston, Massachusetts
Concepts of Fluid and Electrolyte Balance

Diana W. Guthrie, PhD, FAAN, CDE
University of Kansas School of Medicine, Wichita
Wichita, Kansas
Interventions for Clients with Diabetes Mellitus

Pamela J. Haylock, RN, MA, ET
Haylock-Cantril Associates
Woodside, California
Concepts of Altered Cell Growth; Interventions for Clients with Cancer

Deborah J. Henderson, RN, BSN
Food and Drug Administration
Rockville, Maryland
Interventions for Clients with Infectious Diseases

Gloria A. Hinderer-Smith, MS, RN, CRRN
Ravenswood Hospital Medical Center
Chicago, Illinois
Rehabilitation for Clients with Disabling or Chronic Conditions; Interventions for Clients with Peripheral Nervous System Disorders

Anne Keane, EdD, MSN, FAAN
University of Pennsylvania
Philadelphia, Pennsylvania
Pain

Victoria Hargrave Koertge, MSN, RN, OCN
Oncology Consultants, Inc.
Cincinnati, Ohio
Interventions for Clients with Hematologic Disorders

Martha L. Larson, MS, RN
Durham Veterans Administration Hospital
Durham, North Carolina
Interventions for Clients with Lower Respiratory Tract Disorders

Debra Laurent-Bopp, MN, RN
University of Washington
Seattle, Washington
Interventions for Clients with Cardiac Disorders

Carolyn F. McCain, RN, MSN
Formerly, University of North Carolina at Chapel Hill
Chapel Hill, North Carolina
Assessment of the Reproductive System

Patricia Ann Meidenbauer, RN, MS
Anne Arundel Community College
Arnold, Maryland
Interventions for Clients with Chronic and Acute Renal Failure

Marie Rafalowski, MSN, MBA
Medical Education Research Corporation
Pensacola, Florida
Interventions for Clients with Cardiac Disorders

Debra L. Spunt, RN, MS
University of Maryland
Baltimore, Maryland
Interventions for Preoperative Clients; Interventions for Intraoperative Clients; Interventions for Postoperative Clients

Thomas J. Szopa, MS, RN, OCN, CETN
Elliot Hospital
Manchester, New Hampshire
Interventions for Clients with Intestinal Disorders

JoAnne Turner, RNCS, MN
Columbia Cardiology Associates
Columbia, South Carolina
Interventions for Clients with Vascular Disorders

Debra Lee Penner Williams, RN, MS
Department of Veterans Affairs Medical Center
Bay Pines, Florida
Interventions for Clients with Upper Respiratory Tract Disorders

Kathy M. Witta, MSN, RN, CCRN
Pulmonary Associates
Wilmington, Delaware;
Hospital of the University of Pennsylvania
Philadelphia, Pennsylvania
Interventions for Clients with Lower Respiratory Tract Disorders

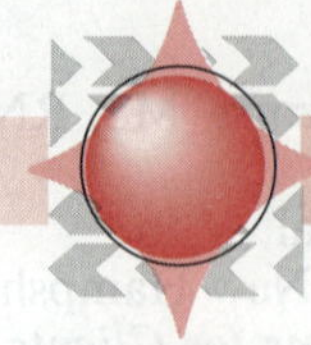

Guide to Special Features

CLINICAL PATHWAYS

CLIENT CARE PLANS

NURSING FOCUS ON THE ELDERLY CHARTS

EDUCATION GUIDE CHARTS

KEY FEATURES CHARTS

NURSING CARE HIGHLIGHT CHARTS

DRUG THERAPY CHARTS

HEALTH PROMOTION GUIDE CHARTS

LAB PROFILE CHARTS

RESEARCH APPLICATIONS FOR NURSING BOXES

RESEARCH APPLICATIONS FOR NURSING BOXES Continued

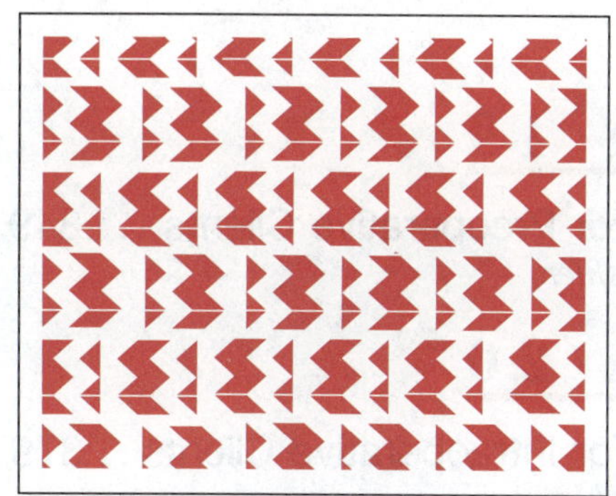

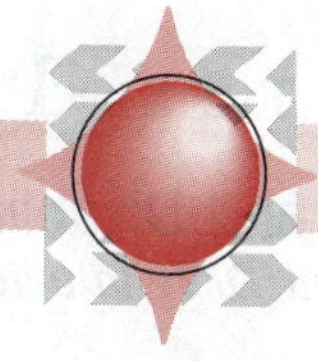

Contents in Brief

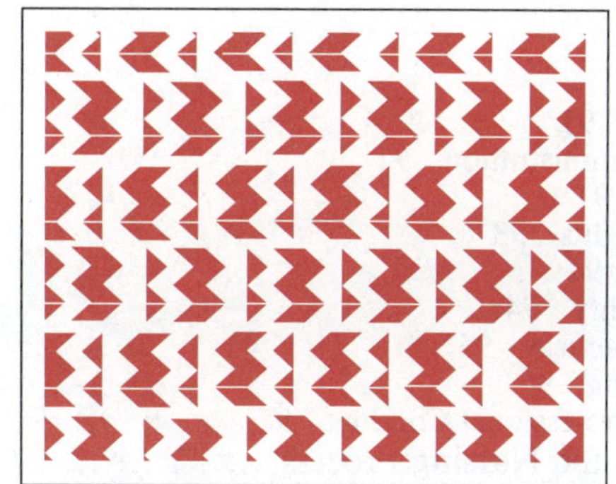

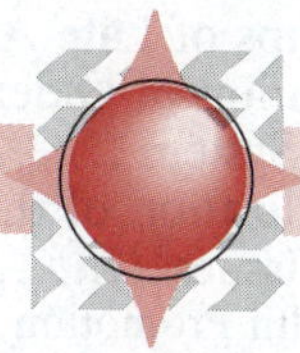

Contents in Detail

CHAPTER 5

UNIT 2

CHAPTER 6

CHAPTER 7

CHAPTER 8

CHAPTER 9

CHAPTER 23

Interventions for Clients with Connective Tissue Disease 459

Donna D. Ignatavicius

CHAPTER 24

Interventions for Clients with Immunologic Disorders 501

Lucille Sanzero Eller

CHAPTER 25

Altered Cell Development and Growth..............................543

M. Linda Workman

CHAPTER 26

Interventions for Clients with Cancer...561

M. Linda Workman

CHAPTER 27

Interventions for Clients with Infection 587

Donna D. Ignatavicius

UNIT 8

Problems of Tissue Perfusion: Management of Clients with Problems of the Hematologic System 1021

CHAPTER 38

CHAPTER 39

UNIT 9

Problems of Mobility, Sensation, and Cognition: Management of Clients with Problems of the Nervous System 1081

CHAPTER 40

CHAPTER 41

UNIT 12

Problems of Digestion, Nutrition, and Elimination: Management of Clients with Problems of the Gastrointestinal System........1487

CHAPTER 52

Assessment of the Gastrointestinal System 1489

Kathleen M. White

CHAPTER 53

Interventions for Clients with Oral Cavity Problems..........................1513

Karin A. Hancher

CHAPTER 54

Interventions for Clients with Esophageal Problems...................1537

Judith K. Sands

CHAPTER 55

Interventions for Clients with Stomach Disorders 1563

Suzanne C. Beyea

CHAPTER 56

Interventions for Clients with Noninflammatory Intestinal Disorders................................1595

Mary K. Kazanowski and Suzanne C. Beyea

CHAPTER 57

CHAPTER 58

CHAPTER 59

CHAPTER 60

CHAPTER 61

UNIT 13

CHAPTER 62

UNIT 16

Problems of Reproduction: Management of Clients with Problems of the Reproductive System 2157

CHAPTER 73

Assessment of the Reproductive System.................................. 2159

Deitra Leonard Lowdermilk

CHAPTER 74

Interventions for Clients with Breast Disorders..................................2191

Lynne Russell Brophy

CHAPTER 75

Interventions for Clients with Gynecologic Problems 2215

Deitra Leonard Lowdermilk

CHAPTER 76

Interventions for Male Clients with Reproductive Problems 2263

Kathleen J. Jones

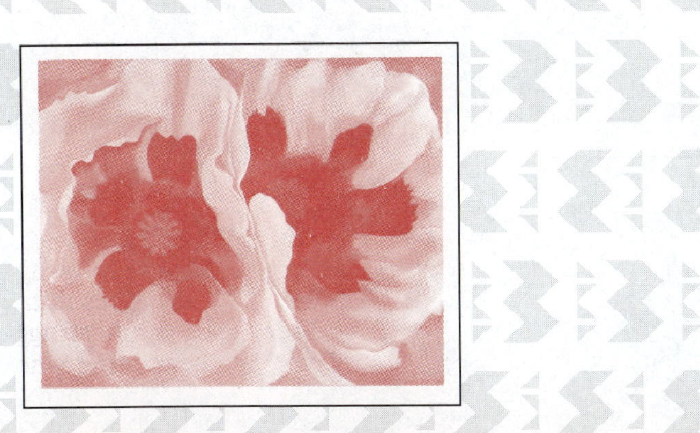

UNIT

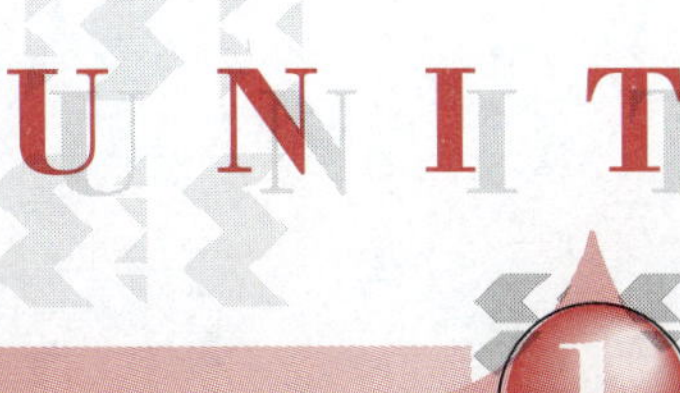

1

Health Promotion and Illness

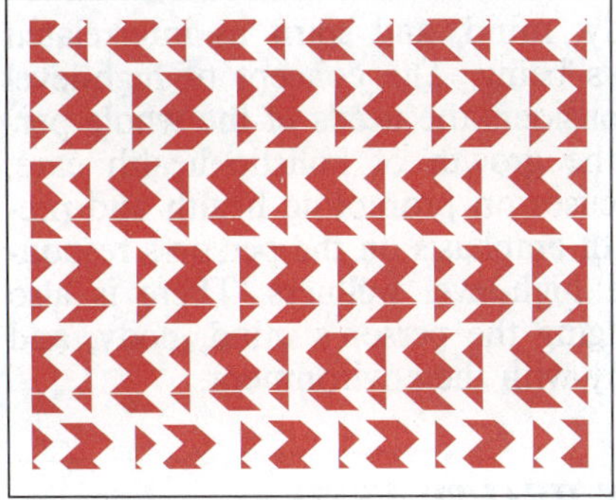

CHAPTER 1

Concepts of Health and Illness

CHAPTER HIGHLIGHTS

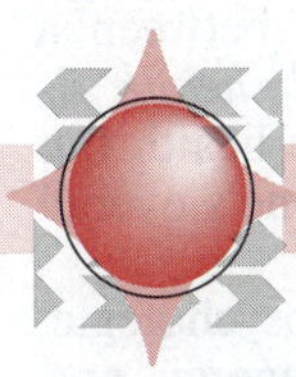

Beliefs about health and illness are a major feature of every known culture. How one views himself or herself as a person and as a part of the environment affects how health is defined. Health is often viewed as a continuum on which optimal wellness, at one end, is the highest level of function, and illness, at the other end, results in death (Fig. 1–1). Every person is somewhere on the continuum. As one's health state changes, the location on the continuum changes.

HEALTH

Although the term *health* is used as part of everyday living, no universally accepted definition has been established. Over time, the focus and expression of health have varied, depending on knowledge, theories, and beliefs. Some people have viewed health and disease as reward or punishment for their actions. Others have considered health as a soundness or wholeness of the body.

Definitions of Health

A typical dictionary may define health in terms of a person's ability to function in society. Some definitions also describe health as a disease-free state or

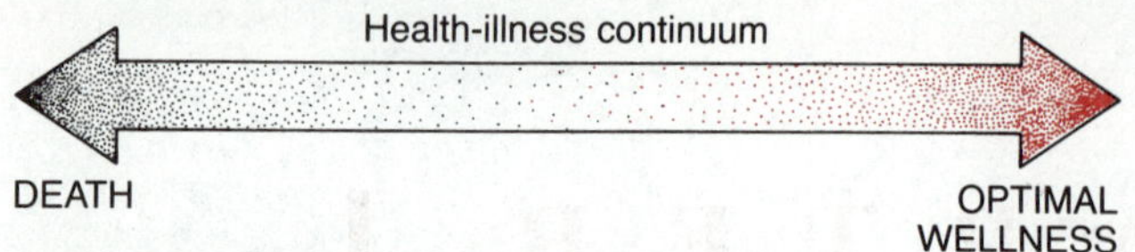

FIGURE 1–1 ◆ Common concept of health as a continuum ranging from optimal wellness at one end to illness culminating in death at the other end.

condition. Definitions such as these are unclear about what constitutes health and illness and seem to present an "either/or" situation—that is, a person is either healthy or ill.

WORLD HEALTH ORGANIZATION DEFINITION OF HEALTH

As science has progressed, the definition of health has evolved. One of the most frequently quoted definitions is the one presented in 1947 by the World Health Organization (WHO). WHO states that health is "a state of complete physical, mental, and social well-being and not merely the absence of disease or infirmity" (WHO, 1947, p. 1). Thus, according to WHO, to be healthy, a person must be in a state of well-being physically, mentally, and socially. Health professionals have found this concept problematic because achieving a state of "health" seems to be an unrealistic goal. This definition does not allow for degrees of health or illness, and it fails to reflect the dynamic, ever-changing nature of health.

A concept related to health is *homeostasis,* or internal equilibrium or balance. When a person experiences a disturbance in homeostasis, he or she is considered to be "unhealthy." Like the WHO definition of health, this concept is losing popularity because "stasis" implies an unchanging state and most theorists today believe that health is always changing.

SOCIOLOGIC DEFINITIONS OF HEALTH

Other definitions of health are found throughout the professional literature. Sociologists view health as a condition that allows for the pursuit and enjoyment of desired cultural values. Studies that have polled laypeople for their definitions of health concur that health is the absence of symptoms and a feeling of well-being. "Good health" includes the ability to carry out "normal," daily activities, such as going to work and performing household chores.

HOLISTIC HEALTH

A term frequently used when health and wellness are discussed is holistic health. The "holistic" view considers the body, mind, and spirit as interrelated parts of a person's being. The concept of high-level wellness, which considers the needs of the whole person, has led to the growth of holistic health care. Holistic health focuses on promoting health and preventing illness, with emphasis on the person's responsibility to achieve high-level wellness. There is also concern with bringing the person's mind, body, and spirit into harmony with the environment.

DEFINITION OF HEALTH USED IN THIS BOOK

In this text, health is defined as a person's level of wellness. This level of wellness is a process in which a person is striving to attain his or her full potential. Health reflects one's biologic, psychologic, and sociologic state (Fig. 1–2). The *biologic* (physical) state refers to the structure of body tissues and organs as well as to the biochemical interactions and functions within the body. The *psychologic* state includes a person's mood, emotions, and personality. The *sociologic* (social) state involves the interaction between a person and the environment. *Spiritual health* is sometimes considered as part of sociologic health but may be described as a separate aspect of one's overall health state.

Factors that affect a person's biologic, psychologic, or social well-being require additional energy and thus alter the level of wellness. Therefore, a high level of wellness is achieved when one's biopsychosocial needs are met.

One of nursing's primary functions is to assist clients in reaching a high level of wellness. Understanding the concept of health and high-level wellness is therefore essential. As nurses assess clients, they must be aware of factors that affect a person's health state and must use nursing interventions to promote and maintain an optimal level of wellness.

Variables Affecting Health

Many variables affect one's level of health (Fig. 1–3):

- Genetic influence
- Cognitive abilities
- Demographic factors
- Environment and lifestyle
- Geographic location
- Culture
- Spirituality and religion
- Standard of living
- Health beliefs and practices
- Previous health experiences
- Support systems

The nurse assesses these variables and incorporates them into the plan of care.

GENETIC INFLUENCE

The biologic make-up of a person is predetermined by his or her genes. Many illnesses and chronic conditions result from genetic composition. As technology and research advance, recognition of the number of genetically influenced diseases is increasing. Examples of health problems that are genetic include diabetes mellitus, sickle cell anemia, and hemophilia.

COGNITIVE ABILITIES

A person's cognitive abilities affect his or her view of health. Educational level and cognitive abilities determine one's capability to reason, use knowledge, and make decisions. The person's understanding of health and the capacity to seek health care resources depend on cognitive abilities.

DEMOGRAPHIC FACTORS

Age and sex can influence a person's state of health. For example, many of today's elderly population will probably live into their 80s and 90s and will experience a high incidence of chronic disease. Some diseases are more common in one sex or the other. For instance, gout and myocardial infarctions are more common in men, and osteoporosis and rheumatoid arthritis are more common in women.

ENVIRONMENT AND LIFESTYLE

The environment in which a person lives can lead to an increased incidence of certain health problems. For example, people living in urban areas with heavy industry are exposed to smog and air pollution. People who live in rural areas are less likely to have this type of health concern, but they may experience other problems, such as decreased access to health care.

The amount of daily activity can also predispose people to certain disease. For example, inactive postmenopausal women are more susceptible to osteoporosis than are physically active women.

Some diseases are associated with occupation. Coal miners and farmers, for example, are prone to lung disease; carpet installers are likely to experience degenerative arthritis of the knees. Certain recreational activities can also be hazardous. Skydiving, skiing, and ice hockey are high-risk sports that frequently result in trauma.

Dietary habits can also influence the likelihood of disease. Research in this area is expanding in an attempt to link dietary intake with certain illnesses. For example, obesity may predispose a person to heart problems and to degenerative arthritis in weight-bearing joints.

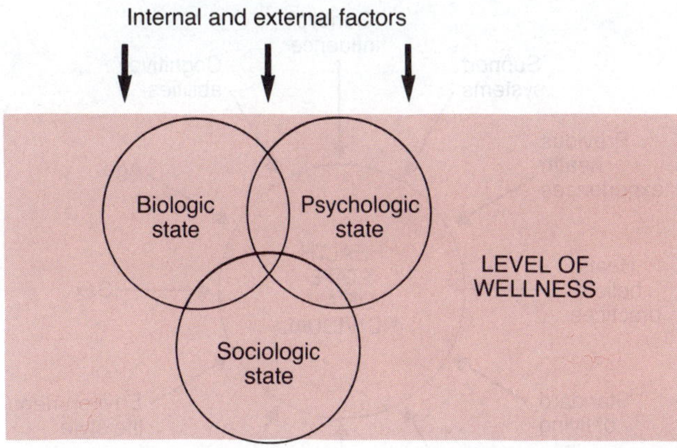

FIGURE 1-2 ◆ Textbook definition of health—one's biologic, psychologic, and sociologic state. Internal and external factors affect a person's level of wellness.

GEOGRAPHIC LOCATION

Where a person lives can affect the incidence of certain health problems. For example, among people living in hot, sunny areas, there is a higher incidence of skin cancer. Those who live around large bodies of water (areas of high humidity) experience a greater incidence of sinusitis.

CULTURE

Each culture defines health and illness in a manner that reflects its previous experience. Culture is the sum of traditions, practices, beliefs, and values developed by a group of people and passed on most often by the family, from generation to generation. Cultural factors determine which health behaviors people perceive as "abnormal." Cultural influence also determines whether or not a person seeks health care and how a person seeks such care. Health practices, as well, are based on cultural beliefs.

This book highlights transcultural (across cultures or subcultures) considerations to help nurses become sensitive to the special needs of many groups of people. In addition, it provides references on transcultural considerations and transcultural nursing care.

SPIRITUALITY AND RELIGION

The term *spirituality* refers to a person's beliefs about a divine being or a higher power or force and related practices. Religion is an organized system of worship often directed toward the divine being, power, or force. Spirituality and religion can affect a person's view of health and health care. For instance, some religious groups regard illness as a form of punishment from God and therefore may refuse medical treatment. A person's health practices may also be influenced by religion. For example, alcohol and drugs are considered "poisons" to the body by some groups and may not be allowed for any purpose.

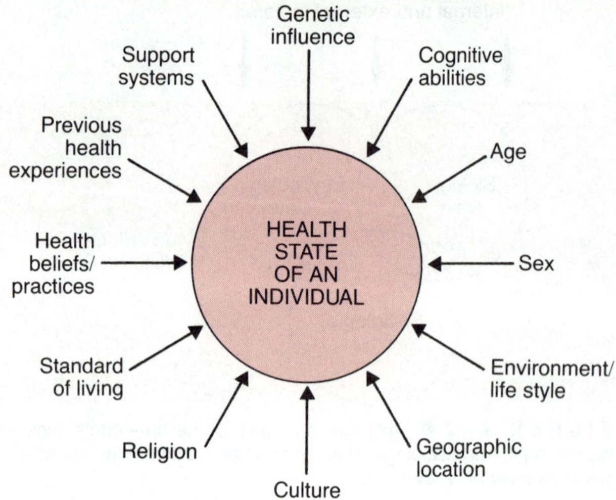

FIGURE 1-3 ◆ Multiple variables influence health and illness.

For some people, spiritual beliefs may have a very positive influence by preventing illness or promoting health. When a person is ill, a strong faith in God or other divine being often helps the person's movement toward wellness.

STANDARD OF LIVING

In many countries, economic status is a major factor affecting health practices and access to the health care system. For instance, in the United States, many people have fixed incomes, such as Social Security benefits, but do not qualify for government funds to help pay health care costs. In countries with socialized health care systems, like Canada and England, access to health care is not limited by a person's ability to pay. However, access may be limited by the availability of health care resources.

Social and economic status may also influence a person's recognition of illness and may affect the way in which one responds to illness. For example, people of upper socioeconomic status report themselves as ill more often than those of lower socioeconomic status. This difference may be related to being able to afford health care and being aware of methods for receiving help.

Home environment can predispose people to various health problems. Crowded, cramped living areas, especially where cleanliness and sanitation are poor, can lead to a higher incidence of disease and illness.

HEALTH BELIEFS AND PRACTICES

Health beliefs are opinions that people hold about health. Health practices are the activities that people carry out as a result of personal health beliefs and may or may not be related to cultural or religious background. These beliefs and practices can affect health positively or negatively. They may lead a person to seek entry into the health care delivery system or to reject treatments that are recommended by health care professionals.

PREVIOUS HEALTH EXPERIENCES

Previous experiences of wellness or illness also contribute to one's reaction when ill. People with limited experience with illness or treatment by health care professionals may be more hesitant to admit illness and to seek treatment. People who have had positive experiences with health care team members may be more likely to seek care when a problem first occurs. On the other hand, those who have had negative experiences with illness or health care (e.g., death of parent or spouse, painful treatments, or unpleasant hospitalizations) may hesitate or refuse to acknowledge the problem or to seek professional care.

SUPPORT SYSTEMS

How a person responds to illness often depends on what support systems are available, both internal and external. Some people cope with stress better than others (see Chapter 7). Family, significant others (friends), and clergy are often helpful as sources of support. If these sources are not available, a person may have more difficulty adapting to the health problem.

ILLNESS

The process of defining oneself as ill is based on one's own perception, the perceptions of others, or both. Each person reacts differently to illness. When assessing the illness experience, the nurse considers the type of illness and the changes that may take place in the client and the family when illness occurs.

Definitions of Illness

Illness may be defined as sickness or a deviation from a health state. Illness has a broader meaning than disease. *Disease* refers to a biologic or psychologic alteration, such as diabetes mellitus or hepatitis, that results in a malfunction of a body organ or system. Disease is usually the term that is used to describe a biomedical condition, and it is supported by clinical manifestations, such as an elevated temperature or inability to move.

The concept of illness includes the perception and response of the client and of those around him or her to not being well. It embraces how the client interprets the source and importance of the disease. Illness can include how the disease affects the client's behavior and relationships with other people and how the client tries to remedy the health problem. In addition to the experience of being ill, the meaning given to that experience is a significant aspect of illness.

A client with rheumatoid arthritis, for instance, has a chronic debilitating disease for which there is no cure. Some clients take a positive attitude and continue to be as active as possible in their daily lives. Others withdraw from their families and significant others. They may seek medically unproven or perhaps unsafe remedies when conventional treatment is unsuccessful in managing their health problem. These aspects and behaviors associated with the presence of a disease are part of the client's illness.

Types of Illness

Acute illness usually refers to a disease or condition that has a relatively rapid onset, high intensity, and short duration. Examples include cholecystitis, pneumonia, and urinary calculi ("stones"). These conditions are usually managed in a hospital or ambulatory setting. If no complications occur, most acute illnesses end in a full recovery and the person returns to the previous or similar level of functioning.

Chronic illness usually refers to conditions that typically have a slower onset, less intensity, and longer duration than acute illnesses. Examples include diabetes mellitus, hypertension, and degenerative joint disease. These conditions are managed in an ambulatory setting, such a as physician's office or health clinic, or in a long-term care facility. The goal of treatment is to help the client attain and maintain the highest possible level of health, although some clients do not return to their previous level of functioning.

Effects of Illness on the Person

Usually, a person experiences one or more changes that signal the presence of illness, for instance:

- Changes in body appearance (weight, skin color)
- Changes in body function (urinary frequency, increased pulse rate)
- Unusual body emissions (blood in urine or stool)
- Changes in the senses (deafness, loss of vision)
- Uncomfortable physical manifestations (headache, backache)
- Changes in emotional state (anxiety, depression)
- Changes in relationships with others (marital conflicts)

Most people experience a mild form of some of these changes in their daily lives. However, when they occur to such a degree that they interfere with usual daily activities, we often consider a person to be ill.

Reactions to Illness

When a person feels ill, his or her reaction to the illness may vary. Some people seek action immediately, whereas others take no action; still others seek counteraction.

TAKING ACTION

When a person responds to illness by taking action, he or she can choose three overlapping sectors of health care: the popular sector, the folk sector, and the professional sector.

The *popular sector* involves a layperson or a nonprofessional. This source of help is usually the first one sought when a person recognizes the presence of an illness and begins health care activities. The health care results from self-treatment or self-medication; advice from relatives, friends, coworkers, or neighbors; activities within a religious or self-help group; or advice from another layperson who experienced a similar type of problem. The main source of primary health care in most societies is the family, and therefore the ill person first seeks assistance from the family when illness occurs.

In some areas of the United States and in non-Western societies, another frequently used source of advice about health care is the *folk sector,* in which certain people specialize in forms of healing. There is a wide variation in types of folk healers, who may include herbalists, spiritual healers, and clairvoyants. Folk healers are not part of the formal medical system.

The third source of help is the *professional sector.* This group includes legally licensed health professionals, such as nurses, physicians, nurse-midwives, and physical therapists. The nurse should accept the client's decision to use more than one sector of health care when illness occurs.

The actions that a person experiencing illness takes are influenced by several factors:

- Availability of health care
- Affordability of health care
- Failure or success of self-prescribed treatment
- Perception of the problem by the client and others

AVAILABILITY OF HEALTH CARE

Access to health care depends on a number of factors. In the United States, if a person lives in an area where health care resources are limited, he or she may not be able to readily find health care services. Even if services are available, the client may have difficulty finding transportation to a physician's office or clinic. *Elderly clients* who no longer drive a car or who live in remote rural areas have to depend on someone else to transport them. Many communities

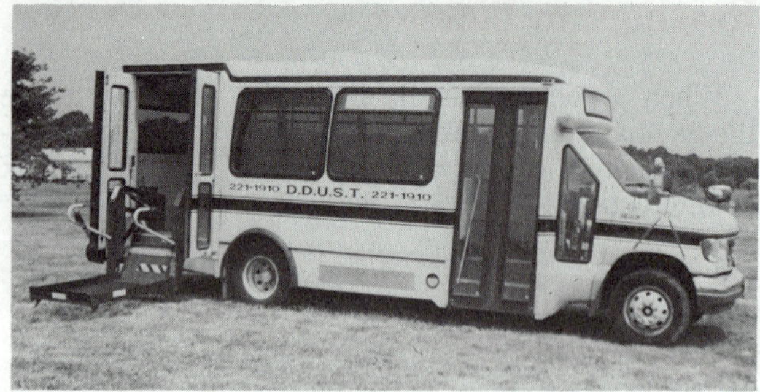

FIGURE 1–4 ◆ A community van that transports elderly clients who cannot drive from their homes to physician offices or clinics.

have Senior Citizens' vans or cars to use for this purpose (Fig. 1–4).

Access to health care has also been a major problem for *homeless people* in the United States. Homeless people usually do not have regular care providers. When the homeless are very ill, they tend to use hospital emergency rooms. In some areas, ambulatory clinics have been established to meet the special needs of this group. The stress of keeping clinic appointments and the fear of being reported for neglect or abuse may prevent the homeless from seeking health care (Berne et al, 1990).

AFFORDABILITY OF HEALTH CARE

Health care in many countries is expensive. In the United States, for example, health care accounts for about 13% of the gross national product. People with health care insurance or adequate finances are more likely than uninsured or poorer people to seek health care for routine physical examinations, preventive health care, or care during illness. Those with more limited budgets necessarily view basic needs of food, clothing, and shelter as more important than health care. Many people cannot afford the high cost of health insurance, and many employers do not offer group health plans to their employees. The number of "working uninsured" in the United States is rapidly growing.

FAILURE OR SUCCESS OF SELF-PRESCRIBED TREATMENT

The results of self-treatment may make further professional help unnecessary. However, when the problem persists despite self-care, the person usually seeks outside assistance for treatment of the illness.

PERCEPTION OF THE PROBLEM

Probably one of the greatest influences on the action of the person in seeking help is his or her perception of the situation. People who do not view themselves as ill are not motivated to seek health care from any source. The severity of the illness, as the client perceives it, may affect the source of help that the client seeks and the speed with which he or she takes action.

The way in which the family or significant others view the health problem also affects the action that the client takes. Agreement with the existence of a problem and its severity may influence the actions that the client takes to seek help.

TAKING NO ACTION

Taking no action is a response to illness. Some people prefer to "wait and see" whether symptoms disappear before deciding to take action. For some short-term illnesses, like indigestion or "colds," taking no action may be appropriate because the body heals itself.

Other people deny the significance of the symptoms or are unwilling to admit that they are ill. Many of the variables that influence people to seek action when illness occurs cause others to take no action. Unavailability of health care resources, unaffordability of health care, failure to recognize the illness, and fear are some of the major reasons why people may not seek needed health care.

TAKING COUNTERACTION

Some people respond to illness by taking counteraction. They engage in certain activities in an attempt to disprove the existence of symptoms. For example, a man with chest pain may increase his activities to prove that he is not having a problem with his heart. Counteraction is an extreme form of denial. The person wants to believe that he or she is healthy even though ill. Because the person is not open to seeking help, the condition may worsen, and severe life-threatening complications may occur.

Stages of Illness

Most people with acute illness follow a pattern of behavior from the onset of illness until recovery. Several theorists have identified a number of stages, but Suchman's (1972) stages are often quoted (Table 1–1).

Effects of Illness on the Family

The presence of illness in a family can have dramatic effects on the function of the family as a unit. The type of effect depends on three factors:

- Which member of the family is ill
- The seriousness and duration of the illness
- The social and cultural customs of the family, with each member of the family having a different role and performing tasks specific to that role

TABLE 1–1 Suchman's Stages of Illness

Stage	Description
Stage 1: Experience of symptoms	• Physical, cognitive, and emotional awareness of illness occurs. The person seeks self-treatment or professional treatment.
Stage 2: Assumption of the sick role	• The person accepts the illness and others validate it.
Stage 3: Contact with the health care system	• The person seeks to verify the illness if it does not improve.
Stage 4: Assumption of the dependent role	• The person may become dependent, but this varies. Some people try to retain control over their lives, but become more passive and concerned about themselves.
Stage 5: Recovery and rehabilitation	• The person returns to usual activities if the illness was acute. Adjustment to a new lifestyle is needed for long-term or chronic illness.

The type of role changes that occur vary, depending on the family member affected. For instance, when the affected family member is the husband, who may have been the primary source of financial support, the wife or children may need to seek employment to supplement the family income. The family makes major role adjustments as the man assumes a dependent role and the woman adapts to a job other than homemaker. When illness affects a woman who is a working single parent, serious economic and child care problems may result. She must depend on support systems to help with the situation or she may experience increased stress.

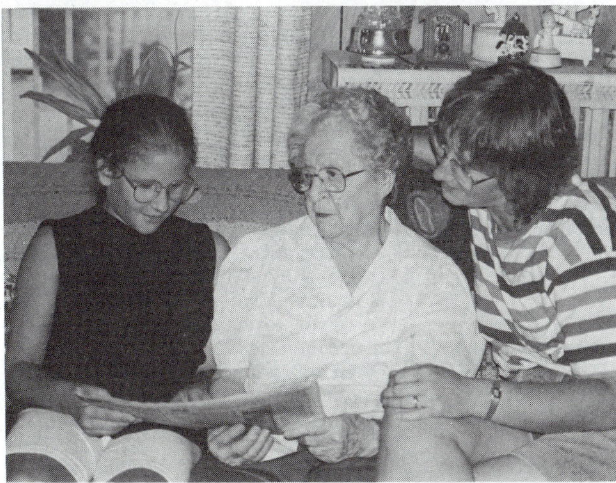

FIGURE 1–5 ◆ A middle-aged woman *(right)* who cares for her child and her mother at home. This caregiver represents someone in the "sandwich generation."

When the sick person is elderly, the family is also affected. An adult child may need to assume parental functions for the parent. As the population becomes older, many young and middle-aged people are caring for their children while caring for their parents. This "sandwich generation" may experience poor health as a result of excessive caregiver responsibilities (Fig. 1–5).

The elderly ill person may have self-care needs related to housing, meals, and assistance with activities of daily living. The added responsibilities on the adult child can cause conflict with personal or other role expectations. Frustrations that are destructive to effective family function may occur.

Economic change related to the loss of a job and the high costs of medical care and hospitalization often has a significant effect on family members. A person's future ability to work and earn income may be affected, depending on the nature of the illness.

HEALTH PROMOTION

Health promotion refers to activities that are directed toward developing a person's resources to maintain or enhance well-being as a protection against illness. Reversing the emphasis from curing the disease to promoting health provides a more positive orientation for health care. Illness no longer needs to be the primary focus of health care. The U.S. Department of Health and Human Services has joined the world mission to promote health in its "Healthy People, 2000" campaign (1990). The expectation is that, by the year 2000, people will be healthier and practicing healthier lifestyles.

Several nursing theorists have developed nursing health promotion models. One of the best known models is that advocated by Pender. In her model, Pender (1987) makes a distinction between health promotion and illness prevention: Health promotion is not "health problem–specific," but prevention is. In addition, she believes that health promotion is a positive activity, whereas illness prevention is an avoidance activity. A number of studies to test her model have been conducted (Research Applications for Nursing).

Although this text integrates illness prevention with health promotion, it recognizes that they are somewhat different. The goal of both types of activities, explained in detail below, is to improve or maintain the client's health. Throughout this text, Health Promotion Guide charts help the nurse in teaching clients about health promotion activities.

Part of the health promotion movement in nursing is reflected in the use of the term *client* rather than *patient.* Although the word patient is associated with a dependent position, the word client suggests an active partnership in the process of health care delivery and maintenance. Client is therefore the term used for the health care consumer in this text.

RESEARCH APPLICATIONS FOR NURSING

Pender's Health Promotion Model Identifies Three Key Factors Predicting a Health-Promoting Lifestyle

Frauman, A. C., & Nettles-Carlson, B. (1991). Predictors of a health-promoting life-style among well adults in a nursing practice. *Journal of the American Academy of Nurse Practitioners, 3*(4), 174–179.

This study was conducted to assess the health-promoting lifestyle of a random sample of 130 well adults in a nurse practitioner's practice. The authors studied the population in relation to the cognitive/perceptual and sociodemographic factors proposed in Pender's Health Promotion Model. The three factors that had a positive effect on self-reported health-promoting lifestyle were the subjects' definition of health, education, and income. The study found that people who have a positive definition of health, who are well educated, and who earn more than $30,000 per year are motivated to engage in health-promoting activities.

Critique This study applied a major nursing model of health promotion to look at factors that affect a person's perception of health and health-promoting behaviors. The sample was randomly selected, although in only one nurse practitioner's practice. Further studies should be conducted to include subjects with other demographic factors, such as more cultural diversity.

Possible nursing implications Nurses should provide clients motivated to engage in health-promoting activities with information that they can use to promote health.

Practices to Promote Health

Researchers have found certain health practices to have a positive correlation with health promotion. Some of these general health practices include:

- Eating well-balanced meals that incorporate foods from the food pyramid as recommended (see Fig. 61–1)
- Moderate eating to maintain ideal weight and prevent obesity
- Moderate exercising on a routine schedule
- Sleeping regularly, about 7 to 8 hours each day
- Limiting consumption of alcohol to a moderate amount
- Not smoking
- Keeping exposure to the sun to a minimum

These practices have been associated with high-level wellness whatever one's sex, age, or economic status. The greater the number of these practices are followed in a consistent, routine manner, the better the health state.

Practices to Prevent Illness

Illness prevention is related to health promotion and maintenance. In an effort to decrease the occurrence of illness, prevention is essential. Preventive health behavior is described as voluntary action taken by a person or group to decrease the potential or actual threat of illness and its harmful consequences. Research has shown that people have to be motivated to make health-related changes (Research Applications for Nursing). Three levels of illness prevention are summarized in Table 1–2: primary, secondary, and tertiary.

PRIMARY PREVENTION

Primary prevention is used to avoid or delay the actual occurrence of a specific disease. Strategies for health maintenance raise the general level of health and well-being of a person, family, or community. Smoking cessation clinics, immunizations, use of seat belts, and use of helmets by motorcyclists are examples of primary prevention strategies.

SECONDARY PREVENTION

Secondary prevention begins after a disease or condition is present, although the signs and symptoms may not be evident. Intervention may lessen the complications and disability resulting from the disease. Emphasis is on early diagnosis and treatment as

TABLE 1–2 Health Behaviors for the Three Levels of Illness Prevention

Level	Examples of Behaviors
Primary prevention	• Wearing seat belts, helmets • Eating well-balanced meals • Not smoking • Consuming no or minimal alcohol • Being immunized • Maintaining ideal body weight
Secondary prevention	• Having yearly Papanicolaou (Pap) smear tests • Doing monthly breast or testicular self-examination • Having mammograms as recommended • Getting skin tests for tuberculosis screening • Having routine tonometry tests to detect glaucoma
Tertiary prevention	• Following a cardiac rehabilitation program • Pursuing rehabilitation programs for stroke, head injury, or arthritis

well as on intervention to prevent or limit permanent disability or death. Screening procedures such as the Papanicolaou (Pap) smear for cervical cancer and purified protein derivative (PPD) skin test for tuberculosis are examples. The purpose is to detect disease early and use preventive measures to avoid further complications, which occur when the disease progresses beyond the early stages.

TERTIARY PREVENTION

Tertiary prevention involves rehabilitation and begins when the disease or condition has stabilized and no further healing is expected, such as cardiac rehabilitation after a myocardial infarction. The goal is to return the person to the highest level of function and to prevent severe disabilities.

Consumer Education and Awareness

Consumer education and awareness have been the major focus in an attempt to influence people and promote wellness. Information about nutrition, exercise, stress management, and routine health examinations is available at schools, work sites, and community centers and in the media. This abundance of information and materials is a major resource for increasing public awareness of the need for health promotion.

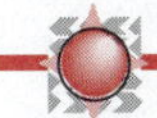

IMPLICATIONS FOR NURSING RESEARCH

Health promotion is an area in which nursing has begun to focus. Some questions for future research include:

- What is the effect of health promotion interventions on the cost of health care?
- What are ways in which nurses can incorporate more health promotion interventions in hospital-based practice?
- How can people be motivated to seek health promotion practices?

SELECTED BIBLIOGRAPHY

Alford, D. M., & Futrell, M. (1992). Wellness and health promotion of the elderly. *Nursing Outlook, 40,* 221–226.

Berne, A. S., Dato, C., Mason, D. J., & Rafferty, M. (1990). A nursing model for addressing the health needs of homeless families. *Image: The Journal of Nursing Scholarship, 22,* 8–13.

Bigbee, J. L., & Jansa, N. (1991). Strategies for promoting health protection. *Nursing Clinics of North America, 26,* 895–913.

*Dunn, H. L. (1980). *High level wellness.* Thorofare, NJ: Charles B. Slack.

Edelman, C. L., & Mandle, C. L. (1990). *Health promotion throughout the lifespan.* Baltimore: C. V. Mosby.

Eubanks, P. (1991). Hospitals offer wellness programs in effort to trim health costs. *Hospitals, 5*(23), 42–43.

Fleury, J. D. (1991). Empowering potential: A theory of wellness motivation. *Nursing Research, 40,* 286–291.

Frauman, A. C., & Nettles-Carlson, B. (1991). Predictors of a health-promoting life-style among well adult clients in a nursing practice. *Journal of the American Academy of Nurse Practitioners, 3*(4), 174–179.

Heidrich, S. M. (1993). The relationship between physical health and psychological well-being in elderly women: A developmental perspective. *Research in Nursing and Health, 16,* 123–130.

Herron, D. G. (1991). Strategies for promoting a healthy dietary intake. *Nursing Clinics of North America, 26,* 875–884.

Lenihan, A. A. (1990). A challenge for nursing: Promotion of self-care among the elderly. *Journal of Gerontological Nursing, 16,* 3–5.

Meleis, A. I., Lipson, J. G., & Paul, S. M. (1992). Ethnicity and health among five Middle Eastern immigrant groups. *Nursing Research, 41,* 98–103.

Melnyk, K. A. C. (1990). Barriers to care: Operationalizing the variable. *Nursing Research, 39,* 108–112.

Palank, C. L. (1991). Determinants of health-promotive lifestyle. *Nursing Clinics of North America, 26,* 815–832.

Peddicord, K. (1991), Strategies for promoting stress reduction and relaxation. *Nursing Clinics of North America, 26,* 867–874.

*Pender, N. J. (1987). *Health promotion in nursing practice* (2nd ed.). Norwalk, CT: Appleton & Lange.

Pruitt, R. H. (1992). Effectiveness and cost efficiency of interventions in health promotion. *Journal of Advanced Nursing, 17,* 926–932.

Rairdan, B., & Higgs, Z. R. (1992). When your patient is a Hmong refugee. *American Journal of Nursing, 92*(3), 52–55.

Spellbring, A. M. (1991). Nursing's role in health promotion. *Nursing Clinics of North America, 26,* 805–814.

*Suchman, E. A. (1972). Stages of medical illness and medical care. In E. G. Jaco (Ed.), *Patients, physicians, and illness.* New York: Free Press.

Tanner, E. K. W. (1991). Assessment of a health-promotive lifestyle. *Nursing Clinics of North America, 26,* 845–854.

U.S. Department of Health and Human Services, Public Health Service. (1990). *Healthy people, 2000: National health promotion and disease prevention objectives.* Washington, D.C.: U.S. Government Printing Office.

*World Health Organization (1947). *Constitution of the World Health Organization: Chronicle of the World Health Organization.* Geneva: Author.

Zhan, L. (1992). Quality of life: Conceptual and measurement issues. *Journal of Advanced Nursing, 17,* 795–800.

SUGGESTED READINGS

Meleis, A. I., Lipson, J. G., & Paul, S. M. (1992). Ethnicity and health among five Middle Eastern immigrant groups. *Nursing Research, 41,* 98–103.

This qualitative research investigated the health beliefs and practices of five Middle Eastern groups who had been in the United States from 1 to 20 years: 16 Arabs, 18 Egyptians, 14 Armenians, 16 Iranians, and 24 Yemenis. The findings showed significant differences among the groups in cultural and social attitudes, family orientation, and perceived health status and morale. The results support the need for nurses and other health professionals to consider ethnic identity as well as country of origin when providing health care.

Rairdan, B., & Higgs, Z. R. (1992). When your patient is a Hmong refugee. *American Journal of Nursing, 92*(3), 52–55.

This article describes the health care beliefs and practices of Hmong families (Southeast Asians) who resettled around Spokane, Washington. The authors present many examples of cultural behavior that nurses should know before providing care to this group. For example, on the basis of an ancient legend, the Hmong consider any blood loss to be extremely dangerous. Therefore, drawing blood samples may be very alarming.

Spellbring, A. M. (1991). Nursing's role in health promotion. *Nursing Clinics of North America, 26,* 805–814.

This article provides an excellent overview of how nurses can promote health. The author discusses the roles of assessment, advocacy, case management, consultancy, promotion of self-care, and health education as they relate to health promotion. (See also Chapter 2 of this textbook.)

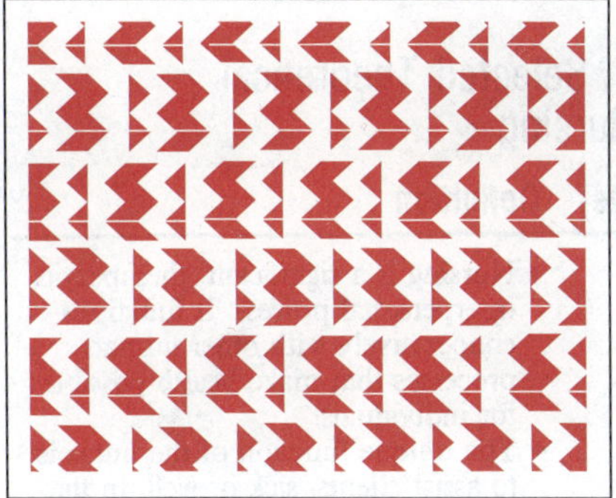

CHAPTER 2

CHAPTER HIGHLIGHTS

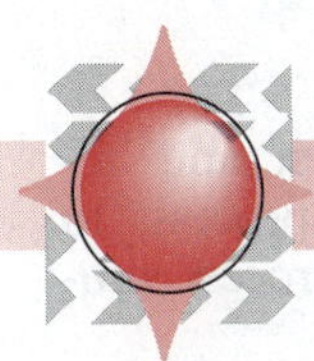

The Nursing Profession and the Role of the Medical-Surgical Nurse

Nursing today is a fast-changing profession that is influenced by increasing knowledge about causes of diseases, rapid advances in science and technology, and lengthening of life expectancy. Nursing is vital to health care and constitutes the largest segment of the total health care delivery system. As changes occur constantly in the health field, nursing continues the processes of defining and describing its role.

DEFINITIONS OF NURSING

Definitions of nursing have been evolving since the time of Florence Nightingale. The question "What is nursing?" is one that has continued to be difficult to answer. Definitions have been developed, analyzed, and reworked.

There are several reasons why it is difficult to state a definition of nursing. First, it is difficult to develop one acceptable definition because the purpose for the definition varies. Defining what nursing is to other professionals requires a different emphasis from that needed for defining nursing to identify the legal scope of practice. Second, the role of nurses is changing as technology, health care consumers, and government influence the practice of nursing.

Legal Definition

Nursing practice varies somewhat from country to country. Each country has its own legislation and guidelines that direct the practice of nursing. In the United States, there was no legal definition of nursing until the 1930s. The early laws did not define nursing; instead, they included descriptions of the nurse and the nurse's functions. In the 1930s, the state nurse practice acts began to define nursing by focusing on the scope of nursing practice. Today, each state has a practice act that legally defines nursing at each level as well as the scope of nursing practice. Because only minor differences exist among the various states, nurses often hold licensure in more than one state. Nurses are held accountable for the performance of activities defined in state nurse practice acts.

Professional Definition

Although nursing is defined legally, professional nursing organizations are also involved in developing a definition and scope of practice for nursing. In the United States, the American Nurses' Association (ANA) defined nursing in its Social Policy Statement of 1980: "Nursing is the diagnosis and treatment of human responses to actual or potential health problems" (ANA, 1980, p. 9).

The ANA also published the *Standards of Clinical Nursing Practice* (1991), which incorporates both standards of care (including the nursing process) and standards of professional performance (including use of research findings and ethics in practice). See the Appendix for the ANA *Standards of Clinical Nursing Practice.* These basic, broad standards apply to nurses in all settings and are supported by most specialty nursing organizations as well as the recently formed Academy of Medical-Surgical Nurses (AMSN). Additional published standards for specialty practice are available through the ANA or specialty nursing organizations.

Definitions by Nursing Theorists

Throughout the history of nursing, definitions by nursing theorists and leaders have evolved. A list of several prominent nursing theorists along with the major points of their definitions is given in Table 2-1. The changing definitions reveal that nursing is progressing from the traditional view of caring for ill people. Today's nurse is a process-oriented, goal-directed professional who cares for individual clients, families, and communities and promotes health maintenance and the prevention of illness.

In addition to having developed a definition of nursing, many nurse theorists have developed conceptual models to describe the unique role of nursing. Because there is no consensus about which, if any, of the models should be accepted by the nursing profession, this text does not adopt a specific model for application. Rather, it uses a well-known and accepted practice framework, the nursing process, to organize the information. The nursing process provides the structure for nursing practice.

TABLE 2-1 Selected Theoretical Definitions of Nursing

Nurse Theorist (Date)	Definition
Peplau (1952)	• Nursing is a significant, therapeutic, interpersonal process. It functions cooperatively with other human processes that make health possible for individuals.
Henderson (1960)	• The unique function of the nurse is to assist clients, sick or well, in the performance of those activities contributing to health, recovery, or peaceful death.
King (1971)	• Nursing is an interpersonal process of action, reaction, interaction, and transaction whereby nurse and client share information about their perceptions in the nursing situation.
Roy (1976)	• As a science, nursing is a developing system of knowledge about human beings used to observe, classify, and relate the processes by which persons positively affect their health status.

ROLES OF MEDICAL-SURGICAL NURSES

As professional nursing meets changing health care needs, the expectations for providing client care have expanded and increased. Medical-surgical nurses assume various roles and functions within the health care setting (Fig. 2-1). Although each role is associated with specific responsibilities, some aspects of each role are interrelated and are common to all nursing positions and specialties.

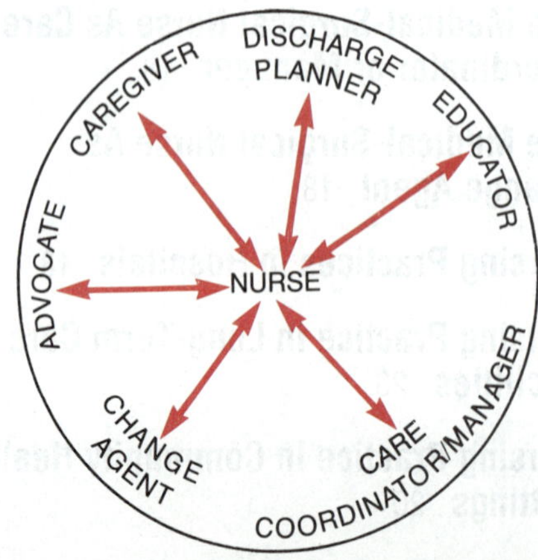

FIGURE 2-1 ◆ Major roles of the medical-surgical nurse.

Caregiver

The role most commonly associated with the medical-surgical nurse is caregiver. In this role, nurses assess clients, analyze collected information to determine clients' needs, develop nursing diagnoses, plan nursing care and carry out the plan, and evaluate the care given. This process, which is referred to as the *nursing process,* is detailed in Chapter 3 and is used throughout this text as an organizational and practice framework.

As a caregiver, the nurse provides physical care through skills such as taking vital signs, changing dressings, or administering medications. The nurse also implements psychosocial interventions, such as encouraging the client to discuss concerns or offering measures to reduce the client's anxiety.

The functions performed by the nurse caregiver are often categorized as collaborative (or interdependent) or independent. *Collaborative* functions include

- Those mutually determined by the nurse and the physician or other health care team member, such as activity limitations or a special diet
- Those directed or prescribed by the physician but requiring nursing judgment to perform, such as giving medications

Independent nursing functions are those initiated and carried out by the nurse without direction from the physician, like weighing a client, listening to bowel sounds, and testing blood glucose with a fingerstick.

This text includes both types of functions—collaborative and independent—in an interrelated framework under the heading Collaborative Management. Charts titled Nursing Care Highlight identify the most important nursing functions for clients with selected health problems.

Discharge Planner

Because the focus of health care continues to emphasize early discharge from the hospital, the role of the medical-surgical nurse as discharge planner has become increasingly important. Discharge planning involves an assessment of the client's health needs before discharge. A large part of this process is assessment of the home or other setting to which the client is discharged for available resources, support systems, and equipment if needed. The nurse then teaches clients how to continue care after discharge.

Discharge planning may be coordinated by a designated discharge planner employed by the hospital in collaboration with the staff nurse. The discharge planner may be a nurse or social worker. If the hospital does not employ designated discharge planners, the staff nurse caring for the client is solely responsible for the discharge planning process. Throughout this text, a section on discharge planning is included to offer guidance to the nurse.

Educator

Client education is a large part of medical-surgical nursing care. The nurse tries to improve health by providing information on health promotion, disease and illness, and specific treatment. As educators, nurses work with individual clients as well as with family members or other caregivers. The role of education has become increasingly important because clients are discharged "quicker and sicker" from the hospital to the home. Nurses often become frustrated when they feel that they do not have as much time as they need to teach in the hospital setting (Research Applications for Nursing).

RESEARCH APPLICATIONS FOR NURSING

Many Nurses See the Importance of Client Education—Yet Fall Short in Providing It

Kruger, S. (1991). The patient educator role in nursing. *Applied Nursing Research, 4,* 19–24.

The author surveyed a stratified random sample of 1230 staff nurses, nurse administrators, and nurse educators for their perceptions of their roles as client educators. Data from 756 questionnaires were usable. The results showed that most nurses in each group thought that client education was an important part of their role. However, they expressed concern that they did not educate their clients as often or as much as they should have. Many nurses in the sample offered suggestions for meeting the expected increasing need for client education in the hospital setting.

Critique The topic of the client educator role for nurses is a timely one in view of one-day hospital stays and early discharges. The author used a large, random sample, which provided adequate data to support her conclusions. She also compared each subgroup for differences in their perceptions.

Possible nursing implications Nurses need to seriously re-evaluate their role as client educators and plan ways to meet the increased need for education in the hospital setting. Nurse educators should examine their curricula to ensure that client education is stressed as a vital role for the nurse. Opportunities for nursing students to incorporate client education into their practice should be provided.

THE TEACHING-LEARNING PROCESS

Before educating clients, the nurse assesses the client's learning needs. A client with a disease of 20 years' duration may need as much teaching as one who is newly diagnosed. The nurse makes no assumptions but, rather, assesses each client individually. The nurse also assesses the client's willingness to learn and determines the client's goals (Redman & Thomas, 1992). If the client has no interest in learning, the nurse waits until another time or setting before beginning client education (if ever). Chart 2–1 summarizes the most important teaching-learning principles for adults.

Teaching may occur in a spontaneous, informal manner, or it may follow a more structured, formal approach based on written plans. Most facilities provide written teaching plans and tools for nurses to use to ensure that every client receives the same accurate information. For particular aspects of teaching, such as therapeutic diets, the nurse requests teaching by the health team member who specializes in that aspect of health care (in this case, the dietitian).

The nurse documents what was taught and what the client learned on the appropriate record (Fig. 2–2). A summary of the teaching-learning process for each client generally becomes a part of the client's medical record. A copy is also given to the client or family or significant other at the time of discharge. Each Discharge Planning section within this text includes a section titled Health Teaching. Education Guides for teaching are also included as appropriate throughout the text.

CHART 2–1

Nursing Care Highlight ♦ Principles of the Adult Teaching-Learning Process

- Assess the client's willingness to learn, and assess the client's goals.
- Before beginning teaching, assess how the client is feeling (e.g., a client in acute pain is unlikely to learn).
- Include family and significant others in teaching as appropriate.
- Assess factors that may influence the client's ability or motivation to learn, such as educational level, socioeconomic status, and cultural background.
- Provide pictures or other types of visual aids to reinforce learning.
- Break complex information or skills into small parts, and teach each part until the client learns it.
- Provide the client with "hands-on" experience for psychomotor skills, and request a return demonstration by the client (e.g., insulin administration, dressing change, colostomy care).
- Provide the client with a health resource contact for follow-up questions or concerns.

FACTORS AFFECTING THE TEACHING-LEARNING PROCESS

As the nurse assesses the teaching-learning needs of each client, the nurse evaluates many factors. Some of the most important factors include the client's educational level, socioeconomic level, support system, age, and transcultural considerations.

EDUCATIONAL LEVEL

The client's educational level directly affects the nurse's plans for teaching. In the United States, it is estimated that more than a third of adults do not have a high school diploma. Consequently, illiteracy in the United States is quite widespread. Information written for the public should therefore not be above the 8th-grade reading level and often needs to be lower. Dixon and Park (1990) found that most hospital education materials are typically written at a level between the 9th and 13th grades.

For clients who cannot read or who have limited reading skills, the nurse uses other types of visual aids, such as pictures and symbols. The nurse explains and interprets information for clients rather than merely offering them a booklet or instruction sheet.

SOCIOECONOMIC LEVEL

When teaching clients how to care for themselves at home, the nurse considers the client's financial resources. For example, if the client needs to perform muscle-strengthening exercises using small weights, the nurse cannot always expect the client to purchase commercial weights because they are expensive. Instead, the nurse suggests the use of 1- or 2-pound coffee cans or bags, bags of sugar or flour, or similar available household items.

Another concern for the nurse is the cost of required medication, equipment, or supplies. For instance, for those clients who do not qualify for medical assistance but work for an employer who does not provide group health insurance, the client may not be able to afford the necessary medically related items or follow-up care. As part of discharge planning, the nurse attempts to locate resources, such as community health organizations like the American Cancer Society, that can provide the necessary resources. In addition, clinics that specialize in providing care for working uninsured clients are beginning to become available in the United States.

SUPPORT SYSTEM

The nurse assesses the client's support system and often includes parts or all of the system in client education. Examples of support systems include families, significant others, churches, and social community clubs and organizations. In general, people tend to be more compliant with their health regimen if they have the encouragement of others (Redman & Thomas, 1992). Support is particularly important if the client must follow many lifestyle restrictions. For instance, a farmer who may be accustomed to fried foods and red meat may find it difficult to change to a low-fat, low-sodium diet. If the farmer's wife has always been the cook in the home, the nurse includes her in the teaching process to help to ensure compliance with the new dietary restrictions.

Teaching-Learning Record for Insulin Self-Administration			
Steps	Taught/Demonstrated (Initial)	Date	Return Demonstration (Initial)
1. Selects correct insulin type.			
2. Selects correct syringe.			
3. Cleans top of vial.			
4. Draws up correct insulin amount(s).			
5. Selects appropriate site for injection.			
6. Cleans skin with alcohol swipe.			
7. Uses 90-degree angle when injecting insulin.			

FIGURE 2–2 ◆ A sample teaching-learning record for self-administration of insulin.

AGE

Age affects the teaching-learning process. An elderly client may take longer to process information or may have visual or hearing deficits (Chart 2–2). The nurse provides small amounts of information at one time and checks with the client before proceeding to make sure that he or she has understood. Too much information is difficult to comprehend and absorb and usually results in the client's frustration and noncompliance.

TRANSCULTURAL CONSIDERATIONS

The nurse considers the client's cultural background before teaching. If the client does not clearly understand the nurse's language, the nurse locates resources that can help with the teaching process. For example, many people who immigrated to the United States in the 1940s have attempted to retain their language and culture and not become too "Americanized." As a result, when they are hospitalized, they often cannot understand what is going on and need someone to interpret for them.

Another aspect to consider is the health practices of various cultures. For example, Mexican-Americans, particularly those living near the Mexican border, often use *curandismo,* or folk medicine, because they cannot afford traditional health care. Another reason that these clients avoid the health care system is that they may have limitations in speaking, reading, or writing English or Spanish (Adams et al., 1992). The nurse needs to know this information so that she or he can incorporate cultural beliefs and practices into the teaching-learning process.

The nurse also considers spiritual and religious differences. A client whose spiritual beliefs forbid taking medication is not likely to comply with instructions about drug therapy.

CHART 2–2

Nursing Focus on the Elderly ◆ Teaching the Older Adult

- Ensure that the client wears glasses or hearing aids if needed.
- Be sure that the area for teaching has ample lighting and results in minimal distraction.
- Provide most of the teaching in the morning (after breakfast), before the client becomes too fatigued.
- Speak slowly, and provide small amounts of new information at a time.
- Ask the client to repeat the information to make sure that he or she has learned it.
- Provide written information so that the client can refer to it later if needed.

Advocate

As a client advocate, the nurse assists the client and family in interpreting information from other health care team members. The nurse offers additional information that the client needs to make decisions about health care. This assistance may include explanations about the implications of the client's decisions about health and ensuring that the client receives appropriate care. For example, a client scheduled for a total knee replacement may not understand that the knee joint will be removed and replaced with a prosthesis. If the nurse determines that the client does not fully understand the operative procedure, he or she notifies the surgeon of the need for additional preoperative education. The nurse reinforces the information even if another health team member has provided it.

Client advocacy is closely associated with the field of ethics. Chapter 6 discusses ethics in detail and illustrates examples of ethical dilemmas that medical-surgical nurses encounter in their practice.

Care Coordinator or Manager

A variety of health care team members provide client care. Although the physician is usually considered the head of the health care team, the nurse serves an important role in coordinating the efforts of all team members in meeting the client's goals. Nurses may conduct team conferences to facilitate communication among members of the team, especially in settings in which the client is institutionalized for an extended period, such as on a rehabilitation unit, or in home care situations.

A fairly new concept in care coordination is *case management,* or *managed care.* Managed care is a way of organizing health care delivery that focuses on coordination among health care team members (Mosher et al., 1992). It provides continuity and consistency of care and promotes communication and client education.

In the hospital setting, the concept of managed care is becoming increasingly popular. The main feature of managed care models is the "commitment of nurses to improve the quality of patient care through the appropriate and efficient use of resources and services . . ." (Smith et al., 1992, p. 47).

Managed care, also called *nursing case management,* may be implemented in a number of ways. One common method requires the nurse to follow pre-established clinical pathways based on medical diagnoses (Zander, 1988; Giuiliano, 1991). A clinical pathway is the tool for tracking client progress in a managed care system. In the example in Figure 2–3, criteria for each postoperative day for the client who has undergone a transurethral resection of the prostate (TURP) are listed. The nurse usually initials each plan when it is implemented. This system not only promotes consistency in nursing care but also decreases the information that the nurse would ordinarily have to record with a traditional system. Ideally, managed care facilitates the client's recovery and discharge from the hospital (Manthey, 1991). Other examples of clinical pathways are located throughout this textbook.

Change Agent

The professional nurse serves as a change agent within the work setting and within the profession. The role of change agent involves planning and implementing a system to change the client's health-related behaviors. In the work setting, the nurse assesses health behaviors of the client and family to identify those that need altering. The most important factor in this process is to assess the client's readiness to change. If the client is not ready, he or she will not comply with the change and the nurse will be ineffective in this role.

Within the community, nurses serve as role models and assist consumers in bringing about changes to improve the environment, work conditions, or other factors that affect health. Nurses also work together to bring about change through legislation. For example, nurses provide and support bills for legislation that can affect a person's health status, such as those mandating seat belts and helmets for motorcyclists.

PRACTICE SETTINGS FOR NURSES

Nurses have opportunities to provide health care in a variety of settings, including hospitals, long-term care facilities, and community health settings.

Hospitals

Hospitals, or acute care facilities, make up the largest employers of nurses; approximately two thirds of all nurses work within hospitals. Most medical-surgical nurses are employed by hospitals.

In the United States, the cost of hospital care is usually paid for by third-party payers, or insurers. Medicare Part A (in-hospital coverage), a federal program, pays for most of the care given to people older than 65 years of age and to any client who is disabled. Private insurers pay for most or part of the care provided to clients with insurance. State medical assistance programs pay for most of the health care provided for clients of any age who are indigent.

In Canada, all people are entitled to free comprehensive health care for life. In the 1960s, the Canadian government started this system with the belief that health care should be accessible to all Canadian citizens.

The Memorial Hospital at Easton, Md., Inc.
CRITICAL PATHWAY – TURP

DRG: 337 LOS 4.0

G O A L S

PATIENT PROBLEM	PRE OP	DOS	PO1	PO2	PO3
1. Knowledge Deficit Related To: 1. procedure 2. post-op care 3. home care	Pre-op education for pt/family to include definition of surgical procedure, and post-operative routine.	Reinforce pre-op teaching emphasizing respiratory care and post-operative routine.	Patient will participate in care by using PCA, assisting with Foley catheter care and increasing ambulation.	Patient can verbalize type of surgical procedure performed, reason for procedure, need for increased fluid intake, and measures to promote bladder control.	Patient can verbalize home care teaching information including sexual activity, activity restrictions, and meds (esp. antibiotics). Patient notes reasons to notify M.D. after discharge including burning on urination, urgency, excessive bleeding.
2. Pain	Appropriate allergy assessment	Patient will report adequate pain control on PCA & anti-spasmodic.	Patient will report adequate pain control with P.O. narcotic & antispasmodic. →	→	→
3. Family/Community Support		Family will be able to state peri-op schedule	Assessment of family functioning noting the need for follow-up care and/or assistive services.	Provide information on the appropriate community support—i.e. Home Health Services.	Formal referral to community support.
4. Post-Op Complications					
A. Blood Loss	Pre-op hematology evaluation	Early detection of excessive blood loss. Expect clear red-pink urinary output →	→	Clear pink urinary output. No clots. H&H within normal range.	Patient will have clear urine—no clots or new bleeding.
B. Infection	Pre-op eval for urinary infection	Evaluation for and early detection of signs and symptoms of sepsis		Patient will be afebrile	
C. Catheter Function		Patient will have a patent urinary catheter with saline irrigation evidenced by clear red urine →	→ clear pink urine →	→ clear yellow urine →	Patient will produce urinary output quantity & frequency sufficient. Patient may experience burning on urination. Clearing kidney rack →

P L A N

	PRE OP	DOS	PO1	PO2	PO3
Consults	Old records to SDS				
Assessment	Evaluation of need for: 1. Medical Consult 2. history of ASA or anti-coagulant therapy 3. history of prosthetic implant	Pre-Op Assessment to include respiratory, C-V & GU systems; I & O; V.S. q 1hr x 4 then q4h x 48h →; Assess blood loss →	→	Assess urinary output frequency, consistency & amount ≥ 100 cc/void with a frequency no greater than one time/hour →	
Tests	Pre-op lab work to include: CBC, SMA 6/60 12/60, Acid Phos. EKG, Chext X-ray PSA T&C – 2u PRBC within 72 hrs of admission	T&C – 2u PRBC's if not T&C as an outpatient	Hgb/HCT 6/60 with creatinine; EKG		
Activity	Elastic stockings		OOB →	→	→
Treatments	IV fluids per anesthesia protocol	Post-op Continuous irrigation with N/S to keep catheter clear →; Irrigate with Toomey syringe pm; Post-Op RL 1 liter KVO at 75 cc/hr	Remove tape and traction D/C IV if stable →	Remove Foley cath if urine is clear yellow. Fill the bladder with irrigation fluid before removing Foley. → Begin kidney rack. →	→
Medications	Antibiotics as necessary. Patient's usual meds as ordered by physician.	Active Post-Op med orders for Senokot, Bentyl, Demerol, Tylenol, MOM, Cascara, sleeping medication and antibiotics.	P.O. pain meds; P.O. antibiotic		Prescription for antibiotics to go home with patient.
Nutrition		NPO Pre-Op; Post-Op clear liquids; After nausea diet as tolerated →	→	→	→
Discharge Planning			Assessment of family function	Send formal referral for home health services if needed	Make follow-up appointment for pateint prior to discharge.
Teaching	Pre-Op instruction to include C&DB, leg exercises, Foley catheter, and pain control. Give the patient a copy of the patient pathway.	Peri-Op & Post-Op teaching including C&DB, leg exercises, Foley catheter, pain control specific to PCA. Encourage fluids.	Institute functional teaching related to pain control. Foley catheter care and ambulation expectations. Bowel teaching to include the possibility of increased bleeding with first BM.	Teach 1, 2, 5, 6 as described on teaching record.	Discharge home instructions to include 3, 4, 7, 8 from teaching record, and the need to call the physician if the patient's perineal skin becomes excoriated. Reinforce teaching. Answer specific questions.
Psycho Social	Pre-Op review of procedure and post-op physical changes	Review with the family the pre-op/post-op O.R. and R.R. process. Reassure family members with information about the post-operative routine.	Reinforce post-op sensations and care the patient will experience →	→	→
Other					

INITIALS	SIGNATURE/TITLE	DATE	TIME	INITIALS	SIGNATURE/TITLE	DATE	TIME

FORM 141855 (5/92)

Physician Signature ________________

FIGURE 2–3 ◆ A clinical pathway used in caring for a client after transurethral resection of the prostate (TURP). (Courtesy of Memorial Hospital at Easton, Easton, MD.)

There are three general types of units in most hospital settings:

- Critical care units
- Intermediate care units
- Long-term care units

Because of the different specialty areas within hospitals, many medical-surgical nursing opportunities are available.

CRITICAL CARE UNITS

Critical care units are areas for the intense care of critically ill clients. Examples are surgical or medical intensive care units, shock trauma and "step-down" units, and neurosurgical intensive care units. Emergency and operating departments are also considered critical care areas because of the acute and intense nature of the care provided in these parts of the hospital. Critical care areas require nurses who thrive in crisis situations and work effectively under high stress. Nurses must be highly skilled in making accurate observations of clients' conditions and interpreting findings quickly and correctly. The nurse-to-client ratio in critical care units is typically 1:1 or 1:2.

INTERMEDIATE CARE UNITS

Intermediate care units have changed dramatically over the past decade. The clients on these units today are much sicker than in the past. Examples of intermediate care areas are neuroscience (neurology) units, renal (urology) units, and orthopaedic units. In hospitals that are too small to separate clients by specialty, intermediate care units provide treatment for a combination of medical and surgical health problems.

Nurses in intermediate care areas must be able to adapt to caring for various types of illness and must be interested in health teaching and discharge planning. As in critical care areas, nurses must also be highly skilled in making accurate assessments and performing technical procedures.

LONG-TERM CARE UNITS

Long-term care (LTC) units are areas within or adjacent to the hospital in which clients have chronic illnesses or health problems requiring constant care and rehabilitation. Examples are rehabilitation and chronic disease units. Some hospitals also offer a skilled nursing facility (SNF), or nursing home, as part of the in-hospital system. In long-term care units, some clients can learn how to help themselves, whereas other clients are at their optimal level of wellness, which must be maintained.

Long-Term Care Facilities

The second largest practice setting for nurses is the long-term care facility, or freestanding nursing home. Roughly 10% of all nurses work in these settings. These health facilities provide long-term nursing care to clients typically older than 65 years of age, although the age range is expanding to include younger clients with chronic and disabling diseases. In the United States, most clients in a long-term care facility pay for care out of pocket. State medical assistance and private insurance pay for part of the care provided for clients who cannot afford to pay otherwise. Medicare Part A pays for only a few selected types of skilled care in a long-term care facility.

A major change in long-term care is the acuity level of the clients. Largely as a result of quicker discharges of clients from hospitals, many long-term care facilities have specialty or subacute units, such as those for head or spinal cord injury and clients using ventilators. Many facilities also have specialized units for clients with dementia.

With the increasing interest in gerontological nursing, nurses are turning to the challenge of long-term care nursing as an alternative to nursing practice in a hospital. The primary advantage of long-term care nursing is the independence to make nursing decisions about client care. The disadvantage is that much of the direct client care in most facilities is given by geriatric nursing assistants, while nurses spend a large amount of time completing government-required paperwork.

Community Health Settings

Community health settings represent the third largest practice setting for nurses and employ about 6.5% of nurses. Examples of community health settings in which nurses practice are:

- Schools
- Physicians' offices
- Industrial centers
- Public health departments
- Visiting nurse organizations
- Health maintenance organizations (HMOs)
- Other ambulatory care centers or clinics

Programs offered in these settings are vast and include family planning, substance abuse intervention, mental illness care, diagnostic and preventive care, and home health care. Nurses in these settings have a great amount of responsibility and influence. In most of these settings, a physician is not readily available and the nurse makes the initial determination about health care needs.

With the increased emphasis on health promotion and maintenance, the number of community health agencies is growing. The early discharge of clients from hospitals to the home is creating a greater need for nurses in the area of home health.

In the United States, payment for home health care depends on the type and frequency of the service required. Some home health care is paid for by Medicare or state medical assistance programs. Clients often have to pay out-of-pocket expenses.

PROFESSIONAL DEVELOPMENT OF NURSES

A critical development related to nursing as a profession is its own specialized body of knowledge on which its skills and services are based. Nursing continually expands this body of knowledge through education, professional association activities, and research.

Education

Formal education programs designed for registered nurses who wish to pursue a baccalaureate degree in nursing or to continue their education through graduate courses at the master's and doctoral levels are becoming more available. Nurses who wish to specialize in particular areas of nursing may elect to take courses in such specialties as gerontology, trauma nursing, and cardiovascular nursing.

In the United States, nurses may also become certified in specialty areas by the American Nurses' Association (ANA) or by nursing specialty organizations that offer a certification examination. The ANA offers certification in medical-surgical nursing. Like continuing education, certification is voluntary. To obtain certification, nurses typically require evidence of experience and continuing education credits and a passing score on a standardized examination (Table 2–2). Some employers recognize certification as validation of expertise and reward nurses who become certified.

Continuing education in nursing is important because of changes occurring in the fields of science and technology. Nurses have a responsibility to expand their knowledge, update their skills, and remain aware of current changes in the health field. Workshops, seminars, and in-service programs within practice settings are a few of the ways by which nurses can continue their education. Professional journals, programmed education texts or computer-assisted instruction, and correspondence courses are other methods by which the nurse can obtain additional knowledge at home.

Professional Organizations

Professional nursing organizations have formed in many countries. For example, in Canada, the largest organization is the Canadian Nurses' Association. In the United States, there are more than one hundred nursing organizations representing many nursing roles and specialties. The purpose of most professional organizations is to continue to define and develop the scope of nursing practice through networking and continuing education. Membership in any nursing organization is voluntary. The two largest organizations in the United States are the ANA and the National League for Nursing (NLN). For nursing students, there is an organization to help meet the special needs of students—the National Student Nurses' Association (NSNA).

AMERICAN NURSES' ASSOCIATION

Founded in 1896, the American Nurses' Association (ANA) is the official professional organization of nursing in the United States. Its purposes are to foster high standards of nursing practice and to promote the professional and educational advancement of nursing. ANA membership is restricted to registered nurses.

NATIONAL LEAGUE FOR NURSING

The NLN was formed to assist in maintaining the purposes and goals of professional nursing within the broader realm of health care. Membership includes registered nurses and licensed practical or vocational nurses, other health professionals, and laypeople. Or-

TABLE 2–2 Selected Nursing Certifications

Organization	Certification	Designation
American Association of Critical-Care Nurses Certification Corporation	• Critical care nurse	• CCRN
Association of Operating Room Nurses Certification Board	• Operating room nurse	• CNOR
American Board of Occupational Health Nurses	• Occupational health nurse	• COHN
American Board of Neuroscience Nurses	• Neuroscience nurse	• CNRN
American Nurses Credentialing Center (ANCC)	• Medical-surgical nurse	• RNC
	• Community health nurse	• RNC
	• Medical-surgical clinical specialist	• CS, RNC
	• Gerontological nurse	• RNC
	• Nursing administrator	• CNAA, CNA
Orthopaedic Nurses Certification Board	• Orthopaedic nurse	• ONC
American Nephrology Nurses Association	• Nephrology nurse	• CHN, CNN
Emergency Nurses Association	• Emergency department nurse	• CEN

ganized in 1952, the NLN promotes the improvement of nursing service and nursing education. One of its major services is the voluntary accreditation of nursing schools to ensure high standards. It also accredits home health agencies on request.

NATIONAL STUDENT NURSES' ASSOCIATION

The NSNA was established in 1952 with the help of the ANA to promote professional development for nursing students. It has encouraged students to become interested in and aware of current issues and trends in nursing. Membership in this organization prepares the nursing student for professional membership in nursing organizations.

OTHER NURSING SPECIALTY ORGANIZATIONS

Many nursing specialty organizations have formed to promote specific areas, such as practice, education, and administration. These organizations offer continuing education, publications, and meetings to keep members informed of advances in their practice areas. Some of the larger specialty groups include the American Association of Critical-Care Nurses (AACN), the Association of Operating Room Nurses (AORN), and the National Association of Orthopaedic Nurses (NAON). (Information on specialty organizations is found in the Appendix.)

Nursing Research

The primary tasks of nursing research are to promote the growth of the science of nursing and to develop nursing theories to serve as a scientific basis for nursing practice. Nurses have a responsibility to become involved in nursing research and to apply research findings in their practice. Although not all nurses are prepared in research methods, each nurse can participate by remaining alert for nursing problems and asking questions about the practice of care. Nurses who give direct care often identify such problems, which serve as a basis for research investigation. Nurses can promote nursing care by incorporating research findings into their practice and by communicating the research to others.

Boxed features called Research Applications for Nursing are found throughout this text to help the student recognize how research can be applied in clinical practice. A brief review and critique of each study is presented, and potential nursing implications that can be used in daily nursing practice are discussed.

MEDICAL-SURGICAL NURSING AS A SPECIALTY

Medical-surgical nursing is one of the many specialties in nursing, yet its scope is much broader than such specialties as cardiovascular and orthopaedic nursing. In 1991 the Academy of Medical-Surgical Nurses (AMSN) was formed as the first specialty organization for this group of nurses. Full membership is available to any registered nurse living in the United States, Canada, or Mexico. The official journal of the AMSN is *MEDSURG Nursing.*

This text explains the diverse roles and responsibilities of the medical-surgical nurse. The nurse who specializes in medical-surgical nursing may be working in any of the health care settings previously described, although most are employed in hospitals.

The focus of medical-surgical nursing is on the adult client with acute or chronic illness. Nurses who specialize in medical-surgical nursing need a broad knowledge of the biologic, psychologic, and social sciences because of the range of clients for whom they care. The goal of care is the same as that for any other specialty—the achievement of an optimal level of wellness and prevention of illness.

Medical-surgical clients range in age from 18 years old to more than 100 years old, and their health problems are usually complex. Because the typical client is usually more than 65 years old, medical-surgical nurses need a strong background in gerontology, or care of the elderly. In this text, boxed features titled Nursing Focus on the Elderly highlight the special nursing interventions that this group of clients requires.

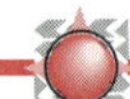

IMPLICATIONS FOR NURSING RESEARCH

Only through continued research can nursing develop theories and establish a scientific basis for practice. The following questions provide areas for further research:

- Are current nursing theories valid in clinical practice?
- What nursing care delivery system can provide high-quality medical-surgical nursing care at an acceptable cost?
- Is managed care effective in ensuring high-quality nursing practice?
- How can the ANA's *Standards of Clinical Nursing Practice* be applied in medical-surgical nursing?
- How does each nursing role affect the care of the medical-surgical client?

SELECTED BIBLIOGRAPHY

Adams, R., Briones, E. H., & Rentfro, A. R. (1992). Cultural considerations: Developing a nursing care delivery system for a Hispanic community. *Nursing Clinics of North America, 27,* 107–116.

Aiken, L. H. (1990). Changing the future of hospital nursing. *Image: The Journal of Nursing Scholarship, 22*(2), 72–78.

Alpert, H. B., Goldman, L. D., Kilroy, C. M., & Pike, A. W. (1992). 7 Gryzmish: Toward an understanding of collaboration. *Nursing Clinics of North America, 27,* 47–59.

American Nurses' Association. (1991). *Standards of clinical practice.* Kansas City: Author.

*American Nurses' Association. (1980). *The nurse practice act: Suggested state legislation.* Kansas City: Author.

*American Nurses' Association. (1980). *Nursing: A social policy statement.* Kansas City: Author.

Carroll-Johnson, R. M. (1991). *Classification of nursing diagnoses: Proceedings of the ninth conference.* Philadelphia: J. B. Lippincott.

Cohen, E. L. (1991). Nursing case management: Does it pay? *Journal of Nursing Administration, 21*(4), 20–25.

Curley, D., & Davis, F. D. (1993). Nursing past, present, and future. *Med-Surg Nursing Quarterly, 1*(3), 98–103.

Funk, S. G., Champagne, M. T., Wiese, R. A., & Tornquist, E. M. (1991). Barriers to using research findings in practice: A clinician's perspective. *Applied Nursing Research, 4,* 90–95.

Giuliano, K. K., & Poirer, C. E. (1991). Nursing case management: Critical pathways to desirable outcomes. *Nursing Management, 22*(3), 52–57.

*Hegyvary, S. (1982). *The change to primary nursing.* St. Louis: C. V. Mosby.

Kelly, K. C., McClelland, E., & Daly, J. M. (1992). Discharge planning. (pp. 265–273). In G. M. Bulachek & J. C. McCloskey (Eds.), *Nursing interventions: Essential nursing treatments.* Philadelphia: W. B. Saunders.

Kruger, S. (1991). The patient educator role in nursing. *Applied Nursing Research, 4,* 19–24.

Lott, T. F., Blazey, M. E., & West, M. G. (1992). Patient participation in health care: An underused resource. *Nursing Clinics of North America, 27,* 61–76.

Manthey, M. (1991). Delivery systems and practice models: A dynamic balance. *Nursing Management, 22*(1), 28–30.

McGuffin, B., & Mariani, M. (1990). Clinical nursing standards: Toward a synthesis. *Journal of Nursing Quality Assurance, 4*(3), 35–45.

Mosher, C., Cronk, P., Kidd, A., McCormick, P., Stockton, S., & Sulla, C. (1992). Upgrading practice with critical pathways. *American Journal of Nursing, 92*(1), 41–44.

Naylor, M. (1990). Comprehensive discharge planning for the elderly: A pilot study. *Nursing Research, 39,* 156–161.

Naylor, M. (1990). Comprehensive discharge planning for the elderly. *Research in Nursing and Health, 13,* 327–347.

Rayfield, C. A. (1991). Later always arrives sooner than you think. *Nursing Management, 22*(3), 84–85.

*Redman, B. K. (1988). *The process of patient education.* St. Louis: C. V. Mosby.

Redman, B. K., & Thomas, S. A. (1992). Patient teaching. (pp. 304–314). In G. M. Bulechek & J. C. McCloskey (Eds.), *Nursing interventions: Essential nursing treatments.* Philadelphia: W. B. Saunders.

Smith, P., Pass, C. M., Pounovich-Stream, C., & Jones, B. (1992). Implementing nurse case management in a community hospital. *MEDSURG Nursing, 1,* 47–52.

Sullivan, P. S., & Goodman, P. S. (1990). Involving practicing nurses in research. *Applied Nursing Research, 3,* 169–173.

Tuazon, N. C. (1992). Discharge teaching: Use this MODEL. *RN, 55*(4), 19–21.

*Zander, K. (1988). Nursing care management: Strategic management of cost and quality outcomes. *Journal of Nursing Administration, 18,* 23–30.

SUGGESTED READINGS

Aiken, L. H. (1990). Changing the future of hospital nursing. *Image: The Journal of Nursing Scholarship, 22*(2), 72–78.

This article addresses a major problem that hospitals are facing—a high turnover and nurses' dissatisfaction. The author makes recommendations that she believes will keep nurses in the hospital setting, including developing realistic career tracks and restructuring support services within the hospital setting.

Rayfield, C. A. (1991). Later always arrives sooner than you think. *Nursing Management, 22*(3), 84–85.

This article presents a case study to illustrate the importance of discharge planning from the acute care setting. In particular, the author discusses client teaching, arrangements for payment of health care, and the need for home health follow-up. Special needs of the elderly client are also addressed.

Tuazon, N. C. (1992). Discharge teaching: Use this MODEL. *RN, 55*(4), 19–21.

The author shares a discharge planning model used by the nurses on a medical-surgical unit in a large medical center in New Jersey. For the acronym MODEL, **M** stands for "Make a written plan"; **O** stands for "Offer resources"; **D** stands for "Devise ways to increase compliance"; **E** stands for "Evaluate your teaching with immediate feedback"; and **L** stands for "Legal implications: Document." This mnemonic device helps the nurses remember the basics of discharge planning, which should begin at the time of admission.

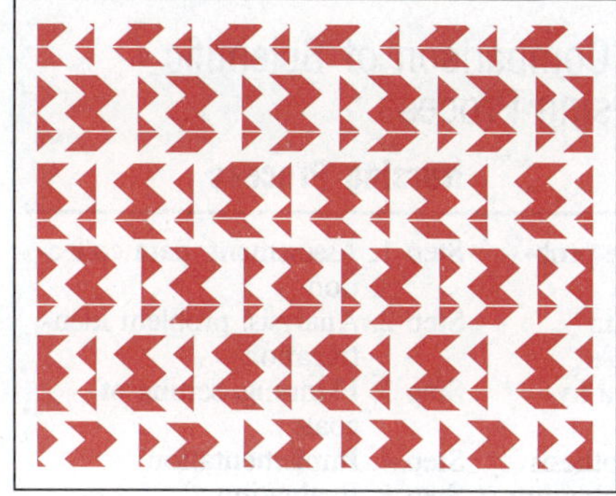

CHAPTER 3

The Nursing Process

CHAPTER HIGHLIGHTS

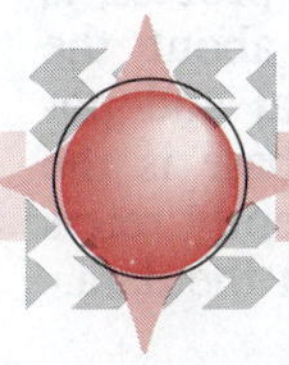

The nursing process is an organized, systematic approach used by nurses to meet the individualized, health care needs of their clients. The term *nursing process* emerged in the mid-1960s. As nursing became more recognized and respected as a profession, there was a growing need to define more clearly what it is that nurses do.

OVERVIEW OF THE NURSING PROCESS

The nursing process is used to describe the care that nurses throughout the world provide for their clients. However, Hiraki (1992) states that some nurses "outside the American culture" do not fully accept the nursing process as a model for nursing practice. For example, Swedish nurses Lundh and coworkers (1988) say that the nursing process is too similar to the model for medical decision-making. Despite this criticism, the nursing process is gaining popularity throughout the international nursing community.

Comparison of the Nursing Process with the Scientific Method

The nursing process is a decision-making approach that promotes critical thinking. Many books compare the nursing process with the scientific method of solving problems. The steps are similar in the two approaches as they proceed from identification of the problem to evaluation of the solution (Table 3–1). One difference, though, is that the scientist identifies the problem first and then collects the data. By contrast, the nurse collects the data first and then determines the problem.

TABLE 3–1 Comparison of Scientific Method and Nursing Process

Scientific Method	Nursing Process
Step 1. Statement of the problem	Step 1. Assessment: data collection
Step 2. Collection of data	Step 2. Analysis: problem identification
Step 3. Formulation of a hypothesis	Step 3. Planning: setting of goals
Step 4. Testing the hypothesis	Step 4. Implementation
Step 5. Analysis and evaluation	Step 5. Evaluation

Intuitive Judgment in Nursing Practice

In the past decade, research has shown that nurses sometimes use (and should use) intuitive judgment in clinical practice (Benner & Tanner, 1987). Intuition is the ability to understand immediately without using formal analysis and is based on experience and knowledge. Rew and Barrow (1987) state that "professional nurses in clinical practice refer to their reliance on intuition as a component of the decision-making process. However, because of difficulty articulating steps of this process, many have discounted the importance of this cognitive skill" (p. 50). Intuition helps the nurse act quickly, if necessary, particularly in critical care settings or emergency situations in which the nurse must assess the client and intervene at once.

The authors of this book use the nursing process as the organizing framework for its content. We do not believe that the nursing process is merely a technical skill with rules that apply in all situations but that nurses also need to use intuition as well as a scientific basis for nursing care.

STEPS OF THE NURSING PROCESS

There are five steps of the nursing process:

- Assessment
- Analysis
- Planning
- Implementation
- Evaluation

The steps initially are followed in sequence, from assessment to evaluation. However, once the nursing process begins, it is continuous or cyclic (Fig. 3–1). For example, if the client's goal is not met on the basis of the initial evaluation, the nurse may need to reassess the client or implement new actions to help the client achieve the desired goal. To understand the nursing process as a whole, it is first necessary to review each step and its associated activities. A more detailed discussion of the nursing process may be found in fundamentals of nursing textbooks.

ASSESSMENT

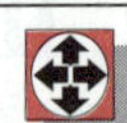

Assessment, the first step of the nursing process, is a systematic method of collecting data about the client for the purpose of identifying actual and potential client health problems. The data base is the organization of assessment data and frequently refers to the tool or chart form used to document the data.

TYPES OF DATA BASES

Jarvis (1992) names four kinds of data bases: complete; episodic, or problem-centered; follow-up; and emergency.

COMPLETE DATA BASE The complete, or total, data base includes a thorough health history and physical assessment. In acute care, the data base is usually completed during the first 8 hours after a client's admission to the hospital. The information collected by the nurse is *not* a repetition of the medical history that the physician records. Rather, the nurse collects additional data on the client's response to health problems, functional ability, ability to perform activities of daily living, usual health behaviors, coping patterns, health goals, and support systems.

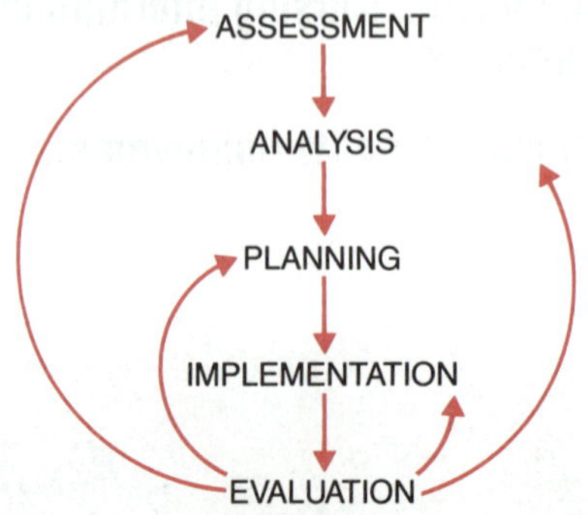

FIGURE 3–1 ♦ The nursing process cycle.

EPISODIC, OR PROBLEM-CENTERED, DATA BASE An episodic data base is collected for a limited or short-term problem. It focuses on one problem, and data collected are associated with the problem. For example, an elderly hospitalized woman falls when trying to get out of bed and complains of hip pain. The nurse's history focuses on how the fall occurred, which parts of the client's body made contact with the floor, and what position she assumed after she fell. The physical assessment is centered on the musculoskeletal system, especially the hip and knee. These data are usually not recorded on a data base form as such, but the information is documented according to agency policy.

In other situations, the nurse documents assessment findings frequently during the day on a flow sheet. For example, the client who is receiving patient-controlled analgesia (PCA) for pain control must be monitored carefully to determine whether the intervention is successful. The Daily Pain/PCA Flow Sheet shown in Figure 3–2 is an episodic data base that requires the nurse to assess and document the client's level of pain and sedation.

EMERGENCY DATA BASE The emergency data base is similar to the episodic data base, in that the nurse focuses on the immediate problem. However, the assessment must be more rapid to prevent life-threatening consequences. For example, a hospitalized client begins to choke on a piece of meat. The nurse quickly assesses whether there is a partial or complete airway obstruction before selecting the appropriate emergency nursing intervention.

FOLLOW-UP DATA BASE The follow-up data base is simply an evaluation of identified problems at regular and appropriate intervals. For example, for the client who was choking in the example just given, the nurse checks on him frequently to make sure that he is still breathing without difficulty and that he doesn't choke again.

SUBJECTIVE AND OBJECTIVE DATA

The information collected by the nurse includes both subjective and objective data. Subjective data include the information that the client states, for example, "I feel very nervous about my new diagnosis of diabetes," and "I'm in terrible pain." Answers by the client to questions such as "What brings you to seek health care?" or "Can you describe your pain?" are other examples of subjective data. If the client cannot communicate, the nurse may obtain subjective data from the family or significant others. Subjective information is information that the nurse cannot independently verify. However, subjective data are just as important as objective data (if not more so) because they reflect the client and family's perception of the health problem.

Objective data are observable, measurable pieces of information about the client. Objective data include measurements (e.g., vital signs or laboratory findings) and information obtained using the senses (e.g., touch or smell). Feeling the warmth of a foot and observing a foul odor from a wound are examples of objective data. Objective data also include clinical manifestations, that is, the signs and symptoms of an illness or disease.

COLLECTION OF DATA

As the nurse begins the task of gathering data, three techniques are commonly used: interview, observation, and physical examination.

INTERVIEW Interviewing is a communication skill by which the nurse can explore the thoughts, feelings, and perceptions of a person, family, or group. The nurse's approach to the client and others greatly affects the amount and quality of the information received. Establishing trust is essential to the development of a relationship in which the client feels comfortable about sharing personal information.

An interview should not be a series of routine questions and answers. Rather, it should flow in a natural progression. The nurse uses cues that the client provides to elicit further information. For instance, if the client seems anxious and nervous during the interview, the nurse explores what the client is feeling and why. It is very important for the nurse to obtain all pertinent data, not just the information needed to complete the nursing assessment form.

The nurse plans the interview carefully, with special attention to the environment, timing of the interview, and demographic data about the client.

Environment Before the interview begins, the nurse should be aware of the surrounding environment and its effect on the interview. Privacy for the client is important but sometimes difficult to achieve in a hospital setting. Often the client is admitted to a semiprivate room. If the roommate is allowed out of bed, the nurse can move him or her out of the room to provide privacy. If the client cannot get out of bed, the nurse selects a time for the interview when there are no visitors and pulls the curtain to attain some privacy. Another option is to find a small area, such as an office, where the client and nurse can talk; however, this is not always possible.

The nurse may also need to make the setting more conducive to sharing information. Factors such as lighting, temperature, background noise, and odors can distract the client. Full attention of both client and nurse is essential for a successful interview.

Timing The nurse plans the timing of the interview with consideration of the client's physical and emotional state. Clients who are experiencing pain, fatigue, hunger, or anxiety may not be able or willing to share information. The nurse postpones the interview until the client is more comfortable.

MEMORIAL HOSPITAL AT EASTON, MD. INC.

DAILY PAIN / PCA FLOW SHEET

Initial Assessment & Plan

1. Has MD told pt. about PCA?

   ____ YES ____ NO

2. Does patient verbalize understanding?

   ____ YES ____ NO

3. BP: ______ PULSE: ______

NOTE: Actual settings in Blue/Black ink.

Nurse Initials & Signature

Init.	Signature	Init.	Signature

ASSESSMENT INFORMATION

DATE/TIME	DRUG NAME & CONC.	PCA DOSE (ML)	LOCKOUT INTERVAL (MIN.)	4 HR LIMIT (ML)	PAIN LEVEL 0 - 5	SEDATION LEVEL 1 - 5	RESPIRATORY RATE	INITIALS	I.E. AMOUNT WASTED, WITNESS, ETC. INJECTOR VIAL CHANGED COMMENTS

LEVEL OF PAIN	SEDATION LEVEL
0 - ASLEEP AT TIME OF CHARTING	1 - ALERT AND AWARE
1 - COMFORTABLE	2 - DROWSY
2 - MILD DISCOMFORT	3 - DOZING INTERMITTENTLY
3 - IN PAIN	4 - MOSTLY SLEEPING
4 - IN BAD PAIN	5 - DIFFICULT TO AROUSE
5 - IN VERY BAD PAIN	

REVISED 1/90

FORM# 140265

FIGURE 3–2 ◆ An example of an episodic data base: a Daily Pain/PCA Flow Sheet. (Courtesy of Memorial Hospital of Easton, Easton, MD.)

Demographic Factors In addition to considering the client's environment and timing for an interview, the nurse assesses demographic factors, such as age, education, and culture, that may affect the interview content or process. Age is a very important consideration. For example, a frail, elderly client may not be able to hear the nurse's questions without a hearing aid. Therefore, the nurse ensures that the client uses mechanical aids, like hearing aids and glasses, during the interview. Chart 3–1 provides nursing tips for interviewing an elderly person.

The nurse also assesses the client's educational level and cultural background. Use of large words or jargon must be avoided for all clients, especially those with an elementary school education. Some words may have different meanings, depending on the person's culture. If the nurse is unsure how a client's culture will affect the interview, he or she should seek resources to assist in the process. For example, many Asians who have recently immigrated to the United States and Canada use their native language as the primary way of communicating and know only a few English words. Family members or other staff members may act as interpreters to help the nurse gather the necessary information. Other examples of transcultural variations and nursing care considerations are discussed throughout this text and are highlighted under the heading Transcultural Considerations.

OBSERVATION The nurse gathers additional data about the client through the highly developed skill of observation. Observation involves the use of the senses of sight, hearing, smell, and touch.

As the nurse interacts with the client, nonverbal cues as well as verbal responses are identified. General appearance, facial expressions, posture, body gestures, movements, and gait provide data to validate findings from the interview. Conflicting nonverbal cues and verbal responses may provide areas for further exploration by the nurse. For example, interactions between the family, significant others, and the client and between the client and health team members can provide information for identifying problems and planning care.

Knowledge from the physical and social sciences provides a foundation for the nurse's understanding of "normal" findings or behaviors. Using that knowledge, the nurse can recognize the significance of abnormal findings and can identify health problems. Although the keen skill of observation is essential to the collection of data, the ability to use all senses and to recognize pertinent data requires practice and experience.

PHYSICAL ASSESSMENT The nurse's qualifications and abilities to perform a physical assessment, also known as a physical examination, vary according to background, education, and experience. The manner by which a nurse collects data during a physical assessment should be logical and organized. Some nurses perform a head-to-toe examination, whereas others choose a body system-by-system approach.

CHART 3–1

Nursing Focus on the Elderly ◆ Interviewing

- Review old records and the medical history, if available, before interviewing the client.
- Provide privacy, as much as possible.
- Ask the client whether family or significant others may be present during the interview.
- Refer to the client by his or her last name unless the client prefers another name.
- Make sure that eyeglasses, contact lenses, and hearing aids are available and working properly, if the client wears these devices.
- Conduct the interview when the client is not experiencing pain and after basic comfort needs have been met.
- Before conducting the interview, allow the client to adjust to a new environment.
- Sit at the client's eye level during the interview.
- Speak clearly and slowly and in a low-pitched voice; do not shout.
- Be aware that the client may not be able to distinguish soft consonant blends, like "sh" or "ch."
- Interview in the morning, after breakfast, or in the early afternoon, after the client has rested.
- Use open-ended questions, when possible, to gather more information; avoid questions that can be answered "yes" or "no."
- Consider the client's education, culture, and age when phrasing questions, especially about sensitive or controversial issues.
- Observe the client's nonverbal behavior as well as what he or she says.

The assessment chapters of this text provide a systematic review of each body system, including the most important components of the physical and psychosocial assessment. (For further information about specific physical assessment skills, refer to one of the physical assessment textbooks listed in the Selected Bibliography.)

Four techniques are usually used to collect data during a physical assessment: inspection, palpation, percussion, and auscultation. These techniques are always performed in the order listed except for the abdominal assessment; for this assessment, auscultation is done immediately after inspection because the other techniques can affect bowel sounds.

Inspection Inspection refers to the visual examination of a client. The nurse performs observations systematically and focuses on one area of the body at a time. For example, the nurse may observe dry, flaky skin on the client's feet.

Palpation Palpation is the use of touch to examine the client's body and to determine characteristics of body structure under the skin. Through palpation, the nurse determines hardness, size, texture, swelling, or mobility of an internal part. For example, the nurse may feel a hard, nonmovable lump in the upper outer quadrant of the client's left breast.

Percussion Percussion involves the tapping of a body surface with a finger or fingers to produce sounds (Fig. 3–3). The sound that results allows the nurse to determine organ size, density, boundaries, and location. For example, the nurse may percuss a distended urinary bladder to the level of the umbilicus.

Auscultation Auscultation is the act of listening for sounds produced by or in organs of the body by means of a stethoscope. For example, the nurse may hear crackles in the bases of both lungs.

SOURCES OF DATA

The nurse obtains and documents data from several sources in the client's medical record according to the policies of the health care agency.

CLIENT The client is the primary source of data. This information is direct and firsthand and is presented in the history.

A medical history differs from a nursing history. A *medical* history is taken by the physician to determine the presence of a pathologic condition and to provide a basis for planning medical care. A *nursing* history is obtained by the nurse and focuses on the meaning of the illness and/or hospitalization to the client and family. It is used as a basis for planning nursing care.

The history is the first part of the data base collected from the client. To enhance organization and completeness of data collection, the nurse uses a systematic plan to gather information. Many guidelines and forms have been devised to assist the nurse in obtaining a history. Formats for the collection of a history vary among health care agencies. If the client is hospitalized, the history should identify the client's perception and expectations related to the illness, hospitalization, and care. Demographic data and the client's understanding of the illness, social and cultural history, usual daily patterns, ability to meet personal needs, and ability to cope with problems should also be included.

The history is typically taken when the client first seeks health care. The history may be obtained by a nurse, nurse practitioner, or physician. Some histories contain closed-ended questions, or checklists, whereas others include a series of open-ended questions. The closed-ended approach is structured and may not allow for documentation of additional collected information or further exploration of problem areas. The open-ended format provides general questions that allow the client the opportunity to elaborate on areas of concern, but it is time-consuming to admin-

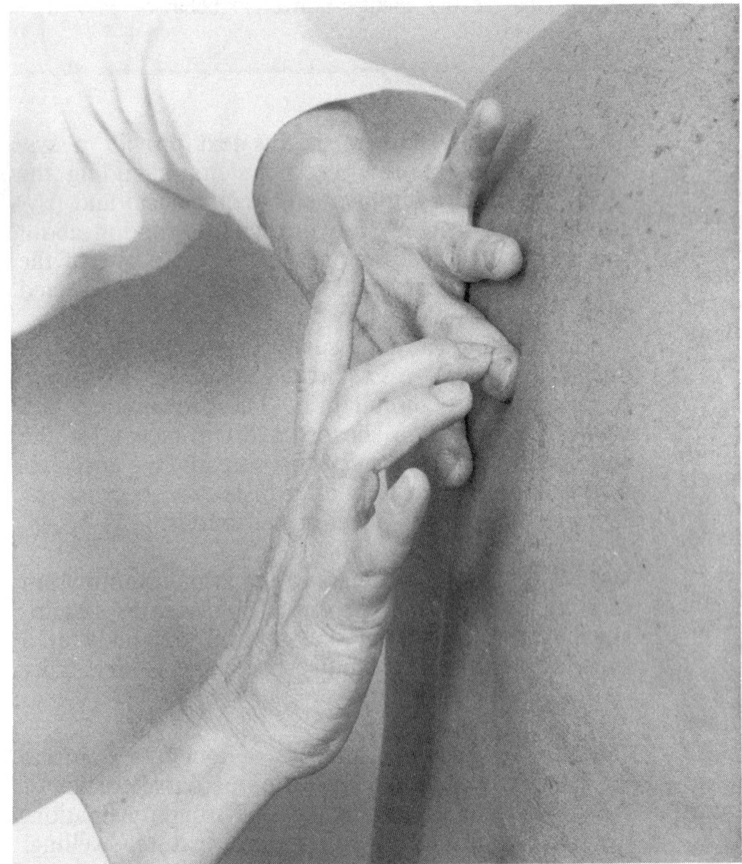

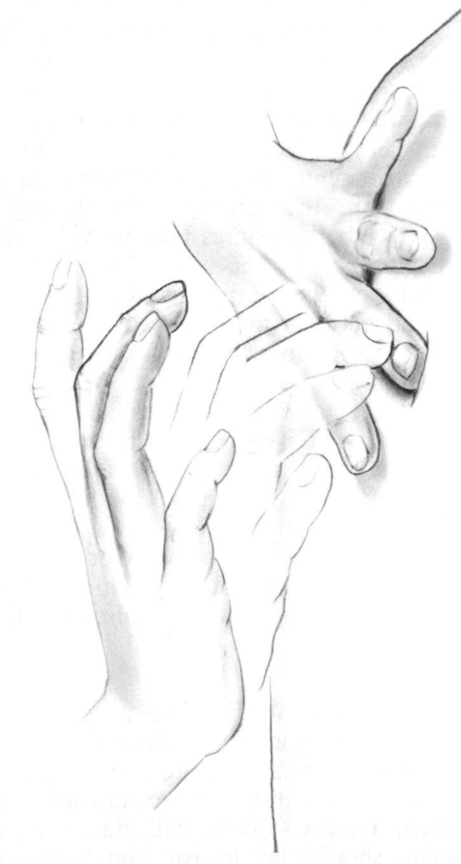

FIGURE 3–3 ◆ Technique for percussion used as part of physical assessment. (From Jarvis, C. [1992]. *Physical examination and health assessment*. Philadelphia: W. B. Saunders.)

ister. Most nursing history forms are a combination of the two types. Whatever the format, collection of these data requires interactions between the nurse and client and family members or significant others. Figure 3–4 illustrates the difference between open-ended and closed-ended questions that may be used in taking a nursing history.

FAMILY AND SIGNIFICANT OTHERS The client's family members or significant others are secondary sources of data. They can often supplement or verify information provided by the client. They may also be able to offer information about the client before the illness, provide family history related to health and illness, and describe the client's home environment.

RECORDS Previous medical histories, laboratory records, vital signs, and diagnostic reports provide pertinent data. These data validate information identified in the current history and physical examination or serve as a comparison to indicate changes in the client's health condition. Records from previous admissions to the hospital also supply additional pieces of information. The client's attending physician usually requests the old records from the hospital's medical records department or other health care facility where the client has sought health care.

CONSULTATION A nurse may supplement client information through consultation with other health care team members who previously had contact with the client. The physician or nurse practitioner is a key source of information. A social worker or community health nurse who has worked with the client can also contribute valuable information.

When a client is admitted to the hospital from another health care facility, such as a nursing home, the nurse in the acute care setting, if possible, should contact the nurse who cared for the client in the facility for specific client information. Most nursing homes supply a nursing transfer form that accompanies the client to the hospital or other facility. The transfer form describes the client's abilities and limitations, drug therapy, diet therapy, and past and current health state. This information is particularly helpful when the client cannot communicate and if no family is available.

ANALYSIS

The second step of the nursing process is the analysis of data. In this phase, the nurse summarizes the data, analyzes the data, and draws conclusions to determine what health problems the client may have or is at risk for. Client data are compared with "normal" findings and behaviors for the client's age, education, and cultural background. Abnormal data are reviewed to determine patterns of altered functioning. Client health problems are identified and categorized as potential problems requiring prevention or actual problems being managed or requiring interventions.

Aspinall and Tanner (1981) state that nurses make two types of judgments or conclusions about the health state of a client:

- Those health problems that nurses, "by virtue of their education and experience, are licensed and able to treat" (p. 4)
- Those problems that are diagnosed and treated by other members of the health team, but require continued nursing assessment and implementation of therapeutic interventions

This textbook uses nursing diagnoses that incorporate both types of client health problems.

EVOLUTION OF NURSING DIAGNOSES

The nursing profession's acknowledgment and endorsement of the term *nursing diagnosis* began in 1973, when the American Nurses' Association (ANA) published its first *Standards of Nursing Practice.* Standard II states: "Nursing diagnoses are derived from the data of the health status of the client" (American Nurses' Association, 1973, p. 3). Since then, other countries have also adopted nursing diagnoses as a way to describe client health problems.

In the early 1980s, the North American Nursing Diagnosis Association (NANDA) was formed to serve

Closed-ended	Open-ended
Have you been hospitalized before? yes ____ no ____	Describe any previous hospitalizations. ____ ____ ____
Do you typically seek health care at a clinic? yes ____ no ____	Where do you typically go for health care? ____
Is your pain continuous or intermittent? ____	Describe the nature of your pain. ____ ____ ____

FIGURE 3–4 ♦ A comparison of closed-ended versus open-ended questions as part of a nursing history. The open-ended format facilitates comprehensive data collection.

as the official organization for the development and dissemination of nursing diagnoses. Nurses from all over the world belong to this organization, although most are from countries within North America. Other countries or continents, like Europe, have formalized nursing diagnosis associations. NANDA is exploring an international union of organizations to meet the needs of nurses throughout the world. The official journal of NANDA is *Nursing Diagnosis,* which is published quarterly.

Although many definitions of nursing diagnosis have been proposed by various nursing leaders, the authors of this book recognize the official definition approved by NANDA at its Ninth Conference in 1990: "A nursing diagnosis is a clinical judgment about an individual, family, or community response to actual or potential health problems/life processes which provides the basis for definitive therapy toward achievement of outcomes for which the nurse is accountable" (Carpenito, 1991a, p. 65).

Unlike medical diagnoses which identify illness, nursing diagnoses identify the *responses* to health problems and life processes, such as aging or death. A medical diagnosis is the basis for medical interventions; a nursing diagnosis is the basis for nursing interventions. Nursing diagnoses are not diagnostic tests, medical treatments, or problems experienced by the nurse while caring for the client. Table 3–2 differentiates medical and nursing diagnoses.

FORMULATING NURSING DIAGNOSIS STATEMENTS

A complete nursing diagnosis is a statement consisting of at least two parts joined by the phrase "related to." The diagnostic statement begins with (1) an actual or potential *health problem* of the client and identifies (2) the *etiology* (probable cause or risk factors). The problem indicates what needs to change, and the etiology reflects factors thought to be related or contributing to the problem. By including the etiology in addition to the problem, one can give greater direction for the planning of nursing interventions to prevent, correct, or alleviate the problem.

TABLE 3–2 Differentiation Between Medical and Nursing Diagnoses

Medical Diagnosis	Nursing Diagnosis
Identifies the pathologic basis for an illness	Identifies a response to illness
Focuses on the physical condition of the client	Focuses on the physical, psychosocial, and spiritual needs of the client
Addresses actual, existing problems	Addresses actual and high-risk problems
Is not validated with the client	Is validated with the client if possible
Uses standardized goals and treatments	Uses individualized goals and interventions
May not be resolvable	Is usually resolvable

For instance, "Pain related to muscle spasm" is a nursing diagnosis. The nurse's interventions should be directed toward relieving the muscle spasm (e.g., with heat application and massage). "High Risk for Aspiration related to impaired swallowing" is a potential nursing diagnosis. The nurse's interventions should be directed toward helping the client swallow and preventing secretions or food from entering the trachea (e.g., placing the client in an upright position during meals, offering thickened foods and liquids, and suctioning the oral cavity to remove excessive secretions).

USING DEFINING CHARACTERISTICS

In addition to the two parts of the diagnostic statement, a third part, defining characteristics, may be included. Defining characteristics are the assessment data that verify the actual nursing diagnosis. Like the other two parts, they have been approved by NANDA for use and testing in clinical practice.

Transcultural Considerations Some researchers believe that the approved defining characteristics need to be expanded to address the needs of culturally diverse clients (Research Applications for Nursing).

Defining characteristics include subjective or objective data, or both, for *actual* nursing diagnoses and are connected to the two-part statement using "as evidenced by" or "as manifested by." An example of a three-part nursing diagnosis with defining characteristics is: Pain related to muscle spasm as evidenced by *moaning and grimacing when moved* (defining characteristics italicized).

Some schools of nursing and health care agencies use a mnemonic to remind nurses of each of the three parts of the nursing diagnostic statement—PES:

P = Problem (actual or high risk [potential])
E = Etiology (or risk factors)
S = Symptoms (defining characteristics)

Throughout this text, the nursing diagnoses are given in two parts—the problem and the etiology, since defining characteristics are individual to each specific client. Only those nursing diagnoses that have been approved by NANDA are included.

PLANNING

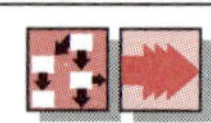

The planning step follows the analysis step of the nursing process. Throughout the planning process, the nurse performs several important functions: setting priorities and goals, selecting nursing interventions, and determining resources.

SETTING PRIORITIES AND GOALS

After analyzing the needs of the client to identify client health problems, the nurse decides on the urgency of the problems. This step is vital because some problems are more critical than others. Problems of higher priority require more immediate inter-

RESEARCH APPLICATIONS FOR NURSING

Some NANDA Nursing Diagnoses May Be Culturally Biased

Geissler, E. M. (1991). Nursing diagnoses of culturally diverse patients. *International Nursing Review, 38,* 150–152.

This study was conducted to determine whether NANDA-approved nursing diagnoses are helpful in caring for clients from diverse cultural backgrounds. A total of 245 RNs from the United States, Canada, Israel, Malawi, Pakistan, the Philippines, Saudia Arabia, and Sweden were asked to rate the usefulness of the defining characteristics of three diagnoses: Impaired Verbal Communication, Impaired Social Interaction, and Noncompliance. The nurses selected only those characteristics that were present at least 50% of the time in culturally diverse clients and suggested 113 additional defining characteristics.

Critique This study is one of the first published papers on the applicability of nursing diagnoses to culturally diverse clients. The sample was from eight countries and represented diverse ethnic and cultural groups.

Possible nursing implications Nurses need to recognize that currently approved diagnoses and defining characteristics do not uniformly meet the needs of clients from various cultures. The North American Nursing Diagnosis Association (NANDA) needs to address this issue as it continues to develop and refine nursing diagnoses for nursing practice.

vention than problems of lower priority. Setting priorities helps the nurse organize and plan care that solves the most urgent problems first.

ESTABLISHING PRIORITIES In determining the priority of the problems, the nurse must consider the impact on the client. Several theorists have presented hierarchies to assist in determining priorities.

Bower (1972) offers a three-level approach, in descending order of priority:

- First priority—problems that threaten life, dignity, and integrity of the client
- Second priority—problems that destructively change the client
- Third priority—problems that affect normal growth and development

Maslow's hierarchy of needs can also serve as a useful guide for establishing priorities. The needs identified by Maslow (1970) form five levels: physiologic basic needs, safety or security, love and belonging, self-esteem, and self-actualization. The client progresses up the hierarchy when attempting to satisfy needs. As shown in Figure 3–5, physiologic needs are of greatest priority and must be met first. Once they are met, the client is more willing and able to seek fulfillment of higher-level needs.

Priorities may fluctuate as the client's level of wellness changes. The nurse should consider both actual and high-risk problems when establishing priorities. Actual problems are usually more important than high-risk problems; at times, however, high-risk problems may be more important. For example, in a client who is asthmatic, the high-risk problem of Ineffective Airway Clearance is more life-threatening than an actual problem of constipation.

The establishment of priorities reflects an agreement between the client and nurse when possible. In addition to the guidelines for priorities that theorists have offered, the nurse must be aware of factors such as the client's health goals, the availability of resources, and the client's knowledge of the problem. The priorities of the client are often more important to the client than the priorities outlined by theoretical guidelines.

ESTABLISHING GOALS After establishing priorities, the client and nurse mutually try to decide on expected goals on the basis of identified nursing diagnoses. In this text, a *client goal* is defined as a desired behavior designed to promote the client's optimal level of wellness. Some nurses use the term *expected outcome* when referring to goals; others make a distinction between the two terms. For this text, expected outcomes and goals are essentially the same statement. Goals serve as guides in selecting nursing interventions and in determining criteria for evaluating nursing interventions. The purpose of writing goals is to assist in the evaluation of the client's progress and to determine resolution, if possible, of the client's problem.

Goals should be:

- Client-centered
- Realistic in terms of the client's potential for achievement and the nurse's ability to help the client achieve them
- Specific and measurable

When writing goals, the nurse should state them in a clear, concise manner that can be understood and measured by all health care team members. Any

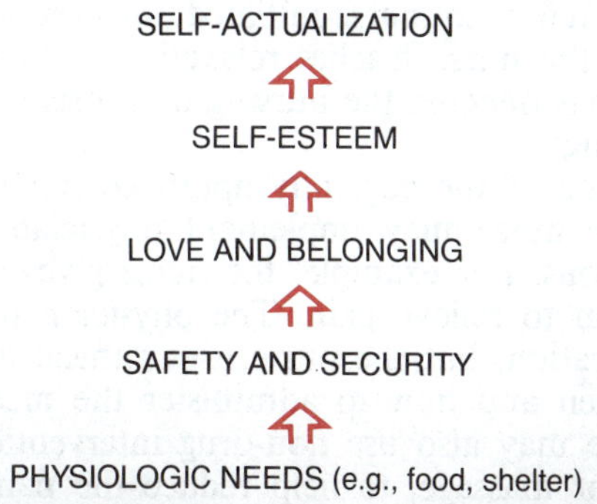

SELF-ACTUALIZATION
SELF-ESTEEM
LOVE AND BELONGING
SAFETY AND SECURITY
PHYSIOLOGIC NEEDS (e.g., food, shelter)

FIGURE 3–5 ♦ Maslow's hierarchy of needs. Needs must be met in ascending order. For example, safety and security must be achieved before love and belonging.

health care professional caring for the client should be able to determine whether the goals have been achieved. For example, "The client will state that anxiety is reduced within 30 minutes after nursing intervention" is a specific goal for one client that can be measured easily. If after 30 minutes, the client states that anxiety is reduced, the goal has been met. This outcome is the expected outcome, or the desired goal, that both the client and nurse want in order to resolve the anxiety.

SELECTING NURSING INTERVENTIONS

After determining the goals, the nurse develops strategies to accomplish them. Nursing interventions, also known as nursing actions or measures, are designed to assist the client in achieving goals. They are based on the client's health problems and define activities required to promote, maintain, or restore the client's health.

Bulachek and McCloskey (1989) define nursing interventions as "any direct care treatment that a nurse performs on behalf of a client. These treatments included nurse-initiated treatments resulting from nursing diagnoses, physician-initiated treatments resulting from medical diagnoses, and performance of the daily essential functions for the client who cannot do these" (p. 25).

Although the definition proposed by these experts in nursing interventions seems to imply that a nurse performs only treatments, or technical skills, these authors have broadened their definition. In a more recent book, Bulachek and McCloskey (1992) discuss interventions that range from physical interventions (positioning, feeding) to psychosocial interventions (therapeutic touch, reminiscence therapy). In 1992 they also published the results of the first phase of the Iowa Intervention Project. This research produced a Nursing Interventions Classification (NIC) system of 336 standardized nursing interventions. Like the development of nursing diagnoses, this list is intended to help nurses standardize their terminology and practice.

Nurse-initiated interventions, also called nurse-prescribed interventions or *nursing orders,* are independent activities that address nursing diagnoses. In the North American Nursing Diagnosis Association (NANDA) definition of nursing diagnosis, "definitive therapy" refers to nurse-initiated interventions. For example, the nurse teaches relaxation techniques for a client experiencing the nursing diagnosis of Ineffective Coping.

For some of the currently approved nursing diagnoses, the nurse may implement physician-initiated interventions. For example, the nurse gives analgesic medication to relieve pain. The physician prescribes the medication, but the nurse uses clinical judgment about when and how to administer the medication. The nurse may also use non-drug interventions, like imagery or massage, to help reduce the pain. Thus, the nurse and physician *collaborate* in an effort to resolve the client's problem of pain.

TABLE 3–3 An Overview of the Nursing Process

Step of the Nursing Process	Nursing Activities and Techniques
Assessment	• Interviewing • Observation • Physical assessment
Analysis	• Summarizing data and drawing conclusions • Nursing diagnosis
Planning	• Setting priorities and goals • Selecting nursing interventions • Developing the care plan • Determining resources
Implementation	• Applying intellectual skills • Applying interpersonal skills • Applying technical skills • Documentation*
Evaluation	• Reassessment • Restating the nursing diagnosis • Revising the goals or action plan

*Although documentation is a part of each step, most of it focuses on implementation.

DEVELOPING THE CARE PLAN

The usual format for recording planned nursing interventions is called a *client care plan.* The plan is a display of specific methods or proposed actions to resolve the problems that have been identified through assessment and analysis.

The client care plan is comprehensive and incorporates actions performed by nurses and coordinated with other members of the health care team. It serves as a tool to inform all health care team members about the client's problems. A well-written client care plan provides a central source of information about the client and can be an effective means to ensure that health problems are addressed. Development of a care plan is a continuous process; revisions are made as new data indicate a need for change. Examples of client care plans are found throughout this text and are listed at the beginning of the book.

The care plan format in this text is included for teaching-learning purposes to help the student or new nurse follow the steps of the nursing process and to identify the rationale for selected nursing interventions. In many clinical practice settings, the format for care plans is changing. For example, the accrediting agency for hospitals and other health care facilities, the Joint Commission on the Accreditation of Healthcare Organizations (JCAHO), no longer requires the use of columnar care plans. Instead, JCAHO requires evidence that nurses plan and implement care based on identified client health problems. Each hospital can decide how the documentation of care planning will be implemented. Some hospitals use nurses' notes, some have unit-based standards, and others use clinical pathways. (See Chapter 2 for a description of clinical pathways.)

To save time and duplication, numerous computer programs and care plan books have been developed to create standardized care plans that nurses can individualize as needed. Although each computer system is different, most programs allow the nurse to enter the client's assessment data, which then cue the computer to list the possible applicable nursing diagnoses for a given client. After the nurse selects the appropriate diagnoses, the computer offers a list of possible nursing interventions for each diagnosis and the nurse again selects those that are suitable for the client. Expected outcomes that can be modified to meet a particular client's needs are also available. As technology advances, these programs should be more widely available to nurses in all health care settings.

DETERMINING RESOURCES

After planning the nursing interventions, the nurse determines which resources are necessary to implement them. The client is a valuable source of information about health care resources that were successful in the past. For example, the client with an irritated stoma may mention that an enterostomal therapist was helpful with previous problems with an ileostomy. Including the client and family while planning care often promotes their cooperation during the implementation phase.

Other nurses and health care team members may also be valuable resources. An interdisciplinary conference during which health care team members identify problems and resources to solve them may be very helpful, especially for discharge planning.

When the feasibility of the plan is explored, the nurse also takes into account the availability of other resources for the client, such as equipment, time, personnel, and money. The client's value system is also considered. For instance, if the client requires dialysis in the home, the type of system implemented depends on the home water supply, electrical capability, space, available money, spiritual beliefs, and personal support system.

IMPLEMENTATION

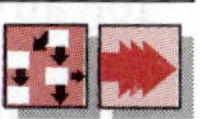

Implementation involves the actual carrying out of a specific, individualized plan. This step of the nursing process is the action phase, as the nurse assumes the responsibility to implement the care plan based on the nursing diagnosis. Interventions are based on scientific principles and, at times, intuitive judgment. Factors involved in selecting appropriate nursing interventions include

- The defining characteristics of the client's nursing diagnoses
- Research knowledge associated with possible interventions
- What interventions have the greatest possibility of success
- The client's acceptance of possible interventions
- What interventions involve the least amount of risk and discomfort for the client
- The capability of the nurse

Because planning and implementation are closely related, this book discusses the two steps under one heading: Planning and Implementation. However, goals and interventions are clearly labeled.

EVALUATION

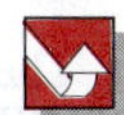

Evaluation, the fifth step of the nursing process, is a cognitive activity that completes the nursing process by indicating the degree to which the client's goals have been met.

Although evaluation is given as the final step of the nursing process, it is an ongoing and integral part of each step of the process (see Fig. 3-1). The nurse reviews the data to determine whether sufficient information was collected and whether the behaviors identified were appropriate. Client health problems are evaluated for their accuracy and completeness. The nurse examines the goals and interventions to determine whether they were realistic, achievable, and effective.

The outcome of evaluation may be one or a combination of the following:

- The client responded as expected and the problem is resolved. No additional nursing actions are needed.
- Client behaviors indicate that the client's problem has not been resolved. Outcomes have been accomplished, but the overall long-term goal has not been achieved. Re-evaluation will continue.
- Client behaviors are similar to those present initially. Little or no evidence is available to show that the problem has been resolved. Reassessment and replanning are needed.
- Client behaviors indicate a new problem. Assessment, planning, and implementation of an additional plan of action are needed to resolve the problem.

In this book, expected outcomes are listed under the evaluation sections and directly relate to the client's goals. For example, if the goal is: "The client will experience less pain," the expected outcome may be: "The client states that pain is lessened after nursing interventions." In this case, the nurse relies on subjective data to verify that the goal was met.

DOCUMENTATION

Documentation of each phase of nursing process is essential and is accomplished by various means. Two general, traditional methods of documentation are still used in many health care settings:

- Source-oriented charting usually includes narrative notes that organize varied data that are entered into the medical record by health care professionals (e.g., nurses' notes, physicians' progress notes, dietary notes).
- In the more popular problem-oriented record (POR), a master health problem list is developed. Each problem is numbered, and all chart entries refer to one of the problems identified on the list.

The notes may be recorded in a SOAP, SOAPIER, or PIE format (or one of its many variations) on the same progress note form in the chart by all health professionals. The initials represent **S**ubjective data, **O**bjective data, **A**nalysis, **P**lan of action, **I**nterventions, **E**valuation, and **R**evision of the plan. This technique of documentation is systematic and limits data to only pertinent information related to the identified problem. Although this system assists the nurse in addressing each step of the nursing process, it is very time-consuming and promotes duplication of record-keeping. Many physicians, social workers, and dietitians still use the SOAP format, but new systems for nursing documentation have been and are being developed.

Nursing Documentation Systems

SPECIALTY NURSING PRACTICE DOCUMENTATION

Some nursing documentation systems are designed for specialty practice. For example, the Cleveland Clinic Foundation Postanesthesia Care Unit (PACU) implemented the PES-EO-IO system, which has greatly improved compliance with the American Society of Post Anesthesia Nursing Standards (Zickuhr, 1992). Chart entries are made using the following initials:

P = Problem
E = Etiology
S = Signs and symptoms
EO = Expected outcome (goal)
I = Interventions
O = Outcome (actual outcome)

FOCUS CHARTING

A more widely used format in documentation is focus charting. Focus charting is not limited to specific client health problems but, rather, encourages nurses to document any significant changes in the client's condition, any client concern, or any significant client event. As seen in Figure 3–6, the nurses' notes have three columns. The actual notes are divided into **D**ata, **A**ction, and **R**esponse information. This technique helps locate desired information but still uses a narrative approach to recording pertinent data.

Date/Time	Focus/Problem	Notes
4/18/94 2:15 P.M.	Fever	D: T = 102.2° (R); face flushed; diaphoretic A: Give Tylenol 2 tab as ordered. Recheck temp. in 1 hr. *R. Jones, RN*
4/18/94 3:15 P.M.	Fever	R: T = 100.2° (R); face not flushed; not diaphoretic *D. Ignas, LPN*
4/19/94 3:30 A.M.	Impaired skin	D: 2-cm reddened area over coccyx; blanches A: Positioned on (L) side *N. Smith, RNC*

FIGURE 3–6 ◆ A sample of focus charting.

CHARTING BY EXCEPTION

One of the newest and widely used systems is charting by exception (CBE). CBE was started at St. Luke's Hospital in Milwaukee, Wisconsin, in an attempt to save nursing time. It incorporates three basic components (Burke and Murphy, 1988):

- Comprehensive flow sheets that list normal findings and require the nurse to initial them if they are present. If the findings are not present, the nurse writes an entry into the notes.
- Reference to pre-established nursing standards. The nurse initials the appropriate space when they are completed.
- Bedside accessibility of forms. All flow sheets are kept at the bedside, which prevents wasting the nursing time in looking for a client's chart. Bedside charting also prevents transcription of data from one form to another, which can lead to errors as well as wasted time. The information is available for any health care professional to read.

Like all charting systems, variations of the concept are being implemented. A portion of a flow sheet used in a CBE system is found in Figure 3–7.

Computerized Nursing Information Systems

A major advantage of documentation systems, such as charting by exception, is the ability to transfer the concept to computerization. Bedside computer charting is beginning to appear in hospitals. At present, about 3% of hospitals in the United States with more than 100 beds have bedside computers, also known as point-of-care (POC) systems. In a 1990 survey, however, another 75% of the U.S. hospitals that responded were looking into POC systems (Meyer, 1992).

		2300-0300	0300-0700	0700-1100	1100-1500	1500-1900	1900-2300
MENTAL	ALERT - ORIENTED X 3						
	COOPERATIVE						
	EMOTIONAL SUPPORT						
CARDIOVASCULAR	RADIAL PULSE REGULAR						
	MONITOR						
	(CIRCLE) COMPRESSION STOCKINGS / TEDS						
	CIRCULATION CHECKS Q ________ HRS TO ________						
	A.V. GRAFT ____________________ THRILL & BRUIT						
RESPIRATORY	RESPIRATIONS EASY AND REGULAR						
	BREATH SOUNDS CLEAR						
	FREQUENT BREATH SOUNDS Q ________						
	DYSPNEA ON EXERTION						
	O_2 ________ L/MIN VIA ________						
	O_2 VIA ________ % VENTI-MASK						
	POST-OP COUGH & DEEP BREATH						
	SUCTIONED VIA ________						
	TRACH CARE						
	COUGH						
	HUMIDIFIER						
	ORAL / NASAL AIRWAY UTILIZED						
IV THERAPY	IV SITE PATENT WITHOUT SIGNS OF INFECTION/ INFILTRATION						
	SOLUTION AND RATE CHECKED						
	IVAC						
	(CIRCLE) HEP LOCK / CENTRAL LINE PATENT W/O SIGNS OF INFECTION/ INFILTRATION						
	PCA						
	BLOOD						
TREATMENT	FINGERSTICK BLOOD SUGAR						
	HYPO/HYPER THERMIA MACHINE						
	ISOLATION						
	PAIN MANAGEMENT						
MUSCULOSKEL	CIRCULATION CHECKS ________						
	CPM						
	TRACTION ________						
	IMMOBILIZATION DEVICE						
	(CIRCLE) CAST / SPLINT LOCATION ________						
	TEMP PUMP						
DIRECTIVES	PLAN OF CARE WRITTEN						
	(CIRCLE) PLAN OF CARE REVIEWED / REVISED						
	ATTENDING PHYSICIAN IN						
	CONSULTING PHYSICIAN IN						
	PATIENT TEACHING ________						
MISC							

FIGURE 3–7 ♦ A portion of a daily flow sheet used for charting-by-exception. (Courtesy of Dorchester General Hospital, Cambridge, MD.)

Illustration continued on following page

DATE	TIME	NURSING PROGRESS NOTES	SIGNATURE

INITIALS	SIGNATURE/TITLE	INITIALS	SIGNATURE/TITLE

FIGURE 3-7 ◆ *Continued*

The literature suggests that the major advantages of POC documentation are accuracy and time savings. Charting at the bedside also increases the time that the nurse spends in the client's room (Meyer, 1992). The goal of any system should be to streamline or diminish paperwork and save valuable nursing time, giving nurses more time for direct client care.

Legal Aspects of Documentation

Regardless of the type of documentation system used, the nurse remembers that the client's chart is a legal document. Chart 3–2 lists basic charting guidelines that all nurses should follow.

Continuous Quality Improvement

Continuous quality improvement (CQI), also called total quality management (TQM) or quality assurance (QA), is a system whereby the health care setting compares the care that it delivers against its pre-established standards. In the nursing department of most hospitals, CQI is unit-based; that is, each nursing unit has its own standards of care that it follows in providing client care. In addition, each unit has designated nursing staff who collect data in coordination with the hospital's CQI department.

The collection of data for quality improvement is called an *audit,* also known as a monitoring and evaluation tool, or *monitor.* Audits may be directed toward structure, process, or outcome.

A *structure* audit looks at the equipment, supplies, and resources available to provide care. Determining whether the unit has adequate teaching materials for a newly diagnosed diabetic is an example.

A *process* audit evaluates whether a policy or procedure is being implemented correctly. For instance, checking all intravenous therapy tubing to make sure that it is properly dated determines whether or not nurses are following nursing policy.

An *outcome* audit evaluates client responses to the care that was provided. For example, keeping records on how many pressure sores were acquired while clients were in the hospital reflects the type of nursing care that was given.

An example of a nursing audit tool is given in Figure 3–8.

Quality improvement does not end after data collection. As in the analysis step of the nursing process, the data must be analyzed to determine whether any problems exist. If a problem is discovered, a plan is developed and implemented. After a set period of time, which varies depending on the aspect of care, another audit is completed to determine whether the problem has resolved. If not, the cycle continues. If the problem is resolved, the aspect of care is still monitored at intervals, but on a less frequent basis.

CHART 3–2

Nursing Care Highlight ◆ Legal Tips for Nursing Documentation

- Write clearly and legibly.
- Do not erase or "white-out" any part of the client's record.
- To correct an error, use one line to cross out the incorrect entry, then initial the change.
- Use only the standard and facility-approved abbreviations and symbols.
- Document significant information as close as possible to the time it is collected instead of waiting until the end of a shift.
- Transcribe physicians' orders carefully and correctly.
- If using nurses' notes or progress notes, do not leave blank spaces between entries.
- Time and date each entry on the client's record.
- Use only blue or black ink (visualizes best for copies or microfilm).
- Document like a reporter, trying to state the facts objectively and avoiding judgment or criticism.
- Do not state that "an incident report has been completed" or refer to any unusual occurrence or special event as an "incident."
- Follow all facility policies for documentation.
- To add one or two words, use a caret (^) and insert the words, then initial the change. If agency policy does not allow this practice, write a late entry.
- To make a late entry, begin by stating that it is a "Late entry for (date and time)." If the entry is more than a day late, state the reason for the entry (e.g., "on vacation for 3 days").
- If an order is discontinued on the record as indicated by a highlighter, be sure that the original can still be read, especially on copies.

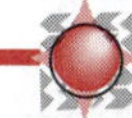

IMPLICATIONS FOR NURSING RESEARCH

Since the evolution of the nursing process, nurses have asked questions about its use in a variety of clinical settings. Within the past decade, research activity in the area of nursing diagnosis has greatly increased, but many questions remain unanswered. For example:

- ◆ How should defining characteristics be identified to ensure that they are appropriate for various cultures?
- ◆ What is the best method for deciding which of the current nursing diagnoses need to be refined, revised, or perhaps removed from the approved list?
- ◆ What are the standardized nurse-prescribed interventions that nurses can use for each nursing diagnosis?
- ◆ Should the concepts of wellness and health promotion be incorporated into the nursing diagnosis framework?

SURGICAL DRESSING QUALITY IMPROVEMENT PROGRAM	Yes	No	N/A	Comments
1. Physician's orders indicate: – materials to be used – timing of changes				
2. Skin sheets done weekly				
3. Isolation/precautions used if indicated				
4. Care plan reflects altered skin status				
5. Dietary consultation on chart				
6. Progress notes indicate: – physician awareness of wound status – healing/nonhealing of wound				
7. Dressing is clean and intact and dated				
8. No items for dressing change kept at bedside				
9. NS and sterile H_2O used for changes are date; discarded after 24 hours				
10. Surrounding skin intact, clear				
11. Preventive measures identified and in use				
COMMENTS				
RECOMMENDATIONS				

FIGURE 3–8 ◆ An example of a nursing audit form for monitoring and evaluating surgical dressings.

- ◆ What is the best nursing documentation system to use?
- ◆ How can computerization enhance nursing practice while maintaining client confidentiality?

SELECTED BIBLIOGRAPHY

Alfaro, R. (1990). *Applying nursing diagnosis and nursing process: A step-by-step guide.* Philadelphia: J. B. Lippincott.

*American Nurses' Association. (1973). *Standards of nursing practice.* Kansas City: Author.

*Aspinall, M. J., & Tanner, C. (1981). *Decision-making for patient care.* Norwalk, CT: Appleton-Century-Crofts.

Avant, K. C. (1990). The art and science in nursing diagnosis development. *Nursing Diagnosis, 1,* 51–56.

Bates, B. (1991). *A guide to physical examination and history taking* (5th ed.). Philadelphia: J. B. Lippincott.

*Benner, P., & Tanner, C. (1987). How expert nurses use intuition. *American Journal of Nursing, 87,* 23–31.

*Bower, F. (1972). *The process of planning nursing care.* St. Louis: C. V. Mosby.

Brider, P. (1991). Who killed the nursing care plan? *American Journal of Nursing, 91,* 35–39.

Bulachek, G. M. & McCloskey, J. C. (1992). *Nursing interventions: Essential nursing treatments* (2nd ed.). Philadelphia: W. B. Saunders.

Bulachek, G., & McCloskey, J. (1989). Nursing interventions: Treatments for potential nursing diagnoses. In R. M. Carroll-Johnson (Ed.), *Classification of nursing diagnoses: Proceedings of the eighth conference* (pp. 23–30). Philadelphia: J. B. Lippincott.

*Burke, L. J., & Murphy, J. (1988). *Charting by exception: A cost-effective, quality approach.* New York: John Wiley.

Carpenito, L. J. (1992). *Nursing diagnosis: Application to clinical practice* (4th ed.). Philadelphia: J. B. Lippincott.

Carpenito, L. J. (1991a). *Nursing care plans and documentation: Nursing diagnoses and collaborative problems.* Philadelphia: J. B. Lippincott.

Carpenito, L. J. (1991b). The NANDA definition of nursing diagnosis. In R. M. Carroll-Johnson (Ed.). *Classification of nursing diagnosis: Proceedings of the Ninth Conference* (pp. 65–71). Philadelphia: J. B. Lippincott.

Geissler, E. M. (1991a). Nursing diagnoses of culturally diverse patients. *International Nursing Review, 38*(5), 150–152.

Geissler, E. M. (1991b). Transcultural nursing and nursing diagnosis. *Nursing and Health Care, 12,* 190–204.

Gordon, M. (1990). Toward theory-based diagnostic categories. *Nursing Diagnosis, 1,* 5–11.

Gordon, M. (1991). *Manual of nursing diagnoses, 1991–1992.* St. Louis: C. V. Mosby.

*Guzzetta, C. E., Bunton, S. D., Prinkey, L. A., Sherer, A. P., & Seifert, P. C. (1989). *Clinical assessment tools for use with nursing diagnoses.* St. Louis: C. V. Mosby.

Haselfeld, D. (1990). Patient assessment: Conducting an effective interview. *AORN Journal, 52,* 551–557.

Hiraki, A. (1992). Tradition, rationality, and power in introductory textbooks: A critical hermeneutics study. *Advances in Nursing Science, 14*(3), 1–12.

Iyer, P. W., & Camp, N. (1991). *Nursing documentation: A nursing process approach.* St. Louis: C. V. Mosby.

Iyer, P. W., Taptich, B. J., & Bernocchi-Losey, D. (1991). *Nursing process and nursing diagnosis.* Philadelphia: W. B. Saunders.

Jarvis, C. (1993). *Physical examination and health assessment* (2nd ed.). Philadelphia: W. B. Saunders.

Kim, M. J., McFarland, G. K., & McLane, A. M. (1991). *Pocket guide to nursing diagnoses.* St. Louis: C. V. Mosby.

Knapp-Spooner, C., & Brett J. (1992). Less is more: A med-surg flow sheet. *RN, 55*(3), 36–39.

Lindsey, A. S. (1990). Identification and labeling of human responses. *Journal of Professional Nursing, 6,* 143–150.

*Lundh, U., Soder, M., & Waerness, K. (1988). Nursing theories: A critical review. *Image: The Journal of Nursing Scholarship, 20,* 36–40.

Lunney, M. (1990). Accuracy of nursing diagnosis: Conceptual development. *Nursing Diagnosis, 1,* 12–17.

*Maslow, A. (1970). *Motivation and personality.* New York: Harper & Row.

McCloskey, J. C., & Bulachek, G. M. (1992). *Nursing interventions classification (NIC).* St. Louis: Mosby Year Book.

Meintz, S. L., & Shaha, S. H. (1992). Our hand-held computer beats them all. *RN, 55*(1), 52–57.

Meyer, C. (1992). Bedside computer charting: Inching toward tomorrow. *American Journal of Nursing, 92*(4), 38–44.

Murphy, J., & Burke, L. J. (1990). Charting by exception. *Nursing90, 20,* 65, 68–69.

North American Nursing Diagnosis Association. (1990). *Taxonomy I revised.* St. Louis: Author.

Pierson, M. A., & Irons, K. (1992). Identification of a cluster of nursing diagnoses for a caregiver support group. *Nursing Diagnosis, 3*(1), 36–41.

*Rew, L., & Barrow, E. (1987). Intuition: A neglected hallmark of nursing knowledge. *Advances in Nursing Science, 10,* 49–68.

Taptich, B. J., Iyer, P. W., & Bernocchi-Losey, D. (1989). *Nursing diagnosis and care planning.* Philadelphia: W. B. Saunders.

Ulrich, S. P., Canale, S. W., & Wendell, S. A. (1990). *Nursing care planning guides: A nursing diagnosis approach* (2nd ed.). Philadelphia: W. B. Saunders.

Zickuhr, M. T. (1992). American Society of Post Anesthesia Nursing. In R. M. Carroll-Johnson (Ed.), *Classification of nursing diagnoses: Proceedings of the Ninth Conference.* Philadelphia: J. B. Lippincott.

SUGGESTED READINGS

Knapp-Spooner, C., & Brett, J. (1992). Less is more: A med-surg flow sheet. *RN, 55*(3), 36–39.

This article describes the experience of medical-surgical nurses in a large northeastern hospital in developing a flow sheet. The flow sheet replaces the traditional nurses' notes and stays at the bedside. The nurses believe that flow sheets save nursing time and improve communication among nursing shifts and with physicians.

Meintz, S. L., & Shaha, S. H. (1992). Our hand-held computer beats them all. *RN, 55*(1), 52–57.

The authors share their experience in evaluating bedside computer systems that are currently available. The preferred system was a hand-held computer, designed by nurses, that nurses could use anywhere on the unit.

Pierson, M. A., & Irons, K. (1992). Identification of a cluster of nursing diagnoses for a caregiver support group. *Nursing Diagnosis, 3*(1), 36–41.

Pierson and Irons facilitate a support group for caregivers of people in the home setting. To help the group focus on their potential problems, they identified a cluster of high-risk nursing diagnoses, such as High Risk for Diversional Activity, Potential for Sleep Pattern Disturbance, and Potential for Social Isolation. A complete list is presented in the article.

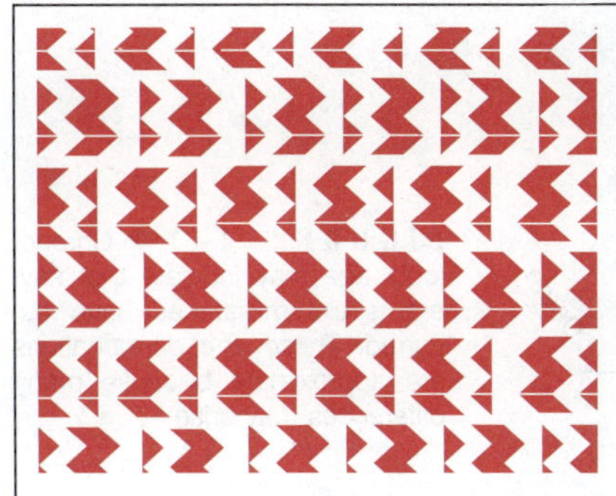

CHAPTER 4

Adult Development

CHAPTER HIGHLIGHTS

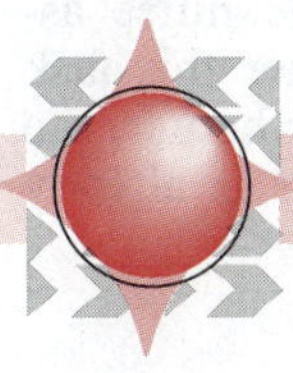

Adulthood is a time of change. It generally requires shifts in how a person defines the situation and his or her interactions and relationships with others. The changes in both body and mind require adjustments in behavior, emotional responses, and patterns of handling life's problems.

The medical-surgical nurse should have an understanding of adult development because it affects the client's response to illness and other stressors. Nurses can be more effective in planning and implementing care if they are aware of the client's somewhat predictable developmental patterns. However, nurses must also remember that each person is unique and therefore may not follow all expected patterns.

THEORIES OF ADULT DEVELOPMENT

The developmental stage of adolescence seems to fade gradually into adulthood. Adulthood is commonly described as having its onset at some point after a person achieves physical maturity. In contrast to earlier periods of the life cycle, adulthood has no established landmarks that precisely characterize its onset or its stages.

People share certain traits with respect to age and the rate of maturation. Age, in years, may indicate that several social milestones have passed (Fig. 4–1).

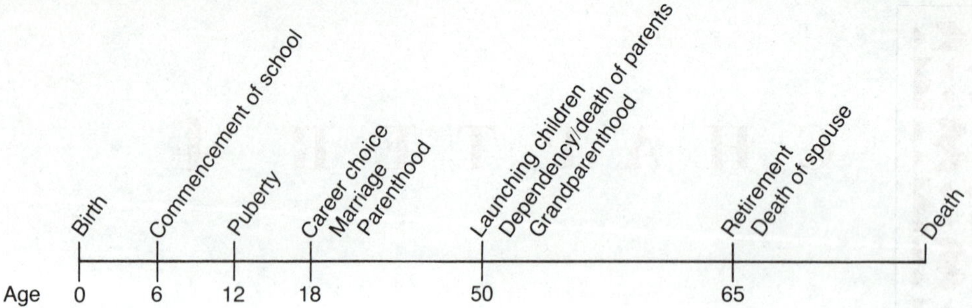

FIGURE 4-1 ◆ Chronologic age may indicate that several social milestones have occurred. These age demarcations are approximate because many differences may arise.

Designating arbitrary ages for the onset of maturity, middle age, and old age, however, may promote a stereotypic view of the stages of adulthood. The nurse should remember that there are many individual differences that result from factors like heredity, gender, health history, and life experience.

A single theory explaining changes during adulthood has been difficult to construct. Thus, many theories have been developed, each representing a different view. Theories of adult development can be divided into two broad areas—developmental theories and theories of aging.

Developmental Theories

Developmental theories imply that certain psychosocial growth mechanisms can be assigned to various ages. The theories expressed by Erikson, Peck, and Havighurst are the most commonly cited. However, these theories were constructed 25 to 30 years ago and may not reflect the developmental patterns of all adults in the 1990s.

ERIKSON'S EIGHT "STAGES OF MAN"

Erikson (1968) proposed that personalities continue to evolve throughout adult life in a gradual, continuous manner. The first five stages of Erikson's theory largely expand on Freud's stages of childhood development. The last three stages provide a useful model for understanding some general issues of adult developmental changes during the adult years. Table 4-1 explains these adult stages and related nursing assessment.

For example, the task of the older adult is ego integrity versus despair. If older adults cannot adjust to the physical, psychologic, and sociologic changes that may occur as they age, they are at risk for despair. The result may be depression. The nurse assesses the older adult to determine whether this task has been accomplished successfully or whether the person is at a high risk for depression or is already depressed.

PECK'S DEVELOPMENTAL TASKS OF ADULTHOOD

The last two of Erikson's stages encompass all the middle adult and late years of the life cycle. This view of adulthood may be too simplistic and general. Using Erikson's model as a foundation, many developmental psychologists have expanded his theory to ones that may more realistically represent adulthood. Peck (1968) identified seven crucial developmental tasks for the last two periods of the life cycle—

TABLE 4-1 Erikson's Adult Developmental Tasks

Developmental Stage	Developmental Task	Nursing Assessment
Young adulthood	• Intimacy versus isolation	• Assess whether the client has meaningful, intimate relationships. • If the client has no intimate relationships, ask whether he or she has had one or more in the past. • Assess other support systems that the client may have.
Middlescence	• Generativity versus stagnation	• Assess whether the client is employed. • Ask the client what he or she does for leisure or recreation. • If the client is not employed or has no regular leisure activity, ask the client what he or she does during a 24-hour day. • Assess for signs of depression, such as excessive sleeping and decreased appetite.
Older adulthood	• Ego integrity versus despair	• Assess what the client does each day. • Ask about the client's family and other relationships. • Ask the client if he or she feels lonely; if so, assess for signs of depression.

TABLE 4–2 Peck's Developmental Tasks of Adulthood

Period of Life Cycle	Developmental Task	Clinical Applications
Middlescence	• Valuing wisdom vs physical powers • Socializing vs sexualizing in human relationships • Cathectic flexibility vs cathectic impoverishment • Mental flexibility vs mental rigidity	• The client is likely to have strong relationships with family or significant others. • The client is likely to be more flexible in his or her lifestyle if necessary. • The client is able to make and adapt to changes as needed.
Old age	• Ego differentiation vs work role preoccupation • Body transcendence vs body preoccupation • Ego transcendence vs ego preoccupation	• The client is able to have a meaningful life after retirement from work. • The client accepts and adapts to changes in body structure and function without difficulty. • The client accepts the inevitability of death and approaches it in a positive manner, feeling that he or she has lived a "good" life.

middlescence (middle adulthood) and late adulthood (Table 4–2). Peck believed that there are four major tasks in middlescence and three tasks in late adulthood that must be confronted for healthy adjustment. If these tasks are not accomplished, a person's state of health may decline.

For example, in the period of "old age," one task is body transcendence versus body preoccupation. Peck included this task because he observed many older adults beginning to focus on the declines in their physical functioning, resulting in a preoccupation with their body. Peck said that in order to age successfully, older adults need to accept these body changes and adapt to them as well as possible. When caring for an older adult, the nurse assesses the person's view of body changes and how he or she has coped with them.

HAVIGHURST'S THEORY OF ADULT DEVELOPMENTAL TASKS

Havighurst's (1972) ideas have also contributed to the understanding of adult development. His theory has a broad definition of successful aging that addresses social competency and adaptation to new roles. He viewed developmental tasks as a continual discovery of new and meaningful roles. This positive view of aging helps people "successfully age." He divided the life cycle into six age periods, each containing six to ten developmental tasks. The tasks for the adult periods are summarized in Table 4–3.

The nurse can use Havighurst's theory in a number of ways. For instance, the nurse may teach the adult what developmental tasks are expected to occur over time and in what general age span. Many of these tasks are stressful to most people. If adults recognize that these tasks are typical and that most people experience them, they should be prepared to cope with them as they occur.

One criticism of Havighurst's ideas is his stereotypic presentation of the tasks in each age period (which were perhaps appropriate for the 1960s and 1970s). For example, he stated that people typically marry and start a family in young adulthood. In the 1990s, it is increasingly common for young adults to postpone marriage or not become married at all. Some adults wait until their middle years, after 35, to have children.

Theories of Aging

In addition to theories of adult development, numerous theories are associated with the aging process. These include biologic (physiologic), sociologic, and psychologic theories. Several of the most commonly cited theories are briefly presented here.

TABLE 4–3 Havighurst's Developmental Tasks of the Adult

Stage	Developmental Task
Early adulthood	• Selecting a mate • Learning to live with a marriage partner • Starting a family • Rearing children • Managing a home • Getting started in an occupation • Assuming civic responsibility • Finding a congenial social group
Middle age	• Achieving adult civic and social responsibility • Establishing and maintaining an economic standard of living • Assisting teenage children to become responsible and happy adults • Developing leisure activities • Accepting and adjusting to the physiologic changes of middle age • Adjusting to the aging of parents
Later maturity	• Adjusting to decreasing physical strength and health • Adjusting to the death of a spouse • Adjusting to retirement and reduced income • Establishing an explicit affiliation with one's age group • Meeting social and civic obligations • Establishing satisfactory physical living arrangements

BIOLOGIC THEORIES OF AGING

Biologists exploring the aging process concluded that aging can be viewed as a progression through a continuum of events that occur from birth to death. From this perspective, the aging process has been defined as the sum total of all changes that occur in a person over the life span. On the basis of this broad definition, it has been proposed that aging can best be understood by studying physiologic development. Although the view of aging as an integral part of human development has opened many avenues of investigation, none has completely explained all the changes associated with aging or why people age at different rates. Over the years, many theories of biologic, or physiologic, aging have emerged, including exhaustion theories, genetic theories, single-organ theories, the free radical theory, and the immunity theory.

EXHAUSTION THEORIES

Early theorists on aging proposed that there is a fixed store of energy available to the body. As time passes, the energy available is depleted, and, because it cannot be restored, the person dies.

Later, other related theories emerged. The *wear and tear theory* stated that the body is like a machine that wears out its parts with repeated use and comes to a grinding halt. Today, the concept of wear and tear is not widely accepted as an explanation for the aging process. However, this theory may explain the development of certain diseases, such as degenerative joint disease, in which the joint cartilage degenerates with prolonged use.

A more popular theory is the *stress theory,* which focuses on the physical and psychologic wear and tear from sudden and unexpected stressors over which a person has no control. This theory maintains that a person copes with stressors through a three-stage process of alarm, resistance, and exhaustion (see Chap. 7). This process eventually leaves the person weakened because of the accumulation of successive stressful events over the life span. Stress theory suggests that as people age, they are no longer capable of fighting off the various stressors as a result of the accumulation of wear and tear.

GENETIC THEORIES

A major breakthrough to help explain biologic development was the identification of deoxyribonucleic acid (DNA) molecules as the information center of the cell. This discovery led to the theory that cellular death results from DNA damage. The possibility that biologic aging results when the wrong information is provided for normal cell function has been considered and is called *error theory* (Burnside, 1988).

Several theories suggest that aging changes may occur as a result of an alteration in cellular genetic information. For example, the *cross-link theory* proposes that a chemical reaction occurs that produces irreparable damage to DNA and consequent cell death (Matteson & McConnell, 1989).

In clinical practice, it is interesting to note the trend for similar life expectancies in families. It is not unusual for a person who is of advanced age to state that he or she had parents who also lived to be very old.

SINGLE-ORGAN THEORIES

Other physiologic theories of aging have attempted to explain aging and the life span on the basis of changes in a single organ or in terms of impairments in control mechanisms. One theory suggests that aging results primarily from lowered oxygen supply delivered to crucial body tissue, such as brain tissue (Burnside, 1988). Other theories suggest that thyroid gland function might be responsible for the slowing of metabolic processes at the cellular level (since cellular metabolism is regulated by the thyroid gland). The slowing of metabolic processes would then promote aging.

FREE RADICAL THEORY

Free radicals are highly reactive cellular components that replace genetic information at the cellular level. Lipofuscin is a material that is associated with free radicals and is rich in lipids and protein. This substance has been found in large quantities in body organs as they age. Some researchers suggest that the accumulation of lipofuscin interferes with cellular metabolism and may play an important role in the aging process (Pryor, 1983; Matteson & McConnell, 1989).

IMMUNITY THEORY

According to the immunity theory, as people age, mutations occur in some cells, resulting in the formation of proteins that the body does not recognize. The immune system then produces antibodies against these new proteins and attempts to destroy them, causing an autoimmune response (Matteson & McConnell, 1989). With increasing age, there would then be a reduction in the function of the immune system. The antibodies fail to recognize abnormal cells, allowing them to divide and multiply. Immune system failure might then promote such late-life diseases as cancer, diabetes, and emphysema.

SOCIOLOGIC THEORIES OF AGING

The concept of socialization during adulthood refers to the process by which people, over the course of their adult lives, acquire ways to perform new roles. Several theories are relevant to how adults learn which roles bring rewards and which roles are considered undesirable, and how they adjust to changing roles and role losses in society. These include Rosow's role theory and the activity theory.

ROSOW'S ROLE THEORY

Rosow (1974) maintained that socialization for roles is a continuous and cumulative process that corresponds to the developmental stages of the life cycle. Socialization for roles begins in infancy and extends through adolescence. However, the actual learning of specific role demands begins and continues as a person moves through the stages of adulthood.

The concept of role continuity suggestes that role demands of the previous stage prepare the person for the responsibilities associated with the next status or position that the adult assumes. Thus, role transitions through the life span progress in a smooth manner from one age level to the next.

ACTIVITY THEORY

The activity theory holds that the maintenance of activities is important to most people as a basis for obtaining satisfaction, self-esteem, and health. Most research has shown the importance of activity as the basis for the promotion of vigor and satisfactory adjustment in the elderly (Fig. 4–2). People who restrict their activities as they age many tend to experience a reduction in overall life satisfaction (Burnside, 1988). The significance of this theory for nurses is that they should encourage older adults to remain active to the extent that they are able. Continued activity includes both physical actions and cognitive stimulation.

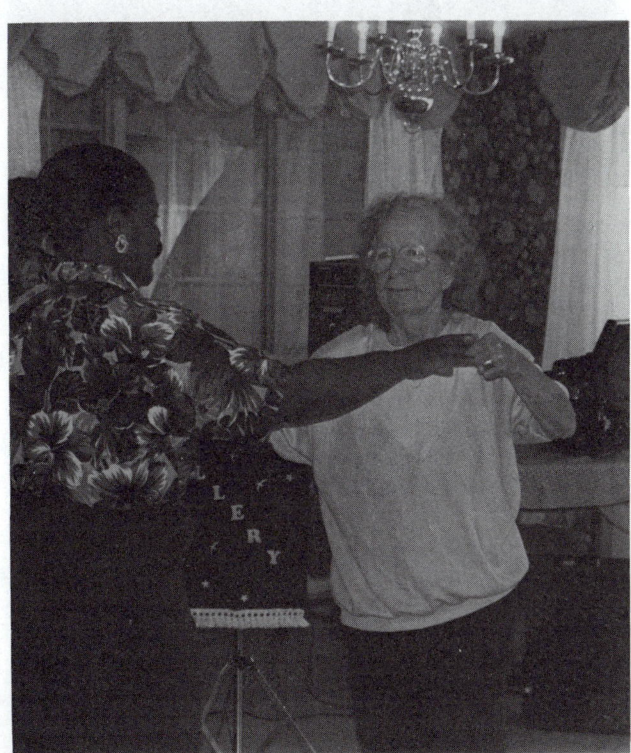

FIGURE 4–2 ◆ An active elderly woman.

PSYCHOLOGIC THEORIES OF AGING

Psychologic theories of aging are often the extension of sociologic and developmental theories. Personality theories usually consider the human needs and forces that motivate thought and behavior within a physical and social environment. The problem with studying personality changes throughout adulthood is that as people pass through life, they become increasingly different rather than more similar. Theorists who have addressed adult personality development have primarily focused on one central issue—whether adult personality is characterized by continuity or by change.

Jung (1928–1971) was one of the first psychologists to consider that the latter half of life has a purpose of its own, quite apart from that of survival—namely, the development of self-awareness through reflective activity. He strongly believed in the importance of the latter half of life. This phase is characterized by inner discovery, as opposed to the first half of life, which is oriented toward biologic and social goals. Butler (1975) and Neugarten (1977) confirmed Jung's views that reflective activity is needed in adulthood. His work regarding the life review process clearly defined the growth potential for aged adults. A review of past events, or reminiscence, helps with personal growth and evolving identity.

STAGES OF ADULTHOOD

Adulthood can be divided into three broad categories: young adulthood, middle adulthood, and older adulthood. In general, experts in adult development do not agree on the age span for each category. Therefore, differences in the professional and popular literature are common.

The medical-surgical nurse should know about normal adult development as a basis for physical and psychosocial assessment. A review of normal development and associated health issues follows.

Young Adulthood

Young adulthood is generally designated as the period between the 20th and 35th year. Many young adults are able today to postpone the tasks of adulthood, to experiment, and to prolong their own transition from childhood by exploring the many choices available to them. This period offers the time needed for the person to grow and make the necessary and complex linkages with adult society.

PHYSIOLOGIC CHANGES

MUSCULOSKELETAL CHANGES

Even though growth essentially ceases at adolescence, minimal growth can continue. Fusion of the epiphyses of long bones occurs approximately at age 18 to 25 years. Muscular efficiency is at its peak level between ages 20 and 30 years. Thereafter, muscular strength declines. Regular exercise is important to maintain a healthy body. People often become more sedentary in the postadolescent years as a result of the lack of a regular exercise plan, changes in work and leisure activities, and alterations in eating patterns.

CARDIOPULMONARY CHANGES

Physical development of the heart, the blood vessels, and the lungs stops in adolescence. Maintaining cardiopulmonary functioning and preventing pathologic changes during the second half of life largely depend on the young adult's lifestyle practices that are carried into middle age and late life.

Although arteriosclerotic disease becomes clinically evident in middle adulthood, it represents the result of progressive changes in the arterial walls that began in childhood. Studies are currently under way to examine the lifestyles of children and to find ways to improve health during childhood to prevent later problems.

Transcultural Considerations Although heart disease is not usually associated with the young adult age group, cardiac-related mortality for young Native Americans is about twice that for all other young adults living in the United States (Jarvis, 1992).

INTEGUMENTARY CHANGES

The abundance of skin care and hair coloring products attests to the aging changes that begin in young adulthood. These changes are often traumatic if a young adult has accepted the youth-oriented value system in Western countries like the United States and Canada.

Wrinkling of the skin occurs with aging and is markedly increased by exposure to the sun. Facial wrinkling becomes obvious in most adults in their 20s and tends to be progressive thereafter. Early wrinkling is usually related to habitual facial expressions, such as frowning and smiling. The skin loses its moisture and gradually dries. In later years, the atrophy of fat accelerates and increases the appearance of wrinkles.

The onset of graying hair and baldness often begins in young adulthood as well. Graying of hair results from the inability of melanocytes to provide hair with pigment granules over time. Hair loss with aging results from a number of factors. Although it is more common in men, it also occurs in women. Early balding is a result of genetic factors and is related to the amount of androgens, such as testosterone, that are produced (Fig. 4–3).

DENTAL CHANGES

The third molars, or wisdom teeth, normally erupt in an adult's early 20s. There are four third molars, although in some adults all four may not develop fully. Wisdom teeth frequently present problems and require dental care. Their eruptions are unpredictable, and it is not uncommon for them to be malaligned or to remain impacted in the gums.

PSYCHOSOCIAL DEVELOPMENT

The central issues of psychosocial development in young adulthood are related to the final resolution of the identity crises begun in adolescence. People work through these issues rather slowly. By the time the adolescent reaches young adulthood, some of these issues are nearing resolution.

The young adult struggles with expanding a sense of self in determining who he or she is within various social roles. In this stage of identity development, the prime concern is the relationship between the person and the social system. Young adults seek to resolve several psychosocial issues in their quest for maturity.

SELF-IDENTITY

In young adulthood, the sense of self usually becomes sharper and clearer, more consistent, and less influenced by others. This identification is quite different from that in the adolescent, who is self-conscious and concerned with seeing the self from the viewpoint of others.

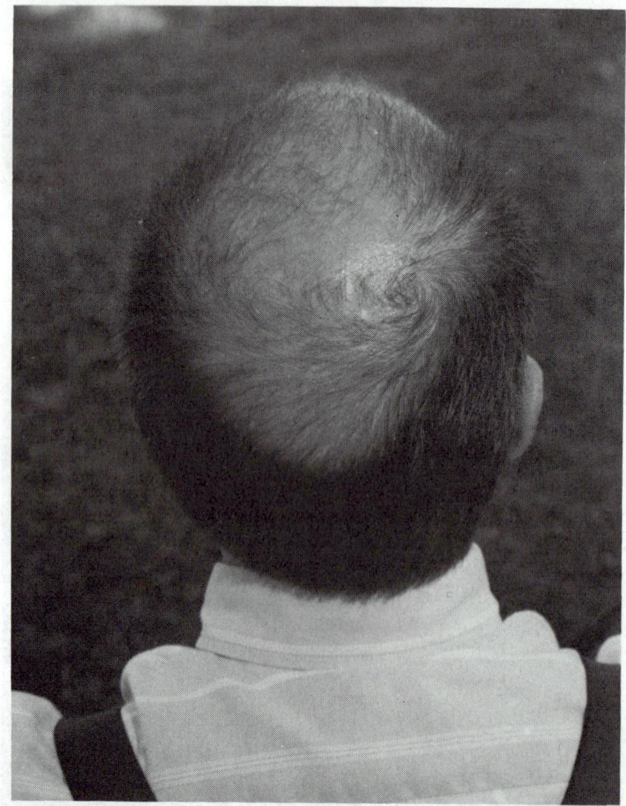

FIGURE 4–3 ◆ Early balding. This man is 34 years old. (Courtesy of Charles A. Henderson III.)

Young adults become increasingly more comfortable with making decisions when faced with unexpected life events. In the mature young adult, coping with the unexpected does not easily disrupt the sense of continuity and integration.

As young adults participate in adult roles, they select lifestyle patterns and role combinations that endure through later life. These decisions solidify their self-identity and enable the young adult to develop a sense of consistency in beliefs, attitudes, and behavior that will continue to develop through their adult years.

SEXUALITY

The development of contraceptive pills, the fear of acquired immunodeficiency syndrome (AIDS), and changes in sexual mores have resulted in a dilemma for many young adults. Much conflict and confusion occurs when one is questioning values related to sexuality.

Change in the sexual aspects of young adulthood relates to more than just sexual behavior. Relationships become increasingly more responsive to understanding and accepting others as they are. Interpersonal relationships depend more on appreciating the uniqueness of others and less on a projection of one's adolescent fantasies, physiologic needs, and a search for a sense of identity. Chapter 11 describes sexuality in detail.

FAMILY STRUCTURE

The major milestones of the transition from childhood to adulthood largely involve the family. These milestones, which typically include leaving one's family of origin, selecting a mate, marrying, and experiencing the birth of the first child, mark the entrance into adult roles and functions (Fig. 4-4). Not all young adults experience all of these milestones. Not everyone marries or has children. Some adults select homosexual rather than traditional heterosexual relationships.

In the United States, there are two general types of family structures: patriarchal (headed by males) and matriarchal (headed by females).

Transcultural Considerations About half of all African-American families are matriarchal, in contrast to one fourth for Hispanic families and one sixth for Caucasian families (Giger and Davidhizar, 1991).

PATRIARCHAL FAMILY STRUCTURE

If the young adult marries and has children, the event of marriage and the establishment of the family bring about many changes and crisis points. The birth of a child requires a major shift from a primarily spouse role to the demands and responsibilities of a parent role. This resocialization requires not only the learning of a new role but also the ability to combine this new role into a set pattern with other roles. The addition of a dependent, demanding third person may disrupt the established couple relationship as well as one's routine patterns of living.

MATRIARCHAL FAMILY STRUCTURE

In the United States, one of every two marriages ends in divorce. More often than not, children of divorced parents live with their mother, which can place a physical, financial, and emotional burden on the single parent. Some single mothers have never been married and/or may not have ongoing contact with the father of their children. Financial or child care support may not be available, and the mother is left with the total responsibility of child rearing. The single mother often ignores personal needs in order to balance child care, work, and home responsibilities. This family structure, rather than the traditional, patriarchal structure described by Havighurst (1972), is becoming increasingly more common in the 1990s.

WORK

Entrance into the work world for the young adult involves a twofold process. The first aspect is the choice of an occupation, followed by socialization into the role demands of the job. The process of selecting and maintaining an occupation is characterized by more flexibility than in years past. The traditional factors of social class, culture, intelligence, gender, aptitudes, role models, and experiences that once operated to limit the range of choices have lost much, but not all, of their impact.

Both partners in a relationship may work outside the home. Not infrequently, one person may need to work at two jobs. Over the past decade, unemployment in the United States has increased. Finding jobs has become more difficult and has greatly increased stress for many adults. Homelessness has increased,

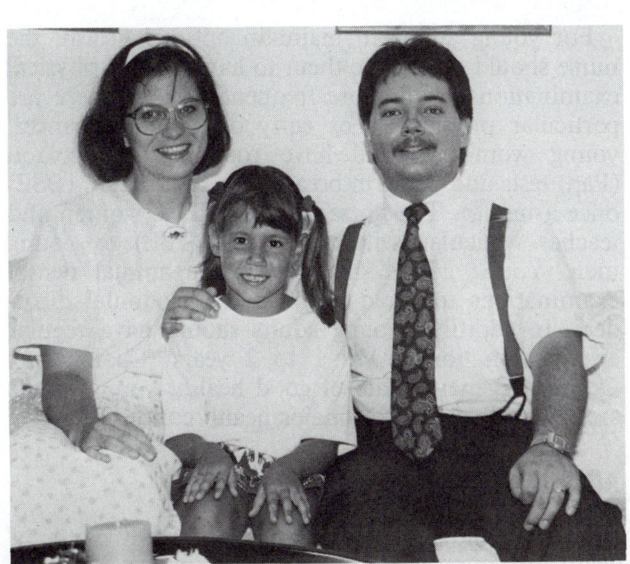

FIGURE 4-4 ◆ A young family.

and an increasing number of people have no health insurance or are underinsured.

Another problem related to employment is the high divorce rate in young adulthood. In the United States, one of two marriages ends in a single-parent family, usually headed by the woman. This has created the need among many young women to ensure their earning ability. Many young adults see prolonged or continuous education as the means to obtain desired standards of living. This often means postponing intimate relationships or combining the roles of student, temporary worker, partner, and parent. Balancing these responsibilities at a time when young adults are still acquiring basic knowledge and skills needed to resolve their developmental tasks can create considerable stress.

LEISURE

Leisure in adulthood is often a difficult concept to define. Most adults consider their work to be the most meaningful activity in their lives. Work provides the necessities of life. It is also the major aspect of one's identity and status. Therefore, to many people, leisure is a negative concept rather than a potentially positive, healthful experience in its own right.

HEALTH ISSUES

The young adulthood years are usually the healthiest years in the life cycle. Most young adults are not seriously ill or incapacitated. As a result, young adults often feel a sense of immunity to illness and neglect health promotion and maintenance activities. The greatest potential for improving health is in what people do and do not do for themselves. Young adults' decisions about diet, exercise, smoking, and drug use are of critical importance to their health status in middle age and later life.

HEALTH PRMOTION

For young adults to maintain optimal health, the nurse should encourage them to have regular physical examinations, with more frequent visits if there are particular problems. For early detection of cancer, young women should have routine Papanicolaou (Pap) tests and perform breast self-examination (BSE) once a month. The nurse teaches BSE to women and teaches testicular self-examination (TSE) to young men. Young adults should schedule annual dental examinations to avoid dental and periodontal disorders. In addition, young adults should have regular eye examinations every 1 to 2 years (Chart 4–1). Despite a general state of good health, young adults are susceptible to a few major health concerns.

CHART 4–1

Health Promotion Guide ◆ Activities to Promote Health and Prevent Illness

- Have regular (yearly) physical examinations.
- For women, have regular Pap tests and perform breast self-examination monthly.
- For men, perform testicular self-examination on a regular basis.
- Have annual dental examinations and prophylaxis.
- Have regular eye examinations (every 1 to 2 years).
- Exercise regularly at least three times a week for 30 minutes.
- Do not smoke; avoid second-hand (passive) smoke.
- Avoid alcohol and so-called recreational drugs.
- Decrease fat and increase fiber in the diet.

ACCIDENTS

In the United States, the most frequent cause of death for young adults is accidents. Injuries occur as a result of work-related incidents, thrill-seeking pleasures, violent crimes, automobile accidents, and war. Men are consistently more frequently involved in accidents than women throughout the life cycle. Between the ages of 15 and 34 years, the male death rate is more than triple that of the female, largely because of the high rate of accidental deaths among males.

The everyday lives of young adults present stressful experiences, such as driving in city traffic or caring for small children, that contribute to accidents. Excessive fatigue occurs in young adults who attempt to balance too many roles. Stress overload combined with excessive fatigue can lead to accidents as well as psychosomatic illnesses.

Young adults should be especially aware of maintaining good health care practices, such as well-balanced diets, regular exercise, and adequate sleep. Because accidents and their consequences present a major threat to the health of young adults, they should take care when engaging in potentially hazardous activities. This care includes using seat belts, avoiding drinking when driving, following speed limits, and observing caution around machinery. In many states in the United States, nurses have advocated for legislation that mandates the use of seat belts and motorcycle helmets to help prevent serious injuries from accidents.

HOMICIDE AND SUICIDE

After accidents, the leading causes of death in young adults are homicide and suicide. The highest incidence of homicide is associated with African-Americans living in urban areas (Giger and Davidhizar, 1991). Some of the deaths are related to abuse of such substances as drugs and alcohol.

DRUG AND ALCOHOL USE AND MISUSE

Few issues have received as much recent attention as drug and alcohol abuse. Use of alcohol and other illicit drugs has increased significantly in the last two decades. Even though the use of tobacco has declined, the use of potentially addictive agents in young adulthood has not decreased, despite the numerous efforts to control this problem. Many law enforcement agencies have joined together in an effort to identify and prosecute drug sellers, buyers, and users. Clinics and programs have also been established to help people wean themselves from drugs. National prevention and awareness programs like DARE (Drug Awareness Resistance Education) have begun in elementary schools (Fig. 4–5).

Regardless of the health care setting, the role of the nurse is affected by the growing problem of substance abuse. In the medical-surgical setting, the nurse often provides care for the client who is or has been a substance abuser. As a result, the planning of nursing interventions is typically more difficult and complicated. For example, the client in pain from a fractured tibia may want pain medication by injection on a regular basis. If the nurse's assessment does not validate that the client is in severe pain, the nurse is faced with an ethical dilemma as well as a care management decision.

Even though alcohol and drug problems are often associated with young adults, this age group is not the only one affected by these addictive agents. Middle-aged and older adults often use addictive agents, but the nurse may have more difficulty in assessing for this problem in these groups.

Middle Adulthood

The time between 35 and 64 years of age is generally considered the period of middle age. This period has been described as the "best years" in the life cycle. During this span of time, adults refer to being in the "prime of life." If healthy development has occurred, the struggles of young adulthood are past and have been resolved, and middle-aged adults should be able to enjoy the results of their labor as established, mature, social, and personally valued people. Yet this time is fraught with its own difficulties.

Middlescense (middle age) is recognized as the midpoint in the life cycle. Most people reflect on and evaluate their lives during this period. Evaluation is not an unusual experience, but it takes on special meaning at this time. The accomplishments of young adulthood shape the life of the middlescent. At this point, people may suddenly realize that this transitional period is the last chance to change life's direction. Many middlescents begin to examine the results of their life work against what they want to do with the rest of their lives. Most of the young adulthood years were spent in working toward achieving goals set in youth. Middlescents reassess their choices and wonder if their chosen directions will progress toward realizing their life goals or desires. This examination may result in massive lifestyle changes for some. This often unsettling time of life, which entails the transition to old age, is often referred to as the "mid-life crisis."

Another problem for some middle-aged adults is that they may not have overcome the struggles of young adulthood. For example, socioeconomic or educational status may interfere with their ability to build a career. As a result, many middlescents are unemployed. Life's goals and desires for these people are not met by this stage in adulthood and may never be met for some.

PHYSIOLOGIC CHANGES

From young adulthood through the middle years, physiologic changes occur gradually.

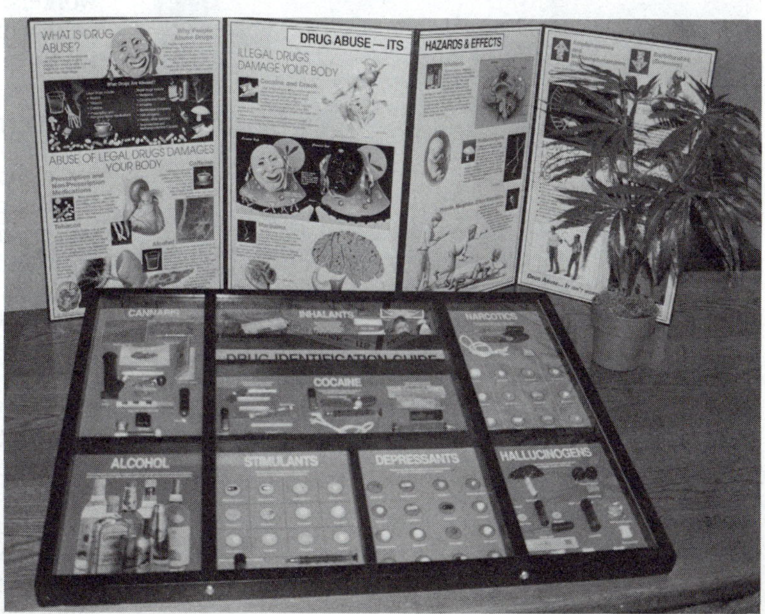

FIGURE 4–5 ◆ Campaigning against substance abuse.

SENSORY CHANGES

VISUAL CHANGES

All people eventually experience a change in visual acuity. The decreased ability of the eyes to accommodate for close and detailed work (presbyopia) becomes evident around age 35 and continues throughout the rest of one's life. Pupil size becomes smaller, which decreases the amount of light that reaches the retina. This change limits the ability of the pupil to constrict and dilate and affects the ability to adapt one's vision in dim light and darkness.

Toward the end of middlescence, the eyes are less able to detect the blues, violets, and greens of the color spectrum and more easily adapt to reds, yellows, and oranges. This change in color perception is linked to the yellowing of the lens with advancing age, but it is not really a color vision impairment (Matteson & McConnell, 1989).

People in their 50s need about twice as much light to see things as they did when they were in their 20s. There is a need for more light for all visual perception with advancing age (Fig. 4–6). The nurse teaches middle-aged and older adults to use extra lighting at home to prevent falls. In the health care setting, the nurse provides adequate lighting, especially at night.

HEARING CHANGES

Hearing loss typically begins in late middlescense. Changes in the efficiency of the cochlea and the hair cells of the organ of Corti are responsible for the impaired transmission of sound waves along the nerve pathways of the brain. These changes are considered to be the most common cause of presbycusis, which is progressive hearing loss associated with aging (Ney, 1993). Presbycusis primarily affects one's ability to hear high-pitched sounds and soft consonants or consonant blends. For example, the "s," "sh," and "ch" sounds are difficult for people with presbycusis to differentiate in conversations. Vowels that have a low pitch are more easily heard. Background noise interferes with conversation so that it is difficult to hear what is being said.

The abilities to see and to hear are major contributors to communication. Age-related changes in these abilities are not only frustrating but also threatening to security and self-esteem. Yet many middlescents are reluctant to get glasses or hearing aids, even when vision or hearing problems significantly affect functioning. Many seem to want to deny the problem rather than to admit to age-related changes. The nurse teaches middle and older adults the importance of wearing assistive devices to help prevent falls or other accidents.

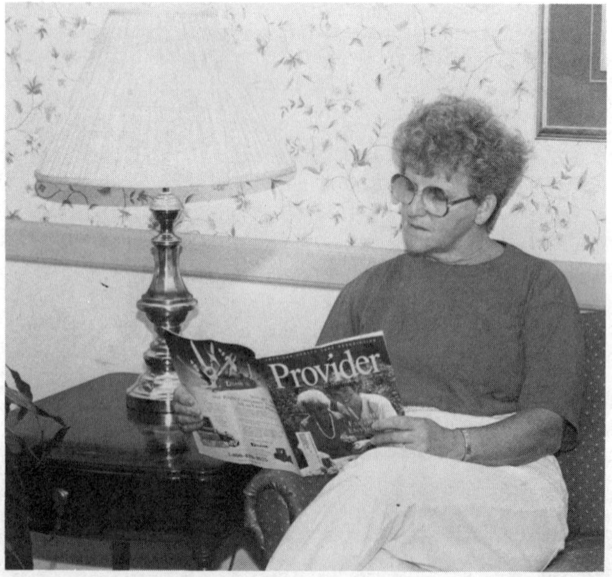

FIGURE 4–6 ◆ A middle-aged adult needs more light while reading.

NEUROMUSCULAR CHANGES

For many middlescents, sedentary or slow-paced lifestyles result in loss of muscle strength and mass. This loss of muscle tone is noticed as waistlines thicken, abdomens protrude, and facial tissue sags.

There is a gradual decline in motor and sensory functioning from its peak during a person's 20s to lower levels in the middle years. Reflexes that entail responses to sudden changes in the environment may be slowed, but for the most part the alterations in function occur gradually and go unnoticed.

Middle-aged adults view neuromuscular changes as relatively insignificant because their progress is so gradual that most people have learned to compensate for them. For example, driving ability is considered to be *better* in middle-aged adults than in younger people, despite declines in coordination, increased reaction time, and sensitivity to glare. It seems that the improvements in judgment and caution compensate for the physical declines. The same is true for manual workers. Middle-aged people usually have fewer disabling injuries and are more conscientious and careful than their younger counterparts.

CARDIOPULMONARY CHANGES

Coronary and pulmonary diseases are among the leading causes of morbidity and mortality in middlescence. These problems are more probably related to lifestyle and genetic factors than to aging per se.

Heart function, rate, and rhythm usually remain unchanged in middlescence. However, when lifestyles become sedentary, anatomic and physiologic changes may occur. Lack of regular exercise over time causes the heart muscle to lose its tone, and changes in rate and rhythm result. Among the most significant factors implicated in atherosclerosis and heart disease are poor nutrition, lack of physical exercise, smoking, and stress.

Pulmonary changes in middlescence are largely related to whether the person is or has been a smoker. Smoking decreases respiratory efficiency and increases the risk of lung disease. Smoking and chronic lung disease largely account for the loss of functioning in lung tissues seen in middlescence. These risk factors, coupled with environmental or occupational pollution, inactivity, and altered cardiac status, can result in decreased breathing capacity. The nurse assesses for risk factors and provides health teaching, such as smoking cessation and regular exercise, to reduce them.

DENTAL CHANGES

Dental problems tend to be a major concern throughout middlescence. Many people older than 55 years of age have lost some of their teeth. This problem is related to lack of dental care throughout the earlier years rather than to the aging process. The nurse teaches the importance of proper dental health care to prevent further problems.

ENDOCRINE CHANGES

Throughout the adult life span, there is a progressive decrease in a person's ability to metabolize glucose efficiently. In fact, this deterioration in performance is so great that nearly all older adults are thought to have increased glucose levels. However, the cause of this change is debatable. Whether the change is physiologic or pathologic is yet to be determined.

The levels of male and female sex hormones decrease in middlescence. Reduced hormone levels result in atrophy of the ovaries, uterus, and vaginal tissues in women. Women lose their ability to have children, but men can father children well into their 70s.

Women are also highly predisposed to osteoporosis, which can lead to painful fractures, and heart disease. The decrease in estrogen production after menopause is associated with these health problems. In men, the development of firmer testes and a tendency for benign prostatic hypertrophy occur during the middle years.

PSYCHOSOCIAL DEVELOPMENT

Middlescence (middle age) is an often unsettling time of questioning former goals, determining what one wants for the future, and making decisions or changes that will influence the second half of life. It is the time when most people acknowledge that they have begun to grow old. Although middle-aged adults recognize that they are in their prime of life, they also realize that time is limited and many accept that they cannot achieve all that they had once hoped. For many people, middlescence is the last chance to identify and pursue new goals and interests. For others, it is merely a plateau into old age.

SELF-CONCEPT

If the maturing years of young adulthood have been handled successfully, middlescents usually have the wisdom and skills to see themselves and their world more realistically. Awareness of their futures assists them to see middlescence as a point in the life cycle when they must make changes, if changes are to be made at all. Typically, middle-aged adults are assessing what they have achieved in the second half of life in their careers, marriages or other intimate relationships, families, lifestyles, social roles, and friendships. For some, this reassessment can result in drastic changes in any or all of the above aspects. Others may elect to continue with their established patterns for the remainder of their lives.

SEXUALITY

Biologically, the most significant milestone in middlescence is the so-called "change of life." This change is signaled by the *climacteric* in both women and men, but it is far less dramatic in men. Climacteric in women, or *menopause,* refers to the process during which menses (menstrual periods) cease, ovaries stop producing ova and female sex hormones, and the genitals atrophy. Other possible signs are sweats, hot flashes, palpitations, dizziness, and emotional changes, such as irritability and depression.

Climacteric for men involves a decrease in the levels of the male sex hormones. This decline is so gradual that most men can produce sperm until well into old age. The male climacteric is not as abrupt or intense as menopause.

FAMILY STRUCTURE

Changes within family relationships, such as children leaving home, separation and divorce, the aging of parents, and the death of a spouse or partner, are often experienced in the middle years. Coping adequately with these changes is a major task of middlescense. Ideally, people should deal with these considerable changes in a manner that helps them grow toward emotional maturity and feel secure and independent rather than depressed, ill, or dependent.

CHILD LAUNCHING

The child-launching phase begins when the first child leaves the parental home and ends when the parents face each other again as a couple. Because of their usually greater emotional and time investments in childrearing, readjustment for women tends to be more critical and profound than for men. The arrival of this change often coincides with menopause, and for family-oriented women the combination of these events may be very stressful. Some women seem unable, for a time, to develop an alternative workable identity, find new ways of nurturing, or find new interests and goals to fill empty time.

Reactions to child launching depend on individual differences and life situations. Women who have combined the work role with motherhood may find it a time of freedom from family responsibilities and financial pressures. Other women may continue to find satisfaction through the roles of wife, partner, and/or grandmother or through work or other activities. Other women may find their lives lonely, frustrating, and generally unsatisfying. To cope effectively, a strong sense of self-identity and an ability to shift roles are crucial.

CHANGE IN INTIMATE RELATIONSHIPS

The stage after active parenting in the family life cycle also greatly influences the marital or intimate relationship. The couple must learn to divert the energy and feelings that flowed to their children back to each other. For many couples, the happiest years of the relationship are the ones before the children are born and the ones after the children are on their own. In these latter years, the couple often experiences a sense of freedom and privacy they have not had for years. This freedom provides an opportunity to get to know each other as people. Divorce or dissolution of an intimate relationship may occur during this time if the relationship has been shaky over the childrearing years. If the relationship has been good, however, it is likely to improve at this time (Fig. 4–7).

CARING FOR AGING PARENTS

During middlescence, a drastic change seems to occur in the relationship between middle-aged children and their parents. Parents suddenly seem old. Aged parents begin to seek their children's help in making decisions and may become dependent for physical and financial support. Middlescents may have to make tough decisions about their parents' living arrangements. Strain is often placed on married middlescents as they weigh their responsibilities toward their parents against those toward their spouse and children. When parents move in with their children, conflict can occur. There may be competition for existing family roles, financial strains, space constraints, or anger over increased responsibilities if the aged person is ill. If the decision to institutionalize the elder is made, the adult child often experiences guilt about the perceived abandonment of the parent. The middle-aged adult who has to care for an older parent while continuing to rear children is sometimes referred to as belonging to the "sandwich generation."

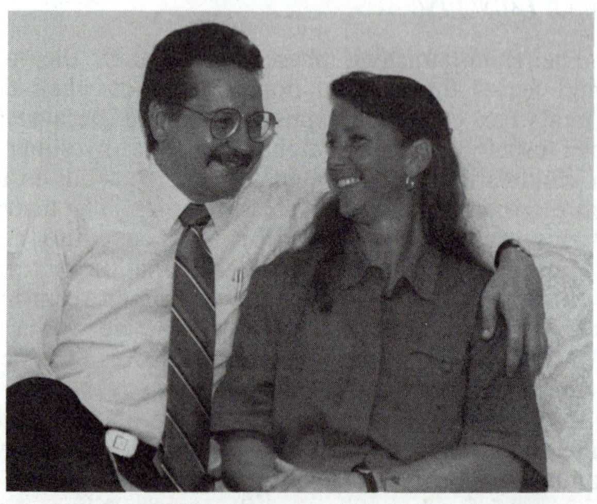

FIGURE 4–7 ◆ A middle-aged couple whose relationship is stronger following active parenting.

Transcultural Considerations The overall institutionalization rate for elderly African-Americans is less than that for Caucasians. A greater number of African-Americans and other minorities choose to care for their elders themselves as a result of a greater sense of responsibility to their older family members and strong religious beliefs (Hines-Martin, 1992).

The medical-surgical nurse needs to be aware that families often are or will be the caregivers after a hospitalized older adult is discharged. Although nursing has been moving toward family-focused care, the family is sometimes not included until discharge planning begins. Schirm and Collier (1992) found that written documentation of family involvement in an older client's care in a hospital setting was sparse (Research Applications for Nursing).

RESEARCH APPLICATIONS FOR NURSING

Nurses Can Improve on Family Involvement in the Care of the Hospitalized Elderly—or at Least Documentation of Family Involvement

Schirm, V., & Collier, J. H. (1992). Nurses' involvement of families in care of hospitalized elders. *Journal of Nursing Care Quality* (Special Report), 36–43.

This study reports the development of an instrument, the Family Nursing Chart Review (FNCR), designed to measure the extent to which nurses involve families in the care of hospitalized elderly relatives. The FNCR contains 16 criteria for family involvement, such as "Health status information shared with family," and "Responses of elders and family documented." The researchers examined 198 medical records from two large urban hospitals. While approximately 32% of the charts showed some evidence of family involvement during data collection on admission, the written documentation on additional family involvement was sparse.

Critique Although the content validity of the instrument was well established, the reliability was not well substantiated. One way to verify the tool might be to use multiple measures of the same concept. The sample in the study was fairly large and probably reflective of many medical records in which family involvement is not well documented.

Possible nursing implications Although nurses do communicate with families about their hospitalized relatives, nurses should document that communication. This is especially important for decision-making during hospitalization and discharge planning.

WORK

For almost all adults, the work role provides a major source of esteem, satisfaction, happiness, and identity. It is a frequently observed phenomenon that career-oriented men and women become increasingly preoccupied with their work as they grow older. This preoccupation with work is a common phenomenon, tending to exclude leisure activities and other roles.

Most adults peak in their careers during middlescence and continue in their chosen fields until retirement. However, there is a new tendency toward changing occupational directions in the middle years. Seeking a second career is an emerging trend within some groups. One such group comprises people who are forced to find new directions because of technologic or economic factors, such as unemployment. Another group includes women who, after devoting their adulthood years to marriage and children, seek a career as an avenue of financial gain and personal growth and satisfaction. Similarly, many people who joined the work force in early adulthood and are eligible for early retirement seek a second career rather than face retirement, which they perceive as boring, idle, and wasteful. Yet another group includes those who made career choices in young adulthood that did not provide them with a sense of satisfaction.

LEISURE

During the later middle adult years, most people find themselves with more time on their hands than their experience or interests can accommodate. Settling into careers, launching children, and retiring result in much unstructured time. Adjustment to this free time is largely related to the person's attitudes toward these events. If the person perceives these losses negatively, fears the loss of accustomed roles or friends, or is uncertain about the future, adjustment may be difficult.

People seek to enhance a positive self-concept through numerous pursuits and interests beyond those of the work and family roles. These alternatives can make the pending loss of roles a means for greater involvement in challenges that are equally important. It is vital for all middlescents to sustain feelings of self-worth by having several alternative life pursuits as the means for achieving a continuing sense of personal growth.

HEALTH ISSUES

Although there are inevitable physical changes and an increasing incidence of chronic conditions as one passes through the middle years, most of the changes from young adulthood are minor ones. Few middlescents are affected by conditions or diseases that necessitate a change in lifestyle or that have a substantial effect on their future. The most common causes of death during the middle years are heart diseases, cancer, strokes, and respiratory tract diseases. People who smoke, drink alcohol, are obese, have high cholesterol levels, and are inactive are at a high risk for these health problems.

General health during middlescence is better than most people expect. Yet it is important for middlescents to engage in preventive and health promotion practices to retain optimal health. The nurse teaches middle-aged adults to schedule annual physical and eye examinations and semiannual dental examinations to detect and treat any significant changes. Because of the relationship of smoking and cardiopulmonary diseases, the nurse encourages smokers to limit or stop their habit. The nurse may refer the person to a smoking cessation program, if available. A regular exercise program and sound nutritional practices, such as reducing the intake of cholesterol and saturated fats, are also effective preventive health measures.

Marital state appears to influence health maintenance as well, with married people often living longer than single or widowed people. When roles are lost in middlescence, it is important for one's mental health to move into another lifestyle that will be satisfying. Prolonged psychologic stress throughout these transition periods can cause injury, illness, and physical and emotional threats.

Middle-aged adults react to stress in a variety of ways. Some endure age changes without psychologic problems. For others, stress can lead to depression, drug abuse, or alcoholism. The nurse working with middle-aged adults assesses the client's level of stress and coping ability. Chapter 7 describes this process in detail.

Late Adulthood

Over the past century, the elderly population (those 65 years of age or older) has increased at rates far higher than those for other segments of the population. The proportion of elderly people in the United States is expected to increase. In 1990, there were 30.1 million older adults, making up 13.3% of the U.S. population. By the year 2030, that proportion is expected to grow to 22% (Walker, 1992). Advances in health care and improved health maintenance habits have resulted in a healthier aged population, with greater numbers of elderly living longer.

The aged person has unique attributes that can be utilized or allowed to remain dormant. Many societies neglect or fail to activate the potential of these people because of stereotypic beliefs about older people. Gerontological research has indicated that there is a systematic stereotyping of and discrimination against people who are old. This is also called *ageism*. It is clear that an accurate understanding of the aged is often lacking.

PHYSIOLOGIC CHANGES

As in every other age cycle, there is no arbitrary dividing line to mark when middle age ends and old age begins. The most popular dividing point is 65 years of age. Physical changes take place at different

CHART 4–2

Nursing Focus on the Elderly ◆ Effects of Aging on Body Systems

System/Function	Normal Changes	Abnormal Changes and Diseases
Cardiovascular	• Increase in the size of the heart • Increase in collagen • Increase in the thickness of valves and blood vessels • Decrease in cardiac output • Decrease in cardiac reserve • Decrease in blood flow to organs	• Hypertension • Coronary artery disease • Congestive heart failure • Peripheral vascular disease • Varicose veins
Endocrine		
Pancreas	• Decreased ability to metabolize glucose • Reduced insulin secretion • Delayed insulin response	• Diabetes mellitus
Gonads	• Decreased hormone levels • Atrophy of the ovaries, uterus, and vagina • Development of firmer testes • Benign prostatic hypertrophy	• Cancer of the uterus, ovaries, or vagina • Cancer of the prostate gland
Integumentary	• Thinning of epithelial cells and subcutaneous fat layers • Lines and wrinkles in the skin • Age spots • Roughness or dryness of the skin • Thinning and loss of color of the hair • Thickening and brittleness of the nails	• Infections: viral, bacterial, fungal • Abnormal cell growth • Tumors: benign and malignant • Skin ulcerations
Musculoskeletal	• Loss of flexibility in the joints • Cartilage degeneration • Bony growths at the edges of joints • Decreased muscle mass	• Osteoporosis • Rheumatoid arthritis • Fracture • Loss of height due to spinal column changes
Neurologic	• General slowing of reaction time • Slow responses to heat and cold • Changing sleep patterns • Decreased cerebral blood flow	• Cerebrovascular disease • Parkinson's disease • Senile dementia and Alzheimer's disease

rates in different people. However, all the body systems are affected somewhat by the aging process. Although some changes become apparent in earlier stages, old age seems to be the time in the life cycle when the progressive changes become more readily apparent and degenerative changes occur more rapidly (Chart 4–2).

In each body system assessment chapter in this text, Nursing Focus on the Elderly charts list major physiologic changes in older people and the nursing implications associated with each change. In addition, normal laboratory values that differ in the elderly are included in Lab Profile charts when appropriate.

INTEGUMENTARY CHANGES

Of all body tissue, the fatty tissue layer fluctuates the most throughout life and with aging is subject to the greatest change. Peripheral body parts display the most striking examples of this alteration, as seen in Clinical Collection 2 in the full-color portion of this textbook. For example, veins and bones of the hand become prominent under a parchment-like, thin layer of skin, and deep hollows appear in the clavicular and axillary areas of the body. The elderly person is susceptible to skin tears, which heal slowly as a result of decreased blood flow to the skin and soft tissues (Resnick, 1993). Breasts sag and become pendulous, and the eyes seem to sink, because of the disappearance of the fat layer around the orbit and decreased skin elasticity.

Subcutaneous tissue has a significant role in the body's adjustment to temperature change. The natural insulation that subcutaneous fat provides is lost. It is not uncommon to hear elderly people say that they are cold, nor is it uncommon to see them wearing a sweater or sitting with a lap blanket when environmental temperatures are comfortable for younger people.

Although subcutaneous tissue does not affect the aged person's tolerance of heat, problems with heat tolerance do exist. Changes in the sweat glands, which diminish in size, number, and activity, cause a decline in the efficiency of the body's cooling mechanism. The elderly do not perspire freely, leaving them at high risk for heat exhaustion. They need to be aware of these changes and learn how to compensate. The nurse teaches them to avoid extreme heat condi-

CHART 4-2

Nursing Focus on the Elderly ◆ Effects of Aging on Body Systems *Continued*

System/Function	Normal Changes	Abnormal Changes and Diseases
Pulmonary	• Increase in the diameter of the chest • Decrease in coughing ability • Decrease in vital capacity and tidal volume • Increase in the production of mucus • Progressive kyphosis • Calcification of the cartilage connecting the ribs to the spinal column and sternum • Decreased strength of the expiratory muscles • Thickening of the alveolar walls; decreased recoil	• Asthma • Bronchitis • Emphysema • Pneumonia • Tuberculosis
Sensory		
Sight	• Presbyopia • Lowered acuity • Altered accommodation to light and dark • Difficulty in color discrimination • Decreased lens clarity	• Cataracts • Glaucoma • Senile ocular degeneration
Hearing	• Decreased discrimination of pitch and acuity • Decreased sensitivity to higher-frequency sounds • Excessive cerumen	• Deafness
Touch	• Decreased receptors • Lowered ability to distinguish temperature and feel pain	• Total loss of feeling
Taste	• Decreased number of taste buds • Diminished ability to distinguish specific tastes	• Total loss of taste
Smell	• Decreased olfactory function • Diminished sensation to distinguish specific odors	• Total loss of smell
Urinary	• Diminished kidney function • Decreased glomerular filtration rate • Decreased number of nephrons • Decreased muscle tone to bladder • Decreased bladder capacity • Decreased sphincter control	• Urinary retention • Urinary tract infection

tions. Sudden changes in room temperature or exposure to overly heated bath water causes the blood vessels in the skin and muscles to dilate. This can result in temporary slowing of blood to the brain, leading to a temporary changes in mental status or to dizziness.

SLEEP CHANGES

The aged take longer to move through the relaxation stages of non–rapid eye movement (non-REM) sleep. The number of awakenings and their duration increase. When asked about the quality of sleep, the aged often respond that they hardly slept all night. Typically, their sleep is more fragmented than that of the young. These interruptions are often due to nocturia (urination at night), leg cramps, and mental stimulation through worry, bereavement, or extraneous noises (Johnson, 1991). It was thought at one time that the elderly needed more sleep, but this is not usually true. The aged seem to sleep less. If one sleeps more, it is usually because of boredom, depression, sedation, or symptoms of disease.

The aged who are not aware that these changes are normal may worry, and the more they worry, the less they sleep. Noisy environments, unresolved fears, worries, and concerns also disrupt sleep quality and patterns. Health care providers often attempt to address the problem by prescribing sleep medications. However, few hypnotic drugs have been found to promote the entire sleep cycle. Instead, these drugs depress REM sleep, or deep sleep, which is necessary for intellectual functioning and for the relief of tension and anxiety. When medications are discontinued, normal sleep patterns usually return, but not until fully re-established dreaming patterns emerge.

NEUROLOGIC AND SENSORY CHANGES

With aging, the central nervous system loses neurons, has a decreased blood supply, and undergoes a decrease in electrical activity. Short-term memory may be affected, but long-term memory is usually intact. For the older adult, these changes may cause altered sensory perception and decreases in reaction time and movement time. It often takes the elder a longer time to respond and initiate action in a given situation.

Visual and hearing changes that started in a person's 30s become much more pronounced in old age. Vestibular (inner ear) functioning decreases, causing dizziness and poor balance. As a result, the elderly person is more prone to falls and accidents.

According to Ney (1993), 25% to 40% of all adults over 65 are hearing-impaired. Ninety percent of people in their 80s have a hearing handicap. Several anatomic changes contribute to hearing loss in the elderly. The cartilage of the auditory canal loses its elasticity and may become narrowed or collapse. In men, stiff coarse hairs in the auditory canal can block the outward flow of cerumen (Ney, 1993). Cerumen impaction sometimes results and can cause hearing impairment.

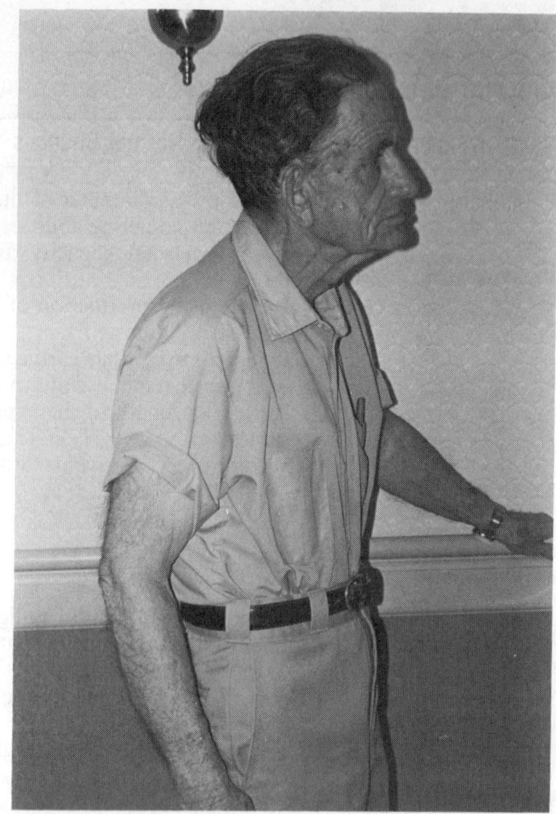

FIGURE 4–8 ◆ Postural changes in an elderly person.

CARDIOPULMONRY CHANGES

All of the body systems and organs change with age, but the most serious changes affect the heart and lungs. The output of the heart is decreased, and the volume of oxygen-carrying blood to all parts of the body is reduced. The continuation of the arteriosclerotic process in the blood vessels ("hardening of the arteries") accentuates this problem.

Respiratory movements of the chest decrease as a result of reduced chest wall muscle activity and deterioration of the alveoli, which alters inspiratory and expiratory volumes. Less oxygen is consumed, and lower respiratory tract infections occur more frequently in older adults. The activity of the cilia diminishes, which allows pathogens and other foreign matter to enter the respiratory tract more easily. The cough reflex, another protective mechanism, is also diminished.

MUSCULOSKELETAL CHANGES

Musculoskeletal problems are very common in old age. The most frequent conditions are:

- Degenerative joint changes
- Osteoporosis resulting from bone atrophy
- Extra-articular pathologic changes of obscure origin, including fibrositis and bursitis
- Fractures caused by trauma and osteoporosis (bone loss)

In addition to these changes, posture and gait changes put the older person at risk for falls (Fig. 4–8). The nurse teaches the older person how to prevent falls at home, by removing scatter rugs, wearing supportive shoes, and using ambulatory devices if needed.

UROLOGIC AND RENAL CHANGES

As a person ages, bladder capacity and muscle tone decrease, sometimes causing urinary retention. As a result, the older adult is prone to urinary tract infections and calculi. The older person typically has to get up in the middle of the night to void (nocturia).

Urinary incontinence is not a normal change associated with aging. However, many elderly people are incontinent. Because the urinary sphincter tone also decreases with age, stress incontinence, particularly in women, is fairly common. Stress incontinence, or urine leakage, occurs when the woman coughs, sneezes, or laughs. Although this can be very embarrassing, many light-weight protective products are available. If the condition worsens, treatment with exercises, medication, or surgery may be necessary (see Chap. 70).

Older men often experience benign prostatic hypertrophy, which causes overflow incontinence. Overflow incontinence is the constant dribbling of urine that results from an overly distended bladder. The enlarged prostate gland causes urine to be retained in the bladder.

The kidneys are also affected by the aging process. Renal nephrons decrease in number, resulting in a decreased ability to concentrate urine. Blood urea nitrogen (BUN) also increases as a result of a decreasing glomerular filtration rate.

GASTROINTESTINAL CHANGES

In older people, the entire gastrointestinal tract undergoes atrophic changes that may interfere with the efficiency of its function. The capacity of the stomach may decrease, and gastric secretions may diminish. The nurse encourages the older adult to eat small, frequent meals. Digestion and absorption of nutrients from the small intestine are also slower. Constipation is a common complaint, usually caused by decreased peristalsis, decreased appetite, inadequate fluid consumption, and lack of exercise. Chronic laxative abuse over the years worsens the problem.

NUTRITIONAL CHANGES

As a result of a lack of proper dental care in earlier years, loss of teeth, gum disease, and bone degeneration may make eating more difficult for the elderly person. Chewing may become more difficult. Poor muscle tone, loss of digestive juices, and impaired circulation often create problems with digestion and elimination. Atrophy of the taste buds coupled with problems related to dentition and digestion diminishes the pleasure of eating for many older adults. Limited incomes and inflationary food costs may prevent some older adults from eating a well-balanced diet.

Changes in eating patterns often lead to anemia, malnutrition, and increased susceptibility to infections. The medical-surgical nurse should be aware that these problems can lead to serious complications when the client is ill or has had surgery.

PSYCHOSOCIAL DEVELOPMENT

The last years of one's life cycle constitute the final stage of development in which adults can grow and change. It is the phase in which the person has the opportunity to make final revisions. How well adults adapt to old age depends in part on how well they have resolved the tasks of the previous stages. People who enter old age with many unresolved crises from prior years experience a difficult time. For others, old age is a time to pass on the wisdom of one's experiences, continue fulfilling productive roles, and enjoy a sense of fulfillment for a life well lived.

SELF-CONCEPT

The way people regard themselves determines their life satisfaction. Self-concept is developed by a continuous interaction between a person and the environment. Loss of a significant other and loss of roles such as parent, spouse, and worker often affect the elder's sense of self and psychologic well-being. The need to be creative and productive is particularly important in old age to gain attention and approval from others.

Other people may attempt to maintain a positive self-concept in several ways. These include such reactions as denial of illness, regression, or retreat into fantasy. Reminiscence may also be used as a defense against present threats to self-esteem. These reactions, while adaptive to conditions or events outside the control of the older person, do not help people to develop their personal potentials. Good health, adequate income, a useful role, opportunities for social interactions, and lively interests are the main determinants of a happy old age. An estimated 10% to 15% of the elderly population in the United States are in poor health and do not have adequate financial support to meet basic needs.

SEXUALITY

Studies of sexual behaviors and interest in these behaviors among the elderly have been limited and inconsistent in their findings. Many studies suggest that elders retain an interest in sexual function and are sexually active. Other studies conclude that there is a decline of sexual interest and behavior among the aged. Reported declines are largely the result of social, cultural, and psychologic factors rather then biologic and physical factors. Factors that determine sexual activity include present health status, past and present life satisfaction, and the status of marital or intimate relationship. For example, many older women are widowed or divorced and lack available sexual partners, which probably accounts for their decline in sexual interest.

Physiologic changes associated with the aging process occur in both men and women. In women, vaginal secretions diminish and the vagina atrophies. In men, the time required to attain an erection increases. With age, men are also able to maintain an erection for an extended period of time without ejaculation. After ejaculation, the older man often cannot have a subsequent erection for 12 to 24 hours. Despite these physiologic changes, both elderly men and women are capable of sexual activity, including intercourse (Fig. 4–9).

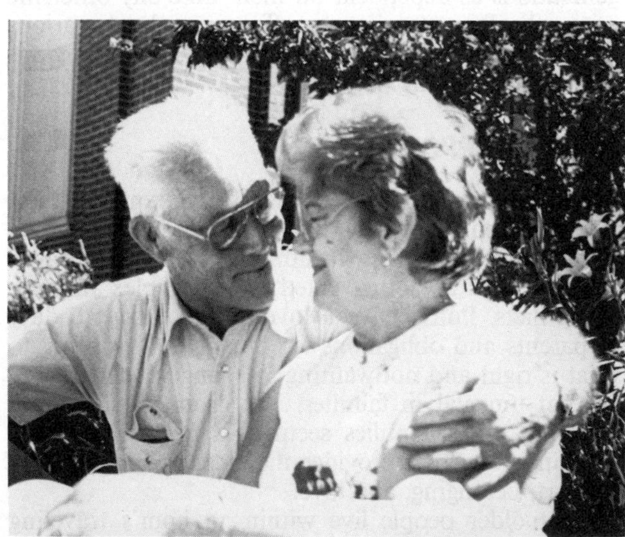

FIGURE 4–9 ◆ Everyone is a sexual being, with individual needs. (Courtesy of St. Anselm College, Manchester, NH.)

FAMILY STRUCTURE

Three principal factors affect family structure and function in late life:

- Health status and expected life span
- Social changes, such as industrialization and urbanization
- Normal aging processes

Most married couples see their last child leave home when the couple are in their 40s or 50s and can expect to live another 30 or more years. This long period that follows active parenting responsibilities presents a variety of problems that elders have not had to deal with in previous generations, such as widowhood.

WIDOWHOOD

Although most elderly men are married, two thirds of all elderly women are widowed. Even when men have been widowed, their chances for remarriage are twice those of women (Matteson & McConnell, 1989).

Because of ill health, poverty, and the normal social losses of old age, the elderly widowed person may confront the prospect of becoming socially isolated. The ability to prevent social isolation may be related to advanced level of education, residence in a small town or a rural area, or, most important, the presence of friends and neighbors with whom one can relate. Older widowed people may adjust better to bereavement because of anticipatory grieving and the tendency to view death as one of the developmental tasks of old age.

Factors other than choice frequently operate to isolate the widowed person. Those who lack skills, money, health, and transportation for engaging in society encounter more difficulties in adjusting to a change in role status. The isolated status of widows may be related to the socialization of women in past generations as dependent on men. Like any other life crisis, the loss of a spouse affects people in various ways. Adjustment is related to the person's previous lifestyle and coping patterns.

FAMILY SUPPORT

The relationship between adult children and their elderly parents depends on a variety of factors, such as distance, economics, health, and emotional health. Relationships are often taxed by a complex mixture of conflicts. Pulls between love and resentment, duty to parents and obligations for others, and wanting to what is right and not wanting to change one's lifestyle are not unusual in families. Yet, from the literature available, most families seem able to resolve problems in a way that provides the elder with a sense of support, belonging, and love.

Most older people live within an hour's traveling distance of their children and manage to see them often. There are, however, some differences according to social class. Upper-class and middle-class adults are likely to live greater distances from their parents than lower-class adults. This difference is more a result of professional career patterns than a desire to be separated. Although patterns of aid and contact vary among the socioeconomic classes, there is no difference in caring. Greater distance results in fewer visits, but the quality of the visits and frequent long-distance communication may compensate for periods of absence. Distance between family members also alters the type of support exchanged. Families living close to one another tend to exchange services, such as shopping and household maintenance tasks, whereas family members who live some distance apart tend to confine their assistance to monetary support.

Fewer than a third of the elderly live with their children. Many elders want their privacy, independence, and freedom rather than having to adjust to their children's lifestyle.

There is a growing proportion of frail, dependent elders. For this group, several options are available. They can live in a retirement community or other group setting or can remain in the community, sustained by families and friends. Most elders prefer to reside in their own communities, but there are problems that make realization of this preference difficult. Families generally attempt to help but may be limited in their ability. Most adult couples are active members of the work force and still have dependent children at home or in school.

GRANDPARENTING

Grandparenting is often the most important role in the life of the elderly, providing them with a sense of purpose, value, and esteem. A relationship with grandparents often brings a sense of stability and perspective to their children's family (Fig. 4–10). Grandparents provide the young with advice, affirmation, and a sense of roots and continuity. For their children, they may relieve some of the parenting burden by assuming actual caretaking responsibilities, especially when both parents are working.

Regardless of the type of role assumed, grandparenting benefits the older adult, the adult child, and the grandchild. Through the role of grandparent, the elder can maintain ego integrity (Erikson) and approach death with a sense of fulfillment and a feeling of extension of his or her influence into future generations. Many schools and senior citizens' centers have joined to help children appreciate the pleasure of forming relationships with other adults other than their grandparents. This intergenerational visiting has also helped the elderly feel wanted and useful (MacPhail, 1993).

WORK AND RETIREMENT

In 1900, two of three older men were employed. In recent years, retirement has become less a matter of choice, with only one of six older men employed. Because women were less likely to be working outside

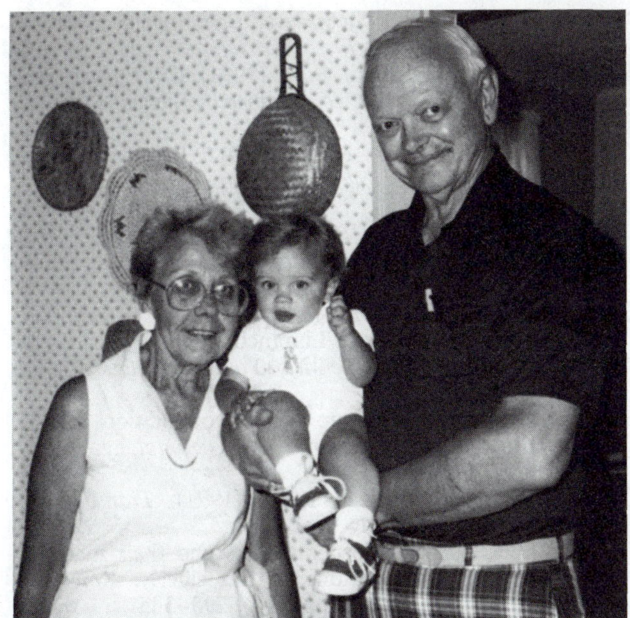

FIGURE 4-10 ◆ Grandparenting roles vary, but everyone involved may benefit from the relationships, regardless of the roles.

the home earlier in the century, the numbers of older female workers were less and have remained stable. This picture may change as the increased numbers of younger women who have entered the labor force become older. Adjustment to retirement remains a significant crisis for a working person. One survey of retirees revealed that one third of all retirees would prefer to work (Ferraro, 1990).

To most elderly people, it comes as a grim surprise that their income may be less than adequate. For those who depend solely on Social Security benefits, their incomes may fall below the poverty levels established by the U.S. government. For some people, therefore, one of the most serious problems retirement creates is inadequate financial resources.

Some older people prefer to work rather than retire. Some need to work to supplement income from other sources. One common emerging pattern is reentry into the work force with part-time employment. Between 10% and 25% of retirees in the United States follow this pattern. Most of the time, these retirees take jobs for wage cuts, change industry or occupation, or become self-employed. Older adults who reenter the labor force after retirement are usually people who retired early, whereas late retirees rarely return to the work force.

LEISURE

Adjustment to time freed from work, family, and social responsibilities in old age depends, to a significant degree, on such factors as prior attitudes toward work, aging, and retirement; health; income; geographic location; and family situation. Favorable adjustment to old age is characterized by a tendency toward substitution. To adequately adjust to the acquired status of retiree, the individual must replace or find substitutes for those satisfactions relinquished with lost roles.

People tend to continue the same patterns of leisure established earlier in life. Some of the most popular activities before and after role losses include visiting friends, watching television, doing odd jobs at home, traveling, and reading. There do not seem to be changes in activities but, rather, an increase in the frequency of customary activities.

Transcultural Considerations In a study by Chin-Sang and Allen (1991), the researchers found that African-American women increased their involvement in their churches as they entered late adulthood. They also frequently attended senior citizens' centers to form relationships and provide service to others (Research Applications for Nursing).

How a person uses leisure time depends on occupation or work role, education, gender, and family status. The success of transitions to retirement and old age relates to educational and occupational background. More highly educated people seem able to more easily structure free time. Similarly, people with

RESEARCH APPLICATIONS FOR NURSING

Church Activities Help Some Elderly African-American Women Cope with Losses

Chin-Sang, V., & Allen, K. R. (1991). Leisure and the older black woman. *Journal of Gerontological Nursing, 17*(1), 30–34.

A convenience sample of 30 elderly African-American women who were living in Florida on fixed incomes and active members of Protestant churches were interviewed to determine how they spend their leisure time. The qualitative analysis of the data revealed four themes: loneliness, church, worship, and duty. During leisure, the women thought about their losses—parents, husbands, pets, and friends. All of the women coped with their loneliness by increasing involvement in their churches. In addition, the women visited and helped others at the local senior citizens' centers.

Critique This study is the first published nursing research to examine leisure in the elderly, especially in African-Americans. The use of an open-ended interview approach permitted the subjects to express their feelings and expand on them.

Possible nursing implications When caring for elderly African-American clients, nurses should incorporate clients' strong religious practices and beliefs in their care, if appropriate. Nurses also need to recognize that these women may be resourceful, as evidenced by the ways in which many of them cope with loss.

higher income status tend to view leisure time more positively and believe that they have a greater degree of control over their lives. A number of studies have reported that life satisfaction in retirement is nearly always higher among professionals or among workers who manifested a positive pre-retirement attitude, although more professionals than other workers do continue working.

Women consistently report an easier adjustment to leisure time in late life than men do. Women generally have consistently developed more social relationships, been more involved with their children and grandchildren, and developed more hobby interests throughout their life spans than men have.

HEALTH ISSUES

Because the population of older adults is growing more rapidly than any other age group, an entire chapter is devoted to health care for the elderly (see Chap. 5). Specific diseases or disorders that commonly occur in the elderly, like arthritis, heart disease, and chronic lung disease, are discussed throughout the book.

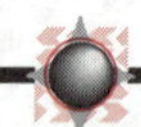

IMPLICATIONS FOR NURSING RESEARCH

As the life expectancy of adults increases, nurses need to be aware of normal development and its impact on health care. However, many questions remain unanswered that could assist the nurse in providing the best possible care to adults in medical-surgical settings. Some of these questions include:

- What impact do socioeconomic and educational factors have on health issues in each developmental stage?
- How does cultural diversity affect adult development?
- How do nontraditional families (e.g., a homosexual couple rearing a child) affect psychosocial development?
- What factors influence health in old age?

SELECTED BIBLIOGRAPHY

Baines, E. (1992). *Perspectives on gerontology nursing.* Boston: Sage.

Bonheur, B., & Young, S. W. (1991). Exercise as a health-promoting lifestyle choice. *Applied Nursing Research, 4,* 2–6.

Burbank, P. M. (1992). An exploratory study: Assessing the meaning of life among older adult clients. *Journal of Gerontological Nursing, 18*(9), 19–28.

Burke, M. M., & Walsh, M. B. (1992). *Gerontologic nursing: Care of the frail elderly.* St. Louis: C. V. Mosby.

*Burnside, I. (1988). *Nursing and the aged: A self-care approach.* New York: McGraw-Hill.

*Butler, R. N. (1975). *Why survive? Being old in America.* New York: Harper & Row.

Chenitz, W. C., & Salisbury, S. A. (1991). *Clinical gerontological nursing: A guide to advanced practice.* Philadelphia: W. B. Saunders.

Chin-Sang, V., & Allen, K. R. (1991). Leisure and the older black woman. *Journal of Gerontological Nursing, 17*(1), 30–34.

Ebersole, P., & Hess, P. (1990). *Toward healthy aging: Human needs and nursing response* (3rd ed.). St. Louis: C. V. Mosby.

Eliopoulos, C. (1990). *Caring for the elderly in diverse care settings.* Philadelphia: J. B. Lippincott.

*Erikson, E. H. (1968). *Identity: Youth and crisis.* New York: W. W. Norton.

Ferraro, K. F. (1990). Group benefit, orientation toward older adults at work. *Journal of Gerontology: Social Sciences, 45,* S220–S227.

Giger, J. N., & Davidhizar, R. E. (1991). *Transcultural nursing.* St. Louis: Mosby-Year Book.

Gottlieb, G. L. (1990). Sleep disorders and their management: Special considerations in the elderly. *American Journal of Medicine, 88* (Suppl. 3A), 295–335.

*Gress, L., & Bahr, R. (1984). *The aging person: A holistic perspective.* St. Louis: C. V. Mosby.

*Havighurst, R. (1972). *Developmental tasks and education.* New York: David McKay.

Heriot, C. S. (1992). Spirituality and aging. *Holistic Nursing Practice, 7*(1), 22–31.

Hines-Martin, V. P. (1992). A research review: Family caregivers of chronically ill African-American elderly. *Journal of Gerontological Nursing, 18*(2), 25–29.

Hogstel, M. O. (1992). *Clinical manual of gerontological nursing.* St. Louis: Mosby-Year Book.

Jarvis, C. (1992). *Physical examination and health assessment.* Philadelphia: W. B. Saunders.

Johnson, J. E. (1991). Progressive relaxation and the sleep of older noninstitutionalized women. *Applied Nursing Research, 4,* 165–170.

*Jung, C. (1971). The stages of life. In J. Campbell (Ed.), *The portable Jung.* New York: Viking. (Original work published 1928).

MacPhail, J. (1993). Intergenerational caring in professional and family life. *Geriatric Nursing, 14,* 104–107.

*Matteson, M. A., & McConnell, E. S. (1989). *Gerontological nursing: Concepts and practices.* Philadelphia: W. B. Saunders.

*Neugarten, B. L. (1977). Personality and aging. In J. E. Birrin & K. W. Schaie (Eds.), *Handbook of the personality of aging.* New York: Van Nostrand Reinhold.

Ney, D. F. (1993). Cerumen impaction, ear hygiene practices, and hearing acuity. *Geriatric Nursing, 14,* 70–73.

Olshansky, S. J. (1993). The human life span: Are we reaching the outer limits? *Geriatrics, 48*(3), 85–88.

*Peck, R. C. (1968). Psychological developments in the second half of life. In B. L. Neugarten (Ed.), *Middle age and aging.* Chicago: University of Chicago Press.

*Pryor, W. (1983). Free radicals and autoxidation in aging. In D. Armstrong et al. (Eds.). *Aging. Vol. 27: Free radicals in molecular biology, aging and disease.* New York: Raven Press.

Resnick, B. (1993). Wound care for the elderly. *Geriatric Nursing, 14,* 26–29.

*Rosow, I. (1974). *Socialization to old age.* Berkeley: University of California Press.

Schirm, V., & Collier, J. H. (1992). Nurses' involvement of families in care of hospitalized elders. *Journal of Quality Care* (Special Report), 36–43.

*Sheehy, G. (1976). *Passages: Predictable crises of adult life.* New York: Bantam Books.

Sheehy, G. (1992). *The silent passage: Menopause.* New York: Random House.

Urinary Incontinence Panel (1992). *Urinary incontinence in adults: Clinical practice guideline.* Agency on Health Care Policy and Research (AHCPR) Pub. No. 92-0038. Rockville, MD: AHCPR, Public Health Service, U.S. Department of Health and Human Services.

Walker, S. N. (1992). Wellness for elders. *Holistic Nurse Practice, 7*(1), 38–45.

SUGGESTED READINGS

Bonheur, B., & Young, S. W. (1991). Exercise as a health-promoting lifestyle choice. *Applied Nursing Research, 4,* 2–6.

This nursing study examines differences between young adults who exercised and those who did not. Of the 105 subjects, those who exercised regularly had higher self-esteem and perceived greater benefits from exercise than those who did not exercise.

Burbank, P. M. (1992). An exploratory study: Assessing the meaning of life among older adult clients. *Journal of Gerontological Nursing, 18*(9), 19–28.

This nursing research presents the components that give meaning to life to older adults. Meaning in life was linked to health, and relationships were felt to give meaning to life. These findings were consistent with those of previous studies.

Olshansky, S. J. (1993). The human life span: Are we reaching the outer limits? *Geriatrics, 48*(3), 85–88.

The author presents two possible models of aging—the risk factor model and the evolutionary model. The first model proposes that eliminating risk factors of disease will prevent aging. The evolutionary model advances the notion that risk factors are not the cause of disease; genetic influence explains diseases which cause aging. In the evolutionary model, which the author supports, risk factors merely affect the course of disease.

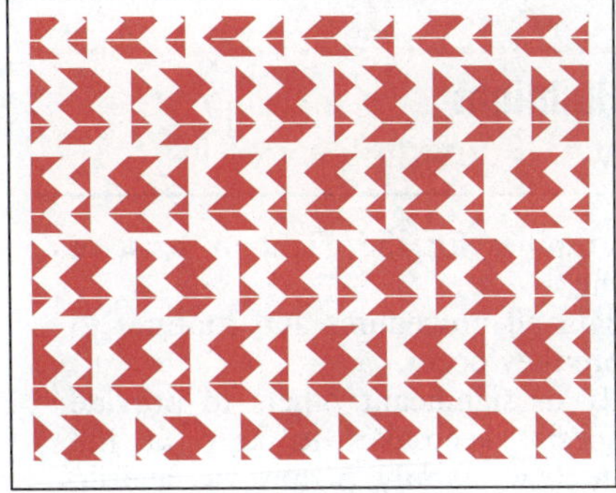

CHAPTER 5

Health Care of Older Adults

CHAPTER HIGHLIGHTS

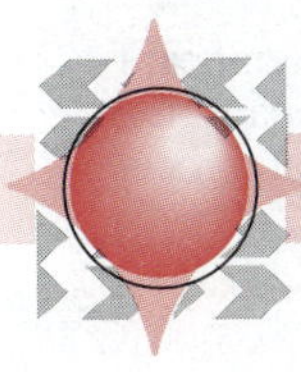

The number of people older than 65 years of age in the Western world is rapidly increasing and will continue to increase well into the 21st century. Nurses have frequent contact with the elderly in both their professional and personal lives. Because much of their professional contact is through health care settings like hospitals, nursing homes, and community health agencies, nurses sometimes have a tendency to stereotype the typical older adult as a confused, dependent person.

This chapter describes major health issues associated with late adulthood. The care of older adults with specific health problems, such as diseases and the need for surgical procedures, is discussed throughout this text under each body system as appropriate. In addition, Focus on the Elderly boxes highlight the most important information related to care of the elderly client with a selected health problem.

SUBGROUPS OF LATE ADULTHOOD

Late adulthood, consisting of people older than 65 years, can be further divided into subgroups:

- Age 65–74 years: the young old
- Age 75–84 years: the middle old
- Age 85–99 years: the old old
- Age 100 years or more: the elite old

The fastest growing subgroup is the old old, sometimes referred to as the frail elderly population. Their needs and problems are generally different from those adults who are between 60 and 74 years old. The incidence of chronic disease increases markedly when a person is over 80. At any age, the older adult is a person with specific needs and problems.

DISTRIBUTION OF OLDER ADULTS IN THE HEALTH CARE SYSTEM

About 80% to 85% of older adults are relatively healthy and living in the community. Another 5% are in long-term care facilities (nursing homes), and another 10% to 15% are ill but are being cared for at home (Matteson & McConnell, 1989). The elderly from any setting usually experience one or more hospitalizations in their lifetime. Seventy percent to 90% of clients on most medical-surgical units in hospitals are older than 65.

HOSPITALIZATION OF THE OLDER ADULT

Being admitted to the hospital is often a traumatic experience for anyone, especially for the older adult. Many elders suffer from *relocation stress,* also known as relocation trauma or relocation syndrome. Most of the early studies on this syndrome examined the increased mortality rate associated with moving elderly people from their own homes to a nursing home or hospital (Coffman, 1981). Other studies have investigated other effects of relocation on behavior and health (Borup, 1983; Patnaik et al., 1974). Few studies have examined the negative impact of relocation on health status and function, although physical and mental changes have been noted (Horowitz & Schulz, 1983; Matteson & McConnell, 1989).

In some cases, the elderly person who is admitted to the hospital from home can become disoriented, confused, agitated, and/or abusive. Risk factors thought to contribute to relocation syndrome are the lack of choice or preparation time and the major environmental change. Men older than age 75 who are physically and mentally impaired are at high risk for relocation syndrome (Coffman, 1981). Chart 5–1 lists nursing interventions that may help minimize the effects of relocation for the elderly client.

CHART 5–1

Nursing Care Highlight ◆ Minimizing the Effects of Relocation Stress in the Elderly

- Provide opportunities for the client to assist in decision-making.
- Carefully explain all procedures and routines to the client before they occur.
- Ask the family or significant others to provide familiar or special keepsakes to keep at the client's bedside (e.g., family picture, a favorite hairbrush).
- Reorient the client frequently to where he or she is.
- Ask the client what his or her expectations are during hospitalization or nursing home placement.
- Encourage the client's family and friends to visit often.
- Establish a trusting relationship with the client as early as possible.
- Assess the client's usual lifestyle and daily activities, including food likes and dislikes and preferred time for bathing.
- Avoid unnecessary room changes.
- If possible, have a family member, significant other, staff member, or volunteer accompany the client when leaving the unit for special procedures or therapies.

HEALTH ISSUES

This book presents many discussions of health problems that are experienced by the elderly, particularly in the institutional health care setting. This portion of the chapter focuses more on health issues and problems that may not warrant hospital or nursing home admission.

Health Promotion

Health is a major concern of most elderly people. An elderly person's health status can affect his or her ability to perform basic activities of daily living and to participate in social roles. An elder's failure in the performance of these activities may increase his or her dependence on others and may have a negative effect on morale and life satisfaction.

The health problems most frequently observed among older clients tend to be chronic and degenerative rather than acute. Further, the health problems of the aged are frequently the result of multiple causes, including physical, psychologic, and social components, in a complex mixture.

For both middle-aged and older adults, heart disease and cancer are the most frequent causes of death. For the older adult, most fatalities are due to disorders resulting from diminished physiologic defenses, such as a severe infection related to cancer or cancer treatment.

Like younger adults, older adults need to practice health promotion and prevention of illness to maintain or achieve a high level of wellness (Chart 5–2). The nurse working with the elderly in any setting needs to teach them the importance of promoting wellness and strategies for accomplishing this goal.

Health is related to a person's level of functioning. In assessing the older person's level of functioning, the nurse considers self-responsibility and self-management, nutritional awareness, physical fitness and mobility, stress management, and environmental factors.

SELF-RESPONSIBILITY AND SELF-MANAGEMENT

An elderly person's ability to maintain a positive self-concept and self-control may be hampered by the loss of resources in the late years of life. The elderly may also experience a number of losses that can affect their sense of control over their lives—the death of a spouse and significant others, the loss of social and work roles, and a decrease in physical mobility. The nurse can support older clients' self-esteem and feelings of competency by encouraging them to maintain as much control as possible over their lives, participate in decision-making, and perform as many tasks as possible.

Regardless of the situation, it is important that elderly clients direct their lifestyle in a manner that encourages them to feel capable and valued. The elderly need to find opportunities to be productive and take care of themselves as well as others.

The nurse in the community health setting often has the opportunity to assess an older adult's self-care or self-management ability. A number of assessment tools are available for this, but most are too long and complex to be used in a hospital setting. When elderly clients are admitted, the nurse also needs to assess their self-management capabilities for discharge planning. Several assessment tools used in acute care have been published (Research Applications for Nursing).

CHART 5–2

Health Promotion Guide ♦ Lifestyles and Practices to Promote Wellness

Health-Protecting Behaviors

- Have yearly influenza vaccinations.
- Obtain a pneumococcal vaccination.
- Wear seat belts when you are in an automobile.
- Use alcohol in moderation or not at all.
- Avoid smoking.
- If you smoke at home, do not smoke in bed.
- Install and maintain working smoke detectors.
- Create a hazard-free environment to prevent falls, such as avoiding scatter rugs and waxed floors.
- Use medications according to your physician's orders.
- Avoid over-the-counter medications unless your physician directs you to use them.

Health-Enhancing Behaviors

- Have a yearly physical examination; see your physician more often if health problems occur.
- Reduce dietary fat to not more than 30% of calories; saturated fat should provide less than 10% of your calories.
- Increase your dietary intake of complex carbohydrate and fiber-containing food to five or more servings of fruits and vegetables and six or more servings of grain products daily.
- Allow at least 10 to 15 minutes of sun exposure two to three times weekly for vitamin D intake.
- Exercise regularly three to five times a week for 30 minutes per session.
- Manage stress through coping mechanisms that you have used successfully in the past.
- Get together with people in different settings.
- Reminisce about your life.

NUTRITIONAL AWARENESS

NUTRITION NEEDS IN THE COMMUNITY

A person's need for adequate nutrition remains constant throughout the life span, yet many elderly people eat an inadequate diet. Inflation, reduced income, and the lack of transportation are factors that may contribute to inadequate nutrition among older adults. Elderly people whose diets consist of inappropriate or unbalanced foods (e.g., an excess of carbohydrates) may also be poorly nourished. Some elders reduce their intake of food to near-starvation levels, even with the availability of assistive programs, such as food stamps, free food, and Meals on Wheels. The lack of transportation, the necessity to travel to obtain such services, and the inability to carry large quantities of groceries prohibit some elders from taking advantage of food programs.

Poor nutrition among the elderly may also be related to loneliness. Elders may respond to loneliness, depression, and boredom by not eating, which can lead to malnutrition. Many elderly who live alone have lost the incentive to prepare or eat balanced diets. Still others respond to stress by overeating, which leads to obesity.

NUTRITIONAL REQUIREMENTS

A person's minimal nutritional requirements from youth through old age remain consistent, with a few exceptions. Older adults need increased dietary intake of calcium, vitamin C, and vitamin A because alterations with age disrupt the ability to store, use, and absorb these substances. Sedentary lifestyles and reduced metabolic rate require a reduction in total caloric intake to maintain ideal body weight.

RESEARCH APPLICATIONS FOR NURSING

A New Assessment Tool May Help Nurses Accurately Assess Their Clients' Ability to Manage Complex Conditions

Snyder, M., Brugge-Wiger, P., Ahern, S., Connelly, S., DePew, C., Kappas-Larson, P., Semmerling, P., & Wyble, S. (1991). Complex health problems: Clinically assessing self-management abilities. *Journal of Gerontological Nursing, 17*(4), 23–27.

Older adults typically have one or more chronic conditions that affect their functional abilities. When these people are hospitalized, they generally have special discharge planning needs for self-management. Snyder and colleagues therefore reviewed existing self-care and functional assessment tools to determine whether any of them would help nurses in acute care settings to assess and plan self-management for clients after discharge. The researchers found that none of the existing tools were helpful in the management of the complex health problems seen in today's acute care setting. The researchers therefore developed and piloted a self-management inventory (SMI) based on Orem's self-care model. The researchers found that this tool had high inter-rater reliability and took only 28 minutes to complete.

Critique The authors looked for a tool that had already been published before developing another, and they based their tool on an accepted theory of self-care. They saw a need in clinical practice and attempted to address it with staff input. Inter-rater reliability was important for the tool, and it was acceptable.

Possible nursing implications With today's early discharge of clients from hospitals, clients need to be able to manage their own care. A tool that can adequately and efficiently assess discharge planning needs helps the nurse determine where to focus his or her interventions.

PHYSICAL CHANGES AFFECTING NUTRITION

Other physical aging changes influence the older adult's nutritional status or ability to take in needed nutrients. Diminished senses of taste and smell often result in a loss of appeal of food. Elderly people experience a greater decline in the ability to taste sweet and salt than in the discrimination of bitter and sour. This phenomenon often results in the elder's overuse of table sugar and salt to compensate. The nurse teaches the elderly client to use herbs and spices to season food or to vary the textures of food substances to achieve satisfaction from food rather than increase the intake of sugar and salt.

The loss of teeth or poorly fitting dentures from inadequate dental care can also cause the elderly to avoid important foodstuffs. The extensive use of prescribed and over-the-counter drugs may affect one's appetite, food tolerances, and food absorption and utilization (Walker, 1992). Older people with dentition problems frequently resort to eating soft, high-calorie foods, like ice cream and mashed potatoes, which lack roughage and fiber. Unless the person carefully chooses more nutritious soft foods, vitamin deficiencies, constipation, and other disorders can result.

The aged person sometimes responds to problems associated with mobility, prescribed diuretics, and limited bladder capacity by limiting fluid intake, especially in the evening. The nurse teaches older adults that fluid restrictions make them prone to dehydration and electrolyte imbalances that can cause serious illness or death.

NUTRITION NEEDS IN THE HOSPITAL

In addition to the nutritional needs that have been described for older adults living in the community, those who are hospitalized or institutionalized have special needs related to their illness and general health state. For example, an elderly client with a pressure sore needs additional protein, vitamin C, and zinc to heal the open skin lesion. The physician, nurse, and dietitian collaborate to determine the best sources of these nutrients. The physician may prescribe a multivitamin tablet with zinc to be given every day. The dietitian may recommend a high-calorie, high-protein supplement like Ensure Plus to be given several times a day. The nurse encourages the client to select and eat high protein foods to promote healing. (See Chapter 61 for further discussion of nutrition in the elderly.)

PHYSICAL FITNESS AND MOBILITY

Exercise and activity are important to the older adult as a means of promoting and maintaining health (Fig. 5–1). Physical activity can help keep the body in shape and maintain an optimal level of functioning. In addition, regular, moderate exercise typically results in feelings of well-being. Numerous studies have shown a lower incidence of coronary artery disease in populations engaged in regular physical activity compared with populations who do not exercise regularly. Karper and Boschen (1993) found that moderate exercise in the elderly also helped to strengthen the immune system and, therefore, prevent the high incidence of acute respiratory infections that are common in this age group.

Without exercise, muscles, organs, and tissues tend to atrophy, and motor, sensory, and cognitive functions can become impaired. It is estimated that 50% of the physical decline of the elderly is caused by disuse rather than by the aging process or illness (Walker, 1992).

The benefits and purposes of regular exercise are to improve circulation, improve blood pressure, improve respiratory function, maintain muscle tone throughout the body, reduce muscle tension, reduce muscle pain, and promote relaxation. One of the best exercises for older adults is to walk three to five times a week for at least 30 minutes each session (Karper &

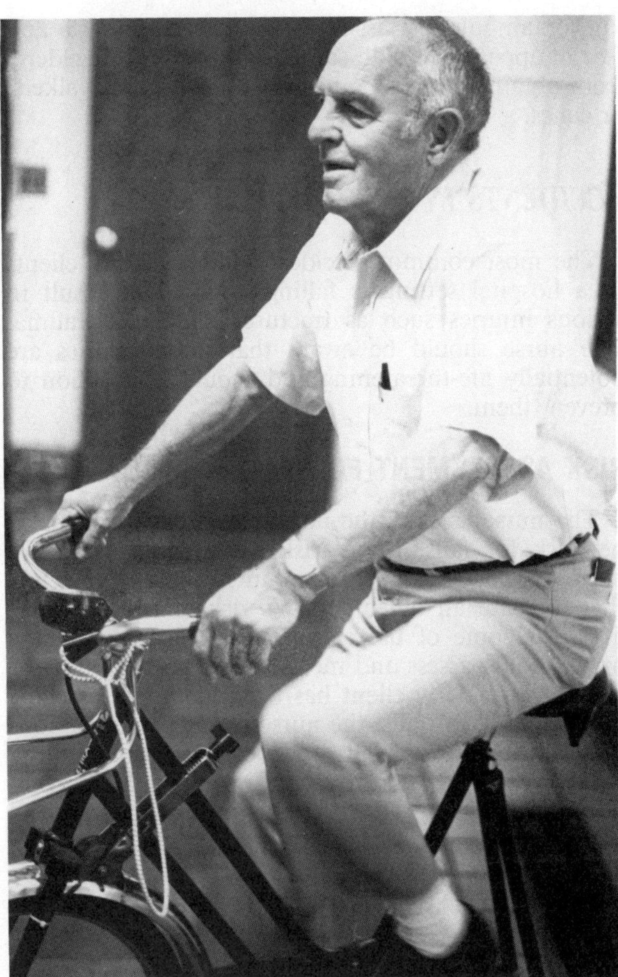

FIGURE 5–1 ◆ Exercise is important to the elderly for health promotion and maintenance. (Courtesy of St. Anselm College, Manchester, NH.)

Boschen, 1993). Swimming is also recommended but does not offer the weight-bearing advantage of walking. Elders who have been sedentary should start their exercise programs slowly and gradually increase the frequency and duration of activity over time (Walker, 1992).

If the older adult is hospitalized, the opportunity for continuing a program of physical fitness is interrupted, at least temporarily. During severe or prolonged illness, the older adult is at a high risk for complications of decreased physical mobility, such as pneumonia, skin impairment, contractures, muscle atrophy, constipation, and renal calculi. These problems are addressed elsewhere in this text.

STRESS MANAGEMENT

FACTORS CONTRIBUTING TO STRESS IN THE ELDERLY

According to many physiologic and psychologic theories of aging, stress and disease play significant roles. Stress can speed up the aging process over time, or it can lead to diseases that increase the rate of degeneration (see Chap. 7). Stress can impair the reserve capacity of the elderly and lessen their ability to respond and adapt to changes in their environment.

Although no period of the life cycle is free from stress, the later years can be a time of especially high risk. Frequently observed sources of stress for the older population include rapid environmental changes that require immediate reaction, changes in lifestyle resulting from retirement or physical incapacity, acute or chronic illness, loss of significant others, financial hardships, and relocation. How people react to these stresses depends on their personal coping skills and support networks. The loss of roles experienced by the elderly often limits the availability of external support networks. For instance, for a number of elderly, successive role losses have left them without friends to whom they can turn for support and help. As a result, many elderly have to rely solely on their personal resources to maintain their mental health. When poor physical health is combined with social problems, older people are susceptible to stress overload, which can result in illness and premature death.

COPING WITH STRESS

The ways in which people adapt to old age largely depend on the personality traits and coping strategies that have characterized them throughout their lives. Establishing and maintaining relationships with others throughout life are especially important to the elder's happiness. Even more important than having friends at all is the nature of the friendships. People who have close, intimate, stable relationships with others in whom they confide are more likely to maintain integrity in times of crises.

In a study to determine the relationship, if any, between self-disclosure and well-being, Nkongho (1990) found that elders who had children *and* friends had a higher well-being than those who had only children. The elders in this study were living independently in their communities. They talked with their children about financial concerns and environmental issues, such as home repairs. With friends, they discussed information about past work experiences, social relationships, and opinions on current issues and events.

ENVIRONMENTAL FACTORS

Most older adults live in and own their own homes. Physical incapacity or economic problems may force some to relocate (Matteson & McConnell, 1989). If an older person must move to a retirement center or a long-term care facility, family members and facility staff need to be aware that the older person needs personal space in the new surroundings. Older people need to participate in deciding how the space will be arranged and what they can keep in the new environment. Such participation helps to offset the feelings of powerlessness and depersonalization that often accompany relocation to an institutional setting. The nurse suggests that the client or family bring in personal items, such as pictures of relatives and friends, favorite clothing, and valued "knick-knacks," to assist in making the new setting seem more familiar and comfortable (Fig. 5–2). The same intervention can be carried out in a hospital setting.

Changes in vision, touch, and motor ability can create difficulties for the elderly in functioning in any environment. For example, decreased vision in old age, especially the poor perception of distance, may make walking more difficult; the person is less aware of where each step is. The reduced sense of touch gives the older person a decreased awareness of body orientation (e.g., whether the foot is squarely on the step). Decreased reaction time that commonly results from age-related changes in the neurologic system may also impair the older adult's ability to recognize or move from a dangerous setting or break a fall.

Accidents

ACCIDENTS IN THE COMMUNITY

The nurse teaches older adults about the need to be aware of safety precautions that should be taken to prevent accidents. The prevention of injury to muscles, bones, and other body parts that have grown fragile with age is not only critically important but also is probably the area in which aging people can do the most to preserve their fitness. Incapacitating accidents are a primary cause of restricted physical fitness and decreased mobility in old age.

Safeguards, such as installing and holding on to hand rails when using steps and getting into and out of the shower or bathtub, securing rugs with slip-proof underpads, and making sure treacherous places are well lighted, are essential. To minimize sensory overload in the elderly, the nurse advises the older person to concentrate on one activity at a time. If needed, the nurse encourages the use of visual, hearing, or ambulatory assistive devices. High costs and fear of appearing "old" sometimes prevent the elderly from obtaining or using hearing aids, glasses, walkers, or canes.

ACCIDENTS IN THE HOSPITAL

The most common accident among elderly clients in a hospital setting is falling. Many falls result in serious injuries such as fractures and head trauma. The nurse should be aware that these injuries are potentially life-threatening and should take action to prevent them.

RISK ASSESSMENT FOR FALLS

The nurse assesses the hospitalized client for his or her risk for falls. Many risk assessment tools have been developed to help the nurse focus on factors that increase an older person's risk of falling. Chart 5–3 lists some of the common risk factors that the nurse should assess and measure to help prevent falls.

Once an elderly client has been identified as being at a high risk for falls, the nurse chooses interventions that help to prevent falls and possible serious injury. One of the most controversial issues in fall prevention is the use of side rails at the bed and physical and chemical restraints.

NURSING INTERVENTIONS TO PREVENT FALLS

In some hospitals and long-term care settings, there are policies that side rails should be up for all clients older than age 65 years, especially at night. This policy does not allow for individual needs and differences. As a result of being in an unfamiliar environment and because of increased nocturia (urination at night), elderly clients commonly get out of bed at night to go to the bathroom. In the darkness and disorientation of a hospital, the client may forget to

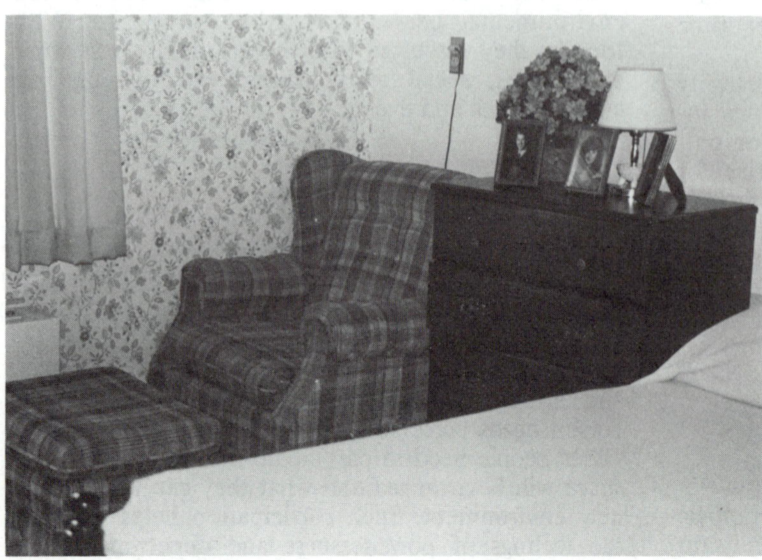

FIGURE 5–2 ◆ Example of the home-like environment of a contemporary nursing home.

CHART 5 – 3

Nursing Care Highlight ◆ Risk Factors and Measures for Preventing Falls in the Elderly

Assess for the presence of these risk factors:
- Advanced age (over 80)
- Multiple illnesses
- Generalized weakness
- Disorientation or confusion
- Use of drugs that can cause increased confusion, mobility limitations, or orthostatic hypotension
- Urinary incontinence
- Communication impairments
- Major visual impairments
- Client's room away from the nurses' station (in the hospital or nursing home)
- Change of shift or mealtime (in the hospital or nursing home)

Implement these nursing interventions:
- Monitor the client's activities and behavior as often as possible, preferably every 30 to 60 minutes.
- Remind the client to call for help before getting out of bed or a chair.
- Help the client to get out of bed or a chair.
- Provide, or remind the client to use, a walker or cane when ambulating.
- Remind the client to wear glasses or a hearing aid if needed.
- Toilet the incontinent client every 1 to 2 hours.
- Clean up spills immediately.
- Arrange the furniture in the client's room or hallway to eliminate clutter or obstacles that could contribute to a fall.
- Provide adequate lighting at all times, especially at night.
- Observe for side effects and toxic effects of drug therapy.

ask for assistance to the bathroom and subsequently fall. In some cases, the client may crawl over the bed rail, which can make the results of a fall more serious. Because of this, some hospitals are reconsidering their policies about side rails and allowing the nurse to use his or her judgment about their use.

Similar considerations are being given to the use of physical and chemical restraints. A restraint is any device or medication that prevents the client from moving freely. The federal government enforced a law in 1990 that gives residents in nursing homes the right to be restraint-free. Although most hospitals have not adopted this policy, most have policies that base the use of restraints on careful nursing assessment.

PHYSICAL RESTRAINTS

Most experts agree that elderly clients should not be placed in a Posey vest or sedated just because they are elderly. However, if other interventions, such as reminding the client to call for assistance when needed, are ineffective in fall prevention, the nurse may need to use a physical restraint for a specified period of time. The nurse checks the client in a restraint every 30 to 60 minutes and releases the restraint every 2 hours. Restraints like Posey vests have caused serious injury and even death.

CHEMICAL RESTRAINTS

Chemical restraints, or psychoactive drugs, are often overused in hospital settings. The client who is noisy, agitated, abusive, or combative often receives or has an "as needed" order for a psychoactive drug. Such medications include:

- Antipsychotic drugs, like haloperidol (Haldol, Peridol✱)
- Antianxiety drugs, like alprazolam (Xanax)
- Antidepressant drugs, like nortriptyline (Pamelor)
- Sedative-hypnotic drugs, like chloral hydrate (Noctec, Novochlorhydrate✱)

These drugs produce serious side and toxic effects and should therefore be reserved for clients who cannot be managed in any other way.

The most potent group of psychoactive drugs is the antipsychotics. These drugs may be appropriate for the control of certain behavioral symptoms, such as hallucinations, delusions, and violent episodes. However, only 40% of clients respond to these drugs, and 10% of the elderly who receive them experience increased behavioral problems (Feinberg, 1993).

If a psychoactive drug is used as a last resort, a low dose should be given. Chapter 41 discusses common psychoactive drugs and appropriate nursing interventions associated with their use.

Drug Use and Misuse

Drug therapy for the elderly population in general is another major health issue. Because of the multiple chronic and acute illnesses that occur in this age group, costs for elderly people account for 25% of all prescription drug costs. The average elderly person receives 13 medication prescriptions a year, and the elderly spend more than $3 billion a year on prescription and nonprescription drugs ("News," 1991).

Older adults frequently use nonprescription drugs, such as analgesics, antacids, cold and cough preparations, laxatives, and vitamins, often without consulting a physician. The occurrence of adverse drug reactions is directly related to the number and frequency of drug exposures. Elders are therefore at high risk for adverse drug reactions or interactions and are often admitted to the hospital for these problems.

PHYSIOLOGIC CHANGES AFFECTING DRUG USE

It has been recognized only recently that older adults may not tolerate the standard dosage of medications traditionally prescribed for younger adults.

The physiologic changes related to aging make drug therapy more complex and challenging. These changes affect the absorption, distribution, metabolism, and excretion of drugs from the body.

Age-related changes that can potentially affect drug absorption from an oral route include an increase in gastric pH, a decrease in gastric blood flow, and a decrease in gastrointestinal motility. Despite these changes, most elderly do not have difficulty with absorption because of age-related changes alone. Age-related changes that affect the distribution of a drug include smaller amounts of total body water, an increased ratio of adipose tissue to lean body mass, a decreased albumin level, and a decrease in cardiac output. Increased adipose tissue in proportion to lean body mass can cause increased storage of lipid-soluble drugs. This leads to a decreased concentration of the drug in plasma but an increased concentration in tissue.

Drug metabolism most often occurs in the liver. Age-related changes affecting metabolism include a decrease in liver size, a decrease in liver blood flow, and a decrease in liver enzyme activity. These changes can result in increased plasma concentrations of a drug. Changes in the kidneys can also result in high plasma concentrations of drugs. Excretion of drugs most often involves the renal system. Age-related changes of the renal system include a decrease in renal blood flow and reduced glomerular filtration rate. These changes result in a decreased creatinine clearance and thus a slower excretion time for medications (Matteson & McConnell, 1989) (see Chap. 71).

EFFECTS OF DRUGS IN THE ELDERLY

Because of age-related physiologic changes, older adults are at a high risk for side and toxic effects from drugs. In 1991, the Geriatric Drug Therapy Research Institute was established to study and make recommendations for drug therapy in the elderly. Currently, the Institute is developing tools that physicians and other health care professionals can use when caring for the older adult ("News," 1991).

When chronic disease is added to the physiologic changes of aging, drug reactions have a more dramatic effect and take a longer time to correct. This is because elders have less reserve capacity in most organ systems. Often a lower dose of medication is necessary to prevent adverse effects. The policy of "start low, go slow" is appropriate when physicians prescribe drugs for the elderly. However, the physiologic changes of aging are highly individual. Thus, alterations in drug therapy should always be individualized according to the actual physiologic changes present and the occurrence and severity of chronic disease.

Common adverse drug reactions in elders include edema, nausea, vomiting, anorexia, dry mouth, fatigue, weakness, dizziness, urinary retention, diarrhea, constipation, and confusion. Many of these signs and symptoms can be mistakenly attributed to a concurrent illness the client might be experiencing or may be assumed to be part of the aging process. The nurse assesses all elderly clients with such symptoms for possible adverse reactions to medications.

SELF-ADMINISTRATION OF MEDICATION

Most people older than 65 years of age live at home and are responsible for taking their own medications. Because the risk of drug toxicity is considerably increased in the elderly population, the nurse should assist elderly clients in assuming this task responsibly. The nurse helps prevent problems through educating clients, providing clear and concise directions, and developing ways to assist elders in overcoming self-administration handicaps or difficulties.

Older adults make errors in self-administration for several reasons. First, they may simply forget. In the rush of daily activities, they may not take the drug at all or may take it too often because of an inability to remember when or whether medications have been taken. It can be helpful if the client associates pill taking with daily events, such as meals, or keeps a simple chart or calendar. Pill boxes have been devised so that a daily, weekly, or monthly supply of medicine can be placed in appropriate compartments (Fig. 5–3). Large print on the drug label assists those clients who have poor visual acuity. Writing the drug regimen on the top of the bottle with large letters and numbers is also helpful.

A second reason that elderly people frequently commit errors in taking medications is poor communication with health care professionals. These difficulties stem from such sources as inadequate explanations to elderly clients or explanations they cannot understand because of educational limitations or language barriers. Health care professionals frequently presume that if they tell the elder about the drugs, the elder has acquired the knowledge. The nurse or other health care provider needs to help older adults plan their medication schedules.

A third reason for medication errors is one's attitude and long-ingrained feelings about taking medicine. Some people are chronic pill takers; they think no physician can help them unless he or she is the one who prescribed medication. These people often

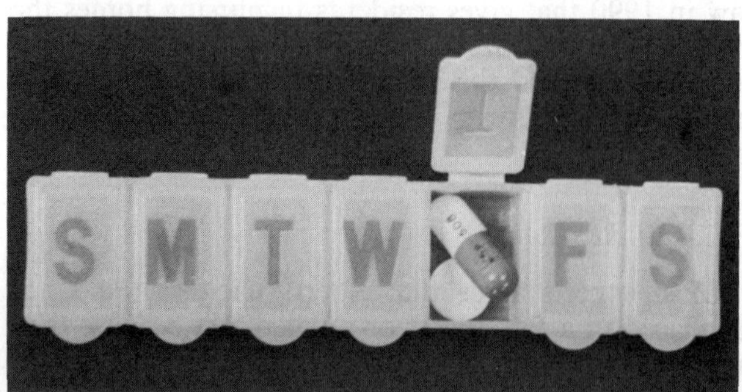

FIGURE 5–3 ◆ A medication system for safe self-administration.

add to their drug regimen by taking over-the-counter drugs that can interact with prescription drugs and cause serious problems. For example, a client receiving warfarin (Coumadin, Warfilone♣) for anticoagulation may take aspirin (Ancasal♣) regularly for arthritis. Aspirin is also an anticoagulant, which can cause overt or occult bleeding.

Conversely, other elderly people avoid taking medication whenever they can. The fear of drug dependency or the cost of the drugs may cause many to discontinue medications too soon. In addition, the action or side effects of some drugs may not be desirable. For example, diuretics may cause incontinence when the client cannot get to the bathroom quickly enough. Others think that two pills will be twice as effective as one; some elders take medication that is left over from a previous illness or a drug that has been prescribed for someone else.

Health care providers can influence the attitudes of elders toward their medication and their health problems. Laypersons of the same socioeconomic or cultural background as the elder can be effective instructors. A method that is being tried in some hospitals and nursing homes is supervised drug self-administration. Clients are allowed to take their own medications under supervision. In this way, the nurse can be sure of a client's understanding and ability to self-administer medications at home or in another health care setting.

Mental Health

A few changes in cognition have been identified as age-related. These changes are linked to specific functions of cognition, as opposed to intellectual capacity. They include a decreased reaction time to stimuli and an impairment of memory of recent events. It is certain, however, that gross cognitive impairment, depression, hallucinations, and delusions are not part of the normal aging process. Most elders are mentally sound.

Losses in income and physical health, the lack of comprehensive health care and social services, the loss of social roles, and the deaths of significant others may affect a person's emotional stability. It is not surprising that mental illness occurs among the aged population. The elder is often unaware of early symptoms of emotional or mental impairments. Symptoms may go unnoticed by family and friends and thus are allowed to progress until the elder is in crisis. The three most common cognitive problems among the elderly are depression, dementia, and delirium.

DEPRESSION

Depression, as a response to multiple life stresses, a single situation (situational depression), or a problem associated with dementia, is one of the major disturbances in cognitive functioning in elders. It is often underdiagnosed by physicians and therefore undertreated. Without treatment, depression can result in suicide.

Transcultural Considerations Caucasian males over 70 years old are at the highest risk for suicide during older adulthood (Antai-Otong, 1990). Older adults contemplating suicide usually do not talk about their plans and choose a method, such as a gun, that will ensure death.

Elderly people with the early clinical manifestations of depression may experience early morning insomnia, excessive daytime sleeping, poor appetite, a lack of energy, and an unwillingness to participate in social and recreational activities. The treatment for depression usually includes drug therapy and psychotherapy. More information on this disorder is available in mental health nursing textbooks.

DEMENTIA

Dementia is a broad term used for a syndrome that is also characterized by a disturbance in cognition occurring in elders. Formerly called organic brain syndrome (OBS) and chronic brain syndrome (CBS), dementia represents global impairment of intellectual function and is generally chronic and progressive. There are many types of dementia, the most common being Alzheimer's disease (senile dementia, Alzheimer type). Multi-infarct dementia, the second most common dementia, is a vascular disorder and accounts for 20% to 25% of all dementias (Cohen-Mansfield et al., 1990). Chapter 41 discusses dementias in detail, with a focus on Alzheimer's disease.

DELIRIUM

Whereas dementia is a chronic, progressive disorder, delirium is an acute state of confusion. Delirium is also different from dementia, in that it is usually short-term and reversible. Delirium is often seen in the hospital setting or in a setting that is unfamiliar to the client. The client may try to climb out of bed, pull out invasive lines (like oxygen or IV cannulas), or become quite agitated and combative.

The nurse should use a calm voice in reorienting the client and try to divert attention away from devices or tubes. A number of innovative nursing interventions have been used with some success. For example, playing tapes of soothing music in the client's room may have a calming effect. Giving the client a doll or stuffed animal to "fidget" with may prevent the client from removing important medical instrumentation. Some nurses believe that providing dolls and stuffed animals is treating the adult like a child, but when used for therapeutic purposes, this intervention can be very effective with some clients. If the client already has a favorite item, such as an afghan or picture, the nurse asks the client's family or significant others to provide it for the same purpose.

There are multiple causes for delirium, including:

- Medication
- Metabolic disturbances
- Infections
- Surgical operations
- Circulatory, renal, and pulmonary disorders
- Nutritional deficiencies

Table 5–1 differentiates delirium and dementia and the major nursing considerations for each. The most difficult challenge is caring for a client with both problems at the same time.

Elder Neglect and Abuse

Another problem that is sometimes encountered by the elderly is neglect and abuse—both verbal and physical. Some elders are very vulnerable to this problem, especially widowed women who may have difficulty being assertive. Studies have shown that older persons who are neglected or abused are often physically dependent. The abuser may be a family member who becomes frustrated or distraught over the burden of caring for the elder (Matteson & McConnell, 1989).

Role theorists propose that prolonged caregiving by a family member is a new, unexpected role for adult children, most often women (Beck & Ferguson, 1981). This new role may result in role fatigue and role conflict (Matteson & McConnell, 1989). Caregiver Role Strain and High Risk for Caregiver Role Strain are problems that have been added to the list of North American Nursing Diagnosis Association (NANDA) approved nursing diagnoses (NANDA, 1992). From their research, McCloskey and Bulechek (1992) identified Caregiver Support as a major nursing intervention (Chart 5–4).

The nurse carefully assesses the elderly client for signs of abuse. If the older adult is too weak or has no other resources or support system, the client may not acknowledge that the abuse is occurring. If physical abuse is suspected, the nurse notifies the physician and social worker to investigate the situation. Some states in the United States and some Western countries have laws requiring health care professionals to report suspected elder abuse.

CHART 5–4

Nursing Care Highlight ◆ Interventions for Family Caregiver Support

- Determine the caregiver's preparation and acceptance of his or her new role.
- Assess the caregiver's level of knowledge about the role and the client's health status.
- Teach stress management techniques to the caregiver (see Chap. 7).
- Monitor for signs of caregiver stress.
- Help the caregiver identify sources of respite care.
- Teach the caregiver health promotion practices for his or her own health.
- Help the caregiver identify caregiver support groups, and encourage participation in them.
- Teach the caregiver about the grieving process.
- Help the caregiver identify financial and other health care resources.
- Encourage the caregiver to share responsibilities with other members of the family or significant others.

ECONOMIC ISSUES

Income

Most adults hope that throughout their life cycle they can provide for their own needs. One of the greatest fears many adults have related to aging is becoming dependent on family, friends, or society. In many cases, older adults have not achieved economic self-sufficiency. One fifth of the total population of the United States is poor, and one fifth of the poor are older than 65 (Brock, 1992).

Most people expect financial resources in their retirement years to decline compared with those in their working years. However, they also expect that the level of their expenses will decline as well, and this may not occur. In the United States, for example, the inflation that began in the 1970s reduced the value of financial assets. The elderly were especially hard hit because most rely on Social Security benefits or pension funds for the bulk of their income. These

TABLE 5–1 Differences in the Characteristics of Delirium and Dementia

	Dementia	Delirium
Description	• A chronic, progressive cognitive decline	• An acute confusional state
Onset	• Slow	• Fast
Duration	• Continuous	• One month or less
Cause	• Unknown, possibly familial, chemical	• Multiple, such as surgery, infection, drugs
Reversibility	• None	• Usually
Treatment	• Treat signs and symptoms	• Remove or treat the cause
Nursing interventions	• Reorientation not effective in the late stages; use validation therapy (agree with the client and don't argue); provide a safe environment; observe for associated behaviors, such as delusions and hallucinations	• Reorient the client to reality; provide a safe environment

assets are usually fixed and cannot be altered by the person. Therefore, many elders are unable to adjust their income to changing economic circumstances and hence are powerless to combat declining real income. Health care purchases are paid for in substantial part by private insurance and federal health and social programs. Yet the rising cost of these programs contributes substantially to rising government costs and may result in more out-of-pocket costs for the aged health care consumer.

Housing

The popular belief that the elderly are frail, dependent, senile people living out their last years in an institution has no factual basis. Only about 5% of the aged population reside in institutions providing long-term care (Brody et al., 1990). Many elders live in their own homes and have paid off their mortgages. Yet, living arrangements are a major problem for some people as they age. The nurse needs to be aware of this issue because it can increase the client's stress level and have an impact on health care planning.

Rising energy and housing costs in many countries have joined the high costs of food and health care as factors that contribute to the economic hardship of aging people. In addition to financial difficulties, housing for the aged may be a problem because environmental supports that would help them to remain residing and participating in the community are lacking.

Deterioration of property, escalation of property taxes, and maintenance service costs create many problems for elder homeowners in keeping their homes. In some areas, elderly renters are extremely vulnerable to high rent fees, real estate speculation, and loss of living quarters because of removal of substandard, low-rent apartment or hotel buildings. Physical impairments and a lack of available, affordable support services, such as household help, transportation, home health care, and assistance with meals, prevent some aged people from being able to manage adequately in their own homes.

The need for special housing for the aged has long been recognized. Numbers of government and privately funded experiments in alternative housing for the aged have been tested. These projects incorporate such variables as personal care services, special health and safety remedies, and recreation and leisure plans. Although most of these projects provide security, improve life satisfaction, and prove cost-effective, in many countries there is no overall plan for alternative living arrangements for the elderly.

RESOURCES FOR THE ELDERLY

In the United States, Canada, and other countries, a broad range of government benefits and services is available to assist older people with problems related to income, health insurance, housing, and social services. The nurse informs older adults and their families about the types of services available to help them achieve a higher quality of life.

Government Resources

INCOME

In the United States, the major portion of federal funds supporting programs for the elderly is devoted to the Social Security programs. The Social Security Act was passed in 1935, after the Depression, when many elderly were economically impoverished. Since that time, there has been a gradual shift from a program that was intended to provide a minimal supplement to retirees' sources of income to one that is the primary source of retirement income for many people. Other provisions of this act that are significant for people younger than 65 years are the disability and survivors' insurance provisions.

HEALTH INSURANCE

Medicare was enacted as part of the amendments to the Social Security Act of 1965. This program was created to help older people meet the cost of health care. Despite its deficiencies, Medicare has provided a means for elders to obtain needed health care in times of escalating costs without decimating their total personal savings.

Medicare provides health insurance to people 65 years of age and older and qualified disabled people. Medicare A primarily pays for most of the in-hospital care and is paid for by the federal government. It pays for a very small portion of care required in long-term care and pays for minimal home health services. Medicare B is an optional insurance and requires payment of a monthly premium. Medicare B pays most of the outpatient costs associated with physicians' visits, medication, and home health services.

Medicaid is a program designed to provide payment for medical services for the poor, including the poor elderly. For eligible people who are age 65 or older, it supplements the Medicare insurance program. Eligibility is related to determination of poverty level, and each state program determines its own criteria for eligibility.

HOUSING PROGRAMS

In the United States, Congress has passed a number of legislative acts designed to alleviate housing problems for older citizens. Among these programs is rental assistance of lower-income families, the elderly, and the disabled. Direct loans at low interest are available to individuals to construct special rental housing facilities for the handicapped and the elderly. The federal government supports construction and rehabilitation of nursing homes. It subsidizes rental facilities, which can be rented by the aged at rates below the existing market price. For information related to these housing programs, nurses can contact the local public housing authority or the Housing and Urban Development Area Office in most communities.

SOCIAL SERVICES

The Older Americans Act of 1965 provided social services to the aged. Under this legislation, each state created an office to provide leadership in the coordination and development of services for the elderly. Some of the more significant programs and services carried out under this legislation are described in Chart 5–5.

RESEARCH AGENCIES

The National Institute on Aging was established in 1974. Its purpose is to conduct research on the biologic, population-related, and sociologic aspects of aging at its Gerontology Research Center in Baltimore. It also supports research by others at universities and laboratories across the United States.

Within the National Institute for Mental Health, one division is devoted exclusively to problems of the aged: the Center for Studies of the Mental Health of the Aging. Its major role is to stimulate, coordinate, and support research training and to offer technical assistance relating to aging and mental health. Although it provides no monies for programs of service delivery to older people, it significantly affects the training of those working with elderly clients in community mental health centers and other service settings.

CHART 5–5

Nursing Focus on the Elderly ◆ Social Services Provided by the Older Americans Act of 1965

- *Senior centers* to meet the need for a central place for older people to congregate, develop new interests, and socialize.
- *Nutrition programs* to provide nutritious meals in a centralized setting as well as to the homebound elderly. Recreation, education, and health activities are incorporated in many sites as a regular part of the program.
- *Transportation services* to accommodate the elderly via special fares on existing public transportation systems and the operation of specially equipped vehicles for the frail and the handicapped elderly.
- *Information and referral services* to direct the elderly to the appropriate agency that provides needed services.
- *In-home services,* such as household help, telephone reassurance, chore maintenance, and visitation by home health aides, to enable the impaired elderly to remain living in the community.

Community Resources

Over the years, it has become evident that government programs cannot provide all services needed by the aged. In many areas, private efforts can supply the same services at lower costs and without the "red tape" that some government programs involve. Transportation is an area in which the private sector, state and local governments, and the federal government all have roles.

In many urban areas, governments have provided Dial-A-Ride or similar services, which provide free transportation. The federal government has subsidized the development and operation of transit systems, but its aid has been focused mainly on high-use systems and routes. For occasional travel, particularly in rural areas, the best solution may be for the elder to rely on a friend or a neighbor. Churches and community groups often help organize this approach by using sign-up sheets and recruiting volunteers to drive 1 day a week.

Education, recreation, and cultural activities help maintain a person's physical condition, mental alertness, and social contact. Education helps older people keep up with a rapidly changing world. Although advances in cable and satellite television systems provide a broad range of new educational experiences at home, the value of person-to-person discussion and the need to focus some educational activities on local issues means that community discussion groups and other informal education will remain important.

Recreation and cultural activities are best managed on a local, nongovernment basis because personal preference plays such a large role in determining individual participation. A variety of activities run by different organizations or informal groups is more likely to please more people than a large program run by a government agency. For example, in the Midwest, elders have formed square dance groups and gourmet groups, which meet frequently for socialization and compete with similar local, regional, and state groups.

Churches and other religious institutions serve the elderly in many ways. In addition to their primary role of providing organized worship, they sponsor many activities that bring the elderly together with their peers as well as with younger people. Clergypersons and other spiritual leaders are often excellent counselors, and other members of the congregation or religious group are sometimes willing to help older members in time of trouble.

Many communities have access to community resource books (e.g., those published by the United Way). Area agencies on aging are excellent referral centers. Some of these agencies publish directories of services that are specifically geared to the elderly. The nurse can help to inform elderly clients about community resources that they may need, depending on their specific life situation.

THE FUTURE OF GERONTOLOGICAL NURSING

Nurses in most adult health care settings encounter the challenges of caring for both well and ill older adults. In view of the rapidly increasing elderly population, especially the over-85 group, nurses in many settings are specializing in gerontological nursing. Nurses can practice gerontological nursing in acute care, long-term care, and community health settings. Just as nurses can achieve certification in medical-surgical nursing, they can become certified in gerontological nursing. The American Nurses' Association (ANA) provides three examinations for certification: gerontological nurse, gerontological clinical specialist, and gerontological nurse practitioner.

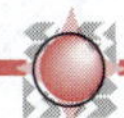

IMPLICATIONS FOR NURSING RESEARCH

As life expectancy continues to increase, nurses will continue to care for large numbers of elderly clients. Gerontology seems destined to be even more important in tomorrow's health care practice. Thus, the physical and psychosocial development of the older adult is an important area of concern for the nurse. Nurses will need to determine specific nursing interventions that address the special needs of the elderly.

Some major research questions that have significance for health care in the older adult years and are of importance to nursing are as follows:

- What factors influence health in old age? Why are some older adults more vulnerable to illness than others?
- What impact do changes of living and household arrangements have on the physical and psychosocial health of the elderly?
- What are the best ways to prevent falls in the elderly?
- What is the most cost-effective way to provide health care to the elderly?
- What treatments or interventions are available as a substitute for drug therapy in the elderly?
- What impact do changes in socioeconomic and marital status have on functional health status in the elderly?
- How can nurses best support family caregivers in the home environment?

SELECTED BIBLIOGRAPHY

Antai-Otong, D. (1990). Suicide risk? *Geriatric Nursing, 11,* 228–230.

*Beck, C. M., & Ferguson, D. (1981). Aged abuse. *Journal of Gerontological Nursing, 7,* 333–336.

*Borup, J. H. (1983). Relocation mortality research: Assessment, reply, and the need to refocus on the issues. *Gerontologist, 23,* 234–242.

Brock, A. M. (1992). Economics and the aged. In E. Baines (Ed.). *Perspectives on gerontology nursing.* Boston: Sage.

Brody, E. M., Dempsey, N. P., & Pruchna, R. A. (1990). Mental health of the institutionalized aged. *The Gerontologist, 30,* 212–219.

Burgener, S., & Barton, D. (1991). Nursing care of cognitively impaired, institutionalized elderly. *Journal of Gerontological Nursing, 17*(4), 37–43.

Burke, M. M., & Walsh, M. B. (1992). *Gerontologic nursing: Care of the frail elderly.* St. Louis: C. V. Mosby.

*Coffman, T. L. (1981). Relocation and survival of institutionalized aged: A re-examination of the evidence. *Gerontologist, 21,* 483–500.

Cohen-Mansfield, J., Marx, M. S., & Rosenthal, A. S. (1990). Dementia and agitation in nursing home residents. *Psychology and Aging, 5,* 3–8.

Ebersole, P., & Hess, P. (1990). *Toward healthy aging: Human needs and nursing response* (3rd ed.). St. Louis: C. V. Mosby.

*Ebert, N. J. (1989). The nursing process applied to the aged person receiving medication. In A. G. Yurick, B. E. Spier, S. S. Robb, N. J. Ebert, & M. H. Magnussen (Eds.), *The aged person and the nursing process* (pp. 709–730). Norwalk, CT: Appleton & Lange.

Feinberg, M. (1993). *Medication use in Alzheimer's disease.* Baltimore: University of Maryland School of Pharmacy.

Ferraro, K. F. (1990). Group benefit, orientation toward older adults at work. *Journal of Gerontology: Social Sciences, 45,* S220–S227.

*Gershon, S., & Herman, S. P. (1982). The differential diagnosis of dementia. *Journal of the American Geriatrics Society, 30,* S58–S65.

*Gress, L., & Bahr, R. (1984). *The aging person: A holistic perspective.* St. Louis: C. V. Mosby.

*Horowitz, M. J., & Schulz, R. (1983). The relocation controversy: Criticism and commentary on five recent studies. *Gerontologist, 23,* 229–233.

Jantz, M. (1990). Clues to elder abuse. *Geriatric Nursing, 11,* 220–222.

Johnson, J. E. (1991). Health-care practices of the rural aged. *Journal of Gerontological Nursing, 17*(8), 15–19.

Karper, W. B., & Boschen, M. B. (1993). Effects of exercise on acute respiratory tract infections and related symptoms. *Geriatric Nursing, 14*(1), 15–18.

Kilpack, V., Boehm, J., Smith, N., & Mudge, B. (1991). Using research-based interventions to decrease patient falls. *Applied Nursing Research, 4,* 50–56.

Lynch-Sauer, J. (1990). When a family member has Alzheimer's disease: A phenomenological description of caregiving. *Journal of Gerontological Nursing, 16*(9), 8–11.

*Matteson, M. A., & McConnell, E. S. (1989). *Gerontological nursing: Concepts and practice.* Philadelphia: W. B. Saunders.

McCloskey, J. C., & Bulechek, G. M. (1992). *Nursing interventions classification (NIC).* St. Louis: Mosby-Year Book.

Miller, C. (1990). When medication harms as well as helps. *Geriatric Nursing, 11,* 301–302.

"News" (1991). *Journal of Gerontological Nursing, 17*(1), 41–42.

Nkongho, N. O. (1990). Talk isn't cheap. *Geriatric Nursing, 11,* 282–284.

North American Nursing Diagnosis Association (1992). *Definitions and classification 1992.* St. Louis: Author.

*Patnaik, B., Lawton, M. P., Kleban, M. H., et al. (1974). Behavioral adaptation to the change in institutional residence. *Gerontologist, 14,* 305–307.

*Sheehy, G. (1976). *Passages: Predictable crises of adult life.* New York: Bantam Books.

Smith, M. A., Plawecki, H. M., Houser, B., et al. (1991). Age and health perceptions among elderly blacks. *Journal of Gerontological Nursing, 17*(11), 13–19.

Snyder, M., Brugge-Wiger, P., Ahern, S., Connelly, S., DePew, C., Kappas-Larson, P., Semmerling, E., & Wyble, S. (1991). Complex health problems: Clinically assessing self-management abilities. *Journal of Gerontological Nursing, 17*(4), 23–27.

Suprock, L. A. (1990). Changing the rules. *Geriatric Nursing, 11,* 288–289.

*U. S. Department of Health and Human Services (1989). *Aging in the eighties: The prevalence of comorbidity and its association with disability.* DHHS, PHS 89-1250. Washington, D. C.: U.S. Government Printing Office.

Walker, S. N. (1992). Wellness for elders. *Holistic Nurse Practice, 7*(1), 39–45.

Yazdanfar, D. J. (1990). Assessing the mental status of the cognitively impaired elderly. *Journal of Gerontological Nursing, 16*(9), 32–36.

*Yurick, A. G., Spier, B. S., Robb, S. S., & Ebert, N. J. (Eds.). (1989). *The aged person and the nursing process* (3rd ed.). Norwalk, CT: Appleton & Lange.

SUGGESTED READINGS

Johnson, J. E. (1991). Health-care practices of the rural aged. *Journal of Gerontological Nursing, 17*(8), 15–19.

This article explores the differences between urban and rural elderly regarding health promotion activities. The findings of this nursing study show that the rural aged are less likely than the urban elderly to practice positive health strategies, such as avoiding alcohol and smoking.

Kilpack, V., Boehm, J., Smith, N., & Mudge, B. (1991). Using research-based interventions to decrease patient falls. *Applied Nursing Research, 4,* 50–56.

This study had been designed to decrease client falls by applying research-based nursing interventions in two hospital units in Dartmouth-Hitchcock Medical Center, a 411-bed tertiary care teaching hospital in the rural Northeastern United States. The fall rate in these two units decreased during the study, but the overall hospital client fall rate increased.

Smith, M. A., Plawecki, H. M., Houser, B., et al. (1991). Age and health perceptions among elderly blacks. *Journal of Gerontological Nursing, 17*(11), 13–19.

The researchers for this study interviewed 20 elderly African-American men and women to determine the relationship between perceived age and health. All subjects were living independently and had access to a number of social support systems. Twelve subjects who felt younger than their chronological age rated themselves as being healthy.

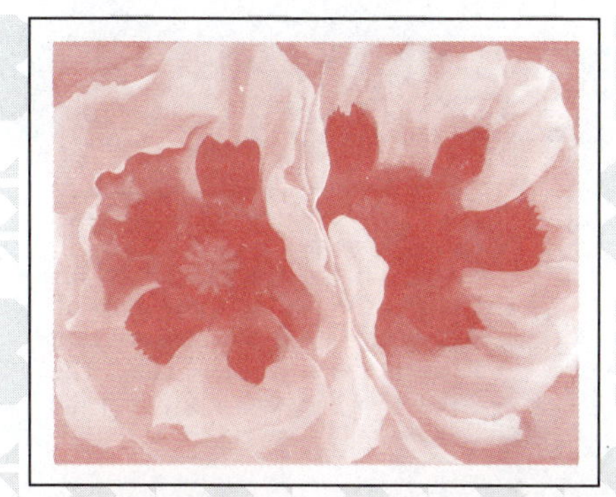

UNIT

Biopsychosocial Concepts Related to Health Care

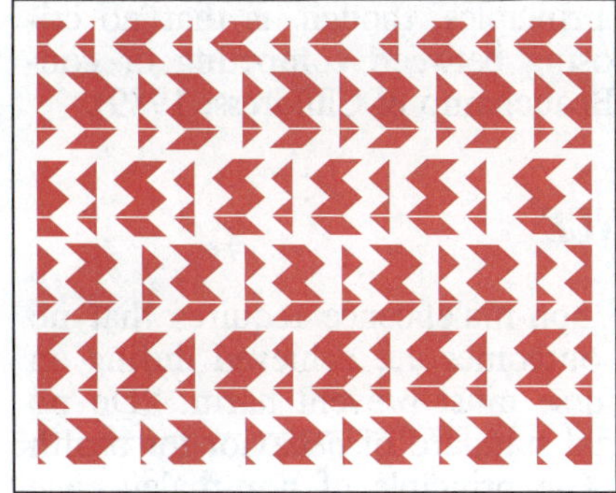

CHAPTER 6

Ethics

CHAPTER HIGHLIGHTS

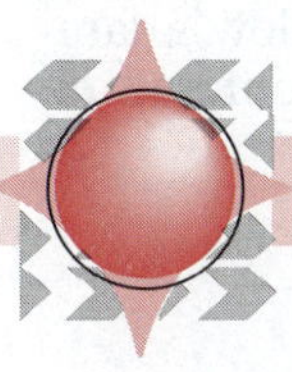

Medical-surgical nurses daily experience a variety of ethical issues. These ethical issues can vary in intensity from seemingly minor issues, such as should a nurse tell a client a "white lie," to extremely emotional issues about euthanasia or how to allocate scarce health care resources. Frequently, nurses realize that they are in the midst of an ethical dilemma when two or more equally unfavorable options exist (Curtin & Flaherty, 1982). At other times, however, the nurse may not recognize that an ethical issue has occurred until after the situation is over.

WHAT IS ETHICS?

Definition

Ethics is the study of what is right or what people ought to do in a specific situation. The nurse decides "what is right" by consulting a variety of resources, including:

- Ethical theories and principles
- Legal statutes
- Decision-making models
- The values of the persons involved
- Professional codes
- Policies
- Nursing and ethics consultants

Thus, a nurse cannot learn the one correct answer for resolving any specific ethical issue because each clinical ethical issue is unique.

Ethical Theories

Ethical theories are a way of approaching ethical problems and determining what is the right action to implement. The two most common ethical theories used for ethical reflections are utilitarianism and deontology.

UTILITARIANISM

The guiding rule in utilitarianism is the Greatest Happiness Principle, which states that "actions are right in proportion that they tend to promote happiness, wrong as they tend to produce the reverse of happiness" (Beauchamp & Walters, 1982, p. 13). The consequences of the possible options are evaluated regarding their ability to promote group happiness or good rather than individual happiness. Utilitarians believe that rules such as "never lie" can be broken if the consequence of lying will bring about the most happiness. For example, if an unstable myocardial infarction client voices concern that his spouse has not visited, a utilitarian would justify not telling the client his spouse had been killed in an automobile accident if telling would cause a setback in recovery (Beauchamp & Childress, 1989; Beauchamp & Walters, 1982; Curtin & Flaherty, 1982; DeWolf, 1989b).

DEONTOLOGY

In contrast, deontologists believe that actions are right or wrong despite their consequences and that a person's intentions to do good should be praised. Deontology emphasizes the importance of the individual person, not the group. Rules are rarely broken. In addition, a deontologist would agree that answers for an ethical issue can be identified and generalized to similar ethical issues (Beauchamp & Childress, 1989; Beauchamp & Walters, 1982; Curtin & Flaherty, 1982; DeWolf, 1989b). As in the example above, a deontologist would tell the unstable myocardial infarction client that his spouse had been killed because truth-telling is always the right action. However, rarely are people purely utilitarian or purely deontological in their approach to ethical decision-making. Generally, ethical decisions reflect a combination of theoretical approaches and ethical principles.

Ethical Principles

Ethical principles can also help the nurse determine what a correct action is for resolving an ethical issue. Four major ethical principles are non-maleficence, beneficence, justice, and autonomy. One difficulty with using ethical principles, though, is that no criteria exist for choosing between competing or conflicting principles (Beauchamp & Childress, 1989).

NON-MALEFICENCE

The principle of non-maleficence requires that no matter what other outcomes are achieved during an ethical issue, the nurse must prevent harm. "Do no harm" is the minimal standard of behavior for health care professionals. The principle of non-maleficence is supported when a nurse follows the "five rights" of medication administration or turns, coughs, and deep breathes a postoperative client.

BENEFICENCE

Beneficence builds on the principle of non-maleficence. Besides doing no harm, the nurse must benefit the client by promoting good. Thus, the principle of beneficence requires the nurse to perform an action. For example, a nurse is acting beneficently when visitation rules in a hospital are relaxed to allow a family member to spend the night with a confused elderly client.

JUSTICE

The principle of justice is concerned with how resources are divided between individual people and/or groups in the society. Typically, justice is concerned only with resources that are in short supply, such as financing or specialized health care services, like organs for transplantation. However, little agreement exists whether resources should be allocated by a person's effort, need, merit, or social contribution or by free market exchange. Nurses make decisions based on justice when they decide how to allocate their time between clients.

AUTONOMY

The principle of autonomy requires that a person be involved in decisions that affect his or her life. Making a decision for a person when he or she could have made the decision is paternalistic and negates the person's autonomy. A nurse promotes client autonomy by advising the client of options in care, ensuring that the client has adequate information to make a decision, and supporting the client's decision.

Ethical Versus Legal Actions

Actions determined to be ethical for a given situation may not be considered legal actions. For example, it may be ethically justifiable to facilitate a client's death based on the principle of beneficence and utilitarian theory. However, assisted suicide is not a legal option in most countries. Typically, legal statutes reflect the ethical mindset held by society 10 to 15 years ago. Thus, new technology can create conflicts between current ethical reasoning and the law.

Because of conflicts between ethical and legal opinions, people may bring suit in the hopes of overturning current law and establishing a new legal precedent. For example, *Cruzan v. Director, Missouri Department of Health,* (1990) addressed the right of a family to have a client's treatment removed, in this case gastrostomy tube feedings. The Helga Wanglie case challenged the physician's ability to remove a ventilator without family consent (Cranford, 1991).

Theorists Who Have Addressed Moral Reasoning

KOHLBERG

Lawrence Kohlberg, a psychologist, built upon the work of Jean Piaget in describing how children develop. Kohlberg focused on moral development and identified six stages in three categories (Table 6–1). The three categories—preconventional, conventional, and post-conventional—reflect the child's maturing abilities to think from the concrete to the abstract. Each category has two stages, again reflecting the child's cognitive ability and social influences at that point in the child's life. Kohlberg believed that people could move into the higher stages, which prescribe ideal behavior based on adherence to principles, not self-gratification or avoidance of punishment. Kohlberg's perspective has been called the justice perspective (Thompson & Thompson, 1985).

GILLIGAN

Carol Gilligan, one of Kohlberg's students, conducted a study on women's decision whether or not to have an abortion (Gilligan, 1982). Her findings challenged Kohlberg's interpretation of moral development. Kohlberg, like Piaget, studied boys and generalized the findings to both sexes. When Kohlberg's findings were generalized to girls, he concluded that girls (and women) had arrested moral development at the conventional level. Gilligan described feminine moral development as a departure from the masculine hierarchical path. Feminine moral development is a web of contexts, relationships, responsibilities, caring, self-sacrifice, and nonviolence.

Gilligan argued that women's moral development is different from that of men. In moral reasoning, Kohlberg's principle-oriented approach excluded consideration of the situation, relationships, and burden. The applicable principles are identified, the overriding principle is determined, and the decision is made with the actions reflecting the overriding principle. However, Gilligan's ethic of care involves consideration of the context of the ethical problem, the concern of prevention of harm or relief of burden, the nature of the relationships, and the responsibilities of all parties. Both Kohlberg's ethic of justice and Gilligan's ethic of care are complex moral reasoning processes. What is important for nurses to recognize is the growing body of research in the nursing literature on feminism in ethics, of which the original work is Gilligan's *In A Different Voice* (1982). However, one cannot assume moral reasoning perspective falls along gender lines. Both perspectives have their merit, and it behooves nurses to be familiar with both.

TABLE 6–1 Kohlberg's Stages of Moral Development

Level I Preconventional Moral Reasoning
- Stage 1: Obey rules to avoid negative consequences
- Stage 2: Personal needs satisfaction is greater than justice

Level II Conventional Moral Reasoning
- Stage 3: Maintain positive, interpersonal relationships
- Stage 4: Maintain law and order

Level III Principled or Postconventional Moral Reasoning
- Stage 5a: Social contract orientation
- Stage 5b: Individualistic orientation
- Stage 6: Individual conscience

Values

A value is a way of looking at life that ultimately directs the person's behavior and gives life meaning. Values are beliefs that have been freely chosen, communicated to others, and acted on repeatedly throughout life. The development of values is influenced by one's family, religion, culture, interpersonal relationships and activities. Despite being of long standing, values do change and are never stagnant (Fromer, 1983; Steele & Harmon, 1983). Examples of personal values include a comfortable life, world peace, happiness, salvation, and love (Rokeach, 1973).

A nurse's personal values serve as the foundation for the development of professional values. Thus, nurses sometimes have difficulty in balancing their personal and professional values. Examples of professional values include promoting health, being truthful with clients, client advocacy, and a nonjudgmental attitude (Fowler & Levine-Ariff, 1987).

Values serve as rationale for determining whether an action is right or wrong. The nurse may experience an ethical quandary when personal and professional values conflict (Fromer, 1987; Steele & Harmon, 1983). For example, when a client requires a valve replacement because of endocarditis caused by intravenous drug abuse, the nurse may experience conflict between professionally believing everyone deserves high-quality health care while personally believing that a person who uses illegal intravenous drugs does not deserve aggressive treatment.

Values clarification is a process of analyzing the actions and exploring the associated feelings and beliefs (Table 6–2). The process serves to identify the conscious and unconscious values that guide behavior. When clarifying values, people ask themselves, "What is important to me?" or "What are my beliefs?" People who have engaged in values clarification are more likely to be insightful, self-confident, and empathetic. Values clarification can facilitate the nurse's understanding of competing values displayed by other health care professionals and clients (Steele & Harmon, 1983).

TABLE 6–2 An Exercise for Clarifying Personal and Professional Values

- Step 1. Choosing freely
  a. Am I sure I've thought about this value and have chosen to believe it for myself?
  b. Who first taught me this value?
  c. How do I know I'm "right"?
- Step 2. Choosing from among alternatives
  a. What other alternatives are possible?
  b. Which alternative has the most appeal for me and why?
  c. Have I thought much about this value/alternative?
- Step 3. Choosing after considering the consequences
  a. What consequences do I think might occur as a result of my holding this value?
  b. What price will I pay for my position?
  c. Is this value worth the price I might pay?
- Step 4. Complement to other values
  a. Does this value "fit" with other values, and is it consistent with them?
  b. Am I sure this value doesn't conflict with other values I deem important?
- Step 5. Prize and cherish
  a. Am I proud of my position and value? Is this something I feel good about?
  b. How important is this value to me?
  c. If this were not my value, how different would my life be?
- Step 6. Public affirmation
  a. Am I willing to speak out for this value?
- Steps 7 and 8. Action
  a. Am I willing to put this value into action?
  b. Do I act on this value? When? How consistently?
  c. Is this a value that can guide me in other situations?
  d. Would I want others who are important to me to follow this value?
  e. Do I think I'll always believe this? How committed to this value am I?
  f. Am I willing to do anything about this value?
  g. How do I know this value is "right"? How do I know? Are my values ethical?

Reprinted with permission from Fowler, M.D.M., & Levine-Ariff, J. (1987). *Ethics at the bedside: A source for the critical care nurse.* Philadelphia: J.B. Lippincott (pp. 160–161).

ETHICAL DECISION-MAKING

Variables Influencing Ethical Decision-Making

Many variables can influence a nurse's ethical decision-making in the medical-surgical setting. The nurse's ethical decision-making can become more complex, depending on the variety and number of variables involved. These variables can be described as nurse, task, or environmental (Newell & Simon, 1972; Simon, 1978).

NURSE VARIABLES

Variables that can influence ethical decision-making processes include those inherent within the nurse, such as values and beliefs, gender, age and maturity, assumptions, and self-image. A nurse's knowledge, education, moral reasoning, and communication skills and previous experiences can also influence how the nurse perceives an ethical issue (DeWolf, 1989a).

TASK VARIABLES

Task variables influence the process used to resolve ethical issues. Ethical decision-making is influenced by the amount of time available to make a decision. The complexity of the decision to be made also influences the decision-making task. Often nurses attempt to use a "rule of thumb," such as "Never give pain medication early," to simplify the decision task. Another variable influencing a decision task is the perceived costs and benefits associated with a possible option (DeWolf, 1989a).

ENVIRONMENTAL VARIABLES

Environmental variables can be classified as either institutional (health care agency) characteristics or community variables.

INSTITUTIONAL CHARACTERISTICS Institutional characteristics identified by nurses during Crisham's (1981) study include:

- Hospital policies
- Time limitations created by work shifts
- Conflicting loyalties between client, profession, and institution
- Difficulties applying knowledge in the clinical setting
- Diversity of expectations of clients, supervisors, and other health care professionals
- Limited awareness by nurses regarding their responsibilities and authority during clinical ethical decision-making

Other institutional characteristics that influence ethical decision-making are philosophy, tolerance for ethical questions, staffing patterns, client acuity, available technology or equipment, economic stability of the institution, the nurse's job description and associated responsibilities, overall quality of working relationships between nurses and other health care professionals, and accessibility of ethics resources (DeWolf, 1989a).

COMMUNITY VARIABLES The ethical decision-making environment is also influenced by changing community variables. For example, the lay public is becoming more informed about health care issues, and community groups are involved in health care reform. Health care decisions are influenced by laws, public beliefs about how resources should be allocated, and current events in the media. Because communities are generally heterogeneous, each community reflects a specific mix of ethnic, religious, and cultural perspectives. Thus, these factors may influence how an ethical issue is resolved.

Normative Ethical Decision-Making Models

A variety of ethical decision-making models have been created to assist the nurse with clinical ethical decision-making. In each model, a specific concept is emphasized, such as rights (Curtin & Flaherty, 1982), biblical principles (Shelly, 1980), or the application of bioethical standards (Husted & Husted, 1991). Each model requires the decision-maker to:

- Identify the ethical problem
- Identify and consider alternatives
- Implement a choice
- Evaluate the decision-making process and its outcome.

Thus, normative decision-making models parallel the nursing process even though some models may require extra steps, such as values clarification or application of ethical principles. Frequently, nurses do not perceive these normative decision-making models as helpful. Nurses have difficulty considering a variety of options and their associated consequences during urgent, time-limited situations. Therefore, these normative models are more useful for retrospective or hypothetical case analysis. The more often nurses use a normative model for retrospective or hypothetical case review, the more familiar they become with the decision-making process. Then in time-limited situations, they can quickly analyze the ethical issues and use the model to guide their ethical decision-making.

Descriptive Ethical Decision-Making Models

The process nurses use to resolve clinical ethical situations in an acute medical-surgical setting has been investigated and is described in the Descriptive Ethical Decision-Making Model (Fig. 6–1). From this model, several difficulties with the nurses' ethical decision-making process have been identified. First, the nurses did not perceive that an ethical situation was occurring until after they:

- Experienced an emotional reaction
- Perceived a limited amount of time available to make a decision
- Considered what they would want done if they were the client
- Experienced a communication failure
- Did not know what was the right thing to do to resolve the ethical situation (DeWolf, 1989a)

Second, the nurses did not identify possible options; instead, they considered options identified by others. The nurses evaluated all possible options on a comfortable-uncomfortable continuum. Comfort was defined as

- The nurse's personal psychologic comfort
- The amount of physical comfort the client would experience as a result of implementing the option

If the nurse was forced to choose between the client's physical comfort and the nurse's psychologic comfort, the nurses always favored their psychologic comfort over the client's physical comfort (DeWolf, 1989a).

Third, nurses often had difficulty putting the ethical issue behind them. Some nurses described their need to keep discussing the ethical issue and how they continued to experience the same emotional reactions years after the issue occurred. Thus, for some nurses, the ethical issue was never resolved (Bosek, 1993a).

ETHICAL RESOURCES

Various ethical resources exist that may facilitate a nurse's ethical decision-making in a medical-surgical setting. These resources may vary among health care agencies. Nurses need to learn what resources are available in their practice setting. These resources may include professional codes, policies and procedures, nursing administrators, and institutional ethics committees or consultants.

Ethical Codes for Nurses

In Canada and the United States, major nursing associations have developed and approved codes of ethics. The Code for Nurses, developed by the American Nurses' Association, is shown in Table 6–3. One of the requirements for a profession is the existence and adherence to an ethical code to regulate professional conduct. Each Code signifies the profession's acknowledgment of the responsibility and faith entrusted by society to the nursing profession. Nurses are expected to follow the Code in their daily practice.

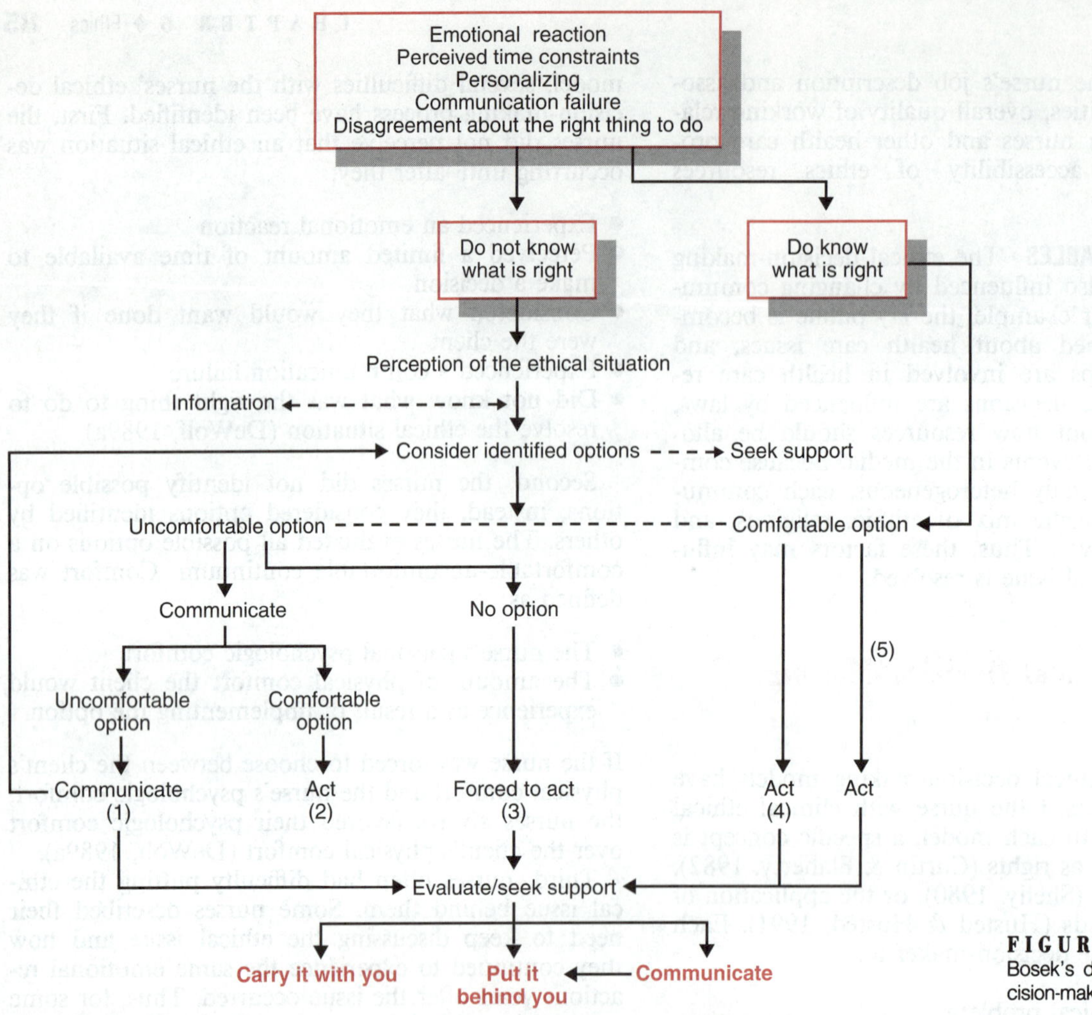

FIGURE 6–1 ♦ Bosek's descriptive ethical decision-making model.

TABLE 6–3 The ANA Code for Nurses

1. The nurse provides services with respect for human dignity and the uniqueness of the client, unrestricted by considerations of social or economic status, personal attributes, or the nature of health problems.
2. The nurse safeguards the client's right to privacy by judiciously protecting information of a confidential nature.
3. The nurse acts to safeguard the client and the public when health care and safety are affected by the incompetent, unethical, or illegal practice of any person.
4. The nurse assumes responsibility and accountability for individual nursing judgments and actions.
5. The nurse maintains competence in nursing.
6. The nurse exercises informed judgment and uses individual competence and qualifications as criteria in seeking consultation, accepting responsibilities, and delegating nursing activities to others.
7. The nurse participates in activities that contribute to the ongoing development of the profession's body of knowledge.
8. The nurse participates in the profession's efforts to implement and improve standards of nursing.
9. The nurse participates in the profession's efforts to establish and maintain conditions of employment conducive to high-quality nursing care.
10. The nurse participates in the profession's efforts to protect the public from misinformation and misrepresentation and to maintain the integrity of nursing.
11. The nurse collaborates with members of the health professions and other citizens in promoting community and national efforts to meet the health needs of the public.

Policies and Procedures

Ethical codes represent standards for ideal behavior. However, the Codes do not tell nurses the exact actions to take in specific ethical situations. One way that health care agencies have addressed this lack of specificity is through the development of policies and procedures that reflect the intents found in the Codes.

Nurses are often faced with ethical issues in practice and have a responsibility to participate in the development and ongoing review of policies and procedures in their agency. For example, with the presurgical hospitalized client, a preoperative policy requires that consent for surgery be obtained prior to the client leaving for the operating suite. This policy reflects the need to respect the client's autonomy and legal right to informed consent. At times, a nurse may experience intense pressure from others to "keep on schedule" and send the client to the operating suite although consent has not yet been obtained. In this situation, the policy provides legal and ethical support for a nurse's refusal to send the client before informed consent is obtained.

Nursing Administrators

Nursing administrators, including unit nurse managers and nurse executives, can be valuable resources when ethical issues arise. Most administrators have had experience as staff nurses and are also familiar with available agency resources and applicable policies and procedures that may assist in resolving an ethical issue. Staff nurses sometimes hesitate to consult a nursing administrator because of fears that they will be perceived as incompetent. However, the opposite is usually true. Nurses should keep nursing administrators informed of any potential or actual ethical situations and should seek an administrator's advice because administrators have the authority to mobilize resources, redistribute responsibilities, and discipline, if necessary, in managing an ethical situation.

Institutional Ethics Committee

Ethical issues arise when a nurse does not know what is a correct course to follow. The Joint Commission on Accreditation of Health Care Organizations (JCAHO) (1990) requires nurses to have a mechanism for dealing with ethical issues. Health care agencies may provide specific ethics resources through institutional ethics committees (IECs), ethics consultants, or a combination of both.

Most health care agencies have a multidisciplinary ethics committee that serves as an advisory group for ethical deliberation. In long-term care agencies, this committee is called the patient care advisory committee (PCAC). This committee has three functions:

- Agency and community education about ethical issues and ethical analysis
- Development of policies relevant to ethical decisions, such as resuscitation, refusal of treatment, or informed consent
- Deliberation of cases

Depending on institutional policy, referral of an ethical issue to an institutional ethics committee may be optional or mandatory. In addition, whether or not a health care professional must follow the recommendations of the institutional ethics committee may be considered optional or mandatory.

Institutional ethics committees may be composed of administrators, physicians, nurses, occupational therapists, physical therapists, dietitians, social workers, laypeople, and someone with an extensive background in ethics (e.g., a philosopher, theologian, ethicist, and/or clinician with advanced education in bioethics). The group process of analyzing a problem reflects the opinions and advice that many minds can contribute on a case. However, institutional ethics committees can be bureaucratic and unwieldy, with outspoken members who intimidate quieter members.

The following is an example of a case referred to the institutional ethics committee: A 78-year-old man with gangrenous feet was refusing amputation. He had not been declared legally incompetent, but the health care team was uncomfortable with his refusal. They referred his case to the committee for advice. After gathering relevant data, the committee concluded that if the client is determined to be competent, his wishes must be respected and the health care team should not amputate his feet. If he is determined to be incompetent, then a legal guardian should be appointed who can decide what treatment is in the client's best interest. The committee also found that the client's refusal for amputation was consistent with earlier expressions of valuing his independence. The health care team considered the committee's conclusions and recommendations. After the health care team followed the protocol to determine the client's competency, they believed that the client was competent to refuse amputation. Although the health care team regretted the client's decision, the committee's recommendation fortified their resolve to respect the client's right to make this difficult decision.

Ethics Consultants

An ethics consultant may be a health care professional, such as a physician, nurse, or hospital chaplain, or a philosopher. This consultant gathers and reviews data and offers an ethical analysis. An ethics consultant model overcomes the bureaucratic problem of coordinating an agency ethics committee meeting, but the multidisciplinary perspectives of a committee are lacking. Nurses should be aware of the various ethics resources in their practice settings.

SELECTED ETHICAL ISSUES

Allocation of Efforts

FUTILITY

One of the major ethical issues to be faced in the future is the concept of futility. Technology can extend human life beyond the point when a person cares to live, has consciousness, or has the possibility of recovery. The determination of futile treatment is made by analyzing the cost of treatment (financial, physical, emotional) and the likely outcome (cure, recovery, prolongation of life, death). The value of the costs and outcomes should be determined by the client or, if the client is unable, by the family and friends closest to the client. This is a gross oversimplification, however. Even if clients request futile treatment (like resuscitation in terminal disease), such requests are not automatically honored. The determination of futility also relies on the clinical judgment of health care professionals. Although treatment is thought to be futile, it may be continued because the health care agency may fear a lawsuit. However, discussion and education must occur to learn the client's values, goals, fears, and motives. A request for futile treatment may represent a client's fear of dying.

QUALITY OF LIFE

Quality of life (QOL) remains an elusive concept; no single definition exists. According to studies by Ferrans and Powers (1985), quality of life is determined by the client's judgment about the importance of certain elements in his or her life and satisfaction with those elements. A client who is confined to a wheelchair, for example, may believe that mobility is very important. Although being in a wheelchair is not as good as walking, using a wheelchair may be better than being immobilized, according to this client. However, other people who believe that walking is crucial for happiness may perceive the client's quality of life as being poor. If clients are unable to communicate, whether they never had this ability or have irreversibly lost this ability, it is impossible to know how they view their quality of life.

UTILITARIAN VERSUS DEONTOLOGICAL APPROACH

From a utilitarian standpoint (for the good of *all*), two perspectives can be taken when evaluating quality of life. First, a person warrants resources on the basis of real or potential productivity that person offers society. Second, humanity is served by protecting vulnerable individuals in society because one never knows when one may be in the vulnerable group. This perspective does not offer guidance in determining how many resources one should expend.

The deontological approach to quality of life is based on respect for an *individual* person's life. Deontologists maintain that human life has intrinsic value and should be preserved at all costs. Certain religions may adopt the deontological approach, but one rarely finds a purely utilitarian or purely deontological approach in determining quality of life. When conflict exists in a specific case of whether or not to continue treatment for someone lacking decisional capacity and the client's wishes are unknown, the health care system turns to the legal system.

LEGAL PERSPECTIVE

Through the legal system, society has grappled with how best to preserve the autonomy of incompetent clients, as in the cases of Nancy Cruzan and Karen Ann Quinlan (Weir, 1989), who were in irreversible comas. In these cases, the central issue was the incompetent person's right to refuse treatment and how this right is exercised. If the person's wishes are unknown, the law presumes that a person, even an incompetent person, prefers to live, and the state has an interest in preserving life; however, society is not in agreement on whether the financial burden of preserving this life is justifiable.

The current health care system in the United States forces allocation based on accessibility to services and ability to pay. The uninsured and underinsured forgo treatment except in emergency care, and then they may receive services only after a lengthy wait. Similarly, some people often must wait for appointments or referrals to specialists when they are in health maintenance organizations (HMOs). In Canada, however, clients are not limited by ability to pay, but they may have to wait for certain procedures or surgeries or they may not have access to some procedures available in the United States. Many groups, especially nursing associations, have worked tirelessly for universal access to health care and believe the health care system should be revamped to focus on preventive care and health maintenance rather than acute inpatient care.

The state of Oregon proposed an allocation of health care dollars based on a quality-of-life-year (QOLY) and probability of medical benefit. A prioritized list of more than 700 treatments was compiled as a method of determining what treatments would be supported and what treatments would not be funded with state dollars (Hadorn, 1991). The Bush administration (1989–1993) opposed this plan, arguing that it potentially discriminated against disabled clients.

PALLIATIVE VERSUS CURATIVE CARE

There may come a point in the course of a disease when a cure may not be possible. Clients with cardiomyopathy, neoplastic diseases, or degenerative diseases may no longer respond to treatment; in such cases, they might perceive continued treatment with poor probability of cure unbearable. These clients may opt for treatment that provides symptom management but does not cure the condition. Palliative care—aimed toward comfort not cure—may involve radiation, chemotherapy, or surgery to reduce tumor mass; administration of analgesics in high and frequent doses; and/or variation in nutrition routes.

Nurses often have an opportunity to practice the art as well as the science of nursing in palliative care. During palliative care, nurses make a commitment to provide relief for the client until death. The nurse becomes a client advocate by negotiating the health care system with the client. A client's comfort is often related to the tenacity of the nurse in advocating and providing client care.

INTENTIONALITY

The doctrine of the "double effect" (May, 1978) is moral reasoning presented by some Catholic theologians in defending the use of analgesics in terminal illness. The double effect doctrine holds that it is morally permissible to medicate a client to relieve pain even though there is a risk that the medication may suppress respirations and cause the client to stop breathing. If the *intent* is to relieve pain, the action is permissible. If the *intent* is to kill the person, it is not permissible. For example, a nurse gives morphine sulfate to a client dying of lung cancer. The nurse realizes that morphine can depress respirations, which are already compromised by the cancer. Nevertheless, the nurse intends to provide pain relief and is aware that an untoward side effect may be death due to apnea. The nurse is ethically justified in giving the morphine because the intent is to relieve pain, not to cause death.

Competency

Two forms of competency exist: legal and clinical competency. A person is considered to be *legally* competent if he or she is:

- 18 years of age or older
- Pregnant or a married minor
- A legally emancipated minor who is self-supporting
- Not declared incompetent by a court of law

If a court determines that a person is legally incompetent, a guardian is appointed to make health care and/or financial decisions.

A person is considered to be *clinically* competent if he or she is legally competent and possesses decisional capacity. Decisional capacity is determined by the person who is the most knowledgeable about the issue. Decisional capacity is determined by assessing the client's ability to:

- Identify the problem
- Recognize options and their potential consequences
- Make a decision
- Provide rationale supporting the chosen option

Thus, a surgeon would determine a client's decisional capacity related to surgery, an internist would assess capacity related to medical treatment, and a nurse would determine the client's ability to make decisions about nursing activities (Bosek, 1993b).

To assist health care professionals in the area of clinical competency, it is very helpful to have a values assessment in which clients express what is most important to them. The nurse includes values assessment questions in the nursing history and updates the information if the client's condition changes, if new diagnoses are made, and/or if long-range treatment goals are discussed (Table 6–4).

TABLE 6–4 Key Questions to Ask in Taking a Values History

- How do you feel about your current health status?
- What goals do you have for the future?
- What are you hoping for at this time?
- What means the most to you right now?
- Do you feel your life is worth living?
- What would make your life more satisfying?
- What would you consider as a life NOT worth living?
- If you were dying, what would be most important to you?
- What is your greatest fear about dying?
- Where would you prefer to die?
- How do you feel about the use of life-sustaining measures if you were dying? In a permanent coma? If you had an irreversible, chronic illness?
- What role do your friends and family play in your life?
- What role do you have in making decisions about your life? Health care?
- What is your faith, tradition, or religious background?
- How do your religious beliefs affect your attitude toward serious illness and death?
- Who do you trust to make decisions on your behalf?
- Have you shared your thoughts with your friends, family and health care team?

Modified from the Values History form, developed at the Institute of Public Law, University of New Mexico in Albuquerque, through a grant from the Ittleson Foundation. Reprinted with permission. Rushton, C.H., & Lynch, M.E. (1992, June). Dealing with advance directives for critically ill adolescents. *Critical Care Nurse,* 31–37.

Written Advance Directives

Written advance directives are "legal documents which provide a mechanism for individuals to indicate their decisions about future medical care" (Bosek & Fitzpatrick, 1992, p. 33). The United States Patient Self Determination Act of 1990 requires health care professionals to inform each client who is admitted to a hospital or nursing home about the availability of advance directives. If the client already has written advance directives on admission, a copy is placed with the medical record so that the directive will be available if needed.

There are two common types of written advance directives: living wills and durable power of attorney for health care.

LIVING WILLS

Living wills, sometimes referred to as "death with dignity" documents, allow persons to document their wishes regarding life-sustaining treatment in case they are ever unable to speak for themselves and are imminently dying of a terminal illness (Fig. 6–2). In the United States, living wills are recognized as legal documents by 38 states and the District of Columbia; however, they are not recognized as legal documents in Canada (Fisher & Meslin, 1990). In most states, "imminent death" refers to when death is expected according to best medical estimates within a few hours or days (Kilner, 1990). In some states, imminent death may be defined as a few months.

DURABLE POWERS OF ATTORNEY FOR HEALTH CARE

A durable power of attorney for health care (DPOA), sometimes called a durable medical power of attorney, is a legal document in the United States. This document allows people to:

DECLARATION UNDER ILLINOIS LIVING WILL ACT

This declaration is made this ______ day of ______ 19___.

I, ______________________________, being of sound mind, willfully and voluntarily make known my desires that my moment of death shall not be artificially postponed.

If at any time I should have an incurable and irreversible injury, disease, or illness judged to be a terminal condition by my attending physician who has personally examined me, and has determined that my death is imminent except for death delaying procedures, I direct that such procedures which would only prolong the dying process be withheld or withdrawn, and that I be permitted to die naturally with only the administration of medication, sustenance, or the performance of any medical procedure deemed necessary by my attending physician to provide me with comfort care.

In the absence of my ability to give directions regarding the use of such death delaying procedures, it is my intention that this declaration shall be honored by my family and physician as the final expression of my legal right to refuse medical or surgical treatment and accept the consequences from such refusal.

Signed ______________________

City, County and State of Residence ______________________

____

____

The declarant is personally known to me and I believe the declarant to be of sound mind. I did not sign the declarant's signature about, for or at the direction of the declarant. At the date of this instrument, I am not entitled to any portion of the estate of the declarant according to the laws of intestate succession or, to the best of my knowledge and belief, under any will of declarant or other instrument taking effect at declarant's death, or directly financially responsible for the declarant's medical care.

Witness ______________________

Witness ______________________

FIGURE 6-2 ◆ An example of a living will.

- Identify someone to make decisions for them if unable to speak for themselves
- Identify how aggressive treatment should be if they should ever be in a coma or a persistent vegetative state (PVS)
- List any medical treatments they would never want performed (Fig. 6-3)

Each state in the United States has legislation that describes the scope and execution of a DPOA.

The following example illustrates the use of advance directives. A client who sustained head trauma in an accident is now in a persistent vegetative state and requires ventilator support. The spouse presents a copy of the client's living will and durable power of attorney for health care to the hospital staff and requests that the ventilator be discontinued. The living will does not apply in this situation because the client is not considered terminally ill. The durable power of attorney, however, does apply and identifies the spouse as the agent to make the health care decisions. In addition, the client has documented the desire to forgo artificial life support in the event of irreversible coma. The health care team respects the client's autonomy, as exercised by the spouse and the written advance directive, and discontinues the ventilator. Nurses should become familiar with applicable laws on advance directives in their state or province.

Verbal Advance Directives

Occasionally, family members, friends, or health care professionals are able to remember conversations with the client when specific comments were made about life-sustaining treatments. These comments may be considered verbal advance directives when the client has no written directives and is unable to communicate his or her wishes. A common myth is that the physician is obligated to follow the next-of-kin consent when the client cannot participate in decision-making. Next-of-kin do not have legal authority to consent or refuse treatment for an adult relative without becoming declared the legal guardian or the agent in a durable power of attorney for health care. Traditionally, however, health care professionals have obtained next-of-kin approval to minimize the chance of being sued.

If a client tells a nurse or other health care professional about his or her wishes regarding health care and life-sustaining treatment, the professional should encourage the client to specifically elaborate on vague phrases, like "do everything" or "when my time comes, let me go." The health care professional helps the client to document these directives in written form when possible. In addition, the nurse should document the conversation in the medical record (Fig. 6–4). All health care professionals should refer to agency policies and procedures about the use of verbal advance directives for guiding clinical ethical decision-making.

Euthanasia

Euthanasia means "good death" (Walters, 1982). Although this concept is an ethical issue, in the United States it is dealt with more from a legal perspective. Chapter 12 includes a complete discussion on euthanasia.

Placebo Administration

A placebo is the intentional administration of an inert substance or benign action as a treatment, usually as a modality for pain relief. For instance, a client may receive a normal saline injection for a complaint of pain. When prescribing a placebo, the physician is intentionally attempting to deceive the client and thus is limiting the client's autonomy. When clients are deceived, they are unable to make informed decisions. In addition, the use of placebos jeopardizes client trust in both the physician's and nurse's motives. When clients seek health care assistance, they are assuming that health care professionals will act in their best interest; thus, the use of a placebo threatens this assumption (Elander, 1991).

When a nurse cannot ethically implement a placebo order, he or she is obligated to explain this position to the physician. According to Beauchamp and Childress (1989) and Elander (1991), nurses may object to the use of placebos because of the conviction that the placebo:

- Results in a denial that the client has pain
- Is deceptive
- Decreases client autonomy
- Threatens client trust in the health care system

If the physician continues the placebo order after this discussion, the nurse is obligated to work toward a resolution of this ethical issue by seeking ethics consultation. When a nurse cannot follow a physician's order, the nurse must follow the health care agency's policy and lines of authority in nursing precisely, documenting each communication.

Many nurses have no moral opposition to using placebos if a client expresses pain relief after receiving the placebo. Oftentimes, clients do experience increased comfort because of personal attention and associated nursing interventions, such as repositioning or relaxation techniques, provided with the placebo (Beauchamp & Childress, 1989; Elander, 1991).

Some nurses rationalize the use of a placebo by not telling any direct lies. For example, if asked what medication is being given, the nurse will state: "This is the injection the physician ordered" (Elander, 1991) or "This is a saline injection" to clients with limited medical knowledge. However, when administering a placebo, the nurse has a basic obligation to prevent harm. The nurse needs to conduct a thorough client assessment before and after administering a placebo. When a client does not experience pain relief, the nurse must notify the physician and request other treatment options. With the patient's permission, alternating pain medication with a placebo as a trial to determine the extent of genuine pain is ethically acceptable.

Restraints

Restraints are interventions that limit a person's freedom to move. Restraints can be physical (e.g., vest, limb, or geri-chairs with lap tables in place) or chemical (e.g., haloperidol [Haldol, Periodol♣]). Because restraints limit movement, they also limit autonomy. Before deciding whether to restrain a client, the nurse needs to identify the desired outcome and consider the related risks and benefits of all possible options (Fig. 6–5).

The nurse may want to achieve the following outcomes when planning client care:

- Preventing harm to the client and to the other clients
- Maintaining the client's autonomy

However, balancing these two outcomes may be difficult when a client's autonomy is compromised by illnesses such as Alzheimer's disease. A client with

DURABLE POWER OF ATTORNEY FOR HEALTH CARE

Power of Attorney made this __________ day of __________, 19______

1. I, the undersigned hereby appoint (insert name and address of agent)

____

as agent to act for me and in my name to make any and all decisions for me concerning my personal care, medical treatment, hospitalization and health care and to require, withhold or withdraw any type of medical treatment or procedure, even though my death may ensue. My agent shall have the same access to my medical records that I have, including the right to disclose the contents to others. My agent shall also have full power to make a disposition of any part or all of my body for medical purposes, authorize an autopsy and direct the disposition of my remains. (Neither the attending physician nor any other health care provider may act as your agent.)

2. The powers granted above shall be subject to the following rules or limitations (if none, leave blank):

____

____

(The subject of life-sustaining treatment is of particular importance. For your convenience in dealing with that subject some general statements concerning the withholding or removal of life-sustaining treatment are set forth below. If you agree with one of these statements, you may initial that statement; but do not initial more than one.)

(I do not want my life to be prolonged nor do I want life-sustaining treatment
(to be provided or continued if my agent believes the burdens of the treatment
(outweigh the expected benefits. I want my agent to consider the relief of
(suffering the expense involved and the quality as well as the possible extension
______(of my life in making decisions concerning life-sustaining treatment.

(I want my life to be prolonged and I want life-sustaining treatment to be
(provided or continued unless I am in a coma which my attending physician
(believes to be irreversible, in accordance with reasonable medical standards at
(the time of reference. If and when I have suffered irreversible coma, I want
______(life-sustaining treatment to be withheld or discontinued.

(I want my life to be prolonged to the greatest extent possible without regard to
______(my condition, the chances I have for recovery or the cost of the procedures.

3. This power of attorney shall become effective on ____________________

____

FIGURE 6-3 ◆ An example of a durable power of attorney for health care.

Alzheimer's disease may be free from harm if he or she has a steady gait, yet wandering may cause harm to other clients. Therefore, on the basis of non-maleficence (preventing harm to others), a nurse would be justified in limiting a client's autonomy by preventing the wandering (Beauchamp, 1982).

When using a restraint, nurses must always consider both the risk and benefits (Table 6-5) and use the least restrictive method possible (Robbins, 1986). For instance, a waist restraint is less restrictive than a vest restraint; a vest restraint is less restrictive than limb restraints. Chemical restraints (drugs) are the most restrictive because they affect the client's physical and mental abilities. As always, a nurse follows both state statutes and the health care agency's policies and procedure when using restraints. A client's mental and physical condition are routinely re-evaluated and documented along with justification for continued use of restraints (also see Chap. 5). Restraints should be discontinued as soon as possible or when an alternate intervention has been implemented (Bosek, 1993b).

4. This power of attorney shall terminate on ______________________________
____

5. If any agent named by me shall die, become legally disabled, resign, refuse to act or be unavailable, I name the following (each to act alone and successively, in the order named) as successors to such agent:
____
____

6. If a guardian of my person is to be appointed, I nominate the following to serve as such guardian (if same as agent, leave blank):
____

7. I am fully informed as to all the contents of this form and understand the full import of this grant of power to my agent.

Signed ______________________________
Principal

The principal has had an opportunity to read the above form and has signed the form or acknowledged his or her signature or mark on the form in my presence.

______________________ Residing at ______________________________
Witness

(You may, but are not required to, request your agent and successor agents to provide specimen signature below. If you include specimen signature in this Power of Attorney, you must complete the certification opposite the signatures of the agents.)

Specimen signatures of agent (and successors)	I certify that the signature of my agent (and successors) are correct.
______________________ (agent)	______________________ (principal)
______________________ (successor agent)	______________________ (principal)
______________________ (successor agent)	______________________ (principal)

FIGURE 6–3 ◆ *Continued*

Personal Rights

A right is a justifiable claim that all persons can make (Curtin & Flaherty, 1982). In the past, health care was acquired through bartering. However, in the late 20th century, health care has evolved into a business industry. When health care is a right, every citizen will be able to access health care services and society will have an obligation to provide health care.

In Canada and several other countries, health care is recognized as a right. National health care programs have been implemented to guarantee that every citizen has equal access to health care; however, not all treatments and procedures are available.

In the United States, many people believe that health care is a right, but no universal health care system exists at this time. At present, health care is available to those who can afford to pay, have insurance, or qualify for Medicare and Medicaid. Emergency care is available to the uninsured, but access to other forms of health care is limited. A growing segment of the U.S. population are uninsurable or unemployed or do not have access to insurance through their employer. There has been much debate about how to deal with this access issue. Many advocate a

Nursing SOAP Note

10/22/93 12 noon Problem A: "Edema"

S: "I won't live much longer...I want all the usual emergency treatments...I wouldn't want a machine continued if there was no hope that I'd get better...I'm not sure if my Mom could actually carry out this request. I'll talk to her today."

O: Increased facial and neck edema. Discussed wishes for emergency treatment for sudden events (arrests). Does not want maintained by machines if no hope for recovery to current level of functioning. Dr. Jones notified.

A: Full code. Potential respiratory distress due to increasing edema

P: Continue to assess respirations. Facilitate autonomy in decision making. *Marcia Bosek, RN*

Nursing Narrative Note

8 am	C/O neck swelling. Left cheek and entire neck obviously swollen. No C/O dysphagia. R=20 and easy. Lungs clear bilaterally. *Marcia Bosek, RN*
8:30 am	Dr. Jones notified of cheek and neck swelling. *Marcia Bosek, RN*
10 am	Informed of O_2 saturation tests q shift, instructed to notify nurse of respiratory distress. Discussion initiated by RN regarding wishes about emergency treatment for respiratory arrest. Stated: "I won't live much longer. I want all the usual emergency treatments. I wouldn't want a machine continued if there was no hope that I'd get better. I'm not sure if my Mom could actually carry out this request. I'll talk to her this afternoon." Provided with copy of DPOA and instructed on use. Verbalized understanding of process. *Marcia Bosek, RN*

FIGURE 6–4 ◆ Sample documentation of verbal directives.

two-tiered system that would provide basic health care to all while allowing each person to purchase additional "high-tech" medical treatment. Others propose a universal, single-payer system emphasizing health promotion and disease prevention.

Obligation

If a person has a specific right to health care, that person also has an obligation to maintain and protect his or her health. Rights and their associated responsibilities are inherently in conflict with autonomy. Life insurance companies often compensate for high correlations between voluntary behavior and disease by charging higher premium rates to people who smoke, drink alcoholic beverages, or engage in high-risk activities, such as auto racing (Veatch, 1980).

Confidentiality

Confidentiality is a major ethical issue. Confidentiality requires that a person has the "right to control

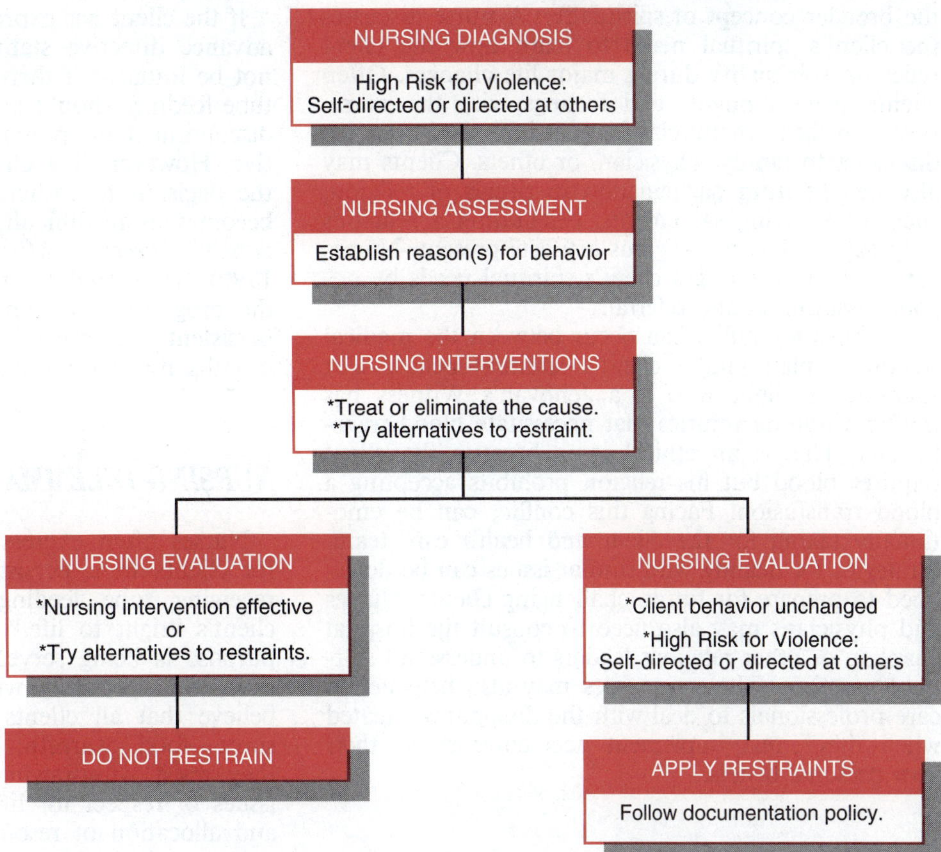

FIGURE 6–5 ◆ A restraint decision tree. (From Morison, J., Crinklaw-Wiancko, F., King, D., et al. [1984]. Formulating a restraint policy. *Journal of Nursing Administration, 17*[3], 39–42.)

information about oneself" (Winslade, 1978, p. 196). Some information may be perceived as sensitive and thus should be shared only on a "need-to-know" basis. For instance, there is an isolation sign on the door to the client's room and a visitor asks the client's nurse about the diagnosis. Realizing that the visitor is asking for confidential information, the nurse explains the isolation procedure but does not divulge any information about the client. Because clients control information about themselves, the nurse directs the visitor to speak directly with the client.

The American Nurses' Association (ANA) and Canadian Code for Nurses require nurses to maintain client confidentiality. Too often, nurses and other health care professionals discuss client cases in elevators, cafeterias, and other public places. Although they do not intend to breach a client's confidentiality, others may overhear the conversations.

TABLE 6–5 Potential Benefits and Risks of Physical Restraints

Potential benefits

- Prevention of falls, which might result in injury
- Protection from other accidents or injuries
- Allowing medical treatment to proceed without client interference
- Protection of other clients or staff from disturbances or physical harm
- Increased client feelings of safety and security

Potential risks

- Injury from falls
- Accidental death by strangulation
- Functional decline
- Skin abrasions or skin breakdown
- Biochemical, physiologic, and psychologic sequelae of prolonged immobilization
- Cardiac arrest
- Reduced appetite and dehydration
- Disorganized behavior
- Emotional desolation
- Possible increased mortality

Reprinted with permission from Evans, L. K., & Strumpf, N. E. (1989). Tying down the elderly: A review of the literature on physical restraint. *Journal of the American Geriatrics Society, 37*, 65–74. Courtesy of the American Geriatrics Association.

Spiritual Practices

Values are critical in ethical issues and are shaped by many influences—family, experiences, culture, and spirituality. Health care decisions involve clarification of values and interpreting the meaning that a client places on illness. Clients often interpret the meaning of their illness through the tenets of their faith. For example, they may view illness as a punishment for wrongdoings or lack of faith and may refuse pain medication because of the belief that suffering leads to redemption.

How clients cope with illness is also affected by their faith. When addressing ethical issues, the nurse assesses the client's spirituality. Often clients are asked to list their religious preference when admitted to a health care agency, but religion is only a part of the broader concept of spirituality. A nurse discusses the client's spiritual needs to learn how the client relies on spirituality during major life changes. Often clients share thoughts and feelings with the nurse, who can help them clarify questions and fears to discuss with family, physician, or others. Clients may also benefit from participation in rituals of religion, such as receiving sacraments, celebrating a religious holy day, or having religious artifacts present. Nurses can facilitate meeting a client's spiritual needs by ongoing assessment and referral.

At times a conflict can occur between the medical treatment plan and a client's spiritual beliefs. For example, a client who is a Jehovah's Witness has multiple trauma injuries that necessitate blood transfusions. This is an ethical issue because the client requires blood but his religion prohibits accepting a blood transfusion. Facing this conflict can be emotionally taxing for the client and health care team. Strategies for dealing with similar issues can be developed to prepare for future challenging clients. Nurses and physicians may also need to consult the hospital chaplain or other religious leaders to understand spiritual practices. These resources may also help health care professionals to deal with the dissonance created when they must implement acts contrary to their own personal beliefs.

Tube Feeding

Certain conditions prevent clients from taking food and fluids orally. For example, the client may have had extensive treatment for cancer of the head and neck or may have a neurologic disorder, such as persistent vegetative state (PVS) or permanent unconsciousness. For clients who hope to recover and take oral feedings again, tube feedings are a temporary intervention to ensure adequate nutrition and hydration. The ethical issue occurs when recovery is unlikely and tube feeding becomes death-delaying instead of life-prolonging treatment. There is controversy over whether tube feeding (nasogastric, gastrostomy, or jejunostomy) is considered a medical treatment or a basic need that must be met.

ETHICAL DEBATE

Some ethicists (Weir, 1989) argue that feeding, whether oral or tube, is a basic need, like oxygen, that must be met regardless of prognosis. One is obligated to feed the client if the client would die of starvation and dehydration, not the underlying disease or disorder. The exception is if the client's condition would actually worsen if feedings were given, as with pulmonary edema, aspiration pneumonia, or renal failure. Other ethicists believe tube feedings are a medical procedure that can be withheld or withdrawn if no medical benefit (improvement or recovery) is foreseen. For clients in a persistent vegetative state, who will not regain consciousness, tube feedings maintain but do not alter their condition.

If the client has expressed wishes in the form of an advance directive stating that tube feedings should not be initiated if there is no hope of recovery, then tube feedings should not be started or they should be discontinued on presentation of this advance directive. However, if a client has no advance directive, the decision to initiate and continue tube feedings becomes more difficult, as in the Cruzan case (*Cruzan v. Director, Missouri Department of Health,* 1990). Tube feedings may have been started before the prognosis was certain because a diagnosis of a persistent vegetative state is usually made 1 to 6 months after an initial injury.

NURSING DILEMMA

Nurses often express ethical discomfort in caring for clients in a persistent vegetative state who are receiving tube feedings. Nurses may respect the client's "right to life," but also may question what purpose is being served by expending resources for those who probably will not benefit—or they may believe that all clients deserve basic comfort measures—food, warmth, protection from harm—and they resist withdrawing feedings. There are deeper issues of respect for life, spirituality, quality of life, and allocation of resources that are involved in the question of whether or not to use tube feedings.

Nurses must first examine their feelings and beliefs about tube feedings, then participate in a team conference that explores the benefits and burdens of this treatment for a particular client. Decisions whether or not to tube feed rest with the client (by advance directive) or family and the physician with input from other health care professionals who know the client and family. Legal requirements may necessitate obtaining a court order to withdraw feedings. In some states, the living will statute specifically mandates that nutrition, hydration, and medication must be provided although all other treatments may be discontinued.

In some states of the United States, laws exist that allow a family and health care team to make the decision to withhold or withdraw feedings without obtaining a court order, provided that specific steps are taken and documented in the medical record. When the nurse does not personally agree with the decision that is made, two courses can be pursued. Even though a nurse may not make the same decision, the nurse should respect the client's autonomy and the process that produced this decision and believe that the best decision was made under these circumstances. On the other hand, if a nurse morally objects to this decision, the nurse should state the objection and rationale to the nursing supervisor and request to be reassigned to another client if necessary. Some health care agencies allow health care professionals who morally object to the management plan to transfer the care for the client to another health care professional who does not have a moral objection.

Unethical Professional Conduct

In the American Nurses' Association Code of Ethics, the third plank addresses the responsibility of nurses to uphold the highest standards and protect clients from health care professionals who engage in illegal, unethical, or incompetent practice. The Code of Ethics for Nursing by the Canadian Nurses Association (1991) lists "Value VIII: Protecting Clients from Incompetence. Value: The nurse takes steps to ensure that the client receives competent and ethical care" (p. 15). In the health care system, however, it is not very easy to report another's unethical conduct ("whistleblowing") without suffering unpleasant and sometimes devastating consequences.

The nurse who observes or discovers an act that jeopardizes a client's safety has an obligation to take steps to protect the client. It may be discovering a medication error or witnessing another health care professional verbally or physically abusing a client. Nurses must take necessary actions, such as notifying the physician if a medication error was made, verifying information as thoroughly as possible, and documenting each incident according to agency policy.

Next, the nurse follows the lines of authority for reporting the incident. Some nurses may wish to discuss the incident with other professional(s) involved, advising them that an incident was discovered and giving them an opportunity to take corrective action or clarify their behavior. In the spirit of collegiality and peer review, nurses can assist each other in keeping the standards of practice of nursing at the highest level.

On a larger scale, nurses have found themselves in situations in which they are made a party to unethical practices. When they have followed channels of communication, they have been threatened with loss of their job or license and even bodily harm (Witt, 1983). Nurses must realistically evaluate the consequences of their actions in whistleblowing. Nursing associations are keenly aware of many pressures nurses experience in these situations and have proposed mechanisms for assisting such nurses. The Illinois Nurses Association House of Delegates (1989) passed a resolution creating an advisory resource for nurses to call regarding reporting incompetent, unethical, or illegal practice. To maintain the public's trust and to self-regulate, nurses must continue to monitor their practice and the practices of others.

APPLICATION TO THE NURSING PROCESS

During every aspect of nursing care, a nurse acts ethically and advocates, when needed, for the client's beliefs, values, and decisions related to health, health care, and medical interventions. Nurses should remember that even though a treatment decision may be clinically sound, the decision may not be ethically justified. For example, a decision to start tube feedings may be appropriate on the basis of nutritional data but may be ethically prohibited if a client does not agree (Wicclair, 1991). Thus, ethical decision-making is not considered a separate process from the nursing process but, rather, a building block on which every nursing decision and action is developed.

ASSESSMENT

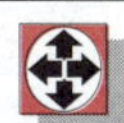

When collecting data, the nurse identifies all persons to be involved in decision-making and notes the ethical issues and concerns being experienced or identified by the various participants. The nurse assesses the decision environment, the time available to make a decision, and the events that preceded this situation. In a study by Corley and Selig (1992), when given an ethical vignette, nurse subjects wanted more data to help make ethical decisions. (Research Applications for Nursing).

ANALYSIS

On the basis of the data collected, the nurse with the various participants identifies the major ethical issue or question to be resolved. For example, is it ethically permissible or does the client's right to confidentiality regarding his or her human immunodeficiency virus (HIV) status outweigh the potential harm to sexual partners? Other common ethical issues experienced by medical-surgical nurses have been discussed in this chapter.

PLANNING AND IMPLEMENTATION

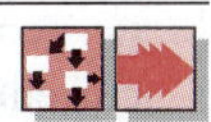

PLANNING: CLIENT GOALS Decision-making outcomes and interventions must be clearly identified. Of the four major ethical principles, non-maleficence, or "do no harm," is a minimum outcome from any intervention. When possible, beneficence toward the client should be fostered. How "good" is accomplished will be determined during a values clarification component in interventions. Finally, client autonomy is promoted to the greatest extent possible. This may be achieved by:

- Identifying the client as *the* decision maker
- Executing the client's advance directive
- Implementing "the best interest" standard on the client's behalf

When the client is incompetent and has not previously identified a durable power of attorney for health care, a designated decision-maker should be identified.

RESEARCH APPLICATIONS FOR NURSING

Contextual Considerations and Adequate Information May Enhance Ethical Decision-Making

Corley, M. C., & Selig, P. M. (1992). Nurse moral reasoning using the Nursing Dilemma Test. *Western Journal of Nursing Research, 14,* 380–388.

Corley and Selig administered the Nursing Dilemma Test to a convenience sample of 75 nurses employed in critical care areas of a large government hospital. The researchers measured each subject's level of moral reasoning based on responses to six common ethical vignettes, such as an adult's request to die, forcing medication, and a medication error. In addition, each subject was encouraged to identify additional moral issues present in the vignettes.

The researchers found that most subjects had familiarity with the ethical vignettes; 81% of the subjects indicated that they would report a medication error, practical considerations were rarely chosen as the most preferable response for resolving the dilemma, and the mean principled thinking score for this sample was lower than scores reported in previous studies. In addition, four additional relevant issues were identified by the subjects: rights, alternative actions, consideration for others, and quality of life issues.

Critique The researchers investigated an important issue that nurses face almost daily. They used a previously tested tool instead of developing another one. However, this tool has been associated with low internal reliability in the past. Efforts to establish internal reliability for this study were also discouraging. The Nursing Dilemma Test was originally developed in 1979 and may need to be updated to reflect current problems with ethical issues.

In addition, the researchers concluded that the Nursing Dilemma Test can accurately measure the moral reasoning of both male and female nurses despite the fact that the tool was developed from Kohlberg's theory of moral reasoning and the absence of supporting data.

Possible nursing implications The inconsistent findings may be accounted for in part by each nurse's values and recent changes in society since the creation of the tool. While the use of hypothetical vignettes may be useful for teaching ethical decision-making skills, the findings from this study suggest that a nurse's moral reasoning is influenced by specific contextual features and the adequacy of information available at the time the ethical decision is made.

INTERVENTIONS A variety of interventions may be necessary before a decision can be made and finally implemented. During the intervention phase, participants need to identify any task, personal, and environmental variables not identified during the assessment phase. When identifying these variables, a nurse must also identify any competing variables, such as justice versus caring perspectives or autonomy versus paternalism. The nurse identifies and consults ethical resources but the designated decision-maker should make the decision. While participants may voice their agreement or objections with the decision, consensus may not occur or be appropriate unless consensus has been identified as a desired outcome.

Health care professionals and clients involved in making an ethical decision must be helped to move beyond the "feels good" test when justifying a decision or action. This test suggests that "if I feel good about the decision, option, or outcome, it must be right." Often "right" ethical decisions are not experienced as comfortable. For example decisions to whistleblow are often not comfortably or easily made.

Nurses need to develop skills in using ethical theories, principles, and decision-making concepts to support and explain decisions. For example, the following comments are not sufficient rationales:

- "I'm uncomfortable with the decision"
- "My church won't let me"
- "That's how it's always done here"

These insufficient comments can be developed into the following useful rationales:

- "I'm uncomfortable with this order because I believe I may be hastening the client's death"
- "My religion believes that life is valuable in any form; therefore, I cannot reject life-sustaining treatment"
- "Traditionally, the attending physician is the person who initiates do-not-resuscitate discussions"

The use of a specific rationale moves the discussion beyond emotions and feelings to concepts, principles, and theories that can be debated logically.

EVALUATION

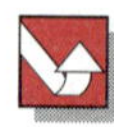

The evaluation of an ethical decision includes the following:

- Were the outcomes achieved? If not, why?
- Did the correct person make the decision?
- What actions will be taken to prevent similar situations from happening?
- How do the various participants feel?

Opportunities may be needed for clients, family, and/or health care professionals to review events, verbalize feelings and fears, and discuss barriers to effective ethical decision-making. Several opportunities may be needed before the ethical issues can be resolved completely.

OTHER ETHICAL ISSUES THAT MEDICAL-SURGICAL NURSES FACE

Some of the ethical issues that nurses in the medical-surgical setting face have been described in this chapter, but many others also exist, especially in the care of the elderly (Chart 6–1). Other ethical issues that occur in the medical-surgical clinical setting include:

- Use of fetal tissue for Parkinson's disease treatment
- Allocation of organs for transplantation
- Mandatory direct observed therapy for tuberculosis or drug abuse treatment
- The impaired nurse
- Confidentiality of computerized records
- Disclosure of the health care professional's human immunodeficiency virus (HIV) status to clients

CHART 6–1

Nursing Focus on the Elderly ♦ Myths and Ethical Issues Related to Care of the Elderly

Myths

- The older the person, the less likely he or she will be competent.
- Adult children have the right to know their parent's medical status or to make health care decisions for their parents.
- The elderly are more likely to have articulated their beliefs about death and life-sustaining treatment than younger persons.
- When a person can no longer control his or her bodily functions, he or she is also unable to make informed decisions about health care.

Ethical Issues

- How should health care resources be allocated for the frail and terminally ill elderly?
- Should health care services be rationed by age?
- Should elderly people be able to choose the time to die?
- Does society have an oblgation to provide for the elderly?
- Should health care treatment decisions be influenced by the elderly person's ability to pay, or by the type of payment (private insurance/Medicare/Medicaid)?
- What is "the best interest" standard for the elderly?
- What constitutes elder abuse?
- Do the elderly have clearly defined values because of life experiences?
- When is it appropriate to provide comfort care for the elderly versus using all available technology?

Many of these issues are presented and discussed elsewhere in this text.

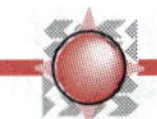

IMPLICATIONS FOR NURSING RESEARCH

The rapid advances in medical technology have created numerous ethical questions. Nurses are in an ideal position to facilitate the scientific inquiry related to ethical issues in the medical-surgical clinical setting. Here are some potential research questions:

- ♦ Does a person's cultural, ethnic or religious background influence his or her perception and use of advance directives?
- ♦ What is the best way to determine a client's clinical competency?
- ♦ Do the use of advance directives promote client autonomy?
- ♦ Do nurses and physicians approach ethical situations from the same moral perspective?
- ♦ Does the form of payment influence the aggressiveness of treatment offered to or selected by a client?
- ♦ Does the client's perception of quality of life influence end-of-life treatment decisions?

SELECTED BIBLIOGRAPHY

* American Nurses' Association. (1976, 1985). The Code for Nurses with Interpretive Statements. Kansas City: Author.

Bandman, E. L., & Bandman, B. (1990). *Nursing ethics through the life span* (2nd ed.). Norwalk, CT: Appleton-Lange.

* Beauchamp, T. L. (1982). Ethical theory and bioethics. In T. L. Beauchamp, & L. Walters (Eds.), *Contemporary issues in bioethics* (2nd ed., pp. 1–43). Belmont, CA: Wadsworth.

* Beauchamp, T. L., & Childress, J. F. (1989). *Principles of biomedical ethics* (3rd ed.). New York: Oxford University Press.

* Beauchamp, T. L., & Walters, L. (1982). *Contemporary issues in bioethics* (2nd ed.). Belmont, CA: Wadsworth.

Benjamin, M., & Curtis, J. (1992). *Ethics in nursing* (3rd ed.). New York: Oxford University Press.

Bosek, M. S. D. (1993a). *Clinical ethical decision-making: The role of gender.* Unpublished manuscript.

Bosek, M. S. D. (1993b). Ethical issues with the use of restraints. *MEDSURG Nursing, 2*(2), 154–156.

Bosek, M. S. D., & Fitzpatrick, J. (1992). A nursing perspective on advance directives. *MEDSURG Nursing, 1*(1), 33–38.

Canadian Nurses Association (1991). *Code of Ethics for Nursing.* Ottawa: Author.

Corley, M. C., & Selig, P. M. (1992). Nurse moral reasoning using the Nursing Dilemma Test. *Western Journal of Nursing Research, 14,* 380–388.

Cranford, R. E. (1991). Helga Wanglie's ventilator. *Hastings Center Report, 21*(4), 23–24.

* Crisham, P. (1981). Decision analysis: A step by step guide for making clinical decisions. *Nursing & Health Care, 7,* 148–154.

Cruzan v. Director, Missouri Department of Health. 110 S. Ct. 2841 (1990).

* Curtin, L., & Flaherty, M. J. (1982). *Nursing ethics: Theory and pragmatics.* Bowie MD: Robert J. Brady Co.

DeWolf, M. S. (1989a). *Clinical ethical decision-making: A grounded theory method.* University Microfilms, Publication 390-06, 043.

DeWolf, M. S. (1989b). Ethical decision making. *Seminars in Oncology Nursing, 5*(2), 77–81.

Elander, G. (1991). Ethical conflicts in placebo treatment. *Journal of Advanced Nursing, 16,* 947–951.

* Evans, L. K., & Strumpf, N. E. (1989). Tying down the elderly: A review of the literature on physical restraint. *Journal of the American Geriatric Society, 36,* 65–74.

* Ferrans, C. E., & Powers, M. J., (1985). Quality of life index: Development and psychometric properties. *Advances in Nursing Science, 8,* 15–24.

Fisher, R. H., & Meslin, E. M. (1990). Should living wills be legalized? *Canadian Medical Association Journal, 142*(1), 23–26.

* Fowler, M. D. M., & Levine-Ariff, J. (1987). *Ethics at the bedside: A source book for the critical care nurse.* Philadelphia: J.B. Lippincott Company.

* Fromer, M. J. (1983). *Ethical issues in health care.* St. Louis: C.V. Mosby.

* Gilligan, C. (1982). *In A Different Voice.* Cambridge: Harvard University Press.

Hadorn, D. C. (1991). The Oregon priority-setting exercise: Quality of life and public policy. *Hastings Center Report, 21*(3, Suppl), 11–16.

Husted, G. L., & Husted, J. H. (1991). *Ethical decision making in nursing.* St. Louis: Mosby Year Book.

Illinois Nurses Association. (1989). Resolution on Reporting Incompetent, Unethical, or Illegal Practice. Chicago: Author.

Joint Commission on Accreditation of Health Care Organizations (1990). *Accreditation manual for hospitals, 1991. Joint Commission Perspectives Insert, 10*(4), B1–B46.

Kilner, J. F. (1990). *Who lives? Who dies? Ethical criteria in patient selection.* New Haven: Yale University Press.

* May, W. E. (1978). Double effect. In W. T. Reich (Ed.), *Encyclopedia of bioethics* (pp. 316–320). New York: Macmillan and Free Press.

* Morrison, J., Crinklaw-Wiancko, D., King, D., Thibeault, S., & Wells, D. L. (1984). Formulating a restraint use policy. *Journal of Nursing Administration, 3,* 39–42.

* Newell, A., & Simon, H. A. (1972). *Human problem solving.* Englewood Cliffs, NJ: Prentice-Hall, Inc.

* Ratzan, R. M. (1987). The use of physical force. *Postgraduate Medicine, 81*(1), 125, 128.

* Robbins, L. J. (1986). Restraining the elderly patient. *Clinics in Geriatric Medicine, 2*(3), 591–597.

* Rokeach, M. (1973). *The nature of human values.* New York: The Free Press.

Rushton, C. H., & Lynch, M. E. (1992, June). Dealing with advance directives for critically ill adolescents. *Critical Care Nurses,* 31–37.

* Shelly, J. A. (1980). *Dilemma.* Downers Grove, IL: Inter-Varsity Press.

* Simon, H. A. (1978). Information-processing theory of human problem solving. In W. K. Estes (Ed.). *Handbook of learning and cognitive processes* (Vol. 5, pp. 271–295). Hillsdale, NJ: Lawrence Erlbaum Associates.

* Steele, S. M., & Harmon, V. M. (1983). *Values clarification in nursing* (2nd ed.). Norwalk, CT: Appleton-Century-Crofts.

* Thompson, J., & Thompson, H. O. (1985). *Bioethical decision-making for nurses.* Norwalk, CT: Appleton-Century-Crofts.

Unkle, D. (1993, Winter). Bioethics of organ transplantation. *Med-Surg Nursing Quarterly,* 1–13.

* Veatch, R. M. (1980). Voluntary risks to health. *Journal of the American Medical Association, 243*(1), 50–55.

* Walters, L. (1982). Euthanasia and the prolongation of life. In T. L. Beauchamp & L. Walters (Eds.), *Contemporary issues in bioethics* (2nd ed., pp. 307–312). Belmont, CA: Wadsworth.

* Weir, R. F. (1989). *Abating Treatment with Critically Ill Patients: Medical and Legal Limits to the Medical Prolongation.* New York: Oxford University Press.

Wicclair, M. R. (1991). Differentiating ethical decisions from clinical standards. *Dimensions of critical care nursing, 10*(5), 280–288.

* Winslade, W. (1978). Confidentiality. In W. T. Reich (Ed.) *Encyclopedia of bioethics* (Vol. 1, pp. 194–200). New York: The Free Press.

* Witt, P. (1983). Notes of a whistleblower. *American Journal of Nursing, 83,* 1649–1651.

SUGGESTED READINGS

Bandman, E. L., & Bandman, B. (1990). *Nursing ethics through the life span* (2nd ed.). Norwalk, CT: Appleton-Lange.

Individual chapters are devoted to the various stages in the life span. In each of these chapters, the authors present selected cases with related ethical principles and identify nursing judgments and actions. Traditional and contemporary models of ethical decision-making and the pitfalls that can occur in moral reasoning are also discussed.

Benjamin, M., & Curtis, J. (1992). *Ethics in nursing* (3rd ed.). New York: Oxford University Press.

Benjamin and Curtis have updated their book in this third edition to include topics on cost containment and health care rationing. In providing cases to illustrate the ethical issues, they address the major issues that medical-surgical nurses will face. Especially helpful is the chapter on recurring ethical issues in nurse-physician relationships.

Unkle, D. (1993, Winter). Bioethics of organ transplantation. *Med-Surg Nursing Quarterly,* 1–13.

This article discusses the weaknesses of the allocation process and donor shortage. Several ethical arguments, including costs, are discussed. The author also presents a table outlining how various religions view organ and tissue donation and transplantation.

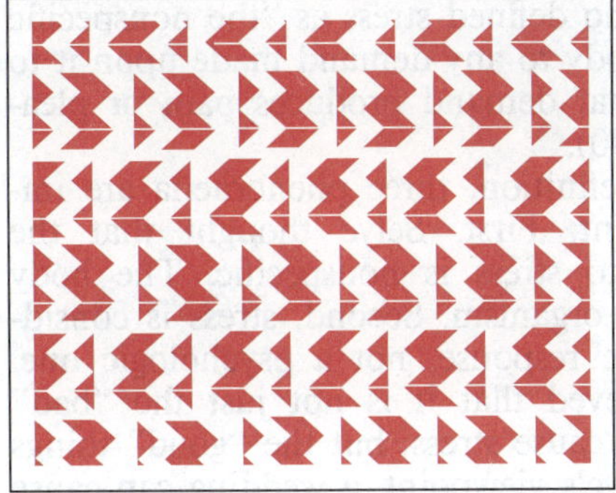

CHAPTER 7

Stress, Coping, and Adaptation

CHAPTER HIGHLIGHTS

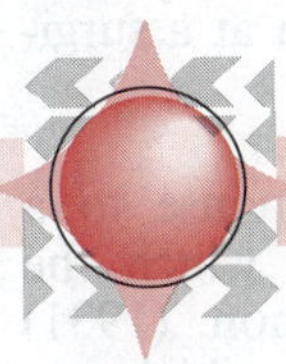

Stress is a familiar concept, yet there is little consensus as to its meaning. Biologists consider stress at a cellular level, whereas engineers speak of stress in structural terms. When laypeople speak of stress, they may say that it is an actual feeling of being overwhelmed: to others, stress is the cause of this feeling. In the social sciences, including nursing, the concept of stress has evolved to include both the feeling and the event.

OVERVIEW

DEFINITIONS

STRESS

Stress is a relationship between a person and the environment that the person perceives as taxing or dangerous (Lazarus & Folkman, 1984). The cognitive evaluation, or thought process, that an event is stressful is called an "appraisal" of stress. A *stressor* is the taxing or dangerous physical, psychologic, social, or environmental event that leads to the appraisal of stress. Following are some examples of stressors:

- *Physiologic:* Injuries; infectious, viral, or fungal agents; radiation; drugs; and alcohol.
- *Psychologic:* Frustrations, loss of control, and anger.

- *Social:* Losses of social support, problems in living arrangements, and the difficulties associated with low economic status.
- *Environmental:* Pollution, the hazards of the workplace, and extremes of temperature.

COPING

To deal with stress effectively, people try to cope by using specific strategies. Coping strategies are the ways by which people try to control the causative problem or stress-related feelings. Some examples of coping strategies are denial, use of social supports, confrontation of the problem, and consideration of the positive aspects of the situation. These strategies are described later in this chapter.

ADAPTATION

Adaptation occurs when a person has mastered, changed, or accepted the stressful event. Adaptation implies that a sense of equilibrium is restored to the person disordered by stress. Adaptation is reflected in one or more changes in a person's psychologic, social, or physical health.

THE IMPORTANCE OF STRESS IN MEDICAL-SURGICAL NURSING PRACTICE

Stress is particularly important in the practice of medical-surgical nursing for adults because its presence may cause, prolong, or aggravate a client's illness. Stress can interfere with other aspects of clients' lives because it may contribute to family, spiritual, and social crises.

Clients use a variety of strategies to deal with stress. Nurses are commonly in positions in which they can aid the clients' coping, either through assisting the clients' self-initiated efforts or by suggesting alternatives. Successful coping and adaptation are the goals of both the client and the nurse. All clients want stress to be reduced to manageable levels or want it to be eliminated.

THEORIES ABOUT STRESS

Stress has been studied from three major viewpoints. First, researchers have viewed stress as the body's physical response to threat. Second, stress has been considered to be a stimulus, or outside force, that causes a reaction. Third, stress has been examined as a transaction between the person and the event.

STRESS AS A RESPONSE

The biologic and medical sciences have traditionally viewed stress as the body's response to an event; that is, stress is the physiologic response or change that occurs within the body. The idea of stress as a response gained prominence through the classic work of Hans Selye, who defined stress as "the nonspecific response of the body to any demand made upon it to adapt, whether that demand produces pain or pleasure" (1946, p. 230).

From Selye's definition, three phenomena are immediately apparent. First, Selye thought that the body's response to stress is nonspecific. The body reacts as a whole organism. Second, stress is considered a physiologic response, not a psychologic one. Third, Selye believed that it is not just the "bad" things in life that cause stress, but the "good" things as well. From Selye's viewpoint, a wedding can cause the same physiologic response as a funeral. Selye called the body's generalized response to a stressor the *general adaptation syndrome* (GAS) (Fig. 7–1). This syndrome has three distinct stages:

1. The alarm stage.
2. The stage of resistance.
3. The stage of exhaustion.

In addition to recognizing the body's *generalized* response, Selye noted a *localized* response. He labeled the body's limited, localized response as the *localized adaptation syndrome* (LAS). Inflammation at a surgical site is an example of the LAS.

THE ALARM STAGE The physiologic response to a stressor begins with the alarm stage, in which the body prepares itself for survival. Cannon (1931) called this initial physiologic response the "fight-or-flight response." As outlined by Cannon, this response process prepares all animals, including humans, for survival. When faced with danger, the body prepares to either fight the danger or flee from it. Either reaction is thought to cause the same changes in the body.

The stress-related changes are coordinated by the central nervous system (CNS). Within the CNS, the limbic system is the emotional response center that triggers the fight-or-flight response. The limbic system then activates the hypothalamus. The hypothalamus in turn initiates the stress response and directs the activities of the autonomic nervous system (ANS), composed of the sympathetic and parasympathetic systems. The ANS controls the body's involuntary responses, such as hormone secretions, metabolism, and fluid regulation.

The sympathetic system of the ANS is responsible for dynamic change, and the parasympathetic system is responsible for restoring the body to its normal resting state. In response to stress, the sympathetic nervous system stimulates the adrenal medulla, which in turn secretes the catecholamines norepinephrine and epinephrine. The adrenal cortex is also stimulated by the pituitary gland's release of adrenocorticotropic hormone (ACTH). The circulating ACTH causes the adrenal cortex to release glucocorticoids (cortisol, corticosterone, and cortisone) and mineralcorticoids (aldosterone and deoxycorticosterone). As a result of the CNS and adrenal activity, seven major changes occur within the body:

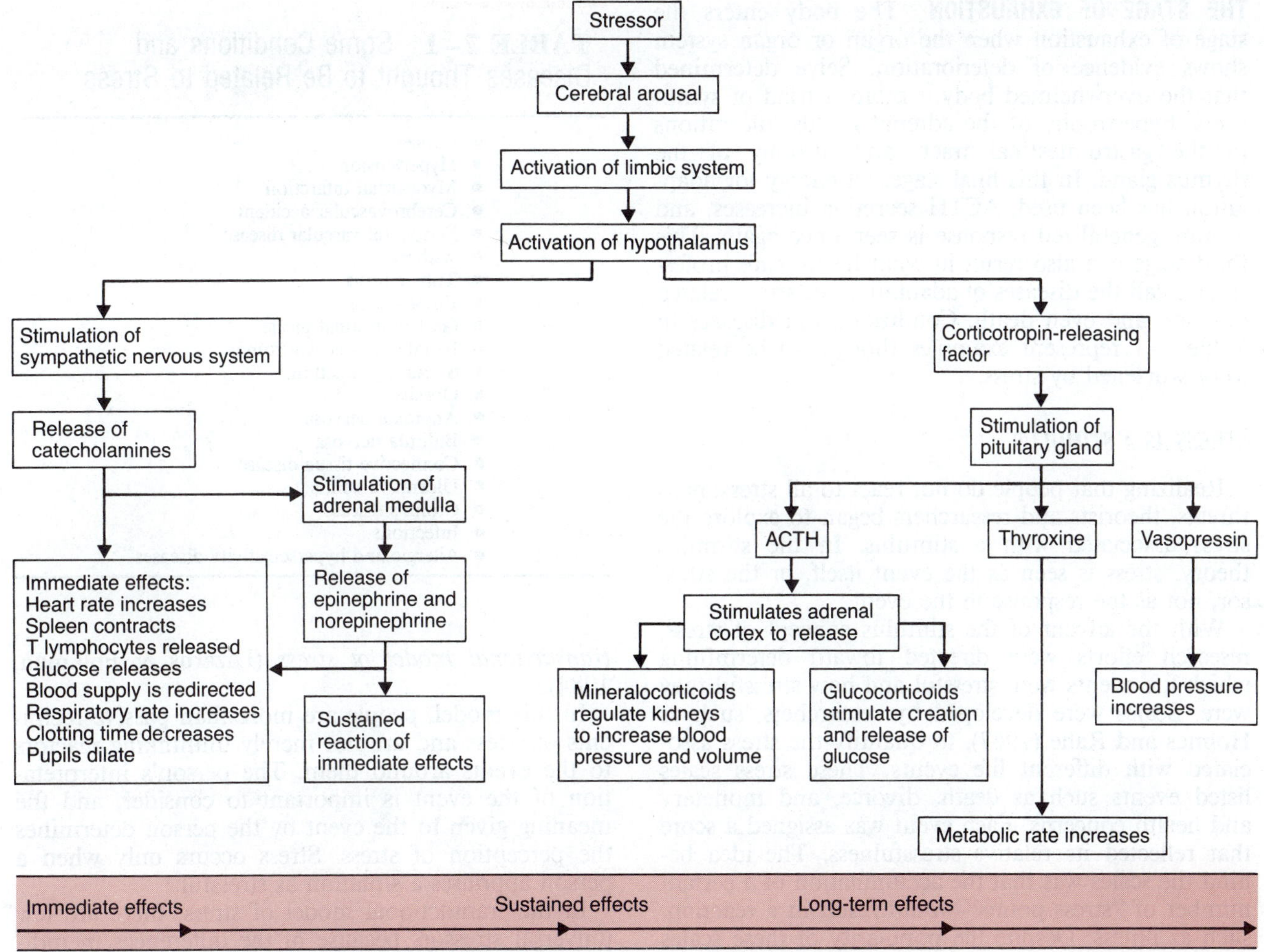

FIGURE 7-1 ◆ The general adaptation syndrome.

- *Increase in heart rate,* to ensure that adequate oxygen and nutrients are available to the muscles and organs.
- *Contraction of the spleen,* to reduce the amount of blood lost from the spleen in case of injury and to release T lymphocytes into the bloodstream for defense.
- *Release of glucose,* to fuel the body for response to danger.
- *Redirection of blood supply,* to ensure blood flow to the vital organs, such as the brain.
- *Changes in the respiratory system* (increased respiratory rate and depth), to provide for effective oxygen–carbon dioxide exchange.
- *Decrease in blood clotting time,* to decrease blood loss in case of body injury.
- *Dilation of pupils,* to enhance vision.

These major changes, plus minor changes, such as increased perspiration and piloerection (hairs standing on end), appear to occur whenever a person is threatened. Selye called these collective processes the alarm stage in the body's preparation for survival. Although these preparations may have been useful in human beings' past, they have limited utility in most of today's threat situations. It is unfortunate that these reactions persist because they result in tremendous wear and tear on the body. If these reactions occur frequently or are sustained, a person may experience damage to the body's systems or illness, such as heart disease and diabetes mellitus.

THE STAGE OF RESISTANCE The second stage in the general adaptation syndrome (GAS) is called the stage of resistance. When the body recognizes continued threat, physiologic forces are mobilized to maintain an increased resistance to stressors. This resistance begins with a decrease in the production of ACTH. The body concentrates its activities on those organs or organ systems that are most involved in the specific stress response. Successful adaptation implies positive growth toward a return to or improvement in physical health. The efforts of the body to resist stress may be ineffectual, leading to a state of maladaptation in which there is deterioration in levels of physical functioning. Chronic resistance eventually causes damage to the involved systems.

THE STAGE OF EXHAUSTION The body enters the stage of exhaustion when the organ or organ system shows evidence of deterioration. Selye determined that the overwhelmed body exhibits a triad of symptoms: hypertrophy of the adrenal glands, ulcerations in the gastrointestinal tract, and atrophy of the thymus gland. In this final stage, all energy for adaptation has been used, ACTH secretion increases, and a more generalized response is seen once again. This third stage can also result in what health care professionals call the diseases of adaptation, or stress-related diseases, and even death. Conditions and diseases in Table 7–1 represent examples thought to be related to or worsened by stress.

TABLE 7–1 Some Conditions and Diseases Thought to Be Related to Stress

- Cancer
- Hypertension
- Myocardial infarction
- Cerebrovascular accident
- Peripheral vascular disease
- Asthma
- Tuberculosis
- Emphysema
- Gastrointestinal ulcers
- Irritable bowel syndrome
- Sexual dysfunctions
- Obesity
- Anorexia nervosa
- Bulimia nervosa
- Connective tissue disease
- Ulcerative colitis
- Crohn's disease
- Infections
- Allergic and hypersensitivity diseases

STRESS AS A STIMULUS

Realizing that people do not react to all stressors as threats, theorists and researchers began to explore the stress associated with a stimulus. In the stimulus theory, stress is seen as the event itself, or the stressor, not as the response to the event.

With the advent of the stimulus concept of stress, research efforts were directed toward determining which life events were stressful and how stressful they were. Scales were developed by researchers, such as Holmes and Rahe (1967), to quantify the stress associated with different life events. These stress scales listed events such as death, divorce, and monetary and health concerns. Each event was assigned a score that reflected its relative stressfulness. The idea behind the scales was that the accumulation of a certain number of "stress points" would result in a reaction, such as illness. Despite the popularity of these scales in both the scientific and the lay literature, they have not proved to be valid as predictors of stress, especially in relation to illness. No research has been able to show more than a limited predictive relation between stressful life events and illness, hospitalization, and mortality.

Although the usefulness of stress scales has not proved valid, common sense indicates that certain events can and do provoke physiologic manifestations and feelings of stress. It seems, however, that the events that provoke stress symptoms may not always be life's major events but, rather, the minor annoyances of everyday life. These daily stresses, or "hassles," have shown more relation to illness than have the major life events (DeLongis et al., 1982). Within the hospital setting, there are many potential hassles that can increase stress. Table 7–2 presents examples of environmental and psychologic hassles common to hospitalization and illness.

STRESS AS A TRANSACTION BETWEEN A PERSON AND THE ENVIRONMENT

Gradually, nurse researchers and others have come to realize that all events have different meanings for different people. The perception of stress appears to be related to the person and event within a certain environment. The view of stress as a relation between the person and the environmental event is called the *transactional model of stress* (Lazarus & Folkman, 1984).

In this model, people are more than passive recipients of stress and are not merely unthinking reactors to the events around them. The person's interpretation of the event is important to consider, and the meaning given to the event by the person determines the perception of stress. Stress occurs only when a person appraises a situation as stressful.

In the transactional model of stress, there are few universal stressors because of the differences in individual appraisal. *Appraisal* is the cognitive evaluation of events (primary appraisal) and available coping resources (secondary appraisal). No event can be considered inherently stressful, not even tornadoes, hurricanes, and other disasters that are generally thought of as stressful. The transactional model states that

TABLE 7–2 Potential Hassles Common to Hospitalization and Illness

- Eating different foods at different times
- Having a stranger for a roommate
- Sleeping in a different bed
- Using a different pillow
- Being awakened at odd hours
- Feeling too hot or too cold
- Smelling hospital odors
- Hearing strange hospital noises
- Having movement restricted
- Being unable to obtain desired objects
- Having too many visitors
- Having no or few visitors
- Worrying about bills, job, or family concerns
- Being uncertain of one's diagnosis
- Not understanding medical language
- Being dependent on others for bathing or toileting
- Being embarrassed about revealing body parts or intimate details
- Having to deal with large numbers of health care workers

there is no way of predicting how a person will respond. Although some people experience a stress reaction to these major events, many others do not. These differences are a result of individual appraisal.

Several factors contribute to a person's perception that an event is stressful. These include factors specific to the person, the environment, or the event itself. Effective nursing care must include an understanding of the many factors that enter into a client's decision that an event is stressful.

APPRAISAL FACTORS RELATED TO THE PERSON

Depth of Feeling One important factor in an appraisal of stress is the depth of feeling that the event arouses in a person. Events about which people feel strongly are more likely to produce stress than events that arouse little or no feeling. For example, if hospitalization interferes with an important life event, such as marriage, the client's appraisal may result in a perception of stress.

Beliefs Along with commitments, beliefs also influence the appraisal of stress. For example, a person with a strongly held religious belief that God can influence the course of life's events may appraise events differently from someone with other spiritual beliefs.

Control Control is also important to the stress-coping response. Many researchers have reported that most people want to maintain a sense of control over their world. For that reason, not having control can be appraised as a stressor. The key to understanding control is the recognition that control means different things to different people and in different situations. Although it is obvious that ill or hospitalized clients cannot control situations such as the course of illness, research has identified a list of areas in which most people seek control even when they are sick (Moos & Tsu, 1977). These areas include:

- Avoidance of pain and incapacitation
- The immediate hospital environment
- Treatments and procedures
- Relationships with hospital personnel
- Emotional balance
- A satisfactory self-image
- Relationships with family and friends
- Preparing for an uncertain future

This list is important for three reasons. First, it alerts nurses that people may seek control over most aspects of their lives, whether they are ill or not. Second, the loss of a sense of control can occur because of the nature of the hospital environment. The loss of a sense of control is stressful to many people. Third, there are some people who do not want active control. People who do not desire control may experience stress when they are given control. Nurses should ascertain how much control clients want before insisting or recommending that they take control.

ENVIRONMENTAL EVENT FACTORS RELATED TO STRESS APPRAISAL Differences in the appraisal of environmental event factors influence whether a person perceives an event as stressful.

Unpredictability of Events One factor that can make a difference in the appraisal of events is their unpredictability. People generally believe that a predictable event is less stressful than a similar unpredictable event. This is partly because with time, people can prepare. Being able to prepare for events appears to be related to a reduction in stress. Without the necessary time or information needed for preparation, events may appear more stressful than they need to be. If possible, the nurse should give clients sufficient information and time to comprehend a potentially stressful event, such as an uncomfortable procedure, before the client experiences it.

Uncertainty of Events The client's uncertainty about an event can also increase its potential stressfulness. It appears that most people like to know what to expect. Although this is true of life events in general, people especially like to know the odds about health-related events. The key to understanding much of the stress experienced by clients with chronic disease may lie in their uncertainty about the disease course. Not knowing how a disease will evolve or the chances of recovery can be very stressful. Clients with cancer often provide a good example of the effects of uncertainty. Despite such treatments as extensive surgery, chemotherapy, and radiation, many clients can never be completely sure of a cure. Thus, the uncertainty of the event enhances its appraisal as stressful.

Timing of Events The timing of events also has an impact on the level of stress. Events that are considered to be in the distant future are usually perceived as less stressful than events that are closer in time. The time that elapses between the client's hearing about an event and its occurrence can also influence appraisal. Although the stress may be manageable for a period of time, the longer a person is kept waiting, the harder it is to control the thoughts about what is to come. Thus, the appraisal of threat can build up when too much time elapses. People need sufficient time to prepare for events. However, too long a period of anticipation can have a negative effect. Unfortunately, there are no set guidelines as to timing for nurses who prepare clients for tests and procedures.

The timing of an event in relation to one's stage of life is also important. Having a heart attack at age 25 may be more stressful than at age 80. Any life event that occurs at an unexpected time can be more stressful than one occurring at a time of life when it is expected.

Duration of Events Another factor related to timing is the duration of events. Chronic, long-term events can sometimes wear down a person's ability to cope. Like Selye's stage of exhaustion, constant demands over a long time can have massive psychologic as well as physical effects. However, people can also become accustomed to long-term events. The difference between the two reactions may lie in a person's appraisal or in the coping strategies used.

Ambiguity of Events Knowing what will happen, when it will happen, and how long it will last is important to the appraisal of stress. Yet, even with this information, there are always unknown elements. The unknown elements contribute to the ambiguity, or vagueness, of the experience. Ambiguity is important to appraisal. Generally, the more vague a situation, the more stressful. Ambiguity can also influence what coping strategies are used. People usually choose their coping strategies on the basis of the information that they have. If information is missing, however, the planning of specific and appropriate coping strategies is not possible.

According to Lazarus and Folkman's theory, the effectiveness of coping mechanisms depends on the accuracy of the appraisal of a stressful situation. Because people may not correctly appraise a situation and because no one can predict the future, misappraisals cannot be avoided—they are part of life. It is the degree of difference between the appraisal of what will happen and the reality of what occurs that makes a difference in coping effectiveness. Because situations are constantly changing, coping effectiveness also depends on the person's ability to reappraise and change strategies as necessary (Fig. 7–2).

THEORIES ABOUT COPING

Coping is any behavioral or cognitive activity that is used to deal with stress. If an event is perceived as taxing or dangerous, coping should occur. The concept of coping implies that most people do not remain passive and allow events to happen; rather, they react. The reactions to a stress-provoking event can be either to use the problem-solving approach to change the event (problem-focused coping) or to change emotional reactions to the event (emotion-focused coping). Coping strategies vary from person to person and event to event. It is thought that people generally use coping strategies that they have found successful in the past. If a strategy is not successful in the current situation, others may be considered.

PROBLEM-FOCUSED COPING

PROBLEM-SOLVING In many cases, the best way to deal with a causative stressor is to try to change or eliminate the problem. A major coping strategy is problem-solving. The inability to use problem-solving was identified by 513 clinical specialists as the major indicator of the nursing diagnosis of Ineffective Individual Coping (Vincent, 1985). In 1992, the North American Nursing Diagnosis Association (NANDA) suggested that "Ineffective" be replaced with "Impaired."

Problem-solving as a coping strategy involves the same skills that are used in the nursing process. In problem-solving coping, a person defines the problem, lists alternatives, chooses the best alternative, and applies it to the problem. When asked about problem-solving coping, people may state that they try to find out more about the problem at hand, analyze the problem, make a plan, and follow it.

Some problem-solving activity is also directed inward. In this case, the coping activity is directed at how the problem is faced. Inward-focused problem-solving solutions might include learning new skills, changing aspirations, or finding other avenues of personal reward.

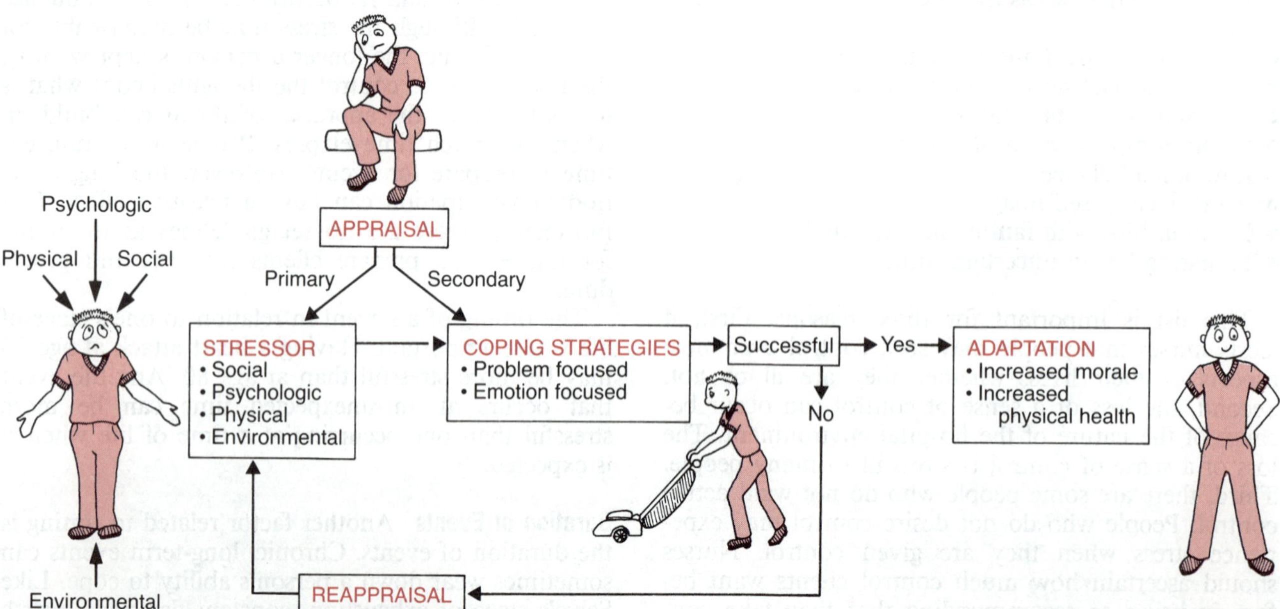

FIGURE 7–2 ◆ Appraisal and coping mechanisms.

When people use problem-solving, they need accurate information and accurate appraisal so that their plans to deal with the stressor are based on reality. Nurses can ask clients if they have made any plans, on what the plans are based, and what is involved in these plans. When plans are unrealistic, the nurse helps the client by sharing his or her expertise and information.

CONFRONTIVE COPING Many people cope by confronting the problem that is causing the stress. Confrontive coping is often used successfully in dealing with life's problems, such as those in the workplace. In addition, confrontive coping may be used when less forceful coping strategies have failed to alleviate the perception of stress. Clients in health care situations may use confrontive coping by aggressively seeking information, refusing treatments, and expressing their anger. Although not all confrontive-type coping activities reflect aggression, many times anger is the primary indicator that the client feels stressed and is attempting to cope. The expressions of anger in confrontive coping often reflect feelings of anxiety and powerlessness in the client.

Although these two problem-focused coping strategies are commonly used, they are not the only ways to cope. Nurses who are interested in supporting the client should find out how the client has coped in the past, how he or she plans to cope with the new stresses, and how other clients with the same problem have coped.

EMOTION-FOCUSED COPING

Some people are more skilled at problem-solving than others, and some problems are easier to resolve than others. When problem-focused strategies are not appropriate or are not sufficient, emotion-focused strategies are used. In some cases, a person may use both problem-focused and emotion-focused coping. Emotion-focused strategies reduce the emotional manifestations of stress, such as anxiety and anger.

DISTANCING STRATEGIES A vast array of distancing strategies are frequently used for coping in health-related situations. Some people deny a problem or blame others, and some people accept responsibility for their contribution to the occurrence of stress—they appear to be seeking a sense of control over life events. The refusal of a person who has had a motor vehicle accident while drinking alcohol to accept some blame is an example of distancing.

DRAWING STRENGTH FROM ADVERSITY A related coping strategy is drawing strength from adversity by growing as a person, finding new faith, and rediscovering what is important in life. At other times, strategies that emphasize the positive aspects of an event can be effective. Trying to have a positive outlook, looking on the bright side, and telling oneself that things could be worse are examples of this form of coping.

TENSION REDUCTION Coping strategies aimed at tension reduction can also be used to deal with stress. Some healthy means of reducing tension may include meditation, yoga exercises, biofeedback, and physical exercise. Other ways of coping, although not healthy, are to reduce tension through the use of alcohol or other so-called recreational drugs. Eating modifications, such as overeating or undereating, can also be used as inappropriate attempts to cope.

HOSTILITY VERSUS HUMOR Hostility may reflect coping activity in some clients. Anger, irritability, childish reactions, or demonstration of temper are reflective of hostility. A more positive expression of feelings that can reflect coping is humor. Humor is a commonly used coping activity (Weinberger, 1991). Many clients make jokes or make light of serious situations when they are under stress.

FATALISM Even fatalism can be used as a coping strategy. When using fatalism, clients say they will take a wait-and-see attitude, leave it in God's hands, or accept what has happened to them. Fatalism is usually accompanied by a sense that there is nothing that can be done about the problem.

SOCIAL SUPPORT Support by family, friends, and the community can be helpful in coping. Social support is often a powerful aid in coping and can be extremely important to those in need of health care. By seeking support from others, people can gain information, physical help, and other forms of assistance. Both the type of help and the number of people willing to help can make a difference to the client's coping success.

Hospital rules and regulations often interfere with a client's ability to obtain the social support he or she needs. The interference with support can be especially acute within ethnic groups with large, close, and supportive families, such as in the Hispanic culture. Loss of social support can result when hospitalization occurs at a physical distance from the client's family, when elderly clients have outlived friends and relatives, or when the client has a socially stigmatizing illness, such as acquired immunodeficiency syndrome (AIDS). The inability to use a coping strategy on which one had previously depended, such as social support, can result in further stress.

FAITH Faith in God, a deity, or an ultimate meaning of life can be an effective aid to coping. For people who have a strong faith, the attitude of relinquishing control to God or believing in transcendence can be beneficial. Prayer, increased religious activity, and even a calm acceptance of God's will or an ultimate purpose are all forms of coping when they help reduce the perception of stress (Fig. 7–3).

EVENT REHEARSAL If time allows, coping often begins before the stress event occurs, through event rehearsal. Event rehearsal is the mental or physical preparation in anticipation of an event or the practice of coping strategies before the event occurs. For ex-

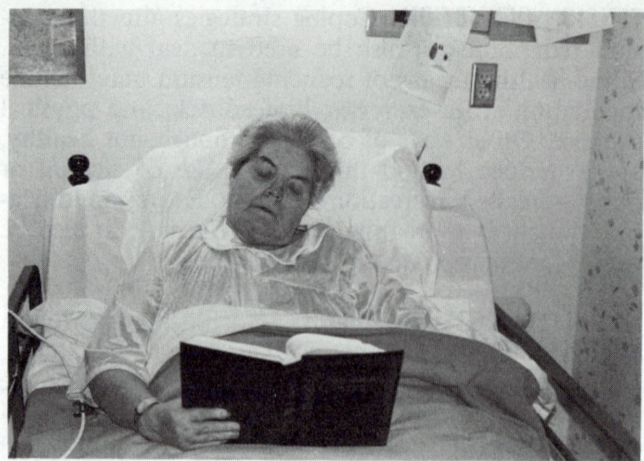

FIGURE 7-3 ◆ A hospitalized client reading the Bible to help her cope with stress.

ample, clients who are to undergo elective surgery begin to plan their coping strategies before the actual surgery occurs. If time allows before a potentially stressful event, clients may mentally envision how they will react or handle the situation. Some authors have called this preparatory coping the "work of worrying" (Janis, 1985). However, that term implies that clients are concerned with only the negative aspects of an upcoming experience and ignores the fact that clients may focus on the positive aspects as well.

EVENT REVIEW After a stressful event, many people cope by reviewing the event. This review can be mental, verbal, or both. Event review probably helps people to cope by giving them the opportunity to understand what has happened to them. Often, during a stress event, there is no time to process the incoming information. Review after an event occurs when there is time and energy available for processing. Nurses aid coping through review by encouraging clients to think or talk about their experiences.

People cope with the same problem in a variety of ways. Most nurses agree that coping in the hospital setting can be successfully accomplished through any one of a number of avenues. Common coping strategies are presented in Table 7-3.

THEORIES ABOUT ADAPTATION

If a client has coped effectively, the stress or the emotional reaction to stress is eliminated or managed and a sense of equilibrium is restored. Restored equilibrium that results from coping is called adaptation. Some nurse theorists, such as Roy and Roberts (1981), have incorporated the concept of adaptation into their theory or model of nursing practice.

Adaptation is dependent on accurate appraisal of a stressful situation and effective coping. Adaptation can have many outcomes. The two results with the most significance to nursing are psychologic and physical well-being.

PSYCHOLOGIC ADAPTATION: MORALE

People who cope adequately, it is hoped, will be satisfied with how they coped and the outcome reached. If a client believes that the correct decision was made with regard to health care issues, such as agreeing to hospitalization, choosing medical professionals, or handling pain or discomfort, the challenge of the stress has been met and coping is viewed as effective. The ability to see stress as a challenge to be overcome is important to the long-term maintenance of morale.

Morale is related to emotional equilibrium and the sense of well-being. In the past, many researchers considered well-being as the absence of depression or other signs of poor psychologic health. More recently, the approach has changed: well-being is assessed through positive indicators, such as happiness and contentment. Healthy psychologic adaptation is reflected in the client's sense of well-being.

PHYSICAL ADAPTATION: SOMATIC HEALTH

Stress is consistently blamed for causing all illness and unhappiness. Diseases in which it can be determined that the mind influences the body's processes are called *psychophysiologic* (previously called psychosomatic). Stress is thought to be a major factor in psychophysiologic disease. Interestingly, the link between stress and illness is far from clear. Some evidence indicates that stress may suppress the effectiveness of the immune system and thus predispose a person to infection, cancer, and other diseases

TABLE 7-3 Common Coping Strategies

Coping Strategy	Examples
Event rehearsal	• Mental and verbal preparation for an event • Practice of coping strategies
Confrontation	• Aggressive information-seeking • Anger • Refusal of treatments
Distancing or denial	• Unwillingness or inability to talk about events • Going on as if nothing has happened
Self-control	• Stoicism • Showing no feelings
Social support	• Seeking out family, friends, or others in similar situations
Accepting responsibility	• Verbally placing responsibility for a situation on oneself
Faith	• Praying • Reading religious material • Seeking out clergy or religious guidance
Problem-solving	• Making plans • Verbally outlining what will be done next
Positive reappraisal	• Speaking of how the situation has fostered growth
Event review	• Discussing situations or coping that has occurred

thought to be related to the immune system (see Table 7–1). Stress may also weaken the body so that any pathogens or toxic agents are more damaging than they would otherwise be. Other evidence indicates that stress may precipitate damage so that it occurs at a faster rate than normal, such as in cardiovascular disease.

At one time, it was hoped that a direct link could be found either between the stress event and illness or between personality type and illness. At that time, it was not uncommon to hear professionals speak of a colitis, ulcer, or arthritis personality. However, none of these theories has held up under study. No research has been able to show a strong relationship among incidence of illness, personality type, and stress.

THE CONCEPT OF HARDINESS

Research into the relationship between illness and personality characteristics is currently focused on hardiness, which is the ability to resist the effects of stress. The attribute of hardiness may be one reason why some people are negatively affected by exposure to stress and others are not. Hardiness is related to three personality characteristics:

1. Hardy people have a sense of *commitment* to work, a way of life, or ideals that provides them with a sense of satisfaction, motivation, and, possibly achievement.
2. Hardy people look at life's occurrences as *challenges,* not threats. These people welcome change for the growth it promotes. They are optimistic and curious about life.
3. Hardy people have a sense of *control* over their lives. They do not feel helpless in the face of what happens to them. On the other hand, people who are low in measures of hardiness usually appear bored, are hopeless, and lack enthusiasm.

Commitment, challenge, and control may be three reasons why differences exist in the ability to adapt to stress. Hardiness may actually help buffer the effects of stress. People who are hardy may be more resilient, or "tougher," in the face of life's ups and downs.

Because hardiness may be a personality characteristic, experts are unsure as to whether people can be taught to be hardy. However, attempts to increase hardiness may be beneficial. Table 7–4 shows a few examples of ways in which clients may increase commitment, challenge, and control in everyday life.

TABLE 7–4 Techniques for Increasing Hardiness

Personality Characteristic	Techniques
Commitment	• Capitalize on skills and interests to develop hobbies. • Reduce time spent watching television. • Develop a list outlining why one's work is important to the community. • Recognize and acknowledge self-worth. • Join a volunteer organization that provides services to help others. • Join political, social, or religious organizations.
Challenge	• Take a controlled physical risk, e.g., become involved in Outward Bound, take a glider flight or parachute jump, or undertake a new sport. • Take a vacation that involves little or no planning. • Take a course or attend a talk on a topic that questions one's own values. • Vary daily activities and change routines.
Control	• Set aside a period of time each week to do exactly what one wants. • Volunteer for leadership positions in clubs and organizations. • Become active in the political process; vote. • Seek work situations in which control is increased. • Recognize the enormous amount of control one can exercise over his or her own life.

COLLABORATIVE MANAGEMENT

ASSESSMENT

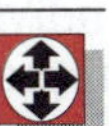

The first step in helping clients to deal with stress is to obtain an accurate assessment of the stress situation. The problem may be in the client's appraisal of the situation, in how the client is coping, or in the inherent stressfulness of the situation, which cannot be controlled or changed. The nurse should assess all aspects of the stress response before determining which nursing interventions are appropriate.

ASSESSMENT OF STRESS

HISTORY

The nurse asks the client to identify possible stressors that may explain or contribute to feelings of stress. The nurse also assesses the client's perception of stress and stress responses. Questions should not be limited to health care history because personal and professional stressors may be more pertinent than health state. The nurse uses careful interviewing techniques to ensure that accurate information is obtained from the client, family, or both.

PHYSICAL ASSESSMENT/CLINICAL MANIFESTATIONS

Within a hospital or ambulatory setting, many situations can serve as major stress initiators. Clients may have illnesses brought on by or aggravated by stress. Because of the potential, serious physical effects of the stress response, nurses are interested in the physiologic signs that identify people experiencing stress (Chart 7-1). One of the most obvious of these signs is heart rate. Although increased heart rate is a stress-related response, heart rate by itself has not proved to be a reliable indicator of the presence of stress. Among the reasons for this unpredictability is that heart rate varies with almost any stimulus, from movement to illness. Thus, heart rate is not specific enough to be a valid sign of stress. The correlation of stress and blood pressure has demonstrated the same problem.

A variety of physical complaints may also reflect stress in the client. Examples of stress-related complaints are headaches, neckaches, stomachaches, muscular cramping, and other signs of muscular tension. Some people perspire, some get pale, and others become flushed under stress. Many people experience alterations in their patterns of elimination, both bowel and urinary. Eating patterns may also reflect change, with some people eating more than usual and others eating less. Sleep patterns may be disrupted, with some clients experiencing insomnia and others wanting to sleep more than usual. The patterns of these changes are as different as the people involved.

CHART 7-1

Nursing Care Highlight ◆ Assessing for Common Signs of Stress

Physical Signs

- Sleep problems
- Headaches
- Shaking
- Inability to sit still
- Muscle tenseness
- Rapid speech, stuttering, or stammering
- Fatigue
- Increased heart rate
- Digestive troubles
- Increased perspiration
- Light-headedness
- Cold chills
- Hot flashes
- Palpitations
- Dry mouth
- Frequent urination
- Menstrual cycle changes
- Crying

Psychosocial Signs

- Resentment toward health care workers
- Anger, loss of temper
- Feelings of helplessness
- Resistance to treatments or tests
- Overuse of drugs, including prescription and over-the-counter drugs
- Withdrawal from friends and family
- Overuse of alcohol
- Excessive excitement
- Confusion and forgetfulness
- Nervousness
- Irritability
- Complaints of anxiety

PSYCHOSOCIAL ASSESSMENT

Nurses use many obvious psychosocial signs to assess stress behavior (see Chart 7-1). Many of the signs used to assess stress actually reflect coping activity. The more common signs attributed to stress include emotional excesses, such as agitation, anxiety, anger, and apathy. Other signs may include inappropriate or ineffectual coping behaviors, such as denial and blaming. Stress in people may be signaled by expressions of hopelessness, powerlessness, or loss of control; alterations in normal communication patterns, such as a change from extreme talkativeness to silence; and changes in thought processes. Even signs that are considered pathologic, such as manipulative behavior, depression, and withdrawal, may only reflect a person's reaction to tremendous stress.

LABORATORY ASSESSMENT

Levels of epinephrine and norepinephrine are somewhat more predictive than other laboratory values. Unlike steroid products, epinephrine and norepinephrine are released almost instantly in response to stress. Initial research has focused on athletes, astronauts, and others exposed to intense, but transient, stress-provoking episodes. Norepinephrine levels almost always rise when a person is subjected to a stressor, but epinephrine levels tend to stabilize after a brief period of elevation. Although these results are promising, they are only preliminary findings. In addition, it is not always possible to obtain blood for laboratory analysis, and this procedure is invasive.

ASSESSMENT OF APPRAISAL AND COPING

The study of coping, including individual appraisal, is a new area of research, and there are many unanswered questions. Until further studies are available, nurses are best guided by the client in the perception of what is stressful and the best coping strategies to be used.

ASSESSMENT OF APPRAISAL

The nurse first tries to determine what the client perceives as stressful. The nurse asks specific questions about which aspects of hospitalization or illness are stressful. The assessment relates specifically to the appraisal process, with the nurse considering such factors as perceived ambiguity, predictability, and uncertainty of events. The nurse also asks specific questions about how much the client knows about diagnosis, diagnostic testing, and expected length of hospitalization.

The nurse next attempts to learn how stressful these items are perceived by the client. Stress is an individual matter, so it is the client's perception, or appraisal, that is important. One way of determining the level of stress is to ask the client to name the most stressful event possible and then compare the new stressor with that event.

After determining the client's appraisal of the event and the coping methods used, the nurse learns the successful coping strategies that the client has used in the past for similar problems.

Figure 7–4 depicts a guide for interviewing clients about stress and coping.

ASSESSMENT OF SPECIFIC COPING STRATEGIES

Nurses should remember that different individuals cope with the same problem in a variety of ways. If the chosen coping strategy is working, the nurse should support the client in that effort. If the coping strategy is not effective, the nurse works with the client to develop alternatives.

The nurse may note that clients are using event rehearsal if they discuss or talk about the upcoming event or if, when asked, say they have been thinking about the situation. If the event rehearsal is to be effective, clients need information about the stressor. Nurses may also make an assessment that clients are using event rehearsal when clients seek information. Many clients actively solicit information from health care providers, friends, or relatives.

Calling friends and family on the telephone, encouraging visitors, and socializing with others who are in the hospital may reflect the client's use of social support as a coping strategy. Talking with others about what has occurred may reflect the use of event review.

Developing a plan to eliminate or reduce the effect of the stressor can be another form of coping that is reflected in information-seeking behavior. When clients use planned problem-solving, they need accurate information so that the plans they make are based on reality.

If clients purposefully appear to keep their emotions or behaviors in check, they may be using self-control to aid their coping. Stoicism can reflect a personality type or even a culturally approved coping

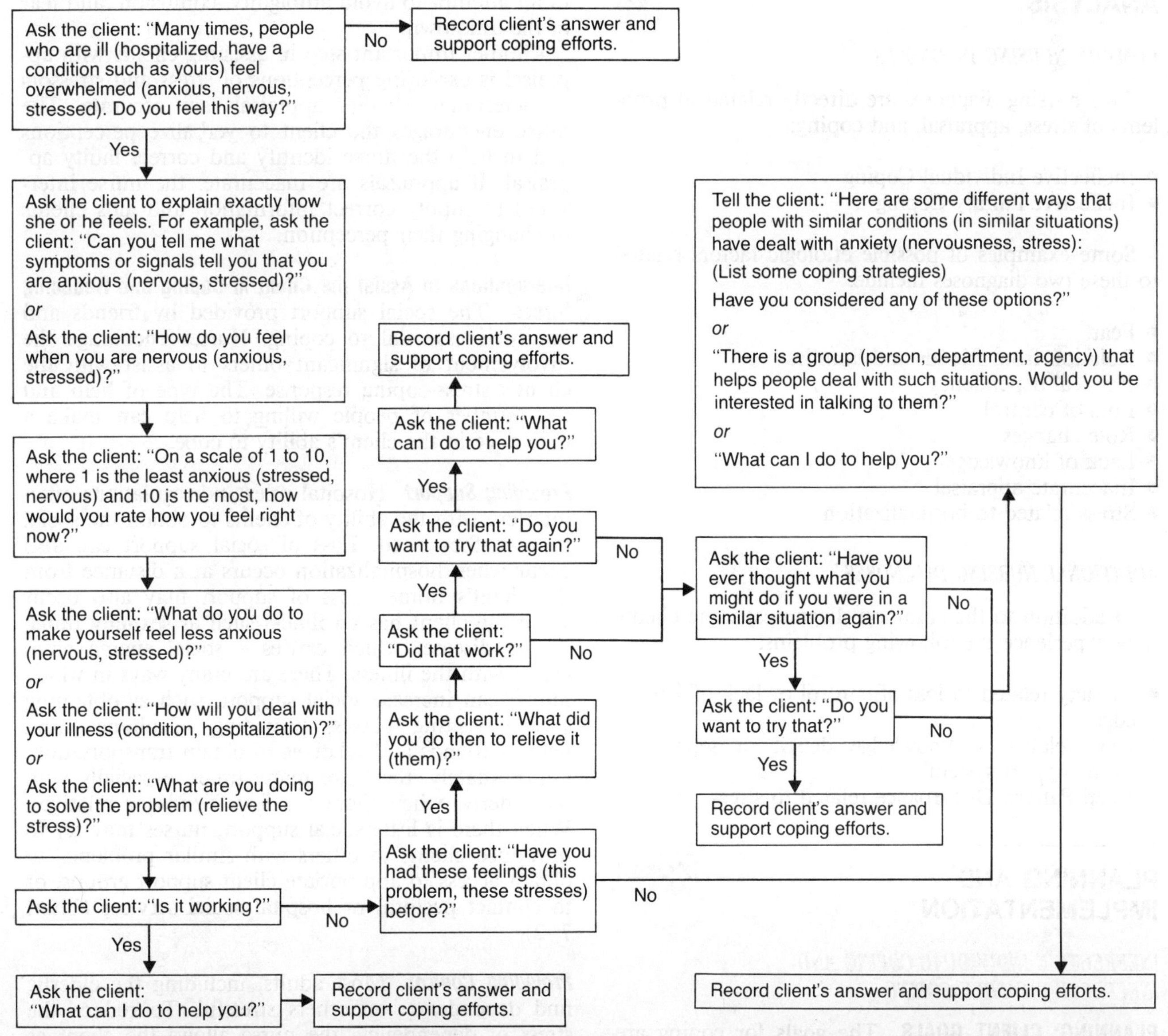

FIGURE 7–4 ◆ A guide for interviewing clients for stress and coping.

strategy. Other more expressive clients may not keep their emotions and feelings in check and may be using confrontive coping strategies. The nurse may also assess anger, hostility, and argumentative behavior in the client as coping strategies.

Nurses may make an assessment of denial or distancing in clients who exhibit avoidance behavior, such as refusing to look at surgical scars or not learning self-care. Clients who do not talk about their conditions, do not prepare for upcoming events, or appear to go on as if nothing had happened to them may also be using denial. Some clients may even exhibit withdrawal behavior by refusing to communicate or by communicating only minimally.

Clients who blame themselves for their illness or hospitalization may be using the coping strategy of self-blame. Clients who use faith as a coping strategy may request clergy visits, use religious articles, and engage in prayer, which are signs that the nurse can observe.

ANALYSIS

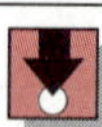

COMMON NURSING DIAGNOSES

Two nursing diagnoses are directly related to problems of stress, appraisal, and coping:

- Ineffective Individual Coping
- Ineffective Family Coping

Some examples of possible etiologic factors related to these two diagnoses include:

- Fear
- Isolation from friends and families
- Physical dependency
- Loss of control
- Role changes
- Lack of knowledge
- Inaccurate appraisal
- Stress related to hospitalization

ADDITIONAL NURSING DIAGNOSES

In addition to the common diagnoses, some clients may experience the following problems:

- Anxiety related to loss of control or lack of knowledge
- Fear related to knowledge deficit or separation from support system
- Sleep Pattern Disturbance related to stress

PLANNING AND IMPLEMENTATION

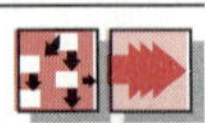

INEFFECTIVE INDIVIDUAL COPING AND INEFFECTIVE FAMILY COPING

PLANNING: CLIENT GOALS The goals for coping are that the client will:

- Develop accurate appraisal of stress situations
- Develop effective coping behaviors
- Experience a reduction in stress

INTERVENTIONS Faulty appraisal or coping may lead to increased stress for the client. Stress may also be the result of the serious nature of health-related problems and hospitalization. After the nurse has assessed that there is a problem in the client's ability to appraise or to cope, many interventions are available. Because of the personal nature of stress, appraisal, and coping, the nurse must remember that there are no universal, standard nursing interventions.

Interventions to Assist the Client in Appraisal Nurses can help clients make more accurate appraisals through client education. Nurses assist clients to recognize and correct faulty appraisal, and they provide positive reinforcement of correct appraisal. Appraisal depends on accurate information. For example, nurses aid clients in appraisal by supplying information about the scheduling and the duration of events in an attempt to avoid ambiguity, confusion, and fear of the unknown.

Another important step in assisting clients with appraisal is exploring perceptions of stress and stressors to determine whether appraisals are accurate. The nurse encourages the client to verbalize perceptions and to help the nurse identify and correct faulty appraisal. If appraisals are inaccurate, the nurse intervenes to supply correct information and aids clients in changing their perception.

Interventions to Assist the Client in Coping and Reducing Stress The social support provided by friends and family is essential to coping. Nurses encourage the involvement of significant others to assist with the client's stress-coping response. The type of help and the number of people willing to help can make a difference in the client's ability to cope.

Providing Support Hospital rules and regulations often interfere with the ability of clients to obtain the social support they need. Loss of social support can also occur when hospitalization occurs at a distance from the client's home. Loss of support may also occur when the client has an illness such as sexually transmitted disease, which carries a social stigma associated with the illness. There are many ways in which nurses can increase social support, such as obtaining special visiting passes, providing telephones, and helping friends and relatives to obtain transportation. Unfortunately, there are many times, especially with the elderly, when there are few friends or relatives. When there is little social support, nurses may try to introduce clients to others with similar problems, to obtain access to appropriate client support groups, or to contact pastoral or hospital social services (Chart 7–2).

Providing Control Most adults, including the elderly, find dependency on others stressful. To reduce the stress of dependency, the nurse allows the client as much physical independence as possible. When phys-

CHART 7-2

Nursing Focus on the Elderly ◆ Reducing Stress

- Assess the client's available social support systems as early as possible.
- Introduce the client to others with similar problems. This may include a change of roommates to match clients to help meet this need.
- Request spiritual support by contacting clergy, requesting religious articles, or saying a prayer, depending on the client's preference. Consider the client's cultural background.
- Take time to listen to the client's concerns.
- Collaborate with the social services department in identifying support systems for the client.
- Allow the client to be as independent as possible, even if it takes more time for a task, such as feeding, to be completed.
- To the extent possible, give the client an opportunity to make decisions about activities of daily living, hospital activities, and nursing interventions.
- Teach information about surgery, procedures, tests, and so forth at a slower pace than for a younger adult.
- Teach the importance of proper rest, sleep, exercise, and nutrition.
- Teach progressive muscle relaxation and guided imagery, if appropriate.

ical independence is not possible, sensitive care by a nurse aware of the client's feelings can be helpful in reducing stress. In most client illnesses, health care personnel expect certain role changes. The client is expected to cooperate, focus on getting well, and be dependent. Each of these role changes can be stressful. If the client finds the change in role to be stressful, the nurse works with the client to develop a plan of care that incorporates maintenance of important role behaviors. Whenever possible, nurses should allow clients who desire it to have control over other activities of daily living, hospital activities, and nursing interventions. Control over such things as times of bathing, food choices, awake and sleep times, and scheduling of therapies and procedures can be very helpful in reducing stress and in maintaining self-esteem.

Providing Information Adequate knowledge may also help clients gain control. Nursing research has shown the importance of client preparation for diagnostic tests and procedures (Johnson, 1972; Johnson & Lauver, 1989). Among the content that should be included in client education are knowledge of the duration of events, expected behaviors, sensations involved, sequencing of activities, and so forth. Nurses should remember that even everyday experiences in the hospital setting, such as the administration of intravenous therapy, can be extremely stressful to the client.

Not all clients want to know about *all* aspects of care and hospitalization (Research Applications for Nursing). For clients who do not know, it is vital that they receive detailed information about those areas in which lack of knowledge is perceived as stressful.

A client's coping strategy of event rehearsal also depends on adequate and correct information about events. Many clients actively seek information from health care providers, friends, relatives, and even comparative strangers who have undergone similar experiences.

After a stress-provoking event, nurses can aid the client's coping through event review by encouraging clients to think or talk about their experiences. Nurses should allow clients to verbally review as much as they need to, even when the account is repetitive. The repetition of thoughts about a threatening event can facilitate coping.

Recognizing Client Feelings When experiencing or responding to stress, clients can have a number of feelings. For example, if the client becomes hostile,

RESEARCH APPLICATIONS FOR NURSING

Clients Who Seek Preoperative Information Seem to Cope Better When They Receive It

Caldwell, L. M. (1991). The influence of preference for information on preoperative stress and coping in surgical outpatients. *Applied Nursing Research, 4,* 177–183.

Previous research has shown that clients differ in their preference for preoperative information. It is not known, however, how preference differences may influence stress and coping ability. This study examined stress and coping using a convenience sample of 69 subjects undergoing outpatient surgery for the first time. Clients with a high preference for preoperative information had significantly lower levels of preoperative stress than those who had a low preference for information. However, preference for information did not influence the number of problem-focused coping strategies used by the sample.

Critique This research examined an area that has not been adequately studied. The researcher used a convenience sample whose age ranged from 19 to 81 years. All of the subjects were Caucasian, and most were married women. The study should be replicated using a larger sample of a mixture of men and women with ethnic and cultural variations.

Possible nursing implications The findings of the study seem to indicate that clients who want preoperative information should receive it to help reduce their stress levels. Nurses need to determine which clients want the information and which ones do not. Further research in this area is needed before generalized conclusions can be made.

nurses should not react personally. Instead, acknowledging the client's feelings of anger and aggression is often helpful. For example, the nurse might say, "I can understand why you're angry. I would be angry too, if that had happened to me." After anger is acknowledged, it often decreases or disappears. If the anger does not diminish, the nurse allows the client to explore his or her anger no matter how irrational it may seem. After the anger has been reduced, the nurse can explore the more logical reasons why the feelings arose.

Occasionally, people become so angry that they become a danger to themselves or others around them. If the client loses control over his or her emotions, the nurse should follow institutional guidelines governing such situations.

The nurse can often best facilitate coping by supporting the client's own coping strategies. For example, when clients use self-controlling mechanisms, they should be supported in those efforts, not forced to express their feelings. Nurses should not force clients to share their feelings or to demonstrate their emotions if they are not comfortable in doing so.

Interventions to Aid Family Coping Families also experience many of the same stressors that the ill or hospitalized client does. Families under stress also use coping strategies, such as seeking social support, reviewing events, and venting hostility. Nurses can aid the family and significant others in appraisal of stress and coping just as they do for the client. The nurse can also refer them to social service agencies and other support services.

Interventions to Reduce the Effects of Stress When clients are facing illness, surgery, and other health-related events, they may experience a high level of stress that is not immediately reducible. The introduction of further stress can inhibit coping effectiveness. Nursing action that eliminates or reduces additional stress allows the clients to concentrate their coping activities on the major stressor and not divert their energies to coping with annoyances.

Although many stressful aspects of illness or hospitalization can be reduced or eliminated, there are still many other aspects with which clients either cannot or will not cope. There may be stressors that cannot be eliminated or avoided. In such cases, effective nursing care may involve teaching the client techniques that may reduce the physical impact of stress on the body as well as provide a means of physical or emotional control to the client. Examples are biofeedback, progressive muscle relaxation (PMR), meditation, and guided imagery. If these techniques are not effective, psychotherapy and/or medication, such as antianxiety drugs, may help.

Biofeedback Biofeedback can be an effective treatment when obvious signs of stress, such as headaches, high blood pressure, muscle tension, and heart palpitations, occur frequently, are debilitating, or may be dangerous. Biofeedback works by training the client to reverse the subtle changes that lead to a somatic, or physical, response. For instance, if a headache is the result of muscle tension in the forehead, the client can be trained to relax that tension before a headache results.

Biofeedback involves using electronic instrumentation to signal the user about selected somatic changes. The machinery is sensitive to minute changes within a body system. For example, if the biofeedback is directed toward sampling muscle activity, the machine detects small changes in the electrical activity of the muscles. If brain wave activity is the variable considered, the machine signals the type of brain waves that are occurring at a given moment. Cardiovascular and skin surface activity can also be monitored. After the physical clues are learned, the client can use them to gain control over and to reduce the undesired activity (Fig. 7–5).

Many hospitals and clinics have biofeedback equipment and trained personnel available. If not, referrals can usually be made to a local practitioner.

Progressive Muscle Relaxation Stress commonly causes muscle tension, which results in many of the nagging physical symptoms of stress, such as headaches and neckaches. Control of muscle tension appears to help reduce the physical effects of such tension as well. Progressive muscle relaxation (PMR) is one method used to reduce muscular tension.

PMR involves the tensing and then the relaxing of all the major muscle groups, usually in sequential steps. In PMR, the nurse guides the client through relaxation of each major body part, having the client first tighten and then relax each part. The following is a suggested sequence: feet, thighs, buttocks, stomach, chest, hands, forearms, shoulders, neck, and head. The nurse instructs the client in PMR until he or she can comfortably perform it alone, without prompting. If time is a problem, the client can use a tape recorder and prerecorded PMR tape after completing the initial instruction (Chart 7–3). PMR is useful in nursing practice because it is easy to teach and can be used for a wide spectrum of clients. It is also inexpensive, unlike methods, such as biofeedback, that use machinery.

Meditation Meditation is a learned process through which a person attempts to quiet the mind. The methods used to quiet the mind involve consciously

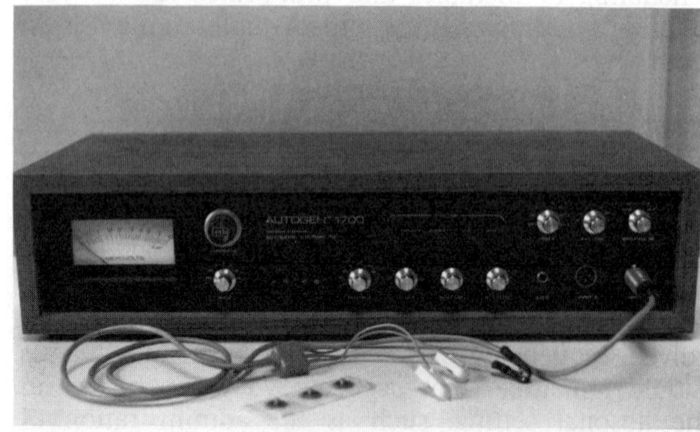

FIGURE 7–5 ◆ An example of a biofeedback system used to reduce stress. (Courtesy of Autogenic Systems, Inc.)

CHART 7 – 3

Education Guide ◆ Progressive Muscle Relaxation

Take a minute and feel your body's different parts. Think about what portions of your body feel tense and which parts feel relaxed.

We are going to do an exercise that will help you to relax and remove the tension from your body. I am going to talk you through this exercise, so just relax and follow my directions.

I am going to ask you to tense one body part at a time. When you tense the body part, try to make the muscle as tight as possible. If you feel pain or a cramp when you tighten, reduce the tightness. This tightening is called tension.

After you hold that muscle tightness for 5 to 10 seconds, I am going to ask you to let all the tightness out of that body part, to let it go limp. This is called relaxation.

First, point your feet and curl your toes. Feel the tension in your feet. Hold that feeling until I tell you to relax.

Relax—let your feet go limp. Feel the difference in going from tension to relaxation. Take a few moments to feel the relaxation.

Now tighten the muscles in your lower legs. Feel the tension in your calves. Feel the tightness of your muscles. Hold that feeling until I say relax.

Now relax your lower legs. Let them go limp. Feel the tightness leave and the feeling of relaxation take over.

Now tighten the muscles of your neck by clenching your lower jaw. Feel the tightness of your muscles. Feel the tenseness as you clench your jaw.

Relax your neck and jaw. Let the tightness go, feel the relaxation take over. Feel the difference between tension and relaxation.

Close your eyes tightly and try to tighten all the other muscles in your face. Feel how tight your face feels.

Now relax your face and let the tenseness flow out.

Finally, I want you to let your whole body go limp, let it all relax. Remember those feelings of relaxation and let those feelings take over. Release any feelings of tension.

Now, it is time to end this exercise. I want you to take your time as you slowly begin to move. When you are ready, you may resume your normal activities.

removing disturbing thoughts or filling the mind with only one thought, such as a *mantra* or prayer. By removing other thoughts, it is believed that stress can be reduced. Meditation is probably best learned through a mentor, although books and other audiovisual aids are available. If clients are interested in learning meditative techniques, they should be referred to an appropriate source.

Guided Imagery Similar to meditation, imagery also attempts to control the mind's thoughts. Imagery seeks to fill the mind with positive and pleasant mental pictures. Usually, imagery involves thinking about a peaceful scene or one in which there is total relaxation. Thinking processes are directed toward the promotion of relaxation rather than stress (see Chap. 8 for more information).

DISCHARGE PLANNING

HOME CARE PREPARATION

Stress is often the result of lack of knowledge or inaccurate knowledge about an upcoming event. For that reason, all clients who are discharged from the hospital should be involved in discharge planning to the extent possible.

HEALTH TEACHING

Every client needs to know what to expect to be able to implement effective coping strategies. For example, clients should be educated about signs and symptoms that are expected as well as those that should be reported. The client and family should know who is to be called if trouble arises.

The nurse also provides both verbal and written directions for home care. Having a written copy of instructions often reduces stress for the client.

Transcultural Considerations The nurse assesses the client's education level to ensure that the information is appropriate. For example, if the client cannot read, the nurse uses pictures or symbols to provide the material. If the client does not speak or understand the nurse's language, the nurse locates a resource to provide the information in the client's primary language.

PSYCHOSOCIAL PREPARATION

If extended care is needed after discharge, the client should be fully aware of what is needed, who will be giving the care, and how to arrange for the care. The family or significant other should understand what is involved in the recovery or convalescent period so that the client's coping efforts are supported and not damaged by unrealistic expectations. Nurses should remember that although discharge is usually a positive event, it is also a stressful one for many clients. Stress related to discharge can be reduced if planning starts early and actively involves the client.

HEALTH CARE RESOURCES

If clients have received education on managing stress or improving coping, the client and the nurse can develop plans that ensure that what was learned is not discarded. Enlisting the help of family or friends may sometimes help clients in adhering to new routines. In other cases, referrals may be made to organizations that deal in stress.

EVALUATION

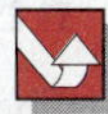

On the basis of the common nursing diagnoses, the nurse evaluates care for the client or the family experiencing stress. The outcomes are that the client and the family:

- Accurately appraise stress situations
- Demonstrate effective coping strategies in stress situations
- Verbalize that the feeling of stress is reduced

NURSING AND STRESS

Nurses as well as clients experience stress. Many nurses are affected by stress that exceeds their ability to cope. Nurses are exposed to tremendous numbers of stressors in their work each day, from exposure to death to sometimes unrealistic expectations of the work environment (Hamilton, 1991). The indicators of stress in clients are also indicators of stress overload in nurses.

People overwhelmed by stress are sometimes referred to as being "burned out." A pilot study by Hildman et al. (1991) showed that daily or frequent hassles contribute to nurse burnout (Research Applications for Nursing). Some of the common symptoms of burnout are resentment toward supervisors and coworkers, loss of temper at small incidents, constant fatigue, reluctance to go to work, and withdrawal from work relationships.

Many programs are available to aid the nurse in reducing stress, and there are also a variety of strategies that the nurse may use. In addition to the strategies outlined for clients, the following stress management techniques may be effective:

- Learn assertiveness techniques to present feelings and thoughts in an honest, direct, and acceptable manner. Remember that hostile expression of anger and aggression usually inflame, rather than reduce, stress feelings.
- Acknowledge the positive aspects of work and do not dwell on the negatives. Happier people have been found to be less "realistic" in their assessments of situations, in that they focus on the funny and the positive aspects of life.
- Develop alternative plans for situations known to cause stress. For example, if transportation is a problem, arrange for a friend or coworker to serve as a back-up when trouble develops.
- Follow the same health care practices that nurses recommend to others. Get adequate sleep, eat a healthy diet, reduce caffeine consumption, get regular exercise, stop smoking, and use alcohol only in moderation, if at all.

RESEARCH APPLICATIONS FOR NURSING

Too Much Paperwork, Too Few Nurses, and Too Little Time May Add Up to Nurse Burnout

Hildman, T. B., Ferguson, G. H., Johnson, J. T., & Thompson, W. R. (1991). Daily hassles cause burnout. *Journal of Nursing Administration, 21*(9), 44–45.

This pilot study examined potential stressors, mediators, and burnout among registered nurses working in a hospital setting. On the basis of the theory that daily hassles cause negative consequences more than major life events, the researchers asked 65 nurses to identify daily or frequent hassles that had occurred within the past 6 months. Working short-staffed and too much paperwork were the top two work-related hassles identified by the sample. The highest ranked home-related hassle item was not having enough time to do everything.

Critique The researchers had intended this study to be a pilot for a larger project. All of the subjects were from one hospital, and their demographic data were not described. The topic of burnout, however, is important for job satisfaction and the recruitment and retention of qualified nursing staff.

Possible nursing implications Although these findings cannot be generalized from a limited sample in one hospital, they validate the anecdotal literature in which nurses are concerned about the inability to provide quality care when short-staffed. This hassle item as well as others, such as too much paperwork, should serve as a guide when staff nurses have input into planning unit budgets and computerized information systems.

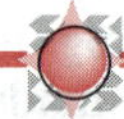

IMPLICATIONS FOR NURSING RESEARCH

The nursing profession continues to make major research contributions in the area of stress and coping. Currently published studies need replication and further development. The following are research questions that need to be addressed.

- ◆ How can nurses accurately assess a client's hardiness level and coping strategies?
- ◆ What nursing interventions help to reduce the client's perception of stress in the acute care setting?
- ◆ What specific coping strategies are effective for clients undergoing special procedures or surgery?
- ◆ How can nurses realistically reduce daily or frequent hassles in their own work environments?
- ◆ Are there transcultural differences in the perception and management of stress? If so, what are the nursing implications for practice?

SELECTED BIBLIOGRAPHY

*Aroian, K. J., & Patsdaughter, C. A. (1989). Multiple-method, cross-cultural assessment of psychological distress. *Image: The Journal of Nursing Scholarship, 21,* 90–93.

Bailey, J. M., & Neilsen, B. I. (1993). Uncertainty and appraisal in women with rheumatoid arthritis. *Orthopaedic Nursing, 12*(2), 63–67.

Caldwell, L. M. (1991). The influence of preference for information on preoperative stress and coping in surgical outpatients. *Applied Nursing Research, 4,* 177–183.

*Cannon, W. B. (1931). *The wisdom of the body.* New York: W. W. Norton.

Davis, L. L. (1990). Illness uncertainty, social support, and stress in recovering individuals and family caregivers. *Applied Nursing Research, 3,* 69–71.

*DeLongis, A., Coyne, J. C., Dakof, G., Folkman, S., & Lazarus, R. S. (1982). Relationship of daily hassles, uplifts and major life events to health status. *Health Psychology, 1,* 119–136.

Hamilton, J. M. (1991). Coping with stress. *Nursing '91, 21*(4), 136.

Hildman, T. B., Ferguson, G. H., Johnson, J. T., & Thompson, W. R. (1991). Daily hassles cause burnout. *Journal of Nursing Administration, 21*(9), 44–45.

*Holmes, T. H., & Rahe, R. H. (1967). The social readjustment rating scale. *Journal of Psychosomatic Research, 11,* 213–218.

*Janis, I. L. (1985). Coping patterns among patients with life-threatening diseases. *Issues in Mental Health Nursing, 7,* 461–476.

*Johnson, J. E. (1972). Effects of structuring patients' expectations on their reactions to threatening events. *Nursing Research, 21,* 499–503.

Johnson, J. E. (1991). Progressive relaxation and the sleep of older noninstitutionalized women. *Applied Nursing Research, 4,* 165–170.

*Johnson, J. E. & Lauver, D. R. (1989). Alternative explanations of coping with stressful experiences associated with physical illness. *Advances in Nursing Science, 11,* 39–52.

Keller, M. L., Jadack, R. A., & Mims, F. (1991). Perceived stressors and coping responses in persons with recurrent genital herpes. *Research in Nursing and Health, 12,* 421–430.

*Kobasa, S. C. (1979). Stressful life events, personality, and health: An inquiry into hardiness. *Journal of Personality and Social Psychology, 37,* 1–10.

*Lazarus, R. S., & Folkman, S. (1984). *Stress, appraisal and coping.* New York: Springer.

Lewis, C., & Randell, B. P. (1992). Alteration in self-care: An instance of ineffective coping in the geriatric patient. In R. M. Carroll-Johnson (Ed.), *Classification of nursing diagnoses: Proceedings of the ninth conference* (pp. 264–265). Philadelphia: J. B. Lippincott.

Mishel, M. H. (1990). Reconceptualization of the uncertainty in illness theory. *Image: The Journal of Nursing Scholarship, 22,* 256–262.

Mishel, M. H., Padilla, G., Grant, M., & Sorenson, D. S. (1991). Uncertainty in illness: A replication of the mediating effects of mastery and coping. *Nursing Research, 40,* 236–240.

*Moos, R. H., & Tsu, V. D. (1977). The crisis of physical illness. In R. H. Moos (Ed.), *Coping with physical illness.* New York: Plenum.

Normal, E. M., Getek, D. M., & Griffin, C. C. (1991). Post-traumatic stress disorder in an urban trauma population. *Applied Nursing Research, 4,* 171–176.

*Peirce, A. G. (1987). Event review in the coping of parous women. (Doctoral dissertation, University of Maryland at Baltimore, 1987). *Dissertation abstracts international, 42,* 705B.

Pellman, J. (1992). Widowhood in elderly women: Exploring its relationship to community integration, hassles, stress, social support, and social support-seeking. *International Journal of Aging and Human Development, 35,* 253–264.

*Pollock, S. E. (1989). The hardiness characteristic: A motivating factor in adaptation. *Advances in Nursing Science, 11,* 53–62.

Pollock, S. E., Christian, B. J., & Sands, D. (1990). Response to chronic illness: Analysis of psychological and physiological adaptation. *Nursing Research, 39,* 300–304.

Pollock, S. E., & Duffy, M. E. (1990). The health-related hardiness scale: Development and psychometric analysis. *Nursing Research, 39,* 218–222.

Robinson, L. (1990). Stress and anxiety. *Nursing Clinics of North America, 25,* 935–943.

*Roy, C., & Roberts, S. (1981). *Theory construction in nursing: An adaptation model.* Englewood Cliffs, N. J.: Prentice-Hall.

*Schroeder, D. H., & Costa, P. T. (1984). Influence of life events on physical illness: Substantive effects or methodological flaws? *Journal of Personality and Social Psychology, 46,* 853–863.

*Selye, H. (1946). General adaptation syndrome and diseases of adaptation. *Journal of Clinical Endocrinology, 6,* 117–230.

Thomas, S. P., & Williams, R. L. (1991). Perceived stress, trait anger, modes of anger expression, and health status of college men and women. *Nursing Research, 40,* 303–307.

*Vincent, K. G. (1985). The validation of a nursing diagnosis: A nurse consensus survey. *Nursing Clinics of North America, 20,* 631–640.

Wagnild, G., & Young, H. M. (1991). Another look at hardiness. *Image: The Journal of Nursing Scholarship, 23,* 257–259.

Weinberger, R. (1991). Teaching the elderly stress reduction. *Journal of Gerontological Nursing, 17*(10), 23–27.

SUGGESTED READINGS

Johnson, J. E. (1991). Progressive relaxation and the sleep of older noninstitutionalized women. *Applied Nursing Research, 4,* 165–170.

Older women often seek help with sleep disturbances from health professionals who typically prescribe medication to induce sleep. This study found a positive effect of progressive muscle relaxation on the promotion of sleep in elderly women. Nurses should encourage this technique as a safe, nondrug intervention.

Norman, E. M., Getek, D. M., & Griffin, C. C. (1991). Post-traumatic stress disorder in an urban trauma population. *Applied Nursing Research, 4,* 171–176.

This descriptive study looked at the incidence of post-traumatic stress disorder (PTSD) in people who experienced physical trauma within the past 6 months. The relationship between severity of the trauma and PTSD was examined, but the findings were not significant. More than half of the 92 clients in the study, however, experienced medium or high levels of PTSD.

Wagnild, G., & Young, H. M. (1991). Another look at hardiness. *Image: The Journal of Nursing Scholarship, 23,* 257–259.

This article discussed the state of the science on the concept of hardiness. The authors reviewed the definitions as they are applied to health and examined the scales used to measure hardiness. The authors also raised many questions for future research, such as whether or not all people have some degree of hardiness.

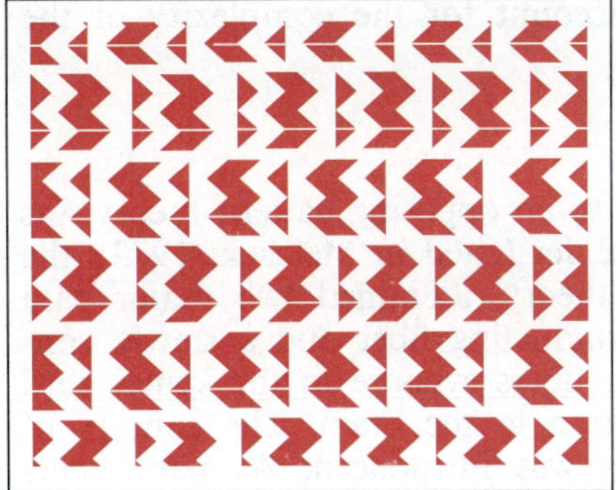

CHAPTER 8

CHAPTER HIGHLIGHTS

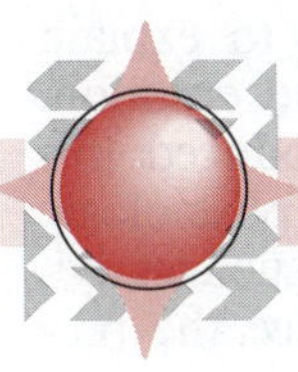

Pain

Pain is a protective mechanism for the body in that it occurs when tissues are being damaged (Guyton, 1991). The person in pain usually takes action to remove the pain or its cause, if possible. Indeed, pain is the number one symptom or complaint that causes people to seek health care. It alters or compromises the quality of life more than any other single health-related problem.

OVERVIEW

Everyone experiences pain, but it is a complex and private experience. Because pain is such an abstract concept, major difficulties arise when one attempts to describe or explain it. Many elements operate to make pain hard to understand or assess. These elements include numerous psychosocial factors and the subjectivity of the pain experience. The interpretation of pain based on a person's behavior is equally cumbersome because the amount of or response to pain is different from person to person.

DEFINITIONS OF PAIN

Several attempts have been made to define pain in descriptive or measurable terms, yet no one definition is more accepted than another. Among the most popular definitions of pain are those of Sternbach (1968), McCaffery (1979), and the International Association on Pain (1979). Sternbach (p. 8) asserted that pain is "an abstract concept which refers to:

- A personal, private sensation of hurt
- A harmful stimulus which signals current or impending tissue damage
- A pattern of responses to protect the organism from harm"

This comprehensive definition serves to explain pain through a physiologic, psychologic, and social approach.

McCaffery (1979) offered a more personal explanation of pain when she stated that pain "is whatever the experiencing person says it is and exists whenever he says it does" (p. 11). This understanding of pain requires that the client be seen as the authority on the pain and the only one who can define the experience.

Finally, the International Association on Pain (1979) described pain as an unpleasant sensory and emotional experience associated with actual or potential tissue damage.

Regardless of the definition, most people agree that pain has both sensory and behavioral components and is strongly influenced by various physiologic, psychologic, and sociologic factors. A comprehensive understanding of pain requires a knowledge of the descriptive definitions, theories, and physiology of pain. The nurse can use this knowledge as a basis to develop an appreciation of the variety of clinical pain situations and skill in pain intervention. This understanding can also help the nurse develop a personal philosophy of pain management.

THEORETICAL BASES FOR PAIN

Several theories have been proposed to explain the complexity of pain. Early theories emphasized the recognition of specific pathways of pain transmission. Later theories attempted to uncover the complexity of central processing of pain in specific areas of the brain. More recently, the concept of a pain-modulating network was introduced. This concept describes the various links and connections in the spinal cord and brain, specifically the medulla and the midbrain. The identification of chemical mediators involved in the pain response has helped in an understanding of pain transmission and perception.

SPECIFICITY THEORY

The specificity theory was proposed in the early 1800s and was accepted for almost 100 years as the most popular theoretical explanation for pain. This theory emphasized the highly specific structures and pathways responsible for pain transmission. Its premise was based on the existence of free nerve endings in the periphery of the body. The nerve endings act as pain receptors that are capable of accepting sensory input and transmitting this information along highly specific nerve fibers. Although this theory set the stage for further research, its major biologic orientation fails to account for the complexity of the pain experience.

PATTERN THEORY

In the early 1900s, an opposing pattern theory was proposed. Goldscheider (cited in Melzack, 1973), the originator of this theory, identified two major pain fibers: a rapidly conducting fiber and a slowly conducting fiber. Both fibers synapse in the spinal cord and relay information to the brain. The concept of central summation was introduced: As pain fibers converge at the level of the spinal cord, the summation of inpulses from these fibers ascends to various levels of the brain. The amount, intensity, and type of sensory input permit the brain to interpret the sensation.

Both the pattern theory and the specificity theory fail to address factors that alter the perception of pain, such as anxiety and depression. Also, neither theory explains the failure of pain to resolve after pain pathways and spinal nerves are cut.

GATE CONTROL THEORY

The gate control theory was proposed to explain the observed relationship between pain and emotion. Melzack and Wall (1982), who first introduced this theory, concluded that pain is not just a physiologic response, but that psychologic variables, such as behavioral and emotional responses, influence the perception of pain.

According to the gate control theory, a gating mechanism occurs in the spinal cord. Pain impulses are transmitted from the periphery of the body by nerve fibers (A delta and C fibers). The impulses travel to the dorsal horns of the spinal cord, specifically to the area of the cord called the *substantia gelatinosa.* The cells of the substantia gelatinosa can inhibit or facilitate pain impulses that are transmitted to the trigger cells (T cells). When T cell activity is inhibited, the gate is closed and impulses are less likely to be transmitted to the brain. When the gate is opened, pain impulses ascend to the brain (Fig. 8–1).

Similar gating mechanisms exist in the descending nerve fibers from the thalamus and cerebral cortex. These areas of the brain regulate a person's thoughts and emotions, including beliefs and values. When pain occurs, a person's thoughts and emotions can influence whether pain impulses reach the level of conscious awareness (Meinhart & McCaffery, 1983).

The gate control theory has helped nurses and other health care professionals recognize the *holistic* nature of pain. As a result, many interventions, such as imagery and distraction (discussed later), are used to help relieve a client's pain.

ANATOMIC AND PHYSIOLOGIC BASES FOR PAIN

SOURCES OF PAIN

Free nerve endings, or receptors capable of responding to painful stimuli, are often referred to as

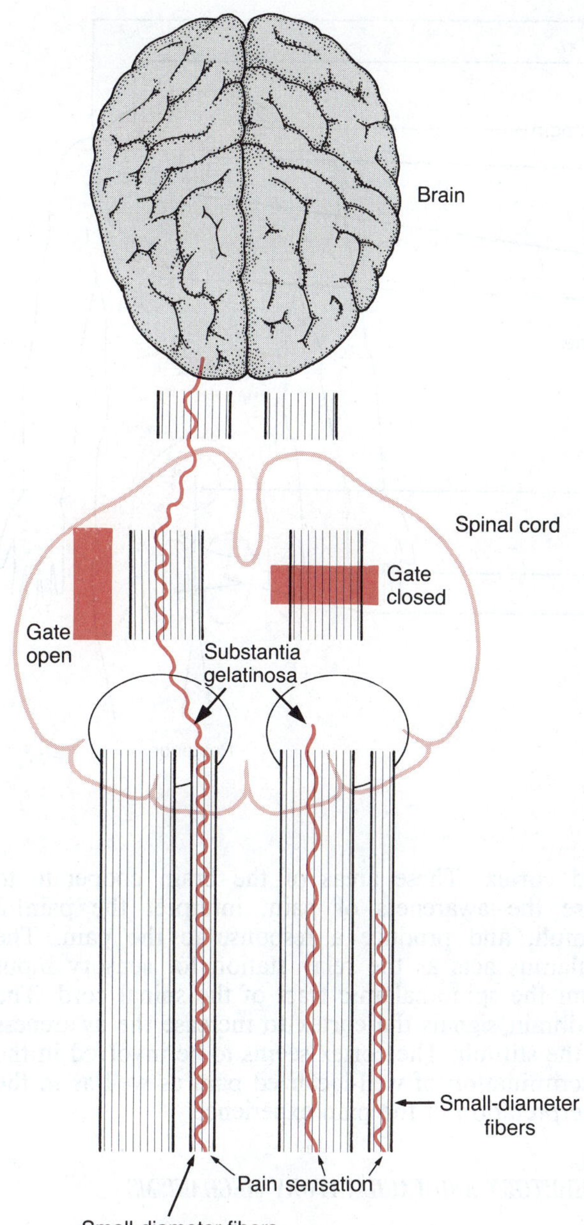

FIGURE 8-1 ♦ The gate control theory of pain.

nociceptors. Nociceptors are located in various body tissues and are activated by thermal, mechanical, and chemical stimuli. In addition to nociceptors, other receptors in the body respond to almost any type of intense stimulation, sometimes resulting in pain.

Pain sources can be classified into three major categories: somatic, visceral, and neuropathic. Nociceptors are located in the somatic and visceral structures.

SOMATIC PAIN Somatic structures are the first source of pain. These structures are further classified as cutaneous and deep. *Cutaneous* structures make up the superficial parts of the body, such as the skin and subcutaneous tissue. The cutaneous structures are well supplied with nerves; therefore, painful stimuli are well defined and localized.

Deep somatic structures include nerve receptors originating in bone, blood vessels, nerves, muscles, and other supporting tissues. Because these structures are poorly supplied with nerves, this pain is usually dull and poorly localized. Deep pain may produce an autonomic nervous system response, including nausea, pulse and blood pressure changes, and sweating.

VISCERAL PAIN The second source of pain is visceral and is defined as pain arising from body organs. The scarcity of nerve receptors in these structures produces poorly localized and diffuse pain. Visceral receptors are sensitive to stretching, inflammation, and ischemia, but they are not sensitive to cuts and extremes of temperature.

Visceral pain is well known for its ability to produce referred pain, which is a type of pain that a person perceives in an area other than the site of the stimuli. Referred pain occurs because visceral fibers synapse at the level of the spinal cord, close to fibers supplying certain subcutaneous tissue areas of the body. A common example of referred pain is pain in the right posterior shoulder that is related to gallbladder disease. The referred pain occurs because the subcutaneous tissue fibers of the scapula are close to the fibers of the gallbladder, which are transmitting the painful stimuli. Other referred pain sites are illustrated in Figure 8-2.

NEUROPATHIC PAIN The third major source of pain is neuropathic. This form of pain is caused by injury or damage to nerve fibers in the periphery or by damage to the central nervous system, resulting in an interruption of the ability for nerve fibers to conduct sensory information.

When a person experiences neuropathic pain, the brain interprets painful stimuli even though there may be no obvious or documented physiologic cause for the pain. This category of pain has been receiving increased attention in the literature because it is believed that neuropathic pain is not easily relieved by analgesics, as is somatic or visceral pain. Phantom limb pain, which may occur after removal of or severe damage to major nerve plexuses that innervate a particular extremity, is one example of neuropathic pain.

PAIN STIMULI

Various types of noxious pain stimuli account for the perception of pain. A wide range of sensory inputs are capable of producing pain. In addition, tissue ischemia and muscle spasm cause pain.

In most circumstances, painful stimuli cause actual tissue damage, which leads to the release of certain chemical substances, such as histamine, bradykinin, serotonin, prostaglandins, and acids. These chemicals are believed to activate pain receptors. For example, the accumulation of lactic acids leads to the pain associated with ischemic tissue damage (Guyton, 1991). Muscle contraction or spasm can also produce ischemic-type pain. The muscle's oxygen demands

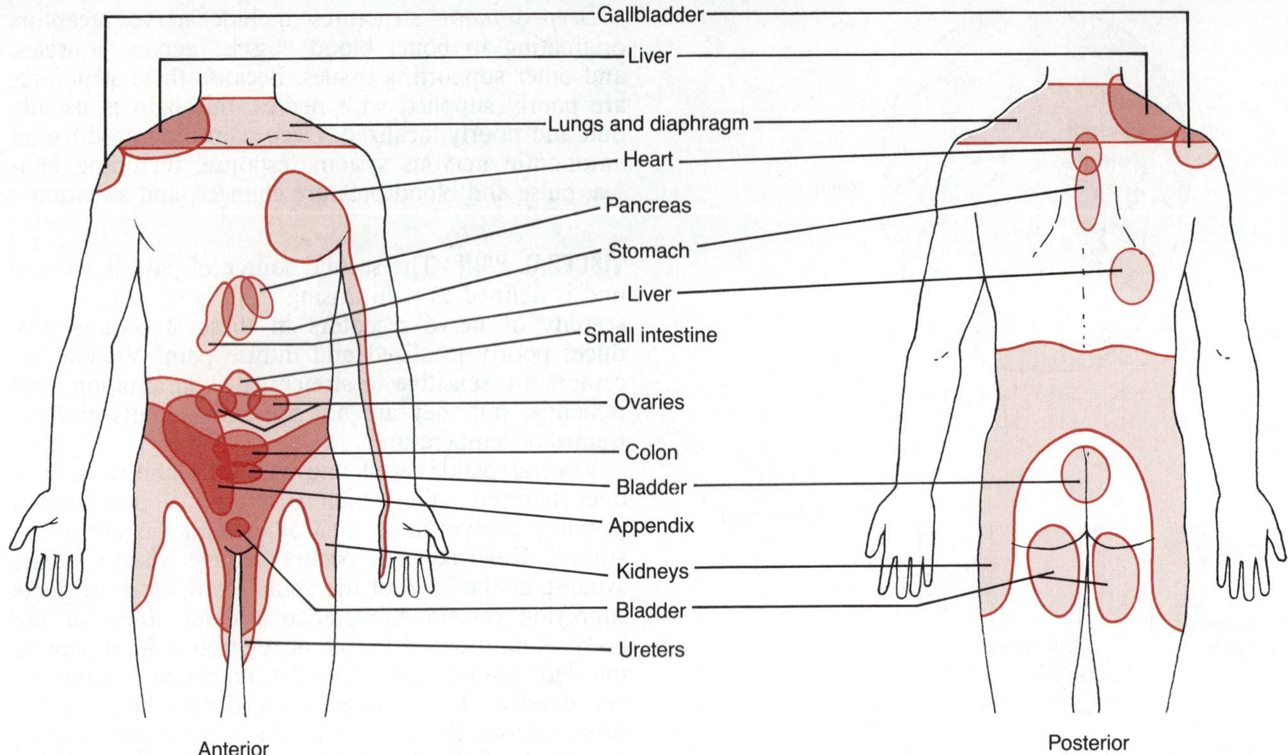

FIGURE 8–2 ♦ Anterior and posterior referred pain sites.

are increased, but the blood supply is limited because of compressed blood vessels.

PAIN PATHWAYS

Usually, painful stimuli originate in the periphery of the body. For the painful stimuli to be perceived, however, they must first be transmitted to the spinal cord and then to the central areas of the brain, as described by the gate control theory of pain (see Fig. 8–1). In the periphery, two specific fibers can transmit stimuli: A delta fibers, which are found primarily in the skin and muscle, and C fibers, which are distributed in muscle, periosteum, and viscera.

A delta fibers are myelinated fibers that carry rapid, sharp, pricking, or piercing sensations. A person feeling these sensations can generally localize them readily to a fairly well-defined area. Because these fibers respond predominantly to mechanical stimuli, rather than to chemical or thermal stimuli, they are called mechanical nociceptors.

C fibers are unmyelinated or poorly myelinated fibers that conduct thermal, chemical, and strong mechanical impulses. Pain conduction from C fibers is more diffuse and dull, burning, or achy—quite different from the sensations of A delta fibers. In contrast to the intermittent nature of A delta sensations, C fibers usually produce continuous, constant pain.

CENTRAL NERVOUS SYSTEM PROCESSING

The central processing of pain occurs at three different levels of the brain: the thalamus, midbrain, and cortex. These areas of the brain cooperate to raise the awareness of pain, interpret the painful stimuli, and produce a response to the pain. The thalamus acts as the relay station for sensory input from the spinothalamic tract of the spinal cord. The midbrain signals the cortex to increase the awareness of the stimuli. The cortex seems to be involved in the discrimination of well-localized pain as well as in the interpretation of the pain experience.

INHIBITORY AND FACILITATORY MECHANISMS

Sensory input to the spinal cord may be influenced by chemical substances known as *neuroregulators.* These are classified as neurotransmitters or neuromodulators.

NEUROTRANSMITTERS Neurotransmitters are chemicals that exert inhibitory or excitatory activity at postsynaptic nerve cell membranes. Acetylcholine, norepinephrine, epinephrine, and dopamine are documented neurotransmitters.

NEUROMODULATORS Neuromodulators, also called endogenous opiates, are protein hormones found in the brain. They have been implicated in the modification of pain. These substances are composed of large amino acid peptides called *alpha-* and *beta-endorphins* and *enkephalins.* The speculation that these natural opiate-like substances were responsible for pain relief was confirmed when induced analgesic effects were reversed with naloxone (Narcan), an opioid antagonist.

Endorphins and enkephalins are similar to morphine-like substances, only more potent. They are believed to play a major role in the biologic response to pain. The larger peptides (endorphins) exert more prolonged analgesic effects than do the enkephalins. Endorphins are produced by the anterior pituitary gland and the hypothalamus. The smaller peptides (enkephalins) tend to be more widespread throughout the brain and the dorsal horn of the spinal cord. Several types of endorphins and enkephalins have been identified. Each acts on highly specific opiate receptors in the central nervous system.

Various factors influence the production of neuromodulators. The activity of endorphins and enkephalins may be enhanced by prolonged strenuous activity (Fig. 8-3), transcutaneous electrical nerve stimulators (see the discussions further on about interventions for pain and chronic pain), and antidepressant therapy, which often increases serotonin levels in the body. Adequate amounts of serotonin, a neurotransmitter, have been shown to enhance analgesia through the activity of endorphins and enkephalins. Similarly, pain and stress are strong activators of the endogenous opiate system.

PAIN PERCEPTION

The subjectivity of the pain experience limits our understanding of the perception and response to pain. This situation is further complicated by the knowledge that even when pain pathways are surgically interrupted, the perception of pain may persist. However, even though the perception of pain is difficult to measure, it can be characterized as the actual awareness of the painful feeling or sensation.

The pain threshold is the amount or degree of noxious stimuli that leads a person to first interpret a sensation as painful. More specifically, this term refers to the point at which a person feels pain and reports it as such.

Even though all pain is real, it sometimes persists without any detectable physical cause. Such pain may be highly influenced by emotional and social factors. In these situations, the lack of a physiologic or organic cause may lead health professionals and clients to doubt the validity of their pain.

Pain tolerance refers to the ability of a person to endure the intensity of pain. Pain tolerance is usually characterized by an overt expression of behavior. Unlike pain perception and pain threshold, the ability to tolerate pain is more a function of psychologic and social variables than biologic characteristics.

The nurse should be aware that many variables affect a person's perception of and response to pain. Demographic factors, such as age, sex, sociocultural background, and personality characteristics, strongly influence the client's ability to process pain sensations and react to them.

AGE

Researchers agree that there are some variations in threshold associated with the chronologic age of the nervous system, but there are no clear trends (Zatzick & Dimsdale, 1990). Some researchers believe that the perceptual acuity of pain diminishes as a result of aging, although this finding has not been validated (Acute Pain Management Guideline Panel, 1992; Neeley, 1993). The perception of cutaneous pain may diminish because of age-related skin changes, but the perception of visceral pain may increase in older adults (Egbert, 1991).

Older adults generally receive less analgesia and tend to report pain less often than do younger adults (Jacques, 1992; Neeley, 1993). These findings may be related to beliefs and concerns that the elderly have about pain and the reporting of pain. Many elderly people hold the following beliefs and concern about pain (Neeley, 1993):

- Pain is something that they must live with.
- Expressing pain is unacceptable or is a sign of weakness.
- Complaining of pain will label them as "bad" clients.
- Nurses are too busy to listen to complaints of pain.
- Pain signifies a serious illness or impending death.

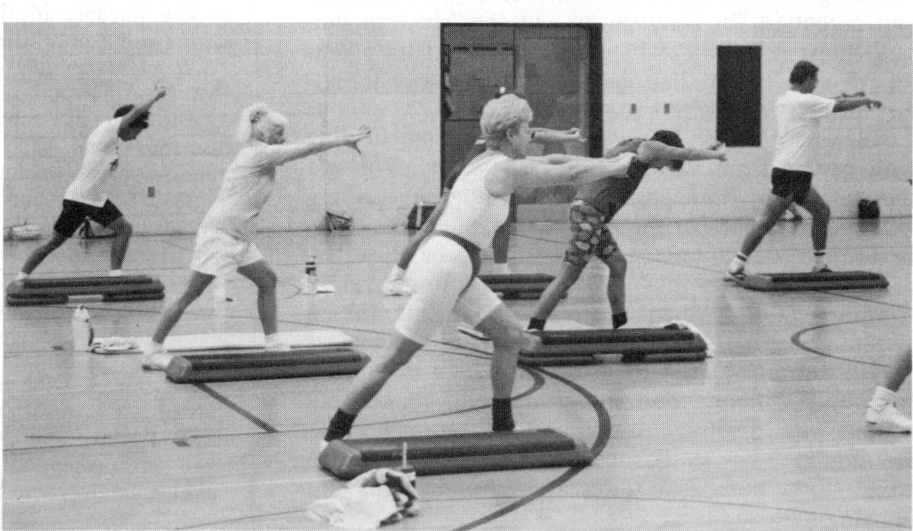

FIGURE 8-3 ◆ Prolonged, strenuous activity, such as sustained aerobic exercise, can enhance the activity of endorphins and enkephalins.

Nurses should be aware of the beliefs that elderly clients hold to manage their pain. Nurses and other caregivers frequently undermedicate elderly clients and are sometimes reluctant to administer prescribed analgesics. Unfounded concerns about overmedication, addiction, and decreases in pain perception may contribute to undermedication (Champlin, 1992; Ferrell et al., 1992b; Greipp, 1992; Haviley et al., 1992). Some nurses may also lack knowledge of pharmacology and pain theory.

SEX

Some investigators have demonstrated that men tolerate pain better than women do, whereas others have found no sex differences. It is widely believed that men exhibit greater stoicism than women do (Zatzick & Dimsdale, 1990). Research has shown that nurses expect men to be stoic but accept more emotional responses from women in pain (Jacques, 1992; Walding, 1991).

TRANSCULTURAL CONSIDERATIONS

Sociocultural groups are sometimes categorized by their ability to tolerate pain. These groups are often stereotyped; for example, "Italian-Americans are very dramatic when they are in pain" or "Mexican-Americans have a low pain tolerance" (Calvillo & Flaskerud, 1991). Many studies have shown a relationship between pain and a person's culture, but the study methods and results have not been consistent (Zatzick & Dimsdale, 1990).

Few nursing studies have examined the transcultural aspects of pain, yet nurses make pain assessments and decisions regarding pain management. For example, many Mexican-American clients, especially women, moan or cry when they are uncomfortable. As a result, they are often identified by nurses as complainers who cannot tolerate pain (Calvillo & Flaskerud, 1991). Nurses who value the stoic model or "norm" for pain response interpret behaviors like moaning and crying as an inability to tolerate pain and a request for intervention. In the Mexican culture, however, these behaviors might help the client relieve pain rather than communicate a need for intervention (Calvillo & Flaskerud, 1991).

Nurses must also consider language when dealing with people from various cultures. If English is not the person's first language within an English-speaking culture, the ability of the person to express pain may be limited, or expressions of pain may be misinterpreted. The nurse may need to rely on nonverbal communication, which can also be misinterpreted (Waldin, 1991). Gaston-Johansson and colleagues (1990) examined the similarities in pain descriptions from four different cultural groups and found that people with diverse cultural and educational backgrounds may use similar words to describe the terms pain, hurt, and ache (Research Applications for Nursing).

PERSONALITY TRAITS

According to the gate control theory of pain, a person's perception of pain and pain tolerance can be influenced by personality and other psychosocial factors. For example, people who are outgoing, or extroverts, may be more likely to express their pain than those who are quiet and shy.

Another personality factor that can influence pain perception and tolerance is anxiety. Many researchers have linked the presence of anxiety with pain. Other associated behaviors are feelings of powerlessness and the inability to cope with anxiety and pain. Nursing interventions to reduce anxiety and increase the ability to cope have also helped to relieve pain (Walding, 1991).

In addition to personality and other factors that cannot be changed, such as age and sex, other factors that are present at a given time may influence a person's experience of pain. Factors that tend to *decrease* the threshold for and tolerance of pain include discomfort, insomnia, fatigue, anxiety, fear, anger, sadness, depression, mental isolation, introversion, and past experience. Factors that tend to *increase* the threshold for and tolerance of pain include relief of symptoms, sleep, rest, sympathy, understanding, diversion, elevation of mood, analgesics, anxiolytic agents, and antidepressants. Because many of these factors can be altered, nursing interventions for pain

RESEARCH APPLICATIONS FOR NURSING

Cultural Differences in the Perception of Pain May Be Nonexistent

Gaston-Johansson, F., Albert, M., Fagan, E., & Zimmerman, L. (1990). Similarities in pain descriptions of four different ethnic-culture groups. *Journal of Pain and Symptom Management, 5*(2), 94–100.

The purpose of this study was to identify pain terms commonly used by four cultural groups living in the United States—Hispanics, Native Americans, African-Americans, and Caucasians. The 153 subjects constituting the convenience sample were asked to use the Visual Analogue Scale and the McGill Pain Questionnaire to indicate their perception of the words "ache," "hurt," and "pain." There were no significant differences among the four groups.

Critique This study was an attempt to continue to examine cultural differences in pain perception. Although the sample was a convenience one, the number of subjects was large enough to obtain meaningful data.

Possible nursing implications Published reports have been inconsistent in defining how various cultures perceive and express pain. This study suggests that pain perception may not be markedly different, at least among these four ethnic-cultural groups.

often include minimizing factors that lower the pain threshold and increasing or maximizing factors that increase the pain threshold.

RESEARCH ON PAIN

NURSING INTERVENTIONS FOR PAIN

Nurse researchers have been concerned with the pain concept, most often in relation to measuring the effects of interventions aimed at relieving pain. A classic study by Wells (1982) provides an example of nursing interventions for pain. Wells studied the postoperative effects of relaxation training in a small sample of clients who had undergone cholecystectomy. Wells found that the training reduced the psychologic discomforts related to pain, but she was unable to demonstrate changes on any physiologic measures, such as blood pressure or pulse rate.

In another evaluation of the effects of nursing intervention, Keller and Bzdek (1986) investigated the effects of therapeutic touch on tension headache pain. In this study, the McGill-Melzack Pain Questionnaire (Fig. 8–4) was used to demonstrate an average 70% pain reduction in the group who received touch intervention compared with the group who did not.

In a more recent nursing study, Ferrel-Torry and Glick (1993) successfully used therapeutic massage as a nursing intervention to modify anxiety and the perception of cancer pain. Music has also been used for clients experiencing cancer-related pain.

ATTITUDES OF NURSES ABOUT PAIN AND PAIN MANAGEMENT

Pain is a personal and subjective phenomenon. The nurse's attitude about pain easily influences the assessment, intervention, and evaluation of the client's pain experience. Studies have documented that both practicing nurses (Ferrell et al., 1992a; Scott, 1992) and nursing faculty (Ferrell et al., 1993) are ill prepared to care for clients in pain.

Nurses may have little personal experience with pain. They may not appreciate how painful a particular treatment or surgery may be. Nurses may expect that clients with chronic pain will react similarly to those with acute pain. They may assume that reactions to pain, including complaints about pain, will fall within a certain norm on the basis of their own cultural values. The more the response of a person with pain varies from these expected norms, the more likely it is that the attitude of the nurse toward the client will be biased, either positively or negatively.

ATTITUDES OF PHYSICIANS ABOUT PAIN AND PAIN MANAGEMENT

Undertreatment of pain, especially cancer pain, is a serious problem in the United States and elsewhere in the world. In 1983, the World Health Organization estimated that on any given day, 3.5 million people in the world experience cancer pain that could be relieved (Haviley et al., 1992).

In spite of increased education about pain, many physicians underprescribe medication for clients in pain, especially opioids like morphine (Hill, 1990). Some investigators have assessed several factors which account for this practice (Abrahm et al., 1993; Von Roenn et al., 1993).

First, there are cultural and societal attitudes about opioid use, especially in the United States. In some states, clients who use these drugs have to register with state regulatory agencies in a manner similar to that required of people enrolled in methadone programs. Requiring this procedure equates the client with drug abusers.

Second, government regulatory agencies do not set practical guidelines for drug use in people with severe or chronic pain. A physician may be reprimanded by the medical board for prescribing what the board considers an inappropriate amount or type of pain medication.

Third, there is still a lack of knowledge about the effects of analgesics. Most of the studies on a person's response to drug therapy have been done with people who were not in pain. Many of the subjects were volunteers who were former drug addicts imprisoned for drug abuse. The fear of respiratory depression that some physicians have is unnecessary because pain prevents or diminishes the respiratory effect of opioids (Haviley et al., 1992; Hill, 1990).

TYPES OF PAIN

There are several ways to classify types of pain. In 1986, the National Institutes of Health Consensus Conference on Pain categorized pain according to its cause. The participants at the conference identified three types of pain: acute, chronic malignant, and chronic nonmalignant. Acute pain results from acute injury, disease, or surgery. Chronic nonmalignant pain is associated with tissue injury that is not progressive or that has healed. Pain that is associated with cancer or another progressive disease is called chronic malignant pain. Although these categories are based theoretically on cause, the nurse is usually concerned with two basic types of pain in practice: acute pain and chronic pain.

ACUTE PAIN

CHARACTERISTICS OF ACUTE PAIN Acute pain is experienced by almost everyone at some time. Certain characteristics distinguish this type of pain from the more chronic, or long-term pain that is often associated with chronic illness. A major distinction between acute and chronic pain is the effect of pain on biologic responses. Acute pain serves a biologic purpose. It acts as a warning signal because it can activate the sympathetic nervous system. This stimulation causes the release of catecholamine neurotransmitters, such as epinephrine, which give rise to various physiologic responses. As a result, clients experiencing acute pain exhibit physiologic responses similar to those found in "fight-or-flight" reactions (see Chap. 7). These responses include increased heart

McGill-Melzack PAIN QUESTIONNAIRE

Patient's name ____________ Age ________

File No. ____________ Date ________

Clinical category (e.g., cardiac, neurologic)

Diagnosis: ____________

____

Analgesic (if already administered):

1. Type ____________
2. Dosage ____________
3. Time given in relation to this test ________

Patient's intelligence: circle number that represents best estimate.

1 (low) 2 3 4 5 (high)

****

This questionnaire has been designed to tell us more about your pain. Four major questions we ask are

1. Where is your pain?
2. What does it feel like?
3. How does it change with time?
4. How strong is it?

It is important that you tell us how your pain feels now. Please follow the instructions at the beginning of each part.

____

Part 1. Where Is Your Pain?

Please mark, on the drawings below, the areas where you feel pain. Put E if external, or I if internal, near the areas you mark. Put EI if both external and internal.

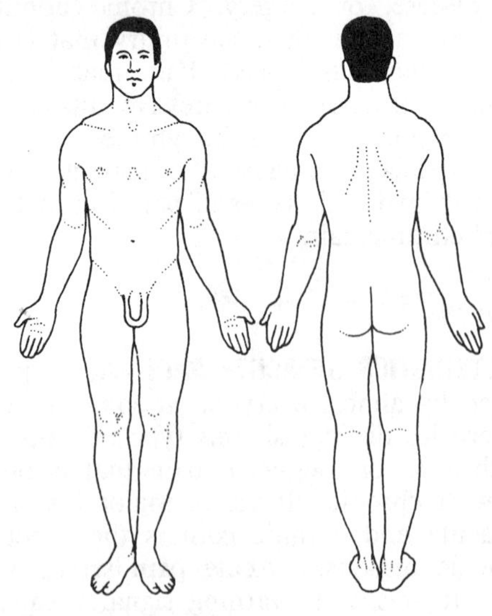

Part 2. What Does Your Pain Feel Like?

Some of the words below describe your *present* pain. Circle *ONLY* those words that best describe it. Leave out any category that is not suitable. Use only a single word in each appropriate category—the one that applies best.

1
Flickering
Quivering
Pulsing
Throbbing
Beating
Pounding

2
Jumping
Flashing
Shooting

3
Pricking
Boring
Drilling
Stabbing
Lancinating

4
Sharp
Cutting
Lacerating

5
Pinching
Pressing
Gnawing
Cramping
Crushing

6
Tugging
Pulling
Wrenching

7
Hot
Burning
Scalding
Searing

8
Tingling
Itchy
Smarting
Stinging

9
Dull
Sore
Hurting
Aching
Heavy

10
Tender
Taut
Rasping
Splitting

11
Tiring
Exhausting

12
Sickening
Suffocat-
ing

13
Fearful
Frightful
Terrifying

14
Punishing
Grueling
Cruel
Vicious
Killing

15
Wretched
Blinding

16
Annoying
Troublesome
Miserable
Intense
Unbearable

17
Spreading
Radiating
Penetrating
Piercing

18
Tight
Numb
Drawing
Squeezing
Tearing

19
Cool
Cold
Freezing

20
Nagging
Nauseating
Agonizing
Dreadful
Torturing

Part 3. How Does Your Pain Change With Time?

1. Which word or words would you use to describe the *pattern* of your pain?

1	2	3
Continuous	Rhythmic	Brief
Steady	Periodic	Momentary
Constant	Intermittent	Transient

2. What kind of things *relieve* your pain?

3. What kind of things *increase* your pain?

Part 4. How Strong Is Your Pain?

People agree that the following 5 words represent pain of increasing intensity. They are:

1	2	3	4	5
Mild	Discomforting	Distressing	Horrible	Excruciating

To answer each question below, write the number of the most appropriate word in the space beside the question.

1. Which word describes your pain right now? ____
2. Which word describes it at its worst? ____
3. Which word describes it when it is least? ____
4. Which word describes the worst toothache you ever had? ____
5. Which word describes the worst headache you ever had? ____
6. Which word describes the worst stomach ache you ever had? ____

FIGURE 8-4 ♦ The McGill-Melzack Pain Questionnaire. (From Melzack, R. [1975]. The McGill Pain Questionnaire: Major properties and scoring methods. *Pain, 1,* 272–281.)

rate, blood pressure, and respiratory rate; dilated pupils; and sweating. Behavioral signs of acute pain may include restlessness, an inability to concentrate, apprehension, and overall distress (Table 8-1).

Acute pain is usually temporary, of sudden onset, and easily localized. The client can frequently describe the pain, which may subside with or without treatment.

Acute pain frequently results from sudden, accidental trauma, such as fractures, burns, and lacerations, or from surgery, ischemia, and acute inflammation. Acute pain is often the result of trauma involving superficial or cutaneous structures. This pain is confined to the affected area. As the painful area heals, the quality or sensation of the pain changes. Acute pain, although possibly severe, is limited over time and generally can be managed successfully clinically. Both the caregiver and the client can see an end in sight which makes coping somewhat easier.

POSTOPERATIVE PAIN Pain accompanying surgery is one of the most common examples of acute pain, but it is poorly understood and not always well managed. It is conservatively estimated that 20% of all clients who undergo surgery experience mild pain, 20% to 40% experience moderate pain, and 40% to 70% experience serve pain (Bonica, 1983). According to some authorities, the alarmingly high number of clients who experience pain after surgery can be attributed to inadequate analgesia (Acute Pain Management Guideline Panel, 1992). As discussed earlier, others believe that inadequate pain control stems from societal attitudes and believe that people in pain should "grin and bear it." Still others identify the fear of addiction as a major factor in physicians prescribing and administering less than optimal amounts of analgesics after surgery. Whatever the reason, some people undergoing surgery suffer needlessly.

Pain is an expected outcome of surgery. Not only is there a sensory component arising from the area of tissue destruction, there is also a major psychosocial component.

TABLE 8-1 Physiologic and Behavioral Responses to Acute and Chronic Pain

Pain Type	Physiologic Response	Behavioral Response
Acute	• Increased blood pressure initially • Increased pulse rate • Increased respiratory rate • Dilated pupils • Perspiration	• Restlessness • Inability to concentrate • Apprehension • Distress
Chronic	• Normal blood pressure • Normal pulse rate • Normal respiratory rate • Normal pupils • Dry skin	• Immobility or physical inactivity • Withdrawal • Despair

Relationship to Type of Surgical Approach According to several studies, the type and site of the operation are the most important predictors in determining the incidence, severity, and duration of postoperative pain. Similarly, the extent of the operation, the degree of tissue trauma, and the positioning of the client during surgery contribute to the overall incidence and severity of postoperative pain.

Intrathoracic and upper intra-abdominal surgical approaches are generally associated with more severe, steady wound pain as well as pain on movement in the postoperative period. Conversely, many clients who undergo superficial surgery of the head and neck, chest wall, or limbs report minimal or no pain postoperatively. Muscle splitting procedures are far more painful than muscle stretching procedures. On the basis of this information, surgeons have modified their techniques over the years in an attempt to reduce or minimize the components of this type of pain.

Influence of Psychosocial Variables A person's postoperative pain experience is not limited to the level of tissue trauma. Postoperative pain is also influenced by many psychosocial variables. Personal factors, such as age and sociocultural group, may be important determinants for predicting patterns of expressing and coping with postoperative pain.

Anxiety is perhaps the best-explored psychologic determinant in predicting postoperative pain. A highly anxious client may appear to be more distressed and affected by pain. Numerous studies have been done in an attempt to correlate preoperative information with postoperative pain (Acute Pain Management Guideline Panel, 1992). Some nursing studies, such as that of Johnson and associates (1978), indicate that clients who receive preoperative procedural information (i.e., a description of the expected sensation as well as techniques to enhance relaxation) seem to cope better with postoperative pain. In addition, these clients recover more quickly than clients given only factual information about the anticipated postoperative experience.

Highly anxious clients, however, may be given minimal procedural information, such as the location of the incision, the sequence of events before surgery (e.g., preoperative sedation and visits from perioperative personnel), and postoperative care regimens. For these clients, too much information can exacerbate fear and pain (Acute Pain Management Guideline Panel, 1992).

The nurse stresses to the client the importance of requesting analgesia when he or she perceives pain. The nurse should repeat these instructions at regular intervals if the client is anxious because anxiety interferes with the ability to process information. The nurse also uses nonpharmacologic interventions, such as distraction and relaxation, to help the highly anxious client (see later).

CHRONIC PAIN

CHARACTERISTICS OF CHRONIC PAIN Chronic pain is a major health problem. It has been estimated that in the United States alone 25% of people, many of them more than 65 years old, are affected with a chronic illness and chronic pain. In contrast to acute pain, chronic pain serves no biologic purpose. After the pain's initial warning signal, the body must learn to adapt to the persistent pain impulses by blocking or adjusting to the activation of the sympathetic nervous system, which causes the fight-or-flight reaction in acute pain. Because of this adaptation, many of the obvious symptoms that are associated with physiologic responses to pain are absent or less obvious in the client with chronic pain.

Chronic pain is defined as pain that persists or recurs for indefinite periods, usually for more than 6 months. Onset is gradual, and the character and quality of the pain changes over time. Because chronic pain frequently involves deep somatic and visceral structures, it is usually diffuse, poorly localized, and often difficult to describe. If the underlying cause of the chronic pain cannot be treated medically, controlling the long-term effects of chronic pain may be a difficult clinical challenge.

Chronic pain is associated with a variety of health problems, such as cancer, connective tissue diseases, peripheral vascular diseases, and musculoskeletal disorders (Fig. 8–5). It is also seen in posttraumatic problems, such as phantom limb pain and low back pain. The degree of chronic pain varies, depending on the type of problem and whether it is progressive, stable, or capable of resolution. Unless the disease process is arrested or reversed, the severity of chronic pain may worsen to the point that the client is physically and emotionally debilitated. Even when the physiologic pain stimuli are eliminated or resolved, the client's perception of pain may linger. This is sometimes called the "chronic pain syndrome." A client's response to chronic pain is influenced by his or her ability to cope, the availability of family support and social resources, and the severity of the physiologic and emotional consequences (see Table 8–1).

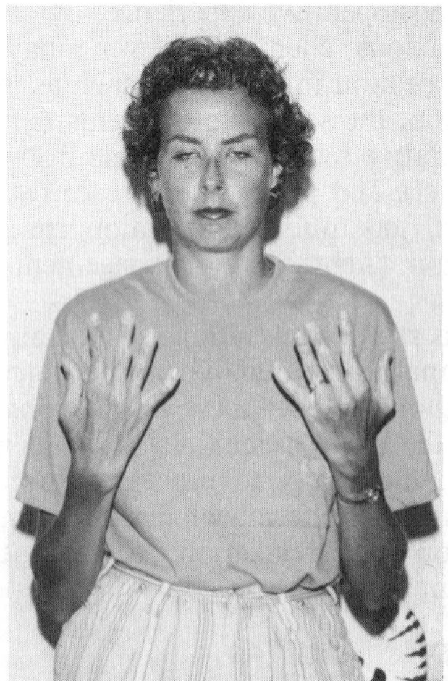

FIGURE 8–5 ◆ For people with such chronic conditions as rheumatoid arthritis, daily pain may be a fact of life.

Because chronic pain persists for extended periods, it can interfere with activities of daily living and personal relationships. It can also result in emotional and financial burdens. Thus, the efforts of an interdisciplinary health care team must manage the situation effectively. If pain is inadequately managed, it is an overwhelming, frustrating experience for both sufferer and caregiver. Although many of the characteristics of chronic pain are similar in different clients, the nurse should be aware that each chronic pain situation is unique and requires a highly specialized plan of care.

CHRONIC PAIN SYNDROME Clients sometimes have chronic pain associated with a physical problem. Eventually, the physiologic alterations resolve or become less detectable. However, the perception or sensation of pain persists. The degree of pain appears to be out of proportion to the physical findings, yet the pain is real to the person experiencing it. Clients in this situation often subject themselves to a variety of medical tests and frequent hospitalization while searching for a cause for or explanation of their pain. So-called doctor shopping is common in this group of clients. Some clients invest an incredible amount of time and energy in the health care system in the hope of uncovering a solution for their pain. As a result, clients with chronic pain syndrome focus on what they cannot do rather than what they can to do. Clients often demonstrate learned helplessness, powerlessness, dependency, and sick role behaviors. When pain persists for long periods, family members are often emotionally drained, frustrated, and in need of help in dealing with the client. A behavioral approach, which includes family therapy coupled with emotional rehabilitation if necessary, is a useful strategy in this situation.

CHRONIC MALIGNANT (CANCER-RELATED) PAIN Although many clients with advanced malignant disease experience severe pain, adequate pain control could be achieved for most of them. Even when the best pain management techniques are used, however, the complexity of this type of pain often limits the success of pain management efforts.

Cancer-related pain arises from a variety of mechanisms. For example, as a malignant tumor invades the bone, chemicals known as prostaglandins are released. These substances sensitize nerve receptors in the bone and increase their sensitivity to painful stimuli. In part, this explains the extreme degree of pain associated with bony metastases.

Other causes of cancer-related pain include arterial ischemia, venous engorgement, nerve compression, infection, inflammation, necrosis, and ulcerations. In addition, the sources of these problems are usually in deep somatic and visceral structures. These types of painful sensations, coupled with the diffuse nature of the pain, hamper the client's ability to describe and localize cancer pain. (For additional information on this type of pain, see Chapter 26.)

COLLABORATIVE MANAGEMENT

ASSESSMENT

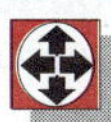

HISTORY

The nurse asks the client about the pain experience, including the sequence of events (precipitating and relieving factors); the nature of adjustments, if any, in the client's life or that of the family; and beliefs about the cause of the pain and what should be done about it (client's expectations). Personal characteristics, such as the client's age and culture, influence attitudes about reporting a pain history. Families and significant others are included in this information-gathering process.

Clients may report pain in the absence of any observable or documented physiologic changes in the body. The nurse keeps in mind that all pain is real and operates from the premise that pain is "whatever the person experiencing it says it is." The nurse respects the client's verbal and nonverbal expressions of pain without making judgments or inferences about the reality of the pain. If clients perceive that health professionals doubt the existence of their pain, mistrust and other negative feelings can arise and interfere with a therapeutic client-nurse relationship.

The nurse also assesses the length of time the client has experienced pain. Clients who experience acute pain may welcome an opportunity to discuss their pain with the nurse because acute pain is a relatively short-term experience and is easily described by clients. However, clients with chronic pain can be frustrated when they are unable to adequately describe their vague, diffuse pain experience. Repeated questioning in this situation can be nonproductive and nontherapeutic for the client.

SPECIAL CONCERNS FOR THE ELDERLY The elderly client's complaints of pain may be ignored by caregivers. Herr and Mobily (1991) found that some elderly clients in a residential center stopped expressing their discomfort because they were treated as "chronic complainers." Other elders stated that the response to their complaints was "What do you expect at your age?" Older adults do not typically have age-related pain (see Chaps. 4 and 5).

Nurses should also consider that when they take a history from elderly clients, the clients may be anxious or temporarily disoriented as a result of pain or because they are in an unusual environment. The nurse observes for nonverbal indicators of pain, such as grimacing, and checks for changes in behavior. For example, if a client becomes restless, hostile, or combative, the nurse considers pain as a possible underlying reason for the behavior. Too often a client who behaves in this manner is labeled with a diagnosis of dementia or other cognitive impairment or is categorized by the nursing staff as "difficult." Chart 8–1 highlights key points for assessing an elderly client in pain.

CHART 8–1

Nursing Focus on the Elderly ♦ The Elderly Client Experiencing Pain

When taking a client history:
- Be sure that the client is wearing glasses and hearing aid(s), if appropriate and available.
- Provide adequate lighting and privacy to avoid distracting background noise.
- Alter a written pain scale to include large lettering, adequate space between lines, and color for increased visualization.

If the client cannot verbally communicate:
- Assess for nonverbal indicators of pain, such as grimacing or crying.
- Observe for changes in the client's behavior, such as increased confusion or combativeness.

Respond to complaints of pain promptly—they are not typically age-related complaints.

Administer the prescribed amount of analgesics for postoperative pain in a timely manner. If pain is not resolved, use nondrug pain relief measures and notify the physician immediately.

ESSENTIAL DATA FOR A COMPLETE PAIN HISTORY Information about a client's pain can be helpful in understanding the factors that are associated with the client's present pain or previous episodes of pain. If the client is in pain when the nurse is taking the history, the nurse should keep the session reasonably short or continue at a later time. Data to obtain include:

- *Precipitating factors.* Does the client associate any activities, ingestion of food, or other environmental factors with the onset of pain? What does the client think causes the present pain? Was the onset of pain sudden or insidious? Has the client done anything or taken anything to relieve the pain? What were the results of the intervention?
- *Aggravating factors.* What factors make the pain worse? What influence has this pain had on the client's activity? What changes in life activity have been affected (e.g., diet, job, sleep)?
- *Localization of pain.* Can the client localize the pain or describe where it travels or radiates?
- *Character and quality of pain.* What words does the client use to describe the pain, its character, quality, or intensity?
- *Duration of pain.* How long has the client experienced this pain?

PHYSICAL ASSESSMENT/CLINICAL MANIFESTATIONS

The overt or observable clinical manifestations of pain include physiologic responses, motor or body movements, and affective behaviors such as crying. Although physiologic changes occur in response to acute noxious stimuli, these changes are usually *not* reliable indicators of chronic pain. Acute pain, with its property of warning an individual about harm, elicits several physiologic signs and symptoms. These signs and symptoms are largely a function of sympathetic nervous system stimulation. Clients with acute pain often manifest pronounced changes in vital body functions, such as tachycardia and blood pressure changes. The blood pressure is usually elevated initially and is then decreased. In addition, clients with acute pain may become diaphoretic, restless, and apprehensive.

Physiologic changes in response to chronic pain are usually masked as the body attempts to compensate for and adapt to the noxious stimuli. The pain no longer serves as a necessary warning. Changes in vital signs related to chronic pain may be evident only when pre-existing pain occurs or as new sites of painful stimuli arise.

Certain motor or body movements may be associated with acute or chronic pain. Some may be more exaggerated or obvious than others. Clients in pain may support or shield ("splint"), holding painful body parts while moving, or lie listlessly because they are afraid to move (Fig. 8–6). The nurse assesses the functional status and degree of impairment in the client with pain (see Chap. 13).

LOCATION OF PAIN The nurse assesses the location of pain from two dimensions:

- The level of pain, either deep or superficial
- The position or location of pain

Most clients, whether they are experiencing acute or chronic pain, can usually describe the depth of pain perceived. However, the actual area or location of the pain may not be as easily identified.

The nurse asks the client whether the pain is superficial or deep. In general, clients who have pain involving superficial or cutaneous structures describe their pain as "superficial" and can often localize the pain to a specific area. These structures have an abundant nerve supply, which contributes to the ease and accuracy of the client localizing the pain. In contrast, clients who perceive pain from deeper somatic or visceral structures within the body may have difficulty localizing their pain (a result of the poor innervation of this area).

Pain may be described as belonging to one of four categories, related to its location:

- Localized pain—pain confined to the site of origin
- Projected pain—pain along a specific nerve or nerves
- Radiating pain—diffuse pain around the site of origin that is not well localized
- Referred pain—pain perceived in an area distant from the site of painful stimuli

A client who has difficulty specifying the exact location of pain can be asked to point to the painful areas on his or her own body or on another person. Sometimes having the client point to or shade in the painful areas on a diagram of the front and back of the human body is helpful (see Fig. 8–2). When clients cannot identify the painful areas and state that they just "hurt all over," the nurse encourages the client to focus on parts of the body that are not painful. The nurse asks the client to concentrate on different body parts, beginning with the hand and fingers of one extremity, while asking him or her to identify the presence or absence of pain. As the nurse focuses attention on selected areas of the body, the client is assisted in localizing painful areas.

Often clients who state that they hurt everywhere begin to realize that some parts of the body are not painful. As painful areas are identified, the nurse helps the client to understand the origin of the pain. This understanding is particularly important for clients with cancer because every new pain often raises the suspicion of metastasis (spread of disease). The pain may be caused by other reasons, such as immobility or constipation.

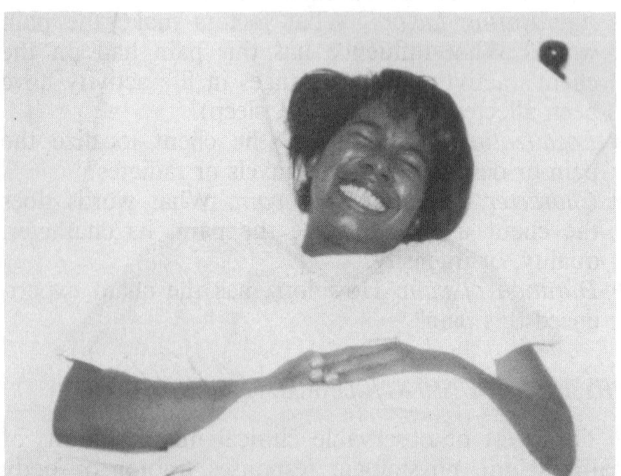

FIGURE 8–6 ◆ A client with severe abdominal pain splinting to reduce her pain.

CHARACTER AND QUALITY OF PAIN After asking the client to locate the pain, the nurse asks him or her to describe how the pain feels. Clients may use a word or group of words to convey the sensations or feelings of the pain. The nurse avoids suggesting descriptive words for the pain. Some clients who are frustrated and are having difficulty describing their pain may benefit from using the McGill-Melzack Pain Questionnaire (see Fig. 8–4). With this measurement tool, the nurse asks the client to circle descriptive terms in the appropriate categories to best describe the pain.

Another useful strategy is to ask the client to describe the sensation by comparing it to a situation or event that may be comparable to the feeling of pain. For example, a man with excruciating diffuse abdominal pain from advanced cancer might say that his pain feels as if a soldier were walking around inside his abdomen, with no set path or destination, stepping on mines. For this man, pain is unpredictable and never-ending, and produces a "blowing-up" sensation.

PATTERN OF PAIN Pain is rarely the same at all times. It is perceived differently over time and is subjected to various precipitating and aggravating factors (see earlier discussion under History).

INTENSITY OF PAIN Subjective measurements of pain intensity are more reliable than the overt or observable parameters of pain. Only the client can determine the amount or severity of pain experienced. Various analog scales and other tools are designed to help the client quantify the degree or intensity of pain and help the nurse assess the pain.

TOOLS TO MEASURE PAIN The nurse may use tools to measure pain in the clinical setting to assess and determine the effectiveness of relief-oriented interventions. This approach involves giving the person in pain a scale, which could be verbal or visual, and asking him or her to rate the pain stimulus by using that scale. Such scales usually indicate pain intensity, although they might also assess the emotional aspects of pain. Verbal descriptive scales typically group words such as "none," "moderate," or "severe" and permit an intensity rating of pain. Visual analog scales (VAS) usually use a 10-cm line to represent a continuum of pain intensity and include verbal anchors that describe the intensity of the stimuli. For examples of such rating scales, see Figure 8-7.

The visual analog scale is the scale most widely used to assess acute postoperative pain. The McGill-Melzack scale is sometimes criticized, though, for lacking a category to indicate no pain.

Variations in the scales are important determinants for selecting the appropriate measurement tool. Clients with chronic, nagging, diffuse pain may have difficulty using broad numeric scales ranging from 0 to 10. Some clients are better able to use word scales and prefer measurements that contain descriptive words or phrases rather than numeric scales.

Most clients find this approach to the clinical evaluation of pain to be reasonably simple, economical, and understandable. However, these types of scales generally allow the client to rate pain only in terms of intensity. In addition, their use may be too difficult for subjects with poor reading or verbal skills.

When using tools to measure pain in elderly clients, the nurse considers possible visual or hearing limitations. The client should wear glasses and one or two hearing aids if appropriate. Increased lighting with non-glare bulbs may improve visual perception. The tools may be altered to include large lettering, adequate spacing between lines, and color on a white background (Herr & Mobily, 1991).

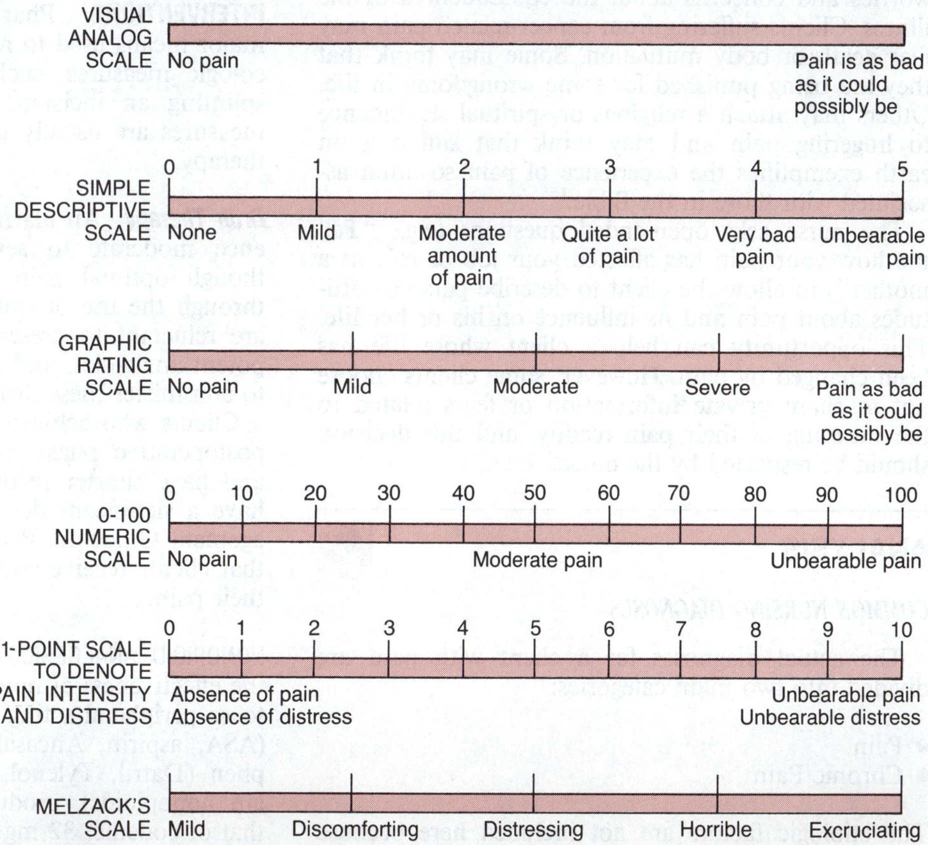

FIGURE 8-7 ◆ Commonly used pain-rating scales.

PSYCHOSOCIAL ASSESSMENT

ACUTE PAIN All pain holds significant meaning for the person experiencing it. For clients experiencing acute pain from surgery, the pain may be interpreted as necessary and expected. The pain may be viewed with relief as a sign that some greater problem has been resolved or alleviated by the surgery. Knowledge that the duration of the pain is limited may allow the client to deal with unpleasant sensations without too much difficulty. In contrast, acute chest pain associated with angina may be the beginning of a life of fear and uncertainty for the client.

CHRONIC PAIN Psychosocial factors that influence chronic pain are varied. Some are similar to those found in the acute pain experience, such as anxiety or fear related to the meaning of the pain for each client. Because pain persists in the chronic situation, or perhaps is only partially relieved, the client may feel powerless, angry, hostile, or desperate. Other people may react to chronic pain with depression, social withdrawal, and preoccupation with physical symptoms. The client with chronic pain is also vulnerable to labels such as "chronic complainer," "fake," or "turkey." Because many of the behavioral manifestations of acute pain (e.g., sweating, writhing, increased blood pressure) are absent in the client with chronic pain, the caregiver might doubt the existence of the pain.

If the pain is chronic and associated with a progressive disease, such as cancer, rheumatoid arthritis, or peripheral vascular disease, the client may have worries and concerns about the consequences of the illness. Clients suffering from cancer-related pain may fear death or body mutilation. Some may think that they are being punished for some wrongdoing in life. Others may attach a religious or spiritual significance to lingering pain and may think that suffering on earth exemplifies the experience of pain so often associated with those in the Bible.

The nurse asks open-ended questions (e.g., "Tell me how your pain has affected your job or role as a mother") to allow the client to describe personal attitudes about pain and its influence on his or her life. This opportunity can help a client whose life has been changed by pain. However, some clients choose not to share private information or fears related to the meaning of their pain readily, and this decision should be respected by the nurse.

ANALYSIS

COMMON NURSING DIAGNOSES

The actual diagnoses for a client with pain are divided into two main categories:

- Pain
- Chronic Pain

The etiologic factors are not included here because they vary, depending on the cause of the pain and each client's response.

ADDITIONAL NURSING DIAGNOSES

In addition to the common nursing diagnoses, the client experiencing acute or chronic pain may have one or more of the following nursing diagnoses:

- Anxiety related to loss of control
- Fear related to pain
- Powerlessness related to illness-related regimen
- Altered Role Performance related to a change in health status and impaired coping
- Altered Sexuality Patterns related to illness and pain
- Impaired Physical Mobility related to pain and discomfort
- Activity Intolerance related to pain and/or depression
- Sleep Pattern Disturbance related to pain
- Self-Care Deficit (total or partial) related to pain
- Altered Health Maintenance related to a feeling of hopelessness

PLANNING AND IMPLEMENTATION

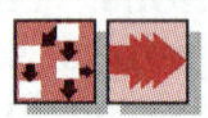

PAIN

PLANNING: CLIENT GOALS The major goal in the management of acute pain is that the client will experience relief of pain.

INTERVENTIONS Pharmacologic measures are the major means used to relieve acute pain. Nonpharmacologic measures, such as the use of a pillow for splinting an incision, are also effective, but these measures are usually used in conjunction with drug therapy.

Drug Therapy An alarming number of clients experience moderate to severe pain after surgery even though optimal pain relief can often be achieved through the use of drugs. However, some physicians are reluctant to prescribe certain drugs, particularly potent analgesics, and nurses are sometimes reluctant to administer these drugs (see earlier discussion).

Clients who achieve adequate analgesia during the postoperative phase experience fewer complications and have shorter recovery periods than clients who have a significant degree of pain (Acute Pain Management Guideline Panel, 1992). Nurses must ensure that clients receive adequate interventions to manage their pain.

NONOPIOID ANALGESICS Many people underestimate the effectiveness of nonopioid analgesics, also referred to as peripheral-acting analgesics. Acetylsalicylic acid (ASA, aspirin, Ancasal✱), 650 mg, and acetaminophen (Datril, Tylenol, Ace-Tabs✱), 650 mg (which are nonopioids), produce pain relief comparable to that of codeine, 32 mg orally, and meperidine (Demerol), 50 mg orally, which are opioids, for mild to moderate pain. Aspirin has direct analgesic effects because it inhibits prostaglandin synthesis in the presence of inflammation.

Over-the-counter (OTC) medications are not given alone for the treatment of severe pain. They are usually administered in conjunction with opioid analgesics. Aspirin must be used with caution after surgery because it can irritate the gastrointestinal tract and interferes with platelet aggregation. The nurse monitors the client carefully for bleeding and bruising.

Nonsteroidal anti-inflammatory drugs (NSAIDs) are also popular nonopioids that possess anti-inflammatory properties by inhibiting prostaglandins. Therefore, they are particularly useful in the management of acute inflammation caused by tissue destruction. Ketorolac (Toradol) is one of the most popular NSAIDs prescribed by physicians for short-term use in cases of acute pain. Unlike other NSAIDs, this drug is available in both oral and parenteral form. The side effects of NSAIDs are similar to those of aspirin, with the additional concern of sodium and water retention. This is a special concern in the elderly, who can easily develop congestive heart failure from fluid retention. The nurse observes for, and teaches the client and family to observe for, these untoward effects of medication.

OPIOID ANALGESICS Opioid analgesics (also called opioids or narcotics) are central-acting analgesics that are the cornerstone of pharmacologic acute pain management (Acute Pain Management Guideline Panel, 1992). These drugs work by binding with opioid receptors both within and without the central nervous system. For acute pain, they may be administered by the oral, rectal, intramuscular, intraspinal, intravenous, or subcutaneous route.

Classification of Opioids. Opioid analgesics are classified as full agonists, partial agonists, or mixed agonist-antagonists. "Full agonists produce a maximal response within the cells to which they bind; partial agonists produce a lesser response . . . ; and mixed agonist-antagonists activate one type of opioid receptor while simultaneously blocking another type" (Acute Pain Management Guideline Panel, 1992, p. 17).

The most important type of opioid receptor is the mu receptor. Commonly used opioids that bind with mu (mu opioids) are morphine (Roxanol, MSIR, Statex♣), hydromorphone (Dilaudid), codeine, oxycodone (Roxicodone), meperidine (Demerol), and fentanyl (Sublimaze) (see Chap. 21). Clients receiving these agonists should not receive agonist-antagonists, such as pentazocine (Talwin) or nalbuphine (Nubain), because they may negate the effect of the agonists (Haviley et al., 1992). Table 8–2 lists common opioid agonists and agonist-antagonists.

Meperidine (Demerol) is a commonly used opioid analgesic prescribed by physicians after surgery. The dose of this drug that is commonly prescribed is insufficient and therefore provides inadequate pain control. Meperidine is effective for 2½ to 3½ hours, and a dose of 75 mg is equivalent to only 5 to 7.5 mg of morphine. In addition, elderly clients and those with renal disease should not take meperidine because of the prolonged half-life of the drug (Acute Pain Management Guideline Panel, 1992). The drug is also contraindicated in the elderly client because it causes cerebral irritation, which leads to seizures, memory loss, hallucinations, paranoia, and depression in these clients (Hofland, 1992).

All mu opioids may cause urinary retention, constipation, sedation, respiratory depression, and nausea and vomiting. These side effects are generally correlated with the blood level of the medication. The nurse observes for these problems and reports their occurrence to the physician. The nurse remembers that pain and the stress and anxiety that are accompany it are potent respiratory *stimulants* that may negate the respiratory depressive action of the drugs. The nurse also keeps in mind that the effect of all opioid analgesics may be potentiated in a client who is small and frail, has reduced blood volume or renal disease, or has received anesthetic agents.

If respirations fall below 10, the physician typically orders naloxone (Narcan), an opioid antagonist, to reverse the respiratory depression. Naloxone also reverses the effects of the analgesic. In the hospital or nursing home setting, this drug is kept in an emergency drug box or cabinet on each unit for use as necessary.

Opioid Analgesic Regimens. Immediately after surgery or traumatic injury, the physician typically prescribes oral or parenteral opioid analgesics on a continuous time schedule or on an intermittent, as needed (PRN) schedule. Oral drugs are the most convenient and least expensive.

When the physician orders an intermittent schedule, the client depends on the nurse to give the medication when requested. If the client cannot communicate the need for analgesia, the nurse must anticipate the client's need by observing for nonverbal clues or behavioral changes.

TABLE 8–2 Opioid Agonists and Antagonists

Opioid Agonists

- Morphine and congeners
  - Morphine (MS Contin, Roxanol, MSIR)
  - Hydromorphone (Dilaudid)
  - Codeine
  - Oxycodone (Roxicodone)
  - Levorphanol (Levo-Dromoran)
  - Fentanyl (Sublimaze, Duragesic)
- Meperidine and congeners
  - Meperidine (Demerol)
- Methadone (Dolophine)

Opioid Agonist-Antagonists

- Morphine-type
  - Butorphanol (Stadol)
  - Buprenorphine (Buprenex)
- Nalorphine-type
  - Pentazocine (Talwin)
  - Nalbuphine (Nubain)
  - Butorphanol (Stadol)

Use of Opioids for Substance Abusers. Acute pain management for clients who are known or suspected substance abusers is a difficult but increasingly common problem. Some hospitals have pain management teams that assist with this type of problem in managing a client's pain. The team members usually represent several disciplines including, but not limited to, nurses, physicians, clinical pharmacists, and social workers.

Clients who are substance abusers often have traumatic injuries and other health problems that cause acute pain. Chart 8–2 lists some recommendations that the nurse can follow when planning and implementing pain management for a client who is a substance abuser.

Adjuvant Drugs for Acute Opioid Analgesia. A relatively common practice in the treatment of acute pain is the administration of adjuvant drugs—drugs that add to the action or effects of opioids. The ones most frequently used are hydroxyzine pamoate (Vistaril) and promethazine (Phenergan, Histanil✱).

These drugs were once thought to potentiate the action of opioids, but evidence has shown that they enhance the sedating effects of the opioid and not the actual pain-relieving effects. They also help to relieve the anxiety and nausea that frequently accompany acute pain. Some analgesic effects have been demonstrated with hydroxyzine alone in the treatment of postoperative pain. The nurse observes clients receiving promethazine or hydroxyzine in addition to opioid analgesics for the side effect of sedation.

Patient-Controlled Analgesia. Patient-controlled analgesia (PCA) is one way to combat the problem of inadequate analgesia in the management of acute and chronic pain. This method allows the client to control the dosage of opioid analgesia received. This approach to pain control can improve pain relief and increase client satisfaction. It can also decrease the amount of opioid consumption per day when compared with intermittent dosing methods.

Clients receiving medication as needed for postoperative pain must sense the pain, report it to the nurse, and wait until the nurse is aware of the client's need and has the time to administer the analgesic. Considerable time may pass in this sequence because the client may wait too long before asking for the medication. Alternatively, the nurse may not understand the need to respond promptly to the request, or the nurse may have other equally pressing responsibilities. Whatever the reasons, the client's pain may be more severe or out of control by the time the analgesic is received. More medication is then required to relieve the pain adequately.

However, clients who have ready access to an analgesic are more likely to medicate themselves before the pain becomes severe, and thus they may require a reduced amount. Having control over when the drug can be administered also reduces the client's anxiety, which helps relieve pain.

PCA is achieved through the use of a PCA infusion pump (Fig. 8–8). Both stationary pole pumps for hospital use and ambulatory pumps for nursing home or home use are available. The infusion pump delivers the desired amount of medication through a conventional intravenous route (for acute pain) or through an implantable intravenous catheter (tunneled catheter) inserted in subcutaneous tissue (for chronic pain) (see Chap. 16). The most commonly used drug for PCA is morphine. However, the use of PCA hydromorphone (Dilaudid) and fentanyl (Sublimaze) is gaining popularity. Meperidine (Demerol) is still reserved for short-term use, usually less than 48 hours.

Drug security (to avoid overdosing) is achieved through a locked syringe pump system or locked drug reservoir system. The device is programmed to deliver a certain amount of drug within a specific interval known as a lockout interval. The physician specifies the interval, usually 5 to 15 minutes, and the nurse programs it into the PCA delivery system. When the client presses the button or pendant (on ambulatory pumps), the appropriate bolus or demand dose is delivered. If the client attempts access to the drug before the designated time interval between doses has elapsed, no drug will be administered. With this system, there is little chance of clients overmedicating themselves.

The nurse's role in caring for clients using PCA is to teach them how to use the device and to report side effects, such as dizziness, nausea and vomiting, and inability to void. As with all opioids, the nurse monitors the client's vital signs frequently, at least every 4 hours. In some cases, the nurse may need to anticipate the client's need for pain medication and administer doses of the drug if the client is unable to do so. For example, the client who is confused or cannot move may need the nurse to push the pump button to administer the drug.

CHART 8–2

Nursing Care Highlight ◆ Pain Management for the Substance Abuser

- Define the exact source(s) of pain and treat them—e.g., heat for muscle spasms, antibiotics for infection.
- Follow the principles of opioid use, such as not giving agonist-antagonists to clients receiving opioid agonists.
- Use nonopioid therapies, including medication, cutaneous stimulation techniques, and cognitive and behavioral strategies.
- Monitor the client for drug abuse while in the health care agency to ensure that drugs are not being stolen or hoarded.
- Set limits and negotiate with the client about drug choices and dosing.
- Provide clear instructions about drug use and dosing schedules.
- Consult with other members of the health care team, such as physicians, psychiatrists, psychologists, pharmacists, and social workers.

Data from the Acute Pain Management Guideline Panel. (1992).

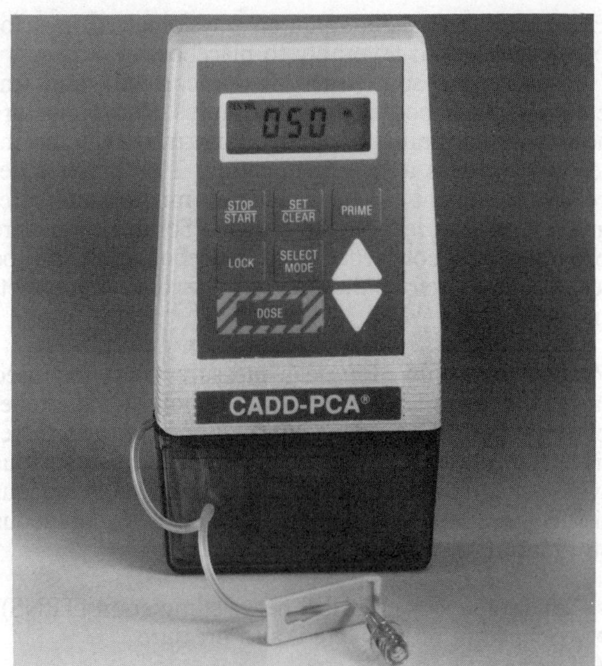

FIGURE 8–8 ◆ An ambulatory patient-controlled analgesia (PCA) infusion pump. (CADD-PCA is a registered trademark of Pharmacia Deltec.)

Continuous Intravenous Opioid Analgesia. Continuous intravenous opioid administration is used for both acute pain, which is usually postoperative pain, and chronic pain, which is mostly associated with cancer. For adequate and consistent pain control, postoperative clients typically receive continuous intravenous infusions coupled with a PCA demand dosing schedule. The continuous rate is sometimes referred to as the basal rate of drug administration. For this type of pain, morphine, hydromorphone (Dilaudid), meperidine (Demerol), and, less frequently, fentanyl (Sublimaze), may be prescribed. Continuous infusion of meperidine is not recommended for more than 48 to 72 hours because its toxic metabolite, normeperidine, is capable of inducing seizures if it accumulates in the blood. The usual morphine dose prescribed by the physician for postoperative pain is 1 to 2 mg per hour, whereas meperidine, at 10 to 25 mg per hour, or hydromorphone, at 0.15 to 0.4 mg per hour, can be administered. Fentanyl doses, prescribed in micrograms, vary.

The physician specifies the PCA demand doses, or bolus amounts, along with the lockout interval.

Intraspinal Opioid Analgesia. There are two major methods for administering intraspinal analgesia: epidural and intrathecal. *Epidural* analgesia, also known as peridural or extradural analgesia, refers to the instillation of a pain-blocking agent, usually an opioid analgesic, into the epidural space (the space between the dura mater and the vertebral column) through a small catheter (Fig. 8–9). It is far more popular than *intrathecal* (subarachnoid) analgesia, in which a pain-blocking agent is introduced into the space between the arachnoid mater and pia mater of the spinal cord, where cerebrospinal fluid is located.

Action of Intraspinal Analgesia. The goal of both types of intraspinal analgesia is to interrupt the conduction of pain at the point that the sensory fibers exit from the spinal cord. Epidural analgesia has been used since the 1950s, but it has become more popular as newer and more innovative approaches to acute pain control are explored. Epidural analgesia is used with clients who are predisposed to respiratory complications, including those undergoing thoracic surgery, those with pre-existing respiratory disease, and those who are obese.

Morphine and fentanyl (Sublimaze) are commonly used drugs that are given intraspinally. A temporary catheter is used for acute pain control. This device is not sutured to the skin and is easily dislodged. The nurse tapes the catheter in two places to anchor it properly. Some clinicians do not recommend transparent dressings, because the catheter may be dislodged when the dressing is removed.

If chronic pain from cancer or nonmalignant causes persists, a tunneled catheter or implanted port (e.g., Porta-Cath Epidural) may be surgically inserted for prolonged use. A tunneled catheter exits onto the abdomen. When the implanted port is used, the port is placed over the lower rib cage for easy access.

Complications of Intraspinal Analgesia. In caring for a client with intraspinal analgesia, the nurse helps to prevent and monitors for complications. Complications associated with intraspinal analgesia are directly related to catheter placement, catheter maintenance, and the type of analgesic used. Complications are more common in intrathecal analgesia.

Pruritus (itching), along with nausea and vomiting, are common side effects of intraspinal opioids. Pruritus is treated with a small amount of naloxone (Narcan) rather than diphenhydramine (Benadryl, Allerdryl✱), which can negate the action of the opioid agonist. The physician usually prescribes an antiemetic for nausea and vomiting.

Infection results from failure to maintain aseptic technique during catheter placement and drug instillation. Infection also results from failure to maintain

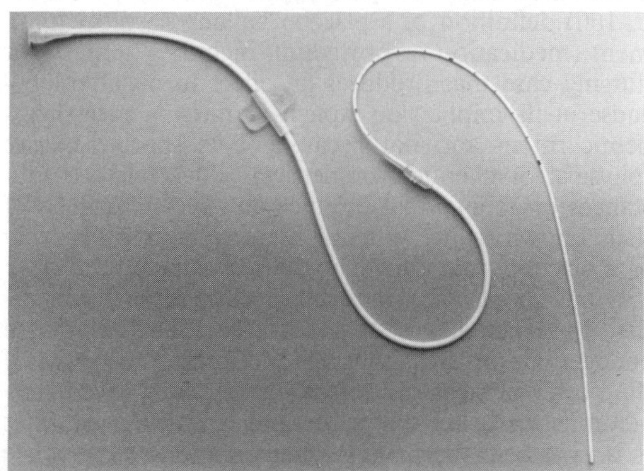

FIGURE 8–9 ◆ A small catheter (SynchroMed Spinal Catheter, Model 8703) is used to instill a pain-blocking agent into the epidural space. (Courtesy of Medtronic, Inc., Minneapolis, MN.)

aseptic conditions for indwelling catheters at the site of insertion or at the site of tube junctions. To prevent infections, the nurse ensures that all catheter line connections are secure and that an occlusive sterile dressing is maintained over the catheter site.

The nurse also observes the elderly or restless client carefully for possible dislodgement of the catheter. The older client may become confused or disoriented as a result of surgery and try to pull out the temporary catheter. The catheter usually stays in place for about 48 to 72 hours, depending on the reason for the analgesia and the hospital policy.

Clients who receive intraspinal analgesics are also at risk for respiratory depression resulting from high plasma and/or cerebrospinal fluid concentrations of the instilled drug. The nurse monitors respirations frequently and reports to the physician immediately respiration rates below 10 per minute during the period after the administration of analgesia. Opioid-induced respiratory depression usually occurs within the first few hours after the administration of fentanyl begins but may not be seen for 12 hours or more when morphine is given. This complication is managed by the administration of naloxone (Narcan), either intravenously or intramuscularly.

Urinary retention is another common problem associated with intraspinal analgesia, although the cause is not clear. This problem usually occurs during the first or second day of analgesia administration and may be treated with bethanecol chloride (Urecholine) or intermittent urinary catheterization. The incidence of this complication is less than 25% and is more likely to occur in men than in women (Wild & Coyne, 1992).

INTRAPLEURAL OPIOID ANALGESIA While not commonly used, opioid analgesia may be administered via the intrapleural route. This method is sometimes used postoperatively for clients who have had a thoracotomy (chest surgery) (Polomano et al., 1993).

PLACEBOS The clinical use of placebos in non–research-based therapies has not been shown to have a sustained effect on pain relief. McCaffery's (1979, p. 160) definition of a placebo is "any medical treatment (medication or procedure, including surgery) or nursing care that produces an effect in a patient because of its implicit or explicit or nursing care therapeutic intent and not because of its specific nature (physical or chemical properties)." Placebos are substances or actions that produce an effect regardless of their known value. When a client responds favorably to a placebo, it is known as the *placebo effect.*

Some clients who receive placebos report pain relief. Evidence has shown that these clients release endogenous opiates, such as endorphins, because of the power of suggestion, trust in the caregiver's interventions, or belief that something, regardless of what it is, will help the pain. A client's favorable response to a placebo does not mean that the pain was not real or was imaginary or faked. Placebos should never be used to determine whether a client's pain is real. Even clients with documented physiologic causes for pain can respond favorably to placebos.

Placebos are sometimes used incorrectly and unethically. Placebos such as intramuscular saline are administered, and the client is informed that the injection contains a pain medication. This practice deceives the client and perpetuates mistrust in caregivers and the health care system. Some health care providers are concerned that placebos may not be legal, and therefore they are not used in many settings.

Physical Measures Physical measures may be used instead of or in addition to drug therapy for the relief of acute pain. Cutaneous stimulation strategies to relieve pain have been in use for many years. Various types of stimulation to the skin and subcutaneous tissue produce pain relief. Methods of cutaneous stimulation include techniques such as:

- Transcutaneous electrical nerve stimulation (TENS)
- Application of heat, cold, and pressure
- Therapeutic touch
- Massage
- Vibration

Whatever the method, several characteristics of cutaneous stimulation must be considered:

- The benefits of these techniques are highly unpredictable and may vary from application to application.
- Pain relief is generally sustained only as long as the stimulation continues.
- Trials may be necessary to establish the desired effects.
- Stimulation itself may aggravate pre-existing pain or may produce new pain.

Despite these drawbacks to cutaneous stimulation, these methods are effective in the management of both acute and chronic pain. These techniques have physiologic as well as psychologic effects on the client. The use of cutaneous stimulation techniques also gives clients an opportunity to participate actively in the management of their pain.

TRANSCUTANEOUS ELECTRICAL NERVE STIMULATION Transcutaneous electrical nerve stimulation (TENS) involves the use of a battery-operated device capable of delivering small electrical currents to the skin and underlying tissues. The first-generation, or conventional, TENS unit is used most frequently. Electrodes connected to a small box are placed over the painful sites. The voltage or current is regulated by adjusting a dial to the point at which the client perceives a prickly, "pins and needles" sensation. The current is adjusted on the basis of the client's degree of pain relief and level of comfort.

The physician, nurse, or physical therapist (depending on the health care setting) assists the client in applying the electrodes either on the painful area or above or below it (Fig. 8–10). A conducting substance (usually a gel) is placed between the electrode and the client's skin.

The advantages of these units are that the client can wear the unit and achieve a level of pain relief while participating in activities of daily living. The unit is easy to use and can be worn for several hours. However, the skin at the site of the electrode placement may become irritated. To prevent this, the nurse teaches the client to rotate electrode sites.

The Pain Suppressor, or second-generation, TENS unit is also available for pain control. This unit works by using electrodes, with water as the conducting substance. The unit delivers a current, which the client generally does not feel. This type of stimulation to the skin and subcutaneous tissues causes an elevation of serotonin levels in the systemic circulation. Serotonin is a neurotransmitter that is associated with enhancing the endogenous opiate activity of endorphins and enkephalins. This type of unit is not worn. Rather, treatments are administered several times per day for 10- to 20-minute periods.

In general, clients use TENS units for the management of acute and chronic pain. The conventional, or first-generation, unit is indicated for localized pain, such as postoperative or local chronic pain, particularly low back pain. The second-generation unit, because of its systemic effects, can be used for diffuse pain syndromes, such as those related to cancer.

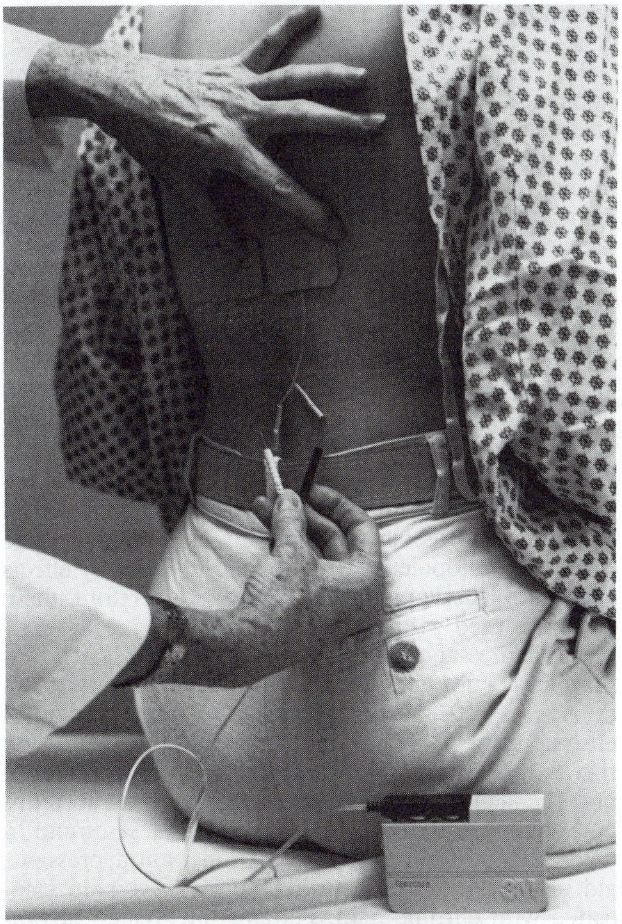

FIGURE 8–10 ◆ Application of a TENS unit.

OTHER CUTANEOUS TECHNIQUES Additional cutaneous stimulation techniques, such as the use of touch, pressure, massage, and vibration, as well as the application of heat and cold, all stimulate the skin and somehow interrupt the pain pathway. These interventions are relatively easy for the client to learn and are fairly economical. Table 8–3 summarizes these techniques.

Cognitive and Behavioral Strategies Cognitive and behavioral strategies to relieve pain, such as distraction, have also been popular for years, either as adjuncts to drug therapy or as alternative interventions. Theoretical explanations for the effectiveness of these measures reflect the beliefs of the gate control theory.

Distraction can be an effective method of acute pain relief. Simple measures such as holding a client's hand, taking him or her for a walk, or encouraging deep breathing exercises can divert attention from the pain. Nurses often observe that clients request less pain medication when family members are present. After visiting hours are over, many clients request something for pain. Instead of viewing distraction as a therapeutic pain relief measure, some nurses may question the presence or severity of the pain if a client is easily distracted from it.

Distraction alters the perception of pain, but it does not influence the cause or peripheral mechanism of pain. It is a transient method of pain relief and is probably best used with other pain control measures.

Nurses can provide several methods of distraction. Visual distractors, such as pictures or television, can divert the client's attention to something pleasant or interesting. Auditory distractors, which include music or relaxation tapes, can have a calming effect. Changing the environment can remove unpleasant stressors or reminders that may enhance the client's pain. Physical distractions, such as deep breathing exercises, help the client concentrate on other physiologic sensations.

Distraction is used for:

- Exacerbations of pain
- Painful procedures (e.g., dressing changes or invasive procedures)
- Interrupting the client's constant perception of pain

CHRONIC PAIN

PLANNING: CLIENT GOALS The major goals are that the client will experience:

- Reduction in or relief of the pain
- Modification of the pain
- Prevention of the recurrence or worsening of the pain

INTERVENTIONS The goals for chronic pain management are accomplished by interrupting the relentless

TABLE 8–3 Cutaneous Stimulation Techniques Used to Interrupt the Pain Pathway

Technique	Method of Application	Comments
Therapeutic touch or "laying on of hands"	• The hands of the caregiver are placed on or close to the client's body.	• The intent to help on the part of the caregiver may contribute to the success of this technique. This technique may extend the nurse-client relationship.
Pressure	• A hand or other object is placed firmly over or around the painful area.	• Pressure seems to relieve pain, decrease bleeding, and prevent swelling. Release of pressure is associated with increased blood flow and return of pain.
Massage	• The hands or fingers are moved slowly or briskly over a body part. A lubricant or other substance is sometimes used.	• Effects include muscle relaxation and sedation.
Vibration	• Electrical and battery-operated vibrators produce a massage effect.	• Vibration may decrease the intensity of the noxious (pain) stimuli.
Application of heat and cold	• Heat may be applied in a variety of ways, including short-wave diathermy, microwave diathermy, sonography, use of melted paraffin and Hubbard tank, use of hot water bottle or heating pad, use of heat cradle and lamp, application of moist pads or towels, use of hot tub or shower, or use of gel packs. • Cold may be applied in a dry or moist way, similar to heat applications. Ice chips, cold towels and packs, and chilled gel packs are commonly used.	• Both heat and cold may reduce muscle spasm and decrease pain. Cold probably slows the conduction velocity of nerves. Heat increases the tendency for bleeding and therefore should not be used after trauma. Heat may also increase edema and is not indicated if circulation is poor. Both heat and cold should be used cautiously if clients have impaired sensation or cannot communicate.

Data from McCaffery, M. (1979). *Nursing management of the patient with pain* (2nd ed., pp. 117–126). Philadelphia: J. B. Lippincott.

cycle of pain, anxiety, and sometimes depression. Nonsurgical methods of pain reduction are generally used before surgical techniques are tried. The client may eventually need a combination of nonsurgical and surgical measures.

Nonsurgical Management A pharmacologic approach to the treatment of chronic pain is the most effective and reliable method of pain management. Other measures may be used in combination with drug therapy.

Drug Therapy Although a number of drugs have been used in the management of chronic pain, the physician most commonly prescribes nonopioid and opioid analgesics.

NONOPIOID ANALGESICS Acetylsalicylic acid (aspirin, Ancasal✱), acetaminophen (Tylenol, Ace-Tabs✱), and nonsteroidal anti-inflammatory drugs (NSAIDs) such as ibuprofen (Motrin, Amersol✱) are effective in the management of mild chronic pain. They are also effective in combination with opioid analgesics. Aspirin and NSAIDs possess anti-inflammatory properties in that they peripherally inhibit prostaglandins. This property makes them particularly useful in treating the inflammation associated with arthritis and cancer. The requirements for opioid analgesics in the client with chronic pain can be reduced by aspirin and NSAIDs. However, both aspirin and NSAIDs can cause gastric disturbances in the client and can have an effect on platelets, which results in a tendency toward bleeding. The nurse observes the client for gastric discomfort or vomiting and bleeding or bruising and reports these problems to the physician immediately. NSAIDs can also cause sodium and water retention and lead to congestive heart failure, especially in the elderly.

The physician also commonly prescribes acetaminophen for chronic pain. Acetominophen exerts its analgesic action by blocking peripheral pain receptors, thus increasing the threshold of these receptors to painful stimuli. Reports of liver toxicity have been associated with higher doses of this drug (1000 mg) taken more frequently than every 4 hours for long-term use.

ADJUVANT DRUGS Other nonopioid drugs that are used to control the pain of certain neuralgias (pain along the distribution of nerves) include carbamazepine (Tegretol, Mazepine✱) and phenytoin (Dilantin). The exact mechanism of action of these drugs is unknown, but it is believed that they inhibit the transmission of pain impulses. Both carbamazepine and phenytoin are associated with a wide variety of side effects (hematopoietic, hepatic, and pulmonary effects and central nervous system toxicity). Therefore, these drugs are used with extreme caution.

Antidepressants, such as amitriptyline (Elavil), imipramine (Tofranil), doxepin (Sinequan), and trazodone (Desyrel), may be beneficial in the treatment of chronic pain. These drugs help treat the depression that can accompany chronic pain. They also stimulate the activity of endogenous opiates (endorphins and enkephalins) by increasing levels of serotonin, a neurotransmitter. In some situations, antidepressants aid in the control of neuropathic or nerve pain associated with chronic pain. Perhaps the greatest advantage of this group of drugs is the sedative effect, which occurs when they are administered at bedtime.

In some cases, antianxiety agents help relax the client and thus help relieve pain. The physician selects the drugs that have the fewest side effects because many of these drugs cause confusion, drowsiness, and hypotension. Examples of drugs that may be ordered include alprazolam (Xanax), clorazepate (Tranxene, Novoclopate✱), and oxazepam (Serax, Zapex✱).

OPIOID ANALGESICS Opioid analgesics are drugs capable of relieving pain by binding to various opiate receptors located in the central nervous system (see the discussion under Nursing Interventions for Pain.) For chronic pain, opioids are commonly administered by the oral, subcutaneous, intravenous, intraspinal, or transdermal route.

The equianalgesic guide (Table 8–4) can help determine the dose and route of one opioid in comparison with another. Equianalgesic refers to the dose and route of administration of one drug that produces approximately the same degree of analgesia as the given dose and route of another drug. Most commonly, 10 mg of morphine is the standard dose that other opioids are measured against. Equianalgesic drug lists should serve only as a guide in determining the comparative analgesic potencies among these drugs. Dose modifications may be necessary according to each client's response to the drugs.

TABLE 8–4 Equianalgesic Guide for Opioids

Analgesic	Oral (PO) Dose (mg)*	Intramuscular (IM) Dose (mg)*
Meperidine (Demerol)†	150	50
Codeine†	100	60
Pentazocine (Talwin)†	90	30
Morphine‡,§	15	5
Oxycodone (Percodan, Tylox)§	10	7.5
Methadone‖	10	5
Diacetylmorphine (heroin)	10	2.5
Oxymorphone (Numorphan)¶	5	1
Hydromorphone (Dilaudid)§	4	2
Levorphanol (Levo-Dromoran)	2	1

* Equianalgesic doses listed are obtained from a variety of sometimes conflicting studies. They are meant only as guidelines for "by-the-clock" standing-order analgesic therapy of chronic pain. No analgesic listed is superior PO to its equianalgesic dose of PO morphine. The dose interval is q3–4 h for all except the following: meperidine, q2–3 h, levorphanol, q4–6 h, and methadone, q6–8 h.

† Of little value in severe pain

‡ Equianalgesic intravenous dosage, 3–4 mg q3–4 h

§ Rectal suppositories are available or can be prepared. The per rectum dose is equal to the PO dose.

‖ Caution: Sedative side effects often accumulate despite inadequate analgesic effect.

¶ Available for nonparenteral use in rectal suppository form only

Problems Associated with Long-Term Use of Opioids. The side effects of opioid analgesics are discussed under Nursing Interventions for Pain. The long-term use of these agents is associated with several problems.

Physical Dependency. Physical dependency is associated with the administration of opioids on a long-term basis. Physical dependency is *not* the same as addiction. However, it is sometimes confused with addiction. Nursing textbooks and resource materials often fail to make the appropriate distinctions (Ferrell et al., 1992a). Physical dependency is a physiologic adaptation of the body tissues that requires continued administration of the drug for normal tissue function. When a client who has become physically dependent on opioid agents abruptly ceases using them, so-called withdrawal symptoms result. These symptoms include nausea and vomiting, abdominal cramping, muscle twitching, profuse perspiration, delirium, and convulsions. When it is necessary to discontinue opioid analgesic therapy in such a client, a slow tapering, or weaning, of the drug dosage lessens or alleviates withdrawal symptoms.

Addiction. Addiction is a common fear of health professionals who administer or prescribe opioids and of clients who receive them. Addiction is a term used to describe persistent craving and abuse of a drug for recreational purposes. Addiction is a psychologic phenomenon. Although physical dependence does occur in many people who become addicted, it should not be used to describe addiction. Although addiction rarely occurs in clients who use opioids for medicinal relief of pain, the fear of addiction is a major factor leading to the inadequate prescription and administration of these drugs.

Clients also worry about becoming addicted to analgesics (Champlin, 1992). They may be concerned about the possibility of drug withdrawal symptoms, which are often seen in the street addict. The nurse clarifies the term addiction with clients while stressing the concept of physical dependency.

Drug Tolerance. The client may also experience drug tolerance from opioid analgesic therapy. Tolerance is characterized by a gradual resistance of the body to the effects of an opioid, including its pain-relieving properties. When tolerance occurs, clients usually require more of the drug to receive the same analgesic effects. This is particularly a problem in clients who are substance abusers (see Chart 8–2). Tolerance to opioid analgesia is measured not only by the analgesic effects but also by the body's ability to adjust to the adverse reactions.

Continuous Intravenous Opioid Analgesia. For chronic cancer pain management, hourly doses of continuous opioid infusions vary, depending on the severity of the pain and the client's ability to tolerate the opioid. If the hourly dose needs to be increased, the physician usually increases it no more than 10% to 20% of the hourly rate and not before 3 to 4 hours has passed. It may be necessary for the nurse to monitor the client's vital signs frequently (at least every hour) until an adequate and safe level of drug is achieved. The physician calculates patient-controlled analgesia (PCA) demand doses on the amount of continuous hourly opioid administration. Usually the PCA demand dose is 33% to 50% of the basal or continuous rate, but sometimes it may be as high as 100% of the hourly rate. The lockout interval, unlike in PCA for acute pain, is usually longer, between 30 and 60 minutes.

Continuous Subcutaneous Opioid Analgesia. Continuous subcutaneous opioid analgesia is best for clients who have comprised venous access or for those whose central venous lines are being used for other fluids (Haviley et al., 1992). Subcutaneous infusion is accomplished through the use of a small (25- or 27-gauge) butterfly-type catheter or a special subcutaneous needle device placed under the skin into the subcutaneous tissue.

Typically, the subclavicular tissue underneath the clavicle or the abdomen is used. Placing the catheter in the extremities should be avoided, if possible, especially in terminally ill clients, since peripheral circulation may be impaired or edema may be present, which could affect absorption of the drug. The nurse applies an occlusive dressing over the site and rotates the site every 3 to 7 days, depending on the drug and the volume delivered. The physician usually orders no more than 3 to 6 mL per hour.

Morphine is the most common drug given by this route. Occasionally, hydromorphone (Dilaudid) or meperidine (Demerol) is used; however, these drugs are more irritating to the tissues, requiring more site changes (Baird et al., 1991). If the physician orders a PCA demand dosing schedule in addition to the continuous infusion, the volume of the bolus dose does not usually exceed 1 mL. In addition, the lockout interval, or time between doses that the client may access more opioids, is usually no more frequent than 30 to 60 minutes. Clients receiving continuous narcotic infusions with a PCA feature may require dose adjustments in their continuous rates if more than 6 to 12 bolus doses per day are used.

The nurse observes for and reports complications of subcutaneous infusion, which include leakage of fluid around the insertion site, inadequate pain relief, and edema around the site (Haviley et al., 1992).

Long-Term Intraspinal Analgesia. Long-term intraspinal opioid administration may be used for the management of chronic, intractable (uncontrollable or unyielding) pain, usually from cancer. A permanent epidural catheter may be inserted. Several catheter devices are available for this purpose. The DuPen Silastic catheter (Davol) is the most commonly used *external* catheter. A portion of the catheter exits the skin, where drugs can be intermittently injected or the catheter can be attached to an infusion device for continuous drug administration.

Implantable devices are also used. The Porta-Cath Epidural is implanted under the skin, and the catheter portion is inserted into the epidural space. Like the DuPen catheter, this device can be injected with drugs intermittently or can be connected to an infusion device for continuous opioid delivery. The SynchroMed pump (Medtronic, Inc.) is a totally implantable system that contains a drug reservoir, which is filled on a routine basis and is capable of continuously administering a certain volume of drug each day (Fig. 8–11).

Clients who receive intraspinal therapy are usually more tolerant of the effects of opioids and may not require the rigorous monitoring needed for postoperative analgesia. In some cases, the client can be managed at home or in a long-term care setting.

Transdermal Opioid Administration. Transdermal opioid administration is now possible with the transdermal fentanyl system (Duragesic). Duragesic is available in patch dose strengths of 25 μg/h, 50 μg/h, 75 μg/h, and 100 μg/h. The system is applied by removing the adhesive backing and placing it on the skin of the client's chest, either front or back, preferably on an area without hair. If hair is present on the chest, the nurse clips and shaves it. Once the patch is applied, it delivers a specified amount of drug into the skin. The drug absorbs over 72 hours. The physician calculates the appropriate dosage from the client's previous opioid requirement; if the requirement is known, the lowest patch strength is used initially. Transdermal administration should be used cautiously when the requirement is *not* known.

The nurse teaches the client and family how to apply the patch and to report side effects, such as dizziness, sedation, nausea, or a decrease in respiratory rate, to the physician or nurse. The nurse also explains that when the patch is first applied, it may take up to 24 hours before pain relief is apparent. Supplemental analgesia with short-acting opioids may be ordered until adequate blood levels of the transdermal drug are reached. The absorption of transder-

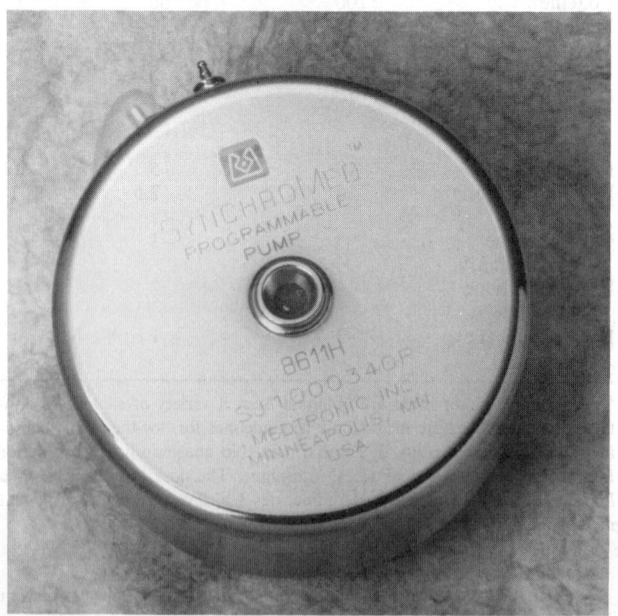

FIGURE 8–11 ◆ A SynchroMed implantable pump for delivery of a certain volume of long-term intraspinal analgesia each day. (Courtesy of Medtronic, Inc., Minneapolis, MN.)

mal analgesics is affected by the client's body temperature. The nurse teaches the client and family that a fever of 102° F (38.9° C) or greater might accelerate absorption of the drug from the skin and increase side effects. Clients should be monitored closely when fever is present. Once the system is removed, the client is monitored for about 24 hours, as the drug may still be released into the bloodstream from the site of application.

Cognitive and Behavioral Strategies Cognitive and behavioral strategies, including imagery, relaxation, hypnosis, biofeedback, and acupuncture, are often effective in the relief of chronic pain. They may be used instead of or in addition to drug therapy.

IMAGERY Imagery is a form of distraction in which the client is encouraged to visualize or think about some pleasant or desirable feeling, sensation, or event. Guided imagery takes place when a person, frequently a nurse, assists the client in sustaining a sequence of thoughts aimed at diverting the client's attention away from pain. Clients require intense concentration to visualize images. Clients who are extremely anxious, agitated, or unable to concentrate may benefit first from mild distraction.

Imagery is particularly useful with clients who experience chronic pain. Clients who practice this technique can mentally experience sights, sounds, smells, events, or other sensations vividly. First, the nurse assesses the client's level of concentration to determine if he or she can sustain a particular thought or thoughts for a desired time. The time interval for mental imagery can vary from 5 to 60 minutes. Behaviors that are helpful in assessing a client's capacity for imagery include the following:

- Reading and comprehending the newspaper
- Listening to music or other auditory stimuli
- Having the ability to follow and participate in sustained conversation
- Having an interest in environmental surroundings

When the client has demonstrated some ability to concentrate, the nurse assists the client in identifying a pleasant or favorable thought. The client is then encouraged to focus on this thought to divert attention away from painful stimuli. Audio tapes may help clients form and maintain images. The nurse, client, or family may wish to create such tapes for the client's use, or commercially available tapes may be used. An example of guided imagery instructions follows: "Imagine yourself on the beach on some deserted island. You can hear the sound of waves rushing onto the shore, the cry of sea gulls flying high above, and the rustling of trees as they are brushed gently by the wind. You can feel the warmth of the sun over your body and the cooling breeze."

RELAXATION TECHNIQUES Clients may use relaxation techniques to reduce anxiety, tension, and emotional stress, which may exacerbate pain. Techniques to help clients relax can be both physical and psychologic. Physical techniques include the following:

- The client receiving a body massage, back rub, or warm or hot bath
- Modifications in the client's environment to reduce distractions
- The client moving into a comfortable position.

Psychologic techniques include:

- The use of pleasant conversation
- The use of music
- The use of relaxation tapes

There are relaxation tapes that assist the client with progressive relaxation of the muscles. Relaxation exercises can be effectively coupled with guided imagery, distraction, and hypnosis. Chapter 7 describes relaxation techniques in detail.

HYPNOSIS Hypnosis is defined as an altered state of consciousness in which a person enters a trance and loses an overall sense of reality. Even though the person is in a trance, there is some sense of awareness and contact with reality and an understanding of what is actually happening. Hypnosis is used to treat a variety of pain syndromes, particularly chronic pain. It is used to help clients overcome the emotional consequences of pain and can promote a positive state of mind. Although nurses do not usually teach clients hypnosis, they are in a key position to help clarify misconceptions, instruct clients about relaxation and distraction, and encourage clients to practice self-hypnosis.

BIOFEEDBACK Biofeedback is used to treat chronic pain, anxiety, and other stress conditions. Biofeedback involves the monitoring of various physiologic responses by an electric device capable of sensing changes in the body and reporting this information to the client (see Fig. 7–4). Certain physiologic signals are transmitted to the feedback unit by electrode sensors, which are placed on the client's skin. The biofeedback unit amplifies and transforms physiologic information into visual signals (usually meter readings or colored lights). Clients are first alerted to stress-related responses, such as increased muscle tension or elevation in blood pressure. Then they are taught to regulate these responses through a combination of techniques, which include deep breathing exercises, progressive relaxation exercises, distraction, and visual imagery.

Biofeedback units vary. Some measure muscle contraction via electromyography and brain activity via electroencephalography. Galvanic skin response and skin temperature, which can reflect changes in blood flow, heart rate, or blood pressure, are also measured. Whatever the technique, physiologic responses that tend to worsen or prolong the client's pain are voluntarily controlled.

The client who is interested in learning biofeedback techniques to control pain is usually trained by a skilled therapist. The client is taught to observe the feedback information, report sensations or feelings that become apparent, and practice stress-reducing or pain-reducing techniques. Clients may need several sessions before they can recognize and control these responses. The client eventually becomes aware of even the most subtle changes in body function that indicate the onset or worsening of pain and automatically responds without the help of the biofeedback unit.

Biofeedback training helps the client gain control over pain. Clients require training and self-discipline if biofeedback and all other cognitive therapy strategies are to be used effectively.

ACUPUNCTURE The practice of acupuncture originated in China. According to ancient beliefs, the body is divided into ten hypothetic sections by parasagittal lines or meridians. Specific acupuncture points are located within these meridians. The acupuncturist inserts tiny needles into the skin and subcutaneous tissues at these points, and manual vibration or electrical stimulation is delivered. This technique is used to relieve pain and is thought to cure certain diseases.

Acupuncture is still widely acclaimed in China, but it is less popular in the Western World. Because the physiologic basis for this technique is unclear, many Western health professionals are skeptical about its usefulness. Nonetheless, acupuncture is practiced for anesthetic purposes during diagnostic procedures, during labor and delivery, during surgery, and for the treatment of pain. It is also used to help clients change behavior, for example, to stop smoking. More than 1000 acupuncture sites have been identified and 14 "lines" exist as *meridians* (Fig. 8–12).

Surgical Management Surgical intervention for chronic pain is used to interrupt the pain pathways when pain is intractable or severely debilitating. Surgery causes tissue destruction and some degree of neurologic deficit. Clients may not experience permanent relief from pain because there may be nerve cell regeneration or the development of alternative pain pathways. When chronic or persistent pain can no longer be adequately controlled with drugs or other pain-reducing methods, various surgical techniques are used (Fig. 8–13).

Nerve Blocks Nerve blocks are usually indicated for pain that is confined to a specific area or nerve distribution. With this procedure, a nerve root (or roots) is destroyed by a chemical agent (e.g., phenol or alcohol). Complications associated with this technique vary. Injections into peripheral nerve roots generally lead to decreased sensation in the area, with no effect on motor function. Injections into the lumbosacral area of the spinal cord may damage motor nerve roots, resulting in lost or impaired bowel, bladder, or sexual function. Although the intent of such procedures is to permanently destroy nerve transmission,

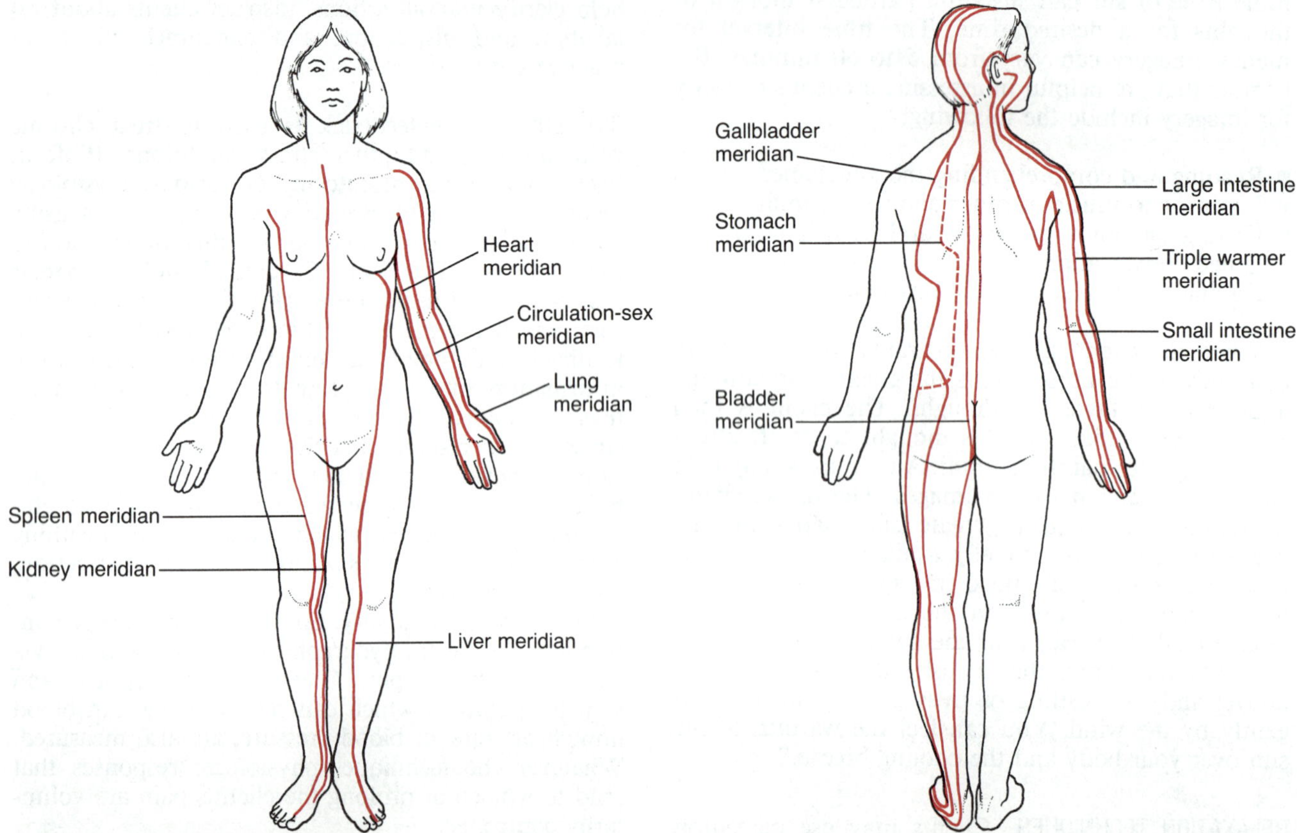

FIGURE 8–12 ◆ Acupuncture meridians.

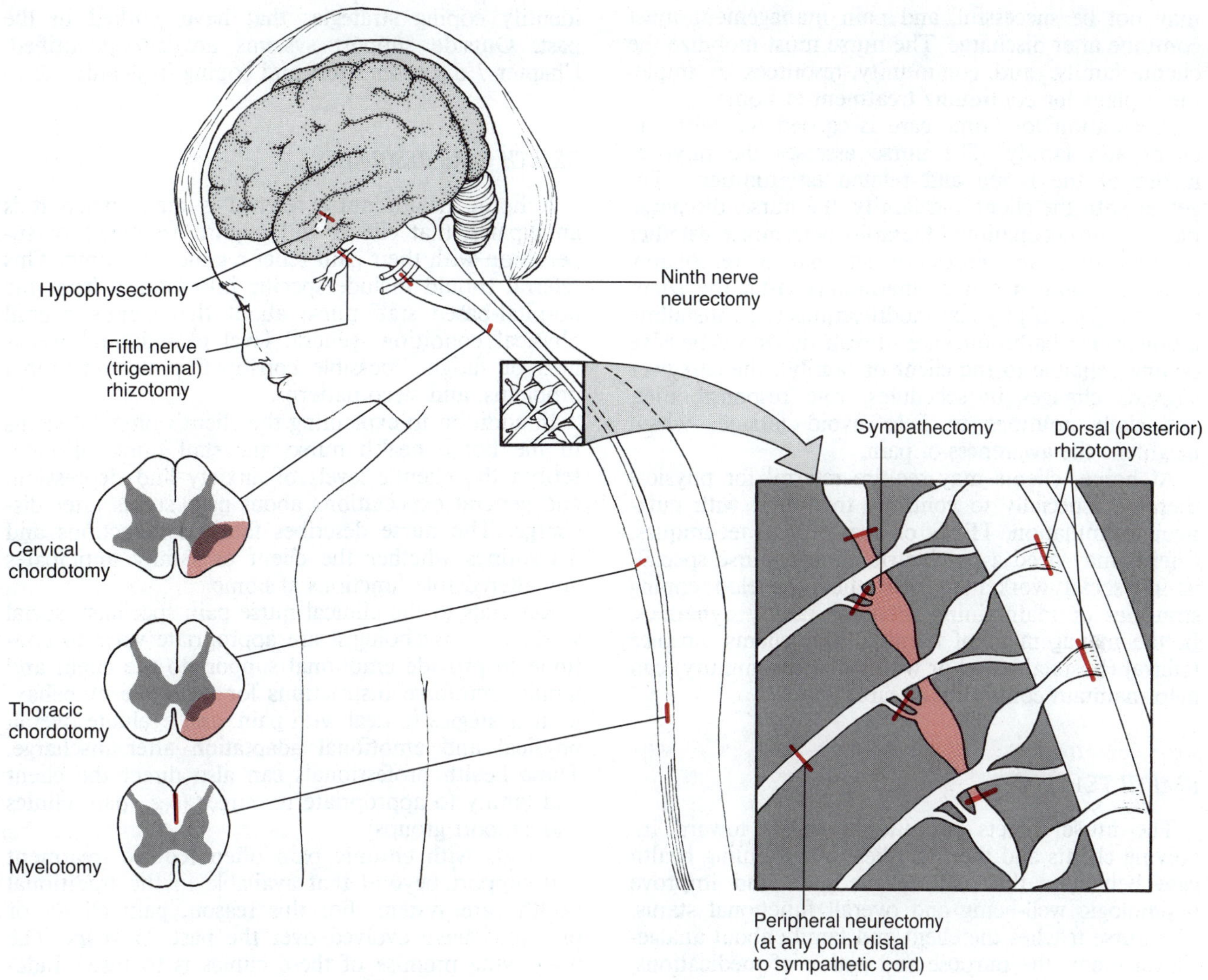

FIGURE 8-13 ◆ Surgical procedures designed to alleviate pain.

clients may experience only transient pain relief from these nerve blocks.

Because a nerve block is a surgical procedure performed by a physician, the physician is responsible for informing the client about the procedure, its risks, and alternative treatments. The nurse reinforces this information with the client and family.

Other Surgical Techniques Other techniques aimed at surgically interrupting the transmission of pain include rhizotomy and cordotomy. With the new, improved pain management measures currently available, these procedures are not performed as commonly today.

In rhizotomy, sensory nerve roots are destroyed where they enter the spinal cord. In a *closed* rhizotomy, a percutaneous catheter is inserted into the area and the sensory nerve roots are destroyed by neurolytic chemicals, coagulation, or cryodestruction (extreme cold). For an *open* rhizotomy, a laminectomy is necessary. During this surgery, the physician isolates the nerve roots and destroys them. With a cordotomy, the surgeon transects the pain pathways at the midline portion of the spinal cord before nerve impulses ascend to the spinothalamic tract. As with the other surgical procedures, clients may experience impaired bowel, bladder, or sexual function. Because of the complexity of the pain experience, the interruption of nerve conduction and pain pathways may not totally interrupt the client's sensation of pain.

After surgical intervention, the nurse assesses the nature of the neurologic deficits, if any, and teaches the client how to adapt to them. If the client has lost sensation in a body area, he or she will need to learn how to protect that area from harm. The nurse also assesses the client's expectations in relation to the surgical interruption of painful sensations and helps the client to express realistic expectations.

DISCHARGE PLANNING

HOME CARE PREPARATION

For some clients, the pain experience extends beyond hospitalization. Efforts to minimize the pain may not be successful, and pain management must continue after discharge. The nurse must mobilize the client, family, and community resources to implement plans for continuing treatment at home.

Preparation for home care is carried out with the client and family. The nurse assesses the physical layout of the home and related environment. Together with the client and family, the nurse, discharge planner, or occupational therapist determines whether modifications are necessary so that a reasonably pain-free regimen can be maintained after the client is discharged. If physical modifications (e.g., installing a downstairs bathroom) are unrealistic (too expensive or unacceptable to the client or family), the caregiver suggests changes in schedules, role responsibilities, and daily routines to help avoid fatigue, which heightens the awareness of pain.

At home, clients may require referral for physical therapy, especially to continue treatment with cutaneous stimulation, TENS, or heat or cold techniques. Clients may need a psychiatric clinical nurse specialist or social worker to help them develop coping strategies or maintaining adequate family dynamics. In the management of terminally ill clients, hospice referral (hospital-based or within the community) can help maintain continuity of care.

HEALTH TEACHING

The nurse directs educational efforts toward involving clients and their families in continuing health care behaviors that will relieve pain and improve psychologic well-being and overall functional status. The nurse teaches the client and family about analgesic regimens, the purpose and action of medications, their side effects or adverse reactions, and the importance of dosage intervals.

The nurse explains that ideally the analgesic regimen should not interfere with the client's sleep, rest, appetite, or level of physical mobility. If such interference occurs, the nurse encourages the family or significant other to consult with the physician or the visiting nurse.

PSYCHOSOCIAL PREPARATION

The nurse evaluates family support systems to assist the client in adhering to and continuing the proposed medical and nursing plans. Family members are informed about and included in activities during and after hospitalization.

To achieve a reasonable level of expectation for the client, the nurse suggests ways to continue participation in household, social, sexual, and work-oriented activities after discharge. The nurse can help the client identify important activities and plan them around adequate rest schedules.

The client with chronic pain needs continued support to cope with the anxiety, fear, and powerlessness that often accompany this type of pain. The nurse helps the client and family or significant others to identify coping strategies that have worked in the past. Outside support systems are also identified. Chapter 7 discusses stress and coping in detail.

HEALTH CARE RESOURCES

A home health nurse referral is made when it is anticipated that clients will require assistance or supervision with their pain relief regimen at home. This referral should include specific information from the hospital-based staff nurse about the client's overall physical condition, general level of sedation, weakness or fatigue, possible constipation or nutritional problems, and sleep patterns.

In addition to explaining the client's physical status to the home health nurse, the staff nurse also describes the client's levels of anxiety and depression, and general expectations about pain status after discharge. The nurse describes family interactions and determines whether the client or family anticipates any altered role functions at home.

Referrals to the clinical nurse pain specialist, social worker, or psychologist are appropriate ways to continue to provide emotional support to the client and family, reinforce instructions for cognitive or behavioral strategies to deal with pain, and evaluate overall physical and emotional adaptation after discharge. These health professionals can also direct the client and family to appropriate resources (e.g., pain clinics and support groups).

Clients with chronic pain often require treatment and support beyond that available in the traditional health care system. For this reason, pain clinics or programs have evolved over the past 25 years. The underlying premise of these clinics is to foster independence and self-care behaviors while promoting pain control and maximizing the client's quality of life. These programs use physical measures, cognitive and behavioral strategies, and surgical interventions as well as individual and group counseling for clients and family. Emphasis on many of the measures differs, depending on the program's orientation.

Some clients receive continuous or intermittent opioid administration at home or in a long-term care facility by any one of the methods described under Drug Therapy. If the nurse in the community health setting is unsure about drug management, a number of companies that manufacture infusion set-ups are available to assist the client and nurse in the home or alternate care setting. If other equipment, such as a TENS unit, is needed, the nurse can arrange for a medical supply company or pharmacy to provide one for the client. Answers to common questions about TENS units are listed in Chart 8-3.

EVALUATION

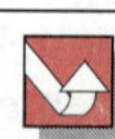

On the basis of the identified nursing diagnoses, the nurse evaluates care for the client with pain. The expected outcomes are that the client will:

CHART 8-3

Education Guide ♦ TENS Units

- The cost of using your TENS unit should be comparable to that for a regimen of prescription drugs or surgery.
- Insurance usually covers the cost of buying or leasing a TENS unit.
- You can get a TENs unit through the physician who prescribed it. TENS units are available by prescription only.
- Whether a TENS unit works for you will depend on your type of pain. These units have been used successfully on back pain, arm and leg pain, pain from neuralgia, arthritis pain, and other types of pain. A trial period under a physician's care is generally advised.
- TENS units are relatively simple to operate. You simply attach color-coded electrodes to your skin over the painful area. You then turn the unit on and, depending on your level of pain, you make day-to-day adjustments.

- State that acute pain is relieved or reduced.
- State that chronic pain is relieved or reduced, or that the pain is not worsened.
- Perform activities of daily living.
- Participate in his or her usual daily lifestyle, with modifications as needed.

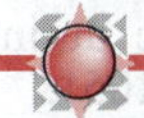

IMPLICATIONS FOR NURSING RESEARCH

Although there has been significant interest in nursing research on pain, a number of questions remain unanswered, for example:

♦ What characteristics of nurses determine their nursing interventions for the client experiencing pain?
♦ What is the best combination of interventions for the client in acute pain, especially after surgery?
♦ What cultural health beliefs and practices determine the response to pain and pain management of members of those cultures?
♦ What are the best guidelines for pain management in the elderly?
♦ What other nonpharmacologic nursing interventions may help relieve or reduce pain and anxiety?

SELECTED BIBLIOGRAPHY

Abrahm, J., Polomano, R. C., Kahn, M., & Tangoren, A. (1993). The Cancer Pain Attitude Scale (CPAS): A tool that assesses physician attitudes toward cancer patients with pain. *American Pain Society Program Book*, Nov. 4–7, p. A118.

Acute Pain Management Guideline Panel. (1992). *Acute pain management: Operative or medical procedures and trauma. Clinical practice guideline.* AHCPR Pub. No. 92-0032. Rockville, MD: Agency for Health Care Policy and Research, Public Health Service, U.S. Department of Health and Human Services.

*Alberico, J. G. (1984). Breaking the chronic pain cycle. *Americal Journal of Nursing, 84,* 1222–1227.

*American Pain Society. (1989). *Principles of analgesic use in the treatment of acute pain and chronic cancer pain: A concise guide to medical practice.* Washington, D.C.: American Pain Society.

Baird, S. B., McCorkle, R., & Grant, M. (1991). *Cancer nursing: A comprehensive textbook.* Philadelphia: W. B. Saunders.

*Barker, E. (1987). Pain. *Journal of Neurosurgical Nursing, 19,* 233–234.

*Bonica, J. (1983). The importance of education and training in pain diagnosis and therapy. In R. Rizzi & M. Visentin (Eds.), *Pain therapy* (pp. 1–10). Amsterdam: Elsevier Biomedical.

Burckhardt, C. S. (1990). Chronic pain. *Nursing Clinics of North America, 25,* 868–870.

*Burke, S. O., & Jerrett, M. (1989). Pain management across age groups. *Western Journal of Nursing Research, 11,* 164–178.

Calvillo, E. R., & Flaskerud, J. H. (1991). Review of literature on culture and pain of adults with focus of Mexican-Americans. *Journal of Transcultural Nursing, 2,* 16–23.

Calvillo, E. R., & Flaskerud, J. H. (1993). Evaluation of the pain response by Mexican-American and Anglo-American women and their nurses. *Journal of Advanced Nursing, 18,* 451–459.

Carroll, K. C., & Magruder, C. C. (1993). The role of analgesics and sedatives in the management of pain and agitation during weaning from mechanical ventilation. *Critical Care Nursing Quarterly, 15*(4), 68–77.

Champlin, L. (1992). Inadequate analgesia: Patients endure pain, fear addiction. *Geriatrics, 47*(8), 71–74.

Clark, I. M. (1993). Management of postoperative pain. *Lancet, 341,* 27.

Dobkin de Rios, M., & Achauer, B. M. (1991). Pain relief for the Hispanic burn patient using cultural metaphors. *Plastic and Reconstructive Surgery, 88*(1), 160–164.

Donovan, M. W. (1990). Acute pain relief. *Nursing Clinics of North America, 25,* 851–861.

Egbert, A. M. (1991). Help for the hurting elderly: Safe use of drugs to relieve pain. *Postgraduate Medicine, 89*(4), 217–228.

*Faherty, B., & Grier, M. F. (1984). Analgesic medication for elderly people post-surgery. *Nursing Research, 33,* 369–372.

Ferrell, B. A., Ferrell, B. R., & Osterweil, D. (1990). Pain in the nursing home. *Journal of the American Geriatrics Society, 38,* 409–414.

Ferrell, B. R., McCaffery, M., & Grant, M. (1991). Clinical decision making and pain. *Cancer Nursing, 14,* 289–297.

Ferrell, B. R., McCaffery, M., & Rhiner, M. (1992a). Pain and education: An urgent need for change in nursing education. *Journal of Pain and Symptom Management, 7*(2), 117–124.

Ferrell, B. R., McCaffery, M., & Ropchan, R. (1992b). Pain management as a clinical challenge for nursing administration. *Nursing Outlook, 40,* 263–268.

Ferrell, B. R., McGuire, D. B., & Donovan, M. I. (1993). Knowledge and beliefs regarding pain in a sample of nursing faculty. *Journal of Professional Nursing, 9*(2), 79–88.

Ferrell-Torry, A. T., & Glick, O. J. (1993). The use of therapeutic massage as a nursing intervention to modify anxiety and the perception of cancer pain. *Cancer Nursing, 16,* 93–101.

Gaston-Johansson, F., Albert, M., Fagan, E., & Zimmerman, L. (1990). Similarities in pain descriptions of four different ethnic-culture groups. *Journal of Pain and Symptom Management, 5*(2), 94–100.

Griepp, M. (1992). Undermedication for pain: An ethical model. *Advances in Nursing Science, 15*(1), 44–53.

Guyton, A. C. (1991). *Textbook of medical physiology* (8th ed.) Philadelphia: W. B. Saunders.

Haviley, C., et al. (1992). Pharmacological management of cancer pain: A guide for the health professional. *Cancer Nursing, 15,* 331–346.

Herr, K. A., & Mobily, P. R. (1991). Complexities of pain assessment in the elderly. *Journal of Gerontological Nursing, 17*(4), 12–19.

Herr, K. A., & Mobily, P. R. (1992). Interventions related to pain. *Nursing Clinics of North America, 27,* 347–370.

Hill, C. S. Jr., (1990). Relationship among cultural, educational, and regulatory agency influences on optimum cancer pain treatment. *Journal of Pain and Symptom Management, 5*(1) (Suppl.), S37–S45.

Hofland, S. L. (1992). Elder beliefs: Blocks to pain management. *Journal of Gerontological Nursing, 18*(6), 19–40.

*International Association on Pain, Mersky, H. (Chairman), Subcommittee of Taxonomy. (1979). Pain terms: A list with definitions and notes on usage. *Pain, 6,* 249.

*Jacox, A. K. (Ed.) (1977). *Pain: A source book for nurses and other health care professionals.* Boston: Little, Brown.

*Johnson, J., Rice, V., Fuller, S., & Endress, M. (1978). Sensory information, information in a coping strategy, and recovery from surgery. *Research in Nursing and Health, 1,* 4–17.

Jones, L., & Brooks, J. (1990). The ABCs of PCA. *RN, 53*(5), 54–60.

Keeney, S. A. (1993). Nursing care of the postoperative patient receiving epidural analgesia. *MEDSURG Nursing, 2*(3), 191–196.

*Keller, E., & Bzdek, V. (1986). Effects of therapeutic touch on tension headache pain. *Nursing Research, 35,* 101–105.

*Kreiger, D. (1975). Therapeutic touch: The imprimatur of nursing. *American Journal of Nursing, 75,* 784–787.

*Kreiger, D. (1981). *Foundations of holistic health practices: The renaissance nurse.* Philadelphia: J. B. Lippincott.

*McCaffery, M. (1979). *Nursing management of the patient with pain.* (2nd ed.) Philadelphia: J. B. Lippincott.

*McCaffery, M. (1980). Relieving pain with noninvasive techniques. *Nursing '80, 10*(12), 54–57.

McCaffery, M. (1990). Pain management: Nurses lead the way to new priorities. *American Journal of Nursing, 90,* 45–50.

*McCaffery, M., & Beebe, A. (1989). *Pain: Clinical manual for nursing practice.* St. Louis: C. V. Mosby.

McCaffery, M., Ferrell, B., O'Neil-Page E., Lester, M., & Ferrell, B. (1990). Nurses' knowledge of opioid analgesic drugs and psychological dependence. *Cancer Nursing, 13*(1), 21–27.

*McGuire, D. B. (1984). The measurement of clinical pain. *Nursing Research, 33,* 152–156.

McGuire, L. (1994). The nurse's role in pain relief. *MEDSURG Nursing, 3*(2), 94–107.

Meinhart, N. T., & McCaffery, M. (1983). *Pain: A nursing approach to assessment and analysis.* Norwalk, CT: Appleton-Century-Crofts.

*Melzack, R. (1973). *The puzzle of pain.* New York: Basic Books.

*Melzack, R. (1975). The McGill Pain Questionnaire: Major properties and scoring methods. *Pain, 1,* 277–299.

*Melzack, R. (1983). The McGill Pain Questionnaire. In R. Melzack (Ed.), *Pain assessment and management* (pp. 41–47). New York: Raven Press.

*Melzack, R., & Wall, P. D. (1982). *The challenge of pain.* New York: Basic Books.

Mooney, N. E. (1991). Pain management in the orthopaedic patient. *Nursing Clinics of North America, 26,* 73–87.

*National Institutes of Health. (1986). *The integrated approach to the management of pain: Consensus Development Conference statement.* Washington, D.C.: U.S. Government Printing Office.

Neeley, M. A. (1993). Pain management in elderly patients. *Med-Surg Nursing Quarterly, 1*(4), 32–51.

Pasero, C. L. (1994). Pain control. *American Journal of Nursing, 94*(2), 22–23.

Pasero, C. L., & McCaffery, M. (1994). Avoiding opioid-induced respiratory depression. *American Journal of Nursing, 94*(4), 25–30.

Polomano, R. C., Blumenthal, N. P., & Riegler, F. X. (1993). Intrapleural analgesia for the management of postoperative pain. *MEDSURG Nursing, 2*(3), 185–190.

Poniatowski, B. C. (1991). Continuous subcutaneous infusions for pain control. *Journal of Intravenous Nursing, 14,* 30–35.

Scott, I. (1992). Nurses' attitudes to pain control and the use of pain assessment scales. *British Journal of Nursing, 2*(1), 11–14, 18.

*Sternbach, R. A. (1968). *Pain: A psychophysiological analysis.* New York: Academic Press.

Stevens, K. (1990). Patients' perceptions of music during surgery. *Journal of Advanced Nursing, 15,* 1045–1051.

Thomas, B. L. (1990). Pain management for the elderly: Alternative interventions (Part 1). *AORN Journal, 52,* 1268–1272.

Turnage, G., Clark, L., & Wild, L. (1990). Spinal opioids: A nursing perspective. *Journal of Pain and Symptom Management, 5*(3), 154–162.

Von Roenn, J. H., Cleeland, C. S., Gonin, R., Hatfield, A. K., & Pandya, K. J. (1993). Physician attitudes and practices in cancer pain management: A survey from the Eastern Cooperative Oncology Group. *Annals of Internal Medicine, 119,* 121–126.

Walding, M. F. (1991). Pain, anxiety, and powerlessness. *Journal of Advanced Nursing, 16,* 388–397.

Walker, J. M., Akinsanya, J. A., Davis, B. D., & Marcer, D. (1990). The nursing management of elderly patients with pain in the community: Study and recommendations. *Journal of Advanced Nursing, 15,* 1154–1161.

*Wells, N. (1982). The effect of relaxation on postoperative pain. *Nursing Research, 31,* 236–238.

Wild, L., & Coyne, C. (1992). The basics and beyond: Epidural analgesia. *American Journal of Nursing, 92*(4), 26–34.

Willens, J. S. (1991). Disconnected epidural catheter. *Nursing, 21*(8), 43.

Willens, J. S. (1994). Giving fentanyl for pain outside the OR. *American Journal of Nursing, 94*(2) 24–28.

Zatzick, D. F., & Dimsdale, J. E. (1990). Cultural variations in response to painful stimuli. *Psychosomatic Medicine, 52,* 544–557.

SUGGESTED READINGS

Ferrell-Torry, A. T., & Glick, O. J. (1993). The use of therapeutic massage as a nursing intervention to modify anxiety and the perception of cancer pain. *Cancer Nursing, 16,* 93–101.

This article describes the authors' research, in which they gave 30 minutes of simple massage on two consecutive evenings to nine hospitalized males. The massage increased relaxation, decreased the perception of pain, decreased anxiety, and decreased heart rate, blood pressure, and respiratory rate.

Haviley, C., et al. (1992). Pharmacological management of cancer pain. A guide for the health professional. *Cancer Nursing, 15,* 331–346.

This article is a complete review of the various drugs used for clients with cancer pain. Typical dosing and nursing implications for each drug group are discussed. Several drug charts help the nurse identify the most important information about each drug.

Neeley, M. A. (1993). Pain management in elderly patients. *Med-Surg Nursing Quarterly, 1*(4), 32–51.

This article reviews nursing assessment and management of elderly clients experiencing acute and chronic pain. The features and practical tips in the article are very useful for daily practice in a medical-surgical nursing setting.

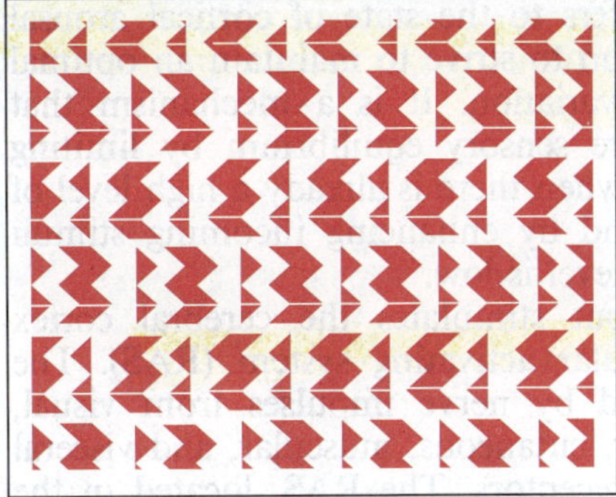

CHAPTER 9

Sensory Deprivation and Sensory Overload

CHAPTER HIGHLIGHTS

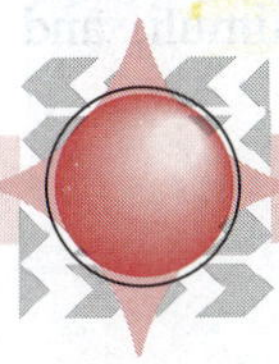

The sensory process allows people to have contact and communication with others and the environment. Sight, hearing, touch, taste, and smell—called the senses—are the components of the sensory process. Each person needs an environment that is responsive to and compatible with the sensory process to support a state of equilibrium and to help maintain health.

Normal sensory changes over a long time are not detrimental as long as the sensory stimuli remain familiar and controllable and the person is able to adapt. When the balance between stimuli and adaptation is disrupted, a person begins to demonstrate behavioral manifestations related to either sensory deprivation (deficit) or sensory overload (excess).

OVERVIEW

People may encounter factors that contribute to sensory deprivation or sensory overload. Understanding the sensory process helps the medical-surgical nurse plan care for clients at risk for sensory problems.

RECEPTION AND PERCEPTION

Two aspects of the sensory process—reception and perception—assist people in maintaining day-to-day contact with the environment. Reception is the biologic component of the sensory process; it involves the function of the sensory organs, such as the eyes and ears. Perception is the psychologic aspect of the process and refers to a person's ability to choose, organize, and give meaning to incoming sensory stimuli. Both reception and perception are essential for people to remain in a state of equilibrium with themselves and the environment.

When a person receives and perceives stimuli, he or she classifies the input and identifies a need or problem. The person takes action according to this interpretation. If the action is effective, the person returns to a state of equilibrium. If the action is not effective, sensory deprivation or overload occurs, leading to major behavioral manifestations (Fig. 9–1).

THE AROUSAL MECHANISM

The concept of arousal is important in understanding how a person copes with changes in the environment. Because of different personalities, inner resources, and lifestyles, an identical environment is perceived differently by each person. In addition, the same stimulus can be monotonous one minute and overwhelming the next. To maintain an optimal level of functioning, clients need to have an optimal level of sensory stimulation.

Sensoristasis refers to the state of cortical arousal that causes a person to strive to maintain an optimal level of sensory variation. It is a mechanism that attempts to restore sensory equilibrium by limiting incoming stimuli when there is already a high level of arousal present and by enhancing incoming stimuli when the arousal level is low.

All sensory input stimulates the cerebral cortex through the reticular activating system (RAS). The RAS is stimulated by nerve impulses from visual, auditory, olfactory, cutaneous, muscular, and visceral (internal organs) receptors. The RAS, located in the core of the brain stem, is composed of ascending and descending pathways that travel to and from the cerebral cortex. Ascending RAS fibers feed the cortex to alert the brain, and descending fibers travel from the cortex to stimulate the RAS.

Disorders in the arousal mechanism occur when the reticular activating system is bombarded with input or when the RAS fails to recognize input because the stimulus lacks meaning. If a person is in an environment that has a low level of stimulation, cortical stimulation is reduced and sensory deprivation occurs. When stimuli are overwhelming, the cortical system is unable to regulate incoming stimuli, and the person experiences sensory overload.

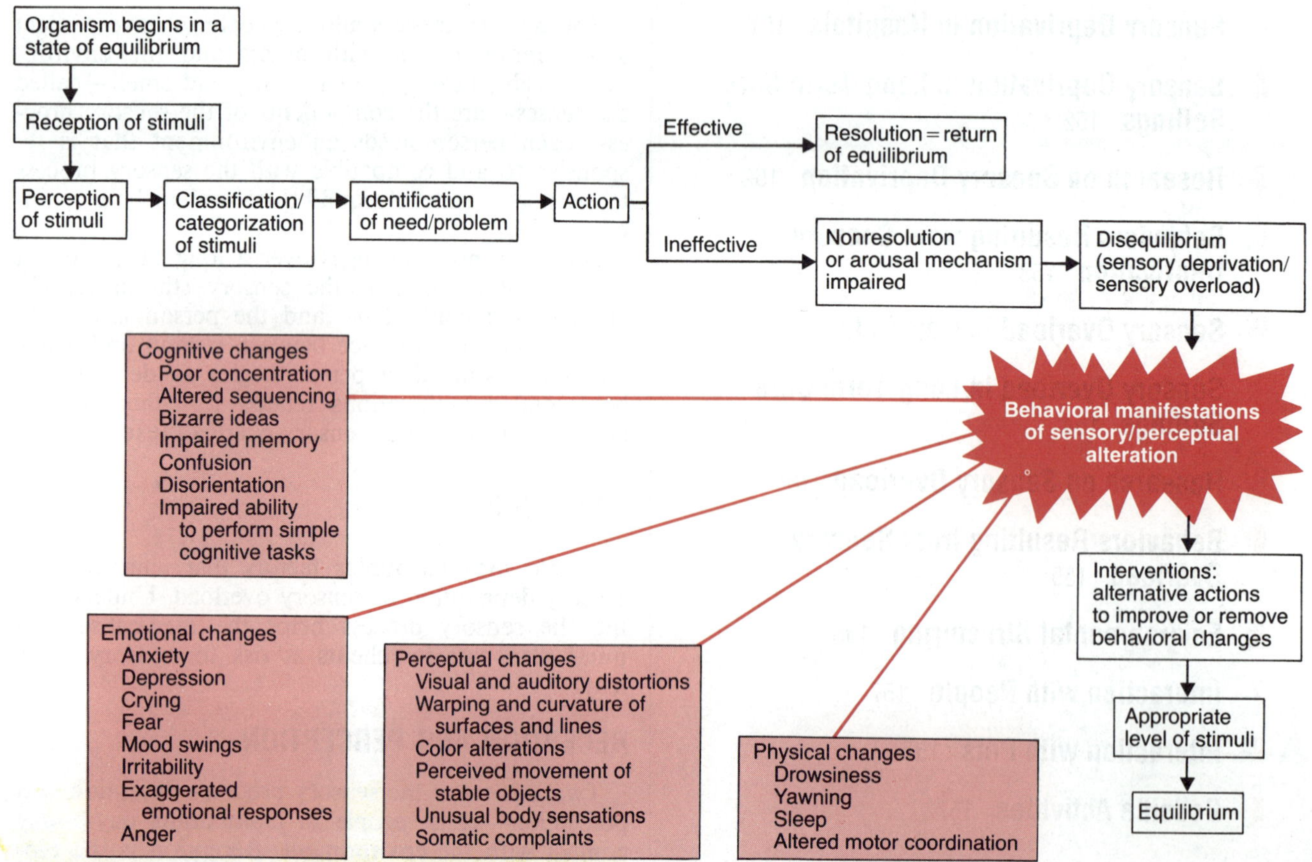

FIGURE 9–1 ◆ The results of sensory deprivation and sensory overload.

SENSORY DEPRIVATION

DEFINITION

Sensory deprivation is a reduction in the variety and intensity of sensory input, with or without a change in the structure or pattern of stimulation. Because many variables affect the occurrence of sensory deprivation, several subtypes of this phenomenon exist:

- Absolute reduction—there are no stimuli in the external environment.
- Reception deprivation—receptor organs are impaired, and either partial or complete loss of sensation occurs.
- Perceptual deprivation—a person cannot recognize and interpret stimuli from the external environment.
- Technologic deprivation—the client is in a highly technical environment in which the nurse focuses on the machines rather than on the person.
- Confinement deprivation—the client is separated from significant others and familiar objects.
- Immobility deprivation—the client shows decreased physical movement and activity (Table 9-1).

Many clients in a hospital or nursing home experience more than one type of sensory deprivation. For example, a paraplegic client with severe hearing loss who is admitted with an acute bowel obstruction has multiple risk factors that predispose him or her to a number of sensory deprivation subtypes.

SENSORY DEPRIVATION IN HEALTH CARE FACILITIES

SENSORY DEPRIVATION IN HOSPITALS Hospital environments have been perceived as being monotonous or "institutional." Traditionally, the walls have been white or pale or without pictures, although this is changing. Hospital rooms, particularly in new facilities, may have wallpaper, with paintings or other artwork on the walls.

TABLE 9-1 Clinical Examples of the Types of Sensory Deprivation

Type	Clinical Example
Absolute reduction	• Complete lack of stimuli in the environment does not occur in a health care setting, but a client in a coma may not perceive the stimuli.
Reception deprivation	• Clients with visual or hearing impairments
Perception deprivation	• Clients with brain injury or stroke
Technologic deprivation	• Clients in critical care environments
Confinement deprivation	• Clients in strict isolation or a private room
Immobility deprivation	• Clients in traction or large casts

Hospital linens and nurses' uniforms may be white in medical-surgical units. In many hospitals, the addition of colored bedspreads and linens has created a more home-like environment.

The lights in hospital rooms or hallways may be dim or glaring. The curtains may be pulled around the client's bed, or the client may be in a private room. Hospital food may be more bland than the client is used to, or the client may not be allowed food by mouth.

Depending on the size of the room, a client's personal space may be restricted by various types of hospital furniture and equipment. Older hospital rooms are typically smaller than newer ones. Contact with significant others is controlled by restricted visiting hours in most units of a hospital. Other factors, such as age, illness, and treatment procedures, may further contribute to sensory deprivation in the hospital setting.

Age As a Contributing Factor In addition to the common environmental findings in a hospital, the client's age may affect the sensory stimuli received (Chart 9-1). The elderly in particular are at high risk of experiencing sensory deprivation because they may have decreased visual, auditory, and gustatory (taste) abilities (reception). Because of the aging process, an elderly person may be less able to process incoming stimuli (perception) as rapidly as a younger adult (also see Chap. 5).

Illness As a Contributing Factor Illness may result in reduced sensory input when one of the senses is affected or when a condition affects the central nervous system. Clients who have had eye surgery, for instance, are at high risk for sensory deprivation if an eye patch is used. The patch reduces visual ability and causes limitations in activity. Another example is the person with a spinal cord injury who is immobile and has no tactile sensation below the level of the injury. Confinement as a result of traction, body casts, or bed rest also enhances the development of sensory deprivation. In addition, clients with long-term chronic or terminal illnesses and clients who are institutionalized for extended periods can experience sensory deprivation (Recker, 1992).

Treatment Procedures As Contributing Factors Treatments used during an illness can result in a change of or reduction in a client's contact with the environment. For instance, clients may be placed in isolation rooms if they have a serious infection that can be spread to others or if they have a low resistance that places them at risk for infection. While the client is in isolation, there may be limited contact with the staff. Health care personnel who enter the room often wear gowns, masks, and gloves, which further reduce visual and tactile stimuli.

Clients who cannot swallow may have nasogastric tubes or may receive total parenteral nutrition, which affects their ability to taste or chew food. The presence of other tubes, such as intravenous fluid systems or urinary catheters, causes restricted movement.

CHART 9 – 1

Nursing Focus on the Elderly ◆ Changes in the Sensory Process Related to Aging

Function	Frequent Changes	Nursing Implications	Rationale
Sight	Decreased response to darkness, size of objects, colors (especially green and blue)	• Place a night light in the client's sleeping area. • Select large print for teaching materials. • Place frequently used objects within the client's reach.	• Abuse and overuse of the eyes can be prevented in the elderly.
Hearing	Decreased response to high-frequency sounds	• Use a light signal to indicate ringing of the telephone. • Avoid having mechanical equipment touch the walls. • Talk to the client in a low-pitched voice.	• Visual cues assist the hearing-impaired elderly. • Sound distortions may produce behavioral reactions in the elderly. • Low-pitched voice is more easily heard and interpreted by the elderly.
Touch	Decreased response to pain (possibly) and different temperatures	• Discuss with the client factors contributing to pain. • Keep the client out of drafts and warm.	• The environment of the elderly can be manipulated to decrease stimuli contributing to sensory alterations.
Taste	Increased response to bitter substances Decreased response to sour and salty substances Decreased response or no change in response to sweet substances	• Assess dietary intake with the client. • Clean the client's dentures (if worn) and have the client rinse his or her mouth daily and after eating.	• A sense of security can be promoted in the elderly when eating is a pleasurable experience.
Smell	Increased response to noxious odors Decreased response to fruity odors	• Provide antibacterial soap for personal hygiene. • Open the window in the client's room daily for a minimum of ½ hour	• Elimination of unpleasant odors can enhance the environment of the elderly.

Specific strategies for assisting the client who is experiencing sensory deprivation are discussed later in this chapter.

SENSORY DEPRIVATION IN LONG-TERM CARE SETTINGS Unlike hospitals, nursing homes and other long-term care (LTC) facilities usually attempt to create a home-like environment for their clients. Recent U.S. legislation mandates that all LTC settings provide an environment that is warm, friendly, and as similar to the client's own home as possible. Clients in these settings wear their own day and night clothes, eat together in brightly painted or wallpapered dining rooms, and bring favorite items to their rooms, including pictures, personal care items, and furniture. Individual and group activities are available during the day and evening, 7 days a week.

RESEARCH ON SENSORY DEPRIVATION

GENERAL RESEARCH Research in the field of sensory deprivation has historically consisted of the effects of long-term sensory and social deprivation. Sensory-deprived persons, such as prisoners in isolation, shipwrecked sailors, and explorers, were studied. People who were in an unchanging environment or people who were placed in isolation or confinement all reported similar findings of oppressive monotony, which led to behavioral changes, such as lack of affect, confusion, and depression.

During the past 25 years, researchers have examined the effects of reduced levels and types of visual, auditory, and tactile stimuli on human behavior. Relatively healthy people were placed in environments in which they could be isolated from sensory input, such as patterned visual or auditory stimuli.

When people were deprived of sensory stimulation, they experienced behavioral changes, such as confusion, inaccurate perception, faulty reasoning, impaired memory, and hallucinations. The problem with most of these studies is that the subjects were healthy, young people. Adding the variables of illness or aging, with their known effects on the sensory process, may cause more drastic alterations in behavior.

NURSING RESEARCH Very little nursing research has been conducted on sensory deprivation. Wood (1977) compared the effect of a private-room and a semiprivate-room (two-bed) environment on clients' sensory stimulation in a hospital. Clients in private rooms experienced more sensory and cognitive disturbances than did clients in rooms with two beds. Visual and auditory acuity and client age had no relationship to these findings, but immobility was a significant factor.

Research is beginning for the validation of nursing diagnoses associated with sensory deprivation. Janken and Cullinan (1991) conducted a study to validate the nursing diagnosis of Sensory/Perceptual Alterations: Auditory. They concluded that further studies are needed to identify the defining characteristics of this diagnosis and other sensory-perceptual diagnoses (Research Applications for Nursing).

BEHAVIORS RESULTING FROM SENSORY DEPRIVATION

Behaviors seen during sensory deprivation fall into several categories: cognitive, emotional, perceptual, and physical (Fig. 9–1). Some nurses might assume that these are normal behaviors for elderly clients, but most elderly clients do not typically experience these changes with aging. The nurse assesses the client's baseline behaviors to determine whether or not he or she is experiencing sensory deprivation.

COGNITIVE CHANGES Cognitive changes range from poor concentration, altered sequencing of thoughts, or unusual ideas to bizarre thinking or hallucinations. Impaired memory, confusion, and disorientation may occur. There may also be an impairment in the client's ability to perform simple cognitive tasks, such as adding a list of numbers.

EMOTIONAL CHANGES Emotional disturbances include anxiety, depression, crying, fear, mood swings, irritability and annoyance over trivial matters, exaggerated emotional responses, and anger. The intensity of emotions displayed by clients varies from mild discomfort to panic.

PERCEPTUAL CHANGES Changes in perception include visual and auditory distortions, warping in the curvature of surfaces and lines, alterations in color, and perceived movement of stable objects. Some people have reported unusual body sensations, such as numbness. Other clients show a preoccupation with internal sensations and complaints, including dry mouth, heart palpitations, difficulty in breathing, and nausea. Olfactory sensory distortions, such as smelling eggs frying, have also occurred in some people with sensory alteration.

PHYSICAL CHANGES Physical behaviors observed during sensory deprivation include drowsiness, excessive yawning, and sleep. Clients may be using sleep as a mechanism to escape the monotony of sensory deprivation. Motor coordination is affected and is seen in the client as impairment of dexterity, hand-eye coordination, movement, and balance.

RESEARCH APPLICATIONS FOR NURSING

Defining Characteristics for Sensory/Perceptual Alteration: Auditory May Not Be Valid

Janken, J., & Cullinan, C. L. (1991). Validation of the nursing diagnosis Sensory/Perceptual Alteration: Auditory. In R. M. Carroll-Johnson (Ed.), *Classification of nursing diagnosis: Proceedings of the ninth conference* (pp. 120–125). Philadelphia: J. B. Lippincott.

This descriptive survey uses a random sample of 250 elderly subjects who had been admitted to non-intensive care units of a large teaching hospital for the first time. Janken and Cullinan wanted to:

- Determine the relationship between hearing ability and psychosocial functioning
- Determine whether age and the presence of impacted cerumen significantly affected hearing ability

Using multiple assessment tools as well as physical assessment, the authors showed that some of the current NANDA-approved defining characteristics do not predict hearing ability. Rather, a client's age, self-reporting of hearing ability, and amount of cerumen accurately reflect the client's level of hearing.

Critique This study attempted to validate one of the Sensory/Perceptual Alterations nursing diagnoses. A random sample was used, but it was limited to English-speaking subjects in one hospital.

Possible nursing implications Although conclusions are not definitive from this single study, this research raises questions about the current defining characteristics for this nursing diagnosis. Nurses working with the elderly should be aware that they need to check the client's ears for cerumen and ask the client to rate his or her hearing ability as part of a hearing assessment.

SENSORY OVERLOAD

DEFINITION

Sensory overload results from an increase in environmental stimuli, in which there is multisensory bombardment of stimuli or an increase in the pattern and intensity of the stimuli so that the input is meaningless. The stimuli are too numerous, too rapid, and too diverse. The behavioral manifestations of sensory overload can have a health-threatening effect.

SENSORY OVERLOAD IN HEALTH CARE FACILITIES

SENSORY OVERLOAD IN HOSPITALS Hospital environments present the risk of overstimulating the client's senses. Noise associated with people and equipment can produce a steady stream of irritating sounds. Various noxious odors mingle with body odors. Invasive and noninvasive tests and examinations occur frequently and may be performed repeatedly and by many different health professionals.

Some clinical conditions also promote the occurrence of sensory overload. For example, clients with intense pain, or those with dressing changes that involve discomfort, may experience an intensity of sensations that is increased above their normal threshold.

Hospital areas such as the postanesthesia care unit (PACU), emergency department, and critical care and medical-surgical units are filled with many stimuli that are foreign and that lack meaning for the client. Clients may react to bright, continuous lights; increased noise levels; monitors or ventilators with alarms; constant interventions by different members of the health care team; lack of privacy; and restrictive equipment, such as chest tubes. The suddenness with which the client is placed in an acute care situation is another factor that affects the client's response. There may be no time for the nurse to prepare the client for the adjustment process required for responding to stimuli. Nursing interventions for sensory overload are discussed later in this chapter.

SENSORY OVERLOAD IN LONG-TERM CARE SETTINGS The problem of sensory overload is increasing in long-term care (LTC) settings for two major reasons. First, the clients they care for are sicker than they were 10 years ago, with many of them undergoing multiple treatment procedures, including infusion therapy. Second, the U.S. government has enacted legislation that greatly restricts the use of psychoactive drugs, including antianxiety agents and hypnotics. As a result, some clients with dementia scream and yell out almost constantly, making it nearly impossible for other clients to rest.

This problem has created a dilemma that is complicated when a client is admitted from the nursing home to a hospital. Because the U.S. federal laws on psychoactive drugs do not yet affect acute care facilities, physicians often prescribe large doses of psychoactive medications while the client is in the hospital but discontinue them when the client returns to the nursing home. Elderly clients cannot tolerate these drastic changes in drug therapy and often display worsened agitated behaviors as a result (Matteson & McConnell, 1988).

RESEARCH ON SENSORY OVERLOAD

The literature is filled with reports of altered behaviors that are observed as a result of sensory overload in critical care areas, such as burn units and coronary care units (Fig. 9–2). These behaviors are often referred to as the syndrome of ICU (intensive care unit) psychosis. Various studies have noted that alterations in cognitive function, as well as confusion, disorientation, and an inability to maintain attention, are a few of the behaviors that may occur on the third to seventh day of a client's stay in the critical care unit. Research on the effects of the ICU envi-

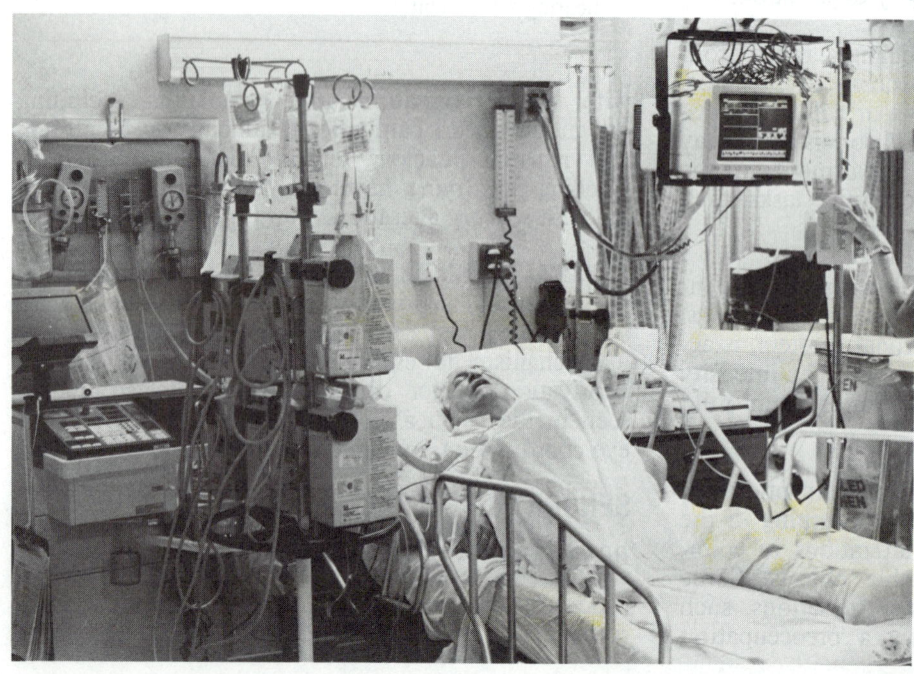

FIGURE 9–2 ◆ A busy critical care unit—a primary setting for sensory overload.

ronment has shown that clients who received less than 50% of their usual amount of sleep experienced hallucinations, disorientation, combativeness, paranoia, and delusions (Thelan et al., 1990).

The effect of the environment on adults in other types of acute care units has not been well studied. The studies that have been done focus on the physical characteristics of the environment (Williams, 1988). For example, almost half of the clients interviewed reported sleep disturbances because of high noise levels in hospitals and nursing homes (Hilton, 1985; Walgenbach, 1990). Besides sleep disturbances, some clients had decreased appetites, altered blood pressure and heart rates (Baker, 1992), and increased anxiety.

BEHAVIORS RESULTING FROM SENSORY OVERLOAD

There are no clear differences between behaviors observed in sensory deprivation and those observed in sensory overload. Most of the clinical findings for sensory overload are similar to those cognitive, emotional, perceptual, and physical alterations discussed for sensory deprivation (see Fig. 9–1).

A distinguishing feature of sensory overload is that the client cannot use sleep as an escape mechanism. Sleep is a vital and basic need. Sensory overload alters the client's specific sleep pattern, and sleep disturbances occur (Hilton, 1985). Conversely, lack of sleep can contribute to sensory overload by causing confusion, memory loss, and other cognitive changes.

COLLABORATIVE MANAGEMENT

ASSESSMENT

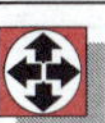

HISTORY

When obtaining a client's history, the nurse asks about and observes the presence of any of the following factors to identify the client at risk of experiencing an alteration in the sensory process:

- Increased age
- Alterations in reception (e.g., decreased sight, hearing, taste, smell)
- Corrective devices required for sensory impairments
- Impaired physical mobility
- Neurologic impairment
- Impaired cognition
- Decreased ability to communicate
- Recent surgery
- Prolonged stay in a health care facility
- Use of medications that affect the senses or mental state
- Substance abuse
- Environment prior to admission to a health care facility (for example, single room living, homelessness)

Data concerning the client's status before hospitalization are very important. However, it is crucial that the nurse continue to assess the client in an ongoing manner. Throughout the client's stay in a health care facility, changes resulting from interventions, such as surgery, activity restrictions, medications, or treatments, greatly affect the sensory status.

The nurse reviews the medications the client is receiving to determine whether symptoms are the result of side effects, toxic effects, or drug interactions. For example, many drugs cause dry mouth and anorexia. The nurse also asks the client about other health problems he or she may have that could be contributing to the present behaviors.

PHYSICAL ASSESSMENT/CLINICAL MANIFESTATIONS

The client whose sensory input is affected displays alterations in activities, such as increased restlessness, drowsiness, increased or decreased sleep, and incoordination. The nurse assesses for behaviors such as dry mouth, heart palpitations, difficulty in breathing, and lack of appetite. Some clients report auditory or visual distortions and a feeling of numbness.

PSYCHOSOCIAL ASSESSMENT

Most clients will not admit to alterations such as bizarre thoughts, delusions, or hallucinations. They fear that expression of such feelings is unusual. Nurses may detect some of these alterations in thought processes after talking to or observing the client. Effects on emotional responses are seen as clients display increased irritability, frequent mood swings, crying, fear, anger, and depression. Cognitive function is often impaired, and the client may report an increased incidence of daydreaming. The nurse may observe a reduced attention span, and the client may exhibit noncompliant behaviors.

For the elderly client, it is especially important that the nurse assess the client's baseline before the changes occurred. Family members or significant others can often provide this information when the client is not able to; they can also validate what the client reports.

LABORATORY ASSESSMENT

Clients with sensory alterations may have increased urinary levels of catecholamines, 17-ketosteroids, and luteinizing hormone. An increase in plasma thyroid-stimulating hormone levels has also been identified. The existence of specific pathologic conditions needs to be determined before the laboratory findings can be considered to be conclusive for sensory problems.

ENVIRONMENTAL ASSESSMENT

The nurse assesses several characteristics of the environmental setting to determine the type of sensory alteration present. For instance, the nurse checks the amount and intensity of stimulation present. Imagining oneself in the client's position helps the nurse to better understand the level of stimulation present and the changes or variability that occurs. Stimuli are assessed for their pattern and meaningfulness. The nurse also carefully considers the degree of social isolation imposed on the client by the environment and the familiarity of the surroundings to the client.

ANALYSIS

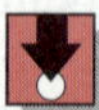

COMMON NURSING DIAGNOSES

Two major diagnoses are related to alterations in the sensory-perceptual process:

1. Sensory/Perceptual Alterations related to altered sensory reception, transmission, or integration; a socially restricted environment; or environmental factors (sensory deprivation)
2. Sensory/Perceptual Alterations related to pain, psychologic stress, or environmental factors (sensory overload)

ADDITIONAL NURSING DIAGNOSES

In addition to the common nursing diagnoses, some clients may experience one or more additional nursing diagnoses:

- Anxiety related to a change in environment
- Fear related to sensory impairment, deprivation, or overload
- Diversional Activity Deficit related to social isolation, effects of chronic illness, or confinement to bed rest
- Altered Thought Processes related to sleep deprivation, sensory overload or deprivation, or social isolation
- Sleep Pattern Disturbance related to sensory overload
- Impaired Verbal Communication related to cognitive impairment, cerebral trauma/lesion, or complex oral surgery
- High Risk for Injury related to sensory/perceptual alterations or impaired physical mobility

PLANNING AND IMPLEMENTATION

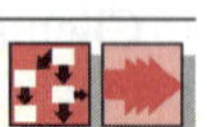

SENSORY/PERCEPTUAL ALTERATIONS (SENSORY DEPRIVATION)

PLANNING: CLIENT GOALS The major goals may include that the client will:

- Receive the optimal level of sensory stimulation
- Interpret sensory input appropriately
- Be consistently oriented to time, person, and place to the extent possible

INTERVENTIONS After assessing and analyzing each client's situation, the nurse identifies factors that contribute to sensory/perceptual deprivation. Nursing interventions are focused on preventing sensory monotony by increasing the level of intensity of the stimulation and increasing the variety of patterns of incoming stimuli (Chart 9–2).

Environmental Structuring Environmental structuring is defined as a group of nursing interventions that directly or indirectly affect the conditions or features within the environment (Mion, 1992). The nurse identifies aspects that are harmful or potentially harmful to the client and alters them to the extent possible.

The nurse tries to create an environment that resembles familiar surroundings for the client and restores meaningful stimulation. Nurses can place "get well" cards on the bedside table; they can also encourage family members to bring in personal objects or photographs of significant others from home to create a more familiar room. Colorful pillowcases, pajamas, and washcloths from home can also reduce monotony for the client. The use of radio and television can help to increase stimulation through sound, but monitoring for content and volume is required to decrease monotony because clients can "block out" these sounds.

CHART 9–2

Nursing Care Highlight ◆ The Client Experiencing Sensory Deprivation

- Place the client in a brightly colored room or a room with wallpaper or wall hangings.
- Ask the family to provide personal items, such as favorite pictures, mementos, or nightwear, if possible.
- Remind the client to wear eyeglasses, dentures, contact lenses, or a hearing aid, if these things are usually worn.
- Ask the client about the use of a radio, tape recorder, or television to provide stimulation (avoid overuse).
- Place the client near a window, if possible.
- Provide a large calendar, clock, or reminder board to help keep the client oriented.
- Reorient the client frequently and talk to him or her while in the room.
- Provide activities that the client can do in bed or at the bedside, such as puzzles, reading, or simple crafts.
- Check on the availability of a recreational or activity therapist in the facility for other creative ideas.
- Request pet visits, if allowed, or provide a stuffed animal or other favorite item for tactile stimulation.

Large clocks, calendars, wrist watches, and windows are effective in orienting the client to time (Fig. 9–3). Name pins worn by staff members assist in orienting the client to people. In some health care facilities, there is a large board in each room on which the nurse writes the current date, day, and name of the nurse assigned to the client.

The nurse also reminds the client to wear assistive devices, such as hearing aids, eyeglasses, or contact lenses, if used. These devices can enhance the reception of sensory input and help the client to feel more in control of the environment. The nurse encourages the client who can perform self-care activities to do so because physical movement serves as a source of stimulation.

Allowing the client to smell the aroma of food, providing foods of different textures, and including warm and cool foods in the diet stimulate the sense of taste. Oral hygiene and properly fitting dentures promote gustatory and chewing abilities.

The nurse uses touch through back rubs, massage, and passive range-of-motion exercises to provide tactile stimuli. Casual touching while talking to a client to demonstrate empathy and foster trust may also provide stimulation. However, the nurse considers the client's age, gender, and cultural beliefs before assuming that the client wants to be touched. Some people are not comfortable with invasion of their personal space.

Interaction with People The nurse acts as a source of stimulation by talking with the client, explaining tests and procedures, and asking simple questions to promote cognitive function. Placing a person in a lounge or hallway where social interactions can occur with other clients or visitors is another means of increasing stimulation.

Interaction with Pets In the home and in long-term care settings, the use of animals to provide companionship and sensory stimulation is becoming popular. Also known as "animal-assisted therapy" or "pet therapy," this intervention involves regular pet visits to allow the client, often an elderly person, the opportunity to establish a human–animal bond (McMahon, 1991). In the hospital setting, stuffed animals may be used instead of live ones.

Bedside Activities The nurse also encourages the client to engage in self-stimulation activities, such as reading, writing, putting a puzzle together, or drawing or painting a picture. In some facilities, art and music therapists implement programs to be used at the bedside. These activities not only provide stimulation but also allow clients to express their feelings, especially through art media. If a therapist is not available, the nurse can suggest that the facility acquire items and activity materials that can be used by clients at high risk for sensory deprivation. If the client cannot use his or her hands, music provided on tape may be beneficial. The nurse assesses the type of activity the client prefers.

SENSORY/PERCEPTUAL ALTERATIONS (SENSORY OVERLOAD)

PLANNING: CLIENT GOALS The major goals are the same as those for sensory deprivation, but interventions are somewhat different. Expected outcomes may include that the client will:

- Receive the optimal level of sensory stimulation
- Interpret sensory input appropriately
- Be oriented to time, person, and place to the extent possible

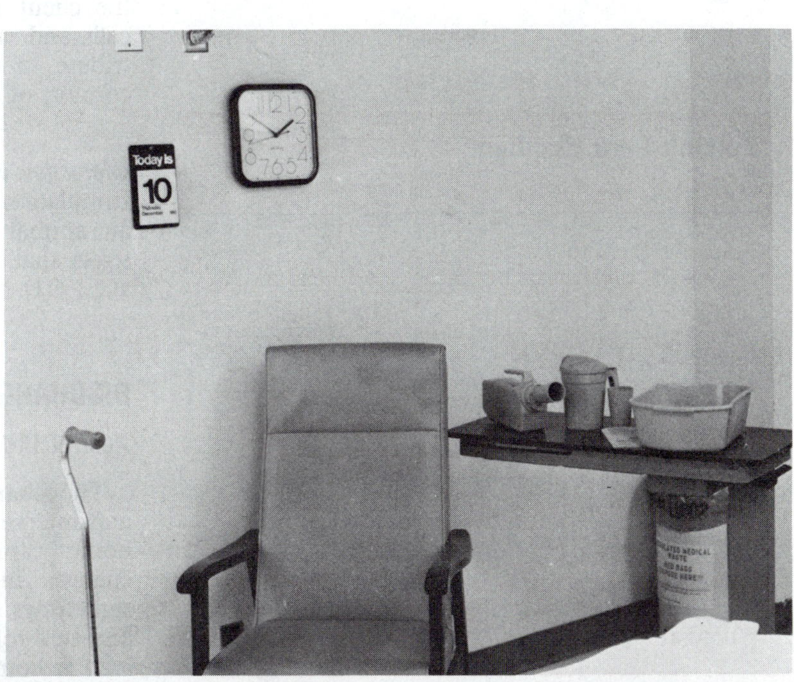

FIGURE 9–3 ◆ A hospital room with items to provide stimulation and reality orientation.

INTERVENTIONS Critical care units or emergency departments are frequent sites in which clients experience sensory overload. Nurses working in these units should reduce the intensity of incoming stimuli and increase the meaningfulness of the stimuli. Clients who are provided with a consistent, predictable pattern of stimulation gain a sense of control over the environment. Without control, clients perceive stimuli as disorganized, irrelevant, and overwhelming.

Environmental Structuring The noise level in a critical care or medical-surgical unit is high. Many of the machines have controls that allow the volume of the alarm signals to be lowered. If this is possible, the nurse may find it valuable to lower the volume, especially during the night when the client's sleep is frequently interrupted. Health care team members should avoid standing in groups by the client's bedside and engaging in simultaneous conversations to reduce the number of voices and conversations that the client hears. In some units, ear plugs may be provided to the client in an attempt to reduce the sound level.

Visual stimulation in a critical care unit is also usually excessive. Bright lights often remain on 24 hours a day, lights on some pieces of equipment constantly blink, cardiac patterns on monitors are visible, and there is much movement as nurses provide care to critically ill clients. At rest and sleep times, the nurse should dim the lights when possible, apply eye shields, post "Do not disturb" signs, and draw the curtain around the client's bed to help reduce visual stimulation. If the client is experiencing a high level of stress, the nurse might suggest progressive muscular relaxation to reduce the stress and thus promote sleep (see Chap. 7). Chart 9–3 lists interventions for the promotion of sleep in health care facilities.

CHART 9–3

Nursing Care Highlight ◆ Interventions to Promote Sleep

Teach the client to
- Avoid caffeinated beverages near bedtime (in some cases, they should be avoided after noon)
- Try not to sleep when hungry or after a heavy meal
- Avoid or decrease smoking or other tobacco use
- Wear comfortable nightwear

Have the room at a comfortable temperature.

Decrease excessive lighting and noise to the extent possible.

Remind the client to try to relax before sleeping; assist the client with progressive muscle relaxation or guided imagery.

Space nursing activities to prevent multiple interruptions at night.

The behaviors of the client who experiences delirium or dementia often worsen in a high-stimulus environment. Strategies for environmental structuring that are specific to these clients are described in Chapter 41 in the discussion on interventions for Alzheimer's disease.

Pain Relief For some clients, intense pain is a source of overstimulation. Use of medications or other pain-relieving techniques may be beneficial (see Chap. 8).

Interaction with People The nurse explains machines, tubes, and monitors to the client in simple, client-oriented terms to help provide meaning to the vast array of unfamiliar items seen in a hospital environment. Clients whose rooms are near the nurses' station, utility rooms, or exit doors often complain of the heavy traffic of personnel. People who work in health care settings should keep their voices lowered and be as quiet as possible when performing activities near clients' rooms.

When interacting with the client, the nurse remains calm, uses an unhurried approach, and speaks in a low, modulated voice. Nurses should also remember to acknowledge the client when coming to the bedside to check on equipment. Scheduling the same nurse to care for the client each day promotes consistency and reduces the number of different caregivers or strangers whom the client meets. In addition, nurses should develop a routine plan of care that establishes times for activities, such as eating, bathing, turning, coughing, and doing range-of-motion exercises. This schedule should allow time for uninterrupted periods of rest.

Nurses can also regulate sensory input by decreasing auditory stimulation while continuing to orient the client to reality, if possible. Limiting telephone calls and visitors may reduce some stimuli that contribute to distress, although some clients need the comfort of these contacts.

Interaction with Pets Pet therapy can provide sensory stimulation while fostering relaxation. The comfort of an animal companion, if allowed, may reduce the stress that contributes to sensory overload (Baun et al., 1991).

DISCHARGE PLANNING

HOME CARE PREPARATION

The changes in health care treatment modalities and interventions are extending to include changes in home care needs and services. The behavioral changes in hospitalized clients are expected and sometimes accepted because it is an arena for care and sick roles. Sensory deprivation and sensory overload at home may also occur.

HEALTH TEACHING

Clients and care providers may need to learn skills related to home treatment using new technology or may need to relearn previously known skills that have been forgotten or have changed because of illness. Use of medications, monitoring health status, and maintaining activities of daily living become the responsibility of the client, who may be overwhelmed by change and new tasks. This feeling of being overwhelmed may lead to sensory overload at home. The home health nurse teaches the new tasks by dividing them into simple steps. The nurse also mobilizes resources to prevent or manage sensory deprivation or overload.

PSYCHOSOCIAL PREPARATION

The client who has had a known sensory/perceptual alteration while in the health care facility is most vulnerable to sensory deprivation and sensory overload at home, but other clients should also be identified as being at risk for these problems. Before the client is discharged, the nurse asks family members or significant others to assess the home for stimuli that may pose sources of difficulty for the client. For example, if the client is living alone, the risk of sensory deprivation is high, especially for an elderly person who may have limited mobility. If the client is living with many members of an extended family, the risk of sensory overload is present until the client becomes healthier.

HEALTH CARE RESOURCES

To prevent or manage sensory deprivation and sensory overload at home, resources for care need to be mobilized and their use maximized. For example, home visits by the home health nurse should include an ongoing assessment and provide continuity in care for effective interventions related to stimuli and behaviors. Strategies that have been successful in the health care facility, such as pet therapy, may be continued at home.

EVALUATION

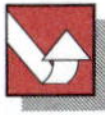

To evaluate nursing care, the nurse considers the subjective and objective data and the goals for the client with alterations in the sensory/perceptual process related to sensory deprivation or sensory overload. The expected outcomes may include that the client:

- Receives an optimal level of sensory stimulation
- Interprets sensory stimuli correctly and meaningfully
- Is oriented to time, person, and place

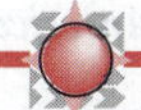

IMPLICATIONS FOR NURSING RESEARCH

Very little nursing research has been done on sensory deprivation. Some research on sensory overload has been undertaken, but most studies have focused on critical care units. Some nursing research questions that need to be addressed are as follows:

- ♦ What are the defining characteristics for each type of sensory/perceptual alteration (e.g., visual, auditory, tactile)?
- ♦ How can nurses best assess a client who is at high risk for sensory/perceptual alterations?
- ♦ What nursing interventions can alter the health care environment so that sensory/perceptual alterations can be prevented or minimized?
- ♦ How can critical care settings be improved to decrease the incidence or severity of "ICU psychosis"?

SELECTED BIBLIOGRAPHY

Baker, C. F. (1992). Discomfort due to environmental noise: Heart rate responses of SICU patients. *Critical Care Nursing Quarterly, 15*(2), 75–90.

Baun, M. M., Oetting, K., & Bergstrom, N. (1991). Health benefits of companion animals in relationship to the physiologic indices of relaxation. *Holistic Nursing Practice, 5*(2), 16–23.

*Bolin, R. (1974). Sensory deprivation: An overview. *Nursing Forum, 13,* 240–258.

*Chodil, J., & Williams B. (1970). The concept of sensory deprivation. *Nursing Clinics of North America, 5,* 453–465.

Cohen, F. L., & Merritt, S. L. (1992). Sleep promotion. In G. M. Bulechek & J. C. McCloskey (Eds.), *Nursing interventions: Essential nursing treatments* (2nd ed.). Philadelphia: W. B. Saunders.

Drury, J., & Akins, J. (1991). Sensory/perceptual alterations. In M. Maas, K. Buckwalter, & M. Hardy (Eds.), *Nursing diagnoses and interventions for the elderly* (pp. 269–386). Redwood City, CA: Addison-Wesley.

Edwards, G. B., & Schuring, L. M. (1993). Sleep protocol: A research-based practice change. *Critical Care Nurse, 13*(2), 84–88.

Griffin, J. P. (1992). The impact of noise on critically ill people. *Holistic Nursing Practice, 6*(4), 53–56.

*Hahn, K. (1989). Think twice about sensory loss. *Nursing '89, 19*(2), 97–99.

*Hilton, B. A. (1985). Noise in acute patient care areas. *Research in Nursing and Health, 8,* 283–291.

*Jackson, C., & Ellis, R. (1971). Sensory deprivation as a field of study. *Nursing Research, 20,* 46–54.

Janken, J., & Cullinan, C. L. (1991). Validation of the nursing diagnosis Sensory/Perceptual Alteration: Auditory. In R. M. Carroll-Johnson (Ed.), *Classification of nursing diagnosis: Proceedings of the ninth conference* (pp. 120–125). Philadelphia: J. B. Lippincott.

*Kopac, C. (1983). Sensory loss in the aged: The role of the

nurse and the family. *Nursing Clinics of North America, 18,* 373–383.
*MacKinnon-Kesler, S. (1983). Maximizing your ICU patient's sensory and perceptual environment. *Canadian Nurse, 79*(5), 41–45.
Manor, W. (1991). Alzheimer's patients and their caregivers: The role of the human-animal bond. *Holistic Nursing Practice, 5*(2), 32–37.
*Matteson, M. A., & McConnell, E. S. (1988). *Gerontological nursing: Concepts and practice.* Philadelphia: W. B. Saunders.
McCloskey, J. C., & Bulechek, G. M. (1992). *Nursing interventions classification (NIC).* St. Louis: Mosby Year Book.
McMahon, S. (1991). The quest for synthesis: Human-companion animal relationships and nursing theories. *Holistic Nursing Practice, 5*(2), 1–5.
Mion, L. C. (1992). Environmental structuring. In G. M. Bulechek & J. C. McCloskey (Eds.), *Nursing interventions: Essential nursing treatments* (2nd ed.). Philadelphia: W. B. Saunders.
Recker, D. (1992). Overcoming the obstacles to caring for the long-term critical care patient. *Critical Care Nurse, 12*(5), 40–48.
Thelan, L., Davie, J., & Urden, L. (1990). *Textbook of critical care nursing: Diagnosis and Management.* St. Louis: C. V. Mosby.
Walgenbach, J. C. (1990). Lullaby and not a good night? *Geriatric Nursing, 11,* 278–279.
*Williams, M. A. (1988). The physical environment and patient care. *Annual Review Nursing Research, 6,* 61–84.
*Wood, M. (1977). Clinical sensory deprivation: A comparative study of patients in single care and two-bed rooms. *Journal of Nursing Administration, 7,* 28–32.

SUGGESTED READINGS

Edwards, G. B., & Schuring, L. M. (1993). Sleep protocol: A research-based practice change. *Critical Care Nurse, 13*(2), 84–88.

This article discusses how staff nurses in a medical intensive care unit (MICU) used their research findings to implement a change in practice. The researchers found that clients in this critical care unit were sleep-deprived. As a result, a sleep protocol was developed and implemented, which increased reports of uninterrupted sleep.

Griffin, J. P. (1992). The impact of noise on critically ill people. *Holistic Nursing Practice, 6*(4), 53–56.

This author reviews the problems resulting from loud and monotonous noises occurring in hospital settings. Hospital noise in particular has been associated with sensory overload, sensory deprivation, ICU psychosis, and reports of increased postoperative pain.

Manor, W. (1991). Alzheimer's patients and their caregivers: The role of the human-animal bond. *Holistic Nursing Practice, 5*(2), 32–37.

This article describes the special benefits of pet therapy for clients experiencing Alzheimer's disease. These clients are prone to loneliness and emotional isolation. Pet therapy provides reminiscence, stimulates memories and socialization, promotes nonverbal and verbal communication, and provides sensory stimulation.

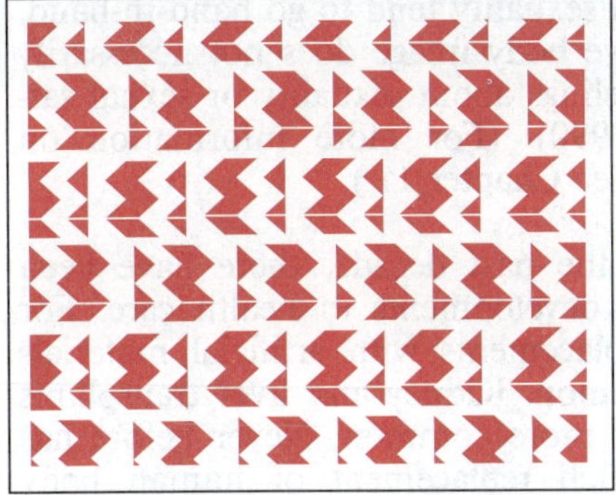

CHAPTER 10

Body Image

CHAPTER HIGHLIGHTS

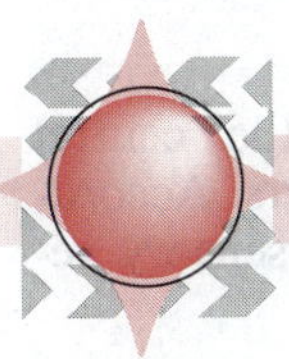

Body image involves both conscious and unconscious information, perceptions, and feelings about one's body. It is part of self-concept, the total collection of feelings a person has about himself or herself. Self-concept is the sum of self-esteem, role performance, and body image (Fig. 10–1).

OVERVIEW

If someone's body image is definite and consistent with reality, the person is likely to feel satisfied with oneself. When illness or chronic disability is present, it is a challenge for someone to integrate the physical changes into his or her body image. Nursing, by diagnosing and treating responses to health problems in a holistic manner, is concerned about the total experience of body image development. Therefore, to assess client responses accurately, medical-surgical nurses must understand how illness can change the body image and how those changes affect practice.

DEFINITION OF BODY IMAGE

Body image includes perceptions of shape, size, mass, function, structure, and significance of the physical, living body in relation to its parts. It also may include inanimate objects that are part of a person's daily contact with the body (e.g., make-up, jewelry, eyeglasses, clothing, wheelchair, crutches, or

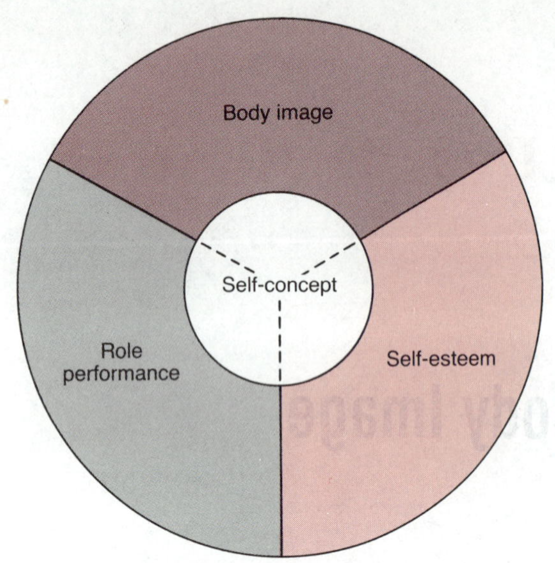

FIGURE 10-1 ◆ Relationship of self-concept to its components. Self-concept is the sum of self-esteem, role performance, and body image.

other appliances). Body image is a complex concept that is difficult to assess in nursing practice and is influenced by many factors.

FACTORS AFFECTING BODY IMAGE

Body image is influenced by several factors, including aging, culture, sex roles, and technology.

AGING The Western World continues to place a major emphasis on the "ideal body"—youth, ideal body weight, beauty, and agility. If a person does not fit this social image, as the older adult *may* not, he or she may receive negative messages about his or her value as a human being. Therefore, the normal aging process can influence body image.

CULTURE The role of culture in the formation of body image can also be significant. People learn to judge themselves by how well they live up to the expectations and demands of their culture. The Western World places a high value on physical appearance and popularity with peers. If a person does not meet these expectations, the culture may perceive him or her less favorably. For example, the adult with anorexia nervosa or obesity may be the brunt of cruel jokes. Therefore, the negative attitudes of a person's culture can contribute to the creation of a poor body image.

SEX ROLES Sex roles play a major role in body image and the way in which it develops. The women's movement in the Western World has emphasized that though the sexes are not identical, they are of equal *value*. Nevertheless, boys and girls learn at an early age that society's expectations of them may differ greatly.

Body image and sexuality tend to go hand-in-hand. However, a positive body image does not necessarily predict positive feelings about sexuality or sexual satisfaction (Rew, 1990). (For more information on human sexuality, see Chapter 11.)

TECHNOLOGY In the past decade, there have been many technologic developments in health care. For example, joint replacements with artificial materials are now very common. Kidney and liver transplants are also becoming more common. Never before has there been so much replacement of human body parts. However, these advances have an impact on body image, although this impact is not clearly understood.

SCHILDER'S THEORY OF BODY IMAGE

Schilder (1950) proposed a holistic approach to body image. He interpreted body image as composed of three separate dimensions:

- Physiologic
- Psychologic
- Social

The *physiologic* dimension involves the central nervous system (CNS) and sensory receptors. According to Schilder, there are three types of sensory receptors:

- *Exteroceptors* detect sensations such as sight, hearing, touch, taste, and smell in the environment or on the body surface.
- *Interoceptors* detect sensations such as pain, hunger, nausea, sensations of excretion and voiding, and sexual excitement within the body.
- *Proprioceptors* detect sensations such as the position of the body in space, stretch, and pressure within the body.

The *psychologic* dimension includes the values that a person ascribes to certain body parts, as well as the attitudes that the person and significant others express toward these parts.

The *social* dimension involves the emotional relationships between people. The closer the relationships, the greater the impact of others on the development of body image.

THE LIFE CYCLE OF BODY IMAGE

The body attempts to achieve consistency throughout the life cycle. Any life experience or change that does not meet or match this established, consistent life model creates increasing anxiety, which results in resistance to change. However, one's body image does readjust and adapt through interaction with significant others and the environment. That is, body image development is an ongoing process of learning and maturation through the cycle of life.

Most developmental theorists say that development of body image does not occur until after birth. According to these theorists, a baby has no body image at birth. That is, the newborn is unable to distinguish clear boundaries between itself and the environment. Therefore, the newborn has no body image. Table 10–1 summarizes body image development from infancy through adolescence. Body image development during adulthood is described below.

YOUNG ADULTHOOD (18 TO 35 YEARS OF AGE)

RELATIONSHIPS Young adults are normally very concerned with developing intimate relationships with others. Over time, body image becomes more stable and positive as a young adult develops these relationships. Without these relationships, the young adult experiences feelings of isolation. A healthy and realistic body image requires positive social reinforcement because people tend to become what others tell them they are. Unfortunately, stereotyping is common during this stage of development. For example, a young, overweight woman may be stereotyped as undisciplined and inactive when she may be just the opposite. This social reinforcement can strongly influence body image development.

PERSONAL CHARACTERISTICS Body image develops and changes as the physical body changes. However, certain personal characteristics seem to be more crucial to body image than others. Sexual identification is central to body image, and any circumstance that alters or threatens this identification can affect it. For example, the woman who experiences a mastectomy may begin to question her sexuality and femininity. "Am I still desirable and attractive?" "Am I still a woman?" "Who am I?"

TABLE 10–1 Development of Body Image from Infancy Through Adolescence

Period of the Life Cycle	Body Image Developmental Task
(Infancy (birth to 1 year of age)	• Develops and uses touch • Perceives the differentiation between self and environment
Toddlerhood (1 to 3 years of age)	• Learns about body parts • Begins to trust feelings
Preschool (3 to 6 years of age)	• Develops a sexual identity • Begins to understand the concepts of normal and different, pretty, and not pretty
Middle childhood (6 to 12 years of age)	• Recognizes differences in body types and structures • Focuses on physical appearance, peer relationships, and adherence to social group norms
Adolescence (12 to 18 years of age)	• Undergoes many internal and external physical changes • Makes comparisons with others and strives for the "perfect" body • Is confused by sexual feelings

WORK The kind of work in which the young adult engages is another characteristic that influences body image. A person's identity may center on a career or occupation, such as nurse, artist, farmer, or homemaker. Injury, illness, or change in career may require a total readjustment of body image. A musician who is no longer able to play an instrument because of amputation must readjust and adapt to the changes in his or her body. A painter who is affected by macular degeneration also faces the developmental task of body image readjustment.

According to Fischer (1964) and others, women seem to have clearer and more accurate images of their bodies than men. Women tend to equate body more with self and are more aware of physical changes, especially around the face. Perhaps these images have related to the historical roles of woman as nurturer and mother, which are closely identified with the body. On the contrary, men have tended to be much less specific in how they view their bodies, perhaps because their roles have traditionally related more toward life accomplishments and attaining power and position in their careers than to their bodies.

MIDDLE ADULTHOOD (35 TO 65 YEARS OF AGE)

The body image of the middle adult (the middlescent) continues to develop as his or her interaction with the environment becomes more complex. During this period, the middlescent must readjust his or her body image to adapt to the psychologic and physical changes of normal aging. This readjustment can be adaptive or maladaptive.

An example of *maladaptive* readjustment of body image is the middlescent who attempts to recapture or mimic youth by applying excessive cosmetics, wearing extremely youthful clothes, or adopting youthful hairstyles. If such an adult continues to perceive his or her physical appearance negatively, the negative body image may result in depression, irritability, and anxiety. The tendency to use maladaptive readjustment strategies depends on a person's personality and level of satisfaction with life up to middlescence.

An example of *adaptive* readjustment is the middle adult who views the changes of this period as evidence of maturity, experience, and knowledge. Such an adult might participate in regular exercise programs, which may slow the normal physical aging process that results in loss of tissue collagen and rearrangement of adipose tissue. The middle-aged adult who has successfully developed a realistic body image accepts the self and the body while realizing that acceptance from others cannot be expected unless self-acceptance is present.

LATE ADULTHOOD (OVER 65 YEARS OF AGE)

No matter when older adults begin to consider themselves as "elderly," they tend to undergo a marked change in body image. For example, sensory deficits resulting from normal aging are common in the older adult and may decrease the ability to enjoy hobbies, such as reading or listening to music. Decreased strength and increased fatigue may reduce the ability to remain a productive, active worker. These reduced abilities may lead to feelings of worthlessness and despair, which influence body image. In addition, events that can affect both body image and self-concept as a whole are retirement, loss of a spouse, and loss of other close family members and friends (see Chap. 5).

BODY IMAGE DISTURBANCE

Illness, whether chronic or acute, can change both external an internal body appearance and function. Changes in *external* body appearance and function can be devastating to body image. Chronic illness is usually more disabling than acute illness because it requires continuous body image reintegration as the disease process continues. For example, a client who has had a stroke is aware each day of the mobility or communication deficits that the illness has caused. As a result, the client continuously attempts to reintegrate not only the current body changes into the body image but also the ever-present fear of future immobility or communication losses that can result from further strokes.

Illness can also affect a person's *internal* function. For instance, a woman who has had a hysterectomy appears physically unchanged but has lost organs that contribute to her image as a woman. The medical-surgical nurse must be aware of these less obvious causes of body image disturbance.

THE THEORY OF READJUSTMENT TO BODY IMAGE DISTURBANCE

Body image readjustment is a lengthy process. Stages of this adaptation process include (1) psychologic shock, (2) withdrawal, (3) acknowledgment, and (4) integration (Fig. 10–2).

PSYCHOLOGIC SHOCK

Psychologic shock is often the initial emotional reaction to the impact of the life change that occurs when a person first becomes aware of a problem. This shock may occur at the time of an injury, illness, or developmental change. Or it may occur later, when body changes are seen or experienced more acutely. Psychologic shock is a defense mechanism that people use in reaction to anxiety. Denial and anger are common reactions during this stage.

WITHDRAWAL

Withdrawal is the next stage of readjustment. Once the person becomes aware of an injury, illness, or developmental change and begins to think about the future, he or she may feel an overwhelming desire to run away from the reality of the situation. Because this is not physically possible, emotional retreat serves as a coping mechanism. This withdrawal provides an opportunity for the person to replenish physical and psychologic energies used during the emotional shock phase. The person may become passive and dependent and lack motivation.

ACKNOWLEDGMENT

Acknowledgment occurs gradually, as the person recognizes the change in body image. Once the loss or change is acknowledged, the person can begin mourning (see Chap. 12, Loss, Death, and Dying). The person may contemplate the meaning of the change and its implications for the future. This acknowledgment allows the person to view the body change itself, and to begin reintegration of the body image.

INTEGRATION

Integration is the long and difficult process of adapting to body changes. The person thinks about future life experiences that will be different as a result of the body change and identifies ways to manage or deal with these changes. Often, the stage of integration can create for the person a new meaning about the change in the body part, and emotional growth occurs. As a result of integration of the body changes into a new image, the person regains a sense of fulfillment. However, the total process of change, from initial impact to adaptation, can be long and painful and is different for everyone.

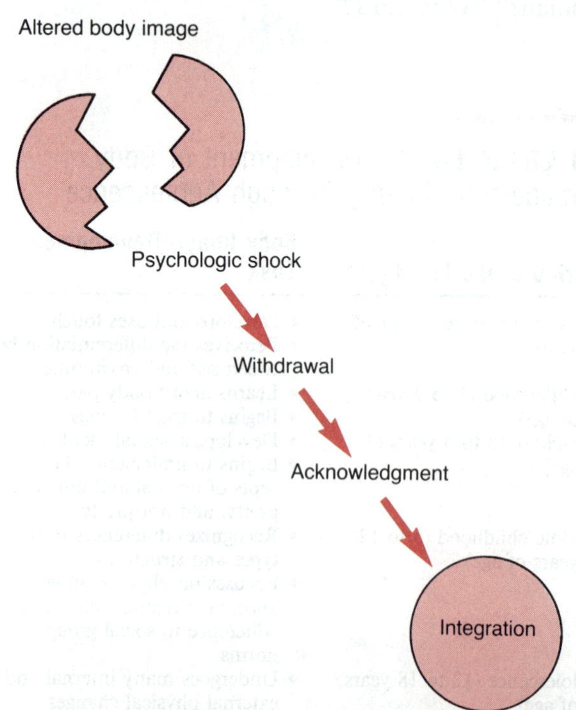

FIGURE 10–2 ◆ Readjustment to altered body image. Stages of the adaptation process include psychologic shock, withdrawal, acknowledgment, and integration.

The adaptation process may also be more successful with the natural, healing passage of time. For example, a study by Samonds and Cammermeyer (1989) showed that some people with multiple sclerosis who were older, had had the disease for a long time, had been affected with the disease at a young age, and were more disabled were more satisfied with their body image than younger, more recently diagnosed, or less disabled people.

RESEARCH ON BODY IMAGE DISTURBANCE

Body image disturbance is most commonly associated with loss of body parts. However, any type of loss (e.g., mobility, independence, or a body function) necessitates some body image readjustment. Research has not clarified how a person perceives the body image after a loss and how this perception relates to the emotional component of body image.

LOSS OF MOBILITY

People value the drive and ability to be mobile. Mobility is of such fundamental importance that healthy adults, even during resting periods, turn or change position frequently. Mobility enables people to exert control or influence over their environment. This control is threatened when mobility is restricted or lost.

People view immobility, whether temporary or permanent, as a loss that can influence body image. This loss, and the lifestyle changes that result, can threaten the survival of the immobilized person. In this respect, body image in relation to immobility can have a considerable impact on nursing practice (see Chap. 13).

PAIN

Pain can play a role in body image development (see Chap. 8, Pain). The impact of illness and pain on body image can be overwhelming. If severe pain continues, the painful body part can become isolated from the rest of the body to the point that it becomes alienated from the body image.

CANCER

Cancer can change the way people feel about their personal appearance. Alopecia (hair loss) that occurs during the treatment of disease is one important factor. Baxley et al. (1984) showed that cancer clients with alopecia have a lower self-image than cancer clients without alopecia. For these clients, alopecia is seen as a constant reminder of their disease. However, the experience of cancer, with or without hair loss, can affect the body image.

CHRONIC ILLNESS

Certain chronic illnesses can affect body image, whether or not pain is involved. For example, people with deforming arthritis, such as the rheumatoid type, are usually very self-conscious about their appearance. Some of these people refuse to socialize or be seen in public. The presence of chronic pain further affects the body image of these people.

Nicholas and Leuner (1992) studied people with another type of chronic illness—chronic obstructive pulmonary disease (COPD). They found that the body image of these people decreased as the disease became more severe (Research Applications for Nursing).

SURGERY

For any client, the anticipation of surgery can create anxiety, a fear of mutilation, and an unrealistic

RESEARCH APPLICATIONS FOR NURSING

Severity of Chronic Lung Disease May Correlate with Negative Changes in Body Image

Nicholas, P. K., & Leuner, J. D. (1992). Relationship between body image and chronic obstructive pulmonary disease. *Applied Nursing Research, 5,* 83–84.

This study explores the relationship between body image and chronic obstructive pulmonary disease (COPD). The researchers studied all clients with a diagnosis of moderate (n = 37) or severe (n = 50) COPD who had visited a pulmonary outpatient clinic during a 1-year period. To each subject the researchers applied the Body Cathexis Scale (BCS) and the Self Cathexis Scale (SCS), which have been used to measure body image for more than 40 years. These tools measure the degree of feeling of satisfaction and dissatisfaction with various parts of the body and with the self as a whole.

The researchers then compared the scores of the clients with COPD against those of 49 healthy subjects who worked in the same hospital. The healthy subjects had the highest score, showing a positive body image perception, followed by the group with moderate COPD. People with severe COPD had the lowest scores. Scores for men and women did not differ significantly.

Critique Although limited to one setting, this study looked at an important concept for nursing assessment and intervention. The researchers used reliable and valid tools to assess body image.

Possible nursing implications Nurses must recognize that most chronic diseases affect body image. In clients with severe COPD, in particular, the functional limitations and impairment in mobility have a marked impact on how the client perceives his or her body.

body image. Facial disfigurement resulting from surgical treatment of head and neck cancer, in particular, can cause severe body image disturbances. Likewise, the deformity that may result from burns or burn surgery can seriously affect a person's body image.

Another procedure that can cause body image disturbances is mastectomy (Frank et al., 1991; Gillies, 1984). For most women, a mastectomy results in the loss of a body part that is viewed as essential for maintaining femininity, attractiveness, and self-esteem. This loss is based on the historical (or traditional) belief that the female breast is a symbol of femininity and maternity.

Body image disturbances are also common after the surgical creation of an ostomy. These disturbances can result from the person's perception of the appearance of the stoma and from the reaction to the stoma by significant others. The person and significant others may equate the stoma with the genital region. Thus, exposure and direct handling of the stoma can be especially damaging to body image (Gillies, 1984; Salter, 1992).

For body image to remain healthy, it must accurately incorporate the actual physical changes of surgery. That is, the person must accept the body as it has become. For example, the client with an ostomy must recognize that the stoma is probably lifesaving and that it serves the same purpose as the bowel tract and rectum. This recognition is realistic.

AMPUTATION, PARALYSIS, AND DEFORMITY

For a person with a limb amputation or any type of paralysis, body image reintegration is required. In clients with an amputation, phantom limb pain creates different body perceptions, which necessitate body image reintegration. In phantom limb pain, the limb is gone but pain continues, *or the limb remains but no feeling is present.*

Deformity, such as a repaired cleft lip, is another physical change that requires adaptation of the body image because of a socially unacceptable change in physical appearance.

Limb amputation, paralysis, and deformity can all limit mobility. For example, the client with a spinal cord injury also experiences serious changes in mobility. These changes in mobility can, in turn, affect body image.

EATING DISORDERS

Obesity, anorexia nervosa, and bulimia nervosa commonly reflect body image disturbances. People with these conditions have a tendency to overestimate their body size, both during and after weight loss. This overestimation results in a feeling of having lost no weight even after dieting has produced a significant weight loss. (Also see Chapters 60 and 61 for more information on body image and eating disorders.)

COLLABORATIVE MANAGEMENT

ASSESSMENT

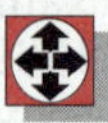

HISTORY

The North American Nursing Diagnosis Association (1992) states that to justify a diagnosis of Body Image Disturbance, the client must have a verbal or nonverbal response to an actual or perceived change in body structure and/or function. To assess and understand a body image disturbance, the nurse collects data about how the client perceives and has adapted to a body change (Chart 10–1).

View of Self The nurse begins the nursing assessment by obtaining data that identify the client's view of self. As the client shares information about body image, the nurse can better diagnose Body Image Disturbance and its cause. The nurse gathers data by inquiring about the client's recent physical body change. Is this perceived positively or negatively? What feelings does this change create? Are current feelings a change from feelings before this illness? Does the client describe herself or himself as hopeful or helpless?

Perception of Body Change After assessing the client's view of self, the nurse identifies the body change as perceived by the client and his or her family or significant others. The nurse must assess both client and family perceptions because they may conflict and/or lend insight into further assessment and intervention. For example, do the client and family understand the actual physiologic surgical alteration? Is the body change perceived a certain way (e.g., lifesaving, positive or negative)? What does this mean to them?

CHART 10–1

Nursing Care Highlight ◆ Specific Factors to Consider When Taking a History of the Client with Body Image Disturbance

- What is the client's view of himself or herself? (e.g., "How would you describe your body to another person?")
- What is the client's or family's perceived body change?
- What is the client's developmental level?
- What are the client's or family's past successful coping strategies?
- What is the client's current occupation or work history?
- What was the client's past experience with pain?
- What is the client's environment?

Developmental Level When assessing body image disturbance, the nurse should take into account the client's developmental level. A young adult client may be functioning only as an adolescent. Therefore, the client's body image may not be developed to the level of an adult, and certain expectations will not be appropriate. The nurse assesses the developmental level of a client by evaluating responses of the client to questions and by noticing the way he or she is affected during an interview. Body language and maturity of responses are important clues to the developmental level of a client. For example, does the client give inconsistent verbal responses to questions? Does he or she have poor eye contact? Is the client unable to answer some questions because he or she does not understand?

Coping Strategies To establish baseline data regarding coping behaviors, nurses should identify the client's and/or family's past successful coping strategies. The nurse can assess these strategies by asking:

- "How have you dealt with hard times in your life in the past?"
- "What did you do in the past that helped you get through them?"
- "Have you been doing some of these same things this time?"
- "Do you think that these things might help you now?"

Chapter 7 discusses the assessment of coping in detail.

Occupation or Work History The client's current occupation or work history can lend further insight into his or her self-image and body image. For example, is the client currently employed, laid off, fired, or retired? Does this work situation create any negative feelings or problems? Does the client anticipate return to work, or is he or she not currently working? Does the client feel useful?

Experience With Pain Body image assessment must also include data about the client's past experience with pain. Has the client ever experienced pain before? Was this pain chronic or acute? Did this pain control the client's life? What caused the pain? How did the client deal with the pain? Were friends or family supportive about the pain? Did the pain change the client's life in any way? The nurse assesses the client's pain experience regardless of whether it is a past or current problem.

Environment As well as assessing the client and family, the nurse also collects data about the client's immediate environment. The environment includes the immediate physical area at home, social supports, and community. Does the client have easy access to follow-up care? Is the home environment conducive to self-care needs (e.g., one-level versus two-level home, steps into home, bathroom and bedroom locations)? Is the community supportive of this client's needs (e.g., are there wheelchair ramps, easy transportation)? By collecting all of this information, the nurse can assess body image disturbances more accurately.

PHYSICAL ASSESSMENT/CLINICAL MANIFESTATIONS

The nurse completes a collection of data concerning body changes. The North American Nursing Diagnoses Association (NANDA) identifies the following *objective* clinical manifestations, or defining characteristics, for assessment of Body Image Disturbance. Although these defining characteristics have not been clinically validated by research, they provide direction for nursing assessment (Hurley, 1986). NANDA's definition and defining characteristics have not been revised or refined since 1986.

- Missing body part
- Actual change in structure or function
- Not looking at body part
- Not touching body part
- Hiding or overexposing body part (intentional or unintentional)
- Trauma to nonfunctioning body part
- Change in social involvement
- Change in ability to estimate spatial relationship of body to environment

Missing Body Part An obvious client characteristic that the nurse considers when assessing body image disturbance is missing body parts. The experience of a loss of any body part, internal or external, can pose definite challenges to the client who is attempting to redefine his or her body image. Therefore, this characteristic may predispose the client to the development of a body image disturbance. Nurses should be aware that a client born without a specific body part has not experienced this loss and may not demonstrate a body image disturbance.

The physical body loss may not always be obvious to the nurse. In this case, the nurse inquires about past surgery experienced and prosthesis used and observes the physical body for scars, disfigurement, or loss of an extremity.

For all clients, the nurse includes an assessment of religious practices. Some religions, for example, may dictate special management of the removed body part. Following this practice can be crucial to the client in the process of readjusting to a new body image.

Actual Change in Structure or Function Specific changes in body structure or function are also major physical losses that the nurse must assess. Any changes in mobility, self-care, or previous level of independence can create difficulty in body image reintegration. The client experiencing recent confinement to a wheelchair or permanent dependence on a walker or cane for mobility may need specific nursing interventions in order to understand the new body image (Fig. 10–3). The nurse should ask about the client's perception of this change in function, since the client may not perceive it as a loss. Is this a recent change for the client? Is this a significant change from previous function before this illness?

Not Looking at or Touching the Body Part The nurse collects objective data about the clients and how they view their bodies. Not looking at or touching the body or body part may indicate an altered body image. However, this characteristic alone is not enough to verify the existence of a body image disturbance. The client may avoid viewing the surgical site of an amputation for some time during the postoperative period because of discomfort related to observing any surgical incision or drainage. As the surgical area begins to heal, the client may have less difficulty viewing or touching the amputation area. Thus, this clinical manifestation must be interpreted carefully.

As another example, a client has experienced a stroke with paralysis of the right arm. The client may ignore the right arm to the extreme that he or she hits it on door frames when entering rooms because of the loss of sensation. This form of ignoring a body part is called *unilateral neglect* and indicates other cognitive or perceptual deficits that may or may not affect body image. Again, the nurse carefully reviews these data.

Feelings of ugliness and mutilation may also be of concern to a client. For example, the client requiring a halo brace for treatment of complex spinal cord problems may experience these feelings until the brace is removed (Olson et al., 1991).

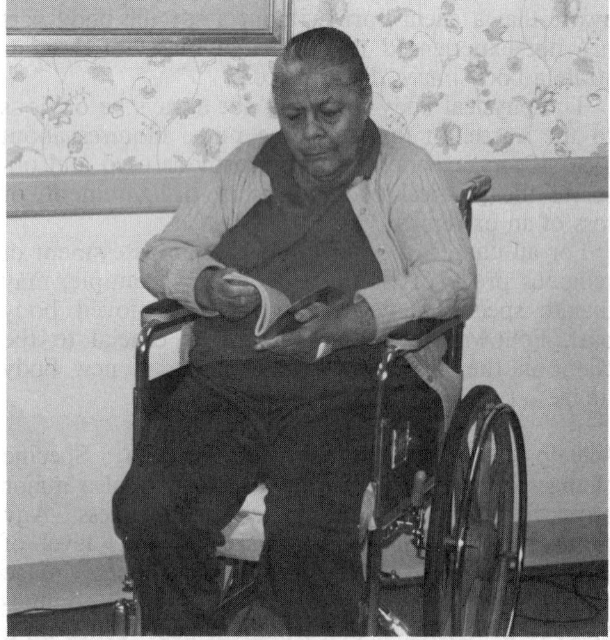

FIGURE 10–3 ◆ A client confined to a wheelchair who must learn to adapt to her new equipment and change in body image.

Hiding or Overexposing a Body Part Hiding or overexposing any body part, whether intentional or unintentional, may also indicate a client's difficulty with body image readjustment. The client recovering from a mastectomy, burn surgery, or limb amputation may experience shame, guilt, anger, or disgust about the body alteration. As a result, the client may hide or even overexpose the changed body area in attempts to deal with this change.

TRAUMA TO A NONFUNCTIONING BODY PART The nurse must also assess the client for any trauma that may have occurred to a nonfunctioning body part. For example, an injury or trauma to a flaccid extremity, originally caused by a past stroke, may cause old or new feelings to surface as a result of the need to adapt to the new body image. The client struggles with these thoughts: "Is my paralyzed arm worse now?" "Has it become more useless?" The client may have been successfully reintegrated past body changes into a new body image. However, the new injury to the past nonfunctioning extremity may pose a new threat to the body image, resulting in a need for further body image adaptation.

CHANGE IN SOCIAL INVOLVEMENT Changes in past social involvement and activities may demonstrate a potential body image disturbance. If the client fails to reintegrate the body changes into a new image, feelings of helplessness, worthlessness, or shame may surface. As a result, the client may choose to reduce social interactions. In addition, the nurse should assess the client's ability to access or attend social functions. If the client is confined to a wheelchair, are there both public transportation and building access for these needs? What are the limitations to wheelchair access in the client's home?

CHANGE IN ABILITY TO ESTIMATE THE SPATIAL RELATIONSHIP OF THE BODY TO THE ENVIRONMENT In cases of a body image disturbance, the client may be unable to estimate the spatial relationships of the body to the rest of the environment. This inability to "separate" the body from environment is a change from a previous ability and is not due to the disease process (e.g., cognitive changes resulting from a stroke). Clients may become so confused about their body boundary (e.g., as in loss of an extremity) that they cannot identify where the body ends and the surrounding environment begins. For example, the client who has experienced a severe stroke with resulting right-sided paralysis and cognitive and visual disturbances may try to move from a bed to a chair. In this attempt, the client misses the chair completely because his or her right visual field is impaired. In addition, because of unilateral neglect, the client cannot perceive his or her right side as separate from the rest of the environment (e.g., chair, bed, or commode). These disturbances also influence the client's coping abilities because cognition is also affected.

THE PRESENCE OF PAIN Although the North American Nursing Diagnosis Association (NANDA) does not identify pain as an additional characteristic for body image assessment, the presence of pain is important to include in data collection. Pain may become incorporated into the body as a normal, day-to-day experience, such as in a client with chronic pain. By assessing a client's pain, the nurse can better understand each client's body image development and the possible impact of illness or injury.

PSYCHOSOCIAL ASSESSMENT

By establishing a trusting, therapeutic relationship with the client, the nurse can thoroughly assess potential body image changes through observation and discussion. The nurse conducts a purposeful interview during which open-ended questions are asked (Fig. 10–4).

The nurse encourages the client to talk about any changes in current lifestyle and role that have occurred as a result of body changes. If usual lifestyle patterns have been interrupted because of the physical changes, the client may have difficulty in body image adaptation. For example, clients with deforming arthritis who are no longer able to perform their jobs may experience a body image disturbance.

NEGATIVE FEELINGS The nurse also discusses with the client any fears related to rejection by or reaction of significant others. For example, a client's perceptions about the family's reaction to the loss of a hand may not be accurate. These fears need to be expressed and assessed in order for the client to cope with this change successfully. In addition, fear itself may interrupt healthy body image adaptation, in that the fear may be unrealistic.

Clients may want to talk about their past strengths, function, or appearance. This focus on past abilities may not be healthy, even though the identification of remaining strengths can be an effective coping strategy. For example, the athlete who has undergone bilateral leg amputation and who continually focuses on past running ability may be experiencing difficulty with body image readjustment.

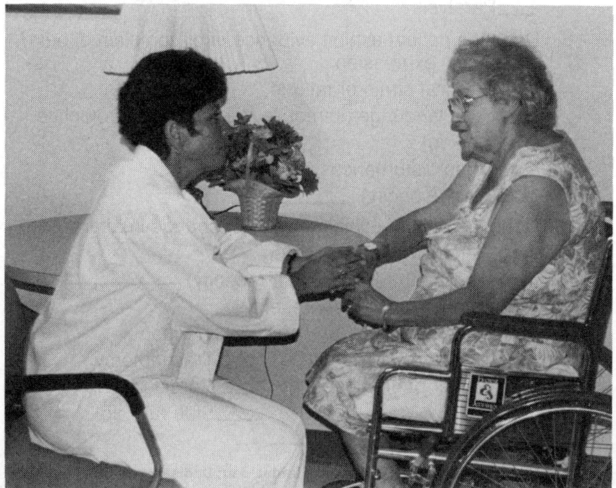

FIGURE 10–4 ♦ A nurse interviewing a client about body image perception and adaptation.

Verbalization of negative feelings about the body may also indicate alteration in body image. Clients commonly experience anger. The nurse can facilitate discussion of these feelings by helping clients to recognize their anger. The nurse then identifies the anger as a common reaction to loss. *Continually* focused anger about the body and any physical changes can become destructive to healthy body image adaptation. The nurse helps the client resolve angry feelings in order to progress through the process of adaptation.

Feelings of helplessness, hopelessness, or powerlessness are common immediate responses to body changes. However, if these feelings continue, body image disturbance can develop. The nurse inquires: "Do you feel as if you have control over what is happening to you?" "Are you hopeful about the future?" "Has the body change left you feeling helpless?"

Any preoccupation with the body change or loss may be characteristic of a body image disturbance. The client may become so focused on the loss of a breast that she plans an entire day's activities around concealing this physical change. This extreme behavior does not facilitate healthy body image adaptation to the loss. Nurses can observe behavior without threatening, invasive questioning.

Identifying remaining strengths can help clients form a healthy body image. However, specific emphasis on all remaining strengths and a sense of heightened achievement may not be healthy behavior. For example, the client may avoid the emotional issue of dealing with an extremity loss by focusing on developing the strength and endurance necessary to walk with a prosthesis. An unrealistic belief about continuing to achieve previous life goals may be destructive. The nurse assists the client in developing realistic goals.

PERSONALIZATION OF A BODY PART The North American Nursing Diagnosis Association (NANDA) has also identified client extension of the body boundary to incorporate environmental objects and personalization of the body part or loss by name as indicative of a body image disturbance. However, research has not established these characteristics as unhealthy behavior. For example, could it be that the client who envisions the body and wheelchair as one has successfully adapted to the new body image? Has the client who calls the colostomy "Sam" successfully incorporated this body change into a healthy image of the body? Future research may clarify these questions.

The client who depersonalizes the body part or loss by the use of impersonal pronouns (e.g., "it") may exhibit difficulty in adapting to the body change. The use of an impersonal pronoun to refer to a mastectomy, colostomy, or stump demonstrates one's inability to perceive the body change as part of the self. Such a reference keeps the body change impersonal and may facilitate denial of the change. By using denial, the client may demonstrate a refusal to verify the actual body change. This refusal then prolongs the grieving and coping process and can interrupt body image reintegration.

COPING AND SUPPORT SYSTEMS The nurse assesses the client's current coping behaviors and the client's attempts at body image adaptation to the change. Current coping behaviors can also be compared with past coping behaviors to assist the client with body image changes. The client who has used anger to cope with past stressful life events may need to demonstrate anger in response to body changes. With the knowledge of these data, the nurse is better prepared to treat a body image disturbance. (Also see Chapter 7.)

Nurses also evaluate the client's current family role to gain an understanding about communication patterns, support systems, and family dynamics. The client's role in the family may be a significant part of the client's identity. If this image of self is interrupted by a body change, major problems with body image may occur. In addition, family members may be significantly influenced by the client's body change and inability to perform previous family roles.

The nurse assesses client and family support systems. The success or failure of a client and family to deal with physical body changes can depend greatly on the existence of support systems. Support systems may be specific people, groups, communities, financial plans, or assistive devices. The nurse initiates this assessment on first contact with the client. However, much of this data collection is ongoing. To develop an effective plan of care, the nurse should know the client and family support systems.

ASSESSMENT TOOLS

Various written tools have been developed, primarily through the efforts of psychology researchers who study self-concept and body image. However, these tools are time-consuming for clients to complete and difficult to evaluate. To assist the nurse in identifying body image disturbances, a clinically useful nursing assessment tool is needed. The Baird Body Image Assessment Tool (BBIAT) attempts to clarify potential versus actual body image disturbances (Fig. 10–5). The client completes the subjective portion, answering each question with "strongly agree" (SA), "agree" (A), "undecided" (U), "disagree" (D), or "strongly disagree" (SD). The nurse asks clients to

Subjective Interview

Points

___ 1. I will be undergoing a major change in my job status as a result of this experience.
___SA ___A ___U ___D ___SD
If so, what?
___Decrease in job status ___Job loss
___Change in job ___Other (specify) ________

___ 2. I do not have someone available to help me or talk to.
___SA ___A ___U ___D ___SD
If someone is available, who?
___Spouse ___Parents
___Close friend ___Children
___Significant other (relative) ___Nurse

___ 3. I think of myself differently as a result of this experience.
___SA ___A ___U ___D ___SD
If so, how?
___Negatively ___Other (specify) ________
___Increased physical complaints

___ 4. My ability to move around by myself has changed as a result of this experience.
___SA ___A ___U ___D ___SD
If so, how?
___Less mobile ___Other (specify) ________
___No change

___ 5. I have definite feelings about specific parts of my body.
___SA ___A ___U ___D ___SD
If so, what?
___Hate ___Fear
___Disgust ___Other (specify) ________

___ 6. I am more fearful now than before this experience.
___SA ___A ___U ___D ___SD
If so, why?
___Fear of falling ___Fear of pain
___Fear of recurrence of problem ___Fear of inability to care for self
___Fear of others' reactions ___Other (specify) ________

Objective Interview

7. Does the patient display any prominent body feature?
___Obesity ___Disfigurement
___Limb loss ___Other (specify) ________
___Paralysis

8. Does the patient exhibit evidence of or complain of pain?
___Facial expression
___Physical strain or fatigue
___Body language (immobile, purposeless, protective, rubbing)
___Sleep disturbances
___Other (specify) ________

9. Does the patient exhibit any major change in affect?
___Withdrawal ___Crying
___Hostility ___Other (specify) ________

10. Is there any equipment present?
___Foley's catheter ___Traction
___NG or other tubes ___Tracheotomy
___Walker or crutches ___Cardiac monitor
___Cast ___Side rails up
___Other (specify) ________

SA, strongly agree; A, agree; U, undecided; D, disagree; SD, strongly disagree, IV, intravenous; NG, nasogastric.

FIGURE 10–5 ◆ The Baird Body Image Assessment Tool. (Courtesy of Susan Baird Holmes.)

respond to questions 1 through 6. Points are then assigned to each answer as follows: SA = 5, A = 4, U = 3, D = 2, SD = 1. The total possible score for the subjective portion of the BBIAT is 30. Reliability and validity of this nursing tool have been established. A score of 23 to 30 points may indicate a serious need for nursing intervention; 19 to 22 points, a potential need that requires nursing intervention; and 18 or lower, no need for nursing intervention or the client has adapted to body changes.

The BBIAT is meant to be used only as a guide or tool to clarify for nurses, in daily practice, the assessment of body image alterations. The nurse uses the objective portion to identify other physical evidence that may have an impact on body image reintegration. No score is given for this portion. However, if many objective variables exist so that the nurse is unsure whether a body image disturbance exists, this portion of the tool may help the nurse clarify the nursing diagnosis, etiology, or both. Further research and tool refinement are needed before one can draw any conclusions.

ANALYSIS

COMMON NURSING DIAGNOSES

The following nursing diagnoses are common in clients with a diagnosis of Body Image Disturbance:

1. Anxiety related to changes in health status and self-concept
2. Ineffective Individual Coping related to changes in lifestyle, loss of body part, or loss of body function
3. Ineffective Family Coping related to effects of major life events or changes

ADDITIONAL NURSING DIAGNOSES

The client may also demonstrate other problems that are related to body image disturbance. These include:

- Sexual Dysfunction related to disturbance in self-esteem or body image
- Social Isolation related to change in physical appearance
- Dysfunctional Grieving related to effects of loss of function or body part
- Impaired Physical Mobility related to neuromuscular impairment, musculoskeletal impairment, perceptual/cognitive impairment, and/or pain/discomfort
- Self Esteem Disturbance related to change in physical appearance
- Hopelessness related to failing or deteriorating physiologic condition or prolonged activity restriction creating isolation

PLANNING AND IMPLEMENTATION

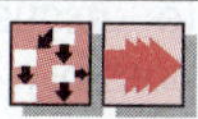

ANXIETY

PLANNING: CLIENT GOALS Major goals are that the client will:

- Verbalize decreased anxiety
- Demonstrate decreased anxiety by participation in the plan of care

INTERVENTIONS Research has established the role of teaching in providing reassurance to clients who are about to undergo surgical body alterations. Preoperative teaching can decrease anxiety before and after surgery (see Chap. 19). In addition, clients may be hospitalized for shorter periods because of reduced anxiety. Visits to clients by people who have had the same health problems have also been effective in assisting the client to adjust to the body image alteration.

If accepted by the client's culture, light touch to an extremity may be used by the nurse during discussion to help clients in re-establishing changed body boundaries. This practice can convey to the client a sense of being valued and that the physical body is still present. Talking to clients at equal eye level can be especially helpful in establishing an open, trusting relationship with those who may be feeling anxious or fearful.

The nurse encourages client verbalization and active thinking by providing for client participation in planning for the client's own needs. A client's sense of independence and responsibility is also enhanced by self-initiated activity. For example, a client with a spinal cord injury usually requires extra time for self-care. The nurse asks the client to suggest the best time for physical therapy appointments according to the client's need to have sufficient time to prepare for the appointment.

INEFFECTIVE INDIVIDUAL COPING

PLANNING: CLIENT GOALS The major goal is that the client will state that he or she accepts the changed body structure or function.

INTERVENTIONS Nursing interventions to help clients cope with alterations in body structure or function focus on teaching and goal setting.

Health Teaching The nurse teaches the client and family or significant other the components of the healthy grieving process. Teaching begins by increasing client and family awareness of the various stages of grieving as well as understanding coping behaviors that are used in response to loss (see Chap. 12). For example, the client, family member, or significant other who responds with anger or denies the body change that has occurred may not be aware of his or her response. The nurse specifically helps the person to discuss feelings, recognize current behaviors, and possibly identify other therapeutic coping strategies. The nurse should also teach an understanding of healthy body image development throughout the life span. Clients and families should be better prepared to understand their fears and concerns and should be more effective in coping by developing an awareness about body image development.

Goal Setting Nursing interventions also focus on setting small, achievable goals; the nurse does this together with the client, family, or both. Goals are established during hospitalization to provide positive reinforcement about remaining strengths as well as effective coping strategies. For example, a client may be convinced that a burn site is noticeable, even under clothing, and may refuse to leave the hospital room. The nurse helps the client set a goal to dress in personal clothes of his or her choice and visit the gift shop in the hospital. The client meets the goal within 3 days and by the end of the week is in the visitors' lounge every afternoon, meeting new people and enjoying social interaction. Meeting the public for the first time after surgery can be threatening, and clients may become progressively desensitized to physical body changes. The nurse helps the client to be aware of his or her feelings about being stared at in public and to plan coping strategies to deal with these feelings.

Clients need to realize their remaining strengths and capabilities. In addition, the nurse can assist the client and/or family with identification of long-term effective coping mechanisms by validating realistic concerns and fears. For example, the amputee who in the past coped with life events by jogging every day needs assistance to identify and practice new coping behaviors. In addition, the nurse may arrange for another client who has experienced similar body changes and has successfully reintegrated these changes into a new body image to visit the client and to discuss concerns. (For more detailed coping and grieving nursing interventions, see Chapter 12.)

INEFFECTIVE FAMILY COPING: COMPROMISED

PLANNING: CLIENT GOALS The primary goal is that the family or significant other will accept the client's body changes with readjustment into the family unit.

INTERVENTIONS Family members and significant others need the same kind of assistance as the client in coping with body changes. Family members need support so that they in turn can be supportive to the client. The family must be able to deal both with any feelings about previous problems concerning the client and with new feelings related to the kind and extent of body changes incurred by the client. For example, family members may feel guilty about a belief that their mother's leg might have been saved if they had gotten her to the doctor sooner. The nurse serves as the client's and family's most consistent health caregiver. This consistency establishes a caring rapport, which increases comfort in discussing these sensitive issues.

Providing empathy, *not* sympathy, can be the single most important intervention when treating body image disturbance. For example, an empathic supporting statement to a client might be, "This must be very difficult for you." A sympathetic statement to a client might be, "I'm so sorry for you." The nurse may convey sensitivity and empathy more clearly to the client and family by the use of a light touch to the arm or hand during these discussions. In addition, the nurse should sit at eye level with the client and family or significant others to facilitate even more open verbalization of concerns (Fig. 10–6).

The nurse may also actively attempt to involve the family in the client's care during hospitalization, but only as they desire. This intervention may increase both the client's and family's sense of control over the situation and may decrease feelings of powerless-

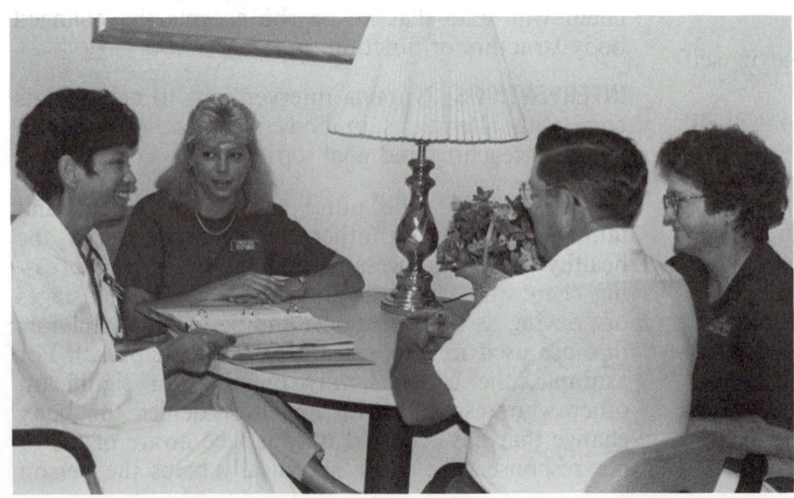

FIGURE 10–6 ◆ A family conference with the nurse to discuss feelings about a change in the client's physical appearance or function.

ness. In addition, with this involvement in care, family members are impressed with the importance for the client to gradually increase responsibility for self-care and other activities. For example, teaching family members how to care for a stump at home after an amputation provides the client with positive reinforcement about the physical change and assists the family in recognizing that the client is still their loved one.

The client and family may need to restructure their relationships, depending on the extent and impact of the body change. The nurse can assist with this restructuring by serving as a buffer between client and family, if necessary. The nurse may also provide knowledge about community or hospital resources if family roles have changed as a result of the body alteration. For example, if the client is unable to maintain the family role as breadwinner, community resources may assist with financial needs. By helping the client and family share concerns or fears and solve problems together, the nurse can alleviate miscommunication problems and can enhance existing support systems.

DISCHARGE PLANNING

HOME CARE PREPARATION

The client returning home faces many challenges concerning continued adaptation to body image changes. The home health nurse can be most effective in helping the client and family cope with these challenges. The nurse can assist with any follow-up care necessary to treat the body change. For example, the amputee client will require future fittings for a prosthesis and continued assessment of the stump after discharge from the hospital. The client with an ostomy may desire future contact with ostomy support groups. The home health nurse can effectively assist these clients with their long-term needs.

HEALTH TEACHING

The nurse provides continued follow-up home care by informing the client and family about new improvements or changes in treatment, medication, and rehabilitation devices or programs (e.g., new prostheses or new procedures). The nurse also presents and reinforces education about long-term care that will be required because of the body change. As hospital stays continue to shorten, it is even more crucial for the nurse to educate the client to ensure client and family understanding with follow-up visits. For example, clients with terminal illnesses are now managing parenteral drug therapy successfully at home. Clients who undergo ostomy procedures are experiencing trial-and-error periods at home with various appliances. The success of these clients' home management abilities depends on effective teaching by the nurse about self-care activities. The nurse teaches and promotes client independence, which assists the body image change to stabilize.

PSYCHOSOCIAL PREPARATION

Psychosocial needs may become even more important as the client returns to the previous environment, and actual losses may become more readily apparent to both the client and family. For example, the client with an ostomy may become discouraged if the ostomy appliance that he or she had been using successfully in the hospital presents problems at home. The home health nurse continues to assess these psychosocial needs and anticipate future client and family experiences in an attempt to help the client and family cope with new feelings. The client who first performs ostomy care at home must not have the unrealistic expectation that the care will always go smoothly.

Another example of a problem arising in transition between the hospital and home can be illustrated by the client who has a spinal cord injury. The family or significant other welcoming the paraplegic or quadriplegic client home after months of hospitalization must also be aware of potential client reactions to returning to the previous environment. The nurse plays a major role in preparing the client and family for the emotional reactions and long-term adaptation to body changes. The client may tend to focus on and re-examine his or her changed body more closely after returning home. Activities of daily living are often completed in a new way. In addition, the familiar home environment may cause the client to remember past activities that he or she can no longer perform. Therefore, the nurse can help prepare the client and family or significant other for possible feelings of depression or anger that can occur after discharge.

HEALTH CARE RESOURCES

Many community support groups and organizations are specially geared to meet the needs of clients with specific body image problems. The nurse can direct the client or family to these agencies for additional help with working through the adjustment process (e.g., Arthritis Foundation, American Cancer Society, National Spinal Cord Association, Multiple Sclerosis Society). The nurse can also refer the client and family to community mental health services or health professionals who provide more in-depth assistance. Clients and their families or significant others must know what resources are available and what to expect from these resources. The nurse serves as the link between clients and families and their support systems.

An awareness of assistive devices or various prostheses that are available can also help the client. Walkers, crutches, wheelchairs, and artificial limbs increase the client's independence in self-care and help to de-emphasize the sense of long-term or permanent disability. Nurses provide this information to clients to assist with long-term body image adaptation. The nurse consults with the discharge planner or social worker to help identify community resources.

EVALUATION

The outcome criteria for the client experiencing body image disturbance are that the client:

- States that anxiety about altered body image is decreased
- Demonstrates acceptance of the change in body image by participating in the plan of care
- Uses specific coping strategies to deal with the body image disturbance

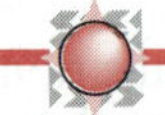

IMPLICATIONS FOR NURSING RESEARCH

Although there was considerable nursing research on body image in the 1980s, very little has been added since that time. Many questions remain unanswered. Some possible nursing research questions include:

- ◆ Is Body Image Disturbance really a component of Self Esteem Disturbance and not a separate nursing diagnosis?
- ◆ What are the most reliable defining characteristics, or clinical manifestations, that indicate a body image disturbance?
- ◆ What is the best way to measure the degree of body image disturbance that a client experiences?
- ◆ What are the most effective nursing interventions for a client experiencing a body image disturbance?

SELECTED BIBLIOGRAPHY

*Baird, S. E. (1985). Development of a nursing assessment tool to diagnose altered body image in immobilized patients. *Orthopaedic Nursing, 4,* 47–54.

*Baxley, K. O., Erdman, L. K., Henry, E. B., & Roof, B. J. (1984). Alopecia: Effect on cancer patients' body image. *Cancer Nursing, 7,* 499–503.

*Cleveland, S. (1976). The place of the head in the body image concept. *Research and Clinical Studies in Headache, 4,* 1–7.

*Corbeil, M. (1971). Nursing process for a patient with a body image disturbance. *Nursing Clinics of North America, 6,* 155–163.

Doolittle, N. D. (1991). Clinical ethnography of lacunar stroke: Implications for acute care. *Journal of Neuroscience Nursing, 23*(4), 235–240.

*Fischer, S. (1964). Sex differences in body perception. *Psychological Monographs,* 1–22.

Frank, A., et al. (1991). Conservative surgery and irradiation for early breast cancer in the older woman. *Nebraska Medical Journal, 76,* 297–306.

French, J. K., & Phillips, J. A. (1991). Shattered images: Recovery for the spinal cord injured client. *Rehabilitation Nursing, 16*(3), 134–136.

*Gellert, E. (1975). Children's constructions of their self images. *Perceptual Motor Skills, 40,* 307–324.

*Gillies, O. A. (1984). Body image changes following illness and injury. *Journal of Enterostomal Therapy, 11,* 186–189.

*Glucksman, M., & Hirsch, J. (1969). The response of obese patients to weight reduction: The perception of body size. *Psychosomatic Medicine, 31,* 1–7.

*Gruendemann, B. J. (1975). The impact of surgery on body image. *Nursing Clinics of North America, 10,* 635–643.

*Harris, M. (1986). Helping the person with an altered self image. *Geriatric Nursing, 7*(2), 90–92.

*Janelli, L. M. (1988). The impact of health status on body image in older women. *Rehabilitation Nursing, 13,* 178–180.

*Koehler, M. L. (1989). Relationship between self-concept and successful rehabilitation. *Rehabilitation Nursing, 14*(1), 9–12.

*Leonard, B. J. (1972). Body image changes in chronic illness. *Nursing Clinics of North America, 7,* 687–695.

*Marten, L. (1978). Self-care nursing model for patients experiencing radical change in body image. *JOGNN, 7*(6), 9–13.

*Morris, C. A. (1985). Self-concept as altered by the diagnosis of cancer. *Nursing Clinics of North America, 20,* 611–630.

*Murray, R. (1972). Body image development in adulthood. *Nursing Clinics of North America, 7,* 617–629.

*Murray, R. L. (1972). Principles of nursing intervention for the adult patient with body image changes. *Nursing Clinics of North America, 7,* 697–707.

Newell, R. (1991). Body image disturbance: Cognitive behavioural formulation and intervention. *Journal of Advanced Nursing, 16,* 1400–1406.

Nicholas, P. K., & Leuner, J. D. (1992). Relationship between body image and chronic obstructive pulmonary disease. *Applied Nursing Research, 5,* 83–84.

Olson, B., Ustanko, L., & Warner, S. (1991). The patient in a halo brace: Striving for normalcy in body image and self-concept. *Orthopaedic Nursing, 10*(1), 44–50.

Rew, L. (1990). Correlates of health-promoting lifestyle and sexual satisfaction in a group of men. *Issues in Mental Health Nursing, 11,* 283–295.

*Rice, M. A., Tate, R. C., Grossberg, G. T., Handal, D. J., Brandeberry, L., & Nakra, R. (1988). Group intervention for reinforcing self-worth following mastectomy. *Oncology Nursing Forum, 15*(1), 33–37.

Salter, M. J. (1992). What are the differences in body image between patients with a conventional stoma compared with those who have had a conventional stoma followed by a continent pouch? *Journal of Advanced Nursing, 17,* 841–848.

*Samonds, R. J., & Cammermeyer, M. (1989). Perceptions of body image in subjects with multiple sclerosis: A pilot study. *Journal of Neuroscience Nursing, 21*(3), 190–194.

*Schilder, P. (1950). *The image and appearance of the human body.* New York: International Universities Press.

Thompson, J. K. (1992). Body image: Extent of disturbance, associated features, theoretical models, assessment methodologies, intervention strategies, and a proposal for a new DSM diagnostic category—body image disorder. *Progress in Behavior Modification, 28,* 3–54.

*Wells, R. W. (1975). Body image and surgical alterations. *AORN Journal, 21,* 812–815.

Willis-Helmich, J. J. (1992). Reclaiming body image: The hidden burn. *Journal of Burn Care Rehabilitation, 13*(1), 64–67.

SUGGESTED READINGS

Doolittle, N. D. (1991). Clinical ethnography of lacunar stroke: Implications for acute care. *Journal of Neuroscience Nursing, 23*(4), 235–240.

This article describes a small study in which 13 clients who experienced lacunar strokes were interviewed on several occasions. The subjects described the stroke as a "bodily event" in which they had loss of control. They considered their affected sides as passive objects and frequently called the affected side "it" or "they."

French, J. K., & Phillips, J. A. (1991). Shattered images: Recovery for the spinal cord injured client. *Rehabilitation Nursing, 16*(3), 134–136.

This article discusses the impact of a spinal cord injury on a person's well-being and body image. The inability to move and have control over one's body is a major contributor to body image disturbance in the client with spinal cord injury.

Willis-Helmich, J. J. (1992). Reclaiming body image: The hidden burn. *Journal of Burn Care Rehabilitation, 13*(1), 64–67.

The author discusses the effect of burns on a person's body image. Health care professionals are usually concerned with the physical problems associated with burns, but body image is an important issue for the burn client.

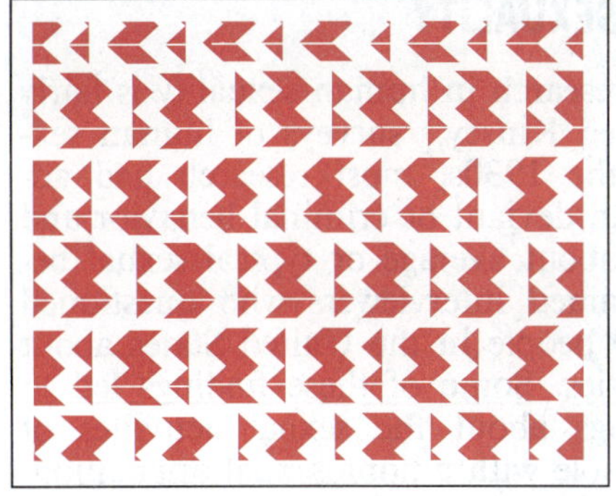

CHAPTER 11

CHAPTER HIGHLIGHTS

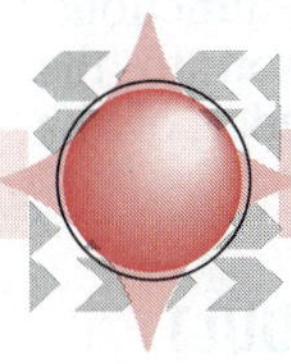

Human Sexuality

Human sexuality is expressed in terms of many factors, such as physical appearance, attitudes and values, knowledge, and behaviors that result from inherited characteristics and social learning. A person's sexual health status is created by the relationships among these factors. Sexual health can be described as a person's freedom from physical and psychologic impairment, the awareness of open and positive attitudes toward sexual functioning, and accurate knowledge about sexuality.

OVERVIEW

Medical-surgical nurses are concerned with issues of sexual health. Through the nursing process, the nurse recognizes the importance of human sexuality and encourages the growth and development of clients as sexual beings. The nurse also intervenes in a variety of situations to promote sexual health and to prevent sexual dysfunctions related to illness and injury throughout a client's life cycle.

CONCEPTUAL MODEL OF SEXUAL HEALTH

As people develop, various factors determine their optimal status of sexual health at a particular time.

- *Physical* factors are associated with changes in one's body; these include age, reproductive history,

level of sexual functioning, past and present illnesses and injuries, the use of medications, and specific sexual behaviors.
- *Psychologic* factors are associated with the mind; these include body image, self-esteem, knowledge of sexuality, attitudes toward gender roles, and preference for sexual partners.
- *Sociocultural* factors include race, ethnicity, social status, marital status, family and social support groups, occupation, and level of education.

External threats—in the form of physical illness, injury, or medical and surgical interventions—may lead to alterations in these factors and can reduce a person's level of sexual health. Similarly, threats to a person's psychologic and sociocultural domains, such as changes in family composition or family violence, may result in alterations that diminish sexual health.

To promote optimal sexual health in clients, the medical-surgical nurse assesses these factors and compares current findings with past patterns that clients have reported. The nurse also evaluates the impact of external threats on these factors and provides nursing interventions that reduce or prevent the negative effects of the threats.

EFFECT OF ANATOMY AND PHYSIOLOGY ON SEXUAL HEALTH

The physical structure and function of the body affect a person's sexual health. Internal reproductive organs, such as the ovaries and uterus in a woman and the testes in a man, constitute one aspect of the anatomy that influences sexual health. In addition, external structures, such as the breasts and external genitalia, affect sexual health. A deformity, injury, disease, or surgical alteration of any of these internal or external structures poses a threat to one's sexual health. The endocrine system also maintains both structure and function of the reproductive organs. For further details on anatomic and physiologic alterations in the reproductive and endocrine systems, see Units 13 and 16.

PSYCHOSEXUAL DEVELOPMENT

A person's psychosexual and physiologic development begins at the moment of conception and continues through young adulthood. Females are generally physically mature by the late teen years, whereas males may continue to mature in terms of secondary sexual characteristics into their early to late 20s. Overt (open) sexual behaviors are observed in adults of all ages. Age, illness or injury, and life experiences have major impacts on an adult's sexuality. Attitudes and values are generally more firmly established in the adult than in the adolescent and influence overt sexual behavior. Although a man may reach his peak of sexual urgency in his 20s, a woman may not reach her peak until her 30s or 40s. This "mismatch" may lead to conflicts within marriage or other intimate relationships.

RESEARCH ON SEXUALITY

The history of research in human sexuality is fairly short. Before Alfred Kinsey's surveys of human sexual behavior in the 1930s, most research had addressed people with deviant or criminal behavior and little was known about average or typical sexual behavior. Kinsey trained interviewers who questioned more than 18,000 people in the United States about their sexual histories. Some of these findings led to new understandings about the sexual activities of women and of people with a homosexual orientation. In addition, the findings enabled the American public to redefine the social code of acceptable sexual activities and to acknowledge more openly the reality of human sexual characteristics.

In the late 1950s and 1960s, the team of Masters and Johnson (1970) began to observe couples engaging in sexual activity and used various instruments to measure the responses of both men and women. In addition to using case studies and clinical and experimental research designs to increase the knowledge base of human sexual response and behavior, this team developed and tested interventions for use with couples who had recognizable sexual dysfunctions. The contributions of Masters and Johnson to the field of sexology as well as to the knowledge of the general public are well documented.

SEXUAL RESPONSE CYCLE OF THE ADULT

As a result of the research of Masters and Johnson in the 1960s, the sexual response cycle of the adult is well documented. This cycle consists of four phases: excitement, plateau, orgasm, and resolution (Table 11–1). The underlying physiology of this cycle consists of vasocongestion and myotonia. *Vasocongestion* refers to blood trapped in tissues of the breast, vulva, and penis. This congestion results in erection of the nipples, clitoris, and penis. *Myotonia* refers to the tension of both voluntary and involuntary muscles that occurs during sexual excitement and orgasm. The differences in male and female sexual response cycles are illustrated in Figure 11–1. The problems of sexual dysfunction in adults are related to the different phases of these cycles.

SEXUAL PREFERENCES

HOMOSEXUALITY

Sexual behavior and preference for partners may change over one's life span. Although most children and many adolescents engage in some types of overt homosexual activities, only a small percentage of adults identify themselves as homosexual. Homosexuality is defined as a person's attraction to one or more persons of the same sex. This preference is the most common of the sexual minorities.

Many stereotypic myths remain about homosexual (gay) men and lesbian women. However, the nurse who is equipped with an appropriate knowledge base

TABLE 11–1 The Adult Sexual Response Cycle

Phase	Male Response	Female Response
Excitement	• Skin flushing begins on the abdomen, then spreads to the neck and face.	• Skin flushing begins on the abdomen and throat, then spreads to the breasts.
	• The nipples become erect.	• The nipples become erect, the veins distend, areolae darken, and the breasts enlarge by 25%.
	• Myotonia of the legs and arms occurs.	• Myotonia of the entire body occurs.
	• Erection of the penis may subside and return.	• The clitoris becomes erect.
	• The testes become elevated.	• The vagina is lubricated.
	• Pulse and blood pressure increase.	• Pulse and blood pressure increase.
Plateau	• Myotonia increases, with carpopedal spasms and facial grimaces.	• Myotonia increases, with carpopedal spasms, flared nostrils, and an arched back.
	• The penis remains erect and darkens.	• The clitoris retracts under its hood.
	• The testes continue to swell and elevate toward the perineum.	• The vaginal barrel distends, and contractions begin.
	• Pulse, respirations, and blood pressure increase.	• Pulse, respirations, and blood pressure increase.
Orgasm	• The skin flush is maximal.	• The skin flush is maximal.
	• Myotonia of the entire body occurs, and the rectal sphincter contracts.	• Myotonia of the entire body occurs.
	• Semen is ejaculated through the penis.	• The clitoris remains retracted.
	• Pulse and blood pressure increase.	• Pulse and blood pressure increase.
	• The respiratory rate doubles.	• The respiratory rate doubles.
Resolution	• The skin flush disappears within 5 minutes in most men, followed by perspiration.	• The skin flush disappears and may be followed by perspiration.
	• The muscles relax.	• The muscles relax.
	• The nipples return to normal.	• The nipples and breasts return to their normal color and size.
	• The penis returns to its normal size in two stages.	• The clitoris returns to its normal position within 10 seconds.
	• The testes return to their normal size and position.	• The vagina collapses and loses its dark color.
	• Pulse, respirations, and blood pressure return to normal.	• Pulse, respirations, and blood pressure return to normal.

can help to dispel these myths and provide nursing care that includes attention to the person's sexual preference or orientation.

Although nursing care of homosexual clients does not differ from care of heterosexuals, there are some similarities and differences. Homosexual women may experience the same concerns about gynecologic and breast problems as heterosexual women but may not have the same needs for contraception, nor are they as likely to become pregnant, as women who are sexually active with heterosexual partners. There is an increasing interest in parenting among homosexual couples, and artificial insemination followed by pregnancy is becoming more frequent in this population. However, many homosexual women have a history of sexual abuse, family violence, or both. Many lesbians approach the health care system cautiously because of widespread homophobia—an aversion or antipathy toward homosexuals or their lifestyle. Because of the lesbian's fear and suspicions about the type of care that she may receive, there may be incomplete attention to minor problems that may become serious.

Similarly, gay men may avoid the traditional health care system and thus may receive inadequate preventive or primary health care. Homosexual men may have the same concerns about genitourinary problems as heterosexual men. Because of the high incidence of anal intercourse among gay men, these clients may seek treatment more frequently for injuries of the rectum and for gastrointestinal infections known as the "gay bowel syndrome." Gay men with this syndrome are infected and reinfected with microorganisms that are causing one or more gastrointestinal infections. The incidence of sexually transmitted diseases (STDs) is also higher among the homosexual population. At this time, gay men also represent the group with the highest incidence of acquired immunodeficiency syndrome (AIDS) (see Chap. 24).

OTHER SEXUAL VARIATIONS

The nurse should be familiar with other sexual variations, such as the following.

BISEXUALITY Bisexuality refers to a person's preference for intimate relationships with members of either sex.

TRANSSEXUALITY A transsexual is a person who is dissatisfied with his or her gender assignment and is convinced that he or she is trapped within the wrong body. Sex reassignment surgery for the man who has a strong urge to live as a woman includes orchiectomy (removal of the testes), penectomy (removal of the penis), and vaginoplasty (construction of a vagina). Hormone replacement treatment is also given. A woman who is reassigned as a man undergoes hysterectomy (uterus removal), oophorectomy (ovary removal), and mastectomy (breast removal) along with hormone replacement therapy.

TRANSVESTISM Also known as cross-dressing, transvestism is more common in men than in women. The person likes to wear clothes associated with the opposite sex for the sake of his or her sexual arousal. Unlike the transsexual, the transvestite does not have a conflict about his or her gender; some transvestites

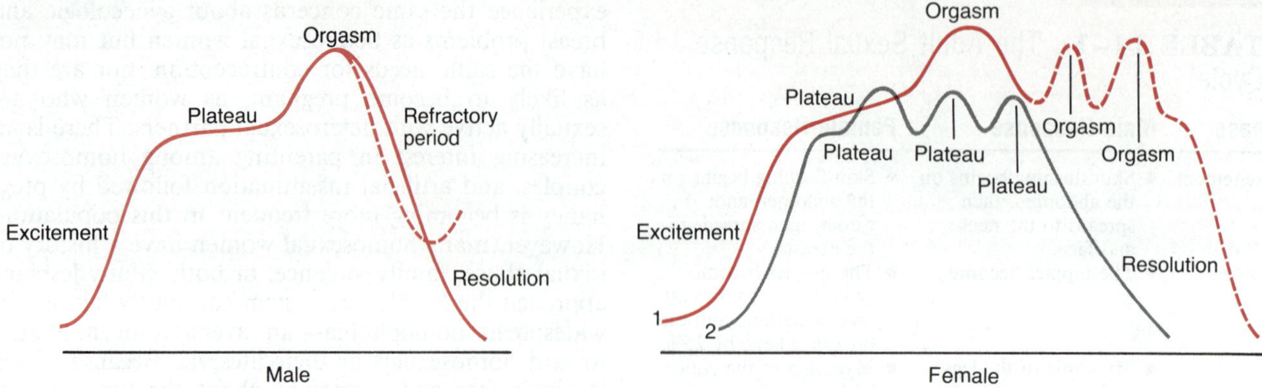

FIGURE 11-1 ◆ The male and female adult sexual response cycles. In the male sexual response cycle, a refractory period usually follows orgasm before another erection occurs. Women respond in various ways to sexual stimulation: Pattern 1 depicts single or multiple orgasms; pattern 2 shows some peaks but no orgasm.

are married, and most engage in this activity in private.

PEDOPHILIA Pedophilia is a sexual preference for children. It is a psychiatric disorder (not discussed in this chapter).

CHANGES IN SEXUAL FUNCTION ASSOCIATED WITH AGING

Physical, social, and psychologic changes affect sexual function throughout a person's life. Chart 11-1 summarizes the major changes in the older adult. For more information on sexuality during each phase of adult development, see Chapter 4.

EFFECTS OF ILLNESS ON SEXUALITY

Many illnesses and injuries can have a negative effect on sexual health. In some cases, sexual dysfunctions may result that can be temporary or permanent.

HOSPITALIZATION

People often perceive the process of hospitalization as impersonal. Elements of sexual identity and behaviors associated with gender roles are frequently denied or seriously curtailed by the social settings that exist in most hospitals. Hospitals provide little privacy; in addition, symbols of sexual identity, such as certain clothing and jewelry, are usually removed. Behaviors associated with sexual arousal and satisfaction are discouraged.

ACUTE ILLNESS

When a person is hospitalized for acute illness or injury, sexual health may be impaired. Not only is the social climate not conducive to sexual health for the reasons just identified, but a client's physical and psychologic conditions may not be consistent with sexual health. Acute medical conditions for which a client may be hospitalized can render the person physically unable to engage in sexual activity because of anxiety, fatigue, pain, malaise, or direct tissue damage or surgery.

Specific acute disorders, such as sexually transmitted diseases (STDs), or complications associated with these disorders may affect the sexuality of the hospitalized person (see Chapter 77). Nurses should consider care that includes assessment of risk factors and sexual contacts when caring for the client with an acute condition requiring hospitalization. Because of the social stigma associated with the diagnosis of STDs, the hospitalized client may also suffer from guilt and low self-esteem, which may impair his or her pursuit of behaviors that would lead to sexual health.

Specific acute bacterial or viral infections, such as pneumonia, hepatitis, gastroenteritis, and prostatitis, affect sexual health. In addition to the fatigue and malaise that are associated with these conditions, specific changes in body function may threaten an ill person's body image and self-esteem.

CHART 11-1

Nursing Focus on the Elderly ◆ Changes Affecting Sexuality

Physical Changes

- In women, vaginal tissue gradually atrophies.
- Women become infertile; male fertility varies.
- Sexual arousal takes longer, and sperm count and the force of ejaculation decrease.

Social Changes

- Both sexes experience a heightened need for human contact and intimacy.

Psychologic Changes

- Both sexes engage in life review and desire to be useful. They may experience low self-esteem.

CHRONIC ILLNESS

The sexual health of the client with a chronic illness or impairment may be threatened in various ways. For example, clients with hypertension, connective tissue disease, cancer, cardiovascular disease, diabetes, end-stage renal disease (ESRD), chronic respiratory disease, chronic liver disease, or spinal cord injury face limitations of previous sexual behavior patterns. These clients must deal with changes in body structure, function, or both in addition to psychologic variables, such as uncertainty, fear, and depression. The client's body image is threatened, and tissue damage may impair the sexual response cycle or may render the client unable to engage in preferred sexual activities. (See also Chapter 10, Body Image.)

HYPERTENSION Adults who experience hypertension are at risk for problems in sexual functioning. Certain antihypertensive drugs, such as methyldopa (Aldomet) and propranolol (Inderal, Novopranol♣), have been associated with decreased libido (sexual desire) in both men and women. In addition, men may experience erectile and ejaculatory failure, whereas women may experience galactorrhea (the presence of milk in the breasts) and an inability to have an orgasm. These adverse effects usually disappear within 2 weeks after medication is discontinued.

Clonidine (Catapres), another antihypertensive agent, may lead to urinary retention, impotence, and gynecomastia (breast enlargement in men), thus affecting the sexual response cycle. Prazosin (Minipress) also causes impotence. The nurse should assess the effects of such drugs in both men and women so that the physician may consider changes in dosages or types of medication if needed.

CONNECTIVE TISSUE DISEASE Clients with connective tissue diseases, like rheumatoid arthritis and systemic lupus erythematosus, face a chronic disabling condition characterized by problems with mobility, pain, and weakness. Although research on the specific incidence of sexual dysfunction among people with arthritis is lacking, obvious physical barriers exist to the usual sexual activities of such clients. Limited joint movement, weakness, fatigue, pain, swelling, and stiffness of extremities make activities of daily living difficult.

In addition to the often deforming nature of some forms of arthritis, large dosages of corticosteroid drugs may alter an arthritic person's physical appearance, which can result in lowered self-esteem and altered body image. Depression and anxiety about the unrelenting course of arthritic conditions may interfere with interpersonal communication and result in decreased sexual desire. Dyspareunia (painful intercourse) may result from changes in secretory function of the vagina, as seen in clients with Sjögren's syndrome (see Chap. 23).

CANCER Various types of cancer may directly affect sexual functioning and body image. Cervical or uterine cancer that results in hysterectomy and breast cancer that results in mastectomy are among the obvious malignancies affecting both sexual functioning and body image in women. In men, testicular and prostatic cancer may result in radical surgery that alters both sexual functioning and body image.

Other primary malignant tumors also contribute to the decline of a person's sexual health. These can include cancers of the gastrointestinal tract, urinary system, and larynx, often necessitating surgical diversion or radical neck dissection. In addition to the damaging effects of malignant growths and surgical procedures, radiation and chemotherapy affect the sexual function, appearance, and self-esteem of a client with cancer. Clients may experience alopecia (loss of hair), fatigue, anorexia, malaise, decline in libido, and secondary ovarian or testicular failure as a result of these therapies.

CARDIOVASCULAR DISEASE Cardiovascular disease affects a person's sexuality because sexual activity makes demands on the cardiopulmonary system. Cardiovascular disease also affects the client's self-concept, self-esteem, and role function. When to resume sexual activity after a myocardial infarction, for example, can be planned and implemented on an individual basis. The conditions under which sexual activity is pursued (relaxing versus anxiety-provoking conditions) and the amount of physical stress that the heart can handle must be considered. The severity of tissue damage and the effects of medications may limit the degree to which people with chronic cardiovascular disease can pursue sexual activity. With physical conditioning programs, regulation of drug therapy, and adequate teaching and support, a client may continue to express sexuality.

DIABETES MELLITUS Diabetes has long been associated with sexual problems. Secondary erectile dysfunction (impotence) in men is often associated with microvascular changes and neuropathy and occurs in more than half of men who have diabetes. A small percentage of diabetic men may experience retrograde ejaculation (the ejaculate is released into the urinary bladder instead of through the urinary meatus). This difficulty and the presence of disease of long duration may contribute to problems with fertility in diabetic men. Comparable changes in women lead to decreased libido, orgasmic dysfunctions, and infertility. A decrease in vaginal lubrication and increased risk of infection contribute to chronic vaginitis in diabetic women. The incidence of sexual problems in people who have had diabetes for longer periods is increased.

END-STAGE RENAL DISEASE The effects of end-stage renal disease (ESRD) are monumental. Every system in the body is affected by impairment of the metabolism and regulation of electrolytes. In addition to the physical limitations resulting from fatigue, pruritus (itching), anorexia, lethargy, and muscle cramping, the client with ESRD faces overwhelming psychosocial changes. The client's self-concept, body image, and self-esteem suffer as a result of the gradual dete-

TABLE 11–2 Effects of Illness on Adult Sexuality

Illness	Effects on Men	Effects on Women
Arthritis	• Decreased libido • Low self-esteem • Altered body image • Depression, anxiety	• Dyspareunia • Low self-esteem • Altered body image • Depression, anxiety
Cancer	• Altered body image • Erectile dysfunction • Decreased libido • Depression, anxiety • Low self-esteem	• Altered body image • Dyspareunia • Decreased libido • Depression, anxiety • Low self-esteem
Cardiovascular disease	• Erectile dysfunction • Low self-esteem • Depression, anxiety	• Decreased libido • Low self-esteem • Depression, anxiety
Diabetes	• Erectile dysfunction • Retrograde ejaculation • Decreased fertility	• Decreased libido • Orgasmic dysfunction • Decreased fertility • Dyspareunia • Chronic vaginitis • Decreased vaginal lubrication
Hepatic disease	• Loss of libido • Sexual unresponsiveness • Erectile dysfunction	• Decreased libido • Orgasmic dysfunction • Amenorrhea
Hypertension	• Decreased libido • Erectile failure • Ejaculatory failure • Gynecomastia	• Decreased libido • Galactorrhea
Renal disease	• Low self-esteem • Altered body image • Loss of libido • Erectile dysfunction • Decreased fertility • Depression, fatigue	• Low self-esteem • Altered body image • Loss of libido • Orgasmic dysfunction • Decreased fertility • Depression, fatigue
Respiratory disease	• Low self-esteem • Decreased libido • Erectile dysfunction	• Low self-esteem • Decreased libido • Orgasmic dysfunction
Spinal cord injury	• Erectile dysfunction • Possible infertility • Retrograde ejaculation • Ejaculatory dysfunction • Orgasmic dysfunction • Low self-esteem • Impaired body image • Loss of libido	• Orgasmic dysfunction • Amenorrhea • Low self-esteem • Impaired body image • Loss of libido

rioration of body functions and structures. Role functions and issues of dependency are altered if the client is forced to stop working or cannot manage usual responsibilities in the home and community. The financial burdens of lost income and expensive treatments add to the stressors for the person with chronic renal disease. As a result of these multiple factors, the person may experience depression, loss of libido, decreased frequency of sexual activity, impotence, and sterility.

CHRONIC RESPIRATORY DISEASE A person with chronic respiratory disease may experience increased levels of fatigue with accompanying threats to self-esteem. For example, people with chronic airflow limitation often report difficulty in continuing sexual intercourse. A review of the adult sexual response cycle indicates that respiratory rates double during plateau and orgasmic phases, which makes coitus difficult for both men and women. Clients may need to learn alternative methods and positions for sexual activity.

LIVER DYSFUNCTION Chronic conditions affecting the liver and immune system frequently lead to impaired sexual health. Clients experiencing anorexia, fatigue, joint pain, nausea, fever, and jaundice associated with chronic hepatitis may become uninterested in sexually overt behavior. In addition, the client may experience complications such as erectile dysfunction or sexual unresponsiveness. Similarly, clients with cirrhosis of the liver related to malnutrition, infection with parasites, or alcohol abuse may experience a loss of libido and specific pathologic conditions, including gynecomastia and erectile dysfunction in men and amenorrhea in women.

SPINAL CORD INJURY Clients with spinal cord injury experience various sexual dysfunctions as a result of altered physical functioning and psychosocial changes. The dysfunctions depend on the extent and location of the injury, and they differ for men and women. Men with injury to the cervical spinal cord usually continue to have reflexive erections of the penis. Men whose injury occurred at lower levels of the spine experience erectile dysfunction because the neural pathways from the spinal cord are damaged or destroyed.

Incomplete injury to the spinal cord permits some sensation and motor function of the genitalia; complete injury results in loss of libido in both men and women, loss of erection and ejaculation in men, and orgasmic dysfunction in women. Men in whom the lumbosacral cord has been completely cut are infertile because of retrograde ejaculation or damaged sperm. Women, however, may experience temporary amenorrhea, may retain fertility, and may be capable of a full-term pregnancy.

Psychosocial problems may contribute to a decline in sexual health for spine-injured clients because of the accompanying change in body image and decrease in self-esteem. However, many people with spinal cord injuries can have satisfying sexual activity when their physical, psychologic, and social problems are addressed.

EFFECTS OF DRUG AND ALCOHOL ABUSE

Nurses should not overlook the possibility of drug abuse or alcoholism as a central factor when suspecting or validating sexual problems in men and women. As middle adulthood approaches, some people turn to alcohol or other drugs to ease their anxieties, including anxiety specifically related to diminished sexual functioning (Table 11–3). The primary effects of limited alcohol intake are often initially stimulating, and both men and women may experience release of inhibitions, relief of anxiety, and an increase in libido. However, as the amount or frequency of alcohol intake increases, clients experience several negative effects. In women, for example, the desire for sexual activity may gradually decrease until there is no interest. Women in the stages of late alcoholism also experience a gradual decrease in vaginal lubrication and sensitivity. It takes more time for such women to have an orgasm, and they experience fewer orgasms.

Men in the late stage of alcoholism experience decreased desire, often accompanied by an increase in aggression and, finally, a total loss of desire and profound aggression. A delay in penile erection leads to an inability to attain an erection even with maximum stimulation, and the man's orgasm may be tentative or may not occur under any circumstances. The man may also experience diminished pleasurable sensations associated with sexual arousal. Although erection is still possible, the resolution stage is prolonged, and the man experiences a loss of sexual satisfaction.

TABLE 11–3 Effects of Alcohol and Other Drugs on Sexual Functioning

Drug	Effects on Men	Effects on Women
Alcohol	• Decreased libido • Increased aggression, possibly leading to sexual abuse • Erectile dysfunction • Decreased fertility • Low sexual satisfaction	• Decreased libido • Increased passivity, possibly leading to sexual abuse from partner • Orgasmic dysfunction • Amenorrhea, sterility • Low sexual satisfaction
Antidepressants	• Erectile dysfunction • Delayed ejaculation	• Delayed orgasm
Antihypertensives	• Decreased libido • Erectile dysfunction • Ejaculatory dysfunction • Retrograde ejaculation	• Decreased libido • Anovulation, amenorrhea • Galactorrhea • Impaired orgasm
Cocaine and amphetamines	• Delayed orgasm • Delayed ejaculation	• Orgasmic dysfunction • Decreased libido
Narcotics	• Decreased libido • Erectile dysfunction • Delayed ejaculation	• Decreased libido • Spontaneous abortion • Amenorrhea
Tranquilizers	• Retrograde ejaculation • Erectile dysfunction	• Galactorrhea • Amenorrhea, anovulation

TRANSCULTURAL CONSIDERATIONS

Many factors affect a person's sexual health and his or her willingness to discuss this very private part of life. Spanish-speaking clients and Native Americans tend to be hesitant to talk about sexually related matters. In some cases, people from these groups may talk more freely to a nurse or other health care professional of the same sex (Giger & Davidhizar, 1991).

Cultural or religious background can also influence one's willingness to discuss sexual matters. This background may permit certain practices and prohibit others. The teachings of the Roman Catholic Church, for instance, prohibit the use of artificial contraception.

The decision to circumcise a male is also culturally based. In the United States, for example, 80 to 90 percent of males are circumcised, although fewer boys today are being circumcised than 20 years ago. In other countries of the world, such as Canada, England, Sweden, and China, circumcision is thought to be unnecessary. Some religious groups, such as Jews and Muslims, include circumcision as part of their practice. Other groups, like Hispanics and Native Americans, do not traditionally practice circumcision (Jarvis, 1992). There is scant scientific evidence that circumcision is necessary, although penile carcinoma occurs more frequently in men who are not circumcised.

NURSES' COMFORT WITH SEXUALITY

Our increased knowledge and awareness of human sexuality throughout the life cycle have led to an increased demand for solutions to problems in sexual functioning. Nursing, as a major provider of health care services, has responded to this demand by developing strategies to prevent the development of sexual problems and to promote sexual health.

In addition to having an adequate knowledge base in human sexuality, the nurse must feel comfortable with applying the nursing process to the sexual health needs of clients. To help clients achieve sexual health, nurses should have an attitude of openness and willingness to approach the subject.

To apply the nursing process to problems of sexual health in clients, nurses must first be aware of their own sexuality. A clarification of one's own values and sexual health is necessary. In her discussion of human sexuality and the nursing process, Lion (1982) identified several characteristics of sexually healthy people and provided a comprehensive overview of clarification exercises related to sexual issues and values for nurses. The use of values clarification exercises, such as the one in Table 11–4, enables nurses to "acknowledge their feelings and thoughts, examine their attitudes and beliefs, consider their convictions and behaviors, and clarify the content and power of their sexual value system" (p. 1).

TABLE 11–4 Values Clarification Exercise

Situation: Mary is a 26-year-old single woman hospitalized for a radical hysterectomy. She has a malignancy. Which of the following responses by nurses is most like your response to assessing, diagnosing, and intervening with regard to her actual and potential sexual problems?

Nurse A: "I hope she doesn't ask about having sexual relations or I'll just die of embarassment!"
Nurse B: "I know how I'll handle any questions about sex. I'll just refer her to the head nurse. She can handle that stuff."
Nurse C: "It's OK if she asks about sex, but I'm not sure I know all the answers. I know I can listen and try to help her find answers if I don't know them."
Nurse D: "It's just fine if she asks about how this will affect her sexually. In fact, even if she doesn't bring it up, I will. I really believe it's an important aspect of her health."

Clarification of values in responses: If you answered that you feel most like one of the nurses above, check below to clarify what this means.

Nurse A: This nurse feels uncomfortable handling concerns about sexual health and needs to do more reading and talking about her feelings with other health professionals.
Nurse B: This nurse also feels uncomfortable and is willing to shirk responsibility, passing it on to one with more authority. Again, more learning and exploration of his or her attitudes are needed.
Nurse C: This nurse feels comfortable. Being able and willing to look for additional information is essential to helping the client.
Nurse D: This nurse also feels comfortable and is willing to take more responsibility for including sexual health in client care.

SEXUAL HARASSMENT

There has been an increased realization of and discussion about sexual harassment in the workplace and other settings. Because most nurses are women, it is possible that they will be harassed at some point while caring for their clients. Sexual harassment by a client can interfere with the nurse's ability to complete a sexual health assessment and effectively intervene for specific sexual problems.

In addition to the possibility of being sexually harassed by clients, the nurse may encounter harassment from other members of the health care team. Several court cases indicate that people should be protected from harassment and the offenders legally punished.

COLLABORATIVE MANAGEMENT

ASSESSMENT

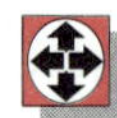

HISTORY

In managing the sexual health of hospitalized clients, the nurse takes a brief sexual history that is integrated with the general health history. Nurses must be sensitive to clients' willingness to discuss this private part of their lives. Factors such as the age of both the client and the nurse may affect the client's willingness to disclose such personal information. For example, elderly clients may be reluctant to discuss sexual health, especially if they were taught that sex should not be discussed openly. An equally embarrassing situation might be one in which a young female nurse interviews a young heterosexual male; both people may feel hesitant about discussing this topic.

Nurses address three areas in taking the sexual health history:

- Physical development and situational changes in sexual functioning
- Alterations in body image, sex role, and self-esteem
- Sociocultural factors, such as ritualistic practices

Here are some examples of questions that the nurse can ask while obtaining a history:

- "Have you ever experienced any injury or disease of the genitourinary system? Is there any history of sexually transmitted diseases?"
- "What was the pattern of development of secondary sexual characteristics (e.g., menstruation)? Have there been any changes in these characteristics (e.g., hirsutism [excessive hair growth in females] or gynecomastia)? What changes do you attribute to your age?"
- "Have you ever experienced any unwanted or traumatic sexual events such as incest or rape?"
- "Have you noticed any changes in sexual functioning in the past related to the use of alcohol or other drugs?"
- "Have you experienced any changes in sexual functioning or desire for sexual activity since your current illness, injury, or surgery?"
- "Has this physical problem (illness, injury, or surgical treatment) changed the way you view your body or feel about yourself as a woman or man?"
- "As a result of this physical problem, have you noticed changes in your usual activities as a woman or man, or changes in your usual roles, such as those of wife or mother, or husband or father?"
- "What are some of your beliefs and practices about sexual functioning? Have any of these been affected by your current illness, injury, or surgery?"

Although some of these questions may be answered easily with "yes" or "no," the nurse should pose them in such a way as to invite the client to discuss his or her sexual identity, roles, or activity. The nurse should phrase questions in language that the client understands, according to his or her educational level and sociocultural background. Beginning each phrase with "Tell me how" may encourage further information. Taking a sexual history is one way to identify misinformation that should be corrected as part of the nursing intervention. Chart 11–2 summarizes the information contained in a brief sexual history and assessment.

PHYSICAL ASSESSMENT/CLINICAL MANIFESTATIONS

The nurse incorporates the sexual health assessment into a general physical assessment. Subjective data concerning body image may be gathered as the nurse palpates various parts of the body, moving from relatively neutral areas, such as the face and extremities, to the breasts and external genitalia. Nurses must always have concern for the client's dignity when assessing these more private areas. The nurse explains what is to be examined, in what manner, and for what reason. As in other physical assessments, the nurse pays attention to external appearance, palpation of internal structures, and any discharges (which may also need to be further assessed in the laboratory).

While assessing the client's genitalia and breasts, the nurse may elicit additional information about sexual activity, knowledge, and attitudes. For example, when inspecting the external genitalia, the nurse might ask the client to describe his or her usual sexual activities and ask whether there is any discomfort or anxiety related to these activities.

Chapter 73 includes a detailed description of the physical assessment of genitalia and breasts. The clinical manifestations described in this chapter relate specifically to sexual *functioning.*

DYSPAREUNIA Dyspareunia (painful intercourse) in women may be related to several factors, such as:

- An intact hymen
- Scarring from an episiotomy
- Infections of the vagina or vulva, including venereal warts or other sexually transmitted diseases (STDs)
- Insufficient vaginal lubrication
- Irritation from chemical products, such as contraceptives, douches, and feminine deodorants

Pathologic conditions of the uterus, cervix, ovaries, and fallopian tubes may also result in dyspareunia. Such conditions should be ruled out through referral to a gynecologist or other physician. In a study by Gloeckner (1991), dyspareunia was the major complaint of women who had undergone a proctocolectomy (surgical removal of the colon and rectum). Dyspareunia may also be related to psychogenic factors, such as trauma from rape, incest, or other unwanted sexual experiences, or to previous experience with an inconsiderate partner.

In men, dyspareunia may be associated with inflammation or infection of the penis, prostate, urinary bladder, urethra, or testes. Men infrequently experience pain related to exposure to vaginal contraceptive creams or foams, irritation from the partner's intrauterine device (IUD), or lubricants on condoms.

HYPOACTIVE SEXUAL DESIRE Hypoactive sexual desire is a loss of interest in sexual activity or a decline in libido. In women it may be related to several factors, including:

- Hormonal replacement therapy
- Use of oral contraceptives

CHART 11–2

Nursing Care Highlight ◆ Brief Sexual History and Assessment Guide

History	Current Assessment
Physical	
• Development of secondary sexual characteristics (onset and pattern of menses in woman)	• Observe and palpate. Note changes over time.
• Use of contraceptives; problems with fertility or pregnancy	• Note current use and problems with contraception; issues of fertility or pregnancy.
• Episodes of STDs	• Note recent changes in sexual activity level or pattern.
• Past genitourinary disease, injury, or surgery	• Note thickening or discharge from the breast or genitalia.
• Past use of alcohol or other drugs	• Note current drug use.
• Past patterns of sexual function	• Note changes in levels of sexual arousal or function.
Psychologic	
• Past sexual dysfunction	• Identify knowledge of sexual function.
• Past problems with body image, gender role, or self-esteem	• Note current feelings about body parts and functions and self-esteem, and current values.
• History of incest, rape, or other unwanted sexual experiences	• Identify recent unwanted sexual experiences.
Social	
• Cultural rituals, beliefs, and inhibitions (e.g., circumcision, menses, marriage)	• Note cultural expectations for sexual behavior.
• Family composition and roles	• Note changes in composition of family or peers.
• Pattern of marital or sexual status and living arrangements	• Note change in living arrangements or marital status.
• Past sexual orientation and preference (e.g., homosexuality, bisexuality, heterosexuality, transsexuality)	• Identify current sexual preference and patterns of sexual activity.

- Eating disorders (e.g., anorexia nervosa or bulimia nervosa)
- Weight gain or loss
- Substance abuse
- Chronic illness (e.g., cancer or end-stage renal disease)

Psychosocial factors, such as abuse, marital or partner discord, depression, anxiety, fear, or other environmental stressors, may be major contributing factors.

In men, hypoactive sexual desire may be related to the use of antihypertensive drugs, substance abuse, or a chronic illness that affects energy levels. The psychosocial factors that affect women are the same for men.

VAGINISMUS In a woman with vaginismus, the muscles of the outer third of the vaginal barrel contract powerfully and prevent insertion of a tampon or other object. This condition may be related to physical factors, such as sexual activity during the healing phase after childbirth, infections of the vagina and vulva, abnormalities of the hymen, and atrophy of the vagina. Other contributing factors include the person's lack of information, anxiety, and fear. Vaginismus is more likely to be related to psychogenic causes, including strong religious teachings, rape trauma, physical or psychosocial abuse, or homosexual experimentation.

For an accurate assessment of vaginismus, the physician or nurse practitioner or nurse specialist must perform a direct pelvic examination.

ORGASMIC DYSFUNCTION Orgasmic dysfunction is defined as the inability to achieve orgasm (primary dysfunction) or as the inability to achieve orgasm with intercourse or at an appropriate time during intercourse (secondary dysfunction). These dysfunctions are the most common sexual complaints of adult women. Orgasmic dysfunctions are related to physical factors, such as adhesions of the clitoris that interfere with stimulation, lack of strength in the pubococcygeal muscles, and diminished contractions of the uterus. The nurse should refer women with these conditions to a physician for confirmation.

Other contributing factors to orgasmic dysfunction are psychogenic and may include:

- Feelings of anxiety or guilt
- Lack of knowledge

- Poor communication skills
- Marital or partner discord

Fear of rejection and conscious withholding of orgasm may lead to secondary orgasmic dysfunctions. General expectations of the culture or society may also be contributing factors.

Assessing the history and environmental circumstances under which orgasmic difficulties are experienced can help the nurse to classify the dysfunction as one of the following:

- Primary (the woman has never experienced orgasm)
- Secondary (the woman has a history of orgasm but is not experiencing it at present)
- Situational (the woman experiences orgasm with manual stimulation but not with penetration of the vagina)

ERECTILE DYSFUNCTION Erectile dysfunction (impotence) is the inability of a man to attain or maintain an erection of the penis of sufficient firmness to permit penetration. This problem can be primary (the man has never been able to sustain an erection) or secondary (he has experienced at least one erection of sufficient firmness to permit penetration). The term erectile dysfunction is preferred to impotence.

Organic causes include spinal cord injury, diabetes mellitus, alcoholism, neurologic disease (such as multiple sclerosis), endocrine disorders, various infections or surgical procedures involving the genitourinary system, and specific drug use and abuse.

Psychosocial factors contributing to erectile dysfunctions include marital or partner discord, anxiety, depression, excessive weight gain or loss, insomnia, and fatigue.

PREMATURE EJACULATORY DYSFUNCTION A man with a premature ejaculatory dysfunction ejaculates after penetration but sooner than either partner desires. Although there are no established norms for the timing of ejaculation during intercourse, this timing is important to the satisfaction of both partners involved in sexual activity. If the man is unable to exercise any voluntary control over the timing of this learned response, premature ejaculation may become a problem.

Organic causes are rare, if they exist at all; psychosocial factors contribute to the learning of this response. A man's feelings of anxiety, guilt, and fear, along with situations in which he may hurry toward a climax, may result in this type of dysfunction.

RETROGRADE EJACULATION Retrograde ejaculation, or "dry orgasm," may sometimes be confused with ejaculatory incompetence because there is no external evidence of the ejaculate. Men experiencing retrograde ejaculation discharge semen in a reverse manner—into the urinary bladder rather than forward through the penis. This may result from prostatic surgery, diabetes, multiple sclerosis, structural defects of the urethra and bladder neck, or the use of tranquilizers. During orgasm, the bladder neck does not close and the semen is forced directly into it. The man experiences the sensation of orgasm but is infertile.

RESEARCH APPLICATIONS FOR NURSING

Clients May Want to Talk About Sexuality After Ostomy Surgery

Gloeckner, M. (1991). Perceptions of sexuality after ostomy surgery. *Journal of Enterostomal Therapy, 18*(1), 36–38.

In her study of 24 men and 16 women who had undergone ostomy surgery at least one year previously, the author examines three aspects of sexual adjustment: physical changes, intrapsychic changes, and interpersonal changes. On the basis of interviews, the author found that the primary physical problem experienced by men was impotence. The major problem reported by women was dyspareunia, probably resulting from scar tissue after surgical procedures like abdominal-perineal resections.

Although most subjects stated that their initial postoperative response to the surgery was shock and repulsion, most (68%) showed an increase in feelings of attractiveness after the first postoperative year. The majority of couples (80%) reported that their relationships changed in a positive direction after surgery.

Almost all of the subjects (97%) stated that either the physician or the enterostomal nurse should discuss issues of sexuality with the client having ostomy surgery. The author presents a model for the nurse to use as a guide when counseling these clients.

Critique The results of this study may be limited by a self-selection bias, in that only subjects who were having sexual problems may have volunteered for the study. However, the topic is important to nurses who care for these clients.

Possible nursing implications Although the subjects specified that they wanted information from the physician or enterostomal nurse, any nurse caring for clients undergoing ostomy surgery should be aware of the importance of sexuality. The nurse can reinforce information provided by the physician or enterostomal nurse and should be available to answer questions and provide emotional support to these clients.

PSYCHOSOCIAL ASSESSMENT

Once a sexual problem is identified or suspected, the nurse must complete a more comprehensive and specific sexual health history. Although the general sexual history described earlier is an essential part of a nursing assessment, the nurse should obtain additional information about the psychologic and social factors related to past and present sexual functioning when making a nursing diagnosis of sexual dysfunction. Subjective responses include the way in which the client perceives the problem as well as how he or she feels, thinks, and acts. The following questions may guide the nurse in making a more complete assessment of past and present factors related to sexual dysfunctions:

- How does the client describe the problem? What specific behaviors, thoughts, feelings, or attitudes are problematic?
- What is the client's perception of what caused the problem or what continues to contribute to the problem?
- What environmental or situational factors were present at the onset of the problem?
- How has the problem changed over time? Has it become more severe or less severe? Does it occur in more than one setting?
- What has the client previously done to seek help from others, both professionals and peers? What forms of self-help has he or she tried?
- What are the client's expectations and goals, both realistic and ideal, for therapeutic intervention and resolution of the problem?

In addition to this direct assessment of the client's sexual health, the nurse may notice problems of sexuality as a result of the client's "acting-out" behaviors. An example would be a client who exhibits inappropriate behaviors, such as exposing genitalia or overtly soliciting sexual favors from the nurse. The nurse should realize that such behavior may represent a coping mechanism on the part of the client, who may be overwhelmed by actual or potential threats to body image, gender identity, gender role, and sexual functioning.

ANALYSIS

COMMON NURSING DIAGNOSES

The major sexual problems addressed through the nursing process are sexual dysfunctions. Common problems related to sexual dysfunctions may affect either men or women or both.

1. Sexual Dysfunction related to dyspareunia or hypoactive sexual desire
2. Sexual Dysfunction related to vaginismus or orgasmic dysfunction
3. Sexual Dysfunction related to erectile dysfunction, premature ejaculatory dysfunction, or retrograde ejaculation

ADDITIONAL NURSING DIAGNOSES

In addition to the common nursing diagnoses, some clients may experience one or more of the following diagnoses:

- Ineffective Individual Coping related to loss of control over body part or body function
- Anxiety related to feelings of failure or loss of control
- Pain related to infectious process, inflammation, or muscle spasm
- Self Esteem Disturbance related to loss of function
- Body Image Disturbance related to change in physical appearance

PLANNING AND IMPLEMENTATION

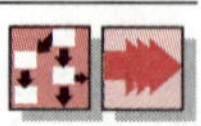

SEXUAL DYSFUNCTION RELATED TO DYSPAREUNIA OR HYPOACTIVE SEXUAL DESIRE

PLANNING: CLIENT GOALS The goals are that the client will:

- Be free from pain or discomfort during sexual intercourse
- Have a return of interest in sexual activity

INTERVENTIONS The Client Care Plan summarizes nursing care for the man or woman who experiences dyspareunia.

Interventions for Dyspareunia in Women Nursing interventions for the woman with dyspareunia depend on the contributing factors. When pain results from physical factors (e.g., an intact hymen, scarring from an episiotomy, or pathologic conditions of the reproductive organs), the nurse refers the client to a gynecologist. Infections of the vagina or vulva also require medical diagnosis and treatment. If infection is present, the nurse administers prescribed antibiotics, provides increased fluid intake, and encourages the client to rest and avoid sexual activity. The nurse can use therapeutic communication and education to reduce further episodes of infection by listening with a nonjudgmental attitude and explaining about the risk of multiple partners, if this is a factor. The nurse also explains the risks associated with the client's usual sexual activities. For example, chronic irritations may result from foreign objects placed into the vagina without adequate lubrication.

When the major contributing factors include inadequate vaginal lubrication or irritation from excessive use of chemical contraceptives, douches, or feminine deodorants, clients need accurate information and specific suggestions for behavioral changes. The nurse reviews anatomy and physiology and emphasizes the ability of the vagina to clean itself. The nurse describes alternative methods of contraception or selection of products without scents and encourages the client to use unscented tampons or sanitary pads. Increasing vaginal lubrication through the use of over-the-counter water-soluble gels or a vaginal dilator may also be suggested.

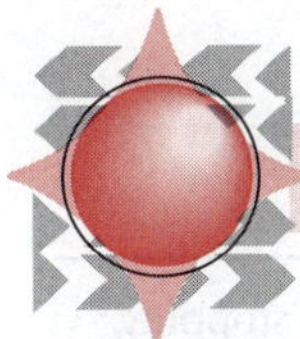

CLIENT CARE PLAN

The Client with an Alteration in Sexuality

Nursing Diagnosis No. 1: Sexual Dysfunction related to dyspareunia: woman

Expected Outcomes	Nursing Interventions	Rationale
The client will express no pain or discomfort associated with sexual intercourse or usual sexual activities.	♦ Instruct the client to use a water-soluble lubricant before sexual intercourse or usual sexual activities.	♦ Water-soluble lubricants do not dry the mucosa as do petroleum products.
	♦ Describe to the client the importance of erotic stimulation for vaginal lubrication; provide examples of visual, auditory, or olfactory sensations associated with sexual arousal.	♦ Adequate arousal and stimulation are prerequisites to adequate lubrication.
	♦ Explain the relationship between use of feminine hygiene products and destruction of the natural cleaning function of vaginal flora and secretions. Discourage the use of products such as feminine deodorant sprays, vaginal douches, and scented perineal pads.	♦ Overuse of feminine hygiene products destroys the natural flora and secretions of the vaginal walls.

Nursing Diagnosis No. 2: Sexual Dysfunction related to dyspareunia: man

Expected Outcomes	Nursing Interventions	Rationale
The client will express no pain or discomfort associated with sexual intercourse or usual sexual activities.	♦ Instruct the client about possible irritation from exposure to vaginal contraceptive cream, jelly, or foam, or from the string of an IUD.	♦ The skin of the external genitalia may be hypersensitive to chemicals in these products.
	♦ Encourage the client to clean under the foreskin if the client is uncircumcised.	♦ Adequate hygiene of the foreskin reduces mechanical irritation.
	♦ Refer the client to a general physician or urologist if symptoms indicate inflammation of the urethra, prostate, or testes.	♦ Treatment with an antibiotic or anti-inflammatory drug may be indicated.

Interventions for Dyspareunia in Men When dyspareunia results from inflammation or infection of organs within the man's genitourinary system, the nurse administers prescribed antibiotics and encourages the client to drink fluids and to rest. The nurse encourages the man with acute inflammation or infection to avoid sexual intercourse with his partner until the acute condition is resolved. Alternative sexual activities that avoid intercourse are suggested and explored with both partners.

When the major contributing factor for dyspareunia in the man is exposure to vaginal contraceptive creams and foams or an intrauterine device (IUD) in the sexual partner, the nurse may suggest alternatives to both partners, such as mutual body massage and caressing.

Interventions for Hypoactive Sexual Desire If hypoactive sexual desire in the woman is related to hormonal replacement therapy or oral contraceptive use, the nurse may present alternatives or refer the client to a gynecologist. For example, contraceptive foams, creams, or patches may be used in place of oral contraceptives. To increase the client's interest and sexual arousal, the nurse may suggest that the client use erotic reading or video materials or change the time and setting of usual sexual activities.

When drug or alcohol abuse or chronic illness is

the major contributing factor in clients with hypoactive sexual desire, medical management of the underlying factor is required before other interventions. If the prognosis for any of these conditions is poor, the outcome for the sexual problem is often poor. The nurse informs the client about the relationship between the underlying causes and the resulting sexual dysfunction.

Psychosocial factors that affect the development of hypoactive sexual desire are similar in both men and women. Marital or partner discord, depression, anxiety, and fear may be sufficiently severe to require the specialized education and experience of a nurse specialist or clinician with expertise in the area of psychology or psychiatry. Nursing interventions include therapeutic communication, encouraging the client to pursue intensive therapy, and referring the client to a competent professional. Often the process involves the client, his or her sexual partner or partners, or all of these people.

SEXUAL DYSFUNCTION RELATED TO VAGINISMUS AND ORGASMIC DYSFUNCTION

PLANNING: CLIENT GOALS The goals are that the client will:

- Relieve or prevent the involuntary spasms of the vagina
- Experience an orgasm by any means

INTERVENTIONS

Interventions for Vaginismus The nursing interventions for an *actual* problem of vaginismus aim to relieve the underlying contributing factors. The interventions for a *potential* problem of vaginismus are directed at educating the woman who is at risk for this response, thus preventing its occurrence.

If the major contributing factor is psychogenic, such as trauma from rape, conflicts surrounding homosexual experimentation, or strong religious teachings, the interventions are similar to those already discussed. Interventions range from giving permission to express anxiety and conflict to providing intensive therapy. If the major contributing factor is a physical one, such as sexual activity too soon after birth trauma, infection, abnormality of the hymen, or atrophy of the vagina, referral to a gynecologist may be indicated. Nursing interventions include encouraging the client to explore alternatives to vaginal intercourse during the healing process. The nurse also educates the woman and her sexual partner about the relationship between physical factors and involuntary muscular response.

Interventions for Orgasmic Dysfunction When the major contributing factors in primary or secondary orgasmic dysfunction are psychogenic, the nurse provides opportunities for the client to talk about this situation. The nurse teaches the client about the relationship between stressors and the physical response of orgasm. The nurse also explains Kegel exercises, which strengthen the pubococcygeal muscles, and encourages general exercise to strengthen the pelvic musculature. Instructions for Kegel exercises are provided in Chart 11–3.

The client may need more intensive therapy, such as marriage counseling or in-depth counseling, for issues of anxiety and guilt. The nurse might refer the client to a nurse specialist or other professional in one or both of these specialties.

If adhesions of the clitoris result in orgasmic dysfunction, the nurse refers the client to a physician for possible surgical intervention and provides encouragement that the condition may be corrected.

CHART 11–3

Education Guide ◆ Kegel Exercises

1. Tighten the muscles as you would when stopping the flow of urine.
2. Hold for 2 to 3 seconds, then release.
3. Contract and relax these muscles 10 to 12 times, and repeat this series several times daily.

SEXUAL DYSFUNCTION RELATED TO ERECTILE DYSFUNCTION, PREMATURE EJACULATORY DYSFUNCTION, OR RETROGRADE EJACULATION

PLANNING: CLIENT GOALS The goals are that the client will:

- Attain or maintain an erection
- Delay ejaculation until the sexual partners are satisfied
- Accept the alteration of retrograde ejaculation and adjust to the resulting possibility of sterility

INTERVENTIONS

Interventions for Erectile Dysfunction For nursing interventions to influence the client's symptoms of erectile dysfunction, underlying diseases (e.g., diabetes mellitus, alcoholism, multiple sclerosis, endocrine disorders, and infections of the genitourinary system) must be under medical supervision. Appropriate nursing interventions include education; specific suggestions, such as the "sensate focus" technique; and alternatives for satisfying sexual activities. The sensate focus technique may also be used when the underlying factors are psychogenic. The nurse instructs the client and his partner in the following steps:

1. Mutual body touching and pleasuring without contact in the area of the genitalia
2. Genital stimulation, resulting in penile erection but not followed by intercourse
3. Orgasm and ejaculation through manual or oral stimulation (not vaginal penetration)
4. Vaginal penetration without orgasm or ejaculation (simple containment)

5. Vaginal penetration with orgasm and ejaculation
6. Dialogue between partners throughout steps

As with all sexual problems in which the major contributing factors are psychogenic, therapeutic communication and intensive therapy are indicated. The nurse makes the appropriate referrals, and the nurse specialist or psychotherapist provides psychotherapy directed at alleviating underlying marital or partner discord, anxiety, or depression.

In the absence of underlying disease or obvious psychologic factors, the use or abuse of various drugs may be the major etiologic factor in erectile dysfunction. The nurse explains the effects of such drugs as antihypertensives, barbiturates, sedatives, and amphetamines on the sexual response cycle. The nurse refers the client to a physician to evaluate the drug regimen so that an alternative drug, dosage, or therapy may be considered.

The client may also need referral to a urologist who treats men by self-injection of papaverine (Pavatine) and phentolamine (Regitine, Rogitine✱). These drugs are vasodilators that allow more blood to flow to the penis and facilitate erection. Many men have found these drugs to be successful. The nurse explains about possible side effects, including prolonged erection, bruising, and liver abnormalities (Althof et al., 1991).

Interventions for Premature Ejaculation Nursing interventions for premature ejaculation include educating the client and sexual partner about the relationship between emotions and the sexual response cycle. The nurse may teach the client, partner, or both systematic relaxation exercises to alleviate anxiety as a major contributing factor. The nurse should be sure to include the client's sexual partner in the treatment because the partner's communication of desires and expressions of distress may be instrumental in maintaining the dysfunction.

With appropriate preparation, the nurse may instruct the client and his partner in the "squeeze technique" for learning voluntary control for premature ejaculatory dysfunction. The man's partner can provide two types of squeezes.

In the *traditional* method, the partner places the thumb and first and second fingers just above and below the head of the penis and applies a squeezing pressure. In the *basilar* method, the thumb and fingers are placed at the base of the penis rather than at the head. Either position is held firmly for approximately 4 seconds, then released. The partner is instructed to always apply the pressure from the front to back of the shaft of the penis and never from side to side because this may result in tissue injury. The nurse should stress the importance of avoiding injury from the fingernails. The partner applies the squeeze shortly after erection occurs, and periodically thereafter, until both partners are ready for penetration to take place. Once the man has been aroused to the point of ejaculatory inevitability, this squeeze technique should not be used; instead, ejaculation should be allowed to continue.

Interventions for Retrograde Ejaculation When the man's problem is retrograde ejaculation, the underlying cause is physiologic. Men who have diabetes, prostatic disease, multiple sclerosis, or abnormalities of the bladder and urethra must be referred to a urologist for further evaluation and medical or surgical intervention. With the exception of a physical abnormality, clients with diabetes, multiple sclerosis, or prostatic disease have an irreversible condition, and nursing interventions are thus directed at assisting them with coping skills. These men have an altered sensation from previous ejaculations and may be rendered sterile.

Education and counseling of the client and his sexual partner are important nursing interventions. The nurse reassures both partners that there are no harmful effects to the ejaculate being deposited in the bladder. Some clients who wish to have children are referred to an infertility clinic. It is possible for semen to be centrifuged from the urine and prepared for in vitro fertilization.

DISCHARGE PLANNING

HOME CARE PREPARATION

When preparing clients to return home after hospitalization for illness, injury, or surgery, the nurse should anticipate plans for follow-up care and sexual counseling.

HEALTH TEACHING

The nurse teaches the client and sexual partner, when appropriate, about the relationship of the illness, injury, or surgery to sexual functioning. For example, when clients receive surgery or chemotherapy for cancer, they may experience temporary alterations in sexual desire. It is appropriate for the nurse to explain this situation and offer suggestions for less strenuous expressions of intimacy. Similarly, the nurse should counsel the client who has had a myocardial infarction about his or her anxiety related to resuming sexual intercourse (see specific health problems).

The nurse teaches clients to report any adverse effects of medications on their sexual functioning. Nurses must be aware of how specific drugs affect sexual functioning and provide appropriate information to clients who will continue to receive these medications after discharge.

PSYCHOSOCIAL PREPARATION

When clients are discharged to home health care, additional follow-up may be directed at the family caregiver. The caregiver who takes primary responsibility for care of a client in the absence of professional home health caregivers is often a spouse whose own health needs must also be considered.

HEALTH CARE RESOURCES

Providing nursing care and being a sexual partner of the client may present conflicts for a spouse who accepts the role of family caregiver. Nurses should anticipate and prevent such conflict by discussing these roles with the family caregiver. The home health nurse can offer counseling or seek more expert assistance as the situation warrants.

EVALUATION

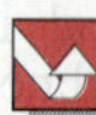

The expected outcomes for the client with common sexual dysfunction problems are that the client:

- Does not experience pain or discomfort associated with intercourse
- Describes restored levels of interest in sexual activity
- States that sexual activity is no longer accompanied by painful involuntary spasms of the vaginal wall
- Experiences orgasm as desired
- Reports satisfaction and enjoyment of orgasm
- Attains or maintains erections of the penis of sufficient firmness to permit vaginal penetration in at least 50% of attempts
- Learns voluntary control over the ejaculatory response

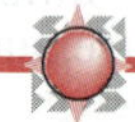

IMPLICATIONS FOR NURSING RESEARCH

Research is needed to identify clients who are at a high risk for sexual problems and to implement nursing interventions that are most appropriate for specific dysfunctions. Because of the sensitive nature of research in the area of human sexuality, special attention to measures for the protection of human subjects must be given.

Here are some specific questions to be answered in future nursing research:

- ♦ What effect does sociocultural background have on the development and management of sexual dysfunction?
- ♦ What nursing interventions offer the most help for clients with specific sexual dysfunctions?
- ♦ What nursing interventions are most helpful in preventing sexual dysfunctions?
- ♦ How can the comfort level of nurses in dealing with clients with sexual dysfunction be enhanced?

SELECTED BIBLIOGRAPHY

Altof, S. E., Turner, L. A., Levine, S. B., Risen, C. B., Bodner, D., Kursh, E. D., & Resnick, M. I. (1991). Sexual, psychological, and marital impact of self-injection of papaverine and phentolamine: A long-term prospective study. *Journal of Sex and Marital Therapy, 17*, 101–112.

*Cardin, S. (1987). Nursing's role in the sexual counseling of critical care patients. *Dimensions of Critical Care Nursing, 6*(2), 67–68.

Cholewinski, J. T., & Burge, J. M. (1990). Sexual harassment of nursing students. *Image: Journal of Nursing Scholarship, 22*, 106–110.

*Engel, N. S. (1987). Menopausal stage, current life change, attitude towards women's roles and perceived health status. *Nursing Research, 36*, 353–357.

Giger, J. N., & Davidhizar, R. E. (1991). *Transcultural nursing: Assessment and intervention.* St. Louis: Mosby Year Book.

*Gilliss, C. L., & Rankin, S. M. (1988). Social and sexual activity after cardiac surgery: A report of the first 6 months. *Progress in Cardiovascular Nursing, 3*(3), 93–97.

Gloeckner, M. (1991). Perception of sexuality after ostomy surgery. *Journal of Enterostomal Therapy, 18*(1), 36–38.

*Haas, K., & Haas, A. (1987). *Understanding sexuality.* St. Louis: C. V. Mosby.

*Higgins, L. P., & Hawkins, J. W. (1984). *Human sexuality across the life span.* Monterey, CA: Wadsworth Health Sciences Division.

Jarvis, C. (1992). *Physical examination and health assessment.* Philadelphia: W. B. Saunders.

Jensen, S. B. (1992). Sexuality and chronic illness: Biopsychosocial approach. *Seminars in Neurology, 12*(2), 135–140.

*Kolodny, R. C. (1978). Ethical issues in the prevention of sexual problems. In C. B. Qualls, J. P. Winczl, & D. H. Barlow (Eds.), *The prevention of sexual disorders: Issues and approaches* (pp. 183–196). New York: Plenum.

*Kolodny, R. C., Masters, W. M., & Johnson, V. E. (1979). *Textbook of sexual medicine.* Boston: Little, Brown.

Kus, R. J. (1991). Sobriety, friends, and gay men. *Archives of Psychiatric Nursing, 5*, 171-177.

Kus, R. J., & Carpenter, M. A. (1991). Lance: A gay recovering alcoholic misdiagnosed as HIV-positive. *Archives of Psychiatric Nursing, 5*, 307–312.

*Lion, E. M. (1982). *Human sexuality in nursing process.* New York: Wiley.

*Lo-Biondo-Wood, G. (1986). Health education for the homosexual female. In V. Littlefield (Ed.), *Health education for women* (pp. 252–267). Norwalk, CT: Appleton-Century-Crofts.

Mackey, T., Sereika, S. M., Weissfeld, L. A., Hacker, S. S., Zender, J. F., & Heard, S. L. (1992). Factors associated with long-term depressive symptoms of sexual assault victims. *Archives of Psychiatric Nursing, 6*, 10–25.

*Masters, W. M., & Johnson, V. E. (1970). *Human sexual inadequacy.* Boston: Little, Brown.

*Masters, W. M., Johnson, V. E., & Kolodny, R. C. (1985). *Human sexuality* (2nd ed.). Boston: Little, Brown.

*McCracken, H. L. (1988). Sexual practice of elders: The forgotten aspect of functional health. *Journal of Gerontological Nursing, 14*(10), 13–18.

*Metcalfe, M. C., & Fischman, S. H. (1985). Factors affecting the sexuality of patients with head and neck cancer. *Oncology Nursing Forum, 12*(2), 21–25.

Rew, L., Esparza, D., & Sands, D. (1991). A comparative study of child sexual abuse among college students. *Archives of Psychiatric Nursing, 5*, 331–340.

Roth, S., & Newman, E. (1991). The process of coping with sexual trauma. *Journal of Traumatic Stress, 4*, 279–297.

Schiavi, R. C. (1992). Normal aging and the evaluation of sexual dysfunction. *Psychiatric Medicine, 10*, 217–225.

*Schover, L. R. (1984). *Prime time: Sexual health for men over 50.* New York: Holt, Rinehart, & Winston.

Segraves, K. B., & Segraves, R. T. (1991). Hypoactive sexual desire disorder: Prevalence and comorbidity in 906 subjects. *Journal of Sex and Marital Therapy, 17*, 55–58.

SUGGESTED READINGS

Cholewinski, J. T., & Burge, J. M. (1990). Sexual harassment of nursing students. *Image: The Journal of Nursing Scholarship*, *22*, 106–110.

This study attempted to explore the type and frequency of sexual harassment among a convenience sample of 277 nursing students in the southeastern United States. Twenty-one students experienced sexual harassment, most often as verbal abuse followed by sexist remarks about the students' clothing, body or sexual activities, and unnecessary touching or leering.

Kus, R. J. (1991). Sobriety, friends, and gay men. *Archives of Psychiatric Nursing*, *5*, 171-177.

This article describes a study of 20 gay men who were recovering alcoholics living in four large cities in the United States. When these subjects attained sobriety, they discovered that people they had thought were friends were only "drinking buddies."

Mackey, T., Sereika, S. M., Weissfeld, L. A., Hacker, S. S., Zender, J. F., & Heard, S. L. (1992). Factors associated with long-term depressive symptoms of sexual assault victims. *Archives of Psychiatric Nursing*, *6*, 10–25.

This article presents a study of 63 women who were sexual assault victims. Nearly two thirds of the subjects experienced symptoms of depression, and 56% reported a history of childhood sexual abuse. Factors associated with high levels of depression were nondisclosure of the assault to significant others, the presence of children in the home, and a pending lawsuit.

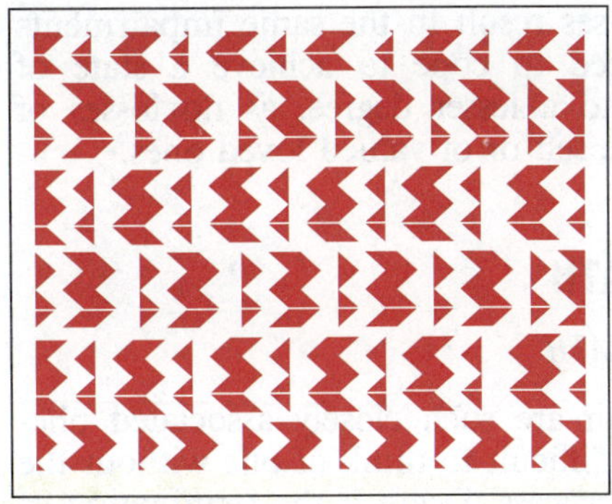

CHAPTER 12

Loss, Death, and Dying

CHAPTER HIGHLIGHTS

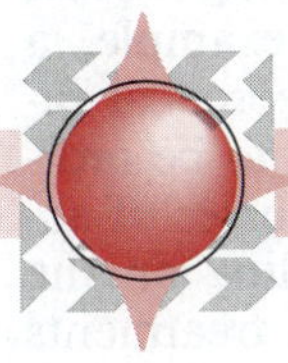

Loss, dying, and death are integral parts of living, yet they are given little thought in the ordinary course of everyday events. People recognize death as inevitable, yet at the same time preserve a belief in their own immortality. However, they cannot escape thinking about loss, dying, and death when confronted by illness. Some diseases, such as cancer and myocardial infarction, give rise to thoughts of death more readily than do other diseases, such as cholecystitis and bronchitis.

OVERVIEW

Feelings of loss, thoughts of death, and fears of dying accompany the normal late developmental stages of adulthood. The ultimate loss is the loss from death—a universal and unique experience. Loss, whatever the cause, can contribute to personal growth if it is accompanied by adaptive coping. Coping is the sum of the cognitive and behavioral strategies a person uses to deal with threatening or challenging situations when normal or routine responses are either unavailable or ineffective. A successful coping process results in the achievement of mastery over the stress, or resolution, and the resumption of equilibrium (see Chap. 7).

Nurses face loss and death daily in the course of their work and must constantly deal with their own reactions along with those of clients, families, and other caregivers. Knowledge of professional theories, principles, and practices helps the nurse to understand, anticipate, and manage these reactions and to develop sound nursing interventions. Although there are no prescriptive rules for caring for dying clients or for people suffering loss, there are helpful guidelines.

LOSS

DEFINITION OF LOSS

Loss is the state of being deprived of or being without something valued that one once had. Some losses, such as the loss of hair in male pattern baldness, are routine and predictable. Others, such as the loss of a limb from an accident, are random and not foreseeable. Losses, then, may occur gradually or suddenly; they may be nonviolent or traumatic, anticipated or unexpected, partial or total, and reversible or irreversible.

TYPES OF LOSS

LOSS OF A LOVED ONE The loss of a significant loved one or valued person is one of the most stressful and disruptive types of loss to endure. Such losses occur through divorce, alienation, death, and other kinds of emotional detachment or through geographic separation. Partial losses can also occur when a loved one is incapacitated by acute or chronic illnesses, such as mental illness or Alzheimer's disease, especially when that illness results in the loss of some special attribute of the person. Change for any reason can produce loss in a valued relationship.

Death also brings about the loss of loved ones. Because of the intimacy, intensity, and interdependency of the bonds, the death of a spouse or a child usually carries the most profound emotional impact.

Chenell and Murphy (1992) concluded that presumptive death was worse for families than confirmed death. In their nursing research involving families of people killed in the Mount Saint Helens' volcanic eruption in 1980, the authors reported that families not finding the bodies of loved ones felt that they were "in limbo."

LOSS OF SELF Another common form of loss is loss of self, or one's own mental image. This image includes feelings about attractiveness, self-worth, physical and mental abilities, roles in life, and impact on the world. Loss of some aspect of self may be temporary or permanent, partial or complete.

Loss of health, for example, is a loss of an aspect of self. The loss of or change in a body part may affect not only a person's capacity to move normally but also one's feeling of one's attractiveness to others. Other aspects of self that may be lost include hearing, sight, memory, intellectual powers, youth, and body functions, like bowel and bladder control.

LOSS OF OBJECTS Another significant form of loss is object loss, or loss of possessions or associations—jewelry, money, furniture, house, job, homeland. These types of losses result in the same impairments and the same need to cope to achieve a state of equilibrium, but to a lesser degree, as do losses of valued parts of the self or of valued loved ones.

DYING AND DEATH

DEFINITIONS OF DEATH

Dying and death are such closely associated phenomena that it is difficult to think of one without the other. Dying is a process. Death is the termination of life.

There was a time when there was little controversy about what was meant by death. Most people accepted that irreversible cessation of respiration and heartbeat and lack of corneal reflexes were sufficient signs of death. This is no longer the case. It is now possible to maintain a person's respiration and circulation through the use of drugs, machines, and artificial and transplanted organs.

Determination of death is important because of its far-reaching legal and ethical consequences. Definitions of death establish a basis for offering clients nursing and medical care options. For example, a clear definition of clinical death is the theoretical rationale for determining what is considered to be ordinary or extraordinary treatment. Many courses of action might be classified as either, depending on the circumstance. Among the more common treatments are experimental drugs, life-sustaining equipment, bone marrow transplants, oxygen, antibiotics, and, in some cases, food and fluids. (Also see Chapter 6 on ethics.)

The definition of death as cessation of brain function rather than cessation of heartbeat is critical to maintaining the viability of donor organs for use as transplants. The term *brain dead,* introduced into clinical medicine in the 1960s, describes a client whose heart and lungs can be maintained functionally by a mechanical life-support system but whose respiratory centers in the brainstem no longer function. If the ventilator were removed, the person would not resume spontaneous breathing.

CRITERIA FOR BRAIN DEATH Many organizations have published various criteria to establish brain death. The apnea test is commonly used to establish brain death in a client who has been in a coma for at least 6 hours with loss of all brainstem reflexes. The usual criteria include:

- Loss of response to external stimuli
- Loss of pupillary response to light
- Loss of corneal reflex
- Loss of eye movement with doll's-eye maneuver or caloric testing
- Loss of gag and cough reflexes

The presence of spinal reflexes does not *exclude* the diagnosis of brain death. The apnea test is performed by assessing the presence or absence of respirations with an arterial carbon dioxide level (PCO_2) of at least 60 mmHg.

Although the cessation of respirations and heartbeat as a definition of death is still sanctioned by Anglo-American common law, many states in the United States have passed brain death statutes. These laws, no matter how stated, are consistent in allowing death to be defined as the irreversible cessation of brain function, as determined by the use of the most reliable clinical method available.

PERSISTENT VEGETATIVE STATE People in a persistent vegetative state (PVS) show no evidence of cortical functioning but have the sustained capacity for spontaneous breathing and heartbeat. This condition has been referred to as *cortical,* or *cerebral, death.* Clients in a PVS must be fed by artificial means, such as a gastrostomy tube placed directly into the stomach. During the past few years, the U.S. courts have permitted health care facilities to discontinue artificial feeding for certain clients and have allowed them to die. This issue is very controversial and involves ethical questions regarding the quality of life that any society must address (see Chap. 6).

NEAR-DEATH EXPERIENCES Numerous descriptions of near-death experiences have appeared in the popular literature, but few have been validated in the professional literature. One of the problems with near-death experiences is that there is no commonly accepted definition.

Few people have had the classic or typical experiences, such as seeing their lives "flashing before their eyes" (Olson, 1992). Greyson (1985) identified and clustered some of the most common findings of near-death experiences reported by people who had had one or more such experiences (Table 12–1).

People who have had a near-death experience seem less anxious about death. They also typically report that they have an increased feeling that life has meaning and purpose (Olson, 1992).

THEORIES OF LOSS, DYING, AND GRIEVING

The theories that are used in discussing loss, dying, and grieving have been derived through research. These theories are not meant to be prescriptive; rather, they serve as general guides to alert the nurse to what may occur and, therefore, what to look for and how to proceed when a response is indicated. Using these findings to help guide client care is similar to using the systematic protocols of signs and symptoms of disease that help guide all nursing observations. For example, not all people with cholecystitis show all of its possible clinical manifestations, nor does the disease follow the same clinical course in all people. Knowing what can occur helps the nurse make observations and devise early interventions to prevent complications.

TABLE 12–1 Characteristics of the Near-Death Experience

Cognitive
- Experiencing life review
- Sensing time and feeling changes
- Having sudden understanding

Affective
- Feeling harmony with the universe
- Sensing peace and tranquility
- Feeling joy and happiness
- Seeing a brilliant light

Paranormal
- Feeling separate from own body
- Seeing scenes from the future
- Having heightened senses, such as hearing
- Being aware of events going on elsewhere

Transcendental
- Seeing deceased people, religious beings, or mystical presence
- Entering an unearthly place
- Coming to a place of no return

Modified from Greyson, B. (1985). A typology of near-death experience. *American Journal of Psychiatry, 142,* 967–969.

RESPONSES TO DYING

In 1969, Elisabeth Kübler-Ross, a psychiatrist, described a series of stages through which people may pass in response to their living through the dying process. She described the first stage as *shock and disbelief.* People could not believe that they were dying. The second stage was described as *denial.* People might say, "Yes, most people with this disease are dying, but not me!" The third stage was called *anger,* often characterized by the question "Why me?" or "What did I do to deserve this?" The fourth stage was termed *bargaining.* In this stage, characteristic responses were, "I'll do anything if . . . " or "Just let me live until my son gets married . . . or my daughter graduates." The next stage, when the person's deteriorating physical condition led to the realization that death was inevitable, was identified as *depression.* The final stage was termed *acceptance.* Acceptance, according to Kübler-Ross, was a stage of self-actualization, of feeling at peace with oneself and with one's imminent death.

PATTERNS OF LIVING-DYING

When death from a known fatal illness is preceded by several years of life, the use of the term "dying" from the time of diagnosis until the moment of death is paradoxical. These people frequently not only look healthy but also enjoy full activity for prolonged periods. They are living, yet dying, and in these cases, the living-dying period has the characteristics of a chronic illness.

Martocchio (1982), a nurse researcher, described four patterns of living-dying that are useful for understanding the uncertainties of living with life-threatening illness:

- *Peaks and valleys,* in which the person experiences hopeful highs and terrible lows
- *Descending plateaus,* in which the person experiences successive cycles of rehabilitation, loss, and rehabilitation
- *Downward slope,* in which there is a lack of time to prepare for death
- *Gradual slant,* in which the person is barely living and presents placement problems

These patterns, which all have a general downward course concluding in death, reflect the natural history of various diseases, such as some cancers and many cardiovascular, renal, and hepatic conditions. They also describe the effects of specific therapeutic regimens. The categories remain consistent regardless of the type of disease or treatment.

PEAKS AND VALLEYS This pattern is characterized by a series of peaks and valleys, or remissions and exacerbations. The peaks represent periods of well-being, and the valleys represent times of loss of well-being. Clients describe "hopeful highs" and "terrible lows." They see previous highs as indicators of hope that they can rally one more time. They see the lows as threats to any expectation of recovery.

DESCENDING PLATEAUS The descending plateaus pattern is a series of steps. Each downward step represents a tangible reduction in functional ability, and each plateau represents a leveling-off or stable period. The plateaus and drop-offs can last for an indeterminate period and may occur any number of times. This pattern creates marked frustration as dying clients and their families try, again and again, to take part in rehabilitation programs to maintain a level of function in the client that is relentlessly but unpredictably declining.

DOWNWARD SLOPE The third pattern of living-dying is the downward slope. This pattern, frequently observed in critical care units, is represented by a continuous and usually rapid downward course. In these cases, in which there are relatively short-term illnesses or unexpected deaths, clients and family members have little time to prepare for death.

GRADUAL SLANT The gradual slant pattern is characterized by a gradual decline over time. Toward the end, it is difficult to know whether the ill person is alive or dead. Difficulties regarding quality of life and definitions of death become issues of concern. Family members and caregivers begin to see the unresponsive client as a biologically living creature but also as a nonexistent person. As there is less meaningful interaction, the client is considered to be socially dead.

Regardless of the pattern, the direction is downward. As the dying person declines and draws nearer to death, all the people involved undergo losses. For each person, the loss is different: The mother loses her son; the wife, her husband; the children, their father; the business partner, his colleague. Each person manifests the loss both in a universally recognized pattern and in his or her unique way.

THE GRIEF RESPONSE

Grieving is the psychologic, social, and physical reaction to the perception of significant loss, which varies from one person to another. In an analysis of the literature on grieving, Cowles and Rodgers (1991) found that there was no single definition of grief. Additionally, the terms *bereavement* and *mourning* were often used interchangeably with grief. Table 12–2 lists the attributes of grief commonly found in the medical and nursing literature.

DEFINITION OF GRIEF The North American Nursing Diagnosis Association (NANDA) recognizes two types of grief—anticipatory grief and dysfunctional grief. Anticipatory grief is the expected form of grief and is defined as "the state in which an individual experiences responses to an actual or perceived loss of a person, relationship, object, or functional abilities before the loss occurs" (Taptich et al., 1989, p. 148). This type of grief is considered normal.

Dysfunctional grieving is defined as "the state in which an individual experiences an exaggerated response to an actual or potential loss of person, relationship, object, or functional abilities" (Taptich et al., 1989, p. 147). This type of grief is sometimes referred to as atypical, abnormal, or troubled.

Although a grief reaction can result from the loss of any precious element in a person's life, loss through the death of a close loved one is used as the major example in the rest of this chapter.

GOALS OF GRIEVING Generally, there are two major goals of grieving. The first is for a person to fully acknowledge the loss and to remember the lost loved one without undue pain. The second is for a person to once more be able to participate in life without losing the capacity to love. Effective grieving is achieved when a person can face the pain of the loss

TABLE 12–2 Attributes of Grief

Attribute	Meaning
Dynamic	• Changing and individualized for each person; a progression through the steps of the grief process
Process	• Clusters or phases of activity, or "work," ranging from 6 months to 2 years
Individualized	• Not the same process for each person; depends on a number of factors, such as cultural and religious backgrounds
Pervasive	• Affects every aspect of a person's existence
Normative	• A general sense of "normal" grief exists; beyond certain boundaries, people experience inappropriate or unacceptable grief

Data from research by Cowles, K. V., & Rodgers, B. L. (1991). The concept of grief: A foundation for nursing research and practice. *Research in Nursing and Health, 14,* 119–127.

and consciously live through its full range of feelings and their expression.

Many people achieve the goals of the grieving process comfortably and rapidly with very little disruption in their lives. For others, the response to loss includes familiar and expected behaviors as well as a wide range of unanticipated feelings and behaviors that may confuse or even frighten them. Nurses should understand these various responses that are sometimes associated with grieving in order to develop the appropriate nursing interventions.

PHASES OF GRIEVING Since Lindemann's (1944) classic account of grieving, many authors have described the general pattern of the grieving process. Most agree that there is a universal grief response that has a more or less predictable course:

- Shock and disbelief, progressing to somatic distress
- Feelings of guilt, anger, and hostility
- Interruption of life's usual activities
- Preoccupation with thoughts of the deceased
- A state of healthy integration

There is no fixed timetable by which a person passes through the grieving process, nor are the stages discrete. There is no rigid order to the progression, nor must each person go through all stages. Manifestations of grief vary widely; people may take one step forward and two steps back, then half steps from side to side as they cycle through their healing journey. Despite this nonlinearity, there are, as in the Kübler-Ross stages of dying, identifiable clusters, or phases, of feelings and behaviors that serve as guides for observation and a description for survivors.

Shock and Disbelief Shock, numbness, and disbelief are the first responses to actual or anticipated loss. People describe a sense of unreality, even though they know intellectually that the person is dead. They may appear outwardly to be accepting the loss. They continue with routine tasks and obligations as if nothing had happened. They are "on automatic pilot."

Some people engage in searching behaviors. They search for the lost, treasured person. They dream that he or she is still alive, or they may have hallucinations about the person. They may see the deceased person in familiar places, hear him or her at the door or on the stairs, or feel his or her touch on waking. These experiences are frightening, and survivors often interpret them as indications of emotional illness.

Grief hurts not only emotionally but also physically. The survivor may experience muscular weakness, tremors, chest pain, tightness in the throat, diaphoresis (excessive sweating), deep sighing, sensations of hot and cold, anorexia, nausea, fatigue, insomnia, and exhaustion. Because the grieving person's immune system is temporarily impaired, the nurse should observe such clients closely because they have a real risk for serious illness.

Yearning and Protest, Anger and Guilt In most instances, in a short time, usually soon after the funeral, a person's feelings of numbness and disbelief give way to feelings of pain and distress at the separation and a powerful sense of longing. During this period, bereaved people may have mood swings and erratic behavior. They may become either hyperactive or hypoactive. Depression, if it occurs, contributes to the bereaved's difficulty in concentrating and fuels excesses of anger, guilt, and extreme sadness. The bereaved may focus exclusively on the deceased and reject all offers of comfort.

Parkes and Weiss (1983), in their classic research on widows, found that feelings of yearning for the return of the relationship and protest at its loss can last for an undetermined period. Clinging behavior may be mild and gradually vanish or can be intense and persist for weeks to months. Survivors may be angry at the deceased for leaving them, at God or fate for allowing the death, and at caregivers for not saving the person's life. The anger can be mild to moderate, severe enough to destroy relationships, or so extreme and bitter that it becomes crippling.

Survivors also feel guilty because they resent others who still have their loved ones, or they envy the deceased because they themselves did not die instead. They may feel guilty about not having done enough for the deceased. Their concerns can range from minor omissions, for example, "Why didn't I start a low-cholesterol diet for the whole family much sooner?" to important perceived errors in decision-making, for example, "Why didn't I insist on that last course of chemotherapy?" or "Why didn't I let them resuscitate her?"

Many survivors who have these feelings may not express them because they question their own mental stability and worry about what others will think of them. When they discover that others have gone through a similar sequence and intensity of emotion, they are more likely to share their feelings and thus gain some comfort from others.

Anguish, Disorganization, and Despair As time goes on and the rage exhausts itself, people being to recognize the permanence of the loss more realistically. Crying and tearfulness become common. The bereaved describe feelings of confusion, aimlessness, and loss of motivation. They worry about their inability to make decisions and their lack of self-confidence. A few people become markedly depressed and apathetic and lose interest in life and its meaning. Some isolate themselves socially. They may avoid activities, such as hobbies, that they had shared with the lost loved one. Many see life as a weighty burden and describe a lack of pleasure. They cannot believe that life will ever hold meaning and joy again. They may talk of suicide during the first year of bereavement and express a strong desire for reunion with the deceased through death.

The intensity of these negative feelings can be frightening. People who have had relatively stable or calm personalities may have a horror of losing emotional control. Their fears can be intensified by memory lapses and difficulty in concentrating. In an attempt to gain control, they center on themselves, which can be interpreted as selfishness by themselves as well as by others.

As time passes, the bereaved experience a new awareness of the precious quality of existence. They see life as fragile; they may display intense fears of being physically or emotionally hurt, or they may worry excessively about the welfare of family members. They may also become overly committed to working for causes related to the cause of the illness. At the same time, they may engage in health-compromising behaviors, such as driving in an unsafe manner or substance abuse (excessive smoking, drinking, or psychoactive drug use).

The need to cry is still strong but erratic. The tears burst through fiercely and unexpectedly. A song, a sunset, the smell of food or flowers, putting on the lights at dusk, or turning a corner into a familiar street may trigger tears. Bereaved people describe this startling experience as similar to being struck by lightning. They realize each time anew that they will never again see the deceased, that the loss is final, irrevocable.

Bereaved people may spend much time reminiscing, thinking about the deceased, and sharing memories with others. During these reminiscences, idealization of the deceased person takes place. In this process, all images and anecdotes about the deceased reveal him or her in only the best light. It is also common for feelings of guilt to resurface in bereaved people during the process of idealization.

Identification with the Deceased During grieving, bereaved people sometimes assume the lost one's characteristics. They may adopt his or her behavior, mannerisms, values, goals, or admired qualities. Some take on the physical symptoms of the deceased's final illness or last days. Family and friends may be alarmed by the appearance of chest pain, shortness of breath, nausea, or joint pain in the bereaved. Although it is always prudent to investigate such physical symptoms, it may be helpful to distinguish symptoms that mimic the deceased's from those that are related to a true organic condition. Symptoms that are associated with loss disappear as the loss approaches resolution.

In some cases, the sexual partners of deceased persons fear having contracted the disease that caused the death. Every pain or ache can be a source of terror for these people.

Reorganization and Restitution There are no time limits for the length of the grieving process. Although the reorganization and restitution associated with integration of the grief can begin within 6 months of the loss, it may take a year or longer for such signs to emerge. Indeed, grieving may not end within 1 or even 2 years of the precipitating event. The feelings and symptoms of grief do not simply stop completely one day. Sadness decreases only gradually, and a new life, based on the new reality, emerges slowly as time passes.

Although life eventually stabilizes, the bereaved person never completely recovers from the loss of a parent, spouse, child, or loved one. Memories persist. Some of the pain of loss may last for a lifetime and resurface with each new loss. The pain of loss can also be precipitated by circumstances that are powerful reminders of the deceased—a special place or activity, a shared important event, music, jokes, birthdays, anniversaries, and holidays. These intense responses, unlike those of early grief, are commonly transitory.

HIGH-RISK BEREAVEMENT

HIGH-RISK REACTIONS Some people are not able to resolve a particular loss satisfactorily. Between 10% and 20% of newly bereaved people can be expected to have serious problems (Martocchio, 1982).

In a few cases, the survivor goes on with life for weeks after a major loss as if nothing serious has happened. This is called delayed grief (Wortman & Silver, 1989). These people do not seem affected by the loss. They do not talk about the death as a loss, nor do they seem disturbed or express grief, sadness, or regret. Delayed grief sometimes occurs when the spouse in a highly conflictual marriage dies.

Another example of a high-risk reaction is the person who experiences uncontrollable weeping and very high levels of distress soon after the death. In some cases, the family tries to prevent these reactions by warning visitors not to talk about the death or the deceased.

Exaggerated expressions of guilt that continue for more than 12 to 18 months can also indicate unresolved grief. In these cases, people have a seemingly endless need to discuss the "if only's" and the "I should have's."

Prolonged anger and hostility are still other signs of troubled grief. The bereaved may express the anger not only in conversations as accusations but also in real or fantasized lawsuits against the health care institutions and health care providers who took care of the deceased during the final stage of illness. The bereaved may also take action against undertakers, insurance companies, and alienated relatives and friends. These people also have difficulty getting along with others in their pre-loss social circle and are not likely to have an easy time developing new relationships.

Successive physical illnesses or complaints for more than 2 years after the loss might be another indication of problems with grief. The same may be true for those who drink too much or who rely heavily on medications for inducing sleep or relieving anxiety.

Death from suicide is a real danger for the excessively bereaved. Because almost all persons who commit suicide talk about it beforehand and because not all those who talk about it really want to succeed, the alert nurse takes any talk of suicide seriously. Elderly white men constitute one of the highest risk groups for suicide but typically do not warn anyone of their intent to kill themselves.

HIGH-RISK GROUPS Some people are at higher risk than others for experiencing troublesome grief reactions. An elderly person who has experienced successive losses of loved ones and friends, with little time in between one loss and another, may not have time to grieve adequately and separately for each loss.

Another high-risk group includes the significant others of those who die of acquired immunodeficiency syndrome (AIDS), who are themselves members of the gay community. These people not only suffer a "bereavement overload" similar to that of the elderly person with multiple losses; many of them also have the added losses of lifestyle and support systems, and they fear for their own health and mortality (Carmack, 1992). They also have deep conflict about the amount of involvement they can tolerate in the active support of gravely ill people who are approaching death.

The survivors of people who die as victims of discrimination or in "social disgrace" (e.g., suicide, AIDS) are also at high risk in bereavement. Because of a society-imposed stigma, survivors fear they will be rejected and judged harshly if the true cause of their loved one's death becomes known. When they offer other explanations, such as cancer or an accident, the deception helps them at the time. In the long run, however, the tension resulting from fear of discovery and anger at having to cover up the true cause of death may negatively affect the survivor (Worden, 1991).

COLLABORATIVE MANAGEMENT

ASSESSMENT

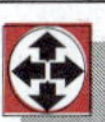

The nurse assesses a variety of factors when working with clients who have experienced the death of a loved one. Guidelines for the nursing assessment are presented in Chart 12–1. Circumstances surrounding the death and the characteristics of the survivor and the deceased have an impact on the client's emotional response.

Nurses must understand that while eliciting the material for a thorough assessment from the bereaved, they will also be engaged in a therapeutic encounter. In all likelihood, the grieving client will not be able to supply all information in a businesslike and straightforward manner. There will be pauses at certain questions for either the control of or expression of feelings. Because it is difficult to predict which parts of the assessment will affect individual clients and in what ways, the nurse moves from topic to topic, not necessarily in the order given but guided by the client's response. The key is for the nurse to keep the information flowing while conferring as much comfort as possible.

REVIEW OF LOSS

Because most newly bereaved people have a need to repeat the circumstances of the terminal episode and the death, items related to this need are placed at the beginning of the assessment. Often, by retelling the story to an empathic listener and possibly discharging tears, guilt, or anger, the client may feel accepted and understood and will not react to the more factual and sensitive assessment items as intrusive or callous.

PHYSICAL ASSESSMENT/CLINICAL MANIFESTATIONS

The questions about physical signs and symptoms are placed near the end of the assessment because many people do not like to emphasize the psychosomatic associations in their lives. This information may be difficult to obtain in a first interview from clients who have used denial as an important defense strategy. Conversely, for people who feel most comfortable talking to the nurse about physical matters, this section of the assessment can be the most effective introduction.

TRANSCULTURAL CONSIDERATIONS

Most of the research on loss, grieving, and death has focused on Caucasian, English-speaking populations. The grieving responses of other cultural groups have not been widely studied, except in relation to religious origin. Table 12–3 lists specific beliefs and customs of various religious groups about death and dying.

SPIRITUAL HEALTH

The items about spiritual matters are placed last in the assessment. This is because the spiritual domain may be volatile. The spiritual layer of a person's life is the one closest to the center of his or her identity. It is thus most difficult, especially in crisis situations, for a person to discuss spiritual matters before establishing a trusting relationship. The nurse who understands this will proceed with subtlety and delicacy. If possible, the nurse should deal with the more sensitive areas of the assessment later.

ANALYSIS

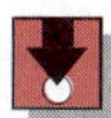

COMMON NURSING DIAGNOSES

The following nursing diagnoses are common to clients who are dying:

1. Anticipatory Grieving related to an actual or perceived loss
2. Fear related to known and unknown factors associated with loss

ADDITIONAL NURSING DIAGNOSES

In addition to the common diagnoses, some clients and their families may experience one or more of the following diagnoses:

CHART 12–1

Nursing Care Highlight ◆ Assessing the Client Undergoing the Loss of a Loved One Through Death

- What was the last illness of the deceased like?
- Was the death timely?
- How long was the preparation for the death?
- What was the age of the deceased?
- What was the relationship of the deceased to the survivor?
  - Spouse
  - Parent
  - Sibling
  - Grandparent
  - Child
  - Other
- What are the survivor's characteristics?
  - Age
  - Education
  - Employment
  - Economic status
  - Ages of dependent children
  - Past depressions or personality problems
  - Diagnosed mental health problems
  - Substance abuse history
  - Past major losses
    - Number recalled
    - When?
    - Were they resolved?
- What coping strategies has the client used with previous losses and setbacks?
- What are characteristics of the relationship with the deceased?
  - Degree of intimacy
  - Dependence (who depended on whom?)
  - Intensity
  - Ambivalence
- What are the relevant cultural and family factors?
  - Ethnic background
  - Family structure (list close members)
    - Are they geographically close?
    - Are they warm and supportive?
    - How often are these close family members seen? talked with?
- What are the physical factors that the client associates with responses to previous losses or stressful events? What physical symptoms has the client had since the most recent loss? Suggested list of signs and symptoms:
  - Headache
  - Appetite: loss, increase
  - Bowel habit changes
  - Bladder habit changes
  - Sleeping and dreaming
  - Tightness in throat or chest
  - Breathlessness
  - Sighing: heavy, frequent
  - Dry mouth
  - Muscle weakness
  - General malaise
- What are the spiritual aspects of the client's life?
  - Is the client a congregant of a formally organized religious group? If yes, document relevant data.
  - What helps the client when he or she is frightened or in need of extra support?
  - What is the client's source of strength and hope in times of crisis?
  - What are the client's ties to the wider community? Beliefs in a hereafter?
  - What is the client's source of a sense of meaning and purpose in life?
  - Is there an unconditional love in the client's life?
  - What does the client hope for now?
- On the basis of this assessment interview, how would the nurse evaluate the client's level of
  - Clinging and pining?
  - Anger and hostility?
  - Guilt and self-reproach?

- Ineffective Individual Coping related to loss of significant other
- Disabling Ineffective Family Coping related to effects of recent or impending death of family member
- Spiritual Distress related to the effect of loss of significant other
- Dysfunctional Grieving related to lack of anticipatory grieving, lack of resolution of previous grieving response, or actual or perceived loss of significant other, health or social status, or valued object
- Hopelessness related to functional loss, terminal illness, or impending death
- Powerlessness related to an inability to control progress of terminal illness and its effects on the body
- Social Isolation related to others' fear of dying person or stigma attached to terminal illness/death

PLANNING AND IMPLEMENTATION

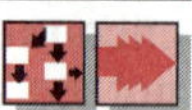

ANTICIPATORY GRIEVING

PLANNING: CLIENT GOALS The major goals are that the client and family or significant others will:

- Accept the reality of the loss
- Share grief with others

INTERVENTIONS

Teaching About the Physical Signs of Death Witnessing the death of a loved one is one of the most effective experiences in helping the family begin to accept the reality of the loss.

ANTICIPATED DEATH If the death is anticipated, the nurse gives the client and family or significant others information about the signs of death. The nurse should use nontechnical language. The nurse describes the physical signs in detail—realistic enough to be unmistakable, yet not so graphic as to alarm the listeners. In one nursing study, Lindley-Davis (1991) identified the defining characteristics of the dying client as a method to determine the most appropriate nursing interventions (Research Applications for Nursing).

Providing Terminal Care. Clients who are awake, yet near death, may be nauseated and may gradually refuse food and fluid. This is a sign that the work of the intestines has stopped. Although the client may still complain of thirst, he or she may have difficulty swallowing. The nurse teaches the family that it is not wise to offer food and fluids in the customary manner. The food or fluids might be regurgitated or aspirated, or both. Clear fluids may be given but only in small amounts. With poor or no fluid intake, the client's mouth becomes uncomfortably dry. The nurse or other caretaker moistens, clears, and rinses the mouth with applicators and saturated gauze. Ice chips may be given, but only if the client is awake. The nurse may apply petrolatum or some other emollient to the lips.

The client may also have difficulty speaking and may lie still much of the time. He or she will sleep deeply for increasingly longer periods and may become difficult to arouse. There are periods when the client does not appear to be breathing or is breathing irregularly. Breathing may become labored, with rapid respirations alternating with very slow and deep ones, then apnea (Cheyne-Stokes respiratory pattern). The client's breathing may become noisy because of the accumulation of mucus in the large bronchi. This noise is known as the "death rattle." The client may be made more comfortable at any time by a change of position. Breathing discomfort may be relieved somewhat if the caregiver places the client on his or her side, with the head slightly elevated and firmly supported on a pillow.

The client's skin may be damp with cold perspiration even though he or she complains of feeling overly warm. The nurse keeps the client dry by frequent sponging if there is a fever. Only a light covering is necessary.

Monitoring Vital Signs. Sensation and strength in the client's arms and legs gradually diminish. As the peripheral circulation lessens, the client's hands, feet, ears, and nose become cold. The client's hands and feet may become mottled and cyanotic. If the nurses have been monitoring blood pressure, they will notice that it becomes lower until it disappears. The dying person's pulse may double its rate, then weaken, gradually decrease, and stop. Meanwhile, respirations become shallow until they too stop. The pupils become fixed and dilated. Bladder and bowels may empty because of relaxation of the sphincters. One can assume death has taken place when there is no breath or heartbeat for a few minutes.

The family and health care professionals should be aware that the client's sense of hearing may remain intact even though it appears that no other stimuli can be perceived by the dying client. Conversation in the room and near the client should be carried on as if the client were alert. Caregivers should be encouraged to talk softly to the client and to touch and gently stroke him or her. The dying person may not respond, but the family will feel better maintaining a semblance of normal interchange. This activity fosters a sense of active, reciprocal communication for everyone right up to the end. Soft music might also be played on a tape recorder.

Interventions Following Death (Postmortem Care). After a client's death in a hospital or nursing home, the physician assesses the client and pronounces death. He or she then completes a death certificate, which must accompany the body to the funeral home. The nurse or other member of the nursing staff prepares the body for immediate postmortem viewing. In some cases, the family or significant others may want to assist with this process.

All tubes and linens are removed or cut according to agency policy, the eyes are closed, dentures are

RESEARCH APPLICATIONS FOR NURSING

Characteristics of Imminent Death May Suggest When the Best Nursing Intervention Is No Intervention

Lindley-Davis, B. (1991). Process of dying: Defining characteristics. *Cancer Nursing, 14,* 328–333.

The study attempted to identify defining characteristics of terminally ill clients as a method of specifying appropriate nursing interventions. The researcher reviewed 11 randomly selected charts of deceased clients in a hospice program. The three most common subjective characteristics were anorexia (82%), lack of pain (55%), and nausea/vomiting (36%). The three most common objective characteristics were an apical pulse of more than 100 per minute (91%); shallow, labored respirations with periods of apnea (73%); and withdrawal with repeated periods of nonverbalization (73%). Many charts documented the clients' desire to be left alone except for the presence of their families.

Critique This study shows an interesting approach to advancing knowledge about terminal care in a hospice setting. However, it is limited by a small sample size, as well as by measurement error due to reliance on documentation by many people.

Possible nursing implications As more studies of dying clients are conducted, increased knowledge can help nurses anticipate clients' needs. Physical care seems to be less important than simply allowing the client and family to be together. Nurses may need to rethink traditional care, such as turning clients every 1 to 2 hours and encouraging nutrition when the client wants to be left alone.

replaced, the bed is leveled, and the body is straightened. The nurse removes all pillows except for one supporting the head, which is kept in place to delay blood pooling and discoloration of the face. Pads are placed under the client's hips and around the perineum to absorb fecal material and fluid. The nurse washes the body as necessary and combs and rearranges the client's hair. The nurse takes care that all dirty linen, apparatus, other clutter, and odors, if possible, are removed from the room. Each health care agency has its own policies and procedures for postmortem care, but a list of typical nursing interventions is provided in Chart 12–2.

The family or significant others may then, in private, join the deceased in the room. The nurse should let the family know that he or she will be near if needed. If the family wishes to see a member of the clergy, the nurse notifies the hospital chaplain or appropriate community religious leader. The nurse may also participate in or initiate general spiritual expression, such as touch, spontaneous prayer, or acknowledgement of the special qualities of the deceased. The family or significant others may want to visit the hospital chapel.

After the client's death, the family can say their last words and perform their farewell gestures freely and naturally around the bed. They can perform any religious or cultural customs they wish (Table 12–3).

After the family or significant others view the body, the nurse follows agency procedure for preparing the client for transfer to either the morgue or a funeral home. The necessary materials, such as a shroud and identification tags, are usually supplied in a packet.

UNANTICIPATED DEATH Unanticipated deaths present a different set of circumstances for survivors than do expected deaths. Unexpected deaths in the hospital, and possibly at home or in the nursing home, may be preceded by resuscitation attempts. Survivors who are not present during resuscitation may not have seen the client when he or she was obviously ill. Survivors of clients who die unexpectedly also have not had time to experience anticipatory grief. The shocking news of the death may be overwhelming. These survivors may not have had the opportunity to interact with nurses or physicians who assisted the dying client at home, in the emergency department, or in a hospital unit.

For these reasons, survivors of clients who experience unexpected death might benefit from viewing

CHART 12–2

Nursing Care Highlight ◆ Postmortem Care

- Ensure that the physician has completed and signed the death certificate.
- Ask the family or significant others if they wish to wash or help wash the client.
- Remove or cut all tubes and lines according to health care agency policy.
- Close the client's eyes.
- Replace dentures or other dental appliances, if worn.
- Straighten the client and lower the bed to a flat position.
- Place a pillow under the client's head.
- Wash the client as needed; comb and arrange the client's hair.
- Place pads under the client's hips and around the perineum to absorb feces and urine.
- Clean up the client's room or unit.
- Allow the family or significant others to see the client in private and perform any religious or cultural customs they wish.
- Notify the hospital chaplain or appropriate community religious leader if requested by the family or significant others.
- Prepare the client for transfer to either a morgue or funeral home; wrap the client in a shroud and attach identification tags per agency policy if the client is to be transferred to the morgue.

TABLE 12–3 Major Religious Groups in the United States: Concepts and Practices Related to Death

Religious Group	Afterlife	Rituals	Handling of the Body After Death	"Extraordinary" Life-Prolonging Measures
Eastern Orthodoxy (including Greek and Russian Orthodoxy)	• Yes; the soul blends into the spiritual cosmos.	• The client's arms are crossed after death, with the fingers set in the shape of a cross. • Special prayers are said for those who have been baptized to bless the sick and dying. • The Last Rites must be delivered while the person is still conscious. • Holy Communion is obligatory.	• Autopsy and embalming are discouraged. • Organ and body donation are discouraged. • Cremation is discouraged.	• Encouraged

TABLE 12–3 Major Religious Groups in the United States: Concepts and Practices Related to Death *Continued*

Religious Group	Afterlife	Rituals	Handling of the Body After Death	"Extraordinary" Life-Prolonging Measures
Judaism	• The dead will be resurrected with the coming of the Messiah. • A person lives on in the memories of his or her survivors. • For Reform Jews, no concept of eternal punishment.	• The dying and dead are never left unattended before burial because the soul should depart in the presence of people. • The body is ritually washed, sometimes by members of a ritual burial society. • Burial is in a wooden casket within 24 hours or as soon as possible after death. • Five stages of mourning extend over a year. • Funerals are very simple, with no flowers because flowers are a symbol of life.	• Orthodox Jews prohibit autopsy and allow no removal of body parts. Conservative and Reform Jews permit autopsy. For Orthodox Jews, no embalming is allowed. • Beliefs about organ and body donation vary. Orthodox Jews generally prohibit both but may agree, with rabbinical consent. • Cremation is largely prohibited, but beliefs vary. Reform Jews allow cremation but recommend burial of ashes in a Jewish cemetery.	• Generally discouraged after irreversible brain damage is determined. Orthodox Jews advocate life support without "heroic measures."
Roman Catholicism	• The faithful go to heaven, but those who reject God's grace go to hell. • The soul goes to Purgatory for a time and is released by prayers and masses. • Resurrection occurs at the second coming of Christ.	• The family and priest choose prayers. • Holy Communion and rites for anointing the sick are mandatory. • Confession may be desired but is not mandatory; however, repentance is recommended.	• Autopsy is permitted, but all body parts must be buried appropriately. • Organ and body donation are unrestricted provided that the donor is not harmed. • Cremation is not restricted.	• Discouraged
Protestantism	• Varies; Episcopalians, Presbyterians, and Lutherans strongly believe in an afterlife, Quakers strongly do not.	• Varies; anointing rites, confession, and communion may be available but are not mandatory. • Healing services may be available, but there are no official sacraments. • The client and family may have a large role in planning services and prayer. Services range from traditional funerals to memorial services. • Clergy may minister through prayer, scripture reading, and counseling.	• Beliefs about autopsy, organ and body donation, and cremation vary by group from no restriction to individual choice to preferred.	• Discouraged
Nonaffiliated	• Varies	• Spontaneous and individualized, possibly including reading of original or traditional prayers or songs such as Psalm 23. • Traditional secular funeral or memorial services are used.	• Autopsy, organ and body donation, and cremation are by individual preference.	• Individual preference

the client's body in the setting where death occurred before the area and the client are cleaned. Tubes, medications, the "crash cart," and other supplies can be left at the scene. When survivors view the deceased client, they see that efforts were made to save their loved one. Survivors also get a more realistic image of how severely ill the client was. Those who advocate this experience for survivors believe that it assists the survivors in accepting the death and eventually resolving their grief.

Offering Physical and Emotional Support The simple presence of the nurse offers a sense of security. Presence implies that the nurse is physically and psychologically with the grieving client to meet his or her health care needs (Gardner, 1992). Physical support, such as being within sound or reach, gentle touching, holding hands, and hugging, are especially important during the first phases of grief. Lending a presence remains important as the weeks or months pass and the funeral crisis supports dissipate. The out-of-town relatives return home, and friends and local relatives resume the activities of their own lives.

The nurse offers physical and emotional support by encouraging the bereaved to eat, drink, rest, and stay as physically active as possible. Exercise to tolerance levels is a wonderful psychic as well as physical energizer.

The nurse informs the family about bereavement groups for persons who have experienced the death of a loved one. It is especially effective if the nurse can help the family locate a group that can meet their special needs.

Facilitating the Expression of Emotion At the same time that nurses help the family to cope in practical ways, they must also give them permission to express their grief. When necessary, nurses should facilitate the expression of grief. They do this by making themselves available to listen and to respond in nonjudgmental ways. The nurse's manner and words show that the expression of grief is not only acceptable and expected but also healthy. The nurse can show acceptance by moving physically closer. A gentle hand is placed on the bereaved's arm, or an arm is placed around the bereaved's shoulder when his or her eyes flood with tears or the voice cracks. Nurses can say something such as, "Just let the tears come. Don't try to hold them back."

Being Realistic The pain of loss cannot be, nor should it be, taken away no matter how committed the nurse may be to the client's comfort. Nurses must recognize the therapeutic value of the "gift of presence." Nurses must avoid pat stereotypic assurances, such as, "Things will be fine. Don't cry" and "Don't be upset. She wouldn't want it that way" or "In a year you will have forgotten." These sorts of comments comfort the nurse, not the client. The nurse accepts whatever the griever says about the situation and remains present, ready to listen attentively and guide gently. In this way, nurses help the bereaved to prepare for the necessary reminiscence and integration of the loss.

Avoiding Explanations of the Loss The nurse should not try soon after the death to explain the loss in philosophical or religious terms. Statements such as, "Everything happens for the best" or "God sends us only as much as we can bear" are not helpful when the bereaved person has yet to express feelings of anguish or anger. Telling someone too soon that they have other children to rely on, or that there are other family members who need them, does not diminish the intensity of the grief. In fact, doing so can create feelings of anger and resentment in the client toward the nurse because it reflects an insensitivity to the acute initial pain.

FEAR

PLANNING: CLIENT GOALS The goals are that the dying client will:

- Identify real reasons for fear and, if necessary, differentiate them from imagined ones
- Gain control over fears

INTERVENTIONS

Interventions for Fear of the Unknown Fear of the unknown is a basic fear of all human beings. Throughout life, all people have some fear of dying and death. This fear, which is amplified when a person is terminally ill, often surfaces in the form of questions. Some of these questions may be philosophical or religious, such as "Where will I be in the hereafter?" Others are more practical. They concern the welfare of those who are left behind, how the survivors will manage, and what will happen to life plans and projects. Many questions revolve around the dying process itself: "What will happen to me?" "Will I be abandoned, alone at my death?" "Will I lose control of myself?" "How will I react?" "Will I have pain?" "What will happen to my body after death?"

Nurses can help the dying person by distinguishing the questions that have answers from those that do not. For questions that have immediate answers, nurses obtain the information. For questions that can be answered in the future, nurses begin to draw together the pertinent resources. For questions that may never have an answer, nurses encourage expression of feeling. The aim is to provide comfort by eliminating as much uncertainty as is realistically possible.

When the dying client questions what will happen to the survivors after his or her death, it might be appropriate to assist with funeral plans and arrangements for religious observations or memorial services. This might also be the time to make sure that wills and advance directives are in order.

The nurse also checks with the client or family about the desire to donate one or more of the client's organs. Some clients have signed donor cards with their personal papers to indicate in advance which organs may be donated. If the client has not thought about organ donation in advance, the physician or nurse may ask the family or significant others if the client's organs, if appropriate for donation, can be removed.

Interventions for Fear of Loneliness, Isolation, and Abandonment All people, and especially dying people, gain reassurance by feeling accepted by others. People who are involved in care can supply this reassurance by simply being with the dying client. Yet, visiting a sick person often produces fear in the visitor. Nurses can prompt family and friends during their visits. Nurses can show them how to participate in the dying client's care and can help them communicate with the client. Nurses can also suggest options such as dying at home, if that is possible, either with or without the support of a participating hospice program. In this way, some of the feeling of abandonment that results from having been removed from home, family, and community to an institution can be relieved.

Some clients are not afraid to die. For example, some elderly clients prefer to withdraw at the end of their lives because they have accepted death. Emotional withdrawal by the person may lead to withdrawal from families and health care providers as well. The nurse helps the family understand that this response is part of normal adult development. Chart 12–3 describes special considerations for caring for an elderly person who is dying.

Interventions for Fear of Loss of Family and Friends Fear of loss of family and friends is closely related to fear of abandonment. Dying people grieve the loss of family and friends just as the family and friends grieve the loss of the dying person.

Interventions for Fear of Loss of Self-Control and Dependency Self-reliance and independence are closely associated with positive self-image and the sense of human dignity. Fear of loss of control and of encroaching dependency, therefore, is a major worry of persons who are becoming progressively more debilitated. Nursing strategies to help in this area include encouraging dying persons to make as many decisions as possible about the details of their lives, such as nursing care and concerns about the future.

Interventions for Fear of Suffering and Pain Many people fear dying in unbearable pain. This may or may not be a realistic concern. Nurses can help by providing information about pain in a way that mitigates fears. The nurse can reassure clients that there are sophisticated combinations of invasive and noninvasive treatments for pain control that were not available 25 years ago. Nurses can also assure clients and families that if pain becomes a problem, the most effective pain relief regimen possible will be devised. Finally, they can assure the client that he or she will not be abandoned, or that the nurse will be present, if pain proves to be a problem.

CHART 12–3

Nursing Focus on the Elderly ◆ The Elderly Client Who Is Dying

- Recognize that the client has probably had experience with death and dying.
- Accept the client's need for emotional or social withdrawal.
- Support the client's need to integrate religious beliefs as part of the grieving process.
- Respect the client's decision to have life-sustaining measures withheld when there is no likelihood of a satisfactory quality of life.
- Assess and accept the client's reaction to death and dying. Many elderly people have accepted death and may wish for death to occur.

EVALUATION

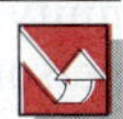

The nurse evaluates the care of the client and family undergoing loss on the basis of identified nursing diagnoses. The expected outcomes for the client and family include that the client and family or significant others:

- State acceptance of the loss
- Share their grief with each other
- Identify the reasons for their fear or fears
- Use coping mechanisms and resources to gain control over fear

Community Resources

OVERVIEW

Nurses play a role in acquainting and linking the bereaved people with helpful community organizations, such as Widow-to-Widow and Compassionate Friends. They may recommend other resources, such as bereavement discussion groups, mental health nurses, psychologists, counselors, social workers, and clergy or religious leaders involved in bereavement counseling.

Nurses can also participate in community and religious educational programs that are designed to assist people in understanding grief and that reach out to the bereaved. Hospice programs are excellent sources of information and referral.

HOSPICE

A hospice is not a building or a place or an institution; it is a concept of care expressed in a centrally coordinated array of services. The aim of hospice care is to enable a dying person to live at home until death to the limit of his or her potential in physical strength; in mental, emotional, and spiritual capacity; and in social relationships. Hospice care offers an alternative to the acute care of a general hospital or the custodial care of a nursing home. Although one of the prominent aspects of hospice care in the United States is the variety of organizational types and sponsoring agencies, a consistent philosophy and a set of core services are common to all accredited and certified or licensed programs.

GENERAL FEATURES

Hospice care is holistic. The interrelationship of the physical and the psychologic is acknowledged and taken into account. Terminal care, provided by an interdisciplinary team, is given to the dying person and his or her family, however the care is defined. The care is directed toward the symptoms and circumstances surrounding the physical, emotional, spiritual, social, and financial spheres. Hospice care is comprehensive and nonfragmented, providing continuity from one service level to another as the dying person's changes in condition and family circumstances call for changes in levels of care. The nursing diagnoses frequently associated with terminal care are as follows:

- Fatigue/Activity Intolerance
- Altered Nutrition: Less than Body Requirements
- Pain and Chronic Pain
- Altered Thought Processes (Delirium)
- Constipation
- Impaired Skin Integrity
- Altered Oral Mucous Membrane
- Spiritual Distress
- Anticipatory Grieving

The four key features of hospice programs are:

- Symptom control or palliation (lessening) for the dying person
- The dying person and his or her "family" as defined by the client
- Care planned and delivered by an interdisciplinary team
- Care supervised and coordinated by the hospice program in a variety of settings

For a model bill of rights for hospice clients, see Figure 12–1.

The hospice's intention is to protect and support the human and legal rights of all in its care by guaranteeing patients and families the right to

- Access to care, regardless of race, religion, ethnicity, sex, age, handicap
- Be treated with dignity and respect at all times
- Full disclosure of the benefits and limitations of the program, including other options for care and costs
- Give (or withhold) informed consent for care; for being treated by others besides program staff, such as students; for being observed by other than staff; for being used as a research subject
- Confidentiality and privacy both in relation to the hospice health care team and the patient's family and attending physician
- Know the truth about diagnosis and prognosis
- Participate in the development and updating of the individualized plan of care
- Continuity of care from home to inpatient facility and through bereavement care
- State-of-the-art management of symptom and pain control
- Know the rules and regulations of the program as well as channels of communication with management and grievance procedures
- Know the program's policies with regard to resuscitation and other "heroic" procedures
- Know the program's usual procedures followed at the time of death
- Choose the place of death: home, inpatient setting
- Choose the time of death, if that becomes necessary
- Determine the disposition of his or her own body both at and after death
- Call on the support of any belief system or cultural practices that will help
- Have sufficient numbers of qualified, competent, compassionate staff to realize these rights

FIGURE 12–1 ◆ A model bill of rights for hospice clients. (From Amenta, M. O., & Bohnet, N. [1986]. *Nursing care of the terminally ill.* Boston: Little, Brown. Reprinted by permission of Scott, Foresman.)

SYMPTOM CONTROL OR PALLIATION

The key clinical feature of hospice care is that it is directed primarily at symptom control or palliation rather than disease control or cure. Invasive diagnostic or therapeutic procedures are seldom used. A diagnosis of terminal illness with a prognosis of less than 6 months to live is an almost universally required criterion for admission to a hospice program, although the time span can vary, depending on the program. Because the psychosocial as well as the physical dimension is emphasized in care, there is a far greater need for intensive personal care than for intensive technical care.

This is not to imply that there is never specific technologic intervention or treatment of the underlying disease; rather, relief of symptoms is the overriding goal. Active intervention in the cancer process with chemotherapy or radiation, for instance, is used only to the extent that it can be expected to contribute to the dying person's quality of life.

In certain instances, reduction of the size of a tumor can relieve an intestinal obstruction or make respiration easier. Chemotherapy can sometimes shrink tumors that are bearing on pain-sensitive tissue, such as nerves or periosteum of the bone. Mild doses of radiation can relieve the pain of bone metastasis. These curative methods, applied with palliative purposes, may then allow several weeks or months of special time to the dying person and his or her loved ones. A wedding might be planned, a will drawn up, or a relationship re-established.

As a practical matter, the problem of considering the use of sophisticated technologic procedures in hospice care arises rarely. When it does become an issue, the best decision will be an individualized one, made in light of all that is known of the client, family, and natural history of the disease.

THE DYING PERSON AND FAMILY AS CLIENT

Family involvement is important in all aspects of health care, but it takes on major significance in caring for the dying. *Family* in hospice care means anyone deeply attached to the dying person—spouse, blood relative, close friend, lover, neighbor—who will take the responsibility of care. Most hospices must identify a primary care person in each family who then acts as the coordinator of care in the program.

The people close to the dying person face problems that may seem insurmountable. Some problems develop from feelings about the impending loss, but more often problems are related to the practical responsibilities as caregivers, to living arrangements, or to financial considerations.

When the family's or primary care person's confidence in his or her ability to manage some of these matters crumbles, the overall care of the dying person can be profoundly affected. As nurses carefully assess families, supporting and teaching them the needed knowledge and skills, the family becomes an important part of the therapeutic and coordinating team.

Hospice involvement with the family does not end with the death of the person. Bereavement follow-up to provide reassurance and support during grieving is a component of most hospice programs. Some functions include:

- Assessing the coping ability of the survivors
- Encouraging and facilitating the expression of the survivors' feelings related to the loss
- Reassuring the survivors that the grieving process, although painful, is normal
- Identifying possible pathologic reactions
- Making referrals if need

AN INTERDISCIPLINARY APPROACH

Because problems in hospice care management arise from a several sources—physical, emotional, social, spiritual, and financial—a team approach is essential. The interdisciplinary team includes physicians, nurses, social workers, clergy or religious or spiritual leaders, and volunteers as key members, with the client and family ideally at the center of decision-making.

Interdisciplinary care is characterized by a lack of sharp distinctions (or blurring) of roles among the functions and decision-making authority of the members of the team. Although each member has expertise in which he or she has primary responsibility and authority, all members must be alert and open to problems and needs in other areas of care. Each member must be prepared to undertake care tasks that are normally in the realm of another. The better welded the team, the more role overlap is tolerated and the better the care of the client and family.

Coordination of all these caregiving participants and levels of care demands leadership and communication. The interdisciplinary team meets regularly on an established schedule to maintain continuity of care.

COORDINATED CARE IN VARIOUS SETTINGS

The dying person must be in the setting that is most appropriate to his or her needs. There must also be continuity of care as the client shifts from one setting or level of care to another as dictated by his or her changing condition. The most usual settings are the person's home, an acute care hospital, and an intermediate care facility.

The most suitable setting for a dying person at any particular time depends on many factors, including:

- The client's physical and emotional condition
- The home situation
- The client and family's attitude toward the illness and impending death
- The dying person's attitude toward the family
- The family's capacity to manage care
- Financial considerations

In addition, the input of the dying person and family, as well as that of the interdisciplinary team, is important in decision-making about where the dying person can best receive care.

In addition to coordinating care in various settings, the hospice program must make services available on a 24-hour basis 7 days a week because problems arise unexpectedly at all hours of the day and night and on weekends. A prompt response is one of the key elements of successful continuity for palliative care. The best pain and symptom control protocols can be useless if they are not maintained without interruption from home to hospital and back to home or nursing home. The accompanying resurgence of pain, anxiety, distorted relationships, and general chaos can undo weeks of careful attention and care.

HOME CARE

Most dying persons and their families who choose hospice care prefer the home to other caregiving environments during the final episodes of the illness. They also wish for death to take place at home, if possible. Although there are exceptions to these preferences, being surrounded by familiar people and things, having ready access to friends and relatives, and the freedom from institutional restriction, no matter how liberal the institution, make the home setting more comfortable and give the client and family more control.

Families who choose home care supported by a Medicare-certified hospice program may also have the advantage of continuous nursing care in the home if the client's condition warrants. Respite care of the client in a hospital or nursing home for a short time may also be available if caregivers need a few days of rest. Home care is much less costly for the family and the overall health care system than any sort of inpatient care. In many cases, hospice home care is reimbursable, either partially or totally, by a third-party payer, such as an insurance company.

There are, however, some disadvantages to home care for the dying client. Families may not be able to manage the physically and psychologically demanding burden of around-the-clock care 7 days a week. Some family members may have crippling anxiety about what to do in a medical crisis. These families may become rapidly exhausted.

Families may be less fearful of attempting home care if they know that they will have the support of the hospice team for physical crises and the assurance of respite time for themselves if they need it. In preparation for home care, there should be meetings between hospice staff and the family to explain such matters as:

- The roles of nurses, volunteers, and other workers
- The on-call system
- Options for readmission to in-service hospice or for respite care
- Use of emergency staff visits
- Continuous care possibilities
- Other available supports

The home must be prepared with supplies and equipment such as disposable pads, hospital bed, water or alternating pressure mattress, oxygen, bed pan and/or urinal, commode, dressings, intravenous poles, and irrigation sets, if needed. The family should be assisted in arranging the home for caregiving comfort, convenience, and privacy.

Euthanasia

Under some conditions, keeping someone alive through technologic life support rather than actively and arbitrarily ending his or her life can provide time—time to try an experimental new therapy or perhaps time for a remission. Unfortunately, an interval like this is not always good or quality time. It may be time fraught with pain, suffering, and confusion rather than peace and growth. The agonizing question emerges, "Is this kind of life worth staying alive for?" It is then that the issue of euthanasia moves to the forefront.

Euthanasia, derived from a Greek word meaning "easy or pleasant death," implies that under some circumstances death is preferable to life. The notion of euthanasia, or "mercy killing" as it is commonly known, is surrounded with controversy in some countries.

The term *assisted suicide* has been used to describe a situation in which a person provides the means for another person to commit suicide. In the United States, the legal system is addressing this situation to determine whether assisted suicide is murder or some other criminal offense. In other countries, such as Sweden, under certain circumstances and on the client's request, a physician may legally perform assisted suicide or give a lethal dose of medication to the client.

Certain agreed-upon distinctions and definitions are used. *Active* euthanasia refers to an act of commission that directly and *intentionally* shortens a person's life. In comparison, *passive* euthanasia is an act of omission (Table 12–4). It usually refers to letting the person die by either withdrawing or withholding a treatment that might prolong life. The distinction between active and passive euthanasia is at best blurred because both are the result of intentional choice. Is it more moral to let someone die than to take measures specifically aimed at ending his or her life? Deciding not to act is a decision. Not acting is an action.

Voluntary euthanasia and *involuntary* euthanasia refer to the amount of the client's involvement in procedures and decisions leading to his or her death. In *involuntary* euthanasia, decisions are made by someone other than the dying person, either with or without his or her knowledge. In *voluntary* euthanasia, the client may actively participate in decision-making or may leave instructions to loved ones about the circumstances under which extraordinary means would or would not be desired.

TABLE 12–4 Classification of Euthanasia

Type of Euthanasia	Type of Action: Active	Type of Action: Passive
Voluntary euthanasia	• Suicide/assisted suicide	• Advance directive, such as a living will (see Chap. 6)
Involuntary euthanasia	• Homicide	• Letting "nature take its course"

Modified from Amenta, M. O., & Bohnet, N. (1986). *Nursing care of the terminally ill.* Boston: Little, Brown. Reprinted by permission of J. B. Lippincott.

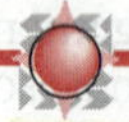

IMPLICATIONS FOR NURSING RESEARCH

Although some nursing research has been conducted in the area of loss, death, and dying, many questions remain unanswered. Some possible questions for research include:

- ♦ How do grief responses differ in various cultures?
- ♦ How can the nurse best anticipate who is at high risk for prolonged or troubled grief?
- ♦ What nursing interventions are most effective in assisting a person who is dying?
- ♦ What nursing interventions are most effective in helping a family or significant others with anticipatory grieving?

SELECTED BIBLIOGRAPHY

*Amenta, M., & Bohnet, N. (1986). *Nursing care of the terminally ill.* Boston: Little, Brown.

*American Nurses' Association. (1987). *Standards and scope of hospice nursing practice.* Kansas City: Author.

Ardery, G. (1992). Terminal care. In G. M. Bulachek & J. C. McCloskey (Eds.), *Nursing interventions: Essential nursing treatments* (2nd ed, pp. 366–378). Philadelphia: W. B. Saunders.

Birenbaum, L. K. (1992). Re: Definitions of grief. *Research in Nursing and Health, 15,* 319.

Callanan, M. (1994). Back from beyond. *American Journal of Nursing, 94*(3), 20–21.
Callanan, M. (1994). Farewell messages. *American Journal of Nursing, 94* (5), 19–20.
Carmack, B. J. (1992). Balancing engagement/detachment in AIDS-related multiple losses. *Image: Journal of Nursing Scholarship, 24,* 9–14.
*Carson, V. B. (1989). *Spiritual dimensions of nursing practice.* Philadelphia: W. B. Saunders.
Chenell, S. L., & Murphy, S. A. (1992). Beliefs of preventability of death among the disaster bereaved. *Western Journal of Nursing Research, 14,* 576–594.
Chidester, D. (1990). *Patterns of transcendence: Religion, death, and dying.* Belmont, CA: Wadsworth.
Cooley, M. E. (1992). Bereavement care: A role for nurses. *Cancer Nursing, 15*(2), 125–129.
Cowles, K. V., & Rodgers, B. L. (1991). The concept of grief: A foundation for nursing research and practice. *Research in Nursing and Health, 14,* 119–127.
Edwards, B. S. (1994). When the family can't let go. *American Journal of Nursing, 94*(1), 52–56.
Farberow, N. L. (1992). Changes in grief and mental health of bereaved spouses of older suicides. *Journal of Gerontology, 47,* 357–366.
Gardner, D. L. (1992). Presence. In G. M. Bulachek & J. C. McCloskey (Eds.), *Nursing interventions: Essential nursing treatments* (2nd ed., pp. 191–200). Philadelphia: W. B. Saunders.
*Greyson, B. (1985). A typology of near-death experience. *American Journal of Psychiatry, 142,* 967–969.
Hudak, C. M., Gallo, B. M., & Benz, J. J. (1990). *Critical care nursing: A holistic approach.* Philadelphia: J. B. Lippincott.
*Kübler-Ross, E. (1969). *On death and dying.* New York: Macmillan.
Levy, L. H. (1991). Anticipatory grief: Its measurement and proposed reconceptualization. *The Hospice Journal, 7*(4), 1–29.
*Lindemann, E. (1944). Symptomatology and management of acute grief. *American Journal of Psychiatry, 101,* 141–149.
Lindley-Davis, B. (1991). Process of dying: Defining characteristics. *Cancer Nursing, 14,* 328–333.
*Martocchio, B. C. (1982). *Living while dying.* Bowie, MD: Robert J. Brady.
Matteson, M. A., & McConnell, E. S. (1989). *Gerontological nursing: Concepts and practice.* Philadelphia: W. B. Saunders.
Mullen, J. T. (1992). The bereaved caregiver: A prospective study of changes in well-being. *Gerontologist, 32,* 673–683.
*National Hospice Nurses' Association (1988). *Quality assurance for hospice patient care.* Escondido, CA: Author.
*National Hospice Organization. (1982). *Standards of a hospice program of care.* Arlington, VA: Author.
Olson, M. (1992). Near-death experiences and the elderly. *Holistic Nursing Practice, 7*(1), 16–21.
Parkes, C. M., & Weiss, R. S. (1983). *Recovery from bereavement.* New York: Basic Books.
*Raphael, B. (1983). *The anatomy of bereavement.* New York: Basic Books.
*Report of the Ad Hoc Committee of the Harvard Medical School to Examine the Definition of Brain Death. (1968). A definition of irreversible coma. *JAMA, 205,* 85–88.
Schoenbeck, S. B. (1993). Exploring the mysteries of near-death experiences. *American Journal of Nursing, 93,* 42–46.
Schoenbeck, S. B., & Hocutt, G. (1991). Near-death experiences in patients undergoing cardiopulmonary resuscitation. *Journal of Near-Death Studies, 3,* 211–218.
*Schraff, S. (1984). *Hospice: The nursing perspective.* New York: National League for Nursing.
*Taptich, B. J., Iyer, P. W., & Bernocchi-Losey, D. (1989). *Nursing diagnosis and care planning.* Philadelphia: W. B. Saunders.
*Worden, J. W. (1982). *Grief counseling and grief therapy: A handbook for the mental health practitioner.* New York: Springer.
Worden, J. W. (1991). Grieving and loss from AIDS. *The Hospice Journal, 7*(1), 143–151.
*Wortman, C. B., & Silver, R. C. (1989). The myths of coping with loss. *Journal of Consulting and Clinical Psychology, 57,* 349–357.

SUGGESTED READINGS

Levy, L. H. (1991). Anticipatory grief: Its measurement and proposed reconceptualization. *The Hospice Journal, 7*(4), 1–29.

This study indicates that anticipatory grief does not serve an adaptive function but, rather, is positively correlated with depression and stress. Therefore, the researcher recommends that nurses should not encourage grieving in spouses of clients in the terminal stages of illness.

Olson, M. (1992). Near-death experiences and the elderly. *Holistic Nursing Practice, 7*(1), 16–21.

This article presents an overview of near-death experience, then focuses on this phenomenon in the elderly. The elderly also have near-death experiences but usually do not have a life review as part of the experience. Elderly people who have had near-death experiences are more prepared for death and feel that their lives have meaning.

Schoenbeck, S. B. (1993). Exploring the mysteries of near-death experiences. *American Journal of Nursing, 93,* 42–46.

This article describes several anecdotes from nurses who have cared for clients who had near-death experiences. These stories have helped nurses become more sensitive to what their clients experience when dying.

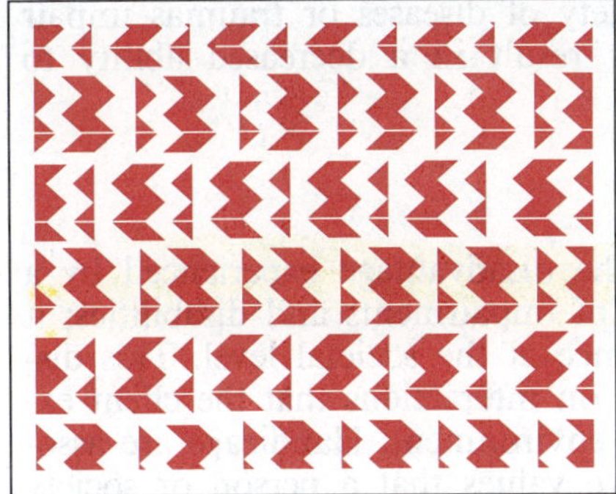

CHAPTER 13

Chronic and Disabling Conditions

CHAPTER HIGHLIGHTS

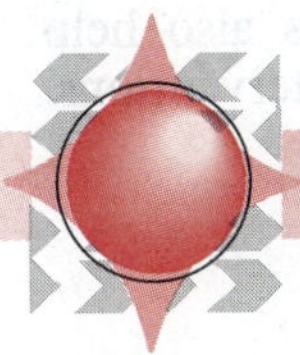

A chronic illness or condition is one that has existed for at least 3 months (Institute of Medicine, 1991). A disabling condition is any physical or mental health problem that can cause disability (Institute of Medicine, 1991). This text focuses on physical health problems; mental health problems are discussed in textbooks on mental health nursing.

Clients with chronic and disabling conditions often participate in rehabilitation programs to prevent disability, maintain functional ability, and restore as much function as possible.

OVERVIEW

Chronic illness is the primary health problem in the United States. Approximately 50% of the population (115 million people) have one or more chronic illnesses. About 35 million people, or one in seven, experience activity limitations owing to their chronic health problems. Of these, 33 million people are in residential settings and the remaining 2 million are in inpatient health care facilities, such as rehabilitation hospitals and nursing homes (Institute of Medicine, 1991). This chapter focuses primarily on the care of adult clients in health care facilities (inpatient settings). For information about community-based rehabilitation (ambulatory care), consult textbooks on community health nursing.

Coronary artery disease, cancer, chronic obstructive pulmonary disease (COPD), and arthritis are some common chronic conditions that may result in varying degrees of disability. Many of these illnesses occur in people older than 65 years of age. A study by Robinson et al. (1993) showed that 49% of clients in inpatient rehabilitation settings were older than 65 and 42% of clients in ambulatory rehabilitation settings were older than 65.

Chronic and disabling conditions are not always diseases such as cancer; they may also result from accidents. Accidents are the leading cause of death among young adults and the third leading cause of death in people 45 to 54 years old. Today increasing numbers of people survive accidents because of advances in medical technology. These survivors are often faced with chronic or disabling conditions, such as head and spinal cord injuries. Therefore, the need for rehabilitation is on the rise. Such survivors may need months to years of follow-up health care after returning to the community.

In the United States, the annual cost of chronic and disabling conditions is almost $200 billion in medical care and lost productivity. Disability occurs slightly more often in men than in women and in families with lower incomes (Institute of Medicine, 1991).

REHABILITATION

Rehabilitation is the process of learning to live with chronic and disabling conditions, often those resulting from trauma. However, rehabilitation is not limited to the return of function in post-traumatic situations. It includes education and therapy for any chronic illness characterized by a change in a body system function or body structure. Rehabilitation programs related to respiratory, cardiac, musculoskeletal, and oncologic disorders are common examples that do not involve trauma. The goal of rehabilitation is to return the client to the fullest possible physical, mental, social, vocational, and economic capacity.

In any discussion of rehabilitation, it is important to define and distinguish the terms impairment, disability, and handicap. These terms have been used interchangeably in some settings; however, for this chapter, the terms are defined according to the *International Classification of Impairments, Disabilities and Handicaps* (World Health Organization, 1980).

IMPAIRMENT

Impairment is an abnormality of a body structure or structures or an alteration in a body system function resulting from any cause; it represents a disturbance at the organ level. Impairments can be temporary or permanent and may or may not be associated with an active pathologic condition.

DISABILITY

Disability is the consequence of an impairment and is usually described in terms of a client's altered functional ability; it represents disturbance at the personal level. A variety of diseases or traumas impair mobility and may result in a decreased ability to function.

HANDICAP

A handicap is the disadvantage experienced by a person as a result of impairments and disabilities; it represents disturbance at the societal level. This disadvantage is based on interactions that the client experiences with the environment. Handicaps are associated with negative values that a person or society ascribes to the person's situation or experience. Handicaps are both preventable and reversible, although impairments caused by pathologic changes in a body organ and the resulting disabilities are often unpreventable or irreversible.

THEORIES RELATED TO CHRONIC AND DISABLING CONDITIONS

Before assessing a client with a chronic or disabling condition, the nurse should be aware of the basic theories that help to explain a client's behavior that results from the disability. These theories also help the nurse to plan appropriate nursing interventions. Six theories are briefly presented:

- Powerlessness theory
- Adaptation theory
- Coping theory
- Self-care theory
- Body image theory
- Family theory

POWERLESSNESS THEORY

Powerlessness is a perception that one's own action will not and cannot affect an outcome. The client perceives a lack of control over a situation. Miller (1991) applied the concept of powerlessness to clients with chronic conditions. Powerlessness can be thought of as the client's perceived inability to be involved in or influence self-care and the quality of life. Because complete alleviation of symptoms and cure may not be realistic goals for the chronically ill client, minimizing powerlessness and enhancing quality of life are appropriate client goals.

Miller (1991) suggested that chronically ill people have deficits in one or several power resources. When one or more power resources are compromised, the client has difficulty coping with problems. For example, an elderly client may have diminished physical strength and reserve, which decreases his or her ability to cope with chronic illness. If nurses can aid the client in restoring power resources, the client's quality of life can be enhanced and powerlessness can be minimized.

ADAPTATION THEORY

Adaptation is defined as the ability to accommodate change. Human beings demonstrate this ability constantly. Accommodation requires energy, motivation, and psychologic support. When assessing the adaptation potential of a client, the nurse should be aware of several factors:

- The previous experiences of the client in adapting to change
- The meaning that change holds for the client
- The inner energy of the client
- The willingness of the client to initiate or implement the change in behavior or beliefs that may accompany adaptation

As a first step in the assessment, the nurse determines whether the client has the ability to adjust to the disability. The nurse may need to listen sensitively to interpret correctly the client's statements.

The nurse should be aware that major adaptive tasks may include coping with pain and becoming comfortable in the rehabilitation setting. Establishing a trusting nurse-client relationship during rehabilitation can be stressful for the client. In addition to developing new relationships with staff, the client must also maintain relationships with family and friends and prepare for an uncertain future. (Chapter 7 discusses adaptation in detail.)

COPING THEORY

The client who has a chronic illness often relies on the nurse for assistance in facing the problems of living with disease. Chronically ill and disabled adults face many coping tasks. Lazarus and Folkman (1984) defined coping in terms of psychologic stress theory. Psychologic stress is a particular relationship between the person and the environment that is appraised by the person as exceeding his or her resources and threatening well-being. The more coping tasks that confront the client, the greater is the likelihood that powerlessness will occur. Coping is a problem-solving process, not a single act. The coping tasks of chronically ill adults are found in Table 13–1.

Lazarus and Folkman's definition limits coping to conditions of psychologic stress. Coping can be more broadly defined as an "effort to manage," which permits coping to include anything a person does to perform everyday activities or to manage stress, regardless of how well it works. The nurse assesses the client's coping strategies—both present and past. (Chapter 7 further describes coping and the role of the nurse.)

SELF-CARE THEORY

Nursing plays a major role in the rehabilitation process by assisting clients to achieve the greatest possible independence and responsibility for self-care. Orem (1980) developed a self-care theory for nursing, which can be a basis for rehabilitation nursing practice. According to Orem, self-care entails the activities that people initiate and perform on their own behalf

TABLE 13–1 Coping Tasks of Chronically Ill Adults

- Maintaining a sense of normalcy
  - Hiding or minimizing the illness and responding to the curious inquiries of others
  - Living as normally as possible, despite daily therapy and obvious symptoms
- Modifying daily routine and adjusting one's lifestyle
  - Including therapy and symptom control in the daily routine
  - Providing for safety
- Obtaining knowledge and skill for continuing self-care
  - Developing internal awareness
  - Monitoring the effects of therapy
- Maintaining a positive concept of self
  - Integrating illness into one's self-concept
  - Maintaining or enhancing self-esteem
- Adjusting to altered social relationships
  - Preserving relationships with friends and family who satisfy dependency needs
  - Maintaining family solidarity
- Grieving over losses concomitant with chronic illness
  - Adjusting to the loss of physical abilities, function, status, income, social relationships, roles, or dignity
  - Dealing with financial losses
- Dealing with role change
  - Adjusting to losing social, work, and family roles; and gaining roles as a dependent help-seeker, self-care agent, and chronically ill client
- Handling physical discomfort
  - Dealing with discomfort that is illness-induced and therapy-induced
- Complying with the prescribed regimen
- Confronting the inevitability of one's own death
- Dealing with the social stigma of illness or disability
- Maintaining a feeling of being in control
  - Maintaining cognitive, behavioral, and decisional control
- Maintaining hope despite uncertain or downward trajectory
  - Looking at the effects of hope and its meaning in physical changes

Adapted from Miller, J. M. (1991). *Coping with chronic illness: Overcoming powerlessness* (2nd ed.). Philadelphia: F. A. Davis.

in maintaining life, health, and well-being. Self-care activities include:

- Universal self-care activities to meet basic human needs
- Age-specific self-care activities related to developmental tasks
- Illness- or disability-related self-care activities to prevent or regulate the effects of deviation from normal body structure or healthy functioning

The nurse can assist clients to maximize their performance of self-care activities. The nurse assesses the self-care deficits of the client and then applies appropriate nursing interventions. The nurse also determines the client's self-care demands and abilities. A difference between demand and ability indicates that nursing interventions are needed. The nurse calculates the self-care deficit and intervenes by acting directly or by guiding, supporting, or teaching the client. The nurse then evaluates the client's movement toward health.

BODY IMAGE THEORY

The term *body image* is used in many different ways. Body image has been linked with self-esteem and self-concept. Schilder (1950) defined body image as the picture of one's own body that is formed in one's mind. This image results from the interaction of perception and experience. Perceptions consist of a person's past and present sensory impressions, and the experiences include past and present memories, events, and activities. Although Schilder's definition has been used for a long time, it is still one of the most graphic and precise definitions of body image.

The nurse assesses alterations in the body image of the chronically ill or disabled client. Factors that should be considered during assessment include the client's developmental level, the effects of treatment, the visibility of the affected body part, the functional significance of the body part involved, and the feasibility of rehabilitation. A change in body image as a result of illness or disability represents a loss for the client undergoing rehabilitation. After assessing the body image changes resulting from a chronic or disabling condition, the nurse can design interventions to help the client cope with the alterations. (See Chapter 10 on body image theory, assessment, and nursing interventions.)

FAMILY THEORY

The family, including relatives and significant others, interacts many times with the health care system when a person becomes chronically ill. The nurse's ability to communicate with the family members helps determine whether the interactions are successful and therapeutic.

The nurse assesses the client and family as a unit. The manner in which the family responds to the disability affects the adjustment of the client. In a study by Hough et al. (1991), the number of stressors that families experienced was predictive of how well they adjusted to the chronic illness of a family member. Stressors not related to the illness had a major impact on the ability of families to cope (Research Applications for Nursing).

When assessing the family, the nurse also determines how decisions are made in the family, who the spokesperson is, and how the family usually copes with crises. The nurse analyzes family structure and roles. Structural assessment includes determining the family's communication patterns and problem-

RESEARCH APPLICATIONS FOR NURSING

Family, Friends, and Religion, in Particular, May Be Sources of Hope in Chronic Illness

Raleigh, E. D. H. (1992). Sources of hope in chronic illness. *Oncology Nursing Forum, 19,* 443–448.

This study identified and explored the sources of hope that clients with chronic illnesses report as being supportive. The theoretical basis of the study was a combination of coping theory and hope theory. Both coping and hope are associated with motivation and goal attainment.

Clients with cancer (group 1) and clients with other types of chronic illnesses (group 2) were studied. Each group was randomly selected from a discharge file of a visiting nurse agency during a 3-month period. Forty-five participants were in each group. Two researchers, using a written guide, interviewed each subject.

There were no significant differences in the findings between the two groups. The main strategies used to raise hope included staying busy, prayer or religion, talking to others, and distractions. The major sources supporting hope were family, religion, and friends.

Critique This research used a qualitative and quantitative approach to obtain data. The sample included women and men, with various religions (although most were Protestant) and various occupations.

Possible nursing implications The use of family and friends as a source of hope has been addressed in other studies. The researchers were surprised, however, at the number of people who relied on religion. They concluded that nurses should be more attentive to spiritual needs and that research is warranted in this area.

solving skills. Family assessment for long-term planning focuses on the status and role of the client in the family and the family's economic status. The nurse should also consider religious and cultural factors.

REHABILITATION AS PART OF THE HEALTH CARE SYSTEM

After a client's acute condition has been stabilized in a hospital, the client is discharged to continue the healing process, generally under the follow-up care of a non-hospital health care provider, such as a family physician. The nurse provides home care preparation, health teaching, psychosocial preparation, and information about various health care resources to help clients resume their usual roles in society.

Some conditions, however, require the intermediate step of rehabilitation, which can take place in a number of settings. Rehabilitation starts in the hospital (sometimes called acute rehabilitation) and continues after discharge from the hospital. The nurse's coordination of care from acute care through extended care and the continuity of care are critical to the success of rehabilitation.

SETTINGS FOR REHABILITATION

Freestanding rehabilitation hospitals or nursing homes, in which the client is usually hospitalized for 6 to 12 weeks, and outpatient (ambulatory) hospital rehabilitation departments are the most common settings for the delivery of rehabilitation services. Some hospitals have converted one or more inpatient units into rehabilitation units. The client can then stay in the same facility for both acute and continuing rehabilitative care. Ideally, this arrangement promotes continuity of care for the client. All clients in these settings receive rehabilitation services.

Transitional living facilities are associated with rehabilitation hospitals or units within hospitals or nursing homes. These units allow the client to begin the move from total supervision in a rehabilitation unit to independent living. The client is monitored but not supervised as closely as in the acute care hospital. These facilities are particularly helpful for young adults with head injury, spinal cord injury, or stroke.

After clients become more confident and independent, they may choose to live in a *group home.* These independent living centers are facilities in which clients live independently, but together with other disabled adults. Each client or group of clients has a care provider, such as a personal care aide, to assist with the activities of daily living (ADL) and decisions requiring accurate judgments. The clients may or may not be employed. The goal of these centers is to provide independent living arrangements outside an institution.

Rehabilitation services are also available in *long-term care settings* (nursing homes) that are certified as skilled nursing facilities and in adult day care centers. A full range of services, including nursing care, physical therapy, occupational therapy, and speech and language therapy, are available (Fig. 13–1). Most skilled nursing facilities and day care centers are not able to provide the special services required for clients with head injuries or spinal cord injuries, unless the facility has specialty units for that purpose. Clients who typically receive rehabilitation in skilled nursing facilities include those with strokes, arthritis, fractures, total joint replacements, and neurodegenerative diseases, such as multiple sclerosis and Parkinson's disease. These clients are typically mixed with other clients who are not receiving rehabilitation care.

THE REHABILITATION TEAM

Successful rehabilitation depends on the coordinated effort of a group of health care professionals—the rehabilitation team—and the involvement of the client in planning and implementing care.

GOALS OF THE REHABILITATION TEAM

The rehabilitation team has two basic aims:

- Prevention of injury
- Restoration of function

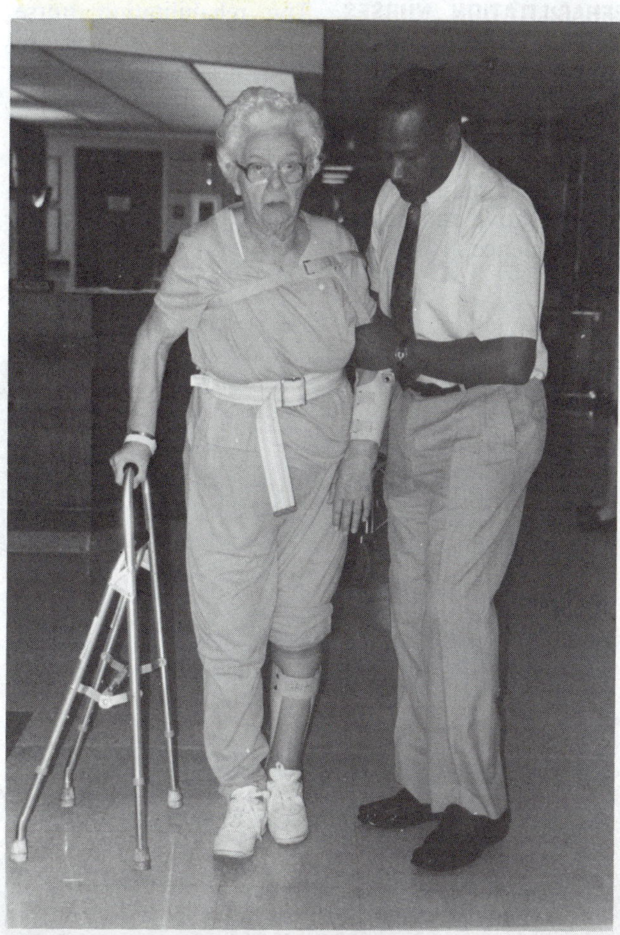

FIGURE 13–1 ♦ A physical therapist in a skilled nursing facility (SNF) helping a client to ambulate with use of a hemi-cane.

The aim of prevention is to maintain the client's activity levels to avoid the deterioration of an unaffected organ or part and to eliminate possible hazards or factors that may contribute to further injury. Prevention is a continuous aspect of care for the chronically ill or disabled client. For example, meticulous skin care is necessary to prevent the formation of pressure sores. The other major goal of the rehabilitation team is restoration of as much function as possible to the injured or diseased body part or system to facilitate the client's independence.

MEMBERS OF THE REHABILITATION TEAM

The interdisciplinary health care team members in the rehabilitation setting include physicians, nurses, physical therapists, occupational therapists, speech/language pathologists, recreational therapists, cognitive therapists, aides, social workers, psychologists, vocational counselors, the clients themselves, and family members or significant others. Not all settings that offer rehabilitation services have all of these members on their team.

PHYSIATRISTS The physician who specializes in rehabilitative medicine is called a physiatrist. Most inpatient rehabilitation settings, except for most skilled nursing facilities, employ physiatrists.

REHABILITATION NURSES The rehabilitation nurse coordinates the efforts of the team members. In clients undergoing rehabilitation, health problems are characterized by an altered functional ability and a diminished quality of life. The goal of rehabilitation nursing is to assist the client in restoring and maintaining optimal health. The rehabilitation nurse must be innovative and patient in helping the client regain independence.

THERAPISTS *Physical therapists* (PTs) intervene to help the client achieve mobility (e.g., by facilitating ambulation and teaching the client to move with braces). Physical therapists teach techniques for performing the activities of daily living such as transferring (e.g., moving into and out of bed), ambulating, and toileting.

Occupational therapists (OTs) work to develop the client's fine motor skills used for activities of daily living, such as those required for eating, maintaining hygiene, dressing, and driving. Occupational therapists may also teach clients skills related to coordination, such as hand movements (Fig. 13–2).

Speech/language pathologists (SLPs) retrain clients with speech or language problems. Speech is roughly defined as the ability to say words, and language is the ability to understand and put words together in a meaningful way. Some clients, especially those with head injury or cerebrovascular accident (CVA, or stroke), have difficulty with both speech and language. The speech/language pathologist also evaluates and treats swallowing disorders.

Recreational, or *activity, therapists* work to help clients continue or develop hobbies or interests. These therapists often coordinate their efforts with those of the occupational therapist.

Cognitive therapists, usually neuropsychologists, work primarily with clients with head injuries who have cognitive impairments. These therapists often use computers to assist with cognitive retraining.

Aides and *health care assistants* work in the nursing or therapy departments to assist in the care of clients. These rehabilitation team members are under the direct supervision of the nurse or the therapist. Special training, ranging from one course to 2 years of vocational or college education, is required to be an aide.

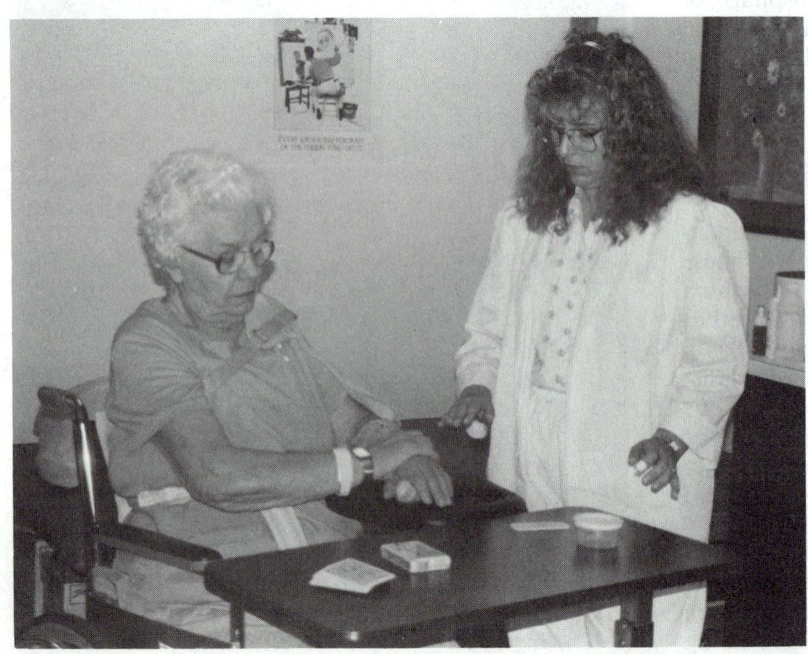

FIGURE 13–2 ◆ An occupational therapist working with a client who has had a stroke.

COUNSELORS Various counselors are helpful in promoting community reintegration of the client and acceptance of the disability or chronic illness. *Social workers* help clients identify support services and resources, including financial assistance. They usually coordinate the client's transfer to or discharge from the rehabilitation setting. *Psychologists* also counsel clients and families on their psychologic problems and on strategies to cope with disability.

Vocational counselors assist clients with job placement, training, or further education. Work-related skills are taught if the client needs to change careers because of the disability. If the client has not yet completed high school, educational tutors may help the client in the rehabilitation setting to complete the requirements for graduation.

Interdisciplinary team conferences for the exchange of ideas are held with the client, family members and significant others, and health care providers on a regular basis. Chart documentation is shared and read by all team members.

COLLABORATIVE MANAGEMENT

ASSESSMENT

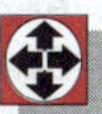

HISTORY

The nurse collects the client's health history, including the history of the present condition, any current medications, and any treatment programs in progress.

GENERAL BACKGROUND DATA The nurse obtains general background data about the client and family. These data include financial status, occupations, educational levels, cultural background, and home situation. Family assessment data include the factors discussed earlier under the heading Family Theory. The nurse addresses architectural features of the environment, such as the layout of the home. The nurse determines whether the physical layout, such as the presence of stairs or the width of doorways, at home will present a problem to the client. The nurse also gathers data on the client's neighborhood, such as the location of shopping centers and available transportation. The nurse determines who does the client's shopping, cooking, and housework. This information is essential for discharge planning.

DAILY SCHEDULE AND HABITS The nurse also assesses the client's usual daily schedule and habits of everyday living. These include hygiene practices, eating, and elimination; sexual activity; and sleep. The nurse asks about the client's preferred method and time of bathing and hygiene activity. In assessing dietary patterns, the nurse notes the client's food likes and dislikes. The nurse also elicits information about bowel and bladder function and the client's normal pattern of elimination.

In the assessment of sexuality patterns, the nurse asks about changes in sexual function since the onset of the disability (see Chap. 11). The nurse assesses the client's current and previous sleep habits, patterns, usual number of hours of sleep, and use of hypnotics. The nurse should also ask whether clients feel well rested after sleep. Sleep patterns have a significant impact on activity patterns. Assessment of activity patterns focuses on work, exercise, and recreational activities.

PHYSICAL ASSESSMENT/CLINICAL MANIFESTATIONS

The nurse collects the physical assessment data systematically according to major body systems (Chart 13–1). The focus of assessment related to rehabilitation and chronic disease is on the functional abilities of the client. The nurse identifies the client's ability to use self-help devices during this portion of the assessment.

CARDIOVASCULAR SYSTEM An alteration in cardiac status may affect the client's cardiac output or cause activity intolerance. The nurse assesses the manifestations of decreased cardiac output, such as chest pain and fatigue. The nurse determines when the client experiences these symptoms and what relieves them. The nurse seeks medical consultation before the client continues activities that provoke these symptoms. The physician may order a change in medications or may prescribe a prophylactic dose of nitroglycerin to be taken before the client resumes the activities. The nurse collaborates with the physician and appropriate therapists to determine whether activities can be modified to be accomplished without these symptoms.

For clients showing fatigue, the nurse and the client together plan methods of using the client's limited energy resources. For instance, the client could take frequent rest periods throughout the day, especially before undertaking activities. Major tasks could be performed in the morning because most people have the most energy at that time.

A great hindrance to rehabilitation for clients with cardiac disorders is fear. A client may have survived a life-threatening experience, such as a myocardial infarction, but now is so afraid of recurrence (and death) that he or she is unable, or unwilling, to resume *any* activity. Clients with cardiac disorders experiencing fear usually benefit from participation in a structured cardiac rehabilitation program. The nurse discusses available programs with the client and the family.

RESPIRATORY SYSTEM The nurse asks the client whether he or she is experiencing shortness of breath during or after activity. It is important to determine the level of activity that the client can accomplish without experiencing shortness of breath. For example, can the client climb one flight of stairs without shortness of breath, or does shortness of breath occur after the client climbs only two steps?

CHART 13–1

Nursing Care Highlight ◆ Physical Assessment of Clients Undergoing Rehabilitation

Body System	Relevant Data
Cardiovascular system	• Chest pain • Fatigue • Fear of cardiac failure
Respiratory system	• Shortness of breath or dyspnea • Activity tolerance • Fear of inability to breathe
Gastrointestinal system and nutrition	• Oral intake, eating pattern • Anorexia, nausea and vomiting • Dysphagia • Laboratory data (e.g., serum albumin level) • Weight loss or gain • Bowel elimination pattern or habits • Change in stool • Ability to get to toilet
Renal/urinary system	• Urinary pattern • Fluid intake • Urinary incontinence or retention • Urine culture or urinalysis
Neurologic system	• Motor function • Sensation • Cognitive abilities
Musculoskeletal system	• Functional ability • Range of motion • Endurance • Muscle strength
Integumentary system	• Risk of skin breakdown • Presence of skin lesions

The fear associated with any inability to breathe normally can render a person dependent in many facets of his or her life. Some problems related to disorders of the respiratory system can be resolved or diminished, but some breathing difficulties must be endured (e.g., in emphysema).

GASTROINTESTINAL SYSTEM AND NUTRITION The nurse assesses the client's oral intake and pattern of eating. The nurse also assesses the client for the presence of anorexia, dysphagia, nausea, vomiting, or discomfort related to or interfering with oral intake. In collaboration with the physician and the dietitian, the nurse assesses the client's height, weight, hemoglobin and hematocrit levels, and serum albumin and blood glucose concentrations. Weight loss or gain is particularly significant and may be related to an associated disease or to the illness that caused disability.

Elimination habits vary from person to person; they are often related to daily job or activity schedules, dietary patterns, and family or cultural background. Elimination habits may be difficult to assess, as many nurses are hesitant to request—and many clients afraid to volunteer—information pertaining to elimination. When assessing the client's elimination status, the nurse first asks what the usual elimination patterns were for that person before the injury or the illness.

The nurse is attuned to any changes in the client's bowel routine or the consistency of the stool. If the client is noticing any change in elimination pattern, the nurse tries to determine whether this alteration can be attributed to a change in diet, activity pattern, or the use of medications that could cause increased or decreased motility of the gastrointestinal tract. Bowel habits are evaluated on the basis of what is normal for that person.

The nurse also determines whether the client can manage bowel functions independently. Independence in bowel elimination requires cognition, manual dexterity, sensation, muscle control, and mobility. If the client requires help, the nurse determines whether there is someone available at home to provide the assistance. The nurse also assesses the client's (and family's) ability to cope with any dependency in bowel elimination.

RENAL/URINARY SYSTEM When assessing the client's urinary system, the nurse determines the client's baseline urinary patterns. The nurse asks about the number of times the client usually voids and whether the client routinely awakens during the night to empty the bladder or has uninterrupted sleep. The nurse determines the client's fluid intake patterns and volume, including the type of fluids ingested and the timing of fluid consumption throughout the day.

The nurse determines whether the client has experienced any problems with incontinence or urinary retention in the past. The nurse and the physician also monitor laboratory reports, especially the results of urine culture and urinalysis.

NEUROLOGIC SYSTEM In rehabilitation, the neurologic assessment identifies the functional aspects of motor ability, sensation, and cognition. The nurse assesses the client's pre-existing problems, general physical condition, and communication abilities.

Motor Ability The movement of an extremity is compared with the function of the opposite extremity to identify paresis (weakness) or paralysis (absence of movement).

Sensation The identification of sensory/perceptual alterations is important in assessing the client's risk for injury. The nurse assesses the client's response to light touch, hot or cold temperature, and position change in each extremity and on the trunk. Levels of decreased sensation are identified. For a perceptual assessment, the nurse evaluates the client's ability to receive and understand what is heard and seen and the ability to express appropriate motor and verbal responses. During this portion of the assessment, the nurse can also begin assessing short- and long-term memory.

Cognitive Abilities The nurse also assesses the client's cognitive abilities, especially if there is a head injury or stroke. Several tools are available to evaluate cognition. One of the most common is the Mini Mental State Examination, which is described in detail in Chapter 41.

MUSCULOSKELETAL SYSTEM As is the case for other body systems, the rehabilitation nursing assessment of the musculoskeletal system focuses on function. The nurse assesses the client's musculoskeletal status, the client's response to the impairment, and the demands of the home, work, or school environment. The nurse determines the client's endurance level and measures both active and passive range of motion (ROM) of joints. The nurse reviews the results of manual muscle testing by physical therapy, which identifies the client's range of motion and resistance against gravity. In this procedure, the therapist determines the degree of muscle strength present in each body segment. The grading system usually ranges from 0 (no evidence of muscle contractility) to 5 (normal muscle contractility) (see Chap. 49).

INTEGUMENTARY SYSTEM In assessing a client's integumentary system, the nurse identifies actual or potential interruptions in the integrity of the skin.

Risk for Skin Breakdown To maintain healthy skin, the body must have adequate food, water, and oxygen intake; intact waste removal mechanisms; sensation; and functional mobility. Changes in any of these variables can lead to rapid and extensive skin breakdown. If the client cannot protect or maintain the skin, the nurse must be able to assess and plan for the client's needs. The nurse monitors the client to determine the risk of skin breakdown before it occurs.

Some rehabilitation settings use special skin assessment tools to identify clients who are at risk for skin breakdown. For example, the Braden Scale for Predicting Pressure Sore Risk (see Chap. 67) assesses six areas: sensory perception, skin moisture, activity level, nutritional status, and the potential for friction and shear.

Several other skin risk assessment tools are available. Some tools also include additional indicators of nutritional status, such as the serum albumin level. When the serum albumin level is low, the client is at high risk for pressure sores. Some tools include incontinence and altered mental state as risk factors. Regardless of which tool is used, Braden and Bergstrom (1992) recommend the following schedule for skin assessment:

- *For clients in critical care units:* during every nursing shift when the client is unstable; at least daily when the client is stable
- *For clients in medical-surgical units:* every other day when the client's condition is stable; and when the condition changes significantly (e.g., after surgery)
- *For clients in nursing homes or rehabilitation units:* weekly for 1 month, then monthly after the first month unless there is a significant change in the client's condition

Actual Skin Breakdown If a pressure sore or other change in skin integrity develops, the nurse accurately assesses the problem and its possible causes. The nurse inspects the client's skin every 2 hours, or more often if needed, until the client has learned to inspect his or her own skin several times a day. The nurse documents the depth and diameter of the open skin area in centimeters or inches, depending on the facility's policy. Chapter 67 presents a widely used classification system for staging skin breakdown. The nurse also assesses the client's understanding of the cause and treatment of skin breakdown as well as his or her ability to inspect the skin and participate in maintaining skin integrity.

In some health care facilities, a skin assessment tool, or "skin sheet," is used to keep track of each area of skin breakdown. A baseline assessment is conducted on admission to the facility, and the form is updated periodically, depending on the agency's policy and the nurse's judgment. In some long-term care or rehabilitation settings, photographs of the client's skin are taken at various intervals to document the skin's condition.

FUNCTIONAL ASSESSMENT

Functional ability refers to the client's ability to perform activities of daily living (ADL) such as bathing, dressing, feeding, and ambulating, and instrumental activities of daily living (IADL), such as using the telephone, shopping, preparing food, and housekeeping. Functional assessment tools are used to assess a person's abilities within the context of a predetermined evaluation process. Rehabilitation nurses, physiatrists, and/or therapists complete one or more of these assessment tools on the basis of the client's abilities and the policy of the health care setting. Some of the commonly used tools are briefly described below. For further information, consult corresponding references in this chapter.

PULSES PROFILE One of the earliest tools used was the PULSES profile. It was developed in 1957 and adapted in 1975 to evaluate and classify functional capacity in the chronically ill and aging client population (Granger et al., 1979). The six categories included for evaluation are:

- *P*hysical condition (basic health status)
- *U*pper limb function (self-care)
- *L*ower limb function (mobility)
- *S*ensory components (sight, communication)
- *E*xcretory function
- *S*upport factors

Scoring uses four numeric grades for each category, with scores increasing as functional ability is diminished. The maximum score is 24. High scores indicate greater levels of dependency for the client. The adapted form of the PULSES profile has been a useful tool in many rehabilitation programs. It indicates the level of independence in life-functioning skills necessary for a person to make adaptations to community living.

KATZ INDEX OF ACTIVITIES OF DAILY LIVING One of the best known and most widely used instruments was developed during the 1950s from observations of clients with fractured hips. The Katz Index of Activities of Daily Living addresses six functional tasks: bathing, dressing, toileting, achieving transfers, level of continence, and feeding (Katz et al., 1963). Each of the six areas is scored as either "dependent" or "independent" on the basis of the client's need for help in performing the task (Table 13–2). The overall functional status is then assigned a grade from A (independent in feeding, being continent, transferring, toileting, dressing, and bathing) through G (dependent in all six functions) from total scores.

The Katz Index has been used for clients with many types of chronic illnesses. It is a valuable tool for evaluating care and developing data about the course of an illness over time.

BARTHEL INDEX The Barthel Index (Mahoney & Barthel, 1965) was designed to measure functional levels and mobility in the physically impaired client. This tool consists of ten variables, in which the clients are scored by their degree of independence in performance. Categories include feeding, bathing, and mobility. The scoring system consists of two descriptive areas: doing an activity with help and performing an activity independently. Scores range from 0, indicating total dependence, to 100, indicating complete independence.

The Barthel Index was intended for use in both immediate and long-term care rehabilitation programs.

LEVEL OF REHABILITATION SCALE The Level of Rehabilitation Scale (LORS), developed by Carey and Posavec (1978), provides a general assessment of the client's functioning for program evaluation rather than clinical assessment. The LORS provides an overview through measurement of function regarding activities of daily living, cognition, home activities, activities outside the home, and social interactions. The LORS was then expanded to include 11 items related to activities of daily living, mobility, and communication (Posavec & Carey, 1982). These items receive a score of 0 to 4, determined through the use of a coding manual ascribing numeric values to behavioral terms.

FUNCTIONAL INDEPENDENCE MEASURE Assessment tools have also been designed for use on a national level; thus, uniform outcome data can be obtained from numerous rehabilitation programs. An example of this kind of system—a uniform data system—is the Functional Independence Measure (FIM), developed by Granger and Gresham (1984). The FIM, as a basic indicator of the severity of a disability, attempts to quantify what the person actually does, whatever the diagnosis or impairment. It does not measure what a person should do or how the person would perform under a different set of circumstances. To eliminate the bias of a particular discipline, the assessment may be done by trained clinicians; the entire assessment may be done by one person, or certain categories may be performed by representatives of various disciplines.

Categories for assessment are self-care, sphincter control, mobility and locomotion, communication, and cognition. Scoring is done with numbers using predetermined criteria for measurement. The evaluation is performed when the client is admitted to and discharged from a rehabilitation institution and at a specified follow-up time.

PSYCHOSOCIAL ASSESSMENT

The nurse must understand the theories of body image and self-esteem to assess the client's psychosocial needs adequately. These concepts serve as a basis for understanding psychologic responses to chronic illness and resulting disability. The client's self-esteem and body image are assessed through the client's verbal indicators and descriptions of self-care. Body image can also be assessed by tools such as the Baird Body Image Assessment Tool (BBIAT) (see Chap. 10).

The nurse assesses the client's use of defense mechanisms and manifestations of anxiety, such as those noted in facial expressions and communication patterns. To assess the client's response to loss, the nurse

TABLE 13–2 Katz Index of Activities of Daily Living

Independence means without supervision, direction, or active personal assistance, except as specifically noted below. This is based on actual status and not ability. A patient who refuses to perform a function is considered as not performing the function, even though he or she is deemed able.

Bathing (sponge, shower, or tub)
Independent: assistance only in bathing a single part (back or disabled extremity) or bathes self completely
Dependent: Assistance in bathing more than one part of body; assistance in getting in or out of tub; does not bathe self

Dressing
Independent: gets clothes from closets and drawers; puts on clothes, outer garments, braces; manages fasteners; act of tying shoes is excluded.
Dependent: does not dress self or remains partly undressed

Going to Toilet
Independent: gets to toilet; gets on and off toilet; arranges clothes, cleans organs of excretion (may manage own bedpan used at night only and may or may not be using mechanical supports)
Dependent: uses bedpan or commode or receives assistance in getting to and using toilet

Transfer
Independent: moves in and out of bed and in and out of chair independently (may or may not be using mechanical supports)
Dependent: assistance in moving in or out of bed and/or chair; does not perform one or more transfers

Continence
Independent: urination and defecation entirely self-controlled
Dependent: partial or total incontinence in urination or defecation; partial or total control by enemas, catheters, or regulated use of urinals and/or bedpans

Feeding
Independent: gets food from plate or its equivalent into mouth (precutting of meat and preparation of food, as buttering bread, are excluded from evaluation)
Dependent: assistance in act of feeding (see above); does not eat at all or parenteral feeding

Evaluation Form

Name ______________________ Date of Evaluation ______________________

For each area of functioning listed below, circle description that applies (the word "assistance" means supervision, direction, or personal assistance).

Bathing—either sponge bath, tub bath, or shower

Receives no assistance (gets in and out of tub by self if tub is usual means of bathing)	Receives assistance in bathing only one part of body (such as back or a leg)	Receives assistance in bathing more than one part of body (or does not bathe self)

Dressing—gets clothes from closets and drawers; puts on clothes, including underclothes, outer garments; manages fasteners (including braces, if worn)

Gets clothes and gets completely dressed without assistance	Gets clothes and gets dressed without assistance except for tying shoes	Receives assistance in getting clothes or in getting dressed or stays partly or completely undressed

Toileting—going to the "toilet room" for bowel and urine elimination; cleaning self after elimination and arranging clothes

Goes to "toilet room," cleans self, and arranges clothes without assistance (may use object for support such as cane, walker, or wheelchair and may manage night bedpan or commode, emptying same in morning)	Receives assistance in going to "toilet room" or in cleansing self or in arranging clothes after elimination or in use of night bedpan or commode	Does not go to room termed "toilet" for the elimination process

Transfer

Moves in and out of bed and in and out of chair without assistance (may use object for support such as cane or walker)	Moves in or out of bed or chair with assistance	Does not get out of bed

Continence

Controls urination and bowel movement completely by self	Has occasional "accidents"	Supervision helps keep urine or bowel control; catheter is used or is incontinent

Feeding

Feeds self without assistance	Feeds self except for getting assistance in cutting meat or buttering bread	Receives assistance in feeding or is fed partly or completely by tubes or intravenous fluids

From Katz, S., et al. (1963). Studies of illness in the aged. The index of ADL: A standardized measure of biological and psychosocial function. *JAMA, 185*, 914–919.

asks the client to describe his or her feelings concerning the loss of a body part or function. The nurse also notes any stress-related physical problems. The client may experience symptoms of depression, such as fatigue, a change in appetite, or feelings of lack of power (also see Chaps. 7 and 12).

The nurse assesses the availability of support systems for the client. The major support system is typically the family or significant others. The family interactions and coping patterns are assessed (see the earlier discussion of family theory).

VOCATIONAL ASSESSMENT

The rehabilitation nurse assists clients in maximizing their functional status, allowing clients to resume many usual activities. The nurse should be aware of appropriate resources for each client in compiling a vocational data base for the client. The nurse works with vocational counselors to help the client find meaningful training, education, or employment after discharge from the rehabilitation setting. The nurse gathers data on the client's educational and employment history, including previous jobs held. The nurse also obtains employers' attitudes toward the disabled client and information on the client's performance on the job, such as absenteeism and work record.

The nurse informs clients who are United States residents about the 1991 Americans with Disabilities Act passed by Congress to prevent employer discrimination against disabled people. Within reason, the employer must offer assistance to the disabled to allow them to perform the job. For example, if a client has a severe hearing loss, the employer may need to hire an interpreter for sign language so that the client can work.

The nurse also notes the cognitive and physical demands of the jobs held and ascertains whether the client can return to the former job or if retraining in another field will be needed. The physical demands of jobs range from light in sedentary occupations (0 to 10 pounds frequently lifted) to heavy (more than 100 pounds frequently lifted). The nurse must also consider other aspects of the job, such as strength, mobility, or senses required in the job (e.g., hearing).

Job analysis also involves assessing the work environment of the client's former job. The nurse works with the vocational counselor to determine whether the environment is conducive to the client's return. Union contracts must also be considered, and any job modifications must be noted. If the injured worker requires vocational rehabilitation, the nurse refers the client to vocational rehabilitation personnel and assists the client to work with the counselors on evaluating present skills and learning new skills for employment (Fig. 13–3). The nurse may also help with job placement in the community.

ANALYSIS

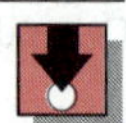

COMMON NURSING DIAGNOSES

Regardless of the client's age or specific disability, the following nursing diagnoses are commonly applicable to clients with chronic illness or disability:

1. Impaired Physical Mobility related to neuromuscular impairment, sensory/perceptual impairment, pain, activity intolerance, fatigue, and/or the effects of trauma or surgery
2. Self Care Deficit (total or partial) related to effects of trauma or chronic illness, muscular weakness, pain, immobility, and/or perceptual or cognitive impairment
3. High Risk for Impaired Skin Integrity related to altered sensation and/or immobility
4. Altered Urinary Elimination related to sensorimotor impairment or immobility
5. Constipation related to neuromuscular or musculoskeletal impairment or immobility
6. Ineffective Individual Coping related to the effects of chronic illness, the loss of control over a body part or a body function, and/or major changes in lifestyle
7. Body Image Disturbance related to a change in body structure or function (see Chap. 10)

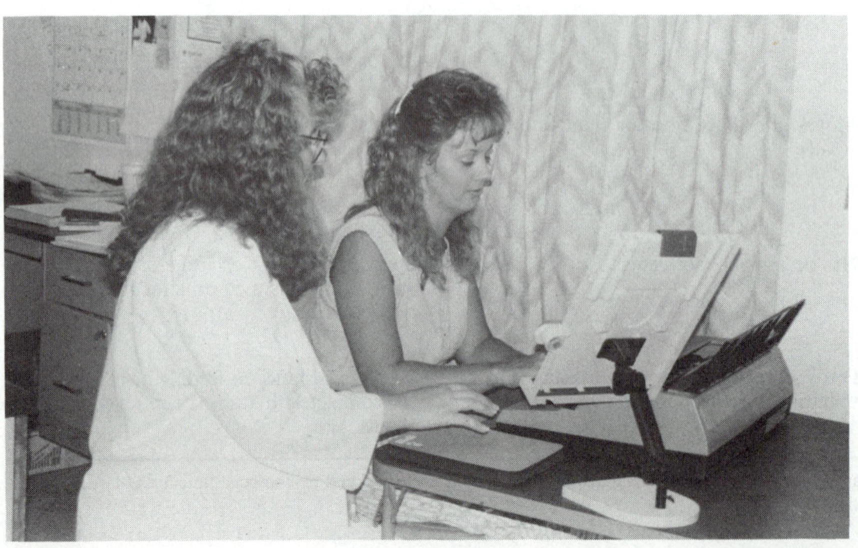

FIGURE 13–3 ◆ A client in vocational training learning to type.

ADDITIONAL NURSING DIAGNOSES

Additional nursing diagnoses may apply, depending on the client's specific disability. For example, a client with rheumatoid arthritis also experiences Chronic Pain. The client with a spinal cord injury may also have Sexual Dysfunction.

PLANNING AND IMPLEMENTATION

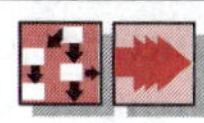

IMPAIRED PHYSICAL MOBILITY

PLANNING: CLIENT GOALS The primary goals are that the client will:

- Achieve the maximal physical mobility possible with the least restriction of activity
- Not experience complications resulting from immobility

INTERVENTIONS Most problems requiring rehabilitation relate to impaired physical mobility. Clients with neurologic disease or injury, amputations, arthritis, severe burns, and cardiopulmonary disease experience some degree of impaired mobility. The physical therapist is the key rehabilitation team member who helps clients to meet mobility goals. Clients often spend several hours every day working in the physical therapy department to regain function and skills. Older clients may not be able to tolerate extensive therapy workouts and may need shorter sessions to prevent extreme fatigue or physical complications. The nurse reinforces the physical therapist's instructions and must be aware of the client's progress and abilities.

Transfer Techniques Clients with decreased mobility may require assistance with transfers, for example, from a bed to a chair, a commode, or a wheelchair. Because the degree of assistance required varies with the client and the specific disability, the nurse carefully assesses the client's mobility status before attempting a transfer. The physical therapist usually specifies how a particular client is to be transferred. For example, a quadriplegic client may use a sliding board for transfer. The client with an above-knee amputation may need a wheelchair with removable arms. In any case, the nurse always plans the transfer technique *before* initiating it. The goal is that the client will eventually be able to transfer independently and safely.

Basic techniques for the nurse to use in assisting in the transfers of clients from a bed to a chair or a wheelchair, and vice versa, are identified in Chart 13–2. These techniques are also taught to the family member or other caregiver who will be caring for the client at home.

ALTERNATIVE TRANSFER TECHNIQUES Some clients cannot bear weight. For example, clients with a spinal cord injury resulting in quadriplegia either use a sliding board (which requires balance skills) or depend on the nurse or the therapist for transfers, using a "bear hug" technique. The sitting client places his or her arms around the nurse's neck while the nurse lifts the client from the bed to the chair, or vice versa. Another person assists with the transfer by stabilizing the wheelchair and holding on to the client's waist. Most physical therapists recommend that clients wear pants or a gait belt so that the assistant can hold on to the belt during the transfer.

POTENTIAL PROBLEMS WITH TRANSFERS Before any client transfer, the nurse carefully observes the client for potential problems. Orthostatic, or postural, hypotension is a common problem for clients in rehabilitation. If the client moves from a lying to a sitting or standing position too quickly, the client's blood pressure drops and he or she becomes dizzy or faints as a result. This complication contributes to falls, which are common in any client with impaired mobility. The problem is worsened when clients, especially elderly clients, are taking antihypertensive med-

CHART 13–2

Nursing Care Highlight ♦ Transfer Techniques

Bed to Wheelchair or Chair

1. Place the chair at an angle to the bed on the client's strong side.
2. Lock the wheelchair brakes or secure the chair position.
3. Assist the client to stand and move his or her strong hand to the armrest.
4. Keep the client's body weight forward and pivot.
5. When the client's legs touch the chair edge, assist the client in sitting.

Wheelchair or Chair to Bed

1. Place the chair with the client's strong side next to the bed.
2. Lock the wheelchair brakes or secure.
3. Assist the client to stand and move the client's strong hand to the armrest.
4. Keep the client's body weight forward and pivot.
5. When the client's legs touch the bed edge, assist the client in sitting and then reclining.

Use of a Sliding Board

1. Place the chair or wheelchair as close to the bed as possible.
2. Remove the armrest from the chair or (if removable) wheelchair.
3. Powder the sliding board.
4. Place the sliding board under the client's buttocks.
5. Instruct the client to reach toward the client's side.
6. Assist the client in sliding gently to the bed.

ications. The nurse helps the client change position slowly with frequent rest periods to allow the blood pressure to stabilize. The nurse may take the client's blood pressure with the client in lying, sitting, and standing positions to examine the differences. More than a 20 mmHg drop in systolic pressure between positions indicates orthostatic hypotension. The nurse notifies the physician about this change.

Another potential problem for the client who requires transfers is weight gain. Because clients undergoing rehabilitation have impaired mobility, many clients tend to gain weight. Excessive weight hinders transfers both for the nurse or the therapist who is assisting and for the client who is learning to transfer independently. The client is usually weighed every week to check for weight gain or loss.

Gait Training The physical therapist works with clients for gait training if they are able to ambulate. While regaining the ability to ambulate, clients may need to use canes or walkers (Fig. 13–4). When working with clients who are using such assistive devices, also known as ambulatory aids, the physical therapist ensures that the client has a level surface on which to walk. The nurse reinforces the physical therapist's instructions and encourages the client to practice. The goal is for the client to walk independently with or without an assistive device. Elderly clients typically use a walker for a broader base of support. Younger clients or clients with minimal impairment often progress to the use of a hemi-cane or straight cane. Chart 13–3 outlines how to use assistive devices for ambulation.

Some clients never regain the ability to walk because of their impairment, such as multiple sclerosis and spinal cord injury. These clients may become wheelchair-dependent and need to learn wheelchair mobility skills. With the help of physical and occupational therapy, most clients can learn to move anywhere they want in the wheelchair.

Prevention of Complications During the rehabilitation phase, clients are vulnerable to complications of immobility. Table 13–3 lists common complications and major strategies that the nurse can use to help prevent each complication. Implementing range-of-motion (ROM) routines, adhering to schedules for turning and repositioning the client, and maintaining skin care are constant components of rehabilitation nursing care to prevent the complications of immobility. The key is to increase the client's mobility.

One way to increase mobility, even with clients who are bedridden, is through range-of-motion exercises. Range-of-motion techniques are beneficial for any client with decreased mobility (Table 13–4). Although basic range-of-motion techniques are presented in basic nursing textbooks, a few key principles are pertinent for rehabilitation nursing care:

1. The human body contains more joints than simply the knees, the hips, the elbows, and the shoulders. For range-of-motion techniques to be effective in preventing musculoskeletal contractures, the client must exercise *all* joints, including each joint of the fingers, hands, toes, and so forth.
2. In performing range-of-motion activities, the nurse or client completes full-range movement of each joint five times or more and completes the entire process at least three times daily.
3. The nurse does not move joints beyond points at which the client expresses pain or the nurse perceives stiffness or difficulty.

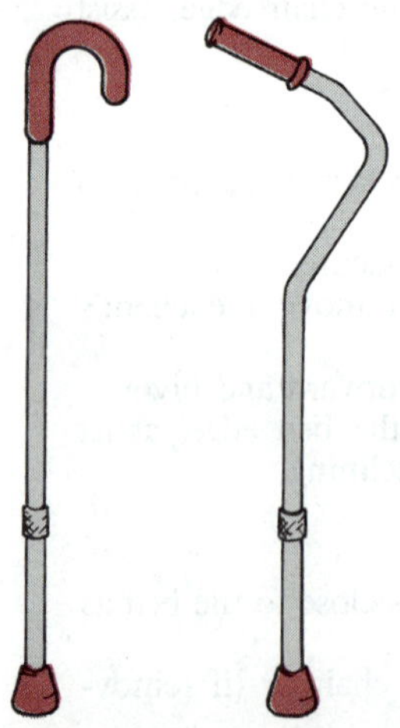

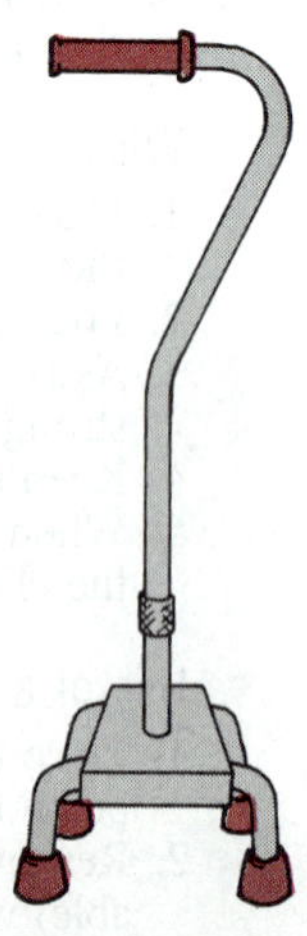

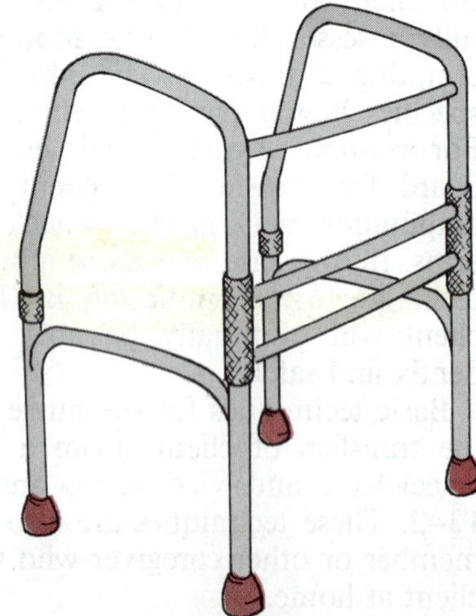

FIGURE 13–4 ◆ Assistive devices for ambulation. Assistive devices vary in the amount of support they provide. A straight cane provides less support than a quadripod cane or walker.

CHART 13–3

Nursing Care Highlight ◆ Gait Training Techniques

Walker-Assisted

1. Apply a gait belt around the client's waist.
2. Assist the client to a standing position.
3. Assist the client in placing both hands on the walker.
4. Ensure that the client is well balanced.
5. Assist the client repeatedly to perform the following sequence:
   a. Lift the walker.
   b. Move the walker 2 ft forward and set it down on all legs.
   c. While resting on the walker, take small steps.
   d. Check balance.

Cane-Assisted

1. Apply a gait belt around the client's waist.
2. Assist the client to a standing position.
3. Assist the client in placing his or her strong hand on the cane.
4. Ensure that the client is well balanced.
5. Assist the client repeatedly to perform the following sequence:
   a. Move the cane forward.
   b. Move the weaker leg one step forward.
   c. Move the stronger leg one step forward.
   d. Check balance.

Clients with decreased mobility who are able to follow directions are taught by the nurse and the physical therapist to perform active or active-assisted range-of-motion exercises.

SELF CARE DEFICIT

PLANNING: CLIENT GOALS The primary goal is that the client will become independent in activities of daily living to the extent possible based on the client's disability.

INTERVENTIONS Activities of daily living, or self-care activities, include eating, bathing, dressing, grooming, and toileting. The nurse encourages clients to perform as much self-care as possible. The nurse consults with the occupational therapist to identify ways in which self-care activities can be modified so that the client can perform them independently. For example, the occupational therapist teaches a hemiplegic client to put a shirt on by placing the affected arm in the sleeve first and putting the unaffected arm in the appropriate sleeve next. The nurse reinforces this dressing technique and encourages the client to practice.

Use of Assistive-Adaptive Devices A variety of assistive-adaptive devices are available for clients with chronic illness and disability. An assistive-adaptive device, or self-care support device, is any item that enables the client to perform all or part of an activity independently. Table 13–5 identifies common devices and describes their use.

TABLE 13–3 Prevention of Some Common Hazards of Immobility

Body System	Complication	Prevention
Musculoskeletal	• Contractures • Foot drop • Osteoporosis • Susceptibility to fractures • Muscular atrophy	• Range-of-motion exercises • Foot support while in bed, range-of-motion activities • Range-of-motion exercises • Weight-bearing exercises • Passive or active range-of-motion exercises
Gastrointestinal	• Constipation	• Increased activity level • Increased fluid intake
Cardiovascular	• Decreased cardiac output • Increased venous stasis • Thrombus formation • Embolism	• Range-of-motion exercises • Exercise, support hose, or antiembolism stockings • Exercise, support hose, or antiembolism stockings • Avoidance of leg massage
Neurologic	• Disorientation • Postural hypotension	• Sleep-wake schedule in accord with light-dark pattern • Reorientation (to person, place, and time) • Control of sensory stimulation • Avoidance of sudden position changes
Renal/Urinary	• Calculi	• Decreased dietary calcium level • Increased fluid intake • Maintenance of acidic urine
Respiratory	• Pneumonia	• Frequent repositioning • Respiratory exercises
Integumentary	• Pressure sores	• Frequent repositioning • Pressure relief devices • Skin care

TABLE 13–4 Types of Range-of-Motion Exercises

Type	Description	Indications
Passive	• Exercises are performed by the nurse for the client.	• The client is too weak to participate actively.
Active	• Exercises are performed by the client.	• The client is able to complete range-of-motion movements.
Assisted, or active-assisted	• Exercises are performed by the client but are guided by the nurse or the therapist.	• The client is weak and needs assistance.
Resistive	• The actions of the client are in opposition to those performed by the nurse or the therapist.	• The client has full range of motion, and an increase in strength is desired.

TABLE 13–5 Uses of Assistive-Adaptive Devices

Device	Use
Buttonhook	• Threaded through the buttonhole to enable clients with weak finger mobility to button shirts. • Alternative uses include serving as a pencil holder or a cigarette holder.
Extended shoe horn	• Assists in the application of shoes for clients with decreased mobility. • Alternative uses include turning light switches off or on while the client is in a wheelchair.
Plate guard	• Applied to a plate to assist clients with weak hand and arm mobility to feed themselves.
Gel pad	• Placed under a plate or a glass to prevent dishes from slipping and moving. • Alternative uses include placement under bathing and grooming items to prevent their moving.
Foam build-ups	• Applied to eating utensils to assist clients with weak handgrasps to feed themselves. • Alternative uses include the application to pens and pencils to assist with writing or over a buttonhook to assist with grasping the device.
Hook and loop fastener (Velcro) straps	• Applied to utensils, a buttonhook, or a pencil to slip over the hand and provide a method of stabilizing the device when the client's handgrasp is weak.
Long-handled reacher	• Assists in obtaining items located on high shelves or at ground level for clients who are not able to change positions easily.

Many department stores carry clothing and assistive-adaptive devices designed for clients with disabilities. The occupational therapist works with the client to determine the client's specific needs with regard to such equipment. In addition, the nurse and the occupational therapist help the client look for creative and inexpensive alternatives to meeting needs. For example, barbecue tongs may be used as "reachers" for pulling up pants or obtaining items on high shelves. A foam curler with the plastic insert removed may be placed over a pencil or eating utensil to make a built-up device. The client might use an extended shoe horn to operate light switches from wheelchair height. Hook and loop fasteners (Velcro) sewn on clothes can prevent the frustrations caused by buttons and zippers.

Energy Conservation Nurses work with occupational therapists to assess the client's self-care abilities and to determine possible ways of conserving energy. Fatigue is commonly associated with chronic and disabling conditions. The nurse and the therapist develop strategies for energy conservation after evaluating the client's self-care routines. Preparation for activities of daily living can be helpful in reducing the client's effort and energy expenditure (e.g., the client gathers all needed equipment before starting grooming routines). The nurse can teach clients with high energy levels in the morning to schedule energy-intensive activities in the morning rather than later in the day or evening. Spacing activities is also helpful for saving energy. Additionally, allowing time to rest before and after eating and toileting decreases the strain on the client's energy level.

HIGH RISK FOR IMPAIRED SKIN INTEGRITY

PLANNING: CLIENT GOALS The primary goal is that the client will have intact skin.

INTERVENTIONS An enormous variety of topical and mechanical remedies have been used to prevent and treat pressure sores, or ulcers, with varying success. Pressure reduction is a nursing intervention that may be achieved when the nurse temporarily repositions the client or alters the physical properties of the mattress surface, such as adding a mattress overlay (Braden & Bergstrom, 1992).

Turning and Repositioning The *best* intervention to prevent skin impairment is frequent position changes in combination with adequate skin care and sufficient nutritional intake. In general, the nurse turns and repositions the client every 2 hours; however, this may not be sufficient for people who are frail and have thin skin, especially elderly people (Chart 13–4). Therefore, the nurse assesses the client's skin condition each time the client is turned and repositioned to determine the best turning schedule. For example, if the client has been sleeping for 2 hours and the nurse decides to postpone turning for 1 hour, reddened areas over the client's bony prominences may be present. If such reddened areas do not fade within

30 minutes after pressure relief, they may be classified as pre-ulcer areas, or stage I pressure areas (see Chap. 67). Some clients need to be turned and repositioned every hour to prevent the development of pressure sores; others may tolerate 2 to 3 hours between turnings.

For the client who sits for prolonged periods in a wheelchair, the nurse repositions the client at least every 1 to 2 hours. Clients who are able are taught to perform "wheelchair pushups" by using their arms to lift their buttocks off the wheelchair seat for 10 seconds or longer every hour, or more often if needed. The physical therapist helps the client strengthen arm muscles in preparation for teaching wheelchair pushups.

Skin Care Adequate skin care is an essential component of prevention. The nurse performs or assists the client in completing skin care each time the client is turned, repositioned, or bathed. Skin care includes cleaning soiled areas, followed by careful drying, massage, and application of body lotion. For clients who are incontinent, topical creams or ointments can help to protect the skin from moisture, which facilitates skin breakdown. If pre-ulcer (reddened) areas are noted, the nurse does not rub these areas because this causes more extensive damage to the already fragile capillary system. Instead, the nurse carefully observes the pre-ulcer areas for further breakdown and relieves pressure on the areas as much as possible.

Nutrition Clients need sufficient nutrition both to repair wounds and to prevent pressure sores. The nurse collaborates with the dietitian to assess the client's food selection and ensure that it contains adequate protein and carbohydrates. Both the nurse and the dietitian closely monitor the client's weight and serum albumin level. If either of these indexes decreases significantly, the client may be given high-protein, high-carbohydrate food supplements, such as milkshakes, or commercial preparations, such as Ensure Plus (also see Chap. 61).

Mechanical Devices Pressure-relieving devices include waterbeds, foam (egg crate) or gel mattresses or pads, air mattresses, alternating-pressure mattresses, and air-fluidized beds. Mattress overlays, such as foam, air, and gel types, are controversial because their effectiveness has not been proven. The nurse and the client usually decide the type of device. The use of any mechanical device (except air-fluidized beds) does not eliminate the need for turning and repositioning.

Specialty beds are categorized as either "low air loss" or "air-fluidized." Air-fluidized therapy (e.g., Clinitron or FluidAir bed) provides the most effective pressure relief. The client is maintained in a nearly pressure-free environment (Fig. 13–5). These beds are generally not used for the prevention of skin breakdown; they are reserved for severe skin problems that have not healed with use of a conventional bed or other mechanical device. If optimal nutrition and healing conditions are maintained, skin breakdowns that have occurred should heal with continued use of air-fluidized therapy. The primary disadvantage is its expense, which may exceed several hundred dollars for each day of use. The cost of air-fluidized therapy may be reimbursed by some health insurance providers, such as Medicare.

CHART 13–4

Nursing Focus on the Elderly ◆ Special Considerations in Rehabilitation

- When getting the client out of bed, move the client or instruct the client to move or sit up slowly to prevent orthostatic hypotension. This problem is most common in elderly clients who take antihypertensive medications.
- Turn the client more often than every 2 hours even if it is just a minor position change. Skin becomes thinner and more fragile with age.
- Determine whether the client had any problem with urinary patterns before the illness or rehabilitation. A client with a previous problem may not have a successful bladder training program.
- Be aware that intestinal motility decreases with age, which leads to constipation.
- Assess the client's support system of family and significant others. Many elderly clients have no spouse or close friends who would usually serve as a support network.

ALTERED PATTERNS OF URINARY ELIMINATION

PLANNING: CLIENT GOALS The primary goals are that the client will:

- Achieve a personally acceptable form of urinary elimination
- Be free from urinary complications

INTERVENTIONS Neurologic disabilities may interfere with successful bladder control in a client undergoing rehabilitation. These disabilities result in three basic functional types of neurogenic bladder:

- Reflex bladder
- Flaccid bladder
- Uninhibited bladder

A *reflex (upper motor neuron) bladder* causes incontinence that is characterized by sudden gushing voids. However, the bladder does not usually empty completely. A reflex bladder is also sometimes referred to as a "spastic" bladder. Neurologic problems affecting the upper motor neuron typically occur with high-level or mid-level spinal cord injuries, above the 12th thoracic vertebra (T-12). These injuries result in a failure of impulse transmission from the lower spinal cord areas to the cortex of the brain. When the bladder fills and transmits impulses to the spinal

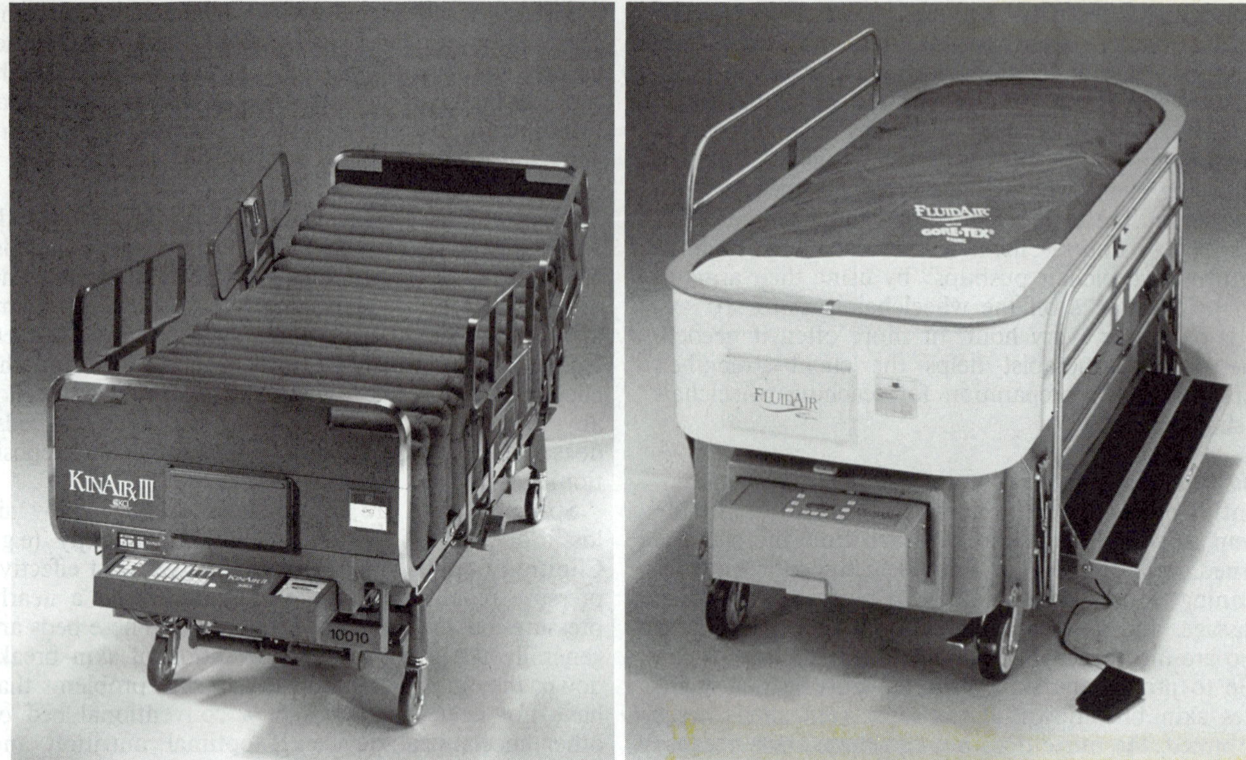

FIGURE 13–5 ♦ Pressure relief devices. *Left,* KinAir beds provide controlled air suspension to redistribute body weight away from bony prominences. *Right,* FluidAir beds use airflow and bead fluidization. Both of these beds are covered with Gore-Tex fabric, which resists tearing. This fabric is also waterproof and acts as a barrier against bacteria. (Courtesy of Kinetic Concepts, Inc., San Antonio, TX.)

cord, the client is not conscious of the filling sensation. However, because there is no injury at the lower spinal cord level and the voiding reflex arc is intact, the efferent (motor) impulse is relayed and the bladder contracts.

A *flaccid (lower motor neuron) bladder* results in urinary retention and overflow (dribbling). Injuries that cause damage to the lower motor neuron at the spinal cord level of S2-4 (e.g., multiple sclerosis and spinal cord injury below T-12) may directly interfere with the reflex arc or may result in inappropriate interpretation of the impulses to the brain. The bladder fills, and afferent (sensory) impulses conduct the message via the spinal cord to the cortical region of the brain. Because of the injury, however, the impulse is not interpreted correctly by the cortical bladder center in the brain, and there is a failure to respond with a message for the bladder to contract.

An *uninhibited bladder* may occur when the client has a neurologic problem that affects the cortical bladder center of the brain (frontal lobe), such as stroke or brain injury. When the bladder needs to empty, the client has little sensorimotor control and cannot wait until he or she is on the commode or bedpan before voiding. Therefore, the client is incontinent, but the bladder may not completely empty.

Bladder Training The nurse can teach three techniques to assist the client in "repatterning" voiding, or bladder training:

- Facilitating, or triggering, techniques
- Intermittent catheterization
- Consistent scheduling of toileting routines

These techniques may not be as effective in a client with physiologic changes associated with aging.

FACILITATING OR TRIGGERING TECHNIQUES The nurse uses facilitating (triggering) techniques to stimulate voiding (Table 13–6). If there is an *upper* motor neuron problem, and the reflex arc is intact (reflex bladder pattern), any stimulus that sends the message to the spinal cord level S2-4 that the bladder might be full can initiate the voiding response. Such techniques include stroking the medial aspect of the thigh, pinching the area above the groin, pulling pubic hair, massaging the penoscrotal area, pinching the posterior aspect of the glans penis, and providing digital anal stimulation.

When the client has a *lower* motor neuron problem, the voiding reflex arc is not intact (flaccid bladder pattern) and additional stimulation may be needed to initiate voiding. Two techniques used to facilitate voiding are the Valsalva maneuver and the Credé maneuver. In teaching the client the Valsalva maneuver, the nurse instructs the client to hold his or her breath and bear down as if trying to defecate. The nurse assists the client to perform the Credé maneuver by placing the client's hand in a cupped position directly over the bladder area, and instructing the client to push inward and downward as if massaging the bladder to empty.

INTERMITTENT CATHETERIZATION Intermittent catheterization is a method of bladder training frequently used for disorders involving a flaccid bladder, generally caused by a lower motor neuron problem. In assisting the client with intermittent catheterization, the nurse inserts a urinary catheter every 2 to 3 hours initially. This is done after the client has attempted voiding and has used the Valsalva and Credé maneuvers. If less than 150 mL of residual urine is obtained, the nurse increases the interval between catheterizations. The interval may be to 3 to 4 hours, according to the physician's order or the health care agency protocol. The interval may be gradually increased to 4 to 6 hours, but the client should not go beyond 8 hours between catheterizations. The exception is when the residual urine volume is less than 150 mL each time with an adequate intake of fluids. If the client will be performing intermittent self-catheterization at home after discharge from the rehabilitation facility, the nurse instructs the client on clean (not sterile) technique.

Intermittent catheterizations may also be done to determine residual urine volumes for clients with a reflex (upper motor neuron) or uninhibited bladder. Clients with these types of neurogenic bladders can void but often do not empty the bladder completely. The nurse catheterizes the client within 10 minutes after the client voids to determine the residual amount of urine in the bladder. For most clients, the desired amount is less than 100 mL of residual urine.

TOILETING SCHEDULE Consistent toileting routines may be the best way of re-establishing voiding continence when the client displays an uninhibited bladder pattern (associated with brain damage or head injury). The nurse assesses the client's previous voiding pattern and determines the client's daily routine. At a minimum, the nurse assists the client with voiding in the morning after rising, before and after meals, before and after physical activity, and at bedtime. The nurse considers the client's bladder capacity, which may range from 100 to 500 mL, as well as the client's mobility limitations and clothing that may be restrictive. The nurse determines bladder capacity by measuring the client's urine output. The nurse ensures that the client is aware of nearby bathrooms at all times or has a call system to contact the nurse for assistance.

Drug Therapy Medications that may be used for urinary elimination problems include cholinergics (to promote bladder emptying), antispasmodics (to prevent incontinence), and skeletal muscle relaxants (to decrease spasticity, which promotes self-care) (Chart 13–5). Medications are not usually prescribed by the physician in the initial management of bladder problems but may be used to assist a bladder training program. The nurse reports the client's progress in bladder training to the physician so that the physician can make the best decision regarding drug therapy. In general, anticholinergics, antispasmodics, and skeletal muscle relaxants help to promote continence in clients with a reflex (upper motor neuron) bladder. Cholinergics, such as bethanechol chloride (Urecholine), may decrease urinary retention problems in clients with a flaccid bladder. This drug type may also facilitate complete bladder emptying in a client with a large residual volume, such as in reflex bladder problems. Clients with an uninhibited bladder do not routinely require medications for bladder training programs unless urinary function is affected by additional pathologic changes.

Fluid Intake The nurse instructs the client to maintain an adequate intake of fluids, at least 2000 to 2500 mL/day. The nurse decreases this amount to prevent complications in clients with congestive heart disease or renal problems, especially elderly clients. Some clients, especially those with flaccid bladder patterns, decrease fluid intake after 6 or 7 PM to avoid the need for catheterization during the night.

The nurse encourages the client to drink fluids that promote an acidic urine, including large amounts of cranberry juice, prune juice, bouillon, tomato juice, and water. Fluids that promote an alkaline urine are discouraged, including citrus juices, excessive amounts of milk and milk products, and carbonated beverages. An acidic urine is preferred to minimize risks of urinary tract infection and calculus (stone)

TABLE 13–6 Management of Altered Urinary Elimination

Functional Type	Neurologic Disability	Clinical Manifestations	Re-establishing Voiding Patterns
Reflex (spastic)	• Upper motor neuron spinal cord injury above T-12	• Urinary frequency, incontinence	• Triggering or facilitating techniques • Medications
Flaccid	• Lower motor neuron spinal cord injury below T-12 (affects S2-4 reflex arc)	• Urinary retention, overflow	• Valsalva and Credé maneuvers • Medications
Uninhibited	• Brain damage from injury or stroke	• Frequency, urgency, incontinence, voiding in small amounts	• Intermittent catheterization • Consistent toileting schedule • Regulation of fluid intake

CHART 13-5

Drug Therapy for Clients in Bladder Training Programs

Drug	Usual Dosage	Nursing Interventions	Rationale
Cholinergics			
Bethanechol chloride (Urecholine)	• 10–50 mg bid–qid PO	• Give 1 hr before or 2 hr after meals. • Instruct clients to change positions slowly. • Give 1 hr before toileting or triggering or facilitating measure.	• This agent may cause nausea and vomiting. • Orthostatic hypotension is a possible side effect. • The drug is effective when using other measures for bladder training.
Antispasmodics			
Oxybutynin chloride (Ditropan)	• 5 mg bid or tid PO	• Instruct the client to avoid driving. • Instruct the client to avoid hot environmental temperatures. • Assess the client for urinary retention.	• Vertigo, drowsiness, and blurred vision may occur. • Sweating is suppressed. • Retention may be a side effect of the drug.
Flavoxate hydrochloride (Urispas)	• 100–200 mg tid or qid PO	• Instruct the client to avoid driving. • Instruct the client to avoid hot environmental temperatures. • Assess the client for urinary retention.	• Drowsiness, mental confusion, and blurred vision may occur. • Sweating is suppressed. • Retention may be a side effect of the drug.
Skeletal Muscle Relaxants			
Dantrolene (Dantrium)	• 25 mg once daily PO initially; increase to 25 mg bid–qid, then by 25-mg increments up to 100 mg	• Instruct the client to avoid driving. • Instruct the client to avoid prolonged sun exposure.	• Fatigue, dizziness, and muscular weakness are side effects. • Photosensitivity may occur.
Baclofen (Lioresal)	• 5 mg tid PO; may increase by 5 mg daily until desired effect attained to maximum of 80 mg	• Instruct the client to avoid alcohol. • Instruct the client to avoid driving.	• Alcohol potentiates the drug's effects. • Drowsiness and dizziness may occur.

formation, although this belief is controversial. Some microorganisms, such as *Escherichia coli,* grow best in acidic environments.

In addition, the nurse discourages high-calorie fluids for overweight clients. The disabled client has more difficulty with mobility and self-care if weight is not controlled.

Prevention of Complications The client with Altered Patterns of Urinary Elimination is at risk for skin breakdown from incontinence, urinary tract infection from urinary retention, and urinary calculi from urinary retention and stasis. The nurse keeps the client clean and dry and provides skin care as described under High Risk for Impaired Skin Integrity earlier in this chapter. (See Chapter 70 for preventive measures for urinary tract infection and calculi.)

CONSTIPATION

PLANNING: CLIENT GOALS The primary goals are that the client will:

- Achieve a personally acceptable form of bowel elimination
- Be free from bowel elimination complications

INTERVENTIONS Neurologic problems often affect the client's bowel pattern by causing:

- A reflex bowel
- A flaccid bowel
- An uninhibited bowel

Upper motor neuron diseases and injuries, such as a high-level or mid-level spinal cord injury, may result in a *reflex* (spastic) bowel pattern, with defecation occurring suddenly and without warning. With a reflex pattern, any facilitating or triggering mechanism may lead to defecation if the lower colon contains stool. Examples of facilitating or triggering techniques include providing anal stimulation (by inserting a finger, using either a finger cot or rubber glove and lubrication, to the first joint), gently pinching the anus, and pulling pubic hair. Digital stimulation should not be used for clients with cardiac disease because of the risk of inducing a vagal response (a rapid decrease in heart rate).

Lower motor neuron diseases and injuries interfere with transmission of the nervous impulse across the reflex arc and may result in a *flaccid* bowel pattern, with defecation occurring infrequently and in small amounts. The use of facilitating and triggering mechanisms in combination with a toileting schedule, suppository use, and disimpaction yields the best results. The client may be able to self-administer the suppository or disimpact if necessary.

Neurologic injuries affecting the brain may cause an *uninhibited* bowel pattern, with frequent defecation, urgency, and complaints of hard stool. Clients may manage uninhibited bowel patterns through a consistent toileting schedule, a high-fiber diet, and the use of stool softeners.

Bowel Training An overview of management techniques for bowel dysfunction is presented in Table 13–7. In many cases, clients are not able to regain control over their bowel function in the manner previously possible. The nurse assists the client in designing a bowel elimination program that accommodates the disability.

The nurse works with the client to schedule bowel elimination as close to the client's previous routine as possible. For example, a client who had stools at noon every other day before the illness or injury should have the bowel program scheduled likewise. An exception is if the client prefers another time that best fits into his or her daily routine. If the client is employed during the day, a time-consuming bowel elimination program in the morning may not be reasonable. The client may prefer to change the bowel protocol until the evening, when there is more time.

Drug Therapy Bowel training programs for clients with neurologic problems are often designed to include the combination of suppository use and a consistent toileting schedule. Although medications should not be a first choice when a bowel training program is being formulated, the nurse routinely considers the need for a suppository if the client does not re-establish defecation habits through consistent scheduling of toileting, dietary modification, anal stimulation, and disimpaction.

The most common agents prescribed by physicians as suppositories in bowel training programs are bisacodyl (Dulcolax) and glycerin. Suppositories must be placed against the bowel wall to stimulate the sacral reflex arc and promote rectal emptying. Both agents are equivalent in effect, with results occurring in 15 to 30 minutes. The suppository is administered by the nurse when the client expects to defecate. For example, if a client had a previous bowel habit of defecating every other day after breakfast, the suppository is administered every other day after breakfast. Ordinarily, administering the suppository every second or third day is effective in re-establishing defecation patterns. Depending on each client's need, other medications, such as laxatives, may be indicated for bowel training programs.

NUTRITION Bowel elimination is directly related to the type and quality of food and fluid ingested. A high-fiber diet is a mainstay of most bowel training programs and includes whole-grain foods, bran, and fresh and dried fruits. Increasing dietary fiber is effective in facilitating defecation only if the client reduces fat intake.

PREVENTION OF COMPLICATIONS Common complications of any bowel training program are constipation, diarrhea, and flatulence. The nurse assesses clients for these complications and modifies the bowel training

TABLE 13–7 Management of Bowel Dysfunction

Functional Type	Neurologic Disability	Dysfunction	Re-establishing Defecation Patterns
Reflex (spastic)	• Upper motor neuron spinal cord injury above T-12	• Defecation without warning	• Triggering mechanisms • Facilitation techniques • High-fiber diet • Suppository use • Consistent toileting schedule
Flaccid	• Lower motor neuron spinal cord injury below T-12 (affects S2-4 reflex arc)	• Infrequent, small stools	• Triggering or facilitating techniques • High-fiber diet • Suppository use • Consistent toileting schedule • Manual disimpaction
Uninhibited	• Brain damage from injury or stroke	• Frequency, urgency, and constipation	• Consistent toileting schedule • High-fiber diet • Stool softener use

program accordingly, in collaboration with the physician and the dietitian.

INEFFECTIVE INDIVIDUAL COPING

PLANNING: CLIENT GOALS The major goal is that the client will learn to cope with the chronic illness or disability and participate in the rehabilitation program.

INTERVENTIONS The client with a disability often has a poor self-concept because of changes in body image from structural or functional changes. The use of an assistive device, such as a wheelchair, also differentiates the client from most other people, and the client may not want to accept that he or she needs the device. The nurse encourages clients to talk about their feelings and asks questions to elicit specific information that can help in assessing the client's acceptance of and coping with the disability.

A disability also affects a person's role in society. For instance, a young medical student may fall from a ladder and become a paraplegic, and plans for a career as a surgeon are altered. A middle-aged farmer may be burned severely when his tractor catches on fire. He can no longer care for his farm and his wife takes over during his rehabilitation process. An elderly woman who cares for her grandchildren is crippled with rheumatoid arthritis and can no longer provide child care. These examples illustrate role changes and losses in the lives of these three people.

In addition to role changes, relationships with people change. Socializing with friends and family when a person feels "different" may be a strain. Intimate relationships are affected because sexual dysfunction may result from disability. The nurse should be sensitive to these issues and should not avoid discussing them.

The nurse assesses coping strategies and support systems that the client has used in the past so that they can be used during rehabilitation if needed. The nurse asks the client what strategies have been used in the past to cope successfully with life crises, if any. Spiritual and religious beliefs are important for some people and should not be overlooked as the nurse helps the client identify sources of support.

In a study by Raleigh (1992), clients with chronic illness reported that family and friends were a chief source of support. These support resources helped the clients have hope, which kept them motivated to help meet their goals (Research Applications for Nursing). (Chapters 7, 10, 11, and 12 provide specific interventions for ineffective coping, body image disorders, disturbances of sexuality, and loss, respectively.)

DISCHARGE PLANNING

HOME CARE PREPARATION

The nurse begins discharge planning at or before client admission. If the client is being transferred from a hospital to a rehabilitation unit or facility, the nurse orients the client to the change in routine and emphasizes the importance of self-care. When the client is admitted to the rehabilitation unit or facility, the nurse assesses the client's current living situation at home. The nurse determines, with the client and family members or significant others, the adequacy of the client's current situation and potential needs after discharge to the home. Clients with chronic illness and disability may require home care, assistance with activities of daily living, nursing care, or physical or occupational therapy after discharge. The nurse as-

RESEARCH APPLICATIONS FOR NURSING

For Families of People with Chronic Illnesses, Look Beyond the Client

Hough, E. E., Lewis, F. M., & Woods, N. F. (1991). Family response to mother's chronic illness. *Western Journal of Nursing Research, 13*, 568–596.

This study examined differences in families' responses to the mother's chronic illness. The study sample included 11 families from a larger sample of families. These 11 families were purposefully selected as representative of the positive and negative extremes in family coping and adjustment. The authors described the differences, reported in five family interviews during an 18-month period, that distinguish the family's coping with and adjustment to the impact of one of three chronic illnesses: breast cancer, diabetes, and fibrocystic breast disease.

The researchers did not find any differences in the degree of physical symptoms reported by the mothers in the two family types. The poorly adjusted families, however, had a greater number of stressors from sources that were unrelated to the chronic illness itself (e.g., unemployment and sickness of other family members). These families were also less likely to report positive experiences as a part of coping and did not perceive that adequate social support was provided by the spouse or friends. By contrast, the well-adjusted families reported positive meaning from their illness experience and felt that there was a great deal of support from spouses and friends.

Critique Although the sample was small and purposefully selected, the topic is an important issue for nurses who care for clients with chronic illness and their families. Only Caucasian middle class families were included in the study, but this may have been to control for other variables that could have affected the study's results.

Possible nursing implications The findings suggest that nurses may use this information in their assessment of families who have a member with a chronic illness. For example, the nurse should assess factors not related to the client's illness (e.g., employment and financial resources) as a source of stress contributing to inability to cope.

sesses these needs and plans with the client, the family or significant other, the social worker, the physical or vocational therapist, and the physician for the best ways to meet identified needs.

Before the client returns home, the nurse assesses the client's readiness for discharge from the rehabilitation facility. The client's home may be assessed in multiple ways.

PRE-DISCHARGE ASSESSMENT The nurse or the occupational therapist may visit the home before discharge to assess the home's layout and accessibility. For example, because of the stress of hospitalization, a client with a fractured hip, who is ambulating well with a walker, may neglect to explain to the nurse that the home has three steps at the entrance and that the bathroom is accessible by stairway only. The client may not consider it important to mention to the nurse that throw rugs, which do not provide a completely level surface on which to use a cane, are scattered throughout the apartment.

During a pre-discharge visit to the home, the nurse or the occupational therapist inspects the accessibility of the home in general and of the bathrooms, bedrooms, and kitchen. If the client will be wheelchair-dependent after discharge from the facility, ramps are needed to replace steps, and doorways should be checked for adequate width. Usually, a doorway width of 36 to 38 inches (slightly less than 1 meter) is sufficient for a standard-sized wheelchair. Any room that the client needs to use is checked. In the bedroom, there should be sufficient room for the client to maneuver transfers to and from the wheelchair and the bed.

Space requirements vary, depending on the client's need to use a wheelchair, a walker, or a cane. In the bathroom, grab bars may need to be installed before the client comes home. Bathtub benches can provide support for clients who have difficulty with mobility and, when used in combination with a hand-held showerhead, can provide easily accessible bathing facilities. Assessment of the kitchen may or may not be critical, depending on whether the client has help with cooking and preparing meals. If the client will be responsible for cooking after discharge from the hospital or facility, the kitchen is assessed for wheelchair or walker accessibility, appliance accessibility, and the need for adaptive equipment.

LEAVE-OF-ABSENCE VISIT A second method of assessing the client's home is through a brief home visit, also called a leave-of-absence (LOA) visit, by the client before discharge. The nurse prepares the client by explaining the need for the trial home visit and by assessing the client's comfort level with this idea. Clients who have been hospitalized for a lengthy period may feel intense anxiety about returning home. The nurse may allay such anxieties with careful preparation. Before the visit, the nurse meets with the client and family members or significant others to set goals for the visit and to identify specific tasks that the client should attempt during the time at home. After the client has been home, the nurse interviews the client to determine the success of the visit and to assess additional education or training needs before final discharge.

Going home may not be an option for all clients. Some clients may not have a support network of family members or significant others. For example, many elderly clients have no spouse or close friends living. Children may reside at a distance, which can make home care difficult. If there is no caregiver available, the family must decide whether care can be provided in the home by an outside resource or if the client needs to be admitted to a 24-hour supervised health care setting, such as a nursing home. Rehabilitation services are available in most long-term care settings (skilled nursing facilities) at least 5 days a week.

HEALTH TEACHING

Education of the client and the family is the cornerstone of nursing care. The nurse assesses every component of the client's care to determine how the client can be taught to perform activities of daily living independently. The nurse assesses the client's learning potential and cognitive capacity. As care is provided, the nurse explains the procedure and its rationale. The client is encouraged to perform or direct the technique independently to verify understanding. The nurse gives written material explaining the steps in the procedure to the client and family members to reinforce learning and to provide support with the technique after discharge. However, before giving the client written material, the nurse assesses the reading level of the material and determines whether it is appropriate for the client's reading ability and language skills.

PSYCHOSOCIAL PREPARATION

Any chronic illness or disability necessitates changes in a client's lifestyle and body image. The nurse assists the client in dealing with such changes by encouraging the client to verbalize feelings and emotions. The nurse also helps the client focus on existing capabilities instead of disabilities.

The client may fail to relate psychologically to the disability during hospitalization. For example, the client may display anger or frustration in attempting to perform self-care routines before discharge from the rehabilitation facility. The nurse encourages the client to be open about such feelings and to talk about ways to prevent worries from becoming realities after discharge.

The leave-of-absence home visit assists the client and family members or significant others in psychosocial preparation for discharge. It allows the client to experience the home situation while being able to return to the hospital environment after a few hours. Clients often find that their fears were not realized during the home visit, but frequently find new problems in the home that must be addressed before discharge. The nurse reviews this information with the client in preparation for discharge to the home.

HEALTH CARE RESOURCES

Various health care resources, such as physical therapy, home health nursing, and vocational counseling, are available to clients with chronic illness and disability after discharge to the home. The nurse assesses the client's need for additional care and support throughout the client's hospitalization and works with the social worker and the physician in arranging for home services.

EVALUATION

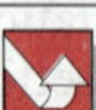

On the basis of the identified nursing diagnoses, the client and the nurse evaluate the rehabilitation interventions for the client with a disabling or chronic condition. Expected outcomes may include that the client will:

- Ambulate independently, with or without assistive devices, or be independent in wheelchair mobility skills
- Perform activities of daily living independently with or without assistive-adaptive devices
- Have intact skin
- Demonstrate effective urinary elimination through an individualized bladder training program
- Demonstrate effective bowel elimination through an individualized bowel training program
- State acceptance of the disability and use coping strategies effectively

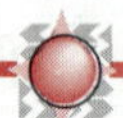

IMPLICATIONS FOR NURSING RESEARCH

Although there has been considerable research in the area of rehabilitation, less attention has been paid to clients with chronic illness or disabling conditions in settings other than rehabilitation units or facilities. Nursing research is beginning to examine the effects of chronic illnesses or disabling conditions on people to better enable them to provide appropriate nursing care.

Future nursing research should address the following questions:

♦ What part does spirituality play in a client's response to a chronic or disabling condition?
♦ What effect does nursing care have on the outcomes of clients with chronic or disabling conditions?
♦ What are the most efficient and cost-effective methods of reducing the occurrence of pressure sores in a rehabilitation setting?
♦ How can nurses keep clients motivated during the rehabilitation phase of health care?
♦ What special needs do elderly clients in rehabilitation programs have and how can they best be met?

SELECTED BIBLIOGRAPHY

*American Nurses' Association and Association of Rehabilitation Nurses. (1988). *Standards of rehabilitation nursing practice.* Kansas City: American Nurses' Association.

*Billhardt, B., & Stewart, A. (1989). Education as the key to rehabilitation. *Nursing Clinics of North America, 24,* 675–680.

Braden, B. J. (1992). Description of learned response to chronic illness: Depressed versus nondepressed self-help class participants. *Public Health Nursing, 9*(2), 103–108.

Braden, B. J., & Bergstrom, N. (1992). Pressure reduction. In G. M. Bulachek & J. C. McCloskey (Eds.), *Nursing interventions: Essential nursing treatments* (2nd ed., pp. 94–108). Philadelphia: W. B. Saunders.

*Carey, R. G., & Posavec, E. J. (1978). Program evaluation of a physical medicine and rehabilitation unit: A new approach. *Archives of Physical Medicine and Rehabilitation, 59,* 330–337.

Cohen, M. H. (1993). The unknown and the unknowable—managing sustained uncertainty. *Western Journal of Nursing Research, 15,* 77–96.

Dilorio, C., & Price, M. E. (1990). Swallowing: An assessment guide. *American Journal of Nursing, 90*(7), 38–41.

Douard, J. (1991). Chronic illness: A problem of passive injustice. *Journal of Clinical Ethics, 2*(3), 153–156.

Glick, O. J. (1992). Interventions related to activity and movement. *Nursing Clinics of North America, 27,* 541–568.

*Granger, C. V., & Gresham, G. E. (1984). *Functional assessment in rehabilitation medicine.* Baltimore: Williams & Wilkins.

Granger, C. V., Hamilton, B. B., Lenacre, J. M., Heinemann, A. W., & Wright, B. D. (1993). Performance profiles of the Functional Independence Measure. *Journal of Physical Medicine and Rehabilitation, 72,* 84–89.

*Hagen, C., & Malkmus, D. (1979). *Intervention strategies for language disorders secondary to head trauma.* Short courses conducted for the American Speech-Language-Hearing Association, Atlanta.

Helgeson, V. S. (1992). Moderators to the relationship between perceived control and adjustment to chronic illness. *Journal of Personality and Social Psychology, 63,* 565–666.

Hickey, J. V. (1992). *The clinical practice of neurological and neurosurgical nursing* (3rd ed.). Philadelphia: J. B. Lippincott.

Hough, E. E., Lewis, F. M., & Woods, N. F. (1991). Family response to mother's chronic illness. *Western Journal of Nursing Research, 13,* 568–596.

Institute of Medicine. (1990). *The second fifty years: Promoting health and preventing disability.* Washington, DC: National Academy Press.

Institute of Medicine. (1991). *Disability in America.* Washington, DC: National Academy Press.

Jensen, S. B. (1992). Sexuality and chronic illness: Biopsychosocial approach. *Seminars in Neurology, 12*(2), 135–140.

*Katz, S., et al. (1963). Studies of illness in the aged. The index of ADL: A standardized measure of biological and psychosocial function. *JAMA, 185,* 914–919.

Kirk, K. (1992). Confidence as a factor in chronic illness care. *Journal of Advanced Nursing, 17,* 1238–1242.
*Lazarus, R. S., & Folkman, S. (1984). *Stress, appraisal and coping.* New York: Springer.
Mayer, D. K. (1992). The health care implications of cancer rehabilitation in the twenty-first century. *Oncology Nursing Forum, 19,* 23–27.
McLane, A. M., & McShane, R. E. (1992). Bowel management. In G. M. Bulachek & J. C. McCloskey (Eds.), *Nursing interventions: Essential nursing treatments* (2nd ed., pp. 73–85). Philadelphia: W. B. Saunders.
Miller, J. M. (1991). *Coping with chronic illness: Overcoming powerlessness* (2nd ed.). Philadelphia: F. A. Davis.
*Orem, D. (1980). *Nursing concepts of practice.* New York: McGraw-Hill.
*Posavec, E. J., & Carey, R. G. (1982). Using a level of function scale (LORS-II) to evaluate the success of inpatient rehabilitation programs. *Rehabilitation Nursing, 7*(6), 17–19.
Raleigh, E. D. H. (1992). Sources of hope in chronic illness. *Oncology Nursing Forum, 19,* 443–448.
Robinson, K. M., Friedman, R. H., Kazis, L. E., Moskowitz, M. A., & Steel, R. K. (1993). Geriatrics training in physical medicine and rehabilitation. *Journal of Physical Medicine and Rehabilitation, 72,* 67–74.
*Schilder, P. (1935). *The image and appearance of the human body.* London: Kegan Paul, Trancy, Trubrer.
Schneider, E. L., & Guralnik, J. M. (1990). The aging of America: Impact on health care costs. *JAMA, 263,* 2335–2340.
Tate, D. G. (1992). Workers' disability and return to work. *American Journal of Physical Medicine and Rehabilitation, 71,* 92–96.
Warren, M. T. (1992). Maintaining identity in elderly couples with chronic illness. *Journal of Psychosocial Nursing and Mental Health Services, 30*(10), 8–11.
*World Health Organization. (1980). *International classification of impairments, disabilities and handicaps.* Geneva: Author.

SUGGESTED READINGS

Institute of Medicine. (1991). *Disability in America.* Washington, DC: National Academy Press.

This book is an excellent resource regarding the scope of problems related to disability in the United States. It discusses how to prevent disability and calls for a national program to focus on prevention.

McClane, A. M., & McShane, R. E. (1992). Bowel management. In G. M. Bulachek & J. C. McCloskey (Eds.), *Nursing interventions: Essential nursing treatments* (2nd ed., pp. 73–85). Philadelphia: W. B. Saunders.

This chapter discusses bowel management for any client who experiences bowel problems. A thorough discussion of diet, general exercise, medications, and pelvic floor exercises is included.

Miller, J. M. (1991). *Coping with chronic illness: Overcoming powerlessness* (2nd ed.). Philadelphia: F. A. Davis.

This book is based on the premise that clients with chronic illness experience powerlessness. The author provides many ideas for nurses in helping clients cope with their health problems.

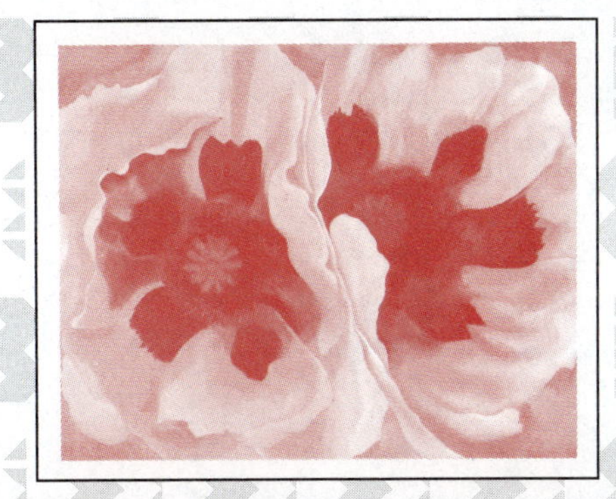

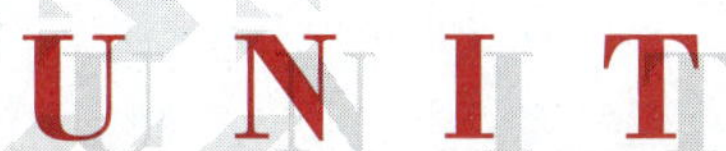

UNIT

3

Management of Clients with Fluid, Electrolyte, and Acid-Base Imbalances

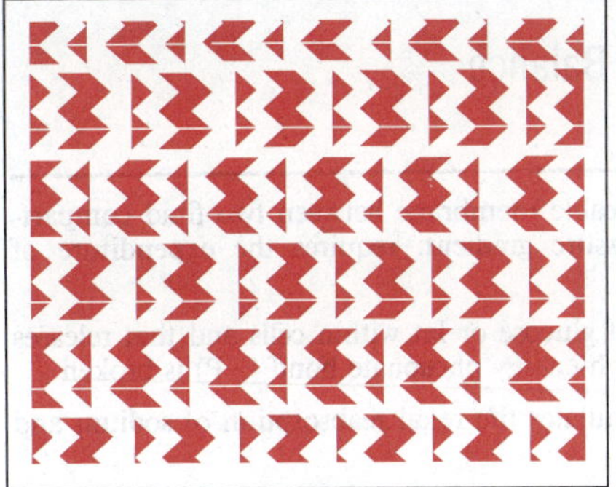

CHAPTER 14

Fluid and Electrolyte Balance

CHAPTER HIGHLIGHTS

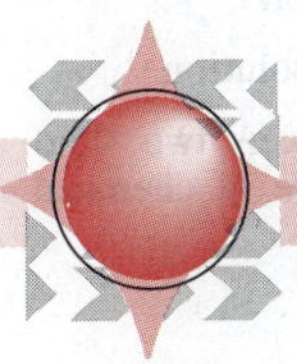

An assessment of fluid and electrolyte status involves examination of the function of every body system. To accomplish this large task, nurses need to understand fluid and electrolyte balance.

ANATOMY AND PHYSIOLOGY REVIEW

Physical and Biologic Influences on Fluid and Electrolyte Balance

Several important physical and biologic processes govern the proper balance of body fluids and electrolytes. These processes work together to regulate homeostasis (equilibrium) so that even when the external environment undergoes dramatic changes, the body's internal environment remains relatively unchanged.

Knowing the specific terminology related to solutions is necessary to understand the processes involved in fluid and electrolyte balance (Table 14-1). Solutions are composed of fluid and particles dissolved or suspended in the fluid. *Solvent* is the fluid portion of a solution (the solvent for human body fluids is always water). *Solutes* are the particles dissolved in the solution. The solutes vary in types

TABLE 14–1 Terminology Associated with Fluid and Electrolyte Balance

Term	Definition
Active transport	• Assisted movement of a substance through a permeable membrane between two fluid compartments against a concentration, electrical, or pressure gradient; requires the expenditure of chemical energy
Adenosine triphosphate (ATP)	• A substance that is generated by the metabolism of glucose or fat within cells and that releases chemical energy for physiologic function when a high-energy phosphate bond (~P) is broken
Aldosterone	• A hormone secreted by the adrenal cortex that stimulates the renal reabsorption of sodium and water and the renal excretion of potassium
Anion	• A molecule (electrolyte) that carries an overall negative charge when dissolved in water
Antidiuretic hormone (ADH)	• A hormone secreted from the posterior pituitary gland that increases the renal reabsorption of pure water and decreases urinary output
Atrial natriuretic peptide (ANP)	• A hormone secreted by cardiac atrial cells that increases renal excretion of sodium and water
Brownian motion	• Inherent molecular motion
Capillary (plasma) hydrostatic pressure	• The force generated by fluid within a capillary that tends to move fluid out from the capillary and into the interstitial space
Capillary (plasma) osmotic pressure	• The force generated by the concentration of plasma solutes (osmotic and oncotic pressures) that tends to retain fluid within the capillary or move fluid from the interstititial space into the capillary
Cation	• A molecule (electrolyte) that carries an overall positive charge when dissolved in water
Cofactor	• A substance required to enhance the activity of an enzyme or a physiologic reaction
Colloidal oncotic pressure	• The osmotic pressure exerted by the concentration of colloids (proteins) within a solution
Diffusion	• Unimpeded movement of a substance through a permeable membrane between two fluid compartments down a concentration gradient; does not require the expenditure of chemical energy
Disequilibrium	• A state in which two fluid compartments are unequal in at least one characteristic
Electrolytes	• Substances that carry an electrical charge when dissolved in water
Electroneutrality	• A state in which a body fluid has an equal number of cations and anions, so that the fluid does not express an electrical charge
Equilibrium	• A state in which two fluid compartments are equal in one or more characteristics
Extracellular fluid (ECF)	• Body fluid present outside of cells; includes plasma, interstitial fluid, and transcellular fluid
Facilitated diffusion	• Assisted movement of a substance through a permeable membrane between two fluid compartments down a concentration gradient; does not require the expenditure of chemical energy
Filtration	• The movement of fluid through a biologic membrane as a result of hydrostatic pressure differences on the two sides of the membrane
Gradient	• A graded difference in some characteristic between two fluid compartments
Hydrostatic pressure	• The force or pressure exerted by static water in a confined space—"water-pushing" pressure
Hypertonic (hyperosmotic)	• Any solution with a solute concentration (osmolarity) greater than that of normal body fluids (>310 mOsm/L)
Hypotonic (hyposmotic)	• Any solution with a solute concentration (osmolarity) less than that of normal body fluids (<270 mOsm/L)
Impermeable membrane	• A membrane separating two fluid compartments that does not permit the movement of one or more substances through the membrane (by diffusion) from one compartment to the other
Insensible fluid loss	• Unregulated fluid losses from the skin, the gastrointestinal tract, wounds, and the pulmonary epithelium
Interstitial fluid	• Fluid present in tissues between cells
Intracellular fluid (ICF)	• Fluid found inside cells
Isotonic (isosmotic)	• Any solution with a solute concentration equal to the osmolarity of normal body fluids or normal saline (0.9% NaCl), ~300 mOsm/L
Obligatory urinary output	• The minimal amount of urinary output necessary to ensure the excretion of metabolic wastes (~400 mL/day)
Osmolality	• The concentration of solute within a solution as measured by the amount of solute osmoles per kilogram of solvent
Osmolarity	• The concentration of solute within a solution as measured by the amount of solute osmoles per liter of solution

TABLE 14–1 Terminology Associated with Fluid and Electrolyte Balance *Continued*

Term	Definition
Osmoreceptor	• Specialized sensory nerve cells in the thalamus or the hypothalamus that are sensitive to changes in the osmolarity of extracellular fluid
Osmosis	• Diffusion of water only through a selectively permeable membrane from an area of lower osmotic pressure to an area of greater osmotic pressure
Osmotic pressure	• The pressure exerted by a solution that contains a relatively high concentration of solute; this pressure draws water from areas or compartments with lower concentrations of solute into the areas or compartments with higher concentrations of solute—"water-pulling" pressure
Permeable membrane	• A membrane separating two fluid compartments that permits movement of one or more substances through the membrane (by diffusion) from one compartment to the other
Solubility	• The degree to which any given solute completely dissolves (dissociates) in water
Solute	• The solid particles dissolved in a solution
Solvent	• The fluid (water) portion of a solution
Tissue hydrostatic pressure (THP)	• The force generated by fluid within the interstitial spaces that tends to move fluid into the capillary from the interstitial space
Tissue osmotic pressure (TOP)	• The force generated by the concentration of interstitial fluid solutes that tend to retain fluid in the interstitial space or move fluid from the capillary into the interstitial space
Transcellular fluid	• Extracellular fluid confined to a specific area or region of the body (cerebrospinal fluid, pericardial fluid, visceral fluid, aqueous humor, peritoneal fluid, and pleural fluid)
Viscosity	• Gumminess or thickness of the molecules in a solution, causing friction within that solution

and concentration from one body fluid compartment to another. Proper body function is highly dependent on maintaining the correct balance of fluid and specific electrolytes within each body fluid compartment.

Important processes involved in fluid and electrolyte balance include:

- Filtration
- Diffusion
- Osmosis
- Active transport
- Capillary dynamics

All of these processes influence the movement of fluids and particles across biologic membranes.

FILTRATION

DEFINITION

Filtration is the movement of fluid through a biologic membrane as a result of hydrostatic pressure differences on both sides of the membrane. Because filtration depends on hydrostatic pressure, knowledge of the factors influencing hydrostatic pressure is necessary.

All fluid has weight resulting from the force of gravity. The weight of the fluid is also related to the amount of fluid present in the confined space. When water molecules are in a confined space, they constantly press outward against the confining boundaries. *Hydrostatic pressure* is the force water molecules exert against the confining walls of the space because of the weight (mass) of the fluid against the walls. Thus, hydrostatic pressure may be thought of as "water-pushing" pressure because it is a major force in moving water outward from a confined space through a membrane.

PHYSIOLOGIC ACTIVITY

Water is the largest component of any body fluid. The amount of water in any fluid compartment is a main factor in determining the hydrostatic pressure of that compartment. The proportion of water present in a fluid is inversely related to the *viscosity* (thickness) of that fluid. Viscosity is a physical property of fluid relating to its density and surface tension. The blood, a viscous fluid (one that is thicker than water), is confined within the blood vessels of the vascular system. Blood has hydrostatic pressure because of its weight and volume and also because of cardiac contraction and ejection of blood into the arterial circulation.

Whenever a permeable (porous) membrane separates two fluid compartments, it is possible to compare the hydrostatic pressures of the two compartments. If hydrostatic pressure is the same in both fluid compartments, a state of *equilibrium* exists for hydrostatic pressure.

If the hydrostatic pressure is not the same in both compartments, a state of *disequilibrium* exists. This means that the two compartments have a gradient, or a graded difference, of hydrostatic pressure. One compartment has a higher hydrostatic pressure than the other compartment. Because the human body is a dynamic biologic system and constantly seeks equilibrium, whenever a gradient exists across a membrane, forces act to rearrange the distribution of substances on both sides of the membrane until an equilibrium is reached (Fig. 14–1).

In most instances, substances are moved or rearranged in the direction from the greater amount (of pressure or concentration) to the lesser amount. Thus, when a hydrostatic pressure gradient exists between two fluid compartments, fluid from the compartment with the higher hydrostatic pressure moves (filters) through the membrane into the fluid compartment with the lower hydrostatic pressure. This filtration continues only as long as the hydrostatic pressure gradient exists. When enough fluid leaves the compartment that initially had the higher pressure and enters the compartment that initially had the lower pressure to make the hydrostatic pressure in both compartments the same, an equilibrium is reached.

When the two compartments are in equilibrium with regard to hydrostatic pressure, a gradient no longer exists between the two compartments. Although water molecules may be exchanged back and forth between two compartments in equilibrium, no net filtration of fluid occurs. Therefore, in equilibrium, neither compartment gains or loses water molecules and the hydrostatic pressure in both compartments remains the same.

CLINICAL FUNCTION AND SIGNIFICANCE

Blood pressure is a hydrostatic filtering force that is measured in millimeters of mercury (mmHg). It moves whole blood from the heart to tissue areas where filtration can occur. Filtration is important for the exchange of water, nutrients, and waste products when blood arrives at the tissue capillaries. One factor that determines whether fluid leaves the vascular system and enters the tissue spaces (interstitial fluid) is the difference between the hydrostatic pressure of the fluid in the capillaries and that of the fluid in the interstitial tissue spaces.

The lining of capillaries is only one cell layer thick, which makes the wall that holds the blood in the capillaries thin. In addition, large spaces, or pores, exist between the cells in the capillary membrane (Fig. 14–2). Water can filter freely through capillary membranes in either direction if a hydrostatic pressure gradient is present. This concept is discussed later in this chapter under the heading Capillary Dynamics.

Edema can develop as a result of changes in normal hydrostatic pressure gradients, such as in clients with right-sided congestive heart failure. In this clinical situation, the volume of blood in the right side of the heart increases greatly because the right ventricle cannot pump blood into the pulmonary vascular system as fast as it receives the blood. As blood volume accumulates, blood backs up into the venous system and the venous hydrostatic pressure rises. The increased venous pressure eventually causes capillary hydrostatic pressures to increase so that they are higher than the pressures in the interstitial spaces. Net filtration of fluid from the capillaries into the interstitial tissue spaces then occurs and results in the formation of visible edema.

DIFFUSION

DEFINITION

Diffusion is the free movement of substances across a permeable membrane down a concentration gra-

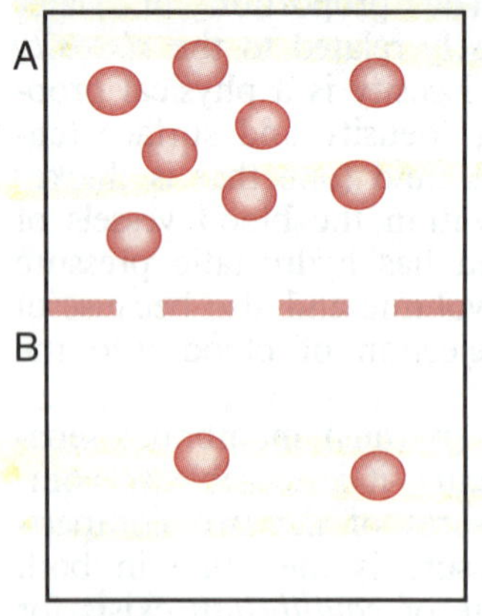

Compartment A has more water molecules and greater hydrostatic pressure than does compartment B.

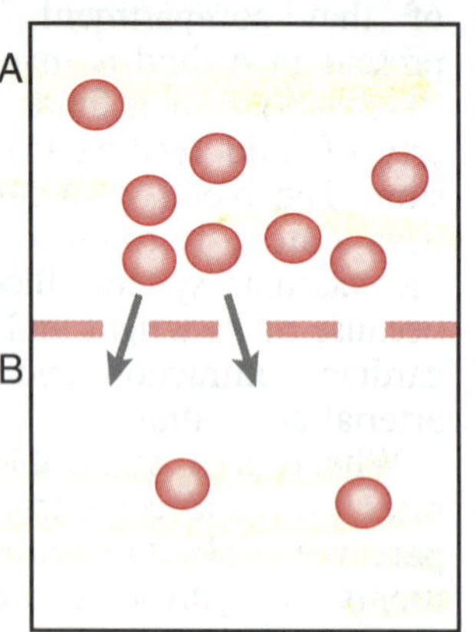

Water molecules move down the hydrostatic pressure gradient from compartment A through the permeable membrane into compartment B, which has a lower hydrostatic pressure.

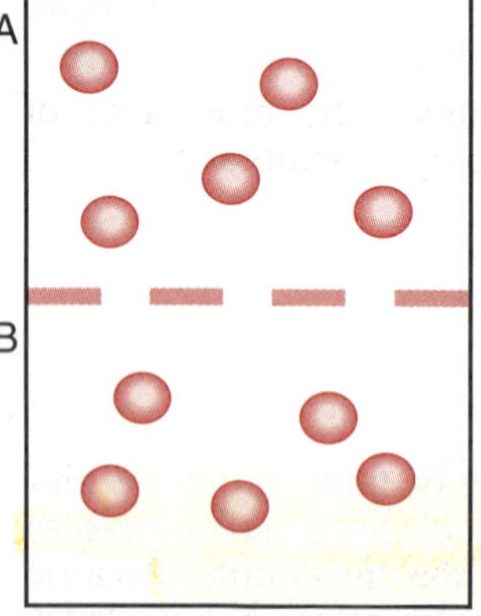

Enough water molecules have moved down the hydrostatic pressure gradient from compartment A into compartment B that both sides now have the same amount of water and the same amount of hydrostatic pressure. An equilibrium of hydrostatic pressure now exists between the two compartments and no further *net* movement of water will occur.

= water molecule
= permeable membrane

FIGURE 14–1 ◆ The process of filtration. (© M. Linda Workman, 1992. All rights reserved.)

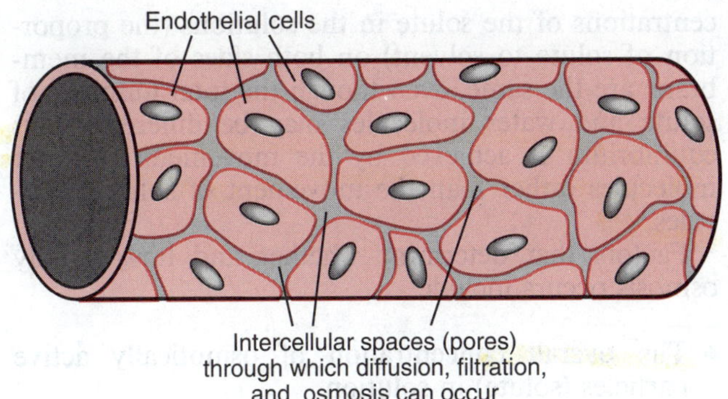

FIGURE 14-2 ◆ The basic structure of a capillary.

dient. Diffusion controls the movement of particles in solution across various body membranes.

PHYSIOLOGIC ACTIVITY

Diffusion of particles into and out of cells and fluid compartments occurs via the kinetic energy of molecular motion known as *brownian motion.* Brownian motion is the vibration of individual molecules caused by electrons orbiting at the core of a molecule. Brownian motion produces totally random movement of molecules. This random movement causes molecules to move and collide with each other within a confined space. The collisions usually result in a temporary increase in the speed of the movement of the molecule that is hit.

As a result of these collisions, molecules in a solution tend to spread out evenly through whatever space is available. They thus move from an area of higher concentration (of atoms and molecules) to an area of lower concentration until a relative equality of concentrations is achieved in all areas.

A concentration gradient exists when two areas have different concentrations of molecules. Brownian motion of the molecules causes them to move down the concentration gradient from the area of the higher concentration to the area of the lower concentration of the same molecules. As a result of the brownian motion, any membrane that separates two areas is struck repeatedly by molecules. When the molecule strikes a pore in the membrane that is large enough for the molecule to pass through, diffusion occurs (Fig. 14–3). The likelihood of any molecule's colliding with the membrane and going through a pore is much greater on the side of the membrane that has a higher concentration of those molecules.

The speed of diffusion is directly related to the degree of concentration difference between the two sides of the membrane. The degree of concentration difference is usually referred to as the steepness of the gradient: the larger the concentration difference between the two sides, the steeper the gradient. Diffusion occurs more rapidly when the concentration gradient is steeper (just as a ball rolls downhill more rapidly when the hill is steep than when the hill is nearly flat). The greater the difference in concentration is, the more rapidly diffusion occurs from the area of higher concentration to the area of lower concentration.

Diffusion of solute particles continues through the membrane as long as there is a concentration gradient between the two sides of the membrane. When the concentration of solute is the same on both sides of the membrane, an equilibrium exists and equal exchange of solute (rather than net movement of solute) continues.

CLINICAL FUNCTION AND SIGNIFICANCE

Diffusion is important in the transport of gases and in the movement of most ions (electrolytes), atoms, and molecules through biologic membranes. Unlike capillary membranes, which permit diffusion of most small-sized substances down a concentration gradient, cell membranes are *selective,* permitting movement of some substances and inhibiting movement of other substances. Some ions and molecules cannot move across a cell membrane, even when a steep "downhill" gradient exists, because the membrane is impermeable (not porous) to that ion or molecule. Thus, the concentration gradient is maintained across the membrane. This impermeability, along with special transport mechanisms, accounts for differences in concentrations of specific ions from one fluid compartment to another. For example, under normal conditions, the extracellular fluid (ECF) contains almost ten times more sodium ions than does the fluid inside the cell, or intracellular fluid (ICF). The relative impermeability of the cell membrane to sodium, coupled with a system of active transport that moves any extra sodium out of the cell "uphill" against its concentration gradient and back into the extracellular fluid, accounts for this extreme concentration difference.

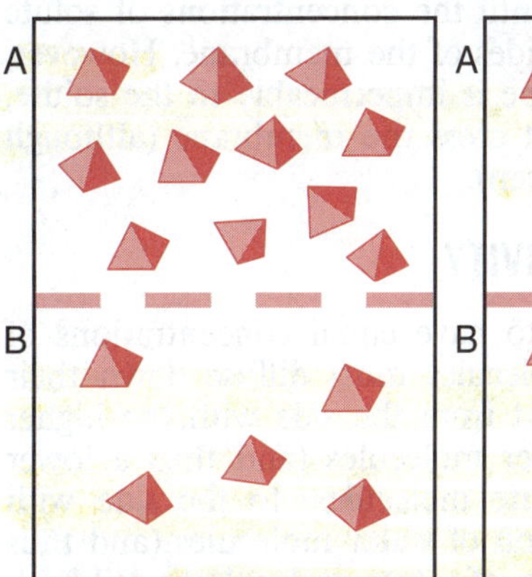

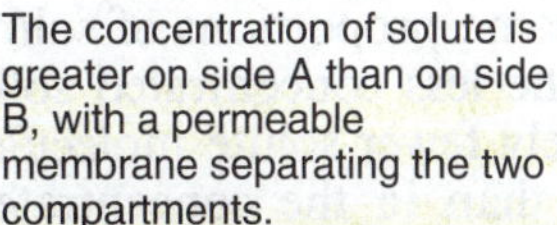
The concentration of solute is greater on side A than on side B, with a permeable membrane separating the two compartments.

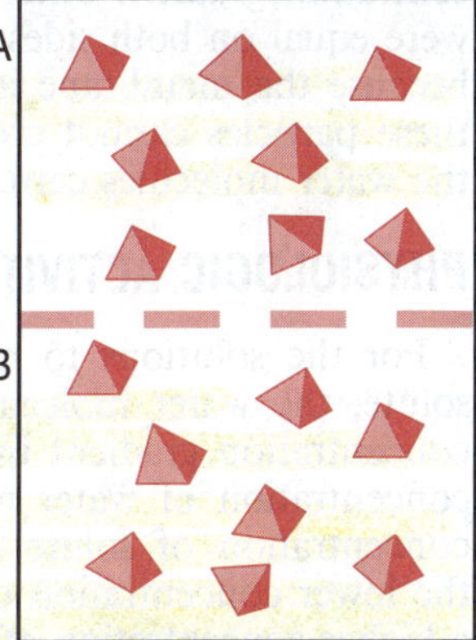

Solute molecules have diffused from side A through the membrane into side B until an equilibrium of solute exists and the concentration of solute is the same on both sides.

FIGURE 14-3 ◆ Diffusion of a solute. (© M. Linda Workman, 1992. All rights reserved.)

In some instances, diffusion cannot occur without assistance, even down steep concentration gradients, because of membrane selectivity. A clinical example is insulin-dependent type I diabetes mellitus. In this disease, there is an absence of or a profound decrease in the levels of the hormone insulin. Insulin binds to cell membranes and facilitates the diffusion of glucose from the extracellular fluid across the cell membrane inside the cell. If there is no insulin, glucose cannot cross the membranes of most cells and the concentration of glucose in the extracellular fluid increases to the point of *hyperglycemia* (an excessive amount of glucose in the blood). Even though the concentration gradient is steep, with a large concentration of glucose in the blood and a low concentration of glucose inside the cell, glucose does not diffuse into some cell types without the presence of insulin.

When diffusion across a cell membrane requires a transport system or carrier (such as insulin, which is a transporter for glucose), the process is called facilitated diffusion or facilitated transport. Because this type of transport occurs down a concentration gradient and requires no energy expenditure by the cell, it is considered a form of diffusion.

OSMOSIS

DEFINITION

Osmosis is the process by which only the solvent (e.g., water molecules) diffuses through a selectively permeable membrane. For osmosis to occur, a membrane must separate two solutions. At least one of these solutions must contain a solute that cannot move through the membrane (the membrane is therefore impermeable to this solute). A concentration gradient of this solute must also exist. If the membrane were permeable to this solute, the solute would diffuse through the membrane down its concentration gradient until the concentrations of solute were equal on both sides of the membrane. However, because the membrane is impermeable to the solute, these particles cannot cross the membrane (although the water molecules can).

PHYSIOLOGIC ACTIVITY

For the solutions to have equal concentrations of solute, the water molecules must diffuse down their concentration gradient from the side with the higher concentration of water molecules (and thus a lower concentration of solute molecules) to the side with the lower concentration of water molecules (and thus a higher concentration of solute molecules) until both compartments contain the same proportions of solute to solvent (Fig. 14–4). In the less concentrated solution, there are proportionately fewer solute molecules and more water molecules than in the concentrated solution. Water therefore moves by osmosis down its concentration gradient from the area of more dilute solute to the area of more concentrated solute until a new equilibrium is achieved. At this point, the concentrations of the solute in the solutions (the proportion of solute to solvent) on both sides of the membrane are the same, even though the total numbers of solute and water molecules may be different. This equilibrium is achieved by the movement of water molecules rather than the movement of solute molecules.

Factors that determine whether and how rapidly osmosis occurs include:

- The overall concentration of osmotically active particles (solute) in solution
- The solubility of the solute
- The amount of membrane available for osmosis

CONCENTRATION OF SOLUTE

The concentration of solutes in human body fluids is expressed as milliequivalents per liter (mEq/L) and milliosmoles per liter (mOsm/L). Osmoles and milliosmoles are used to express the total concentration of solute particles (including electrolytes) contained within a solution. The number of milliosmoles present in body fluids can be expressed as either osmolarity or osmolality.

Osmolarity is defined as the number of milliosmoles in a liter of solution; *osmolality* is defined as the number of milliosmoles in a kilogram of solution. The normal osmolarity value for plasma and other body fluids ranges between 270 and 300 mOsm/L (Guyton, 1991).

Because the body functions best when the osmolarity of the fluids in all compartments is about 300 mOsm/L, many mechanisms function to maintain solute concentration homeostasis. When all body fluids have this solute concentration, the osmotic pressures (water pulling) of the various fluid compartments are essentially equal and no *net* water movement occurs. In such a situation, the body fluids are said to be *isosmotic* to each other. Another term that has essentially the same meaning is *isotonic* (sometimes called normotonic). Examples of specific solutions that contain overall concentrations of specific substances to equal 270 to 300 mOsm/L include 0.9% sodium chloride in water and the complex formula of Ringer's lactate in water (Trissel, 1992). Because these substances are isotonic, or isosmotic, to plasma, their addition to plasma does not change plasma osmolarity or plasma osmotic pressure.

Fluids that have osmolarities (solute concentrations) greater than 300 mOsm/L are said to be hyperosmotic, or hypertonic, when compared with isosmotic fluids. Hyperosmotic fluids have a greater osmotic pressure than do isosmotic fluids and tend to pull water from the isosmotic fluid compartment into the hyperosmotic fluid compartment until an osmotic balance is achieved.

Fluids that have osmolarities (solute concentrations) of less than 270 mOsm/L are said to be hyposmotic, or hypotonic, when compared with isosmotic fluids. Hyposmolar fluids have a lower or smaller osmotic pressure than do isosmotic fluids. As a result, water tends to be pulled from the hyposmotic fluid

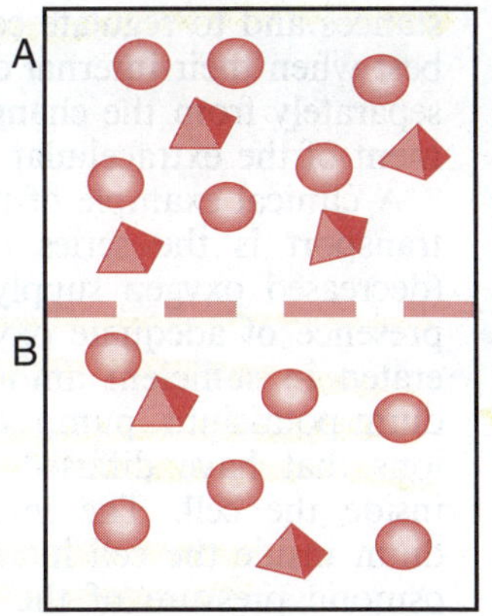

Side A has more solute molecules than does side B, even though the number of water molecules is the same on both sides. Thus, side A has a greater osmotic (water pulling) pressure than does side B.

DISEQUILIBRIUM
side A 1.5:1 ratio of water to solute
side B 3:1 ratio of water to solute

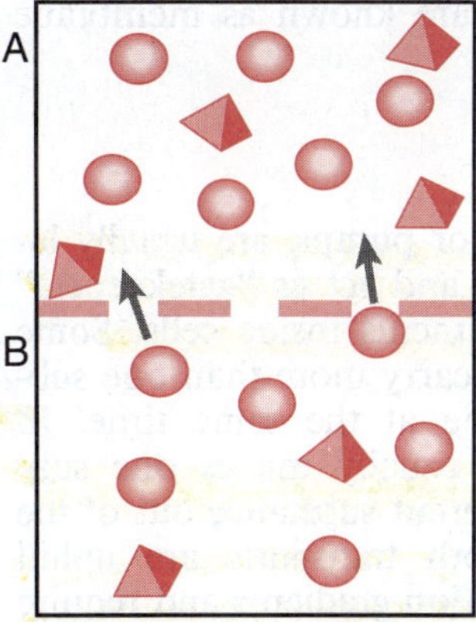

Movement of water occurs by osmosis toward side A because it has greater osmotic pressure. The membrane is *not* permeable to the solute molecules, so the actual number of solute molecules in side A and side B does not change. *Only the water molecules move because the membrane is not permeable to the solute molecules.*

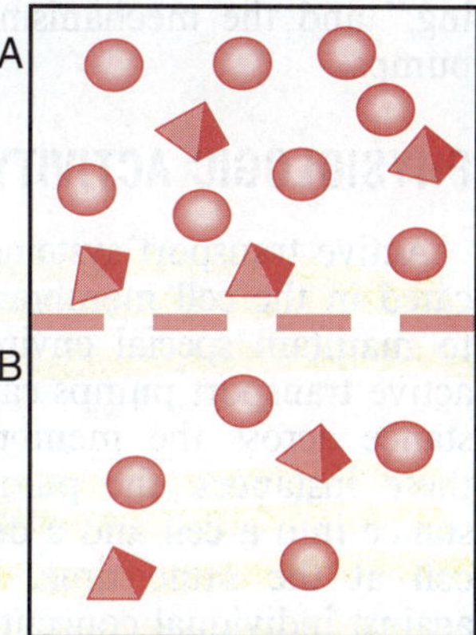

Enough water molecules have moved from side B into side A that the actual concentration of solute is now the same on both sides, with a ratio of water to solute of 2:1. An equilibrium of osmotic pressure now exists between the two compartments, and no further *net* movement of water molecules or solute molecules will occur.

EQUILIBRIUM
side A 2:1 ratio of water to solute
side B 2:1 ratio of water to solute

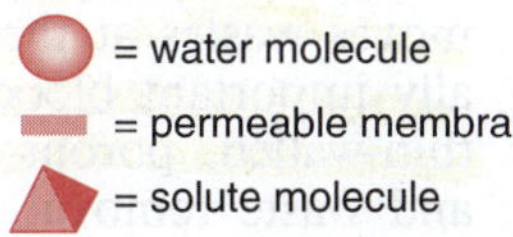

FIGURE 14-4 ◆ The process of osmosis. (© M. Linda Workman, 1992. All rights reserved.)

compartment into the isosmotic fluid compartment until an osmotic balance is achieved (Metheny, 1992).

SOLUBILITY OF SOLUTE

The *solubility* refers to the degree to which a solute dissolves or dissociates completely in water. Solubility is directly related to osmotic pressure: the greater the solubility of the solutes in a fluid, the higher the osmotic pressure of that fluid.

AMOUNT OF AVAILABLE MEMBRANE

The greater the amount of membrane available for osmosis, the faster the rate of osmosis. More membrane increases the chances that water molecules will strike the membrane at a point where penetration is possible.

CLINICAL FUNCTION AND SIGNIFICANCE

The process of osmosis acts together with the process of filtration in capillary fluid dynamics to regulate extracellular and intracellular fluid volumes. A clinical example of the importance of osmosis in the maintenance of homeostasis is the thirst mechanism (Burns, 1992; Porth & Erickson, 1992). Thirst is the result of activation of cells in the hypothalamus of the brain that respond to changes in extracellular fluid osmolarity. These cells are so sensitive to changes in extracellular fluid osmolarity that they are called osmoreceptors. When a person experiences a loss of body fluids, such as that seen with excessive sweating during prolonged heavy exercise, the extracellular fluid volume is decreased and the osmolarity is increased (hypertonic conditions exist). The cells in the thirst center shrink as water moves from the cells into the hypertonic extracellular fluid. Shrinking of these cells stimulates the awareness of the sensation of thirst and its resultant behavioral responses. The person usually drinks enough fluid to replace what was lost through sweating and restore the extracellular fluid osmolarity to its normal value. After the extracellular fluid volume and osmolarity return to normal levels, the osmoreceptors resume their normal size and no longer send stimulatory messages.

ACTIVE TRANSPORT

DEFINITION

A cell must expend energy to move a substance across a cell membrane against a concentration gradient (uphill). Such movement is called *active transport* because the cell must make active efforts for the net movement to occur. Because of its energy demands, active transport is sometimes called "pumping," and the mechanisms are known as membrane pumps.

PHYSIOLOGIC ACTIVITY

Active transport systems, or pumps, are usually located in the cell membrane and act as "gatekeepers" to maintain special environments inside cells. Some active transport pumps can carry more than one substance across the membrane at the same time. In these instances, the pump usually moves one substance into a cell and a different substance out of the cell at the same time. Both transports are uphill against individual concentration gradients and require energy. The sodium-potassium pump is an example of such a double active transport system.

Sodium tends to diffuse slightly down its concentration gradient into the intracellular fluid because it has such a high extracellular fluid concentration compared with its intracellular fluid concentration. Similarly, because potassium has such a high concentration inside the cells compared with its concentration in extracellular fluid, it tends to diffuse slightly down its concentration gradient into the extracellular fluid. The action of the sodium-potassium pump moves the extra sodium out of the cell, while returning the lost potassium to the cell. The sodium-potassium pump requires cellular energy expenditure.

Usually, the cellular energy used for this process is derived from breaking a high-energy bond (~P) when splitting off a phosphate group from an adenosine triphosphate (ATP) molecule. Optimal functioning of active transport pumps depends on the presence of adequate amounts of cellular ATP.

CLINICAL FUNCTION AND SIGNIFICANCE

The process of active transport is used by cells to control the intracellular concentration of many substances and to regulate cell volume. All cells function best when their internal environments are maintained separately from the changes occurring in the environment of the extracellular fluid.

A clinical example of the results of failure of active transport is the series of events following hypoxia (decreased oxygen supply in the body). Without the presence of adequate oxygen, ATP is no longer generated in sufficient amounts. Without ATP, the sodium-potassium pump cannot remove the sodium ions that have diffused from the extracellular fluid inside the cell. The increased concentration of sodium inside the cell increases the osmolarity and the osmotic pressure of the fluid inside the cell. Water moves into the cell in response to the increased osmotic pressure, which causes the cell to swell and perhaps to lyse (break open) and die if oxygen is not provided.

Table 14–2 summarizes the processes involved in fluid and electrolyte balance.

CAPILLARY DYNAMICS

The circulatory system distributes nutrients and removes wastes at the tissue level. The most functionally important blood vessels for this purpose are the thin-walled, porous capillaries. Nutrient distribution and waste removal depend on capillary fluid movement.

Fluid movement at the capillary level is dynamic not only because it is continuous but also because relative homeostasis of vascular and interstitial fluid volumes must be maintained. Opposing processes must occur to accomplish the tasks of nutrient distribution, waste removal, and the maintenance of vascular and interstitial fluid volumes. In these processes, some fluid with nutrients must leave the

TABLE 14–2 Summary of Membrane-Fluid Actions

Action	Definition	Specific Characteristics
Filtration	• The movement of fluid through a biologic membrane as a result of hydrostatic pressure differences on both sides of the membrane	• Does not require energy • Is limited to solvent and low-molecular-weight solute • Usually occurs from capillaries to the interstitial fluid • Depends on hydrostatic pressure differences
Diffusion	• Free movement of substances across a permeable membrane down a concentration gradient	• Does not require energy • Is not pressure dependent • Moves solute as well as solvent down their individual gradients • Occurs more rapidly with steep gradients • Is directly related in speed to the amount of membrane available • Occurs in both directions across capillary and cell membranes • Is responsible for maintaining tissue nutrition
Osmosis	• The process by which only the *solvent* diffuses through a selectively permeable membrane	• Does not require energy • Involves movement of water only • Depends on hydrostatic and osmotic pressures
Active transport	• The movement of a substance across a selectively permeable membrane against a concentration, electrical, or pressure gradient	• Requires energy • Requires a transport system (pump) • Helps maintain a special intracellular environment

capillary and enter the interstitial (tissue space) fluid compartment for a short period, which temporarily expands the interstitial fluid volume. The nutrients in the interstitial fluid are then taken up by the cells through various membrane transport processes. Water may be exchanged between the intracellular compartment and the interstitial compartment, but under normal circumstances, no net change in water volume occurs. Metabolic wastes created in the cells are moved into the interstitial fluid. Any extra fluid in the interstitial space, together with the excreted metabolic waste products, must be returned via the capillary to the systemic circulation. Without a provision for the return of the fluid originally lost to the interstitial compartment, the vascular volume would become progressively depleted to the point of circulatory failure and the interstitial fluid compartment would become greatly expanded.

CAPILLARY FORCES INFLUENCING FLUID MOVEMENT

Starling's forces at the capillary level permit capillary fluid loss followed by a return of fluid to the capillary so that a near-equilibrium of fluid distribution is maintained at the capillary-tissue level. These forces are outlined in Figure 14–5. The equilibrium is based on the forces that tend to move fluid out from the capillary at the arterial end being nearly equal to the forces that tend to move fluid from the interstitial compartment back into the capillary at the venous end.

Capillary blood normally flows from the arterial to the venous end:

Venous end of capillary

Arterial end of capillary

Plasma hydrostatic pressure (PHP) 17 mmHg

Plasma hydrostatic pressure (PHP) 32 mmHg

Plasma colloidal oncotic pressure (PCOP) 22 mmHg

Tissue hydrostatic pressure (THP) 6 mmHg
Tissue osmotic pressure (TOP) 4 mmHg

Tissue hydrostatic pressure (THP) 4 mmHg
Tissue osmotic pressure (TOP) 4 mmHg

At the arterial end, the forces that tend to move fluid from the capillary into the tissue space are

Plasma hydrostatic pressure 32 mmHg
+
Tissue osmotic pressure 4 mmHg
Total forces moving fluid out = 36 mmHg

At the arterial end, the forces that tend to move fluid from the tissue spaces into the capillary are

Tissue hydrostatic pressure 4 mmHg
+
Plasma colloidal oncotic pressure 22 mmHg
Total forces moving fluid in = 26 mmHg

The total forces tending to move fluid out at the arterial end are 10 mmHg higher than the total forces tending to move fluid in at the arterial end (36 − 26 = 10). Thus, at the arterial end, fluid leaks out of the capillary into the tissue (interstitial) spaces.

At the venous end of the same capillary, the forces that tend to move fluid from the capillary into the tissue space are

Plasma hydrostatic pressure 17 mmHg
+
Tissue osmotic pressure 4 mmHg
Total forces moving fluid out = 21 mmHg

At the venous end of the capillary, the forces that tend to move fluid from the tissue spaces back into the capillary are

Tissue hydrostatic pressure 6 mmHg
+
Plasma colloidal oncotic pressure 22 mmHg
Total forces moving fluid in = 28 mmHg

The total forces tending to move fluid out at the venous end are 7 mmHg lower than the total forces tending to move fluid into the capillary at the venous end (28 − 21 = 7). Thus, at the venous end, fluid moves from the tissue spaces back into the capillary.

Because the pressures tending to move fluid out of the capillary at the arterial end (10 mmHg) are greater than the pressures that tend to move fluid back into the capillary at the venous end (7 mmHg), more fluid is lost from the capillary than is returned to it. Lymph drainage eventually returns this extra lost fluid.

FIGURE 14–5 ◆ Capillary dynamics.

Blood flowing from the arterial end of the capillary to the venous end is controlled by:

- Pressure of blood
- Dynamic ejection of blood from the left ventricle of the heart
- Patency of the capillaries

The blood entering the arterial end of the capillary has a blood pressure, or a capillary (plasma) hydrostatic pressure (PHP), of about 32 mmHg. The capillary membrane is thin and permeable. The usual tissue hydrostatic pressure is low. These factors create a natural tendency for filtration to occur from the blood outward into the tissue spaces. The fluid portion of the blood, along with most of the smaller substances dissolved in the blood, filters through the capillary membrane into the tissue spaces. By this process, nutrients and other essential substances can reach the cells.

If net filtration, as a result of plasma hydrostatic pressure, were the only force or factor involved at this level, blood volume would be progressively lost from the vascular space and would reappear in the tissues. Fortunately, other mechanisms that favor the reabsorption of tissue fluid into the capillaries are also part of capillary dynamics. Those forces are plasma osmotic and tissue hydrostatic pressure.

Osmosis (of water) through the capillary membrane (in either direction) occurs in response to differences in the concentrations of osmotically active substances in the capillary blood and the tissue fluid. Tissue osmotic pressure tends to draw fluid out of the capillary. Plasma osmotic pressure (POP) in the capillary tends to keep fluid in the capillary and to draw fluid from the interstitial space into the capillary. Under normal conditions, capillary plasma osmotic pressure is greater than tissue (interstitial fluid) osmotic pressure because of the higher concentration of proteins in the blood compared with that in the interstitial fluid.

The capillary membrane does not allow blood proteins to pass freely through it into the tissue space because the capillary membrane is highly impermeable to proteins. Thus, blood proteins remain in the capillary and add to the osmotic pressure. The specific type of osmotic pressure exerted by plasma proteins is called *colloidal oncotic pressure* because it is due to the presence of proteins (colloidal substances) rather than dissociated ions such as sodium (crystalloid substances). The average colloidal oncotic pressure in capillary blood is about 22 mmHg.

Blood pressure (hydrostatic pressure) is greater than colloidal oncotic pressure at the arterial end of the capillary. Capillary hydrostatic pressure favors the filtration of fluid from the capillary into the tissue spaces, and colloidal oncotic pressure favors the reabsorption of fluid from the interstitial space into the capillary. The difference between these two capillary pressures at the arterial end of the capillary indicates that there is a greater filtering force outward than a reabsorbing force inward.

TISSUE FORCES INFLUENCING FLUID MOVEMENT

Tissue forces are also present and influence the movement of solutions at the capillary level. These forces are tissue hydrostatic pressure (THP) and tissue osmotic pressure (TOP). Usually, both are relatively small forces. However, in some diseases, these forces increase greatly and significantly alter capillary dynamics.

To determine the direction of fluid movement in any one area of the capillary, it is necessary to compare the forces that move fluid out of the capillary with the forces that move fluid into the capillary. Two forces at the arterial end that move fluid out of the capillary are the plasma hydrostatic pressure (normally about 32 mmHg) and the tissue osmotic pressure (normally about 4 mmHg). The pressures at the arterial end that return fluid to the capillary are the plasma colloidal oncotic pressure (normally about 22 mmHg) and the tissue hydrostatic pressure (normally about 4 mmHg). Because the outward filtration force is 10 mmHg higher than the inward reabsorbing force, the overall result at the arterial end of the capillary is the outward filtration of fluid and small solute particles into the tissue spaces.

Plasma hydrostatic pressure decreases along the length of the capillary as blood flows through it. As filtration proceeds along the capillary, water is lost from the capillary and the plasma hydrostatic pressure gradually decreases. Therefore, the pressures that create the outward filtration force (from the capillary into the interstitial fluid) become smaller, while the pressures that create the inward reabsorption force (from the interstitial fluid into the capillary) remain the same. Eventually, the outward filtration pressures and the inward reabsorption pressures become equal.

Finally, at the venous end of the capillary, the inward reabsorption forces exceed the outward filtration forces. The venous end of the capillary has a much lower hydrostatic pressure than does the arterial end. This decreased hydrostatic pressure has two causes:

- Because much of the water in the blood was filtered out of the capillary at the arterial end, the volume of water remaining in the blood at the venous end of the capillary is greatly diminished.
- The venous portion of the capillary is farther away from the heart than the arterial end, so that blood pressure is lower in the venous end.

Because hydrostatic pressure in the venous end of the capillary is low and the interstitial fluid (tissue) hydrostatic pressure is high (because water moved from the arterial end of the capillary into the interstitial space), some water returns from the interstitial space back into the capillary at the venous end.

Lymph

Usually, not all the fluid that leaves the capillary at the arterial end and enters the interstitial space is returned to the capillary at the venous end. A small amount remains in the tissues. If this situation were not balanced by another mechanism to return the fluid to the systemic circulation, the circulating volume would become depleted and the interstitial areas would constantly be edematous. Instead, this extra fluid leaking out from the capillaries is returned to systemic circulation as lymph.

Lymph fluid is similar to blood plasma (from which it is derived) but contains far less protein. It is returned to systemic circulation by the auxiliary venous system known as lymph vessels, or *lymphatics.* Lymphatics begin as small, thin-walled, vein-like vessels that merge to form larger lymphatic vessels. Two large groups of lymphatic vessels connect the entire lymph system with the general circulatory system. The left thoracic lymph duct drains lymph from the abdomen, the gastrointestinal tract, the pelvis, the lower extremities, the left side of the thorax, the left arm, and the left side of the head and neck into the left subclavian vein at the point where it joins the left internal jugular vein. Lymph from the right arm, the right side of the thorax, and right side of the head and neck drains into the right subclavian vein through three lymph ducts. Lymph nodes are situated along the lymphatic paths and act as lymph fluid filters.

Lymphatics carry lymph fluid in only one direction—toward the heart. Lymph flow is slower than blood flow because there is no pump and no direct connection between the arterial blood circulation and the lymphatic system. The physical mechanisms that enhance lymph flow are skeletal muscle contractions, intrathoracic pressure changes that occur during pulmonary ventilation, and an intrinsic peristalsis-like motion in lymph vessels.

Hormonal Influences on Fluid and Electrolyte Balance

Many endocrine mechanisms assist in the regulation of fluid and electrolyte balance. Two hormones that help control these critical balances are aldosterone and antidiuretic hormone (ADH). An additional substance that influences fluid and electrolyte balance is atrial natriuretic peptide (ANP).

ALDOSTERONE

Aldosterone is a mineralocorticoid secreted by the adrenal cortex. This hormone directly influences sodium balance by preventing sodium loss. Because sodium in solution exerts osmotic pressure (water-pulling pressure), water attempts to follow sodium, in physiologically proportionate amounts (Guyton, 1991). As a result of this sodium-water relationship, aldosterone secretion also indirectly regulates water balance. Aldosterone secretion is stimulated by events that occur in response either to decreased levels of sodium in the extracellular fluid or to increased amounts of sodium in tubular urine. The events surrounding aldosterone secretion and function are outlined in Figure 14–6.

In the kidney, blood is supplied to the glomerulus of nephrons via the afferent arteriole. Specialized cells (juxtaglomerular cells) inside the afferent arteriole near the glomerulus are sensitive to changes in the serum concentrations of sodium. This area of the afferent arteriole comes into direct contact with a specialized area of the distal convoluted tubule (the macula densa). Together, the juxtaglomerular cells and the macula densa form a functional group called the *juxtaglomerular complex.* When this complex senses that actual serum sodium concentrations are lower than normal or that the total blood volume is low, the macula densa stimulates special juxtaglomerular cells to secrete renin.

Renin catalyzes intrarenal or systemic reactions, depending on the body's needs. Renin acts enzymatically on an inactive plasma protein called angiotensinogen (also known as renin substrate), converting it to a smaller substance called angiotensin I. Angiotensin I causes some vasoconstriction but the effects are minimal because this substance is immediately further degraded by an enzyme called converting enzyme. Converting enzyme is produced in the lung and secreted into the blood. It catalyzes the conversion of angiotensin I to angiotensin II.

Angiotensin II causes massive vasoconstriction of many blood vessels and increases blood flow to the kidney. In addition, angiotensin II causes selective constriction of either the afferent arteriole or the efferent arteriole of the nephron, depending on the overall state of hydration. If the serum sodium concentration is low and the blood volume is greater than normal, the efferent arteriole is constricted. Efferent arteriolar constriction causes an elevation of the effective filtration pressure in the glomerulus, increasing glomerular filtration and urinary output. If serum sodium levels are low and blood volume is normal or low, angiotensin II causes constriction of the afferent arteriole so that blood flow to the glomerulus is diminished and effective filtration pressure is low, decreasing glomerular filtration and urinary output (Guyton, 1991). This action preserves vascular volume, while restoring the serum sodium concentration. At the same time, angiotensin II stimulates the release of aldosterone from the adrenal cortex.

Aldosterone acts on the distal convoluted tubules of the nephrons. When the serum osmolarity is too low, aldosterone secretion stimulates these areas to reabsorb sodium (in exchange for potassium) from the filtrate (urine) back into systemic circulation, thus increasing the serum osmolarity. Aldosterone secretion increases when the blood osmolarity or serum sodium levels are low, and its presence is normally required to prevent excessive renal excretion of sodium. In addition, secretion of aldosterone helps to prevent serum potassium levels from becoming too high. Secretion of aldosterone is inhibited when the serum sodium level or blood osmolarity is greater than normal.

ANTIDIURETIC HORMONE

Antidiuretic hormone (ADH) is synthesized in specific areas of the brain and stored in the posterior pituitary gland. The release of ADH from the posterior pituitary gland is controlled by the hypothalamus in response to changes in blood osmolarity. The hypothalamus contains specialized cells (osmoreceptors)

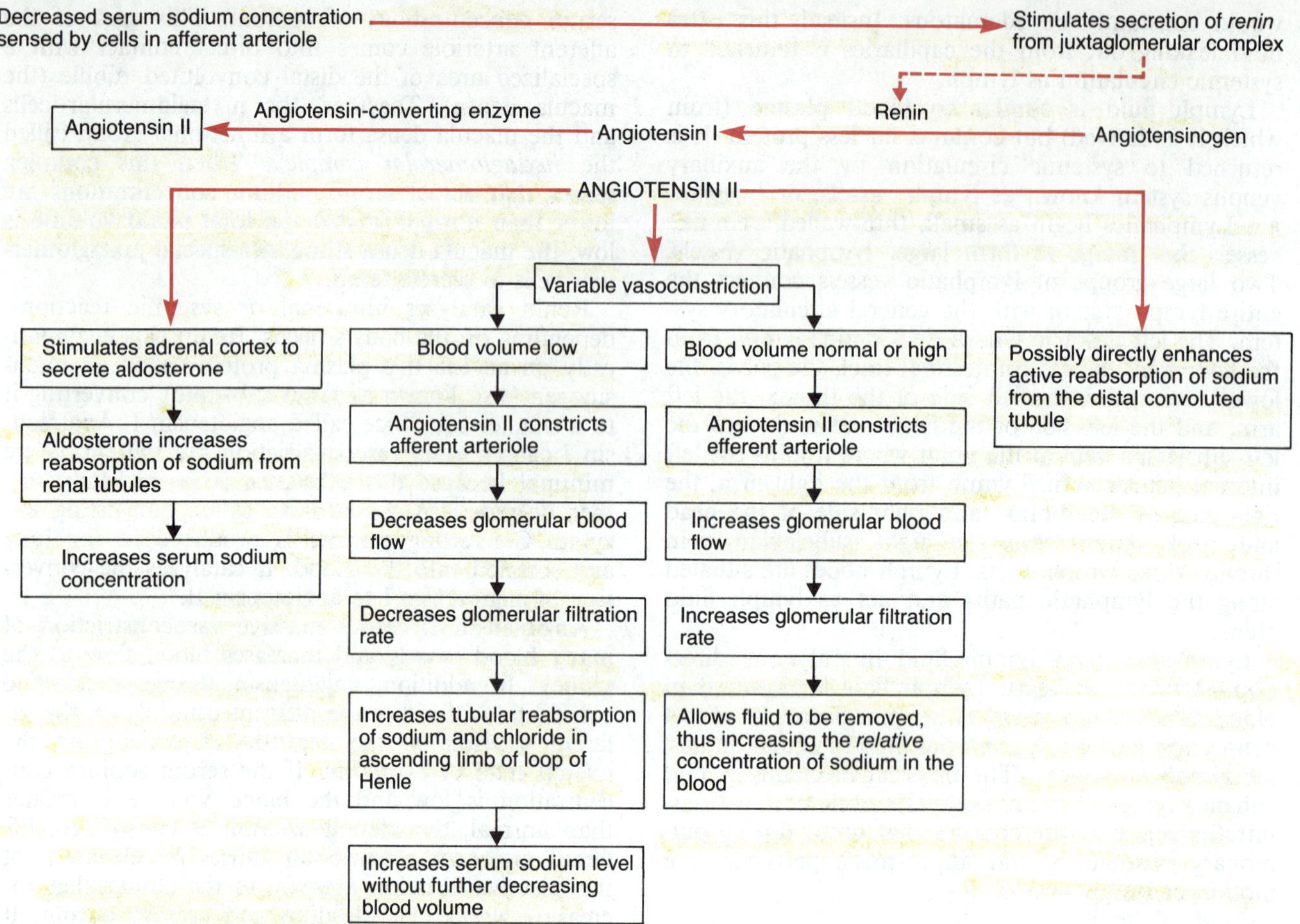

FIGURE 14–6 ◆ The role of aldosterone, angiotensinogen, angiotensin I, and angiotensin II in the renal regulation of water and sodium.

that are sensitive to changes in the osmolarity of blood. Increased blood osmolarity, especially an increase in the plasma sodium concentration, results in slight shrinkage of these cells and causes the hypothalamus to stimulate the posterior pituitary to release ADH.

The ADH acts directly on the renal tubules and collecting ducts, making them more permeable to water. As a result, more water is reabsorbed by these tubules and returned to the systemic circulation, causing the blood to have decreased osmolarity by becoming more dilute. When the osmolarity of the blood is decreased, especially when the plasma sodium concentration is below normal, the osmoreceptors swell slightly and inhibit the release of ADH. Then, less water is reabsorbed and more is lost from the body in the urine. As a result, the amount of water in the extracellular fluid decreases, causing an increase in osmolarity.

ATRIAL NATRIURETIC PEPTIDE

Atrial natriuretic peptide (ANP) is under investigation to determine its exact mechanism of action and characteristics. This hormone-like substance is believed to be secreted by special cells lining the atria of the heart in response to increased blood volume and blood pressure. ANP has effects that are opposite to those of aldosterone. In the presence of ANP, glomerular filtration is greatly increased and the tubular reabsorption of sodium is inhibited. The outcome is increased output of urine with a high sodium content, which results in a decreased circulating blood volume and a decreased blood osmolarity.

Body Fluids

Fluids constitute approximately 55% to 60% of total adult weight and consist of the extracellular fluid and intracellular fluid. The extracellular compartment comprises the plasma volume (blood) and the interstitial fluid (IF). Extracellular fluids constitute approximately 15 L (40%) of total body water and include interstitial fluid, blood plasma, lymph, bone and connective tissue water, and the fluid within special spaces (called transcellular fluid), such as cerebrospinal fluid, synovial fluid, peritoneal fluid, and pleural fluid. The remaining 25 L (60%) of total body water is intracellular fluid. Figure 14–7 shows the normal distribution of total body water.

The person's age, sex, and lean mass to body fat ratio influence the amounts and distribution of body fluids. An elderly adult has less body water than does a younger adult. Men have more body water than do women. Because fat cells contain practically no water compared with other cells, obesity is a factor, with obese people having less water than lean people of the same body weight.

Body fluids are solvents and transport substances. They enable the nutrition of cells and transport biologic molecules (such as hormones) that are important in the regulation of normal physiologic functions. Most biochemical reactions and nutrient transport processes require a liquid medium. The body fluids are constantly renewed, purified, and replaced when fluid balance is maintained through intake and output. Even though the total amount of water within each fluid compartment is stable, water movement occurs continuously among all compartments. Thus, the water in any compartment is not static but is exchanged continuously while maintaining a volume equilibrium. Table 14–2 summarizes key points regarding fluid and electrolyte balance.

SOURCES OF FLUID INTAKE

The intake of fluid is regulated through the thirst drive. Fluids enter the body primarily as liquids (Table 14–3). Because solid foods contain up to 85% water, some fluid also enters the body in ingested solid foods. In addition, water is a by-product of cellular metabolism. This by-product is called the water of oxidation. Approximately 10% (300 mL) of daily water requirements are met by the water of oxidation. A rising plasma osmolarity or a decreasing plasma volume stimulates the sensation of thirst. Other sensory inputs to the hypothalamus, such as dryness of the oral mucosa and sensorimotor input from higher cortical centers, are also important. An adult consumes an average of 1500 mL of fluid per day and obtains an additional 800 mL of fluid from the water of ingested foods.

ROUTES OF FLUID LOSS

The body has several routes by which excessive water and waste products are removed (Table 14–3).

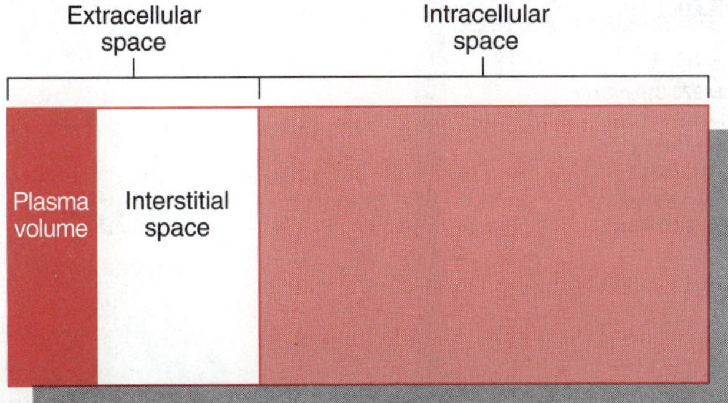

FIGURE 14–7 ◆ Normal distribution of total body water. (© M. Linda Workman, 1992. All rights reserved.)

TABLE 14–3 Routes of Fluid Ingestion and Excretion

Intake	Output
Measurable	
Oral fluids	Urine
Parenteral fluids	Emesis†
Enemas*	Feces†
Irrigation fluids*	Drainage from body cavities
Not Measurable	
Solid foods	Perspiration
Metabolism	Vaporization through the lungs

* Measured by subtracting the amount returned from the amount instilled.
† Measurement accurate only when these substances are excreted in liquid form.

Of all the water loss pathways, the renal route is the most important and most sensitive, being the major adjustment mechanism to preserve fluid and electrolyte balance. Fluid loss via the renal route is closely regulated and adjustable. The volume of urine varies, depending on the amount of fluid intake and the body's need to conserve fluids.

The minimum amount of urine per day needed to dissolve and excrete the toxic waste products of metabolism ranges between 400 and 600 mL. This minimal volume is called the *obligatory urinary output.* If the 24-hour urine volume falls below the obligatory output amount, metabolic wastes are retained and problems can occur. This urine is maximally concentrated, with a specific gravity (weight of a liquid compared with weight of pure water) of 1.032 or higher, and an osmolarity of at least 1200 mOsm/L.

The urine can also become maximally dilute, with a specific gravity of 1.005 and an osmolarity of 200 mOsm/L. This dilution can result from a large fluid intake and is reflected in a large volume of urinary output. The concentrating and diluting capacity of the renal tubules is a response to the changes in the osmolarity of the extracellular fluid, the volumes and pressures of the extracellular fluid compartments, and variation in the secretion of aldosterone, antidiuretic hormone, and atrial natriuretic peptide.

Other normal water loss occurs through the skin, the lungs, and the gastrointestinal tract. Additional water losses can occur via salivation, drainage from fistulas and drains, and gastrointestinal suction.

Water loss from the skin and lungs, termed *insensible water loss,* can be significant. In the healthy adult, insensible water loss is about 15 to 20 mL/kg per day. Insensible water loss can increase dramatically in hypermetabolic states such as thyroid crisis, trauma, burns, states of extreme stress, and fever. For every degree Celsius of increase in body temperature, insensible water loss increases by 10%. When atmospheric conditions are hot and dry, insensible water loss is also increased. Examples of clients at risk for increased insensible water loss include clients undergoing mechanical ventilation and those with rapid respirations (tachypnea). Insensible water loss (not including sweat) is pure water and does not contain electrolytes. Therefore, excessive amounts of insensible water loss result in a more hypertonic extracellular fluid of a smaller volume. If this loss is not balanced by intake, the hypertonic extracellular fluid and accompanying dehydration can lead to the pathophysiologic state of hypernatremia (an elevated serum sodium level).

Loss by sweating is variable and can reach a maximal rate of about 2 L/hour. Sweat, although it contains electrolytes, is slightly hypotonic to the plasma. The amount of sweating is regulated by the autonomic nervous system, the body temperature, and the skin blood flow.

Water loss through stool is normally minimal. However, in severe diarrhea or excessive fistula drainage, this loss can increase significantly. Clients with ulcerative colitis can have diarrheal fluid loss that amounts to several liters per day. Diarrheal fluid contains water, potassium, sodium, bicarbonate, and chloride. Thus, with diarrhea, hypotonic fluid containing some electrolytes is lost.

Electrolytes

Electrolytes, or ions, are substances in body fluids that carry an electrical charge. Cations are positively charged ions, and anions are negatively charged ions. The body fluids are electrochemically neutral: positive ions are balanced by negative ions. However, the composition and distribution of ions differ in the extracellular fluid and the intracellular fluid (Fig. 14–8).

Most electrolytes have different concentrations inside cells compared with those of the extracellular fluid. This concentration difference is important to maintain membrane excitability and transmit impulses. The electrolyte concentration ranges in these fluid compartments are extremely narrow. Even small changes in these concentrations can result in major pathologic alterations.

Table 14–4 lists the major body fluid electrolytes together with their normal serum concentrations and primary functions. The concentration of most electrolytes is reported in milliequivalents per liter. However, the concentration of calcium may be reported as milligrams per deciliter. Most electrolytes enter the body in the form of ingested food.

Electrolyte homeostasis is controlled by balancing the dietary intake of electrolytes with the renal excretion or reabsorption of electrolytes. For example, the plasma potassium concentration is maintained between 3.5 and 5 mEq/L. Potassium in common foods could theoretically increase the extracellular fluid potassium concentration dramatically and lead to major pathologic consequences. However, the renal excretion of potassium keeps pace with potassium intake and prevents major changes in the plasma potassium concentration.

SODIUM

Sodium (Na^+) is the major cation in the extracellular fluid and is the main factor responsible for maintaining extracellular fluid osmolarity. The activity of the sodium-potassium pump keeps the sodium concentration of the intracellular fluid low (about 14 mEq/L) while maintaining high sodium concentrations in the plasma and other extracellular fluids. Preserving this difference in sodium concentration is extremely important for these normal physiologic functions:

- Initiation of skeletal muscle contraction
- Initiation of cardiac contractility
- Transmission of neuronal impulses
- Maintenance of extracellular fluid osmolarity
- Maintenance of extracellular fluid volume
- Maintenance of the renal urine-concentrating system

The concentration of sodium in the extracellular fluid determines whether water is retained, excreted, or moved from one body compartment to another.

The concentration of sodium, a cation, within a body fluid must be matched by an equal concentra-

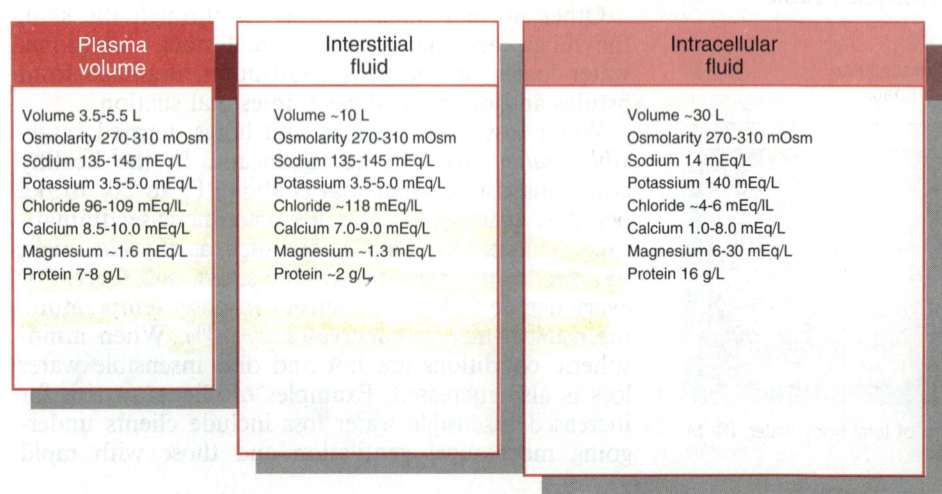

FIGURE 14–8 ◆ Comparison of the composition of various body fluids. (© M. Linda Workman, 1992. All rights reserved.)

TABLE 14–4 Major Body Fluid Electrolyte Concentrations and Functions

Electrolyte	Serum Concentration (mEq/L)	Major Functions
Sodium (Na^+)	• 136–145	• Maintenance of plasma osmolarity • Generation and transmission of action potentials • Maintenance of acid-base balance • Maintenance of electroneutrality
Potassium (K^+)	• 3.5–5.0	• Regulation of intracellular osmolarity • Maintenance of electrical membrane excitability • Maintenance of plasma acid-base balance
Calcium (Ca^{2+})	• 4.5–5.5 • 8.0–10.5 mg/dL	• Cofactor in blood-clotting cascade • Excitable membrane stabilizer • Provision of strength and density to teeth and bones • Essential element in contractile processes in cardiac, skeletal, and smooth muscle
Chloride (Cl^-)	• 96–106	• Maintenance of plasma acid-base balance • Maintenance of plasma electroneutrality • Formation of hydrochloric acid

Data from Keyes, J. (1990). *Fluid, electrolyte, and acid-base regulation* (2nd ed.). Belmont, CA: Wadsworth.

tion of anions to maintain electrical balance. Each cation in the extracellular fluid must be balanced by an anion so that the fluid does not carry either an overall positive or an overall negative charge. When such a balance is maintained, a state of electroneutrality exists in that fluid. Changes in the plasma sodium concentration profoundly affect the fluid volume and the distribution of other electrolytes.

The normal concentration of plasma sodium ranges between 136 and 145 mEq/L (see Table 14–4). Sodium enters the body from ingestion of many foods and fluids (Table 14–5). The average dietary intake of sodium is about 6 to 12 g/day (Keyes, 1990). Sodium is also stored in interstitial fluid areas deep within the renal tissues and can be released to extracellular fluids as needed. Despite great variations in sodium intake, the serum concentration of sodium usually remains within the normal range. Plasma sodium balance is regulated by the kidney under the influences of aldosterone, antidiuretic hormone (ADH), and atrial natriuretic peptide (ANP).

Low serum sodium levels inhibit ADH and ANP while stimulating the secretion of aldosterone. These actions together increase the serum sodium concentration by increasing renal reabsorption of sodium and enhancing renal loss of water.

High serum sodium levels inhibit secretion of aldosterone and directly stimulate the secretion of ADH. Because high serum sodium levels are usually accompanied by an increased circulating volume, ANP secretion is indirectly stimulated. Together, these hormones cause an increase in the renal excretion of sodium and an increase in the renal reabsorption of water.

POTASSIUM

In contrast to sodium, potassium (K^+) is the major cation of the fluid inside the cells. The normal plasma concentration of potassium ranges between 3.5 and 5 mEq/L (see Table 14–4). The normal intracellular concentration of potassium is about 140 mEq/L. Because of its high concentration inside cells, potassium exerts some control over intracellular osmolarity and volume. Maintaining this large difference in potassium concentration between the fluid inside the cell and the extracellular fluid is critical for excitable tissues to generate action potentials and to transmit impulses. Intracellular and extracellular functions of potassium include:

- Regulation of protein synthesis
- Regulation of glycolysis and glycogen synthesis
- Maintenance of action potentials in excitable membranes

TABLE 14–5 Common Food Sources of Sodium*

Food Source	Amount (mg)
Table salt (1 tsp)	2000
Cheddar cheese (1 oz)	176
Cottage cheese (4 oz)	457
American cheese (1 oz)	439
Whole milk (8 oz)	120
Skim milk (8 oz)	126
Butter (1 tsp)	123
White bread (1 slice)	123
Whole-wheat bread (1 slice)	159
Soy sauce (1 tbsp)	1029
Ketchup (1 tbsp)	156
Mustard (1 tbsp)	188
Beef, lean (4 oz)	60
Pork, lean, fresh (4 oz)	60
Pork, cured (4 oz)	850
Chicken, light meat (4 oz)	70
Chicken, dark meat (4 oz)	70

Data from Pennington, J. (1992). *Bowe's and Church's food values of portions commonly used* (16th ed.). Philadelphia: J. B. Lippincott.

* U.S. Department of Agriculture recommended daily allowance for adults: 1100–3300 mg.

Because extracellular fluid potassium levels are so low, any alteration in the extracellular fluid potassium concentration is poorly tolerated by the body and profoundly changes physiologic activities. For example, a decrease in plasma potassium of only 1 mEq/L (from 4 mEq/L to 3 mEq/L) represents a significant difference (25%) in the total extracellular potassium concentration, whereas a decrease in plasma sodium of 1 mEq/L (from 140 mEq/L to 139 mEq/L) represents a much smaller change (less than 1%) in the total extracellular sodium concentration.

Potassium drifts out of cells down its concentration gradient into the extracellular fluid. In addition, almost all ingested foods contain potassium (Table 14–6). The average potassium intake is about 2 to 20 g/day. Despite heavy potassium ingestion and the drifting of potassium from cellular storage sites into the extracellular fluid, the healthy body keeps plasma potassium levels within the narrow range of normal values required for optimal physiologic function.

The primary controller of extracellular potassium concentration is the sodium-potassium pumps within the membranes of all body cells. The cells of excitable tissues (such as nerves, skeletal muscle cells, and cardiac muscle cells) have greater numbers of these membrane-bound pumps. The pump removes three sodium ions from the fluid inside the cells for every two potassium ions that it returns to the cell. Thus, the concentration differences for both ions are maintained.

Some potassium regulation also occurs through renal function. The kidney is the excretory route for ridding the body of extracellular potassium (80% of potassium removal from the body occurs via the kidney). Unlike the situation with sodium, no hormone has been identified that directly controls renal reabsorption of potassium, and thus, the kidney does not conserve potassium directly.

TABLE 14–6 Common Food Sources of Potassium*

Food Source	Amount (mg)
Corn flakes (1¼ c)	26
Cooked oatmeal (¾ c)	99
Egg (1 large)	66
Codfish, raw (4 oz)	400
Salmon, pink, raw (3½ oz)	306
Tuna fish (4 oz)	375
Apple, raw with skin (1 medium)	159
Banana (1 medium)	451
Cantaloupe (1 c pieces)	494
Grapefruit (½ medium)	175
Orange (1 medium)	250
Raisins (½ c)	700
Strawberries, raw (1 c)	247
Watermelon (1 c pieces)	186
White bread (1 slice)	27
Whole-wheat bread (1 slice)	44
Beef (4 oz)	480
Beef liver (3½ oz)	281
Pork, fresh (4 oz)	525
Pork, cured (4 oz)	325
Chicken (4 oz)	225
Veal cutlet (3½ oz)	448
Whole milk (8 oz)	370
Skim milk (8 oz)	406
Avocado (1 medium)	1097
Carrot (1 large)	341
Corn (4-inch ear)	196
Cauliflower (1 c pieces)	295
Celery (1 stalk)	170
Green beans (1 c)	189
Mushrooms (10 small)	410
Onion (1 medium)	157
Peas (¾ c)	316
Potato, white (1 medium)	407
Spinach, raw (3½ oz)	470
Tomato (1 medium)	366

Data from Pennington, J. (1992). *Bowe's and Church's food values of portions commonly used* (16th ed.). Philadelphia: J. B. Lippincott.

* U.S. Department of Agriculture recommended daily allowance for adults: 1875–5625 mg.

CALCIUM

Calcium (Ca^{2+}) is a mineral whose presence and functions are closely related to the activities of phosphorus and magnesium. Calcium is a divalent cation (an ion that expresses two positive charges) that exists in the body in two forms: bound and ionized (unbound or free).

Bound calcium is usually connected to specific serum proteins, especially albumin. Ionized calcium is present in the blood and other extracellular fluids as free calcium. The free calcium is physiologically active, and it is this form that must be maintained in the extracellular fluid within narrow ranges. The body functions best when plasma calcium concentrations are maintained at 5 mEq/L (it may also be calculated as 8 to 10.5 mg/dL). Because the intracellular fluid concentration of calcium is low, a steep gradient exists for calcium between extracellular fluid and intracellular fluid. Calcium functions in many ways and in many specialized body systems, including:

- Biochemical cofactor (a substance required to enhance the activity of enzymes or reactions)
- Skeletal muscle contraction
- Cardiac contractility
- Regulation of neural impulse transmission
- Blood clotting
- Bone strength and density

Calcium enters the body by dietary intake and absorption through the intestinal tract (Table 14–7). For dietary calcium to be absorbed by the intestines, the active form of vitamin D must also be present. Calcium is stored in the bones. When both plasma calcium levels and stored calcium levels are adequate, gastrointestinal absorption of dietary calcium is inhibited and urinary excretion of excess calcium increases. When more plasma calcium is needed, parathyroid hormone (PTH, or parathoromone) is secreted and released from the parathyroid glands (Table 14–8). PTH causes extracellular fluid calcium levels to increase through the following processes:

TABLE 14–7 Common Food Sources of Calcium*

Food Source	Amount (mg)
Cheddar cheese (1 oz)	204
Cottage cheese (4 oz)	68
American cheese (1 oz)	174
Whole milk (8 oz)	288
Skim milk (8 oz)	302
Yogurt, low-fat (1 c)	415
Broccoli, raw (½ c)	75
Carrot (1 large)	37
Collard greens, raw (3 oz)	200
Green beans (1 c)	62
Rhubarb (1 c)	266
Spinach, raw (3½ oz)	93
Tofu (3 oz)	100

Data from Pennington, J. (1992). *Bowe's and Church's food values of portions commonly used* (16th ed.). Philadelphia: J. B. Lippincott.
* U.S. Department of Agriculture recommended daily allowance for adults: 800–1200 mg.

- Release of free calcium from bone storage sites directly into the extracellular fluid (resorption)
- Stimulation of vitamin D activation, thus increasing intestinal absorption of dietary calcium
- Inhibition of renal excretion of calcium and stimulation of renal tubular reabsorption of calcium

When excesses of calcium are present in the plasma, secretion of PTH is inhibited and secretion of calcitonin (a hormone secreted by the thyroid gland) is increased. Calcitonin causes the plasma calcium level to decrease through the following processes:

- Inhibition of bone resorption of calcium
- Inhibition of activation of vitamin D; decreased gastrointestinal uptake of calcium
- Increase of renal excretion of calcium in the urine

PHOSPHORUS

Phosphorus (P) is present in the body in both inorganic and organic forms. Normal plasma levels of phosphorus range between 2.5 and 4.5 mg/dL. The majority of phosphorus (80%) can be found in the bones. Phosphorus is the major anion in the intracellular fluid, and its concentration inside cells is much higher than that in extracellular fluid. Phosphorus has more intracellular functions than plasma functions. Phosphorus acts intracellularly as a cofactor, participating in the following activities:

- Activation of B-complex vitamins
- Formation and activation of high-energy substances, including adenosine triphosphate
- Cell division
- Carbohydrate metabolism
- Protein metabolism
- Lipid (fat) metabolism

Extracellular fluid phosphorus functions include acid-base buffering and calcium homeostasis. Phosphorus is present in a variety of foods, such as nuts, legumes, dairy products, red meat, organ meat, bran, and whole grains (Table 14–9), and the average diet is high in phosphorus (1 to 2 g/day) (Pennington, 1992).

Phosphorus balance and calcium balance are intertwined. Normally, plasma concentrations of calcium and phosphorus exist in a reciprocal relationship in that the product of the plasma concentrations remains a constant. Therefore, a change in the concentration of phosphorus results in an equal and opposite change in the concentration of calcium (and vice versa).

The regulation of extracellular fluid phosphorus occurs through the activity of parathyroid hormone (PTH). Increased secretion of PTH results in a net loss of phosphorus. Reduced PTH levels enhance the renal reabsorption of phosphorus, resulting in increased extracellular fluid concentrations of phosphorus.

MAGNESIUM

Magnesium (Mg^{2+}) is another mineral that forms a cation when it is dissolved in water. The adult human body has an average of 25 g of magnesium, most of which (60%) is stored in bones and cartilage. Little magnesium is present in the extracellular fluid, and more than 25% of that is bound to albumin. Plasma levels of ionized magnesium range between

TABLE 14–8 Hormonal Regulation of Calcium

Hormone	Action
Parathyroid Hormone (PTH)	
Secreted in response to low or low-normal serum calcium levels Secretion results in a rise in serum calcium concentration.	• Increases bone resorption of calcium (leaching of stored calcium) • Increases the absorption of ingested calcium from the gastrointestinal tract into extracellular fluid • Increases renal reabsorption of calcium at the proximal convoluted tubule
Thyrocalcitonin (TCT)	
Secreted by the thyroid gland in response to high or high-normal serum calcium levels Secretion results in a reduction of the serum calcium concentration.	• Increases bone uptake of calcium • Inhibits the absorption of calcium from the gastrointestinal tract so that ingested calcium is excreted from the body in feces • Inhibits renal reabsorption of calcium at the proximal convoluted tubule so that more calcium is excreted in the urine

TABLE 14–9 Common Food Sources of Phosphorus*

Food Source	Amount (mg)
Rolled oats, cooked (¾ c)	133
Egg (1 large)	90
Codfish (3 oz)	175
Tuna fish, white, canned (6½ oz)	405
Raisins (½ c)	75
White bread (1 slice)	26
Whole-wheat bread (1 slice)	23
Cheddar cheese (1 oz)	145
American cheese (1 oz)	211
Whole milk (8 oz)	228
Skim milk (8 oz)	247
Yogurt, low-fat (8 oz)	326
Beef (4 oz)	215
Beef liver (4 oz)	375
Pork, fresh (4 oz)	325
Chicken (4 oz)	200
Almonds (1 oz)	141
Peanuts (1 oz)	110

Data from Pennington, J. (1992). *Bowe's and Church's food values of portions commonly used* (16th ed.). Philadelphia: J. B. Lippincott.

* U.S. Department of Agriculture recommended daily allowance for adults: 800 mg.

1.5 and 2.5 mEq/L (Metheny, 1992). Much more magnesium is present in the intracellular fluid, and it is the second most common cation inside the cells. Magnesium has more functions inside the cells than in the plasma. Magnesium's intracellular functions center on its role as a cofactor. Magnesium is critical for the following reactions or activities:

- Muscle contraction
- Carbohydrate metabolism
- Activation and use of adenosine triphosphate
- Activation of many B-complex vitamins
- DNA synthesis
- Protein synthesis

Extracellular magnesium regulates blood coagulation and skeletal muscle contractility.

Magnesium is abundant in many foods, such as nuts, vegetables, fish, and whole grains (Table 14–10). The daily magnesium requirement for adults is about 300 mg.

Although magnesium is similar to calcium in many respects and its presence in the plasma must be maintained within a narrow range of normal values, little is known about its regulation. Magnesium is absorbed from the intestinal tract at the same point at which calcium is absorbed, and both electrolytes can be absorbed simultaneously. The absorption of phosphorus inhibits magnesium absorption to the same degree that it inhibits calcium absorption. Parathyroid hormone stimulates the release of magnesium from bone in much the same way that it stimulates the release of calcium. The renal tubule is the site of magnesium excretion and absorption.

CHLORIDE

Chloride (Cl^-) is the major anion of the extracellular fluid. It cooperates with sodium in maintaining osmotic pressure in the extracellular fluid. Chloride is also important in the formation of hydrochloric acid in the stomach. The normal plasma concentration of chloride ranges between 96 and 106 mEq/L.

Only a small quantity of chloride is present inside the cells because negatively charged particles on the cell membrane repel chloride and prevent it from crossing the cell membranes. However, extracellular chloride can enter cells when it is exchanged for another anion that is leaving the cell. This situation is called a chloride shift, resulting in a decrease in plasma chloride concentration but with no net loss of chloride. The anion most commonly exchanged for chloride in this way is bicarbonate (HCO_3^-). Chloride enters the body through dietary intake. Because chloride exists as part of a salt, with sodium, potassium, and many other minerals, most diets contain enough chloride to meet the body's normal need.

Fluid and Electrolyte Changes Associated with Aging

Elderly people have only 45% to 50% of their body weight in the form of water; for younger adults, the amount is 55% to 60%. This decrease represents a loss of muscle mass in the elderly person and a reduced ratio of overall lean body weight to total body weight. The decrease in total body water places elderly people at greater risk for water deficit states.

Skin turgor is not always an accurate assessment of extracellular fluid volume deficit in the elderly person

TABLE 14–10 Common Food Sources of Magnesium*

Food Source	Amount (mg)
Rolled oats (¾ c)	42
Tuna fish, white, canned (6½ oz)	59
Raisins (½ c)	25
Beef (4 oz)	24
Pork (4 oz)	30
Chicken (4 oz)	26
Whole milk (8 oz)	33
Skim milk (8 oz)	28
Yogurt, low-fat (8 oz)	40
Peanut butter (1 tbsp)	22
Avocado (1 medium)	70
Broccoli (1 stalk)	24
Cauliflower (1 c pieces)	24
Peas (¾ c)	35
Potato (1 medium)	34
Spinach, raw (3½ oz)	88

Data from Pennington, J. (1992). *Bowe's and Church's food values of portions commonly used* (16th ed.). Philadelphia: J. B. Lippincott.

* U.S. Department of Agriculture recommended daily allowance for adults: 300–350 mg.

because the natural aging process is associated with decreased turgor (Chart 14–1). Furthermore, the elderly person may have a diminished thirst sensation and decreased renal function, both of which contribute to risk of fluid volume deficit and make assessment more difficult. Accurate documentation of intake and output and accurate weight measurement are extremely important when nurses work with elderly clients because these measurements reflect hydration status more accurately in this population than does skin turgor. In addition, the very old person may be confused or forgetful and unable to give a reliable history.

Electrolyte balance may be more difficult to maintain in older people. Although the plasma and intracellular fluid electrolyte ranges may remain normal, the electrolyte balance is fragile and more easily disturbed. Part of the fragility of the balance is related to decreased regulatory functions that occur with aging. Age-related renal changes include decreased renal blood flow, decreased glomerular filtration rate, and decreased numbers of functional nephrons. Renal and membrane changes that are associated with hypertension may also be present in the elderly person. Variations in the responses of excitable membranes to electrical changes may also influence fluid and electrolyte balance in elderly clients. Small changes in the concentrations of potassium and calcium, in particular, may produce unexpectedly profound results.

HISTORY

The nurse collects data to assess the status of fluid and electrolyte balance by obtaining a thorough and detailed history. Because fluid and electrolyte imbalances can develop rapidly and occur in a variety of conditions, the nurse asks pertinent questions to elicit information that the client may not know has critical relevance. For example, a client with dehydration caused by hyperosmolarity of the extracellular fluid might have either diabetes or renal disease. Because the hyperosmolar state may have been caused by excessive ingestion of cola soft drinks and snack cakes that lead to hyperglycemia (an excessive plasma glucose level), the client's nutritional history can often reveal the underlying pathophysiologic processes influencing the condition. The client may not understand the connection between dietary intake and the onset of fluid and electrolyte imbalances and thus may not volunteer this important information.

The guidelines for obtaining a thorough fluid and electrolyte history do not differ from those usually used for assessing any other system; however, the kind of information collected is more quantitative. For example, intake and output volumes are often extremely important, as are serial daily weights. The nurse may need to guide clients in making an accurate report of the amount of fluid ingested and of changes in voiding patterns. The nurse assesses the types of fluids and foods ingested to determine osmolarity as well as amount. In addition, many clients do not consider solid food to contain liquid. Solid foods such as ice cream, gelatin, and ices are liquids at body temperature, and the nurse includes them when calculating fluid intake.

Output fluids include not only urine but also losses through significant diaphoresis and diarrhea and insensible loss during fevers. The nurse asks specific questions about prescribed and over-the-counter medications the client has taken and ascertains the dosage, the length of time taken, and the client's compliance with the medication regimen. A client taking diuretics can have an imbalance of fluid, potassium, sodium, or hydrogen ions if additional threats to water balance, such as vomiting and excessive sweating, also occur.

Laxatives are frequently used by elderly people and can disturb fluid and electrolyte balance. Misuse and overuse of these drugs can lead to serious imbalances.

Other pertinent areas of the client history include body weight changes, thirst or excessive drinking, exposure to environmental heat, and the presence of other pre-existing disorders such as renal or endocrine

CHART 14–1

Nursing Focus on the Elderly ◆ Impact of Changes Related to Aging on Fluid and Electrolyte Balance

System	Change	Result
Integumentary	• Loss of elasticity • Decreased turgor • Decreased oil production	• An unreliable indicator of fluid status • Dry, easily damaged skin
Renal	• Decreased glomerular filtration • Decreased concentrating capacity	• Poor excretion of waste products • Increased water loss
Muscular	• Decreased muscle mass	• Decreased total body water • Greater risk of dehydration
Neurologic	• Diminished thirst reflex	• Decreased fluid intake, increasing risk of dehydration
Endocrine	• Adrenal atrophy	• Poor regulation of sodium and potassium, predisposing the client to hyponatremia and hyperkalemia

diseases (Cushing's disease, Addison's disease, diabetes mellitus, and diabetes insipidus). The nurse should make a general assessment of the client's level of consciousness and mental status because changes in mental status may further support findings of imbalance. In such cases, the nurse may need to verify the accuracy of historical data.

PHYSICAL ASSESSMENT

Hydration is defined as the normal state of fluid balance (Metheny, 1992). A normally hydrated adult is alert, has moist eyes and mucous membranes, has a urinary output appropriate for the amount of fluid ingested (with a specific gravity of urine of approximately 1.015), and has an adequate state of skin hydration as measured by skin turgor.

Turgor is the normal resiliency of a pinched fold of skin. This pinched fold should return immediately to its original shape after it is released. Decreased turgor, a sign of dehydration, is present when the fold remains in a pinched shape after being released and rebounds slowly *(tenting)* (Fig. 14–9). The nurse can best assess skin turgor in body areas that contain little adipose tissue, such as over the sternum or on the back of the hand. The elderly person may have poor skin turgor because of the loss of tissue elasticity that is related to the aging process; thus, a true state of hydration may be more difficult to assess than in a younger adult. Areas in which to assess turgor in the elderly are over the sternum and on the forehead.

Skin hydration assessment also includes an examination for dryness. The mucous membranes and the conjunctiva are normally moist. An assessment of fluid balance always includes an examination of the eyes, the nose, and oral mucous membranes. A dry, sticky, "cottony" mouth; the absence of tearing; the presence of weight loss; and a decreased urinary output indicate an actual fluid volume deficit.

A major criterion used in assessing fluid and electrolyte status is the accurate measurement of a client's fluid intake and output. Accurate assessment of actual fluid intake and output is the nurse's responsibility, and volumetric measuring devices should be used. However, even when daily measuring and recording of intake and output are prescribed, many nurses only estimate these volumes and are not always accurate in the estimation, as shown in Research Applications for Nursing. In addition, data on intake and output are not always recorded; therefore, the assessment of a client's thirst, renal function, and fluid and electrolyte status on the basis of these variables may not be valid.

Behavioral and neurologic assessments are included in fluid assessment because changes in fluid balance can result in alteration of neurologic function. In hypertonic states, neuronal cell shrinkage may induce serious nervous system excitability and hyperactivity, and convulsions may occur. Another variable to as-

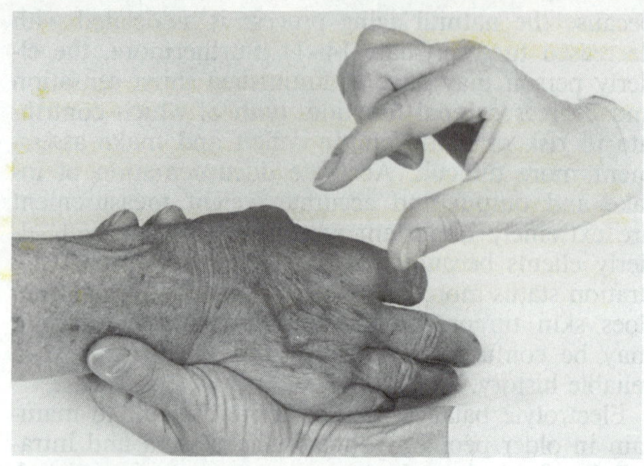

FIGURE 14–9 ◆ Tenting of the skin during testing for skin turgor. (From Jarvis, C. [1992]. *Physical examination and health assessment*. Philadelphia: W. B. Saunders.)

RESEARCH APPLICATIONS FOR NURSING

Estimates of Fluid Intake and Output May Be Grossly Inaccurate

Burns, D. (1992). Working up a thirst. *Nursing Times, 88*(26), 44–45.

Many nurses do not take the time to measure the exact fluid intake or output, even when assessment of fluid volume is critical for the client. Instead, nurses often estimate the amount of fluid that a specific container holds and how much the client has ingested or excreted. This technique is open to significant error.

Burns therefore sought to determine how accurately nurses estimate the volume of specific food and beverage containers. The subjects of the study were 48 registered nurses on a medical-surgical nursing unit. Burns asked each nurse to estimate the volume of four different standard food and beverage containers (soup bowl, porcelain coffee cup, drinking glass, and plastic water pitcher). Out of a possible 192 correct answers, 103 answers (53%) were incorrect. The nurses either underestimated or overestimated the container volumes.

Critique. Although this article did not include enough detail to determine the validity of the results, it identified an important issue: that estimates of intake and output may be grossly inaccurate.

Possible nursing implications. If estimations are not accurate, interventions that are based on fluid intake or fluid output may be inappropriate and even dangerous. Nurses must accurately measure fluid intake and output for clients at risk for fluid imbalances. Surveys to determine how common is the practice of estimating fluid volume could be helpful in establishing policies for the precise measurement of intake and output.

sess is the degree of thirst. With an elderly client who is confused, thirst may be difficult to determine accurately.

The nurse approximates insensible water loss (e.g., sweat) in every client. In addition, special situations require an assessment of fluid loss from other routes, including:

- Fluid losses from wounds
- Gastric or intestinal drainage
- Blood loss from hemorrhage
- Drainage of body secretions, such as bile and pancreatic juices, through surgical fistulas

Electrolytes control the activity of excitable membranes, and electrolyte imbalances are associated with alterations in the function of these membranes. Electrolyte assessment includes a complete neuromuscular assessment for muscle tone and strength, movement, coordination, and the presence of tremors. An assessment of other systems, including cardiac (assess the heart rate, the strength of contractions, and the presence of arrhythmias) and gastrointestinal (assess the activity of peristalsis) systems, may indicate alterations of excitable membrane function.

Part of the nurse's assessment focuses on changes from previous findings (including mental status, physical examination data, and laboratory data). Fluid and electrolyte imbalances can arise quickly; therefore, the nurse must be familiar with the client's baseline assessment data to determine what changes have occurred.

PSYCHOSOCIAL ASSESSMENT

The psychosocial assessment of a client for fluid and electrolyte status includes both psychologic and cultural factors that might influence balance. Depressed clients may refuse fluids or forget to drink adequate amounts of fluid. Clients with bulimia or anorexia nervosa (eating disorders) may use laxatives to excess, which results in fluid and electrolyte imbalances.

Nurses should also assess social practices. Excessive alcohol or drug use may lead to fluid or electrolyte imbalance.

DIAGNOSTIC ASSESSMENT

Laboratory results, along with the history and physical assessment, are necessary to identify specific fluid and electrolyte imbalances or the presence of disorders that alter fluid and electrolyte status. Normal serum electrolyte values are presented in Table 14-4. Other laboratory values that may assist in assessing a client's fluid and electrolyte status include blood urea nitrogen level, glucose concentration, creatinine level, pH, bicarbonate level, and osmolarity as well as hemoglobin level and hematocrit.

The urine test results are important in assessing fluid status. When a laboratory report is not available, the nurse can perform various tests using a dipstick-type technique to help determine fluid and electrolyte status, including presence of substances that should not be present in the urine, such as glucose, acetone, protein, and blood. Urine measurements such as pH and specific gravity can be determined in this way and abnormal or unusual findings recorded.

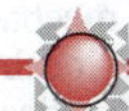

IMPLICATIONS FOR NURSING RESEARCH

The nurse has direct control over and responsibility for the client's fluid and electrolyte balance. However, an assessment of hydration and electrolyte balance can be difficult, particularly in elderly clients. Some questions appropriate for nursing research include:

- ♦ Should clients taking high-ceiling diuretics follow sodium-restricted diets?
- ♦ What specific assessment techniques accurately reflect the hydration status in elderly people?
- ♦ Is a video approach to teaching sodium intake calculation effective in the older adult population?

SELECTED BIBLIOGRAPHY

Birney, M., & Penney, D. (1990). Atrial natriuretic peptide: A hormone with implications for clinical practice. *Heart & Lung, 19*(2), 174.

Burns, D. (1992). Working up a thirst. *Nursing Times, 88*(26), 44-45.

Carlson, K., Snyder, M., LeClair, H., Underhill, A., Ashwood, E., & Detter, J. (1990). Obtaining reliable plasma sodium and glucose determinations from pulmonary artery catheters. *Heart & Lung, 19*(6), 613-619.

* Chenevey, B. (1987). Overview of fluids and electrolytes. *Nursing Clinics of North America, 22*(4), 749.

Gilmour, J., & Penny, S. (1991). Hydration and aging. *New Zealand Nursing Journal, 84*(10), 15-17.

Guyton, A. (1991). *Textbook of medical physiology* (8th ed.). Philadelphia: W. B. Saunders.

Jones, A., Moseley, M., Halfmann, S., Heath, A., Henkelman, W., Ciaccio, J., & Bolcas, B. (1991). Fluid volume dynamics. *Critical Care Nurse, 11*(4), 74-76.

Keyes, J. (1990). *Fluid, electrolyte, and acid-base regulation* (2nd ed.). Belmont, CA: Wadsworth.

Kokko, J., & Tannen, R. (1990). *Fluids and electrolytes* (2nd ed.). Philadelphia: W. B. Saunders.

Metheny, N. (1992). *Fluid and electrolyte balance: Nursing considerations* (2nd ed.). Philadelphia: J. B. Lippincott.

Norris, M. K. (1992). Evaluating sodium levels. *Nursing92, 21*(7), 20.

Pennington, J. (1992). *Bowe's and Church's food values of portions commonly used* (16th ed.). Philadelphia: J. B. Lippincott.

Porth, C., & Erickson, M. (1992). Physiology of thirst and drinking: Implication for nursing practice. *Heart & Lung, 21*(3), 273–284.

Terry, J. (1991). The other electrolytes: Magnesium, calcium and phosphorus. *Journal of Intravenous Nursing, 14*(3), 167–76.

Trissel, L. (1992). *Handbook on injectable drugs* (7th ed.). Bethesda, MD: American Society of Hospital Pharmacists.

Watt, S. (1991). Quenching the body's thirst. *New Zealand Nursing Journal, 84*(10), 18–19.

SUGGESTED READINGS

Gilmour, J., & Penny, S. (1991). Hydration and aging. *New Zealand Nursing Journal, 84*(10), 15–17.

This brief but interesting article summarizes the basic mechanisms of normal fluid balance and describes how these mechanisms become less effective as a result of aging. Practical guidelines for nurses to use in assessing the fluid and electrolyte status of older adults and suggestions for fluid replacement options are presented.

Jones, A., Moseley, M., Halfmann, S., Heath, A., Henkelman, W., Ciaccio, J., & Bolcas, B. (1991). Fluid volume dynamics. *Critical Care Nurse, 11*(4), 74–76.

This easy-to-read article uses a unique approach for teaching the principles of fluid balance. Fifteen true-false questions are asked about specific aspects of fluid balance. The questions are presented in a client situation format. The answers include not only the correct response, but also an in-depth explanation of why a response is correct.

Porth, C., & Erickson, M. (1992). Physiology of thirst and drinking: Implication for nursing practice. *Heart & Lung, 21*(3), 273–284.

This article provides detailed explanations of how the thirst mechanism influences fluid balance, hydration status, and the client's comfort. The types of thirst are defined and explained. Drugs that alter the sensation of thirst are listed. The article also addresses nursing assessment for thirst and implications for nursing care of clients who are experiencing dry mouth or thirst discomfort.

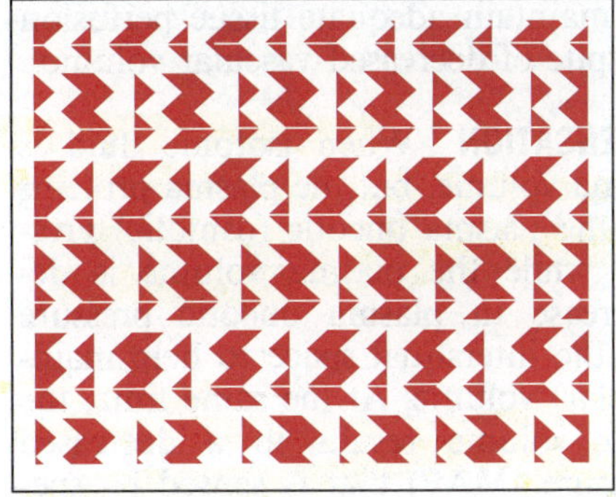

CHAPTER 15

Interventions for Clients with Fluid Imbalances

CHAPTER HIGHLIGHTS

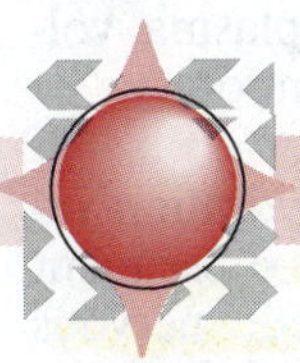

Fluid and electrolyte imbalances are common in clients in all settings. Physiologic homeostasis depends heavily on normal fluid balance. Because any health problem can upset fluid balance to some degree, virtually every client is at some risk. Specific imbalances are discussed separately in this text, although fluid levels and the concentrations of most electrolytes are so interrelated that fluid imbalances rarely occur without an accompanying electrolyte imbalance.

Dehydration

OVERVIEW

In dehydration, the body's fluid intake is not sufficient to meet the body's fluid needs, resulting in a fluid volume deficit. Three basic types of dehydration (Fig. 15–1) are possible:

- Isotonic dehydration, in which isotonic fluids are lost
- Hypertonic dehydration, in which a greater proportion of fluid is lost compared with solute loss
- Hypotonic dehydration, in which a greater proportion of solute is lost compared with fluid loss

Dehydration may be an actual decrease in total body water, which is caused by either inadequate

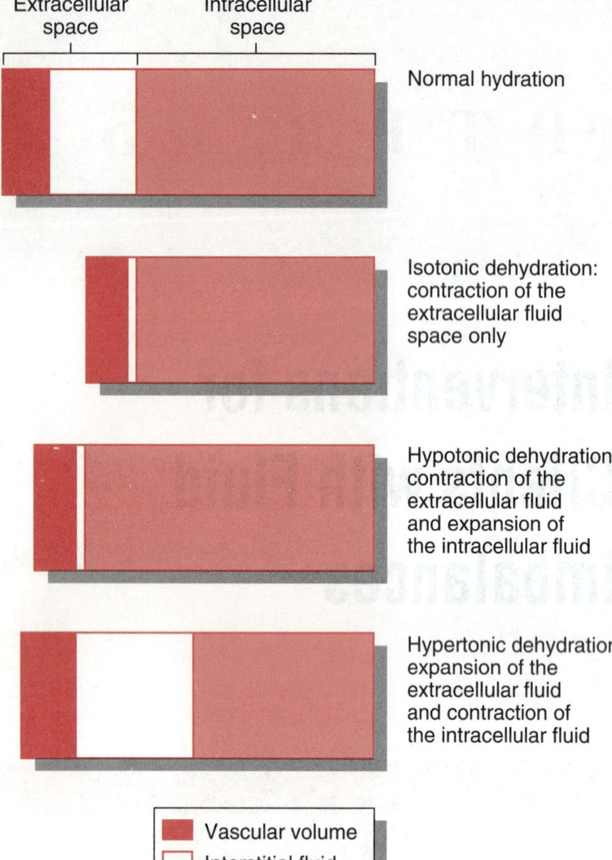

FIGURE 15-1 ◆ Three types of dehydration. (© 1992 M. Linda Workman. All rights reserved.)

fluid intake or excessive fluid loss. Dehydration can also be present without an actual decrease in total body water, such as when water shifts from the plasma into the interstitial space. Dehydration is a clinical state rather than a disease and can be caused by many underlying pathologic changes.

ISOTONIC DEHYDRATION

Isotonic dehydration, or hypovolemia, is the most common type of dehydration. Problems associated with isotonic dehydration result from a reduction in plasma volume.

PATHOPHYSIOLOGY

Isotonic dehydration involves loss of isotonic fluids from the extracellular fluid (ECF) compartment (both the plasma and the interstitial space). Because isotonic fluid is lost, plasma osmolarity remains normal. This type of dehydration does not result in a shift of fluids between compartments; thus the intracellular fluid (ICF) volume remains normal. The overall result of isotonic dehydration is an inadequate circulating volume. Compensatory mechanisms (Fig. 15-2) attempt to maintain adequate tissue perfusion to vital organs in spite of decreased vascular volume.

HORMONAL COMPENSATION When isotonic fluid is lost from the plasma volume, but the plasma proteins and cells remain, the plasma oncotic (osmotic) pressure is increased, while the plasma volume is decreased. This increase in plasma oncotic pressure draws water from the interstitial space to help maintain plasma (vascular) volume. At the same time, the decreased vascular volume results in a decreased mean arterial pressure (MAP) that is sensed by special cells in the kidney. The low MAP stimulates the secretion of renin and initiates the renin-angiotensinogen cascade, which causes the formation of angiotensin II and the release of aldosterone from the adrenal cortex. The angiotensin II causes vasoconstriction, and the aldosterone increases renal reabsorption of water and sodium (see Fig. 14-6). These two mechanisms together increase plasma volume and MAP, thus assisting to maintain adequate tissue perfusion (Guyton, 1991). However, without additional fluid intake, this mechanism increases plasma volume by depleting the fluid volume of the interstitial space. Therefore, restoration of the plasma volume by this mechanism is limited and temporary.

SYMPATHETIC COMPENSATION When dehydration involves a 3% loss of plasma volume, the subsequent drop in the MAP activates the sympathetic nervous system (SNS). Activation of the SNS inhibits the parasympathetic division and causes the release of catecholamines (epinephrine and norepinephrine). Catecholamines increase cardiac output by increasing heart rate and contractility. At the same time, SNS stimulation causes selective systemic vasoconstriction (constriction of small arteries and arterioles). This action shunts blood away from the skin, the gastrointestinal (GI) tract, and the kidneys, making more blood available to the central vascular space. These compensatory mechanisms adequately maintain circulation and perfusion until 25% to 30% of the vascular volume is lost. At that point, compensatory mechanisms are inadequate to maintain perfusion, even to vital organs, and symptoms of severe hypovolemic shock are manifested. (See Chapter 36 for a discussion of hypovolemic shock.)

ETIOLOGY

Isotonic dehydration has many causes (Table 15-1):

- Excessive losses of isotonic fluids
- Inadequate intake of fluids and solutes
- Fluid shifts between compartments

Excessive losses of isotonic fluids occur through hemorrhage or abnormal losses through the gastrointestinal tract, the kidneys, and the skin. Severe losses of extracellular fluid and solutes can result from excessive vomiting, diarrhea, profuse salivation, pro-

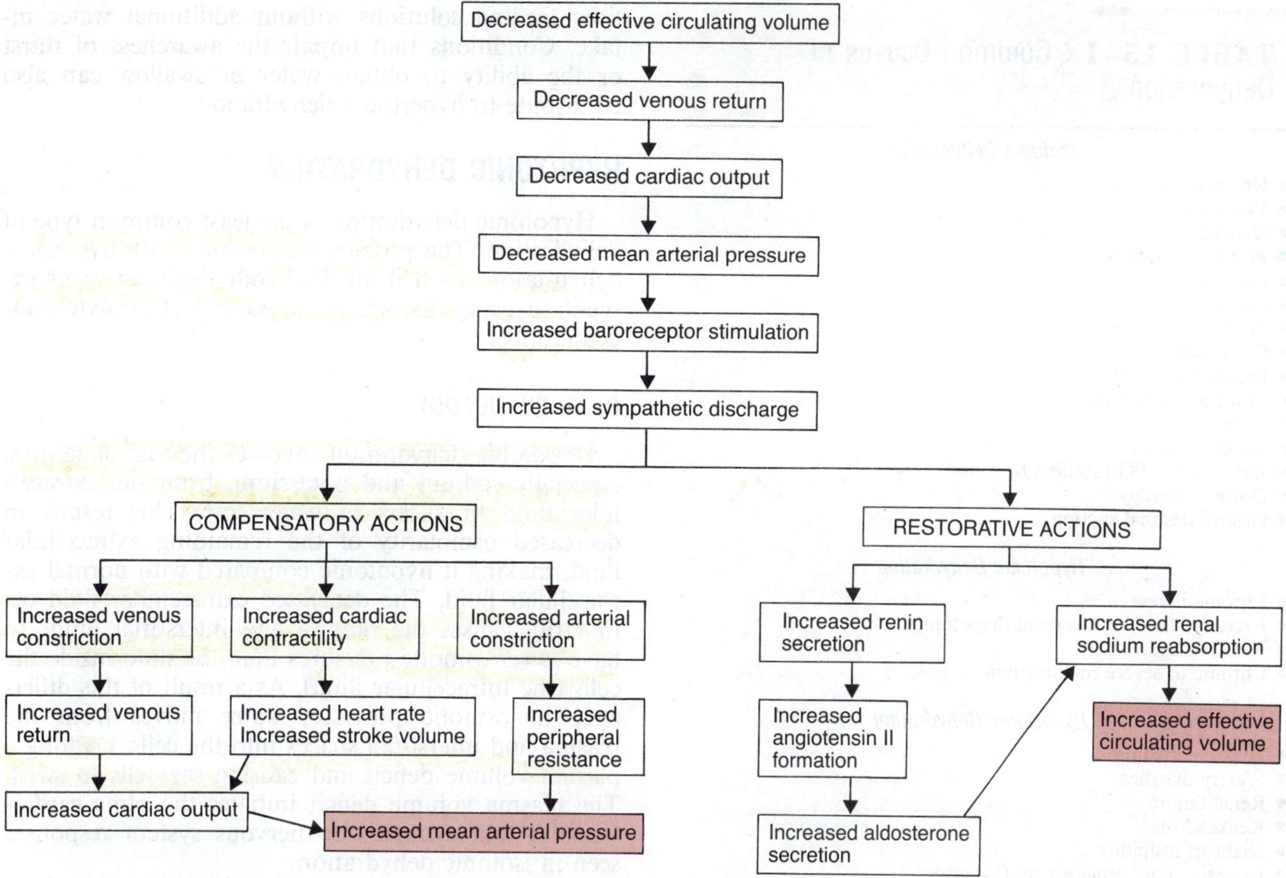

FIGURE 15–2 ◆ Compensatory mechanisms associated with isotonic dehydration.

longed nasogastric suctioning, and drainage from wounds. Additional causes of isotonic dehydration include the excessive diuresis that accompanies the high-output stage of renal failure, decreased secretion of aldosterone (such as in Addison's disease or after adrenalectomy), and diuretic therapy.

Decreased fluid intake can also produce isotonic dehydration. This cause is most common among clients with motor impairments, those with decreased level of consciousness, and clients who receive nothing by mouth (NPO) for several days. The risk increases among clients who also have conditions, such as infection or fever, that increase the body's fluid need.

Fluid shifts from the plasma (vascular) space to the interstitial space (also known as "third spacing") can produce isotonic dehydration. These shifts occur with increased capillary hydrostatic pressure or increased capillary permeability often associated with extensive trauma, burns, sepsis, peritonitis, intestinal obstruction, and cirrhosis of the liver.

HYPERTONIC DEHYDRATION

Hypertonic dehydration is the second most common type of fluid volume deficit. The problems associated with hypertonic dehydration result from alterations in the concentrations of specific plasma electrolytes.

PATHOPHYSIOLOGY

Hypertonic dehydration occurs when water loss from the extracellular fluid exceeds solute loss. This water loss increases the osmolarity of the remaining plasma, making it hypertonic or hyperosmolar compared with normal extracellular fluids. The hyperosmolar plasma has an increased osmotic pressure that causes fluid to move rapidly from the intracellular fluid into the plasma and interstitial fluid spaces. This fluid shift results in cellular dehydration and shrinkage. The fluid shift causes the plasma volume to approach normal levels (or perhaps even be elevated). Thus, the compensatory mechanisms and signs and symptoms of hypovolemic shock are not present. However, the stability of excitable membranes, particularly cardiac contractility, may be profoundly affected by accompanying alterations in the plasma levels of specific electrolytes (especially potassium and calcium).

Compensatory mechanisms for hypertonic dehydration are responses to the increased extracellular fluid osmolarity (Fig. 15–3). These mechanisms begin as soon as either an increase in osmolarity or a decrease in vascular volume occurs. The thirst reflex is stimulated by the hypothalamus in an attempt to increase fluid intake. In addition, the secretion of antidiuretic hormone increases, which promotes renal reabsorption of water back into the body.

TABLE 15–1 Common Causes of Dehydration

Isotonic Dehydration

- Hemorrhage
- Vomiting
- Diarrhea
- Profuse salivation
- Fistulas
- Abscesses
- Ileostomy
- Cecostomy
- Frequent enemas
- Profuse diaphoresis
- Burns
- Severe wounds
- Long-term NPO (nothing by mouth)
- Diuretic therapy
- Gastrointestinal suction

Hypotonic Dehydration

- Chronic illness
- Excessive fluid replacement (hypotonic)
- Renal failure
- Chronic or severe malnutrition

Hypertonic Dehydration

- Hyperventilation
- Watery diarrhea
- Renal failure
- Ketoacidosis
- Diabetes insipidus
- Excessive fluid replacement (hypertonic)
- Excessive sodium bicarbonate administration
- Tube feedings
- Dysphagia
- Impaired thirst
- Unconsciousness
- Fever
- Impaired motor function
- Systemic infection

ETIOLOGY

Hypertonic dehydration results from the loss of any body fluid that is hypotonic (low osmolarity, or decreased concentration of solute particles compared with that in isotonic body fluid). Common causes of hypertonic dehydration are conditions that increase insensible fluid loss. Such conditions include excessive perspiration, hyperventilation, ketoacidosis, and excessive skin water evaporation loss during high or prolonged fevers (see Table 15–1). Losses of hypotonic body fluids also contribute to hypertonic dehydration, including copious secretions from tracheostomies, watery diarrhea, renal failure in which water reabsorption is impaired, diabetes insipidus, and ketoacidosis in the diuretic phase.

Additionally, any condition that increases the body's metabolic rate also increases the body's need for water. Other causes of hypertonic dehydration include excessive intravenous (IV) infusions of hypertonic fluids (especially fluids containing sodium bicarbonate) and long-term intake of high-osmolarity tube feeding solutions without additional water intake. Conditions that impair the awareness of thirst or the ability to obtain water or swallow can also contribute to hypertonic dehydration.

HYPOTONIC DEHYDRATION

Hypotonic dehydration is the least common type of dehydration. The problems associated with hypotonic dehydration result from fluid shifts between compartments causing disruption in normal electrolyte concentrations.

PATHOPHYSIOLOGY

Hypotonic dehydration involves the loss of solutes, especially sodium and potassium, from the extracellular fluid in excess of water loss. This results in decreased osmolarity of the remaining extracellular fluid, making it hypotonic compared with normal extracellular fluid. The decreased extracellular fluid osmolarity causes the plasma and interstitial fluids to have *lower* osmotic pressures than the fluid inside the cells (the intracellular fluid). As a result of this difference in osmotic pressure, water moves from the plasma and interstitial spaces into the cells, creating a plasma volume deficit and causing the cells to swell. The plasma volume deficit initiates the same cardiovascular and sympathetic nervous system responses seen in isotonic dehydration.

Intracellular swelling causes several problems and symptoms, depending on which organs sustain the influx of fluid. Because brain cells are more sensitive to cellular fluid changes than are the cells of other tissues, neurologic dysfunction usually accompanies hypotonic dehydration. In addition, the hypotonic fluid can dilute the normal electrolyte concentrations and can result in sodium and potassium imbalances.

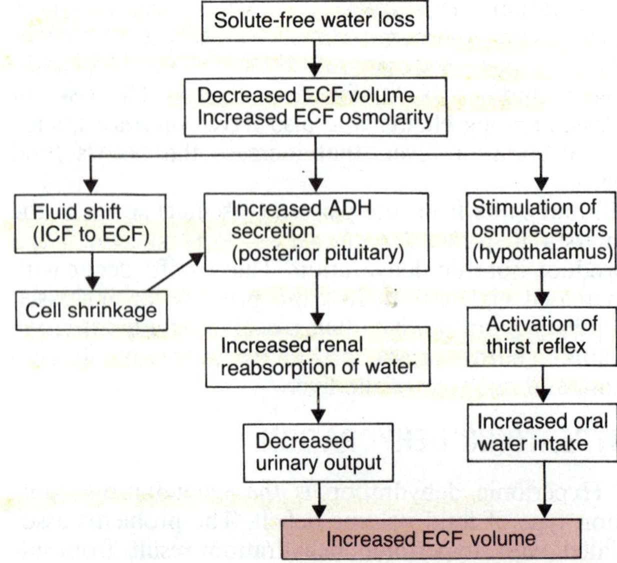

FIGURE 15–3 ◆ Compensatory mechanisms associated with hypertonic dehydration.

ETIOLOGY

Hypotonic dehydration is usually associated with chronic illness. Chronic renal failure, in which the kidneys waste sodium, leads to hypotonic dehydration. Chronic malnutrition and excessive ingestion of hypotonic fluids also cause hypotonic dehydration.

INCIDENCE/PREVALENCE

Although the actual incidence of dehydration is not known, virtually every ill client is at risk. Elderly clients are at high risk because they have less total body water than younger adults. Additionally, the average fluid requirement of well elderly people is 1500 to 2000 mL/day of hypotonic fluid (such as water). Conditions that may contribute to an inadequate fluid intake among elderly people include a diminished thirst sensation and possible difficulty with ambulation or other motor skills necessary for taking fluids.

COLLABORATIVE MANAGEMENT

ASSESSMENT

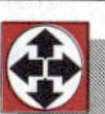

HISTORY

The nurse collects data on risk factors and factors causing dehydration (Table 15–2).

AGE Age is an important consideration, because dehydration in the elderly develops in response to relatively small fluid losses. In addition, elderly people are more likely to have chronic illnesses or to be taking medications that can lead to fluid and electrolyte imbalances.

HEIGHT AND WEIGHT Measurement of height and weight is important for calculating approximate fluid needs. If this information is not known or if the client is confused, the nurse obtains these measurements directly. Because weight and liquid measurements are related, changes in daily weights are good indicators of fluid losses or excesses. One liter of water weighs approximately 1 kg (2.2 pounds). Therefore, a weight change of 1 pound corresponds to a fluid volume change of 475 to 500 mL.

OTHER CHANGES The nurse questions the client about changes in the tightness of clothing, rings, and shoes. A sudden decrease in the tightness may indicate dehydration; an increase in the tightness may reflect a fluid shift to the interstitial space with an accompanying deficit in the vascular space. Other relevant findings include the presence of palpitations or a feeling of lightheadedness on moving from a lying or a sitting position to a standing position (caused by orthostatic, or postural, hypotension).

The nurse asks about any abnormal or excessive fluid losses, such as perspiration, diarrhea, bleeding, vomiting, urination, salivation, and wound drainage.

TABLE 15–2 Risk Factors for Dehydration

Illnesses	Other Situations
• Vomiting	• Extremes of age: elderly, infants
• Diarrhea	• Unconsciousness
• Burns	• Motor limitations
• Large draining wounds	***Therapies***
• Liver dysfunction	• Surgery
• Diabetes mellitus	• Diuretics
• Diabetes insipidus	• Nothing by mouth (NPO)
• Renal disease	• Excessive hypertonic enemas
• Hemorrhage	• Nasogastric suction
• Major venous obstruction	
• Prolonged febrile state	

The nurse questions clients about chronic illnesses, recent acute illnesses, recent surgery, and medications. Not only does this information indicate potential risk or possible causes of dehydration, but it may also indicate the presence of specific problems that affect how the type of dehydration should be corrected.

The nurse asks specific questions about urinary output, including the frequency and amount of voidings. The nurse also asks about the client's usual fluid intake and the intake during the previous 24 hours. It is just as important to determine the types of fluids ingested as the amount of fluids ingested. The nurse inquires about the amount of strenuous physical activity the client may have engaged in recently and asks whether the activity took place in hot or dry environmental conditions.

PHYSICAL ASSESSMENT/CLINICAL MANIFESTATIONS

The clinical manifestations of dehydration depend on which fluid compartments lose fluid, although all body systems are affected to some degree (Chart 15–1). There is controversy about the manifestations that are consistent indicators of dehydration (Research Applications for Nursing). The most obvious and life-threatening clinical manifestations are seen when the dehydration involves significant fluid loss from the vascular (plasma) portion of the extracellular space.

CARDIOVASCULAR MANIFESTATIONS Cardiovascular changes are the most reliable indicators of changes in the plasma volume. The heart rate increases with plasma volume deficits. Peripheral pulses are weaker, are difficult to find, and are easily blocked with light pressure. If interstitial edema accompanies the dehydration, the peripheral pulses may not be palpable. Blood pressure decreases, as does the pulse pressure, with a greater decrease being present in the systolic blood pressure. Hypotension is more profound with the client in the standing position than in the sitting or the lying position. This type of unstable blood pressure is called orthostatic, or postural, hypoten-

CHART 15-1

Key Features of Dehydration

Manifestations of Dehydration in General*

Cardiovascular

- Increased pulse rate
- Thready pulse quality
- Decreased blood pressure
- Postural hypotension
- Flat neck and hand veins in dependent positions
- Diminished peripheral pulses

Respiratory

- Increased respiratory rate
- Increased depth of respirations

Neuromuscular

- Decreased central nervous system activity (lethargy to coma)
- Fever

Renal

- Decreased urinary output
- Increased specific gravity

Integumentary

- Skin dry and scaly
- Turgor poor, tenting present
- Mouth dry and fissured, paste-like coating present

Gastrointestinal

- Decreased motility
- Diminished bowel sounds
- Constipation
- Thirst

Manifestations of Hypotonic Dehydration

- Skeletal muscle weakness

Manifestations of Hypertonic Dehydration

- Hyperactive deep tendon reflexes
- Increased sensation of thirst
- Pitting edema

* These manifestations are most severe with hypotonic dehydration.

sion. Because the blood pressure with the client in the standing position may be much lower than that in other positions, blood pressure is measured first with the client in the lying position, then in the sitting position, and last in the standing position.

Another cardiovascular indicator of hydration status is the degree of neck and hand vein filling. Normally, hand veins fill and become engorged when the hands are lower than the level of the heart. As the hand is raised above the level of the heart, the veins flatten or collapse (Fig. 15-4). Neck veins are normally distended when a client is in the supine position. These veins tend to flatten when the client moves to a sitting position. When dehydration in-

RESEARCH APPLICATIONS FOR NURSING

Most Defining Characteristics of Fluid Volume Deficit Appear to Be Valid, and Other Clinical Indicators May Be Valid As Well

Gershan, J. A., Freeman, C. M., Ross, M. C., Greenlee, K., Smejkal, C., Brukwitzki, G., Schneider, K., Jiricka, M., Johnson, D., & Anderson, C. (1990). Fluid volume deficit: Validating the indicators. *Heart & Lung, 19*(2), 152-156.

Gershan and colleagues studied the defining characteristics of the nursing diagnosis Fluid Volume Deficit to determine which clinical signs accurately reflect the presence of the diagnosis. The researchers first developed an instrument that listed 72 clinical indicators of Fluid Volume Deficit cited in the literature. The investigators then used this instrument to conduct a three-phase survey of clinical nurse specialists and other nurses with specialized knowledge of fluid balance. The 53 participants agreed on 17 critical clinical indicators, which they organized into four categories:

- Changes in fluid balance: decreased urinary output and negative input-output balance
- Clinical and physical assessment cues: weight loss, other changes in body weight, increased heart rate, thready pulse, decreased pulse volume and pressure, diminished venous filling, and poor skin turgor
- Changes in laboratory values: increased hematocrit and urine osmolality
- Hemodynamic changes: decreased blood pressure, postural blood pressure changes, decreased central venous pressure, and decreased pulmonary artery wedge pressure

Of the seven original defining characteristics approved by the North American Nursing Diagnosis Association (NANDA) for the nursing diagnosis Fluid Volume Deficit, this study validated six. The NANDA-approved defining characteristic "increased serum sodium concentration" was not validated. In addition, the study validated 11 other consistent clinical indicators of Fluid Volume Deficit as defining characteristics.

Critique The researchers accomplished the first stage of validation of the defining characteristics of an important nursing diagnosis. Future studies are needed to verify the relevance of these indicators in various settings.

Possible nursing implications Some of the critical indicators of Fluid Volume Deficit are subtle. However, failure to recognize early changes in fluid volume status may have serious consequences. Nurses unfamiliar with these indicators may find the four-part classification presented by the researchers helpful. In time, and with experience, clinicians will learn to quickly recognize and diagnose alterations in fluid balance.

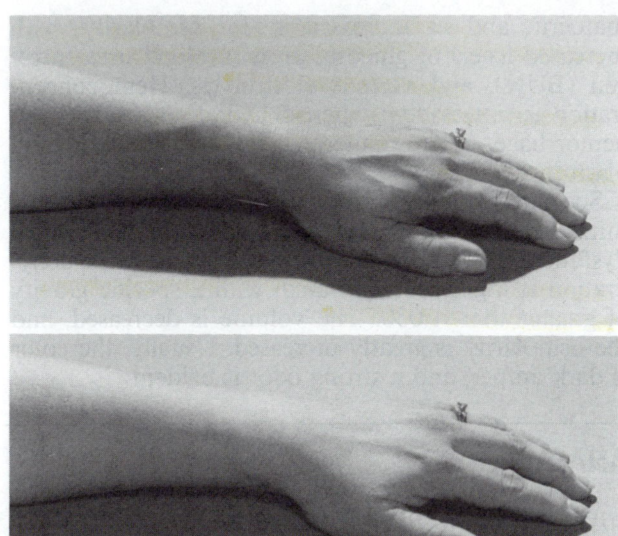

FIGURE 15-4 ◆ *Top,* The hand veins full and bulging in the dependent position. *Bottom,* The hand veins collapsed.

volves a plasma volume deficit, neck and hand veins are flat, even when these structures are dependent to the heart. The cardiovascular changes listed earlier are not seen in states of dehydration in which plasma volume is normal or above normal, such as hypertonic dehydration.

RESPIRATORY MANIFESTATIONS Respiratory rate increases directly with the degree of fluid loss from the plasma volume. When ketoacidosis causes or accompanies dehydration, respirations become deep and rapid. This type of respiratory pattern is called *Kussmaul breathing.*

INTEGUMENTARY MANIFESTATIONS Integumentary changes may be useful indicators of hydration. The nurse assesses the integumentary system for changes in the skin and mucous membranes that may indicate dehydration. Specific factors to assess include skin color, the degree of moisture, skin turgor, and the presence of edema. In elderly clients, this information is less reliable because of poor skin turgor due to the loss of elastic tissue and the loss of tissue fluids with aging.

The nurse assesses skin turgor by noting:

- How easily the skin over the back of the hand and arm can be gently pinched between the thumb and the forefinger to form a "tent"
- How soon the pinched skin resumes its normal position after release
- Whether depressions (pits) remain in the skin after a finger is pressed firmly but gently (over the shin, over the sternum, and over the sacrum)
- How deep the depression is (in millimeters)
- How long the depression remains

In generalized dehydration, skin turgor is poor, with the tenting remaining for minutes after pinching up the skin, and skin depressions do not occur with gentle pressure. The skin appears dry and scaly in dehydrated clients. The nurse assesses skin turgor in an elderly client by pinching the skin over the sternum, the forehead, or the abdomen because these areas tend to indicate hydration more reliably. As a person ages, the skin loses elasticity and tents on extremities even if the person is well hydrated.

In addition, oral mucous membranes are not moist when dehydration is present. They may be covered with a thick, sticky, paste-like coating and may have cracks and fissures. The surface of the tongue may have deep furrows.

NEUROLOGIC MANIFESTATIONS Clients with dehydration may show changes in body temperature and mental status. The client with dehydration typically has a fever. The fever may cause or result from dehydration. Clients with temperature elevations of greater than 39° C (102° F) for longer than 6 hours are especially at risk. The nurse determines the client's baseline body temperature to estimate the severity of temperature elevation. For example, elderly clients typically have a normal body temperature range of 35.4° to 36.6° C (96° to 98° F). A prolonged temperature elevation of 38° to 38.6° C (100° to 101° F) may cause severe dehydration in an elderly client.

The nurse assesses the client's neurologic status by first determining the level of consciousness and orientation to time, place, and person. The nurse notes whether the client is asleep or awake. If the client is asleep, the nurse gently awakens him or her and documents the ease with which the client arouses. When the client is awake, the nurse establishes whether the client is oriented. The nurse avoids asking questions that can be answered with a "yes" or "no" response and documents the manner in which the client responds to the questions. Is it necessary to repeat questions to obtain a response? Does the response answer the question asked? Does the client have difficulty with word choices in forming responses? Is the client irritated or upset by the questions? Can the client concentrate on a question long enough to provide an appropriate response or is the attention span short? (Other useful questions and techniques to assess mental status can be found in Chapter 40.)

The nurse observes the client closely and documents the presenting behavior. The nurse asks family members whether the presenting behavior and mental status are typical for this client.

RENAL MANIFESTATIONS The volume and the composition of urinary output indicate the hydration status of the renal system. The nurse closely monitors urinary output, comparing the total output with the total fluid intake and daily weight. Accurate measurements of intake and output are a major nursing responsibility. A urinary output below 500 mL/day for any client without renal disease is cause for concern. Clients with fluid imbalance are weighed each day, at the same time and with the same scales. When possible, the client should be wearing the same amount and type of clothing for each weigh-in. Usually, metabolic tissue loss (even in starvation) accounts for only about ½ pound of weight loss each day. Therefore, any weight loss in excess of this amount is considered fluid loss.

PSYCHOSOCIAL ASSESSMENT

The nurse observes the client for behavioral changes that accompany dehydration. Initially, the dehydrated client may have a flat affect and may seem unconcerned or indifferent about the state of health and possible treatment regimens. As dehydration worsens, the client's psychosocial activities reflect abnormal functioning of the central nervous system (CNS). The client may be apprehensive, restless, lethargic, and confused. These behavioral changes are more obvious with hypertonic and hypotonic dehydration because of intracellular fluid shifts in brain cells, resulting in shrinkage or swelling of the cells. If the conditions causing the dehydration continue, circulation to cerebral tissues becomes so impaired that delirium and coma can occur.

LABORATORY ASSESSMENT

No single laboratory test result confirms or rules out dehydration. Instead, a diagnosis of dehydration must be made from several laboratory findings along with the presenting signs and symptoms. Changes in serum laboratory values depend on the type of dehydration present (Chart 15–2). Isotonic and hypotonic dehydration states with accompanying plasma volume deficits are manifested as hemoconcentration, with elevated levels of hemoglobin and increased hematocrit, and as increased serum osmolarity, with increased levels of glucose, protein, blood urea nitrogen (BUN), and various electrolytes. Hemoconcentration is not evident when dehydration results from hemorrhage, because there is loss of all blood and plasma products.

Specific urine laboratory values can help to determine dehydration if the client does not have renal dysfunction. Usually, the urine of clients with dehydration is highly concentrated, with a specific gravity of greater than 1.030. The volume is decreased, and the osmolarity is greatly increased. Usually, the color is dark amber, and a strong odor is evident.

ANALYSIS

COMMON NURSING DIAGNOSES

The priorities for nursing diagnoses to be considered when the nurse is caring for a client with dehydration are:

1. Fluid Volume Deficit related to excessive fluid loss or inadequate fluid intake
2. Decreased Cardiac Output related to insufficient plasma volume
3. Altered Oral Mucous Membrane related to inadequate oral secretions

ADDITIONAL NURSING DIAGNOSES

In addition to the common nursing diagnoses, the client who is dehydrated may have one or more of the following nursing diagnoses:

- Constipation related to decreased body fluids
- High Risk for Injury (fall) related to orthostatic (postural) hypotension

CHART 15–2

Lab Profile ◆ Dehydration

Values*	Isotonic Dehydration	Hypotonic Dehydration	Hypertonic Dehydration
Blood Values			
BUN	• Normal or increased	• Increased	• Increased
Creatinine	• Normal or increased	• Increased	• Increased
Sodium	• Normal	• <120 mEq/L (mmol)	• >150 mEq/L (mmol)
Osmolarity	• Normal	• Decreased	• Increased
Hematocrit	• Increased	• Increased	• Normal or decreased
Hemoglobin	• Increased	• Increased	• Normal or decreased
WBC	• Increased	• Increased	• Normal or decreased
Protein	• Increased	• Increased	• Increased
Urine Values			
Specific gravity	• >1.010	• <1.010	• >1.010
Osmolarity	• Increased	• Decreased	• Increased
Volume	• Decreased	• Increased	• Decreased

* All values reflect dehydration states alone and not the underlying pathologic changes or disease states contributing to the dehydration.

- Knowledge Deficit related to medication regimen and preventive measures
- High Risk for Impaired Skin Integrity related to deficiencies of interstitial fluid and inadequate tissue perfusion
- Ineffective Airway Clearance related to thick, tenacious secretions

PLANNING AND IMPLEMENTATION

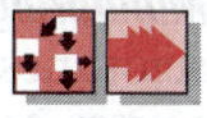

FLUID VOLUME DEFICIT

PLANNING: CLIENT GOALS The major goal is that the client will have normal body fluid levels.

INTERVENTIONS Interventions attempt to:

- Restore normal fluid balance
- Provide supportive care until the imbalance is resolved
- Prevent future fluid deficits

Management of dehydration is aimed at preventing further fluid losses and increasing fluid compartment volumes to normal ranges. Drugs and diet therapy are the methods of choice.

Diet Therapy Mild-to-moderate dehydration may be successfully treated with oral fluid replacement if the client is alert enough to swallow and can tolerate oral fluids.

The nurse encourages and measures all fluid intake. The specific type of fluid needed for replacement varies with the type of dehydration.

The client's compliance with the ingestion of oral replacement fluids can be enhanced by using fluids the client enjoys at fluid temperatures that the client is comfortable with and carefully timing the intake schedule. Dividing the total amount of fluids needed by nursing shifts helps to meet fluid needs more evenly with less danger of overhydration. The nurse offers the client small volumes of fluids every hour to increase client compliance. Usually, alert clients who are dehydrated have some sensation of thirst and require minimal encouragement to meet fluid needs.

Clients who ingest solid foods obtain some fluid from these foods; however, the amount of fluid in solid food is not enough to increase the client's fluid volume to normal levels during dehydration. In addition, specific foods, because of their electrolyte content, may need to be restricted if an electrolyte imbalance is also present. For example, hypernatremia often accompanies hypertonic dehydration. In this situation, the client should avoid foods and fluids with a high sodium content.

Oral Rehydration Therapy Oral rehydration therapy (ORT) is the most cost-effective way to replace fluids and treat the client with diarrhea. Specifically formulated solutions containing glucose and electrolytes cause water to be absorbed even in the presence of diarrhea and vomiting. Fluid losses from diarrhea are usually 2 to 3 L/day and should be replaced liter for liter, especially in elderly clients. A typical physician's order might be "Resol 1 L every 8 hours." Table 15–3 lists several commercially available ORT solutions.

Drug Therapy Drug therapy for dehydration is directed at restoring the fluid balance and controlling the conditions causing the dehydration. Whenever possible, fluids are replaced by the oral route. When dehydration is severe or life-threatening, intravenous (IV) fluid replacement may be necessary. Calculation of the volume of replacement fluids needed is based on both the weight loss and the presenting symptoms. The rate of fluid replacement depends on the client's degree of dehydration and the presence of pre-existing cardiac, pulmonary, or renal problems.

The type of fluid ordered by the physician varies with the type of dehydration and the client's cardiovascular status. The desired outcome of the therapy is both appropriate fluid replacement and normal volumes in all body fluid compartments. Usually, the

TABLE 15–3 Commercial Solutions for Oral Rehydration Therapy

Brand Name	Na^+ (mEq/L)	K^+ (mEq/L)	Cl^- (mEq/L)	Citrate (mEq/L)	Sugar or Starch	Calories (kcal) per Liter
Ricelyte (Mead-Johnson)	50	25	45	34	Rice syrup (30 g)	126
Resol (Wyeth-Ayerst)	50	20	50	34	Dextrose (20 g)	84
Rehydralyte (Ross Labs)	75	20	65	30	Dextrose (25 g)	100
Pedialyte (Ross Labs)	45	20	35	30	Dextrose (25 g)	100
Gastrolyte (Rorer)	60	20	60	10	Dextrose (17.8 g)	75
Rapolyte✱ (Richmond)	90	20	80	30	Dextrose (20 g)	84

client receives IV infusions of water with whatever solutes (especially electrolytes) are determined necessary on the basis of laboratory values. Table 15–4 lists the electrolyte content of common IV fluids. Generally, isotonic dehydration is treated with isotonic fluid solutions; hypertonic dehydration, with hypotonic fluid solutions; and hypotonic dehydration, with hypertonic fluid solutions.

Drug therapy includes the use of medications to correct the underlying cause of the dehydration. Antidiarrheal medications, such as diphenoxylate hydrochloride (Lomotil, Diarsed♣), are ordered when excessive diarrhea causes dehydration. Antimicrobial therapy is used in selected clients with bacterial diarrhea, such as that due to *Clostridium difficile*. Antiemetics, such as prochlorperazine (Compazine, Stemetil♣), to control vomiting may be necessary when excessive vomiting produces dehydration. Antipyretics to reduce body temperature are helpful when fever contributes to dehydration.

DECREASED CARDIAC OUTPUT

PLANNING: CLIENT GOALS The major goals are that the client will:

- Have cardiac output restored to normal levels
- Maintain adequate oxygenation to vital organs

INTERVENTIONS Interventions aim at:

- Increasing the circulating fluid volume
- Supporting the client's compensatory mechanisms
- Preventing ischemic complications

Drug Therapy Drug therapy to increase body fluid volume and prevent excessive fluid loss is the same as that for the client with Fluid Volume Deficit. Drugs to increase venous return or improve cardiac contractility are used only when a coexisting cardiac problem is present.

Oxygen Therapy Oxygen can be delivered by mask, hood, nasal cannula, nasopharyngeal tube, endotracheal tube, and tracheostomy tube. Usually, masks and nasal cannulas are used to administer oxygen to clients with dehydration. The nurse administers water-nebulized oxygen to the client at the rate or amount specified by the physician's prescription.

Monitoring Monitoring vital signs and level of consciousness (LOC) is an important responsibility of nurses caring for dehydrated clients. The nurse monitors the client's pulse, blood pressure, pulse pressure, central venous pressure, respiratory rate, skin and mucous membrane color, and urinary output at least every hour until the fluid imbalance is resolved.

ALTERED ORAL MUCOUS MEMBRANE

PLANNING: CLIENT GOALS The major goals are that the client will:

- Experience less discomfort
- Not experience complications, such as infections or altered nutrition, related to dry oral mucosa

INTERVENTIONS Interventions are:

- Fluid replacement
- Good oral hygiene
- Early diagnosis of complications

Diet and drug therapies to resolve the dehydration also result in resolution of the altered oral mucous membranes.

Drug Therapy Drug therapy to increase body fluid volume and prevent excessive fluid loss is the same as that discussed earlier for Fluid Volume Deficit. Some pharmacologic agents that reduce the sensation of mouth dryness are commercial preparations of artifi-

TABLE 15–4 Characteristics of Common Intravenous Therapy Solutions

Solution	Osmolarity (mOsm/L)	pH	Calories* (kcal)	Tonicity
0.9% saline	308	5	0	Isotonic
0.45% saline	154	5	0	Hypotonic
5% dextrose in water (D_5W)	272	3.5–6.5	170	Isotonic†
10% dextrose in water ($D_{10}W$)	500	3.5–6.5	340	Hypertonic†
5% dextrose in 0.9% saline	560	3.5–6.5	170	Hypertonic†
5% dextrose in 0.45% saline	406	4	170	Hypertonic†
5% dextrose in 0.225% saline	321	4	170	Isotonic†
Ringer's lactate	273	6.5	9	Isotonic
5% dextrose in Ringer's lactate	525	4.0–6.5	179	Hypertonic†

Data from Trissel, L. (1992). *Handbook on injectable drugs* (7th ed.). Bethesda, MD: American Society of Hospital Pharmacists.

*Calories are calculated on the basis of a volume of 1000 mL.

†*Solution tonicity at the time of administration.* Within a short time after administration, the dextrose is metabolized and the tonicity of the infused solution decreases in proportion to the osmolarity or tonicity of the nondextrose components (electrolytes) within the water.

cial saliva. The nurse avoids the use of such agents when clients are not conscious.

Oral Hygiene Nursing actions to promote oral hygiene can increase the client's comfort. The nurse keeps the client's lips clean and moistens them with a petrolatum-based lubricant. The thick, sticky coating of the oral cavity during episodes of dehydration increases the client's discomfort. Frequent use of oral hygiene measures can remove this coating. Mouth care includes brushing and flossing, but is not limited to these activities. The client brushes and flosses gently so as not to damage tender oral tissues. The use of focused water pressure to clean the mouth (as with a water pick), is controversial because some dentists believe that the pressure can force debris into tissues and under the gums, where decay can occur undetected.

Another technique clients can use to clean the mouth is to rinse the mouth every hour. Clients should avoid commercial mouthwashes that contain alcohol and glycerin-containing washes and swabs because these products dry the oral mucosa further and may cause increased discomfort by stinging or burning open fissures in the mucosa. Rinsing the mouth with dilute solutions of hydrogen peroxide two or three times per day is a good form of oral hygiene; however, when used more frequently, this treatment increases oral dryness. Other solutions that can safely be used as frequently as the client wishes for oral hygiene are tap water and normal saline. Clients may experience increased relief if these solutions are at room temperature or lukewarm rather than cold.

Prevention of Complications A dry mouth contributes to the development of sores and fissures in the mucosa, providing a portal of entry for many pathogens. In addition, the thick, sticky coating is an excellent breeding ground for microorganisms. A major complication of mouth dryness is a wide variety of oral infections. Nursing management of oral hygiene includes an assessment of the integrity of the oral mucosa every 8 hours. The nurse reports the presence of any suspicious open lesion and obtains a physician's order for a culture.

A dry mouth can also interfere with adequate nutrition. Not only do fissures and sores cause pain and discomfort during chewing and swallowing, but also the coating may alter taste sensation and decrease appetite. To help maintain the client's nutrition at an appropriate level, the nurse offers oral hygiene right before meals or snacks. The nurse assists the client in menu selection to avoid foods that are highly spiced or hard. Bland, soft, cool foods are most easily tolerated by clients with mouth dryness.

Chart 15-3 summarizes important nursing interventions for mouth care.

CHART 15-3

Nursing Care Highlight ◆ Mouth Care for Clients with Dehydration

- Examine the client's mouth (including under the roof, on the tongue, and between the teeth and cheek) every 4 hours.
- Document the location, size, and character of fissures, blisters, sores, or drainage.
- Obtain an order to culture sores or drainage.
- Brush the client's teeth and tongue with a soft-bristled brush or sponges every 8 hours.
- Rinse the client's mouth with a 50:50 solution of ½ peroxide and ½ normal saline every 12 hours.
- Avoid the use of alcohol or glycerin-based mouthwashes.
- Assist the conscious client to swish and spit room-temperature tap water or normal saline PRN.
- Apply petrolatum jelly to the client's lips after each episode of mouth care and PRN.
- Assist the client to use artificial saliva.
- Assist the client in menu choices to avoid spicy or hard foods.
- Offer complete mouth care before and after every meal.

DISCHARGE PLANNING

HOME CARE PREPARATION

No extensive home care preparations are necessary for clients with mild dehydration or for those with dehydration of sudden onset. The imbalance is corrected before the client is discharged from the facility and, with minimal precautions, is unlikely to recur. Clients who are most likely to be discharged before the imbalance is completely corrected and who are susceptible to recurrent episodes of imbalance have chronic pathologic conditions, such as renal insufficiency, diabetes, malignancy, adrenal insufficiency, and specific endocrine disorders. These clients often require long-term diet and drug therapy.

HEALTH TEACHING

Education is important in the prevention and early detection of dehydration. The teaching plan for any client at risk for dehydration includes diet, drug regimens, and the signs and symptoms of dehydration.

PSYCHOSOCIAL PREPARATION

For clients whose dehydration is caused by acute illness or alterations in fluid volumes, psychosocial preparation is usually minimal. The client may be concerned about the possibility of recurrent episodes. The nurse reassures the client that such a recurrence is unlikely unless the causative conditions are repeated. In addition, the nurse instructs the client in actions to prevent dehydration when precipitating conditions exist.

Clients whose dehydration results from chronic health problems may have learned to cope well and may require minimal psychosocial support. However, this situation cannot be assumed. The nurse assesses each client's psychosocial needs individually for new factors, established support patterns, changes in lifestyle, previous and current coping patterns, and stability of the chronic disease or underlying pathologic condition.

HEALTH CARE RESOURCES

Clients with severe chronic health problems may be discharged to a nursing home or extended care facility on a permanent or a temporary basis. The hospital nurse uses the transfer chart to communicate all important information about the client's individual needs and special care problems.

EVALUATION

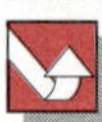

On the basis of the identified nursing diagnoses, the nurse evaluates the care of clients with dehydration. The expected outcomes include that the client

- Ingests at least 1500 mL of hypotonic fluids each day
- Maintains a fluid output that is approximately equal to the fluid intake
- States that oral mucosal discomfort is relieved
- Experiences no oral mucosal complication

Overhydration

OVERVIEW

Overhydration, also referred to as fluid overload, is body fluid excess. It is not an actual disease but, rather, is a clinical manifestation of a physiologic problem in which fluid intake or retention exceeds the body's fluid need. Overhydration may be characterized as either an actual excess of total body fluid or a relative fluid excess in one or more fluid compartments. Three basic types of fluid volume excess are possible:

- Isotonic overhydration
- Hypotonic overhydration
- Hypertonic overhydration

Figure 15–5 illustrates the three types of overhydration.

PATHOPHYSIOLOGY

Most problems associated with overhydration are related to fluid volume excesses in the vascular space or to dilution of specific electrolytes and blood components. Clinical manifestations vary with the type and degree of overhydration (Chart 15–4).

ISOTONIC OVERHYDRATION

Isotonic overhydration is also called hypervolemia because the problems associated with it result from

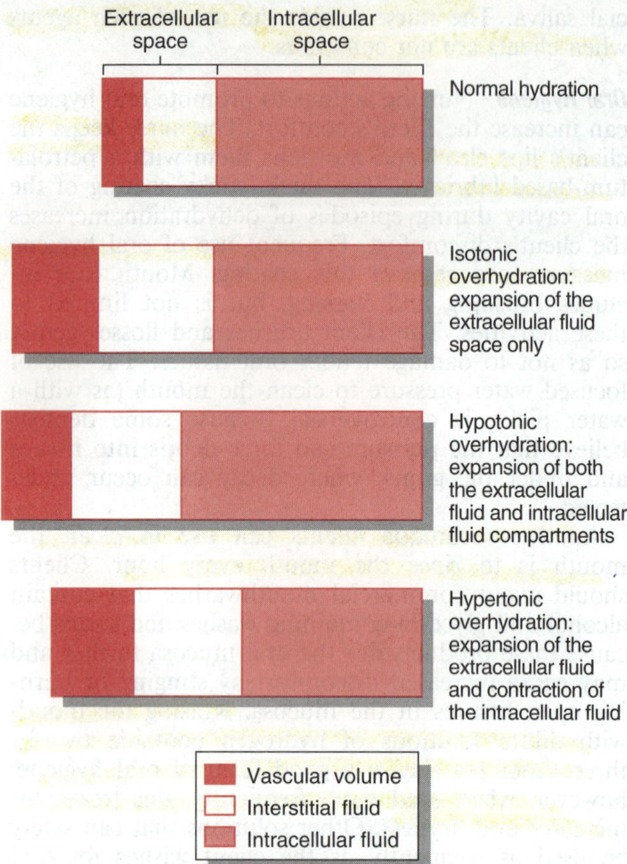

FIGURE 15–5 ◆ Three types of overhydration. (© 1992 M. Linda Workman. All rights reserved.)

excessive fluid in the extracellular fluid compartment. In isotonic overhydration, isotonic fluids are ingested or retained so that osmolarity remains normal. Only the extracellular fluid compartment is expanded, and fluid does not shift between the extracellular and intracellular compartments. The effects of severe isotonic overhydration are circulatory overload and the formation of interstitial edema.

MILD-TO-MODERATE ISOTONIC OVERHYDRATION Mild-to-moderate acute overhydration in healthy people rarely has serious consequences because the body has several compensatory mechanisms to handle the extra fluid. As shown in Figure 15–6, when blood volume increases and osmolarity remains normal, mean arterial pressure (MAP) and vascular hydrostatic pressure both increase. The increased volume, along with an elevated MAP, results in an increased venous return and stretching of the myocardium, increasing the cardiac output. In addition, the elevated MAP stimulates an increase in renal blood flow and glomerular filtration. This reaction causes both water and sodium to be excreted, assisting in preventing overhydration.

SEVERE OR PROLONGED ISOTONIC OVERHYDRATION When isotonic overhydration is severe, or when it occurs in a person with a poor cardiac status such as an elderly person, overhydration results in congestive

CHART 15–4

Key Features of Overhydration

Manifestations of Overhydration in General

Cardiovascular

- Increased pulse rate
- Bounding pulse quality
- Peripheral pulses full
- Elevated blood pressure
- Decreased pulse pressure
- Elevated central venous pressure
- Distended neck and hand veins
- Engorged venous varicosities

Respiratory

- Respiratory rate increased
- Shallow respirations
- Dyspnea increases with exertion or in the supine position
- Moist crackles present on auscultation

Integumentary

- Pitting edema in dependent areas
- Skin pale and cool to touch

Neuromuscular

- Altered level of consciousness
- Headache
- Visual disturbances
- Skeletal muscle weakness
- Paresthesias

Gastrointestinal

- Increased motility

Manifestations of Isotonic Overhydration

- Liver enlargement
- Ascites formation

Manifestations of Hypotonic Overhydration

- Polyuria
- Diarrhea
- Nonpitting edema
- Cardiac arrhythmias associated with electrolyte dilution
- Projectile vomiting

heart failure and pulmonary edema. Cardiac output decreases as the myocardium stretches beyond the desired point. Damming of venous blood causes an increase in the hydrostatic pressure of the venous system. This increase in hydrostatic pressure leads to the formation of edema in interstitial tissues as fluid is forced from the plasma space into the interstitial space. (Chapter 34 describes the pathophysiology of congestive heart failure and pulmonary edema in detail.)

HYPOTONIC OVERHYDRATION

In hypotonic overhydration (water intoxication), the excess fluid is hypotonic to normal body fluids, so that the osmolarity of the extracellular fluid decreases and hydrostatic pressure increases. The excessive fluid moves into the intracellular space because of the decreased vascular osmotic pressure. Thus, with hypotonic overhydration, all body fluid compartments experience expansion. Because the excessive fluid is hypotonic, electrolyte imbalances due to dilution accompany hypotonic overhydration.

ETIOLOGY

The conditions leading to overhydration, or fluid overload, are related to excessive intake or inadequate excretion of fluid. Conditions that produce excessive fluid intake include:

- Excessive oral ingestion of water
- Poorly controlled IV therapy
- Excessive irrigation of any body cavity or organ with hypotonic fluids
- The replacement of isotonic fluid losses with hypotonic fluids

Conditions in which inadequate excretion of fluids leads to hypotonic overhydration include:

- Certain types of renal failure
- Any condition in which cardiac output and mean arterial pressure cannot maintain renal blood flow (such as in congestive heart failure)
- Syndrome of inappropriate antidiuretic hormone (SIADH) secretion (see Chap. 26)

COLLABORATIVE MANAGEMENT

ASSESSMENT

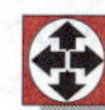

The clinical manifestations of overhydration vary with the specific type, the fluid compartments involved, and the degree of overhydration. Clients with isotonic overhydration or hypertonic overhydration have signs and symptoms associated with circulatory overload. Clients with hypotonic overhydration have problems associated with intracellular fluid increase and electrolyte dilution. Chart 15–4 summarizes the common clinical manifestations of overhydration.

The physician does not use one laboratory test to diagnose overhydration. Instead, a diagnosis of overhydration is based on physical assessment findings together with the results of several laboratory tests. In isotonic overhydration, serum electrolyte values are normal, but decreased hemoglobin levels, hematocrit, and serum protein levels may result from hemodilution (excessive water in the vascular compartment). Elevated levels of most electrolytes, along with increased blood urea nitrogen (BUN) and creatinine levels, are associated with overhydration caused by renal failure. Hypotonic overhydration is accompanied by a decreased complete blood count (CBC) and decreased protein and electrolyte levels.

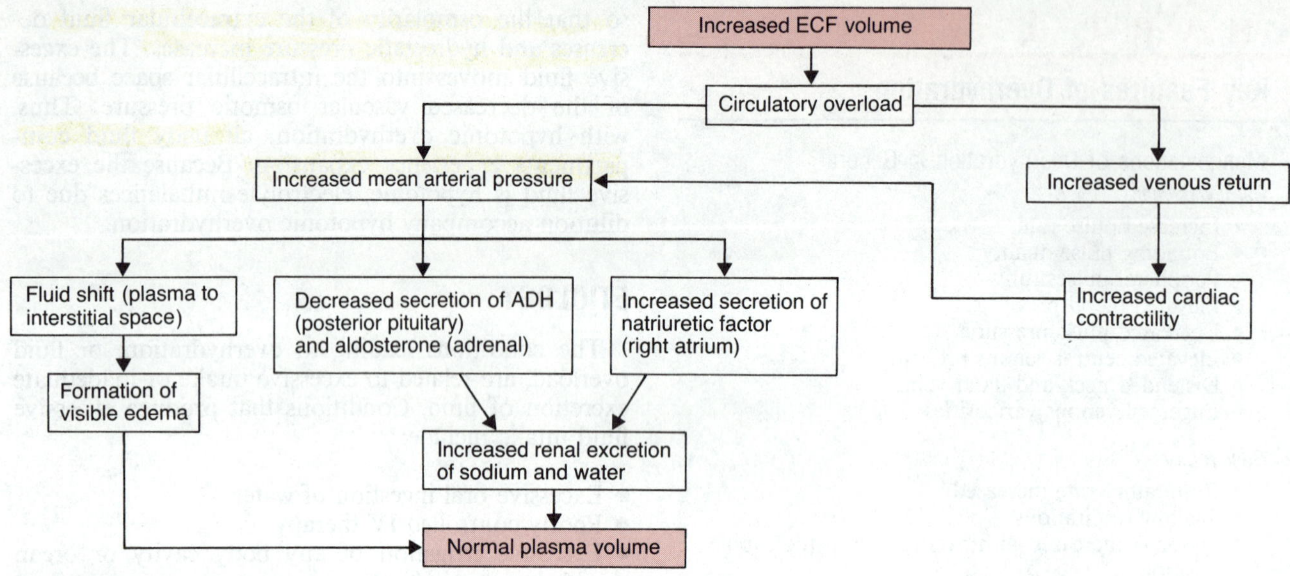

FIGURE 15-6 ◆ Compensatory mechanisms associated with hypervolemia.

INTERVENTIONS

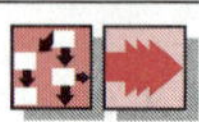

Interventions for clients with fluid volume excesses include actions to:

- Restore normal fluid balance
- Provide supportive care until the imbalance is resolved
- Prevent future fluid overload

The physician may prescribe diet and drug therapy to restore fluid balance.

DRUG THERAPY

The physician may order diuretics for clients with overhydration, provided that renal failure is not the cause of overhydration. Diuretics work on the kidneys to increase the excretion of water or sodium from the body. Osmotic diuretics, such as mannitol, are typically prescribed first to prevent severe electrolyte imbalances. Osmotic diuretics primarily cause renal excretion of water rather than excretion of sodium or potassium. If osmotic diuretics are not effective, the physician may prescribe high-ceiling (loop) diuretics, such as furosemide (Lasix, Furoside♣).

The nurse monitors the client for response to medication, especially weight loss and increased urinary output. The nurse also observes the client for signs and symptoms of electrolyte imbalance and assesses laboratory findings every 8 hours.

DIET THERAPY

For mild or chronic overhydration, long-term diet therapy may be valuable in controlling fluid volume through restrictions of both fluid and sodium intake. The client's serum sodium concentration should be considered whenever overhydration is present.

INTAKE AND OUTPUT MEASUREMENT

The nurse accurately measures fluid intake and output and explains the reason for any fluid restriction. In addition to regulating the total amount of fluid ingested in a 24-hour period, the nurse carefully schedules fluid offerings throughout the 24 hours. The nurse also monitors the client's urine for color, character, and specific gravity.

If the client is receiving IV therapy, the nurse administers the exact amount ordered by the physician and monitors the client for increased fluid overload. (Nursing care for clients with IV therapy is addressed later in this chapter.)

WEIGHT MONITORING

Fluid retention may not be visible. However, a sudden weight gain or loss indicates that fluid is retained or lost from the body. The nurse weighs the client at the same time every day (before breakfast) using the same scale. Whenever possible, the client wears the same type of clothing for each weigh-in.

Principles of Intravenous Therapy

OVERVIEW

Intravenous therapy is a major component of medical treatment and the most common invasive procedure experienced by hospitalized clients. It can also be performed routinely in ambulatory and home care settings. Although it is a common procedure, IV therapy presents potential hazards to the client's health. These hazards are preventable when the nurse uses appropriate techniques and provides ongoing client assessment.

COLLABORATIVE MANAGEMENT

Nursing responsibilities for IV therapy extend from obtaining a physician's order to begin therapy through the discontinuing of IV therapy.

TYPES OF INTRAVENOUS THERAPY ADMINISTRATION

IV therapy can be administered by two major routes—peripheral and central.

PERIPHERAL INTRAVENOUS THERAPY

Peripheral IV therapy is usually given through a cannula (a small, hollow metal or plastic tube) inserted into a vein in the arm. The nurse skilled in venipuncture (the insertion of a cannula into the vein) may place IV cannulas in peripheral veins.

CENTRAL INTRAVENOUS THERAPY

Central IV therapy is given through a long catheter known as a central venous catheter (CVC). The physician inserts the catheter at the bedside or in the operating room. The physician generally uses the subclavian or internal jugular vein to allow the catheter to enter the central venous system—the superior vena cava or the right atrium of the heart. Another term that is used for the central venous catheter is venous access device (VAD).

Central venous catheters are used for clients who need multiple infusions of hyperosmolar solutions and blood, prolonged antibiotic therapy, or total parenteral nutrition. Most central venous catheters are inserted percutaneously (through the skin) at the bedside to provide central venous access for a short time, usually less than 4 weeks. Most short-term catheters used today have more than one lumen (opening) and are made of flexible material, such as polyurethane or elastomeric hydrogel (Viall, 1990). The nurse assists the physician with the insertion procedure as needed.

When the client requires therapy for more than 4 weeks, a long-term CVC is usually inserted. There are two major types of catheters for long-term use—tunneled and implanted. Both types are inserted by the surgeon in the operating room.

TUNNELED CENTRAL VENOUS CATHETERS A tunneled central venous catheter is inserted into the subclavian or internal jugular vein and advanced into the superior vena cava or the right atrium. The proximal end of the catheter is then tunneled from the entrance site through a subcutaneous pocket of the chest wall and brought out through an exit site below the nipple line (Fig. 15–7). Examples of tunneled catheters are the Hickman and Broviac catheters (Fig. 15–8).

IMPLANTED PORTS An implanted central venous catheter, or port, is a central venous catheter for long-term use with no external parts; it is surgically placed entirely under the skin. A silicone or polyurethane catheter is first inserted into the subclavian or internal jugular vein. Then a plastic, titanium, or stainless steel port is implanted in a subcutaneous pocket of the chest wall. When the incision is closed, the port cannot be seen, but a small bulge under the skin indicates its location (Fig. 15–9). Access to the client's vascular system is made by inserting a special needle (Huber needle) through the skin and into the rubber septum on the top of the port. Some ports have a side entry access (S.E.A. Port). Examples of implanted ports are the MediPort and Port-A-Cath (Fig. 15–10). Because implanted ports are often used for chemotherapy, specific nursing care associated with implanted ports is discussed in Chapter 26 under Chemotherapy.

OTHER TYPES OF CENTRAL VENOUS CATHETERS Two other types of central catheters are available. The Groshong catheter is similar to the Hickman catheter in appearance, with two important differences. First, it has an internal valve that omits the need for the catheter to be clamped. Second, the catheter does not

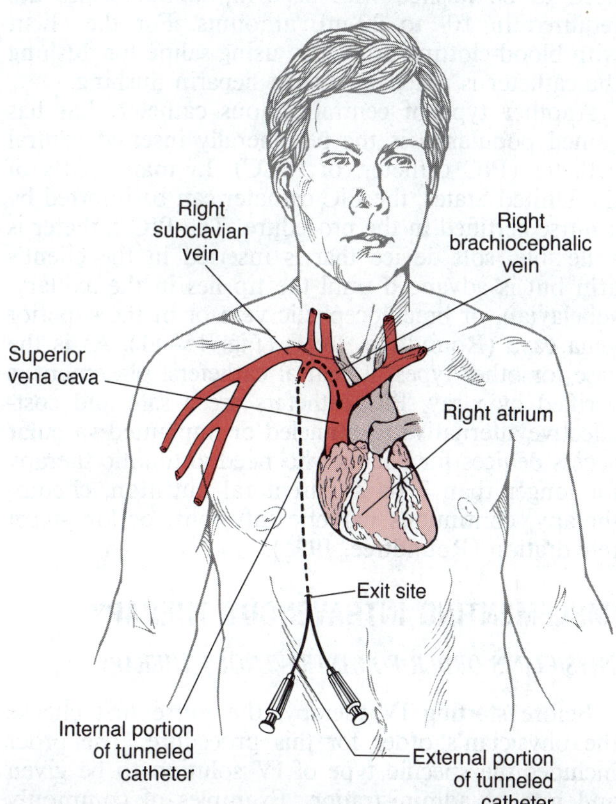

FIGURE 15–7 ◆ The usual anatomic position of tunneled catheters.

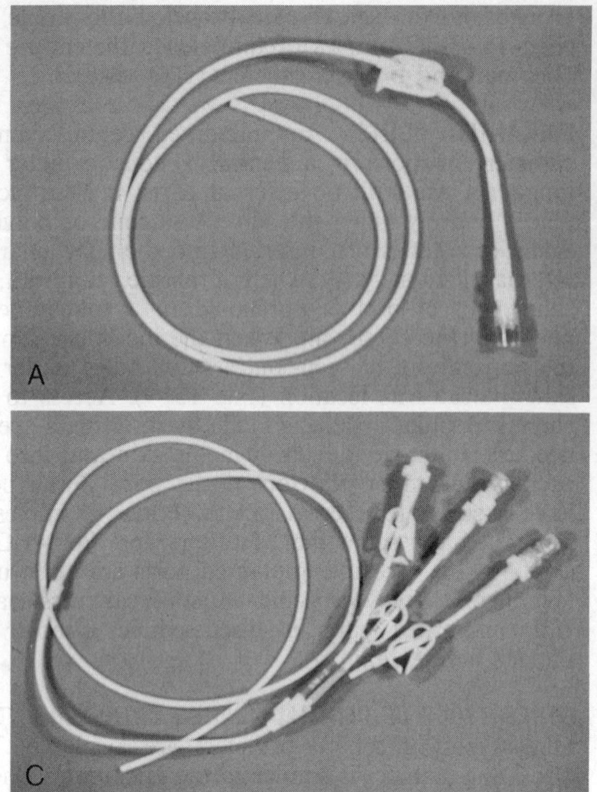

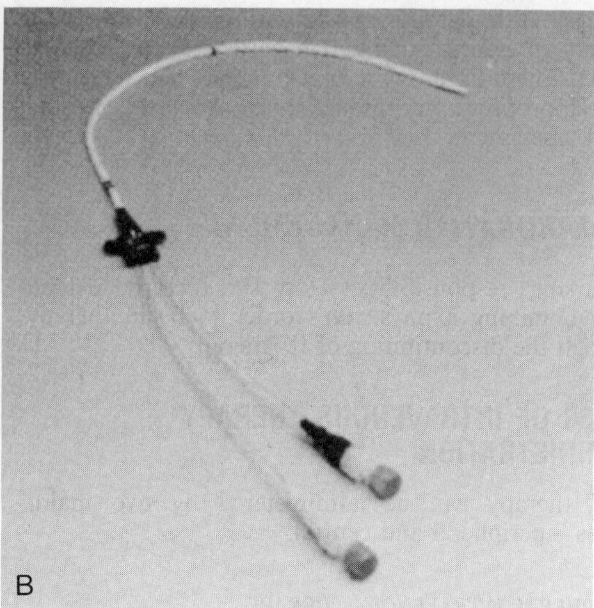

FIGURE 15-8 ◆ *A–C*, Hickman intravenous catheters.

need to be flushed with heparin; saline flushes are required in 10- to 20-mL amounts. For the client with blood-clotting problems, using saline for flushing the catheter is much safer than heparin flushing.

Another type of central venous catheter that has gained popularity is the peripherally inserted central catheter (PIC catheter, or PICC). In many parts of the United States, the PIC catheter can be inserted by a nurse certified in the procedure. The PIC catheter is a flexible, soft device that is inserted in the client's arm but is advanced until the tip lies in the axillary, subclavian, or brachiocephalic vein or in the superior vena cava (Roundtree, 1991) (Fig. 15–11). As is the case for other types of central catheters, placement is verified by x-ray. PIC catheters are a safe and cost-effective alternative to tunneled or implanted vascular access devices for clients who need antibiotic therapy for longer than 7 days, parenteral nutrition, chemotherapy, continuous narcotic infusions, or long-term rehydration (Roundtree, 1991).

IMPLEMENTING INTRAVENOUS THERAPY

PHYSICIAN'S ORDER FOR INTRAVENOUS THERAPY

Before starting IV therapy, the nurse first checks the physician's order for this procedure. The order includes the specific type of IV solution to be given and rate of administration. Examples of commonly used IV solutions and their compositions are listed in Table 15–4.

If the physician orders medication for IV administration, the dosage, volume, and frequency are also specified. When the client has more than one IV line, the physician may indicate which one to use for a particular solution or medication.

PURPOSE OF INTRAVENOUS THERAPY

IV therapy may be ordered for several reasons, such as:

- Continuous or intermittent medication administration
- Correction of an actual fluid or electrolyte imbalance
- Prevention of a fluid or electrolyte imbalance, and
- Provision of long-term nutritional support

The site and the equipment used to begin IV therapy depend on the purpose of the therapy. For example, a large-bore cannula may be placed in the antecubital fossa (at the bend of the elbow) during an emergency. This site is inappropriate for long-term IV therapy as described below.

SITE SELECTION FOR INTRAVENOUS THERAPY

The purpose and the duration of the prescribed therapy, as well as the age and physical condition of

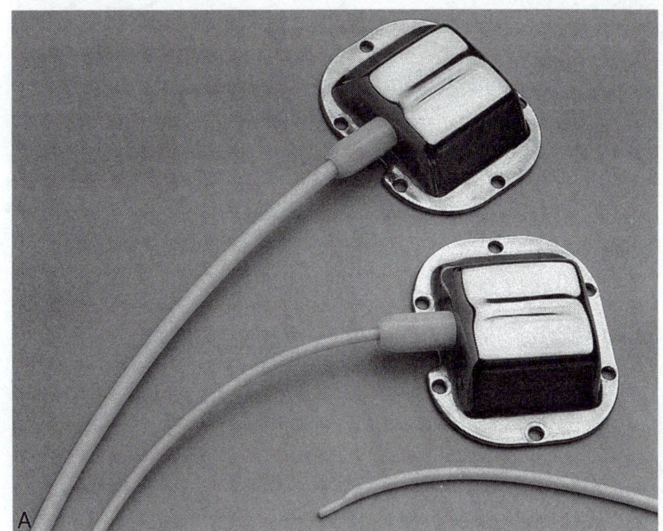

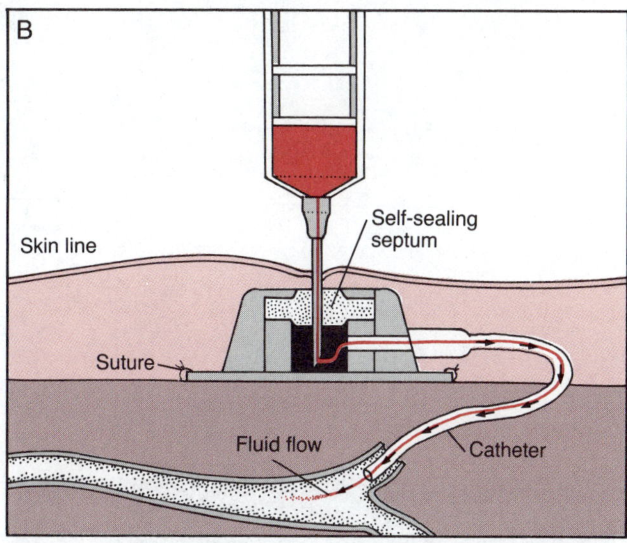

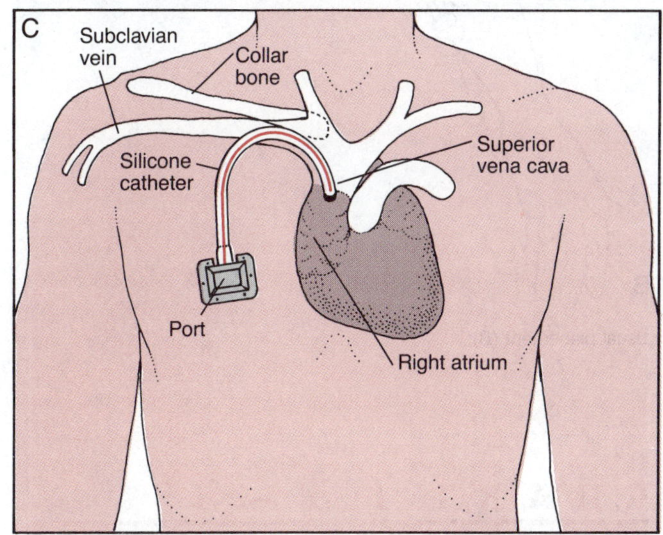

FIGURE 15-9 ◆ *A*, A dual-access implantable port for venous access. *B*, A needle puncture through the skin into the port allows drugs, fluids, and blood to be administered. *C*, For systemic drug and fluid delivery, the catheter is placed in the subclavian vein. (*A*, Courtesy of Harbor Medical Devices, Inc., Boston. *B* and *C*, redrawn from Winters, B. [1984]. Implantable vascular access devices. *Oncology Nursing Forum, 11*[6], 25–30.)

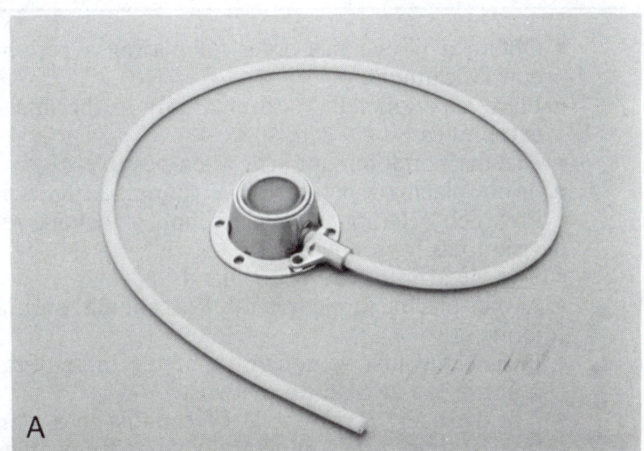

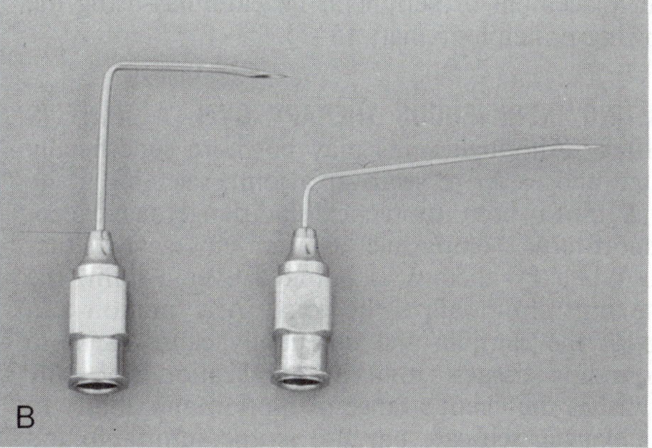

FIGURE 15-10 ◆ An implanted port (*A*) and Huber (right-angle) needles (*B*).

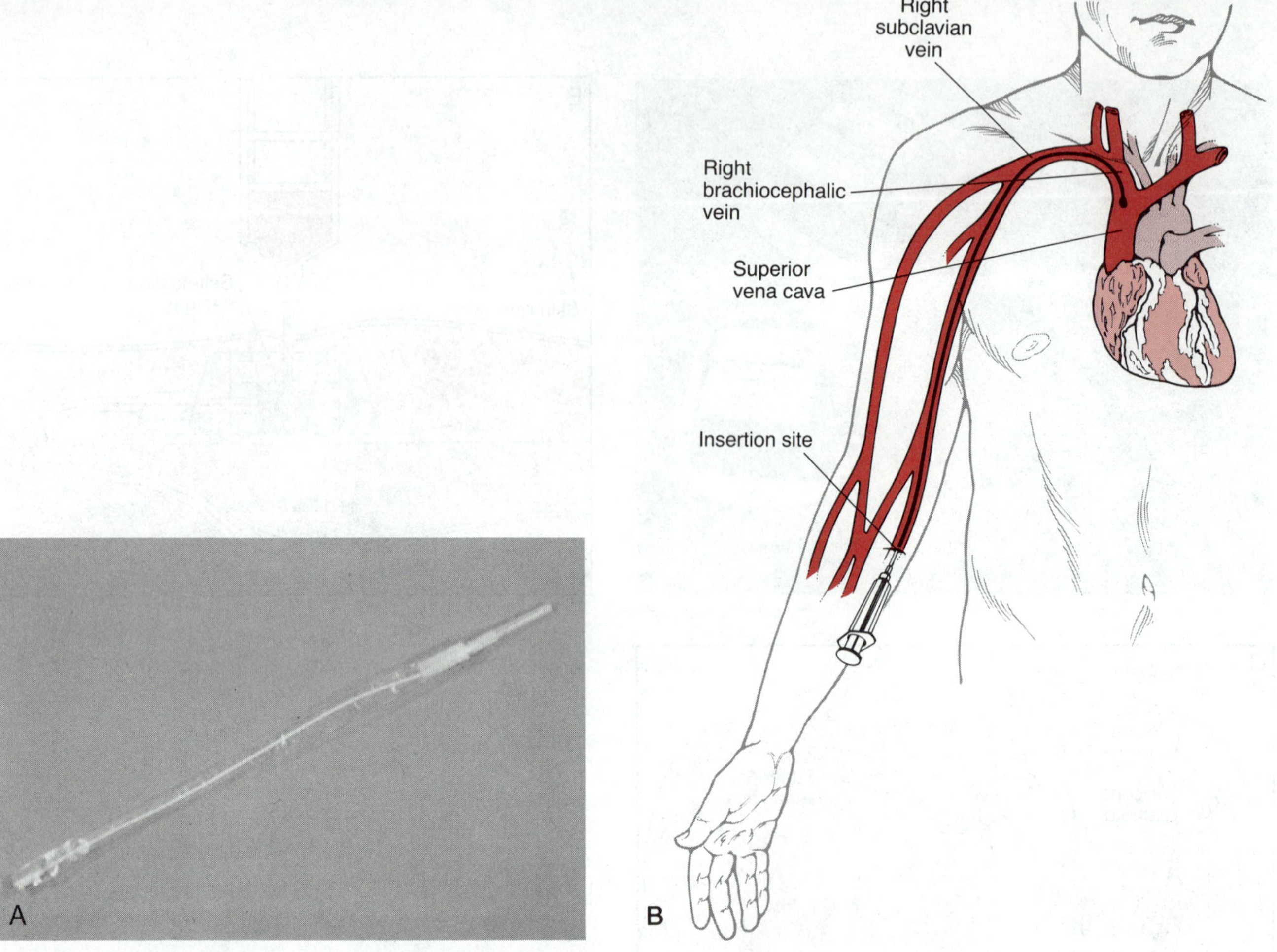

FIGURE 15-11 ◆ A peripherally inserted central catheter (*A*) and its usual placement (*B*).

the client, determine whether a particular site is appropriate for IV therapy. For central venous therapy, the physician typically decides on the site of the IV catheter unless the nurse is using a peripherally inserted central catheter. The nurse usually decides about placement of peripheral IV cannulas using the following principles (Chart 15-5).

STARTING INTRAVENOUS THERAPY OVER A JOINT IS AVOIDED Although veins may be more superficially located and easier to see over a joint, selecting a site over a joint is both impractical and dangerous, except for short-term therapy such as in an emergency situation. When IV therapy is initiated over a joint, the nurse must immobilize the joint. Any motion can dislodge the cannula and potentially cause harm to surrounding tissues. Joint immobilization not only diminishes the client's range of motion and ability to participate in self-care but also is uncomfortable and difficult to achieve for some clients, especially those with contractures. In addition, the volar (palm) side of the wrist is not used because the radial nerve

CHART 15-5

Nursing Care Highlight ◆ Criteria for Placement of Peripheral Venous Access Devices

- Obtain a physician's order for placing a peripheral IV cannula.
- Place a peripheral IV cannula only in the upper extremities.
- Use the nondominant arm when possible.
- Avoid placing a peripheral IV cannula in an arm in which a lymph node dissection or venous revision has been done.
- Use the arm instead of the hand.
- Avoid placing a peripheral IV cannula over a joint.
- Initiate the first venipuncture at the most distal point of the arm above the wrist.
- Avoid placing a peripheral IV cannula in a vein that is bruised, has puncture wounds from other venipunctures, is streaked, is hard, has a palpable cord, or is tender when touched.

causes pain during cannula insertion (Hadaway, 1991).

INTRAVENOUS THERAPY IS STARTED IN UPPER EXTREMITIES WHEN POSSIBLE In most clients, venous return is better in the upper extremities than in the lower extremities. Gravity and distance from the heart contribute to the decreased flow rate in the superficial and deeper veins of the legs. This decreased flow rate impairs venous return, diminishes nutrient exchange at the tissue level, and increases the risk of thrombus or embolus formation, especially in elderly clients. Using veins in the lower extremities for IV therapy greatly increases the risk of these problems. Unless no other veins can be used, the veins of the lower extremities of an adult are not used for IV therapy.

Whenever possible, IV therapy is started in the nondominant arm. The nurse asks the client, family member, or significant other which arm is the dominant one or observes which arm the client uses for eating or bathing. An exception to this guideline is the use of peripherally inserted central catheters. Some nurses and physicians prefer the dominant arm for insertion of this device because arm movement promotes blood flow and prevents dependent edema (Roundtree, 1991).

INTRAVENOUS THERAPY IS STARTED IN ARM VEINS—NOT HAND VEINS Because the veins of the hand tend to be more visible than the veins of the arm (often evident without a tourniquet), some health care professionals may select hand veins for IV therapy. Hand veins are not the best choice unless there are no other possible sites for therapy. The dorsal surface of the hand has little subcutaneous supportive tissue; thus the veins are more prominent. However, these veins are small and thin-walled. The lack of subcutaneous tissues also makes IV therapy at this site more painful and increases the risk of serious tissue damage if extravasation or infiltration occurs. In addition, the use of this site for IV therapy limits the client's use of the hand. Because clients tend to change hand positions frequently, IV cannulas in the hand are dislodged frequently and are susceptible to variation in infusion rate.

THE FIRST VENIPUNCTURE IS IN THE DISTAL PORTION OF THE ARM When the arm is used, the site should be as distal as possible and the wrist joint area is avoided. Using the most distal sites first or earlier in venipuncture attempts allows the later use of proximal (upward) sites, if necessary. The nurse uses dorsal veins in preference to ventral veins for their size, straightness, and decreased susceptibility to mechanical damage. For an elderly client, however, the skin on the forearm may be thin and fragile from sun exposure and age. Preferred sites for starting IV therapy in elderly clients include the cephalic vein, the basilic vein, and the veins of the dorsal forearm (Hadaway, 1991) (Fig. 15-12).

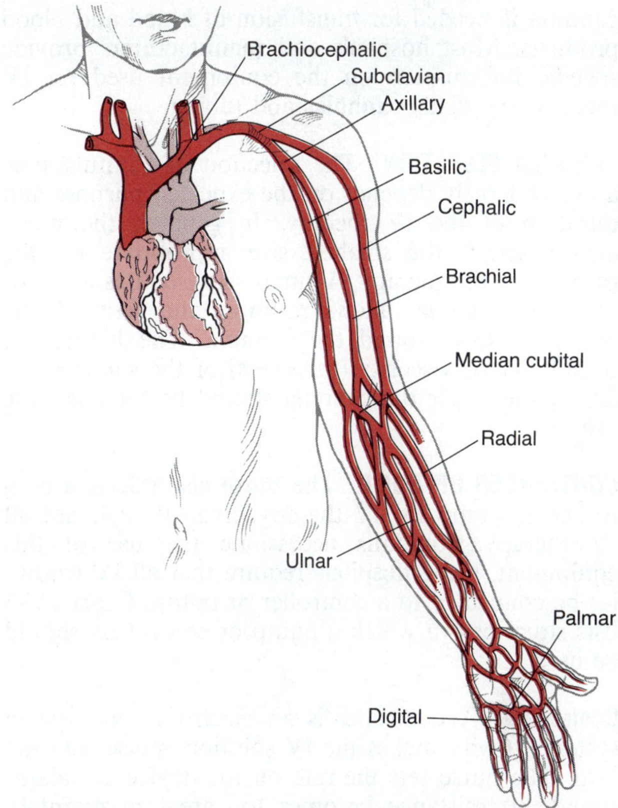

FIGURE 15-12 ♦ The superficial veins of the arm.

INTRAVENOUS THERAPY IS STARTED IN A HEALTHY VEIN As a person ages, veins lose elasticity and become fragile. Healthy veins feel soft and elastic. Veins that feel hard and sclerosed should not be used.

INTRAVENOUS THERAPY IS STARTED IN THE ARM WITH THE BETTER VENOUS AND LYMPHATIC CIRCULATION Because the cannula slows blood flow to some degree through a vein, the nurse takes precautions to avoid using a vein or a limb that has venous or lymphatic flow problems. Sites to be avoided include the arm on the same side on which a mastectomy or lymph node resection has been performed. The nurse also avoids an arm in which veins have been removed, shunt procedures have been performed, large varicosities are present, or thrombosed or sclerosed veins are present.

EQUIPMENT SELECTION FOR INTRAVENOUS THERAPY

Equipment selection includes the type and size of cannula; the type of tubing; the type of controller or pump, if needed; and the materials for starting IV therapy, such as preparation solution and tourniquet. The physician prescribes the specific type of fluid to be used. The fluid composition and the expected purposes of the therapy determine the selection of tubing style and cannula. For example, a large-gauge cannula is needed for transfusion of blood and blood products. Most hospitals and manufacturers provide specific information on the equipment used for IV therapy, especially cannulas and tubing.

CANNULA SELECTION The selection of cannula type and size largely depends on the expected purpose and duration of the IV therapy. In general, the nurse always selects the smallest size appropriate for the purpose of the therapy. A small size (such as a 24- or 26-gauge cannula) allows room in the vein for the blood to flow around the cannula. The higher the osmolarity or viscosity (thickness) of the solution ordered, the larger the cannula should be for adequate infusion.

CONTROLLER OR PUMP The nurse also selects a controller or pump for IV therapy. Even though not all IV therapy situations necessitate the use of this equipment, some hospitals require that all IV cannulas be connected to a controller or pump. Chart 15–6 lists situations in which a pump or controllers should be used.

Controllers A controller is an electronic gravity-run system; gravity makes the IV solution infuse into the arm. The nurse sets the rate on the device; an alarm sounds if resistance becomes too great to maintain the desired rate. Controllers can be set at a maximum of about 400 mL/hour (Lorenz, 1990). The advantage of a controller is that the device alarm is activated when the wrong rate is being given to the client. However, the device is so sensitive that the nurse may spend so much time checking the controller that it becomes a nuisance. Examples of controllers are the Abbott 1050 and the IVAC 280.

Pumps A pump is better than a controller when the client requires a precise amount of fluid or medication, such as a dopamine drip, or receives hyperosmolar solutions, such as total parenteral nutrition. The pump pushes the fluid into the client at a rate greater than gravity. Most models can deliver as much as 999 mL/hour or more (Lorenz, 1990). A disadvantage is that an extravasation (infiltration) may not be detected by the machine until it has become serious. Examples of commonly used pumps are the AVI 200, IMED 960, the IVAC 560, and the Baxter Flo-Gard 6201 (Fig. 15–13).

CHART 15–6

Nursing Care Highlight ◆ Criteria for the Use of Pumps and Controllers in Intravenous Therapy

- The client has poor cardiac or respiratory function.
- The client is on severe fluid restriction.
- The IV fluid contains potassium chloride concentration greater than 40 mEq/L (mmol).
- The client is receiving continuous infusions of:
  - Alprostadil
  - Aminocaproic acid
  - Aminophylline
  - An antidysrhythmic (lidocaine, procainamide, verapamil, diltiazem, labetalol)
  - Antihypertensive agents
  - Antilymphocyte globulin
  - Antithymocyte globulin
  - Barbiturates
  - Benzodiazapines
  - Calcium
  - Chemotherapeutic agents
  - Cimetidine
  - Cyclosporine
  - Diuretics
  - Dobutamine
  - Dopamine
  - Epinephrine
  - Heparin
  - Insulin
  - Immune globulin
  - Isoproterenol
  - Narcotics
  - Nitroglycerin
  - Nitroprusside
  - Pancuronium
  - Phenylephrine
  - Ranitidine
  - Streptokinase
  - Tissue plasminogen activator
  - Urokinase
  - Vasopressin

SITE PREPARATION FOR INTRAVENOUS THERAPY

After an appropriate site is selected and the proper equipment is assembled and prepared, the nurse prepares the skin area to reduce the risk of tissue damage, the client's discomfort, and infection as a result of IV therapy. Jewelry and restrictive clothing are removed from the area. If there is a lot of hair at the site that would interfere with proper anchoring or make tape and cannula removal painful, the nurse uses scissors to clip excessive hair from the area. Shaving is not recommended because it impairs skin integrity and allows possibly infectious microorganisms to enter the skin (Corrigan et al., 1990).

ANTIMICROBIAL PREPARATION According to the intravenous nursing standards of practice (Corrigan et al., 1990), only tincture of iodine 1% to 2%, iodophors, 70% alcohol, or chlorhexidine should be used for cleaning the IV site. Because alcohol tends to dry the skin, the nurse uses one of the other solutions for the elderly client. The nurse applies the preparation solution in a circular motion starting at the actual IV cannula insertion site and cleans outward for an area of 2 to 3 inches in diameter. When alcohol is used for younger clients, the nurse applies gentle friction for a minimum of 30 seconds or until the applicator is clean. Commercial cleaning solutions, such as I.V. Prep, are also available. This solution contains alco-

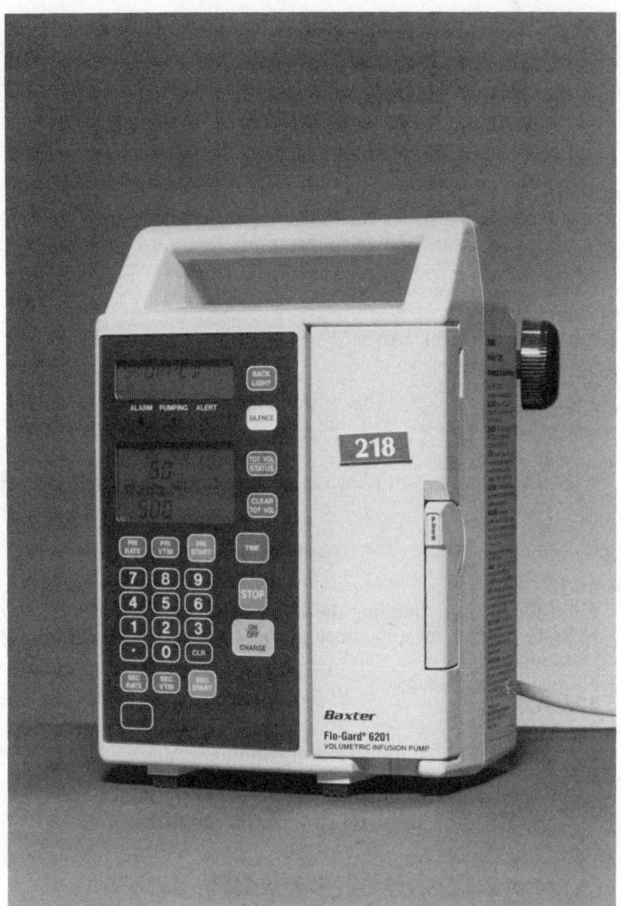

FIGURE 15–13 ◆ The Baxter Flo-Gard 6201 volumetric infusion pump.

hol, an antibacterial agent, and two film-forming agents to protect the skin and help keep transparent dressings in place.

TOURNIQUET USE Another component of site preparation is increasing the accessibility of the vein. Well-filled veins are most prominent and allow easier access. These veins bulge through subcutaneous tissues and are more easily palpated or viewed through the skin.

The use of a tourniquet above the site causes partial obstruction of venous flow and allows backfilling or overfilling of the veins below the tourniquet. After a tourniquet is applied, the nurse ensures that arterial blood flow is not obstructed by checking for the radial pulse.

Having the client open and close the hand also assists in venous filling by moving blood from muscle tissues into the veins. To decrease the risk of tissue damage, the tourniquet should be at least 1 inch wide, should be applied only tightly enough to interfere with venous flow, and should not remain in place for longer than 3 minutes.

VENIPUNCTURE

The technique of performing successful venipuncture varies with the type and purpose of the cannula, the location of the vein, the cooperativeness of the client during the procedure, and the skill of the person performing the venipuncture. Skill in technique is gained through instruction and practice. Many hospitals have a team consisting of nurses certified in venipuncture and IV therapy. Clients should not be subjected to repeated venipunctures by an unskilled or ill-prepared health care professional.

In keeping with universal precautions, the nurse wears disposable gloves during the venipuncture. The wearing of eye protection is also recommended in some settings. The nurse uses aseptic technique to keep the cannula and the prepared skin site sterile during the procedure. The cannula is placed into the vein going with the direction of blood flow. If it is necessary to stick the client more than once, a new cannula is used each time. After the cannula is properly placed in the vein (as evidenced by backflow of blood without tissue swelling at the site), the tourniquet is removed and solution flow is established. (For more detailed procedures for inserting IV cannulas, see skills textbooks and hospital procedure manuals.)

ANCHORING METHODS FOR CANNULAS

Because successful IV therapy involves maintaining the cannula in position, proper anchoring of the cannula (also known as cannula stabilization) after insertion is essential. Anchoring reduces the risk of phlebitis (vein inflammation), infection, extravasation (infiltration), and cannula movement or migration. Materials commonly used for anchoring include tape, transparent semipermeable membrane (TSM) dressings (such as Op-Site and Tegaderm), and sutures (for central venous catheters). Methods of taping vary, but the nurse never applies the tape directly to the skin-cannula junction site.

DRESSINGS FOR CANNULAS

After the cannula is anchored, the nurse applies a sterile occlusive dressing over the cannula site to reduce the risk of infection. Sterile gauze pads and tape or TSM dressings such as Op-Site and Tegaderm may be used (Fig. 15–14). For peripheral and central IV sites, gauze dressings are usually changed every 48

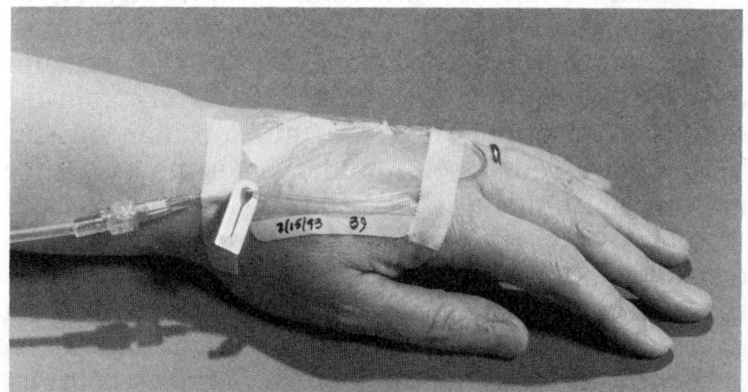

FIGURE 15–14 ◆ An intravenous therapy site anchored with a transparent dressing.

hours, or immediately if the dressing becomes wet, is soiled, or loosens. Protocols vary depending on specific agency policy. The optimal time for changing TSM dressings is not known and is still being studied (Corrigan et al., 1990). The range for changing TSM dressings is 2 to 5 days, depending on agency policy.

The advantage of TSM dressings is that they allow the nurse to see the site when monitoring for complications such as infection and phlebitis. The disadvantage is that, as is the case for tape, they can damage fragile, thin skin, especially in the elderly client. The nurse applies protective polymer solutions, such as Skin Prep, under the tape or TSM dressing to protect the skin.

For clients who pull or pick at their dressing or IV tubing, the nurse *loosely* applies a rolled, nonelastic gauze bandage, such as Kerlix, around the arm. The site and area around the site is not covered to allow frequent nursing observation. The nurse may need to obtain a physician's order for wrist restraints or mitts if the client is likely to pull out the IV cannula.

MAINTAINING INTRAVENOUS THERAPY

When a hospitalized client is receiving IV therapy, the nurse frequently assesses the flow rate, equipment function, and site condition. The frequency of nursing assessment depends on the type of solution and equipment used but may be as often as every hour. The nurse determines how much solution has been infused since the last assessment. In addition, the nurse maintains the flow rate and volume delivered within the limits of the physician's order.

A major nursing responsibility when caring for clients receiving IV therapy is prevention, assessment, and management of complications (Table 15–5). These complications can be severe enough to cause significant health problems and even death. There are three major types of complications of IV therapy:

- Infection
- Tissue damage
- Rapid changes in fluid volume and composition and electrolyte balance

INFECTION

Because IV therapy interrupts the integrity of the skin and provides a direct entrance for microorganisms, infection is always possible. The skin remains open, with a cannula or catheter penetrating from the outer surface through the skin into subcutaneous tissues and a blood vessel. Another factor increasing the risk of infection during IV therapy is that most IV therapy systems are open. Access to solution containers, tubing, and cannulas or catheters is achieved in the external environment. The risk of introducing microorganisms into the internal environment increases in direct proportion to the number of times that access to the system is obtained and how often the cannula or catheter is handled.

TABLE 15–5 Complications of Intravenous Therapy

Tissue Damage

- Skin
  - Hematomas at the needle penetration site
  - Abrasions from the skin preparation
  - Abrasion or desquamation from tape or adhesives
  - Allergic reactions
- Veins
  - Thrombus formation
  - Phlebitis
  - Fibrotic scarring
- Subcutaneous tissue
  - Edema
  - Hypoxia
  - Tissue necrosis from ischemia or the extravasation of vesicants or irritants

Infection

- Local
  - On the skin surrounding the site
  - In the skin, vein, and subcutaneous tissue at the needle penetration site
  - Deep tissue abscess
  - Cellulitis
- Septicemia
  - Bacterial (most common among immunocompetent clients)
  - Fungal (most common among neutropenic clients)

Fluid Volume Overload*

Electrolyte Imbalance

- Hyponatremia (most common among hospitalized clients)
- Hyperkalemia (potentially lethal)

* Most common in hospitalized clients.

The solutions used for IV therapy also increase the risk of infection. Although the solutions are sterile when administered, their essential composition promotes the growth of microorganisms.

Time critically influences the risk of infection from IV therapy. The longer the therapy is continued, the greater is the risk of infection.

PREVENTION OF INFECTION Because clients receiving IV therapy are at a high risk for infection, the nurse uses specific interventions to prevent infection. These interventions are listed in Chart 15–7.

ASSESSMENT OF INFECTION Signs and symptoms of IV therapy–related infections may not be obvious for more than 24 hours after the infection begins. The nurse observes the cannula or central catheter site for redness, heat, and discomfort. Purulent drainage may be present. If the infection becomes systemic, the client may experience chills and a low-grade fever. The most common microorganisms causing IV therapy–related infections are *Staphylococcus aureus* and *Staphylococcus epidermidis.*

MANAGEMENT OF INFECTION If infection is suspected, the nurse removes the cannula immediately. A physi-

CHART 15–7

Nursing Care Highlight ◆ Interventions to Prevent Infection

- When inserting a cannula, clean the skin with an antimicrobial solution in an inward-to-outward, circular motion.
- Maintain sterile, occlusive dressings over the cannula or central catheter site, and change them according to agency policy.
- When changing cannula to a new site, use new tubing.
- Change the tubing every 48 hr using sterile technique, and label the tubing with the date and time of the change.
- Do not let IV solution containers hang for more than 24 hr.
- Do not leave a contaminated cannula attached to IV tubing.
- Do not allow any part of the tubing to touch the floor.
- Do not handle cannulas and catheters while they are in place.
- You may use a 0.22-μm (sometimes referred to as 0.2-μm) filter as an extra safeguard against contaminants and air embolism.
- Swab access sites (latex injection ports) for adding medication or solutions for 30 to 60 sec with 70% alcohol, tincture of iodine 1% to 2%, iodophors, or chlorhexidine before inserting the needle. Use the smallest and shortest needle possible.

cian's order is not required for this action, but the nurse notifies the physician about why the IV cannula was removed. The physician may order antibiotic therapy. The nurse restarts the IV therapy in the other arm if possible. Ice or heat may be applied to the infected area, depending on how red and painful the area is. A sterile dressing with antibiotic ointment may be applied to a draining cannula site.

TISSUE DAMAGE

The tissues most commonly damaged by IV therapy include skin, blood vessels, and subcutaneous tissues. Tissue damage may be temporary or permanent. All tissue damage causes the client to experience some degree of discomfort, and most tissue damage can be avoided by proper technique and nursing observation.

SKIN The skin can be damaged when the IV therapy is started by the tourniquet application, skin preparation, cannula insertion, and anchoring techniques. When the tourniquet used to fill the vein is too narrow, is applied too tightly, or is left in place too long, hematomas, contusions, and abrasions can result. In addition, some nurses attempt to "bring up" a vein by tapping the skin over the vein site. Tapping the area can damage both the skin and the vein, especially in areas where there is little soft tissue beneath the skin to absorb the blow.

Elderly clients typically have fragile and thin skin. Therefore, the nurse is careful not to use excessive pressure to clean the skin site or to use harsh chemicals that can abrade or burn the skin. Chart 15–8 presents specific tips for safe administration of IV therapy to elderly clients.

The skin is also traumatized when the needle penetrates it. The larger the needle is and the more pressure applied during the penetration, the greater is the chance of causing skin damage. The nurse observes for ecchymosis (bruising) around the cannula insertion site. Ecchymosis is especially common when the client is receiving steroids or anticoagulants. The nurse informs the client and family members that the bruises will disappear in 1 to 2 weeks.

Skin is also susceptible to damage by anchoring materials. Some people are allergic to tape adhesives or react to adhesives when these agents are present on the skin for hours or days. The nurse observes every 4 hours for skin reactions, including erythema and blister formation. Removal of tape and adhesive dressings also can result in skin abrasion, especially in the elderly client. Protective materials such as Skin Prep help prevent this problem.

CHART 15–8

Nursing Focus on the Elderly ◆ Intravenous Therapy

- Assess the client's mental status every 4 hr.
- Explain that the IV route is common for administering medication and is not limited to very ill clients.
- Use the smallest gauge needle and catheter that can safely deliver the fluid.
- Use the shortest needle or cannula possible (24 gauge is preferable if blood is not being administered).
- Use a flexible catheter with a "winged" hub rather than a metal needle with a round hub whenever possible.
- Keep the angle of insertion less than 15 degrees.
- Do not tap to bring up a vein.
- Follow standard practice guidelines for IV therapy initiation, administration, and maintenance (see Charts 15–5 and 15–7).
- Place the IV cannula in the client's lower forearm on the nondominant side.
- Anchor the IV cannula with transparent dressing material rather than tape.
- Use flexible elastic netting to stabilize tubing connected to the needle or catheter.
- Use pumps, controllers, or volume-limited dispensing equipment (buretrols).
- Avoid circumferential restraints on the extremity with the IV cannula.
- Assess the site at least every 2 hr.

Another skin problem associated with IV therapy is hematoma (clot) formation at the IV site resulting from improper cannula removal. To prevent a hematoma, the nurse removes the cannula quickly and applies direct pressure immediately with a sterile gauze for 1 to 2 minutes. The nurse also elevates the client's arm while applying pressure to slow bleeding. After bleeding stops, the nurse applies a sterile gauze over the site.

VEINS Tissue damage to veins usually is the result of either mechanical or chemical trauma. Mechanical trauma is produced by the cannula or results when veins are tapped and broken. The insertion of the needle not only punctures the vein but also can tear away several membrane layers. After the needle is in place, it damages the innermost endothelial lining of the vein (tunica intima) by continuously exerting mechanical pressure against blood vessel walls. The nurse helps to prevent this problem by using the smallest possible cannula for the solution being administered. If possible, cannulas smaller than a 22 gauge are inserted.

Tissue damage to veins as a result of chemical trauma is related to the type and concentrations of IV therapy solutions, as well as to the rate of the infusion. Agents capable of causing chemical trauma to veins irritate the endothelium and cause postinfusion phlebitis (vein inflammation) or thrombophlebitis (inflammation with clot formation). Common IV agents or solutions capable of causing chemical trauma to veins include hypertonic solutions, potassium chloride, antibiotics, calcium, magnesium, ethyl alcohol, and chemotherapeutic drugs. In general, the more acidic or hyperosmolar the solution is the greater the risk of phlebitis is.

The nurse minimizes chemical trauma by diluting the agents administered intravenously and infusing the agent slowly into a large vein with a high-volume blood flow. Many solutions are given through a central venous catheter to avoid the risk of postinfusion phlebitis. The most likely persons to experience phlebitis from IV therapy are debilitated and elderly clients with thin skin.

The nurse assesses for phlebitis by looking for one or more reddened and warm areas or hard streaks that follow the vein path. The client usually complains of discomfort. Several scales have been developed to standardize assessments of the degree of inflammation. These range from assigning a value of 0 (no signs and symptoms) to 1+ to 3+ (all signs of inflammation present) (Corrigan et al., 1990). An example of the recommended scale is presented in Table 15-6.

If postinfusion phlebitis occurs, the nurse removes the IV catheter immediately and notifies the physician. The nurse applies ice or heat, depending on the amount of inflammation present. The client may have relief of discomfort from ice on a reddened area, followed by heat after the inflammation decreases. The nurse restarts the IV therapy in the other arm if possible, or the physician may insert a central venous catheter.

TABLE 15–6 Postinfusion Phlebitis Scale

Score	Defining Criteria
0	• No skin or vein abnormalities observed
1+	• Pain at site • Erythema present • Edema may be present
2+	• Pain at site • Erythema present • Edema may be present • Streak is visible
3+	• Pain at site • Erythema present • Edema may be present • Streak is visible • Vein cord palpable

Data from Corrigan, A., Delisio, N., Lonsway, R., Pelletier, G., & Rutherford, C. (1990). *Intravenous nursing standards of practice.* Belmont, MA: Intravenous Nurses Society.

SUBCUTANEOUS TISSUE Subcutaneous tissues sustain damage during IV therapy in two ways: by hypoxia and by extravasation, or infiltration.

Hypoxia Specific problems occurring during IV therapy can result in diminished oxygenation of local subcutaneous tissues, or hypoxia. Improper anchoring techniques that involve taping or the encircling the entire circumference of the arm with the IV catheter can lead to restriction of blood flow into and out of the area below the IV site. Another situation that leads to local tissue hypoxia is the leakage of IV fluids into the interstitial space, causing the formation of edema. Edema increases the diffusing distance for oxygen and other essential nutrients at the tissue and capillary levels so that tissue hypoxia develops.

Extravasation Extravasation, also called infiltration, occurs when chemically irritating IV solutions, often called vesicants, escape into the subcutaneous tissues, causing mild to severe tissue damage. Some solutions can cause tissue necrosis and sloughing wherever they contact healthy tissue (Table 15-7). Usually, the problem is discovered early enough to confine the damage to superficial, local subcutaneous tissues. This damage is painful and may require grafting for complete and functional healing. When vesicants penetrate into deeper tissues, such as muscles, nerves, and even bones, these tissues can be permanently damaged, with significant loss of function.

Prevention of Extravasation Clients who have steel cannulas instead of plastic cannulas are at a higher risk for extravasation (Wood & Gullo, 1993). The nurse prevents this problem from becoming serious by checking the IV catheter frequently to ensure that

TABLE 15–7 Common Tissue Vesicants Administered Intravenously

Chemotherapeutic Agents
- Dactinomycin
- Doxorubicin
- Daunorubicin
- Mitomycin C
- Mechlorethamine
- Vincristine
- Vinblastine

Antibiotics
- Vancomycin
- Nafcillin

Vasopressors
- Epinephrine
- Dopamine
- Dobutamine
- Norepinephrine

Electrolyte Solutions
- Potassium chloride
- Calcium chloride
- Calcium gluconate

Other Agents
- Diazepam
- Phenytoin
- Total parenteral nutrition
- Radiopaque contrast material

the cannula is completely in the vein. The nurse uses several methods for checking for blood return (backup), which include the following:

- Lowering the IV solution container (bag or bottle) below the level of the IV site and looking for blood return. When the IV catheter is in a small vein or the client has a low blood pressure, blood return may not be evident, even when the cannula is in the vein.
- Stopping the IV infusion, wrapping a tourniquet around the arm above the IV site, and looking for blood return.
- Using a syringe to aspirate blood back into the tubing.

The nurse does not depend solely on blood return for assurance that the cannula is in the vein. If the cannula is partly in the vein and partly in the tissues, a blood return may be present. Another way to check for proper placement is to apply pressure on the vein about 2 inches above the IV site. The IV rate should decrease when pressure is applied.

Assessment and Management of Extravasation The nurse assesses for signs and symptoms of early extravasation, which include discomfort at the IV site, blanching, coolness or warmth around the site, and leakage around the cannula. The IV rate is not always affected by extravasation, especially when an IV pump is used. The alarm on a pump may not be sensitive to the problem until it is severe. The nurse stops the IV therapy immediately and removes the cannula if there is any doubt that the cannula is in the vein. Compresses may be applied to the IV site area for 2 to 3 days. Whether the compresses are hot or cold depends on the specific solution extravasated.

A major nursing responsibility when extravasation occurs is documentation. The nurse describes the area thoroughly and accurately when the extravasation is discovered and every 8 hours after until the client is discharged from the facility. Depending on the institution's policies, serial photographs may be taken and become part of the client's permanent record. Other details for the nurse to document are presented in Chart 15–9.

CHART 15–9

Nursing Care Highlight ◆ Documentation of Extravasation

- Document the date and time when extravasation was suspected or identified.
- Note the date and time when the infusion was started.
- Record the time when the infusion was stopped.
- Note the exact contents of the infusion fluid and the volume of fluid infused.
- Document the estimated amount of fluid extravasated.
- Note the needle type and size.
- Diagram the exact insertion site.
- Indicate on the diagram the location and number of venipuncture attempts.
- Record the time between the extravasation and the last full blood return.
- Identify all agents administered in the previous 24 hr through this site (list the agent administered, the dosage and volume, and order of administration).
- Note the client's symptoms (at the site and systemic).
- Record the client's vital signs.
- Take a photograph of the site.
- Document the administration of neutralizing or antidote agents.
- Note the application of compresses.
- Note other nursing interventions.
- Record the client's responses to nursing interventions.
- Document the physician notification (including the time).
- Document the written and oral instructions given to the client about follow-up care.
- Note any consultation request.
- Sign the documentation.

FLUID AND ELECTROLYTE IMBALANCES

Because IV therapy involves infusion of fluids directly into the bloodstream, the potential risk for rapid changes in blood volume and composition is great. The overall effects of these changes depend on what degree of change is present, how rapidly the change occurs, and what specific electrolytes are out of balance.

FLUID IMBALANCE Fluid volume excess is the most common imbalance that occurs among clients receiving IV therapy. Often, this situation occurs because the excessive fluid is infused too rapidly. Factors contributing to rapid IV infusion include position changes of the client or the solution container, administration of solutions without the use of a controller or a pump, and the change in infusion rate (accidentally or intentionally) by clients, ancillary personnel, or visitors. The nurse monitors IV administration carefully and frequently.

Fluid volume excess can result in circulatory overload when the client's cardiopulmonary or renal status is compromised to the extent that he or she cannot adequately handle the fluid load. The elderly client is at increased risk for this complication. The nurse carefully monitors intake and output, and observes for signs and symptoms of fluid volume excess as described earlier in this chapter.

Another problem that can occur with IV therapy is inaccurate calculation of fluid volume when IV medications are added to an IV container. Not only does the addition of the actual medication increase the amount of fluid being infused, but the added medication is diluted and dosage delivery can be miscalculated. The recommended intervention to avoid additional fluid and prevent overdilution of medication is to remove (decant) from the IV container the exact volume of medication solution to be added before actually adding the medication solution (Research Applications for Nursing).

ELECTROLYTE IMBALANCES In addition to fluid volume change, too much IV solution can also result in dilution of serum electrolytes. Some electrolyte imbalances have serious consequences and can be life-threatening.

If the rapidly infused solution contains specific electrolytes in concentrations greater than normal physiologic amounts (for example, 40 mEq of potassium chloride in 1000 mL of 0.9% saline), the rapid infusion can greatly increase the serum electrolyte concentration to dangerous or even lethal levels (see Chap. 16).

DISCONTINUING INTRAVENOUS THERAPY

IV therapy is discontinued when the purpose of the therapy is accomplished or when specific IV-related problems occur. Because IV therapy is an invasive

RESEARCH APPLICATIONS FOR NURSING

We Still Do Not Know the Best Way to Mix Intravenous Medications

Sulzbach, L. M., & Munro, B. H. (1991). Survey of nursing practice related to decanting intravenous solutions. *Heart & Lung, 20*(6), 624–630.

Nurses frequently prepare IV medications so that, when mixed with the base IV solution, 1 mL of fluid equals a specific amount of medication. Often mixed in either 250- or 500-mL bags, these IV medications are titrated for an effective client response. Despite current practice, however, no research has determined the best way to prepare these potent medications. For example, how does the nurse determine whether the IV medication bag contains overfill (a quantity of fluid greater than the labeled amount)? If it does, should the nurse decant (remove the overfill) before adding medication? For example, if a medication requires reconstitution in 50 mL of normal saline, should the nurse remove an equal volume from the base solution?

Sulzbach and Munro conducted a survey of 1000 critical care nurses from 47 states of the United States and the District of Columbia. Of the 475 respondents, 91% were staff nurses and 72% worked in community hospitals. Of the total sample, 71% did not decant. The remaining 29% used a needle and syringe to withdraw a volume of fluid from the bag equal to the amount of medication to be added.

Critique This study addresses an important problem with direct implications for the client's well-being. The generalizability of the findings would have been strengthened by a randomized and stratified sampling design that included a greater proportion of responses from nurses working in university-affiliated, government, and military hospitals. Thus, future studies are needed.

Possible nursing implications Some participants in this study disagreed with the premise that accurate knowledge of the drug concentration is necessary. They reasoned that the dosage of the IV medications is titrated to desired effects for the client, such as optimal systolic blood pressure. But what if several new bags are hung throughout the day, each with supposedly the same (but actually different) concentrations? If the drug must be titrated upward to sustain the client's blood pressure, is this because the client is more critically ill or because the actual drug concentration has changed? The authors recommended decanting when the added amount is equal to or greater than 20% of the base solution. Also, they suggested that nurses work on hospital committees to develop protocols for IV medication preparation and that nurses encourage drug manufacturers to develop research-based guidelines for practice.

procedure, the nurse checks the physician's order to discontinue therapy before removing the needle. When the nurse determines that a problem with the infusion exists (such as extravasation or phlebitis), a physician's order is not needed, but the physician is notified.

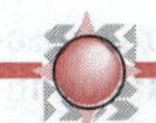

IMPLICATIONS FOR NURSING RESEARCH

No one has more influence over the client's fluid status than the nurses administering oral and parenteral fluids. Because these activities are within the domain of nursing, they are relevant for nursing research. Nursing research needs to be conducted to answer the following questions about the care of clients at risk for fluid imbalance:

- What assessment criteria are best for determining the client's hydration status?
- Which assessment criteria of hydration status are accurate for elderly clients?
- What effect does health care teaching have on the prevention of dehydration in clients at high risk?
- Are heat applications more or less beneficial than cold applications in reducing the discomfort associated with phlebitis at IV sites?
- What skin preparation techniques are best for reducing skin flora for the initiation of IV therapy?
- Are video presentations as effective as direct in-person presentations in teaching clients self-care of vascular access devices?
- Can volume-controlled containers be used in place of controllers or pumps for careful fluid volume administration in IV therapy?
- Are transparent dressings more cost-effective than gauze dressings at IV sites?

SELECTED BIBLIOGRAPHY

Burns, D. (1992). Working up a thirst. *Nursing Times, 88*(26), 44–45.

Camp-Sorrell, D. (1992). Implantable ports: Everything you always wanted to know. *Journal of Intravenous Nursing, 15*(5), 262–273.

Corrigan, A., Delisio, N., Lonsway, R., Pelletier, G., & Rutherford, C. (1990). *Intravenous nursing standards of practice.* Belmont, MA: Intravenous Nurses Society.

Coulter, K. (1992). Intravenous therapy for the elder patient: Implications for the intravenous nurse. *Journal of Intravenous Nursing, 15*(Suppl.), S18–S23.

Dellasega, C., & Shellenbarger, T. (1992). Discharge planning for cognitively impaired elderly adults. *Nursing and Health Care, 13*(10), 526–531.

Dennison, R., & Blevins, B. (1992). Myths and facts about fluid imbalance. *Nursing92, 22*(3), 22.

Fry, B. (1992). Intermittent heparin flushing protocols: A standardization issue. *Journal of Intravenous Nursing, 15*(3), 160–163.

Gershan, J., Freeman, C., Ross, M., Greenlee, K., Smejkal, C., Brukwitzki, G., Schneider, K., Jiricka, M., Johnson, D., & Anderson, C. (1990). Fluid volume deficit: Validating the indicators. *Heart & Lung, 19*(2), 152–156.

Gilmour, J., & Penny, S. (1991). Hydration and aging. *New Zealand Nursing Journal, 84*(10), 15–17.

Guyton, A. (1991). *Textbook of medical physiology* (8th ed.). Philadelphia: W. B. Saunders.

Hadaway, L. (1991). IV tips. *Geriatric Nursing, 12*(2), 78–81.

Hirschorn, N., & Greenough, W. (1991). Progress in oral rehydration therapy. *Scientific American, 264*(5), 50–56.

Holder, C., & Alexander, J. (1990). A new and improved guide to I.V. therapy. *American Journal of Nursing, 90*(2), 43–47.

Jones, A., Moseley, M., Halfmann, S., Heath, A., Henkelman, W., Ciaccio, J., & Bolcas, B. (1991). Fluid volume dynamics. *Critical Care Nurse, 11*(4), 74–76.

Keyes, J. (1990). *Fluid, electrolyte, and acid-base regulation* (2nd ed.). Belmont, CA: Wadsworth.

Kokko, J., & Tannen, R. (1990). *Fluids and electrolytes* (2nd ed.). Philadelphia: W. B. Saunders.

Kuc, J. (1993). When herparin causes clots. *RN, 56*(3), 34–37.

Lorenz, B. (1990). Are you using the right IV pump? *RN, 53*(5), 31–36.

Metheny, N. (1992). *Fluid and electrolyte balance: Nursing considerations* (2nd ed.). Philadelphia: J. B. Lippincott.

Millam, D. (1990). Electronic infusion devices: Controlling the flow. *Nursing90, 20*(8), 65–68.

Millam, D. (1993). How to teach good venipuncture technique. *American Journal of Nursing, 93*(7), 38–41.

Newton, M., Newton, D., & Fudin, J. (1992). Reviewing the "big three" injection routes. *Nursing92, 22*(2), 34–41.

Porth, C., & Erickson, M. (1992). Physiology of thirst and drinking: Implication for nursing practice. *Heart & Lung, 21*(3), 273–284.

Roundtree, D. (1991). The PIC catheter: A different approach. *American Journal of Nursing, 91*(8), 22–26.

Siek, A., & Brentin, L. (1993). A little light makes venipuncture easier. *RN, 56*(3), 40–43.

Smith, R. (1993). A nurse's guide to implanted ports. *RN, 56*(4), 48–53.

Sterns, R., & Spital, A. (1990). Disorders of water balance. In J. Kokko & R. Tannen (Eds.), *Fluids and electrolytes* (2nd ed., pp. 139–194). Philadelphia: W. B. Saunders.

Sulzbach, L., & Munro, B. (1991). Survey of nursing practice related to decanting intravenous solutions. *Heart & Lung, 20*(6), 624–630.

Trissel, L. (1992). *Handbook on injectable drugs* (7th ed.). Bethesda, MD: American Society of Hospital Pharmacists.

Viall, C. (1990). Your complete guide to central venous catheters. *Nursing90, 20*(2), 34–41.

Watt, S. (1991). Quenching the body's thirst. *New Zealand Nursing Journal, 84*(10), 18–19.

Whitehouse, M. (1992). Nursing assessment of the elderly patient. *Journal of Intravenous Nursing, 15*(Suppl.), S14–S17.

Wickham, R. (1990). Advances in venous access devices and nursing management strategies. *Nursing Clinics of North America, 25,* 345–364.

Wood, L., & Gullo, S. (1993). IV vesicants: How to avoid extravasation. *American Journal of Nursing, 93*(4), 42–46.

SUGGESTED READINGS

Coulter, K. (1992). Intravenous therapy for the elder patient: Implications for the intravenous nurse. *Journal of Intravenous Nursing, 15*(Suppl.), S18–S23.

The author describes physical and psychologic characteristics of the geriatric client that should be considered whenever nursing care is provided to an elderly person receiving intravenous therapy. Suggestions for starting IV treatment in the elderly person are presented (along with appropriate rationale), as are specific problem areas to be assessed.

Hirschorn, N., & Greenough, W. (1991). Progress in oral rehydration therapy. *Scientific American, 264*(5), 50–56.

This excellent article provides a complete description of the mechanisms underlying the success of oral rehydration therapy as well as historical information on its impact on world health. Drawings underscore the osmotic influences of different solutions in their effectiveness for gastrointestinal absorption. In addition, serial photographs showing the resuscitation of a dehydrated child provide visual proof of clinical effectiveness.

Wood, H., & Gullo, S. (1993). IV vesicants: How to avoid extravasation. *American Journal of Nursing, 93*(4), 42–46.

This concise yet detailed article describes the problems associated with extravasation of vesicants and specific nursing interventions to avoid this complication of intravenous therapy. Photographs graphically show the tissue damage associated with extravasation.

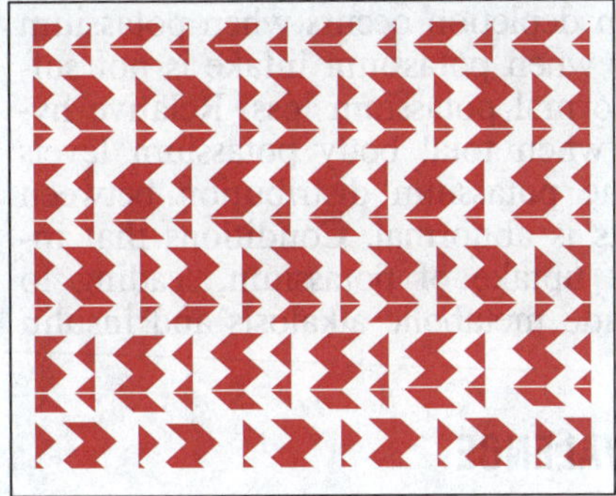

CHAPTER 16

Interventions for Clients with Electrolyte Imbalances

CHAPTER HIGHLIGHTS

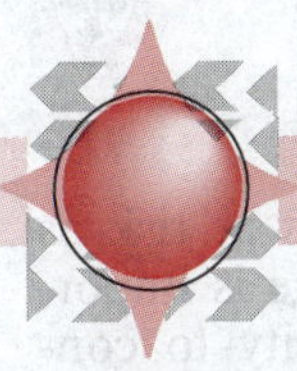

Electrolyte imbalances occur frequently among hospitalized clients. Because many imbalances can be life-threatening, all nurses should have basic understanding of the pathophysiology, clinical manifestations, and interventions associated with specific electrolyte imbalances.

POTASSIUM IMBALANCES

Hypokalemia

OVERVIEW

Because 98% of the total body potassium (K^+) is intracellular, small changes in extracellular potassium levels cause major changes in cell membrane excitability as well as in other processes within the cell. Hypokalemia is indicated by a serum potassium level of less than 3.5 mEq/L. Hypokalemia is a relatively common electrolyte imbalance and is potentially life-threatening because every body system can be affected.

PATHOPHYSIOLOGY

When the serum potassium level decreases, there is an *increased* potassium concentration gradient (difference) between the fluid inside the cells, or intracellular fluid (ICF) and the extracellular fluid (ECF). This increased gradient reduces the excitability of cells. Consequently, the cell membranes of all excitable tissues, such as nerve and muscle, are less responsible to normal stimuli.

The degree of pathologic changes associated with hypokalemia is directly related to how rapidly the serum potassium level decreases. When extracellular potassium loss is slow, intracellular potassium also decreases in proportion to the extracellular fluid potassium level. In this situation, the potassium concentration gradient between the two fluid compartments is essentially unchanged and symptoms of hypokalemia may not appear until the potassium loss is extreme. Rapid changes in extracellular potassium levels (representing a more rapid loss of potassium) are not compensated for quickly, and result in dramatic changes in body function.

ETIOLOGY

Hypokalemia may result from actual total body potassium depletion or abnormal movement of potassium from the extracellular fluid to the intracellular fluid, causing a relative decrease in the extracellular potassium level. Table 16–1 summarizes the common causes of hypokalemia.

TABLE 16–1 Common Causes of Hypokalemia

Actual Potassium Deficits
Excessive Loss of Potassium
• Inappropriate or excessive use of drugs
• Diuretics
• Digitalis
• Corticosteroids
• Increased secretion of aldosterone
• Cushing's syndrome
• Diarrhea
• Vomiting
• Wound drainage (especially gastrointestinal)
• Prolonged nasogastric suction
• Heat-induced excessive diaphoresis
• Renal disease impairing reabsorption of potassium
Inadequate Potassium Intake
• Nothing by mouth (NPO)
Relative Potassium Deficits
Movement of Potassium from Extracellular Fluid to Intracellular Fluid
• Alkalosis
• Hyperinsulinism
• Hyperalimentation
• Total parenteral nutrition
Dilution of Serum Potassium
• Water intoxication
• IV therapy with potassium-poor solutions

Actual potassium depletion occurs when potassium loss is excessive or when potassium intake is not sufficient to match normal potassium loss. Relative hypokalemia occurs when total body potassium levels are normal but the potassium distribution between fluid compartments is abnormal. Conditions that increase the cellular uptake of potassium, leading to hypokalemia, include metabolic alkalosis and insulin administration.

INCIDENCE/PREVALENCE

Although exact statistics about the incidence of hypokalemia are not available, this imbalance occurs frequently in both hospitalized clients and in those receiving ambulatory care. Hypokalemia may be associated with virtually all illnesses. Elderly clients are especially at high risk for hypokalemia that results from chronic illness or prescribed medications.

COLLABORATIVE MANAGEMENT

ASSESSMENT

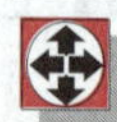

HISTORY

AGE The nurse collects data from clients at risk as well as those with actual hypokalemia. Age is important to consider because the renal capacity to concentrate urine decreases, increasing potassium loss. Elderly clients are more likely to use medications, such as diuretics and laxatives, that promote the renal or gastrointestinal loss of potassium.

MEDICATION USE The nurse questions the client about the use of all medications, especially diuretics and corticosteroids. These drugs increase potassium loss through the kidneys. One of the most common causes of hypokalemia is the use and misuse of diuretics. For clients taking digitalis preparations such as digoxin (Lanoxin, Novodigoxin✱), hypokalemia increases the sensitivity of the myocardium to the drug and may result in digitalis toxicity, even when the dosage is within the therapeutic range.

The nurse questions whether the client takes a prescribed potassium supplement, such as potassium chloride (KCl). The client may not be taking the potassium chloride as prescribed owing to its unpleasant taste.

OTHER FACTORS Any acute or chronic disease state may lead to hypokalemia. The nurse asks about recent illnesses and medical or surgical interventions. A thorough diet history, including a typical day's food and beverage intake, helps the nurse identify clients at risk for hypokalemia.

PHYSICAL ASSESSMENT/CLINICAL MANIFESTATIONS

Clinical manifestations of hypokalemia are associated with altered function of many systems (Chart 16–1).

CHART 16–1

Key Features of Hypokalemia

Cardiovascular

- Variable pulse rate, more often rapid
- Pulse quality thready and weak
- Peripheral pulses difficult to palpate
- Orthostatic (postural) hypotension
- Electrocardiographic abnormalities
  - ST depression
  - Inverted T wave
  - Prominent U wave
  - Heart block

Respiratory

- Shallow, ineffective respirations due to profound weakness of the skeletal muscles of respiration
- Diminished breath sounds

Neuromuscular

- Anxiety, lethargy, confusion, coma
- Loss of tactile discrimination
- General skeletal muscle weakness
- Deep tendon hyporeflexia
- Eventual flaccid paralysis

Gastrointestinal

- Decreased motility
- Hypoactive-to-absent bowel sounds
- Nausea
- Vomiting
- Abdominal distention
- Paralytic ileus
- Constipation

Renal

- Decreased ability to concentrate urine
- Polyuria
- Decreased specific gravity

RESPIRATORY SYSTEM The respiratory system can be profoundly affected by hypokalemia through depression of the nerves and muscles used during inhalation and exhalation. Contraction of specific muscle groups causes respiratory movement and permits breathing. Weakness of the skeletal muscles of respiration results in shallow and ineffective respirations. The nurse assesses breath sounds, the ease of respiratory effort, and the color of nail beds and mucous membranes, as well as the rate and depth of respiration. *The nurse assesses the client's respiratory status at least every 2 hours, because respiratory insufficiency frequently accompanies hypokalemia and is a major cause of death* (Tannen, 1990).

CARDIOVASCULAR SYSTEM Cardiovascular changes often accompany hypokalemia. The nurse assesses the cardiovascular system by first palpating peripheral pulses. In the client with hypokalemia, the pulse is usually thready and weak. Palpation is difficult, and the pulse is easily blocked with light pressure. The pulse rate ranges from excessively slow to excessively rapid, depending on whether a dysrhythmia (irregular heart beat) is present. The nurse measures blood pressure with the client in lying, sitting, and standing positions, because orthostatic (postural) hypotension accompanies hypokalemia.

NERVOUS SYSTEM Neurologic manifestations of hypokalemia include changes in mental status. The client may experience short-term irritability and anxiety followed by lethargy that progresses to confusion and coma as hypokalemia worsens. Severe hypokalemia affects sensory nerves by decreasing the awareness of sensations. For example, clients may not be able to identify mild sensations of pain, touch, heat, and cold.

MUSCULOSKELETAL SYSTEM Skeletal muscles become weak in response to hypokalemia, and a stronger stimulus is needed to begin muscle contraction. Clients may be so weak that they are unable to stand. Handgrasps are weak, and clients have hyporeflexia (a decreased response to deep tendon reflex stimulation). Severe hypokalemia can lead to flaccid paralysis. The nurse assesses the degree of muscle weakness and determines the client's ability to perform activities of daily living (ADL).

GASTROINTESTINAL SYSTEM Hypokalemia results in decreased smooth muscle contractility within the gastrointestinal system, leading to decreased peristalsis. Clients have hypoactive bowel sounds and may experience nausea, vomiting, constipation, and abdominal distention. The nurse assesses distention by measuring abdominal girth. The nurse also assesses bowel sounds in all four abdominal quadrants to determine the extent of decreased peristalsis. Severe hypokalemia can result in a paralytic ileus (the absence of peristalsis).

PSYCHOSOCIAL ASSESSMENT

Because hypokalemia is seldom a long-term problem, the behavioral changes usually occur within a short period of time. The nurse's knowledge of the client's usual mental status and mood is useful in assessing changes that may be due to hypokalemia. Information about the client's behavior may need to be obtained from close family members or friends, depending on the client's condition.

The nurse collects data about the onset and duration of behavioral changes as well as their association with any other physical signs and symptoms. These data are important and need to be as accurate as possible. The client may be lethargic and unable to perform simple problem-solving tasks that require concentration, such as counting backward from 100 by threes. As hypokalemia progresses, the client may become increasingly confused, especially being disoriented to time and place. In severe hypokalemia, coma may develop.

LABORATORY ASSESSMENT

The definitive laboratory test result that confirms hypokalemia is a serum potassium value of less than 3.5 mEq/L. However, this value does not indicate whether a true potassium deficit exists or there has been a shift of potassium from the blood to the intracellular fluid. Urine laboratory values generally are not helpful in determining potassium loss, because the kidneys do not normally conserve potassium.

OTHER DIAGNOSTIC ASSESSMENT

The physician usually orders a baseline electrocardiogram (ECG) followed by continuous cardiac monitoring for clients with severe hypokalemia. Hypokalemia causes electrical conduction abnormalities, including ST segment depression, flat or inverted T waves, and increased U waves. Dysrhythmias can result in death, particularly in elderly clients taking digitalis medications.

ANALYSIS

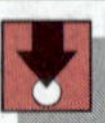

COMMON NURSING DIAGNOSES

Common nursing diagnoses among clients experiencing hypokalemia are:

1. High Risk for Injury related to skeletal muscle weakness
2. High Risk for Ineffective Breathing Pattern related to neuromuscular impairment
3. Constipation related to smooth muscle atony

ADDITIONAL NURSING DIAGNOSES

In addition to the common nursing diagnoses, clients with hypokalemia may have one or more of the following nursing diagnoses:

- Impaired Mobility related to skeletal muscle weakness
- Total Self Care Deficit related to skeletal muscle weakness
- Decreased Cardiac Output related to dysrhythmia

PLANNING AND IMPLEMENTATION

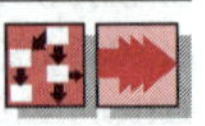

HIGH RISK FOR INJURY

PLANNING: CLIENT GOALS The major goals are that the client will:

- Avoid experiencing injury
- Have a return of serum potassium level to normal

INTERVENTIONS Interventions are aimed at preventing potassium loss, increasing serum potassium levels, and providing a safe environment for the client. Drug and diet therapies help restore normal serum potassium levels.

Drug Therapy Potassium supplements (oral or intravenous [IV]) are commonly given for the treatment and prevention of hypokalemia.

POTASSIUM SUPPLEMENTS Most postassium supplements (replacements) are composed of potassium chloride. The amount and the route of potassium replacement are based on the degree of potassium loss. A client with a serum potassium level of 3 mEq/L needs 100 to 200 mEq of potassium supplement. A client with a serum potassium level of 2 mEq/L needs 500 to 600 mEq (Tannen, 1990).

For severe hypokalemia, potassium is given IV. A dilution of no more than 1 mEq/10 mL of solution is recommended. The maximum recommended rate of infusion is 5 to 10 mEq/hour—*never to exceed 20 mEq/hour under any circumstances.* Elderly clients may not be able to handle this rate. Rapid infusion of potassium can cause cardiac arrest; therefore, the nurse never gives potassium by IV push (DeAngelis & Lessig, 1991).

Potassium is a severe tissue irritant and is never administered as an intramuscular (IM) or subcutaneous (SC) injection. Tissues damaged by potassium can become necrotic (dead) and slough (shed from the body), leading to loss of function and requiring reconstructive surgery. IV potassium solutions irritate veins and can cause phlebitis (vein inflammation). The nurse checks the physician's orders carefully to ensure that the client receives the correct amount of potassium. The nurse assesses the IV site every 2 hours and asks the client whether burning or pain at the site is felt. The IV is stopped immediately if it is infiltrated.

Most oral preparations of potassium contain a potassium chloride base, but brands may vary in dosage. Therefore, potassium products should not be switched without a physician's order. Oral potassium preparations may be administered as liquids or solids. Potassium chloride has a strong, unpleasant taste that is difficult to mask. Because potassium chloride can cause nausea and vomiting, it should not be taken on an empty stomach.

POTASSIUM-SPARING DIURETICS Diuretics that increase the renal excretion of potassium commonly cause hypokalemia. These classes of diuretics include high-ceiling, or loop, diuretics, such as furosemide (Lasix, Furoside✱), bumetanide (Bumex), and ethacrynic acid (Edecrin), and the thiazide diuretics, such as chlorothiazide (Diuril), hydrochlorothiazide (Esidrex, Nefrol✱), and quinethazone (Hydromox, Aquamox✱). Therefore, the physician avoids the use of these drugs for clients with actual hypokalemia or those who are susceptible to hypokalemia. When the client with hypokalemia requires diuretic therapy, a potassium-sparing diuretic may be appropriate. Potassium-sparing diuretics cause diuresis without increasing potassium excretion. Diuretics with this action include spironolactone (Aldactone, Novo-spiroton♣), triamterene (Dyrenium), and amiloride (Midamor).

Diet Therapy The nurse consults with the dietitian in teaching the client how to increase dietary potassium intake. Eating food naturally rich in potassium helps to restore normal potassium levels, and also prevents further loss. Table 14-6 lists foods with a high potassium content. Foods eaten raw or baked contain more potassium than those prepared by boiling, poaching or frying.

Safety Measures While the client is experiencing muscle weakness, the nurse employs safety measures and eliminates hazards. The nurse assists the client with ambulation. Before the client ambulates, the nurse ensures that the path is free from obstacles or slippery areas and that the client is wearing nonslip footgear. When ambulating with assistance, the client wears a gait belt around the waist.

INEFFECTIVE BREATHING PATTERN

PLANNING: CLIENT GOALS The goal is that the client's breathing pattern will be adequate to maintain gas exchange.

INTERVENTIONS The nurse monitors the client's rate and depth of respiration at least once per hour, particularly noting increases in rate and decreases in depth. The effectiveness of respiratory muscles can also be determined by the client's ability to cough. If clients are conscious, the nurse asks them to cough and notes how deeply the clients can cough. The nurse examines the client's face, oral mucosa, and nail beds for signs of pallor or cyanosis. The nurse assesses the arterial blood gases for the presence of hypoxemia (decreased blood oxygen concentration) or hypercapnia (increased arterial carbon dioxide concentration). (Chapters 28 and 29 discuss respiratory assessment and interventions in more detail.)

CONSTIPATION

PLANNING: CLIENT GOALS The major goal is that the client's normal bowel elimination pattern will be restored.

INTERVENTIONS Interventions are aimed at restoring normal serum potassium levels and inducing gastric motility. Specific interventions include drug and diet therapies to restore serum potassium levels to normal values (discussed earlier under drug and diet therapies for High Risk for Injury) and stimulate intestinal peristalsis as well as interventions to avoid conditions that contribute to constipation.

Drug Therapy Laxatives that add bulk or fiber may be used to stimulate peristalsis. Other drugs, such as metoclopramide (Reglan, Maxeran♣), that enhance gastric emptying and stimulate gastrointestinal motility are used to treat the constipation associated with hypokalemia.

Diet Therapy The nurse questions the client about normal bowel functions and what specific interventions have worked well for the client in the past to prevent or alleviate constipation. Whenever possible, the nurse uses these familiar techniques with the client experiencing constipation. The nurse provides meals that contain high-fiber foods and plenty of liquids for clients who are not on fluid restrictions. To ensure client cooperation, the nurse prepares a list of foods that contain high concentrations of fiber and asks the client to select favorite items from that list.

Comfort Measures The nurse can help the client maintain normal bowel elimination patterns in several ways. When the client is using the toilet or bedpan, the nurse provides as much privacy as possible. The nurse closes the door, pulls privacy curtains, and asks visitors to step out of the room. Physical activity and exercise promote gastric motility. The nurse encourages the client to ambulate whenever the client's condition permits. The nurse assists bedridden clients with frequent position changes and mild bed exercises.

DISCHARGE PLANNING

HOME CARE PREPARATION

When hypokalemia is resolved and the causative conditions are controlled, home care preparations are individualized to the client's baseline physical and mental functioning.

HEALTH TEACHING

The nurse instructs clients at risk (especially those receiving diuretics or corticosteroids) in the proper use of medications, the signs and symptoms of hypokalemia, when to seek medical help, and which food sources are rich in potassium. The nurse teaches clients to measure the rate, rhythm and quality of their peripheral pulses. The nurse instructs clients to take their pulse at least once each day and whenever any signs or symptoms of hypokalemia are present. The nurse discusses with chronically ill clients how potassium is lost from the body so that the client can act to reduce potassium loss before actual deficits occur. The nurse reinforces how often the client should have serum potassium levels assessed.

PSYCHOSOCIAL PREPARATION

Clients at risk for repeated episodes of hypokalemia are those with chronic conditions requiring specific drugs that induce potassium loss. For these clients, discharge planning must include assessment of the client's knowledge level and ability to adhere correctly to prescribed drug regimens.

HEALTH CARE RESOURCES

Because hypokalemia is a manifestation of other health problems rather than a distinct disease, necessary health care resources vary with the underlying health problem.

EVALUATION

On the basis of the identified nursing diagnosis, the nurse evaluates the care of the client experiencing hypokalemia. The expected outcomes for the client with hypokalemia include that the client:

- Returns to and maintains a normal serum potassium level (between 3.5 and 5 mEq/L)
- Complies with drug and diet therapy as prescribed
- States the early signs and symptoms of hypokalemia
- Does not experience injury
- Has normal bowel elimination patterns
- Maintains adequate gas exchange
- Maintains regular cardiac rate and rhythm

Hyperkalemia

OVERVIEW

Hyperkalemia is a serum potassium level greater than 5 mEq/L. Because the range of normal serum potassium values is narrow, even slight increases above normal values can have serious adverse effects on the physiologic function of excitable tissues, especially the myocardium.

PATHOPHYSIOLOGY

When the serum potassium level increases, there is a *decreased potassium concentration gradient* between the fluid inside the cells and the extracellular fluid. This decreased gradient increases cell excitability so that excitable tissues respond to less intense stimuli and may even discharge spontaneously.

Hyperkalemia alters the function of all excitable membranes to some degree. However, the myocardium is more sensitive to increases in serum potassium levels than are other excitable membranes, so that the more serious complications of hyperkalemia are associated with alterations of cardiac function.

The degree of pathologic changes associated with hyperkalemia is directly related to how rapidly extracellular fluid potassium levels increase. Sudden increases in serum potassium levels cause profound function changes at potassium levels between 6 and 7 mEq/L. When increases in serum potassium levels occur slowly or chronically, problems with excitable membrane function may not be obvious until potassium levels reach 8 mEq/L (Innerarity, 1992).

TABLE 16–2 Common Causes of Hyperkalemia

Actual Potassium Excesses

Excessive Potassium Intake

- Overingestion of potassium-containing foods or medications
  - Salt substitutes
  - Potassium chloride
- Rapid infusion of potassium-containing IV solution
- Bolus IV potassium injections

Decreased Potassium Excretion

- Adrenal insufficiency (Addison's disease, adrenalectomy)
- Renal failure
- Potassium-sparing diuretics

Relative Potassium Excesses

Movement of Potassium from Intracellular Fluid to Extracellular Fluid

- Tissue damage
- Acidosis
- Hyperuricemia
- Hypercatabolism

ETIOLOGY

Hyperkalemia may result from an actual increase in the amount of total body potassium. Such conditions include renal impairment, adrenalectomy, Addison's disease, and the use of potassium-sparing diuretics. Hyperkalemia may also result from abnormal movement of potassium from the cells to the extracellular fluid. Table 16–2 summarizes the causes of hyperkalemia.

INCIDENCE/PREVALENCE

Hyperkalemia is rare in persons with normally functioning kidneys. Therefore, most cases of hyperkalemia occur among hospitalized clients or those who are undergoing medical treatment. Clients at greatest risk for hyperkalemia are chronically ill, debilitated, or elderly.

COLLABORATIVE MANAGEMENT

ASSESSMENT

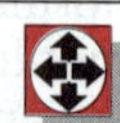

HISTORY

When documenting the client's history, the nurse collects data about risk factors, as well as causative factors, for hyperkalemia. Age is important, because decreased renal function occurs in elderly people. The nurse asks about the presence of chronic illnesses, particularly renal disease and diabetes mellitus. The nurse also asks questions concerning recent medical

CHART 16–2

Key Features of Hyperkalemia

Cardiovascular

- Irregular heart rate, usually slow
- Decreased blood pressure
- Electrocardiographic abnormalities
  - Tall T waves
  - Widened QRS complexes
  - Prolonged PR intervals
  - Flat P waves
- Ectopic beats
- Late: arrhythmias, ventricular fibrillation, cardiac arrest in diastole

Respiratory

- Unaffected until late, when profound weakness of the skeletal muscles causes respiratory failure

Neuromuscular

- Early phase, or mild hyperkalemia
  - Muscle twitches, cramps
  - Paresthesias
- Late phase, or severe hyperkalemia
  - Profound weakness
  - Ascending flaccid paralysis in distal-to-proximal direction involving the arms and the legs

Gastrointestinal

- Increased motility
- Hyperactive bowel sounds
- Diarrhea

or surgical interventions. Clients are questioned about urinary output, such as the frequency and amount of voidings. The nurse also inquires about medication use, particularly potassium-sparing diuretics. The nurse obtains a diet history to pinpoint possible causative factors, such as the intake of potassium-containing foods, especially those eaten raw. The nurse specifically asks the client about the use of salt substitutes; many of these substitutes contain potassium salts.

The nurse collects data indicating the presence of symptoms related to hyperkalemia. The client is asked if palpitations, skipped heartbeats, or other cardiac irregularities have been experienced. Information about the presence of muscle twitching, weakness in leg muscles, and unusual sensations of tingling followed by numbness in the hands, the feet, or the face is obtained. The nurse inquires about recent changes in bowel habits, especially diarrhea, colic, and explosive bowel movements.

PHYSICAL ASSESSMENT/CLINICAL MANIFESTATIONS

The clinical manifestations of hyperkalemia are summarized in Chart 16–2.

CARDIOVASCULAR SYSTEM Cardiovascular changes are the most severe results of hyperkalemia and are the most common cause of death in clients with hyperkalemia (Tannen, 1990). The nurse assesses the cardiac status of all clients with hyperkalemia through careful observation and cardiac monitoring. Conduction changes indicative of hyperkalemia include gradual worsening of bradycardia; heart block; the presence of tall, peaked T waves; prolonged PR intervals; flattening or disappearance of P waves; and widening of QRS complexes (Fig. 16–1).

As serum potassium levels rise, impulse conduction through the cardiac Purkinje system slows and may be blocked at the atrioventricular (AV) node. The heart muscle dilates and becomes flaccid. As electrical conduction is blocked at the AV node, ectopic beats (beats generated outside the normal conduction system in the ventricles) may appear. Complete heart block, ventricular standstill, or ventricular fibrillation are major life-threatening complications of severe hyperkalemia (Innerarity, 1992).

In addition to noting specific ECG changes, the nurse also assesses cardiac status through peripheral pulse and blood pressure measurements. The client with hyperkalemia usually has a slow, weak pulse and low blood pressure.

NEUROMUSCULAR SYSTEM The neuromuscular response to hyperkalemia has two phases. During the early stages of hyperkalemia, skeletal muscles twitch and the client may be aware of unusual nerve sensations, such as tingling and burning, followed by numbness in the hands, in the feet, and around the mouth. As hyperkalemia progresses, muscle twitching changes to weakness and is followed by flaccid paralysis. The weakness ascends from distal-to-proximal areas and affects the muscles of the arms and the legs. Trunk, head, and respiratory muscles are not affected until serum potassium levels reach lethal levels.

GASTROINTESTINAL SYSTEM The smooth muscle of the gastrointestinal tract responds to hyperkalemia by increasing peristaltic movement. The nurse assesses the gastrointestinal system by listening to bowel sounds and observing stools. The client may experience diarrhea and spastic colonic activity. Bowel sounds are hyperactive, with frequent audible rushes and gurgles. Bowel movements may be frequent, watery, and explosive.

PSYCHOSOCIAL ASSESSMENT

Behavioral changes are not usually associated with hyperkalemia because cardiac problems cause the client to seek medical assistance before serum potassium levels become high enough to produce neurologic manifestations.

LABORATORY ASSESSMENT

The laboratory test result that confirms the condition of hyperkalemia is a serum potassium value

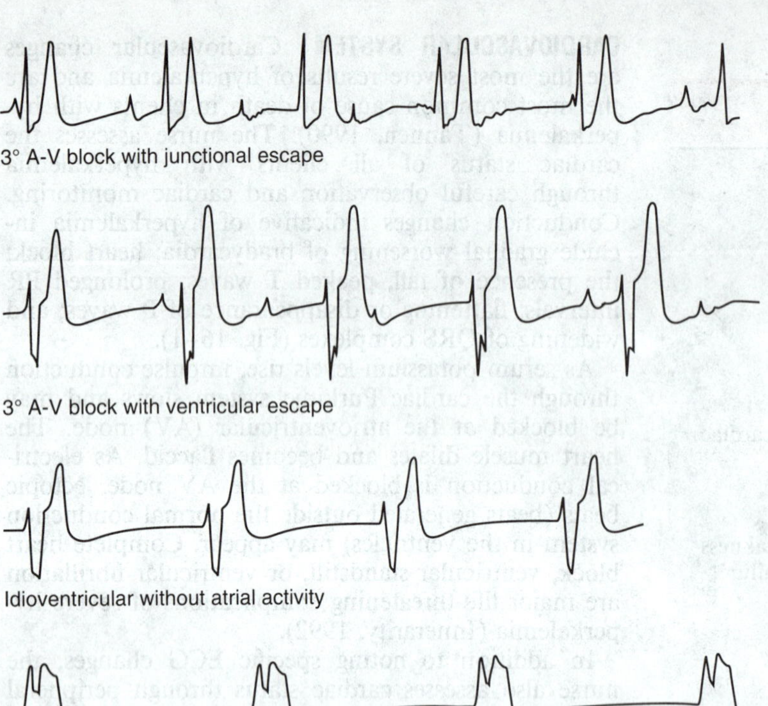

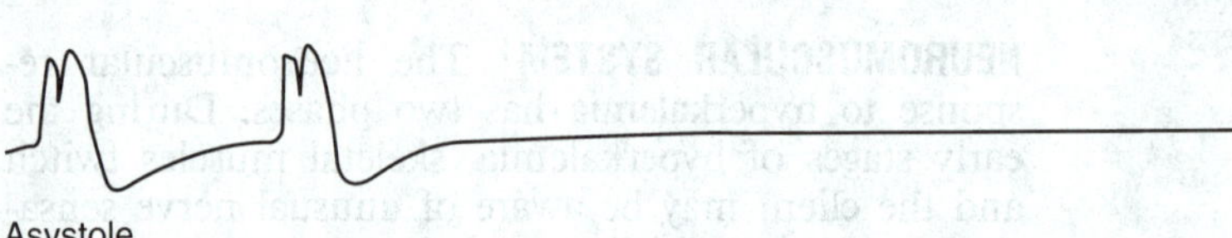

FIGURE 16-1 ◆ Electrocardiographic (ECG) changes associated with hyperkalemia. (Modified with permission from John M. Clochesy.)

greater than 5 mEq/L. If the hyperkalemia results from dehydration, levels of other serum electrolytes may be elevated, as are hematocrit and hemoglobin levels. Hyperkalemia associated with renal failure is usually accompanied by elevations of serum creatinine and blood urea nitrogen levels, a decreased blood pH, and normal or low hematocrit and hemoglobin levels.

ANALYSIS

COMMON NURSING DIAGNOSES

The most significant problem experienced by clients with hyperkalemia is Decreased Cardiac Output related to altered electrical conduction.

ADDITIONAL NURSING DIAGNOSES

Clients experiencing hyperkalemia may have one or more of the following nursing diagnoses:

- Pain related to muscle cramps
- Diarrhea related to increased smooth muscle irritability

PLANNING AND IMPLEMENTATION

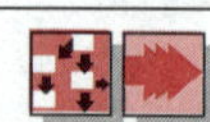

DECREASED CARDIAC OUTPUT

PLANNING: CLIENT GOALS The goals are that the client will:

- Have serum potassium levels restored to normal values
- Avoid experiencing lethal cardiac dysrhythmias

INTERVENTIONS Although identifying the causes of hyperkalemia is important, interventions are aimed at immediately reducing the serum potassium level. Drug therapy is useful for restoring normal potassium balance.

Drug Therapy The aims of drug therapy are to prevent further increases in serum potassium levels by:

- Eliminating potassium administration
- Enhancing potassium excretion
- Promoting the movement of potassium from the extracellular fluid into the cells

ELIMINATING POTASSIUM ADMINISTRATION When hyperkalemia occurs, the nurse stops infusions of potassium-containing IV solutions, but the IV catheter is kept open. Oral potassium supplements are withheld, and the physician may order a potassium-restricted diet. When hyperkalemia is accompanied by dehydration, bolus administration of IV fluids that do not contain potassium may help dilute the serum potassium level to less dangerous levels.

INCREASING POTASSIUM EXCRETION If renal function is not impaired, the physician orders the administration of potassium-excreting diuretics, such as furosemide (Mendyka, 1992). For clients with renal problems, drug therapy to increase the excretion of potassium includes the use of cation exchange resins, such as sodium polystyrene sulfonate (Kayexalate). Sodium polystyrene sulfonate releases sodium (a cation) and, in exchange, absorbs potassium (another cation). The potassium remains bound to the resin and is excreted through the feces. This treatment can be administered orally or rectally. If the client is able to retain the polystyrene enema for the required 45 minutes, the rectal route is preferred, because the action of polystyrene is more pronounced in the large intestine. Although sodium polystyrene sulfonate reduces potassium levels, the effect can take many hours. Therefore, if potassium levels are dangerously high, additional measures, such as dialysis and ultrafiltration, are necessary.

PROMOTING THE MOVEMENT OF POTASSIUM Potassium movement from the extracellular fluid to the cells is enhanced by the presence of insulin. Insulin increases the activity of the membrane-bound sodium-potassium adenosinetriphosphatase (ATPase) pumps (see Chap. 14), resulting in movement of potassium from the blood and other extracellular fluids into the cell (Tannen, 1990). Therefore, the physician may order IV fluids that contain substantial amounts of glucose and insulin to help decrease the serum potassium levels (usually 250 mL of 10% to 20% glucose with 10 to 20 units of regular insulin). These IV solutions are hypertonic and are administered through a central venous catheter in a vein with a high blood flow to avoid local vein inflammation. The nurse observes the client for signs and symptoms of hypokalemia and hypoglycemia during this therapy.

Cardiac Monitoring Prevention of lethal dysrhythmias depends not only on reducing potassium levels but also on recognizing early signs and symptoms of the adverse response of cardiac muscle. The nurse compares recent electrocardiographic (ECG) tracings with the client's baseline tracings or tracings obtained when the client's serum potassium level was close to normal. The nurse is responsible for reporting and recording these findings.

Diet Therapy Dietary limitation of potassium is useful when hyperkalemia is chronic or related to renal disease. However, when hyperkalemia is sudden or severe, diet therapy is of little benefit.

DISCHARGE PLANNING

HOME CARE PREPARATION

Although the hyperkalemic state is usually corrected or reduced before clients are discharged from the hospital or facility, clients most likely to experience hyperkalemia have other chronic pathologic conditions that may remain. Consequently, these clients are chronically at risk for hyperkalemia. Special equipment and training are required for clients with chronic renal failure or end-stage renal disease who choose home dialysis (see Chap. 72). Usually, these clients are followed by a nephrology team. However, the primary nurse caring for the client during hospitalization is responsible for contacting the team coordinator and providing information about the client's condition and needs at the time of hospital discharge.

HEALTH TEACHING

Education is a key factor in the prevention of hyperkalemia and in the early detection of its life-threatening complications. The teaching plan for the client at risk for hyperkalemia includes diet, medications, and how to recognize the signs and symptoms of hyperkalemia. Diet education includes foods to avoid (those high in potassium) and permissible foods containing little potassium (Chart 16–3). The nurse instructs the client to examine medication and food package labels to determine the potassium content. The client is instructed to avoid salt substitutes, because these preparations usually contain potassium. It is important to teach the person who actually pur-

CHART 16–3

Education Guide ◆ Dietary Management of Hyperkalemia

- You should avoid
  - Organ meats
  - Fish
  - Fresh fruits
  - Dried fruits
  - Beef
  - Chicken
  - Pork
  - Milk
  - Vegetables
- You may eat
  - Eggs
  - Breads
  - Cereals
  - Butter
  - Sugar

chases or prepares meals, as well as the client, whenever possible.

The nurse instructs the client and family members about the signs and symptoms of hyperkalemia as well as what information should be reported immediately to the primary health care provider. It is especially critical to teach the client how to take a pulse accurately and determine its rate, regularity, and quality. The nurse reinforces how often the client should have serum potassium levels assessed. The nurse also stresses adherence to prescribed medical regimens.

PSYCHOSOCIAL PREPARATION

Psychosocial preparation needs vary not only with the individual client's background but also with the different underlying pathologic conditions contributing to the risk of hyperkalemia. Clients with newly diagnosed chronic health problems may require counseling before acceptance and participation in self-care can begin. Local support groups can ease the process of adjustment to living with a chronic illness. The nurse provides the client with information about and local telephone numbers for specific support groups. Such information is available in telephone directories and through hospital social services departments.

If hyperkalemic episodes are the result of long-term health problems, clients may have learned to cope and require less psychosocial support. However, this situation cannot be assumed. The nurse assesses the psychosocial needs of each client individually in terms of new factors, established support systems, previous and current coping patterns, and stability of the chronic disease.

A major psychosocial issue for clients at risk for hyperkalemia resulting from chronic disease is compliance. The nurse must convey to the client that quality of life depends to a great extent on the client's compliance with the planned treatment regimen. Some aspects of the regimen may be unpleasant or require significant self-control by the client. Assisting the client and family members to understand the disease process may increase the client's sense of control and willingness to cooperate. In conveying this information, the nurse focuses on the potential positive outcomes of good compliance rather than the negative effects of noncompliance.

HEALTH CARE RESOURCES

For the client with chronic health problems that increase the risk of hyperkalemia, the appropriate health care resource people include the physician, the home care nurse, the pharmacist, and the nutritionist or dietician. When special equipment needs or financial problems interfere with the client's ability to obtain necessary food or medications, the nurse contacts the social services department of the facility. The client with chronic health problems frequently requires assistance with self-care. If no one is able to perform these functions, either home care nursing may be necessary or the client may have to be placed in an extended-care facility. Specific organizations related to the chronic disease or organ problem causing the hyperkalemia may be helpful. Such organizations include the Kidney Foundation and the American Diabetes Association.

EVALUATION

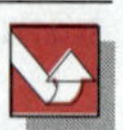

On the basis of the identified nursing diagnoses, the nurse evaluates the care of the client with hyperkalemia. The expected outcomes include that the client will:

- Have a serum potassium level between 3.5 and 5 mEq/L
- Not experience life-threatening dysrhythmias
- Comply with prescribed drug and diet therapy
- Re-establish his or her normal pattern of bowel elimination

SODIUM IMBALANCES

Hyponatremia

OVERVIEW

Hyponatremia is a serum sodium (Na^+) level less than 135 mEq/L. Because sodium is the major cation of the blood and interstitial fluid and is primarily used for maintaining the osmolarity of these fluids, imbalances of sodium levels are usually associated with imbalances of fluid volume.

PATHOPHYSIOLOGY

The pathophysiologic changes underlying hyponatremia have two mechanisms:

- The first mechanism is a change in cell excitability or activity. As the concentration of sodium in the blood and other extracellular fluids decreases, the sodium concentration gradient between the extracellular fluid and the fluid inside the cells also decreases. Less sodium is available to move across the excitable membrane. This situation results in delayed and slower membrane depolarization.
- The second mechanism is the movement of water from the extracellular fluid space into the intracellular fluid space. Cells swell and function decreases. The tissues most sensitive to hyponatremia are in the central nervous system (CNS).

ETIOLOGY

Various conditions can lead to hyponatremia by causing either an actual or a relative decrease in so-

TABLE 16–3 Common Causes of Hyponatremia

Actual Sodium Deficits
Increased Sodium Excretion
• Excessive diaphoresis
• Diuretics (high-ceiling diuretics)
• Wound drainage (especially gastrointestinal)
• Decreased secretion of aldosterone
• Hyperlipidemia
• Renal disease (scarred distal convoluted tubule)
Inadequate Sodium Intake
• Nothing by mouth (NPO)
• Low-salt diet
Relative Sodium Deficits
Dilution of Serum Sodium
• Excessive ingestion of hypotonic fluids
• Psychogenic polydipsia
• Freshwater drowning
• Renal failure (nephrotic syndrome)
• Irrigation with hypotonic fluids
• Syndrome of inappropriate antidiuretic hormone secretion (SIADH)
• Hyperglycemia
• Congestive heart failure

dium content (Table 16–3). Hyponatremia can represent a loss of total body sodium, movement of sodium from the serum to other fluid spaces, or dilution of serum sodium by the presence of excessive water in the plasma.

Total body sodium is deficient when excessive amounts of sodium are lost through normal and abnormal routes. Conditions causing excessive loss are heavy diaphoresis, vomiting, hemorrhage, wound drainage, use of high-ceiling (loop) diuretics, renal disease (especially with scarring of the ascending limb of the loop of Henle), and Addison's disease. Hyponatremia can also be present when sodium loss is normal but sodium intake is insufficient, such as with clients who are taking nothing by mouth (NPO) or who are on sodium-restricted diets.

Hyponatremia also occurs when total body sodium levels are normal but diluted by excessive fluids. Conditions causing sodium dilution include polydipsia, irrigation of body cavities with hypotonic solutions, IV administration of sodium-free solutions, and movement of water from the intracellular fluid space into the extracellular fluid space.

COLLABORATIVE MANAGEMENT

ASSESSMENT

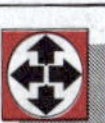

The clinical manifestations of hyponatremia are associated with its effects on excitable cellular activity. The cells especially affected are involved in cerebral, neuromuscular, and gastric smooth muscle functions (Chart 16–4).

CEREBRAL FUNCTION

Changes in cerebral function are the most obvious signs and symptoms of hyponatremia. Because these changes may be seen as either depressed activity or excessive activity (and sometimes both), establishing the client's usual cerebral function and behavioral patterns is important to detect changes associated with hyponatremia. Behavioral changes result from cerebral edema and increased intracranial pressure (Norris, 1992).

The nurse observes the client closely and documents the client's behavior. The nurse assesses the

CHART 16–4

Key Features of Hyponatremia

Cardiovascular*
- Normovolemic
  - Rapid pulse rate
  - Normal blood pressure
- Hypovolemic
  - Rapid pulse rate
  - Pulse quality thready and weak
  - Hypotensive
  - Central venous pressure normal or low
  - Flat neck veins
- Hypervolemic
  - Rapid, bounding pulse
  - Central venous pressure normal or elevated
  - Blood pressure normal or elevated

Respiratory
- Late manifestations related to skeletal muscle weakness
  - Shallow, ineffective respiratory movements
- Hypervolemia
- Pulmonary edema
  - Rapid, shallow respiration
  - Moist rales

Neuromuscular
- Generalized skeletal muscle weakness
- Diminished deep tendon reflexes
- Personality changes
- Headache

Renal
- Increased urinary output
- Decreased specific gravity

Gastrointestinal
- Increased motility
- Nausea
- Hyperactive bowel sounds
- Diarrhea

* Symptoms vary with changes in vascular volume.

client's current mental status, starting with the level of consciousness, in the same manner described under neurologic manifestations of dehydration, p. 269.

NEUROMUSCULAR SYSTEM

The nurse assesses the client's neuromuscular status during each nursing shift for changes from baseline values. The neuromuscular response to hyponatremia is generalized muscle weakness. Muscle tone and deep tendon reflex responses diminish. The nurse assesses muscle strength by having the client:

- Squeeze the nurse's hands
- Attempt to keep the arms flexed while the nurse pulls downward on the lower arms
- Push both feet against a flat surface while the nurse applies resistance

Muscle weakness associated with hyponatremia occurs bilaterally and is worse in the extremities. The nurse assesses deep tendon reflexes by lightly tapping the patellar (knee) tendons and Achilles (heel) tendons with a reflex hammer and documenting the degree of reflex movement. The technique for assessment of motor strength and reflexes is described in depth in Chapter 40.

GASTROINTESTINAL SYSTEM

The smooth muscle of the gastrointestinal system responds to decreases in serum sodium levels with increased gastrointestinal motility, causing nausea, diarrhea, and abdominal cramping. The nurse assesses the gastrointestinal system by listening to bowel sounds and observing stools. Bowel sounds are hyperactive, with frequent rushes and gurgles, especially over the splenic flexure and in the lower left quadrant. Bowel movements are frequent, watery, and explosive. Peristaltic movements may be palpated through the abdominal wall and may even be visible on the abdominal surface.

CARDIOVASCULAR SYSTEM

Hyponatremia has little direct effect on cardiac muscle contractility; however, alterations in cardiac output are associated with hyponatremia. When hyponatremia is accompanied by changes in the plasma volume, these fluid changes alter cardiac function. Generally, cardiac responses to hyponatremia with an accompanying hypovolemia (decreased plasma volume) are manifested as a rapid, weak, thready pulse. Peripheral pulses are difficult to palpate and are easily blocked with light pressure. Neck veins are flat with the client in the upright position and also may be flat in the supine position. Blood pressure is decreased, especially diastolic pressure. The client may experience severe hypotension when moving from a lying or sitting position to a standing position. The central venous pressure is normal or low.

When hyponatremia is accompanied by plasma hypervolemia (increased plasma volume), cardiac manifestations include a rapid, full pulse. Blood pressure is normal or elevated. The central venous pressure is normal or elevated, depending on how well the left ventricle is handling the extra fluid. Peripheral pulses are full and difficult to block; however, if edema is present, peripheral pulses may not be palpable.

Accurate laboratory assessment of serum sodium levels is needed to plan appropriate interventions. When obtained directly from a venipuncture, blood values of sodium are accurate. However, when blood for serum electrolyte evaluation is drawn through pulmonary arterial catheters, adjustment in technique is necessary to ensure accurate blood levels (Research Application for Nursing).

INTERVENTIONS

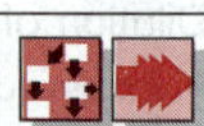

Interventions are aimed at restoring serum sodium levels to normal values and preventing further decreases in serum sodium levels.

Drug Therapy The purpose of drug therapy is to restore the serum sodium level to normal.

DRUG THERAPY FOR HYPONATREMIA WITH FLUID DEFICIT

When hyponatremia occurs with a fluid deficit (hypovolemia), the physician orders IV saline infusions to restore both sodium content and fluid volume. Depending on the severity of the hyponatremia, IV saline solutions may be isotonic (0.9%) or hypertonic (3% to 5%). In general, the rate of IV infusion is determined by the rate of the sodium or fluid loss. When sodium is replaced too rapidly, excitable cells, especially those in the brain, may over-respond to the fluid and electrolyte changes with severe adverse reactions. The nurse monitors the infusion rates and the client's responses. The infusions are delivered through a controller or a pump to prevent accidental alterations in infusion rates.

DRUG THERAPY FOR HYPONATREMIA WITH FLUID EXCESS

When hyponatremia is accompanied by fluid excess, drug therapy includes the administration of diuretics that primarily promote the excretion of water rather than sodium. These drugs are osmotic diuretics, such as mannitol (Osmitrol✱). When cerebral edema is severe, the physician may prescribe drugs that promote intracranial fluid loss, such as dexamethasone (Decadron, Dexasone✱). The nurse assesses the client hourly for signs that indicate excessive loss of fluids and potassium or dramatic increases in sodium levels.

Drug therapy for hyponatremia as a result of inappropriate or excessive secretion of antidiuretic hormone (ADH) includes agents that antagonize ADH, such as lithium and demeclocycline (Declomycin).

Diet Therapy For mild hyponatremia, diet therapy can help restore normal sodium balance. Table 14–5 in Chapter 14 lists the sodium content of common

RESEARCH APPLICATIONS FOR NURSING

Discarding a Certain Volume of Blood from Pulmonary Artery Catheter Blood Samples May Yield More Accurate Results

Carlson, K., Snyder, M., LeClair, H., Underhill, S., Ashwood, E., & Detter, J. (1990). Obtaining reliable plasma sodium and glucose determinations from pulmonary artery catheters. *Heart & Lung, 19*(6), 613–619.

Critically ill clients often have pulmonary artery catheters placed for clinical management of hemodynamic and fluid volume status. An advantage of this catheter is easy access for blood samples and the elimination of the need for venipuncture. Most often, a pressurized infusion of heparinized saline is used to maintain patency of the catheter. To prevent contamination of the blood sample by this solution, the nurse must aspirate and discard a certain volume of the saline solution before obtaining the client's blood sample. This study of 30 people undergoing cardiac surgery compared the accuracy and the reliability of sodium and glucose determinations in 15 consecutive blood samples (per person) taken from the pulmonary artery catheter with those of a blood sample drawn by venipuncture. For sodium plasma values, there was no significant difference between samples. The glucose plasma values, however, were significantly higher in the samples aspirated from the pulmonary artery catheter; on average, they were 6 mg/dL greater than the control samples obtained from venipuncture. Sodium values remained stable over time when the pulmonary artery dwell volume (i.e., the blood visible in the catheter tubing between the catheter insertion site and the blood drawing port) plus an additional milliliter was aspirated. For glucose determinations, an additional milliliter of blood needed to be aspirated from the catheter to produce reliable results.

Critique These investigators should be commended for executing this well-designed study because so few studies of this kind have been done. Reports of the types of IV infusions, as well as indications of whether any clients had diabetes mellitus, would have been helpful in determining why plasma glucose results were higher in the pulmonary artery. Although the researchers found a difference of 6 mL to be statistically significant, this difference is unlikely to affect nursing practice and therefore may be considered clinically insignificant.

Possible nursing implications More studies are needed to determine volumes to be discarded for accurate and reliable determination of the client's hemoglobin concentration, coagulation times, and electrolyte status. Studies of heparin locks in peripheral venous sites are also needed to determine discard volumes. On the basis of this study, the nurse should aspirate and discard 2 mL of blood plus the dwell volume in the pulmonary artery catheter before obtaining a blood sample for determinations of sodium and glucose.

foods. The nurse collaborates with the dietitian in teaching the client about which foods to increase in the diet. The therapy consists of increasing the oral sodium intake and restricting the oral intake of fluids to some degree. When overhydration with oral hypotonic fluids is the underlying cause of the hyponatremia, or when renal fluid excretion is impaired, fluid restriction may be a long-term regimen. The nurse measures fluid intake and output. The nurse also reinforces the purpose of the fluid restriction. Diet therapy has little effect on severe hyponatremia or hyponatremia due to chronic illness other than renal disease.

Hypernatremia

OVERVIEW

Hypernatremia is represented by a serum sodium level greater than 145 mEq/L. Increases in serum sodium levels can be caused by changes in fluid volumes and can also cause changes in fluid volumes. Table 16–4 lists the common causes of hypernatremia.

As the extracellular sodium level rises, there is a larger sodium concentration gradient (difference) between the extracellular fluid and the intracellular fluid. More sodium is available to move rapidly across cell membranes. With mild hypernatremia, almost all excitable tissues are excited more easily, a condition called irritability. This irritability causes excitable tissues to over-respond to stimuli. However, as the extracellular sodium concentration increases, the

TABLE 16–4 Common Causes of Hypernatremia

Actual Sodium Excesses

Decreased Sodium Excretion

- Hyperaldosteronism
- Renal failure
- Corticosteroids
- Cushing's syndrome

Increased Sodium Intake

- Excessive oral sodium ingestion
- Excessive administration of sodium-containing IV fluids

Relative Sodium Excesses

Decreased Water Intake

- Nothing by mouth (NPO)

Increased Water Loss

- Increased rate of metabolism
- Fever
- Hyperventilation
- Infection
- Excessive diaphoresis
- Watery diarrhea
- Dehydration

osmolarity and the osmotic pressure of the extracellular fluid also increase. This situation causes osmosis of water from the cells into the extracellular fluid as a compensatory action to dilute the hyperosmolar extracellular fluid. When hypernatremia persists or becomes more severe, the compensatory action causes severe intracellular dehydration and excitable tissues may no longer be able to respond to stimuli. Excitable tissues in the brain are the most sensitive to changes in serum sodium concentration.

COLLABORATIVE MANAGEMENT

ASSESSMENT

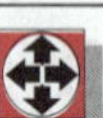

The clinical manifestations of hypernatremia vary with the degree of imbalance and whether a fluid imbalance is also present. Rapid increases in serum sodium level generally produce more obvious and severe symptoms. Gradual increases in serum sodium levels may produce no observable physical changes, even when sodium levels are increased to well above normal ranges. Clinical manifestations of hypernatremia are primarily associated with changes in cell membrane activity, especially among excitable tissues involved in cerebral, neuromuscular, and cardiac functions (Chart 16–5).

CENTRAL NERVOUS SYSTEM

Cerebral function is the most likely to be altered during episodes of hypernatremia. Therefore, the nurse assesses the client's mental status in terms of attention span, recall of recent events, and ability to perform cognitive functions. In the presence of hypernatremia with normal or decreased fluid volumes, the client may be agitated and somewhat confused about the sequence of recent events. The client's attention span is short, and the client may not be able to concentrate on simple tasks, such as counting backward from 100 by threes. The client's perception of noise and other environmental stimuli may be increased. If the serum sodium concentration continues to increase, the client may become manic or experience convulsions. When hypernatremia is accompanied by an extracellular volume overload, the client may exhibit symptoms of lethargy, drowsiness, stupor, or coma.

NEUROMUSCULAR SYSTEM

Skeletal muscles respond differently to various degrees of hypernatremia. Mild hypernatremia causes muscle twitches and irregular muscle contractions. As the hypernatremia worsens, the ability of skeletal muscle and nerves to respond to a stimulus diminishes. Muscles become progressively weaker and demonstrate rigid paralysis. Deep tendon reflexes are diminished or absent. The nurse assesses the neuromuscular status by looking for twitching among muscle groups. The nurse also assesses the client's muscle strength by having the client perform handgrasps and arm flexion against resistance. Muscle weakness associated with hypernatremia occurs bilaterally and has no specific progressive pattern. The nurse assesses the response of the peripheral nerves by lightly tapping the patellar (knee) tendons and Achilles (heel) tendons with a reflex hammer, and measuring the degree of movement. (For an in-depth description of nursing assessment of mental status, deep tendon reflexes, and muscle strength, see Chapter 40.)

CARDIOVASCULAR SYSTEM

Increases in serum sodium levels prevent movement of calcium into the myocardium, thus decreasing the ability of the myocardium to contract (Briggs et al., 1990). The nurse assesses the cardiovascular status by taking the client's blood pressure and measuring the rate and quality of apical and peripheral pulses. Pulse rate and blood pressure may be normal, above normal, or below normal during hypernatremic episodes, depending on the fluid volume and the

CHART 16–5

Key Features of Hypernatremia

Cardiovascular
- Decreased myocardial contractility
- Diminished cardiac output
- Heart rate and blood pressure respond to vascular volume

Respiratory
- Problems associated with pulmonary edema when hypernatremia is accompanied by hypervolemia

Neuromuscular*
- Hypernatremia and normovolemia or hypovolemia
  - Increased neural activity
  - Agitation, confusion, seizures
- Hypernatremia and hypervolemia
  - Decreased neural activity
  - Lethargy, stupor, coma
- Mild or early hypernatremia
  - Spontaneous muscle twitches
  - Irregular contractions
- Severe or late hypernatremia
  - Skeletal muscle weakness
  - Deep tendon reflexes diminished or absent

Renal
- Decreased urinary output
- Increased specific gravity

Integumentary
- Dry, flaky skin
- Presence or absence of edema related to accompanying fluid volume changes

* Upper neural function changes are related to volume changes as well as sodium increases.

speed with which the imbalance occurs (Dennison & Blevins, 1992). In clients with hypernatremia and hypovolemia, the pulse rate is increased. Peripheral pulses may be difficult to palpate and are easily blocked with light pressure. The client is hypotensive, with severe orthostatic (postural) hypotension, and the pulse pressure is greatly diminished.

Clients with hypernatremia and hypervolemia have slow-to-normal bounding pulses. Peripheral pulses are full and difficult to block. Neck veins are distended, even with the client in the upright position. Blood pressure, especially diastolic pressure, is increased.

INTERVENTIONS

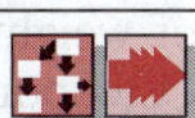

Interventions are aimed at preventing further increases in serum sodium levels and decreasing elevated serum sodium levels. Drug administration and diet therapy play important roles in restoring normal sodium balance. Other interventions that the physician may use when hypernatremia becomes life-threatening include hemodialysis, peritoneal dialysis, and blood ultrafiltration techniques.

Drug Therapy When hypernatremia is caused by fluid loss, drug therapy for the treatment of hypernatremia focuses on restoring fluid balance. The physician orders IV infusions of glucose and water (e.g., 5% dextrose in water). When hypernatremia is caused by fluid and sodium losses, it may be necessary to replace the fluid with IV administration of isotonic sodium chloride (NaCl) solutions. When hypernatremia is caused by inadequate renal excretion of sodium, drug therapy with diuretics promoting sodium loss, such as furosemide (Lasix, Furoside✱), bumetanide (Bumex), and ethacrynic acid (Edecrin), is ordered. The nurse assesses the client hourly for symptoms that indicate excessive loss of fluids, sodium, or potassium.

Diet Therapy Dietary restrictions of sodium are useful in preventing hypernatremia. Clients with renal disease must have their intake of sodium rigidly restricted from 200 mg to 2000 mg/day, depending on the degree of renal impairment. Often, fluids must be restricted as well. The nurse collaborates with the dietitian in helping the client to understand how to determine the sodium content of foods, beverages, and medications and the importance of complying with the diet.

CALCIUM IMBALANCES

Hypocalcemia

OVERVIEW

Hypocalcemia is defined as a serum calcium (Ca^{2+}) level of less than 9 mg/dL, or 4.5 mEq/L. Calcium is stored in bone, and only a small fraction of the total body calcium is present in extracellular fluid. Because the normal serum level of calcium is so low, small changes in serum calcium levels have major effects on body function.

PATHOPHYSIOLOGY

The presence of measurable hypocalcemia indicates either that the normal protective and regulatory mechanisms are not functioning properly, or that the conditions causing the hypocalcemia have been present so long that compensatory mechanisms are exhausted and no longer adequate to maintain homeostasis. Calcium ions decrease excitable membrane permeability to sodium ions, preventing spontaneous depolarization. Thus, calcium is considered a membrane stabilizer, regulating depolarization and the generation of action potentials. Low serum calcium levels increase the permeability of excitable membranes to sodium so that depolarization occurs more easily and at inappropriate times (Pak, 1990).

Excitable tissues vary in their sensitivity to low serum calcium levels. The excitable tissues that demonstrate the most obvious responses to decreased serum calcium levels are peripheral nerves, skeletal muscles, cardiac muscle, and the smooth muscle of the gastrointestinal system. The severity of the signs and symptoms associated with hypocalcemia depends on the degree of the calcium imbalance.

Hypocalcemia can also cause pathologic effects on bone. Bone is the primary storage site for calcium and can release calcium into the bloodstream when needed. Excessive calcium loss from bone can cause bone to weaken its supporting structure. Chronic hypocalcemia leads to progressive osteoporosis, resulting in bones that are less dense and more susceptible to fracture or deformity. (See Chapter 50 for a discussion of osteoporosis.)

ETIOLOGY

Hypocalcemia can result from a variety of chronic and acute pathologic states as well as from specific medical or surgical treatment. Table 16–5 lists the common causes of hypocalcemia.

ACTUAL CALCIUM LOSS

Actual calcium loss, (a reduction in total body calcium) occurs in response to conditions that:

- Inhibit calcium absorption from the gastrointestinal tract
- Increase the loss of calcium from the body

Examples of conditions that inhibit calcium absorption are Crohn's disease and lactose intolerance. Examples of conditions that increase calcium excretion are the polyuric phase of renal failure and severe diarrhea.

TABLE 16–5 Common Causes of Hypocalcemia

Actual Calcium Deficits

Inhibition of Calcium Absorption from the Gastrointestinal Tract

- Inadequate oral intake of calcium
- Lactose intolerance
- Malabsorption syndromes
  - Celiac sprue
  - Crohn's disease
- Inadequate intake of vitamin D
- End-stage renal disease

Increased Calcium Excretion

- Renal failure—polyuric phase
- Diarrhea
- Steatorrhea
- Wound drainage (especially gastrointestinal)

Relative Calcium Deficits

Conditions That Decrease the Ionized Fraction of Calcium

- Hyperproteinemia
- Alkalosis
- Calcium chelators or binders
  - Citrate
  - Mithramycin
  - Penicillamine
  - Sodium cellulose phosphate (Calcibind)
  - Aredia
- Acute pancreatitis
- Hyperphosphatemia
- Immobility

Endocrine Disturbances

- Removal or destruction of parathyroid glands
  - Thyroidectomy
  - Radiation to thyroid
  - Strangulation
  - Neck injuries

RELATIVE CALCIUM LOSS

Relative calcium loss in which total body calcium concentration is normal but serum calcium levels are low occurs in response to conditions that:

- Decrease the free, or ionized (unbound), calcium in the body
- Affect the parathyroid glands

Acute pancreatitis, immobility, and alkalosis decrease the ionized fraction of calcium.

The primary hormone for maintaining adequate amounts of ionized serum calcium is parathyroid hormone (PTH). Therefore, conditions that interfere with production of PTH can cause hypocalcemia. For example, thyroid surgery or radiation to the neck area can cause removal or destruction of parathyroid tissue.

Transcultural Considerations Many African-American clients have a lactose intolerance related to a genetic deficiency of the enzyme lactase. These clients cannot use the nutrients present in milk, and they experience cramping, diarrhea, and abdominal pain after ingesting dairy products. Dairy products, especially milk, are a common, rich source of both calcium and vitamin D. Clients with lactose intolerance may have difficulty obtaining enough calcium and vitamin D from other sources to maintain normal calcium levels in the blood and storage sites.

HYPOCALCEMIA AND WOMEN

Postmenopausal women are susceptible to hypocalcemia. This occurrence appears to be related to lack of weight-bearing and sex hormone (estrogen) action. Osteoporosis occurs when weight-bearing activity decreases or is limited. Because women generally are smaller framed than men, the female skeleton does not experience as much weight-bearing as the male skeleton. In addition, many women decrease weight-bearing activities, such as running and walking, as they get older. As women age, the estrogen secretion that protects against osteoporosis also diminishes. All of these factors increase the risk of hypocalcemia among women, particularly elderly women.

HYPOCALCEMIA AND THE ELDERLY

Elderly people are at risk for most electrolyte imbalances for many reasons. Major organs and body systems undergo changes with aging. For example, an older adult has a smaller fluid volume per body weight than a younger adult, so that any variation in fluid volumes or electrolyte levels leads to imbalances more quickly. The elderly client is more likely to be taking prescription or over-the-counter (OTC) medications that affect fluid or electrolyte balance. Some elderly clients have nutritional deficits for calcium or vitamin D because of economic conditions or general problems with obtaining, preparing, or eating food.

COLLABORATIVE MANAGEMENT

ASSESSMENT

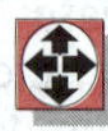

The most critical factor in assessing for the risk of actual or potential hypocalcemia is the diet history. The nurse also identifies whether the client uses a calcium supplement on a regular basis. The nurse questions clients regarding the intake of calcium-containing foods (see Chap. 14, Table 14–7). In addition, the nurse asks the client how much time is spent outdoors with the skin exposed to sunlight.

An indicator of hypocalcemia is the report of frequent painful muscle spasms (charley horses) in the calf or foot during periods of inactivity or sleep. Other information that can alert the nurse to a possible risk of hypocalcemia is a history of recent orthopedic surgery or bone healing. Although the nurse should note presence of any disease state, diseases related to endocrine disturbances are significant for

CHART 16–6

Key Features of Hypocalcemia

Cardiovascular

- Increased heart rate
- Decreased myocardial contractility
- Diminished peripheral pulses
- Hypotension
- Electrocardiographic abnormalities
  - Prolonged ST interval
  - Prolonged QT interval

Respiratory

- Not affected directly
- Respiratory failure or arrest can result from decreased respiratory movement due to muscle tetany or seizure activity

Neuromuscular*

- Anxiety, irritability, psychosis
- Paresthesias followed by numbness
- Irritable skeletal muscles—twitches, cramps, tetany, seizures
- Hyperactive deep tendon reflexes
- Positive Trousseau's sign
- Positive Chvostek's sign

Gastrointestinal

- Increased gastric motility
- Hyperactive bowel sounds
- Abdominal cramping
- Diarrhea

* The neuromuscular system is most profoundly affected by hypocalcemia.

hypocalcemia. A previous history of thyroid surgery, therapeutic radiation to the upper middle chest and neck area, or a recent anterior neck injury predisposes the client to hypocalcemia.

The most common clinical manifestations of hypocalcemia are related to overstimulation of nerves and muscles (Terry, 1991; Walpert, 1990). Chart 16–6 lists the clinical manifestations of hypocalcemia.

NEUROMUSCULAR SYSTEM

Although all nerves and muscles are affected by hypocalcemia to some degree, the client usually notices symptoms first in the limbs, with distal-to-proximal movement from the hands and feet. At first, paresthesia may be noted, with sensations of tingling alternating with sensations of numbness. If hypocalcemia continues or worsens, these sensations may progress to actual muscle twitchings or painful cramps and spasms. Paresthesias may affect the lips, nose, and ears. These symptoms signal the approach of serious neuromuscular overstimulation, or muscle tetany.

The nurse assesses for hypocalcemia by testing for two signs:

- Trousseau's sign
- Chvostek's sign

Testing for Trousseau's sign is accomplished by placing a blood pressure cuff around the upper arm, inflating the cuff to greater than the client's systolic pressure, and keeping it inflated for 1 to 4 minutes. Under these hypoxic conditions, the hand and fingers go into spasm in palmar flexion (Fig. 16–2). A positive Chvostek's sign also may indicate the presence of hypocalcemia. The nurse taps on the face just below and anterior to the ear (over the facial nerve) to trigger facial twitching that includes one side of the mouth, nose, and cheek (Fig. 16–3).

CARDIOVASCULAR SYSTEM

The heartbeat may be slightly faster than normal, but the myocardial contractility is weaker, resulting in a diminished pulse quality. For hypocalcemia to produce significant changes in cardiac activity and function, the degree of hypocalcemia must be either severe or chronic. Under these conditions, the client has severe hypotension and electrocardiographic (ECG) changes, including a prolonged ST interval, leading to a prolonged QT interval.

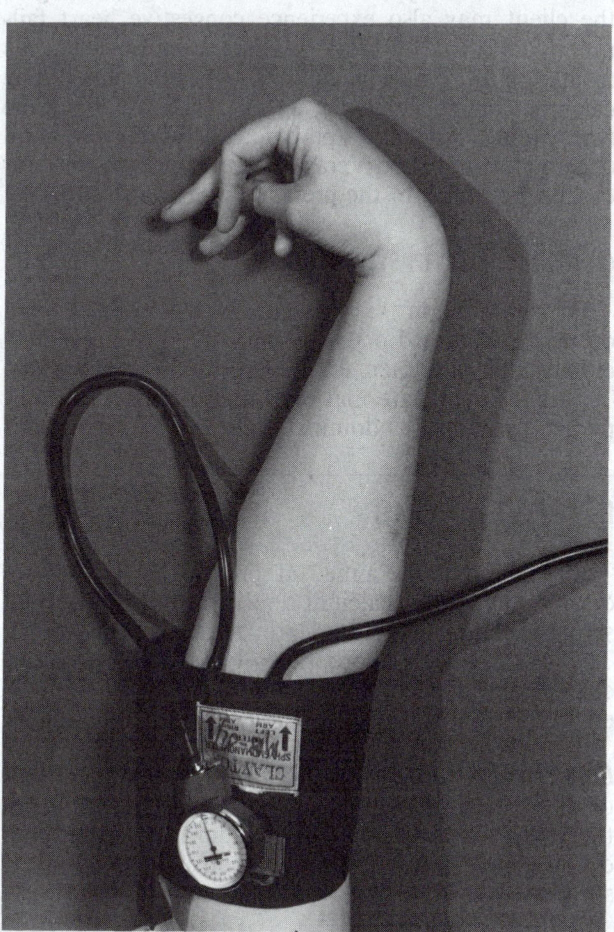

FIGURE 16–2 ◆ Palmar flexion—positive Trousseau's sign in hypocalcemia.

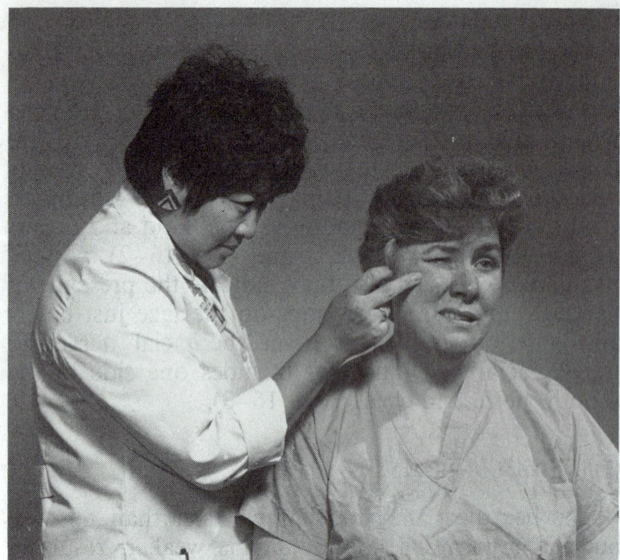

FIGURE 16–3 ♦ Facial muscle response—positive Chvostek's sign in hypocalcemia.

The nurse measures the blood pressure with the client in the lying, sitting, and standing positions, because postural changes make the hypotension more pronounced. If hypocalcemia is severe or prolonged, the client may also experience congestive heart failure, manifested by weak peripheral pulses and the formation of visible edema. Clients who are taking calcium channel–blocking agents, such as nifedipine (Procardia, Adalat, Apo-Nifed♣) and verapamil (Calan, Isoptin, Apo-Verap♣), are at greater risk for cardiac problems in the presence of hypocalcemia.

GASTROINTESTINAL SYSTEM

Overstimulation associated with hypocalcemia occurs as increased peristaltic activity. The nurse auscultates the abdomen for hyperactive bowel sounds. The client may state that intestinal motion is accompanied by painful abdominal cramping and diarrhea.

INTERVENTIONS

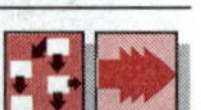

Interventions are aimed at preventing further decreases in serum calcium levels, restoring normal serum calcium levels, and preventing complications. The interventions appropriate for hypocalcemia include drug therapy, diet therapy, and reduction of environmental stimuli.

Drug Therapy Drug therapy for hypocalcemia consists of direct calcium supplements or replacements, drugs that enhance absorption of calcium, and drugs that decrease nerve and muscle responsiveness to overstimulation.

CALCIUM SUPPLEMENTS The physician orders oral supplements of calcium carbonate, calcium gluconate, or calcium lactate for clients with mild hypocalcemia. The nurse administers these medications 1 to 2 hours after meals to ensure maximal intestinal absorption.

Parenteral (IV) calcium is administered when the hypocalcemia is severe (as evidenced by tetany or cardiovascular complications) or when intestinal absorption is impaired. The preferred route of administration is by slow IV drip, unless hypocalcemia is life-threatening. Rapid IV calcium administration can cause hypercalcemia, which can be equally life-threatening. Common agents used are solutions containing either calcium chloride or calcium gluconate. Nursing responsibilities during the IV administration of calcium include continuous assessment of cardiovascular status (ideally, the client should be evaluated via continuous cardiac monitoring), hourly assessments of Chvostek's and Trousseau's signs, hourly drawing of blood for a determination of serum calcium levels, and assessment of the infusion site every 15 minutes.

DRUGS THAT INCREASE CALCIUM ABSORPTION The physician may prescribe additional drugs to correct hypocalcemia. These medications do not directly add calcium to the bloodstream. Rather, they indirectly increase extracellular calcium concentrations by altering the concentrations of other electrolytes that influence serum calcium regulation. For example, the administration of vitamin D helps to increase serum calcium levels by promoting the intestinal absorption of calcium. Aluminum hydroxide can increase serum calcium levels by reducing serum phosphorus levels.

DRUGS THAT DECREASE NERVE AND MUSCLE RESPONSIVENESS In addition to drugs previously mentioned for treatment of hypocalcemia, some drugs may be prescribed to decrease nerve and muscle responsiveness and overstimulation. Drugs that reduce membrane excitability and result in skeletal muscle relaxation are sometimes used. These drugs include methocarbamol (Robaxin, Delaxin), metaxalone (Skelaxin), orphenadrine (Banflex, Flexoject, Myolin), carisoprodol (Soma, Rela), and diazepam (Valium, Rival, E-Pam♣). Magnesium sulfate may be given to decrease the responsiveness of skeletal muscles.

Diet Therapy A high-calcium diet is indicated for clients with mild hypocalcemia and for those with chronic conditions that cause them to be at continuous risk for hypocalcemia. The nurse consults with the dietitian to assist the hospitalized client in selecting foods that are calcium-rich (common sources of calcium are listed in Table 14–7 in Chapter 14).

Vitamin D intake must also be adequate for dietary calcium to be beneficial. Skin exposure to sunlight enhances the body's synthesis of active vitamin D. Thus, increasing skin exposure to sunlight is an inexpensive way to increase vitamin D content. However, environmental or personal health conditions may make increased skin exposure to sunlight impractical or dangerous. Other sources of vitamin D include fortified milk, liver, eggs, fatty fish, and butter. Dairy products other than milk, such as cheese and yogurt, usually are *not* fortified with vitamin D.

Reduction of Environmental Stimuli The excitable membranes of both the nervous system and the skeletal system are overstimulated in hypocalcemia. Therefore, in addition to increasing serum calcium levels, the nurse should provide an environment that reduces extraneous stimulation of these systems.

Client activity is restricted, because any nerve or muscle stimulation can increase muscle twitching, cramps, and tetany. If Chvostek's sign or Trousseau's sign is positive, the client is kept on complete bed rest with total care provided by the nurse. Prolonged or intermittent physical contact that allows stimulation of the deeper tissues (such as rubbing the back) or unexpected touching of the client can stimulate muscle tetany or even seizure activity. Thus, actual touching of the client must be limited to the minimum necessary to maintain safety and hygiene.

The nurse minimizes environmental stimulation by providing a quiet, relatively dark, private room for the client. Diagnostic and therapeutic activities not vital to the immediate well-being of the client are postponed. The telephone is removed from the room or its bell adjusted so that it does not ring. The nurse providing direct care to this client speaks softly and no more frequently than necessary. Care is taken to avoid bumping the bed and other furniture. The nurse avoids shining a light into the client's face.

Prevention of Injury The nurse places the client on seizure precautions, which include padding the side rails of the bed and having emergency equipment such as oxygen and suction at the bedside. The emergency cart equipped with emergency drugs and an endotracheal tray is positioned near the client's room.

Clients with long-standing calcium loss may have brittle, fragile bones that are easily fractured. When lifting or moving clients with fragile bones, the nurse uses a lift sheet rather than pulling or grasping the client directly. Because fragile bones may fracture at slight provocation and cause little pain, the nurse observes the client for the presence of any unusual surface projections or depressions over bony areas as well as for normal range of joint motion.

Hypercalcemia

OVERVIEW

Hypercalcemia is a serum calcium ion level greater than 11 mg/dL, or 5.5 mEq/L. Because the normal range for serum calcium is extremely narrow, even small increases can have severe effects on body function. Although the effects of hypercalcemia are most noticeable in body systems that depend on cell excitability, all body systems are affected to some degree.

PATHOPHYSIOLOGY

The presence of hypercalcemia indicates either that the amount of serum calcium is so great that the normal calcium-regulating mechanisms are overburdened or that at least one calcium-regulating mechanism is not functioning properly. Because extracellular calcium ions function as stabilizers of excitable cell membranes, hypercalcemia causes excitable tissues to be less sensitive to normal stimuli and require a stronger stimulus to function.

Excitable tissues that demonstrate obvious and serious immediate responses to hypercalcemia are cardiac muscle tissue, nerve tissue, skeletal muscle, and gastrointestinal smooth muscle. The severity of the signs and symptoms associated with hypercalcemia depends on the degree of the imbalance and how quickly the imbalance occurs.

Calcium is also a critical cofactor for many of the enzymes involved in the blood-clotting process. Hypercalcemia usually results in faster clotting times. This condition may cause clots to form at inappropriate times and places. Excessive clotting related to hypercalcemia is more likely to occur in vessels or organs in which blood flow is slow or blocked.

ETIOLOGY

The underlying causes of hypercalcemia generally include increased absorption of calcium, decreased excretion of calcium, and increased bone resorption of calcium (Table 16–6).

TABLE 16–6 Common Causes of Hypercalcemia

Actual Calcium Excesses

Increased Absorption of Calcium

- Excessive oral intake of calcium
- Excessive oral intake of vitamin D

Decreased Excretion of Calcium

- Renal failure
- Use of thiazide diuretics

Relative Calcium Excesses

Increased Bone Resorption of Calcium

- Hyperparathyroidism
- Malignancy
  - Direct invasion (cancers of breast, lung, prostate, and osteoclastic bone and multiple myeloma)
  - Indirect resorption (liver cancer, small cell lung cancer, and cancer of the adrenal gland)
- Hyperthyroidism
- Immobility
- Use of glucocorticoids

Hemoconcentration

- Dehydration
- Use of lithium
- Adrenal insufficiency

CONDITIONS THAT DECREASE RENAL EXCRETION OF CALCIUM

Although the kidney is not the primary regulator of the body's calcium content, the kidney can either reabsorb or excrete calcium at the proximal convoluted tubule (PCT). In renal failure, the nephrons may not be able to excrete excessive calcium ions, thus contributing to the development of hypercalcemia (although renal failure usually is associated with hypocalcemia).

Many diuretics exert their effects within the tubular system of the nephron. Thiazide diuretics, such as chlorothiazide (Diuril) and hydrochlorothiazide (Esidrex, Nefrol✱), alter the function of the distal convoluted tubule. These diuretics *enhance* the reabsorption of calcium in the proximal convoluted tubule and their prolonged use may cause hypercalcemia.

CONDITIONS THAT INCREASE BONE RESORPTION OF CALCIUM

Bones are large storage sites for calcium. Any condition that causes bone resorption of calcium (calcium removed from the bone into systemic circulation) can cause hypercalcemia. The causes of hypercalcemia through excessive bone resorption include hyperparathyroidism, cancer, immobility, and prolonged use of glucocorticoids.

CONDITIONS THAT INCREASE ABSORPTION OF CALCIUM

Excessive intake of calcium can lead to hypercalcemia. People who ingest large amounts of calcium-containing antacids are at an increased risk for hypercalcemia. People who ingest large quantities of milk and other dairy products may develop hypercalcemia.

The gastrointestinal absorption of calcium is highly dependent on the presence of the active form of vitamin D. Hypercalcemia associated with an increased absorption of calcium can occur when a person ingests normal amounts of calcium and excessive amounts of vitamin D.

COLLABORATIVE MANAGEMENT

ASSESSMENT

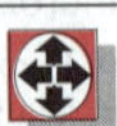

The onset of clinical manifestations of hypercalcemia is related to both the severity of the imbalance and how quickly the imbalance occurred. Thus, clients with mild excesses of serum calcium levels that occurred rapidly usually experience more severe signs and symptoms than do clients whose hypercalcemic states are severe but developed slowly over a long period. The clinical manifestations of hypercalcemia are primarily associated with alterations of excitable membrane activity (Chart 16-7). Therefore, the body systems most affected by hypercalcemia include the cardiovascular, neuromuscular, gastrointestinal, and renal/urinary systems.

CHART 16-7

Key Features of Hypercalcemia

Cardiovascular
- Increased heart rate
- Increased blood pressure
- Bounding, full peripheral pulses
- ECG abnormalities
  - Shortened ST segment
  - Widened T wave
- Potentiation of digitalis-associated toxicities
- Decreased clotting time
- Late phase
  - Bradycardia
  - Cardiac arrest, sinus arrest

Respiratory
- Ineffective respiratory movement related to profound skeletal muscle weakness

Neuromuscular
- Disorientation, lethargy, coma
- Profound muscle weakness
- Diminished or absent deep tendon reflexes

Renal
- Increased urinary output
- Dehydration
- Formation of renal calculi

Gastrointestinal
- Decreased motility
- Hypoactive bowel sounds
- Anorexia, nausea
- Abdominal distention
- Constipation

CARDIOVASCULAR SYSTEM

The most serious and life-threatening clinical manifestations of hypercalcemia are involved with alterations of cardiac function. Increased extracellular calcium levels disturb cardiac muscle function and electrical conduction through the heart. Mild hypercalcemia initially causes an increased heart rate and blood pressure. Severe or prolonged hypercalcemia affects electrical conduction.

The nurse assesses cardiac status by measuring pulse and blood pressure and observing for indications of inadequate tissue perfusion (such as cyanosis and pallor). In addition, when the client is being monitored, the nurse observes the tracings for indications of dysrhythmias, especially shortening of the QT interval.

Although hypercalcemia does not directly cause blood clots to form, increased calcium levels produce clot formation more easily whenever abnormal conditions are present. Thus, the client with hypercalcemia may be at an increased risk for thrombus (clot) formation in locations where blood vessel or tissue damage have occurred and in vessels or organs in which blood flow is blocked. Blood clotting is more likely to occur in the lower legs, the pelvic region, anywhere that blood flow is blocked by internal or external constrictions, and places where internal blood vessel obstructions are present.

The nurse assesses each client at risk for hypercalcemia for indications of slow or impaired blood flow. Calf circumferences are measured with a soft tape measure and recorded. The nurse asks the client to alternately dorsiflex and plantar flex the ankles and state whether calf pain is present in either position. The nurse assesses the lower legs for temperature, color, and capillary refill to determine the adequacy of blood flow to and from the area.

NEUROMUSCULAR SYSTEM

The neuromuscular clinical manifestations of hypercalcemia are severe muscle weakness, without accompanying paresthesia, and greatly diminished deep tendon reflexes. Central nervous system manifestations of hypercalcemia include an altered level of consciousness that ranges from disorientation and lethargy to coma.

GASTROINTESTINAL SYSTEM

Decreased peristalsis, or gastrointestinal motility, is an early manifestation of hypercalcemia. The nurse assesses the gastrointestinal tract by auscultating for bowel sounds in all four abdominal quadrants. Bowel sounds are hypoactive or absent. The abdomen increases in size because intestinal contents remain in the gastrointestinal tract instead of being propelled to the outside. The nurse assesses abdominal size by measuring abdominal girth with a soft tape measure in a line circling the abdomen at the level of the umbilicus. The client may have constipation, anorexia, nausea, vomiting, and abdominal pain.

RENAL SYSTEM

Excessive serum calcium levels affect renal function. Hypercalcemia causes increased urinary output and leads to serious dehydration. Chronic hypercalcemia results in the formation of renal calculi (stones) in the kidney tubular system because the excessive calcium precipitates out of solution into a solid form. Stones can block the flow of filtrate and urine through different parts of the renal system. When these stones reach the ureter, bladder, and urethra, they cause intense pain (see Chap. 70). The nurse assesses the renal system for changes associated with hypercalcemia by measuring intake and output, assessing voided urine for blood or cloudiness, and straining the urine for the presence of renal calculi.

INTERVENTIONS

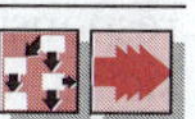

Interventions for hypercalcemia are aimed at preventing further increases in serum calcium levels and decreasing excessive serum calcium levels.

Drug Therapy The purpose of drug therapy for the treatment of hypercalcemia is to restore normal calcium balance by preventing additional calcium administration and promoting calcium excretion. IV infusions of solutions containing calcium are stopped. In addition, the administration of oral drugs containing calcium or vitamin D, such as calcium-based antacids, is discontinued.

INTRAVENOUS FLUID THERAPY Fluid volume replacement alone can help to restore normal serum calcium levels. This therapy is appropriate when renal function is normal and the client's cardiopulmonary status can tolerate the extra fluid load. The physician usually orders IV normal saline (isotonic sodium chloride) in this situation, because it does not contain calcium. The administration of sodium also prevents tubular reabsorption of calcium, so that saline infusions promote calcium excretion.

DIURETIC THERAPY The physician also discontinues thiazide diuretic administration. Diuretics that enhance the excretion of calcium such as furosemide (Lasix, Furoside♣) are prescribed.

THERAPY WITH OTHER CALCIUM-REDUCING DRUGS Agents that act as calcium chelators (calcium binders) can be useful in lowering the serum calcium levels. Such drugs include mithramycin (Mithracin) and penicillamine (Cuprimine, Pendramine♣).

Other drugs that may be useful in treating hypercalcemia include agents that inhibit calcium resorption from the bone, such as phosphorus, calcitonin (Calcimar), biphosphonates (etidronate), and prostaglandin synthesis inhibitors (aspirin, nonsteroidal anti-inflammatory drugs).

Dialysis When hypercalcemia is so severe that life-threatening cardiac problems are present, drug therapy may not reduce serum calcium levels quickly enough to prevent death. In this situation, dialysis (either hemodialysis or peritoneal dialysis) or blood ultrafiltration may be necessary. (For a discussion of nursing responsibilities during dialysis and ultrafiltration, see Chapter 72.)

Cardiac Monitoring Clients with hypercalcemia usually undergo continuous cardiac monitoring to identify possible dysrhythmias and decreased cardiac output. The nurse compares recently obtained electrocardiographic (ECG) tracings with the client's baseline tracings or tracings obtained when the client's serum calcium level was normal. The nurse observes the ECG for changes in the T waves and the QT interval as well as changes in rate and rhythm. The nurse is responsible for reporting all ECG changes to the physician immediately.

PHOSPHORUS IMBALANCES

Hypophosphatemia

OVERVIEW

Hypophosphatemia is a serum phosphorus level less than 2.5 mg/dL. Even though the serum concentration of phosphorus has a narrow range of normal values (2.5 to 4 mg/dL), body functions are not significantly impaired as a result of rapid, wide changes in serum phosphorus levels. Alterations in function are more obvious when hypophosphatemia is chronic.

PATHOPHYSIOLOGY

Most of the pathophysiologic effects of hypophosphatemia are related to decreased energy metabolism and altered levels of other electrolytes and body fluids. Because of the reciprocal relationship between phosphorus and calcium, decreases in serum phosphorus levels are accompanied by increases in serum calcium levels.

ETIOLOGY

Three main processes underlie decreased serum phosphorus levels: decreased absorption of phosphorus, increased excretion of phosphorus, and intracellular phosphorus shift (Table 16–7).

DECREASED ABSORPTION OF PHOSPHORUS

Intestinal absorption of phosphorus is decreased indirectly during periods of malnutrition or starvation. Poor nutrition with inadequate phosphorus intake is also seen in clients with severe alcoholism. Inadequate vitamin D synthesis or intake can also contribute to poor intestinal absorption of phosphorus.

Ingested phosphorus can bind to substances in the gastrointestinal tract and be eliminated in the feces rather than absorbed through the intestinal mucosa. Antacids containing either aluminum hydroxide or magnesium (Alternagel, Amphojel, Bisodol, milk of magnesia) bind phosphorus in the intestinal tract and inhibit its absorption. In addition, when large concentrations of calcium are present in the intestinal tract, the calcium combines with the phosphorus to form an insoluble calcium-phosphate compound that is not absorbed. Other conditions interfering with intestinal absorption of phosphorus include diarrhea, laxatives, and loss or destruction of intestinal tissue.

TABLE 16–7 Common Causes of Phosphorus Imbalance

Hypophosphatemia
Insufficient Intake of Phosphorus
• Malnutrition
• Starvation
• Use of aluminum hydroxide–based antacids
• Use of magnesium-based antacids
Increased Renal Excretion of Phosphorus
• Hyperparathyroidism
• Hypocalcemia
• Renal failure
• Malignancy
Intracellular Shift
• Hyperglycemia
• Hyperalimentation
• Respiratory alkalosis
Hyperphosphatemia
• Decreased renal excretion due to renal insufficiency
• Tumor lysis syndrome
• Increased intake of phosphorus
• Hypoparathyroidism

INCREASED EXCRETION OF PHOSPHORUS

Parathyroid hormone (PTH) regulates serum phosphorus levels by causing phosphorus to be resorbed from the bones and, at the same time, greatly increases renal excretion of phosphorus. Because phosphorus excretion occurs more efficiently than bone resorption of phosphorus, when PTH is present phosphorus is lost from the body. Conditions that increase the amount of PTH include hyperparathyroidism and hypocalcemia.

Any condition that increases the flow of urine along the renal tubule also increases renal excretion of phosphorus. Osmotic diuresis increases renal phosphorus excretion by increasing the flow rate. In addition, ethanol ingestion appears to inhibit phosphorus reabsorption in the proximal convoluted tubule.

SHIFTING OF PHOSPHORUS TO THE INTRACELLULAR SPACE

Whenever the demand for intracellular adenosine triphosphate (ATP) is high (see Chapter 14), extracellular phosphorus shifts to the intracellular space. Although the serum phosphorus levels are below normal under these conditions, total body phosphorus levels are usually normal. Conditions that increase the amount of glucose in the blood tend to increase intracellular glycolysis and cause shifting of extracellular phosphorus into the intracellular space. These conditions include hyperglycemia, rapid or constant administration of total parenteral nutrition or hyperalimentation fluids, excessive carbohydrate ingestion (carbohydrate loading), and insulin administration. Respiratory alkalosis also results in a shift of extracellular phosphorus to the intracellular space.

COLLABORATIVE MANAGEMENT

ASSESSMENT

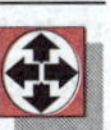

The onset of clinical manifestations of hypophosphatemia occurs when the decrease in serum phosphorus levels is severe or prolonged. Acute clinical manifestations of hypophosphatemia are related to the decreased availability of high-energy compounds (such as ATP) necessary to perform normal cellular metabolic functions. These clinical manifestations include alterations in the function of the cardiac, musculoskeletal, hematologic, and central nervous systems (Chart 16–8).

CARDIOVASCULAR SYSTEM

The cardiac manifestations of hypophosphatemia include decreased stroke volume and decreased cardiac output. Peripheral pulses are slow, difficult to find, and easy to block. The myocardial depression is caused by low intracellular energy stores. Without sufficient quantities of energy in myocardial cells, contractions are weak and ineffective. Prolonged hypophosphatemia can lead to progressive but reversible myocardial damage (Peppers et al., 1991).

CHART 16–8

Key Features of Hypophosphatemia

Cardiovascular
- Decreased contractility
- Cardiomyopathy (reversible)

Respiratory
- Shallow respirations

Musculoskeletal
- Weakness
- Rhabdomyolysis
- Decreased deep tendon reflexes

Central Nervous
- Irritability
- Confusion
- Seizures

Hematologic
- Increased bleeding
- Decreased platelet aggregation
- Immunosuppression

MUSCULOSKELETAL SYSTEM

The mechanism of hypophosphatemia that weakens cardiac muscles also appears to be responsible for weakening the skeletal muscles. The weakness is generalized, and paresthesias usually are not present. When the skeletal muscle weakness becomes profound, respiratory movements are ineffective, which can lead to respiratory failure. The nurse assesses for muscle strength and observes respiratory ability. The nurse reports significant changes to the physician immediately.

The clinical manifestations of chronic hypophosphatemia are most evident in the skeletal system. Bone density is decreased, and fractures and alterations in bone shape may occur. These changes result from the calcium resorption that often accompanies hypophosphatemia. The nurse assesses the client for unusual lumps, projections, or depressions over bony areas indicating fracture of demineralized bone.

HEMATOLOGIC SYSTEM

The metabolic activity of all blood cells is diminished in hypophosphatemia. Erythrocytes are less able to release oxygen at the tissue level, causing generalized tissue hypoxia, although clinical signs of hypoxia may not be evident.

Leukocytes are unable to perform their specific immune functions. As a result, even though the numbers of leukocytes may be within the normal range, the client is immunosuppressed and at an increased risk for infection.

Platelets demonstrate a reduced ability to aggregate (clump together) and secrete substances important for blood clotting. The client is susceptible to episodes of prolonged bleeding in response to relatively slight trauma or tissue injury. The nurse observes for bruises and bleeding of the gums.

CENTRAL NERVOUS SYSTEM

Central nervous system manifestations of hypophosphatemia usually are not apparent until hypophosphatemia is severe. The central nervous system manifestations first appear as increased irritability and may progress to seizure activity, followed by coma.

INTERVENTIONS

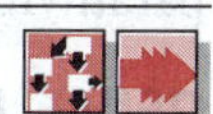

Drug Therapy The physician discontinues the administration of drugs that contribute to the development of hypophosphatemia, such as antacids, osmotic diuretics, and calcium supplements. Generally, oral replacement of phosphorus along with a vitamin D supplement is sufficient to correct the hypophosphatemia. IV phosphorus administration is initiated only when serum phosphorus levels are less than 1 mg/dL and the client has serious clinical manifestations. IV

CHART 16–9

Education Guide ◆ Dietary Management of Hypophosphatemia

- You should avoid
  - Milk
  - Cheese
  - Yogurt
  - Collard greens
  - Rhubarb
- You may eat
  - Fish
  - Beef
  - Chicken
  - Pork
  - Organ meats
  - Nuts
  - Whole-grain breads and cereals

phosphorus is administered slowly, because problems associated with hyperphosphatemia are equally serious.

Diet Therapy Diet therapy for hypophosphatemia primarily consists of increasing the intake of phosphorus-rich foods, while decreasing the intake of calcium-rich foods (Chart 16–9).

Hyperphosphatemia

OVERVIEW

Hyperphosphatemia is defined as a serum phosphorus level greater than 4.5 mg/dL. Elevations of serum phosphorus levels above normal are tolerated well by most body systems.

The health problems associated with hyperphosphatemia center on the hypocalcemia that results when serum phosphorus levels increase. These problems include increased sensitivity of excitable membranes, to the extent that they may depolarize spontaneously and inappropriately.

The underlying causes of increased serum phosphorus levels are renal insufficiency, some cancer treatments, increased phosphorus intake and hypoparathyroidism (see Table 16–7).

RENAL INSUFFICIENCY

The kidney is the primary site of phosphorus excretion from the body when the serum concentration of phosphorus is greater than normal levels. In renal insufficiency, phosphorus excretion is decreased and phosphorus is retained.

TREATMENT OF CANCER

Phosphorus is the primary anion of the intracellular fluid of all cells, including cancer cells. When cancer cells are destroyed, the cell membranes break and intracellular substances are released into the extracellular spaces. Aggressive treatment of cancer resulting in massive destruction of cancer cells causes rapid release of intracellular products (including phosphorus) into the blood. This process is known as the tumor lysis syndrome (see Chap. 26). Cancers most likely to respond to treatment rapidly enough to cause hyperphosphatemia are the leukemias, the lymphomas, and small cell lung cancer.

INCREASED INTAKE OF PHOSPHORUS

Phosphorus is present in many foods. However, unless renal insufficiency is present, dietary ingestion of phosphorus is not a common cause of hyperphosphatemia. Many laxatives have a phosphorus base. Clients who excessively use phosphate-containing laxatives and enemas are at risk for hyperphosphatemia.

HYPOPARATHYROIDISM

Less phosphorus is excreted in the urine and more is reabsorbed into the systemic circulation when hypoparathyroidism occurs. Conditions causing hypoparathyroidism include thyroid surgery, thyroid radiation, partial parathyroidectomy, and cancer.

COLLABORATIVE MANAGEMENT

Hyperphosphatemia produces few direct problems with body function. However, hypocalcemia is usually present as well because the calcium and phosphorus ions exist in the blood in a balanced reciprocal relationship—when one increases, the other decreases. The accompanying hypocalcemia dramatically alters the physiologic functioning of many body systems and has the potential for causing serious and life-threatening side effects. Thus, the management of hyperphosphatemia entails the management of hypocalcemia.

MAGNESIUM IMBALANCES

Hypomagnesemia

OVERVIEW

Hypomagnesemia is a serum magnesium (Mg^{2+}) level less than 1.5 mEq/L. Because most conditions resulting in hypomagnesemia are related either to decreased magnesium intake or increased magnesium loss, measurable hypomagnesemia reflects a decrease in the total body magnesium concentration.

The direct pathophysiologic effects of hypomagnesemia are related to alterations in the function of excitable membranes and accompanying imbalances of serum calcium and potassium. These problems in-

TABLE 16–8 Common Causes of Magnesium Imbalance

Hypomagnesemia
Insufficient Intake of Magnesium
• Malnutrition
• Starvation
• Diarrhea
• Steatorrhea
• Celiac disease
• Crohn's disease
Increased Renal Excretion of Magnesium
• Drugs (diuretics, aminoglycoside antibiotics, cisplatin, amphotericin B, cyclosporine)
• Citrate (blood products)
• Ethanol ingestion
Intracellular Movement of Magnesium
• Hyperglycemia
• Insulin administration
• Sepsis
• Alkalosis
Hypermagnesemia
• Increased magnesium intake
• Magnesium-containing antacids and laxatives
• IV magnesium replacement
• Decreased renal excretion of magnesium due to renal insufficiency

clude increased sensitivity of excitable membranes, especially nerve cell membranes, to the extent that they may depolarize spontaneously and inappropriately.

The major causes of hypomagnesemia are due to either decreased absorption of dietary magnesium or increased renal excretion of magnesium (Table 16–8). Insufficient intake of magnesium can account for some instances of hypomagnesemia. Situations that contribute to this condition include malnutrition, starvation, and prolonged nasogastric suctioning.

Other conditions decrease intestinal absorption of magnesium by interfering with the selective uptake of magnesium by the intestinal villi. Conditions that speed up passage of feces through the intestines decrease intestinal absorption of magnesium. These include diarrhea, steatorrhea, and loss or destruction of the intestinal mucosa. Alcoholism, especially when accompanied by liver disease, also decreases intestinal absorption of magnesium.

Specific drugs increase renal excretion of magnesium as either a primary action or a side effect. These drugs include high-ceiling (loop) diuretics such as furosemide (Lasix, Furoside♣) and bumetadine (Bumex), osmotic diuretics such as mannitol and urea, aminoglycosides such as kanamycin (Kantrex), gentamicin (Garamycin, Cidomycin♣), and tobramycin (Nebcin), and some antineoplastic agents such as Cisplatin (Platinol). Other conditions that increase renal magnesium excretion include *hypoparathyroidism* and *primary hyperaldosteronism.*

COLLABORATIVE MANAGEMENT

ASSESSMENT

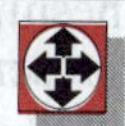

Most of the clinical manifestations of hypomagnesemia result from alterations in the activity of excitable cell membranes. The most frequent clinical manifestations are seen in the neuromuscular, central nervous, and gastrointestinal systems (Chart 16–10).

NEUROMUSCULAR SYSTEM

The neuromuscular manifestations of hypomagnesemia result from increased nerve impulse transmission at some synaptic areas. Normally, the presence of magnesium inhibits the release of the neurotransmitter acetylcholine from the presynaptic cell. Decreased levels of magnesium allow greater release of acetylcholine, which increases the transmission of impulses from nerve to nerve or nerve to skeletal muscle. Therefore, clients with hypomagnesemia have hyperactive deep tendon reflexes (+4) accompanied by painful paresthesia (numbness and tingling) and tetanic muscle contractions. Positive Chvostek's and Trousseau's signs may be present, because hypomagnesemia may be accompanied by hypocalcemia (see discussion of these assessment signs earlier under Hy-

CHART 16–10

Key Features of Hypomagnesemia

Cardiovascular
- Electrocardiographic changes
  - Tall T waves
  - Depressed ST segments
- Dysrhythmias
  - Ectopic beats
  - Ventricular tachycardia
  - Ventricular fibrillation
- Hypertension

Respiratory
- Shallow respirations

Neuromuscular
- Fasciculations
- Twitches
- Paresthesias
- Positive Trousseau's sign
- Positive Chvostek's sign
- Hyperreflexia
- Tetany
- Seizures

Central Nervous
- Irritability
- Confusion
- Psychosis

pocalcemia). If intracellular magnesium levels are also decreased in an attempt to restore normal magnesium balance, skeletal muscle weakness may be present. As hypomagnesemia progresses, the client may develop tetany and seizures.

CENTRAL NERVOUS SYSTEM

The central nervous system manifestations of hypomagnesemia are related to a general increase in the transmission of nerve impulses. The client experiences an increase in central nervous system irritability that may manifest as psychologic depression, psychosis, and confusion.

GASTROINTESTINAL (GI) SYSTEM

Gastrointestinal manifestations are associated with decreased contractility of the intestinal smooth muscle. Clients have decreased gastric motility with anorexia, nausea, and abdominal distention. If the hypomagnesemia is severe, a paralytic ileus may occur.

INTERVENTIONS

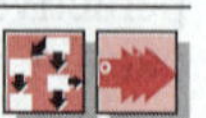

The interventions for hypomagnesemia are aimed at correction of the electrolyte imbalance and management of the specific conditions that caused the hypomagnesemia. In addition, because hypocalcemia frequently accompanies hypomagnesemia, some interventions are aimed at restoring normal serum calcium levels.

Drug Therapy The physician discontinues the administration of drugs that contribute to the development of hypomagnesemia, such as high-ceiling (loop) diuretics, osmotic diuretics, aminoglycosides, and drugs containing phosphorus. Generally, when hypomagnesemia is severe, the magnesium is replaced IV in the form of magnesium sulfate ($MgSO_4$). The IV route is selected, because magnesium sulfate causes pain and tissue damage when injected intramuscularly. Oral preparations of magnesium frequently cause diarrhea and increase magnesium loss. If hypocalcemia is also present, the physician prescribes drug therapy to increase the serum calcium concentration.

Diet Therapy Diet therapy for hypomagnesemia consists of increasing the intake of foods that contain high concentrations of magnesium (see Chap. 14, Table 14–10).

Hypermagnesemia

OVERVIEW

Hypermagnesemia is a serum magnesium level greater than 2.5 mEq/L.

Magnesium is a membrane stabilizer. Thus, when excesses of magnesium are present, excitable membranes require a stronger-than-normal stimulus to respond. Excitable membranes are less sensitive, or less excitable, when hypermagnesemia is present. If hypermagnesemia is severe, excitable membranes may not respond to any stimulus.

Hypermagnesemia results from an increased intake of magnesium coupled with decreased renal excretion of magnesium. For example, many antacids and laxatives, such as Maalox and milk of magnesia, have a high concentration of magnesium. People who overuse these agents are at risk for hypermagnesemia if renal function is inadequate. Clients who are receiving parenteral magnesium as a treatment for hypomagnesemia are also at risk for hypermagnesemia.

The most common condition producing decreased excretion of magnesium is renal insufficiency. Conditions that decrease the synthesis of aldosterone, such as Addison's disease, also decrease the renal excretion of magnesium (see Table 16–8).

COLLABORATIVE MANAGEMENT

ASSESSMENT

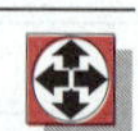

Most clinical manifestations associated with hypermagnesemia occur as a result of alterations in the activity of excitable cell membranes. Usually, clinical manifestations are not apparent until serum magnesium levels are greater than 4 mEq/L. The most frequent clinical manifestations are seen in the cardiac, central nervous, and neuromuscular systems.

CARDIOVASCULAR SYSTEM

Cardiac manifestations of hypermagnesemia are related to bradycardia, peripheral vasodilation, and hypotension. Manifestations are progressive and become more severe as the serum magnesium concentration increases. The nurse looks for electrocardiographic changes that include a prolonged PR interval with a widened QRS complex. Bradycardia can be severe, with cardiac arrest occurring during diastole of the cardiac cycle. Hypotension with a wide pulse pressure is severe; the diastolic pressure is much lower than normal. Clients with severe hypermagnesemia are in grave danger of cardiac arrest (Van Hook, 1991).

CENTRAL NERVOUS SYSTEM

Central nervous system clinical manifestations of hypermagnesemia are related to depression of the transmission of nerve impulses at specific synaptic points. Clients may be drowsy to the point of lethargy. Coma may occur if the hypermagnesemic condition is prolonged or becomes severe.

NEUROMUSCULAR SYSTEM

Neuromuscular clinical manifestations of hypermagnesemia are related to decreased transmission of impulses from nerves to skeletal muscles. The nurse observes that deep tendon reflexes are greatly diminished or even absent. Voluntary skeletal muscle contractions become progressively weaker and finally stop.

RESPIRATORY SYSTEM

Hypermagnesemia has no direct effect on the organs of respiration. However, when the skeletal muscles of respiration are involved, respiratory insufficiency may occur, leading to respiratory failure and death from anoxia.

INTERVENTIONS

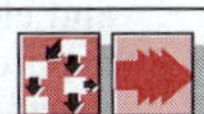

Interventions for hypermagnesemia are aimed at reducing the serum magnesium level and correcting the underlying pathologic change that initiated or contributed to the development of hypermagnesemia.

Drug Therapy All oral and parenteral administration of magnesium is discontinued. When renal failure is not a contributing factor, the administration of magnesium-free IV fluids can assist in reducing serum magnesium levels. Further reduction in serum magnesium levels can occur through the administration of high-ceiling (loop) diuretics such as furosemide (Lasix, Furoside✱). When cardiac manifestations are severe, administration of calcium may reverse the cardiac effects of hypermagnesemia.

Diet Therapy Diet therapy is most effective in the prevention of hypermagnesemia when other chronic pathologic conditions predispose the client to the development of excess serum magnesium levels. Dietary restrictions involve limiting the ingestion of meat, nuts, legumes, fish, vegetables, and whole-grain cereal products.

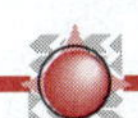

IMPLICATIONS FOR NURSING RESEARCH

Electrolyte imbalances can have life-threatening consequences; therefore, prevention and early recognition of actual imbalances are critical to preventing complications. More clinically descriptive data are needed to establish identifiable clinical manifestation patterns of specific electrolyte imbalances.

Nursing research may answer the following questions regarding the care of clients at risk for electrolyte imbalances:

- What effect does health teaching have on the prevention of specific electrolyte imbalances among clients at risk?
- What effect does health teaching have on the early detection of specific electrolyte imbalances among clients at risk?
- What nursing actions are most helpful in the management of the side effects of electrolyte imbalances?
- Which assessment tool is best in determining the presence of skeletal muscle weakness?

SELECTED BIBLIOGRAPHY

Briggs, J., Sawaya, B., & Schnermann, J. (1990). Disorders of salt balance. In J. Kokko & R. Tannen (Eds.), *Fluids and electrolytes* (2nd ed., pp. 70–138). Philadelphia: W. B. Saunders.

Bryce, J. (1994). S.I.A.D.H. *Nursing94, 24*(4), 33.

Carlson, K., Snyder, M., LeClair, H., Underhill, S., Ashwood, E., & Detter, J. (1990). Obtaining reliable plasma sodium and glucose determinations from pulmonary artery catheters. *Heart & Lung, 19*(6), 613–619.

*Chenevey, B. (1987). Overview of fluids and electrolytes. *Nursing Clinics of North America, 22*(4), 749.

Cronin, R. (1990). Magnesium disorders. In J. Kokko & R. Tannen (Eds.), *Fluids and electrolytes* (2nd ed., pp. 631–646). Philadelphia: W. B. Saunders.

Daily, W., Tonnesen, A., & Allen, S. (1990). Hypophosphatemia—incidence, etiology, and prevention in the trauma patient. *Critical Care Medicine, 18*(11), 1210–1214.

Davis, K., & Attie, M. (1991). Management of severe hypercalcemia. *Critical Care Clinics, 7*(1), 175–190.

DeAngelis, R., & Lessig, M. L. (1991) Hypokalemia. *Critical Care Nurse, 11*(7), 71–75.

Dennison, R., & Blevins, B. (1992). Myths and facts about electrolyte imbalance. *Nursing92, 22*(2), 26.

Guyton, A. (1991). *Textbook of medical physiology* (8th ed.). Philadelphia: W. B. Saunders.

Hawthorne, J., Schneider, S., & Workman, M. L. (1992). Common electrolyte imbalances associated with malignancy. *AACN Clinical Issues in Critical Care Nursing, 3*(3), 714–723.

Hutchinson, R., Barksdale, B., & Watson, R. (1992). The effects of exercise on serum potassium levels. *Chest, 101*(2), 398–400.

Innerarity, S. (1992). Hyperkalemic emergencies. *Critical Care Nursing Quarterly, 14*(4), 32–39.

Keyes, J. (1990). *Fluid, electrolyte, and acid-base regulation* (2nd ed.). Belmont, CA: Wadsworth.

Kokko, J., & Tannen, R. (1990). *Fluids and electrolytes* (2nd ed.). Philadelphia: W. B. Saunders.

Lau, K. (1990). Phosphate disorders. In J. Kokko & R. Tannen (Eds.), *Fluids and electrolytes* (2nd ed., pp. 505–595). Philadelphia: W. B. Saunders.

Mendyka, B. (1992). Fluid and electrolyte disorders caused by diuretic therapy. *AACN Clinical Issues in Critical Care Nursing, 3*(3), 672–680.

Metheny, N. (1992). *Fluid and electrolyte balance: Nursing considerations* (2nd ed.). Philadelphia: J. B. Lippincott.

Norris, M. K. (1992). Evaluating sodium levels. *Nursing92, 22*(7), 20.

Pagana, K., & Pagana, T. (1990). *Diagnostic testing and nursing implications* (3rd ed.). St. Louis: C. V. Mosby.

Pak, C. (1990). Calcium disorders: Hypercalcemia and hypocalcemia. In J. Kokko & R. Tannen (Eds.), *Fluids and electrolytes* (2nd ed., pp. 596–630). Philadelphia: W. B. Saunders.

Peppers, M., Geheb, M., & Desai, T. (1991), Hypophosphatemia and hyperphosphatemia. *Critical Care Clinics, 7*(1), 201–214.

Salem, M., Munoz, R., & Chernow, B. (1991). Hypomagnesemia in critical illness. *Critical Care Clinics, 7*(1), 225–252.

Strong, P., Jewell, S., Rinker, J., Hoch, D., & Crapo, L. (1991). Thiazide therapy and severe hypercalcemia in a patient with hyperparathyroidism. *Western Journal of Medicine, 154*(3), 338–340.

Tannen, R. (1990). Potassium disorders. In J. Kokko & R. Tannen (Eds.), *Fluids and electrolytes* (2nd ed., pp. 195–300). Philadelphia: W. B. Saunders.

Terry, J. (1991). The other electrolytes: Magnesium, calcium and phosphorus. *Journal of Intravenous Nursing, 14*(3), 167–176.

Van Hook, J. (1991). Hypermagnesemia. *Critical Care Clinics, 7*(1), 215–223.

Walpert, N. (1990). An orderly look at calcium metabolism disorders. *Nursing90, 20*(7), 60–64.

Workman, M. L. (1992). Magnesium and phosphorus: The neglected electrolytes. *AACN Clinical Issues in Critical Care Nursing, 3*(3), 655–663.

Yarnell, R., & Craig, M. (1991). Detecting hypomagnesemia: The most overlooked electrolyte imbalance. *Nursing91, 21*(7), 55–57.

SUGGESTED READINGS

DeAngelis, R., & Lessig, M. L. (1991). Hypokalemia. *Critical Care Nurse, 11*(7), 71–75.

This article presents a detailed summary of potassium action on the cell membranes. The authors graphically describe specific ECG changes associated with mild-to-severe hypokalemia. An excellent summary of nursing responsibilities during IV administration of potassium is presented.

Mendyka, B. (1992). Fluid and electrolyte disorders caused by diuretic therapy. *AACN Clinical Issues in Critical Care Nursing, 3*(3), 672–680.

This article presents in text and tables the mechanisms of action and electrolyte effects of the major diuretic categories. Normal nephron function is reviewed. Nursing care considerations for specific electrolyte disturbances are summarized.

Workman, M. L. (1992). Magnesium and phosphorus: The neglected electrolytes. *AACN Clinical Issues in Critical Care Nursing, 3*(3), 655–663.

Detailed presentations of magnesium and phosphorus functions and regulations are presented. Information about the causes, pathophysiology, complications, and management of hypomagnesemia and hypophosphatemia is highlighted.

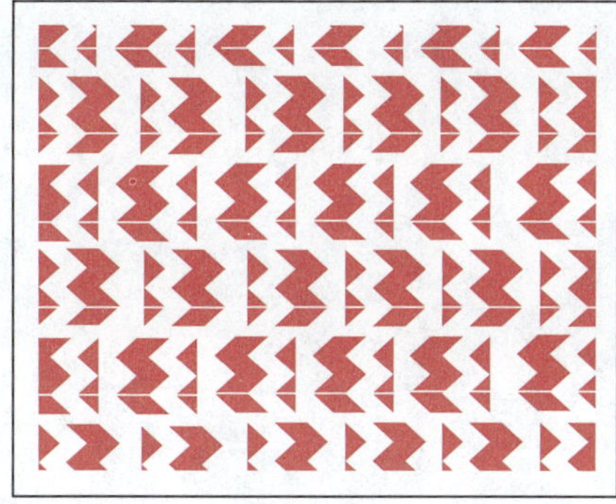

CHAPTER 17

Acid-Base Balance

CHAPTER HIGHLIGHTS

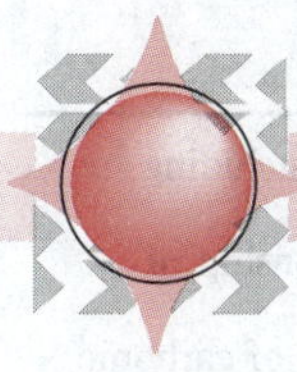

The human body functions best when the concentrations of specific ions in body fluids remain within narrow ranges of normal. This is especially true for the hydrogen ions (H^+). Even small changes in body fluid hydrogen ion concentration (pH) for short periods of time can disrupt vital functions. Because the processes of binding and releasing hydrogen ions are performed by acids and bases, control of pH is called *acid-base balance.* Table 17-1 summarizes the terminology used to describe acid-base balance.

The normal hydrogen ion concentration of the blood and other body fluids is quite low (<0.0001 mEq/L) compared with the body fluid concentrations of other electrolytes (see Chapters 14 and 16). Because the hydrogen ion concentration is so low, it is measured in pH units, calculated as the negative logarithm of the concentration in milliequivalents per liter (Fig. 17-1). The normal hydrogen ion concentration (pH) ranges from 7.34 to 7.45 for arterial blood and from 7.31 to 7.42 for venous blood (Keyes, 1990).

Because pH is calculated in negative logarithm units, the value of the pH is *inversely* related to the concentration of hydrogen ions. Thus, the lower the pH value of a fluid, the higher the concentration of hydrogen ions present in that fluid. With the pH scale (a 14-point scale), *a change of 1 pH unit actually represents a tenfold difference in the hydrogen ion concentration.* Therefore, even a pH unit change of one tenth (e.g., a change from a pH of 7.4 to a pH of

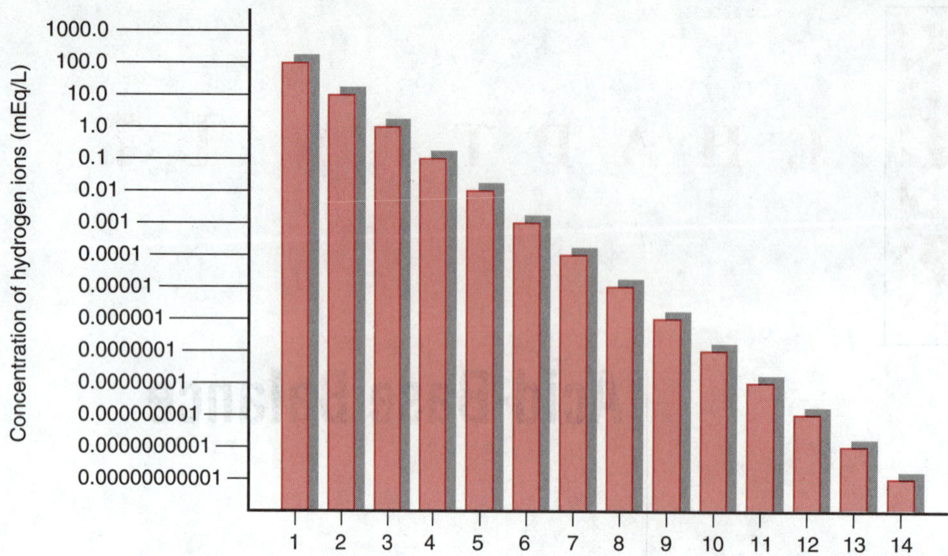

FIGURE 17-1 ◆ Relationship between pH and concentration of hydrogen ions.

7.3) represents a dramatic increase in the hydrogen ion concentration of a given solution (Ganong, 1991).

Changes in body fluid hydrogen ion concentration (pH) interfere with many normal physiologic functions. Some of the ways in which imbalances of hydrogen ions disrupt normal function include:

- Altering the shape or position of hormones and enzymes to the extent that they can no longer perform their designated functions
- Changing the distribution of other electrolytes, causing fluid and electrolyte imbalances
- Altering the responses of excitable membranes, so that the heart, nerves, skeletal muscles, and gastrointestinal tract are less active or more active than normal
- Decreasing the uptake, activity, and distribution of many hormones and drugs, possibly making them ineffective

TABLE 17-1 Terminology Pertinent to Acid-Base Balance

Term	Definition
Acid	• Any substance releasing a hydrogen ion when dissolved in water
Anaerobic metabolism	• Cellular metabolism occurring without the presence of oxygen
Base	• Any substance binding a hydrogen ion when dissolved in water
Buffer	• A substance capable of binding a hydrogen ion from body fluids (acting as a base) or releasing a hydrogen ion into body fluids (acting as an acid)
Chemoreceptors	• Special cells in the respiratory center of the brain sensitive to changes in the carbon dioxide concentration of extracellular fluid
pH	• The concentration of hydrogen ions in a solution calculated as the negative log of the milliequivalent concentration per liter

TABLE 17-2 Key Concepts of Acid-Base Balance

- The normal pH of the body's extracellular fluids (including blood) is 7.35–7.45.
- The pH in the body can be described as the relationship of bicarbonate to carbonic acid, or a 20:1 ratio.
- Carbon dioxide is the most changeable component of carbonic acid.
- The concentration of carbon dioxide is directly related to the concentration of hydrogen ions.
- An acid gives up hydrogen ions in solution; a base binds hydrogen ions in solution.
- Acids are formed in the body as a result of metabolism and incomplete oxidation of glucose and fats.
- Acid-base balance is regulated by chemical, respiratory, and renal mechanisms.
- Chemical buffers are the immediate way that acid-base imbalances are corrected.
- The lungs control the amount of carbon dioxide that is retained or exhaled.
- The kidneys regulate the amount of hydrogen and bicarbonate ions that are retained or excreted by the body.
- Compensation is the process in which the body uses its three regulatory mechanisms to correct for changes in the pH of body fluids.

Fortunately, the body has many well-regulated mechanisms to ensure minimal changes in hydrogen ion concentration. Table 17-2 lists the key concepts of acid-base balance.

Acid-Base Balance

As discussed in Chapters 14 and 16, body fluids are electrically neutral even though they contain ions having an overall positive charge (cations or protons) and ions having an overall negative charge (anions). When fluids contain an equal number of positive and negative charges, the electrical charge remains neutral. The system maintains a body fluid hydrogen ion concentration pH between 7.35 and 7.45 in a similar manner; however, this value is not strictly neutral (7.0 is actual neutral pH) but is slightly alkaline. Normal body fluid hydrogen ion concentration (pH) remains at a near-neutral value when the numbers of acid and base components are in relative balance, thus limiting the total number of free hydrogen ions. That is, acid-base balance concerns regulation of the overall concentration of free hydrogen ions by matching the rate of hydrogen ion production with the activity of mechanisms for hydrogen ion removal and uptake.

ACID-BASE CHEMISTRY

ACIDS

Acids are substances that donate, or release (set free), a hydrogen ion when the substance is dissolved in water. Thus, an acid in a solution increases the concentration of free hydrogen ions in that solution. The strength of an acid is determined by how easily it releases a hydrogen ion in solution. A strong acid, such as hydrochloric acid (HCl), dissociates (separates) completely in water and readily releases all its hydrogen ions:

HCl	$+ H_2O \longrightarrow$	H^+	$+ Cl^-$	$+ H_2O$
Hydrochloric acid	Water	Hydrogen ion	Chloride ion	Water

A weak acid does not completely dissociate in water; it releases only a small number of its total hydrogen ions. In the following example, each molecule of acetic acid (CH_3COOH) (a weak acid) contains a total of four hydrogen molecules. When acetic acid combines with water, it releases only *one* of its four hydrogen molecules. The other three hydrogen molecules remain bound to the acetic acid molecule

$$CH_3COOH + H_2O \longrightarrow H^+ + CH_3COO^- + H_2O$$

BASES

A base is a substance that binds free hydrogen ions in solution. Thus, bases are hydrogen acceptors—they reduce the concentration of free hydrogen ions in solution. Strong bases bind hydrogen ions easily, and some may bind more than one hydrogen ion to one molecule of base. Examples of relatively strong bases are sodium hydroxide (NaOH) and ammonia (NH_3). Examples of weak bases are aluminum hydroxide (AlOH) and bicarbonate (HCO_3^-).

Weak bases bind hydrogen ions less readily. Although bicarbonate is a relatively weak base, bicarbonate ions in the body are crucial in preventing major disturbances in body fluid pH.

BUFFERS

Buffers are special substances that can either release a hydrogen ion into a fluid or bind a hydrogen ion from a fluid. Most substances, when dissolved in water, react in only one way: They either release a hydrogen ion (this an acidic substance) or bind a free hydrogen ion (this is a basic substance). Buffers, when dissolved in water, can react in two ways: They can act either as an acid (and release a hydrogen ion) or as a base (and bind a hydrogen ion).

The way in which a buffer reacts when dissolved in water or other fluid depends on the existing acid-base balance of that fluid. Buffers always try to bring the fluid as close as possible to neutral (or a normal body fluid pH of 7.35 to 7.45). Thus, if the fluid is basic (with few free hydrogen ions present), the buffer will release hydrogen ions into the fluid (Fig. 17–2). If the fluid is acidic (with many free hydrogen ions), the buffer substance will act as a base and will bind some of the hydrogen ions. In a sense, buffers are considered hydrogen ion "sponges," soaking up hydrogen ions when too many are present in a fluid and squeezing out hydrogen ions when too few are present in a fluid. Because of this flexibility, buffers are important regulators of body fluid hydrogen ion concentration (acid-base balance).

Solutions with a pH of 7.0 are considered neutral; they contain a set concentration of hydrogen ions as a result of an equilibrium of the number and strength of acid and base components. Figure 17–3 is an artificial, yet concrete, representation of the concept of neutral pH. The representation indicates that the strength as well as the amount of all acid components is equal to strength as well as the amount of all the base components in a given solution. Although this is never the actual case in human physiology, if there is acid-base homeostasis, the relative amounts and strengths of acids (A) and bases (B) are approximately equal, so that the overall hydrogen ion concentration remains constant.

Solutions with a pH ranging from 1.0 to 6.99 contain an excess in the amount or strength (or both) of the acid components compared with the amount or strength (or both) of the base components. Such solutions are considered *acidic* (see Fig. 17–3). This situation results in more hydrogen ions being released than bound, thus greatly increasing the number of free hydrogen ions.

Solutions with a pH ranging from 7.01 to 14.0 have an excess in the amount or strength (or both) of the base components compared with the amount or strength (or both) of the acid components. These solutions are considered *basic*. This situation results in more hydrogen ions being bound than released, causing a deficit in the number of free hydrogen ions (Fig. 17–4).

BODY FLUID CHEMISTRY

BICARBONATE IONS

Body fluids contain many different acidic substances and a few bases. The most common base in human body fluid is bicarbonate (HCO_3^-); the most common acid is carbonic acid (H_2CO_3). Under normal conditions, the body maintains these substances

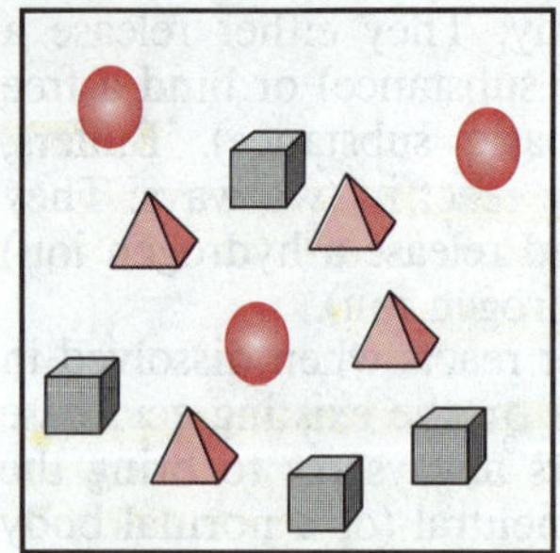

Fluid pH 7.38 (normal). The number and strength of acid components are equal to the number and strength of base components. Hydrogen ion concentration is limited and constant.

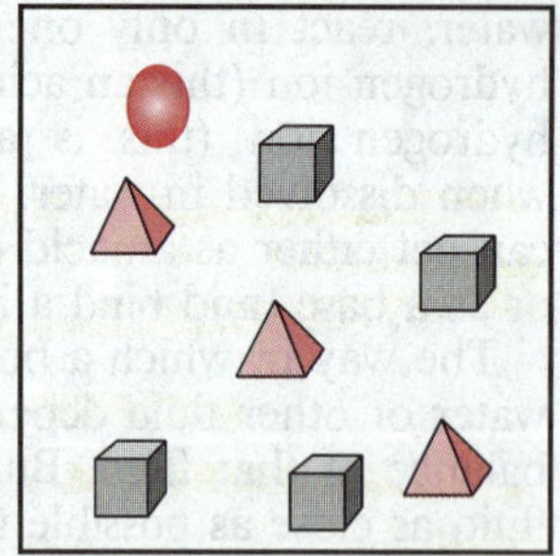

Fluid pH 7.51 (alkaline). The number and strength of base components are greater than the number and strength of acid components. Hydrogen ion concentration is below normal.

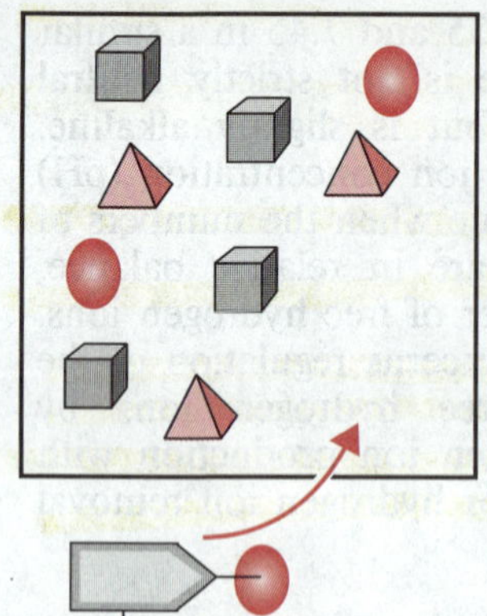

Buffer is added to the alkaline fluid.

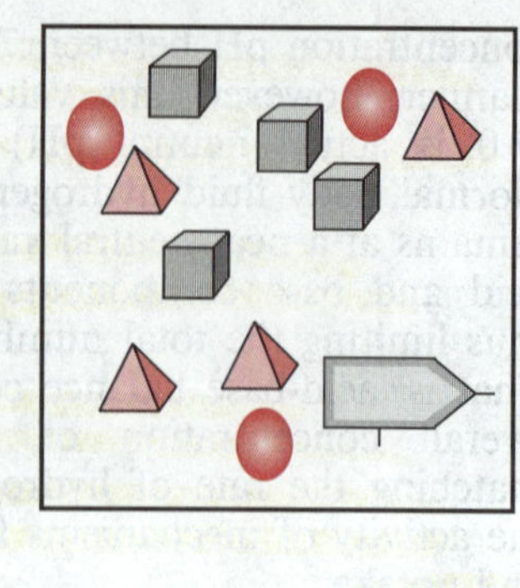

The buffer acts as an acid, releasing a hydrogen ion.

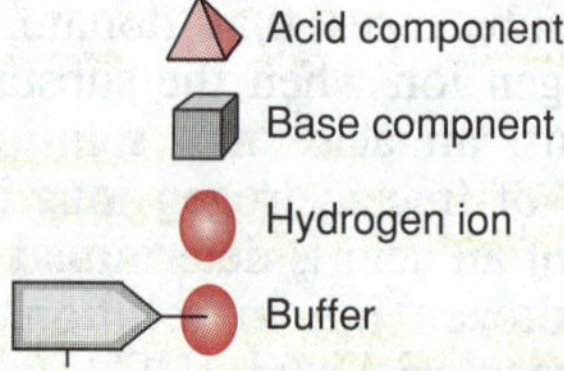

FIGURE 17–2 ◆ Action of buffer in solution.

within extracellular fluids (ECF) at a constant ratio of 1 molecule of carbonic acid to 20 free bicarbonate ions (1:20) (Fig. 17–5). To maintain this ratio, both carbonic acid and bicarbonate must be well controlled. Both of these substances and the constant ratio between them are related to the production and elimination of both carbon dioxide (CO_2) and the hydrogen ion (H^+).

A key concept that aids in understanding acid-base balance is the *carbonic anhydrase equation* (shown below). This equation, driven by an enzyme called carbonic anhydrase, demonstrates how H^+ concentration and CO_2 concentration are directly related to each other, so that an increase in one causes a corresponding increase in the other:

$$\underset{\text{Carbon dioxide}}{CO_2} + \underset{\text{Water}}{H_2O} \longleftrightarrow \underset{\text{Carbonic acid}}{H_2CO_3} \longleftrightarrow \underset{\text{Hydrogen ion}}{H^+} + \underset{\text{Bicarbonate ion}}{HCO_3^-}$$

Carbon dioxide (CO_2) is a gas that, when combined with water, forms carbonic acid (H_2CO_3). Carbon dioxide then, is the changeable part of carbonic acid. Because carbonic acid is not stable and because the body needs to maintain a 1:20 ratio of carbonic acid to bicarbonate, as soon as carbonic acid is formed from water and carbon dioxide, it immediately dissociates (separates) into free hydrogen ions and bicarbonate ions. *Therefore, the carbon dioxide content of a fluid is directly related to the hydrogen ion concentration of that fluid. Whenever conditions cause the*

AAABBB	AAAABBB	AAABB
AAABBB	AAAABBB	AAABB
AAABBB	AAAABBB	AAABB
Neutral	Acidic (acid excess)	Acidic (base deficit)

FIGURE 17–3 ◆ The concept of acidic versus normal pH.

AAABBB	AAABBBB	AABBB
AAABBB	AAABBBB	AABBB
AAABBB	AAABBBB	AABBB
Neutral	Alkaline (base excess)	Alkaline (acid deficit)

FIGURE 17–4 ◆ The concept of alkaline versus normal pH.

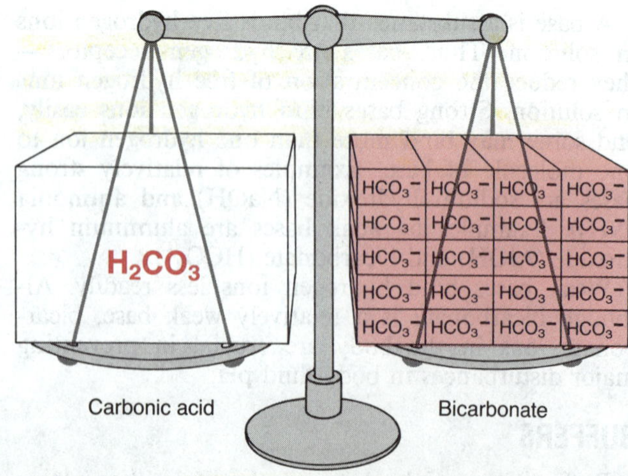

FIGURE 17–5 ◆ The normal ratio of carbonic acid to bicarbonate is 1:20.

amount of carbon dioxide made to be increased, more hydrogen ions are also created. Likewise, whenever hydrogen ion production increases, more carbon dioxide is also produced.

INCREASES IN CARBON DIOXIDE CAUSE INCREASES IN HYDROGEN IONS

When excess carbon dioxide is produced, the concentration of carbon dioxide is increased and the carbonic anhydrase equation is shifted to the right, demonstrating an increase in the hydrogen ion concentration (and a decrease in pH):

$$CO_2 + H_2O \longleftrightarrow H_2CO_3 \longleftrightarrow H^+ + HCO_3^-$$
$$\longrightarrow \qquad \longrightarrow$$

When very little carbon dioxide is produced, no hydrogen ions are generated by the carbonic anhydrase equation.

INCREASES IN HYDROGEN IONS CAUSE INCREASES IN CARBON DIOXIDE

When excess hydrogen ions are produced or brought into the body, the carbonic anhydrase equation is shifted to the left, demonstrating the creation of more carbon dioxide.

$$CO_2 + H_2O \longleftrightarrow H_2CO_3 \longleftrightarrow H^+ + HCO_3^-$$
$$\longleftarrow \qquad \longleftarrow$$

When the body fluids are low on hydrogen ions, no extra carbon dioxide is produced.

CALCULATION OF HYDROGEN ION CONCENTRATION

The pH is a calculated measurement of hydrogen ion concentration for body fluids because the actual number or percentage of hydrogen ions in these fluids cannot be measured directly. The pH calculations are derived from the Henderson-Hasselbalch equation, a mathematical formula that expresses the interrelatedness of three factors:

- The concentration of free hydrogen ions
- The concentration of bases
- The concentration of acids in a solution

When other influences (such as temperature and pressure) remain constant, if two of the three factors are known, we can calculate the third factor.

$$pH = 6.1 + \log \frac{[HCO_3^-]}{[H_2CO_3 + CO_2]}$$

Because the concentrations of carbonic acid and bicarbonate in extracellular fluid are present in a ratio of 1:20 under normal physiologic conditions, the major factor in the preceding equation that tends to fluctuate is the concentration of carbon dioxide. As a result, whenever the concentration of carbon dioxide changes, a corresponding change in pH also occurs.

In the Henderson-Hasselbalch formula, the concentration of carbon dioxide is the divisor (on the bottom of the equation), making the concentration of carbon dioxide *inversely related to pH* while it is *directly related to the hydrogen ion concentration.* Thus, when the carbon dioxide concentration of a solution increases, the pH *drops,* indicating an *increase* in the hydrogen ion concentration. Conversely, when the carbon dioxide concentration of a solution decreases, the pH *rises,* indicating a *decrease* in the hydrogen ion concentration.

An increase in the bicarbonate concentration causes the hydrogen ion concentration to decrease and the pH to *increase,* or become more alkaline (basic). Conversely, an increase in the carbon dioxide concentration, causes the hydrogen ion concentration to increase and the pH to *decrease* or become more acidic. In either case, the normal 1:20 ratio is changed and the pH of the blood is also changed.

Because the kidneys control bicarbonate concentration and the lungs control carbon dioxide concentration in the body, pH can also be described as the function of the kidneys divided by the function of the lungs, or

$$pH = \frac{\text{kidneys (bicarbonate)}}{\text{lungs (carbon dioxide)}}$$

SOURCES OF ACIDS

Acids are formed in the body as by-products of normal metabolism. Common sources of hydrogen ions are (1) carbon dioxide production, (2) metabolism of proteins and fats, (3) anaerobic metabolism of glucose or fats, and (4) destruction of cells.

PRODUCTION OF CARBON DIOXIDE

Carbon dioxide (CO_2) is a by-product of glucose breakdown and many other metabolic reactions. (The complete breakdown of one molecule of glucose results in the formation of 36 molecules of adenosine triphosphate [ATP], 6 molecules of water, and 6 molecules of CO_2.) Because of the relationship between carbon dioxide and hydrogen ions through the carbonic anhydrase equation, any increase in carbon dioxide concentration in body fluids always leads to the formation of increased amounts of hydrogen ions in those fluids, with a resulting decrease in pH.

Carbon dioxide leaves the body in air exhaled during breathing. Therefore, one determinant of blood pH is how much carbon dioxide is produced by body cells during metabolism versus how rapidly carbon dioxide is removed from the body by the lungs.

METABOLISM OF FATS AND PROTEINS

The catabolism (breakdown) of food for energy results in the formation of "fixed acids." Protein catabolism creates sulfuric acid. Fat catabolism creates fatty acids.

ANAEROBIC METABOLISM OF GLUCOSE AND FATS

Incomplete oxidation—as occurs whenever cells continue to metabolize substances under anaerobic (no oxygen) conditions—of glucose leads to the formation of lactic acid. Incomplete breakdown of fatty acids, either because excessive amounts of fatty acids are being metabolized or because insufficient oxygen is present during any fatty acid breakdown, results in the formation of ketoacids (Guyton, 1991).

DESTRUCTION OF CELLS

Whenever cells are damaged or destroyed, plasma membranes are broken and intracellular contents are released. Some cell structures contain acids that are released into the extracellular fluid when the cell is damaged or destroyed (Keyes, 1990).

SOURCES OF BICARBONATE IONS

Bicarbonate is the principal buffer of the extracellular fluid (ECF). Sources of bicarbonate in the extracellular fluids of the body, according to Guyton (1991), include:

- The breakdown of carbonic acid
- Gastrointestinal absorption of ingested bicarbonate
- Pancreatic synthesis and secretion of bicarbonate
- The movement of intracellular bicarbonate into the extracellular fluid
- Renal reabsorption of filtered bicarbonate

Once bicarbonate is in the extracellular fluids, it is maintained at a concentration that is 20 times greater than the fluid concentration of carbonic acid.

Homeostasis

The production of various acids, carbon dioxide, and hydrogen ions is a normal and continuous process as long as body cells are capable of metabolism. Despite this production, homeostasis of body fluids with regard to hydrogen ion concentration, bicarbonate, oxygen, and carbon dioxide concentrations is maintained under normal physiologic conditions. Chart 17–1 gives normal values for these substances in arterial and venous blood. This homeostasis depends on three factors:

- Hydrogen ion production must be consistent and not excessive.
- Carbon dioxide loss from the body through breathing must occur at a rate that keeps pace with hydrogen ion production.
- The ratio between carbonic acid and bicarbonate must be maintained at a 1:20 ratio.

ACID-BASE REGULATORY MECHANISMS

To maintain the hydrogen ion concentration (pH) of the extracellular fluid within the narrow ranges of normal, the body has three well-regulated mechanisms for acid-base balance: chemical, respiratory, and renal (Table 17–3).

CHEMICAL MECHANISMS

Buffers are the first line of defense against changes in hydrogen ion concentration. Because they are constantly present in body fluids, buffers can engage in immediate actions to reduce or raise the hydrogen

CHART 17–1

Lab Profile ◆ Acid-Base Assessment

Test	Normal Range for Adults: *Arterial*	*Venous*	Significance of Abnormal Findings
pH	• 7.34–7.45	• 7.31–7.42	• *Increased:* alkalosis • *Decreased:* acidosis
PaO_2 (mmHg)	• >80	• 30–50	• *Increased:* not significant • *Decreased:* acidosis
$PaCO_2$ (mmHg)	• 32–45	• 39–52	• *Increased:* acidosis • *Decreased:* alkalosis
HCO_3^- (mEq/L)	• 20–26	• 22–28	• *Increased:* renal compensation of respiratory acidosis • Metabolic alkalosis • *Decreased:* metabolic acidosis

TABLE 17–3 Acid-Base Regulatory Mechanisms

Chemical Mechanisms	
Protein buffers Extracellular Albumin Globulins Intracellular Hemoglobin Chemical buffers Extracellular Bicarbonate Intracellular Phosphate Bicarbonate	• Very rapid • Provide immediate response to changing conditions • Can handle relatively small fluctuations in hydrogen ion production and elimination encountered under normal metabolic and health conditions
Respiratory Mechanisms	
Increased hydrogen ions Increased carbon dioxide Stimulates central respiratory neurons, leading to increased rate and depth of breathing, causing more carbon dioxide to be lost and decreasing the hydrogen ion concentration Decreased hydrogen ions Decreased carbon dioxide Inhibition of central respiratory neurons, leading to decreased rate and depth of breathing, causing normally produced carbon dioxide to be retained, increasing the hydrogen ion concentration	• Primarily assist buffering systems when the fluctuation of hydrogen ion concentration is acute
Renal Mechanisms	
Mechanisms to decrease pH Increased renal excretion of bicarbonate Increased renal reabsorption of hydrogen ions Mechanisms to increase pH Decreased renal excretion of bicarbonate Decreased renal reabsorption of hydrogen ions	• The most powerful regulator of acid-base balance • Respond to large or chronic fluctuations in hydrogen ion production or elimination

ion concentration to normal. By acting as hydrogen ion "sponges," buffers can bind hydrogen ions when the concentration is too high or they can release hydrogen ions when the concentration is too low. Fluid buffers are composed of chemicals or proteins.

CHEMICAL BUFFERS

Chemical buffers are paired mixtures, usually consisting of a weak base and the conjugated salt of an acid. The two most common chemical buffer systems are:

- Bicarbonate buffers, which are active in both the extracellular and intracellular fluids
- Phosphate buffers, which are active in the intracellular fluid

PROTEIN BUFFERS

Proteins constitute the largest buffer store. Although most proteins in solution in the human body tend to carry an overall negative charge, they can either bind or release hydrogen ions as needed. Both intracellular and extracellular proteins serve as buffers.

The major intracellular protein buffer is hemoglobin. Hemoglobin buffers hydrogen ions directly and also buffers whole acids formed during synthesis and transport of carbon dioxide (Keyes, 1990). When the hydrogen ion concentration of the blood increases, some of the excess hydrogen ions cross the plasma membrane of red blood cells and bind to the large numbers of hemoglobin molecules present in each red blood cell.

Extracellular buffering proteins include albumins and globulins. These proteins buffer both carbonic acid and the fixed acids that are present in the extracellular fluid as a result of catabolism.

RESPIRATORY MECHANISMS

When chemical buffers alone cannot prevent the changes in body fluid pH, the respiratory system is the second line of defense against changes. Breathing controls hydrogen ion concentration by regulating the concentration of carbon dioxide in arterial blood. Carbon dioxide is converted into hydrogen ions through the carbonic anhydrase reaction; therefore, the concentration of carbon dioxide is directly related to the concentration of hydrogen ions. Breathing is a major physiologic mechanism for ridding the body of carbon dioxide, which is created as a by-product of metabolism.

The concentration of carbon dioxide in venous blood increases during normal metabolism. This carbon dioxide is transported to the capillaries of the lungs. Because the partial pressure (concentration) of carbon dioxide is far higher in the capillary blood than in the atmospheric air in the alveoli, carbon dioxide diffuses freely from the blood into the alveolar air. Once in the alveoli, carbon dioxide is exhaled during breathing and is lost from the body. Because the partial pressure (concentration) of carbon dioxide in atmospheric air is so low as to be nearly zero, carbon dioxide usually continues to be exhaled at an appropriate rate even when alveolar gas exchange is impaired to some degree.

HYPERVENTILATION

Respiratory regulation of acid-base balance is under the control of the nervous system (Fig. 17–6). Special chemoreceptors in the areas of the brain that directly regulate the rate and depth of respiration are sensitive to changes in the concentration of carbon dioxide in the cerebral extracellular fluid. As the concentration of carbon dioxide begins to rise in cerebral blood and tissues, these central chemoreceptors stimulate the neurons that control the rate and depth of respira-

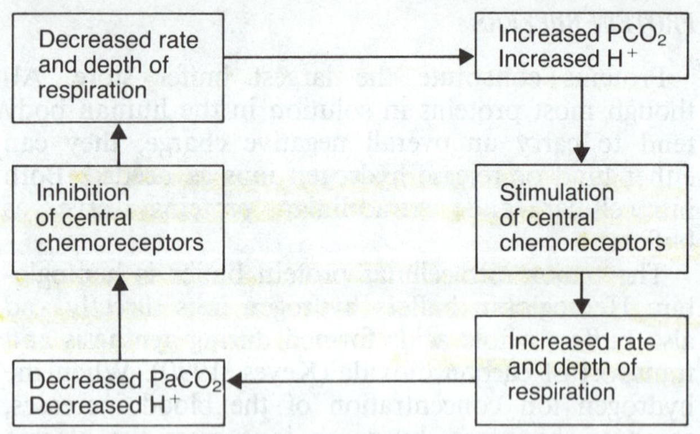

FIGURE 17-6 ◆ Neural regulation of respiration and hydrogen ion concentration.

tion. Under this stimulation, both the rate and the depth of respiration increase so that more carbon dioxide is exhaled ("blown off") from the alveoli and the carbon dioxide concentration of the extracellular fluid decreases. When the arterial carbon dioxide concentration returns to normal, the rate and depth of respiration return to levels normal for the particular person.

HYPOVENTILATION

If the hydrogen ion concentration of the extracellular fluid is too low, the carbon dioxide concentration is also too low. The low carbon dioxide levels are sensed by the central chemoreceptors, which inhibit stimulation of neurons in the respiratory control centers. As a result of this lack of stimulation, the rate and depth of respiration dramatically diminish so that less carbon dioxide is lost through the lungs and more carbon dioxide is retained in arterial blood. This retention, coupled with the normal carbon dioxide-generating metabolic reactions, results in a rapid return of the arterial carbon dioxide concentration (and hydrogen ion concentration) to normal levels. When these levels are normal, the rate and depth of respiration also return to basal levels.

The respiratory system's response in regulating acid-base balance is rapid. Changes in the rate and depth of respiration occur within minutes after changes in the hydrogen ion concentration and/or carbon dioxide concentration of the extracellular fluid have occurred.

RENAL MECHANISMS

The kidneys are the third line of defense against fluctuations in body fluid pH. Renal mechanisms are the most powerful mechanism for regulating acid-base balance but take longer to start than the chemical and respiratory mechanisms. When changes in body fluid pH are persistent, renal mechanisms that increase rates of excretion and reabsorption of acids or bases (depending on the direction of the pH changes) begin to operate (Fig. 17-7). These mechanisms include (1) renal tubular movement of bicarbonate, (2) formation of acids, and (3) formation of ammonium (Keyes, 1990, Schrier, 1992).

TUBULAR MOVEMENT OF BICARBONATE

The first renal mechanism—tubular movement of bicarbonate—is accomplished in the kidney tubules in two ways. The first way is renal movement of bicarbonate made elsewhere in the body. The second way is renal movement of bicarbonate made in the kidneys. Much of the bicarbonate made in other body areas is absorbed into the blood and is filtered from the blood into early urine at the level of the glomerulus (see Chap. 14). When blood hydrogen ion levels are high, this filtered bicarbonate is reabsorbed from the tubules back into systemic circulation, where it can help buffer the excess hydrogen ions. When blood hydrogen ion levels are low, the filtered bicarbonate remains in the urine and is excreted. In addition to renal bicarbonate excretion and reabsorption, when a hydrogen ion excess is evident, the kidney tubules can respond by making additional bicarbonate that will be reabsorbed.

FORMATION OF ACIDS

The second renal mechanism, formation of acids, occurs through the phosphate-buffering mechanism inside the cells of the kidney tubules. When the newly created bicarbonate made in the tubule cells is reabsorbed into systemic circulation along with the sodium, the urine has an excess of anions, including phosphate (HPO_4^{2-}). This negatively charged environment draws hydrogen ions into the urine (Keyes, 1990). Once the hydrogen ion is in the urine, it combines with the phosphate ion, forming an acid, H_2PO_4, which is then lost from the body in the urine.

FORMATION OF AMMONIUM

In the third renal mechanism, ammonium (NH_4^+) is formed from ammonia (NH_3). Ammonia is a by-product of normal amino acid catabolism (Guyton, 1991). Ammonia is excreted into the tubular urine, where it can combine with free hydrogen ions and form ammonium. Afterward, it is excreted from the body in the urine. This trapping of free hydrogen ions in ammonium prevents the tubular urine hydrogen ion concentration from becoming so high that it inhibits diffusion or transport of free hydrogen ions from the blood and other extracellular fluids into the urine. The overall result of this process is a loss of hydrogen ions and an increase in blood pH.

COMPENSATION

In the process of compensation, the body attempts to correct for changes in body fluid (blood) pH. A pH below 6.9 or above 7.8 is usually fatal (the normal pH range for human extracellular fluids is 7.35 to 7.45).

1. TUBULAR MOVEMENT OF BICARBONATE

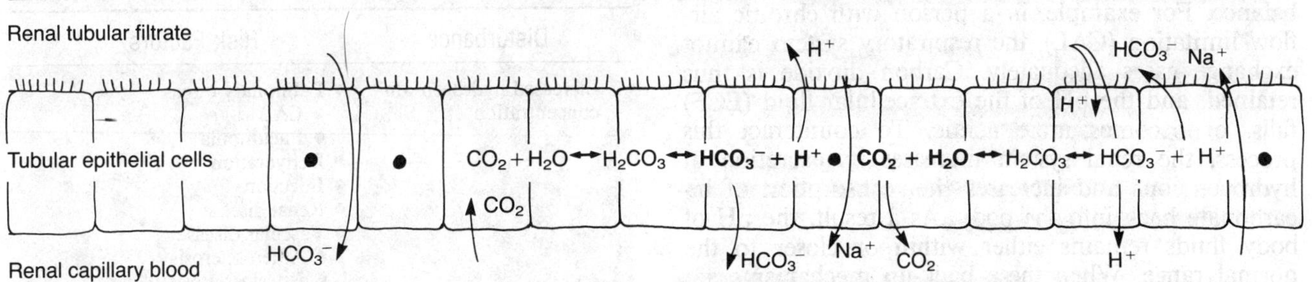

Bicarbonate filtered at the glomerulus into the filtrate ("early urine") is reabsorbed across the renal tubular epithelium into the renal capillaries and returned to the systemic circulation. This movement of bicarbonate into the systemic circulation increases blood pH (makes blood less acidic).

If Blood CO_2 Levels Are High
Carbon dioxide enters the tubular epithelium, shifting the carbonic anhydrase equation to the right to form bicarbonate and hydrogen ions. Bicarbonate moves into the renal capillaries. Hydrogen moves into the tubular filtrate in exchange for sodium. The loss of hydrogen ions from blood reduces its pH (makes it less acidic).

To prevent excess hydrogen in the renal tubular filtrate, hydrogen ions must combine with other substances. The second and third renal mechanisms of acid-base balance now come into play.

If Blood CO_2 Levels Are Low
Hydrogen ions from the tubular filtrate are reabsorbed into the renal capillaries in exchange for sodium. This flow of hydrogen may be direct, or it may shift the carbonic anhydrase equation to the left so that carbon dioxide is reabsorbed into the systemic circulation and bicarbonate moves into the renal tubular filtrate. Retention of acids and excretion of bases reduce blood pH (makes blood more acidic).

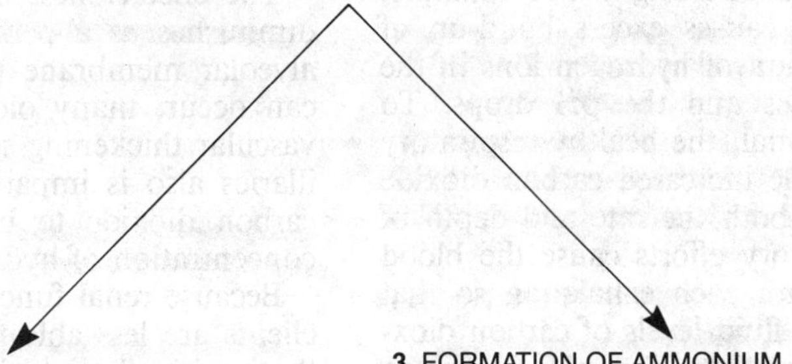

2. FORMATION OF ACIDS

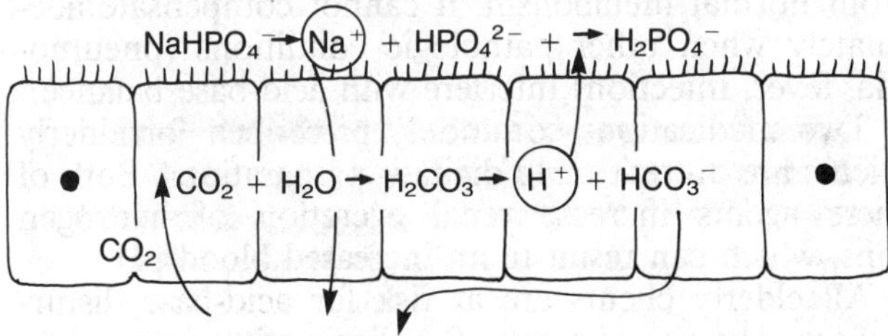

After the newly generated bicarbonate and the cation sodium are passed into the systemic circulation, the renal tubular filtrate has an excess of anions, including phosphate. The cation hydrogen is attracted to the negatively charged environment of the renal tubular filtrate. There, hydrogen binds with phosphate to form the acid H_2PO_4, which is excreted in urine.

3. FORMATION OF AMMONIUM

$H^+ + NH_3 \rightarrow NH_4$

$CO_2 + H_2O \rightarrow H_2CO_3 \rightarrow H^+ + HCO_3^-$ NH_3

Ammonia produced by amino acid (glutamine) catabolism is excreted into the renal tubular filtrate. There, ammonia combines with hydrogen cations to form ammonium, which is excreted in urine.

FIGURE 17-7 ◆ Renal mechanisms of acid-base balance.

RENAL COMPENSATION

The healthy renal system can correct or compensate for changes in pH when the respiratory system is either overwhelmed or is actually a cause of the imbalance. For example, in a person with chronic airflow limitation (CAL), the respiratory system cannot exchange gases adequately. Carbon dioxide is thus retained, and the pH of the extracellular fluid (ECF) falls, or becomes more acidic. To counteract this process, the renal system increases its excretion of hydrogen ions and increases the reabsorption of bicarbonate back into the body. As a result, the pH of body fluids remains either within or closer to the normal range. When these back-up mechanisms are completely effective, the respiratory problems are *fully compensated* and the pH of the blood is normal, even though the concentration of other substances (such as oxygen and bicarbonate) may be abnormal.

Sometimes, however, the respiratory factors contributing to the acid-base imbalance are so severe that renal actions can only *partially compensate* and thus the pH is not normal. Even partial compensation is critically important to acid-base balance because it prevents the imbalance from becoming more severe (and possibly life-threatening).

RESPIRATORY COMPENSATION

The respiratory system can compensate for acid-base imbalances of a metabolic origin. For example, when prolonged running causes excess build-up of lactic acid, the concentration of hydrogen ions in the extracellular fluid increases and the pH drops. To bring the pH back to normal, the healthy respiratory system is stimulated by the increased carbon dioxide concentration to increase both the rate and depth of respiration. These respiratory efforts cause the blood to lose carbon dioxide with each exhalation so that gradually the extracellular fluid levels of carbon dioxide and hydrogen ions decrease. The pH returns to normal when this mechanism is capable of full or complete compensation.

Although both the renal and respiratory systems can compensate for acid-base imbalances, they are not equal in their compensatory actions and reactions. The respiratory system is much more sensitive to acid-base changes and can begin compensation efforts within seconds to minutes after a change in pH. However, these efforts are limited and can be overwhelmed easily. The renal compensatory mechanisms are much more powerful and result in dramatic changes in extracellular fluid composition. However, these more powerful mechanisms are not stimulated fully until the acid-base imbalance is sustained for a significant time (hours to several days).

Changes in Acid-Base Balance Associated with Aging

Elderly people are more susceptible to pH disturbances than younger people because their normal physiologic mechanisms are less able to respond to minor fluctuations in hydrogen ion production or elimination. In addition, an elderly person may be taking medications that alter the activity of normal pH compensating mechanisms (Chart 17–2).

CHART 17–2

Nursing Focus on the Elderly ◆ Age-Related Risk Factors for Acid-Base Disturbances

Disturbance	Risk Factors

Increased hydrogen ion concentration	• Pulmonary diseases
	  • CAL
	  • Pneumonia
	• Dehydration
	• Infection
	• Renal disease
	• Vascular disease
	  • Atherosclerosis
	  • Arteriosclerosis
	  • Angiitis

Decreased hydrogen ion concentration	• Overhydration
	• Congestive heart failure
	• Drugs
	  • Diuretics (loop and thiazide)
	  • Digitalis preparations
	  • Insulin
	  • Antibiotics
	  • Chemotherapeutic agents

The effectiveness of gas exchange during breathing diminishes as a person ages. Not only is there less alveolar membrane present through which exchange can occur; many older people have some degree of vascular thickening so that gas diffusion through capillaries also is impaired. These conditions can cause carbon dioxide to be retained, which increases the concentration of hydrogen ions.

Because renal function diminishes with age, elderly clients are less able to excrete hydrogen ions or synthesize bicarbonate ions. Although the renal system may be able to handle ordinary changes resulting from normal metabolism, it cannot compensate adequately when other pathologic conditions (pneumonia, fever, infection) interfere with acid-base balance.

Two medications commonly prescribed for elderly clients are diuretics and digitalis preparations. Both of these agents increase renal excretion of hydrogen ions, which can result in an increased blood pH.

All elderly clients are at risk for acid-base disturbances. The risk is greater for clients with pulmonary, vascular, cardiac, or renal impairments.

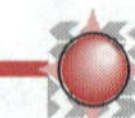

IMPLICATIONS FOR NURSING RESEARCH

Few studies conducted by nurses address issues related to acid-base balance. Nursing research is needed to answer the following questions:

- What specific assessment findings are associated with renal compensation of respiratory acidosis?
- How well do peripheral pulse oximetry findings correlate with arterial blood gas partial pressure of oxygen values?
- Is there a consistent relationship between changes in hydration status and the presence of specific acid-base problems in older clients?
- To what degree does oral ingestion of basic substances alter blood pH?
- Can increased intake of water dilute the serum hydrogen ion concentration?

SELECTED BIBLIOGRAPHY

Anderson, S. (1990). ABGs: Six easy steps to interpreting blood gases. *American Journal of Nursing, 90*(8), 42–45.

*Brenner, B., Coe, F. L., & Rector, F. C., Jr. (1987). *Renal physiology in health and disease.* Philadelphia: W. B. Saunders.

England, B., & Mitch, W. (1990). Acid-base, fluid, and electrolyte aspects of parenteral nutrition. In J. Kokko & R. L. Tannen (Eds.), *Fluid and electrolytes* (pp. 1024–1042). Philadelphia: W. B. Saunders.

Ganong, W. (1991). *Review of medical physiology*, 15th ed. Norwalk, CT: Appleton and Lange.

Guyton, A. C. (1991). *Textbook of medical physiology* (8th ed.). Philadelphia: W. B. Saunders.

Keyes, J. (1990). *Fluid, electrolyte, and acid-base regulation.* Boston: Jones & Bartlett.

Kokko, J. (1990). Overview of renal physiology. In J. Kokko & R. L. Tannen (Eds.), *Fluid and electrolytes* (pp. 1043–1068). Philadelphia: W. B. Saunders.

Metheny, N. (1992). *Fluid and electrolyte balance: Nursing considerations* (2nd ed.). Philadelphia: J. B. Lippincott.

Morris, L. (1990). The POLK method of ABG interpretation. *Critical Care Nurse, 10*(1), 18–20.

Russell, J. (1991). Successful method for arterial blood gas interpretation. *Critical Care Nurse, 11*(5), 14–19.

Scherer, P. (1990). Get true blood gas values with less blood loss. *American Journal of Nursing, 90*(2), 28.

Schrier, R. (1992). *Renal and electrolyte disorders* (4th ed.). Boston: Little, Brown & Co.

Tasota, F., & Wesmiller, S. (1994). Assessing A.B.G.s: Maintaining the delicate balance. *Nursing94, 24*(5), 34–46.

SUGGESTED READINGS

Morris, L. (1990). The POLK method of ABG interpretation. *Critical Care Nurse, 10*(1), 18–20.

This article describes a simplistic approach to describe the relationship between blood gas values and the efficiency of renal and pulmonary function. The reader is encouraged to use the acronym "POLK," with P = pH, O = oxygen, L = lungs, and K = kidney. This method is most appropriate for beginning practitioners and does not address mixed acid-base disorders or actions.

Russell, J. (1991). Successful method for arterial blood gas interpretation. *Critical Care Nurse, 11*(5), 14–19.

This article presents a system of formulas for quickly interpreting arterial blood gas values. The physiologic bases for the formulas and case studies illustrating formula use are discussed. The author also lists situations in which use of the formulas is not appropriate.

Scherer, P. (1990). Get true blood gas values with less blood loss. *American Journal of Nursing, 90*(2), 28.

The author reviews the findings of previous nursing research that established the minimal blood discard for obtaining undiluted blood gas values through central arterial lines (A-lines). Values after a 2-mL discard were consistent with those obtained after discards of 5 mL and 10 mL.

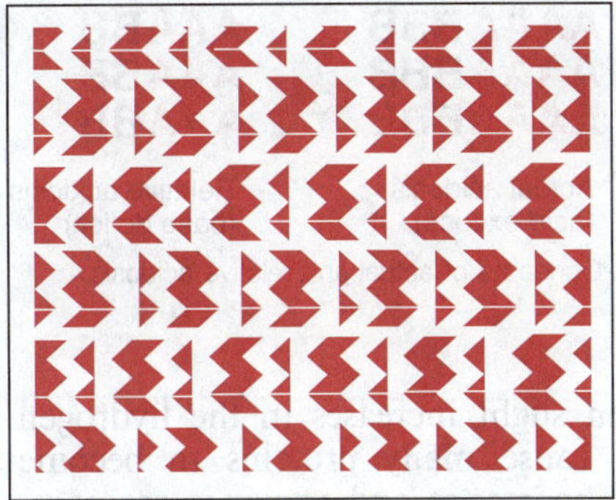

CHAPTER 18

Interventions for Clients with Acid-Base Imbalances

CHAPTER HIGHLIGHTS

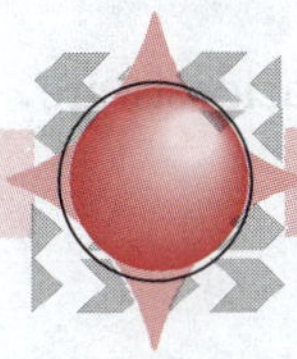

The most carefully regulated electrolyte in body fluids is the hydrogen ion concentration, or acid-base balance, as measured by pH. The normal range for pH of body fluids is 7.35 to 7.45. Some pathologic conditions directly impair the actions of specific acid-base regulatory mechanisms. Other conditions, not directly associated with acid-base regulatory mechanisms, can change the concentrations of acids or bases at a rate that exceeds the body's normal capacity for regulation. The result of either type of action is an acid-base imbalance that can alter many physiologic functions, possibly causing serious or even fatal side effects. Table 18-1 summarizes key points associated with acid-base imbalance.

Acidosis

OVERVIEW

In a person with acidosis, the acid-base balance of the blood and other extracellular fluid (ECF) is disturbed and is characterized by an excess of hydrogen ions (H^+), or an arterial blood pH below 7.35. The concentration and/or strength of acid components are proportionately higher than normal compared with the concentration and/or strength of the base components.

Acidosis is not a specific disease; rather, it is a manifestation of a disease or pathologic process. Acidosis can be caused by metabolic problems, respiratory problems, or both (Cotran et al., 1989).

TABLE 18–1 Key Points Related to Acid-Base Imbalances

- Acidemia is defined as an increase in the hydrogen ion concentration (pH) of the blood and is reflected by an arterial blood pH below 7.35.
- Acidemia can result from an actual acid excess or a relative base deficit.
- Metabolic acidosis usually results from a lack of bicarbonate or an excess acid production in the body.
- Respiratory acidosis results from retention of carbon dioxide in the body causing increased carbonic acid production.
- Manifestations of acidemia are related to fluid and electrolyte imbalances that accompany acid-base imbalance, such as hyperkalemia.
- Chronic respiratory acidosis is common in the medical-surgical setting as a result of chronic obstructive pulmonary disease, such as emphysema.
- Alkalemia is defined as a decrease in the hydrogen ion concentration of the blood and is reflected by an arterial blood pH above 7.45.
- Alkalemia can result from an actual base excess or an acid deficit.
- Metabolic alkalosis most often occurs when body acids are lost, such as in prolonged vomiting or nasogastric suctioning.
- Respiratory alkalosis most often occurs when hyperventilation causes an excessive loss of carbon dioxide from the body.
- Dehydration and hypokalemia are associated with metabolic alkalosis, and they account for most of the clinical manifestations seen in this acid-base imbalance.
- The goal of management for any type of acid-base imbalance is to restore fluid, electrolyte, and acid-base balance to normal or near-normal.

PATHOPHYSIOLOGY

Acidosis can result from an actual or relative increase in the concentration and/or strength of acid components. In an actual acid excess, acidosis results from processes that cause either an overproduction of acids (and release of hydrogen ions) or an underelimination of normally produced acids (retention of hydrogen ions).

In a relative acidosis, the actual amount or strength of acid components does not increase. Instead, the concentration or strength (or both) of the base components has decreased (base deficit), which makes the fluid relatively more acidic than basic (Keyes, 1990). A relative acid excess acidosis (actual base deficit) results from processes that cause either an overelimination of base components (usually in the form of bicarbonate ions, HCO_3^-) or an underproduction of base components (Fig. 18–1).

Regardless of its origin, acidosis causes significant changes in physiologic function. The primary pathologic effects are related to the fact that hydrogen ions are cations (positively charged electrolytes). An increase in hydrogen ion (H^+) concentration creates imbalances of other electrolytes, especially potassium, that disrupt functions of excitable membranes, such as nerve and cardiac tissue. Therefore, many of the early signs and symptoms associated with acidosis appear in the neuromuscular, cardiac, respiratory, and central nervous systems (Metheny, 1992).

AAABBB AAABBB AAABBB	AAAABBB AAAABBB AAAABBB	AAABB AAABB AAABB
Acid-base balance	Actual acidosis (acid excess)	Relative acidosis (base deficit)

FIGURE 18–1 ◆ Concepts of actual and relative acidosis.

In addition, even slight increases in the hydrogen ion concentration cause many proteins to become inactive. All body hormones and enzymes are composed of proteins, and many are essential for maintaining specific life-sustaining physiologic processes. Therefore, if these proteins are inactivated for even a short period, the client may die.

ETIOLOGY

Acidosis can be caused by:

- Metabolic disturbances
- Respiratory disturbances
- Combined metabolic and respiratory disturbances

The causes of metabolic and respiratory acidosis are summarized in Table 18–2.

METABOLIC ACIDOSIS

Four processes can result in metabolic acidosis:

- Overproduction of hydrogen ions
- Underelimination of hydrogen ions
- Underproduction of bicarbonate ions
- Overelimination of bicarbonate ions

OVERPRODUCTION OF HYDROGEN IONS Metabolic processes that increase body fluid hydrogen ion concentration include:

- Excessive breakdown of fatty acids
- Hypermetabolism (anaerobic lactic acidosis)
- Excessive ingestion of acidic substances

Excessive Breakdown of Fatty Acids Excessive breakdown of fatty acids is usually a result of diabetic ketoacidosis or starvation. For example, the client in diabetic ketoacidosis does not have sufficient amounts of insulin available to move glucose from the blood into cells to use as fuel for generating energy. Instead, liver and fat cells release fatty acids into the blood and other extracellular fluid. The fuel-starved cells take up these fatty acids and make high-energy substances from them. However, the metabolites (end products) from fatty acid breakdown form strong acids called *ketoacids*. These acids release large amounts of hydrogen ions.

Hypermetabolism (Anaerobic Lactic Acidosis) Hypermetabolism occurs whenever intracellular glucose is not completely metabolized to carbon dioxide, water,

TABLE 18–2 Common Causes of Acidosis

Pathology	Condition
Metabolic Acidosis	

Overproduction of hydrogen ions	• Excessive oxidation of fatty acids
	  • Diabetic ketoacidosis
	  • Starvation
	• Hypermetabolism
	  • Heavy exercise
	  • Seizure activity
	  • Fever
	  • Hypoxia, ischemia
	• Excessive ingestion of acids
	  • Ethanol intoxication
	  • Methanol ingestion
	  • Salicylate intoxication

Underelimination of hydrogen ions	• Renal failure
Underproduction of bicarbonate	• Renal failure • Pancreatitis • Liver failure
Overelimination of bicarbonate	• Diarrhea • Dehydration • Buffering of organic acids
Respiratory Acidosis	

Underelimination of hydrogen ions	• Respiratory depression
	  • Anesthetics
	  • Drugs (especially narcotics)
	  • Poisons
	  • Electrolyte imbalance
	  • Trauma
	  • Cerebral edema
	  • Spinal cord injuries
	  • Neuritic diseases
	    • Guillain-Barré
	    • Polio
	    • Myasthenia gravis
	• Inadequate chest expansion
	• Skeletal deformities
	  • Muscle weakness
	  • Nonpulmonary restriction
	    • Obesity
	    • Fluid
	    • Tumor
	• Airway obstruction
	• Alveolar-capillary block
	  • Thrombus or embolus
	  • Vascular occlusive disease
	  • Pneumonia
	  • Pulmonary edema
	  • Tuberculosis
	  • Cystic fibrosis
	  • Atelectasis
	  • ARDS
	  • Emphysema
	  • Cancer

and energy. Intracellular oxygen must be present for complete metabolism of glucose. This process is known as aerobic metabolism. When cells are forced to use glucose without adequate oxygen (anaerobic metabolism), glucose is incompletely metabolized and forms lactic acid. Lactic acid molecules leave the cell, enter the extracellular fluid, and release hydrogen ions, causing acidosis. Anaerobic metabolism that results in lactic acidosis occurs whenever oxygen is inadequate in the body. Lactic acidosis may result after heavy exercise of skeletal muscles, seizure activity, fever, and whenever there is a condition in which insufficient oxygen reaches metabolizing body tissues (Kokko & Tannen, 1990).

Excessive Intake of Acidic Substances Excessive ingestion of acidic substances floods the body directly with hydrogen ions. Some of the most common substances that cause acidosis when ingested in excess include ethyl alcohol, methyl alcohol (poison), and acetylsalicyclic acid (aspirin).

UNDERELIMINATION OF HYDROGEN IONS The major routes for hydrogen ion elimination are respiratory (via the lungs) and renal (via the kidneys). Renal failure causes acidosis when the renal tubules cannot secrete hydrogen ions into the urine. As a result, too many hydrogen ions are retained.

UNDERPRODUCTION OF BICARBONATE IONS As discussed in Chapter 17, bicarbonate (HCO_3^-) is the most common base in the fluid outside the cells and is responsible for buffering carbonic acid (H_2CO_3). When body fluid levels of bicarbonate are too low, a base deficit state exists. Base deficit acidosis occurs when hydrogen ion production and elimination are normal but too few molecules of bicarbonate ions are present to balance the hydrogen ions. Such base deficits occur when bicarbonate ions are not produced at the normal rate. Because bicarbonate is made in the kidney tubules and in the pancreas, renal failure and diminished hepatic or pancreatic function can result in a base deficit acidosis (Guyton, 1991).

OVERELIMINATION OF BICARBONATE IONS A base deficit acidosis also occurs when hydrogen ion production and elimination are normal but too many bicarbonate ions have been eliminated (overelimination). The most common example is diarrhea. The increased intestinal motility that accompanies diarrhea causes the bicarbonate-containing intestinal fluid to be lost from the body rather than absorbed.

A base deficit acidosis also can occur when bicarbonate is produced and eliminated in normal amounts but is combined with other substances instead of being freely available. For instance bicarbonate buffers other organic acids in addition to carbonic acid (Keyes, 1990). When large amounts of bicarbonate buffer substances other than carbonic acid, a base deficit acidosis may result.

RESPIRATORY ACIDOSIS

Respiratory acidosis results from an impairment in any area of respiratory function, thus causing an inadequate exchange of oxygen (O_2) and carbon dioxide (CO_2). Such impairment causes carbon dioxide to be retained. Because any increase in carbon dioxide concentration causes a corresponding increase in hydrogen ion concentration, carbon dioxide retention leads to acidosis, as demonstrated in the carbonic anhydrase equation

$$CO_2 + H_2O \longleftrightarrow H_2CO_3 \longleftrightarrow H^+ + HCO_3^-$$

An excess of carbon dioxide forces this equation to the right, first increasing the production of carbonic acid. The carbonic acid then rapidly dissociates (separates) into hydrogen ions and bicarbonate ions. This increase in the free hydrogen ion concentration of the blood is the acidosis.

Unlike metabolic acidosis, respiratory acidosis results from only one primary mechanism: the underelimination of hydrogen ions through the retention of carbon dioxide. Virtually all causes of respiratory acidosis result in an "acid-excess" acidosis. Four types of respiratory problems can cause respiratory acidosis:

- Respiratory depression
- Inadequate chest expansion
- Airway obstruction
- Interference with alveolar-capillary diffusion

RESPIRATORY DEPRESSION Respiratory depression involves a change in the function of the neurons stimulating inhalation and exhalation. The overall result is a reduced rate and depth of respiration, causing inadequate gas exchange and a retention of carbon dioxide. Respiratory depression may be chemical or physical.

Chemical Depression Chemical depression of respiratory neurons in the brain can occur as a result of the action of anesthetic agents, drugs (especially opioids), and poisons that cross the blood-brain barrier. In addition, specific electrolyte imbalances (hyponatremia, hypercalcemia, and hyperkalemia) also slow or inhibit respiratory neurons.

Physical Depression Physical depression of respiratory neurons can occur in response to many conditions. Respiratory neurons can be damaged or destroyed by trauma or when problems in other areas of the brain cause an increase in intracranial pressure. Such an increase causes edema of brain tissues, which then press on the respiratory centers (located in the brain stem). Conditions causing cerebral edema with resultant respiratory depression include brain tumors, cerebral aneurysm, cerebral vascular accidents, overhydration, and hyponatremia.

INADEQUATE CHEST EXPANSION Any condition that restricts or limits chest expansion can result in inadequate gas exchange. Inadequate chest expansion can result from skeletal trauma or deformities, respiratory muscle weakness, or nonrespiratory-associated movement restrictions.

Skeletal Problems Respiratory movements of the chest wall will be restricted if broken or malformed bones distort the shape of the chest. Broken ribs restrict chest movement by failing to provide the rigid structure needed for pressure changes to occur (as in flail chest). Pain from broken ribs may cause the client to voluntarily restrict chest movement.

Respiratory Muscle Weakness Some conditions causing respiratory muscle weakness to the degree that chest expansion may be inadequate are (Cotran et al., 1989):

- Electrolyte imbalances (especially hyperkalemia and hyponatremia)
- Fatigue
- Muscular dystrophy
- Rhabdomyosarcoma
- Inflammatory myositis

Nonrespiratory Conditions Nonrespiratory conditions also can restrict the chest movement necessary for full lung expansion. Some external causes of restricted chest movement include:

- Body cast enclosure of the thoracic cavity
- Tight scar tissue formation around the chest
- Severe obesity

Internal conditions that either displace lung tissue or increase the intrathoracic pressure may also restrict chest movement, such as:

- Thoracic or abdominal masses
- Ascites (abnormal peritoneal fluid accumulation)
- Hemothorax (blood in the thoracic cavity)
- Pneumothorax (air in the thoracic cavity)

AIRWAY OBSTRUCTION Prevention of air movement in and out of the lungs through airway obstruction can lead to ineffective gas exchange, carbon dioxide retention, and acidosis. Upper airways can be obstructed externally or internally. Conditions causing external upper airway obstruction include:

- Extreme pressure on the neck
- Use of restrictive clothing
- Nuchal (neck) edema
- Regional lymph node enlargement

Conditions causing internal upper airway obstruction include:

- Inhalation of foreign objects
- Constriction of bronchial smooth muscles
- Edema

Lower airway obstruction occurs through constriction of smooth muscle, edema, and excessive mucus. Some causes include:

- Emphysema
- Asthma
- Chronic exposure to inhalation irritants (cigarette smoke, coal dust, asbestos fibers).

Interference with Alveolar-Capillary Diffusion Most pulmonary gas exchange occurs by diffusion at the point where the alveolar membrane and the capillary membranes meet. Any condition that prevents or slows this diffusion process can cause retention of carbon dioxide and acidosis. Diffusion problems can occur at several sites:

- At the alveolar membrane
- At the capillary membrane
- In the area between the two membranes

Alveolar Membrane Problems A blocked or thickened alveolar membrane can prevent or slow diffusion of gases. Any condition that blocks the alveolar membrane increases the distance through which gases must diffuse and slows the rate of diffusion (Guyton, 1991). Such conditions include pneumonia, pulmonary edema, and aspiration of fluids.

Conditions that increase the actual thickness of the alveolar membrane create a physical barrier to diffusion. These conditions include radiation pneumonitis, tuberculosis, and emphysema.

When alveoli are collapsed, gas exchange cannot occur. Some causes of alveolar collapse include emphysema, asthma, adult respiratory distress syndrome (ARDS), near-freshwater drowning, high concentration oxygen therapy, chest trauma, and sepsis (Cotran et al., 1989).

Capillary Membrane Problems A problem in the capillary membrane inhibits gas exchange and causes acidosis by blocking blood flow through the capillaries. Such conditions include hypovolemic shock with vascular collapse and the formation of thrombi or emboli (blood clots).

Problems Between the Alveolar and Capillary Membranes Problems between the alveolar and capillary membranes increase the distance between these membranes and slow the rate of diffusion. Some conditions that increase the distance between the alveolar and capillary membranes include pulmonary edema, interstitial fibrosis, and cancer.

COMBINED METABOLIC AND RESPIRATORY ACIDOSIS

Metabolic and respiratory acidosis processes can occur at the same time. An uncorrected acute respiratory acidosis always leads to anaerobic (lacking molecular oxygen) metabolism and lactic acidosis (Metheny, 1992). The resulting acidosis is more profound than that caused by either metabolic acidosis or respiratory acidosis alone. Cardiac arrest is an example of a condition leading to combined metabolic and respiratory acidosis. Another example is the development of severe diarrhea in a client with chronic obstructive lung disease.

INCIDENCE/PREVALENCE

Because acidosis is a manifestation of many pathologic conditions rather than a separate disease state, its actual incidence is not known. However, mild metabolic acidosis that results from lactic acidosis is common among healthy persons. Normal respiratory compensation usually prevents this problem from becoming severe or prolonged, and no intervention is necessary. Clients particularly at risk for acidosis are those with conditions that impair any aspect of respiratory function to any degree, as in the elderly.

COLLABORATIVE MANAGEMENT

ASSESSMENT

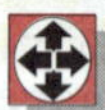

HISTORY

When obtaining a history from any client, the nurse collects data related to risk factors as well as causative factors related to the development of acidosis.

AGE Age is an important factor because the elderly are more vulnerable to conditions that may cause an acid-base imbalance. Such conditions include impairments of cardiac, renal, and pulmonary functions. In addition, elderly persons are more likely to be taking prescribed or over-the-counter medications that interfere with acid-base, fluid, and electrolyte balance, especially diuretics, aspirin, and products containing alcohol. The nurse asks about specific risk factors such as the presence of any type of respiratory problem, renal failure, diabetes mellitus, persistent diarrhea, pancreatitis, or fever.

NUTRITION The nurse obtains a detailed diet history to determine total caloric intake as well as the approximate proportions of carbohydrates, fats, and proteins of the foods ingested. The nurse specifically asks the client if he or she has fasted or followed a strict diet during the preceding week. Such questions on food and alcohol intake as well as the previous 24-hour dietary recall, can be helpful for the nurse in the client assessment.

SYMPTOMS The nurse also asks the client about any symptoms that might indicate the presence of acidosis. Because a person's central nervous system is frequently depressed in acidosis, the nurse may question a close family member or the client's significant other. The nurse should ask the client whether he or she has experienced headaches, behavior changes, increased drowsiness, reduced alertness, reduced attention span, lethargy, anorexia, abdominal distention, nausea or vomiting, muscle weakness, or increased fatigue. Having the client relate activities of the previous 24 hours may disclose additional information about activity intolerance, changes in behavior, and the presence of unexplained fatigue.

PHYSICAL ASSESSMENT/CLINICAL MANIFESTATIONS

The clinical manifestations of acidosis are similar whether the cause is metabolic or respiratory (Chart 18-1). Clinical manifestations are associated primarily with changes in activity of excitable membranes involved in cerebral, neuromuscular, and gastric smooth muscle functions.

CHART 18-1

Key Features of Acidosis

Central Nervous System Manifestations

- Depressed activity (lethargy, confusion, stupor, and coma)

Neuromuscular Manifestations

- Hyporeflexia
- Skeletal muscle weakness
- Flaccid paralysis

Cardiovascular Manifestations

- Delayed electrical conduction
  - Bradycardia to block
  - Tall T-waves
  - Widened QRS complex
  - Prolonged PR interval
- Hypotension
- Thready peripheral pulses

Respiratory Manifestations

- Kussmaul respirations (in metabolic acidosis with respiratory compensation)
- Variable respirations (generally ineffective in respiratory acidosis)

Integumentary Manifestations

- Warm, flushed, dry skin in metabolic acidosis
- Pale to cyanotic and dry skin in respiratory acidosis

CENTRAL NERVOUS SYSTEM MANIFESTATIONS Depression of central nervous system functions is common in acidosis and may be manifested as lethargy that progresses to confusion, especially in elderly clients. As the acidosis worsens or if it is accompanied by hyperkalemia, the client may become stuporous and unresponsive. The nurse assesses the client's level of consciousness (see Chap. 40).

NEUROMUSCULAR MANIFESTATIONS The actual increase in the serum hydrogen ion concentration as well as any accompanying hyperkalemia causes a decrease in muscle tone and deep tendon reflexes. The nurse assesses muscle strength by having the client:

- Squeeze the nurse's hand
- Attempt to keep arms flexed while the nurse pulls downward on the lower arms
- Push both feet against a flat surface while the nurse applies resistance

Muscle weakness associated with acidosis is bilateral and can progress to flaccid paralysis. Respiratory movements diminish when skeletal muscles become weak.

CARDIOVASCULAR MANIFESTATIONS Early cardiac manifestations of acidosis include increased heart rate and cardiac output. However, as acidosis worsens or if it is accompanied by hyperkalemia, electrical conduction through the myocardium is reduced and bradycardia (slow heart rate) results. The nurse monitors for clinical as well as electrocardiographic (ECG) changes. As a result of cardiac changes, peripheral pulses may be hard to find and are easily blocked with light pressure. The client may experience hypotension as a result of vasodilation.

RESPIRATORY MANIFESTATIONS The nurse assesses the client's respiratory system by observing the rate, depth, and ease of respirations.

Metabolic Cause When the acidosis has a metabolic origin, the rate and depth of respiration increase in proportion to the increase in the hydrogen ion concentration. Respirations are deep and rapid and are not under voluntary control. This pattern is called *Kussmaul respiration.*

Respiratory Cause When the acidosis has a respiratory origin, the effectiveness of respiratory efforts is greatly diminished. Respirations are usually shallow and quite rapid.

INTEGUMENTARY MANIFESTATIONS In metabolic acidosis, respiration is unimpaired and respiratory rate is increased. The increased gas exchange, coupled with a vasodilation, makes the client's skin and mucous membranes warm, dry, and pink. Because respirations are ineffective in respiratory acidosis, skin and mucous membranes are pale to cyanotic.

PSYCHOSOCIAL ASSESSMENT

It is important for the nurse to complete a psychosocial assessment because behavioral changes resulting from central nervous system effects may be the first observable clinical manifestations of acidosis. The nurse observes and documents the client's presenting behavior by description (objectively) rather than by interpretation (subjectively). For example, the nurse may state that "the client is unable to recognize close family members" rather than "the client is confused"; or "the client spit out the oral medication" rather than "the client is uncooperative." The nurse questions family members and significant others to determine whether the presenting behavior and mental status are typical for this client.

LABORATORY ASSESSMENT

The most definitive laboratory value to confirm the presence of acidosis is the arterial blood pH. When arterial blood pH is less than 7.35, acidosis is present. However, this test alone does not indicate the underlying pathologic condition or the origin of the acidosis. Because the clinical manifestations of metabolic acidosis and respiratory acidosis are similar and the effective treatments are different, it is critical that the nurse obtain and interpret additional laboratory data, such as arterial blood gas (ABG) values and measurements of certain serum electrolytes (Chart 18–2).

METABOLIC ACIDOSIS The presence of a pure metabolic acidosis is indicated by:

- A low pH
- A low bicarbonate level
- A normal $PaCO_2$
- An elevated serum potassium level

pH The pH is low because buffering and respiratory compensation are not adequate to maintain the hydrogen ion concentration at a normal level.

Bicarbonate The decreased bicarbonate level, coupled with the normal carbon dioxide level, indicates that the acidosis process is metabolic. The bicarbonate level is below normal for any one (or all) of the following reasons:

- Bicarbonate has been lost from the body, creating the actual base deficit acidosis.

CHART 18–2

Lab Profile ♦ Acid-Base Imbalances

Imbalance	pH	HCO_3^-	PaO_2	$PaCO_2$	K^+	Ca^{2+}	Cl^-
	Laboratory Value Changes*						
Metabolic acidosis	↓	↓	∅	∅	↑	∅	↑
Respiratory acidosis	↓	↑	↓	↑	↑	∅	↓↑
Combined acidosis	↓	↑	↓	↑	↑	∅	↑
Metabolic alkalosis	↑	↑	∅	↑	↓	↓	↓
Respiratory alkalosis	↑	↓	∅	↓	↓	↓	↑
Combined alkalosis	↑	↑	∅	↓	↓	↓	↓

* ↑ indicates above normal; ↓, below normal; ∅, normal.

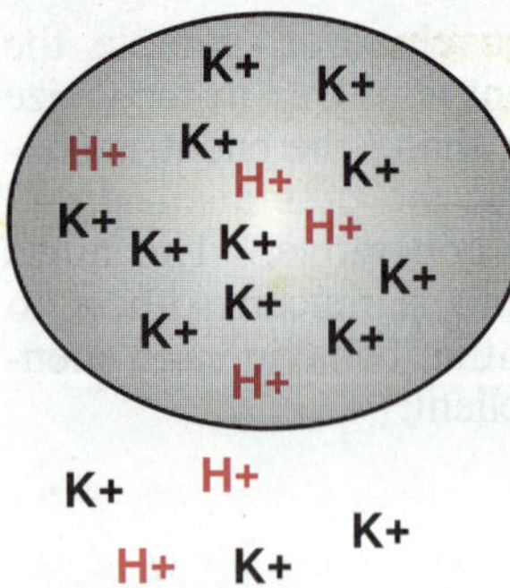

Under normal conditions, the intercellular potassium content is much greater than that of the extracellular fluid. The concentration of hydrogen ions is low in both compartments.

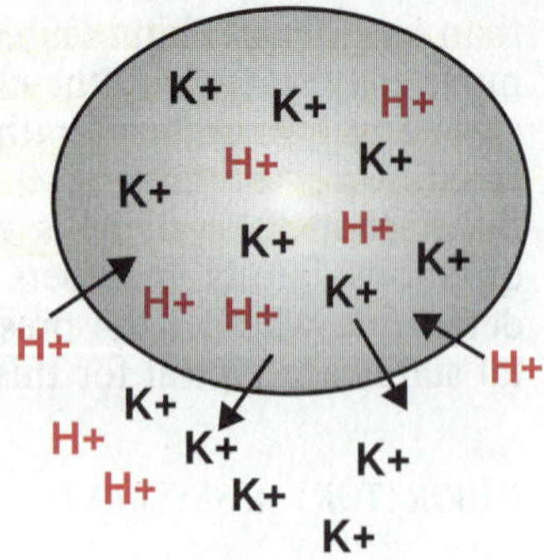

In acidemia, the extracellular hydrogen ion content increases, and the hydrogen ions move into the intracellular fluid. To keep the intracellular fluid electrically neutral, an equal number of potassium ions leave the cell, creating a relative hyperkalemia.

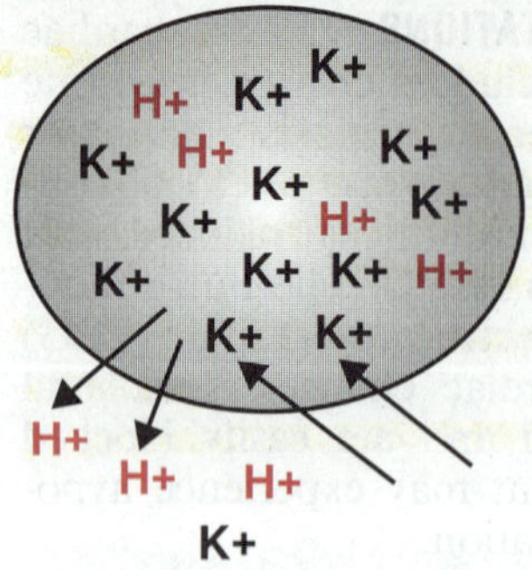

In alkalemia, more hydrogen ions are present in the intracellular fluid than in the extracellular fluid. Hydrogen ions move from the intracellular fluid into the extracellular fluid. To keep the intracellular fluid electrically neutral, potassium ions move from the extracellular fluid into the intracellular fluid, creating a relative hyperkalemia.

FIGURE 18–2 ◆ Movement of potassium response to changes in extracellular hydrogen ion concentration. (© 1992 M. Linda Workman. All rights reserved.)

- Bicarbonate has not been produced in sufficient quantities, creating the actual base deficit acidosis.
- Bicarbonate may be bound to other substances during the buffering of organic acid-stimulated acidosis.

Carbon Dioxide and Oxygen The carbon dioxide level is normal (or even slightly decreased) because gas exchange is adequate and retention of carbon dioxide is not a factor in this process. The oxygen level is normal because gas exchange is adequate.

Potassium The serum potassium level is frequently elevated in metabolic acidosis as a result of the body's attempt to maintain electroneutrality during buffering. In some cases, prolonged elevation of potassium in the blood may contribute to the development of metabolic acidosis.

Figure 18–2 demonstrates movement of potassium ions associated with changes in serum pH. As the hydrogen ion concentration of the blood increases, some of the excess hydrogen ions enter cells (especially red blood cells), the site of intracellular buffering mechanisms. The movement of hydrogen ions into the cells creates an intracellular excess of positive ions. To prevent intracellular charge imbalances, an equal number of potassium ions move from the cells into the blood. This increases the extracellular potassium concentration and causes an associated hyperkalemia.

RESPIRATORY ACIDOSIS The presence of respiratory acidosis is indicated by:

- A low pH
- Elevated $PaCO_2$
- A decreased PaO_2

Changes in bicarbonate and serum potassium levels vary with the duration of the acidosis and the degree of renal compensation (see Chap. 17).

pH The pH is low because an increase in the extracellular fluid hydrogen ion concentration is present. If the renal system partially compensates for this acidosis, the pH is low but not as abnormal as could be expected, considering the degree of derangement apparent in the retention of carbon dioxide.

Carbon Dioxide and Oxygen The $PaCO_2$ is elevated and the PaO_2 is decreased because the cause of this acid-base disturbance is an impairment of gas exchange. The impairment causes carbon dioxide to be retained, along with an inability of the client to take in adequate amounts of oxygen.

Bicarbonate When the onset of respiratory acidosis is acute, the bicarbonate level is normal because no bicarbonate has been lost from the body and it is buffering only carbonic acid. When the respiratory acidosis persists for at least 24 hours or longer, renal compensation for the acidosis results in increased generation and reabsorption of bicarbonate. Thus, an elevated bicarbonate level, coupled with the increased $PaCO_2$, indicates the presence of chronic respiratory acidosis.

Potassium Other electrolyte values change when respiratory acidosis is chronic. During acute respiratory acidosis, serum potassium levels are elevated. When respiratory acidosis is chronic and renal compensation is present, serum potassium levels are normal or low.

OTHER DIAGNOSTIC ASSESSMENT

The client with acidosis typically should undergo one or more electrocardiographic (ECG) evaluations, primarily to detect changes caused by an increased potassium level. Such changes include the presence of tall T waves, a widened QRS complex, and a prolonged PR interval (see Fig. 16–1). Ventricular dysrhythmias are common. The nurse compares these findings with the client's healthy baseline ECG if available.

ANALYSIS

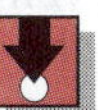

COMMON NURSING DIAGNOSES

1. Ineffective Breathing Pattern related to decreased lung expansion, alveolar inflammation, and lower airway obstruction
2. Activity Intolerance related to an imbalance between oxygen supply and demand
3. Altered Thought Processes related to lack of oxygen to the brain

ADDITIONAL NURSING DIAGNOSES

In addition to the common diagnoses, the client experiencing acidosis may present with one or more of the following diagnoses:

1. Altered Nutrition: Less than Body Requirements related to fatigue and increased metabolic needs
2. High Risk for Injury related to alterations in thought processes
3. Self Care Deficit: Total related to fatigue
4. High Risk for Infection related to increased pulmonary secretions

PLANNING AND IMPLEMENTATION

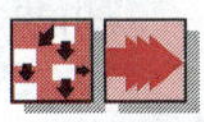

INEFFECTIVE BREATHING PATTERN

PLANNING: CLIENT GOALS The major goals are that the client will:

- Have a patent airway
- Increase the effectiveness of respiratory efforts
- Not experience respiratory complications

INTERVENTIONS The interventions for ineffective breathing patterns in clients with chronic acidosis are aimed at maintaining a patent airway and enhancing gas exchange. Interventions include:

- Drug therapy
- Oxygen therapy
- Positioning, breathing techniques
- Prevention of complications

(For a complete discussion of chronic obstructive pulmonary diseases [COPD] also known as chronic airflow limitations [CAL], see Chapter 30.)

Drug Therapy Drug therapy includes the use of agents that increase the diameter of upper and lower airways and that thin the pulmonary secretions. Drug therapy is not aimed directly at altering the arterial pH.

DRUGS THAT INCREASE AIRWAY DIAMETER Drugs that increase airway diameter induce relaxation of bronchial smooth muscle. Many of these agents are adrenergic agonists, sympathomimetic agents, antimuscarinic drugs, and methylxanthines. These drugs include albuterol (Novosalmol♣, Proventil, Ventolin), ephedrine, fenoterol (Berotec), isoproterenol (Isuprel), metaproterenol (Alupent), pributerol (Maxair), terbutaline (Brethine, Bricanyl), ipratropium (Atrovent), atropine, aminophylline (Amoline, Palaron♣, Somophyllin), and theophylline (Bronkodyl, Theo♣-Dur).

Clients may take agents that increase bronchodilation by reducing inflammation of bronchial luminal tissues. These agents are primarily cortisol (steroid)-based, such as beclomethasone (Vanceril, Beclovent), dexamethasone (Decadron Respihaler, Dexasone♣), flunisolide (Aerobid, Bronalide♣), and triamcinolone (Azmacort).

DRUGS THAT THIN BRONCHIAL SECRETIONS Some drugs can break up mucus when thick, tenacious pulmonary secretions contribute to airway obstruction. These agents are classified as mucolytic; an example is acetylcysteine (Airbron♣, Mucomyst, Respaire). (For a discussion of drugs used for clients with COPD or CAL, see Chapter 30.)

Oxygen Therapy Oxygen therapy can help promote gas exchange for the client with acidosis. However, the nurse must use caution when administering oxygen to clients with CAL and carbon dioxide retention, as evidenced by a high $PaCO_2$ level in arterial blood. (For a detailed description of the nursing responsibilities of administering oxygen, see Chapter 30.)

Pulmonary Hygiene To promote gas exchange, the nurse considers client positioning, techniques to enhance excretion of pulmonary secretions, and specific breathing techniques to change airway resistance and maintain inflated alveoli. To help the client increase lung expansion, the nurse helps the client assume a Fowler's or semi-Fowler's position. (For techniques to help with excretion of pulmonary secretions, including chest physiotherapy and deep breathing exercises, see Chapter 30.) Increasing the client's fluid intake also may reduce the thickness of pulmonary secretions and assist in improving their excretion.

At least every 2 hours, the nurse assesses the respiratory status of the client who is experiencing chronic respiratory acidosis. In addition to assessing the rate and depth of respiration, the nurse performs auscultation of breath sounds. The nurse notes the ease with which the client moves air in and out of the lungs, including the presence of any muscle retractions, use of accessory muscles, and whether respiratory effort produces a sound that can be heard without a stethoscope. The nurse notes the color of the nail beds and mucous membranes.

ACTIVITY INTOLERANCE

PLANNING: CLIENT GOALS The major client goals are that the client will:

- Not experience an increase in fatigue
- Increase activity as tolerated, including participation in self-care activities

INTERVENTIONS Interventions are aimed at preventing increased acidosis resulting from respiratory problems and at conserving the client's energy. Drug therapies and oxygen therapy are used to enhance gas exchange and are described under the nursing diagnosis Ineffective Breathing Pattern.

Nutrition The client must ingest enough calories to meet energy requirements, but this can be difficult when the client is fatigued. In collaboration with the dietitian, the nurse provides small, frequent meals high in protein and carbohydrate.

Energy Conservation The nurse assesses the client's schedule of activities during hospitalization. The nurse than evaluates activities that do not have a direct positive effect on the client's condition in terms of their usefulness to the client. If the benefit of the activity does not outweigh its actual or potential aggravation of the client's fatigue, the nurse consults with other members of the health care team about eliminating or postponing the activity. Examples include physical therapy and specific invasive diagnostic tests not required for assessment or treatment of presenting problems.

ALTERED THOUGHT PROCESSES

PLANNING: CLIENT GOALS The major goal is that the client will remain oriented to person, time, and place.

INTERVENTIONS The nurse assesses changes in central nervous system activity from normal or from baseline activity. This assessment serves as a basis for initiating specific interventions.

The nurse assesses the client's mental status at least every 4 hours to evaluate the effectiveness of current interventions and to determine whether the acid-base imbalance continues to exist. This assessment includes the client's:

- Level of consciousness
- Orientation to time, place, and person
- Past and recent memory
- Ability to concentrate
- Cognitive function

The nurse is sensitive to the elderly person who may seem disoriented because of an abrupt change in his or her environment. Therefore, the nurse makes the assessment when the client is fully awake and after the client has had time to adjust to the hospital setting. In this way, the nurse can distinguish normal, temporary disorientation due to unfamiliarity from disorientation due to an acid-base or electrolyte imbalance. Other nursing interventions for the elderly client experiencing acid-base imbalances are presented in Chart 18–3.

If the client is disoriented, the nurse initiates interventions to promote orientation, such as prompting the client or providing cues (hints) about the environment. Use of large calendars and clocks also can

CHART 18–3

Nursing Focus on the Elderly ◆ The Elderly Client Experiencing Acid-Base Imbalance

When Taking a Client's History:

- Assess the risk factors for acid-base imbalance including medications, chronic health problems (especially renal disease, pulmonary disease), and acute health problems.
- Take the history when the client is awake and more familiar with surroundings.
- Ask the client to list all prescribed and over-the-counter medications (especially diuretics and antacids). If the client cannot recall this information or seems confused, ask the significant other to bring medications from home to show the nurse.
- Ask the client to recall what liquids she or he has taken in the past 24 hours and whether the client has urinated as much as usual.

When Assessing the Client:

- Compare the client's mental status with what the family, significant other, or health record states is the client's baseline.
- Observe the rate and depth of respiration:
  - Can the client complete a sentence without stopping to take a breath?
  - Examine the color of the client's nail beds and mucous membranes.
- Obtain a specimen of urine and observe for color and character. Test for specific gravity and pH.
- Examine skin turgor to determine whether dehydration is present. Attempt to pinch the skin up to form a tent over the sternum and on the forehead. If a tent forms, record how long it remains.
- Measure the rate and quality of the pulse.

Observe the client's clinical responses and laboratory values carefully while the acid-base imbalance is being corrected.

Administer intravenous therapy by pump or controller.

help reorient clients. (Chapter 40 details the mental status assessment and interventions for client reorientation.)

DISCHARGE PLANNING

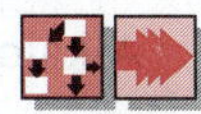

HOME CARE PREPARATION

Acidosis that results from chronic respiratory acidosis may be resolved before the client's discharge from the hospital, but the underlying contributing factors may remain problematic and may become more severe with time. Usually, the severity of the pathologic condition increases the chances that acidosis will recur. Many clients with chronic obstructive pulmonary disease (COPD), or chronic airway limitation (CAL), and chronic respiratory acidosis cannot work or live alone.

If the client is being discharged to the home, the hospital nurse contacts a home health nurse to assess the physical home environment to meet the client's needs for safety and activities of daily living. Special equipment (e.g., an electric hospital bed or portable oxygen) may be needed.

Because respiratory illnesses are chronic, clients may already be participating in a long-term follow-up program. In this case, the hospital staff nurse contacts the follow-up team to update the team about the client's current health status.

HEALTH TEACHING

The nurse instructs the client and family in the signs and symptoms of acidosis; in addition, the nurse asks them to pay close attention to symptoms such as increased sleepiness, headache, increased irritability, or disorientation. Family members are instructed to regard as significant any persistent behavior change or the onset of lethargy.

PSYCHOSOCIAL PREPARATION

Clients whose episodes of acidosis are related to long-standing chronic obstructive pulmonary disease (COPD), or chronic airway limitation (CAL), may have learned to cope with their health problems and require little intensive psychosocial support. However, the nurse cannot assume that this is the case. The nurse assesses each client's psychosocial needs in terms of new factors, established support systems, previous and current coping patterns, and the progression of the chronic disease. Most clients with COPD have changed their lifestyles because of activity intolerance. As a result, many of these clients lack social interactions and many fear being alone.

HEALTH CARE RESOURCES

For the client with chronic respiratory acidosis who is discharged home, the appropriate health care resources include the physician, pharmacist, respiratory therapist, nutritionist, and home health care nurse. Social services personnel are helpful if the client cannot obtain the necessary medication and oxygen support.

When a client cannot return home after discharge, placement in an extended care facility may be necessary. Chapter 30 covers the discharge planning for the client with chronic obstructive pulmonary disease or chronic airway limitation.

EVALUATION

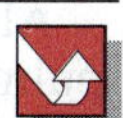

On the basis of identified nursing diagnoses, the nurse evaluates the care for the client experiencing acidosis. The expected outcomes are that the client will

- Maintain a patent airway
- Minimize respiratory effort through specific interventions
- Increase activity tolerance to include participation in self-care activities
- Be oriented to person, time, and place

Alkalosis

OVERVIEW

In a person with alkalosis, the acid-base balance of the extracellular fluid (ECF) is disturbed and is characterized by an excess of bases, especially bicarbonate (HCO_3^-). The concentration and/or strength of base components are proportionately higher than normal compared with the concentration and/or strength of the acid components. Alkalosis is defined as a decrease in the hydrogen ion concentration of the blood and is reflected by an arterial blood pH above 7.45.

Alkalosis is not a disease; instead, it is a manifestation of a disease or pathologic process. Alkalosis can be caused by metabolic problems, respiratory problems, or both.

PATHOPHYSIOLOGY

Alkalosis can result from an actual or relative increase in the concentration and/or strength of base components. In an actual base excess, alkalosis is the result of processes that cause either an overproduction of base components or an underelimination of normally produced base components (usually bicarbonate).

In a relative alkalosis, the actual amount or strength of base components does not increase. Instead, the concentration or strength (or both) of the acid components has decreased (acid deficit), which makes the fluid relatively more basic than acidic. A relative base excess alkalosis (actual acid deficit) results from processes that cause either an overelimination of acid components (usually as hydrogen ions) or an underproduction of acid components (Fig. 18–3).

AAABBB AAABBB AAABBB	AAABBBB AAABBBB AAABBBB	AABBB AABBB AABBB
Acid-base balance	Actual alkalosis (base excess)	Relative alkalosis (acid deficit)

FIGURE 18-3 ◆ Concepts of actual and relative alkalosis.

Alkalosis causes disturbances in metabolism and in pulmonary respiration. Consequences can be serious and life-threatening. Because alkalosis is the manifestation of another abnormal process (or processes), treatment is most effective when it is directed at the underlying abnormal processes. Treatment that is effective for metabolic alkalosis is different from treatment that is effective for respiratory alkalosis. Therefore, one must be able to distinguish between metabolic and respiratory alkalosis in order to prevent and manage this condition.

Whether its origin is metabolic, respiratory, or both, alkalosis greatly affects specific physiologic functions. The pathologic effects are related to the accompanying electrolyte imbalances that occur in response to decreased blood cation concentration. The most common manifestations of alkalosis are associated with increased stimulation of the central nervous, neuromuscular, and cardiovascular systems.

ETIOLOGY

Alkalosis can be caused by:

- Metabolic disturbances
- Respiratory disturbances
- Combined metabolic and respiratory disturbances

The causes of alkalosis are summarized on Table 18-3.

METABOLIC ALKALOSIS

Most conditions that result in metabolic alkalosis create the acid-base disturbance through either of two mechanisms:

- An actual increase of base components
- An actual decrease of acid components

INCREASES IN BASE COMPONENTS Increases in base components (base excesses) occur as a result of oral or parenteral ingestion of bicarbonates, carbonates, acetates, citrates, and lactates. Excessive use of oral

TABLE 18-3 Common Causes of Alkalosis

Pathology	Condition
Metabolic Alkalosis	

Increase of base components	• Oral ingestion of bases
	  • Antacids
	  • Milk-alkali syndrome
	• Parenteral base administration
	  • Blood transfusion
	  • Sodium bicarbonate
	  • Total parenteral nutrition (TPN)

Decrease of acid components	• Prolonged vomiting • Nasogastric suctioning • Cushing's syndrome (hypercortisolism) • Hyperaldosteronism • Thiazide diuretics
Respiratory Alkalosis	

Excessive loss of carbon dioxide	• Hyperventilation
	  • Fear
	  • Anxiety
	  • Mechanical ventilation
	  • CNS stimulation
	    • Salicylates
	    • Catecholamines
	    • Progesterone
	• Hypoxemia
	  • Asphyxiation
	  • High altitudes
	  • Shock
	  • Early-stage pulmonary problems
	    • Pneumonia
	    • Asthma
	    • Pulmonary emboli

antacids containing sodium bicarbonate or calcium bicarbonate can cause a metabolic acidosis. Other base excesses can occur as a result of some medical treatments, such as:

- Citrate excesses during rapid and/or massive blood transfusions
- Acetate and lactate excesses during hyperalimentation
- Intravenous sodium bicarbonate administration for correction of lactic acidosis or ketoacidosis

DECREASES IN ACID COMPONENTS Decreases in acid components (acid deficit) can occur in response to disease processes or medical treatment. Contributing conditions include prolonged vomiting, Cushing's syndrome (hypercortisolism), and hyperaldosteronism. Medical treatments that promote acid loss and can cause a metabolic alkalosis include the use of thiazide diuretics and prolonged nasogastric suctioning (Mendyka, 1992).

RESPIRATORY ALKALOSIS

The primary mechanism responsible for respiratory alkalosis is the excessive loss of carbon dioxide through hyperventilation (increased, shallow respirations).

Clients may hyperventilate in response to anxiety, fear, or improper settings on mechanical ventilators. Hyperventilation can also result from direct stimulation of the central chemoreceptors in the brain.

Conditions that stimulate the central chemoreceptors directly include fever, respiratory compensation for metabolic acidosis, central nervous system lesions, and certain drugs (e.g., salicylates, catecholamines, and progesterone).

CHART 18–4

Key Features of Alkalosis

Central Nervous System Manifestations

- Increased activity
- Anxiety, irritability, tetany, seizures
- Positive Chvostek's sign
- Positive Trousseau's sign
- Paresthesias

Neuromuscular Manifestations

- Hyperreflexia
- Muscle cramping and twitching
- Skeletal muscle weakness

Cardiovascular Manifestations

- Increased heart rate
- Normal or low blood pressure
- Increased digitalis toxicity

Respiratory Manifestations

- Increased rate and depth of ventilation in respiratory alkalosis
- Decreased respiratory effort associated with skeletal muscle weakness in metabolic alkalosis

COLLABORATIVE MANAGEMENT

ASSESSMENT

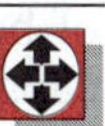

PHYSICAL ASSESSMENT/CLINICAL MANIFESTATIONS

Whether its origin is metabolic or respiratory, clinical manifestations of alkalosis are consistent. Many symptoms are the result of the hypocalcemia (low calcium levels) and hypokalemia (low potassium levels) that usually accompany alkalosis. These manifestations are associated with changes in central nervous system, neuromuscular, and cardiovascular functions (Chart 18–4).

CENTRAL NERVOUS SYSTEM MANIFESTATIONS Overexcitement of the central and peripheral nervous systems is the major cause of symptoms associated with alkalosis. Clients experience lightheadedness, agitation, confusion, and hyperreflexia that may progress to seizure activity. Paresthesias may be present as tingling or numbness around the mouth and in the toes. Other reliable indicators of alkalosis with accompanying hypocalcemia are positive Chvostek's and Trousseau's signs (see Chapter 16).

NEUROMUSCULAR MANIFESTATIONS Alkalosis with hypocalcemia or hypokalemia increases the activity of the nervous system. Nerve stimulation results in nonvoluntary skeletal muscle contractions that are manifested as cramps, twitches, and "charley horses." Deep tendon reflexes are hyperactive. *Tetany* (continuous spasms) of isolated muscle groups may be present. Tetany is painful and indicates a rapidly worsening condition.

Although skeletal muscles may contract as a result of overstimulation by the nerves, the skeletal muscles themselves become weaker because of the alkalosis and hypokalemia. Hand-grasp strength diminishes, and the client may be unable to walk or support his or her own weight. The client's respiratory efforts become less effective as the skeletal muscles of respiration become weaker.

CARDIOVASCULAR MANIFESTATIONS Alkalosis causes an increase in the irritability of the myocardium, especially in the presence of an accompanying hypokalemia. The heart rate increases, and the pulse is "thready." When hypovolemia also is present, the client may experience profound hypotension. Alkalosis also causes the myocardium to be more sensitive to digitalis derivatives, resulting in an increased risk for digitalis toxicity.

RESPIRATORY MANIFESTATIONS Alterations in the rate and depth of respiration are the underlying causes of respiratory alkalosis. Tidal volume (the volume of air inhaled and exhaled with each breath) is nearly normal, but minute respiratory volume (the total volume of air inhaled and exhaled in one minute's time) rises in proportion to the increase in rate. The increase in minute respiratory volume may result from other physiologic changes or from anxiety.

LABORATORY ASSESSMENT

The most definitive laboratory value to confirm the presence of alkalosis is the arterial blood pH. When arterial blood pH is above 7.45, alkalosis is present. However, this test alone does not identify the underlying pathologic condition or the origin of the alkalosis. Because the clinical manifestations of metabolic alkalosis are similar to those of respiratory alkalosis, it is critical that the nurse obtain additional laboratory data, especially arterial blood gas (ABG) values and measurements of specific serum electrolytes (see Chart 18–2).

METABOLIC ALKALOSIS The presence of a metabolic alkalosis is indicated by:

- A high pH (above 7.45)
- An elevated bicarbonate level (above 28 mEq/L)
- A normal PaO_2
- A rising $PaCO_2$
- Decreased serum potassium levels
- Decreased serum calcium levels

The pH is high because buffering and respiratory compensation are not adequate to maintain the hydrogen ion concentration at a normal level.

The increased bicarbonate level, coupled with a rising $PaCO_2$, is the hallmark of metabolic alkalosis. The rising $PaCO_2$ compensates for the decreased hydrogen ion concentration. The serum potassium level is decreased as a result of the body's attempt to maintain electroneutrality during acid-base imbalances (see Fig. 18–2). As the pH increases, calcium binding increases and the concentration of serum calcium decreases, creating an accompanying state of hypocalcemia. Most of the serious clinical manifestations of alkalosis are attributed to this accompanying hypocalcemia.

RESPIRATORY ALKALOSIS Arterial blood data that demonstrate the presence of a respiratory alkalosis are as follows:

- A high pH
- A reduced bicarbonate level
- A reduced $PaCO_2$
- A reduced serum potassium level
- A reduced serum calcium level

The pH is high because buffering and renal compensation cannot maintain the hydrogen ion concentration at a normal level.

The classic picture of respiratory alkalosis is the reduced bicarbonate level (not usually below 15 mEq/L) coupled with a very low $PaCO_2$. The carbon dioxide level is low because it is being exhaled through hyperventilation more rapidly than it is being made. The bicarbonate level is reduced in response to the pH increase. A variety of blood and intracellular buffers generate hydrogen ions, which immediately combine with the serum bicarbonate ions and form carbonic acid, thus reducing the serum concentration of bicarbonate.

As in metabolic alkalosis, the serum potassium level is reduced as a result of the body's attempt to maintain electroneutrality during acid-base imbalances. Again, as the pH increases, calcium binding increases, and the concentration of serum calcium decreases, resulting in hypocalcemia.

INTERVENTIONS

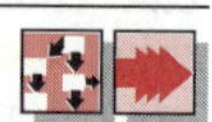

Interventions are aimed at:

- Preventing further losses of hydrogen, potassium, calcium, and chloride ions
- Restoring fluid balance

Drug therapy is the intervention of choice for alkalosis. Drug therapy is prescribed to resolve the underlying causes of alkalosis and to restore normal fluid, electrolyte, and acid-base balance. For example, the client with metabolic alkalosis that has resulted from diuretic therapy receives fluid and electrolyte replacement and is then re-evaluated by the physician for the need to resume a diuretic. The physician may prescribe a different type of diuretic, perhaps one that is potassium-sparing, to prevent potassium loss. For the client who is experiencing prolonged vomiting, the physician orders antiemetic medications to halt the problem. In addition, fluids and electrolytes are replaced, orally, parenterally, or in some combination of both. The nurse carefully monitors and records the client's intake and output. Serum electrolyte values are monitored daily or every other day until a return to normal or near-normal.

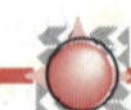

IMPLICATIONS FOR NURSING RESEARCH

Nursing research is needed to answer the following questions about the care of clients at risk for or with an actual acid-base imbalance:

- ◆ What is the relationship between hydration status and tenacity of pulmonary secretions?
- ◆ Does external mechanical chest vibration increase excretion of pulmonary secretions?

- How long should pressure be applied to an arterial puncture site to prevent the formation of a hematoma?
- What mental status changes are associated with acid-base imbalance?
- When pulmonary problems are unilateral, does positioning make a difference in oxygenation?

SELECTED BIBLIOGRAPHY

Anderson, S. (1990). ABGs: Six easy steps to interpreting blood gases. *American Journal of Nursing, 90*(8), 42–45.

*Brenner, B., Coe, F. L., & Rector, F. C. (1987). *Renal physiology in health and disease.* Philadelphia: W. B. Saunders.

*Cotran, R., Kumar, V., & Robbins, S. (1989). *Robbins pathologic basis of disease* (4th ed). Philadelphia: W. B. Saunders.

Guyton, A. C. (1991). *Textbook of medical physiology* (8th ed). Philadelphia: W. B. Saunders.

Hamm, L. (1990). Mixed acid-base disorders. In J. Kokko & R. L. Tannen (Eds.), *Fluids and electrolytes* (pp. 485–504). Philadelphia: W. B. Saunders.

Janusek, L. (1990). Metabolic alkalosis. *Nursing90, 20*(6), 49–50.

Janusek, L. (1990). Metabolic acidosis. *Nursing90, 20*(7), 52–53.

Keyes, J. (1990). *Fluid, electrolyte, and acid-base regulation.* Boston: Jones & Bartlett.

Kokko, J., & Tannen, R. L. (1990). *Fluids and electrolytes* (2nd ed.). Philadelphia: W. B. Saunders.

Mendyka, B. (1992). *AACN Clinical Issues in Critical Care, 3*(3), 672–680.

Metheny, N. (1992). *Fluid and electrolyte balance: Nursing considerations* (2nd ed.). Philadelphia: J. B. Lippincott.

Molony, D., Schiess, M., & Evanoff, G. (1990). Respiratory acid-base disorders. In J. Kokko & R. L. Tannen (Eds.), *Fluids and electrolytes* (pp. 391–484). Philadelphia: W. B. Saunders.

Morris, L. (1990). The POLK method of ABG interpretation. *Critical Care Nurse, 10*(1), 18–20.

*Robbins, S. L., & Kumar, V. (1987). *Basic pathology* (4th ed). Philadelphia: W. B. Saunders.

Russell, J. (1991). Successful method for arterial blood gas interpretation. *Critical Care Nurse, 11*(5), 14–19.

Scherer, P. (1990). Get true blood gas values with less blood loss. *American Journal of Nursing, 90*(2), 28.

Schrier, R. (1992). *Renal and electrolyte disorders* (4th ed). Boston: Little, Brown & Co.

Tasota, F., & Wesmiller, S. (1994). Assessing A.B.G.s: Maintaining the delicate balance. *Nursing94, 24*(5), 34–46.

Taylor, D. L. (1990). Respiratory alkalosis. *Nursing90, 20*(8), 60–61.

Taylor, D. L. (1990). Respiratory acidosis. *Nursing90, 20*(9), 52–53.

Toto, R. (1990). Metabolic acid-base disorders. In J. Kokko & R. L. Tannen (eds.), *Fluids and electrolytes* (pp. 301–390). Philadelphia: W. B. Saunders.

Yeaw, E. (1992). Good lung down? How position affects oxygenation. *American Journal of Nursing, 92*(3), 27–29.

SUGGESTED READINGS

Janusek, L. (1990). Metabolic acidosis. *Nursing90, 20*(7), 52–53.

This brief article uses color pictures to describe the sequence of physiologic events occurring during metabolic acidosis. The author provides tips on when signs and symptoms are apparent and when laboratory data change.

Taylor, D. L. (1990). Respiratory acidosis. *Nursing90, 20*(9), 52–53.

This brief but clinically applicable article summarizes the clinical manifestations and pathophysiology associated with respiratory acidosis. Color diagrams help to reinforce understanding of cellular mechanisms operating under conditions of acidosis.

Yeaw, E. (1992). Good lung down? How position affects oxygenation. *American Journal of Nursing, 92*(3), 27–29.

This comprehensive article reviews the basic physiology regarding pulmonary ventilation and perfusion and suggests client positions according to specific breathing problems. The author presents case studies and very specific assessment techniques.

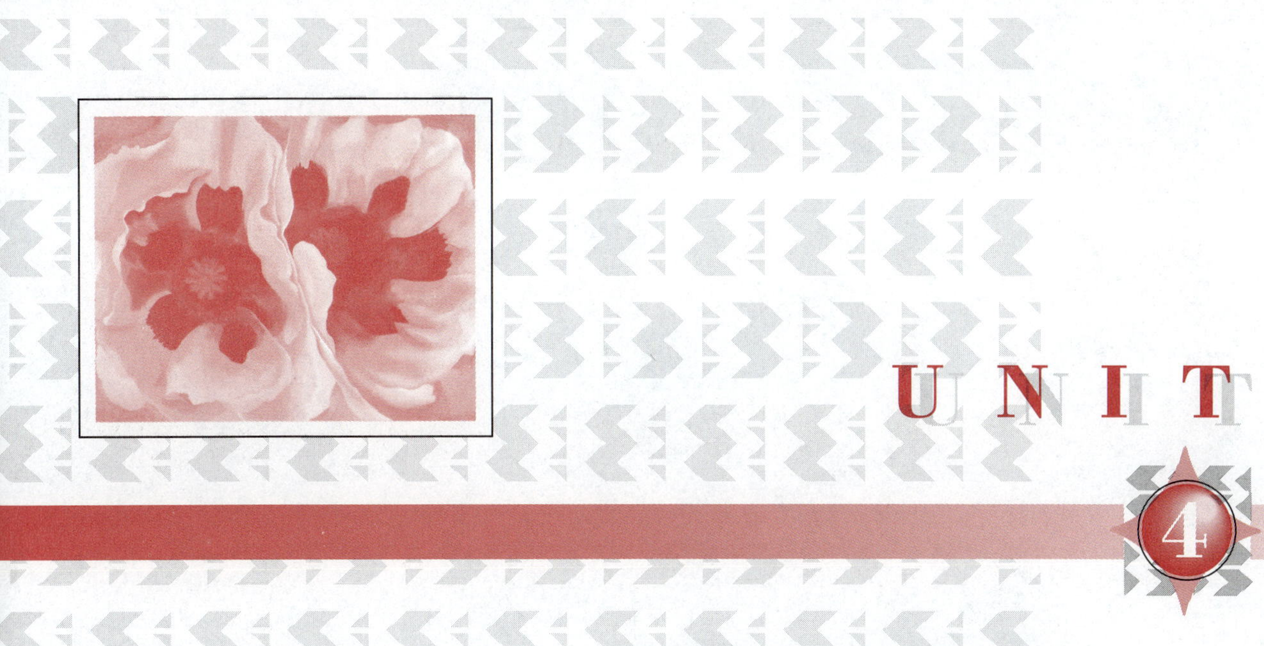

UNIT 4

Management of Perioperative Clients

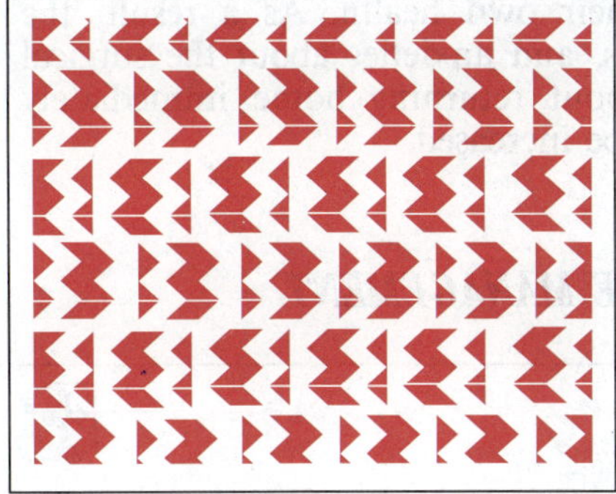

CHAPTER 19

Interventions for Preoperative Clients

CHAPTER HIGHLIGHTS

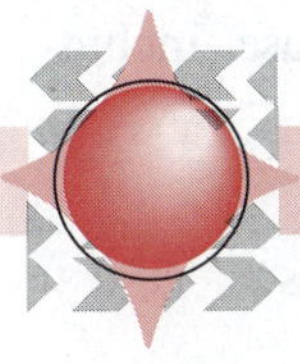

The nurse's role in caring for surgical clients has changed in response to emerging trends in health care. With increased emphasis on reducing the length of the hospital stay and using ambulatory care services, the role of the nurse has intensified in the inpatient setting and has expanded in the outpatient setting. Perioperative, or surgical, nursing focuses on client care before (preoperative), during (intraoperative), and after surgery (postoperative).

OVERVIEW

The preoperative period begins when the client is scheduled for surgery and ends at the time of transfer to the surgical suite. Primarily, the nurse acts as an educator, an advocate, and a promoter of health. Perioperative nursing places special emphasis on safety.

After a thorough assessment, the nurse develops an individualized teaching care plan to help the client and family through the surgical experience. Preoperative care mainly consists of education to reduce anxiety and postoperative complications and to promote cooperation in postoperative procedures. In preoperative teaching, the nurse uses adult teaching and learning principles and validates and clarifies information that the physician has provided.

CATEGORIES AND PURPOSES OF SURGERY

The nurse understands the terminology for surgical procedures to provide the client and family members with comprehensive information. Procedures are usually categorized according to:

- The reason for the surgery
- The urgency of the procedure
- The degree of risk
- The anatomic location
- The extent of surgery required

The primary purposes, or reasons, for surgery can be divided into five general subcategories: diagnostic, curative, restorative, palliative, and cosmetic. For example, palliative surgery makes the client more comfortable, and cosmetic surgery reconstructs the skin and underlying structures. The urgency of the procedure can be divided into three subcategories: elective, urgent, and emergent. The degree of risk is classed as minor or major. Location means the bodily area being operated on, such as abdominal surgery, intracranial surgery, and heart surgery. The extent can be simple, modified, or radical. Table 19–1 explains the categories and gives examples of surgical procedures.

SURGICAL SETTINGS

In response to United States government regulations, the economic concerns of third-party payers (e.g., insurance companies), and public awareness of health care costs, changing trends in surgical settings have emerged. Surgery continues to be performed under aseptic conditions, although the setting may now be other than the classic hospital operating room (OR). The use of surgical settings, such as hospital-based ambulatory surgical centers, freestanding surgical centers, physicians' offices, and ambulatory care centers, is becoming more common. The term *inpatient* refers to a client who is admitted to a hospital. The client may be admitted the day before or the day of surgery (often termed same-day admission [SDA]), or may already be an inpatient when the need for surgical intervention is identified. In contrast, the term *outpatient* refers to a client who goes to the surgical area the day of the surgery and returns home on the same day (i.e., same-day surgery [SDS]).

One of the many advantages of outpatient surgery is that clients are not separated from the comfort and security of their home and family. With continuous improvements in surgical techniques and anesthesia, more procedures are being safely performed on an outpatient basis. However, changes in the surgical experience present particular challenges for the client without an adequate or available support system. An elderly spouse may be unable to assist in the preoperative and postoperative care of the client. A client who is primarily responsible for others may be unable to perform his or her usual tasks within the family. Clients may try to continue their family role, but then jeopardize their own health. As a result, the client's stress, fears, and anxieties about the surgical experience and about returning home immediately after surgery may be increased.

COLLABORATIVE MANAGEMENT

ASSESSMENT

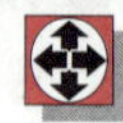

HISTORY

Collection of data about the client before surgery begins in various settings (e.g., in the surgeon's office, the preadmission or admission office, and the inpatient unit and over the telephone). The nurse provides privacy to increase the client's comfort with the interview process. The anesthesia and the surgery are both physical and emotional stressors for the client. The nurse collects the following data from the preoperative client:

- Age
- Tobacco, alcohol, and illicit substance use, including marijuana
- Current medications
- Medical history
- Prior surgical procedures and experiences
- Prior experience with anesthesia
- Autologous or directed blood donations
- Allergies
- General health
- Family history
- Type of surgery planned
- Knowledge and understanding about events during the perioperative period
- Support system adequacy and availability

When taking a history, the nurse screens the preoperative client for risks that may contribute to complications during the perioperative period. Some conditions that could either increase the surgical risk or increase the possibility of postoperative complications are outlined in Table 19–2.

AGE Elderly clients are at increased risk. The normal aging process decreases immune system functioning and delays wound healing. There is an increased frequency of chronic illness in elderly clients. See Chart 19–1 for other physiologic changes in elderly clients.

MEDICATION AND SUBSTANCE USE The use of tobacco products increases the risk of pulmonary complications because of the changes they cause to the lungs and thoracic cavity. Excessive alcohol and illicit substance use can alter the effects of anesthesia and response to pain medication. Withdrawal of alcohol in preparation for surgery may precipitate delirium tremens. Prescription and over-the-counter medications may also affect how the client reacts to the

TABLE 19–1 Selected Categories of Surgical Procedures

Category	Description	Condition or Surgical Procedure
Reasons for Surgery		
Diagnostic	• Performed to determine the origin and cause of a disorder or the cell type for cancer	• Breast biopsy • Exploratory laparotomy
Curative	• Performed to resolve a health problem by repairing or removing the cause	• Cholelithiasis • Mastectomy • Hysterectomy
Restorative	• Performed to improve a client's functional ability	• Total knee replacement • Finger reimplantation
Palliative	• Performed to relieve symptoms of a disease process, but does not cure	• Colostomy • Nerve root resection • Tumor debulking • Ileostomy
Cosmetic	• Performed primarily to alter or enhance personal appearance	• Liposuction • Revision of scars • Rhinoplasty • Blepharoplasty
Urgency of Surgery		
Elective	• Planned for correction of a nonacute problem	• Cataract removal • Hernia repair • Hemorrhoidectomy • Total joint replacement
Urgent	• Requires prompt intervention; or may be life-threatening if treatment delayed more than 24–48 hr	• Intestinal obstruction • Bladder obstruction • Kidney or ureteral stones • Bone fracture • Eye injury • Acute cholecystitis
Emergent	• Requires immediate intervention because of life-threatening consequences	• Gunshot or stab wound • Severe bleeding • Abdominal aortic aneurysm • Compound fracture • Appendectomy
Degree of Risk of Surgery		
Minor	• Procedure without significant risk, often done with local anesthesia	• Incision and drainage (I&D) • Implantation of a venous access device (VAD) • Muscle biopsy
Major	• Procedure of greater risk, usually longer and more extensive than a minor procedure	• Mitral valve replacement • Pancreas transplant • Lymph node dissection
Extent of Surgery		
Simple	• Only the most overtly affected areas involved in the surgery	• Simple/partial mastectomy
Radical	• Extensive surgery beyond the area obviously involved; is directed at finding a root cause	• Radical prostatectomy • Radical hysterectomy

perioperative experience. The potential effects of specific medications are noted in Table 19–3.

MEDICAL HISTORY The nurse asks the client about his or her medical history. The presence of certain chronic illnesses increases perioperative risks and is considered when planning care. For example, a client with systemic lupus erythematosus may need additional medication to offset the physical and emotional stress of the surgery. A diabetic client may need a more extensive preoperative bowel preparation because of decreased gastrointestinal motility. An infection may need to be treated before surgery.

PRIOR CARDIAC HISTORY The nurse obtains a history of cardiac disease because complications from anesthesia could occur. Cardiac disorders that increase risks associated with surgery include coronary artery disease, angina pectoris, myocardial infarction (MI) within 6 months before surgery, congestive heart fail-

TABLE 19–2 Selected Factors That Increase Surgical Risk or Increase the Risk of Postoperative Complications

Age

- Older than 65 yr

Medications

- Antihypertensives
- Tricyclic antidepressants
- Anticoagulants
- Nonsteroidal anti-inflammatory drugs (NSAIDs)

Medical History

- Decreased immunity
- Diabetes
- Pulmonary disease
- Cardiac disease
- Hemodynamic instability
- Multisystem disease
- Coagulation disorder
- Anemia
- Dehydration
- Infection
- Hypertension
- Hypotension
- Any chronic disease

Prior Surgical Experiences

- Less-than-optimal emotional reaction
- Anesthesia reactions or complications
- Postoperative complications

Health History

- Malnutrition or obesity
- Medication, tobacco, alcohol, or illicit substance use or abuse
- Altered coping ability

Family History

- Malignant hyperthermia
- Cancer
- Bleeding disorder

Type of Surgical Procedure Planned

- Neck, oral, or facial procedures (airway complications)
- Chest or high abdominal procedures (pulmonary complications)
- Abdominal surgery (paralytic ileus, deep vein thrombosis)

ure, hypertension, and dysrhythmias. These disorders impair the client's ability to withstand and respond to both anesthesia and the hemodynamic changes during surgery. The risk of intraoperative MI is also higher in clients with pre-existing heart problems.

PULMONARY HISTORY Adults with chronic respiratory problems, elderly people, and smokers are all at risk for pulmonary complications because of physiologic pulmonary changes. Increased rigidity of the thoracic cavity and loss of lung elasticity reduce the efficiency of anesthesia excretion. Smoking increases the level of circulating carboxyhemoglobin (carbon monoxide in the oxygen-binding sites of the hemoglobin molecule), which in turn decreases oxygen delivery to organs. Concurrently, mucociliary transport decreases, which leads to increased secretions and predisposes the client to pulmonary infection (pneumonia) and atelectasis (collapse of alveoli). Atelectasis prevents the exchange of oxygen and carbon dioxide and causes intolerance of anesthesia. Chronic pulmonary conditions such as asthma, emphysema, and chronic bronchitis also reduce the elasticity of the lungs, which causes an ineffective exchange of carbon dioxide and oxygen. As a result, these clients have decreased oxygen diffusion to and oxygenation of the tissues.

PREVIOUS SURGERY AND ANESTHESIA The number and type of previous surgeries and previous surgical experiences affect the preoperative client's readiness for surgery. Previous perioperative complications may contribute to the client's fears and concerns about the scheduled surgery. The nurse asks about the client's experience with anesthetic agents and all allergies. These data provide the nurse with information about tolerance of and possible fears about the use of anesthesia. The client's sensitivity or allergy to certain substances alerts the nurse to a possible reaction to anesthetic agents or to substances that are used for preoperative skin preparation. For example, povidone-iodine used for skin preparation contains some of the same components as those found in shellfish. The family medical history and problems with anesthetics may indicate possible intraoperative needs and reactions to anesthesia, such as malignant hyperthermia.

AUTOLOGOUS OR DIRECTED BLOOD DONATIONS Clients may donate their own blood (autologous donations) in the few weeks immediately before the scheduled surgery date. If clients then need blood because of their surgery, an autologous blood transfusion can be given. This practice eliminates the possibility of transfusion reactions and the transmission of disease.

Clients may be candidates for autologous blood donations up to 5 weeks preoperatively if they are afebrile, have a hemoglobin level greater than 11 g/dL, and have a physician's recommendation. If clients are to give their own blood, the physician usually orders supplemental iron beginning before the first donation. Autologous donations can be made as frequently as every 3 days if the other criteria can be met. Usually, a total of 2 to 4 units are donated. The last donation cannot be less than 72 hours before surgery.

A special tag is affixed to the transfusion bag when an autologous blood donation has been made. The blood donor center gives the client a matching tag that he or she brings to the surgical area preoperatively. This procedure helps to ensure that the client receives only his or her own blood. If the client does not use the blood, the blood goes to the blood bank to be used as any other unit of donated blood would be used.

Clients may wish to have family and friends donate blood exclusively for their use, if needed. This practice of directed blood donation is possible only if the

CHART 19–1

Nursing Focus on the Elderly ◆ Changes of Aging as Surgical Risk Factors

Physiologic Change	Nursing Interventions	Rationale
Cardiovascular System		
Decreased cardiac output Increased blood pressure Decreased peripheral circulation	• Determine normal activity levels and note when the client tires. • Monitor vital signs and peripheral pulses.	• Knowing limits helps prevent fatigue. • Having baseline data helps detect deviations.
Respiratory System		
Reduced vital capacity Loss of lung elasticity Decreased oxygenation of blood	• Teach coughing and deep breathing exercises. • Monitor respirations and breathing effort.	• Pulmonary exercises help prevent pulmonary complications. • Having baseline data helps detect deviations.
Renal/Urinary System		
Decreased blood flow to kidneys Reduced ability to excrete waste products Decline in glomerular filtration rate Nocturia common	• Monitor intake and output. • Assess overall hydration. • Monitor electrolyte status. • Assist frequently with toileting needs, especially at night.	• Ongoing assessment helps detect dehydration, fluid overload, decreased renal function, and electrolyte imbalances. • Frequent toileting helps prevent incontinence and falls.
Neurologic System		
Sensory deficits Slower reaction time Decreased ability to adjust to changes in the surroundings	• Orient the client to the surroundings. • Allow extra time for teaching the client. • Provide for the client's safety.	• An individualized preoperative teaching plan is developed on the basis of the client's orientation and any neurologic deficits. • Safety measures help prevent falls and injury.
Musculoskeletal System		
Increased incidence of deformities related to osteoporosis or arthritis	• Assess the client's level of mobility. • Teach turning and positioning. • Encourage ambulation. • Place on fall precautions, if indicated.	• Interventions help prevent complications of immobility. • Safety measures help prevent injury.

blood types are compatible and the donor's blood is acceptable. Clients may fear disease transmission from unknown blood and feel more comfortable knowing who gave the blood. Some blood collection centers and other health care personnel are discouraging the practice, stating it gives the client a false sense of security. As with autologous blood donations, a special tag is affixed to the blood. This tag notes the names of the client and the donor and has the client's signature.

The nurse asks whether autologous or directed blood donations have been made and documents this information in the client's chart. It may be important to know the specific blood collection center and whether the blood has arrived before the client has surgery.

DISCHARGE PLANNING The nurse also assesses the client's home environment, self-care capabilities, and support systems. The nurse anticipates the client's postoperative needs during the preoperative period. All clients should have discharge planning. Elderly people and dependent adults may need referrals for transportation to and from the physician's office. They may also need the help of a home care nurse to monitor their postoperative recovery and to provide instruction on wound care. All clients with inadequate support systems may need follow-up care at home.

PHYSICAL ASSESSMENT/CLINICAL MANIFESTATIONS

The preoperative client may be of any age, with a health status that varies from well to debilitated. The nurse performs a complete preoperative physical assessment on all clients before surgery to obtain baseline data. In addition, during the physical assessment, the nurse identifies current health problems, potential complications related to the administration of anesthesia, and potential postoperative complications.

TABLE 19–3 Effects of Routine Medications Taken Preoperatively

Drug	Implications for the Perioperative Experience	Nursing Interventions	Rationale
Antiarrhythmics			
Quinidine gluconate (Quinate🍁, Quinaglute Dura-Tabs) Procainamide hydrochloride (Pronestyl, Procan-SR)	• Antiarrhythmic medications affect the client's tolerance of anesthesia and potentiate anesthetics that are neuromuscular blockers. • Antiarrhythmics depress cardiac function by decreasing cardiac output and slowing the pulse rate. • Antiarrhythmics may cause peripheral vasodilation.	• Communicate the use and type of antiarrhythmics to the anesthesia personnel. • Monitor vital signs. • Obtain a baseline electrocardiogram, as ordered. • Assess the client's peripheral circulation.	• Cardiac complications during surgery can be life-threatening. • Ongoing monitoring helps to detect deviations and potential complications.
Antihypertensives			
Methyldopa (Aldomet, Novomedopa🍁) Captopril (Capoten) Clonidine hydrochloride (Catapres)	• Antihypertensive agents alter the client's response to muscle relaxants and opioid analgesics by inhibiting synthesis and storage of norepinephrine. • Antihypertensives may cause a hypotensive crisis intraoperatively and postoperatively.	• Monitor blood pressure and pulse frequently. • Assess for hypotension during transfer and turning.	• Ongoing monitoring helps to detect deviations and potential complications. • Hypotensive crisis can occur and may be prevented through timely assessments.
Corticosteroids			
Dexamethasone (Decadron, Dexasone🍁) Hydrocortisone sodium (Solu-Cortef) Prednisone (Deltasone, Winpred🍁)	• Surgery increases the demand for corticosteroids in the client with no adrenal function. • Steroids delay wound healing because of blockage of collagen formation. • Steroids increase the serum glucose level and block fibroblast formation. • Steroids increase the risk of hemorrhage. • Steroids mask the signs and symptoms of infection.	• Continue steroid therapy during surgery. • Monitor vital signs. • Assess for signs of hyperglycemia. • Assess for subtle signs of infection and bleeding. • Monitor wound healing, support the incision area with binders, and splint the wound when the client is turning, coughing, and deep breathing.	• Continuation of steroid therapy avoids problems associated with abrupt withdrawal. • Ongoing monitoring helps to detect deviations and potential complications. • It is important to detect early signs and symptoms of infection. • Specific wound and incision care helps to prevent complications.
Anticoagulants			
Warfarin sodium (Coumadin, Warfilone sodium🍁) Heparin sodium (Lipo-Hepin, Hepalean🍁) Aspirin (acetylsalicylic acid, Ancasal🍁, Astin🍁, Coryphen🍁)	• Anticoagulant therapy increases the risk of hemorrhage intraoperatively and postoperatively	• Monitor coagulation studies (PTT, PT). • Monitor for signs of bleeding. • Gradually discontinue anticoagulants 24–48 hr before surgery, as ordered. • Have an antidote (protamine sulfate for heparin and vitamin K [Mephyton] for warfarin sodium) available to reverse the effects of the anticoagulant.	• Coagulation studies help detect bleeding disorders. • Anticoagulant administration is discontinued to avoid hemorrhage. • An antidote needs to be available to prevent complications of bleeding in an emergency situation.
Antiseizure Medications			
Phenobarbital (Luminal🍁, Gardenal🍁)	• Seizure activity can cause injury to the surgical wound. • Antiseizure medications alter the metabolism of anesthetic agents.	• Maintain use of the drug. • Inform the anesthesiologist or anesthetist to allow for adjustment of the dosage of the anesthetic. • Assess for seizure activity. • Pad the side rails of the bed. • Place suction equipment at the bedside.	• Antiseizure medications prevent seizures. • Safety measures prevent injury.

TABLE 19–3 Effects of Routine Medications Taken Preoperatively *Continued*

Drug	Implications for the Perioperative Experience	Nursing Interventions	Rationale
Glaucoma Medications			
Demecarium bromide (Humorsol) Echothiophate (Phospholine iodide) Pilocarpine hydrochloride (Isopto-Carpine, Pilocar, Miocarpine✱) Timolol maleate (Timoptic)	• Glaucoma medications have cumulative systemic effects and can cause respiratory and cardiovascular collapse, especially during surgery.	• Consult the physician about stopping Humorsol at least 2 weeks before surgery. • Monitor respiratory status and cardiac output. • Assess for increased intraocular pressure.	• Collaboration with the physician helps prevent complications. • Ongoing monitoring helps to detect complications.
Antidiabetic Agent			
Insulin	• Insulin needs decrease preoperatively when the client is on NPO status. • Postoperative insulin demands increase because of IV administration of dextrose. • Insulin levels may fluctuate during healing because of dietary and activity restrictions and the physical stress of surgery.	• Monitor serum glucose levels. • Administer antibiotics and other intermittent medications in normal saline instead of dextrose when possible, as ordered, or as per facility policy.	• Monitoring will detect an increased or a decreased need for insulin. • The use of normal saline prevents complications.

When beginning the assessment, the nurse obtains a complete set of vital signs. The nurse may need to obtain vital signs several times for accurate baseline values. Abnormal vital signs may cause the postponement of surgery until the underlying problem is treated and the client's condition is stable. The nurse also assesses for anxiety, which could increase the client's blood pressure, pulse, and respiratory rate and documents this in the client's chart as part of the overall assessment.

Throughout the physical assessment, the nurse focuses on problem areas that have been identified from the client's history and on all body systems affected directly or indirectly by the surgical procedure. The elderly (Chart 19–2; see also Chap. 6) or chronically ill client is at increased risk for intraoperative and postoperative complications. Perioperative morbidity and mortality are higher in elderly and chronically ill clients owing to their preoperative physical condition.

The nurse reports any abnormalities found on physical assessment to the physician and anesthesiology personnel. In this manner, the nurse functions as a proactive client advocate and is exercising the nurses' legal responsibility.

CARDIOVASCULAR SYSTEM Alterations in cardiac status are responsible for as many as 30% of perioperative deaths. The nurse evaluates the client for hypertension, which is common and often undiagnosed in adults and can affect surgery. Cardiovascular assessment also includes auscultation of heart sounds for rate, regularity, and abnormalities. The nurse evaluates the client's extremities for temperature, color, peripheral pulses, capillary refill, and edema. Any physical alterations, such as absent peripheral pulses and pitting edema, or cardiac symptoms such as chest pain, shortness of breath, and dyspnea, are reported to the physician for further assessment and evaluation. (Chapter 32 further discusses cardiovascular assessment.)

RESPIRATORY SYSTEM In assessing the client's respiratory status, the nurse considers the client's age, history of smoking, and the presence of chronic illness. The nurse observes the client's posture; respiratory

CHART 19–2

Nursing Focus on the Elderly ◆ Specific Considerations When Planning Care for the Elderly Preoperative Client

- Greater incidence of chronic illness
- Greater incidence of malnutrition
- More allergies
- Increased incidence of impaired self-care abilities
- Inadequate support systems
- Decreased ability to withstand the stress of surgery and anesthesia
- Increased risk of postoperative cardiopulmonary complications
- Risk of a change in mental status when admitted (related to unfamiliar surroundings, change in routine, medications administered, and so forth)
- Increased risk of a fall and resultant injury

rate, rhythm, and depth; overall respiratory effort; and lung expansion. Clubbing of the fingertips (swelling at the base of the nailbeds caused by a chronic lack of oxygen) or any cyanosis is noted. The nurse auscultates the lungs to determine the quality and presence of any adventitious (crackles, wheezes, rubs) or abnormal breath sounds. (More information is found in Chapter 28.)

RENAL/URINARY SYSTEM Renal and urinary function affects the filtration and eventual excretion of waste products. If renal and urinary function is not optimal, fluid and electrolyte balance can be altered, especially in the elderly client. The nurse asks the client about the presence or absence of symptoms such as urinary frequency, dysuria (painful urination), nocturia (awakening during nighttime sleep because of a need to void), difficulty starting urine flow, and oliguria (scant amount of urine). The nurse also asks about the appearance and odor of the urine. Equally important is an assessment of the client's usual fluid intake and degree of continence. If the client is suspected of having underlying renal or urinary problems, the nurse consults with the physician about further client work-up. (Chapter 69 further discusses renal/urinary assessment.)

Abnormal renal function can decrease the excretion rate of preoperative medications and anesthetic agents. As a result, the drug's effectiveness may be altered. Scopolamine (Buscopan✱), morphine, meperidine (Demerol), and barbiturates frequently cause confusion, disorientation, apprehension, and restlessness when administered to clients with decreased renal function.

NEUROLOGIC SYSTEM The nurse should assess the client's overall mental status, including level of consciousness, orientation, and ability to follow commands, before planning preoperative teaching and postoperative care. A deficit in any of these areas affects the type of care required during the perioperative experience. The nurse determines the client's baseline neurologic status to be able to identify changes that may occur later. The nurse also assesses for any motor or sensory deficits. (See Chapter 40 for complete nervous system assessment.)

The usual neurologic status of a mentally impaired or elderly client may be difficult to assess. The client who has been independent and oriented while in the home environment may become disoriented in an unfamiliar hospital setting. Family members and significant others can often provide information about what the client was like at home.

Often, as part of the neurologic assessment, the nurse assesses the client's risk of falling, especially for elderly clients. Factors such as mental status, muscle strength, steadiness of gait, and sense of independence are evaluated to determine the client's risk of falling. The client's ability to ambulate and his or her steadiness of gait are noted preoperatively as baseline data.

MUSCULOSKELETAL SYSTEM Deformities of the musculoskeletal system may interfere with intraoperative and postoperative positioning of the client. For example, clients with arthritis may be able to assume conventional intraoperative positions but then have unnecessary discomfort postoperatively from prolonged immobilization of joints. Other anatomic characteristics, such as the shape and length of the client's neck and the shape of the thoracic cavity, may interfere with respiratory and cardiac function and positioning during surgery.

The nurse asks about a history of joint replacements. It is particularly important during surgery to ensure that electrocautery pads are not placed near the area of the prosthesis and cause an electrical burn.

NUTRITIONAL STATUS Malnutrition and obesity can increase surgical risks. Surgery usually increases the body's metabolic rate and consequently depletes potassium, ascorbic acid, and B vitamins, all of which are needed for wound healing and fibrin formation. In malnourished clients, hypoproteinemia retards postoperative recovery. Negative nitrogen balance may result from depleted protein stores. This situation increases the risk of perioperative morbidity and mortality from delayed wound healing, possible dehiscence or evisceration (see Chap. 21), fluid volume deficit, and sepsis.

Some elderly clients are susceptible to nutritional imbalances because of chronic illness, the use of diuretics or laxatives, poor dietary planning or habits, anorexia, lack of motivation, and financial limitations. Clinical indications of alterations in the fluid and nutritional status of the client preoperatively include brittle nails, muscle wasting, dry or flaky skin, hair alterations (dull, sparse, dry), decreased skin turgor, orthostatic (postural) hypotension, decreased serum albumin levels, and abnormal serum electrolyte values.

The obese client is often malnourished because of poor eating habits and an imbalanced diet. These clients have an increased chance of poor or incomplete wound healing because of excessive adipose tissue. Fatty tissue lacks nutrients, is not as vascular, and has little collagen, all of which are important for wound healing. Obesity causes increased stress on the heart and reduces the available lung volumes, which can affect the client's intraoperative experience and postoperative recovery.

PSYCHOSOCIAL ASSESSMENT

The nurse performs a psychosocial assessment and preparation of the client in order to:

- Determine the client's level of anxiety, coping ability, and support systems
- Provide information
- Offer support

A client scheduled for surgery experiences some preoperative anxiety and fear. The extent and type of these reactions vary for each client according to the kind of surgery, the perceived effects of the surgery and its potential outcome, and the client's basic personality. Surgery may be seen as a threat to the client's biologic integrity, body image, self-esteem, self-concept, or lifestyle. Clients may fear death, pain, helplessness, decreased socioeconomic status, a diagnosis of life-threatening conditions, possible disabling or crippling effects, and the unknown.

The client's anxiety and fear affect his or her ability to learn, cope, and cooperate with preoperative teaching and perioperative procedures. Anxiety and fear may also influence the amount and type of anesthesia that is needed and may retard postoperative recovery. The nurse is aware of potential fears and anxieties when interviewing the client and planning preoperative teaching.

The nurse assesses coping mechanisms used by the client under similar situations or in the past when the client had been confronted with a stressful situation. The nurse asks open-ended questions pertaining to the client's feelings about the entire perioperative experience. The nurse assesses factors that influence coping. These factors include age, previous surgical and sick-role experiences, emotional and physical signs of fear, anxiety, and discomfort. Signs of fear and anxiety include anger, crying, restlessness, diaphoresis (sweating, usually profusely), increased pulse rate, palpitations, sleeplessness, diarrhea, and urinary frequency. (For more information on stress and coping, see Chapter 7.)

LABORATORY ASSESSMENT

Preoperative laboratory tests provide baseline data about the client's health and help predict potential complications. The client who is scheduled for surgery in a surgical center or who is admitted to the hospital on the morning of or day before surgery may have preadmission testing performed 48 hours to 21 days before the scheduled surgery, depending on the facility's policy. The results of prior testing are usually valid unless there has been a change in the client's condition that warrants repeated testing. Depending on the test needed, the hospitalized client has testing done under similar time guidelines.

The choice of routine preoperative laboratory tests varies among facilities and depends on the client's age and medical history and the type of anesthesia planned. The most common tests are:

- Urinalysis
- Blood type and crossmatch
- Complete blood count or hemoglobin level and hematocrit
- Coagulation studies (prothrombin time [PT], partial thromboplastin time [PTT], and platelet count)
- Electrolyte levels
- Serum creatinine

Depending on a female client's age, a pregnancy test may also be ordered.

A preoperative urinalysis is done to assess for the presence of protein, glucose, blood, and bacteria, all of which are abnormal constituents of the urine. If renal disease is suspected or the client is elderly, the physician may order other tests to determine the type and degree of disease present.

The nurse reports electrolyte imbalances or other abnormal results to the surgeon before surgery. Hypokalemia (decreased serum potassium level) increases the risk of digitalis toxicity (if the client is receiving a digitalis preparation), slows recovery from anesthesia, and increases cardiac irritability. Hyperkalemia (increased serum potassium level) increases the risk of cardiac dysrhythmias, especially with the use of anesthesia. Both hypokalemia and hyperkalemia should be treated before the surgery.

The physician may order other studies, depending on the client's medical history. For example, baseline arterial blood gas (ABG) values are assessed before surgery for clients with chronic pulmonary problems. Chart 19–3 presents abnormal laboratory findings and their possible causes.

RADIOGRAPHIC ASSESSMENT

A chest x-ray, when ordered by the physician or the anesthesiologist, is commonly obtained to determine the size and contour of the heart, lungs, and major vessels and to determine the presence of any infiltrates that could indicate pneumonia or tuberculosis. A chest x-ray also provides baseline data in the event of postoperative complications. Abnormal x-ray results alert the physician to potential cardiac or pulmonary complications. The presence of congestive heart failure, cardiomyopathy, pneumonia, or infiltrates may cause cancellation or delay of elective surgery. For emergency surgery, x-ray results assist the anesthesiologist in the selection of anesthesia. In many facilities, chest x-ray results are valid when done within 6 months before surgery, provided that there has not been a change in the client's condition.

Other radiographic studies are based on the individual client's needs, the medical history, and the nature of the surgical procedure. For example, a client with back pain may have computed tomography (CT) or magnetic resonance imaging (MRI) done before a laminectomy to identify the exact location of the abnormality.

OTHER DIAGNOSTIC ASSESSMENT

An electrocardiogram (ECG) may routinely be required for all clients older than a specific age who are to have general anesthesia. The age varies among facilities but is often older than 40 to 45 years. An ECG may also be ordered for clients with a history of cardiac disease or those at risk for cardiovascular complications. An ECG provides baseline information on new or pre-existing cardiac conditions, such

CHART 19-3

Lab Profile ◆ Perioperative Assessment

Test	Normal Range for Adults	Significance of Abnormal Findings: Increased in	Significance of Abnormal Findings: Decreased in
Potassium (K^+)	• 3.5–5 mEq/L, or 3.5–5 mmol/L	• Dehydration • Renal failure • Acidosis • Cellular damage	• Excessive use of diuretics • Vomiting • Malnutrition • Diarrhea
Sodium (Na^+)	• 136–145 mEq/L, or 136–145 mmol/L	• Cardiac or renal failure • Hypertension • Excessive amounts of IV fluids containing normal saline • Edema • Dehydration	• Nasogastric drainage • Vomiting or diarrhea • Excessive use of laxatives or diuretics • Syndrome of inappropriate antidiuretic hormone secretion (SIADH)
Chloride (Cl^-)	• 90–110 mEq/L, or 98–106 mmol/L	• Respiratory alkalosis • Dehydration • Renal failure • Excessive amounts of IV fluids containing sodium chloride (NaCl)	• Excessive nasogastric drainage • Vomiting • Excessive use of diuretics • Diarrhea
Carbon dioxide (CO_2)	• 23–30 mEq/L, or 23–30 mmol/L	• Chronic pulmonary disease • Intestinal obstruction • Vomiting or nasogastric suctioning	• Hyperventilation • Diabetic ketoacidosis • Diarrhea • Lactic acidosis • Renal failure • Salicylate toxicity
Glucose (fasting)	• 70–105 mg/dL, or 3.9–5.8 mmol/L • **Elderly:** increased normal range after age 50 yr	• Hyperglycemia • Excess amounts of IV fluids containing glucose • Stress • Steroid use • Pancreatic or hepatic disease	• Hypoglycemia • Excess insulin
Creatinine	• Females: 0.5–1.1 mg/dL, or 44–97 μmol/L • Males: 0.6–1.2 mg/dL, or 53–106 μmol/L • **Elderly:** may be slightly increased	• Renal damage with destruction of large number of nephrons	• Atrophy of muscle tissue
Blood urea nitrogen (BUN)	• 10–20 mg/dL, or 3.6–7.1 mmol/L • **Elderly:** may be as high as 69 mg/dL	• Dehydration • Renal failure • Excessive protein in diet • Liver failure	• Overhydration • Malnutrition
Prothrombin time (Protime, PT)	• 11–12.5 sec, 85%–100%, or 1–1.1 client/control ratio	• Coagulation defect (bleeding disorder) • Liver disease • Anticoagulant therapy (aspirin, warfarin)	• Coagulation (clotting) disorder such as thrombophlebitis or pulmonary embolus • Extensive cancer
Partial thromboplastin time (PTT), activated (aPTT)	• PTT: 60–70 sec • aPTT: 30–40 sec	• Coagulation defect (bleeding disorder) • Anticoagulant therapy (heparin) • Liver disease	• Coagulation (clotting) disorder such as thrombophlebitis or pulmonary embolus • Extensive cancer

CHART 19-3

Lab Profile ♦ Perioperative Assessment *Continued*

Test	Normal Range for Adults	Significance of Abnormal Findings: Increased in	Significance of Abnormal Findings: Decreased in
White blood cell count	• Total: 5000–10,000 cells/mm³	• Infection	• Immune disorder • Immunosuppressant therapy
Hemoglobin	• Females: 12–16 g/dL, or 7.4–9.9 mmol/L • Males: 14–18 g/dL, or 8.7–11.2 mmol/L • **Elderly:** slightly decreased	• Dehydration • Polycythemia • Chronic pulmonary disease • Congestive heart failure	• Blood loss • Anemia • Renal failure
Hematocrit	• Females: 37%–47% • Males: 42%–52% • **Elderly:** may be slightly decreased	• Dehydration	• Renal failure • Blood loss

as an old anterior wall myocardial infarction. A client with a known cardiac condition may require a preoperative consultation with a cardiologist. Prophylactic medication, such as nitroglycerin and antibiotics, may be needed during the perioperative period to reduce or prevent stress on the cardiovascular system. Abnormal or potentially life-threatening ECG results may cause the cancellation of surgery until the client's cardiac status is stable.

ANALYSIS

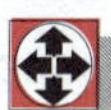

COMMON NURSING DIAGNOSES

Two nursing diagnoses are common to the preoperative client:

1. Knowledge Deficit related to a lack of education and lack of exposure to the specific perioperative experience
2. Anxiety related to the threat of a change in health status or fear of the unknown

ADDITIONAL NURSING DIAGNOSES

In addition to the common diagnoses, other nursing diagnoses may apply:

- Sleep Pattern Disturbance related to internal sensory alterations (e.g., illness and anxiety)
- Ineffective Individual Coping related to the impending surgery
- Anticipatory Grieving related to the effects of surgery
- Body Image Disturbance related to anticipated changes in the body's appearance or function
- Ineffective Family Coping: Compromised related to temporary family disorganization and role changes
- Powerlessness related to the health care environment, loss of independence, and loss of control of one's body
- Altered Family Processes related to situational crisis

PLANNING AND IMPLEMENTATION

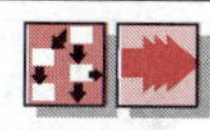

KNOWLEDGE DEFICIT

PLANNING: CLIENT GOALS The two major goals are that the client will:

- Verbalize and comply with preoperative procedures
- Demonstrate techniques to prevent postoperative complications

INTERVENTIONS Because the perioperative experience is foreign to many people, the nurse focuses on preoperative education of the client and family members as shown in the Client Care Plan. Preoperative teaching typically begins in the surgeon's office for planned or elective surgery. Pamphlets and written instructions may be given and sent to the client as well. More teaching may occur when the client has preadmission testing. Some facilities conduct preoperative classes for groups of clients who are having the same or similar surgical procedures. A tour of the operating suite and the postanesthesia care unit (PACU) may be included. Information about informed consent, dietary restrictions, preoperative preparation (bowel and skin preparations), and postoperative exercises and procedures promotes the client's participation in

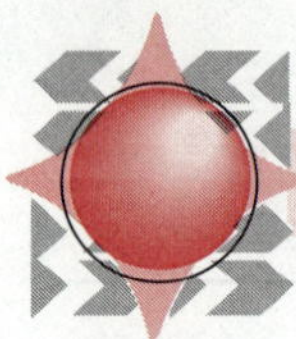

CLIENT CARE PLAN

The Preoperative Client

Nursing Diagnosis No. 1: Knowledge Deficit related to lack of exposure to the specific perioperative experience

Expected Outcomes	Nursing Interventions	Rationale
The client will: Verbalize an understanding of the perioperative routine. State the reasons for the postoperative exercises. State the expected frequency of the postoperative exercises. Demonstrate the correct use of an incentive spirometer (IS). State the goals to achieve with the IS. Demonstrate splinting of the anticipated surgical area.	♦ Assess the client's current level of knowledge. ♦ Provide information about the perioperative routine, as necessary. ♦ Discuss with the client and significant others the reasons for the postoperative exercises. ♦ Discuss and demonstrate correct breathing and leg exercises. ♦ Discuss and demonstrate the technique for splinting. ♦ Encourage the client to practice the exercises. ♦ Supplement instructions with written materials, videos, and so on, as available.	♦ By assessing the client's knowledge base, the nurse is able to individualize the preoperative teaching. ♦ Clients are more likely to comply when they understand the reasons for the activities. ♦ Significant others are able to reinforce instructions and encourage the client postoperatively. ♦ Repetition helps the learning process. ♦ Reinforcement of instructions in more than one format facilitates learning.

Nursing Diagnosis No. 2: Anxiety related to the threat of a change in health status or fear of the unknown

Expected Outcomes	Nursing Interventions	Rationale
The client will: Use successful coping mechanisms. Verbalize the reasons for anxieties or fears, if possible. State that anxiety is reduced or manageable. Demonstrate relaxation breathing exercises.	♦ Assess the client's level of anxiety. ♦ Assess the client's support systems and coping mechanisms. ♦ Encourage the client to verbalize concerns and fears. ♦ Incorporate the client's methods of reducing stress, as indicated. ♦ Review perioperative events and routines. ♦ Teach relaxation breathing. ♦ Provide distractions such as music and television.	♦ By assessing the client's anxiety level, support systems, and coping mechanisms, the nurse is able to individualize the plan for anxiety reduction. ♦ When the client is able to continue familiar activities and actions, anxiety is reduced. ♦ Familiarity with the usual perioperative events decreases the unknown, which is often a source of anxiety. ♦ Focused thoughts and distractions help to decrease anxiety.

health care. Figure 19–1 is a sample comprehensive preoperative educational checklist. Because education of the client takes place in a variety of settings, coordination of client teaching efforts is particularly challenging. The nurse who cares for the client immediately before surgery (same-day, ambulatory surgery outpatient or inpatient hospital unit) assesses the client's knowledge and provides additional information as needed.

Ensuring Informed Consent Surgery of any type involves invasion of the body and requires informed consent from the client or legal guardian (Fig. 19–2). Consent implies that one has been provided with information necessary to understand the following:

- The nature of and reason for surgery
- All available options and the risks associated with each option
- The risks of the surgical procedure and its potential outcomes
- The risks associated with the administration of anesthesia

Signed permission helps protect the client from any unwanted procedures and the physician and the facil-

PRE-OPERATIVE TEACHING DOCUMENTATION FORM

*Key
P = Patient
SO = Significant Other

Indicate N/A (not applicable) in comments section if communication assessment of patient is abnormal.

Preoperative teaching will include, but will not be limited to, the following learning objectives:

EVIDENCE OF LEARNING Behavior Objectives	* LEARNER P	SO	COMMENTS	DATE Initials
1. Verbalizes understanding of surgical procedure to be performed.				
2. Expresses fears and anxieties over impending surgery.				
3. Discusses pain management.				
4. Verbalizes importance of nothing by mouth.				
5. Verbalizes understanding of invasive procedures as explained by attending physician (IV's, NGT, urinary catheters, etc.).				
6. Demonstrates coughing and deep breathing techniques.				
7. Verbalizes the importance of turning/early ambulation.				
8. Other (specify)				
9. Other (specify)				

/pap/3087N

FIGURE 19–1 ◆ A preoperative teaching documentation form. (Courtesy of Northwest Hospital Center, Randallstown, MD.)

ity from lawsuit claims related to unauthorized surgery or uninformed clients.

The physician is usually responsible for having the consent form signed before preoperative sedation is given and before surgery is performed. The nurse is not responsible for providing detailed information about the surgical procedure. Rather, the nurse clarifies facts that have been presented by the physician and dispels myths that the client and family may have about the perioperative experience. The nurse ensures that the consent form is signed and serves as a witness to the signature, not to the fact that the

NORTHWEST HOSPITAL CENTER

REQUEST AND AUTHORIZATION FOR MEDICAL AND/OR SURGICAL TREATMENT

1. I HEREBY REQUEST AND AUTHORIZE DR.______________________ AND/OR ASSOCIATES AND WHOMEVER THEY MAY DESIGNATE AS THEIR ASSISTANTS, TO ADMINISTER SUCH TREATMENT AS IS NECESSARY, AND TO PERFORM THE FOLLOWING OPERATION______________________ ______________________ AND SUCH ADDITIONAL OPERATIONS OR PROCEDURES AS ARE CONSIDERED NECESSARY ON THE BASIS OF CONDITIONS THAT MAY BE REVEALED DURING THE COURSE OF SAID OPERATION OR TREATMENT.

2. I REQUEST AND AUTHORIZE THE ADMINISTRATION OF SUCH ANESTHETICS AND/OR OTHER MEDICATIONS AS ARE NECESSARY.

3. FINAL DISPOSITION OF ANY TISSUES OR PARTS SURGICALLY REMOVED IS TO BE HANDLED IN ACCORDANCE WITH THE CUSTOMARY PRACTICES OF THE HOSPITAL.

4. REASONS WHY THE ABOVE NAMED SURGERY AND/OR TREATMENT IS CONSIDERED NECESSARY, ITS ADVANTAGES, PROBABILITY OF SUCCESS, POSSIBLE COMPLICATIONS, AND RISKS, AS WELL AS POSSIBLE ALTERNATIVE MODES OF TREATMENT WERE EXPLAINED TO ME BY DR. ______________________.

5. I AM AWARE THAT THE PRACTICE OF MEDICINE AND SURGERY IS NOT AN EXACT SCIENCE AND I ACKNOWLEDGE THAT NO GUARANTEES HAVE BEEN MADE TO ME CONCERNING THE RESULTS OF THE OPERATION OR PROCEDURE.

6. I HEREBY ACKNOWLEDGE THAT I HAVE READ AND FULLY UNDERSTAND THE ABOVE REQUEST AND AUTHORIZATION FOR MEDICAL AND/OR SURGICAL TREATMENT.

DATE:______________________ TIME: ______________________

SIGNED: ______________________
Patient

OR: ______________________
Legal Representative

____
Relationship (if any)

____
WITNESS

/PL/2736N
702/1019-E-R-5/90 40-1331

FIGURE 19–2 ◆ A surgical consent form. (Courtesy of Northwest Hospital Center, Randallstown, MD.)

client is informed. The surgeon is contacted and requested to see the client for clarification of information if the nurse believes that the client has not been adequately informed. The nurse documents this action in the client's chart.

Clients who cannot write may sign with an "X," which must be witnessed by two people. In an emergency, telephone or telegram authorization is acceptable and should be followed with written consent as soon as possible. The number of witnesses (usually two) and the type of documentation vary according to the facility's policy. In a life-threatening situation in which every effort has been made to contact the person with medical power of attorney, consent is desired but not essential. In lieu of written or oral consent, written consultation by at least two physicians who are not associated with the case may be requested by the physician. This formal consultation legally supports the decision for surgery until the appropriate person can sign a consent form. If the client is not capable of giving consent and has no family, the court can appoint a legal guardian to represent the client's best interests.

A blind client is capable of signing his or her own consent form, which usually needs to be witnessed by two people. Clients who speak a language other than the general language in the agency require a translator and a second witness. Some facilities have consent forms written in more than one language.

Some surgical procedures require a special permit in addition to the standard consent. National and local governing bodies and the individual surgical facility determine which procedures require a separate permit. Intraocular lens implants, sterilization, and experimental procedures are examples of procedures for which the extra form is usually required. Separate consents for anesthesia and the administration of blood products may be required as well.

Implementing Dietary Restrictions For any type of surgery and regardless of whether the client is to receive any kind of anesthetic, he or she is restricted to nothing by mouth (NPO) for 6 to 8 hours before surgery. NPO means no eating of food, drinking (including water), or smoking (nicotine stimulates gastric secretions). It is common practice to begin NPO status for all preoperative clients at midnight on the night before surgery. This extra precaution ensures that the stomach contains a limited volume of gastric secretions, which helps decrease the possibility of aspiration. Outpatients and clients who are scheduled for admission to the hospital on the same day that surgery is performed must receive written and oral instructions about remaining NPO after midnight. The nurse emphasizes the importance of compliance; failure to comply can result in cancellation of surgery or an increased risk of intraoperative or postoperative aspiration.

Administering Regularly Scheduled Medications On the day of surgery, the client's usual medication schedule may need to be altered. The nurse consults the client's medical physician for instructions about the administration of medications, such as those used for diabetes mellitus, cardiac disease, and glaucoma, as well as regularly scheduled anticonvulsants, antihypertensives, anticoagulants, antidepressants, and corticosteroids. The physician may order the administration of some medications to be stopped until after surgery. The physician may order other medications intravenously (IV) to maintain the client's blood level of the medication. Medications for cardiac disease and hypertension are commonly allowed with a sip of water if taken at least 2 hours before surgery. Some antihypertensive or antidepressant medications may be withheld on the day of surgery because of a possible adverse affect on the blood pressure intraoperatively.

The diabetic client who is taking insulin may be given a reduced dose of intermediate- or long-acting insulin on the basis of the serum glucose level, or the client may be given regular (fast-acting) insulin subcutaneously in divided doses on the day of surgery (see Chapter 65 for information on medication for diabetes). An alternative method of diabetes management is an IV infusion of 5% dextrose in water given with the insulin to prevent hypoglycemia intraoperatively. Because of numerous treatment approaches to diabetes, the nurse clarifies medication and IV orders with the physician. (More information about the surgical client with diabetes is found in Chapter 65.)

Gastrointestinal Preparation Bowel or gastrointestinal preparations are done to prevent injury to the colon and to reduce the number of intestinal bacteria. Evacuation of the gastrointestinal tract is done when a client is having major abdominal, pelvic, perineal, or perianal surgery. The surgeon's preference and the type of surgical procedure determine what type of bowel preparation is to be done. Table 19–4 shows typical gastrointestinal preparation regimens for common surgical procedures and complications of the regimens. An enema ordered to be given until return flow is clear is a physically stressful procedure for anyone, but especially for the elderly client. Repeated enemas can cause electrolyte imbalance (especially potassium depletion), fluid volume deficit, vagal stimulation, and postural (orthostatic) hypotension. Enemas also cause severe anorectal discomfort in clients with hemorrhoids. To prevent complications, some physicians prescribe the newer, more potent laxatives (e.g., GoLYTELY) instead of enemas, especially for elderly clients. Bowel preparation procedures can be exhausting, and the nurse takes safety precautions to prevent client falls.

Skin Preparation The skin preparation may be embarrassing to or uncomfortable for the client, especially if the surgical site is in a sensitive or generally private area. The nurse provides a warm, comfortable, private, and safe environment for the client during the procedure.

The skin is the body's first line of defense against infection. A break in this protective mechanism in-

TABLE 19–4 Complications of Common Bowel Preparations for the Surgical Client

Surgical Site	Preparation	Complications
Stomach, duodenum, and proximal jejunum	• Oral laxative (e.g., castor oil preparation or bisacodyl [Dulcolax, Laxit🍁]) • Clear liquid diet the evening before surgery • NPO after midnight	• Abdominal cramping • Dehydration • Electrolyte imbalance • Fatigue
Small intestine	• Oral laxative (e.g., magnesium citrate) • Clear liquid diet the evening before surgery • Multiple-position enema the evening before surgery • NPO after midnight	• Abdominal cramping • Dehydration • Electrolyte imbalance • Fatigue
Large intestine to rectum	• Multiple or combination of oral laxatives 12–24 hr before surgery • Multiple-position tap water or antibiotic (neomycin) enemas (three times or until the return flow is clear) the evening and morning before surgery • Oral antibiotics to sterilize the bowel (e.g., neomycin and erythromycin) 24 hr before surgery • Clear liquid diet the day before surgery • NPO after midnight	• Abdominal cramping • Fatigue and weakness • Fluid excess or deficit • Potassium or sodium deficit • Decreased cardiac output from vagal stimulation • Irritation of bowel and rectal mucosa from enemas

creases the risk of infection, especially for elderly clients. Preoperative skin preparation is the initial step in the prevention of wound infection. One or 2 days before the scheduled surgery, the surgeon may require the client to shower using an antiseptic solution such as povidone-iodine (Betadine) and hexachlorophene. The physician may want the client to be especially attentive to cleaning around the proposed surgical site. If the patient is hospitalized before surgery, the showering and cleaning is often repeated the night before surgery or in the morning before the client is transferred to the surgical suite. This cleaning reduces contamination of and the number of microorganisms on the surgical field. After the final cleaning procedure, especially for an orthopedic surgery, the area may be covered with sterile towels or drapes to prevent contamination.

A controversial step in preoperative skin preparation after the cleaning or showering is the shave. Many health care practitioners believe that the shaving procedure itself is a possible source of contamination of the surgical area and traumatizes the skin around the area where the incision will be made. Those factors believed to predispose the client to wound contamination include bacteria found in hair follicles, disruption of the normal protective mechanisms of the skin, and nicks in the skin (e.g., from shaving). Shaving of hair creates the potential for infection. Clipping of the hair with electrical surgical clippers is becoming increasingly popular to decrease the complications associated with traditional razors. In the United States, the Centers for Disease Control and Prevention recommend that, if shaving is necessary, the hair should be removed by using disposable sterile supplies and aseptic principles immediately before the start of the surgical procedure. Thus, shave preparations are performed in the treatment room, the holding area of the operating suite, or the operating room. Figure 19–3 shows areas shaved for various surgical procedures. Shaving of hair, especially from the head or genital area, can be emotionally upsetting to the client, and regrowth of this hair can be uncomfortable.

Preparing the Client for Tubes, Drains, and Intravenous Access The nurse prepares the client for possible insertion of tubes, drains, and IV access devices. Preparation reduces the client's postoperative anxiety and fear. The nurse is careful not to scare the client while providing information about the purpose of each tube.

TUBES The client may require an indwelling urinary catheter (Foley) before, during, or after surgery to keep the bladder empty and to enable monitoring of renal function. The client having major abdominal or genitourinary surgery usually has a Foley catheter.

A nasogastric tube may be inserted before emergency surgery or major abdominal surgery for decompressing or emptying the stomach and the upper bowel. However, it is more often inserted after the induction of anesthesia, when insertion is less disturbing to the client and is easier to perform

DRAINS Drains are frequently inserted during surgery to promote the evacuation of fluid from the surgical site. Some drains are under the dressing, whereas others are visible and require emptying. Drains come in various shapes and sizes (see Chap. 21). The nurse informs the client that drains are often used routinely and that they are not painful. The nurse further discusses with clients the reasons why they should not kink or pull on the drain.

INTRAVENOUS ACCESS An IV access (line) is placed by the nurse or anesthesia personnel for all clients receiving general anesthesia and some clients receiving other types of anesthesia. An access is needed to administer medication and fluids before, during, and after surgery. Clients who are dehydrated or who are

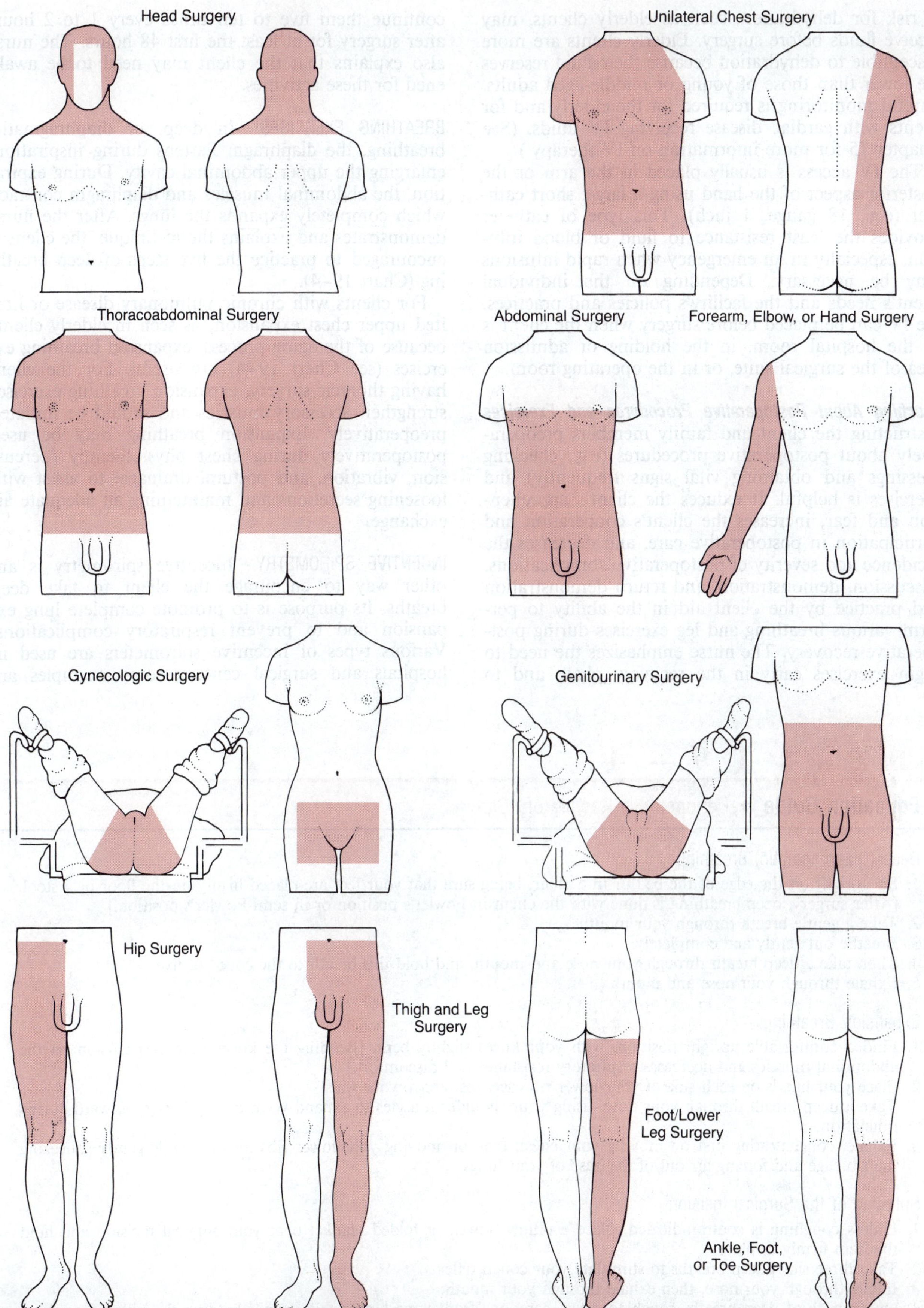

FIGURE 19-3 ◆ Skin preparation of common surgical sites. Shaded areas indicate areas of hair removal.

at risk for dehydration, such as elderly clients, may receive fluids before surgery. Elderly clients are more susceptible to dehydration because their fluid reserves are lower than those of young or middle-aged adults. Careful monitoring is required for the elderly and for clients with cardiac disease receiving IV fluids. (See Chapter 15 for more information on IV therapy.)

The IV access is usually placed in the arm or the posterior aspect of the hand using a large, short catheter (e.g., 18 gauge, 1 inch). This type of catheter provides the least resistance to fluid or blood infusion, especially in an emergency when rapid infusions may be necessary. Depending on the individual client's needs and the facility's policies and practices, the IV can be placed before surgery when the client is in the hospital room, in the holding or admission area of the surgical suite, or in the operating room.

Teaching About Postoperative Procedures and Exercises
Instructing the client and family members preoperatively about postoperative procedures (e.g., checking dressings and obtaining vital signs frequently) and exercises is helpful. It reduces the client's apprehension and fear, increases the client's cooperation and participation in postoperative care, and decreases the incidence and severity of postoperative complications. Discussion, demonstration, and return demonstration and practice by the client aid in the ability to perform various breathing and leg exercises during postoperative recovery. The nurse emphasizes the need to begin exercises early in the recovery phase and to continue them five to ten times every 1 to 2 hours after surgery for at least the first 48 hours. The nurse also explains that the client may need to be awakened for these activities.

BREATHING EXERCISES In deep, or diaphragmatic, breathing, the diaphragm flattens during inspiration, enlarging the upper abdominal cavity. During expiration, the abdominal muscles and diaphragm contract, which completely expands the lungs. After the nurse demonstrates and explains the technique, the client is encouraged to practice the five steps of deep breathing (Chart 19-4).

For clients with chronic pulmonary disease or limited upper chest expansion, as seen in elderly clients because of the aging process, expansion breathing exercises (see Chart 19-4) are useful. For the client having thoracic surgery, expansion breathing exercises strengthen accessory muscles and should be initiated preoperatively. Expansion breathing may be used postoperatively during chest physiotherapy (percussion, vibration, and postural drainage) to assist with loosening secretions and maintaining an adequate air exchange.

INCENTIVE SPIROMETRY Incentive spirometry is another way to encourage the client to take deep breaths. Its purpose is to promote complete lung expansion and to prevent respiratory complications. Various types of incentive spirometers are used in hospitals and surgical centers; some examples are

CHART 19-4

Education Guide ◆ Perioperative Respiratory Care

Deep (Diaphragmatic) Breathing

1. Sit upright on the edge of the bed or in a chair, being sure that your feet are placed firmly on the floor or a stool. [After surgery, deep breathing is done with the client in Fowler's position or in semi-Fowler's position.]
2. Take a gentle breath through your mouth.
3. Breathe out gently and completely.
4. Then take a deep breath through your nose and mouth, and hold this breath to the count of five.
5. Exhale through your nose and mouth.

Expansion Breathing

1. Find a comfortable upright position, with your knees slightly bent. [Bending the knees decreases tension on the abdominal muscles and decreases respiratory resistance and discomfort.]
2. Place your hands on each side of your lower rib cage, just above your waist.
3. Take a deep breath through your nose, using your shoulder muscles to expand your lower rib cage outward during inhalation.
4. Exhale, concentrating first on moving your chest, then on moving your lower ribs inward, while gently squeezing the rib cage and forcing air out of the base of your lungs.

Splinting of the Surgical Incision

1. Unless coughing is contraindicated, place a pillow, towel, or folded blanket over your surgical incision and hold the item firmly in place.
2. Take three slow, deep breaths to stimulate your cough reflex.
3. Inhale through your nose, then exhale through your mouth.
4. On your third deep breath, cough to clear secretions from your lungs while firmly holding the pillow, towel, or folded blanket against your incision.

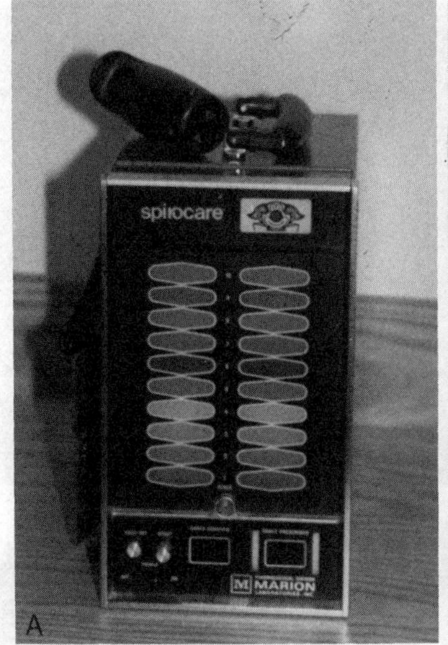

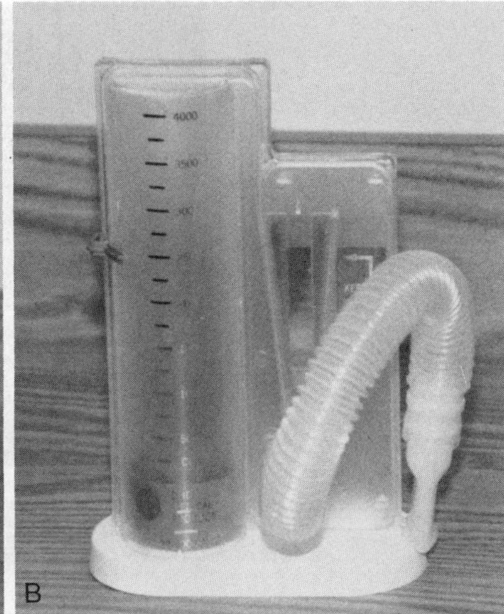

FIGURE 19–4 ◆ Examples of incentive spirometers for lung expansion. *A*, A volume incentive spirometer. *B*, A volume or flow incentive spirometer.

shown in Figure 19–4. With all types, the client must be able to seal his or her lips tightly around the mouthpiece, inhale spontaneously, and hold his or her breath for 3 to 5 seconds to achieve effective lung expansion. Goals (e.g., attaining specific volumes) can be set according to the client's ability and the type of incentive spirometer. Visualization by seeing a light move up a column or a bellows expanding often reinforces and motivates the client to continue performance.

COUGHING AND SPLINTING Coughing may be performed in conjunction with deep breathing every 1 to 2 hours postoperatively. The purposes of coughing are to promote expectoration of secretions, keep the lungs clear, allow full aeration, and prevent pneumonia and atelectasis (lung collapse). Coughing may be uncomfortable for the client, but when performed correctly, it should not harm the surgical area. Splinting (e.g., holding) the incision area provides support, promotes a feeling of security, and reduces pain during coughing. The proper technique for splinting the incision site and coughing is described in Chart 19–4. A folded bath blanket is helpful to use as a splint.

Some practitioners think that coughing exercises should no longer be encouraged routinely. Their belief is that coughing has the potential to harm the surgical wound and that it would be better to emphasize other, safer measures for pulmonary hygiene such as the deep breathing and incentive spirometer exercises. When routine coughing exercises are contraindicated for a client, however, such as after a hernia repair, the physician usually writes a "do not cough" order.

LEG PROCEDURES AND EXERCISES Antiembolism stockings (T.E.D. stockings or Jobst hose), elastic (Ace) wraps, or pneumatic compression devices (e.g., "sequentials" and "boots") may be used perioperatively in combination with leg exercises and early ambulation to promote venous return. Venous stasis can lead to deep vein (venous) thrombosis (DVT) or a pulmonary embolus (PE) if the blood clot breaks off and travels to the lungs. Interventions depend on the client's risk factors. Clients at greater risk for deep vein thrombosis:

- Are obese
- Are older than 40 years of age
- Have a concurrent cancer diagnosis
- Have decreased mobility or immobility
- Have a fracture or leg trauma
- Have a history of deep vein thrombosis, pulmonary embolus, varicose veins, or edema
- Are taking estrogen or oral contraceptives
- Smoke
- Have decreased cardiac output
- Are undergoing pelvic surgery

Antiembolism Stockings and Elastic Wraps. T.E.D.s and elastic wraps provide graduated compression of the lower extremities starting distally at the foot and ankle. The nurse measures the client's leg length and circumference and orders the appropriate stocking size. Elastic wraps are used when the client's leg is too large or too small for the T.E.D.s. The nurse assists the client in applying the T.E.D.s or elastic wraps and ensures that they are neither too loose (are ineffective) nor too tight (inhibit blood flow). The T.E.D.s or elastic wraps also need to be worn as ordered to be effective and should be removed one to three times per day for 30 minutes for skin care and inspection.

Pneumatic Compression Devices. Pneumatic compression devices enhance venous blood flow by providing intermittent periods of compression on the lower extremities. As is the case with T.E.D.s, the nurse measures the client's leg and orders the appropriate size. The nurse places the boots on the client's

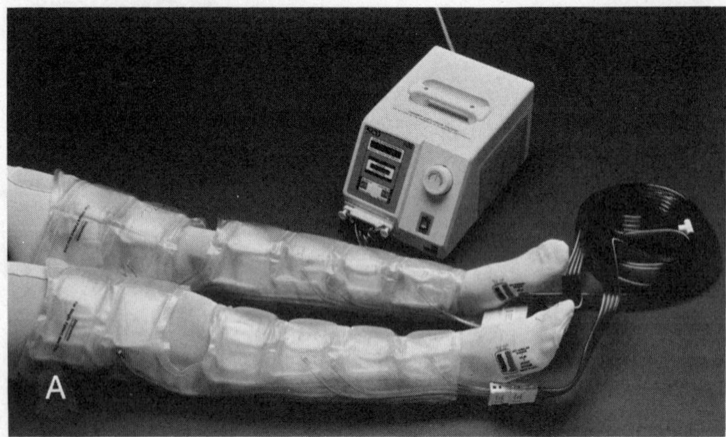

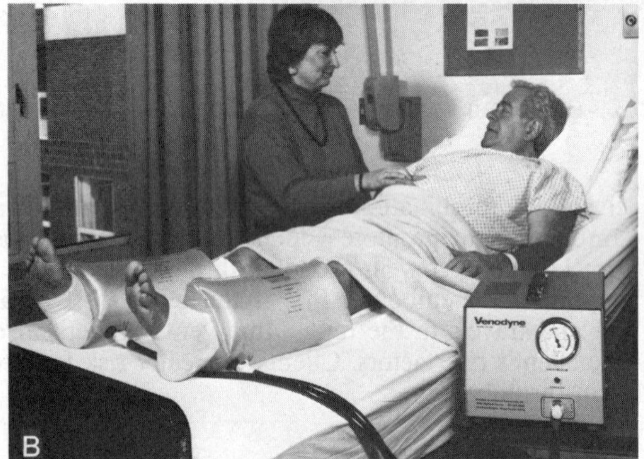

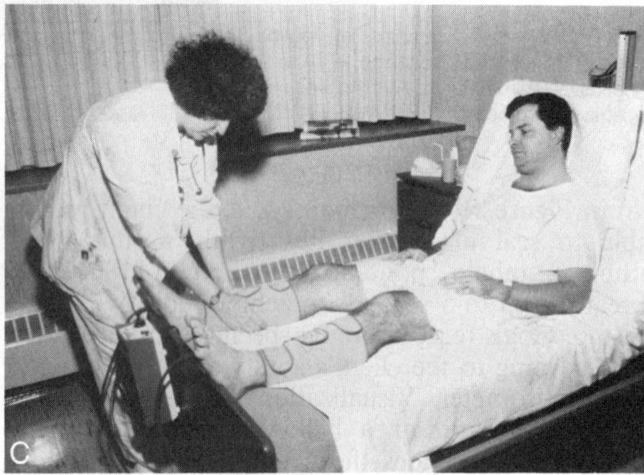

FIGURE 19–5 ◆ Examples of external pneumatic compression devices used to promote venous return and prevent deep vein thrombosis (DVT). *A*, Kendall SCD machine, sleeves, and T.E.D. stockings. *B*, Venodyne pneumatic compression system. *C*, Flowtron DVT calf garments.

legs and sets and checks the prescribed or recommended compression pressures (often 35 to 55 mmHg). Figure 19–5 shows various types of sequential devices. Antiembolism stockings may be worn in addition to the boots and may alleviate some of the uncomfortable sensations associated with the boots (itching, sweating, heat).

Leg Exercises. Leg exercises also promote venous return. The nurse teaches the client the postoperative leg exercises outlined in Chart 19–5 and then encourages the client to practice these exercises preoperatively. The exercises are important, even when the other devices are being used.

EARLY AMBULATION Mobility soon after surgery (early ambulation) stimulates gastrointestinal motility, enhances lung expansion, mobilizes secretions, promotes venous return, prevents rigidity of joints, and relieves pressure.

In general, the nurse instructs the client that he or she should turn at least every 2 hours after surgery while confined to bed. To aid clients, the nurse teaches them how to use the bed side rails safely for turning and how to protect the surgical wound (splinting) when turning. The nurse assures clients that assistance will be given as needed to alleviate any anxiety they may have about this activity.

For certain surgeries, such as some brain, spinal, and orthopedic surgeries, the physician may order turning restrictions. The nurse discusses with the physician other interventions to prevent deep vein thrombosis in clients with turning restrictions. The nurse informs the client of anticipated turning restrictions during preoperative teaching.

Many clients are allowed and encouraged to get out of bed the day of or the day after surgery. The client is often moved into a chair or helped to ambulate the evening after the surgery or the next day, depending on the type of surgery and the physician's preference. If clients must remain in bed, they must turn, deep breathe, and perform leg exercises every 2 hours to prevent the complications of postoperative immobility.

RANGE-OF-MOTION EXERCISES Passive or active range-of-motion exercises to prevent rigidity of joints and muscle contractures are also appropriate postoperative exercises. The client should do these exercises three to five times each, three to four times a day while bedridden. The nurse instructs the client in these procedures and informs the client that he or she will receive assistance as needed postoperatively. (Guidelines for range-of-motion exercises are found in Chapter 23.)

CHART 19-5

Education Guide ◆ Postoperative Leg Exercises

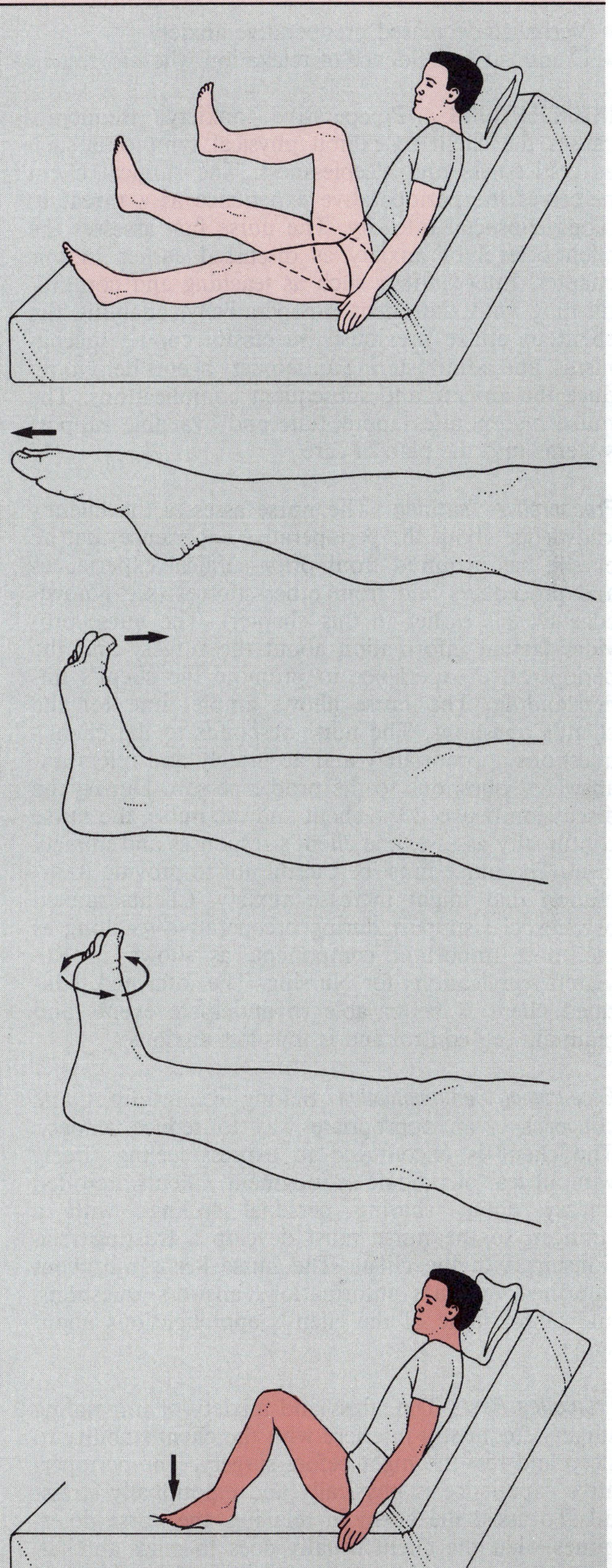

Exercise No. 1

1. Lie in bed with the head of your bed elevated to about 45 degrees. [Using semi-Fowler's position during postoperative leg exercises improves peripheral circulation, prevents thrombus formation, and strengthens muscles.]
2. Beginning with your right leg, bend your knee, raise your foot off the bed, and hold this position for a few seconds.
3. Extend your leg by unbending your knee, and lower the leg to the bed.
4. Repeat this sequence four more times with your right leg, then perform this same exercise five times with your left leg.

Exercise No. 2

1. Beginning with your right leg, point your toes toward the bottom of the bed.
2. With the same leg, point your toes up toward your face.
3. Repeat this exercise several times with your right leg, then perform this same exercise with your left leg.

Exercise No. 3

1. Beginning with your right leg, make circles with your ankles, first to the left, then to the right.
2. Repeat this exercise several times with your right leg, then perform this same exercise with your left leg.

Exercise No. 4

1. Beginning with your right leg, bend your knee and *push* the ball of your foot into the bed or floor until you feel your calf and thigh muscles contracting.
2. Repeat this exercise several times with your right leg, then perform this same exercise with your left leg.

ANXIETY

PLANNING: CLIENT GOALS The goals are that the client will:

- Verbalize decreased preoperative anxiety
- Demonstrate evidence of relaxation when at rest

INTERVENTIONS Preoperative anxiety frequently causes the client to exhibit physical symptoms such as restlessness and sleeplessness. The surgical client perceives the perioperative experience as a threat to biopsychosocial integrity. The nurse first assesses the client's level of anxiety as discussed earlier in this chapter. Interventions such as teaching and communicating with the client preoperatively, enabling the client to utilize previously successful coping mechanisms, and administering antianxiety agents help to reduce the anxiety and subsequent complications. The nurse incorporates appropriate and available support systems into the plan of care.

Preoperative Teaching The nurse assesses the client's knowledge about the perioperative experience that he or she has acquired from prior surgical experiences and procedures and from other sources (see Knowledge Deficit earlier in this chapter). The nurse provides factual information about the surgery and the perioperative experience to promote the client's understanding. The nurse allows ample time for the client's questions. The nurse responds to the client's questions appropriately and accurately and refers unanswered questions to the proper person. During the discussion between the client and the nurse, the nurse continually assesses the client's responses and anxiety level. The nurse must be careful not to provide information that might increase anxiety. Clients ranked psychosocial support during preoperative teaching as the most important component, as shown in Research Applications for Nursing. The informed, educated client is better able to anticipate events and maintain self-control and is thus less anxious.

Encouraging Communication Stating feelings, fears, and concerns is an appropriate way to reduce anxiety. The client is encouraged to express feelings freely without fear of ridicule or judgment. Clients are often uneasy about sharing personal feelings with a stranger, so the nurse must develop a trusting relationship with the client. The nurse keeps the client informed, clarifies information, answers questions, and allays some of the client's apprehensions about surgery.

Promoting Rest The stress and anxiety of impending surgery frequently interfere with the client's ability to sleep and rest the night before surgery. The perioperative experience is physically and emotionally stressful. To assist the client in relaxing, the nurse determines what the client usually does to relax and fall asleep. If permitted and able, the client is encouraged to continue these methods of relaxation. A back rub

RESEARCH APPLICATIONS FOR NURSING

Nurses and Clients May Not Have the Same Priorities for Preop Teaching

Yount, S., & Schoessler, M. (1991). A description of patient and nurse perceptions of preoperative teaching. *Journal of Post Anesthesia Nursing, 6*(1), 17–25.

Preoperative teaching improves the chances of a positive surgical outcome. Clients who receive preoperative teaching experience fewer postoperative complications, a shortened length of stay, enhanced satisfaction, and a quicker return to work. With the increase in same-day surgery, however, nurses have fewer opportunities for assessment, teaching, and client preparation. With so little time to teach, nurses should teach what clients need to learn. Yount and Schoessler therefore conducted a descriptive study of 116 postsurgical clients and 159 hospital nurses to determine how closely the clients and nurses agreed on the relative importance of five dimensions of preoperative teaching:

- Psychosocial support
- Situational information
- Client role
- Sensation/discomfort
- Skills training

Clients ranked the order of importance of these dimensions as listed above. Both clients and nurses rated psychosocial support as the most important component of preoperative teaching. In contrast, however, nurses ranked skills training second whereas clients relegated this category to last place. Both clients and nurses agreed that all five components should be addressed before surgery.

Critique This convenience sample included many clients (25%) scheduled for gynecologic surgery and many others (22%) scheduled for urologic surgery. This kind of sampling may have skewed the results. The investigators suggested that the high client ranking of psychosocial support may have been due to the nature of the surgery. Further studies are needed to determine whether client ranking of the importance of the components of preoperative teaching remains the same regardless of the type of surgery.

Possible nursing implications Health care professionals caring for clients before admission to the hospital may need to determine the client's learning requirements at that time. These professionals should assess the client's prior knowledge, readiness to learn, and priorities for learning content. They should then communicate the results to the admitting hospital nurse. Prehospital teaching programs could also initiate skills training (such as training in coughing and deep breathing) before admission. With that teaching accomplished before the morning of surgery, the admitting nurse may have more time to provide the psychosocial support that surgical clients in this study wanted.

is a relaxing and therapeutic measure that should be offered to all clients in the hospital setting. A sedative or short-acting hypnotic may be prescribed to ensure that the client is well rested for surgery. The nurse offers the medication to the client. If the client refuses, the nurse informs him or her that the sedative is available anytime before midnight.

Using Distraction The nurse may use distraction as an intervention for anxiety. Especially in the 24 hours immediately before surgery, listening to humorous or comedy audiotapes may decrease anxiety (Gaberson, 1991) as may watching television (Friedman et al., 1992).

Teaching Family and Significant Others The nurse assesses the readiness and desire of the family or significant others to take an active part in the client's care. The involved family provides support for the client and helps to reduce anxiety. A positive sign of family members' interest is their initiation of questions about the perioperative experience. After the family members' readiness is determined, the nurse keeps them informed and encourages their involvement in all aspects of preoperative education with the client. The nurse emphasizes the important role of the family preoperatively, but guides discussions and practice sessions so that family members do not dominate the sessions. Family members can practice postoperative exercises with the client and encourage continued practice after the session with the nurse.

The nurse informs the family of the time for surgery, if known, and of any schedule changes. The family is encouraged to visit the client briefly preoperatively to support the client. The nurse reminds the family that the client may be anxious at that time and may have received preoperative sedation.

Most families are anxious about the surgery planned for their loved one. To aid in reducing their anxiety, the nurse explains the intraoperative and postoperative routine to them. The nurse explains that, after the client leaves the hospital room or admission area, there is usually a 30- to 60-minute preparation period in the operating area (holding room, treatment area, and so on) before the surgery actually begins. After surgery, the client is taken to the postanesthesia care unit (PACU) for 1 to 2 hours before returning to the hospital room or the discharge area. The nurse instructs the family about the best place to wait for the client or the surgeon according to the facility's policy and the physician's preference. Many hospitals and surgical centers have designated surgical waiting areas so families can wait in comfortable surroundings and be easily located when the procedure is completed.

PREOPERATIVE CHART REVIEW

The nurse reviews the client's chart to ensure that all documentation, preoperative procedures, and orders are completed. The nurse checks the surgical informed consent form and, if indicated, any other special consent forms, to see that they are signed and dated and contain the witnesses' signatures. Allergies should be noted on the front of the chart. Accurate documentation of height and weight is important for proper dosage calculation of the anesthetic agents. The results of all laboratory, radiographic, and diagnostic tests should be on the chart; any abnormal results are documented and reported to the physician and the anesthesiologist or anesthetist. If the client was an autologous blood donor or had directed blood donations made, those special slips must be included in the chart. The nurse records a current set of vital signs (within an hour or two of the scheduled surgery time) and documents any significant physical or psychosocial observations. The nurse reports special needs and concerns of the client to the surgical team. For example, the nurse advises the surgical team whether the client is a member of Jehovah's Witnesses and does not accept blood products, or whether the client is hard of hearing and does not have his or her hearing aid. This information assists the surgical team in providing continuity of care while the client is in the surgical area.

PREOPERATIVE CLIENT PREPARATION

Facilities generally require that the client remove most clothing and wear a hospital gown into the operating room. Underwear may be permitted for surgery above the waist; socks may be worn, except for foot or leg surgery. The gown prevents the possible introduction of contaminants and provides easy access to the operative area. If ordered by the surgeon, antiembolism stockings are applied preoperatively.

The client's valuables, including jewelry, money, and clothes, are locked in a safe place, according to the facility's policy. The nurse tapes in place rings that cannot be removed and notes that on the preoperative checklist. Religious emblems may be pinned or fastened securely to the client's gown; in some facilities, paper emblems are available from a religious leader.

The client wears an identification band that clearly gives first and last names and hospital number. A bracelet designating that a blood sample for type and crossmatch has been drawn may be worn, depending on the facility's policy.

Dentures, including partial dental plates, are removed and placed in a labeled denture cup. The removal of dentures is a safety measure to prevent aspiration and obstruction of the airway. If a client has any capped teeth, the nurse documents this finding on the preoperative checklist.

All prosthetic devices, such as artificial eyes and limbs, are removed and safely stored, as are contact lenses, wigs, and toupees. The nurse checks for hairpins and clips, which, if not removed, can conduct electrical current used during surgery and cause scalp burns.

Some facilities allow hearing aids in the surgical suite to facilitate communication before and after surgery. If the client is sent to surgery with a hearing aid, the nurse communicates this to the surgical nurse to prevent accidental loss of or damage to the aid. Some facilities allow dentures, wigs, glasses, and so on to be worn by the client into the operating suite to prevent embarrassment to the client. These items can then be removed when absolutely necessary.

The removal of fingernail polish or artificial nails is controversial. This procedure permits assessment of nail bed color as an indicator of oxygenation and circulation during surgery. Currently, pulse oximetry or blood gas analysis is being used more frequently in the operative setting to assess oxygenation. Artificial nails may affect the accuracy of pulse oximetry readings, however. In some facilities, at least one artificial nail must be removed for this reason.

After the client is prepared for surgery and the operating suite is ready to receive the client, the nurse asks the client to empty his or her bladder to prevent incontinence or overdistention and to provide a starting point for intake and output measurement. An overly full bladder may hinder access to the surgical site. The nurse answers any final questions that the client has, offers reassurance as needed, and administers any ordered preoperative medication.

PREOPERATIVE MEDICATIONS

Preoperative medication may be ordered for clients, regardless of the type of planned anesthesia. Various preoperative medications reduce anxiety, promote relaxation, reduce pharyngeal secretions, prevent laryngospasm, inhibit gastric secretions, and decrease the amount of anesthetic required for the induction and maintenance of anesthesia. The selection of medication is based on the client's age, physical and psychologic condition, medical history, and height and weight; the medications that the client takes routinely; the results of preoperative tests; and the type and extensiveness of the surgical procedure. If more than one pharmacologic response is required, combination therapy is usually ordered. A typical combination consists of a sedative or tranquilizer, a narcotic, and an anticholinergic agent. Chart 19–6 gives important information about common preoperative medications.

The preoperative medication is often ordered when the client is "on call" to the surgical suite. After the nurse positively identifies the client (using the arm band) and makes sure that the operative permit is signed, he or she administers the correct medication.

CHART 19–6

Drug Therapy for Preoperative Clients

Drug	Usual Preoperative Dosage	Nursing Interventions	Rationale
Sedatives and Hypnotics			
Pentobarbital sodium (Nembutal, Novopentobarb✱)	• 50–200 mg PO	• Monitor respiratory status.	• Sedatives and hypnotics can cause respiratory depression.
Secobarbital sodium (Seconal sodium, Novosecobarb✱)	• 200–300 mg PO	• Monitor level of anxiety; encourage verbalization and relaxation.	• Reduced anxiety and fear increase the effectiveness of the medication and can lower the amount of anesthesia needed.
Chloral hydrate (Novochlorhydrate✱)	• 0.5–1 g PO		
Tranquilizers			
Chloropromazine hydrochloride (Thorazine, Chlorpromanyl✱)	• 25–50 mg PO • 12.5–25 mg IM	• Maintain NPO status and assess for gastrointestinal upset or nausea.	• NPO status prevents postoperative nausea, decreases intraoperative and postoperative vomiting, and reduces the need for postoperative antiemetics.
Hydroxyzine hydrochloride (Vistaril, Multipax✱)	• 50–100 mg PO • 25–100 mg IM		
Diazepam (Valium, E-Pam✱)	• 5–10 mg PO/IM/IV		
Promethazine hydrochloride (Phenergan, Histanil✱)	• 50 mg PO • 25–50 mg IM	• Promote relaxation by dimming the lights and instructing the client on the importance of relaxation.	• Relaxation allows easier intubation and visualization of the surgical wound.
Lorazepam (Ativan, Novolorazem✱)	• 1–4 mg IM/IV		
Midazolam hydrochloride (Versed)	• 2.5–5 mg IM	• Monitor blood pressure and psychomotor activity.	• Hypotension, drowsiness and decreased coordination are possible and

CHART 19-6

Drug Therapy for Preoperative Clients *Continued*

Drug	Usual Preoperative Dosage	Nursing Interventions	Rationale
		• See additional interventions for Promethazine on p. 374.	monitoring protects the client from injury.
Opioid Analgesics			
Meperidine hydrochloride (Demerol) Morphine sulfate Hydromorphone hydrochloride (Dilaudid)	• 50–100 mg SC/IM • 5–15 mg SC/IM/IV • 2–4 mg PO/SC/IM/IV	• Give as a deep intramuscular injection with a 1- or 1½-inch needle.	• Opioids can be irritating to subcutaneous tissue, and deep injection provides increased effectiveness.
		• Monitor blood pressure and respiratory status.	• Opioid analgesics can cause respiratory and circulatory depression. Reduced doses may be used in elderly or debilitated clients.
		• Inform the client that these medications will decrease the discomfort of treatments, procedures, and so on.	• Positive reinforcement enhances the desired effect.
Anticholinergics			
Atropine sulfate Glycopyrrolate (Robinul)	• 0.4–0.6 mg SC/IM/IV • 0.002 mg/lb (0.004 mg/kg) of body weight IM (0.1–0.3 mg)	• Monitor blood pressure and heart rate.	• Palpitation or bradycardia can occur with low doses; tachycardia can occur with higher doses.
Scopolamine (hyoscine)	• 0.3–0.6 mg SC/IM	• Monitor hydration and maintain NPO status.	• Anticholinergics inhibit secretions before and during surgery, which could cause aspiration, nausea, and vomiting postoperatively.
		• Inform the client of a dry mouth sensation to follow.	• Keeping clients informed decreases anxiety.
		• Scopolamine can cause restlessness and confusion in the elderly; monitor closely.	• Monitoring protects the client from injury.
H_2-Receptor Antagonists			
Cimetidine (Tagamet)	• 300 mg IV	• Infuse slowly over at least 15 min.	• A too-rapid infusion may cause bradycardia.
		• Assess for mental status changes, especially in the elderly.	• Confusion and other mental status changes are indications to discontinue the drug.
Ranitidine hydrochloride (Zantac)	• 50 mg IV	• Give cautiously with renal or hepatic dysfunction. • Assess for burning and itching, at the IV site.	• Ongoing assessment permits early intervention to prevent complications.
Famotidine (Pepcid)	• 20 mg IV	• Store in a refrigerator.	• Proper storage prevents drug breakdown.
		• Administer at bedtime.	• Efficacy increases when the drug is given at bedtime.

Chart continued on following page

CHART 19–6

Drug Therapy for Preoperative Clients *Continued*

Drug	Usual Preoperative Dosage	Nursing Interventions	Rationale
Antiemetics			
Metoclopramide (Reglan, Maxeran✱)	• 10 mg IV	• Monitor for central nervous system effects, especially in the elderly.	• Elderly clients are more susceptible to extrapyramidal effects and tardive dyskinesia.
		• Monitor blood pressure.	• Transient hypertension has occurred.
Droperidol (Inapsine)	• 0.625–2.5 mg IM	• Monitor blood pressure.	• Hypotension is common.
		• Assess respirations.	• Laryngospasm and bronchospasm have occurred.
		• Use with caution in the elderly.	• Elderly are more susceptible to the side effects of droperidol.
Scopolamine (Transderm-Scōp, Transderm-V✱)	• 1.5 mg transdermal patch	• Apply the patch 12–24 hours preoperatively.	• It takes time for the drug to be absorbed.
Promethazine hydrochloride (Phenergan, Histanil✱)	• 25–50 mg PO/IM/IV	• Do not use with monoamine oxidase inhibitors or phenothiazides.	• Drug interactions occur, resulting in increased effects.
		• Give with caution with other central nervous system depressants.	• Can get increased anticholinergic effects with MAO inhibitors.

Then the nurse raises the side rails of the bed or stretcher, places the call system within easy reach of the client while reminding him or her not to try to get out of bed, and places the bed in a low position. The nurse tells the client that he or she may become drowsy and have a dry mouth owing to the medication.

An increasingly common practice is for the premedication to be given *after* the client is transferred to the operating area. This practice permits the operating and anesthesia personnel to make more accurate assessments and have last-minute discussions with a client not yet affected by medication. In addition, after the client is in the operating area, medications can be given via the IV route. The oral (PO) or intramuscular (IM) route is less desirable because of unpredictable absorption rates.

CLIENT TRANSFER TO THE SURGICAL SUITE

In the immediate preoperative preparation, the nurse reviews and updates the client's chart, reinforces preoperative teaching, ensures that the client is appropriately dressed for surgery, and administers preoperative medication, if ordered. The nurse uses a preoperative checklist to assist in the smooth, efficient transfer of the client to the surgical suite (Fig. 19–6). The client, along with the signed consent form, the completed preoperative checklist, the chart, and the addressograph plate, is transported to the surgical suite.

Most clients in the hospital setting are transferred to the surgical suite on a stretcher with the side rails up. In special circumstances (e.g., clients requiring traction, those having orthopedic surgery, and those who should be moved as little as possible immediately after surgery), the client is transferred in his or her hospital bed. Other factors that influence the nurse's decision to transfer the client in a bed are the client's age, size, and physical condition.

EVALUATION

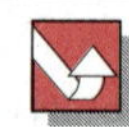

The nurse evaluates the care of the preoperative client according to the identified nursing diagnoses. The outcomes for the client in the preoperative phase of the perioperative experience include that the client:

- States that he or she understands informed consent as it applies to surgery
- Complies with the NPO requirement before surgery
- Verbalizes an understanding of and the reason for a bowel preparation, if applicable
- States the purpose of the skin preparation
- Verbalizes an understanding of how tubes, drains, and IV lines and catheters may be used during and after surgery
- Demonstrates postoperative exercises: turning, deep breathing, splinting, coughing, and performing specific leg exercises

NORTHWEST HOSPITAL CENTER
PRE-OPERATIVE CHECKLIST

Date of Surgery__________________

ALLERGIES

Addressograph Plate

CLINICAL DATA:	Yes	No	Comments
Authorization for Surgical Treatment Completed			
Height & Weight Charted			
History and Physical			
Chest X-Ray			
EKG Report			
Urine Report -			
Blood Sugar Within Range of (75-250mg%)			
Hematocrit Within Range of (27-55%)			
Potassium Within Range of (3.2-5.5mEq/L)			
Results Out of Range Reported to Dept. of Anesthesia			
Anesthesiologist	Time:		By:

PATIENT PREPARATION:	Yes	No	Comments
Jewelry Removed			
Hair Piece, Wig, Hairpin, Barrettes, Beads, Rubberbands Removed			
Loose Teeth or Caps Noted			
Dentures Removed			
Artificial Eye, Contact Lenses, Glasses Removed			
Any Prosthetic Appliance Removed			
Voided or Catheterized - I&O Sheet on Chart			
Identification Bracelet in Place			
Parenteral Fluids Patent & Infusing at cc/hr			
B/P, T.P.R. Charted			
Premedication Given As Ordered			
Side Rails Up-Pt. Care Data & Care Plan on Chart			

COMMUNICATION ASSESSMENT:	Normal	Abnormal	Comments
Vision			
Hearing			
Mental			
Speech			
Other			
Patient's Preferred Name:			

NURSE-TO-NURSE REFERRAL:

Limb For Burial ☐ Yes ☐ No at ______________________ Funeral Home

702/1091-3-R-5/91 (40-1471) 3133N

(O V E R)

FIGURE 19-6 ◆ A preoperative checklist. (Courtesy of Northwest Hospital Center, Randallstown, MD.)

- Demonstrates the use of an incentive spirometer
- States that preoperative anxiety is lessened after preoperative teaching

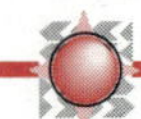

IMPLICATIONS FOR NURSING RESEARCH

Surgery is, and will continue to be, common treatment of many conditions. New perioperative settings are emerging and preoperative nursing is changing as well. Further research will contribute to the continuous quality improvement focus in the health care industry. Some specific preoperative research that could be conducted includes:

- ♦ Does group versus individual preoperative instruction affect the incidence of postoperative complications?
- ♦ What effect does the client's educational level have on the retention of preoperative teaching?
- ♦ How does the timing of preoperative teaching affect the client's recall of instructions in the postoperative period?
- ♦ What is the most effective method of teaching postoperative breathing exercises?
- ♦ What is the relationship between a client's prior surgical experiences and preoperative anxiety?
- ♦ What are the most common causes of preoperative anxiety?
- ♦ How do family members affect a client's level of preoperative anxiety?
- ♦ How does preoperative anxiety affect the postoperative complication rate?

SELECTED BIBLIOGRAPHY

Barrett, J. B., Deehan, R. M. (1992). Preoperative patient teaching: A video approach. *Nursing92, 22*(2), 32F, 32H.

Caldwell, L. M. (1991). The influence of preference for information on preoperative stress and coping in surgical outpatients. *Applied Nursing Research 4*(4), 177–183.

Chana, C. H. (1992). Documenting the nursing process. *AORN Journal, 55*(5), 1231–1235.

Dellasega, C., & Burgunder, C. (1991). Perioperative nursing care for the elderly surgical patient. *Today's OR Nurse, 13*(6), 12–17, 30–31.

Drago, S. S. (1992). Banking on your own blood. *American Journal of Nursing, 92*(3), 61–64.

Eddy, M. E., & Coslow, B. I. (1991). Preparation for ambulatory surgery: A patient education program. *Journal of Post Anesthesia Nursing, 6*(1), 5–12.

Friedman, S. B., Fitzpatrick, S., & Badere, B. (1992). The effects of television viewing on preoperative anxiety. *Journal of Post Anesthesia Nursing, 7*(4), 243–250.

Gaberson, K. B. (1991). The effect of humorous distraction on preoperative anxiety. *AORN Journal, 54*(6), 1258–1263.

Haines, N. (1992). Same day surgery: Coordinating the education process. *AORN Journal, 55*(2), 573–576, 578–580.

Johnson, G. M., & Bowman, R. J. (1992). Autologous blood transfusion: Current trends, nursing implications. *AORN Journal, 56*(2), 281–285, 288–293, 296–298.

Kapp, M. B. (1990). Informed, assisted, delegated consent for elderly patients. *AORN Journal, 52*(4), 857–862.

Keene, A. (1991). Perioperative assessment and nursing implications for the elderly. *Plastic Surgical Nursing, 11*(4), 143–150, 163–167.

Leckrone, L. (1991). Preparing your patient for surgery. *Nursing 91, 21*(7), 46–49.

Leske, J. S. (1992). Practice-based perioperative research. *AORN Journal, 55*(2), 581–590.

Litwak, K. (1991). What you need to know about administering preoperative medications. *Nursing 91, 21*(8), 44–47.

Meckes, P. F. (1991). Geriatric surgery. In Meeker, M. H. & Rothrock, J. C. (Eds.), *Alexander's care of the patient in surgery* (9th ed., pp. 1004–1017). St. Louis: Mosby Year Book.

Meeker, B. J., Rodriguez, L. S., & Johnson, J. M. (1992). A comprehensive analysis of preoperative patient education. *Today's OR Nurse, 14*(3), 11–18, 33–34.

Meeker, M. H., & Rothrock, J. C. (1991). *Alexander's care of the patient in surgery* (9th ed.). St. Louis: Mosby Year Book.

Miner, D. (1990). Preoperative outpatient education in the 1990s. *Nursing Management, 21*(12), 40, 44.

Oetker-Black, S. L., Hart, F., Hoffman, J., et al. (1992). Preoperative self-efficacy and postoperative behaviors. *Applied Nursing Research, 5*(3), 134–139.

Parfitt, J. (1990). Humorous preoperative teaching: Effect on recall of postoperative exercise routines. *AORN Journal, 52,* 114–120.

Persson, A. V., Davis, R. J., & Villavicencio, J. L. (1991). Deep vein thrombosis and pulmonary embolism. *Surgical Clinics of North America, 71*(6), 1195–1209.

Peterson, K. J. (1992). Nursing management of autologous blood transfusion. *Journal of Intravenous Nursing, 15*(3), 128–134.

Recommended practices: Skin preparation of patients (standards). (1992). *AORN Journal, 56*(5), 937–941.

Roberts, S. (1991). Operation reassurance . . . pre-operative visiting program. *Nursing Times, 87*(40), 70–71.

Rost, C. (1991). Preparing for surgery: A pre-admission testing and teaching unit. *Nursing Management, 22*(2), 66.

Ryan, M. E. (1991). Surgical nurse liaison: Expediting the surgical admission process. *AORN Journal, 53*(6), 1529–1532.

Sangermano, C. A. (1991). Practice and principles of ambulatory surgery. In M. H. Meeker & J. C. Rothrock (Eds.), *Alexander's care of the patient in surgery* (9th ed., pp. 964–978). St. Louis: Mosby Year Book.

Shea, S. I. (1992). Our patients face recovery with confidence. *RN, 55*(6), 17–18, 20.

Tappen, R. M. (1991). Alzheimer's disease: Communication techniques to facilitate perioperative care. *AORN Journal, 54*(6), 1279–1286.

Which presurgical tests are worthwhile? (1992). *Emergency Medicine, 24*(14), 88–90.

Yount, S., & Schoessler, M. (1991). A description of patient and nurse perceptions of preoperative teaching. *Journal of Post Anesthesia Nursing, 6*(1), 17–25.

SUGGESTED READINGS

Keene, A. (1991). Perioperative assessment and nursing implications for the elderly. *Plastic Surgical Nursing, 11*(4), 143–150, 163–167.

The first half of this article is a comprehensive review of mental, physical, and functional changes associated with the aging process. Then specific nursing implications related to the elderly preoperative and postoperative client are discussed. A 45-item continuing education post-test is included.

Meeker, B. J., Rodriguez, L. S., & Johnson, J. M. (1992). A comprehensive analysis of preoperative patient education. *Today's OR Nurse, 14*(3), 11–18, 33–34.

The authors wanted to determine whether structured preoperative teaching would have an effect on the incidence of postoperative atelectasis. Their review of the literature is comprehensive, and each study is summarized in this article. An outline of content for the preoperative class is included. Although there was an increase in the frequency of atelectasis in one group of clients, the authors could not show statistical significance. A ten-item continuing education quiz is included.

Peterson, K. J. (1992). Nursing management of autologous blood transfusion. *Journal of Intravenous Nursing, 15*(3), 128–134.

This article reviews the historical development of autologous blood transfusion as well as its current advantages, disadvantages, and contraindications. Five types of autologous transfusions are discussed, and photographs are included. Nursing care and anticoagulation are included.

Tappen, R. M. (1991). Alzheimer's disease: Communication techniques to facilitate perioperative care. *AORN Journal, 54*(6), 1279–1286.

This article reviews pathophysiologic changes in Alzheimer's disease as well as the cognitive changes associated with the disease. The author identifies specific interventions to increase effective communication with the preoperative client who has Alzheimer's disease.

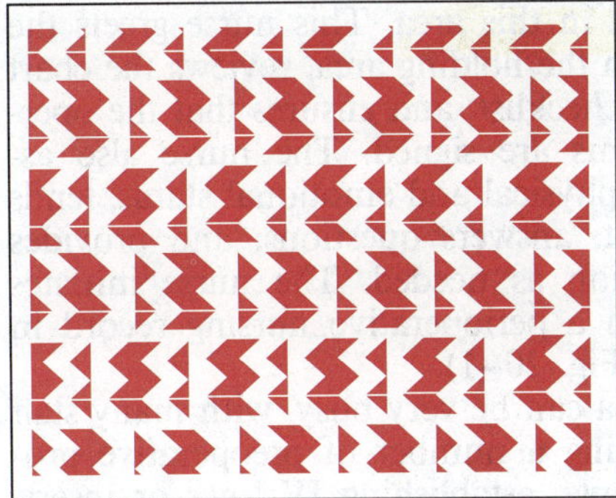

CHAPTER 20

Interventions for Intraoperative Clients

CHAPTER HIGHLIGHTS

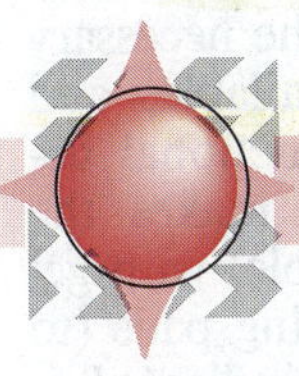

The intraoperative phase of the perioperative experience begins as the client enters the surgical suite. This is an anxious time for the client, as he or she enters into unfamiliar experiences involving unknown outcomes. Nursing care during the intraoperative period addresses all of the client's physical needs as well as the client's comfort, safety, dignity, and psychological status. Specific procedures and policies may differ among agencies, but similarities are evident and reflect the standards and recommended practices for perioperative nursing, as published by the Association of Operating Room Nurses (AORN, 1993).

OVERVIEW

MEMBERS OF THE SURGICAL TEAM

The surgical team consists of the following:

- The surgeon
- One or more surgical assistants
- The anesthesiologist and/or nurse anesthetist
- Operating room nurses

Operating room nurses include the holding area nurse, circulating nurse, scrub nurse, and any specialty nurses. The number of assistants, circulating nurses, and scrub nurses depends on the complexity and projected length of the surgical procedure. For some minor diagnostic or outpatient procedures, only a scrub nurse or a circulating nurse may be required in addition to the surgeon.

SURGEON AND SURGICAL ASSISTANT

The surgeon is a physician who assumes responsibility for the surgical procedure and any surgical judgments about the client. The surgical assistant might be another surgeon (or physician, such as a resident or intern), a physician's assistant, nurse, or surgical technologist. Under the direction of the surgeon, the assistant may hold retractors, suction the wound (to allow visualization of the operative site), cut tissue, suture, and dress wounds. Regulating agencies determine who may qualify to be a surgical assistant and usually delineate the functions of the surgical assistant.

ANESTHESIOLOGIST AND NURSE ANESTHETIST

The anesthesiologist is a physician who specializes in the administration of anesthetic agents. A certified registered nurse anesthetist (CRNA) is a specially trained registered nurse with additional credentials who administers anesthetics under the supervision of an anesthesiologist, surgeon, dentist, or podiatrist. The anesthesiologist or CRNA administers anesthetic drugs to induce and maintain anesthesia and administers other medications as indicated to support the client's physical status during surgery.

The anesthesiologist or nurse anesthetist usually monitors the client intraoperatively by measuring, assessing, and monitoring the following:

- Vital signs
- Cardiopulmonary function (via ECG monitoring, pulse oximetry, end-tidal CO_2 monitoring, arterial blood gases, and hemodynamic parameters via arterial lines and/or pulmonary artery catheters)
- Intake and output

Depending on the client's needs, anesthesia personnel administer intravenous (IV) fluids, including blood and blood components, to maintain the client's physiologic homeostasis.

(See Units 3, 6, and 7 for further discussion on fluid balance; acid-base balance; oxygenation; and cardiac monitoring, assessment, and function.)

OPERATING ROOM NURSES

Operating room (OR) nurses assume several roles within the operating suite, depending on their education, experience, skill, and job responsibilities.

HOLDING AREA NURSE Some operating suites feature a private area adjacent to the main operating rooms, known as the presurgical holding area. The client waits in this area until the operating room is ready. The holding room nurse manages the client's care while the client is in this area. This nurse greets the client on arrival in the holding area, reviews the chart and preoperative checklist, and ensures that the operative consent forms are signed. The nurse also assesses the client's physical and emotional status, lends emotional support, answers questions, and provides additional education as needed. The nurse initiates documentation on a perioperative nursing record in the holding area (Fig. 20–1).

The holding area can be very busy, with many staff members performing a number of preoperative procedures (for example, establishing IV lines or inserting nasogastric tubes). The holding area nurse should maintain an atmosphere conducive to the client's overall well-being. The holding area nurse intervenes on behalf of the client to maintain comfort, privacy, and confidentiality.

CIRCULATING NURSE The circulating nurse (who must be a registered nurse) coordinates, oversees, and participates in the client's nursing care while the client is in the operating room. The circulating nurse's actions are vital to the smooth flow of events before, during, and after the operation. The circulator sets up the operating room, ensures that the necessary supplies and equipment are readily available, and checks that all equipment is safe and functional before the surgery. The circulating nurse makes the operating bed (formerly called the OR table) with gel pads (to prevent pressure sores) and heating pads (to prevent hypothermia) under the sheets as indicated.

If there is no holding room nurse, the circulator assumes the responsibilities of that nursing role as well. Even when there is a holding room nurse, the circulator also greets the client and reviews findings with the holding area nurse, since the circulator is responsible for continuity of client care.

Once the client is ready to move into the operating room, the circulating nurse assists the OR team in transferring the client onto the operating bed. The nurse then positions the client, protecting bony prominences with extra padding as indicated while comforting and reassuring the client. The nurse continues to document interventions and events. The circulating nurse also assists the anesthesiologist or CRNA with the induction of anesthesia, and then may "prep" (scrub) the surgical site before the client is draped with sterile drapes.

Throughout the surgery, the circulating nurse:

- Monitors the traffic in the room
- Assesses the amount of urine and blood loss
- Reports findings to the surgeon and anesthesia personnel
- Ensures that the surgical team maintains sterile technique and a sterile field
- Documents care, events, and findings

Depending on facility policy, the circulating nurse may obtain and record medications, blood, and blood components (or this may partially be a function of anesthesia personnel). Before the surgical procedure is

PRE-OPERATIVE

Date:______ Surgeon:______ Procedure:______

______

Arrival: ______ AM/PM Identification:______ Verbally:______ Nameband______

Verbalization: Name of Surgeon ___Yes ___No Procedure to be done ___Yes ___No

Allergies: ___ No Known Allergies Drugs: ______

N.P.O. Status: ___ Yes ___ No Comment:______

Prosthesis: ___ None ___ Dentures ___ Hearing Aid ___ Glasses/Contact Lens ___ Jewelry

Disposition of Prosthesis: ______

Implants: ___ None ___ Yes Type:______

Equipment: ___ I.V. ___ Foley ___ Ventilator ___ Cardiac Monitor ___ IABP:______

Other: ______

Handicaps: ___ None ___ Language ___Mobility ___Hearing ___ Other:______

Level of Consciousness: ___ Awake ___ Oriented ___ Sedated ___ Confused ___ Agitated ___Crying

Blood: ___Type & Screen ___ Type & Cross ___ Units in O.R. ___Units in Blood Bank

Available on Chart:

___ Permit ______ ___ Blood Consent ______

___ History & Physical ______ ___ Electrocardiogram ______

___ Complete Blood Count ______ ___ Chest X-Ray ______

___ Urinalysis ______ ___ Coag Profile ______

___ Other ______

R.N. Signature: ______

INTRA OPERATIVE

Identification: ___Verbally ___ Nameband Scrub Sees Permit: ___Yes ___No

Scrub Nurse Aware of Allergies if Applicable: ___Yes

Position: ___ Supine ___ Prone ___ Lithotomy ___ Lateral ___ Jackknife ___ Fracture Table

Other: ______

Positioned By: ______

Padding/Supports/Restraints:

___ Safety Belt ___ Arm Secured on Armboard L/R ___ Pillows

___ Kidney Rest ___ Stirrups ___ Axilliary Roll

___ Shoulder Roll ___ Sandbag ___ Blankets

___ Heel/Elbow Pads ___ Mayfield: ___ Horseshoe ___ Chest Roll

___ Arm Secured at Side L/R ___ 3 Pt. Skeletal

___ Action Pads

OUR LADY OF LOURDES MEDICAL CENTER
PERIOPERATIVE NURSING RECORD

PREOP:C

7220.12A 2/92

FIGURE 20–1 ◆ A perioperative nursing record with areas for charting preoperatively upon the client's arrival in the operating room (OR) suite, intraoperatively, and postoperatively before transfer out of the operating room. (Courtesy of Our Lady of Lourdes Medical Center, Camden, NJ.)

Illustration continued on following page

Skin Condition:________ Prep: ________ Betadine_____ Hibiclens______ Other________

Tourniquet: Location:____________ Time Inflated_____:_____ AM/PM

P.S.I.____________ Time Deflated_____:_____ AM/PM

Applied By:____________ Hospital #____________

Electrocautery: None____________ Hospital #____________

Coag Setting:____________ Cut Setting:____________

BiPolar:________ Hospital #____________ BiPoplar Setting:____________

Warming Blanket: ________ None Hospital #__________ Temp Set__________

Time on:________ AM/PM Time off:________ AM/PM

Other Equipment Used:____________________________

Irrigation:____________________________

Medications: Time Drug Dose Route Prepared By Given By

Specimens: ______ None Cultures: ______ Aerobic ______ Anaerobic

______ Frozen Section:____________________

______ Routine:____________________

______ Other:____________________

Drains/Catheters: ___ None ___ Foley Inserted By:____________ Immediate Urine Output______

_____Other:_____ ______ Hemovac ______ Penrose ______ Jackson Pratt ______ Chest Tube

Intraoperative X-Ray: ______ Yes ______ No Type:____________

R.N. Signature: ____________________________

IMMEDIATE POST OPERATIVE

Level of Consciousness: _____ Awake _____Sedated _____ Sedated & Responsive to Verbal Stimuli

Skin Condition:____________________ Dressing Site:____________________

Airway Status: ______ Intubated ______ Extubated

Accompanying Personnel:____________________________

Receiving Unit:____ ICU/CCU____ CVU ____ PACU ____ SDS ____ Nursing Unit:__________

Comments: ____________________________

Report Given To:____________________ By Phone:__________

R.N. Signatue ____________________ Date: __________

OUR LADY OF LOURDES MEDICAL CENTER
PERIOPERATIVE NURSING RECORD

PREOP:C

7220.12B 2/92

FIGURE 20-1 ◆ *Continued*

over, the circulating nurse completes documentation (Fig. 20–2; see also Fig. 20–1). The nurse notes drains or catheters in place, the length of surgery, and the count of all sponges, "sharps" (needles, blades), and instruments. The nurse notifies the postanesthesia care unit (PACU) of the client's estimated time of arrival and any special needs of the client (e.g., a ventilator).

SCRUB NURSE AND SURGICAL TECHNOLOGIST The scrub nurse sets up the sterile field (Fig. 20–3), assists with draping of the client, and hands sterile supplies and instruments to the surgeon and the assistant. Knowledge of anatomy and physiology and familiarity with the surgical procedure allow the scrub nurse to anticipate which instruments and types of sutures the surgeon will need; the nurse's ability to anticipate these needs reduces the duration of anesthesia for the client. Throughout the surgical procedure, the scrub nurse (with the circulating nurse) maintains an accurate account of sponges, sharps, instruments, and the amounts of irrigation fluid used.

The scrub role may be performed by a specially trained person who is not a nurse. Such people are called operating room technicians (ORTs) or surgical technologists. (The term CST may be used for those who are certified surgical technologists.)

SPECIALTY NURSES The specialty coordinator nurse is educated in a particular type of surgery (e.g., orthopedic, cardiac, ophthalmologic) and is responsible for intraoperative nursing care specific to clients needing that type of surgery. The specialty coordinator nurse also cares for and maintains equipment and instruments used in the specialty and maintains needed supplies. During surgery, the specialty nurse may function as the scrub or circulating nurse.

If the facility has laser technology, nurses specially trained in the use, care, and maintenance of the laser should be on hand. Such a nurse may be called a *laser specialty nurse* or *a laser nurse coordinator.* "Laser" is an acronym for *l*ight *a*mplification by the *s*timulated *e*mission of *r*adiation. A laser emits a high-powered beam of light that cuts tissue more cleanly than scalpel blades do. This process produces intense heat for rapid coagulation of blood vessels or tissue and can turn tissue (such as a tumor) into vapor. It is essential for all personnel to observe safety measures (e.g., eye shields, door signs) during laser procedures.

PREPARATION OF THE SURGICAL SUITE AND TEAM

SAFETY

During the intraoperative phase, safety of the client is a primary concern of all members of the surgical team. The operating room layout is designed to prevent infection by limiting the source of contaminants. The staff uses safety straps for the client and securely locks the operating bed in place. Heating pads are used to prevent hypothermia, and interventions are instituted to prevent skin breakdown.

The nurse ensures electrical safety through the proper placement of grounding pads and the use of electrical equipment that meets safety standards. All equipment that might be used during surgery must be appropriately cleaned and sterilized and in proper working condition. The nurse ensures a correct count of surgical instruments and sponges before, during, and after surgery.

Fire prevention is of utmost concern to OR personnel, as is prevention of complications associated with the use of hazardous and potentially toxic substances. A cool room temperature and low humidity are optimal, and staff and clients must be protected against thermal or chemical burns caused by fire or spills. The nurse should be aware of appropriate emergency measures to take in the event of a fire or spill.

LAYOUT

The surgical suite should be located out of the mainstream of the hospital or facility and adjacent to the postanesthesia unit (PACU), support services (e.g., blood bank, pathology and radiology departments, and the supply, processing, and distribution [SPD] department). Traffic flow should be such that contamination from outside the suite is minimal. Within the suite, there must be separation of clean and contaminated areas. Traffic flow is controlled by designating areas as unrestricted, semirestricted, and restricted (AORN, 1993).

The size of a surgical suite depends on the size and surgical capabilities of the facility. The average suite contains staff changing rooms (staff locker rooms) and staff lounges, an admission (or preoperative holding) area, a scrub area (for staff), a number of operating rooms, designated cabinets for sterile supplies, separate utility rooms for clean and soiled equipment, and a clean linen room.

Figure 20–4 shows a typical operating room. The exact number of tables and specialized equipment used in the room are based on the needs of each client. A reliable communication system provides the vital link between the operating room and the main desk of the surgical unit or suite. The system should include an intercom and the capability to differentiate between routine and emergency calls.

HEALTH AND HYGIENE OF THE SURGICAL TEAM

Everyone has a large number of potentially pathogenic bacteria on the skin and hair and in the respiratory tract. Because these pathogens can be transmitted to the client, special health requirements and dress are required. Health standards require that all members of the surgical team and other support personnel in the surgical suite be free from communicable diseases. Anyone who has an open wound, cold, or other infection should not participate in surgery.

O.R. SUITE# 1 2 3 4 5 6 7 ____ Scheduled ____ Emergency

Date: Chart Checked By: ____

Time Sched: ____ A/P in Room: ____ A/P Began: ____ A/P End: ____ A/P Out: ____ A/P

Wound Classification: ____ I Clean ____ II Clean Contaminated ____ III Contaminated ____ IV Dirty

Surgeon: ____ Assistant: ____

Anesthesiologist/Anesthetist: ____

Perfusionist: ____ Type Anesthesia: ____

Scrub: ____

Relief Scrub: ____

Circulator: ____

Relief Circulator: ____

Pre-operative Diagnosis: ____

Post-Operative Diagnosis: ____

Operation: ____

Estimated Blood Loss: ____

Clamptime: On: Off:

Vein Graft Taken From: ____ Internal Mammary ____ Right Leg ____ Left Leg ____ Other: ____

Implants: ____

Counts	Original	Relief	First	Second
Sponge				
Instrument				
Needle				

Count Aborted: X-Ray Taken ____ Yes ____ No

Comments: ____

Signature/Operating Surgeon: ____

Signature/Circulator: ____ Signature/Scrub: ____

OUR LADY OF LOURDES MEDICAL CENTER
OPERATIVE RECORD

OR SUITE: C

7220.04 7/91

FIGURE 20–2 ◆ An interdisciplinary operative record. Names of all personnel involved are listed, and numerous signatures are required for completion. (Courtesy of Our Lady of Lourdes Medical Center, Camden, NJ.)

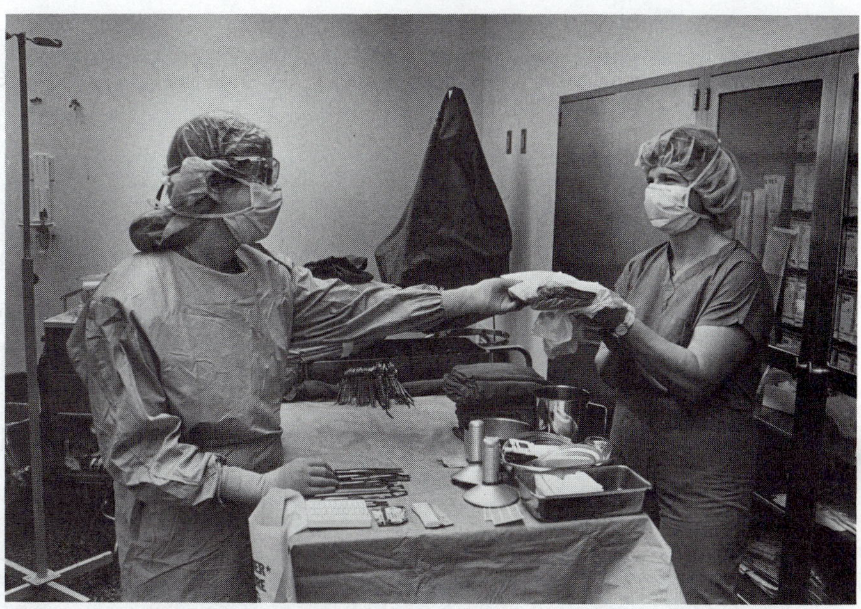

FIGURE 20–3 ◆ Setting up the sterile table.

Good personal hygiene aids in the control of infection, as does frequent and appropriate hand washing. Because the shedding of microorganisms and skin debris is greatest immediately after showering, surgical staff should bathe a few hours before changing into operating room attire. Personnel should wear only a minimum of jewelry, which can carry multiple microorganisms.

In preparing for surgery, all personnel must wash their hands between procedures and more frequently

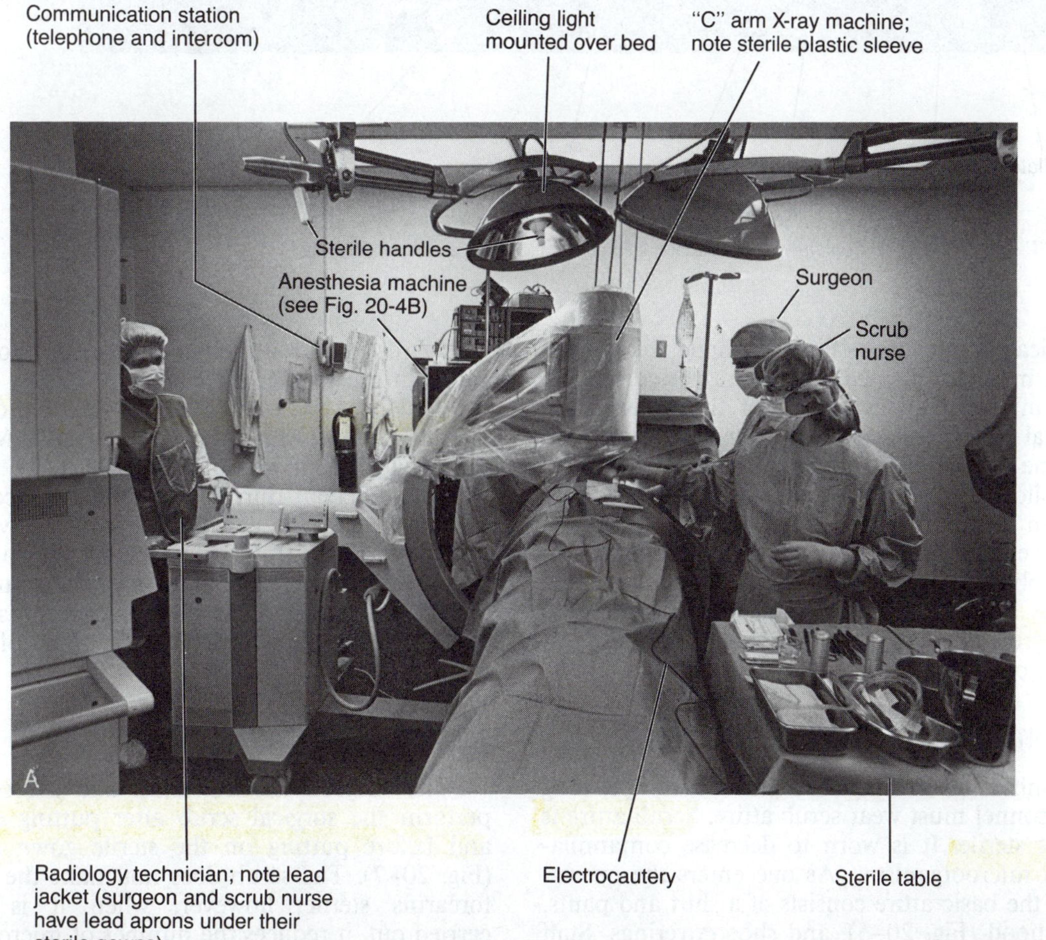

FIGURE 20–4 ◆ *A*, A typical operating room.

Illustration continued on following page

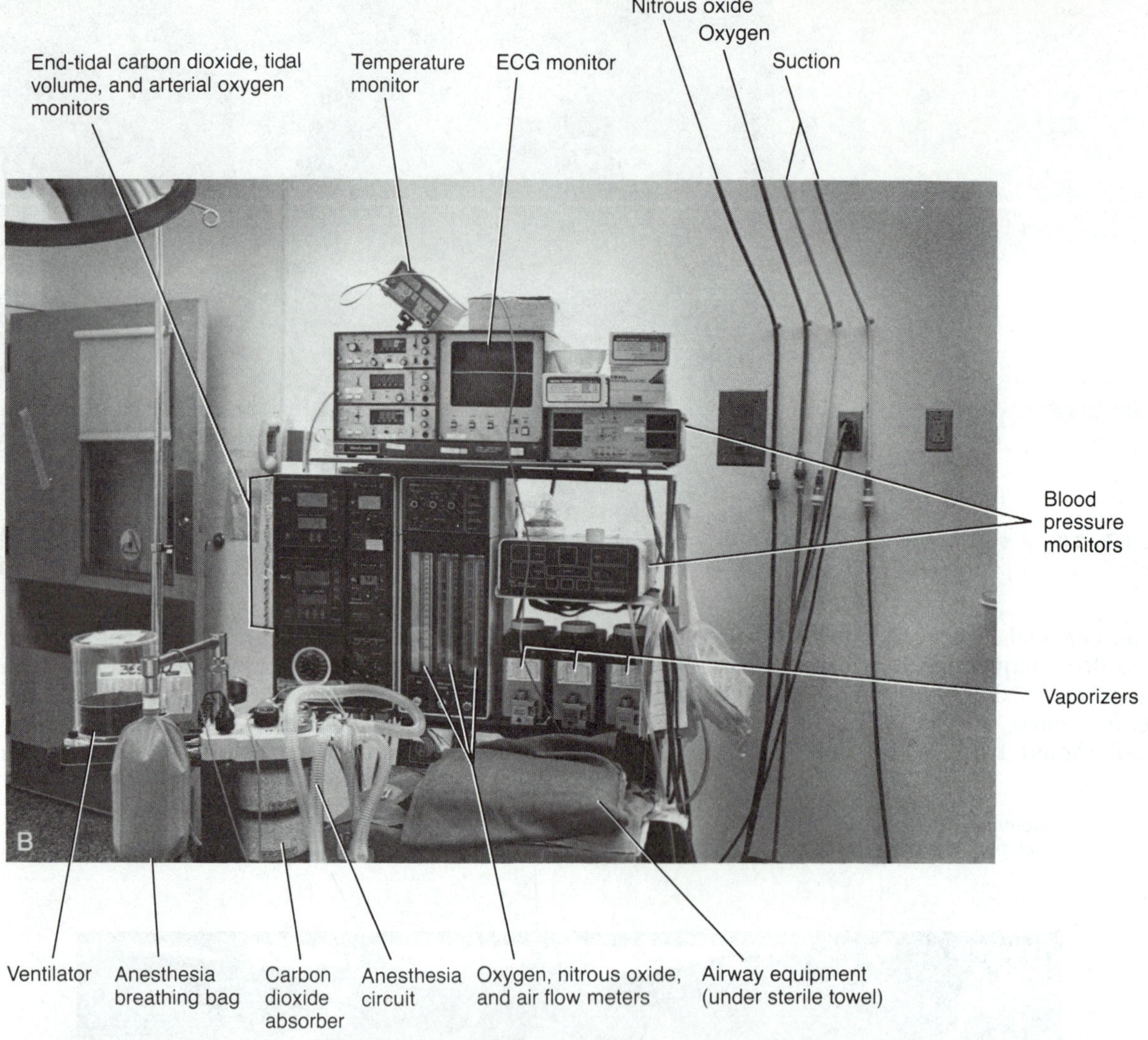

FIGURE 20–4 ◆ *Continued B,* A typical anesthesia station with an anesthesia machine.

when indicated. Specimens from the hands of surgical personnel may be obtained for culture periodically in order to maintain an awareness of the potential of nosocomial (hospital-acquired) infections and to identify the source of pathogenic invasion. Personnel should follow agency policy and should participate more often if quality reports (e.g., through the Quality Improvement Program or Quality Reviews) indicate a problem. The average time between routine cultures is 3 to 6 months. Surgical attire and the surgical scrub are additional interventions that help to prevent contaminations.

SURGICAL ATTIRE

All members of the surgical team and all operating room personnel must wear scrub attire. Scrub attire is clean, not sterile. It is worn to decrease contamination from microorganisms. As one enters the operating *suite,* the basic attire consists of a shirt and pants, a cap or hood (Fig. 20–5), and shoe coverings. Staff change into clean surgical attire in the operating locker rooms, not at home. All members of the surgical team must cover their hair.

In addition to basic attire, anyone who enters an operating *room* must also wear a mask. Members of the surgical team who are scrubbed to be at the bedside of the client during the surgical procedure must also be in a sterile gown, with sterile gloves and eye protectors (Fig. 20–6). Members of the surgical team in the operating room who are *not* scrubbed (e.g., anesthesiologist and circulating nurse) usually wear cover scrub jackets to prevent shedding of organisms from bare arms.

SURGICAL SCRUB

The surgeon, all assistants, and the scrub nurse perform the surgical scrub after putting on a mask and before putting on the sterile gown and gloves (Fig. 20–7). The scrub does not make the hands and forearms sterile; however, when it is effectively carried out, it reduces the number of microorganisms.

A disposable scrub brush or sponge, impregnated

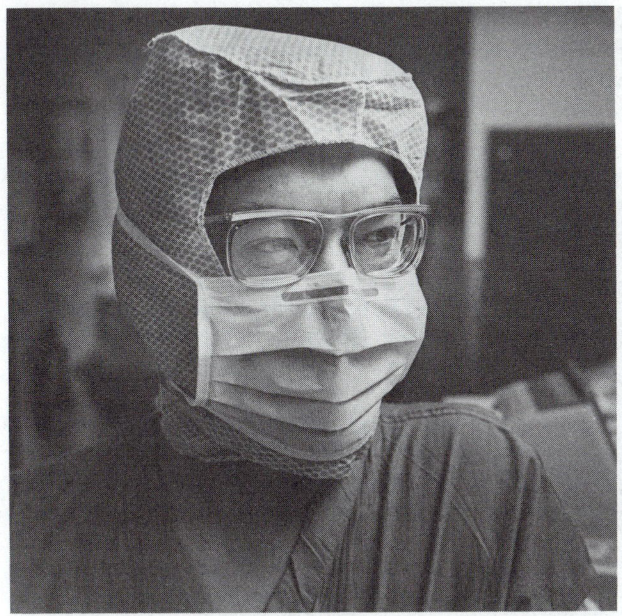

FIGURE 20-5 ♦ An example of a hood-type hair covering that adequately covers facial and scalp hair.

with an antimicrobial solution, and a nail cleaner are used. As with hand washing, the effectiveness of the scrub depends on the application of friction from the fingertips to the elbow. The surgical scrub continues for 5 to 6 minutes, followed by a rinse. During the rinse, surgical personnel position their hands and arms in such a way that water runs off, rather than up or down, their arms. After scrubbing, personnel enter the operating room with their hands held higher than the elbows and thoroughly dry their hands and forearms with a sterile towel. After drying, the scrubbed staff member is assisted into a sterile gown ("gowning") and puts on sterile gloves ("gloving").

Gowns, gloves, and materials that are used at the operative field must be sterile, and they are changed between surgical procedures. The areas of the surgical gown considered sterile are the front of the gown from 2 inches below the neck to the waist area, and the elbow to wrist area. Only when they are properly scrubbed and attired should members of the surgical team handle sterile drapes and other equipment.

ANESTHESIA

The word anesthesia comes from the Greek word *anesthesis,* meaning "negative sensation." The administration of anesthesia is an exact and sophisticated science requiring the skill of a licensed anesthesiologist or a certified registered nurse anesthetist (CRNA).

Anesthesia is an artificially induced state of partial or total loss of sensation, occurring with or without loss of consciousness. The purpose of anesthesia is to block the transmission of nerve impulses, suppress reflexes, promote muscular relaxation, and, in some cases, achieve a controlled level of unconsciousness. Anesthesia personnel use a separate Anesthesia Record for documentation (Fig. 20-8).

The choice of anesthesia is determined primarily by the anesthesiologist or CRNA on the basis of consultation with the surgeon and consideration of other specific client-related factors. The nurse or client or both communicate the client's preference and fears related to a particular type of anesthesia to the anesthesiologist or CRNA. Specific problems noted in the client history as well as the client's preoperative physical and mental status are major factors in the selection and dosage of anesthesia. Selection is also influenced by the following factors:

- The type and duration of the procedure
- Whether or not the procedure is an emergency
- How long it has been since the client ate
- The surgical site
- The client position indicated for the surgical procedure

The administration of anesthesia begins with the selection and administration of preoperative medication (see Chap. 19).

The nurse should know the pharmacologic characteristics of commonly used agents and their effects on

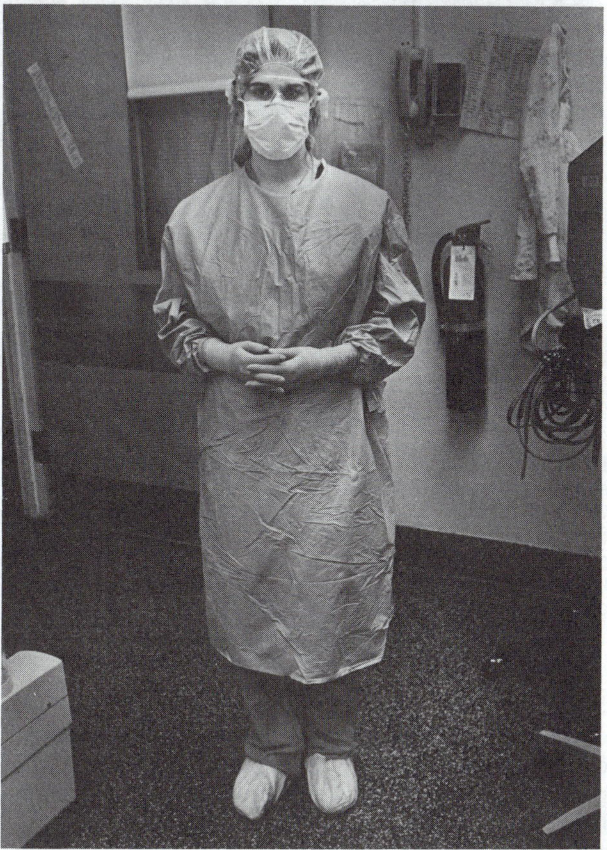

FIGURE 20-6 ♦ Typical attire for all scrubbed personnel. Note complete hair covering, eye shields, mask, sterile gloves over the sleeves of the sterile gown, and shoe coverings. Note that when not in use, the hands are typically folded in front of the body, never below the waist.

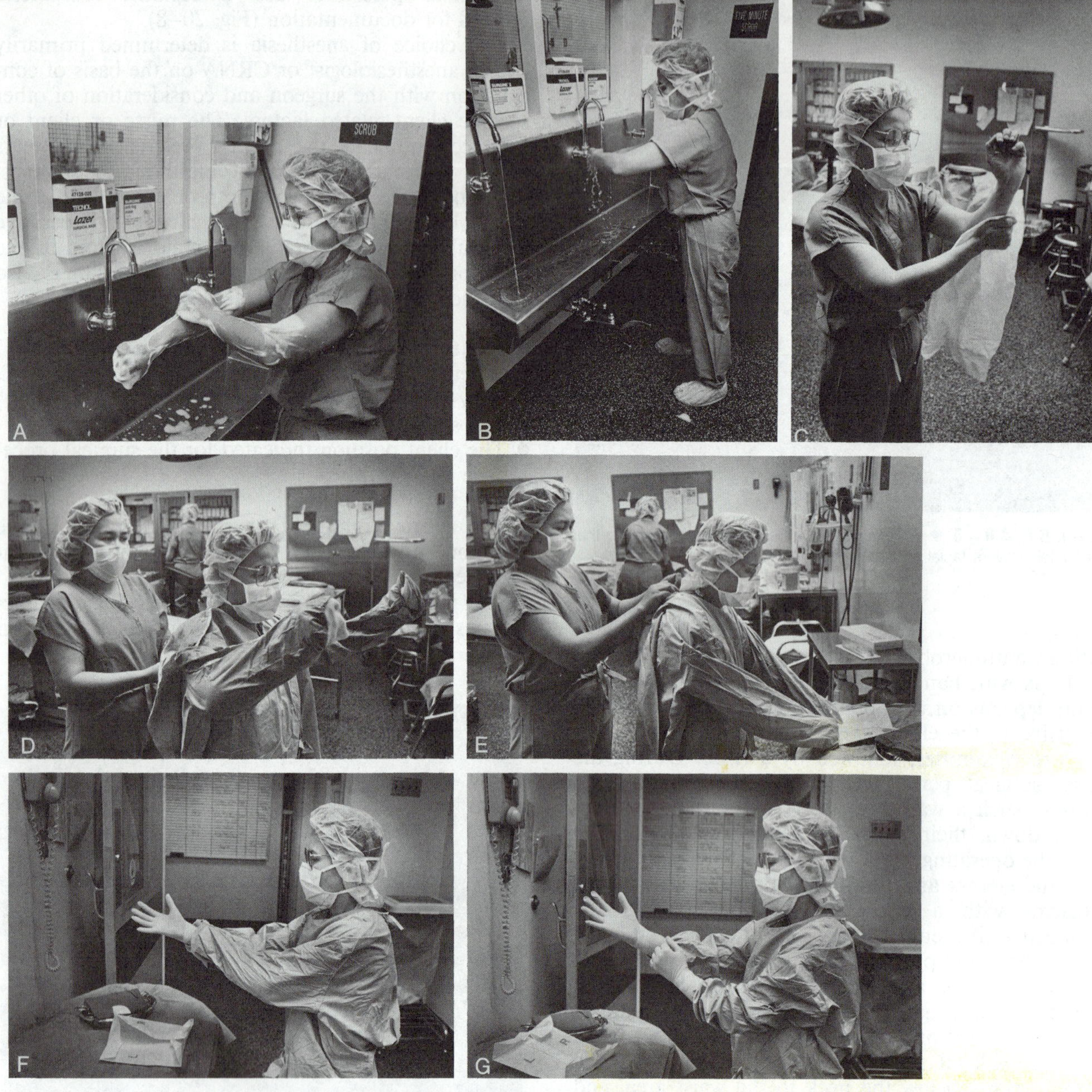

FIGURE 20–7 ◆ The scrubbing, gowning, and gloving process. *A*, The surgical scrub. *B*, Rinsing. Note the water falling off the hands and arms. Also note the leg-operated handle that controls the water flow. *C*, After scrubbing and rinsing, the scrub nurse dries her hands and arms with a sterile towel inside the operating room. *D*, The scrub nurse is assisted into a sterile gown. *E*, The scrub nurse prepares sterile gloves while the sterile gown is being tied in the back. Note that the scrub nurse's hands are *inside* the sleeve of the gown and that she is touching the sterile gloves only with the sterile sleeve. *F*, With her sterile gown securely tied in the back, the scrub nurse puts on her first sterile glove. Note again that her hand never emerges from under the sterile sleeve. *G*, With both gloves on and over the sleeves of the sterile gown, the nurse adjusts the gloves until they fit snugly.

the client during and after surgery. Anesthesia produces multiple systemic effects, which can affect the client's care and can compound other coexisting problems. For example, most anesthetics are metabolized by the liver and excreted by the kidneys. Hepatic or renal dysfunction can significantly enhance anesthetic effects and toxicity. In addition, there may be drug interactions between the anesthetic agents and other medications the client has been receiving.

The state of anesthesia may be produced in a number of ways (Table 20–1):

- General or balanced anesthesia
- Local or regional anesthesia
- Hypnosis or hypnoanesthesia
- Cryothermia
- Acupuncture

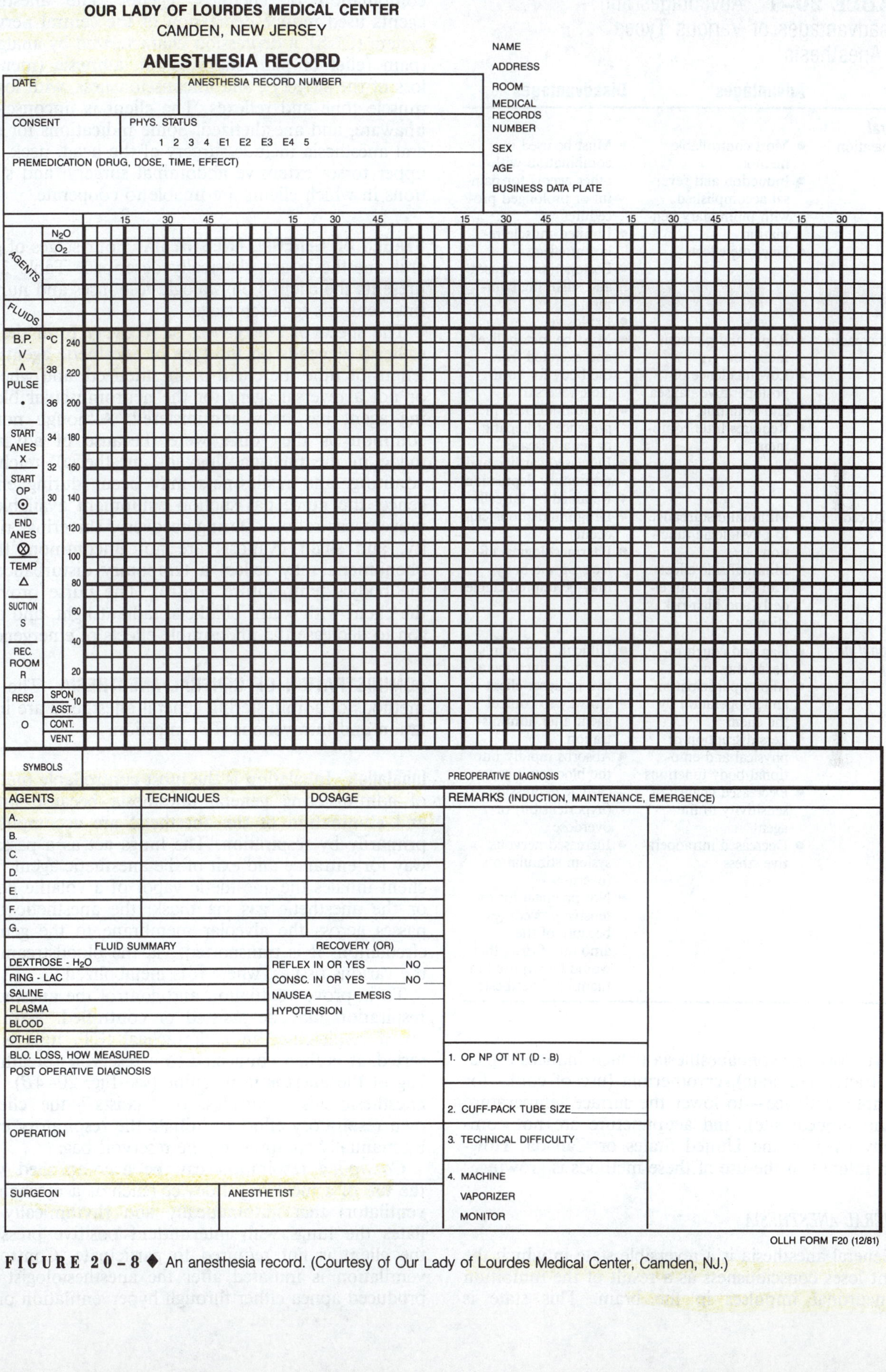

OUR LADY OF LOURDES MEDICAL CENTER
CAMDEN, NEW JERSEY
ANESTHESIA RECORD

NAME
ADDRESS
ROOM
MEDICAL RECORDS NUMBER
SEX
AGE
BUSINESS DATA PLATE

DATE	ANESTHESIA RECORD NUMBER
CONSENT	PHYS. STATUS 1 2 3 4 E1 E2 E3 E4 5
PREMEDICATION (DRUG, DOSE, TIME, EFFECT)	

15 30 45 15 30 45 15 30 45 15 30 45 15 30

AGENTS: N_2O, O_2
FLUIDS

B.P. V Λ
PULSE •
START ANES X
START OP ⊙
END ANES ⊗
TEMP △
SUCTION S
REC. ROOM R

°C: 38, 36, 34, 32, 30
240, 220, 200, 180, 160, 140, 120, 100, 80, 60, 40, 20, 10

RESP. O: SPON, ASST., CONT., VENT.

SYMBOLS

PREOPERATIVE DIAGNOSIS

AGENTS	TECHNIQUES	DOSAGE
A.		
B.		
C.		
D.		
E.		
F.		
G.		

REMARKS (INDUCTION, MAINTENANCE, EMERGENCE)

FLUID SUMMARY	
DEXTROSE - H_2O	
RING - LAC	
SALINE	
PLASMA	
BLOOD	
OTHER	
BLO. LOSS, HOW MEASURED	

RECOVERY (OR)
REFLEX IN OR YES ______ NO ______
CONSC. IN OR YES ______ NO ______
NAUSEA ______ EMESIS ______
HYPOTENSION

POST OPERATIVE DIAGNOSIS

OPERATION

SURGEON
ANESTHETIST

1. OP NP OT NT (D - B)
2. CUFF-PACK TUBE SIZE
3. TECHNICAL DIFFICULTY
4. MACHINE
VAPORIZER
MONITOR

OLLH FORM F20 (12/81)

FIGURE 20-8 ◆ An anesthesia record. (Courtesy of Our Lady of Lourdes Medical Center, Camden, NJ.)

TABLE 20–1 Advantages and Disadvantages of Various Types of Anesthesia

Type	Advantages	Disadvantages
General		
Inhalation	• Most controllable method • Induction and reversal accomplished with pulmonary ventilation • Few side effects	• Must be used in combination with other agents for painful or prolonged procedures • Limited muscle relaxant effects • Postoperative nausea and shivering common • Explosive
Intravenous	• Rapid and pleasant induction • Low incidence of postoperative nausea and vomiting • Requires little equipment	• Must be metabolized and excreted from the body for complete reversal • Contraindicated in presence of hepatic or renal disease • Increased cardiac and respiratory depression • Retained by fat cells
Balanced	• Minimal disturbance to physiologic function • Minimal side effects • Can be used with elderly and high-risk clients	• Drug interactions can occur • Pharmacological effects on the body may be unpredictable
Regional or Local	• Gag and cough reflexes stay intact • Allows participation and cooperation by the client • Less disruption of physical and emotional body functions • Decreased chance of sensitivity to the agent • Decreased intraoperative stress	• Difficult to administer to an uncooperative or upset client • No way to control agent after administration • Absorbs rapidly into the blood and causes cardiac depression (hypertension) or overdose • Increased nervous system stimulation (overdose) • Not practical for extensive procedures because of the amount of drug that would be required to maintain anesthesia

Hypnosis or hypnoanesthesia (which induces a passive trance-like state), cryothermia (use of cold—for example, with ice—to lower the surface temperature of the surgical site), and acupuncture are not commonly used in the United States or Canada. However, interest in the use of these methods is growing.

GENERAL ANESTHESIA

General anesthesia is a reversible state in which the client loses consciousness as a result of the inhibition of neuronal impulses in the brain. This state is achieved by the administration of a single agent or a combination of chemical agents. The anesthetic agents used induce depression of the central nervous system (CNS), a depression characterized by analgesia (pain relief or pain suppression), amnesia (memory loss of the surgery), and unconsciousness, with loss of muscle tone and reflexes. The client is unconscious, unaware, and anesthetized. Some indications for general anesthesia include surgery of the head, neck, and upper torso; extensive abdominal surgery; and situations in which clients are unable to cooperate.

STAGES OF GENERAL ANESTHESIA Four stages of general anesthesia are classically described. Table 20–2 presents the client's physiologic responses and nursing interventions for each stage.

The speed of *emergence*, or recovery from the anesthesia, depends on the type of anesthetic agent, the length of time the client is anesthetized, and whether or not a reversal agent for the neuromuscular blocking agent has been administered. Although not as common as they once were (because of advances made in the pharmacology of anesthesia), retching, vomiting, and restlessness may occur during emergence; the nurse has suction equipment available to prevent aspiration. During recovery, shivering, rigidity, and slight cyanosis are not uncommon; these phenomena may reflect a temporary disturbance in the body's temperature control. The nurse provides the client with warm blankets, radiant light, and oxygen to decrease the undesirable effects of emergence.

ADMINISTRATION OF GENERAL ANESTHESIA The two methods of administering general anesthesia are inhalation and intravenous (IV) injection.

Inhalation Inhalation is the most controllable method of administering general anesthesia because intake and elimination of the anesthetic are accomplished primarily by respiration. The lungs act as a passageway for entrance and exit of the anesthetic agent. The client inhales the anesthetic vapor of a volatile liquid or the anesthetic gas via mask; the anesthetic then passes across the alveolar membrane to the general circulation. It is transported, via the bloodstream, to the various tissues, where it is metabolized.

To improve ventilation and control the anesthesia, respiration may be assisted or controlled. With *assisted* respiration, an endotracheal (ET) tube is inserted. It is then connected to a reservoir (breathing) bag of the anesthesia machine (see Fig. 20–4*B*). The anesthesiologist overrides, or "assists," the client's own respiratory effort to initiate the respiratory cycle by manually compressing the reservoir bag.

Controlled respiration can be accomplished with the use of a mechanical device (such as a mechanical ventilator) that automatically and rhythmically inflates the lungs with intermittent positive pressure; the client is not required to participate. Controlled ventilation is initiated after the anesthesiologist has produced apnea either through hyperventilation or by

TABLE 20–2 The Four Stages of General Anesthesia and Related Nursing Interventions

Stage	Description	Nursing Interventions	Rationale
Stage 1 (analgesia and sedation, relaxation)	• Begins with induction and ends with loss of consciousness. • Client feels drowsy and dizzy, has a reduced sensation to pain, and is amnesic. • Hearing is exaggerated.	• Close operating room doors, dim the lights, and control traffic in the operating room. • Position client securely with safety belts. • Keep conversation and discussions about the client to a minimum.	• Avoiding external stimuli in the environment promotes relaxation. • Using safety measures in stage 1 prepares for stage 2. • Being sensitive to the client maintains his or her dignity.
Stage 2 (excitement, delirium)	• Begins with loss of consciousness and ends with relaxation, regular breathing, and loss of the eyelid reflex. • Client may have irregular breathing, increased muscle tone, and involuntary movement of the extremities during this stage. • Laryngospasm or vomiting may occur. • Client is susceptible to external stimuli.	• Avoid auditory and physical stimuli. • Protect the extremities. • Assist the anesthesiologist or CRNA with suctioning as needed. • Stay with client.	• Sensory stimuli can contribute to the client's response. • Safety measures help to prevent injury. • Staying with the client is emotionally supportive.
Stage 3 (operative anesthesia, surgical anesthesia)	• Begins with generalized muscle relaxation and ends with loss of reflexes and depression of vital functions. • The jaw is relaxed, and there is quiet, regular breathing. • The client cannot hear. • Sensations are lost (i.e., to pain).	• Assist the anesthesiologist or CRNA with intubation. • Place client into operative position. • Prep (scrub) the client's skin over the operative site as directed.	• Providing assistance helps promote smooth intubation and prevent injury. • Performing procedures as soon as possible promotes time management to minimize total anesthesia time for the client.
Stage 4 (danger)	• Begins with depression of vital functions and ends with respiratory failure, cardiac arrest, and possible death. • Respiratory muscles are paralyzed, apnea occurs. • Pupils fixed and dilated.	• Prepare for and assist in treatment of cardic and/or pulmonary arrest. • Document occurrence in the client's chart.	• Teamwork and preparedness help decrease injuries and complications, and promote the possibility of a desired outcome for the client.

administering respiratory depressant or neuromuscular blocker drugs.

The anesthesiologist or CRNA inserts the ET tube with the assistance of the circulating nurse. A laryngoscope is used to visualize the vocal cords, and the tube is placed in the trachea (Fig. 20–9). With the ET tube safely in place, the client has an open airway (through the tube) and an avenue for the safe administration of the inhaled anesthetic and oxygen.

Inhalation anesthetic agents are divided into two categories: gases and volatile agents. Table 20–3 lists the advantages, disadvantages, and related nursing implications of various inhalation anesthetic agents.

Gaseous Agents In the past, gaseous agents included ether and cyclopropane gas. *Nitrous oxide* (N_2O) is now the most commonly used gaseous anesthetic agent and is usually administered with oxygen. It is a colorless, odorless, nonirritating gas and provides analgesia equivalent to 10 mg of morphine sulfate. It is a relatively weak anesthetic agent and, except for short procedures, requires the addition of other agents. Nitrous oxide can produce hypoxia if the concentration of the gas is too high.

Volatile Agents Liquids that are vaporized for inhalation are considered volatile agents. Oxygen acts as a carrier, flowing over or bubbling through the liquid in the vaporizer system on the anesthesia machine. All volatile agents can produce postoperative shivering in the client because of an effect on the hypothalamus.

HALOTHANE (FLUOTHANE) Halothane is a halogenated hydrocarbon that depresses the cardiovascular system, resulting in hypotension and bradycardia. It can sensitize the myocardium to dysrhythmias. The intraoperative use of epinephrine to control bleeding may exacerbate or precipitate a dysrhythmia when halothane is used.

ENFLURANE (ETHRANE) Enflurane is an inhalation anesthetic agent that reduces the client's ventilations and decreases blood pressure as the depth of anesthesia increases. The heart rate and rhythm remain stable.

ISOFLURANE (FORANE) Isoflurane is another halogenated compound and appears to be a preferred inhala-

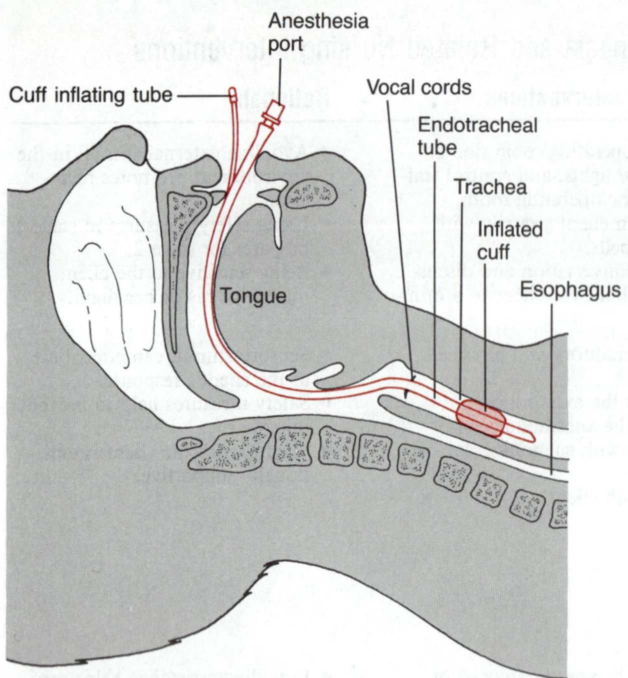

FIGURE 20–9 ◆ An oral endotracheal tube in position. The cuff of the tube was placed just below the vocal cords, then inflated to seal off the airway.

tion agent. Because it is not significantly metabolized, the cardiovascular system remains stable and there is no renal or hepatic damage.

Intravenous (IV) Injection Intravenous anesthetic agents are injected, usually via a peripheral IV line, into the circulation. A pleasant, rapid, and smooth dissipation of the agent occurs. The drug is diluted by the blood, but it travels in high concentration to the organs of high blood flow (brain, liver, and kidneys). The reversal and removal of the agent from circulation are not possible with IV injection, and the recovery from the agent is directly related to the client's metabolism. Table 20–4 lists advantages, disadvantages, and related nursing implications of various intravenous anesthetic agents.

Barbiturates Barbiturates are often used for IV induction of anesthesia. These drugs act directly on the central nervous system, producing a reaction ranging from mild sedation to unconsciousness. The principal barbiturate used is thiopental sodium (Pentothal). It acts rapidly, resulting in unconsciousness in 30 seconds. Because thiopental is a potent respiratory and cardiovascular system depressant, the client's vital signs must be monitored continuously during administration.

Ketamine (Ketalar) Ketamine is a dissociative anesthetic agent (one that promotes a feeling of dissociation from the environment). It acts by selectively interrupting various pathways in the brain. There is rapid onset of a trance-like, analgesic state. It is commonly used for diagnostic and short surgical procedures or to supplement weaker agents, such as nitrous oxide.

During the client's recovery from ketamine, emergence reactions are expected. The operating room nurse reports the use of the drug to the postanesthesia nurse so that safety precautions can be implemented. If the client is combative or restless, the nurse pads the side rails of the bed to prevent injury. The nurse minimizes external stimuli until the client awakens naturally. For severe reactions during the recovery phase, small doses of diazepam (Valium, Vivol✱, Novodipam✱) may be given as needed. The medical-surgical nurse continues interventions until the effects of the drug have worn off.

Propofol (Diprivan) Propofol is the first of a new classification of intravenous anesthetic agents, the alkylphenols. Its short action makes it desirable as an anesthetic agent. Hypnosis occurs in less than 1 minute from the time of injection, and because it is so rapidly metabolized, it does not accumulate during maintenance of the anesthesia. The client becomes responsive quickly after the infusion is ended (within 8 minutes). Propofol is also used to supplement nitrous oxide during short procedures and is used as a hypnotic agent with regional anesthesia.

Innovar Innovar is a 50:1 combination of the tranquilizer droperidol with the potent opioid analgesic fentanyl citrate. Innovar has been used in small doses to supplement nitrous oxide or regional anesthesia. It has a long duration, requiring close observation of the client for respiratory depression, hypoventilation, apnea, and hypotension during the postoperative period. The nurse maintains an open airway and a patent IV access and has vasopressors available to counteract anesthetic side effects, especially hypotension. In the initial postoperative period, the physician usually orders reduced doses of opioid analgesics when Innovar has been used.

ADJUNCTS TO THE GENERAL ANESTHESIA AGENTS
Other drugs, such as hypnotics, opioid analgesics, and neuromuscular blocking agents, may be used as part of the anesthesia regimen.

Hypnotics The benzodiazepines may be used for various effects. Common drugs in this classification include midazolam (Versed), lorazepam (Ativan, Novolorazem✱), and diazepam (Valium, Vivol✱, Novodipam✱). All have hypnotic, sedative, anti-anxiety, muscle relaxant, and amnesic effects. Generally, lower doses are ordered for preoperative sedation. Each may be used as part of an intravenous conscious sedation regimen for diagnostic or endoscopic procedures. Higher doses of midazolam may be used to induce general anesthesia. The benzodiazepines may also be used intraoperatively in conjunction with regional or local anesthesia. Adverse reac-

TABLE 20–3 Advantages, Disadvantages, and Related Nursing Implications of Various General Inhalation Anesthetic Agents

Agent	Advantages	Disadvantages	Nursing Implications	Rationale
Nitrous oxide (N_2O)	• Rapid induction and recovery • Useful for short procedures • When used with other agents, reduces the required concentration of the other agents • Minimal cardiovascular and respiratory depression	• Relatively weak anesthetic agent • May produce hypoxia if the concentration is high • Needs addition of other agents for longer procedures	• Assess oxygenation via pulse oximetry, physical assessment.	• Ongoing assessment leads to early detection and treatment of potential complications.
Halothane (Fluothane)	• Rapid and smooth induction • Low incidence of postoperative nausea and vomiting • Less irritating to the respiratory tract than other inhalation agents • Sweet smell makes it easy to use in children • Tolerated well by children	• Shivering common postoperatively • Malignant hyperthermia is possible in susceptible clients. • Metabolized by the liver • Hypotension and bradycardia may occur. • Can sensitize the myocardium to dysrhythmias	• Monitor heart rate for bradycardia. • Monitor blood pressure for hypotension. • Provide warm blankets, radiant heat.	• Ongoing assessment leads to early detection and treatment of potential complications. • Warmth helps promote client comfort and decrease shivering.
Enflurane (Ethrane)	• Rapid induction and recovery • Does not alter heart rate	• Respiratory depression and hypotension may occur. • Malignant hyperthermia is possible in susceptible clients. • Lowers seizure threshold	• Monitor respiratory rate and depth for hypoventilation. • Assess oxygenation via pulse oximetry, physical assessment. • Monitor blood pressure for hypotension.	• Ongoing assessment leads to early detection and treatment of potential complications.
Isoflurane (Forane)	• Rapid induction and recovery • Has some muscle relaxant properties • Stimulates heart, which helps keep a stable heart rate • Is not significantly metabolized; no renal or hepatic damage	• Respiratory depression may occur. • Malignant hyperthermia is possible in susceptible clients.	• Monitor respiratory rate and depth for hypoventilation.	• Ongoing assessment leads to early detection and treatment of potential complications.

tions include respiratory depression, apnea, and oversedation.

Opioid Analgesics Common opioid analgesics used to supplement inhalation anesthesia include morphine sulfate (Statex✱), meperidine hydrochloride (Demerol), fentanyl citrate (Sublimaze), and sufentanil (Sufenta). The use of opioids during surgery contributes to postoperative analgesia. All opioid analgesics decrease alveolar ventilation and are respiratory depressants. The nurse monitors respirations and maintains an open airway. Reduced dosages are prescribed for the elderly, for the client with a circulatory problem (such as heart failure), and for the debilitated client.

Fentanyl has a potency 80 to 100 times greater than that of morphine. Sufentanil has five to ten times the analgesic potency of fentanyl and produces a more rapid onset of central nervous system effects than fentanyl does. It is often used in open heart surgery when the sternum must be opened. The nurse monitors the client who has received sufentanil for bradycardia and decreased cardiac output.

Neuromuscular Blocking Agents The neuromuscular blockers are used to produce muscle relaxation so that the anesthesiologist or CRNA can pass the endotracheal tube. These drugs are also used throughout the surgical procedure to provide continued overall muscle relaxation. Neuromuscular blocking agents act on the striated muscles of the body by interfering with impulse transmission at the neuromuscular junction. The drugs are administered intravenously in small amounts and may cause circulatory alterations and decreased respirations or apnea from muscle paralysis. The nurse ensures the client's safety by securing the client on the operating bed with safety straps and assists the anesthesiologist or CRNA with intubation. Throughout the surgery, the anesthesiologist

TABLE 20–4 Advantages, Disadvantages, and Related Nursing Implications of Various General Intravenous Anesthetic Agents

Agent	Advantages	Disadvantages	Nursing Implications	Rationale
Barbiturates				
Thiopental sodium (Pentothal), methohexital sodium (Brevital), thiamylal-sodium (Surital)	• Rapid, pleasant induction and recovery • Acts directly on the central nervous system • Short-acting • Low incidence of postoperative nausea and vomiting	• Strong respiratory and cardiovascular depressant effect • No antagonist medication available • Mild to severe local tissue reaction with extravasation • Poor analgesic, muscle relaxant effects	• Monitor respiratory rate and depth for hypoventilation. • Monitor heart rate for bradycardia. • Monitor blood pressure for hypotension. • Assess IV site.	• Ongoing assessment leads to early detection and treatment of potential complications.
Nonbarbiturates				
Ketamine hydrochloride (Ketalar)	• Rapid induction • Short-acting • Can be given IM or IV • No respiratory depression or loss of muscle tone (protects the airway) • Protective reflexes remain intact • Stimulates the cardiovascular system • Can use for clients with respiratory or cardiac disorders • Good amnesic effect • Postop emergence reactions generally last only 24 hr.	• Emergence reactions are common: hallucinations, irrational behaviors, distorted images, unpleasant dreams, restlessness • Increased heart rate • Increased blood pressure • Increased cardiac output • Poor muscle relaxant effect • Nausea, vomiting, and aspiration can occur.	• Minimize external stimuli: noise, light, touch, movement. • Speak in a calm, soothing voice. • Reassure client and family that emergence reactions are common and temporary. • Have suction equipment near. • Monitor blood pressure for hypertension. • Monitor heart rate for tachycardia.	• Stimuli increases the severity of the emergence reaction. • Quiet promotes comfort, decreases anxiety. • Reassurance decreases anxiety. • Suction may be needed in the event of vomiting to prevent aspiration. • Ongoing assessment leads to early detection and treatment of potential complications.
Propofol (Diprivan)	• Short-acting • Rapidly metabolized • Client becomes responsive quickly postoperatively. • Minimal postoperative nausea, vomiting, or sedation	• Allergic skin reactions have occurred. • Client becomes aware of postoperative pain and discomfort sooner than with other anesthetics.	• Be prepared to administer analgesic medications as ordered early in the postoperative period. • Plan for nonpharmacologic pain interventions (see Chap. 8).	• Awareness of pain very early in the postoperative period can be frightening. • Pain can increase blood pressure and increase anxiety.
Fentanyl citrate with droperidol (Innovar) (50:1 ratio)	• Excellent postoperative analgesia • Long-acting analgesia • Has antiemetic effects • Has antiarrythmic effects • Combination agent • Can be given IM or IV • Client has psychological indifference to the environment before the onset of anesthesia.	• Significant respiratory depression can occur several hours after administration. • Prolonged somnolence • Cardiovascular depression can occur. • Laryngospasm and bronchospasm can occur. • Slow onset of anesthesia • Extrapyramidal side effects can occur.	• Monitor respiratory rate and depth for hypoventilation. • Monitor blood pressure for hypotension. • Have atropine, naloxone (Narcan), vasopressors, and resuscitative equipment nearby.	• Ongoing assessment leads to early detection and treatment of potential complications. • Having necessary supplies and equipment available provides for prompt response to an emergency.

or CRNA checks the effectiveness of the blocker agent by using a peripheral nerve stimulator (Davidson, 1991; Jarpe, 1992). There are two types of neuromuscular blocking agents: non-depolarizing and depolarizing.

Non-depolarizing Blocker Agents The non-depolarizing blockers block acetylcholine at the neuromuscular junction. Only skeletal muscles are blocked, and the drug is easily reversed with an antidote of neostigmine and atropine. Examples of non-depolarizing blockers include pancuronium (Pavulon), atracurium (Tracrium), vecuronium (Norcuron), doxacurium (Nuromax), tubocurarine (Tubarine✱), and mivacurium (Mivacron). Pancuronium has been in use for a long time and has a relatively long effect (45 to 60 minutes) compared with the newer agent mivacurium (15 to 20 minutes). The longer the effect of the drug, the longer it takes for the client to recover.

Depolarizing Blocker Agents The depolarizing blocker agents, also called "noncompetitive" blockers, depolarize the motor end plate at the neuromuscular junction. In the process, potassium is forced out of the muscle cells and into general circulation, which can cause hyperkalemia. Clients often experience transient intraoperative muscle twitching, which can result in generalized muscle aches after awakening. There is no specific antidote. Other side effects include increased salivation, which puts the client at risk for aspiration, and increased intraocular pressure, which may be contraindicated in a client with glaucoma. An example of a depolarizing blocker is succinylcholine (Anectine). Anectine is frequently used to relax the jaw and vocal cords immediately after induction to facilitate placement of the endotracheal tube.

BALANCED ANESTHESIA Balanced anesthesia is widely used. It provides a safe and controlled anesthetic experience, especially for elderly and high-risk clients. A combination of agents is used to provide hypnosis, amnesia, analgesia, muscle relaxation, and relaxation of reflexes with minimal disturbance of the client's physiologic function. An example of balanced anesthesia is the use of a barbiturate (such as thiopental) administered intravenously for induction, nitrous oxide for amnesia, morphine for analgesia, and a muscle relaxant (such as pancuronium) to provide additional relaxation of the muscles.

A second example of balanced anesthesia is the use of 70% nitrous oxide for induction and maintenance (to prevent awareness throughout the procedure and to prevent recall afterward), 30% oxygen to maintain the client's oxygenation saturation greater than 90%, along with an opioid and a muscle relaxant. Many combinations are possible, and selection reflects assessment of the individual client and the specific surgical procedure.

COMPLICATIONS FROM GENERAL ANESTHESIA Complications can range from minor and annoying to the most severe, which is death.

Malignant Hyperthermia Malignant hyperthermia (MH) is an acute, life-threatening complication of general anesthesia. The client with a genetic predisposition for MH is at risk for this complication from MH-triggering general anesthetic agents. Anesthetic agents that may trigger MH include halothane, enflurane, isoflurane, and succinylcholine. Stressors, such as severe fatigue, strenuous exercise, muscle injury, and emotional stress, may also trigger this crisis. A biochemical reaction occurs as a result of a defect in the muscle cell membrane, causing a rise in the circulating calcium level, an increase in metabolic rate, hyperkalemia, and metabolic and respiratory acidosis.

Signs of malignant hypothermia include tachycardia or other dysrhythmia; muscle rigidity, especially of the jaw (masseter muscle rigidity) and upper chest; hypotension; tachypnea; and cola-colored urine. Extremely elevated temperature, perhaps as high as 44° C (111.2° F), is a late sign of MH. Treatment and survival of the client depend on early diagnosis and cooperation of the entire surgical team.

Once a client or family history of MH is known, close family members can undergo a muscle biopsy to determine whether they are at risk. In the case of a known history or predetermination, the person can be treated preoperatively, intraoperatively, and postoperatively with dantrolene to prevent this complication. Chart 20–1 summarizes the nursing care of the client with malignant hyperthermia.

Overdose An anesthesia overdose can occur if the client's pharmokinetics do not react or respond as

CHART 20–1

Nursing Care Highlight ◆ Malignant Hyperthermia

The Susceptible Client

- Assess client and family history preoperatively for signs and symptoms of MH or of muscular dystrophy.
- Counsel client regarding muscle biopsy test that would determine his or her predisposition to MH.
- Assist client in finding the muscle biopsy testing center.
- Provide information about MH and the MH Association of the United States (MHAUS).
- Reassure the client that surgery can still be performed safely.

The Client in Malignant Hyperthermia Crisis

- Call for help!
- Assist the physician and anesthesiologist and/or CRNA with the immediate discontinuation of surgery.
- Reconstitute dantrolene (Dantrium) with sterile *distilled* water.
- Give 2.5–4.0 mg/kg of dantrolene (Dantrium) intravenously as ordered.
- Cool the client with external ice packs, iced intravenous (IV) saline; iced lavages of the bladder, rectum, stomach, and wound; and a hypothermia blanket as ordered.
- Collect urine and blood specimens as ordered.
- Have sodium bicarbonate, mannitol (Osmitrol✱), procainamide (Pronestyl), hydrocortisone (Solu-Cortef), furosemide (Lasix, Furoside✱), IV insulin in dextrose, and heparin (Hepalean✱) available.
- Assist with monitoring as indicated.
- Document the event, detailing times, interventions, and client response.

expected. Drugs (e.g., antihypertensive medications) also alter the pharmokinetics, and drug interactions can occur between the anesthetic agents and other regularly administered medications. Accurate, accessible information about the client, such as height, weight, and history, is vital in determining anesthetic type and dosage. Intraoperative death, however, is most often related to the client's premorbid condition, not overdosage of anesthetics.

Complications Related to Specific Anesthetic Agents Specific complications have been discussed earlier in the chapter. The elderly or debilitated client may be more susceptible to complications of anesthesia because of an intolerance to the agent, decreased metabolism, or general physical condition. (For preoperative risk factors, see Chapter 19.)

Complications of Intubation Many complications can occur from intubation, for example, broken or injured teeth and caps, swollen lip, or trauma to the vocal cords. Intubation may be difficult because of the individual client's anatomy or disease process (e.g., a small oral cavity, a tight mandibular joint, a tumor). Improper extension of the client's neck during intubation may also cause injury. The surgeon should be in the operating room in case an emergency arises (e.g., a tracheostomy is needed) when the endotracheal tube is placed. Placement of the endotracheal tube causes some degree of irritation and edema of the trachea and accounts for the client's sore throat postoperatively.

LOCAL OR REGIONAL ANESTHESIA

Local or regional anesthesia temporarily interrupts the transmission of sensory nerve impulses from a specific area or region. Motor function may or may not be affected, and the client does not lose consciousness. Thus, the client is able to follow instructions throughout the procedure. Because the gag and cough reflexes remain intact, there is little risk of aspiration or other respiratory complications. Local or regional anesthesia is typically supplemented with sedatives, opioid analgesics, and/or hypnotics.

The OR nurse provides the client with information, directions, and emotional support before, during, and after the procedure. Table 20–5 describes various local or regional anesthetic agents and related nursing interventions.

LOCAL ANESTHESIA The techniques used to administer local anesthesia include topical anesthesia and local infiltration. Sometimes when the term "local" is used, it means *any* form of anesthesia that is not general anesthesia. The client could be receiving regional anesthesia, but local anesthetic agents are used.

Topical Anesthesia Topical anesthesia refers to an anesthetic that is applied *directly* to the surface of the area to be anesthetized. Often the anesthetic is in the form of an ointment or spray. This method is often used for respiratory intubation or for diagnostic procedures, such as laryngoscopy, bronchoscopy, or cystoscopy. The onset of action is 1 minute, and the duration is 20 to 30 minutes. Collapse or depression of the cardiovascular system may occur after the topical anesthetic is applied to the respiratory tract.

Local Infiltration Local infiltration is the injection of an anesthetic agent intracutaneously and subcutaneously *into* the tissue surrounding an incision, wound, or lesion. The anesthetic agent blocks peripheral nerve stimulation at its origin. Local infiltration is commonly used during the suturing of superficial lacerations.

TABLE 20–5 Advantages, Disadvantages, and Related Nursing Implications of Local or Regional Anesthetic Agents

Agent	Advantages	Disadvantages	Nursing Implications	Rationale
Procaine (Novocain) Tetracaine (Pontocaine) Lidocaine (Xylocaine) Mepivacaine (Carbocaine) Bupivacaine (Marcaine)	• Easily administered • Rapid onset (4–17 min) • Can be administered topically or by injection • Excellent muscle relaxant effects • Protective reflexes (cough, gag) remain intact • Client does not lose consciousness • Many are available with epinephrine added	• Absorbs into the bloodstream • Can cause cardiac depression and dysrhythmias with absorption • Difficult to control dosage • Drug interactions with monoamine oxidase (MAO) inhibitors can cause hypertension. • Tremors, twitching, shivering, respiratory arrest can occur with absorption.	• Assess for return of movement and sensation in the area anesthetized. • Monitor blood pressure and pulse. • Assess administration site for pallor, drainage. • Protect area anesthetized until full sensation has returned.	• Movement returns first, then sense of touch, pain, warmth, and cold, in that order. • Ongoing assessment leads to early detection and treatment of potential complications. • Protection prevents injury to the area. • Duration of the anesthetic is 3–6 hr.

REGIONAL ANESTHESIA Regional anesthesia—a type of local anesthesia—may be used:

- When general anesthesia is contraindicated because of the presence of medical problems (e.g., dysrhythmias and respiratory disease)
- When the client has experienced previous adverse reactions to general anesthetic agents
- When the client has a preference and a choice is possible

If the client has eaten and the surgery is an emergency, it may be possible to perform the procedure with the client under regional anesthesia (depending on the procedure) to decrease the risks associated with gastric contents (e.g., aspiration). Types of regional anesthesia include field block, nerve block, spinal, and epidural.

Field Block A field block is produced by a series of injections *around* the operative field. Injecting around a specific nerve or group of nerves depresses the entire sensory nervous system of a localized area. This type of blocking is used for thoracic procedures, herniorrhaphy (hernia repair), dental procedures, and plastic surgery.

Nerve Block A nerve block is achieved by injection of the local anesthetic agent *into or around* a nerve or nerves supplying the involved area. Nerve blocks interrupt sensory, motor, or sympathetic transmission. They are used surgically to prevent pain during a procedure, diagnostically to identify the cause of pain, and therapeutically to relieve chronic pain and increase circulation in some vascular diseases.

Figure 20–10 shows common nerve block sites. Lidocaine (Xylocaine) or bupivacaine (Marcaine) is frequently the agent used. A nerve block takes effect within minutes after the injection, and the anesthesia lasts longer than is achieved with local infiltration. Epinephrine added to the anesthetic agent potentiates the drug, causing a prolonged effect. Seizures, cardiac depression, dysrhythmias, and/or respiratory depression may occur if the nerve-blocking agent is injected into the bloodstream. The nurse observes for signs of systemic absorption, sensitivity, or overdose.

Spinal Anesthesia Spinal anesthesia—intrathecal block—is achieved by injection of the anesthetic agent into the subarachnoid space (Fig. 20–11). The drug acts on the nerves as they emerge from the spinal cord and before they leave the spinal canal through the intervertebral foramen, thereby inhibiting conduction in the autonomic, sensory, and motor systems. The drug is rapidly absorbed into the nerve fibers and produces analgesia with relaxation, which is effective for lower abdominal and pelvic surgical procedures.

Epidural Anesthesia The anesthetic is injected into the epidural space so that the protective coverings of the spinal cord (dura mater and arachnoid mater) are never entered. Because the anesthetic can diffuse or float up the vertebral column, the client can achieve anesthetic effects as high as the T-4 level; however, potential respiratory complications may make injection at this high a level undesirable.

Epidural anesthesia is used for anorectal, vaginal, and perineal procedures as well as for hip and lower extremity operations, such as total hip or knee replacements. Two important advantages are associated with this type of anesthesia:

- Decreased cardiopulmonary complications, which is particularly important for the elderly client
- Ability to retain the epidural catheter for the administration of analgesics postoperatively (see Chap. 8)

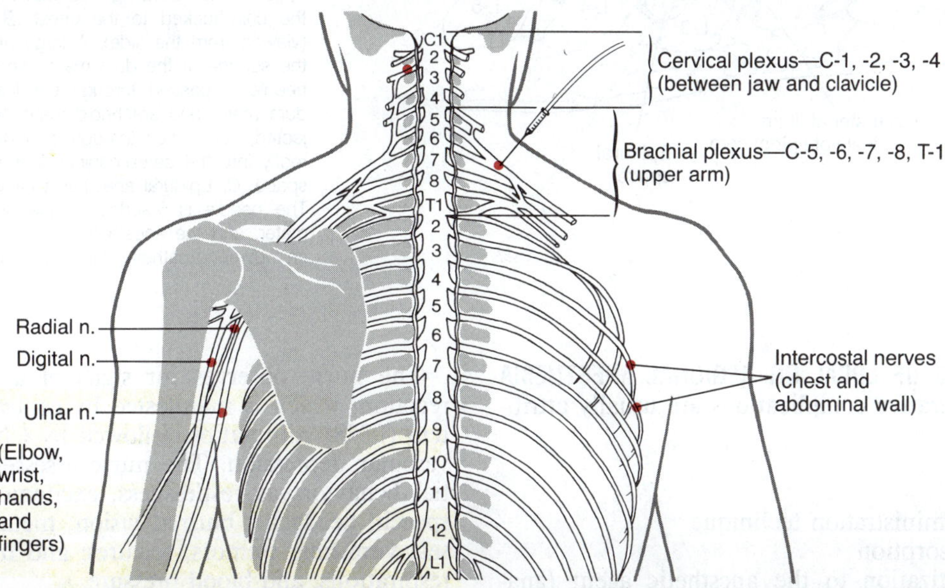

FIGURE 20–10 ◆ Nerve block sites.

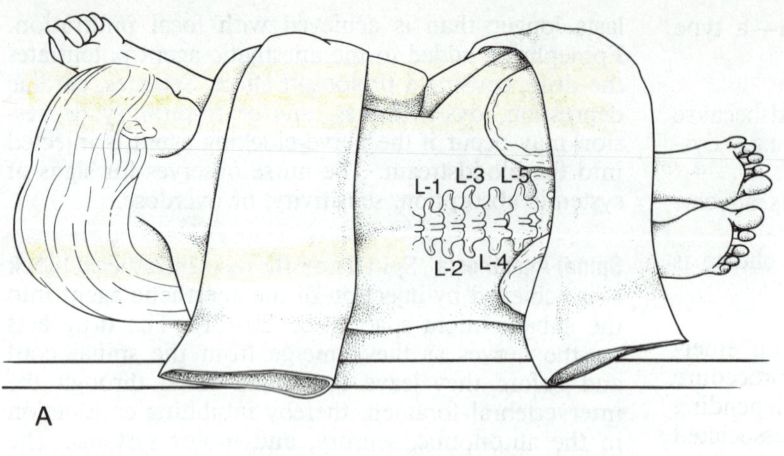

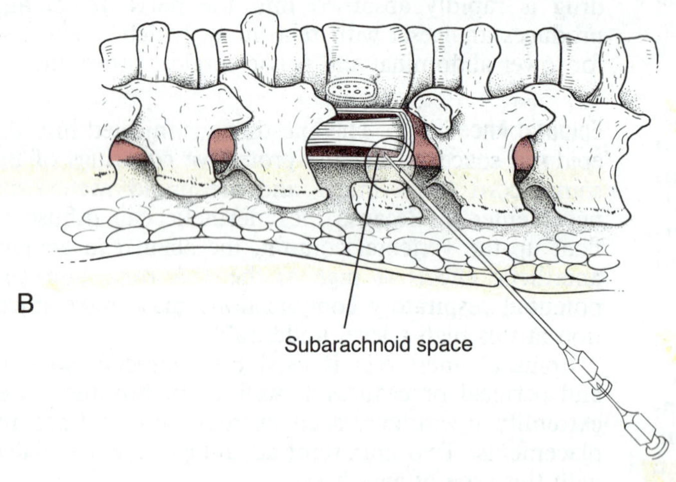

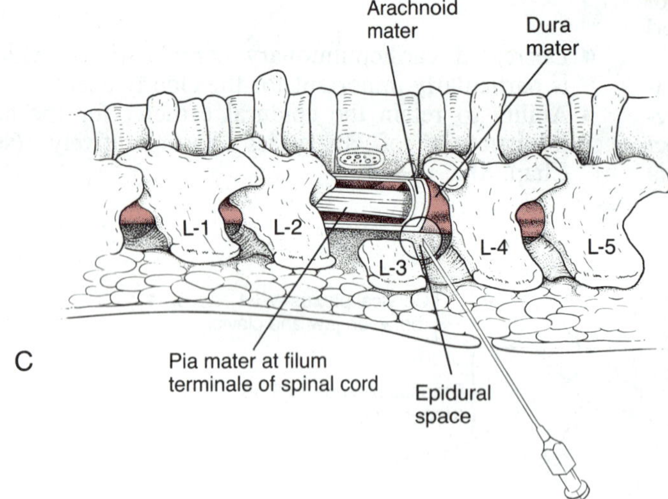

FIGURE 20-11 ◆ Administration of spinal and epidural anesthesia. *A*, Spinal or epidural anesthesia is administered by inserting a spinal needle between the second and third or the third and fourth lumbar vertebrae (L2-3 or L3-4). The client is placed in the flexed lateral (fetal) position (shown here) or seated on the edge of the operating bed with the back arched and the chin tucked to the chest. *B*, Spinal anesthesia (viewed from the side). A large needle is inserted to the surface of the dura mater, and a second, smaller needle is passed through the first to penetrate the dura mater and arachnoid mater. An anesthetic is injected, sometimes through an indwelling catheter, directly into the cerebrospinal fluid in the subarachnoid space. *C*, Epidural anesthesia (viewed from the side). The needle is inserted to the surface of the dura mater, and the anesthetic is injected, usually through an indwelling catheter, into the epidural space.

COMPLICATIONS OF LOCAL OR REGIONAL ANESTHESIA
Major intraoperative complications are usually attributable to:

- Overdosage
- Incorrect administration technique
- Systemic absorption
- Client sensitization to the anesthetic agent (anaphylaxis)

The nurse observes for signs of a systemic toxic reaction, which is manifested by central nervous system (CNS) stimulation followed by CNS and cardiovascular depression. The nurse assesses for such initial behaviors as restlessness; excitement; incoherent speech; headache; blurred vision; metallic taste; nausea; vomiting; tremors; seizures; and increased pulse, respirations, and blood pressure.

Nursing interventions include the following:

- Establishing and maintaining an open airway
- Administering oxygen
- Notifying the surgeon

It is usually necessary to administer a fast-acting and short-acting barbiturate. If the client's toxic reaction remains untreated, unconsciousness, hypotension, apnea, cardiac arrest, and death may result.

Localized complications include edema and inflammation initially, with possible abscess, necrosis, and/or gangrene later. Inflammation and abscess usually result from a break in sterile technique occurring at the time of injection of the anesthetic agent. Necrosis and gangrene are rare but may occur as a result of vasoconstriction in the area of the injection.

The nurse's role in the administration of regional anesthesia consists of:

- Assisting the anesthesiologist or certified registered nurse anesthetist (CRNA)
- Observing for breaks in sterile technique
- Providing physical and emotional support for the client
- Staying with the client
- Providing the client a chance to verbalize feelings
- Offering information, encouragement, and reassurance
- Positioning the client comfortably and safely

CONSCIOUS SEDATION

Conscious sedation, usually administered by direct intravenous (IV) injection ("IV push"), is given to dull or reduce the intensity of pain or awareness of pain during a procedure without loss of defensive reflexes. Diazepam (Valium, Vivol, Novodipam), midazolam (Versed), meperidine (Demerol), fentanyl (Sublimaze), and morphine sulfate are the most commonly used drugs for IV conscious sedation. Conscious sedation is typically used for procedures such as endoscopy, cardiac catheterization, closed fracture reduction, percutaneous transluminal cardiac angiography (PTCA), cardioversion, and other special procedures.

The physician determines whether the client is a candidate for IV conscious sedation and administers the first dose of the selected drug. In some states, a credentialed registered nurse may give subsequent doses under physician supervision. The nurse monitors the client during and after the procedure for his or her response to drug administration. The nurse carefully monitors the client's airway, level of consciousness, oxygen saturation via pulse oximetry, electrocardiographic (ECG) status, and vital signs every 15 to 30 minutes until the client is alert and oriented.

Clients receiving IV conscious sedation may be discharged to go home with a responsible adult. If the client returns to the general medical-surgical nursing unit, the unit staff nurses continue to monitor the client. The client is expected to be sleepy but arousable for several hours after the procedure. The nurse usually does not permit oral intake until 30 minutes after the client has received medication or, in other cases, according to physician order. When fluids are permitted, the nurse makes sure that the client is awake and positioned to avoid aspiration.

COLLABORATIVE MANAGEMENT

ASSESSMENT

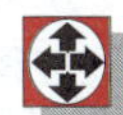

CLIENT INTERVIEW

On arrival in the surgical suite, the client is taken to the holding area or directly into the operating suite. The holding area nurse and/or the circulating nurse greets the client on arrival. The nurse verifies the client's identity with his or her identification bracelet and asks, "What is your name?" This practice prevents errors that may occur, for example, if a client is asked, "Are you Mr. James?" Clients may respond inappropriately if they are drowsy, anxious, or sedated. The nurse always validates the identification obtained using the chart, the client's name, and the client's identification number. Correct identification of the client is the responsibility of every member of the health care team.

After completing the identification process, the nurse validates that the surgical consent form has been signed and witnessed. The nurse asks the client, "What kind of operation are you having today?" The nurse checks to ascertain that the client's perception of the procedure, the operative permit, and the operative schedule coincide. This practice is especially important when the nurse is validating the side on which a procedure is to be performed (e.g., for amputation, cataract extraction, or hernia repair). Before proceeding, the nurse thoroughly investigates *any* discrepancy in information and notifies the surgeon and anesthesiologist and/or certified registered nurse anesthetist (CRNA).

The nurse checks the client's attire to ensure compliance with hospital policy. The nurse checks to see that dentures and dental prostheses (e.g., bridges and retainers), jewelry, eyeglasses, contact lenses, hearing aids, wigs, and other prostheses are removed for the client's safety during surgery. The nurse pays special attention to the removal of dentures because the denture plate could become loose and obstruct the client's airway during surgery. Occasionally, the anesthesiology team may request that the dentures be left in place to ensure a snug fit of the anesthesia mask. In some facilities, clients may be permitted to retain their eyeglasses and hearing aids until after the induction phase of anesthesia.

CHART REVIEW

The circulating nurse and anesthesia personnel review the client's chart in the holding area (or in the operating room if there is no holding area). The chart provides information needed to identify potential and actual needs of the client during the intraoperative period and allows the circulating nurse to assess and plan for the client's needs during and after surgery. The client's chart is a primary source of information on the type and location of the planned surgical procedure. A check of the chart ensures that all required data are present in the record before the procedure is begun.

ALLERGIES AND PREVIOUS REACTIONS TO ANESTHESIA OR TRANSFUSIONS In reviewing the chart, the nurse asks the client about allergies and previous reactions to anesthesia or blood transfusions. Allergies or sensitivity to iodine products or shellfish may indicate the potential for a reaction to the antimicrobial agents used to clean the surgical area. The nurse clearly indicates the allergies on the chart and notifies the operating room (OR) team. The client's previous experience with anesthesia helps the nurse and anesthesiologist or CRNA plan and anticipate the client's needs. For example, if a client is restless or agitated as a reaction to anesthesia, the nurse can have padding for the stretcher side rails and protective restraints available. The use of blood and blood products during surgery may be influenced by the client's history, religious beliefs or preferences, and type of transfusion reaction in the past.

AUTOLOGOUS BLOOD TRANSFUSION Increasingly, autologous blood transfusion (reinfusing the client's own blood) is being used for surgery. This method of blood transfusion eliminates the risk of acquiring blood-borne infections, such as hepatitis B and human immunodeficiency virus (HIV), from another person. Chapter 19 discusses autologous blood transfusion in more detail, and Chart 20–2 outlines key points of intraoperative autologous blood transfusion.

LABORATORY AND DIAGNOSTIC TEST RESULTS The OR nurse checks reports of preoperative laboratory and diagnostic test results. The nurse assesses the most recent laboratory results (usually obtained within 24 to 48 hours before surgery) to inform the surgical team about the client's medical condition and to alert them to potential intraoperative and postoperative interventions. The nurse reports all abnormalities to the surgeon and the anesthesiologist or CRNA. Laboratory values that are significantly greater than or less than the normal range are potentially life-threatening for any client, but especially for the client undergoing surgery (see Chap. 19). For example, if the hemoglobin concentration is less than 10 g/dL, the client's oxygen transport capacity is lessened; this condition affects the amount and type of anesthesia used and the potential impact of blood loss during surgery.

MEDICAL HISTORY AND PHYSICAL EXAMINATION FINDINGS The OR nurse checks that the client's medical history and examination findings, including normal pulse and blood pressure, are recorded. This information provides the circulating nurse, surgeon, anesthesiologist and/or CRNA, and postanesthesia care unit (PACU) nurse with baseline data to assess the client's reaction to the surgical procedure and anesthesia. Medications that the client has routinely taken preoperatively may affect the client's reaction to surgery and wound healing. For example, aspirin has an anticoagulant effect and can cause increased clotting time and danger of hemorrhage.

Knowing the client's medical history and age (Chart 20–3) allows the nurse to take special precautions and plan appropriate interventions for the care and safety of high-risk clients. Arthritic and osteoporotic clients need special padding and extra protection

CHART 20–2

Nursing Care Highlight ◆ Intraoperative Autologous Blood Salvage and Transfusion

- Be aware of the cell-processing method to be used.
- Make sure that collection containers are labeled for the client.
- Assist with sterile set-up as necessary.
- Assist with processing and reinfusing procedures as needed.
- Document the transfusion process.
- Monitor the client's vital signs during the transfusion procedure.

CHART 20–3

Nursing Focus on the Elderly ◆ Intraoperative Nursing Interventions

- Allow clients to retain eyeglasses and hearing aids until anesthesia has been administered.
- Use a small pillow under the client's head if his or her head and neck is normally bent slightly forward.
- Lift clients into position to prevent shearing forces on fragile skin.
- Position arthritic and artificial joints carefully to prevent postoperative pain and discomfort from strain on those joints.
- Pad bony prominences to prevent pressure sores.
- Provide extra padding for those clients with decreased peripheral circulation.
- Use head caps to prevent heat loss through the scalp.
- Place stockinette on extremities to conserve body heat.
- Warm prepping solutions and intravenous and irrigation fluids as indicated.
- Follow strict aseptic technique.
- Carefully monitor intake and output, including blood loss.

of joints during surgery. The nurse carefully monitors elderly clients and those with cardiac disease for potential fluid overload, which can be life-threatening.

After completing the chart review, the nurse may insert an intravenous catheter and perform a surgical shave. The circulating nurse provides additional emotional support and explains procedures to the client. The client is never left unattended. If the client is in the holding area, he or she is transferred to the operating room after the preoperative routine is completed.

ANALYSIS

COMMON NURSING DIAGNOSES

Two nursing diagnoses commonly applicable to intraoperative clients include:

1. High Risk for Injury related to adverse effects of anesthesia and intraoperative positioning
2. Impaired Skin Integrity and Impaired Tissue Integrity related to pressure, immobility, and the surgical incision.

ADDITIONAL NURSING DIAGNOSES

Additional nursing diagnoses may apply to intraoperative clients:

- High Risk for Injury related to fire and electrical hazards within the operating environment
- High Risk for Disuse Syndrome related to decreased level of consciousness, or immobilization
- Hypothermia related to evaporation from skin and exposed tissue in a cool environment, body heat loss, alteration in the hypothalamus from anesthetic agents, inadequate body covering, or aging
- Ineffective Thermoregulation related to sedation, fluctuating environmental temperature, medications, or age extremes
- Fear related to threat of death, actual or perceived; or anticipation of events posing a threat to self-esteem
- Anxiety related to loss of control, or threat of death
- Fluid Volume Deficit related to decreased intake, evaporative fluid loss through the skin and exposed tissue, or blood loss

PLANNING AND IMPLEMENTATION

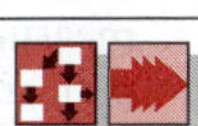

HIGH RISK FOR INJURY

PLANNING: CLIENT GOALS The primary goal is for the client to be free of injury.

INTERVENTIONS Interventions are directed toward preventing injury resulting from anesthesia, positioning, or operating room equipment use.

Appropriate Use of Anesthesia Appropriate preparation for and use of anesthesia are necessary (see earlier).

Positioning Because of preoperative medication, anesthetic agents, and the narrowness of the bed, the client's normal defense mechanisms cannot guard against nerve or joint damage and muscle stretch and strain. Proper positioning, therefore, is important. The circulating nurse pads the operating bed with foam and/or silicone gel pads, properly places the grounding pads, coordinates the transfer of the client to the operating bed, and helps the client obtain a comfortable position. The circulating nurse assesses the skin, especially of the elderly, for bruising or injury, placing extra padding as indicated.

The client is usually in a dorsal recumbent (supine) position after transfer to the operating bed. Anesthesia may be administered with the client supine, and the client may be repositioned for surgery. When general anesthesia is used, the nurse repositions the client after he or she is in stage 3 (see Table 20–2).

The circulating nurse coordinates repositioning of the client for surgery and modifies the position according to the client's safety and special needs. Factors influencing the *timing* of repositioning include:

- The surgical site
- The age and size of client
- Anesthetic administration technique
- Pain experienced by the conscious client on movement

Factors influencing the actual *position* include:

- The specific procedure being performed
- The surgeon's request
- The client's age, size, and weight
- Any respiratory, skeletal, or neuromuscular limitations, such as rheumatoid arthritis, joint replacements, or emphysema

Table 20–6 presents possible complications related to prolonged surgical immobility and preventive nursing actions.

The dorsal recumbent, prone, lithotomy, and lateral positions are frequently used for surgery. Figure 20–12 illustrates common surgical positions and the use of protective padding. When general anesthesia is used, the nurse positions the client slowly to prevent neurogenic shock. The nurse ensures proper positioning by assessing for:

- Physiologic alignment
- Minimal interference with circulation and respiration
- Protection of skeletal and neuromuscular structures
- Optimal exposure of the operative site and intravenous line
- Adequate access to the client for the anesthesiologist or CRNA
- The client's comfort and safety
- Preservation of the client's dignity

TABLE 20–6 Interventions to Prevent Neuromuscular Complications Related to Intraoperative Positioning

Anatomic Area	Complications	Interventions
Brachial plexus	• Paralysis • Loss of sensation in the arm and shoulder	• Pad the elbow. • Avoid excessive abduction. • Secure the arm firmly on an arm board, positioned at shoulder level.
Radial nerve	• Wrist drop	• Support the wrist with padding. • Do not overtighten wrist straps.
Medial or ulnar nerves	• Hand deformities	• Place a safety strap above or below area.
Peroneal nerve	• Foot drop	• Place pillow or padding under knees. • Support lower extremities. • Do not overtighten leg straps.
Tibial nerve	• Loss of sensation on the plantar surface of the foot	• Place a safety strap above the ankle. • Do not place equipment on lower extremities.
Joints	• Stiffness • Pain • Inflammation	• Place pillow or foam padding under bony prominences. • Maintain good body alignment. • Slightly flex joints and support with pillows, trochanter rolls, or pads.

The nurse must be aware of potential complications related to specific positions and modifies care as indicated (Research Applications for Nursing). Throughout the intraoperative period, the nurse assists in preventing obstruction of circulatory, respiratory, or neurologic systems caused by tight straps, improperly placed pads and pillows, or position of the bed.

Operating Room Equipment The OR nurses ensure the proper functioning and use of all equipment and supplies in the operating room. The nurse ensures that he or she is properly trained or educated to use specific pieces of equipment. Competency prevents injury to clients as a result of improper technique or use.

IMPAIRED SKIN INTEGRITY AND IMPAIRED TISSUE INTEGRITY

PLANNING: CLIENT GOALS The primary goal is that the client will experience minimal skin and tissue impairment and contamination as a result of surgery.

INTERVENTIONS Surgery is an invasive procedure that places the client at risk for complications related to:

- The surgical wound, such as incisional tears and lacerations
- Bacterial contamination
- Loss of body fluids from the wound during and after surgery

RESEARCH APPLICATIONS FOR NURSING

Complications May Occur As a Result of the Lithotomy Position

Graling, P. R., & Colvin, D.B. (1992). The lithotomy position in colon surgery. *AORN Journal, 55*(4), 1029–1039.

The lithotomy position provides simultaneous surgical access to the client's abdomen and perineum during colon surgery. In some instances, it is difficult to position the client into the lithotomy position appropriately because of the type of stirrups or because of the client's age, weight, and/or degree of musculoskeletal flexibility. Improper positioning, however, may stretch peripheral nerves or place excessive pressure on muscle and neurovascular bundles. Backache, muscle strain, nerve palsy, and obstruction of blood flow to the legs can occur.

A nurse-physician team studied the incidence of complications in 60 clients confined to the lithotomy position for 2 or more hours during colon surgery. Postoperative complications occurred in 20 clients, including postoperative leg swelling; pain in the legs, hip, and back; a change in sensation; diminished pedal pulses; and impaired ambulation. All clients who stayed in the lithotomy position for more than 6 hours experienced complications. Back pain was most prevalent on postoperative day 4, although the researchers acknowledge that reductions in the prescribed opioid analgesic also commonly occur on this day.

Critique The findings in this study could have been strengthened by using more refined and objective measures of complications. For example, pulse strength could have been measured using a Doppler ultrasound flowmeter, and pain could have been measured by using a reliable tool, such as the McGill pain instrument.

Possible nursing implications To prevent intraoperative complications from use of the lithotomy position, adequately pad the stirrups and position the client in correct body alignment. Using two people, raise both legs simultaneously into position. Bring the client's buttocks to the edge of the operating bed to prevent lordosis. Do not lean on the inner aspects of the client's thighs during surgery. Two people should remove the client from the lithotomy position.

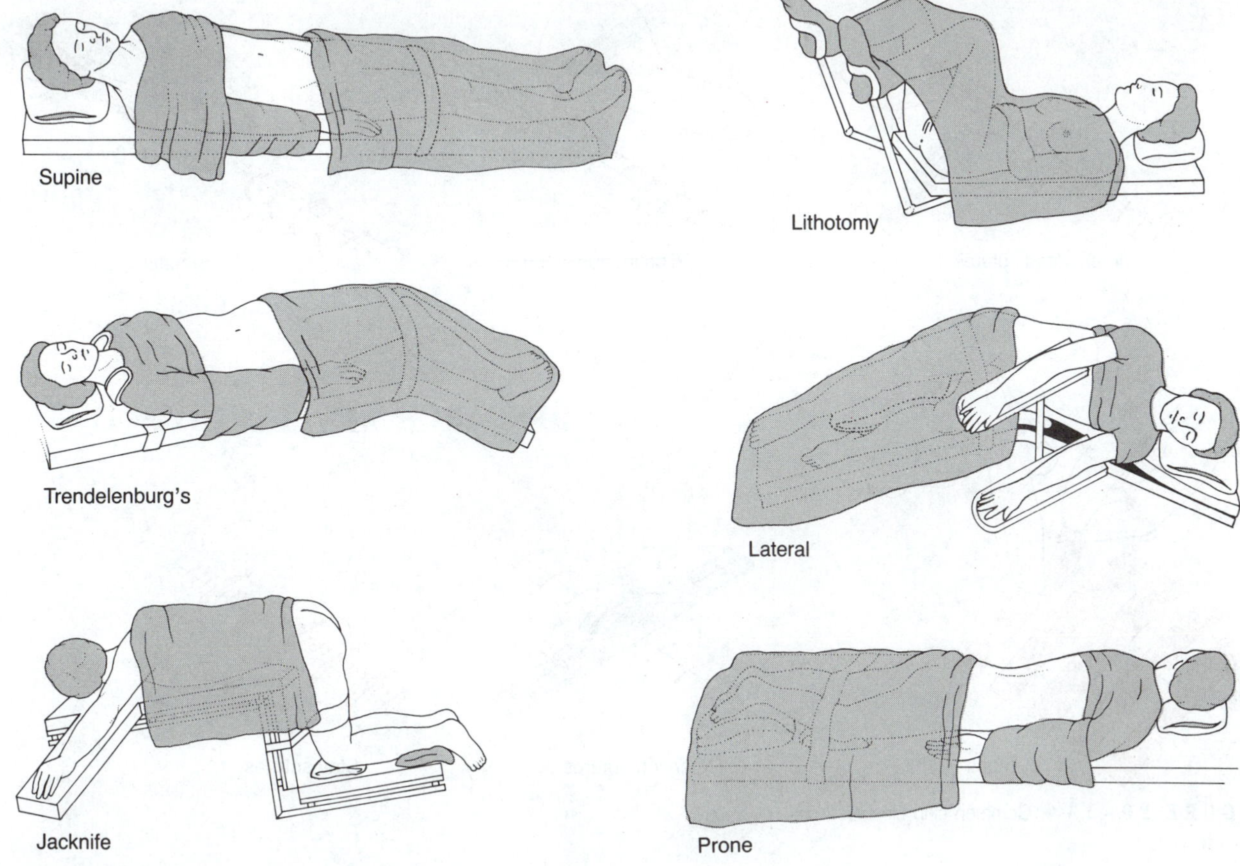

FIGURE 20-12 ◆ Common surgical positions.

Sterile surgical technique and the use of protective drapes, skin closures, and dressings help to minimize complications and promote wound healing.

Plastic Adhesive Drapes If a sterile plastic adhesive drape is used, the scrub nurse helps the surgical assistant apply the drape after the surgical site has been cleaned and dried. The plastic drape is applied directly to the client's skin to prevent shifting and exposure of skin edges. The surgeon makes the incision through the plastic drape. The cut edge remains adherent to the skin and keeps the surgical incision sealed from the migration of bacteria into the wound. The scrub nurse and surgical assistant *gently* remove the drape after closure of the surgical incision. The nurse pays special attention to the elderly and to clients with fragile skin to prevent skin tearing when the adhesive drape is removed.

Skin Closures Skin and tissue closures, such as sutures and staples, are used for several reasons:

- To approximate wound edges until wound healing is complete
- To occlude the lumen of blood vessels, preventing hemorrhage and loss of body fluids
- To prevent wound contamination

The quality of the approximated tissue and the type of closure material are two factors that determine the strength and integrity of the closure. The wound is usually closed in layers to maintain tissue integrity and promote healing with minimal scarring. The surgeon selects the method and type of closures to be used on the basis of the surgical site, the tissue involved, the size and depth of the surgical wound, and the age and medical history of the client. A combination of sutures and clips is commonly used for closure of internal layers of the wound. Staples, stay and retention sutures, and skin closure tapes (Steri-Strips) are used for closure of superficial wounds of the epidermis. Figure 20-13 illustrates commonly used wound closures.

A suture consists of one or more strands of material and is designated by its size or gauge. The size designation sequence, from largest diameter to smallest, is 5, 4, 3, 2, 1, 0, 2-0, 3-0, 4-0, and so forth, to 11-0. Size 5 may be used to close the deep layers of an abdominal wound; 11-0 is the smallest-diameter suture and is used in plastic surgery and ophthalmology. Other characteristics of the suture material, such as type (nylon, silk, vicryl), color (e.g., green, blue, black, white, violet), and structure (twisted, braided) are often listed on the package.

Suture material can be absorbable or nonabsorbable. *Absorbable* sutures are digested over time by

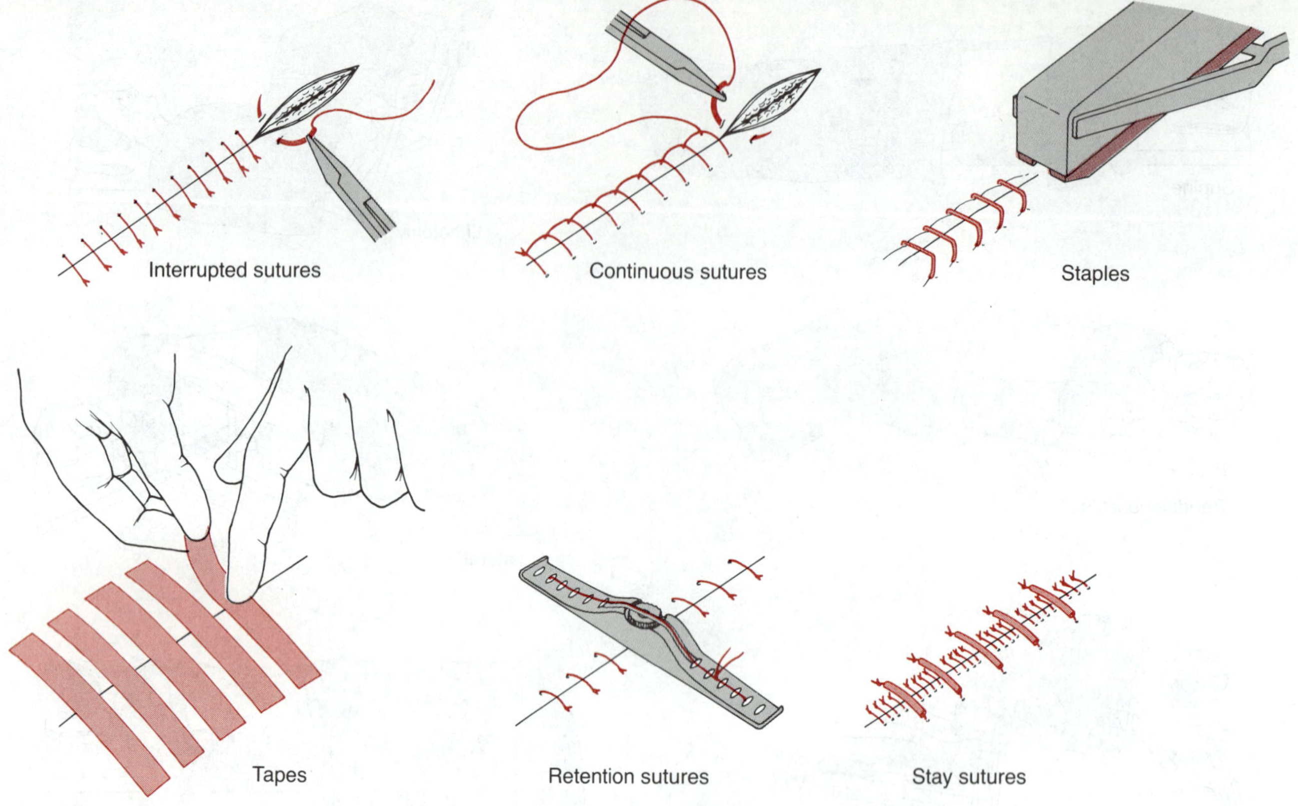

FIGURE 20–13 ◆ Common skin closures.

body enzymes. These sutures first lose strength and then gradually disappear from the tissue. Catgut suture, such as "plain gut" and "chromic gut," was a common type of absorbable suture material that is still in use today, although not as frequently as it once was. Other absorbable sutures are made of synthetics and are labeled as such on the package. The client's physical status, the presence of inflammation, and the type of suture used all influence the rate of absorption, usually up to about 2 weeks.

Nonabsorbable sutures are not affected by body enzymes. Nonabsorbable sutures become encapsulated in the tissue during the healing process and remain embedded in the tissue unless they are removed. These sutures are made of silk, cotton, steel, nylon, polyester, or other synthetic material. Nonabsorbable sutures are used for vascular anastomosis, "wiring" the sternum together after open heart surgery, and closing external wounds. The surgeon may use a double or interlocking stitch to increase the integrity of the closure. Retention and stay sutures (see Fig. 20–13) may be used in addition to standard suture material for high-risk clients (those having major abdominal surgery, obese clients, diabetic clients, and clients taking steroids, which inhibit wound healing).

After the incision is closed, the physician may inject a local anesthetic or instill an antibiotic into the wound. A gauze or spray dressing may be applied to protect it from contamination. A variety of dressings may also be used to absorb drainage and provide support to the incision. A pressure dressing may be applied to prevent or stop a vascular area from bleeding postoperatively. One or more drains (see Chap. 21) may be inserted to prevent the accumulation of secretions within tissues around the surgical area. These secretions, if not drained, impede healing and serve as a medium for bacterial growth, which could result in wound infection.

After the dressing is secure, the nurse coordinates the surgical team in repositioning and transferring the client as indicated. A roller board or a lift sheet is used to transfer the client safely from the operating bed to a stretcher or bed. The circulating nurse and anesthesiologist or CRNA accompany the client to the postanesthesia care unit (PACU) and give a report of the client's intraoperative experience to the PACU nurse. Important information to be relayed includes the following:

- The client's level of anxiety before anesthesia
- The type and length of the surgical procedure
- The location of incisions and drains
- Blood loss
- Intravenous fluids infused
- Medications given
- The client's previous reactions to anesthesia
- Respiratory dysfunctions
- Joint or limb immobility
- The client's primary language
- Any special requests the client may have verbalized

EVALUATION

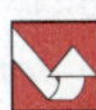

On the basis of identified nursing diagnoses, the nurse evaluates the care of the intraoperative client and ensures that the client:

- Is safely anesthetized without complications
- Does not experience any injury related to intraoperative positioning or equipment
- Is free of skin or tissue contamination during surgery
- Is free of skin tears, bruises, redness, abrasion, or maceration over pressure points and elsewhere

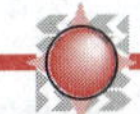

IMPLICATIONS FOR NURSING RESEARCH

Changing technology and trends and more interest in ambulatory surgery and same-day admission, along with increasing numbers of elderly clients, are providing the nurse with new challenges related to the intraoperative client. Some questions for nursing research that could impact client care include the following:

- Is there a change in the client's level of anxiety when premedication is given before the client is transferred into the holding or operating area?
- Is there a role for the family or significant other(s) in the holding area? What is that role?
- How has ambulatory surgery affected clients who are without adequate support systems?
- How does knowledge of intraoperative procedures and routines affect client anxiety?
- What are the special needs of the elderly during the intraoperative period?
- Which intraoperative interventions help to decrease a client's postoperative pain, discomfort, nausea, hypothermia, shivering, and other complications?
- In light of the technology explosion, how do nursing personnel maintain competency in caring for intraoperative clients?
- What is the role of the operating room nurses with regard to the anesthetic agents being administered?

SELECTED BIBLIOGRAPHY

AORN quality improvement standards for perioperative nursing (1992). *AORN Journal, 55*(1), 212–221+.

AORN revised statement on the patient and health care workers with human immunodeficiency virus (HIV) and other bloodborne diseases (1992). *AORN Journal, 55*(6), 1415–1416.

Atkinson, L. J. (1992). *Berry & Kohn's Operating Room Technique* (7th ed.). St. Louis: Mosby Year Book.

Ball, K. A. (1990). *Lasers: The perioperative challenge*. St. Louis: C. V. Mosby.

Ball, K. A. (1990). The basics of laser technology. *Nursing Clinics of North America, 25*(3), 619–634.

Bateman, B. (1992). One solution for pressure sores. *AORN Journal, 56*(5), 832.

Bauer, P. (1991). Universal precautions in OR practice: Risks and regulations. *Nursing Management, 22*(6), 56Q–R,V,X.

Bauer, P. (1991). Universal precautions in OR practice: People and perceptions. *Nursing Management, 22*(7), 101–104.

Bauer, P. (1991). Universal precautions in OR practice: Compliance and knowledge. *Nursing Management, 22*(8), 48 Q–S,V,X.

Beaudet, D. S. (1991). Documenting nursing care in the operating room. *Canadian Operating Room Nursing Journal, 9*(4), 13–14.

Blitt, C. D. (1990). *Monitoring in anesthesia and critical care medicine* (2nd ed.). New York: Churchill Livingstone.

Bruton-Maree, N. (1990). Anesthesia and the aging population. *CRNA, 1*(1), 25–31.

*Burden, N. (1988). Post-anesthesia: While the patient is unconscious. *RN, 51*(4), 34–44.

Campbell, C., & Iwamoto, R. (1992). Intraoperative radiation therapy. *Today's OR Nurse, 14*(9), 19–23, 39–40.

Chana, C. H. (1992). Documenting the nursing process: A perioperative nursing care plan. *AORN Journal, 55*(5), 1231–1235.

Chiarella, M. (1991). The role of the nurse in today's operating room. *AORN Journal, 4*(4), 15–16.

Crow, S. (1990). It's second nature to me now . . . surgical aseptic practices used today. *Today's OR Nurse, 12*(10), 6–8, 50–51.

Cruz, L. D. (1991). A history of the RN first assistant. *AORN Journal, 53*(6), 1536–1537.

Davidhizar, R. (1992). When patients die in the operating room. *Today's OR Nurse, 14*(1), 4.

Davidhizar, R., & Bowen, M. (1992). Managing stress in the OR. *Today's OR Nurse, 14*(5), 24–29.

Davidson, J. E. (1991). Neuromuscular blockade. *Focus on Critical Care—AACN, 18*(6), 512–520.

Dellasega, C., & Burgunder, C. (1991). Perioperative nursing care of the elderly surgical patient. *Today's OR Nurse, 13*(6), 12–17.

DeLong, D. L. (1992). Preoperative holding area. *AORN Journal, 55*(2), 563–566.

Drescher, N. I. (1991). An integrated care plan: Developing an innovative guideline for patient care. *AORN Journal, 54*(6), 1265–1270.

Eccleston, S. B. (1992). Gloving: Clinical question demands further research. *AORN Journal, 56*(2), 265–269.

Entrup, M. H. (1991). Perioperative complications of anesthesia. *Surgical Clinics of North America, 71*(6), 1151–1173.

Fiesta, J. (1992). Anesthesia-related liability. *Nursing Management, 23*(10), 28–30.

Gallagher, M. T., & Kahn, C. (1990). Lasers: Scalpels of light. *RN, 53*(5), 46–53.

Garber, N. (1993). OSHA regulations for the OR nurse. *Today's OR Nurse, 15*(1), 27–30.

Graling, P. R., & Colvin, D. B. (1992). The lithotomy position in colon surgery. *AORN Journal, 55*(4), 1029–1039.

Gruendemann, B. J. (1990). Surgical asepsis revisited. *Today's OR Nurse, 12*(10), 10–14, 50–51.

Hussar, D. A. (1992). New drugs (mivacurium chloride). *Nursing92, 22*(12), 61.

*Jackson, M. F. (1989). Implications of surgery in very elderly patients. *AORN Journal, 50*(4), 859–869.
Jarpe, M. B. (1992). Nursing care of patients receiving long-term infusion of neuromuscular blocking agents. *Critical Care Nurse, 12*(7), 58–63.
Jespen, O. B., & Bruttomesso, K. A. (1993). The effectiveness of preoperative skin preparations. *AORN Journal, 58*(3), 477–479, 482–484.
Johnson, G. M., & Bowman, R. J. (1992). Autologous blood transfusion. *AORN Journal, 56*(2), 282–298.
Keene, A. (1991). Perioperative assessment and nursing implications for the elderly. *Plastic Surgical Nursing, 11*(4), 143–167.
Kelsey, M. (1992). Ophthalmic medications, glaucoma, and the surgical patient. *Journal of Post Anesthesia Nursing, 7*(5), 312–316.
Kemp, M. G., Keithley, J. K. & Morreale, B. (1991). Coordinating clinical research: A collaborative approach for perioperative nurses. *AORN Journal, 53*(1), 104–109.
Lafountain, J. (1992). The RN first assistant in surgery. *Nursing Management, 23*(12), 51–53.
Lambert, D. H. (1992). Continuous spinal anesthesia. *Anesthesiology Clinics of North America, 10*(1), 87–102.
Lehr, P. S., & Pashley, H. S. (1991). Surgeons, nurses, anesthesiologists discuss current issues for the OR. *AORN Journal, 54*(1), 109–110, 112–117.
Leske, J. S. (1992). Practice-based perioperative research. *AORN Journal, 55*(2), 581–590.
Longinow, L. T., & Rzeszewski, L. B. (1993). The holding room: A perioperative advantage. *AORN Journal, 57*(4), 914–924.
Mandy, P. (1992). The regulated health professions act: The keynote address to the Operating Room Nurses Association of Ontario. *Canadian Operating Room Nursing Journal, 10*(2), 11–12, 24–25.
Marco, A. P., & Furman, W. R. (1993). Anesthetic problems: Venous air embolism, airway difficulties, and massive transfusion. *Surgical Clinics of North America, 73*(2), 213–228.
Mathis, J. M. (1992). Collaborative practice eases OR problems. *OR Manager, 8*(3), 8–9.
McLaughlin, A. (1991). Operating in Canada. *Nursing Times, 87*(4), 23–29, 44–46.
Meckes, P. F. (1991). Geriatric surgery. In M. H. Meeker & J. Rothrock (Eds.), *Alexander's care of the patient in surgery* (9th ed., pp. 1004–1017). St. Louis: Mosby Year Book.
Meeker, M. H., & Rothrock, J. (1991). *Alexander's care of the patient in surgery* (9th ed.). St. Louis: Mosby Year Book.
Miller, R. D. (1990). *Anesthesia* (Vols. 1–3, 3rd ed.). New York: Churchill Livingstone.
Moore, J. L., & Rice, E. L. (1992). Malignant hyperthermia. *American Family Physician, 45*(5), 2245–2251.
Murphy, E. K. (1991). Liability for injury resulting from poor patient positioning. *AORN Journal, 53*(6), 1361–1365.
Operating room nurses: On the "cutting edge" of change (1993). *Nursing93, 23*(2), 73–83.
Pereira, L. J., Lee, G. M., & Wade, K. J. (1990). The effect of surgical handwashing routines on the microbial counts of operating room nurses. *American Journal of Infection Control, 18*(6), 354–364.
Peterson, K. J. (1992). Nursing management of autologous blood transfusion. *Journal of Intravenous Nursing, 15*(3), 128–134.
Polis, S. L. (1992). Competency-based laser education: Its implementation in the OR. *AORN Journal, 55*(2), 567–572.
Poss, C. (1991). Outpatient surgery documentation. *AORN Journal, 53*(1), 81–92.
Proposed recommended practices—disinfection (1991). *AORN Journal, 54*(1), 75–80.
Proposed recommended practices—sterilization (1991). *AORN Journal, 54*(1), 82, 84–9, 92–94+.
Ratner, L. E., & Smith, G. W. (1993). Intraoperative fluid management. *Surgical Clinics of North America, 73*(2), 229–241.
Recommended practices: Aseptic technique (1991). *AORN Journal, 54*(4), 819–824.
Recommended practices: Care of instruments, scopes, and powered surgical instruments (1992). *AORN Journal, 55*(3), 838–846+.
Recommended practices: Laser safety in the practice setting (1993). *AORN Journal, 58*(5), 1027–1031.
Recommended practices: Monitoring the patient receiving IV conscious sedation (1993). *AORN Journal, 57*(4), 978–983.
Recommended practices: Positioning the surgical patient (1990). *AORN Journal, 52*(5), 1035–1039.
Recommended practices: Sanitation in the surgical practice setting (1992). *AORN Journal, 56*(6), 1089–1095.
Recommended practices: Skin preparation of patients (1992). *AORN Journal, 56*(5), 937–941.
Recommended practices: Traffic patterns in the surgical suite (1993). *AORN Journal, 57*(3), 730–734.
Recommended practices: Universal precautions in the perioperative practice setting (1993). *AORN Journal, 57*(2), 554–558.
Reeder, J. M. (1993). Do-not-resuscitate orders in the operating room. *AORN Journal, 57*(4), 947–951.
Revised AORN official statement on RN first assistants (1993). *AORN Journal, 57*(1), 47–51.
Rowell, C. C. (1990). The nosocomial wound infection report: Its impact in the OR. *Today's OR Nurse, 12*(10), 21–23, 50–51.
Sangermano, C. A. (1991). Practice and principles of ambulatory surgery. In M. H. Meeker & J. Rothrock (Eds.), *Alexander's care of the patient in surgery* (9th ed. pp. 964–978). St. Louis: Mosby Year Book.
Schild, S. M. (1991). Negligence in the operating room: Understanding the law. *Today's OR Nurse. 13*(11), 11–16.
Scott, S. M. (1992), Mayhew, P. A., & Harris, E. A. Pressure ulcer development in the operating room: Nursing implications. *AORN Journal, 56*(2), 242–250.
Smalley, P. J. (1992). Laser nursing—a perioperative challenge. *Canadian Operating Room Nursing Journal, 10*(1), 18–22+.
Smith, K. A. (1990). Positioning principles: An anatomical review. *AORN Journal, 52*(6), 1196, 1198, 1200–1202+.
Standards and recommended practices for perioperative nursing (1993). Denver, CO: Association of Operating Room Nurses, Inc.
Standards of perioperative nursing: Clinical practice/professional performance (1992). *AORN Journal, 55*(4), 1047–1056.
Stephens, G. (1992). Technology and its effect on OR nursing. *Canadian Operating Room Nursing Journal, 10*(1), 6–7.
Takes, K. L. (1992). Cost-effective practice: Do OR nurses care? *Nursing Management, 23*(4), 96Q–R, V–X.
Tappen, R. M. (1991). Alzheimer's disease: Communication techniques to facilitate perioperative care. *AORN Journal, 54*(6), 1279–1286.
*Thomas, S. D. (1989). Malignant hyperthermia. *Critical Care Nurse, 9*(6), 58–69.
Treat, M. R., Oz, Mehmet C., & Bass, L. S. (1992). New

technologies and future applications of surgical lasers: The right tool for the right job. *Surgical Clinics of North America, 72*(3), 705–742.

Vance, A., & Davidhizar, R. (1992). The element of care in the operating room. *Today's OR Nurse, 14*(11), 24–27.

Walsh, J. (1993). Postop effects of OR positioning. *RN, 56*(2), 50–57.

Watson, D. S. (1991). Safe nursing practices involving the patient receiving local anesthesia. *AORN Journal, 53*(4), 1055, 1058–1059.

Who has responsibility to monitor O.R. blood loss? (1992). *Regan Report on Nursing Law 33*(4), 2.

Wilhelm-Hass, E., Rowley, S., & Robinson, M. (1991). The OR record: Developing a format for documenting care. *AORN Journal, 53*(3), 754–755.

Wound closure manual (1994). Somerville, NJ: Ethicon, Inc. (Pub. No. EPB010).

Young, M. A., Meyers, M., McCulloch, L. D., et al. (1992). Latex allergy: A guideline for perioperative nurses. *AORN Journal, 56*(3), 485–497.

SUGGESTED READINGS

Davidson, J. E. (1991). Neuromuscular blockade. *Focus on Critical Care—AACN, 18*(6), 512–520.

The beginning of this article reviews various aspects of physiology and pharmacology related to the use of nondepolarizing neuromuscular blocking agents in the clinical setting. The remainder of the article discusses peripheral nerve stimulation in conjunction with the use of the blocker agents and related nursing care.

Gallagher, M. T., & Kahn, C. (1990). Lasers: Scalpels of light. *RN, 53*(5A), 46–53.

This article defines and describes lasers and laser therapy. The authors list many procedures that are performed with lasers. An operating room checklist of safety and general preoperative and postoperative nursing care and teaching are included. The article also presents a continuing education test.

Johnson, G. M., & Bowman, R. J. (1992). Autologous blood transfusion. *AORN Journal, 56*(2), 282–298.

Perioperative autologous blood transfusions are the focus of this article. The authors review selection criteria for each collection—preoperative, intraoperative, and postoperative. Intraoperative blood salvage and subsequent transfusion are described in detail. The article also addresses complications, costs, equipment, and quality assessment. A home study test is included.

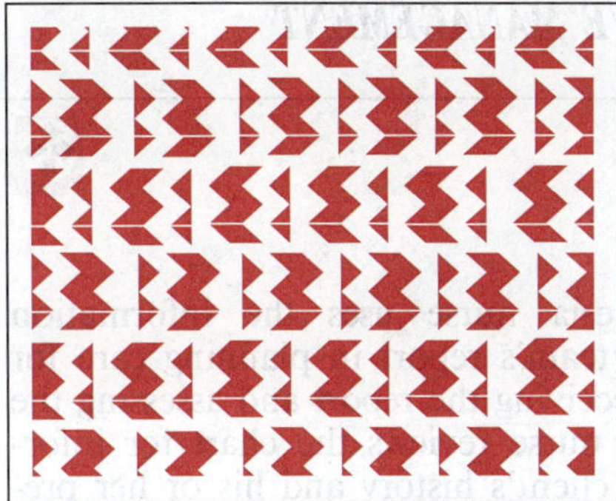

CHAPTER 21

Interventions for Postoperative Clients

CHAPTER HIGHLIGHTS

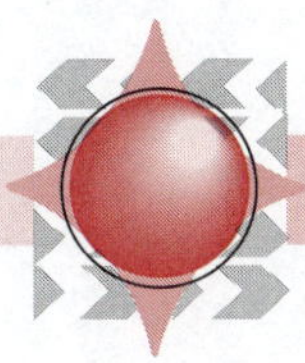

The third and final stage of the perioperative experience is the postoperative period. It begins when the client's surgical procedure has been completed. The client is transferred from the operating room (OR) to another area for specialized nursing care (often a postanesthesia care unit [PACU]), until his or her condition stabilizes. The postoperative period continues after the client's condition is stabilized and after the client is discharged from the hospital or the ambulatory surgery facility. The actual time spent in the hospital or the facility after surgery varies according to the client's age and physical health, the type and length of surgical procedure, anesthesia, and complications (if any).

OVERVIEW

The postanesthesia care unit (PACU) is usually located close to the operating department. The unit is usually a large and open room in order to provide maximal visibility of clients, appropriate ventilation and lighting, and easy access to supplies and emergency equipment. The client area in the unit is often divided into individual cubicles. Curtains or screens for privacy are available, but are usually closed only during bedside procedures. Each cubicle is stocked with equipment and supplies commonly used by the nurse to monitor and care for clients, such as oxygen, suction equipment, cardiac monitors, airway equipment, and emergency medications.

After the surgical procedure is completed, the circulating nurse and the anesthesiologist or nurse anesthetist (certified registered nurse anesthetist, or CRNA) accompany the client to the PACU. In some situations, such as when the client is in critical condition, he or she may go directly from the operating department to the intensive (critical) care unit.

The postanesthesia nurse is a specialist who is skilled in the care of clients of all ages with multiple medical and surgical problems immediately after surgery. The postanesthesia nurse has in-depth knowledge of anesthetic agents, analgesics, pain management, and surgical procedures. He or she is skilled in physical and psychosocial assessment and can make quick decisions if emergencies or complications occur. The postanesthesia nurse monitors the client closely and consults with the anesthesiology personnel and the surgeons as needed.

On the client's arrival in the PACU, anesthesiology personnel give the postanesthesia nurse a verbal report and explain the following:

- The type and extent of the surgical procedure
- The type of anesthesia
- The client's tolerance of anesthesia and the surgical procedure
- The client's allergies
- The pathologic condition
- The status of vital signs
- The type and amount of fluids and medications administered
- Estimated blood loss (EBL)
- Any intraoperative complications, such as a traumatic intubation

The circulating nurse adds information related to:

- The client's level of anxiety before receiving anesthesia
- The client's preoperative and intraoperative respiratory function and dysfunction
- Pertinent medical history
- The location and type of dressings, catheters, tubes, drains, or packing
- Intake and output, including current intravenous (IV) fluid administration and estimated blood loss
- Joint or limb immobility while in the operating room, especially in the elderly client
- Other intraoperative positioning that may be relevant in the postoperative phase
- Special requests that were verbalized by the client preoperatively
- The client's primary language spoken and any sensory impairments
- Any other important intraoperative occurrences

COLLABORATIVE MANAGEMENT

ASSESSMENT

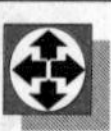

HISTORY

The postanesthesia nurse uses the information from the surgical team's report in planning care for the client. After receiving the report and assessing the client, the PACU nurse reviews the chart for information about the client's history and his or her presurgical physical and emotional status. In ideal situations, the postanesthesia nurse reviews pertinent information before the client arrives in the unit. The nurse on the medical-surgical unit later incorporates all of the surgical and postanesthesia information into the client's postoperative plan of care. Chapter 19 identifies clinical situations that put a client at risk for postoperative complications, such as:

- Allergic reactions
- Hypothermia
- Hyperthermia
- Hypertension
- Hypotension
- Hypovolemic shock
- Renal failure
- Electrolyte imbalances
- Dysrhythmias
- Congestive heart failure
- Paralytic ileus
- Acute urinary retention
- Deep vein (venous) thrombosis
- Pulmonary embolism
- Atelectasis or pneumonia
- Laryngeal edema
- Ventilator dependence
- Gastrointestinal (GI) bleeding
- Disseminated intravascular coagulation (DIC)
- Anemia
- Wound evisceration

PHYSICAL ASSESSMENT/CLINICAL MANIFESTATIONS

The postanesthesia nurse assesses the client and compiles data on a postanesthesia care unit (PACU) record form (Fig. 21–1). Assessment data include the client's temperature, pulse, respiration, and blood pressure. The nurse examines the surgical area for bleeding. The postanesthesia nurse initiates assessments, and the medical-surgical nurse continues assessments after the client is discharged to the medical-surgical nursing unit. The frequency of vital signs measurement is based on the facility's policy and the surgeon's orders. Vital signs are often recorded every 15 minutes for four times, every 30 minutes for four times, every 2 hours for four times, and then every 4 hours for 24 to 48 hours if the client's condition is stable. Thereafter, vital signs are assessed according to the facility's policy, the client's condition, and the nurse's judgment.

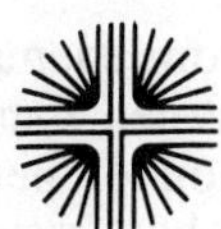

OUR LADY OF LOURDES MEDICAL CENTER
POST ANESTHESIA CARE UNIT RECORD

DATE: ____________ TIME: ____________ OPERATION: ____________

ANESTHESIA: ____________ AIRWAY: ____________ SURGEON: ____________

DRESSING ON ARRIVAL: ____________ OXYGEN: ________ TIME ON: ________ TIME OFF: ________

260
240
220
200
180
160
140
120
100
80
60
40
20

NURSES NOTES

POST ANESTHESIA RECOVERY SCALE

		ARRIVAL	D/C
Activity	2-Able to move 4 extremities 1-Able to move 2 extremities 0-Able to move 0 extremities		
Respiration	2-Able to cough & deep breath 1-Dyspnea or limited breathing 0-Apneic		
Circulation	2-BP =20% Preanesthesia 1-BP=20-50% Preanesthesia 0-BP=50% Preanesthesia		
Consciousness	2-Fully awake 1-Rousible on calling 0-Not responding		
Color	2-Pink 1-Pale, dusky, blotchy, etc. 0-Cyanotic		
Total			

DRESSINGS AT DISCHARGE: ____________
VERBAL REPORT TO: ____________
DISCHARGE TIME: ____________
P.A.C.U. NURSE SIGNATURE: ____________

INTAKE RECORD

FLUIDS	OR	PACU	TOTAL	AMOUNT REMAINING
D5 .2NS				
LR				
D5W				
PSS				
D5 .45NS				
BLOOD				
ORAL				

MEDICATIONS

TIME	DRUG	DOSE	ROUTE	SIGNATURE

OUTPUT RECORD

	OR	PACU	TOTAL
URINE			
GASTRIC			
EBL			

FORM G88/Rev. 7/88 7010.06

FIGURE 21–1 ◆ Example of a postanesthesia care unit record. (Courtesy of Our Lady of Lourdes Medical Center, Camden, NJ.)

The health care team determines the client's readiness for transfer or discharge from the postanesthesia area by noting a postanesthesia recovery score (see Fig. 21-1) of at least 10. In addition, the facility may have specific criteria for discharge (e.g., stable vital signs, normothermia, no overt bleeding, and return of gag, cough, and swallow reflexes). After the nurse determines that all criteria have been met, the client is discharged by the anesthesiologist to the hospital unit or the home (as in the case of outpatient surgery).

Physical assessment continues from the PACU to the medical-surgical nursing unit. If the client is to be discharged from the PACU to the home, physical assessment is continued by home care nurses or by the client or family members themselves after adequate instruction.

RESPIRATORY SYSTEM

Airway Assessment When the client is admitted to the PACU, the nurse immediately assesses the client for a patent airway and adequate respiratory exchange. An artificial airway, such as an endotracheal (ET) tube, a nasal trumpet, or an oral airway, may be in place. If the client is also receiving supplemental oxygen, the nurse notes the type of delivery device and the concentration or liter flow of the oxygen. The nurse usually maintains continuous pulse oximetry (see Chap. 28) for monitoring the client's oxygen saturation while in the PACU.

To determine airway patency, the nurse places a hand above the client's mouth, nose, or artificial airway to feel exhalation. The nurse assesses the rate, pattern, and depth of respirations to measure the adequacy of air exchange. A respiratory rate of fewer than 10 breaths per minute may indicate anesthetic or opioid analgesic depression. Rapid, shallow respirations signal cardiovascular compromise, increased metabolic rate, or pain.

Breath Sounds The nurse auscultates the lungs bilaterally over all lung fields to determine the quality and adequacy of breath sounds. The nurse also assesses for symmetry of breath sounds. If the client has an endotracheal tube, it could move farther down into the right mainstem bronchus, thus preventing left lung expansion. In this case, lung sounds on the left are absent or significantly decreased and the nurse observes only the right chest wall rise and fall with respirations.

Other Respiratory Assessments Respiratory assessment by the postanesthesia nurse includes ongoing inspection of the chest wall for the use of accessory muscles, sternal retraction, and diaphragmatic breathing. These signs could indicate an excessive anesthetic effect, airway obstruction, and neurologic complications such as paralysis, all of which could result in hypoxia. The nurse also listens for snoring and stridor (a high-pitched crowing sound). Snoring and stridor are signs of upper airway obstruction resulting from tracheal or laryngeal spasm or edema, mucus in the airway, or occlusion of the airway from edema or relaxation of the tongue (Table 21-1). When there is a delayed metabolism of and elimination of neuromuscular blocking agents, the client has residual muscle weakness, which could affect pulmonary ventilation. The nurse assesses the client for the inability to sustain a head lift, weak handgrasps, and an abdominal breathing pattern.

After the client returns to an inpatient medical-surgical nursing unit, the nurse completes an initial assessment on arrival and then continues to assess for signs and symptoms of respiratory depression or hypoxemia. The medical-surgical nurse also auscultates the lungs for effective expansion and for adventitious or other abnormal breath sounds. This auscultation is usually performed every 4 hours during the first 24 hours postoperatively and then during every nursing shift, or more frequently, as indicated. Elderly clients, smokers, and clients with a history of respiratory disease are more susceptible to postoperative respiratory complications (see Chap. 19 for more detail).

CARDIOVASCULAR SYSTEM

Vital Signs The nurse assesses the client's blood pressure, pulse, and heart sounds on admission to the

TABLE 21-1 Significance of Abnormal Postoperative Respiratory Assessment Findings

Abnormal Findings	Possible Significance
Inspection	
Loud snoring, grunting, or stridor	• Narrowing of the airway • Vocal cord or tracheal edema
Unequal chest wall movement	• Obstruction in one side of the bronchi • Pneumothorax
Irregular depth, rate, or rhythm of respirations	• Ineffective respirations
Cyanosis of lips, ears, or extremities	• Ineffective respirations • Hypoxemia
Palpation	
Crepitation	• Leakage of air into the subcutaneous tissue
Unequal tactile fremitus	• Obstruction or narrowing of the bronchi
Percussion	
Dullness over lung fields	• Pulmonary edema • Pleural effusion • Pneumonia
Auscultation	
Crackles	• Pulmonary edema • Pneumonia
Wheezes	• Narrowing of the airways • Bronchospasm • Mucosal edema
Pleural friction rub	• Pleural inflammation • Pulmonary embolus

postanesthesia care unit (PACU) and then at least every 15 minutes until the client's condition stabilizes. Automated blood pressure cuffs and continuous cardiac monitoring assist the nurse in making frequent assessments.

Both the PACU and medical-surgical nurses review postoperative vital signs for upward or downward trends. The nurse reports blood pressure fluctuations of more or less than 25% of preoperative values (15- to 20-point difference, systolic or diastolic) to the anesthesiologist or the surgeon. A decrease in the client's blood pressure, pulse pressure, and heart sounds indicates possible myocardial depression, fluid volume deficit, shock, hemorrhage, or the effects of medication (see Chaps. 15, 36, and 8). Bradycardia (slow heart rate) could indicate an anesthesia effect or hypothermia (decreased body temperature). Elderly clients are especially predisposed to hypothermia because of aging changes in the hypothalamus (the temperature regulation center), loss of subcutaneous tissue, and coolness of the operating suite. An increased pulse rate could indicate hemorrhage, shock, or pain.

Cardiac Monitoring Cardiac monitoring is maintained until the client is discharged from the PACU. For clients at risk for dysrhythmias, monitoring may continue until the client returns to the medical-surgical unit. Many facilities have telemetry available on either specialized telemetry units or on general medical-surgical units.

In assessing the vital signs of a client who is not undergoing continuous monitoring, the medical-surgical nurse determines the rate, rhythm, and quality of the client's apical pulse compared with those of a peripheral pulse such as the radial pulse. A pulse deficit (a difference between the apical and peripheral pulses) could indicate a dysrhythmia.

Peripheral Vascular Assessment Anesthesia and positioning during surgery (e.g., the lithotomy position for genitourinary procedures) may compromise the client's peripheral circulation. Both the postanesthesia and medical-surgical nurses assess the client's peripheral circulation. The nurse performs this assessment by comparing distal pulses bilaterally for the presence and quality of pulsation, noting the color and temperature of extremities, evaluating sensation, and determining the speed of capillary refill. Palpable dorsalis pedis pulses indicate adequate circulation and tissue perfusion of the distal lower extremities.

As part of the ongoing assessment, the medical-surgical nurse assesses the lower extremities for redness, pain, warmth, swelling, and the presence of Homan's sign, any of which could indicate the presence of deep vein thrombosis (DVT), a life-threatening condition. Assessment of the lower extremities may be performed once during a nursing shift or once daily, depending on the risk of complications and the facility's policy. (Chapters 19, 35, and 51 have further information on deep vein thrombosis.)

NEUROLOGIC SYSTEM

General Cerebral Functioning Regardless of the type of surgical procedure, the postanesthesia nurse assesses cerebral function and the level of consciousness or awareness of all clients who have received general anesthesia (Table 21–2) or any type of sedation. To assess the client's level of consciousness, the nurse observes the client's lethargy, restlessness, or irritability and tests coherence and orientation. The nurse determines awareness by observing responses to calling the client's name, touching the client, and giving simple commands, such as "Open your eyes" and "Take a deep breath." Eye opening in response to a command indicates wakefulness or arousability but not necessarily awareness. The nurse determines the degree of orientation to person, place, and time by asking the conscious client to answer simple questions, such as "What is your name?" (person), "Where are you?" (place), and "What day is it?" (time).

For an elderly client, a rapid return to his or her prior level of orientation may not be realistic. The preoperative, intraoperative, and postoperative medications and anesthetic agents often affect the elderly client's reorientation ability (see Chaps. 19 and 20).

The nurse compares the client's preoperative baseline neurologic status with the postoperative assessment findings. Clients with altered cerebral functioning preoperatively due to a pre-existing condition continue to have that alteration postoperatively. After the client has returned to a satisfactory consciousness level (and all other criteria have been met), he or she is either discharged to home or transferred to the nursing unit. The medical-surgical nurse continues to assess the client's level of consciousness every 4 to 8 hours or as indicated by the client's condition and the facility's policy.

Motor/Sensory Evaluation For all clients receiving general and regional anesthesia, motor and sensory function is assessed. General anesthesia renders

TABLE 21–2 Immediate Postoperative Neurologic Assessment: Return to Preoperative Level

Order of Return to Consciousness After General Anesthesia

1. Muscular irritability
2. Restlessness and delirium
3. Recognition of pain
4. Ability to reason and control behavior

Order of Return of Motor and Sensory Functioning After Local or Regional Anesthesia

1. Sense of touch
2. Sense of pain
3. Sense of warmth
4. Sense of cold
5. Ability to move

clients unconscious and depresses voluntary motor function; regional anesthesia alters the motor and sensory function of only part of the body. (See Chapter 20 for more information on types of anesthesia.) Motor and sensory assessment is especially important after the client has had epidural or spinal anesthesia. The postanesthesia nurse evaluates motor function by instructing the client to move each extremity. The client who had epidural or spinal anesthesia remains in the postanesthesia care unit until sensory function (feeling) and voluntary motor movement of the lower extremities have returned (see Table 21–2). In addition, the nurse assesses the strength of each limb and compares the results bilaterally.

The postanesthesia nurse also tests for the return of sympathetic nervous system tone by gradually elevating the client's head and monitoring for hypotension. This evaluation begins after the client's sensation has returned to at least the spinal dermatome level of T-10. (See Chapter 40 for further neurologic assessment.) After the client is transferred to the nursing unit, the medical-surgical nurse continues neurologic assessment as indicated.

FLUID AND ELECTROLYTE BALANCE Fasting before and during surgery, the loss of fluid during the procedure, and the type and amount of blood or IV fluid administered affect the client's postoperative fluid and electrolyte balance. Either fluid volume deficit or fluid volume overload may occur after surgery. Sodium, potassium, chloride, and calcium imbalances may also result, as may alterations in other electrolyte levels. Complications of fluid and electrolyte imbalances occur more often in elderly or debilitated clients or in clients with medical problems such as diabetes mellitus, Crohn's disease (especially after major intestinal surgery), and heart failure.

Intake and Output Intraoperative intake and output measurement is part of the operative record and part of the circulating nurse's report to the postanesthesia nurse. The postanesthesia nurse records any intake or output, including IV fluid intake, vomitus, urine, and nasogastric (NG) tube drainage. When the postanesthesia nurse gives a report, the medical-surgical nurse needs to know the total intake and output from both the operating room and the postanesthesia care unit to assess fluid balance accurately and to complete the 24-hour intake and output record.

Hydration Assessment The medical-surgical nurse continues to assess the client's hydration. The nurse inspects the color and moist appearance of mucous membranes; the turgor, texture, and "tenting" of the skin (test over the sternum or forehead of an elderly client); the amount of drainage on dressings; and the presence of axillary sweat, which indicates adequate hydration. The nurse measures total output (e.g., nasogastric tube drainage, urinary output, and wound drainage) and compares it with total intake to identify a possible fluid imbalance. The nurse considers insensible fluid loss when reviewing total output. The nurse continues to assess the client's intake and output while the client is at risk for fluid imbalances. Some facilities have policies that require intake and output to be measured if the client receives IV fluids or has a catheter, drains, or a nasogastric tube.

Intravenous Fluids The nurse administers and closely monitors IV fluids to promote fluid and electrolyte balance. Standard isotonic solutions such as lactated Ringer's (LR) and 5% dextrose with lactated Ringer's (D5/LR) are used for IV fluid replacement and maintenance in the PACU. After the client returns to the medical-surgical unit, the type and rate of administration of IV solutions are based on the individual client's need. An example of a typical IV solution for the client when admitted to the nursing unit is 5% dextrose with 0.45% (D5/½ NSS) normal saline. (See Chapters 15 and 16 for further discussion of IV fluid administration, electrolyte balance, and assessment of hydration.)

ACID-BASE BALANCE Acid-base balance may be affected by preoperative, intraoperative, and postoperative respiratory status, intraoperative metabolic changes, and losses of acids or bases in drainage. For example, nasogastric tube drainage or vomitus represents a loss of hydrochloric acid. The postanesthesia and medical-surgical nurses assess acid-base status mostly through arterial blood gas measurement and other laboratory values (e.g., the anion gap). (See Laboratory Assessment later in this chapter and Chapter 18 for more detailed information on acid-base imbalances.)

RENAL/URINARY SYSTEM Voluntary control of urinary function may return immediately after surgery or may not return for 6 to 8 hours or longer after inhalation, IV, and epidural or spinal anesthesia. The effects of preoperative medications and anesthetic agents and manipulation during surgery, in combination or alone, can cause urinary retention. Both the postanesthesia and medical-surgical nurses assess for this complication by inspection, palpation, and percussion of the client's lower abdomen for bladder distention. Assessment may be difficult to perform when the client has had lower abdominal surgery. Urinary retention is common in the early postoperative period and requires appropriate intervention, often one or more intermittent (straight) catheterizations to empty the bladder.

When the client has an indwelling urinary (Foley) catheter, the nurse assesses the urine for color, clarity, and amount. If the client is voiding, the nurse also assesses the urinary frequency, associated amount per void, and any symptoms. Urinary output should correlate with total input for a 24-hour period, but other sources of output need to be considered. The nurse reports a urinary output of less than 30 mL/hour (240 mL/8-hour nursing shift) to the physician. Decreased urinary output may indicate hypovolemia or renal complications. (Refer to Chapter 69 for complete information on the assessment of renal/urinary function, including the interpretation of specific gravity, electrolyte values, and osmolality of urine.)

GASTROINTESTINAL SYSTEM

Nausea and Vomiting One of the most common postoperative reactions is nausea and vomiting. Approximately 30% of clients receiving general anesthesia have some form of gastrointestinal upset within the first 24 hours after surgery. Clients with a history of motion sickness are more likely to develop postoperative nausea and vomiting. Obese individuals may be at risk because many anesthetics are retained by fat cells and therefore have a lingering effect. Abdominal surgery and the use of opioid analgesics reduce intestinal peristalsis after surgery. These situations predispose the client to nausea and vomiting for longer than the first 24 hours after surgery. Research Applications for Nursing addresses the effect of intraoperative steroid administration on postoperative nausea and vomiting.

Postoperative nausea and vomiting can cause stress and irritation of abdominal and gastrointestinal (GI) wounds, increase intracranial pressure in clients who had head and neck surgery, elevate intraocular pressure in clients who had eye surgery, and increase the risk of aspiration and aspiration pneumonia. Both the postanesthesia and medical-surgical nurses assess for nausea and vomiting continuously. Often, a client experiences nausea as the head of the bed is raised in the early postoperative period. This symptom may occur with or without associated dizziness.

Gastrointestinal Peristalsis The nurse in the postanesthesia care unit and later on the medical-surgical unit assesses for the return of peristaltic function. Peristalsis may be delayed because of the length of time under anesthesia, the amount of bowel handling intraoperatively, and opioid analgesic use.

Assessment The nurse auscultates for bowel sounds in all four abdominal quadrants and at the umbilicus. If the client is undergoing nasogastric suctioning, the suction must be turned off before auscultation of the abdomen. Otherwise, the nurse could mistake the sound of the suction for bowel sounds. In addition, the nurse asks the client whether flatus has been passed. Both bowel sounds and flatus passage indicate peristalsis, but abdominal cramping denotes trapped, nonmoving gas and not peristalsis.

Complications Decreased peristalsis can occur in clients with a paralytic ileus. The walls of the intestine are distended and there is no movement of the intestinal wall (aperistalsis). The nurse assesses the postoperative client for the clinical manifestations of paralytic ileus. These include few or absent bowel sounds, distended abdomen, diffuse abdominal discomfort (due to the distention), vomiting, lack of flatus, and no passage of stool.

The client may also experience constipation postoperatively owing to anesthesia, analgesia (especially codeine [Paveral✱] and other opioid analgesics), decreased activity, and decreased oral intake. The nurse assesses the client's abdomen by inspection, palpation, percussion, and auscultation and records the client's elimination pattern to determine whether interventions are needed. Increased dietary fiber intake, the administration of mild laxatives or bulk-forming agents, or the use of enemas may be necessary.

Nasogastric Tube Drainage A nasogastric tube may be inserted intraoperatively to decompress and drain the stomach, to promote gastrointestinal rest, to allow the lower gastrointestinal tract to heal, or to provide an enteral feeding route. It may also be used to monitor

RESEARCH APPLICATIONS FOR NURSING

Intraoperative Steroid Administration May Help Prevent Postoperative Nausea and Vomiting

Mataruski, M. R., Keis, N. A., Smouse, D. J., & Workman, M. L. (1990). Effects of steroids on postoperative nausea and vomiting. *Nurse Anesthesia, 1*(4), 183–188.

About 30% of postoperative clients experience nausea and vomiting because of the effects of anesthetics and, in some cases, the surgery itself. Many of the antiemetics used to treat nausea and vomiting have side effects, ranging from cerebral depression to hypotension. The use of antiemetics can therefore contribute significantly to postoperative morbidity. Mataruski and colleagues studied the effects of prophylactic intraoperative steroid administration on nausea and vomiting during the first 24 hours after surgery. The authors retrospectively examined 61 adult clients who had undergone lumbar laminectomy, some of whom routinely received intraoperative steroids because of their anti-inflammatory effects on neuroskeletal dysfunction. Thirty-four (56%) of the clients studied had received intraoperative steroids, and 27 (44%) had not. The clients who had received intraoperative steroids experienced significantly less nausea, vomiting, and pain than those who had not received these agents. The incidence of vomiting in the nonsteroid group was 26%, compared with 8.8% in the steroid group.

Critique The sample groups were homogeneous for age, gender, height, weight, anesthetic agents, and time under anesthesia. The study examined only the number of episodes of nausea and vomiting—not the degree of nausea and vomiting.

Possible nursing implications The preliminary nature of these findings does not allow firm guidelines for nursing practice. However, this study suggests that the prophylactic use of intraoperative steroids may reduce the incidence of postoperative nausea and vomiting in clients undergoing lumbar laminectomy and similar procedures.

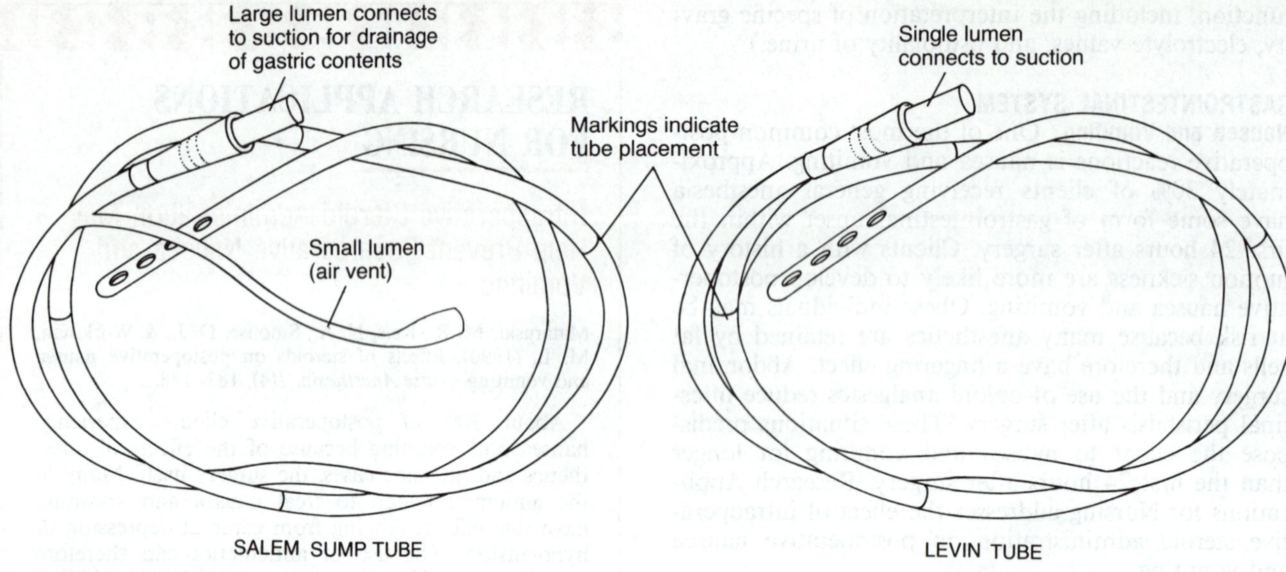

FIGURE 21-2 ◆ Two types of nasogastric tubes.

the occurrence of bleeding and prevent intestinal obstruction. The Levin tube and the Salem sump are the two most common tubes used (Fig. 21-2). The Salem tube is a double-lumen tube with an air vent to keep the tube from adhering to the gastric mucosa. This feature allows easy drainage of the stomach and prevents gastric mucosal damage. The Levin tube is a single-lumen tube with no air vent. To promote drainage, varying degrees of suction (high, medium, or low) are applied to the nasogastric tube. Suction is either continuous (recommended for the Salem tube) or intermittent on the basis of the surgeon's preference and the tube type.

Assessment The nurse records the color, consistency, and amount of the drained material every 8 hours (Table 21-3). In some instances, the results of an occult blood test (Hemoccult or guaiac test) may also be recorded. Normal nasogastric drainage fluid is greenish-yellow; red drainage fluid indicates active bleeding, and brown liquid or coffee-ground drainage indicates the possibility of old bleeding.

Complications The nurse assesses the client for possible complications related to nasogastric tube use, which include fluid and electrolyte imbalances, aspiration, and nares discomfort. To prevent aspiration, the nurse checks the tube placement every 4 to 8 hours and before the instillation of irrigation solution into the tube (see Chap. 55 for information on tube placement and care). After gastric surgery, the nasogastric tube should not be manipulated or irrigated without an order from the physician. Fluid and electrolyte imbalances can result from nasogastric drainage and nasogastric tube irrigation with water instead of saline. Imbalances include fluid volume deficit (see Chap. 15), hypokalemia and hyponatremia (see Chap. 16), hypochloremia, and metabolic alkalosis (see Chap. 18).

INTEGUMENTARY SYSTEM The surgical or clean wound heals itself at skin level in approximately 2 weeks in the absence of infection, trauma, connective tissue disease, malnutrition, or the use of some medications such as steroids. Smokers, elderly clients, obese clients, and those with diseases that decrease immunity have delayed wound healing. Complete healing of underlying tissue and return to presurgical integrity may take 6 months to 1 year. The physical condition and age of the client, the size and location of the wound, and the stress on the surgical wound also affect the length of time for wound healing. Because of the rich blood supply, wounds of the face and head heal more quickly than do abdominal and leg wounds.

TABLE 21-3 Calculating Nasogastric Tube Drainage

Formula

$$\text{drainage in collection device} - \text{amount of irrigant} = \text{true (actual) amount of drainage}$$

Example

A client's drainage container was marked at 150 mL at 7 AM. At 3 PM, there were 525 mL in the container. During the nursing shift, the nurse instilled 30 mL of saline as an irrigant into the tube four times, as ordered by the physician.

525 mL − 150 mL = 375 mL of drainage

30 mL × 4 = 120 mL of irrigant

375 mL − 120 mL = 255 mL of actual drainage

Normal Wound Healing The nurse uses a knowledge of wound healing (Clinical Collection 1 in the full-color portion of this textbook) to plan care and protection of the incision area. During the first few days of normal wound healing, the incised tissue regains blood supply and begins to bind together. After 3 to 4 days, connective tissue cells strengthen the wound. By the ninth or tenth day, the wound appears to be healed; however, healing is not complete until the scar is strengthened. (See Chapter 67 for discussion of wound healing and wound infection.)

After the surgeon removes the original postoperative dressing (usually on the first or second postoperative day), the medical-surgical nurse assesses the incision on a regular basis, usually every 8 hours, for redness, increased warmth, swelling, tenderness or pain, and the type and amount of drainage. Some drainage is normal during the first few days, changing from sanguineous (bloody) to serosanguineous to serous (serum-like or yellow). Serosanguineous drainage continuing beyond the fifth postoperative day should alert the nurse to the possibility of dehiscence, and the surgeon should be notified. Slight crusting on the incision line is normal, as is a pink color to the line itself owing to inflammation from the surgical procedure. Slight swelling under the sutures or staples is also normal. Redness or swelling of or around the incision line, excessive tenderness or pain on palpation, and purulent or odorous drainage could indicate wound infection and is reported to the surgeon.

Ineffective Wound Healing Ineffective wound healing may be caused by wound infection, distention from edema or paralytic ileus, stress at the surgical site, and pre-existing conditions that cause delayed wound healing. Wound *dehiscence* is a partial or complete separation of the outer layers of the wound, sometimes described as a "splitting open of the wound" (Fig. 21–3). *Evisceration* is the total separation of the layers and extrusion of internal organs or viscera (usually abdominal) through the open wound (see Fig. 21–3). Both of these alterations in wound healing are more often seen between the fifth and the tenth postoperative day and occur more frequently in obese clients or others predisposed to delayed wound healing. Wound dehiscence or evisceration may be preceded by excessive coughing, not splinting the surgical site, vomiting, or straining. The client may state, "Something gave way" or "I feel as if I just split open."

Dressings and Drains All dressings, including casts and elastic (Ace) bandages, are assessed for bleeding or other drainage on admission to the postanesthesia care unit and then frequently until the client is discharged to home or transferred to the inpatient unit. The medical-surgical nurse assesses the client's dressing each time vital signs are taken. When inspecting the dressing, the nurse checks for drainage and notes the amount, color, consistency, and odor of the drainage fluid. The nurse also checks underneath the client, as drainage (often blood from hemorrhage) may leak from the side of the dressing, yet not appear on the dressing itself. The dressing should not restrict circulation or sensation.

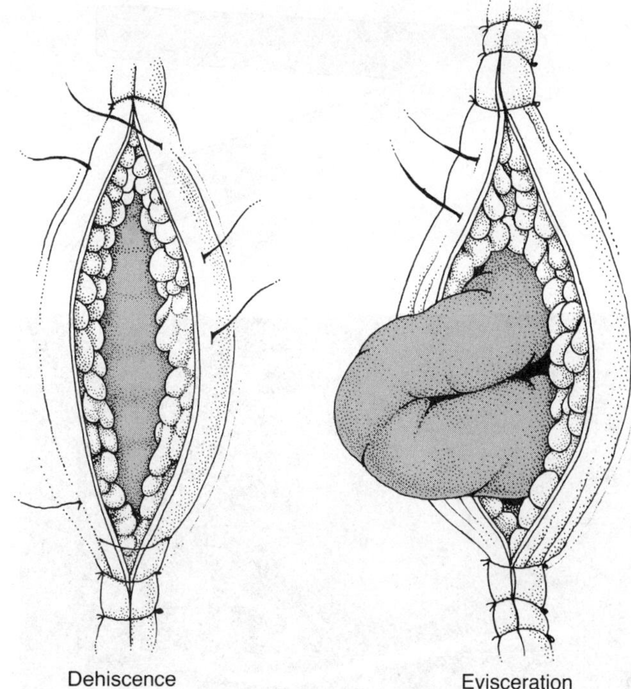

FIGURE 21–3 ◆ Complications of wound healing.

To confine or contain drainage, the surgeon inserts a drain into or close to the wound if more than a minimal amount of drainage is expected. A Penrose drain (a single-lumen, soft latex tube) is a gravity-type drain under the dressing. The nurse assesses closed-suction drains such as Hemovac, VacuDrain, and Jackson-Pratt drains to ensure maintenance of compression and thus suction. The surgeon may place a T tube after abdominal cholecystectomy to drain bile. Figure 21–4 shows commonly used drains.

The nurse assesses all drains for patency when the client is admitted to the postanesthesia care unit (PACU) and every time vital signs are taken during the postoperative period. The nurse monitors the amount, color, and consistency of the drainage while the client is in the postanesthesia care unit and at least every 8 hours after the client is transferred to the medical-surgical nursing unit. For example, large amounts of sanguineous drainage may indicate internal bleeding.

DISCOMFORT/PAIN ASSESSMENT The surgical client almost always reports pain. Postoperative pain is related to the surgical wound, tissue manipulation, the presence of drains, and intraoperative positioning. In assessing the client's discomfort or pain and need for medication, the nurse considers the type, extent, and length of the surgical procedure. The nurse assesses for physical and emotional signs of pain such as increased pulse and blood pressure, increased respiratory rate or hyperventilation, diaphoresis (profuse perspiration), restlessness, increased confusion (in the

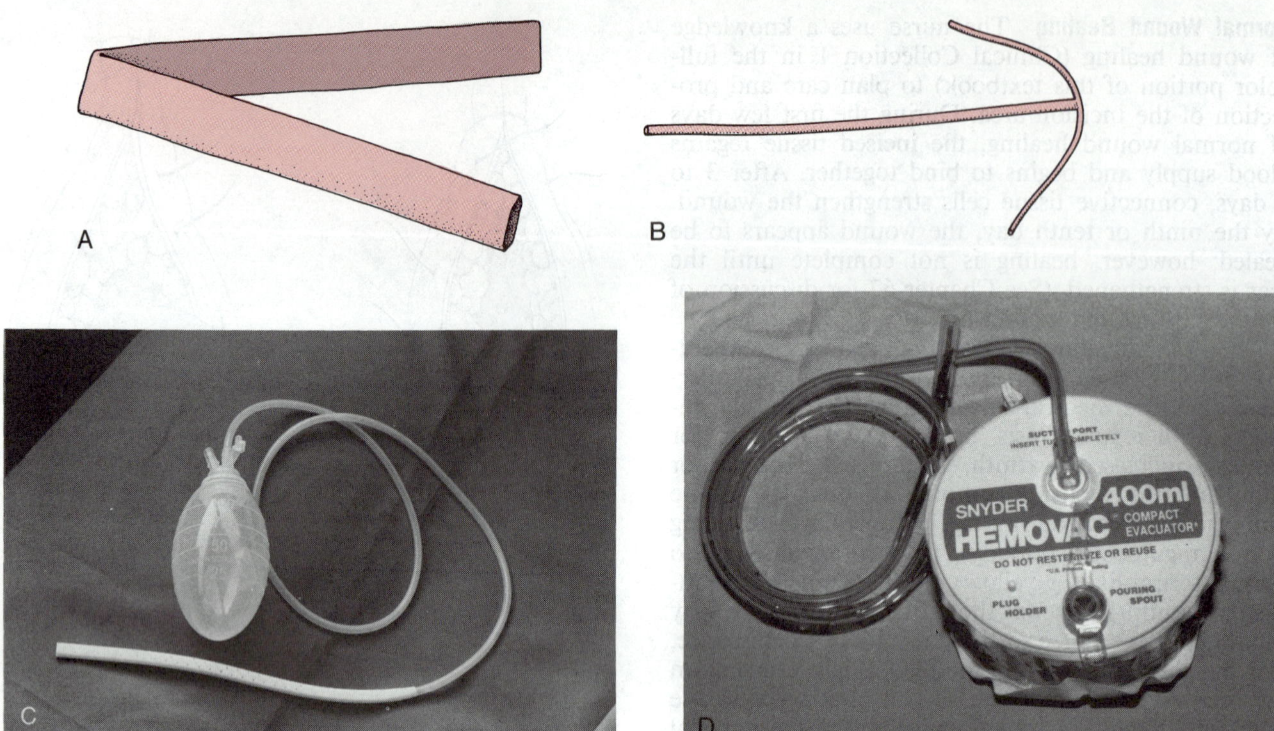

FIGURE 21-4 ◆ Types of surgical drains. Gravity drains, such as the Penrose (*A*) and the T tube (*B*), drain directly through a tube from the surgical area. In closed wound drainage systems, such as the Jackson-Pratt (*C*) and Hemovac (*D*), drainage collects in a collecting vessel by means of compression and re-expansion of the system.

elderly), wincing, moaning, and crying. When possible, the nurse asks the client to quantify or rate the discomfort or pain before and after medication is given (e.g., on a scale of 1 to 10, with 1 being least intense and 10 being extreme pain). In addition, the nurse observes for a return of the client's normal (baseline) physical behaviors. (See Chapter 8 for further discussion of pain assessment.)

Discomfort or pain assessment is initiated by the postanesthesia nurse. After the client is transferred out of the PACU, the medical-surgical nurse continues to assess the client's comfort level. Postoperative pain generally reaches its peak on the second postoperative day, when the client is more awake and the anesthetics and analgesics given intraoperatively have been metabolized and excreted.

PSYCHOSOCIAL ASSESSMENT

As the nurse completes the physical aspects of postoperative assessment, the psychologic, social, and cultural characteristics of the client are considered. This assessment may be delayed or difficult to do in the postanesthesia care unit when the client is drowsy or incoherent. The nurse considers the client's age and medical history, the surgical procedure, and the impact of the procedure on the client's recovery, body image, roles, and lifestyle.

Physical signs that may indicate anxiety include restlessness; increased pulse, blood pressure, and respiratory rate; and crying. The client may be anxious and ask questions about the results or findings of the surgical procedure. The nurse reassures the client that the surgeon will speak with him or her after the client is fully awake. If the surgeon has already spoken with the client, the nurse reinforces what was said. (Chapter 7 has further information on stress.)

After the client returns to the medical-surgical unit, the medical-surgical nurse continues the psychosocial assessment of the client and assesses significant others as well.

LABORATORY ASSESSMENT

Postoperative laboratory tests are performed to monitor the client for complications. Tests are based on the surgical procedure and the client's medical history and postoperative clinical manifestations. Common postoperative serum tests include analysis of electrolytes and a complete blood count. A change in laboratory test results (e.g., electrolyte levels, hematocrit, and hemoglobin levels) commonly occurs during the first 24 to 48 hours postoperatively because of blood and fluid loss and the body's reaction to the surgical process. Fluid loss without significant blood loss may result in hemoconcentrated laboratory values (decreased fluid in the blood with resultant increased concentration). The laboratory test result is reported as increased, but actually represents a concentrated normal value (Chart 21-1).

A subtle early indication of infection is an increase in the band cells (immature neutrophils) in the white

CHART 21-1

Lab Profile ◆ Postoperative Assessment

Test	Normal Range for Adults	Significance of Abnormal Findings
Hemoglobin	• Male: 14–18 g/dL, or 8.7–11.2 mmol/L • Female: 12–16 g/dL, or 7.4–9.9 mmol/L • **Elderly:** values are slightly decreased	• *Increased* in hemoconcentration • *Decreased* early postoperatively owing to blood loss
Hematocrit	• Male: 42–52% • Female: 37–47% • **Elderly:** values may be slightly decreased	• *Increased* in hemoconcentration • *Decreased* with bleeding
Sodium (Na^+)	• 136–145 mEq/L, or 136–145 mmol/L	• *Increased* in hemoconcentration • *Decreased* with body water overload, excess antidiuretic hormone level, nasogastric suction, vomiting, or IV fluid with water administration
Potassium (K^+)	• 3.5–5 mEq/L, or 3.5–5 mmol/L	• *Increased* with massive tissue damage, acidosis, infection, acute renal failure, hemolysis of the blood specimen • *Decreased* in NPO states when K^+ replacement is inadequate, diarrhea, use of non–K^+-sparing diuretics, and alkalosis
White blood cell count	• 5000–10,000/mm^3	• Slight *increase* with inflammatory process from surgery • Greater *increase* in infection, stress, and tissue necrosis
Anion gap	• 6–16	• *Increased* in metabolic acidosis

cell differential count. This increase is termed a "shift to the left." The source of the infection may be the respiratory system, the urinary tract, the wound, or the IV site. The medical-surgical nurse obtains the appropriate specimen for culture and sensitivity testing and monitors the culture results reported from the microbiology laboratory at 24, 48, and 72 hours. The nurse notifies the physician of positive culture results. (See Chapter 27 for more information on infection.)

Arterial blood gas (ABG) determinations may be indicated for clients with a history of respiratory or cardiac disease, those undergoing prolonged mechanical ventilation postoperatively, and those having had surgery involving the thoracic cavity. Both the postanesthesia and medical-surgical nurses interpret arterial blood gas results and notify the surgeon of any deviation from the expected normal for that client (acid-base imbalance or hypoxemia). The anion gap can be calculated from serum electrolyte values or recorded by the chemistry laboratory. An increase in the anion gap alerts the nurse to the possibility of metabolic acidosis. (For more discussion on arterial blood gases and acidosis, see Chapters 17 and 18.)

Urine and renal laboratory studies are ordered as indicated (e.g., urinalysis, urinary electrolyte levels, and serum creatinine levels). Other laboratory studies performed depend on the client's diagnosis, the type of surgical procedure, and so on. Examples are serum amylase level for a client who had pancreatic surgery and blood glucose level for a diabetic client.

ANALYSIS

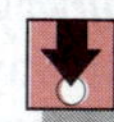

COMMON NURSING DIAGNOSES

The following nursing diagnoses are common when caring for the postoperative client:

1. Impaired Gas Exchange related to the residual effects of anesthesia, pain, the use of opioid analgesics, and immobility
2. Impaired Skin Integrity related to surgical wounds, inflammatory processes, drains and drainage, and tubes
3. Pain related to the surgical incision and positioning during surgery

ADDITIONAL NURSING DIAGNOSES

Depending on the type and extent of surgery, the family structure, and so on, there may be additional nursing diagnoses for the postoperative client (see the discussion of surgical management in other chapters as appropriate). Possible diagnoses are:

- High Risk for Aspiration related to decreased mobility, anesthesia, and opioid analgesic use
- Ineffective Airway Clearance related to ineffective or absent cough
- Fluid Volume Deficit related to decreased oral intake and abnormal fluid loss

- Constipation related to decreased mobility, anesthesia, and opioid analgesic use
- High Risk for Infection related to surgery and invasive lines, tubes, and catheters
- Urinary Retention related to anesthesia, surgical procedures, and decreased mobility
- Sleep Pattern Disturbance related to the use of medications and hospitalization
- Self Care Deficit related to surgical procedures and decreased mobility
- Body Image Disturbance related to surgical procedures, the loss of a body part or function, and pain
- Altered Family Processes related to the impact of surgery and illness on the family system
- Altered Sexuality Patterns related to surgery, pain, and hospitalization
- Spiritual Distress related to hospitalization as evidenced by separation from religious or cultural ties

PLANNING AND IMPLEMENTATION

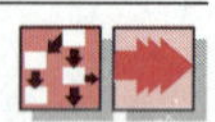

IMPAIRED GAS EXCHANGE

PLANNING: CLIENT GOALS The goal is that the client will attain or maintain optimal lung expansion and respiratory function.

INTERVENTIONS

Airway Maintenance Depending on the status of the airway, the postanesthesia nurse may need to insert an oral airway if the client does not already have one. This type of airway pulls the tongue forward and holds it down to prevent obstruction. If the client has clenched teeth, a large tongue, or upper airway obstruction, the nurse could insert a nasal airway (nasal trumpet) to keep the airway open. The nurse keeps the manual resuscitation bag and emergency equipment for intubation or tracheostomy nearby. For clients whose only airway is a tracheostomy or laryngectomy stoma, the nurse alerts other staff members by posting signs in the room, notes on the chart, and so forth.

Positioning Immediate care by the nurse in the postanesthesia care unit includes positioning the client in a side-lying position or turning the client's head to the side to prevent aspiration of secretions (or vomitus) while the client is still unreactive and vulnerable to aspiration. The nurse suctions the mouth, nose, and throat to keep the airway clear of mucus or vomitus as necessary.

The postanesthesia nurse keeps the head of the stretcher or bed flat to prevent hypotension and possible shock, unless this position is contraindicated by the client's condition or surgical procedure. (For example, after intracranial surgery, the head of the bed or stretcher is elevated to promote respiratory function and prevent postoperative cerebral edema.) The nurse administers oxygen via face tent, nasal cannula, or mask to facilitate the excretion of inhalation anesthetic agents, to increase arterial oxygen levels, and to raise the level of consciousness. After the client is fully reactive and stable, the postanesthesia nurse raises the head of the bed to promote respiratory function.

Breathing Exercises After the client regains the gag and cough reflex and meets the agency's criteria for extubation (if intubated), the airway or endotracheal tube is removed. Examples of extubation criteria are the client's ability to raise and hold his or her head up and evidence of thoracic breathing. The nurse encourages the client to cough (with the incision splinted) and deep breathe to expand the lungs, promote gas exchange, and hasten the elimination of inhalation anesthetic agents. Chart 19–4 reviews the teaching of postoperative breathing exercises and splinting of the surgical wound area to the client. As soon as the client is awake enough to follow commands, and throughout the postoperative period, the postanesthesia and medical-surgical nurses encourage the client to cough, use the incentive spirometer, and take deep breaths. The client who is unable to expectorate mucus or sputum voluntarily may require oral or nasal suctioning. Meticulous mouth care is important after the removal of secretions.

Mobilization The client is out of bed and ambulating as soon as possible to help mobilize secretions and promote lung expansion. Even for hospitalized clients with extensive surgery, the goal may be to get the client out of bed the same day as surgery or the first postoperative day. If this is not possible, given the individual client's situation, the nurse turns the client at least every 2 hours (side to side) and ensures that the client performs his or her respiratory exercises and leg exercises (see Chart 19–5). Early ambulation minimizes the risk of pulmonary complications, including a pulmonary embolism, which could arise from impaired venous circulation in the legs. The client may report pain and resist getting up, but the nurse stresses the importance of activity to prevent postoperative complications. When indicated, the nurse offers pain medication 30 to 45 minutes before the client gets out of bed.

IMPAIRED SKIN INTEGRITY

PLANNING: CLIENT GOALS The goal is that the client will have incision healing without postoperative wound complications.

INTERVENTIONS Nursing assessment of the surgical area postoperatively is critical (see the discussion of integumentary system assessment earlier in this chapter). Although most wound complications can be treated without additional surgical intervention, emergency surgical procedures may be necessary.

Nonsurgical Management Postoperative nonsurgical wound care usually includes changing and care of the dressing, assessment of the wound for signs of infection, and care of drains, including emptying, measuring, and documenting characteristics of the drainage. The nurse emphasizes to the client the importance of early deep breathing exercises (see Chap. 19) to prevent respiratory complications that could cause forceful coughing. The nurse encourages hip flexion when the client is in the supine position to reduce tension on the wound. The nurse also reminds the client always to splint the incision when coughing. The nurse promotes an atmosphere conducive to wound healing and protective of the skin in general, especially for the elderly client (Chart 21–2).

Dressings The surgeon performs the first dressing change so that he or she can assess the wound, remove any packing, and advance (pull partially out) or remove drains as indicated. Before the first dressing change, the nurse reinforces the dressing if it becomes wet from drainage. The nurse documents the reinforcement, as well as the color, type, amount, and odor of drainage fluid and the time of observation, in the client's chart. The nurse assesses the surgical area frequently and reports any unexpected findings to the surgeon.

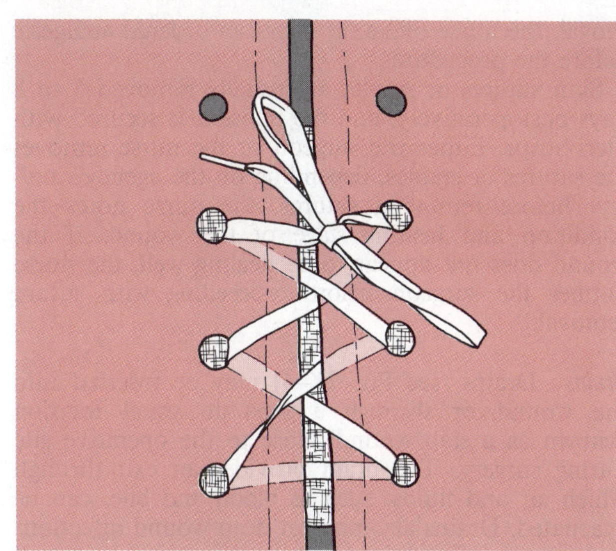

FIGURE 21–5 ◆ Montgomery straps may be used when frequent dressing changes are anticipated. They help to prevent skin irritation from frequent removal of tape.

CHART 21–2

Nursing Focus on the Elderly ◆ Postoperative Skin Care

- Improve perfusion to the wound to promote wound healing:
  - Keep the client adequately hydrated to maintain cardiac output.
  - Keep the airway patent and provide adequate oxygenation.
  - Keep the client's oxygen saturation on pulse oximetry at greater than 90%.
- Conserve the client's energy:
  - Allow the client to sleep in darkened, quiet room.
  - Administer medication to combat pain and sleeplessness, as ordered.
  - Provide rest periods throughout the day.
  - Control the client's room temperature.
  - Assist in activities of daily living.
- Place the client on a safety program to prevent falls, if indicated.
- Maintain strict aseptic technique in caring for breaks in the integument (IV or other catheters, indwelling urethral catheter, wound).
- Maintain the client's psychosocial health:
  - Prevent unnecessary stressors.
  - Allow the client liberal visitation of supportive others.
  - Enable the client to utilize individual successful coping mechanisms.
  - Keep the client well groomed and bathed.
- Protect fragile skin:
  - Minimize the use of tape on the skin.
  - Use hypoallergenic tape or Montgomery straps.
  - Change dressings as soon as they become wet.
  - Lift the client during transfer or repositioning.

Data from Jones, P. L., & Millman, A. (1990). Wound healing and the aged patient. *Nursing Clinics of North America, 25*(1), 263–277.

After removal of the surgical dressing, the surgeon may wish to leave the suture or staple line open to the air, which allows easy assessment of the wound and early detection of poor approximation, drainage, swelling, or redness. Some surgeons believe that air-drying promotes healing. A draining wound, however, is always covered with a dressing.

Dressing changes are generally ordered by the surgeon, but the facility or unit may have established standards or policies that dictate specific protocols for postoperative dressing changes and incision care. An unchanged wet or damp dressing becomes a source of infection. The nurse performs dressing changes under aseptic conditions until the sutures or staples are removed.

Dressings vary, depending on the surgical procedure and the surgeon's preference. The standard postoperative dressing for a large incision consists of gauze or nonadherent pads covered with a larger absorbent pad held in place by tape or by Montgomery straps (Fig. 21–5). In other cases, the incision may be covered with a transparent plastic surgical dressing (such as Op-Site) or a spray in the operating room. This type of dressing stays intact for 3 to 6 days and allows visualization (observation) of the wound while preventing contamination and eliminating the need for dressing changes.

Wound or suture line care generally consists of changing gauze dressings at least once during a nursing shift or daily and may include cleaning the area with sterile saline or some other solution. The hospital's policy, the unit's standards, and the surgeon's preference determine what solution, if any, is used on the wound and also the frequency of the dressing changes. For extensive dressing changes or drain removal, the nurse offers the client an ordered analgesic before the procedure.

Skin sutures or staples are usually removed 6 to 8 days postoperatively, and the incision is secured with Steri-Strips. Either the surgeon or the nurse removes the sutures or staples, depending on the agency's policy. Before removing sutures, the nurse notes the condition and healing stage of the wound. If the wound does not appear to be healing well, the nurse notifies the surgeon before proceeding with suture removal.

Drains Drains (see Fig. 21–4) may be inserted into the wound or through a separate small incision (known as a stab wound) close to the operative site during surgery. The drain provides an exit through which air and fluids, such as blood and bile, can be evacuated. Drains also prevent deep wound infections and abscess formation within the surgical wound during healing.

The Penrose drain is a superficial device that is placed into the external aspect of the incision and drains directly onto the client's dressing and perisurgical area (the skin around the incision). In caring for a client with a Penrose drain, the nurse changes a damp or soiled dressing by carefully cleaning under and around the drain. The nurse then pads the area distal to the drain with absorbent pads to prevent skin irritation and contamination of the surgical wound. Whether sutured in place or not, the drain can easily be dislodged or accidentally pulled out during a dressing change. As the wound heals, the surgeon shortens (advances) the drain by pulling it out and removing the excess external portion until drainage stops.

Jackson-Pratt and Hemovac drains are two commonly used self-contained drainage systems by which the wound drains directly through a tube via gravity, suction, or vacuum. These drains are commonly sutured in place with a pursestring suture that seals the area when the drain is removed. The nurse empties the reservoir of the drain and records the amount and color of drainage during every nursing shift or more frequently if ordered by the surgeon. After emptying and compressing the reservoir, the nurse secures the drain to the client's gown or pajamas (never to the sheet or mattress) to prevent pulling and stress on the surgical wound.

Drug Therapy Wound infection is a major postoperative complication. It usually results from contamination during surgery, preoperative infection, or the debilitated or immunosuppressed state of the client. A client at risk for a wound infection may receive prophylactic antibiotic therapy with a broad-spectrum antibiotic or one that is effective in fighting organisms common to the specific surgical site. These antibiotics are usually continued for 24 to 72 hours postoperatively to ensure that adequate antibiotic levels are reached in this critical time period. The first dose may be administered IV before or during the surgery.

Wounds that become infected and open (without intact sutures) are usually treated with a specific dressing change and prolonged systemic antibiotic administration. Depending on the physician's order, the nurse irrigates the wound (e.g., with sterile saline, hydrogen peroxide, povidone-iodine, or acetic acid), loosely packs it with solution-soaked gauze (e.g., with neomycin, gentamicin, iodoform, povidone-iodine, or acetic acid), and covers the wound with dry, sterile dressings. This procedure (wet-to-dry dressings) may be ordered one to three times daily. The packing promotes healing from within the wound and debridement (removal) of the infected tissue as the wound heals.

Surgical Management

Management of Dehiscence If dehiscence (wound opening) occurs, the nurse applies a sterile nonadherent or saline dressing to the wound and notifies the surgeon. A wound that becomes infected dehisces by itself, or it may be opened by the surgeon through an incision and drainage (I&D) procedure. In either case, the wound is left open rather than resutured and is treated as described previously.

Management of Evisceration An evisceration (a wound opening with the protrusion of internal organs or viscera) is considered a surgical emergency. One nurse tends to the client while another nurse immediately notifies the surgeon. Chart 21–3 outlines emergency care. The nurse provides emotional support by explaining what happened and reassuring the client that the emergency can, and will, be handled by competent, capable individuals.

The surgeon may order a nasogastric tube to decompress the stomach and relieve some of the pressure internally or to remove the stomach's contents if the client has been eating and general anesthesia is planned. The nurse prepares the client for surgery (see Chap. 19) to close the wound. Regional or local anesthesia may be used, depending on the location of the wound and the surgeon's or the anesthesiologist's preference. Postoperative nausea and vomiting, which places undue stress on the already fragile incision, is minimized when regional or local anesthesia is used. To increase the incision's integrity, stay or retention sutures of wire or nylon are used over the standard suture or staple line (see Fig. 20–13).

PAIN

PLANNING: CLIENT GOALS The primary goal is that the client will attain or maintain optimal comfort levels throughout the postoperative phase. This entails the alleviation or reduction of pain or discomfort associated with the surgical wound and positioning during surgery.

INTERVENTIONS Postoperative pain management usually includes drug therapy and other methods such as positioning, massage, relaxation techniques, and di-

CHART 21–3

Nursing Care Highlight ◆ Surgical Wound Evisceration

1. Call for help! Instruct the person who responds to notify the surgeon *immediately* and to bring any needed supplies into the client's room.
2. Stay with the client.
3. Cover the wound with a nonadherent dressing premoistened with *warmed sterile normal saline.* Note: The supplies needed for this emergency should be in the client's room, especially if the client is at high risk.
4. If premoistened dressings are not available, moisten sterile gauze or sterile towels in a sterile irrigation tray with sterile saline, then cover the wound.
5. If saline is not immediately available, cover the wound with gauze, then moisten with sterile saline using a sterile irrigation tray *as soon as* someone brings saline.
6. Do *not* attempt to reinsert the protruding organ or viscera.
7. While covering the wound, note the client's response and assess for signs and symptoms of shock.
8. Place the client in a supine position with the hips and knees bent.
9. Take and document vital signs. Note: If the person who answered the call for help is back in the room before this, instruct that individual to take vital signs while you focus on covering the wound and repositioning the client.
10. Provide support and reassurance to the client.
11. Continue assessing the client, including vital signs assessment every 5 to 10 min until the surgeon arrives.
12. Keep dressings continuously moist by adding warmed sterile saline to the dressing as often as necessary. Do *not* let the dressing become dry.
13. When the surgeon arrives, report your findings and your interventions, then follow his or her directions.
14. Document the incident, the activity the client was engaged in at the time of the incident, your actions, and your assessments.

version. Often, the client achieves greater benefit from a combination of approaches. The nurse assesses the client's comfort level and the effectiveness of the therapies. (Chapter 8 provides a comprehensive discussion of pain assessment and management for the postoperative client.) The client who has optimal pain control is better able to cooperate with the therapies and exercises designed to prevent postoperative complications and promote the postoperative rehabilitation process.

Drug Therapy The use of opioids or other analgesics for the management of pain may mask or increase the amount and severity of symptoms of an anesthesia reaction. Therefore, these drugs must be administered with caution. This is especially true in the postanesthesia care unit when the client's condition is not stabilized. Pain medication, when administered in the postanesthesia care unit, is usually given IV in small doses. After the nurse administers medication for pain, the client remains in the postanesthesia care unit for a defined period (often, 30 to 45 minutes). The postanesthesia nurse can assess for hypotension, respiratory depression, or other side effects. Approximately 5 to 10 minutes after an IV injection, the nurse assesses the effectiveness of the medication (i.e., on a rating scale) in relieving the client's pain.

Opioid analgesics are routinely given during the first 24 to 48 hours after surgery to control acute pain. Round-the-clock administration is generally more effective than medicating on client demand because more constant blood levels can be obtained. Drugs commonly used include meperidine hydrochloride (Demerol), morphine sulfate (Statex✱), hydromorphone hydrochloride (Dilaudid), ketorolac (Toradol), codeine sulfate, butorphanol tartrate (Stadol), and oxycodone hydrochloride with aspirin (Percodan), or oxycodone hydrochloride with acetaminophen (Tylox, Percocet). The nurse assesses the type, location, and intensity of the pain before and after the administration of medication (see also Discomfort/Pain Assessment earlier in this chapter). The nurse monitors the client's vital signs closely, especially for hypotension and hypoventilation, after the administration of opioid analgesics. Chart 21–4 has further information on various analgesics utilized during the postoperative period.

Patient-controlled analgesia (PCA) via IV or internal pump (the catheter is sutured into or proximal to the surgical area) and epidural analgesia are becoming more common to achieve better pain control. In PCA, the client adjusts the rate or dosage of infusion of an opioid analgesic on the basis of his or her pain level and physical response to the drug. This method allows more consistent pain relief and more control by the client. The maximal dose per hour is "locked in" to the pump so the client cannot accidentally overdose. Drugs commonly used by the PCA method include morphine, meperidine, and hydromorphone.

Epidural analgesia can be administered intermittently by the anesthesiologist or via continuous drip with or without PCA through an epidural catheter left in place after epidural anesthesia. Drugs commonly given by epidural catheter include the opioids fentanyl citrate (Sublimaze) and preservative-free morphine (Duramorph), and the local anesthetic bupivacaine (Marcaine).

The nurse uses care not to overmedicate or undermedicate the client, especially the elderly client. In assessing for *overmedication,* the nurse monitors the client's vital signs, especially blood pressure and respiratory rate, and level of consciousness. Complications from the use of opioid analgesics include respiratory depression, hypotension, nausea, vomiting, and constipation. An opioid antagonist such as naloxone

CHART 21–4

Drug Therapy for Management of Postoperative Pain

Drug	Usual Dosage	Nursing Interventions	Rationale
Meperidine hydrochloride (Demerol)	• 50–150 mg q3–4h PO or IM • 12.5–25 mg IV • Maximum 6–8 doses	• Monitor blood pressure. • Move and ambulate the client slowly. • Monitor pulse rate. • Assess for decreased GI motility or GI upset.	• Common side effects include decreased blood pressure, orthostatic (postural) hypotension, and bradycardia. • Constipation, nausea, and vomiting can occur.
Morphine sulfate (Epimorph*, Statex*)	• 5–15 mg IM or IV incrementally • 30–60 mg q4h PO • Maximum 6 doses	• Monitor respiratory status. • Monitor blood pressure. • Assess for GI motility and urinary output.	• Respiratory depression can be severe and need medical intervention. • Hypotension, constipation, and urinary retention can occur.
Hydromorphone hydrochloride (Dilaudid)	• 1–2 mg q3–4h IV • 1–10 mg q3–4h PO	• Monitor respirations. • Monitor blood pressure. • Monitor for food intolerance. • Monitor fluid and electrolyte balance. • Assess GI motility.	• Respiratory depression, hypotension, anorexia, nausea, vomiting, and constipation can occur.
Codeine sulfate, codeine phosphate (Paveral*)	• 15–60 mg q4h IM or PO • Maximum 6 doses	• Monitor respiratory status. • Monitor for food intolerance. • Monitor fluid and electrolyte balance. • Assess GI motility.	• Respiratory depression, nausea, and vomiting can occur. • Constipation is common; prophylactic interventions may be indicated.
Butorphanol tartrate (Stadol)	• 1–4 mg q3–4h IM • 0.5–2 mg IV • Maximum 6–8 doses	• Monitor neurologic status and changes in level of consciousness. • Monitor respiratory status.	• Butorphanol can cause increased intracranial pressure and respiratory depression.
Oxycodone hydrochloride and aspirin (Percodan, Endocan*, Oxycodan*)	• 1–2 tablets (5–10 mg) q3–4h PO • Maximum 80 mg	• Assess GI tolerance of medication. • Assess for GI bleeding. • Monitor GI motility. • Monitor coagulation respiratory studies (PT, PTT).	• The aspirin component can irritate the stomach and could cause GI bleeding. • Bleeding times and other coagulation study results may be increased be-

hydrochloride (Narcan) may be administered to reverse the acute effects of opioid depression. Because of the short effect of the opioid antagonist, the nurse monitors the blood pressure and respirations closely (i.e., every 15 to 30 minutes) until the full effect of the opioid analgesic has passed. The nurse may need to give more doses of the opioid antagonist during this time. See Chart 21–5 for more information on the opioid antagonists. In addition, the client has breakthrough pain after the opioid antagonist is administered, so the nurse initiates other interventions to promote comfort.

The nurse assesses for *undermedication* by questioning the client about the effects of the medication and observing for nonverbal cues that indicate pain (e.g., restlessness, increased confusion, "picking" at bedcovers, and aggressive behaviors). The nurse offers pain medication after checking for hypotension and respiratory depression.

As the client's recovery progresses, the nurse administers pain medications in reduced doses and frequency. The medications are changed from injectable or PCA to oral as soon as the client can tolerate oral administration. Nonopioid analgesics, such as acetaminophen (Tylenol, Atasol*), and nonsteroidal anti-inflammatory drugs (NSAIDs), such as ibuprofen (Mortrin, Novoprofen*, Amersol*) and ketorolac (Toradol), are used during convalescence or can be given with an opioid analgesic as an adjunct. Antianxiety drugs, such as hydroxyzine (Vistaril, Novohydroxyzin*), may be given in combination with an opioid analgesic. This combination decreases pain-related anxiety and alleviates muscle tension that could contribute to the client's pain or discomfort, and controls nausea.

Other Methods of Pain Control The nurse provides comfort measures that may lower the amount of pain

CHART 21–4

Drug Therapy for Management of Postoperative Pain *Continued*

Drug	Usual Dosage	Nursing Interventions	Rationale
		• Monitor respiratory status.	cause of the aspirin component. • Respiratory depression and constipation can be caused by the oxycodone component.
Oxycodone hydrochloride and acetaminophen (Tylox, Percocet, Endocet♣, Oxycocet♣)	• 1–2 tablets q3–4h PO • Maximum 16 tablets	• Monitor blood pressure and respiratory status. • Assess for GI motility.	• Respiratory depression, hypotension, and constipation can occur.
Ketorolac tromethamine (Toradol)	• 15–60 mg IM or IV q6h • Maximum 120 mg	• Monitor for GI bleeding. • Monitor for renal effects, especially in the elderly.	• GI bleeding, ulceration, and perforation can occur. • Decreased urinary output, increased serum creatinine, hematuria, and proteinuria can occur. • Ketorolac is cleared more slowly in the elderly. • The elderly are more sensitive to the renal effects of NSAIDs.
Ibuprofen (Motrin, Amersol♣, Novoprofen♣)	• 300–600 mg q4–6h PO • Maximum 2400 mg daily	• Monitor upper GI tolerance of medication. • Give with food or milk • Monitor coagulation studies (PT, PTT). • Assess for signs of bleeding or delayed clotting.	• Food or milk helps decrease irritation of the stomach. • Bleeding times and other coagulation study results may be increased. • Monitoring leads to early detection of complications.

PT, prothrombin time; PTT, partial thromboplastin time; NSAID, nonsteroidal anti-inflammatory drug.

medication needed. These measures reduce anxiety and allow the client to relax and rest (Chart 21–6).

POSITIONING In positioning the client, the nurse considers the client's position during surgery, the location of the surgical incision and drains, and medical problems such as arthritis and chronic pulmonary disease. The nurse assists the client in achieving a position of comfort, while enabling the client to maintain optimal function. The client's extremities are supported with pillows. No pillows are placed under the client's knees, and the knee gatch of the bed is not raised because this position could restrict circulation and increase the risk of thrombophlebitis. The nurse turns the client or helps the client to turn at least every 2 hours while the client is bedridden to prevent stiffness and the pulmonary complications sometimes caused by immobility.

On the basis of the surgeon's orders and the nurse's assessment of the client's tolerance, the nurse encourages the client progressively to increase activity. Activity decreases stiffness, promotes lung expansion, and promotes venous circulation. When the client is initially allowed out of bed, the nurse assists him or her to the side of the bed and into a chair. The client splints the surgical wound for support and comfort during the transfer.

MASSAGE The nurse uses gentle massage of stiff joints or a sore back to decrease postoperative discomfort. The nurse positions the client in a side-lying position and applies lotion with smooth, gentle strokes to increase blood flow to the area and promote general relaxation. The legs, especially the calves, are *not* massaged because of the increased risk of loosening a thrombus and causing a pulmonary embolus, which can be life-threatening.

OTHER INTERVENTIONS Relaxation and diversion are also used to control acute episodes of pain. These

CHART 21–5

Drug Therapy for Management of Opioid Overdose

Drug	Usual Dosage*	Nursing Interventions*	Rationale
Levallorphan tartrate (Lorfan) Nalorphine (Nalline) Naloxone hydrochloride (Narcan)	• 0.01 mg/kg IV* • 0.1 mg/kg IV • 0.4–2 mg IV, SC, and IM • Repeat every 2– 3 minutes PRN up to 10 mg	• Maintain an open airway. • Have suction available. • Monitor vital signs closely until the client responds. • Do not leave the client unattended until fully responsive. • Observe for significant reversal of analgesia.	• A patent airway maximizes respiratory effort. • Suction prevents aspiration. • Monitoring leads to early detection of cardiovascular emergencies. • Staying with the client promotes safety. • Nausea, vomiting, and circulatory stress may be caused by too rapid a reversal.

* Repeat doses as necessary every 2–3 min on the basis of the client's response.

techniques are used effectively by the client during painful procedures such as dressing changes and injections. Chapters 7 and 8 discuss how the nurse instructs and guides the client through these pain control methods. Research Applications for Nursing discusses the use of music therapy. Chart 21–6 lists examples of other interventions that may help to reduce pain and promote comfort.

DISCHARGE PLANNING

Many clients are discharged after a brief hospital stay or directly from the postanesthesia care unit to home. Because of the shortened length of hospitalization, discharge planning, teaching, and referral begin preoperatively and continue postoperatively.

HOME CARE PREPARATION

If the client is discharged directly home, the nurse reviews data to help assess the home environment for safety, cleanliness, and the availability of caregivers. The nurse uses the data base that was completed when the client was admitted to the hospital or the ambulatory surgical unit to ascertain the client's needs. For example, if the client is unable or not allowed to climb stairs and lives in a two-story house with only one bathroom, the nurse advises the client to rent a bedside commode. The social worker or discharge planner, in collaboration with the nurse, helps the client identify needs related to postoperative care, including meal preparation, dressing changes, and personal hygiene. A referral to a home care nursing agency may be indicated.

HEALTH TEACHING

The teaching plan for the postoperative client and appropriate others includes:

- Prevention of infection
- Care and assessment of the surgical wound
- Diet therapy
- Drug therapy
- Progressive increase in activity

If dressing changes are needed, the client and family members are instructed on the importance of proper hand washing to prevent infection. The nurse thoroughly explains and demonstrates wound care to the client and the family. The client or a family member performs a return demonstration of that care. During

CHART 21–6

Nursing Care Highlight ◆ Examples of Nonpharmacologic Interventions to Reduce Postoperative Pain and Promote Comfort

- Control or remove noxious stimuli.
- Cushion and elevate painful areas; avoid tension or pressure on those areas.
- Provide adequate rest to increase pain tolerance.
- Encourage the client's participation in diversional activities.
- Instruct the client in relaxation techniques; use audiotapes and breathing exercises.
- Provide opportunities for meditation.
- Help the client to stimulate sensory nerve endings near the painful areas to inhibit ascending pain impulses.
- Use ice to reduce and prevent swelling, as indicated.
- Find a general position of comfort for the client.
- Help the client to stimulate the area contralateral (opposite) to the painful area.

RESEARCH APPLICATIONS FOR NURSING

Music in the Postanesthesia Care Unit May Help Relieve Postoperative Discomfort

Heitz, L., Symreng, T., & Scamman, F. L. (1992). Effect of music therapy in the postanesthesia care unit: A nursing intervention. *Journal of Postanesthesia Nursing, 7*(1), 22–31.

Heitz and colleagues examined the effects of postoperative music on pain level and analgesic requirements. The researchers studied these effects among 30 people undergoing thyroidectomy and parathyroidectomy and 30 women undergoing mastectomy. The researchers provided 20 clients with headphones that delivered music of their choice, 20 clients with headphones that did not deliver music but filtered out environmental noise, and 20 clients with no headphones at all. Although the pain levels and analgesic requirements among the three groups did not differ, clients who listened to music waited significantly longer (6½ hours, on average) than the control group (4½ hours) before requesting pain medication after transfer to the postoperative floor. Interestingly, clients who received headphones without music waited an average of only 3½ hours before requesting analgesics. Clients who listened to music postoperatively were also more likely than those in the other groups to characterize their experience as pleasant one day and one month after surgery. Among the clients who listened to music, 94% reported that music had been beneficial, 80% reported that they felt more relaxed, 60% reported that they had less anxiety, and 33% reported that they perceived less pain or discomfort. All of those who listened to music reported that they would choose to listen to music postoperatively if given the opportunity.

Critique In this well-designed study, music therapy appears to have provided adjunctive relief of postoperative pain. It would have been helpful if the study had addressed the finding that reducing the environmental noise level alone was not associated with a prolonged period of comfort.

Possible nursing implications In surgical populations such as those studied, music may help to relieve discomfort by providing a familiar experience in an unfamiliar setting.

the teaching sessions, the nurse evaluates learning and promotes compliance after discharge. At the same time, the nurse teaches the signs and symptoms of complications such as wound infection. The nurse also discusses with the client and family members appropriate measures to take if complications occur.

A diet that is high in protein, calories, and vitamin C promotes wound healing. A dietary consultation before the client is discharged helps him or her to select a balanced diet to promote healing. Supplemental vitamin C, iron, and multivitamins are often prescribed after surgery to aid in wound healing and the formation of red blood cells. Often, these supplements are prescribed for 10 to 14 days postoperatively. The nurse instructs clients with prior dietary restrictions about the importance of following the prescribed diet during convalescence. Elderly or debilitated clients are encouraged to continue using dietary supplements, if ordered, between meals until the wound is completely healed and their energy level is restored.

The nurse instructs clients about taking pain medication, with special attention to the proper dosage and frequency of administration. The nurse instructs the client to notify the surgeon if the medication does not control the pain or if the pain suddenly increases. If antibiotics or other medications are prescribed, the client is instructed to finish the entire prescription as ordered by the surgeon.

Surgery places physical and emotional stress on the body, and time and rest are required for healing. The nurse instructs the client to increase his or her activity level slowly, balance rest with activity (e.g., plan rest periods), and avoid straining the surgical wound or the surrounding area. Depending on the type of surgery and the client's occupation and usual activities, the surgeon decides when the client may climb stairs, return to work, drive, and resume other usual activities such as sexual intercourse. The amount of weight a client may safely lift after discharge from the facility needs to be specifically defined by the surgeon (i.e., in pounds or kilograms, as appropriate) and interpreted and reinforced as necessary by the nurse (grocery bags, laundry baskets, children, books, and so on).

The nurse also instructs the client in the use of proper body mechanics. A client whose work involves a moderate amount of physical labor may be allowed back to work 6 weeks after nonlaser abdominal surgery. The client may be eager to return to work or to other activities and may not follow activity restrictions. The nurse emphasizes the importance of compliance to prevent complications or disability. It is imperative that clients receive written discharge instructions for reinforcement at home. A visiting nurse may be necessary for follow-up.

PSYCHOSOCIAL PREPARATION

Clients are usually apprehensive about postoperative complications, pain, and changes in their usual activity level; thus, the nurse must allay their fears. The more extensive the surgical procedure is, the more fearful clients are of assuming self-care. The nurse supports the client and family members as they make discharge plans. The client whose surgical procedure has left visible scars may require more emotional support from his or her family for acceptance. (See Chapter 10 for further discussion of body image.) The client may express anger about the surgical outcome or temporary or permanent role changes and concern about financial matters and work. The surgical outcome may not have met the client's expectations, and further interventions may be necessary to assist the client in resolving his or her feelings. Referrals are made for additional counseling as indicated.

HEALTH CARE RESOURCES

After returning home, the client may need equipment and assistance with dressing changes, activities of daily living (ADL), and meal preparation. Referral to a home care agency is made and may be paid for by third-party insurance payers, including Medicare, if the client is homebound and requires skilled care. The home care nurse provides skilled nursing assessments, dressing supplies, education in self-care, and referrals for services as needed by the client. Such referrals include Meals on Wheels, support groups, and homemaker services (e.g., for housecleaning and food shopping).

EVALUATION

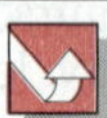

On the basis of the identified nursing diagnoses and desired outcomes, the nurse evaluates the care of the postoperative client. The outcomes include that the client:

- Maintains a patent airway
- Maintains adequate lung expansion and respiratory function as evidenced by clear breath sounds
- Has stable vital signs
- Returns to baseline arterial blood gas values
- Returns to preoperative mental state
- Has complete wound healing without complications
- States that postoperative pain is reduced or alleviated by interventions

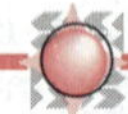

IMPLICATIONS FOR NURSING RESEARCH

In the postoperative period, the client is primarily faced with recovery and reintegration into roles and functions that may have been temporarily interrupted. This presents numerous opportunities for nursing research. Some questions that could be studied include:

- How effective are various nursing interventions in promoting postoperative respiratory function?
- Which nursing interventions affect the incidence of postoperative nausea and vomiting?
- What memories and feelings do clients have during emergence from anesthesia and in the immediate postoperative period?
- Which nursing interventions affect the client's sense of safety and security in the postoperative period?
- Do different types of dressings or local wound care affect the incidence of postoperative wound infections?
- What is the effect of surgery on the individual's role in the family?
- What factors determine whether clients comply with discharge instructions?
- How do clients perceive nurses and their nursing care during the postoperative period?

SELECTED BIBLIOGRAPHY

Acute pain management in adults: Operative procedures (AHCPR Pub. No. 92-0019). (1992). Rockville, MD: Agency for Health Care Policy and Research, U.S. Department of Health and Human Services.

Anderson, K., & Harris, A. (1992). Is there a statistically significant difference in two post-surgical rewarming methods: Convection versus radiation. *Journal of Post Anesthesia Nursing, 7*(3), 219.

Barnes, W. H., et al. (1991). The effect of routine vs. p.r.n. post-operative analgesia on pulmonary complications: A multicenter trial. *Canadian Journal of Nursing Research, 23*(4), 7–22.

Berels, D. J., et al. (1991). SaO2 monitoring in the postanesthesia care unit. *Journal of Post Anesthesia Nursing, 6*(6), 394–401.

Bowman, A. M. (1992). The relationship of anxiety to development of postoperative delirium. *Journal of Gerontological Nursing, 18*(1), 24–30.

Cahill-Wright, C. (1991). Managing postoperative pain. *Nursing91, 21*(12), 42–45.

Campbell, A., & Johnston, C. A. (1991). OR-PACU reports: What they should tell you about your postoperative patient. *Nursing91, 21*(10), 49–51.

Carroll, P. (1992). Using cuffs to prevent clots. *RN, 55*(4), 57–59.

Chana, C. H. (1992). Documenting the nursing process: A perioperative nursing care plan. *AORN Journal, 55*(5), 1231–1235.

Cormier, S., Pickett, S. J., & Gallagher, J. (1992). Comparison of nurses' and family members' perceived needs during postanesthesia care unit visits. *Journal of Post Anesthesia Nursing, 7*(6), 387–391.

Cushing, M. (1992). Back to (PACU) basics . . . the legal side. *American Journal of Nursing, 92*(7), 21–22.

Ehrlichman, R. J., Seckel, B. R., Bryan, D. J., & Moschella, C. J. (1991). Common complications of wound healing. *Surgical Clinics of North America, 71*(6), 1323–1351.

Ellis, L. M. (1991). Perioperative nutritional support. *Surgical Clinics of North America, 71*(3), 493–507.

Elmquist, L. (1992). Decision making for extubation of the post-anesthesic patient. *Critical Care Nursing Quarterly, 15*(1), 82–86.

Fuller, P. B. (1992). The relationship between preintubation lidocaine and postanesthesia sore throat. *AANA Journal, 60*(4), 374–378.

Giuffre, M., et al. (1991). Rewarming postoperative patients: Lights, blankets, or forced warmed air. *Journal of Post Anesthesia Nursing, 6*(6), 387–393.

Gliniecki, A. M. (1992). Postanesthesia shaking: A review. *Journal of Post Anesthesia Nursing, 7*(2), 89–93.

Graff, B. M., Thomas, J. S., Hollingsworth, A. O., et al. (1992). Development of a postoperative self-assessment form. *Clinical Nurse Specialist, 6*(1), 47–50.

Heffline, M. S. (1992). Managing PACU emergencies. *Journal of Post Anesthesia Nursing, 7*(3), 215.

Heitz, L., Symreng, T., & Scamman, F. L. (1992). Effect of music therapy in the postanesthesia care unit: A nursing intervention. *Journal of Post Anesthesia Nursing, 7*(1), 22–31.

Hershey-Hannan, J., Valenciano, C., Williams, D., et al. (1992). A comparison study of three interventions to warm patients and reduce the duration of hypothermia in the PACU. *Journal of Post Anesthesia Nursing 7*(3), 223–224.

Hinojosa, R. J. (1992). Nursing interventions to prevent or relieve postoperative nausea and vomiting. *Journal of Post Anesthesia Nursing, 7*(1), 3–14.

Hogenson, K. D. (1992). Acute postoperative hypertension in the hypertensive patient. *Journal of Post Anesthesia Nursing, 7*(1), 38–44.

Hutcheson, H. A. (1991). Epidural analgesia in the postoperative patient: A nursing perspective. *Plastic Surgical Nursing, 11*(1), 6–10, 27.

Hypoxemia on the general care floor. (1992). Newport Beach, CA: Communicore.

Jones, P. L., & Millman, A. (1990). Wound healing and the aged patient. *Nursing Clinics of North America, 25*(1), 263–277.

*Kearns, P. C. (1986). Exercises to ease pain after abdominal surgery. *RN, 49*(7), 45–48.

Lassen, K., Epstein-Stiles, M., & Olsson, G. L. (1992). Ketorolac: A new parenteral nonsteroidal anti-inflammatory drug for postoperative pain management. *Journal of Post Anesthesia Nursing, 7*(4), 238–242.

Lawler, M. (1991). Preventing postop complications: Managing other complications. *Nursing91, 21*(11), 33, 40–48.

Leske, J. S. (1992). Practice-based perioperative research: Meeting the challenges. *AORN Journal, 55*(2), 563–566.

Litwak, K. (1991). Managing postanesthesia emergencies. *Nursing91, 21*(9), 49–51.

Marshall, M. (1993). Postoperative confusion: Helping your patient emerge from the shadows. *Nursing93, 23*(1), 44–47.

Mataruski, M. R., Keis, N. A. Smouse, D. J. & Workman, M. L. (1990). Effects of steroids on postoperative nausea and vomiting. *Nurse Anesthesia, 1*(4), 183–188.

McConnell, E. A. (1990). Determining the cause of postoperative fever. *Nursing90, 20*(8), 82–83.

McConnell, E. A. (1991). Preventing postop complications: Minimizing respiratory problems. *Nursing91, 21*(11), 33–39.

McConnell, E. A. (1992). Assessing postoperative chills and tremors. *Nursing92, 22*(4), 110–114.

McConnell, E. A. (1992). Assessing wound drainage. *Nursing92, 22*(7), 66.

McConnell, E. A. (1992). Diagnosing postoperative fatigue. *Nursing92, 22*(3), 70–74.

Metzler, D. J., & Fromm, C. G. (1993). Laying out a care plan for the elderly postoperative patient. *Nursing93, 23*(4), 67–74.

Moore, F. A., Feliciano, D. V. Andrassy, R. J., et al. (1992). Early enteral feeding, compared with parenteral, reduces postoperative septic complications. *Annals of Surgery, 216*(2), 172–183.

Mullen, C. (1992). Hypoxemia during transfer to the PACU. *Journal of Post Anesthesia Nursing, 7*(3), 220.

Neal, J. M. (1992). Management of postdural puncture headache. *Anesthesiology Clinics of North America, 10*(1), 163–178.

Oetker-Black, S. L. (1992). Preoperative self-efficacy and postoperative behaviors. *Applied Nursing Research, 4*(4), 177–183.

Peden, L. (1992). Helping postop patients to sleep. *RN, 55*(4), 24–26.

Perioperative total parenteral nutrition in surgical patients. *New England Journal of Medicine, 325*(8), 525–532.

Ready, L. B. (1992). Intraspinal opioid analgesia in the perioperative period. *Anesthesiology Clinics of North America, 10*(1), 145–162.

Rowland, M. A. (1990). Myths—and facts—about postop discomfort. *American Journal of Nursing, 90*(5), 60–64.

Shade, P. (1992). Patient-controlled analgesia: Can client education improve outcomes? *Journal of Advanced Nursing, 17*(4), 408–413.

Study finds that gastric aspiration during surgery does not reduce—but actually increases—the incidence of postoperative nausea and vomiting. (1992). *Canadian Operating Room Nursing Journal, 10*(1), 36.

Summers, S. (1991). Axillary, tympanic, and esophageal temperature measurement: Descriptive comparisons in postanesthesia patients. *Journal of Post Anesthesia Nursing, 6*(6), 420–425.

*Treloar, D. M. (1984). When a surgical wound bursts. *RN, 47*(6), 20–30, 78.

Veterans Affairs Total Parenteral Nutrition Cooperative Study Group. (1991).

Vogelsang, J. (1992). Butorphanol tartrate (Stadol) relieves postanesthesia shaking more effectively than meperidine (Demerol) or morphine. *Journal of Post Anesthesia Nursing, 7*(2), 94–100.

Vogelsang, J. (1992). Research in the PACU. *Journal of Post Anesthesia Nursing, 7*(3), 218.

Vogelsang, J. (1992). The Bair Hugger System does not stop shaking. *Journal of Post Anesthesia Nursing, 7*(3), 222.

Walhout, M. F. (1992). Treat for hypothermia. *RN, 55*(4), 50–55.

Whitman, G. R. (1991). Hypertension and hypothermia in the acute postoperative period. *Critical Care Nursing Clinics of North America, 3*(4), 661–673.

Wild, L., & Coyne, C. (1992). The basics and beyond: Epidural analgesia. *American Journal of Nursing, 92*(4), 26–35.

Woodin, L. M. (1993). Cutting postop pain. *RN, 56*(8), 26–34.

SUGGESTED READINGS

Jones, P. L., & Millman, A. (1990). Wound healing and the aged patient. *Nursing Clinics of North America, 25*(1), 263–277.

This comprehensive article discusses normal changes in the integumetary system related to aging, followed by a discussion on chronologic age versus physiologic age. The causes of poor or delayed surgical wound healing are considered in detail, as are related nursing interventions.

Marshall, M. (1993). Postoperative confusion: Helping your patient emerge from the shadows. *Nursing93, 23*(1), 44–47.

Four main causes of postoperative confusion in the elderly client are discussed in this article: hypoxia, anesthetics and other medications, infection or sepsis, and fluid and electrolyte imbalances. A case example and nursing interventions are included for each of the four causes of confusion.

McConnell, E. A. (1991). Preventing postop complications: Minimizing respiratory problems. *Nursing91, 21*(11), 33–39.

After an introduction on risk factors, the author presents four main postoperative respiratory complications: hypoventilation, atelectasis, pneumonia, and aspiration. The pathophysiology and the signs and symptoms of each are discussed. Prophylactic nursing interventions are then considered in detail.

Walhout, M. F. (1992). Treat for hypothermia. *RN, 55*(4), 50–55.

Although not written specifically for the postoperative situation, this article presents an excellent, comprehensive discussion of hypothermia. Normal body temperature regulation is reviewed, including a description of core body temperature and methods of measuring core temperature. The signs and symptoms of mild, moderate, and severe hypothermia, including "cold diuresis," are discussed. Rewarming techniques, as well as other treatments, are also presented.

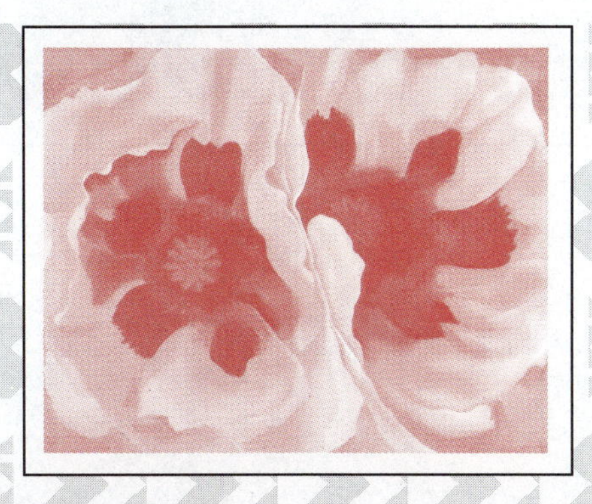

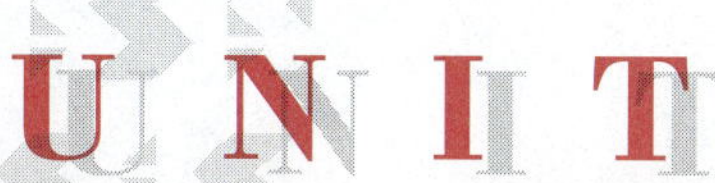

UNIT 5

Problems of Protection: Management of Clients with Problems of the Immune System

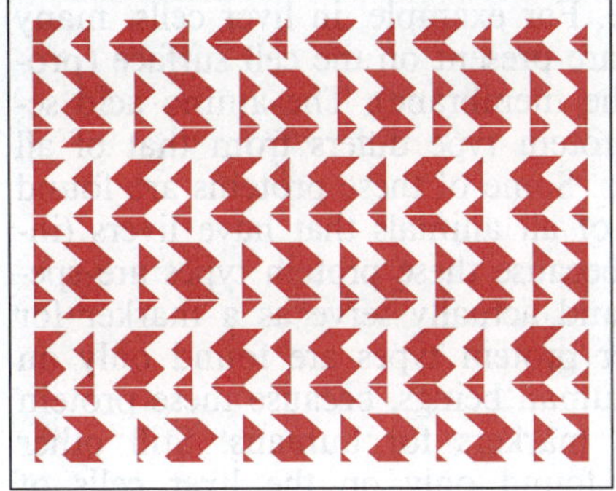

CHAPTER 22

Inflammation and the Immune Response

CHAPTER HIGHLIGHTS

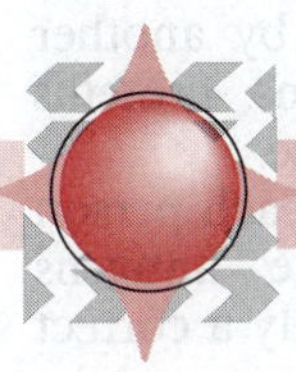

Inflammation and immunity have critical roles in preventing infectious diseases and in maintaining good health. Many diseases, injuries, and medical therapies alter immune function to some degree. These alterations in immune function may be temporary or permanent, but they always have an impact on the overall health and well-being of the client. Nurses need a strong working knowledge of immune function to provide a safe environment, adequate client support, and appropriate interventions for minimizing the risk of complications when altered immune function is present.

BASIC CONCEPTS OF INFLAMMATION AND IMMUNITY

Immunity is composed of functions that protect people against the effects accompanying injury or invasion of the body. People interact with many other living organisms in the environment. The size of these organisms varies from large (other humans and animals) to microscopic (bacteria, viruses, molds, spores, pollens, protozoa, and cells from other people or animals). People are in harmony with these organisms as long as the organisms do not enter the human body's internal environment. The human body has many defenses to prevent such organisms from gaining access to the internal environment. However, these defenses are not perfect, and invasion of the body's internal environment by microorganisms occurs often. Invasion occurs much more frequently than does an actual disease or illness because of the immune system's proper functioning.

Purpose

The ultimate purpose of the immune system is to neutralize, eliminate, or destroy microorganisms that invade the internal environment. To accomplish this purpose without harming the body, immune system cells use defensive actions only against *nonself* proteins and cells. Therefore, immune system cells can differentiate between the body's own, healthy *self* cells and other *nonself* proteins and cells.

Self Versus Nonself

Nonself proteins and cells include infected or debilitated body cells, self cells that have undergone malignant transformation into cancer cells, and all foreign cells and microorganisms (Workman et al., 1993). This ability to recognize self versus nonself, which is necessary so that healthy body cells are not destroyed along with the invaders, is called *self-tolerance.* The immune system cells are the only body cells capable of recognizing self and nonself.

All organisms are made up of cells. Each cell is surrounded by a plasma membrane (Fig. 22–1). In all cells, many different proteins protrude through the plasma membrane. For example, in liver cells, many different proteins are present on the cell surface (protruding through the membrane). The amino acid sequence of each protein type differs from that of all other protein types. Some of these proteins are found on the liver cells of all animals that have livers (including humans) because these protein types are specific to the liver and actually serve as a marker for liver tissues. Other protein types are found only on the liver cells of human beings, because these protein types are specific markers for humans. Still other protein types are found only on the liver cells of humans with a specific blood type. In addition, each human's liver cells have surface protein types that are specific to that human.

These proteins are unique to the person and would be identical only to the proteins of an identical twin. These unique proteins, found on the surface of all body cells of that individual, serve as a "universal product code" or a personal identification code for that person (Workman et al., 1993). The proteins that make up the universal product code for one person are recognized as "foreign" by the immune system of another person. Because the cell-surface proteins would be recognized as foreign by another person's immune system, they are antigens, proteins capable of stimulating an immune response.

This unique universal product code for each person is composed of the human leukocyte antigens (HLAs). "Leukocyte" antigen is not actually a correct term because these antigens are also present on the surfaces of all nucleated body cells, not just on leukocytes. HLAs are a normal part of the person and act as antigens only if they enter another person's body. These antigens specify the tissue type of an individual. Humans have about 40 major leukocyte

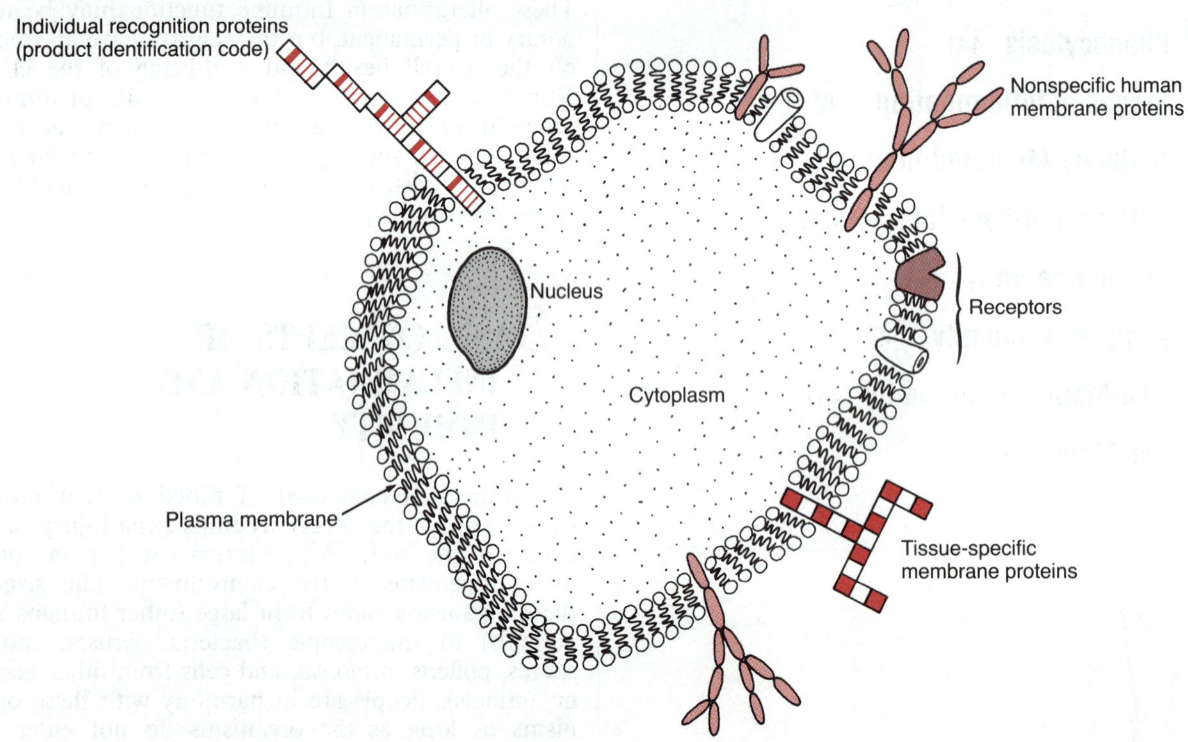

FIGURE 22–1 ◆ Properties of human cell membranes.

antigens (known as *histocompatibility antigens*) that are determined by a series of genes collectively called the major histocompatibility complex (MHC), but the exact number of minor human leukocyte antigens that any person has is not known. The specific antigens any person has (of a large number of possible antigens) are genetically determined by which MHC genes were inherited from his or her parents.

This universal product code (HLA) is a key feature for recognition and self-tolerance. The immune system cells constantly come into contact with other body cells and with any invader that happens to enter the body's internal environment. At each encounter, the immune system cells compare the surface protein universal product codes (HLAs) to determine whether the encountered cell belongs in the body's internal environment (Fig. 22-2). If the encountered cell's universal product code (HLA) perfectly matches the code of the immune system cell, the encountered cell is considered self and is not further molested by the immune system cell. If the encountered cell's universal product code (HLA) does not perfectly match the code of the immune system cell, the encountered cell is considered nonself or foreign. The immune system cell takes actions to neutralize, destroy, or eliminate the foreign invader.

Immune function changes during a person's life, according to:

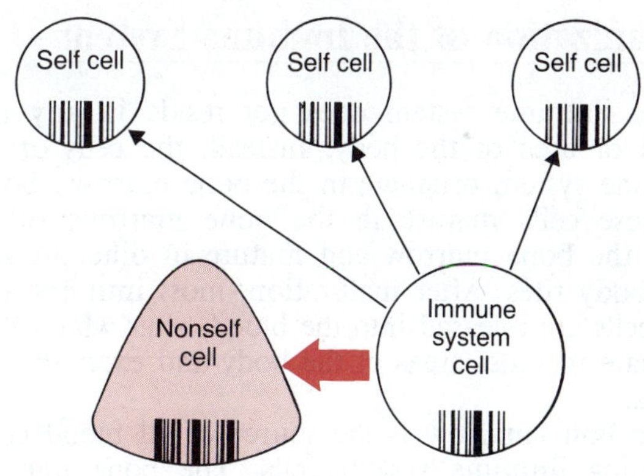

FIGURE 22-2 ◆ Determination of self versus nonself.

- Nutritional status
- Environmental conditions
- Medications
- Presence of disease
- Age

Immune function is generally most efficient when people are in their 20s and 30s; it slowly declines with increasing age. The elderly have marginal immune function causing increased susceptibility to a variety of pathologic conditions (Chart 22-1).

CHART 22-1

Nursing Focus on the Elderly ◆ Changes in Immune Function Related to Aging

Immune Component	Functional Change	Nursing Implications
Inflammation	• Probable defect in neutrophil function	• Neutrophil counts may be normal, but activity is reduced or impaired.
	• Leukocytosis does not occur during episodes of acute infection	• Clients may have an infection but not show standard changes in white blood cell counts.
	• Elderly persons may not have a fever during inflammatory or infectious episodes	• Not only is there potential loss of protection through inflammation, but minor infections may be overlooked until the client becomes severely infected or septic.
Antibody-mediated immunity	• The total number of colony-forming B lymphocytes and the ability of these cells to mature into antibody-secreting cells are diminished.	• The elderly are less able to make new antibodies in response to the presence of new antigens. Thus, the elderly should receive immunizations, such as "flu shots" and the pneumococcal vaccination.
	• There is a decline in natural antibodies, decreased response to antigens, and reduction in the amount of time the antibody response is maintained	• Elderly people may not have sufficient antibodies present to provide protection when they are re-exposed to microorganisms against which they have already generated antibodies. Thus, elderly clients need to avoid people with viral infections and receive "booster" shots for old vaccinations and immunizations.
Cell-mediated immunity	• Thymic activity decreases with aging, and the number of circulating T lymphocytes decreases	• Skin tests for tuberculosis may be falsely negative. • Elderly clients are more at risk for bacterial and fungal infections, especially on the skin and mucous membranes, in the respiratory tract, and in the genitourinary tract.

Organization of the Immune System

The immune system does not reside in any one organ or area of the body. Instead, the cells of the immune system originate in the bone marrow. Some of these cells mature in the bone marrow; others leave the bone marrow and mature in different specific body sites. After maturation, most immune system cells are released into the blood, after which they circulate to most areas of the body and exert specific effects.

The bone marrow is the source of all blood cells, including immune system cells. The bone marrow produces an immature, undifferentiated cell called a stem cell (Abbas et al., 1991). This immature stem cell is also described as pluripotent, multipotent, totipotent, and even omnipotent. These adjectives describe the potential future of the stem cell. When the stem cell is first created in the bone marrow, it is undifferentiated. The cell is not yet committed to differentiating into a specific blood cell type. At this stage, the stem cell is flexible and has the potential to become any one of a variety of mature blood cells. Figure 22-3 presents a scheme showing the major possible maturational outcomes for the pluripotent stem cell. The specific cell type of mature blood cell the stem cell becomes depends on which maturational pathway it follows.

The maturational pathway of any stem cell depends, to some extent, on body needs at the time and also on the presence of specific hormones (termed cytokines, factors, or poietins) that stimulate specific commitment and induce maturation. For example, erythropoietin is made in the kidney. When immature stem cells are exposed to erythropoietin, the immature stem cells commit to the erythrocyte maturational pathway and eventually become mature red blood cells.

White blood cells (leukocytes) are cells that protect the body from the effects of invasion by foreign microorganisms. These cells are the immune system cells. Table 22-1 summarizes the functions of different immune system cells. The leukocytes can provide protection through a variety of defensive actions (Abbas et al., 1991). These actions include:

- Recognition of self versus nonself
- Phagocytic destruction of foreign invaders, cellular debris, and unhealthy or abnormal self cells
- Lytic destruction of foreign invaders and unhealthy self cells
- Production of antibodies directed against foreign invaders
- Activation of complement
- Production of hormones that stimulate increased formation of leukocytes in bone marrow
- Production of hormones that increase specific leukocyte growth and activity

The three processes necessary for immunity and the cells involved in these responses can be categorized as

- Inflammation
- Antibody-mediated immunity (humoral immunity)
- Cell-mediated immunity

These three processes represent diverse defense actions (Fig. 22-4). Full immunity, or immunocompetence, requires the adequate function and interaction of all three processes, even though some functions of each overlap functions of the others.

TABLE 22-1 Immune Functions of Specific Leukocytes

	Leukocyte	Function
Inflammation	Neutrophil	• Nonspecific ingestion and phagocytosis of microorganisms and foreign protein
	Macrophage	• Nonspecific recognition of foreign proteins and microorganisms; ingestion and phagocytosis
	Monocyte	• Destruction of bacteria and cellular debris; matures into macrophage
	Eosinophil	• Weak phagocytic action; releases vasoactive amines during allergic reactions
	Basophil	• Releases histamine and heparin in areas of tissue damage
Antibody-Mediated Immunity	B lymphocyte	• Becomes sensitized to foreign cells and proteins
	Plasma cell	• Secretes immunoglobulins in response to the presence of a specific antigen
	Memory cell	• Remains sensitized to a specific antigen and can secrete increased amounts of immunoglobulins specific to the antigen
Cell-Mediated Immunity	T lymphocyte helper/inducer T cell	• Enhances immune activity through secretion of various factors, cytokines, and lymphokines
	Cytotoxic/cytolytic T cell	• Selectively attacks and destroys nonself cells, including virally infected cells, grafts, and transplanted organs
	Natural killer cell	• Nonselectively attacks nonself cells, especially body cells that have undergone mutation and become malignant; also attacks grafts and transplanted organs

INFLAMMATION

Inflammation provides immediate protection against the effects of tissue injury and invading foreign pro-

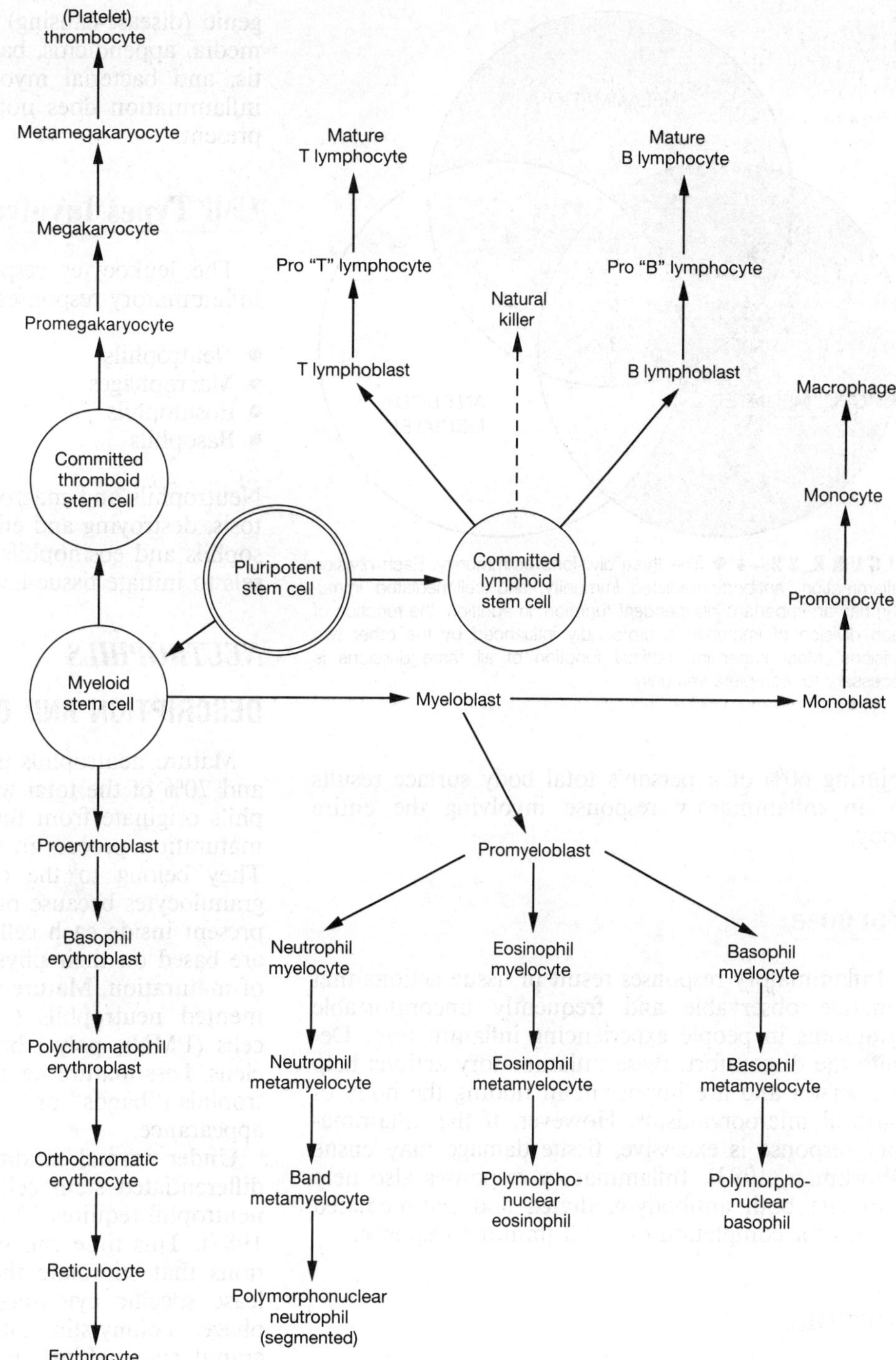

FIGURE 22-3 ◆ Stem cell differentiation and maturation. (From Workman, M. L., Ellerhorst-Ryan, J., & Koertge, V. [1993]. *Nursing care of the immunocompromised patient* [p. 9]. Philadelphia: W. B. Saunders.)

teins. The capacity of a person to generate an inflammatory response is a critical component of overall health and well-being. Inflammation differs from antibody-mediated immunity and cell-mediated immunity in two important ways:

1. Inflammatory responses provide immediate but short-term protection against the effects of injury or foreign invaders rather than sustained, long-term immunity on repeated exposure to the same foreign invaders.
2. Inflammation is a nonspecific body defense to invasion or injury.

Inflammation is nonspecific because the same tissue responses occur with any type of injury or invasion, regardless of the location on the body or the specific initiating agent. Therefore, the inflammatory processes stimulated by a scald burn to the hand are the same as the inflammatory processes stimulated by either excessive acid in the stomach or the presence of bacteria in the middle ear. How widespread the symptoms of inflammation are in the body depends on the intensity, severity, duration, and extent of exposure to the initiating injury or invasion. For example, a splinter in the finger triggers an inflammatory response only at the splinter site, whereas a burn

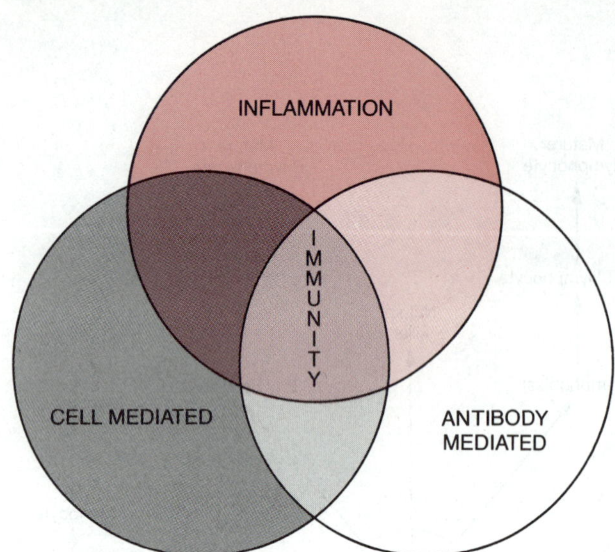

FIGURE 22-4 ◆ The three divisions of immunity. Each division (inflammation, antibody-mediated immunity, and cell-mediated immunity) has an important independent function. In addition, the function of each division of immunity is profoundly influenced by the other two divisions. Most important, optimal function of all three divisions is necessary for complete immunity.

injuring 60% of a person's total body surface results in an inflammatory response involving the entire body.

Purpose

Inflammatory responses result in tissue actions that generate observable and frequently uncomfortable symptoms in people experiencing inflammation. Despite the discomfort, these inflammatory actions help the person and are important in ridding the body of harmful microorganisms. However, if the inflammatory response is excessive, tissue damage may ensue (Workman, 1993). Inflammatory responses also help stimulate both antibody-mediated and cell-mediated actions for completion of a full immune response.

Infection

A confusing issue about inflammation is that this process occurs in response to tissue injury as well as to invasion by microorganisms or other foreign proteins. Infection is usually accompanied by inflammation; however, inflammation can occur without the presence of foreign proteins or microorganisms. For example, inflammatory responses not associated with infection occur with sprain injuries to joints, myocardial infarction, sterile surgical incisions, thrombophlebitis, and blister formation caused by temperature extremes. Examples of inflammatory responses associated with noninfectious invasion by foreign proteins include allergic rhinitis, contact dermatitis, and other immediate-type allergic reactions. Inflammatory responses associated with invasion by pathogenic (disease-causing) microorganisms include otitis media, appendicitis, bacterial peritonitis, viral hepatitis, and bacterial myocarditis, among others. Thus, inflammation does not always mean an infection is present.

Cell Types Involved in Inflammation

The leukocytes responsible for the generation of inflammatory responses are:

- Neutrophils
- Macrophages
- Eosinophils
- Basophils

Neutrophils and macrophages participate in phagocytosis, destroying and eliminating foreign invaders. Basophils and eosinophils act on cells within blood vessels to initiate tissue-level inflammatory responses.

NEUTROPHILS

DESCRIPTION AND ORIGIN

Mature neutrophils usually constitute between 55% and 70% of the total white blood cell count. Neutrophils originate from the stem cells and complete the maturation process in the bone marrow (Fig. 22-5). They belong to the class of leukocytes known as granulocytes because of the large number of granules present inside each cell. Other names for neutrophils are based on their physical characteristics and degree of maturation. Mature neutrophils are also called segmented neutrophils ("segs") or polymorphonuclear cells (PMNs, polys) because of their segmented nucleus. Less mature neutrophils are called banded neutrophils ("bands" or "stabs") because of their nuclear appearance.

Under normal conditions, maturation from the undifferentiated stem cell to the functional segmented neutrophil requires 12 to 14 days (Werb & Goldstein, 1987). This time can be shortened by certain conditions that stimulate the body to synthesize and release specific cytokines such as granulocyte-macrophage colony-stimulating factor (GM-CSF) and granulocyte colony-stimulating factor (G-CSF). The purpose and action of cytokines are described later in this chapter under the heading Cytokines.

In the immunocompetent, healthy person, more than 100 billion fresh, mature neutrophils are released from the bone marrow into the systemic circulation daily (Abbas et al., 1991). This massive generation of neutrophils is necessary because the life span of a circulating neutrophil is extremely short, averaging only about 12 to 18 hours.

FUNCTION

Although the neutrophils, as a group, compose the largest number of circulating leukocytes, the individual cell is small. This army of powerful small cells

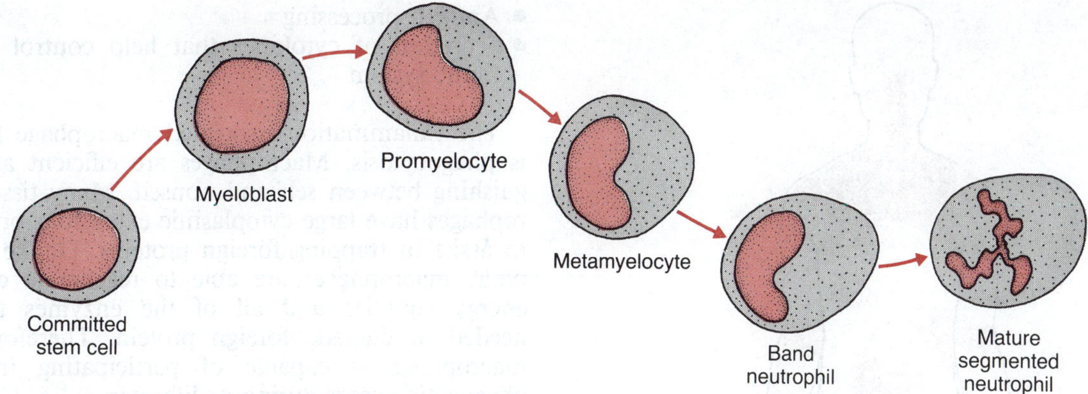

FIGURE 22–5 ♦ Neutrophil maturation.

provides the first internal line of defense, via phagocytosis, against foreign invaders (especially bacteria) in blood and extracellular fluid. It is the granules inside the neutrophils that complete the phagocytic destruction of foreign invaders. The mature neutrophil is filled with large numbers of granules containing a variety of enzymes that can degrade different parts of foreign invaders.

Neutrophils have a small energy supply and no internal way of replenishing either the energy supply or the enzymes used in degradation. For this reason, each neutrophil is capable of only one episode of phagocytic destruction before its supplies are exhausted and its death ensues.

The mature, segmented neutrophil is the only neutrophil stage that is capable of effective phagocytosis. Because this cell is responsible for providing continuous, instant, nonspecific protection against invasion by microorganisms, the percentage and actual number of circulating white blood cells that are mature neutrophils reliably measure a client's susceptibility to infection: The higher the numbers, the greater the resistance to infection. This measurement is the absolute neutrophil count (sometimes called the absolute granulocyte count [AGC] or total granulocyte count).

The differential of a normal white blood cell count indicates that most of the neutrophils released into the blood from the bone marrow are segmented neutrophils, with only a small percentage being banded neutrophils (Fig. 22–6). The less mature neutrophil

differential	%	/mm³
Total WBC	100	10,000
segs	62	6,200
bands	5	500
monos	3	300
lymphs	28	2,800
eosin	1.5	150
baso	0.5	50

FIGURE 22–6 ♦ Example of a laboratory slip showing the differential of a normal white blood cell count.

forms should not be present in the blood. Some infectious conditions cause the major population of neutrophils in the blood to change from mostly segmented neutrophils to less mature forms. This situation is termed a *left shift* because the segmented neutrophil, which is seen at the far right of the neutrophil maturational pathway (see Fig. 22–5), no longer represents the greatest number of circulating neutrophils. Instead, the major population is made up of one of the cell types found farther left on the neutrophil maturational pathway.

This situation is an ominous clinical sign. It indicates that the client's bone marrow cannot produce enough mature neutrophils to keep pace with the continuing presence of microorganisms and releases immature neutrophils into the blood. Unfortunately, most of these immature neutrophils are of no benefit to the client because they are not functional phagocytic cells and cannot continue to mature in the blood.

MACROPHAGES

DESCRIPTION AND ORIGIN

Macrophages originate from the committed myeloid stem cell in the bone marrow and form the mononuclear phagocyte system. This cell first begins to differentiate into a monocyte and is released into the blood at this stage. Until they mature, monocytes have only limited immune activity. Most monocytes migrate into various tissues, where they complete the maturation process into macrophages. Some macrophages become "fixed" in position within the tissues, and others remain mobile in the tissue's interstitial fluid. Macrophages in various tissues have slightly different appearances and different names. Table 22–2 summarizes the names of the different tissue macrophages. Figure 22–7 shows the distribution of tissue macrophages throughout the body. The liver and spleen contain the greatest concentration of these cells.

Tissue macrophages have relatively long life spans lasting from months to years. Macrophages are the largest of all the leukocytes and have granules containing a wide variety of degradative enzymes.

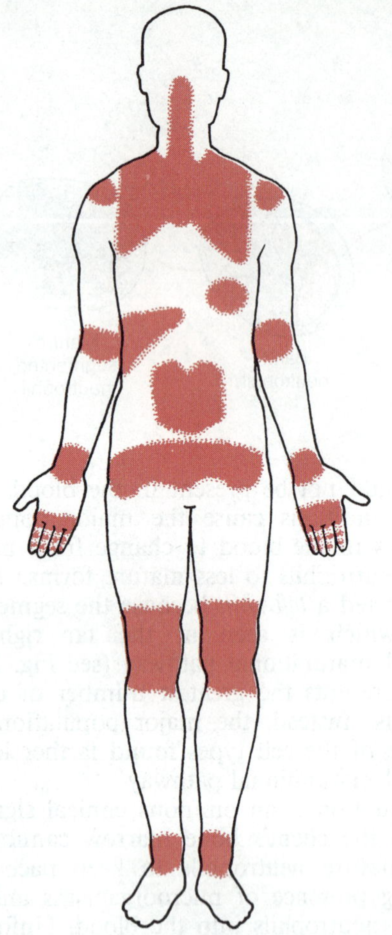

FIGURE 22–7 ◆ The areas of highest concentration of tissue macrophages.

FUNCTION

Macrophage activity is complex. These cells have more than one role in providing protection against invasion and tissue injury. Macrophages are critically important in immediate inflammatory responses and can also participate in the stimulation of the longer lasting immune responses associated with antibody- and cell-mediated immunity (Werb & Goldstein, 1987). Specific macrophage functions include:

- Phagocytosis
- Repair of injured tissues
- Antigen processing
- Secretion of cytokines that help control the immune system

TABLE 22–2 Tissue Macrophages

Tissue	Macrophage
Lung	• Alveolar macrophage
Connective tissue	• Histiocyte
Brain	• Microglial cell
Liver	• Kupffer cell
Peritoneum	• Peritoneal macrophage
Bone	• Osteoclast
Joints	• Synovial type A cell
Kidney	• Mesangial cell

The inflammation-associated macrophage function is phagocytosis. Macrophages are efficient at distinguishing between self and nonself. Many tissue macrophages have large cytoplasmic extensions or "arms" to assist in trapping foreign proteins. Unlike neutrophils, macrophages are able to regenerate chemical energy supplies and all of the enzymes that are needed to degrade foreign protein. Therefore, each macrophage is capable of participating in many phagocytic events during its life span.

BASOPHILS

DESCRIPTION AND ORIGIN

Of all the leukocytes, basophils are the smallest and the rarest. They are derived from myeloid stem cells and are released from the bone marrow after a short maturation period. Even though they are rare, basophils are associated with the obvious signs and symptoms that often accompany inflammation. Basophils contain enormous numbers of cytoplasmic granules.

FUNCTION

Basophilic granules contain heparin and various chemicals (vasoactive amines) that act on blood vessels, including histamine, serotonin, kinins, and leukotrienes. Most of these vasoactive amines, when released into the blood, act on smooth muscle and blood vessel walls. Heparin inhibits coagulation of blood and other protein-containing extracellular fluids. Histamine constricts the smooth muscles of the respiratory system and small veins. Constriction of respiratory smooth muscle narrows the lumen of airways and restricts breathing. Construction of venular smooth muscle inhibits blood flow through small veins and decreases venous return. This effect causes blood to collect in capillaries and small arterioles. Kinins cause slow vasodilation of arterioles. Together, kinins and serotonin increase capillary permeability, which permits the plasma portion of the blood to leak into the interstitial space. This chemical-induced process is called vascular leak syndrome (VLS).

EOSINOPHILS

DESCRIPTION AND ORIGIN

Eosinophils originate from the myeloid line and are similar to neutrophils in their abilities. Usually only 1% to 2% of the total white blood cell count is made up of eosinophils.

FUNCTION

Eosinophils are not efficient phagocytes, although they can act against infestations of parasitic larvae.

Cytoplasmic granules of eosinophils contain many substances with vastly different actions. Some of these substances are vasoactive amines, which produce inflammatory and often severe tissue-damaging reactions when released. This action may be the cause of some of the uncomfortable and damaging effects associated with exposure to allergens in sensitive people. Certain enzymes from eosinophils degrade vasoactive amines and in this way may control or modulate the extent of inflammatory reactions.

Phagocytosis

The key mechanism for the successful outcome of inflammation is phagocytosis—the destruction of nonself cells. Phagocytosis is the process by which leukocytes engulf foreign proteins and destroy them by enzymatic degradation. Phagocytosis rids the body of debris after tissue injury and destroys foreign invaders. Of all the leukocytes, neutrophils and macrophages perform phagocytosis the most efficiently. Phagocytosis occurs in a predictable manner and involves seven steps (Fig. 22-8):

1. Exposure and invasion
2. Attraction
3. Adherence
4. Recognition
5. Cellular ingestion
6. Phagosome formation
7. Degradation

EXPOSURE AND INVASION

Leukocytes that engage in phagocytosis and stimulate inflammation are present in the blood and most other extracellular fluids. For phagocytosis to be initiated, these leukocytes must first be exposed to debris from damaged tissues or foreign proteins (antigens). Therefore, the initiating event for phagocytosis is injury or invasion.

ATTRACTION

Phagocytosis is effective only when the phagocytic cell comes into direct contact with the target or victim cell (antigen or foreign protein). Because tissue injury or invasion by foreign proteins can occur at sites remote from either neutrophils or macrophages, mechanisms to unite phagocytic cells with their intended targets are necessary.

Special chemical substances can act as chemical magnets that attract a variety of leukocytes, including neutrophils and macrophages. These substances are called chemotaxins or leukotaxins. Damaged tissues secrete chemotaxins. Substances present in plasma and other extracellular fluids as a result of blood vessel injury also attract neutrophils and macrophages. These substances include fibrin, collagen, and plasminogen activator. Bacterial endotoxins are often powerful chemotaxins. In addition, substances that combine with surface components of invading foreign proteins serve as chemotaxins. This combining (and attracting) mechanism is detailed under the heading Adherence.

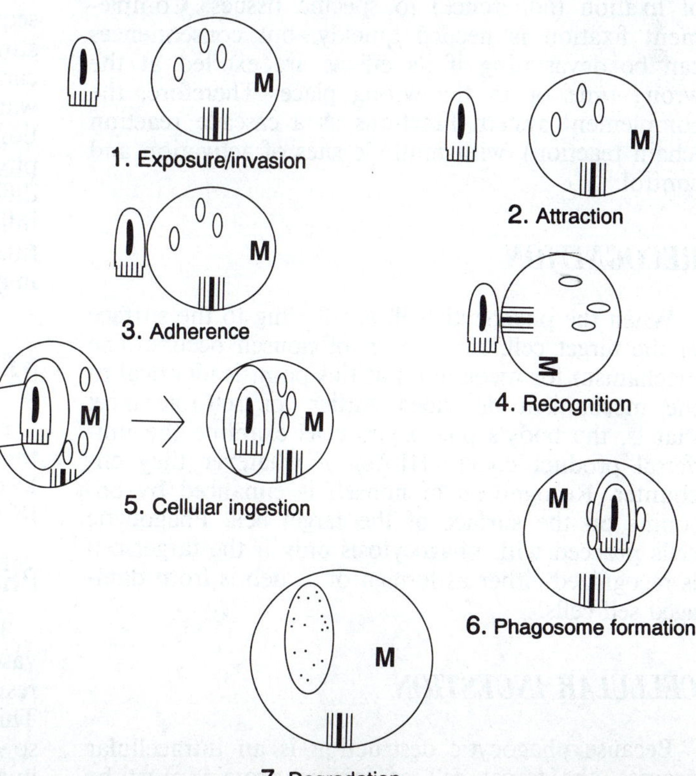

FIGURE 22-8 ◆ The steps of phagocytosis. (Modified from Workman, M. L., Ellerhorst-Ryan, J., & Koertge, V. [1993]. *Nursing care of the immunocompromised patient* [p. 23]. Philadelphia: W. B. Saunders.)

ADHERENCE

Because phagocytosis requires direct contact of the phagocyte with its intended target, the phagocytic cell must first bind to the surface of the target. A special process called *opsonization* helps to ensure the direct contact of the phagocyte with its target.

OPSONIZATION

The word *opsonin* is derived from the Greek and literally means "to cover food with a sauce in preparation for eating." In biologic processes, opsonins coat a target cell (antigen or foreign protein); this changes the target cell's surface charge and makes it easier for phagocytic cells to stick to it. Several substances can act as opsonins. Some of these substances are residual particles from dead neutrophils, antibodies, and activated (fixated) complement components.

COMPLEMENT ACTIVATION AND FIXATION

One mechanism of opsonization and enhancement of phagocytic adherence to target cells is complement activation and fixation. About 20 different inactive protein components of the complement system are present in the blood. The major complement proteins are labeled C1 through C9. Some of these major proteins have subsets (e.g., the C1 protein complex can be separated into C1q, C1r, and C1s), so that the number of known complement components is approximately 20 (Abbas et al., 1991). These components are made by the liver. With proper stimulation, individual complement proteins become activated and act together to cause dramatic actions as a result of fixation (adherence) to specific tissues. Complement fixation is needed quickly, but consequences can be devastating if its effects are exerted at the wrong time or in the wrong place. Therefore, the complement system functions as a cascade reaction (chain reaction), with multiple sites of activation and control.

RECOGNITION

When the phagocytic cell is adhering to the surface of the target cell, recognition of nonself occurs. The mechanism for recognition at this point is identical to the mechanism described earlier for self-tolerance; that is, the body's phagocytic cells examine the universal product codes (HLAs) of whatever they encounter. Recognition of nonself is enhanced by opsonins on the surface of the target cell. Phagocytic cells proceed with phagocytosis only if the target cell is recognized either as foreign or as debris from damaged self cells.

CELLULAR INGESTION

Because phagocytic destruction is an intracellular process, the target cell or foreign protein must be brought inside the phagocytic cell through absorptive endocytosis. The phagocytic cell changes its shape and bends its membrane (invaginates) around to enclose the target cell. Once the target is surrounded, the touching edges of the phagocytic cell's membrane fuse. The target is sealed within a vesicle inside the phagocytic cell; thus, a vacuole is formed.

PHAGOSOME FORMATION

If some of the phagocyte's granules are inside the vacuole, the structure is called a phagosome (or phagolysosome). When these granules break open and release enzymes into the fluid of the phagosome, destruction of the ingested target begins. Assistance from enzyme-containing lysosomes enhances this intracellular destruction.

DEGRADATION

The granular and lysosomal enzymes within the phagolysosome exert their specific effects on different parts of the ingested target. The target is broken down into progressively smaller pieces until only minute particles are left to be removed from the body as debris.

Sequence of Inflammatory Responses

Inflammatory responses for protecting the body against the effects of tissue injury or invasion by foreign proteins occur in a predictable sequence. The sequence is the same regardless of the initiating stimulus. Responses at the tissue level elicit the five cardinal physical manifestations of inflammation: warmth, redness, swelling, pain, and decreased function. Tissue and cellular events that cause these physical manifestations are described as part of the different stages of inflammation (Table 22–3). The inflammatory response can occur in three distinct functional stages, although the timing of the stages may overlap.

STAGE I (VASCULAR)

In stage I of the inflammatory response, most of the early effects involve changes at the blood vessel level. When inflammation is an effect of tissue injury, this stage has two phases.

PHASE I

The first phase is an immediate but short-term vasoconstriction of arterioles and venules as a direct result of physical trauma to vascular smooth muscle. This phase lasts only seconds to minutes and may be so short that the person undergoing the response is unaware of the vasoconstriction.

TABLE 22–3 Stages of Inflammation

Stage	Onset	Cells Involved	Actions
Stage I: Vascular stage	• Minutes after injury or invasion	• Tissue macrophages	• Limited phagocytosis of invading microorganisms or cell debris from injured tissues • Secretion of vasoactive amines (histamine, bradykinin, serotonin) to dilate blood vessels and increase capillary leak; this action results in redness, warmth, swelling, and pain at the site but also increases blood flow to the area; more nutrients are available to the tissues; plasma proteins moved into the tissues clot and "wall off" microorganisms, limiting their spread • Secretion of chemotaxins to draw more leukocytes into the area to sustain the inflammatory response • Secretion of cytokines to increase bone marrow production of granulocytes
Stage II: Cellular exudate stage	• Hours after injury or invasion	• Granular myeloid cells • Neutrophils • Basophils • Eosinophils	• Increased phagocytosis • Secretion of slow-acting vasoactive amines to ensure a sustained inflammatory response • Secretion of substances to increase the rate of neutrophil maturation and macrophage maturation
Stage III: Tissue repair and replacement stage	• Begins at initial injury and continues until new tissues are formed and mature or are functional	• Neutrophils • Macrophages	• Stimulation of mitotically active cells to divide; stimulation of fibroblasts in blood vessels to grow and release collagen to form scaffold on which to build scar tissue

PHASE II

The second phase is characterized by increased blood flow to the area (hyperemia) and swelling (edema formation) at the site of injury or invasion. Injured tissues and the leukocytes in this area secrete vasoactive amines (histamine, serotonin, and kinins) that cause constriction of the small veins and dilation of the arterioles in the immediate area. The effects of these changes in blood vessel dilation cause the symptoms of redness and increased warmth of the tissues. This response increases the supply of nutrients at the tissue level by increasing the blood flow.

Some of these vasoactive amines increase capillary permeability, allowing blood plasma to leak into the interstitial space. This response causes the symptoms of swelling and pain. Pain, although an uncomfortable sensation, is somewhat beneficial to the person experiencing inflammation. Pain increases the person's awareness that a problem exists and encourages action to avoid further injury or inflammation. Edema formation at the site of injury or invasion is an overall helpful event. This swelling protects the area from further injury by creating a cushion of fluid. The extra fluid can also dilute the concentration of any toxins or microorganisms that entered the area. The duration of these responses depends on the severity of the initiating event.

The major leukocyte involved in stage I of inflammation is the tissue macrophage. The response of tissue macrophages is immediate because they are already in place at the site of injury or invasion. However, this response is limited because the number of such macrophages is so small. In addition to functioning in phagocytosis, the tissue macrophages secrete several cytokines to enhance the inflammatory response. One cytokine is colony-stimulating factor, which stimulates the bone marrow to reduce the time of leukocyte production from 14 days to a matter of hours. In addition, tissue macrophages secrete substances that increase the release of neutrophils from the bone marrow and attract them to the site of injury or invasion, which leads to the next stage of inflammation.

STAGE II (CELLULAR EXUDATE)

Stage II of inflammation is characterized by neutrophilia (an increase in the percentage and number of circulating neutrophils), secretion of many factors into the interstitial fluid, and formation of exudate.

The most active leukocyte in this stage is the neutrophil. Under the influence of chemotactic agents and substances that increase the number and rate of maturation of neutrophils, the neutrophil count can increase up to five times within 12 hours after the onset of inflammation. At the site of inflammation, the neutrophils attack and destroy foreign materials and remove dead tissue. Both of these functions are accomplished through phagocytosis.

During acute inflammatory responses, the healthy person can synthesize enough mature neutrophils to keep pace with the effects of injury and invasion and to eventually overcome the ability of invaders to multiply. At the same time, the leukocytes secrete *cytokines,* which increase reproduction of tissue macrophages and bone marrow production of monocytes.

Although this reaction is slower to start, its effects are long lasting.

When infectious processes stimulating inflammation are longer or chronic, the bone marrow cannot synthesize and release enough mature neutrophils into the blood to keep pace with the ability of microorganisms to multiply. In this situation, the bone marrow begins to release immature neutrophils, many of which cannot complete maturation and phagocytose. Such a reduction in the number of functional phagocytic neutrophils limits the effectiveness of the inflammatory response and increases the susceptibility of the person to microbial infections.

STAGE III (TISSUE REPAIR AND REPLACEMENT)

Although stage III is completed last, it begins at the time of injury and is critical to the ultimate function of the inflamed area.

Some of the leukocytes involved in inflammation are capable of stimulating replacement and repair of lost or damaged tissues by inducing the remaining healthy tissue to divide. In tissues that are not mitotically active (nondividing tissues), leukocytes stimulate revascularization and the laying down of different types of collagen to form scar tissue. Because scar tissue does not behave like normal differentiated tissue, functional loss occurs where damaged tissues are replaced with scar tissue. The extent of the functional loss is determined by the percentage of tissue that is replaced by scar tissue.

Inflammation alone cannot confer immunity; however, the interaction of specific components of inflammation with other leukocytes and tissues assists in providing long-lasting immunity against re-exposure to the same microorganisms. Long-lasting immune actions are those generated by antibody-mediated immunity and cell-mediated immunity.

ANTIBODY-MEDIATED IMMUNITY

Antibody-mediated immunity (AMI), also known as humoral immunity, involves antigen-antibody actions to neutralize, eliminate, or destroy foreign proteins. Antibodies for these actions are produced by populations of B lymphocytes.

Purpose

The primary functions of B lymphocytes are to become sensitized to a specific foreign protein (antigen) and to synthesize an antibody directed specifically against that protein. The antibody (rather than the actual B lymphocyte) then participates in one of several actions to neutralize, eliminate, or destroy that antigen.

Cell Types Involved in Antibody-Mediated Immunity

The leukocytes that play the most direct role in antibody-mediated immunity are the B lymphocytes. Because they are not efficient at recognition of self versus nonself, B lymphocytes must cooperate with macrophages to initiate and complete antigen antibody actions. In addition, special T lymphocytes, helper/inducer T cells (discussed later under Cell Mediated Immunity), secrete products that regulate the activity of B lymphocytes and assist with recognition of nonself. Therefore, for optimal antibody-mediated immunity, the entire immune system must function adequately.

B lymphocytes start life as pluripotent stem cells in the bone marrow, the primary lymphoid tissue. The pluripotent stem cells destined to become B lymphocytes commit early to the lymphocyte maturational pathway (see Fig. 22–3), possibly under the influence of a specific poietin for lymphocyte development. At the point of commitment, these stem cells are no longer pluripotent but are limited to differentiation into lymphocytes. The committed lymphocyte stem cells are released from the bone marrow into the blood; they then migrate into various secondary lymphoid tissues, where maturation is completed.

In humans, the secondary lymphoid tissues for B-lymphocyte maturation are the spleen, germinal centers of lymph nodes, tonsils, and Peyer's patches of the intestinal tract. Once maturation is complete, the B lymphocytes are released into the general circulation.

Antigen-Antibody Interactions

The body learns to make enough of any specific antibody to provide long-lasting immunity against specific microorganisms or toxins. Seven steps in a series of special interactions are required for the production of a unique and specific antibody that is directed against a unique and specific antigen whenever the person is exposed to that antigen (Fig. 22–9):

1. Exposure and invasion
2. Antigen recognition
3. Lymphocyte sensitization
4. Antibody production and release
5. Antigen-antibody binding
6. Antibody-binding reactions
7. Sustained immunity/memory

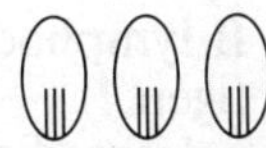

1. Invasion of the body by new antigens in sufficient numbers to stimulate an immune response.

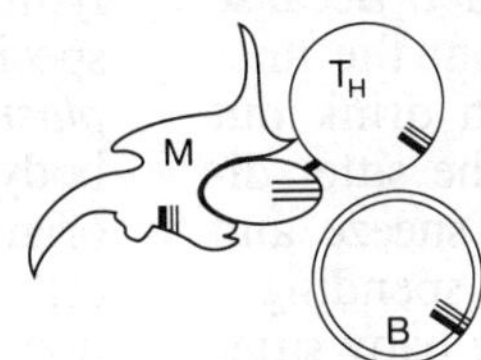

2. Interaction of macrophage (M) and T helper (T_H) cell in the processing and presenting of the antigen to the unsensitized "virgin" B lymphocyte (B).

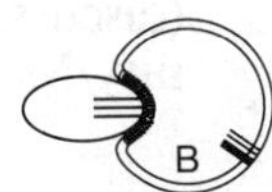

3. Sensitization of the virgin B lymphocyte to the new antigen.

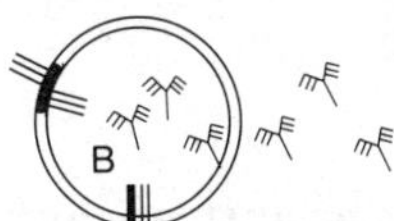

4. Antibody production by the B lymphocyte. These antibodies are directed specifically against the initiating antigen. The antibodies are released from the B lymphocyte and float freely in the blood and some other fluids.

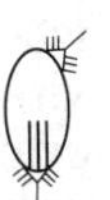

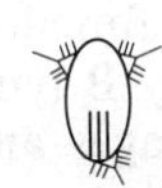

5. Antibodies bind to the antigen, forming an immune complex.

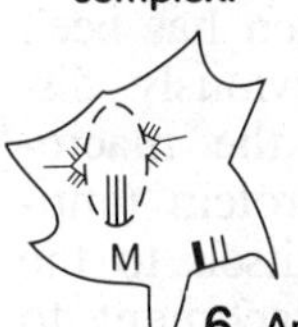

6. Antibody binding causes cellular events and attracts other leukocytes to the complex. The interaction of other leukocytes along with the cellular events results in the neutralization, destruction, or elimination of the antigen.

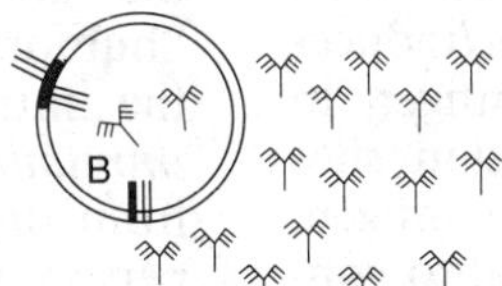

7. On reexposure to the same antigen, the sensitized lymphocytes and their progeny produce large quantities of the antibody specific to the antigen. In addition, new "virgin" B lymphocytes become sensitized to the antigen and also begin antibody production.

FIGURE 22–9 ◆ The sequence of events stimulating antibody-mediated immunity. (Modified from Workman, M. L., Ellerhorst-Ryan, J., & Koertge, V. [1993]. *Nursing care of the immunocompromised patient* [p. 35]. Philadelphia: W. B. Saunders.)

EXPOSURE AND INVASION

Antigen-antibody interactions occur in the body's internal environment. To make an antibody that can exert its effects on a specific antigen, the body must first be exposed to that antigen to the degree that the antigen enters the body. Even when exposure includes penetration, not all exposures result in the stimulation of antibody production. Invasion by the antigen must occur in such large numbers that some of the antigen either evades detection by the normal nonspecific defenses or overwhelms the abilities of the inflammatory response to neutralize, eliminate, or destroy the invader.

For example, a person has never contracted or even been exposed to the childhood viral disease chickenpox. This person baby-sits for three children who show chickenpox lesions within the next 10 hours. These children, in the pre-eruption stage, shed many millions of live chickenpox virus particles via the droplets from the upper respiratory tract. Because small children are often unconcerned about the finer points of infection control, these children drink out of the baby sitter's soft drink can, kiss the sitter directly (and wetly) on the lips, and both sneeze and cough directly into the sitter's face. After spending 5 hours with the children at close range, the baby sitter has been overwhelmingly invaded by the chickenpox virus (varicella-zoster) and will become sick with this disease within 14 to 21 days. While the virus is incubating and the disease is developing, the body's leukocytes are participating in the next steps in the series of antibody-antigen interactions to prevent the development of chickenpox more than once.

ANTIGEN RECOGNITION

To begin to make antibodies against an antigen, the "virgin" or previously unsensitized B lymphocyte must first recognize the antigen as nonself. B lymphocytes cannot carry out this important function alone. For this reason, antigen recognition by B lymphocytes requires the assistance of macrophages and helper/inducer T cells.

This cooperative effort is initiated by the macrophages. After the membrane of the antigen has been altered somewhat by opsonization (previously discussed under the heading Adherence), the macrophage recognizes the invading foreign protein (antigen) as nonself and physically attaches itself to the antigen. This particular macrophage attachment to the antigen does not result in phagocytosis or in immediate destruction of the antigen. Instead, the macrophage brings the attached antigen in contact with a helper/inducer T cell. At this time, the helper/inducer T cell and the macrophage process the antigen in some way to expose the antigen's recognition sites (universal product code). After processing the antigen, the helper/inducer T cell brings the antigen into contact with the B lymphocyte so that the B lymphocyte can recognize the antigen as nonself.

LYMPHOCYTE SENSITIZATION

Once the B lymphocyte recognizes the antigen as nonself, the B lymphocyte becomes sensitized to this antigen. An individual virgin B lymphocyte can undergo sensitization only once. Therefore, in theory, each B lymphocyte can be sensitized to only one antigen.

As a result of sensitization, this B lymphocyte can respond to any substance that carries the same antigens (universal product codes) as the original antigen. Once it is sensitized to a specific antigen, the B lymphocyte always remains sensitized to that specific antigen. In addition, all daughter cells of that sensitized B lymphocyte are sensitized to that same specific antigen.

Immediately after it is sensitized, the B lymphocyte (or B blast) divides and forms two different types of lymphocytes, each one remaining sensitized to that specific antigen (Fig. 22–10). One new cell becomes a *plasma cell* and immediately starts to produce antibody directed specifically against the antigen that originally sensitized the B lymphocyte. The other new cell becomes a *memory cell.* The plasma cell functions immediately and has a short life span. The memory cell remains sensitized but functionally dormant until the next exposure to the same antigen (discussed later under the heading Sustained Immunity/Memory).

ANTIBODY PRODUCTION AND RELEASE

Antibodies are produced by the plasma cell. When it is fully stimulated, each plasma cell can produce as much as 300 molecules of antibody per second. Each plasma cell produces antibody specific only to the antigen that originally sensitized the parent B lymphocyte. For example, in the case of the baby sitter who was exposed to and invaded by chickenpox virus, the plasma cells derived from the B lymphocytes sensitized to the chickenpox virus can produce only antichickenpox antibodies. The exact antibody type that the plasma cell can produce (e.g., IgG or IgM) may vary, but the specificity of that antibody remains forever directed against chickenpox virus (explained later in the chapter under the heading General Antibody Classification).

Antibody molecules produced by the plasma cells are secreted into the blood and other extracellular fluids as free antibody. Individual molecules of free antibody remain in the blood 3 to 30 days. Because the antibody circulates in body fluids (or body "humors") and is separate from the B lymphocytes, the immunity provided is sometimes called *humoral immunity.* Circulating antibodies can be transferred from one person to another to provide the receiving person with immediate immunity of short duration.

ANTIGEN-ANTIBODY BINDING

An antibody is basically a bilaterally symmetric Y-shaped molecule (Fig. 22–11). The different parts of the antibody molecule are named for the fragments that are formed when antibodies are digested with protein-degrading enzymes.

The tips of the short arms of the Y are the areas that recognize the specific antigen and bind to it. These tips form two fragments (called Fab fragments) when the whole molecule is digested with enzymes. Because each individual antibody molecule has two Fab fragments, antibody molecules are bivalent and can bind to either two separate antigen molecules or two areas of the same antigen molecule (Cooper, 1987).

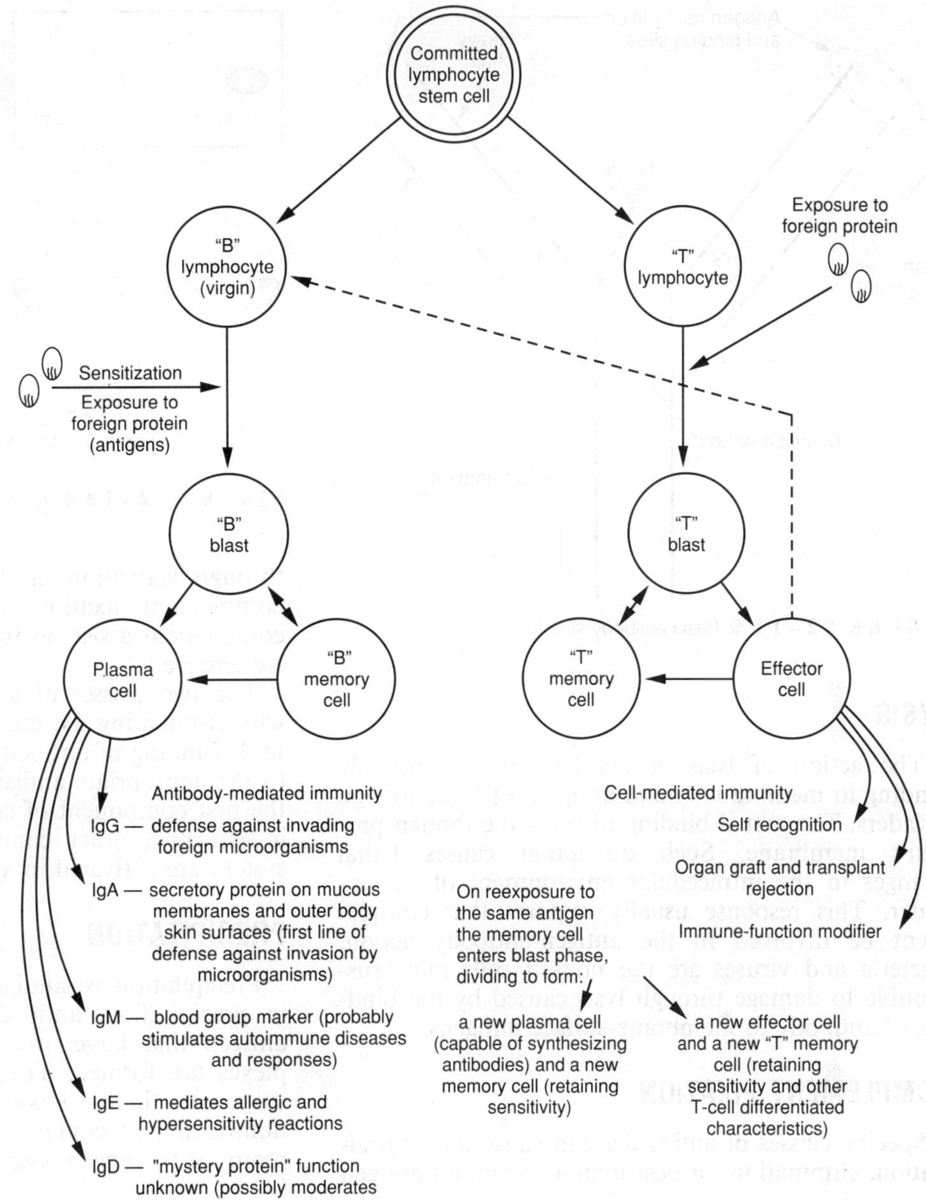

FIGURE 22-10 ◆ Differentiated functions of lymphocytes. (From Workman, M. L., Ellerhorst-Ryan, J., & Koertge, V. [1993]. *Nursing care of the immunocompromised patient* [p. 38]. Philadelphia: W. B. Saunders.)

The stem of the Y forms what is called the Fc fragment when the antibody molecule is digested with enzymes. This area of the antibody molecule can bind to Fc receptor sites on leukocytes so that the leukocyte then has not only its own mechanisms of attacking or destroying antigens but also the added power of having antibodies on its surface that stick to antigens (Fig. 22-12).

The actual binding of antibody to antigen is not usually lethal to the antigen. Instead, the physical binding of the antibody to the antigen initiates other actions that result in the neutralization, elimination, or destruction of the antigen.

ANTIBODY-BINDING REACTIONS

The action of binding antibody to antigen allows or triggers specific reactions to cause the neutralization, elimination, or destruction of the antigen. These reactions include agglutination, lysis, complement fixation, precipitation, and inactivation/neutralization.

AGGLUTINATION

Agglutination is an antibody action that results from an antibody molecule's having at least two antigen binding sites. The binding of more than one antigen molecule to each antibody does not directly destroy the antigen. Agglutination permits defensive effects by at least two mechanisms. First, it slows the movement of the antigen through the extracellular fluids. Second, the irregular shape of the antigen-antibody complex (Fig. 22-13) increases the likelihood that this complex will be attacked by other leukocytes, including macrophages, neutrophils, and cytotoxic/cytolytic T cells (discussed later under Cell-Mediated Immunity).

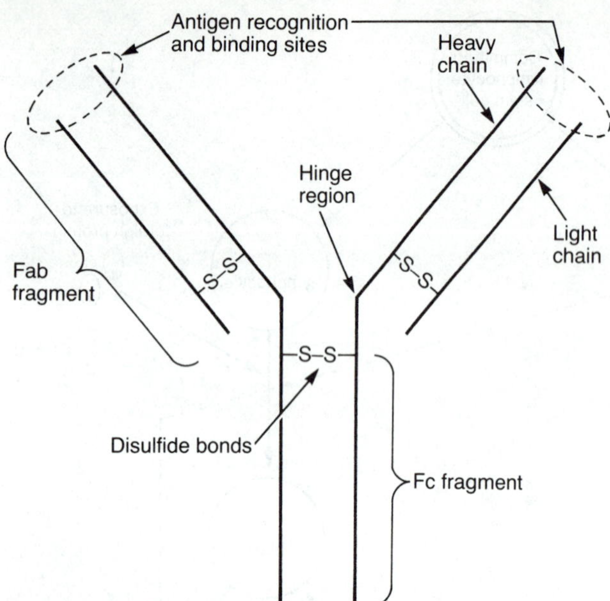

FIGURE 22–11 ◆ Basic antibody structure.

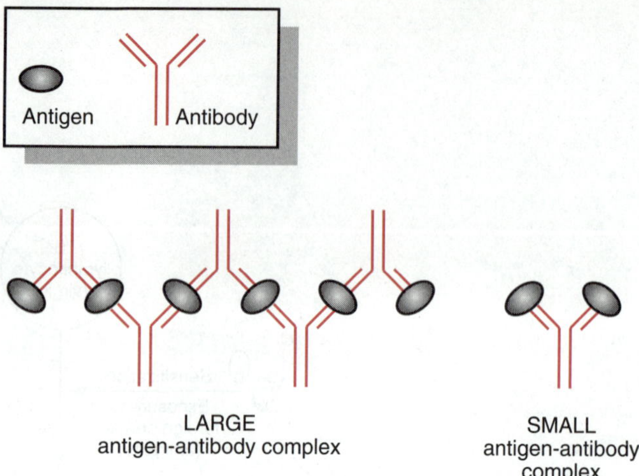

FIGURE 22–13 ◆ Antibody-antigen complexes.

LYSIS

The action of lysis occurs because of antibody binding to membrane-bound antigens of some foreign invaders. The actual binding disrupts the foreign protein's membrane. Such disruption causes lethal changes in the intracellular environment of the invader. This response usually requires that complement be involved in the antigen-antibody action. Bacteria and viruses are the nonself cells most susceptible to damage through lysis caused by the binding of antibody to membrane-surface antigens.

COMPLEMENT FIXATION

Specific classes of antibodies can cause the neutralization, elimination, or destruction of nonself antigen through activation of the complement cascade and complement fixation. (The mechanism by which complement assists in immunity was discussed under Adherence.)

The two classes of antibody frequently associated with stimulating the complement system are IgG and IgM. Binding of antibody from either of these classes to the appropriate antigen provides a binding site for the first component of complement (C1q). Once C1q is activated, other components of the complement system are activated in a cascade.

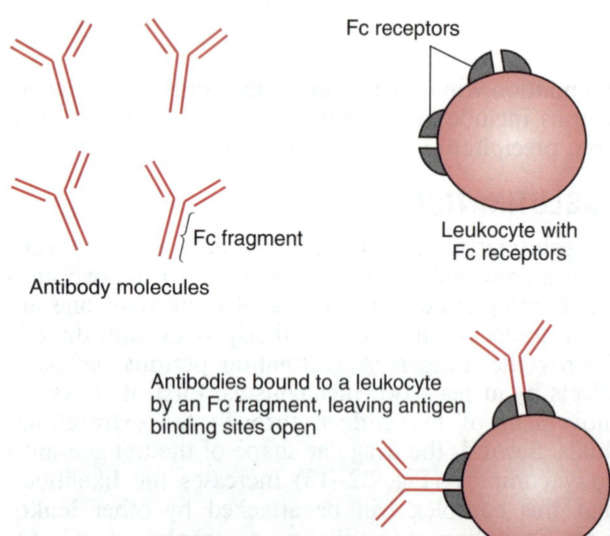

FIGURE 22–12 ◆ Antibody Fc receptors on leukocytes.

PRECIPITATION

Precipitation is similar to agglutination. However, in precipitation, antibody molecules bind so much antigen that large, insoluble antigen-antibody complexes are formed. These complexes cannot stay in suspension in the blood. Instead, they form a large, nonmoving precipitate, which can be acted on and removed by other nonspecific leukocytes.

INACTIVATION/NEUTRALIZATION

Inactivation/neutralization is unique in that it does not result in the immediate destruction of the antigen. An antigen usually has a relatively small area that is actually responsible for exerting harmful effects. The rest of the antigen is not harmful to the host. Binding of antibody can interfere with the function of the active site by covering it up or changing its shape. Either mechanism inhibits the activity of the antigen and renders it harmless without destroying it or eliminating it.

SUSTAINED IMMUNITY/MEMORY

The sustained immunity/memory function of antibody-mediated immunity provides humans with long-lasting immunity to a specific antigen. Sustained immunity is provided by the action of the B-lymphocyte memory cells that are generated during the lymphocyte sensitization stage. These memory cells remain sensitized to the specific antigen to which they were originally exposed. On re-exposure to the same antigen, the memory cells are stimulated into rapid response. First, the cells divide and form new sensitized blast cells and new sensitized plasma cells. The blast cells continue to divide to generate even more sensitized plasma cells. The sensitized plasma cells begin to rapidly make and secrete large amounts of the antibody specific for the sensitizing antigen.

This ability of the sensitized memory cells to initiate events on re-exposure to the antigen that originally sensitized the B lymphocyte allows a rapid and widespread immune *(anamnestic)* response to the antigen. This response usually eliminates the invading antigen completely so that the person does not become ill. Because of this process, most people do not become ill with chickenpox or other viral diseases more than once, even though they are exposed many times to the causative organism. Without the process or action of memory, people would remain susceptible to specific diseases on subsequent exposure to the antigen and no sustained immunity would be generated.

General Antibody Classification

All antibodies are referred to as immunoglobulins (abbreviated Ig) and gamma globulins. These names are based on the structure, location, and function of antibodies. A globulin is a type of protein structure that is globular rather than straight. Because antibodies are composed of this type of protein, they are globulins. The name immunoglobulin is appropriate for antibodies because they are globular proteins that assist in immune function. Antibodies are called gamma globulins because during the process of electrophoresis, different groups of proteins in blood plasma separate out at different times, depending on how they move in response to electrical charge (Fig. 22–14). The protein groups are named according to when they emerge. The first group to emerge are the plasma albumins, which make up a large group. Three smaller groups emerge at specific times after the albumins. The fourth group, or protein fraction (gamma fraction), contains all five different types of antibody proteins. The five antibody types are classified by differences in antibody structure, molecular weight, and patterns of association (Table 22–4).

Acquiring Antibody-Mediated Immunity

Two broad categories of immunity are innate immunity and acquired immunity.

INNATE IMMUNITY

Innate immunity is a genetically determined characteristic of an individual, group, or species. A person either has or does not have innate immunity. For example, people have many innate immunities to viruses and other microorganisms that cause specific diseases in animals. As a result, humans are not susceptible to such diseases as mange, distemper, hog cholera, or any of a variety of animal afflictions. This type of immunity cannot be developed or transferred from one person to another and is not an adaptive response to exposure or invasion by foreign proteins.

ACQUIRED IMMUNITY

Acquired immunity is the immunity that every person's body makes (or can receive) as an adaptive response to invasion by foreign proteins. Antibody-mediated immunity is an acquired immunity. Acquired immunity occurs either naturally or artificially and can be either active or passive.

ACTIVE IMMUNITY

Active immunity occurs when antigens enter the body and the body responds by making specific antibodies against the antigen. This type of immunity is active because the body takes an active part in making the antibodies. Active immunity can occur under conditions that are either natural or artificial.

NATURAL ACTIVE IMMUNITY

Natural active immunity occurs when an antigen enters the body, without human assistance, and the body responds by actively making antibodies against that antigen (e.g., chickenpox virus). Most of the time, the first invasion of the body by this antigen results in the person's manifesting signs and symptoms of the disease. However, processes occurring in the body at the same time allow the person to acquire immunity to that antigen so that he or she will not become ill after a second exposure to the same antigen. This type of immunity is the most effective and the longest lasting.

ARTIFICIAL ACTIVE IMMUNITY

Artificial active immunity is a type of protection developed against illnesses that produce such serious side effects that total avoidance of the disease is most desirable. Small amounts of specific antigens are deliberately placed (as a vaccination) in the body so that the body responds by actively making antibodies against the antigen. Because antigens used for this procedure have been specially processed to make them less likely to proliferate within the body, this exposure does not in itself cause the disease.

Examples of diseases for which artificially acquired active immunity can be obtained include tetanus, diphtheria, measles, smallpox, mumps, and rubella, among others. This type of immunity lasts many years, although repeated but smaller doses of the

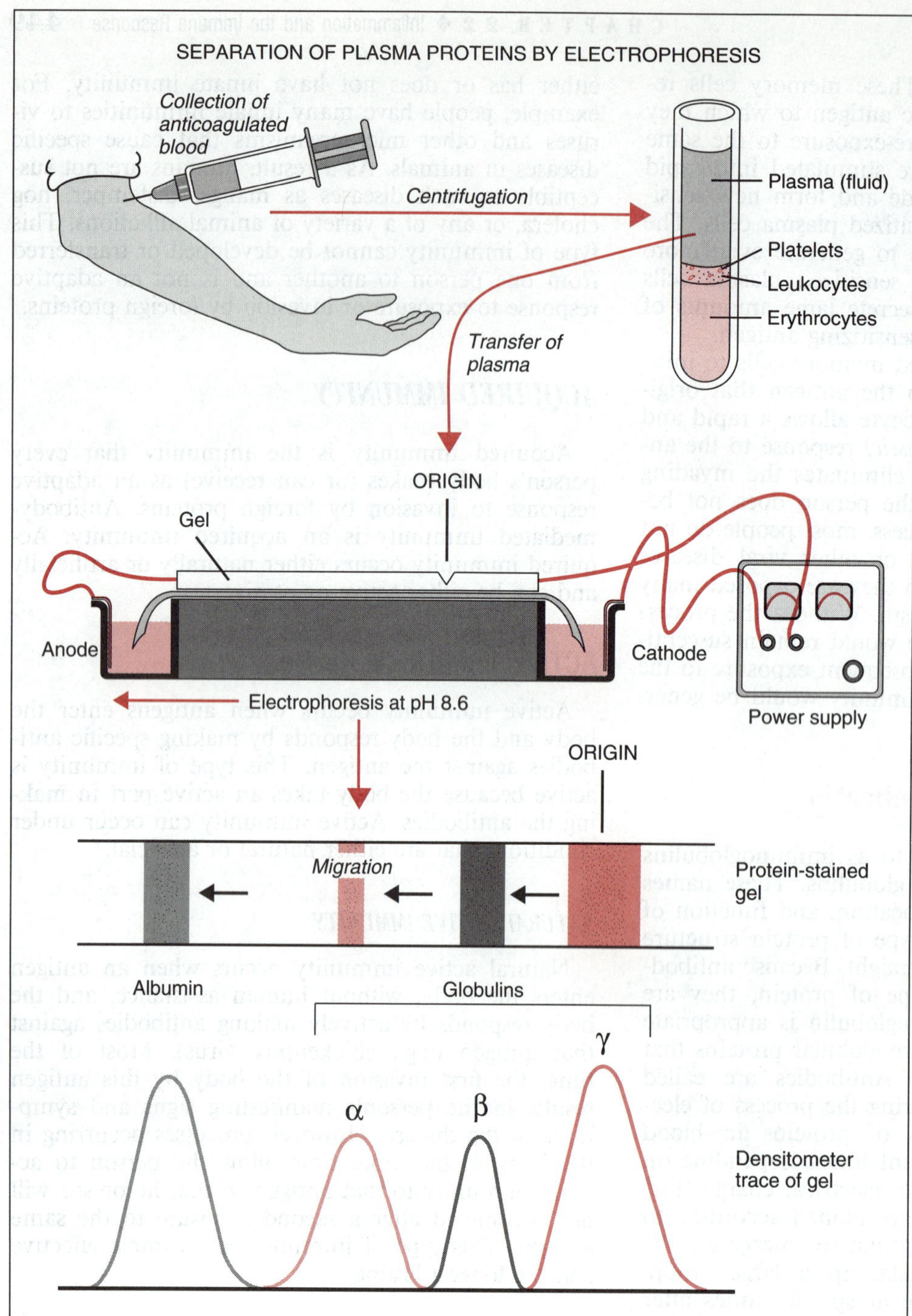

FIGURE 22-14 ◆ Electrophoresis of plasma proteins, including gamma globulin. (From Abbas, A., Lichtman, A., & Pober, J. [1991]. *Cellular and molecular immunology* [p. 42]. Philadelphia: W. B. Saunders.)

original antigen are required as a "booster" for maintaining complete protection against the antigen.

PASSIVE IMMUNITY

Passive immunity occurs when antibodies against a specific antigen are in a person's body but the person did not actively generate these antibodies. These antibodies are made in the body of another person or animal and then transferred to the body of a specific individual. Because these antibodies are foreign to the individual, the body recognizes the antibodies as nonself and takes steps to eliminate them relatively quickly. For this reason, passive immunity can provide only immediate, short-term protection against a specific antigen.

NATURAL PASSIVE IMMUNITY

Natural passive immunity occurs when antibodies are passed from the mother to the fetus via the placenta or to the infant through colostrum and breast milk.

ARTIFICIAL PASSIVE IMMUNITY

Artificial passive immunity involves deliberately injecting one person with antibodies that were produced in another person or animal. This type of immunity is used when a person is exposed to a serious disease or illness for which he or she has little or no known actively acquired immunity. Instead, the injected antibodies are expected to inactivate the anti-

TABLE 22–4 Classification and Characterization of Antibodies

Type	Configuration	Content in Blood (%)	Function
IgA	• Dimer	• <15%	• "Secretory"—present in body secretions, such as tears, mucus, saliva • Inhibits bacteria and viruses from adhering to skin and mucous membranes, making penetration into the internal environment more difficult
IgD	• Monomer	• <1%	• Modification of IgM activity
IgE	• Monomer	• <1%	• Degranulation of basophils and mast cells during inflammatory responses • Assists in clearance of parasites and prevention of pulmonary infections • Mediates many types of allergic reactions
IgG	• Monomer	• 75%	• Activates complement • Neutralizes toxins • Enhances phagocytosis • Provides significant sustained immunity against viral and bacterial infections
IgM	• Pentomer	• 10%	• Activates complement • Clears antigens through precipitation • Possibly mediates autoimmune reactions • Mediates ABO incompatibility reactions in blood transfusions

gen. This type of immunity provides only temporary protection lasting for days to a few weeks. Some of the conditions or diseases for which artificial passive immunity may be used include exposure to rabies, tetanus, and poisonous snake bites.

Antibody-mediated immunity (AMI) works with the inflammatory responses in providing protection to the person against infection. However, AMI can provide the most effective, long-lasting immunity only when its actions are combined with the processes of cell-mediated immunity.

CELL-MEDIATED IMMUNITY

Cell-mediated immunity (CMI) or cellular immunity, involves many leukocyte actions, reactions, and interactions that range from the simple to the complex. This type of immunity is provided by committed lymphocyte stem cells that mature in the secondary lymphoid tissues of the thymus and pericortical areas of lymph nodes. Certain CMI responses influence and regulate the activities of antibody-mediated immunity and inflammation by producing and releasing cytokines. Therefore, for total immunocompetence CMI must function optimally.

Cell Types Involved in Cell-Mediated Immunity

The leukocytes playing the most important roles in cell-mediated immunity include several specific T-lymphocyte subsets along with a special population of cells known as natural killer cells (NK cells). T lymphocytes further differentiate into a variety of subsets, each of which has a specific function.

One way of identifying different T-lymphocyte subsets is to determine the presence or absence of certain "marker proteins" (antigens) on the cell membrane's surface. Fifty different T-lymphocyte proteins have been identified on the cell membrane, and 11 of these (named T1 through T11) are commonly used in clinical situations to identify various immune system components. Antibodies have been made against each of these 11 proteins so that each T-lymphocyte subset can be identified by how the T lymphocyte reacts to the commercial antibodies. Most T lymphocytes have more than one antigen on their cell membranes. For example, all mature T lymphocytes contain T1, T3, T10, and T11 proteins. Certain subsets of T lymphocytes also contain other specific T-lymphocyte membrane antigens.

The nomenclature used to identify specific T-lymphocyte subsets includes the specific membrane antigen and the overall functional activities of the cells in a subset. The three T-lymphocyte subsets that are critically important for the development and continuation of cell-mediated immunity are:

- Helper/inducer T cells
- Suppressor T cells
- Cytotoxic/cytolytic T cells

HELPER/INDUCER T CELLS

DESCRIPTION

The cell membranes of these T lymphocytes contain the T4 protein. Usually, these cells are called T4 cells or T_H cells. A newer name for helper/inducer T cells is CD4 (for cluster of differentiation 4). Several companies have made antibodies to the T4 cell membrane protein. These antibodies include OKT4 and LEU-3; thus, the helper/inducer T cells may also be referred to as the cells that are OKT4-positive or LEU-3–positive.

FUNCTION

Helper/inducer T cells are efficient in the recognition of self versus nonself. These important cells indirectly participate in cell-mediated immunity by stimulating the activity of many other leukocytes. In response to the recognition of nonself (antigen), helper/inducer T cells secrete lymphokines that can regulate the activity of other leukocytes.

In general, the lymphokines secreted by the helper/inducer T lymphocytes have overall stimulatory effects on immune function. These lymphokines increase bone marrow production of stem cells and speed up the maturation of cells of myeloid and lymphoid origin. In effect, the helper/inducer T lymphocyte acts as an organizer in calling to arms various squads of leukocytes involved in inflammatory, antibody, and cellular defensive actions to destroy, eliminate, or neutralize antigens.

SUPPRESSOR T CELLS

DESCRIPTION

The cell membranes of suppressor T lymphocytes contain the T8 lymphocyte antigen, and these cells are commonly called T8 cells, or T_S cells. Suppressor T cells participate in the regulation of cell-mediated immunity.

FUNCTION

Suppressor T cells prevent continuous overreaction or hypersensitivity reactions to exposure to nonself cells or proteins. This function is important in preventing the formation of autoantibodies directed against normal, healthy self cells, the basis for many autoimmune diseases.

The suppressor T cells secrete substances that have an overall inhibitory action on most and perhaps all cells of the immune system. These substances inhibit both the proliferation of immune system cells and the activation of immune system cells.

In general, suppressor T cells directly oppose the activity of helper/inducer T cells. Therefore, for optimal function of cell-mediated immunity, a balance between helper/inducer T-cell activity and suppressor T-cell activity must be maintained. This balance is usually provided when the helper/inducer T cells outnumber the suppressor T cells by a ratio of 2 to 1. When this ratio increases, overreactions can be expected to occur (some of these overreactions are tissue-damaging, as well as unpleasant). When the helper-to-suppressor ratio decreases, immune function is suppressed profoundly and the body is much more vulnerable to invasion by nonself cells and infections of all types.

CYTOTOXIC/CYTOLYTIC T CELLS

DESCRIPTION

Cytotoxic/cytolytic T lymphocytes are also called T_C cells. Because they have the T8 protein present on their surfaces, they are a subset of suppressor cells. Cytotoxic/cytolytic T cells function in cell-mediated immunity by lysing or destroying cells that contain a processed antigen-MHC complex. This activity is most effective against self cells that are infected by parasitic organisms, such as viruses or protozoa.

FUNCTION

Parasite-infected self cells have both self MHC proteins (universal product code) and the parasite's antigens on the cell surface. This allows the person's immune system cells to recognize the infected self cell as abnormal, and the cytotoxic/cytolytic T cell can bind to it.

The binding of the cytotoxic/cytolytic T lymphocyte to the infected cell's antigen-MHC complex stimulates activities that result in the death of the infected cell. The cytotoxic/cytolytic T cell bores a hole in the membrane of the infected cell and delivers a "lethal hit" of enzymes to the infected cell, causing it to lyse and die. Once the lethal hit has been administered to the infected cell, the cytotoxic/cytolytic T lymphocyte releases the dying infected cell and can go attack and destroy other infected cells that carry the same antigen-MHC complex.

NATURAL KILLER CELLS

DESCRIPTION

Natural killer (NK) cells are extremely important in providing cell-mediated immunity. The actual site of differentiation and maturation of NK cells is unknown. Although this cell population has some T-lymphocyte characteristics, it is not considered a true T-lymphocyte subset (Abbas et al., 1991).

FUNCTION

NK cells direct cytotoxic/cytolytic effects on target nonself cells. Unlike cytotoxic/cytolytic T cells, NK cells can exert these cytotoxic effects without first undergoing a period of sensitization to nonself cell membrane antigens. In addition, NK cells do not need to share any of the major histocompatibility complex (MHC) proteins in common with the nonself cell to initiate defensive actions against the nonself cell. The defensive actions of NK cells appear to be totally unrelated to either antigen sensitivity or the interactions of other leukocytes. NK cells essentially conduct "seek and destroy" missions throughout the body to eliminate foreign proteins and unhealthy self cells.

NK cells are most effective in destroying unhealthy or abnormal self cells. The nonself cells most susceptible to defensive actions of NK cells are (1) self cells that are virally infected and (2) cancer cells (Gallucci, 1987).

CYTOKINES

The inducing and regulatory aspects of cell-mediated immunity are controlled through the selected production and activity of cytokines. Cytokines are small protein hormones synthesized by the various leukocytes. Cytokines synthesized by the mononuclear phagocytes (macrophages, neutrophils, eosinophils, and monocytes) are termed monokines; cytokines produced by T lymphocytes are *lymphokines* (Van Snick, 1990).

Cytokine activity is similar to the action of any other kind of hormone: One cell produces and secretes a cytokine, which then exerts its effects on other cells of the immune system (Guyton, 1991). The cells responding to the cytokine may be right next to the cytokine-secreting cell or remote from the cytokine-secreting cell. The cells that change their activity in response to the cytokine are known as "responder" cells. For a responder cell to respond to the presence of a cytokine, the membrane of the responder cell must have a specific receptor for the cytokine to bind to and initiate changes in the responder cell's activity (Nicola, 1989) (Fig. 22–15).

Cytokines induce and regulate a wide variety of inflammatory and immune responses. Most cytokines are produced as they are needed and are not stored to any great extent (Balkwill & Burke, 1989). The actions of some cytokines are pleiotropic in that the effects are widespread within the immune system, setting into motion a variety of immunomodulating actions. Other cytokines have specific actions limited to only one type of cell. Table 22–5 summarizes the origins and activities of the currently known cytokines.

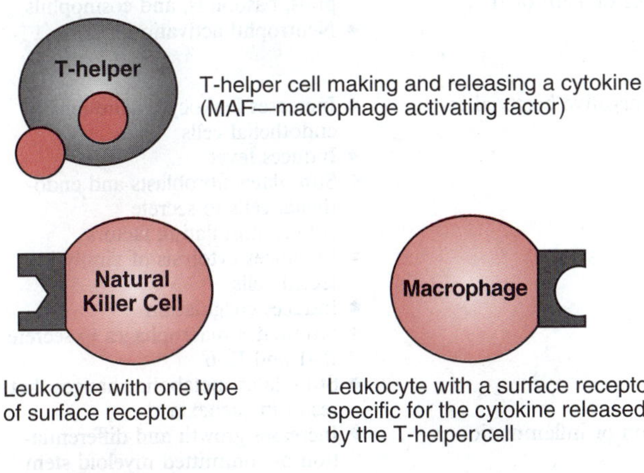

FIGURE 22–15 ◆ Cytokine receptors on leukocytes.

Protection Provided by Cell-Mediated Immunity

Specific components of cell-mediated immunity (CMI) assist in providing protection to the body by their highly developed abilities to differentiate self from nonself. The nonself cells most easily recognized by CMI are those self cells that are infected by organisms that live within host cells and those self cells mutated at the DNA level and no longer normal. CMI provides a surveillance system for ridding the body of self cells that might potentially harm the body. CMI is critically important in preventing development of cancer and metastasis after exposure to carcinogens.

Transplantation Rejection

Natural killer cells and cytotoxic/cytolytic T cells also destroy cells from other people or animals. Although this action is generally helpful, it is also responsible for rejection of grafts and transplanted organs. Because the solid organ transplanted into the host is seldom a completely identical match of universal product codes (HLAs) between the donated organ and the recipient host, the client's immune system cells recognize a newly transplanted organ as nonself. Without intervention, the host's immune system initiates standard inflammatory and immunologic actions to destroy, eliminate, or neutralize these nonself cells. This activity causes rejection of the transplanted organ. Graft rejection is the result of a complex series of responses that change over time and involve different components of the immune system. Graft rejection can be hyperacute, acute, or chronic.

HYPERACUTE REJECTION

Hyperacute graft rejection begins immediately on transplantation and is an antibody-mediated response (Abbas et al., 1991). Antigen-antibody complexes form within the blood vessels of the transplanted organ. The host's blood has pre-existing antibodies to one or more of the antigens (including blood group antigens) present in the donated organ. The antigen-antibody complexes adhere to the lining of blood vessels and stimulate complement activation. The activated/fixated complement in the blood vessel linings initiates the blood clotting cascade, with microcoagulation occurring throughout the organ vasculature. Widespread coagulation and occlusion lead to ischemic necrosis, inflammation with phagocytosis of the necrotic blood vessels, and release of lytic enzymes into the transplanted organ (Smith, 1990). These enzymes cause massive cellular destruction and graft loss.

Hyperacute rejection occurs primarily in trans-

TABLE 22–5 Summary of Cytokine Activity

Cytokine	Cellular Origin	Inducing Event	Cytokine Action
Interleukin-1 (IL-1)	• Macrophage	• Contact with gram-negative bacterial products • Contact with CD4 cell • Presence of TNF	• Stimulates increased production of prostaglandins • Induces fever • Increases proliferation of CD4 cells • Stimulates growth and differentiation of B lymphocytes • Induces further secretion of IL-1 and IL-6
Interleukin-2 (IL-2)	• T helper/inducer cells ($CD4^+$) • $CD8^+$ T cells	• T-cell activation by antigens	• Increases the growth and differentiation of T lymphocytes • Stimulates increased production of IL-2 from activated lymphocytes
Interleukin-3 (multilineage colony-stimulating factor, IL-3)	• T helper/inducer cells ($CD4^+$)	• Infection or invasion	• Stimulates production of immature bone marrow stem cells (pluripotent)
Interleukin-4 (B-cell stimulatory factor, IL-4)	• T helper/inducer cells ($CD4^+$) • Activated mast cells	• Presence of anti-Ig antibody	• Stimulates growth and proliferation of B lymphocytes • Stimulates increased production of IgE • Induces further secretion of IL-4, IL-5, and IL-6 • Acts as a macrophage-activating factor
Interleukin-5 (B-cell growth factor, IL-5)	• T helper/inducer cells ($CD4^+$) • Activated mast cells	• Helminth infections	• Stimulates growth and differentiation of eosinophils • Stimulates mature B lymphocytes to increase the synthesis of immunoglobulins (especially IgA)
Interleukin-6 (IL-6)	• Macrophage • Vascular endothelial cells • Fibroblasts • Activated T cells	• Infection or inflammation • Presence of IL-1 and TNF	• Stimulates hepatocytes to make fibrinogen, macroglobulin, and C protein • Stimulates the growth of activated B lymphocytes • Serves as a cofactor in stimulating production of bone marrow hematopoietic stem cells
Interleukin-7 (IL-7)	• Bone marrow stromal cells	• Presence of antigen	• Stimulates growth and differentiation of committed B-lymphocyte stem cells
Interleukin-8 (monocyte chemotactic factor, IL-8)	• Activated T cells, macrophage endothelial cells, platelets, fibroblasts, and epithelial cells	• Infection or inflammation • Presence of TNF or IL-1	• Chemotactic factor for neutrophils, basophils, and eosinophils • Neutrophil activation
Tumor necrosis factor (TNF)	• LPS-activated macrophage • Antigen-stimulated T cells • Activated NK cells • Activated mast cells	• Gram-negative bacterial infection	• Increases leukocyte adhesion to endothelial cells • Induces fever • Stimulates fibroblasts and endothelial cells to secrete colony-stimulating factors • Enhances cytolysis of virally infected cells • Induces coagulation • Stimulates macrophages to secrete IL-1 and IL-6 • Stimulates metabolic changes that result in cachexia
Granulocyte-macrophage colony-stimulating factor (GM-CSF)	• Activated T cells • Macrophages • Vascular endothelial cells • Fibroblasts	• Infection or inflammation	• Increases growth and differentiation of committed myeloid stem cells • Minor activator of macrophages
Monocyte-macrophage colony-stimulating factor (M-CSF)	• Macrophages • Vascular endothelial cells • Fibroblasts	• Infection or inflammation	• Enhances proliferation and maturation of the committed progenitor cells for monocytes-macrophages (CFU-M)

TABLE 22–5 Summary of Cytokine Activity *Continued*

Cytokine	Cellular Origin	Inducing Event	Cytokine Action
Granulocyte colony-stimulating factor (G-CSF)	• Macrophages • Vascular endothelial cells • Fibroblasts	• Infection or inflammation	• Enhances neutrophil maturation and release from bone marrow
Interferon (INF-alpha, -beta, -gamma)	• Macrophages (INF-alpha) • Fibroblasts (INF-beta) • T helper/inducer cells (INF-gamma) • CD8$^+$ cells (INF-gamma) • NK cells	• Viral infection	• Limits viral infection by inhibiting viral replication, increasing NK-mediated lysis, and increasing cytolytic T-lymphocyte recognition of virally infected cells • Activates macrophages (INF-gamma) • Promotes differentiation of T and B lymphocytes (INF-gamma) • Activates neutrophils (INF-gamma) • Activates NK cells (INF-gamma)

From Workman, M. L., Ellerhorst-Ryan, J., & Koertge, V. (1993). *Nursing care of the immunocompromised patient.* Philadelphia: W. B. Saunders.
TNF, tumor necrosis factor; Ig, immunoglobulin; LPS, lipopolysaccharide; CFU-M, colony-forming unit—monocyte-macrophage; NK, natural killer.

planted kidneys. According to Smith (1990), people at greatest risk for hyperacute rejection are:

- Those who have received donated organs of an ABO blood type different from their own
- Those who have received multiple blood transfusions at any time in life before transplantation
- Those who have a history of multiple pregnancies
- Those who have received a previous transplant

The manifestations of hyperacute rejection are apparent within minutes of attachment of the donated organ to the host's blood supply. *The process cannot be stopped once it is initiated, and the rejected organ must be removed as soon as hyperacute rejection is diagnosed.*

ACUTE REJECTION

Acute graft rejection occurs within 3 months of transplantation and can occur as soon as 1 week after transplantation. Two mechanisms are responsible.

The first mechanism is *antibody-mediated* and results in vasculitis within the transplanted organ. This reaction differs from that of hyperacute rejection in that blood vessel necrosis (rather than thrombotic occlusion) leads to the organ's destruction (Abbas et al., 1991).

The second mechanism is *cellular.* Host cytotoxic/cytolytic T cells and natural killer cells enter the transplanted organ through the blood, infiltrate the organ cells (rather than the blood vessel cells), and cause lysis of the organ cells.

A diagnosis of acute rejection is made by laboratory tests indicating impaired function of the specific organ along with biopsy of the grafted organ. Manifestations of acute rejection vary with each client and with the specific organ transplanted. For example, when acute rejection occurs in the presence of transplanted kidneys, the host usually experiences some tenderness in the kidney area and may experience other general symptoms of inflammation.

An episode of acute rejection after solid organ transplantation does not automatically mean that the host will lose the transplant. Pharmacologic manipulation of host immune responses at this time can limit the damage to the organ and allow the graft to be maintained.

CHRONIC REJECTION

The origin of chronic rejection is not clear, but it resembles the aftermath of chronic inflammation and scarring. Functional tissue of the transplanted organ is replaced with fibrotic, scarlike tissue. Because this fibrotic tissue does not resemble the organ tissue in either structure or function, the ability of the transplanted organ to perform differentiated tasks diminishes in proportion to the percentage of normal tissue replaced by fibrotic tissue. This type of reaction is long-standing and occurs continuously as a response to chronic ischemia caused by blood vessel injury (Abbas et al., 1991).

Good control over host immune function can delay the manifestations of this type of rejection, but the process probably occurs to some degree with all solid organ transplants. Because the fibrotic changes are permanent, there is no cure for chronic graft rejection. When the fibrosis increases to the extent that there is significant interference with the functional capacity of the transplanted organ, the only recourse is retransplantation.

IMMUNOSUPPRESSIVE AGENTS

Rejection of transplanted solid organs involves all three components of immunity, although cell-mediated immune responses are most significant in the rejection process.

MAINTENANCE THERAPY

Three pharmacologic agents are generally used for routine immunosuppressive therapy after solid organ transplantation. These agents are azathioprine (Imuran); cyclosporine (Sandimmune); and one of the corticosteroids, such as prednisone (Apo-Prednisone✱, Deltasone) or prednisolone (Delta-Cortef). The drug doses are adjusted for the immune responses of each client. A regimen of these agents increases the client's risk for bacterial and fungal infections.

RESCUE THERAPY

The following agents are used not to maintain the graft within the host but to reduce the host's immunologic responses during rejection episodes, especially acute rejection. These agents may be used in addition to or in place of any of the maintenance drugs in the host's post-transplantation treatment regimen.

ANTILYMPHOCYTE GLOBULIN

Antilymphocyte globulin (ALG) is an antibody (or group of antibodies) generated in another animal after exposure of the animal to human lymphocytes. The globulin can be made more specific by exposing the animal to human T lymphocytes instead of mixed lymphocytes. When these anti–human lymphocyte antibodies are administered to humans, the antibodies selectively attack and clear lymphocytes from the blood, extracellular fluids, and tissues into which they have infiltrated (such as the transplanted organ). This agent is given only for a short time to combat the acute rejection episode.

Most clients receiving ALG have some associated immunologic response ranging from low-grade fever and malaise to serum sickness and anaphylaxis. The response usually increases with intensity on repeated exposure to ALG.

OKT3

OKT3 is an antibody directed specifically against the human T-lymphocyte cell-surface antigen CD_3. OKT3 is generated with a murine (mouse) model rather than an equine (horse) model. Because the agent is generated in mice, the humans receiving it rapidly develop antimouse antibodies. These antimouse antibodies attack the OKT3 and prevent its anti–T-cell activities. Thus, OKT3 has the best action against rejection during the first episode for which it is used. Its utility in combating graft rejection decreases at each subsequent use.

FK 506

FK 506, a new immunosuppressive agent, has been approved for use in maintenance therapy and rescue therapy, primarily after liver transplantation. It is similar in chemical composition to erythromycin and specifically suppresses T-lymphocyte actions, including the synthesis of interleukin-2. These effects are achieved through a variety of mechanisms. In the presence of FK 506, receptor sites for interleukin-2 (IL-2) are inhibited on helper/inducer T cells and cytotoxic/cytolytic T cells. Without continuous stimulation by IL-2, these lymphocytes are slow to reproduce and do not perform their designated differentiated functions. In addition, FK 506 is able to prevent activation of immature or unsensitized cytotoxic/cytolytic T lymphocytes. Because the cytotoxic/cytolytic T cell is primarily responsible for immunologic destruction of transplanted cells and tissues, and because the helper/inducer T cells boost the activity of cytotoxic/cytolytic T cells, selective suppression of the activity of these two cell populations allows the transplanted organ to remain free from immunologic destruction yet does not result in so profound an immunosuppressive state that the host is excessively susceptible to infection.

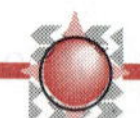

IMPLICATIONS FOR NURSING RESEARCH

Nursing research is beginning to explore interventions to prevent complications when clients experience an alteration in immune function. Little attention has been paid to nonpharmacologic influences on immune function. Future nursing research may focus on the following questions:

- ◆ What effect does a program of regular physical exercise have on immune function?
- ◆ Do supplemental vitamins increase specific populations of leukocytes?
- ◆ Is there a relationship between "positive thinking" and immune function?

SELECTED BIBLIOGRAPHY

Abbas, A., Lichtman, A., & Pober, J. (1991). *Cellular and molecular immunology.* Philadelphia: W. B. Saunders.

*Balkwill, F., & Burke, F. (1989). The cytokine network. *Immunology Today, 10,* 299.

*Cooper, N. (1987). The complement system. In D. Stites, J. Stobo, & J. Wells (Eds.), *Basic and clinical immunology* (6th ed.). Norwalk, CT: Appleton & Lange.

*Gallucci, B. (1987). The immune system and cancer. *Oncology Nursing Forum, 14*(Suppl.), 3.

Gawlikowski, J. (1992). White cells at war. *American Journal of Nursing, 92*(3), 44–51.

Guyton, A. C. (1991). *Textbook of medical physiology* (8th ed.). Philadelphia: W. B. Saunders.

Hooks, M. (1990). Immunosuppressive agents used in transplantation. In S. Smith (Ed.), *Tissue and organ transplantation: Implications for professional nursing practice* (pp. 48–75). St. Louis: C. V. Mosby.

Jackson, R. (1991). The immune system: Basic concepts for understanding transplantation. *Critical Care Nursing Quarterly, 13*(4), 83–88.

*Nicola, N. (1989). Hematopoietic cell growth factors and their receptors. *Annual Review of Biochemistry, 58,* 45.

Payne, J. (1992). Immune modification and complications of immunosuppression. *Critical Care Clinics of North America, 4*(1), 43–61.

Pezze, J. (1990). RATG: Implications for nursing care in organ transplantation. *Critical Care Nurse, 10*(9), 18–19, 22, 24.

Pillon, L. (1990). Cyclosporine: A nursing focus on immunosuppressive therapy. *Dimensions in Critical Care Nursing, 10*(2), 68–73.

Roitt, I. (1991). *Essential immunology* (7th ed.). London: Blackwell Scientific Publications.

Smith, S. (1990). Immunologic aspects of transplantation. In S. Smith (Ed.), *Tissue and organ transplantation: Implications for professional nursing practice* (pp. 15–47). St. Louis: C. V. Mosby.

*Stites, D. (1987). Clinical laboratory methods for detection of cellular immune function. In D. Stites, J. Stobo, & J. Wells (Eds.), *Basic and clinical immunology* (6th ed.). Norwalk, CT: Appleton & Lange.

*Stites, D., Stobo, J., & Wells, J. (Eds.). (1987). *Basic and clinical immunology* (6th ed.). Norwalk, CT: Appleton & Lange.

Van Snick, J. (1990). Interleukin-6: An overview. *Annual Review of Immunology, 8,* 253.

Vaska, P. (1991). OKT3 monoclonal antibody in cardiac transplant patients. *Dimensions of Critical Care Nursing, 10*(3), 126–132.

*Werb, Z., & Goldstein, I. (1987). Phagocytic cells: Chemotaxis and effector functions of macrophages and granulocytes. In D. Stites, J. Stobo, & J. Wells (Eds.), *Basic and clinical immunology* (6th ed.). Norwalk, CT: Appleton & Lange.

Workman, M. (1993). The immune system: Your defensive partner and offensive foe. *AACN Clinical Issues in Critical Care, 4*(3), 568–593.

Workman, M., Ellerhorst-Ryan, J., & Koertge, V. (1993). *Nursing care of the immunocompromised patient.* Philadelphia: W. B. Saunders.

SUGGESTED READINGS

*Gallucci, B. (1987). The immune system and cancer. *Oncology Nursing Forum, 14*(Suppl.), 3.

Although this is an older article, it remains a classic for its concise explanation of the relationship between immune function and cancer development. The author presents concepts about immunosurveillance and surveillance failure in a "user friendly" fashion.

Gawlikowski, J. (1992). White cells at war. *American Journal of Nursing, 92*(3), 44–51.

This well-written article provides a basic overview of immune function and common conditions of altered immune function. Hints on interpreting laboratory data are included, as is practical clinical information. A self-assessment test using a case study presentation format is included.

Workman, M. (1993). The immune system: Your defensive partner and offensive foe. *AACN Clinical Issues in Critical Care, 4*(3), 568–593.

The major focus of this article is the tissue-damaging actions of uncontrolled immune system activity. The pathophysiologic mechanism of chronic inflammation, autoimmunity, and hypersensitivity reactions is explained, and clinical examples are presented for illustration.

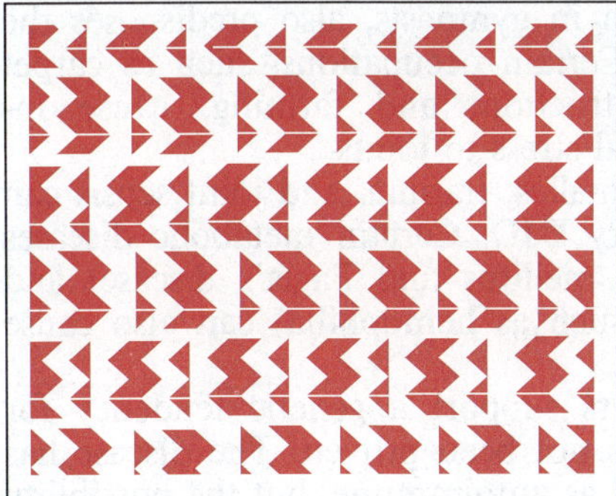

CHAPTER 23

Interventions for Clients with Connective Tissue Disease

CHAPTER HIGHLIGHTS

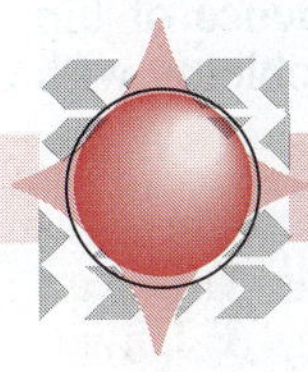

Connective tissue disease (CTD) is the major focus of *rheumatology,* the study of rheumatic disease. According to the American Rheumatism Association classification, any disease or condition involving the musculoskeletal system is categorized as a *rheumatic disease* (Schumacher, 1988). In this text, CTDs are discussed separately from musculoskeletal conditions because most CTDs are classified as probably autoimmune.

More than 37 million people in the United States, or 1 in 7, have one or more of over 100 CTDs. The primary clinical manifestation of most of these diseases is *arthritis,* the inflammation of one or more joints. Consequently, the diseases are often incorrectly referred to as arthritis. Some CTDs present with additional localized clinical manifestations, whereas others are systemic. Management of clients with CTDs requires an interdisciplinary approach, including medicine, surgery, nursing, and physical and occupational therapy.

Degenerative Joint Disease

OVERVIEW

Several terms describe the most common connective tissue disease, degenerative joint disease (DJD). *Osteoarthritis* (OA) and *osteoarthrosis* are used interchangeably with DJD; however, this condition is not a primary inflammatory disease, and thus osteoarthritis is not the most accurate term.

PATHOPHYSIOLOGY

Degenerative joint disease (DJD) is characterized by the progressive deterioration of and loss of articular cartilage in peripheral and axial joints. It is caused by prolonged or excessive use of these joints. Weight-bearing joints (hips and knees), the vertebral column, and hands are primarily affected because they are used most often and/or bear the stress of body weight. Therefore, DJD is also known as the "wear and tear disease." Most clients have the *primary* form of the disease, but *secondary* DJD can result from other musculoskeletal conditions or from trauma.

In the affected joints, the normal bluish, translucent cartilage becomes soft, opaque, and yellow. Fissures and pitting develop, and the cartilage thins. As cartilage and bone beneath the cartilage begin to erode, the joint space narrows and osteophyte (bone spur) formation occurs (Fig. 23–1). Inflammatory enzymes enhance tissue deterioration as a result of the alteration in cartilage metabolism. As a result, the repair process is unable to overcome the rapid process of degeneration. Bone cysts and secondary synovitis are common in advanced disease. Eventually, subluxation and joint deformities cause marked immobility, pain, and muscle spasm.

ETIOLOGY

Although the causative mechanisms of degenerative joint disease (DJD) at the cellular level have not been well identified, the risk factors for DJD are known. Aging causes degenerative changes in all tissues of the body; joints that are used most often are affected. Obesity also contributes to the likelihood of degeneration, particularly in the hips and knees, the weight-bearing joints. Overuse or abuse of certain joints causes chronic pain and degeneration. Joint hyperextensibility, as seen in gymnasts, also predisposes the person to DJD. Certain occupations, such as carpet installation, construction, and farming, cause increased mechanical stress to joints.

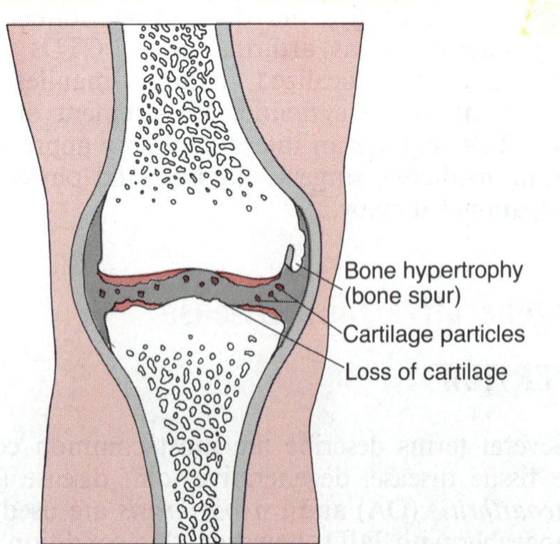

FIGURE 23-1 ◆ Joint changes in degenerative joint disease.

Congenital anomalies, trauma, and joint sepsis can result in secondary DJD. Certain metabolic diseases (such as diabetes mellitus and Paget's disease) and blood disorders (such as hemophilia) can also cause joint degeneration.

Some researchers support a genetic tendency for DJD, but this has not been proven. The disease has not been classified as autoimmune, but the possibility of immune system involvement in its development is being studied.

INCIDENCE/PREVALENCE

More than 20 million people in the United States have symptomatic degenerative joint disease, but probably more than 40 million have degenerative joint changes that can be seen on x-ray examinations. Prevalence increases with age; almost everyone older than age 60 has some degree of symptomatic joint degeneration. Women are affected more often than men. Men usually have the greatest incidence of hip problems, whereas women have more problems with hands.

Transcultural Considerations. Native Americans are affected more often than non–Native American groups, but the reason is unknown (Giger & Davidhizar, 1991; Schumacher, 1988).

COLLABORATIVE MANAGEMENT

ASSESSMENT

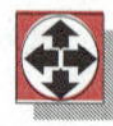

HISTORY

At the initial interview, the nurse collects information from the client that is specifically related to degenerative joint disease (DJD). Because this disease is observed more often in older women, age and sex are important factors for the nursing history. The nurse asks about the client's occupation, nature of work, history of trauma, and current or previous involvement in sports. Even if the client appears to be within the ideal range for body weight, the nurse asks the client about a possible history of obesity. The nurse should also note a family history of "arthritis" because many connective tissue diseases seem to have familial tendencies.

Finally, the nurse determines whether the client has a current or previous medical condition that may cause joint manifestations. As with all musculoskeletal disorders, the nurse asks questions about the course of the disease.

PHYSICAL ASSESSMENT/CLINICAL MANIFESTATIONS

In the early stage of the disease, the clinical manifestations of degenerative joint disease (DJD) may

TABLE 23–1 Differential Features of Rheumatoid Arthritis and Degenerative Joint Disease

Characteristic	Rheumatoid Arthritis	Degenerative Joint Disease
Typical onset	• At 35–45 yr	• At >60 yr
Sex affected	• Female (3:1)	• Female (2:1)
Risk factors or etiology	• Probably autoimmune Emotional stress	• Aging • Obesity • Trauma • Occupation
Disease process	• Inflammatory	• Degenerative
Disease pattern	• Bilateral, symmetric, multiple joints • Usually affects upper extremities first • Distal interphalangeal joints of hands spared • Systemic	• May be unilateral, single joint • Affects weight-bearing joints and hands, spine • Metacarpophalangeal joints spared • Nonsystemic
Laboratory findings	• Elevated rheumatoid factor, antinuclear antibody, ESR	• Normal or slightly elevated ESR
Drug therapy	• Salicylates • NSAIDs • Gold or penicillamine • Corticosteroids • Immunosuppressive agents • Other analgesics	• NSAIDs • Acetaminophen • Other analgesics

ESR, erythrocyte sedimentation rate; NSAIDs, nonsteroidal anti-inflammatory drugs.

appear similar to those of rheumatoid arthritis (RA). As the disease progresses, the distinction between DJD and RA becomes more evident. Table 23–1 differentiates the major characteristics of both diseases and their treatments.

JOINT PAIN The major complaint of the client with DJD is typically joint pain, which early in the course of the disease diminishes after rest and intensifies after activity. Later, the pain occurs with slight motion or even when the person is at rest. Because cartilage has no nerve supply, the pain is probably due to joint and soft-tissue involvement and to spasms of surrounding muscles. During examination of the joints, the nurse can often elicit pain or tenderness by palpation or by putting the joint through range of motion. Crepitus, a continuous grating sensation, may be felt or heard as the joint is put through range of motion. One or more joints are affected. The client may also complain of joint stiffness that lasts *less* than 30 minutes after a period of inactivity.

JOINT CHANGES On inspection, the nurse notes that the joint is frequently enlarged because of bony hypertrophy; rarely does a joint appear to be hot and inflamed. The presence of inflammation in a client with degenerative joint disease usually indicates a secondary synovitis. Approximately 50% of clients with hand involvement display the characteristic Heberden's nodes (at the distal interphalangeal joints) and Bouchard's nodes (at the proximal interphalangeal joints). Although DJD is not a bilateral, symmetric disease, these large bony nodes appear in that pattern, especially in women. The nodes may be painful and red, but some clients do not experience discomfort from their presence. The nodes have a familial tendency and are usually a cosmetic concern to the client. The nodes feel hard when the nurse palpates them; the client may complain of tenderness on palpation.

OTHER CLINICAL MANIFESTATIONS Joint effusions are common when the knees are involved. When trying to differentiate the presence of fluid from subcutaneous tissue, the nurse is able to move fluid from the infrapatellar notch (the area directly below the knee) into the suprapatellar notch (the area directly above the knee). Subcutaneous tissue cannot be relocated.

The nurse also observes skeletal muscle atrophy from disuse. The vicious pain cycle of the disease discourages movement of painful joints, which then results in contractures, muscle atrophy, and further pain.

Degenerative joint disease can also affect the spine, especially the lumbar region at the L3-4 level, or the cervical region at C4-6. Compression of spinal nerve roots may occur as a result of vertebral facet bone spurs. The client typically complains of radiating pain, stiffness, and muscle spasms in one or both extremities. Spinal and vertebral arteries may also become compressed.

In addition to performing a musculoskeletal assessment, the nurse performs a physical assessment of the client with DJD to determine the client's level of mobility and ability to perform activities of daily living (ADL). Severe pain and deformity interfere with ambulation and self-care. (Chapter 13 describes activities of daily living and functional assessment in depth.)

PSYCHOSOCIAL ASSESSMENT

Degenerative joint disease is a chronic condition that may cause permanent changes in the client's lifestyle. A person's inability to care for oneself in advanced disease prevents socialization and results in role changes and other losses. Therefore, the client may exhibit a variety of behaviors indicative of the grieving process, such as anger and depression (see Chap. 12).

The client may experience a role change in the family, workplace, or both. The nurse asks the client about his or her roles before the disease developed to identify changes that have been or need to be made. The nurse and client mutually determine problem areas and adjustment in lifestyle that may still be needed as a result of the disease.

In addition to role change, joint deformities and bony nodules often cause an alteration in body image and self-esteem. The nurse observes the client's response to body changes: Does the client ignore them or seem overly occupied with them? How does the client refer to the changes—with anger, degradation, or humor? These clues help the nurse to assess the client's acceptance of body alterations. (For further discussion of the assessment of body image, see Chap. 10.)

LABORATORY ASSESSMENT

There are no significant laboratory tests for degenerative joint disease. The erythrocyte sedimentation rate (ESR) may be slightly elevated when secondary synovitis occurs (see Table 49–2).

RADIOGRAPHIC ASSESSMENT

Routine x-rays are useful in determining structural joint changes. Specialized views are obtained when the disease cannot be visualized on standard x-ray but is suspected. A computed tomography (CT) scan may be used to determine vertebral involvement.

OTHER DIAGNOSTIC ASSESSMENT

The physician may order magnetic resonance imaging (MRI) studies of the vertebral column to detect degenerative bony changes in the spine.

ANALYSIS

COMMON NURSING DIAGNOSES

The priority for nursing diagnoses when the nurse is caring for a client with degenerative joint disease (DJD) is:

1. Chronic Pain related to muscle spasm and/or inflammation
2. Impaired Physical Mobility related to pain and muscle atrophy

ADDITIONAL NURSING DIAGNOSES

In addition to the common diagnoses, the client may have secondary problems caused by the pain and immobility common in DJD. These include:

- Activity Intolerance related to pain and fatigue
- Self Care Deficit (partial) related to pain, fatigue, and immobility
- Body Image Disturbance related to effects of loss of body function

PLANNING AND IMPLEMENTATION

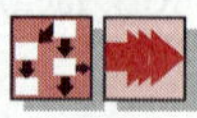

CHRONIC PAIN

PLANNING: CLIENT GOALS The major concern of the client with degenerative joint disease (DJD) is pain control. Therefore, the goal is that the client will experience a reduction in chronic pain.

INTERVENTIONS Pain control may be accomplished by drug and nondrug measures. If these measures become ineffective, surgery may be performed to reduce pain.

Nonsurgical Management Management of chronic joint pain is difficult for both the client and the health care professional. A combination of modalities is often used. Chapter 8 elaborates on methods of pain control for chronic pain.

Drug Therapy The purpose of drug therapy is to reduce pain, relieve muscle spasm, and reduce secondary inflammation if present. The drug class of choice is usually nonsteroidal anti-inflammatory drugs (NSAIDs) (Chart 23–1). Acetaminophen (Tylenol, Atasol*) may also be used. For temporary relief of pain in a single joint, the physician may inject the joint with a corticosteroid, such as cortisone. Muscle relaxants, such as cyclobenzaprine HCl (Flexeril), are sometimes given for severe muscle spasms, especially spasms occurring in the back. Potent analgesics are not usually appropriate for the client with DJD because of the chronic nature of the pain.

Rest Several types of rest are used to treat clients with DJD:

- *Local* rest involves the immobilization of a joint with a splint or brace. If a joint becomes acutely inflamed, the joint is rested until inflammation subsides. The nurse or physician consults the occupational therapist (OT), who fits the client for the appropriate device and explains its use.
- *Systemic* rest refers to the immobilization of the entire body, such as a nap. The nurse teaches the client about the importance of sleeping about 10 hours and, if possible, resting an additional 1 to 2 hours each day.
- *Psychologic* rest is equally important because it allows relief from daily stresses that can enhance pain.

Chapter 7 describes methods for relaxation and strategies for coping that the nurse can use to teach clients.

CHART 23-1

Drug Therapy for Connective Tissue Disease

Drug	Usual Dosage	Nursing Interventions	Rationale
Salicylates, e.g., aspirin, buffered aspirin (Ecotrin, Ascriptin, Ancasal*)	12–18 tablets/d (4–6 g) are given in divided doses to achieve therapeutic effect.	• Give with meals or snacks.	• Aspirin products can cause gastrointestinal problems, including bleeding and ulcers, because of increased stomach acid production. Drugs can damage eighth cranial nerve and prevent platelet aggregation, which causes clotting.
		• Instruct client to observe for tinnitus, bleeding, or bruising (especially seen in *elderly* clients). Teach client to use soft-bristled toothbrush.	• Gums may bleed easily because of decreased clotting.
NSAIDs, e.g., naproxen (Naprosyn, Apo-Naproxen*), sulindac (Clinoril), indomethacin (Indocin, Apo-Indomethacin*), ibuprofen (Motrin, Advil, Amersol*), mefenamic acid (Ponstel, Ponstan*), phenylbutazone (Butazolidin, Novobutazone*), piroxicam (Feldene, Apo-Piroxicam*), diclofenac sodium (Voltaren), flurbiprofen (Ansaid)	Dose varies depending on which drug is used. Piroxicam and naproxen are given in fewer doses because of longer half-life. Indomethacin and phenylbutazone are not as commonly used because of tendencies to cause peptic ulcer and CNS changes.	• Same as for salicylates above.	• Same as for salicylates above.
		• In addition, observe for fluid retention, increased blood pressure, and changes in renal function.	• Most NSAIDs cause sodium retention, which can lead to edema formation, hypertension, renal damage, and/or congestive heart failure. Drugs should be used with caution in *elderly* population.
		• Monitor electrolyte and complete blood count values.	• Most NSAIDs cause increased sodium levels and can cause bone marrow suppression.
		• Observe for CNS changes, e.g., dizziness or confusion.	• Most NSAIDs can cause CNS effects, especially in the *elderly*.
		• If a client is taking aspirin *and* an NSAID or is taking two NSAIDs, observe carefully for side effects or toxic effects.	• Drugs are often used in combination, especially in clients with rheumatoid arthritis. Additive effects can cause serious complications.
Gold			
Auranofin (Ridaura)	Dose is 3 mg bid PO.	• Observe for and instruct client to report gastrointestinal problems, such as diarrhea, nausea/vomiting, abdominal cramping.	• This side effect causes discomfort and can lead to electrolyte imbalance.
Gold sodium thiomalate (water-based gold) (Myochrysine)	After a 10-mg test dose, 25 mg and then 50 mg is given every week until monthly maintenance of 50 mg IM is reached.	• Observe for rash or other skin change and for mouth ulceration (stomatitis).	• Drug may be discontinued for a short period, then restarted.
Aurothioglucose (oil-based gold) (Solganal)	Same as for gold sodium thiomalate. If total of 1000 mg is used and no clinical change is seen, gold is discontinued.	• Instruct client to expect metallic taste in mouth; teach importance of proper mouth care.	• Proper, frequent mouth care reduces risk of stomatitis and metallic taste.
		• Monitor urine for pro-	• These changes indicate

Chart continued on following page

CHART 23-1

Drug Therapy for Connective Tissue Disease *Continued*

Drug	Usual Dosage	Nursing Interventions	Rationale
		tein and serum for CBC. If CBC is markedly decreased or if proteinuria is present, discontinue drug.	serious toxic effects, and drug needs to be discontinued.
		• Give *deep* IM, preferably by Z-track technique.	• Drug is locally irritating to soft tissue.
		• After IM administration, observe for nitroid crisis, a form of anaphylactic reaction.	• Flushing, dyspnea, and anxiety may occur shortly after drug administration.
Hydroxychloroquine sulfate (Plaquenil)	200 mg PO each day is given.	• Instruct client to have frequent (every 3–6 mo) ophthalmologic examination.	• Drug can cause retinal damage.
Penicillamine (Cuprimine)	125–250 mg PO each day is used (may be given in two divided doses).	• Same as for IM gold, except no nitroid crisis occurs.	• Same as for IM gold.
Immunosuppressive agents, e.g., azathioprine (Imuran), cyclophosphamide (Cytoxan, Procytox✱), methotrexate (Mexate)	Dose varies depending on disease activity and route of drug administration.	• Observe for side effects and toxic effects, including, but not limited to, nausea/vomiting, bone marrow suppression, and alopecia.	• Side effects and toxic effects of these drugs can be devastating. Drugs are reserved for severe forms of CTDs in which organ involvement is potentially life-threatening.
		• Teach client to avoid crowds and people with infections such as influenza.	• Bone marrow suppression or immune suppression increases risk of infection.
Prednisone (Deltasone, Apo-Prednisone✱)	Dose is 10–150 mg PO each day. For maintenance, attempt to give dose every *other* day (to allow client's adrenal glands to function).	• Observe for cushingoid changes, e.g., moon-face, buffalo hump, striae, acne, thin skin, bruising, fluid retention, and increased blood pressure.	• These changes are expected and tend to be dose-related. Changes diminish as dose decreases.
		• Monitor electrolyte and glucose levels.	• Chronic steroid therapy can cause sodium or fluid retention, potassium depletion, and elevated glucose level.
		• Observe for long-term effects of chronic steroid therapy, such as osteoporosis, cataracts, hypertension, diabetes, or impaired healing.	• These complications may need to be treated with other drugs or modalities.
		• Teach client to avoid crowds and individuals with infections such as influenza.	• Drug suppresses immune system (lymphocytes) and increases risk of infection or decreased healing.

Positioning Joints should be placed in their functional position, which may not be the position of comfort. When the client is in a supine position (recumbent), the nurse places a small pillow under the client's head or neck but avoids the use of other pillows. The client may quickly experience flexion contractures from the use of large pillows under the knees or head. If needed, the client's legs may be elevated 8 to 12 inches (20.3 to 30.5 cm) to reduce back discomfort. Lying prone twice a day is recommended if the client can tolerate that position. The nurse also reminds the client to use proper posture when standing and sitting to reduce undue strain on the vertebral column.

Heat The client with degenerative joint disease generally uses heat instead of cold to reduce pain. Cold application is usually reserved for acutely inflamed joints. The nurse can provide comfort to the client with hot showers and baths, hot packs or compresses, and moist heating pads. Regardless of treatment, the nurse ensures that the heat source is not too heavy or so hot as to cause burns. A temperature just above the body's temperature is adequate to promote comfort. The nurse also controls the temperature of the client's room so that the client does not experience a chill. A physical therapist provides special heat treatments, such as paraffin dips, diathermy (use of electrical current), and ultrasound (use of sound waves). Usually a 15- to 20-minute heat application is sufficient to temporarily reduce pain, spasm, and stiffness.

Diet Therapy There is no "arthritis diet," as has been proposed by the media and uninformed authors. The nurse explains which foods are high in protein and vitamin C to promote tissue healing. In addition, the nurse encourages obese clients to lose weight to lessen stress on weight-bearing joints. Less weight reduces pain and slows the disease process in affected joints. If needed, the nurse collaborates with the dietitian to provide more in-depth client teaching about nutrition and meal planning.

Other Pain Relief Measures Additional measures may be used for pain reduction. A transcutaneous electrical nerve stimulator (TENS) may be particularly helpful for vertebral involvement. The physician collaborates with the nurse and physical therapist to determine whether the client might benefit from this pain management modality. The client must be able to control the TENS unit for pain relief.

Clients may also use acupuncture, hypnosis, music therapy, and imagery for pain relief (see Chap. 8).

Surgical Management When all other measures are inadequate to provide pain control for clients with DJD, surgery may be indicated. The two major surgical procedures performed for these clients are osteotomy and total joint replacement (TJR).

Osteotomy During an osteotomy, the surgeon cuts the bone to correct joint deformity and promote realignment. Joint deformity causes pain and abnormal stress on bone ends in people with DJD.

Preoperative Care. The preoperative care for a client undergoing an osteotomy is similar to that provided for the client who is having an open reduction internal fixation (ORIF) (see Chap. 51).

Operative Procedure. As shown in Figure 23-2, in an osteotomy, the surgeon removes or inserts a bone wedge or rotates the bone to correct weight-bearing abnormalities. Hip and knee operations are performed most often.

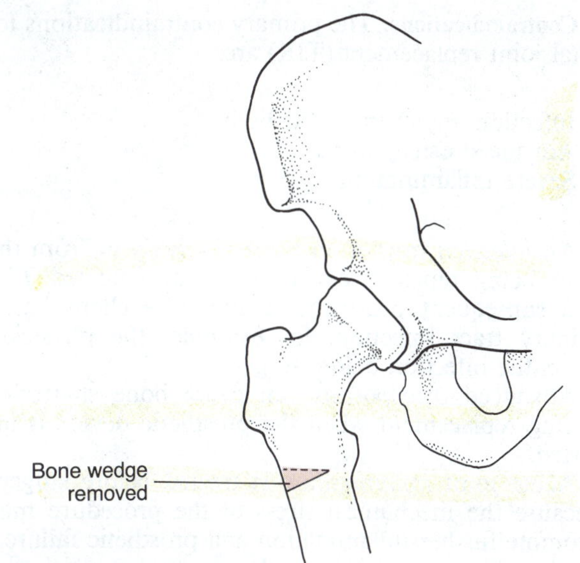

FIGURE 23-2 ♦ An intertrochanteric (hip) osteotomy accomplished by removal of bone wedge.

Postoperative Care. If the client has a hip osteotomy the postoperative care is similar to that described in Chapter 51 for open reduction internal fixation of the hip. A client undergoing knee surgery generally has a tibial osteotomy to correct valgus (bowleg) or varum (knock-knee) deformities. The affected leg is wrapped with an elastic bandage from groin to heel, and one or two surgical drains remain in place until the bulky pressure dressing is removed. A knee immobilizer prevents the knee from flexing. The surgeon may use a hard or soft cast instead of the bandage and immobilizer. The surgeon and physical therapist determine the type of weight bearing and exercise. The client typically uses crutches for ambulation.

Total Joint Replacement (TJR) Any synovial joint of the body can be replaced with a prosthetic system consisting of at least two parts, one for each joint surface. A TJR is the major type of arthroplasty (surgical creation of a joint) that is performed.

Indications. Total joint replacement is a procedure of last resort for pain management; it is used when all other methods of pain relief have been unsuccessful. Hips and knees are most commonly replaced, but replacements of finger and wrist joints, elbows, shoulders, and toe joints and ankles have become more popular in the past 20 years.

Although TJRs are performed most often for clients with degenerative joint disease, other conditions causing joint damage may also require surgery. These disorders include rheumatoid arthritis, congenital anomalies, trauma, and avascular necrosis—bony necrosis secondary to lack of blood flow, usually from trauma or chronic steroid therapy.

Contraindications. The primary contraindications for total joint replacement (TJR) are:

- Infection anywhere in the body
- Advanced osteoporosis
- Severe inflammation

An *infection* from a source in the body or from the joint being replaced can result in an infected TJR and subsequent prosthetic failure. If a client has a urinary tract infection, for example, the physician treats the infection before surgery.

Advanced *osteoporosis* can cause bone shattering during replacement when the prosthetic device is inserted.

Acute joint *inflammation* is treated before surgery because the mechanical stress of the procedure may promote further inflammation and prosthetic failure.

As a group, total joint replacements are quite successful. Many clients who have lived with chronic, unbearable pain for years and who could not function independently at home or in the workplace no longer experience pain in the diseased joint. The pain relief and psychologic benefit may outweigh the perioperative risks, but the surgeon and client must make that decision. When the client is of advanced age, this decision may become an ethical issue in addition to a physical risk-versus-benefit decision.

TOTAL HIP REPLACEMENT (THR) The most commonly replaced joint is the hip. Clients of any age have the surgery, but the procedure is done most often for clients older than 60. The special needs and normal physiologic changes of elderly clients often complicate the perioperative period and may result in additional postoperative complications. (See Chapters 19 to 21 for routine perioperative care and the special considerations needed for care of the elderly client.)

Preoperative Care. As with any surgical procedure, preoperative care begins with assessment of the client's level of understanding about the impending replacement. The physician explains the procedure and postoperative care expectations during the office visit, but this explanation may have occurred weeks or months before the surgery was scheduled. Elderly clients, in particular, may forget some of the information or may not know what questions to ask. Many orthopedic surgeons employ nurses in the office who can follow up and address any of the client's special concerns.

In addition, nurse educators or orthopedic nurses may lead formal classes in the hospital several weeks before surgery to answer questions and clarify information. During class, the client is shown the prosthesis or a picture of the device and receives written instructions or teaching booklets to reinforce the information.

In some hospitals, the physical therapist can meet the surgical candidate before surgery to explain ambulation and postoperative exercises.

Most clients are admitted on the morning of surgery and do not come to the orthopedic, surgical, or medical-surgical unit until after surgery.

Operative Procedure. Before the start of the procedure, the operating room may be specially cleaned to reduce the risk of infection. The surgery is usually scheduled early in the morning, if possible, and movement into and out of the room is kept to a minimum. The client is given the first dose of intravenous antibiotics, usually a cephalosporin, such as cefotetan (Cefotan), at least an hour before the initial surgical incision is made.

The anesthesiologist or nurse anesthetist places the client under general, epidural, or spinal anesthesia. Epidural or spinal induction reduces the risk of cardiopulmonary complications for which the elderly are at high risk. The 8- to 10-inch (20.3- to 24.5-cm) incision is usually longitudinal on the lateral or anterolateral thigh. A posterior incision may be used instead to preserve muscle, but postoperatively the client is more likely to experience hip dislocation with this incision.

After the client is anesthetized, the surgeon dislocates the hip and removes the natural acetabulum in the pelvis. The area is prepared for the prosthetic acetabular cap, which is usually a metal cup with a plastic insert.

If the prosthesis is *cemented*, polymethyl methacrylate (an acrylic fixating substance) is used. During the surgical procedure, the operative area is irrigated with a cool solution. To help prevent infection, the surgeon may mix an antibiotic with the cement or may use antibiotic impregnated beads to plant deep into the wound. The surgeon also inserts one or two wound drains to remove exudate from the tissues that might serve as a medium for pathogenic growth and cause wound infection.

Advances in Technology. A major advance in joint replacement surgery is the increased use of *noncemented* prostheses. Although polymethyl methacrylate is an excellent initial fixator, it has a finite life span and deteriorates over time, which causes loosening of the implant and pain. The average life span of a cemented hip is 10 years. When a prosthesis eventually loosens and causes pain, it is replaced; this procedure is called a *revision arthroplasty.* To prevent repeated replacements, several devices that do not require a fixating substance have been designed.

The most common mechanism that is used to avoid polymethyl methacrylate is a porous metal coating on the shaft of the femoral component and the back of the acetabular cap. By using a tight fit, known as a "press fit," the surgeon places the implant (prosthesis) snugly against the client's bone tissue. Most of the prostheses used today are custom-designed by computers to match the size of the prosthesis with the size of the client's own joint. Figure 23-3 illustrates a typical noncemented hip replacement system.

New bone tissue grows between the pores of the prosthesis and "grafts" to the device within 6 to 12 weeks. The older the client, the longer the bone grafting may take. This bony ingrowth serves as the

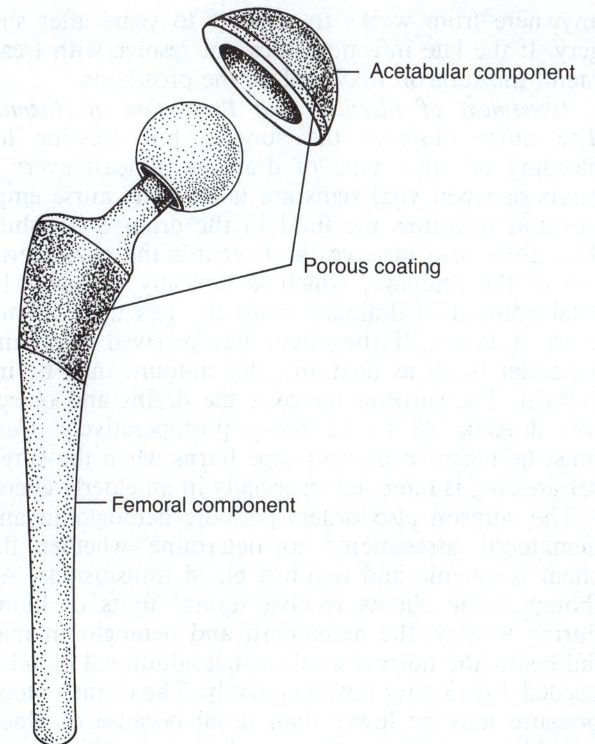

FIGURE 23–3 ◆ Noncemented, porous-coated hip replacement system.

fixating mechanism and, ideally, lasts a lifetime. However, the earliest noncemented total joint systems, which were inserted in the 1970s and 1980s, have needed revisions, primarily because of undersizing of the prosthesis. As a result, the device loosens and is replaced with a new noncemented device. Freeze-dried bone grafts (*allografts*) are used to fill in bony defects that result from removing the old prosthesis. During the healing process, the essentially dead bone revascularizes and grafts with the client's own bone. Clients over the age of 75 and/or those who do not have sufficient bone mass are usually not candidates for the noncemented hip.

Postoperative Care. In addition to providing the routine postoperative care discussed in Chapter 21, the nurse assesses for and assists in the prevention of postoperative complications that could occur after a joint replacement. Table 23–2 summarizes common postoperative complications of total hip replacement surgery, including nursing measures for prevention, assessment, and intervention. Chart 23–2 highlights special concerns for the care of the elderly in the postoperative period.

Prevention of Dislocation. The most common complication of total hip replacement is subluxation (partial dislocation) or total dislocation. Therefore, correct positioning is maintained at all times. When the client returns from the postanesthesia care unit (PACU), the nurse places the client in a supine position with the head slightly elevated. The nurse may place a trapezoid-shaped abduction pillow, wedge, or splint, with or without straps, between the client's legs to prevent adduction beyond the body's midline. In some hospitals, this device is no longer used because it is uncomfortable for the client and not necessary in most cases. Abduction devices are reserved for clients who are very restless or who are unable to follow instructions, especially the elderly. One or two regular bed pillows are used instead for most clients.

The nurse may place and support the affected leg in neutral rotation by using a device such as the cradle boot. The cradle boot not only prevents rotation but also elevates the leg to the desired functional position and keeps the client's heel off the bed linen to prevent heel tissue breakdown. Keeping the heels off the bed is particularly important for the elderly client who is at a high risk for pressure sores.

The nurse turns the client toward either side as long as the abduction or other pillow is in place. Some surgeons allow turning directly onto one side or the other. This policy varies, depending on the surgeon's preference and the policy of the hospital unit.

The nurse observes the client for possible signs of hip dislocation, which include increased hip pain, shortening of the affected leg, and leg rotation. If any

TABLE 23–2 Nursing Interventions to Prevent Complications of Total Joint Replacement Surgery

Complication	Prevention/Interventions
Dislocation	• Position correctly. • For hip, keep legs slightly abducted. • For hip, prevent hip flexion beyond 90 degrees. • Assess for pain, rotation, and/or extremity shortening. • Keep client in bed. • Report immediately to physician.
Infection	• Use aseptic technique for wound care and emptying of drains. • Wash hands thoroughly when caring for client. • Culture drainage fluid. • Monitor temperature. • Report excessive inflammation and/or drainage to physician.
Deep vein thrombosis/ pulmonary embolism	• Have client wear elastic stockings and/or sequential compression stockings. • Teach leg exercises to client. • Encourage fluid intake. • Observe for signs of thrombosis (redness, swelling, or pain). • Test for Homans' sign with client's legs flexed. • Observe client for changes in mental status. • Keep client in bed. • Do not massage legs. • Do not use knee gatch on bed.
Hypotension, bleeding, or infection caused by use of polymethyl methacrylate	• Take vital signs at least every 4 h. • Observe client for bleeding. • Report excessively low blood pressure or bleeding to physician.

CHART 23–2

Nursing Focus on the Elderly ♦ Total Hip Replacement

- Use an abduction pillow or splint to prevent adduction after surgery if the client is very restless or has an altered mental state.
- Keep the client's heels off of the bed to prevent pressure sores.
- Do not rely on fever as a sign of infection; elderly clients often have infection without fever. Decreasing mental status typically occurs when the client has an infection.
- When assisting the client out of bed, move the client slowly to prevent orthostatic (postural) hypotension.
- Encourage the client to deep breathe and cough, and use the incentive spirometer every 2 hours to prevent atelectasis and pneumonia.
- As soon as permitted, get the client out of bed to prevent complications of immobility.
- Anticipate the client's need for pain medication, especially if the client is unable to verbalize the need for pain control.
- Expect a temporary change in mental state immediately after surgery as a result of the anesthesia and unfamiliar sensory stimuli. Reorient the client frequently.

of these clinical manifestations occurs, the nurse keeps the client in bed and notifies the surgeon immediately. The surgeon relocates the affected hip after the client is anesthetized. The hip is then immobilized by an abduction splint or other device until healing occurs.

Prevention of Infection. The second most common potential complication of hip replacement is infection, although this is the *most* common problem when all types of total joint replacements are considered. As soon as the client's bowel sounds return and the client is voiding in sufficient quantity, the nurse converts the intravenous catheter to a heparin or saline lock for the intermittent administration of antibiotics for 24 hours to prevent infection per the physician's order.

The nurse also monitors the surgical incision and vital signs carefully—every 4 hours for the first several days and every 8 hours thereafter. The nurse observes for signs of infection, such as elevated temperature and excessive or foul-smelling drainage from the incision. An elderly client may not have a fever with infection but may experience an altered mental state instead. The nurse obtains a sample of the drainage for culture and sensitivity to determine the offending organisms and the antibiotics that may be needed for treatment.

An infection that occurs during hospitalization is referred to as an "early" infection. If an early infection occurs, the surgeon usually prescribes intravenous antibiotic therapy. "Late" infection can occur anywhere from weeks to months to years after surgery. If the late infection does not resolve with treatment, the surgeon may replace the prosthesis.

Assessment of Bleeding and Prevention of Anemia. The nurse observes the surgical hip dressing for bleeding or other type of drainage at least every 4 hours or when vital signs are taken. The nurse empties and measures the fluid in the drain every shift. The nurse also observes and records the characteristics of the drainage, which is typically bloody. The total amount of drainage is usually less than 50 mL every 8 hours. If the client has received a plasma expander (such as dextran), this amount may be increased. The surgeon removes the drains and operative dressing 48 to 72 hours postoperatively. Care must be taken to prevent tape burns when the surgical dressing is removed, especially in an elderly client.

The surgeon also orders periodic hemoglobin and hematocrit assessments to determine whether the client is anemic and requires blood transfusions. Although some clients receive several units of blood during surgery, the hematocrit and hemoglobin may fall below the normal level so that additional blood is needed 2 or 3 days postoperatively. The client's blood pressure may be lower than usual because of blood loss during surgery or the use of cement, which tends to dilate blood vessels and cause hypotension. Because total joint replacements are elective procedures, autologous blood transfusions are common (see Chap. 20).

The cell saver may also be used during surgery or in the early postoperative period. With this device, the client's drainage can be reinfused to prevent anemia (see Chap. 20).

Assessment for Neurovascular Compromise. As with other bone surgery, frequent neurovascular assessments, which are performed at the same time as vital signs are checked, are necessary to monitor for possible compromise in circulation to the distal extremity (see Chart 51–3).

Management of Incisional Pain. Although hip replacement is performed to relieve joint pain, the client experiences pain related to the surgical procedure. Many clients state that they have pain after surgery but that it is a different type and less excruciating than the pain before surgery. Pain control may be achieved by epidural analgesia, patient-controlled analgesia (PCA), intramuscular opioid analgesia, or a combination of techniques.

(Chapter 8 details these techniques as well as the nursing care associated with each type. Chapter 21 contains a chart of commonly used opioid analgesics and related nursing interventions.)

The nurse anticipates the elderly client's need for pain medication if he or she cannot verbalize the need. Many elderly clients experience several days of increased disorientation or delirium as a result of surgery and anesthesia.

Regardless of the pain management method used, most clients do not require parenteral analgesia after the first few days. Oral opioids, such as oxycodone (Supeudol✱), or oxycodone plus acetaminophen (Percocet, Tylox) are then commonly prescribed until the client's pain can be controlled by nonsteroidal anti-inflammatory drugs, such as ibuprofen (Motrin, Apo-Ibuprofen♣).

Progression of Activity. The client with a total hip replacement is usually allowed to get out of bed the day after surgery. Activities that are permitted differ among surgeons and hospitals, but prolonged bed rest can cause numerous complications, such as atelectasis and pneumonia, especially in the elderly. When getting the client out of bed, the nurse stands on the same side of the bed as the client's affected leg. After achieving a sitting position, the client stands on the unaffected leg and pivots to the chair with assistance. To prevent hip dislocation (Fig. 23–4), the nurse at all times ensures that the client does not flex the hips beyond 90 degrees. Raised toilet seats, straight-back chairs, and reclining wheelchairs help prevent hyperflexion.

The surgeon, the type of prosthesis, and the surgical approach all determine the resumption of weight bearing on the affected leg. A client with a cemented implant is usually allowed partial weight bearing (PWB) or weight bearing to tolerance immediately. A client with an uncemented prosthesis cannot tolerate weight until bony ingrowth occurs. Toe-touch weight bearing only is typically permitted for the first 6 weeks or until there is x-ray evidence of bony ingrowth. Toe-touch weight bearing is usually defined as less than 20% weight bearing on the affected leg.

The physical therapist (PT) teaches the client how to follow these weight-bearing restrictions and, if possible, helps the client progress to full-weight-bearing (FWB) status. Most clients generally use a walker, although young clients may use crutches.

Prevention of Thromboembolitic Complications. Because the client does not resume full activity for several weeks, the risk of developing lower extremity or pelvic thrombi is high. Elderly clients are especially at increased risk for thrombi because of age and compromised circulation before surgery. Obese clients or those with a history of deep vein thrombi are also at high risk for thrombi. In clients with total hip replacement, thrombi usually develop in the thigh; these thrombi become life-threatening emboli more readily than calf and other thrombi. For this reason,

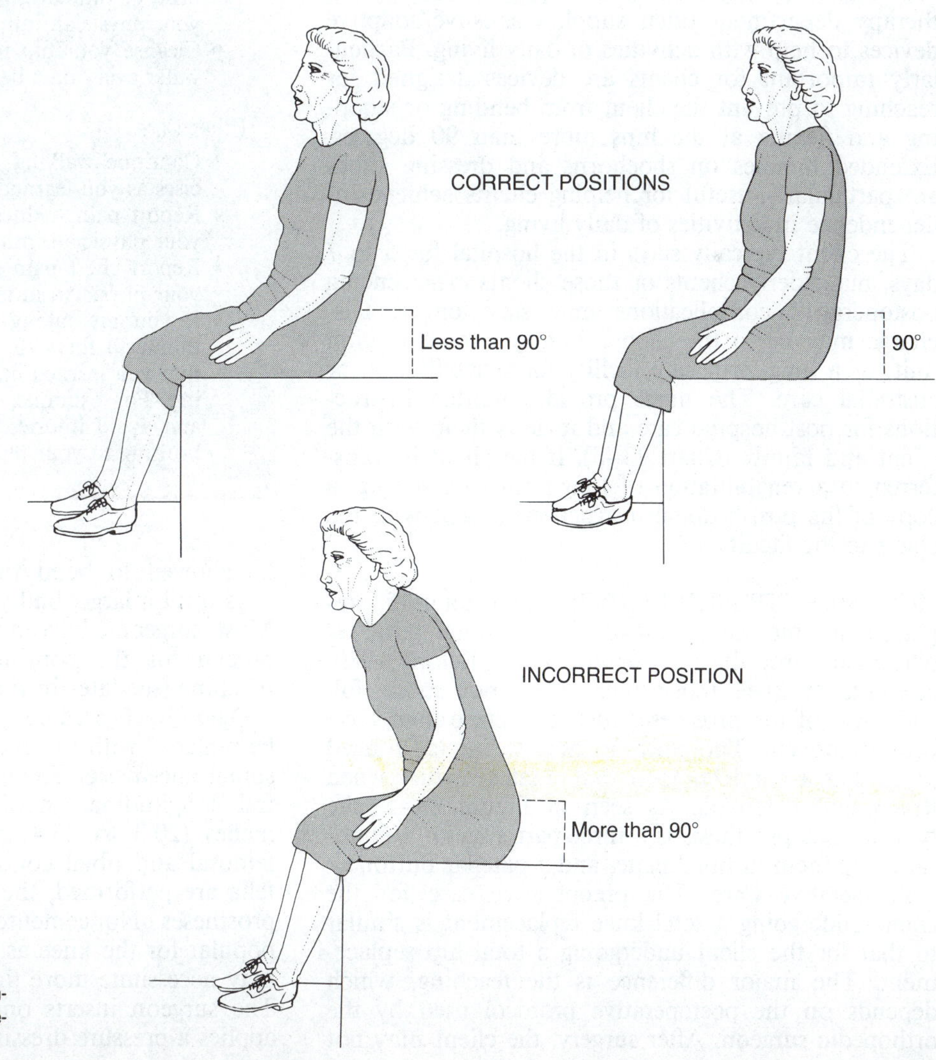

FIGURE 23–4 ◆ Correct and incorrect hip flexion after a total hip replacement.

thigh-high stockings, elastic bandages, and/or sequential compression devices (SCDs) are used during the hospital stay (see Chap. 19).

Anticoagulants, such as aspirin (Ecotrin or buffered aspirin), warfarin (Coumadin, Warfilone♣), or subcutaneous heparin (Hepalean♣), are prescribed in maintenance doses. The nurse and physician monitor the prothrombin time (PT) if the client is taking warfarin and monitors partial thromboplastin time (PTT) if the client is receiving heparin.

The physical therapist or nurse or both teach leg exercises, which are begun in the immediate postoperative period and continue until the client is fully ambulatory. These exercises include plantar flexion and dorsiflexion (heel pumping), circumduction (circles) of the feet, gluteal and quadriceps muscle setting, and straight-leg raises (SLRs). The client performs gluteal exercises by pushing the heels into the bed. The client achieves quadriceps-setting exercises ("quad sets") by straightening the legs and pushing the back of the knees into the bed. In addition to preventing clots, these exercises improve muscle tone, which aids in restoration of function of the extremity.

(Prevention of thrombi is discussed in detail in Chapter 35.)

Promotion of Self-Care. The hospital's occupational therapy department often supplies assistive/adaptive devices to help with activities of daily living. Particularly important for clients are devices designed for reaching to prevent the client from bending or stooping and flexing at the hips more than 90 degrees. Extended handles on shoehorns and dressing sticks are particularly useful for helping clients achieve independence in activities of daily living.

The client typically stays in the hospital for 5 to 7 days, but elderly clients or those clients experiencing postoperative complications may stay longer. Discharge may be to the client's home, a rehabilitation unit, or a long-term care facility for rehabilitation or custodial care. The nurse provides written instructions for post-hospital care and reviews them with the client and family (Chart 23–3). If the client is transferred to a rehabilitation or long-term care setting, a copy of the post-hospital instructions is sent with the client to the facility.

CHART 23–3

Education Guide ◆ Total Hip Replacement

Hip Precautions

- Do not sit or stand for prolonged periods.
- Do not cross your legs beyond the midline of your body.
- Do not bend your hips more than 90 degrees.
- Use an ambulatory aid, such as a walker, when walking.
- Use assistive/adaptive devices for dressing, such as for putting on shoes and socks.
- You can resume sexual intercourse as usual, but when doing so, use the hip precautions that you learned in the hospital.

Pain Management

- Report increased hip pain to the physician immediately.
- Take oral analgesics, as prescribed, only as needed.
- Do not overexert yourself; take frequent rests.

Incisional Care

- Inspect your hip incision every day for redness, heat, or drainage; if any of these are present, call your physician immediately.
- Cleanse your hip incision with a mild soap and water every day; be sure to dry it thoroughly.

Other Care

- Continue walking and performing the leg exercises as you learned in the hospital.
- Report pain, redness, or swelling in your legs to your physician immediately.
- Report chest pain and/or shortness of breath to your physician immediately.
- If you are taking an anticoagulant (or "blood thinner") for 4–6 weeks, follow the precautions that you learned in the hospital to prevent bleeding. For example, avoid using a straight razor; and avoid injuries. Report bleeding or excessive bruising to your physician immediately.

TOTAL KNEE REPLACEMENT (TKR) After total hip replacement, the second most common total joint replacement procedure is for the knee. Before 1980, attempts at knee replacement were not successful, and most of the prostheses inserted before then have been removed. The knee is not a simple, hinged joint; it is a condylar joint that rotates slightly when flexed and extended. As seen in Figure 23–5, the typical knee prosthesis is a three-part system: a femoral component, a tibial plate, and a patellar button.

Preoperative Care. The preoperative care for the client undergoing a total knee replacement is similar to that for the client undergoing a total hip replacement. The major difference is the teaching, which depends on the postoperative protocol used by the orthopedic surgeon. After surgery, the client may not be allowed to bend the operative knee for several days until a large, bulky pressure dressing is removed. Most surgeons have abandoned this traditional approach for the continuous passive motion (CPM) machine (see later in this chapter).

Operative Procedure. As with the hip, the knee can be replaced with the client under general, epidural, or spinal anesthesia. The surgeon typically makes a central longitudinal incision, approximately 8 to 10 inches (20.3 to 25.4 cm) long. Osteotomies of the femoral and tibial condyles and of the posterior patella are performed; the surfaces are prepared for the prostheses. Noncemented implants are becoming as popular for the knee as they are for the hip, but they may necessitate more time for the surgical procedure. The surgeon inserts one or two surgical drains and applies a pressure dressing to prevent bleeding.

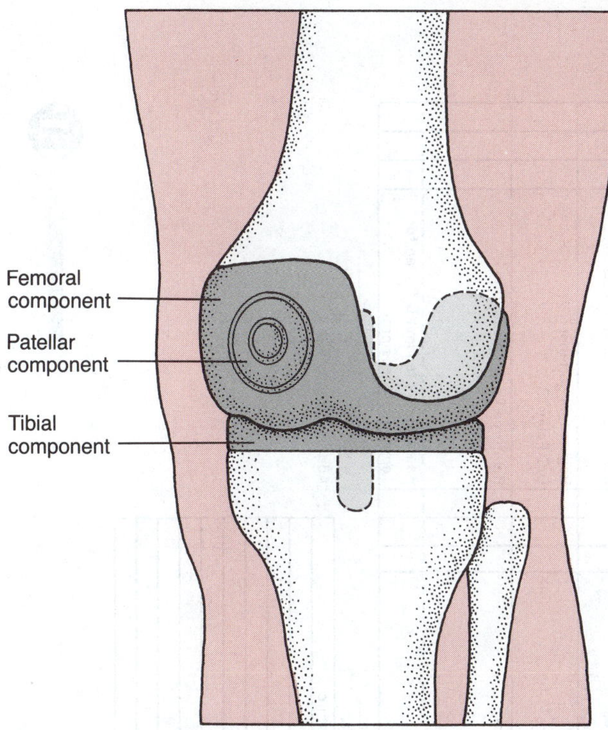

FIGURE 23-5 ◆ Typical three-part condylar knee replacement system.

CHART 23-4

Nursing Care Highlight ◆ The Client Using a Continuous Passive Motion (CPM) Machine

- Ensure that the machine is well padded with sheepskin or other similar material.
- Check the cycle and range-of-motion settings at least once per shift (every 8 hours).
- Ensure that the joint being moved is properly positioned on the machine.
- If the client is confused, place the controls to the machine out of the client's reach.
- Assess the client's response to the machine.
- Turn off the machine while the client is having a meal in bed.
- When the machine is not in use, do not store it on the floor.

Postoperative Care. Postoperative nursing care of the client with a total knee replacement is similar to that for the client with a total hip replacement, but maintaining abduction is not necessary. The surgeon orders a continuous passive motion (CPM) machine, which is usually applied in the postanesthesia care unit (PACU), but may not be used until 1 to 2 days after surgery (Fig. 23-6). The CPM keeps the prosthetic knee in motion and prevents scar tissue formation, which could impede mobility of the knee and exacerbate postoperative pain.

The surgeon, physical therapist, or technician presets the CPM machine for the appropriate range of motion and cycles per minute. A typical initial setting is 20 to 30 degrees range of motion at 2 cycles/minute, but this setting varies according to surgeon preference. The machine is generally used for 8 to 12 hours/day, and the range of motion is increased gradually. The current trend is intermittent use for several hours at a time. Each day the nurse notes the client's response to the use of the device.

Some machines do not allow the leg to achieve full extension, thus promoting flexion contractures; however, one solution is for the client to use the CPM machine during the day and sleep in a knee immobilizer at night to achieve the desired extension. Chart 23-4 outlines the nurse's responsibility when caring for a client who is using the CPM machine.

Some facilities have created clinical pathways for clients undergoing total knee replacement. For an example, see pages 472 and 473.

Because dislocation is a rare problem for a client with a total knee replacement, special positioning is not required. Other complications affecting total hip replacement clients may affect these clients as well.

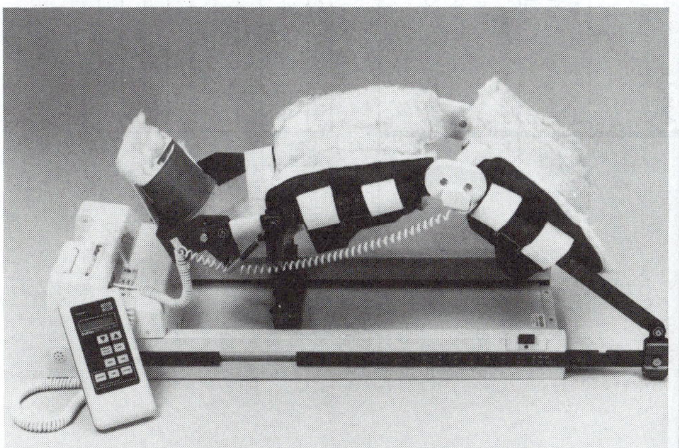

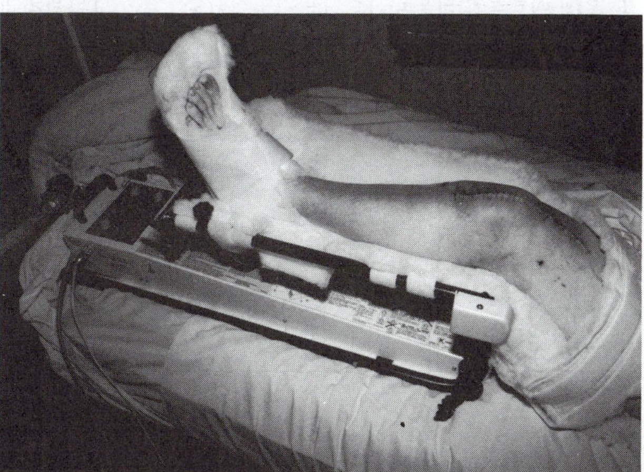

FIGURE 23-6 ◆ Two types of continuous passive motion (CPM) machines, one shown in use after a total knee replacement. (*Left*, Courtesy of Sutter Corporation.)

TOTAL KNEE REPLACEMENT

DATE CARE NEEDED	PREADMISSION	Variance D	Variance E	Variance N	DAY 1 DOS	Variance D	Variance E	Variance N	DAY 2 POD 1	Variance D	Variance E	Variance N
PAIN	Teach: PCA/Epidural/IM Pain Scale				PCA/IM/EPIDURAL				PCA/IM/EPIDURAL			
RESPIRATION	Assess: Actual/Potential inspiration on I.S. (if ordered) Baseline B.S. Teach: C & DB Incentive spirometer (if ordered)				Check BS I.S. per protocol (check for order) TCDB q 2-3 hrs, W.A. O2 prn				Check BS I.S. per protocol (check for order) TCDB q 2-3 hrs, W.A. O2 D/C'd 7-3			
NUTRITION	Assess: Baseline nutrition Teach (Flipchart bklt): NPO pre-op Diet in hospital & post D/C				IV Clear liquids post-op I&O				DAT, with HS supplement if < 50 % tray eaten Decrease IV to TKO			
SELF CARE N	Assess: Present status Teach/Discuss: Pathway routine, consent form				Total Care				Self oral care, hands, face, bedbath			
MOBILITY N	Assess: Upper arm strength, ROM, etc. Teach/Discuss: Positioning, bed exercise, CPM (if ordered)				Active/passive ROM non-op side q 4 hrs Reposition q 2 hrs Trapeze If CPM: Check for CPM position				Transfer to BSC prn If CPM: Check position/settings			
PT	Patient seen by PT for pre-op assessment and teaching ___PT				Review bed exercises & "post" on bed If CPM: Check for CPM set-up ___PT				Exercises per protocol OOB to recliner Ambulate if approp If CPM: Check set-up if started POD1 Increase CPM if started DOS ___PT			
MENTATION	Assess: Baseline mentation				A + O x 3 or baseline				A + O x 3 or baseline			
LABS	CBC with diff and Labs per MD orders				RN check for baseline PT/PTT, if on prophyl.				PT or PTT, if on prophylaxis			
NEUROVASC	Assess: Per NS assessment Measure for TED/SCD hose				Neurovasc check per protocol TED/SCD hose				Neurovasc check per protocol TED/SCD hose			
SKIN/ INFECTION	Assess: For skin breaks Teach: Betadine scrub protocol pre-op				T < 38 Dressing dry & intact Skin intact at pressure sites Call MD if >400cc drainage in 4hrs				T < 38 Dressing dry & intact Skin intact at pressure sites			
ELIMINATION	Assess: Bowel/urine habits Discuss: High fiber diet post-op (Flipchart Booklet)				Cath if O void in 8-12 hrs 2 x ---> insert Foley				Begin stool softener D/C Foley			
DISCHARGE PREPARATION N	Assess: Need for SWS referral per screening criteria Notify SWS if indicated Flipchart Booklet given and reviewed				Reinforce knee precautions				Reinforce knee precautions			
SWS/ VNS									Re-evaluate preadmit D/C plan for appropriateness prn			

___ D ___ E ___ N   ___ D ___ E ___ N   ___ D ___ E ___ N

Init.	Signature	Init.	Signature	Init.	Signature

Addressograph

Variance Codes
A-Not indicated
B-Patient condition
C-Physician order override
D-Equipment/supplies
E-Pt/family decision
F-Family unavailable
G-Scheduling
H-Service not provided
I-Department closed
J-Placement availability
K-Docum. for DC
L-Physician DC plan
Z-Other

CP

DATE CARE NEEDED	DAY 3 POD 2	Variance D	 E	 N	DAY 4 POD 3	Variance D	 E	 N	DAY 5 POD 4	Variance D	 E	 N	DAY 6 POD 5	Variance D	 E	 N
PAIN	D/C PCA @ 0600 or have Anesthesia d/c epidural Begin PO pain meds				PO				PO				PO			
RESPIRATION	Check BS I.S. prn TCDB while awake prn				BS clear or baseline I.S. prn TCDB while awake prn				BS clear or baseline				Assess as indicated			
NUTRITION	RD consult prn. _____RD Heplock IV if PO tolerated DAT, with HS supplement if < 50 % of tray eaten				75% regular diet taken or HS supplement D/C IV as appropriate				75% regular diet taken or HS supplement							
SELF CARE N	ADL's with assist for LE's				Up to sink for ADL's				Shower if approp/Up for ADL's				Shower if approp/Up for ADLs			
OT					OT consult if indicated Assess for D/C assistive device prn ____OT				Order D/C equip prn ____OT							
MOBILITY N	OOB to recliner for 2 meals Ambulate to BR if approp w/crutches, walker, splint per PT If CPM: Check position/settings				Increase ambulation OOB to chair for meals x 2 If CPM: Check position/ settings				Increase ambulation Ambulate to BR & hall OOB to recliner for meals x2 If CPM: Check position/ settings				If CPM: Check position/ settings			
PT	Exercises per protocol Ambulate to recliner/BR Order OT per criteria __Y __N ROM w/pulley or If CPM: Increase CPM __PT				Exercises per protocol Increase ambulation Bathroom transfer Start home exercise program If CPM: Increase CPM __PT				Crutches if approp Increase ambulation Pt (caregiver) in/out CPM & adjust controls indep Home exercise program If CPM: Increase CPM ___PT				Gait training Stairs, if appropriate Home exercise program _____PT Active flexion ____ Active extension ____			
MENTATION	A + O x 3 or baseline				A + O x 3 or baseline				A + O x 3 or baseline				A + O x 3 or baseline			
LABS					PT or PTT if on prophylaxis											
NEUROVASC	Neurovasc check per protocol TEDs/Assess need for SCD's				Neurovasc check per protocol TEDs, D/C SCD's 7-3				Neurovasc check per protocol TEDs				Assess as indicated			
SKIN/ INFECTION	T < 38 Dressing dry & intact Skin intact at pressure sites MD: D/C drain				Afebrile MD to change dressing				Monitor closely for s/s infection Dressing change per orders				Afebrile Assess for s/s infection Dressing change			
ELIMINATION	Stool softener Laxative @ hs if no BM				Stool softener, suppos 3-11; enema if no BM				Continue bowel program							
DISCHARGE PREPARATION N	Notify VNS of TKR patient 7-3 HUC to send message to SWSP1				Review s/s infection, pre-cautions w/pt & caregiver				Review D/C teaching with booklet				D/C instructions: __s/s infection __wound care __precautions __D/C meds (give Med info sheets prn)			
PT	If CPM: Review CPM operation w pt/caregiver ____PT								Order equip prn/home PT referral per criteria/pool prog referral prn ____PT				Review CPM use @ home if approp ______PT			
SWS VNS					Evaluate/revise D/C plan prn VNS review for home PT potential				VNS review for home PT needs							

Variance Codes

A-Not indicated			
B-Patient condition	F-Family unavailable	J-Placement availability	
C-Physician order override	G-Scheduling	K-Docum. for DC	
D-Equipment/supplies	H-Service not provided	L-Physician DC plan	
E-Pt/family decision	I-Department closed	Z-Other	tkr/pathway2

___ D ___ E ___ N (Day 3) ___ D ___ E ___ N (Day 4) ___ D ___ E ___ N (Day 5) ___ D ___ E ___ N (Day 6)

Init	Signature	Init	Signature	Init.	Signature

Clinical Pathway: Total knee replacement. (© Overlake Hospital Medical Center, Bellevue, WA 1994.)

CP

After discharge from the hospital, the client should not hyperflex the knee or kneel for prolonged periods.

TOTAL SHOULDER REPLACEMENT Replacement of the shoulder has not been performed as often as other types of replacement techniques. Because the joint is complex with many articulations, subluxation, or dislocation, is a major complication. The Neer prosthesis is commonly used, with or without cement.

Postoperatively, the client's affected arm is placed in a sling and swathed for 2 to 3 days until the client begins an exercise program to regain range of motion. An alternative to this protocol is use of the continuous passive motion (CPM) machine shortly after surgery (see Chart 23–4). During the first few postoperative days, frequent neurovascular assessments are important.

TOTAL ELBOW REPLACEMENT The elbow replacement is usually successful in increasing range of motion, but infection is common because of extensive tissue cutting during surgery. The Ewald prosthesis is commonly inserted, and the CPM device is often used postoperatively.

FINGER AND WRIST REPLACEMENTS Any joint of the hand can be replaced. The flexible, silicone prostheses are implanted without the use of polymethyl methacrylate because no weight bearing is required for the prostheses.

Postoperatively, a bulky dressing is used for 2 to 4 days, when it is replaced by a dynamic splint, brace, or cast or by a very small CPM machine. Edema formation is controlled if the client elevates the arm as much as possible. The rehabilitation program for finger arthroplasties lasts for months, until normal function and strength return. These procedures are typically performed in specialized hand centers.

Any bone of the wrist can be replaced, including the heads of the radius and ulna. The postoperative pressure dressing is removed in 2 to 3 days, and a splint or short arm cast is applied. The client usually regains full function within 6 to 12 weeks, but lifting may be restricted for a longer period. Occupational therapists are usually involved with upper extremity rehabilitation.

ANKLE AND TOE REPLACEMENTS Because the ankles support approximately 25% of the body's weight, developing an implant that is both small and strong enough to withstand the weight of the body has been difficult. When the ankle is replaced, usually an *arthrodesis,* or bone fusion, is performed for added stability. Replacing the ankle is not a common procedure.

The metatarsal implants are made of silicone and cannot bear excessive weight. Typically, the client has one or more osteotomies and fusions, which are immobilized by wires and a cast while healing occurs. Chapter 50 discusses foot osteotomies and their associated nursing care.

IMPAIRED PHYSICAL MOBILITY

PLANNING: CLIENT GOALS The primary goal is that the client will function independently in performing activities of daily living (ADL) and ambulation.

INTERVENTIONS Management of the client with degenerative joint disease is an interdisciplinary effort. The nurse collaborates with the physical and occupational therapists to meet the goal of independent function. The major interventions include therapeutic exercise and promotion of ADL and ambulation through teaching about health and use of assistive/adpative devices.

Exercise Two types of exercise are recommended for the client with DJD: recreational and therapeutic. Recreational exercise includes hobbies and sports, with no planned purpose other than relaxation. Therapeutic exercise includes carefully planned activities that are designed to improve muscle strength and tone and the range of motion of the joint. Therapeutic exercise can also reduce pain and improve the client's psychologic health.

Certain recreational activities may also be therapeutic, such as doing the breast stroke during swimming to enhance chest and arm muscles. Usually, the physical therapist prescribes exercises for the client with DJD, but the nurse reinforces their techniques and principles. The ideal time for exercise is immediately after the application of heat. To prevent further joint damage, clients should rigorously follow the instructions for exercise outlined in Chart 23–5.

Use of Assistive/Adaptive Devices The physical therapist evaluates the client's need for ambulatory aids,

CHART 23–5

Education Guide ◆ Exercises for Clients with Degenerative Joint Disease or Rheumatoid Arthritis

- Follow the exercise instructions that have been specifically prescribed for you. There are no universal exercises; your exercises have been specifically tailored to your own needs.
- Do your exercises on both "good" and "bad" days. Consistency is important.
- Respect pain. If pain increases as you exercise, stop exercising and report this occurrence to your physician.
- Use active rather than active-assist or passive exercise whenever possible.
- Reduce the number of repetitions when the inflammation is severe (when you have more pain).
- Do not substitute your normal activities or household tasks for the prescribed exercises.
- Avoid resistive exercises when your joints are severely inflamed.

such as canes, walkers, or platform crutches. Although many clients do not like to use these aids or may forget how to use them, these aids help prevent further joint deterioration and pain. An occupational therapist evaluates the client's ability to perform activities of daily living and can provide ideas and devices for assistance. (Chapter 13 describes these assistive/adaptive devices and their uses.)

DISCHARGE PLANNING

HOME CARE PREPARATION

The client with degenerative joint disease (DJD) is not usually hospitalized for the disease itself but for surgical management. However, the client may be admitted for another medical or surgical reason. The nurse considers the problems that are present as a result of arthritis before the client is discharged home. If weight-bearing joints are markedly involved, the client may have difficulty going up or down stairs. Making arrangements to live on one floor with accessibility to all rooms is often the best solution. A home health nurse, physical therapist, and/or occupational therapist assesses the need for structural alterations to the home to accommodate ambulatory aids and to enable the client to perform activities. For example, a kitchen counter may need to be lowered or a seat and handrails to be installed in the shower. If the client has a total hip replacement, an elevated toilet seat is necessary to prevent excessive hip flexion.

HEALTH TEACHING

Learning how to protect the joint is the most important feature of client education. Preventing further damage to joints slows the progression of degenerative joint disease and minimizes pain. The nurse explains general rules of joint protection and cites examples, as in Chart 23–6.

As with other diseases in which drugs and diet therapy are used, the nurse teaches the drug protocol, side effects, and toxic effects to the client and family. The nurse also emphasizes the importance of reducing weight and eating a well-balanced diet to promote tissue healing.

Many clients with "arthritis" become frustrated and desperate about the course of the disease and treatment, and they look for a cure. Unfortunately, there is no cure for these joint diseases, even though tabloids, books, and the media frequently cite "curative" remedies. People spend billions of dollars each year on quackery, including liniments, special diets, and copper bracelets. More hazardous substances, such as snake venom and industrial cleaners, are also advertised as remedies. The nurse instructs the client to always check with The Arthritis Foundation about new "cures." For example, if a client believes that wearing a copper bracelet or eating more foods with a high vitamin C content is helpful, the nurse may encourage the continuation of the practice as long as it is not harmful. If there is a potential for harm, the nurse instructs the client to avoid the modality and provides the rationale for doing so.

CHART 23–6

Education Guide ◆ Instructions for Joint Protection

- Use large joints instead of small ones; for example, place your purse strap over your shoulder instead of grasping the purse with your hand.
- Do not turn a doorknob clockwise. Turn it counterclockwise to avoid twisting your arm and promoting ulnar deviation.
- Use two hands instead of one to hold objects.
- Sit in a chair with a high, straight back.
- When getting out of bed, do not push off with your fingers; use the entire palm of both your hands.
- Do not bend at your waist; bend your knees instead, while keeping your back straight.
- Use long-handled devices, such as a hairbrush with an extended handle.
- Use assistive/adaptive devices, such as Velcro closures and built-up utensil handles, to protect your joints.
- Do not use pillows in bed, except a small one under your head.
- Avoid twisting or wringing your hands.

PSYCHOSOCIAL PREPARATION

With most types of connective tissue disease, clients must live with a chronic, unpredictable, and painful disorder. The client's roles, self-esteem, and body image may be affected by these diseases. Body image is often not as devastating in degenerative joint disease as in the inflammatory arthritic diseases, such as rheumatoid arthritis. The psychosocial component is discussed in more detail under the heading Rheumatoid Arthritis.

HEALTH CARE RESOURCES

The client who has undergone surgery is most likely to need help from community resources. After a joint replacement, the client needs extensive assistance with mobility. The client may be discharged to home, a long-term care facility, or a rehabilitation unit. The nurse collaborates with the social worker and physician to find the best placement for each client. If the client is discharged to home, home health nurses should visit frequently for the first 6 weeks. A nursing assistant may visit the home to help with hygiene-related needs; a physical therapist works with the client on ambulatory and mobility skills. In addition, a client who has had a total hip or knee replacement should not be discharged to home alone. A family member or significant other must be in the home at all times for at least the first 6 weeks, when the client needs the most assistance.

The nurse provides written instructions about the care that is required, regardless of whether the client goes home or to another inpatient facility. For continuity of care, communication with the new care provider is ideal. Arrangements are made so that the client can return to the same acute care hospital if needed.

The Arthritis Foundation is an important community resource for all clients with connective tissue disease. This organization provides information to lay people and health professionals and refers clients and their families to other resources as needed. Local support groups can help clients and their families cope with these diseases.

EVALUATION

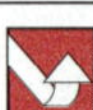

The nurse evaluates the care provided by determining whether the client:

- States that chronic pain is reduced as a result of interdisciplinary interventions
- Ambulates without personal assistance (although a mechanical aid such as a walker may be used)
- Is independent in activities of daily living (may use assistive/adaptive devices)

Rheumatoid Arthritis

OVERVIEW

Rheumatoid arthritis (RA) is the second most common connective tissue disease but is the most destructive to joints. It is a chronic, progressive, systemic inflammatory process that affects primarily synovial joints (see Table 23-1).

PATHOPHYSIOLOGY

The onset of RA is characterized by synovitis, or inflammation of the synovial tissue in joints. The synovium thickens and becomes hyperemic, fluid accumulates in the joint space, and a pannus forms. The pannus is vascular granulation tissue, composed of inflammatory cells, that erodes articular cartilage and eventually destroys bone. As a result, fibrous adhesions, bony ankylosis, and calcifications occur; bone loses density and secondary osteoporosis occur.

If the client is diagnosed early in the course of the disease, permanent joint changes may be avoided. Treatment can cause a remission of the disorder; about 25% of clients experience a remission, which may last as long as 20 years. Clients may also experience spontaneous remissions and exacerbations without treatment.

Rheumatoid arthritis is a systemic disease; that is, areas of the body—in addition to synovial joints—can be affected. Inflammatory responses similar to those occurring in synovial tissue may be seen in any organ or body system in which connective tissue is prevalent. If blood vessel involvement (*vasculitis*) occurs, the organ that is supplied by that vessel can be affected. The result is malfunction and eventual failure of an organ or system. These pathologic changes occur late in the disease process and cause life-threatening problems (see Physical Assessment/Clinical Manifestations).

ETIOLOGY

A number of theories have been formed to explain the pathogenesis of rheumatoid arthritis (RA). The most popular theory to date—the *immune complex hypothesis*—states that unusual antibodies of the immunoglobulin (Ig) G and/or IgM type (rheumatoid factor) develop against IgG antigenic determinants to form complexes that lodge in synovium and other connective tissues. Local and systemic inflammatory responses result. RA has been found to be strongly associated with the human leukocyte antigen (HLA) DRw4. Other antigens have been identified but are observed less frequently. (See Chapter 22 on inflammation and the immune response.)

Although RA is probably an autoimmune disease, the origin of rheumatoid factor is unclear. A *genetic predisposition* for RA is most likely because the disease affects people with a family history of RA two to three times more often than the rest of the population.

Some researchers suspect that female reproductive hormones influence the development of RA because it affects women more often than men. Others suspect that a virus, such as Epstein-Barr, may trigger the autoimmune process. Studies have failed to support these theories. Physical and emotional *stresses* have been linked to exacerbations of the disorder and may be contributing factors in its development.

INCIDENCE/PREVALENCE

Rheumatoid arthritis affects 3% of the world's population and affects women three times more often than men. Women who are taking or who have taken oral contraceptives are less likely to have RA. The *onset* of the disease is typically between ages 35 and 45 years, but it can occur at any age. The sex difference is not as great in the elderly population. There are no significant differences among geographic locations, despite the common lay belief that warmer, drier climates can be beneficial to people with RA. Although joint pain may be less severe in these locales, the disease occurs as frequently.

Transcultural Considerations With the exception of Native Americans, there are no major differences among races or ethnic groups. Studies of several northern Native American groups revealed RA prevalence rates that were three to seven times higher that those in non–Native American groups (Giger & Davidhizar, 1991; Schumacher, 1988).

COLLABORATIVE MANAGEMENT

ASSESSMENT

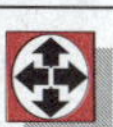

HISTORY

The nurse considers the age and sex of the client because rheumatoid arthritis most often begins in young women. The nurse also assesses other risk factors, such as family history and previous viral infections. The nurse asks the woman whether she has taken oral contraceptives because clients who are taking this medication seem less likely to have the disease. The nurse also ascertains the client's ability to cope with stress because increased physical and emotional stress *may* be correlated with the onset or exacerbation of RA.

PHYSICAL ASSESSMENT/CLINICAL MANIFESTATIONS

The onset of rheumatoid arthritis may be acute and severe, or it may be insidious; clients may have vague complaints lasting for several years before diagnosis. The manifestations of RA can be categorized as "early" or "late" disease and as articular or extra-articular (Chart 23–7).

CHART 23–7

Key Features of Rheumatoid Arthritis

Early Manifestations

Joint

- Inflammation

Systemic

- Low-grade fever
- Fatigue
- Weakness
- Anorexia
- Paresthesias

Late Manifestations

Joint

- Deformities, e.g., swan neck or ulnar deviation
- Moderate to severe pain and morning stiffness

Systemic

- Osteoporosis
- Severe fatigue
- Anemia
- Weight loss
- Subcutaneous nodules
- Peripheral neuropathy
- Vasculitis
- Pericarditis
- Fibrotic lung disease
- Sjögren's syndrome
- Renal disease

EARLY DISEASE MANIFESTATIONS The client with RA typically complains of fatigue, generalized weakness, anorexia, and a weight loss of about 2 or 3 pounds (1 kg) early in the disease process. Persistent low-grade fever may accompany these complaints because RA is an inflammatory disease. In clients with early disease, the nurse notes that the upper extremity joints are involved initially, typically the proximal interphalangeal (PIP) and metacarpophalangeal (MCP) joints of the hands. These joints may be slightly reddened, warm, stiff, swollen, and tender or painful, particularly on palpation. The typical pattern of joint involvement in RA is *bilateral* and *symmetric* (e.g., both wrists), and the number of joints involved usually increases as the disease progresses.

LATE DISEASE MANIFESTATIONS As the disease worsens, the joints become progressively inflamed and quite painful. The client complains of morning stiffness (also called the gel phenomenon), which lasts between 30 minutes and several hours after awakening. On palpation, the nurse notes that the joints feel soft because of synovitis and effusions. The fingers often appear spindle-like. The nurse may observe muscle atrophy, which can result from disuse secondary to joint pain, and a decreased range of motion in affected joints.

Eventually, most or all synovial joints are affected. In severe disease, the temporomandibular joint (TMJ) may be involved, but this involvement is infrequent. When the TMJ is affected, the client typically complains of pain when chewing or opening the mouth.

When the spinal column is involved, the cervical joints are most likely to be affected. The nurse palpates the posterior cervical spine to elicit pain or tenderness. Cervical disease may result in subluxation, especially the first and second vertebrae. This is a life-threatening complication because branches of the phrenic nerve that supply the diaphragm can be compressed and respiratory function may be subsequently compromised. The client is also in danger of becoming quadriparetic or quadriplegic.

JOINT MANIFESTATIONS Joint deformity occurs as a late, articular manifestation, and secondary osteoporosis can cause bone fractures. The nurse observes common deformities, especially in the hands and feet (Fig. 23–7). Extensive wrist involvement can result in carpal tunnel syndrome (see Chap. 51 for assessment and management).

The nurse palpates the tissues around the joints to elicit pain or tenderness associated with other rheumatoid complications. For example, Baker's cysts, enlarged popliteal bursae, may occur and cause tissue compression and pain. Tendon rupture is also common, particularly rupture of the Achilles tendon.

SYSTEMIC MANIFESTATIONS Numerous extra-articular clinical manifestations are associated with advanced disease. Consequently, the nurse assesses other body systems to ascertain systemic involve-

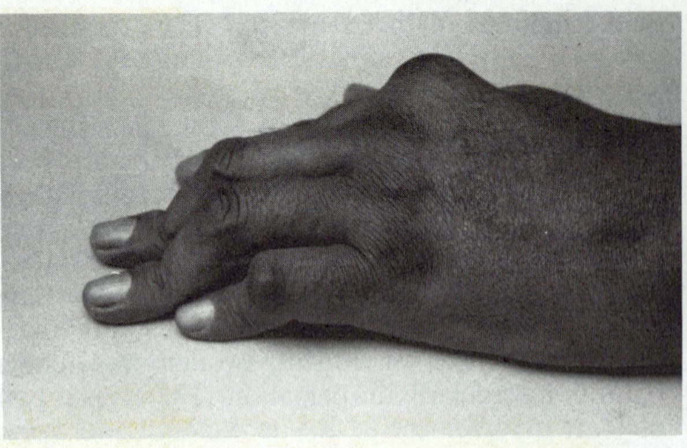

A

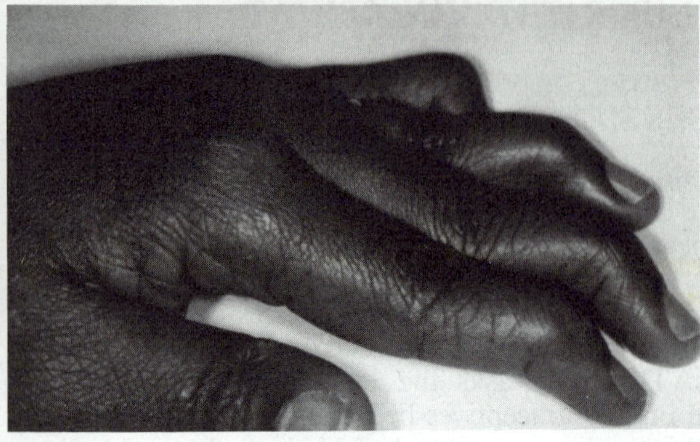

B

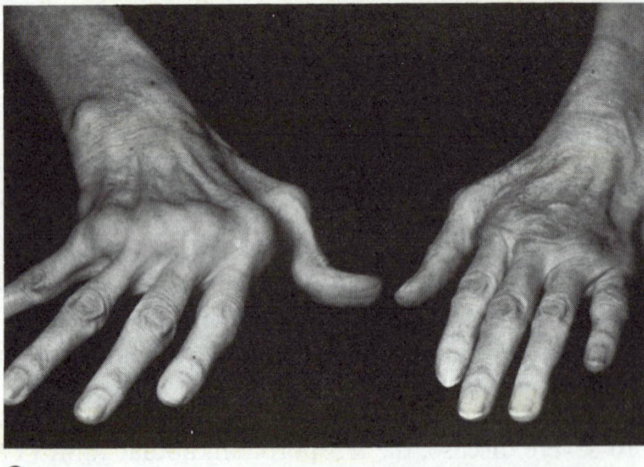

C

FIGURE 23-7 ◆ Common joint deformities seen in rheumatoid arthritis. *A*, Boutonniére, or buttonhole. *B*, Swan neck. *C*, Ulnar deviation (on left). (From the Arthritis Teaching Slide Collection, copyright 1980. Used by permission of the Arthritis Foundation.)

ment. Moderate to severe weight loss, fever, and extreme fatigue are common in late disease exacerbations, often called "flares." Approximately 25% of clients have the characteristic round, movable, nontender subcutaneous nodules, which most often appear on the ulnar surface of the arm. These nodules disappear and reappear at any time and are associated with severe, destructive disease. They occasionally open and become infected, but otherwise they do not usually cause a problem.

Inflammation of the blood vessels results in vasculitis, particularly of small to medium-sized vessels. When arterial involvement (rheumatoid arteritis) occurs, major organs and body systems become ischemic and malfunction. Ischemic skin lesions appear in groups as small, brownish spots, most commonly around the nail bed (periungual lesions). The nurse and physician monitor the number of lesions and note their location each day. An increased number of lesions indicates increased vasculitis; a decreased number indicates decreased vasculitis. The nurse also carefully assesses any larger lesions that appear on the lower extremities; they often lead to ulcerations, which heal slowly as a result of decreased circulation. Peripheral neuropathy associated with decreased circulation can cause foot drop and paresthesias (burning and tingling sensations), most often in the elderly.

Respiratory complications manifest as pleurisy, pneumonitis, diffuse interstitial fibrosis, and pulmonary hypertension. Cardiac complications include pericarditis and myocarditis. The nurse also assesses for ocular involvement, which typically manifests as iritis and scleritis. If either of these complications is present, the nurse notes that the sclera of one or both eyes is reddened and the pupils have an irregular shape.

ASSOCIATED SYNDROMES Several syndromes are seen in clients with advanced RA. The most common is *Sjögren's syndrome*, which includes a triad of:

- Dry eyes (keratoconjunctivitis sicca [KCS], or the sicca syndrome)
- Dry mouth (xerostomia)
- Dry vagina (in some cases)

In Sjögren's syndrome, immune complexes and inflammatory cells are thought to obstruct secretory glands and ducts. The syndrome is usually associated with connective tissue diseases such as RA but may occur alone. The nurse notes the client's complaint of dry mouth or dry eyes. Some clients state that their eyes feel "gritty," as if sand were in their eyes. The nurse also inspects the mouth for dry, sticky membranes and the eyes for redness and lack of tearing.

Less commonly observed is *Felty's syndrome*, which is characterized by RA, hepatosplenomegaly (enlarged liver and spleen), and leukopenia.

Caplan's syndrome is characterized by the presence of rheumatoid nodules in the lungs and pneumoconiosis, which is noted primarily in coal miners and asbestos workers. The physician diagnoses these syndromes by physical examination and diagnostic testing.

PSYCHOSOCIAL ASSESSMENT

Rheumatoid arthritis *can* be a crippling disease. After 10 to 15 years of having the disease, fewer than 50% of clients are totally independent in activities of daily living. These physical limitations result in role changes in the family and society. For example, the person may not be able to cook for the family or be an active sexual partner. In addition, extreme fatigue often causes clients to desire an early bedtime and may result in a reluctance to socialize. In a nursing study by Crosby (1991), 52% of 101 people with RA stated that they consistently lacked energy and 32% indicated that they were too tired to work for more that 4 hours without resting. In some cases, the client may not be able to work at all and support the family financially.

Body changes may also cause poor self-esteem and body image. Because many societies value people with physically fit, attractive bodies, the client with RA may be embarrassed to be seen in public places. The client may grieve, may experience depression, and may attempt suicide. The client may experience a feeling of helplessness, accompanied by a loss of control over a disease that can "consume" the body.

Living with a chronic disease and the pain that results is difficult for the client, family, and significant others (Peeters, 1992). The nurse assesses the client's emotional and mental status in relation to the disease and its problems and evaluates the client's support systems and resources. Ward and Leigh (1993), studying the relationship of marital status to the progression of functional disability, found that being married was associated with decreased progression of disability, regardless of the RA client's income or gender.

(For further information on psychosocial assessment for this type of client, see Chapters 7, 12, and 13 on stress, coping, loss, and disabling and chronic disease, respectively.)

LABORATORY ASSESSMENT

Laboratory tests help to support a diagnosis of rheumatoid arthritis, but no single test or group of tests can confirm it. Chart 23–8 summarizes the common laboratory tests that the physician uses for diagnosis of connective tissue disease.

CHART 23–8

Lab Profile ♦ Connective Tissue Disease

Test	Normal Range for Adults	Significance of Abnormal Findings
Rheumatoid factor		
Rose-Waaler	• <1:80	• *Elevations* of either titer (increase in number at right of colon) indicative of possible CTD • *Increased* Rose's titer indicative of RA (seropositive); not a sensitive test
Latex agglutination	• <1:120	• Latex titer not as specific to one disease, but quite sensitive test
ANA (total)	• <1:8 (if positive, types of ANA identified, e.g., anti-DNA, anti-DNP, anti-RNA, to indicate what part of cells involved)	• *Elevations* common in SLE, PSS, RA, and other inflammatory CTDs (5% of healthy adults have positive ANA results)
Serum complement (C′ or CH_{50})	• Varies greatly among laboratories	• *Decreased* value indicative of active autoimmune disease such as SLE
LE preparation	• <1:8	• A type of ANA (anti-DNP); not reliable because negative result does *not* rule out SLE; can be used as screening test
SPEP		
Albumin	• 52–68*	• *Increased* levels of gamma globulins indicative of CTD (inflammatory type) • *Increased* level of alpha globulins possible in RA
Globulin	• 32–48	
$Alpha_1$ globulin	• 2.4–5.3	
$Alpha_2$ globulin	• 6.6–13.5	
Beta globulin	• 8.5–14.5	
Gamma globulin	• 10.7–21.0	
HLA testing (HLA-B27)	• None	• *Presence* of HLA-B27 indicative of Reiter's syndrome or ankylosing spondylitis
ESR	• Described in Table 49–3	

* SPEP values given as a percentage of total protein.

ANA, antinuclear antibody; CTD, connective tissue disease; DNP, dinitrophenol; SLE, systemic lupus erythematosus; PSS, progressive systemic sclerosis; LE, lupus erythematosus; SPEP, serum protein electrophoresis; RA, rheumatoid arthritis; HLA, human leukocyte antigen; ESR, erythrocyte sedimentation rate.

RHEUMATOID FACTOR The test for rheumatoid factor (RF) measures the presence of unusual antibodies of the IgG and/or IgM type that develop in a number of connective tissue diseases. Two methods are used most commonly to ascertain the degree to which these antibodies are present in the body: Rose-Waaler and latex agglutination. In both procedures, values are reported as titers.

The Rose-Waaler test is more specific for a diagnosis of RA than the latex but is not as sensitive. A client with a positive Rose-Waaler result probably has RA and is seropositive; a client with a negative test result may or may not have the disease and is seronegative. About 60% of RA clients are seropositive and have a titer higher than 1:80 as assessed by this test.

The latex agglutination test is sensitive but is not as specific for RA. Its normal value is less than 1:120. Generally, the higher the titer, the more active the disease process.

ANTINUCLEAR ANTIBODY TITER The antinuclear antibody (ANA) test measures the titer of unusual antibodies that destroy the nuclei of cells and cause tissue death. When the fluorescent method is used, the test is sometimes referred to as FANA. If this test result is positive (a value higher than 1:8), various subtypes of this antibody are identified and measured. As with the rheumatoid factor, the higher the titer, the more active the disease process.

ERYTHROCYTE SEDIMENTATION RATE The "sed rate," as the ESR is sometimes called, can confirm inflammation or infection anywhere in the body. It is particularly useful in connective tissue disease because the value directly correlates with the degree of inflammation and, later, with the severity of the disease.

Because several laboratory procedures are used to measure ESR, normal values vary; women have higher normal values than men. Generally, a value of 20 to 40 mm/hour indicates mild inflammation; 40 to 70 mm/hour, moderate inflammation; and 70 to 150 mm/hour, severe inflammation.

The ESR is also used to monitor a client's response to anti-inflammatory drug therapy. The value should decrease if the drug dosage is effective.

SERUM COMPLEMENT In an attempt to destroy the immune complexes, complement (C′) attaches to the complex. If a large amount of complement is used in this lytic process, the concentration of free-floating complement in the blood diminishes. Normal values vary considerably, depending on the laboratory technique used. An abnormal finding is indicated by a decrease in serum complement and is seen primarily in clients with vasculitis.

SERUM PROTEIN ELECTROPHORESIS In SPEP, the protein fractions of the plasma are measured using electrical current to separate them. In acute inflammation, the level of alpha globulin is raised, but in chronic inflammatory conditions such as rheumatoid arthritis, the level of gamma globulin is increased because of the increase in immunoglobulins.

IMMUNOGLOBULINS The serum immunoglobulins can be separated into subtypes. In chronic inflammation, IgG is needed to combine with rheumatoid factor. Thus, in rheumatoid arthritis the IgG value is typically elevated.

OTHER LABORATORY TESTS The presence of most chronic diseases usually causes mild to moderate anemia, which contributes to the client's fatigue. Therefore, the client's complete blood count (CBC) is monitored for a low hemoglobin, hematocrit, and red blood cell (RBC) count. An increase in white blood cell (WBC) count is consistent with an inflammatory response. A decrease in the WBC count may indicate Felty's syndrome. Additional laboratory tests may be performed, depending on the body systems and organs that may be affected by the disease. For example, if heart involvement is suspected, the physician may order cardiac enzymes.

RADIOGRAPHIC ASSESSMENT

The standard x-ray is used to visualize the joint changes and deformities that are typical of rheumatoid arthritis. The computed tomography (CT) scan may help to determine the presence and degree of cervical spine involvement.

OTHER DIAGNOSTIC ASSESSMENT

An *arthrocentesis* is a common diagnostic procedure used for clients with joint involvement. It may be done at the bedside or in a physician's office or clinic. After administering a local anesthetic, the physician inserts a large-gauge needle into the joint, usually the knee, to aspirate a sample of synovial fluid, which may also relieve pressure. The fluid is analyzed by use of tests described in Chart 23–8. After the procedure, the nurse monitors the insertion site for bleeding or leakage of synovial fluid. If either of these problems occur, the nurse notifies the physician.

A *bone scan* or *joint scan* can also assess the extent of joint involvement (see Other Diagnostic Assessment in Chapter 49). *Magnetic resonance imaging (MRI)* may be performed to assess spinal column disease.

Because rheumatoid arthritis can affect multiple body systems, tests to diagnose specific systemic manifestations are performed as necessary. For example, electromyography helps to confirm peripheral neuropathy. Pulmonary function tests help to determine the presence of lung involvement.

ANALYSIS

COMMON NURSING DIAGNOSES

The client with rheumatoid arthritis disease typically presents with the following nursing diagnoses:

1. Chronic Pain related to joint inflammation
2. Impaired Physical Mobility related to fatigue, inflammation, and pain
3. Self Care Deficit (partial) related to fatigue, pain, stiffness, and joint deformity
4. Fatigue related to states of discomfort, sleep pattern disturbance, and increased energy requirement to perform activities of daily living
5. Body Image Disturbance related to effects of loss of body function

ADDITIONAL NURSING DIAGNOSES

In addition to the common nursing diagnoses, some clients experience one or more of the following nursing diagnoses:

- Ineffective Individual Coping related to effects of chronic illness
- Altered Sexuality Patterns related to effects of illness, pain, and extreme fatigue
- Sleep Pattern Disturbance related to pain, lifestyle disruptions, and/or depression
- Altered Nutrition: Less than Body Requirements related to decreased appetite and fatigue
- Impaired Home Maintenance Management related to effects of chronic debilitating disease or inadequate support systems

PLANNING AND IMPLEMENTATION

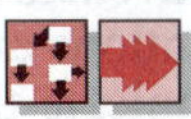

CHRONIC PAIN

PLANNING: CLIENT GOALS The primary goal is that the client will experience a reduction in joint pain. Total relief of pain may not be realistic in this chronic disease.

INTERVENTIONS As in other types of arthritis, the health care team manages pain by using a combination of drug and nondrug measures. When these measures are no longer effective, surgery may be indicated. The accompanying Client Care Plan highlights the most important nursing interventions for the client with rheumatoid arthritis.

Nonsurgical Management Although numerous pain relief modalities are available, the client with RA often needs a variety of medications to relieve pain and/or slow the progression of the disease.

Drug Therapy Medications that are prescribed for clients with RA have analgesic, antipyretic, and/or anti-inflammatory actions.

SALICYLATES The first drug type of choice is often salicylates, although the selection of drugs varies by physician and geographic area. As seen in Chart 23–1, any one of several agents may be used. Large doses of aspirin (ASA, Ancasal✱) may be prescribed unless gastrointestinal distress (nausea, vomiting, or ulcers) occurs or the client has a history of one or more of these symptoms.

The initial dosage of aspirin is typically 12 to 18 tablets each day in divided doses (usually four times a day) until a therapeutic serum salicylate level of 20 to 25 mg/100 mL (25 mg/dL) is achieved, usually in 3 to 6 weeks. The physician regulates the dosage so that side effects are minimized and the serum level is less than 30 mg/100 mL. A level higher that this often results in signs of toxicity, such as tinnitus. The nurse asks the client whether he or she has experienced this symptom. If so, the physician usually reduces the daily dosage of the drug. Once the client's pain and other clinical manifestations are alleviated or reduced, the dosage can be adjusted to a maintenance level, which usually falls between 15 and 20 mg/100 mL (not >1.45 mmol/L).

NONSTEROIDAL ANTI-INFLAMMATORY DRUGS (NSAIDS) If pain and inflammation are not decreased within 6 to 12 weeks after the initiation of salicylates, other NSAIDs may be given instead of or in combination with aspirin. The choice of which drug to administer depends on the client's needs and the physician's preference. If after 6 weeks or so there is no clinical change, the physician may discontinue the NSAID and another NSAID may be tried instead. This process may be repeated until the appropriate drug is found to be effective for that client.

Side effects and toxic effects of NSAIDs are similar to those of aspirin. In addition, many of these agents cause retention of sodium and water, which poses a life-threatening risk to clients with hypertension, renal disease, or congestive heart failure. Elderly clients are especially vulnerable to side and toxic effects of NSAIDs. The nurse carefully monitors these clients and reports problems as early as possible to the physician.

REMITTIVE AGENTS When pain and inflammation are not reduced by aspirin and NSAIDs, gold therapy is usually added to the drug regimen. Unlike the former drugs, gold can induce disease remission as well as reduce pain and inflammation. The most commonly used parenteral preparation is gold sodium thiomalate (Myochrysine). After a small test dose of 10 mg intramuscularly to detect an allergy to the drug, weekly gold injections are given. The dosage increases from 25 to 50 mg/week until improvement is evident or until a cumulative total of 1000 mg is administered.

If the client responds to gold without having toxic effects, such as rash, blood dyscrasias, or renal involvement, the injections are slowly tapered to every 2 weeks, then to every 3 weeks, and then to once a month. Before each drug administration, the client's urine is tested for protein level and a complete blood count is taken. If remission does not occur after a total of 1000 mg has been given, the drug is usually discontinued.

Because intramuscular administration of gold preparations is painful, auranofin (Ridaura), an oral gold product, may be used. The client must take this drug daily to achieve a therapeutic serum level. Its major

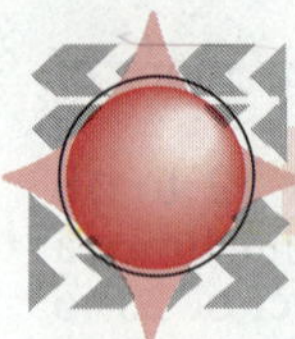

CLIENT CARE PLAN

The Client with Rheumatoid Arthritis

Nursing Diagnosis No. 1: Chronic Pain related to joint inflammation

Expected Outcomes	Nursing Interventions	Rationale
The client will experience a reduction in joint pain.	◆ Give prescribed drugs, as ordered, on time.	◆ Giving drugs on time ensures a consistent blood level (e.g., salicylates).
	◆ Give analgesic drugs as needed, if ordered, and periods of rest, especially after periods of *increased* activity (e.g., physical therapy).	◆ Supplemental analgesics may be needed to control chronic pain; rest is necessary to prevent overuse of joints and help decreased inflammation.
	◆ Provide a warm shower, tub bath, and/or hot compresses after periods of *decreased* activity or rest.	◆ Heat application increases blood flow to the joints to decrease pain and increase joint mobility.
	◆ Provide nonpharmacologic pain relief measures, such as imagery, massage, and music therapy. (Determine which of these measures are effective for each client.)	◆ Independent nursing interventions help reduce pain and decrease the amount of analgesics needed for pain relief.
	◆ Evaluate the effectiveness of all pain relief interventions and document/communicate the outcome to the physician and other involved health care team members. (Also see Chapter 8 for additional interventions and pain assessment tools.)	◆ Evaluation of the effectiveness of pain relief interventions helps the health care team plan care for the client. Changes may be necessary if the plan is not effective in meeting the expected outcome.

Nursing Diagnosis No. 2: Impaired Physical Mobility related to fatigue, inflammation, and pain

Expected Outcomes	Nursing Interventions	Rationale
The client will ambulate independently, with or without ambulatory aids.	◆ Reinforce the importance of and techniques for therapeutic joint and muscle exercises as taught by the physical therapist.	◆ Therapeutic joint and muscle exercises increase joint mobility, decrease pain, and increase muscle strength.
	◆ Teach the importance of recreational exercises, such as walking and swimming.	◆ Certain recreational exercises, such as walking and swimming, increase muscle tone and enhance psychologic well-being.
	◆ Reinforce the importance of and techniques for use of ambulatory aids, such as a cane or walker; allow rest periods during ambulation.	◆ Ambulatory aids help reduce stress on affected joints and therefore reduce pain and inflammation.
	◆ Emphasize the client's abilities and strengths in mobility skills.	◆ Focusing on the client's abilities rather than deficits builds the clients self-esteem and confidence.

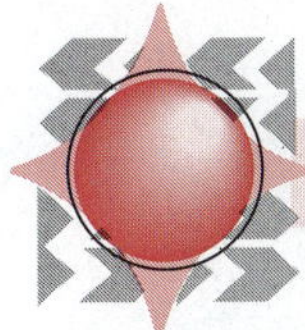

CLIENT CARE PLAN

The Client with Rheumatoid Arthritis *Continued*

Nursing Diagnosis No. 3: Self Care Deficit (Partial) related to fatigue, pain, stiffness, and joint deformity

Expected Outcomes	Nursing Interventions	Rationale
The client will independently perform activities of daily living (ADL) with or without the use of assistive/adaptive devices	♦ In collaboration with the occupational therapist, assess the client's abilities in ADL.	♦ The nurse allows the client to perform all ADL independently. If the client needs assistance, the nurse plans ways to promote independence in these areas.
	♦ Set up the client's tray, if needed, by opening packages and cartons and cutting food; assess the need for assistive/adaptive devices.	♦ The client may be able to self-feed if the tray is set up and/or if assistive devices, such as a plate guard, are obtained.
	♦ For dressing activities, assess the need for long-handled assistive/adaptive devices and other mechanical aids.	♦ The client may be able to dress independently if assistive/adaptive devices are available.
	♦ Encourage the client to use large muscle groups and joints instead of smaller ones, if possible.	♦ Using larger joints helps prevent stress and pain in small joints (joint protection).
	♦ Emphasize the client's abilities in performing ADL.	♦ Focusing on the client's abilities builds self-esteem and confidence.
	♦ Teach the client to allow rest periods during ADL.	♦ Rest reduces fatigue that contributes to a decreased ability to perform ADL.
	♦ Assess the client's pain level, and intervene appropriately (see Nursing Diagnosis No. 1).	♦ Pain and stiffness contribute to a decreased ability to perform ADL.

side effect is gastrointestinal (GI) symptoms, especially diarrhea, nausea, and vomiting. The nurse teaches the client to report any GI problems to the physician or clinic.

Other remittive agents may be prescribed, such as the antimalarial drug hydroxychloroquine (Plaquenil) and penicillamine (Cuprimine). These drugs are not used as often as gold in rheumatoid disease because they produce numerous side effects and toxic effects and are often not as effective. The physician recommends that clients receiving hydroxychloroquine have an eye examination every 3 to 6 months to detect changes in vision because retinal toxicity may occur. Retinal toxicity results in decreased visual acuity. If this complication occurs, the physician discontinues the drug. The side and toxic effects of penicillamine are similar to those of gold.

Methotrexate (MTX) and azathioprine (Imuran) can also cause RA remission. These drugs are immunosuppressive agents that are also used to treat certain cancers. In smaller doses, these agents may be of benefit to clients with RA. Weinblatt and colleagues (1993) found that methotrexate was more effective than Auranofin in slowing the progression of rheumatoid arthritis. In some cases, cyclosporine A and methotrexate may be given together.

The nurse observes for the side and toxic effects of methotrexate, which include mouth sores, acute dyspnea from pneumonitis, chronic liver inflammation, and bone marrow suppression (Fries et al., 1993). Lymphoma and bone marrow suppression may also occur with azathioprine administration. Cyclophosphamide (Cytoxan, Procytox✱) is also sometimes given to control RA vasculitis; however, this drug may cause leukemia or other types of malignancy.

For clients who do not experience relief of symptoms from the commonly administered medications, steroids, usually prednisone (Deltasone, Winpred✱, Apo-Prednisone✱), are given for their anti-inflammatory and immunosuppressive effects. Unfortunately, chronic steroid therapy can result in devastating complications, such as diabetes mellitus, infection, fluid and electrolyte imbalances, hypertension, osteoporosis, and glaucoma. As shown in Chart 23–1, some drug effects are dose-related whereas others are not. The nurse observes the client for complications associated with chronic steroid therapy and reports them to the physician. For example, if the client's blood pressure becomes elevated or significant laboratory values change, the nurse notifies the physician.

ANALGESIC DRUGS Other analgesic drugs may be prescribed to supplement the anti-inflammatory drugs that are specific for RA. Some analgesics include acetaminophen (Tylenol, Exdol*), propoxyphene (Darvon, Novopropoxyn*), and propoxyphene napsylate (Darvocet-N). Propoxyphene and its associated products can cause headache, dizziness, and drowsiness. Over a long period, in clients with decreased metabolic rates, this slow-excreting drug may accumulate in the body and may cause death. The nurse teaches the client about the side and toxic effects of these drugs and advises the client to report any unusual symptom or complaint to the physician.

Rest, Positioning, Ice, and Heat Adequate rest, proper positioning, and ice and heat application are important in pain management (see Chronic Pain in the discussion of degenerative joint disease). If acute inflammation is present, the nurse or physical therapist (PT) applies ice to the "hot" joints for pain relief until the inflammation lessens. The nurse or PT takes precautions to prevent the ice pack from being too heavy.

To relieve morning stiffness or the pain of late-stage disease, the nurse recommends a hot shower for the client rather than a sponge bath or a tub bath. It is often difficult for the client with rheumatoid arthritis to get into and out of the bathtub, although special hydraulic lifts and tub chairs may be available. Hot packs applied directly to involved joints are also beneficial. Most physical therapy departments have Hydrocollators that keep hot packs ready any time they are needed (Fig. 23–8).

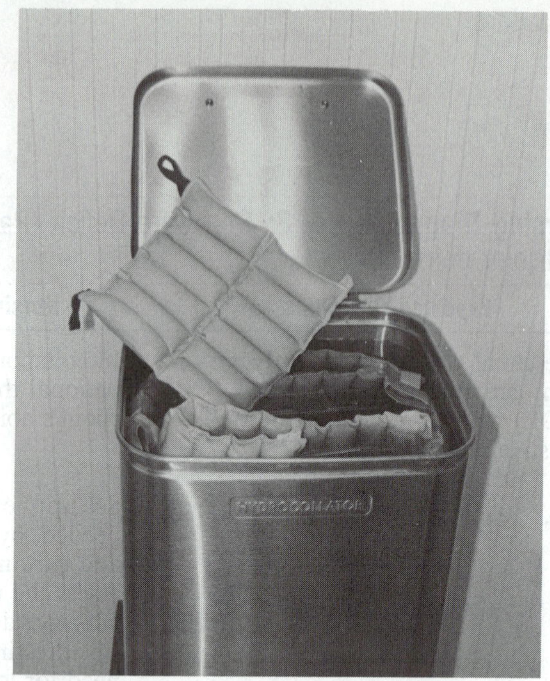

FIGURE 23–8 ◆ A Hydrocollator used for keeping hot packs warm.

Other Pain Relief Measures As in any client with arthritis, other nonpharmacologic pain relief techniques are available. For example, some clients may achieve relief with transcutaneous electrical nerve stimulation (TENS), hypnosis, acupuncture, imagery, or music therapy. Stress management is also becoming more popular as a pain relief intervention. Chapters 7 and 8 describe these interventions in detail.

Experimental Therapies In addition to the drug regimens described earlier, two newer techniques—pulse therapy and plasmapheresis—are being tried and evaluated to treat severe rheumatoid arthritis. In pulse therapy, the client receives rapid infusions of high-dose steroids or chemotherapeutic agents, usually over a period of several days. Plasmapheresis is a procedure in which the client's plasma is treated to remove the antibodies that are causing the disease. Sometimes called a plasma exchange, this procedure may be combined with pulse therapy.

Surgical Management When nonsurgical pain management techniques are not effective in reducing pain, the physician may refer the client to a surgeon. In early disease, a synovectomy may be performed to remove excess synovial tissue, thus decreasing pressure on nerve endings in and around joints. In advanced disease, other surgical procedures (osteotomy and total joint replacement) are used. (For a description of these procedures and their associated nursing care, see Surgical Management in the discussion of chronic pain in degenerative joint disease.)

Because of the joint deformity and joint destruction caused by rheumatoid arthritis, clients having a joint replacement may not achieve increased mobility, but they usually experience pain relief or reduction.

IMPAIRED PHYSICAL MOBILITY

The goals and interventions that apply to the client with rheumatoid arthritis (RA) who has impaired physical mobility are the same as those for the client with a nursing diagnosis of degenerative joint disease (DJD). Clients with RA are more likely to become restricted to a wheelchair or to bed than clients with DJD, but an aggressive mobilization program may prevent total dependence. Of special importance to the client is the need for assistive/adaptive devices, such as elevated toilet seats or chairs, and wheelchairs to facilitate transfers.

SELF CARE DEFICIT

PLANNING: CLIENT GOALS The primary goal is that the client will independently perform activities of daily living (ADL) with or without the use of assistive/adaptive devices. The nurse collaborates with physical and occupational therapists to accomplish this goal.

INTERVENTIONS Although the physical appearance of a client with severe rheumatoid arthritis (RA) may lead the nurse to think that independence in activities of daily living is not possible, the client can use a number of alternative methods to perform these activities. The nurse should not automatically perform activities for the client; clients with RA do not want to be dependent. For example, hand deformities frequently prevent a client from opening packages of food, such as a box of crackers. The client may prefer to use his or her teeth to open the crackers rather than depend on someone else.

In the hospital or long-term care facility, a client may not eat because of the barriers of heavy plate covers, milk in cartons, small packages of condiments, and heavy containers. Styrofoam or paper cups may bend and collapse as the client attempts to hold them. A china or heavy plastic cup with handles may be easier to manipulate. The nurse and client collaborate with the dietitian to allow the client access to food and total independence in eating activity.

When fine motor activities (such as squeezing a tube of toothpaste) become impossible, larger joints or body surfaces can substitute for smaller ones. In this case, the nurse teaches the client to use the palm of the hand to press the paste onto the brush. Devices such as long-handled brushes can allow clients to brush their hair; dressing sticks can facilitate putting on pants. These examples illustrate the need for the nurse to assess the problem area, suggest alternative methods, and refer the client to an occupational therapist for special assistive and adaptive devices if necessary.

Chapter 13 describes additional interventions for clients with self-care deficits.

FATIGUE

PLANNING: CLIENT GOALS The goal is that the client will experience a decrease in fatigue.

INTERVENTIONS Nursing interventions depend, in part, on identifying the factors contributing to fatigue. For example, Crosby (1991) found that increases in pain, sleep disturbance, and weakness were positively associated with increased fatigue (Research Applications for Nursing). Anemia may also be a contributing factor and may be treated with iron (if an iron deficiency anemia is present), folic acid, and/or vitamin supplements, prescribed by the physician. Chronic normochromic or chronic hypochromic anemia frequently occurs in most chronic, systemic diseases. The nurse also assesses for drug-related blood loss, such as that caused by salicylate therapy or other nonsteroidal anti-inflammatory drugs, by checking the stool for gross or occult blood. Elderly Caucasian women are the most likely clients to experience gastrointestinal bleeding from these medications.

When a client's fatigue results from muscle atrophy, the physician prescribes an aggressive physical therapy program to strengthen muscles and to prevent further atrophy. Clients experience increased fatigue when pain prevents them from getting adequate rest and sleep. Measures to facilitate sleep include promoting a quiet environment, giving warm beverages, and administering hypnotics or relaxants as pre-

RESEARCH APPLICATIONS FOR NURSING

Fatigue in Clients with Rheumatoid Arthritis May Be Related to Pain, Sleep Fragmentation, and Functional Ability

Crosby, L. (1991). Factors which contribute to fatigue associated with rheumatoid arthritis. *Journal of Advanced Nursing*, *16*, 974–981.

Although fatigue is a primary clinical feature of rheumatoid arthritis (RA), the physiologic basis for this sensation is not well understood. The researcher measured walking time, hand grip strength, joint pain, and electroencephalographic sleep variables in 27 clients with RA. She determined that, when compared with control subjects and RA clients in remission, RA clients in flare had significantly more joint pain, more fragmented sleep, reduced walking time, and decreased hand grip strength. Increases in these objective measures were positively associated with increases in subjective complaints of fatigue. In contrast, fatigue levels of control subjects and RA subjects in remission either were not associated or were negatively correlated with increases in these objective measures.

Critique Correlations between measures neither explain nor find a cause for the relationships between factors. However, this exploratory study provides initial evidence for the relationship between fatigue and pain, sleep fragmentation, and functional ability of clients with RA flare. Future research should include a larger sample size and a method of distinguishing between acute and chronic fatigue.

Possible nursing implications As in pain assessment, evaluation of fatigue is often difficult because of the subjective nature of fatigue. Nurses should acknowledge and accept the client's perception of the fatigue and realize that fatigue increases when clients with RA experience an exacerbation of their disease.

scribed, if necessary. Pain relief measures have been discussed.

In addition to identifying and managing specific reasons for fatigue, the nurse assesses the client's daily activities and teaches principles of energy conservation, including:

- Pacing activities
- Allowing rest periods
- Setting priorities
- Obtaining assistance when needed

Chart 23–9 lists specific suggestions for conserving the client's energy and thus increasing activity tolerance.

BODY IMAGE DISTURBANCE

PLANNING: CLIENT GOALS The goal is that the client will demonstrate behaviors that indicate an improved body image, such as participating in social activities.

INTERVENTIONS A client's body image may be affected by the disease process and drug therapy as well. Steroids, for instance, can cause a moon-faced appearance, acne, striae, "buffalo humps," and weight gain. The nurse determines the client's perception of these changes and the impact of family and significant others' reactions to them. The most important intervention for the nurse is communicating acceptance of the client. When a trusting relationship is established, the nurse encourages the client to express his or her feelings.

Another way to improve body image while the client is in the hospital or nursing home is the use of personal items. The client's use of a hospital gown reinforces the sick role. The nurse encourages clients to wear their own clothes, to brush their hair, and to use make-up if desired. The nurse assists in making the client as presentable as possible. The use of colored bows for hair, nail polish, and perfume may improve the female client's image and self-concept. Chapter 10 identifies additional strategies for care of a client with an altered body image.

CHART 23–9

Education Guide ◆ Energy Conservation for the Client with Arthritis

- Balance activity with rest. Take one or two naps each day.
- Pace yourself; do not plan too much for one day.
- Set priorities. Determine which activities are most important, and do them first.
- Delegate responsibility and tasks to your family and friends.
- Plan ahead to prevent last-minute rushing and stress.
- Learn your own activity tolerance and do not exceed it.

As a reaction to body image disturbance and the presence of a chronic, painful disease, the client may display behaviors indicative of loss. Clients may use coping strategies ranging from denial or fear to anger or depression. In an attempt to regain control over the effects of the disease process, the client may appear to be manipulative and demanding and may sometimes be referred to as having an "arthritis personality." This personality, which has negative connotations, is a myth. Clients are trying to cope with the effects of their illness and should be treated with patience and understanding. The nurse continually assesses and accepts these behaviors but remains realistic in discussing goals to improve self-esteem. The client's strengths are emphasized, and previously successful coping strategies are identified. Further interventions for coping and loss are discussed in Chapters 7 and 12.

DISCHARGE PLANNING

HOME CARE PREPARATION

Clients with rheumatoid arthritis are usually managed at home but may be institutionalized in a long-term care setting if they become restricted to bed or a wheelchair. Some clients may be discharged to a rehabilitation facility for several weeks to aid in developing strategies, techniques, and skills for independent living at home.

The amount of home care preparation depends on the severity of the disease. Structural changes may be necessary if there are deficits in activities of daily living or mobility. Doors must be wide enough to accommodate a wheelchair or a walker if one is used. Ramps are needed to prevent the client in a wheelchair from being homebound. If the client cannot negotiate stairs, the client must have access to facilities for all activities of daily living on one floor.

To promote continued homemaking functions, structural changes of countertops and appliances may be needed. The client may also require handrails and elevated chairs and toilet seats, which facilitate transfers (Fig. 23–9).

HEALTH TEACHING

Health teaching is the most important nursing intervention for promoting the client's compliance with a treatment plan. The nurse should take precautions regarding myths and quackery to protect the client from harm. The nurse reviews information about drug therapy, joint protection, energy conservation, rest, and exercise with the client, family, and significant others. This information is summarized in Charts 23–1, 23–5, 23–7, and 23–9.

PSYCHOSOCIAL PREPARATION

The client with rheumatoid disease often complains of being on an "emotional roller coaster" from coping with a chronic illness every day of life. Control over one's life is an important human need. The

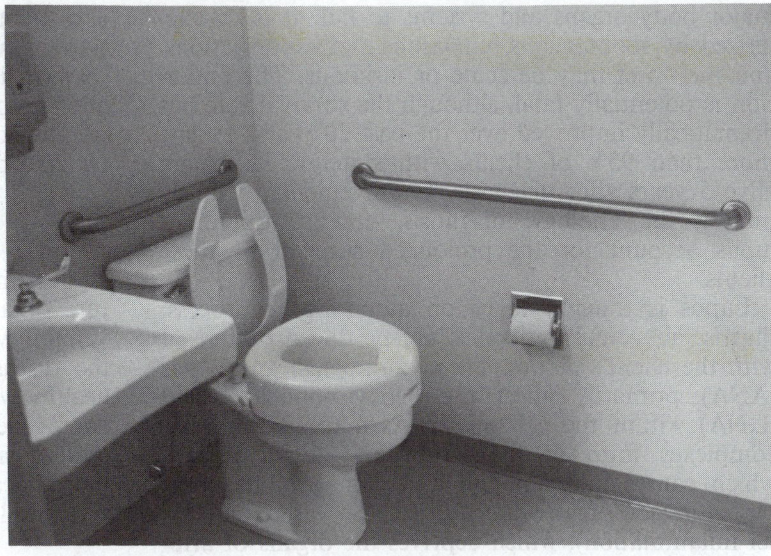

FIGURE 23–9 ◆ Handrails and an elevated toilet seat make transfers easier for the client.

client with an unpredictable chronic disease may lose this control, which lowers self-esteem. Health providers must allow the client to make decisions about care. Families and significant others must also include the client in decision-making. Although the client's behavior may be perceived as demanding or manipulative, the client's self-esteem cannot be improved without this important aspect of interpersonal relationships.

Increased dependency also affects the client's sense of control and self-esteem. Some clients ignore their health needs and portray a tough image for others by insisting that they need no assistance. The nurse emphasizes to the client and family that asking for help may be the best decision at times to prevent further joint damage and disease progression.

Social and work roles are dramatically affected by rheumatoid arthritis. The client may find new friends among others who have the same problem to be a support system to cope with these changes. Becoming an active member of and volunteering for The Arthritis Foundation can help the client to meet social and work needs. Loss of income from being unable to be gainfully employed can also be a major source of stress. The client may qualify for disability benefits through the federal Social Security program. If possible, the client can learn new skills for a less stressful career.

In addition to the interventions just described for self-esteem disturbance, the nurse may need to refer the client to a counselor or to a religious or spiritual leader for emotional support and guidance during times of crisis. The nurse should identify and recommend other support systems within the family and community when necessary.

HEALTH CARE RESOURCES

The need for health care resources for the client with rheumatoid arthritis is similar to that for the client with degenerative joint disease. A home health nurse or aide, physical therapist, and/or occupational therapist may be indicated. In collaboration with the discharge planner, the nurse in the hospital or nursing home identifies these resources and makes sure that they are available before the client is discharged.

EVALUATION 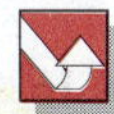

The nurse evaluates the care provided for the client with rheumatoid arthritis. The desired outcomes are that the client:

- States that pain and stiffness are reduced after intervention
- Ambulates without personal assistance (may use an ambulatory aid such as a walker)
- Is independent in all activities of daily living (may use assistive/adaptive devices)
- States that fatigue is decreased
- Participates in daily activities at his or her own pace
- Demonstrates a positive self-esteem as evidenced by participation in daily activities and decision-making

Lupus Erythematosus

OVERVIEW

The word lupus is the Latin term for "wolf." In the mid-19th century, the facial rash that was seen in clients with the disease was thought to look like bites caused by a wolf. The rash was usually red, and thus the term *erythematosus,* a Latin word meaning reddened, was added to describe the disease.

There are two main classifications of lupus: discoid lupus erythematosus (DLE) and systemic lupus erythematosus (SLE). A small percentage of clients with lupus have the DLE type, which affects only the skin.

The systemic disorder is a chronic, progressive, inflammatory connective tissue disorder that can cause major body organs and systems to fail. It is characterized by spontaneous remissions and exacerbations, and the onset may be acute or insidious. The condition is potentially fatal, although the survival rate has dramatically improved over the past 20 years. Today, more than 95% of clients with systemic lupus are alive 5 years after diagnosis. Improvements in determining the etiology, diagnosis, and treatment of lupus account for the prolonged survival of these clients.

Lupus is thought to be an autoimmune process; that is, abnormal antibodies are produced that react with the client's tissues. These antinuclear antibodies (ANA) primarily affect the deoxyribonucleic acid (DNA) within the cell nuclei. As a result, immune complexes form in the serum and organ tissues, which causes inflammation and damage. The complexes invade organs directly or cause vasculitis (vessel inflammation), which deprives the organs of arterial blood and oxygen.

Many clients with SLE have some degree of kidney involvement—the leading cause of death. Other causes of death from SLE are cardiac and central nervous system involvement.

In kidney disease, renal biopsies show progressive changes within the glomeruli:

- In *minimal lupus nephritis,* the glomeruli are slightly irregular; immunoglobulins and complement are seen by electron microscopy.
- *Focal, or mild, lupus nephritis* is characterized by further glomerular changes, and immune complex deposits are common. In this type of lupus, the client begins to show clinical signs of renal impairment.
- In *diffuse, severe proliferative nephritis,* more than 50% of the glomeruli are affected and the client is in renal failure.

Lupus affects women between the ages of 15 and 40 years at a rate eight to ten times more often than men. The onset of the disease is most often during the childbearing years, but it has been reported in young children and the elderly.

Transcultural Considerations About 1 in 700 women between the ages of 15 and 64 years have the disease; 1 in 250 African-American women of this age group are affected.

COLLABORATIVE MANAGEMENT

ASSESSMENT

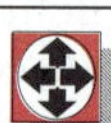

HISTORY

In view of the incidence and etiologic factors associated with lupus, the nurse notes the sex and age of the client. The nurse asks about a family history of lupus or other related connective tissue diseases and asks whether the client is pregnant. The client's reaction to ultraviolet light is also important because many clients report burns or "splotches" develop after exposure to bright sunlight. A complete medication history is valuable because the client may be taking a drug that may cause drug-induced lupus.

PHYSICAL ASSESSMENT/CLINICAL MANIFESTATIONS

It is impossible to describe a typical textbook picture of a client with lupus because of the extreme variability of symptoms among affected clients. When the disease is in remission, the client may appear healthy with no activity limitations. When the disease flares, the client may be so ill that admission to a critical care unit is required. Chart 23–10 highlights the clinical manifestations that occur in clients with systemic lupus.

CHART 23–10

Key Features of Systemic Lupus Erythematosus (SLE) and Progressive Systemic Sclerosis (PSS)

SLE	PSS
Skin Manifestations	
• Inflamed, red rash	• Inflamed
• Discoid lesions	• Fibrotic
	• Sclerotic
	• Edematous
Renal Manifestations	
• Nephritis	• Renal failure
Cardiovascular Manifestations	
• Pericarditis	• Myocardial fibrosis
• Raynaud's phenomenon	• Raynaud's phenomenon
Pulmonary Manifestations	
• Pleural effusions	• Interstitial fibrosis
Neurologic Manifestations	
• CNS lupus	• Not common
Gastrointestinal Manifestations	
• Abdominal pain	• Esophagitis
	• Ulcers
Musculoskeletal Manifestations	
• Joint inflammation	• Joint inflammation
• Myositis	• Myositis
Other Manifestations	
• Fever	• Fever
• Fatigue	• Fatigue
• Anorexia	• Anorexia
• Vasculitis	• Vasculitis

SKIN INVOLVEMENT The major and usually only manifestation of discoid lupus is a dry, scaly, raised rash appearing on the face ("butterfly" rash) and/or upper body, or individual round lesions, sometimes referred to as discoid (coin-like) lesions (Color Figure 23–1). The nurse observes all skin changes and monitors changes daily while the client is in an acute care setting.

MUSCULOSKELETAL CHANGES In addition to skin changes, articular involvement occurs in most clients with systemic lupus erythematosus (SLE). The initial joint changes are similar to those seen in rheumatoid arthritis, but severe deformities are not common (Kaplan et al., 1992). Avascular necrosis (bone necrosis from lack of oxygen) is often seen in clients with SLE who have been treated for at least 5 years, usually with steroids. Chronic steroid therapy may cause constriction of small blood vessels supplying the joint causing the tissue to die. The hip is most commonly affected, and the client complains of pain and decreased mobility as a result.

The nurse observes for muscle atrophy, which can result from disuse or from skeletal muscle invasion by the immune complexes (myositis). Myalgia (muscle pain) may also occur. The nurse inspects and palpates major muscles, especially those in the extremities.

SYSTEMIC MANIFESTATIONS Because SLE is an inflammatory condition, fever is a common finding. The presence of fever is the classic sign of a flare, or exacerbation. Various degrees of generalized weakness, fatigue, anorexia, and weight loss occur. These signs may be the only evidence of impending disease, which makes diagnosis by the physician difficult. Consequently, some clients have a diagnosis of "probable SLE."

Any or all body systems may be affected by SLE. Because lupus nephritis is the leading cause of death, the nurse carefully assesses for signs of renal involvement, for example, changes in urinary output, proteinuria, hematuria, and fluid retention. About 50% of clients with systemic lupus have some type of nephritis.

Pleural effusions are found in almost half of clients with SLE, but this complication is usually not life-threatening. Pulmonary restrictive or obstructive changes may not result in overt clinical signs. However, progressive involvement can lead to dyspnea and arterial blood gas abnormalities. The nurse performs a complete respiratory assessment to determine any abnormalities in respiratory pattern or breath sounds.

Pericarditis is the most common cardiovascular manifestation and causes tachycardia, chest pain, and myocardial ischemia. The nurse monitors the client's vital signs at least every 4 hours while the client is in the hospital and reports chest pain immediately to the physician.

Raynaud's phenomenon is noted in 15% of clients with lupus. On exposure to cold or extreme stress, the client complains of the characteristic red, white, and blue color changes and severe pain in the digits caused by arteriolar vasospasm. The nurse may not observe these episodes but should ask clients whether color changes occur when their hands or feet are exposed to cold or when these clients are extremely stressed.

Neurologic manifestations are varied. Central nervous system effects include psychoses, paresis, seizures, migraine headaches, and cranial nerve palsies. Peripheral neuropathies are also common. The nurse performs a neurologic assessment (see Chap. 40).

The nurse also monitors for reports of abdominal pain. Recurrent abdominal pain occurs frequently, but its cause may not be identified. Mesenteric arteritis, pancreatitis from arteritis of the pancreatic artery, and colonic ulcers can cause abdominal pain in the client with lupus. The nurse may note liver enlargement on assessment of the abdomen, but jaundice is rare. More than 50% of clients have lymph enlargement, and 10% have splenomegaly. The nurse palpates lymph nodes and documents findings.

PSYCHOSOCIAL ASSESSMENT

The psychosocial results from lupus can be devastating. In either discoid or systemic disease, the rash can be disfiguring and embarrassing to the client. Young adult women who never had a blemish are confronted with a rash that cannot be completely covered with make-up. If chronic steroid therapy is used, side effects such as acne, striae, fat pads, and weight gain intensify the problem of an already altered body image.

Chronic fatigue and generalized weakness may prevent the client from being as active as in the past. The client may avoid social gatherings and may withdraw from family activities. The unpredictability and chronicity of SLE can cause fear and anxiety. Fear may heighten if the client knows another person with the disease, particularly if the other person has more advanced, severe disease. The myth that lupus is always a fatal condition is still common.

The nurse assesses the client's feelings about the illness to identify areas that require intervention. The nurse should assess the person's usual coping mechanisms and support systems before developing a plan of care.

(For additional information about psychosocial assessment of clients with chronic illness, see Rheumatoid Arthritis in this chapter as well as Chapter 13.)

LABORATORY ASSESSMENT

Because discoid lupus is not a systemic condition, the only test that is significant is a skin biopsy. The physician gently scrapes skin cells from the rash for microscopic evaluation. The characteristic lupus cell and a number of inflammatory cells confirm the diagnosis.

The immunologic-based laboratory tests that are used to diagnose systemic lupus are the same as those performed for rheumatoid arthritis (RA): rheumatoid factor, antinuclear antibody, erythrocyte sedimentation rate, serum protein electrophoresis, serum complement, and immunoglobulins. The lupus cell preparation (LE cell prep) may also be performed, but this assay is a poor indicator of disease; rather, the test is best used for screening. (See the corresponding heading under Rheumatoid Arthritis as well as Chart 23–8.)

In addition to immunologic testing, several tests are performed to evaluate possible involvement of major organs and body systems. A complete blood count (CBC) commonly shows pancytopenia (a decrease of all cell types), probably caused by direct attack of the blood cells or bone marrow by immune complexes. Serum electrolyte levels, renal function, cardiac and liver enzymes, and clotting factors are also routinely assessed to determine other body system functioning.

INTERVENTIONS

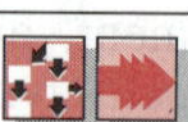

The physician often prescribes potent drugs that are used topically and systemically. In addition, the client takes precautions to prevent further skin impairment and exacerbations (flare-ups) of the disease. Many of the skin lesions do not disappear, even with treatment, but they usually fade when the disease is in remission.

Drug Therapy In discoid lupus, the client's major concern is the rash or discoid lesions. Clients with systemic lupus may also have concern about skin changes. Topical cortisone preparations help reduce inflammation and promote fading of the skin lesions. In addition, the physician may prescribe the antimalarial hydroxychloroquine (Plaquenil) for some clients to decrease the inflammatory response, but other systemic medications are usually not used (see Chart 23–1).

For clients with systemic lupus, the aim of management is to treat the disease aggressively until remission. In addition to medications for skin lesions, the physician often prescribes chronic steroid therapy to treat the systemic disease process. For clients with renal or central nervous system lupus, the physician may also order immunosuppressive agents, which are sometimes used for clients with rheumatoid arthritis (see Chart 23–1). Although clinical manifestations improve during remission, maintenance doses of these drugs are usually continued to prevent further exacerbations of disease. The nurse observes for side and toxic effects of these medications and reports their occurrence to the physician.

Skin Protection The client with lupus should avoid prolonged exposure to sunlight and other forms of ultraviolet lighting, including certain types of fluorescent light. The nurse instructs clients that they may need to wear long sleeves and a hat with a large brim outdoors. The client should use sun-blocking agents with an SPF (sunburn protection factor) of 30 or higher on exposed skin surfaces.

In addition, the nurse teaches the client to clean the skin with mild soap (such as Ivory) and to avoid harsh, perfumed substances. The client rinses and dries the skin well and applies lotion. Excess powder and other drying substances are avoided. The client carefully selects cosmetics and should include moisturizers and sun protectors. The nurse may refer the client to a medical cosmetologist who specializes in applying make-up for clients with skin lesions of all types.

The client's hair should receive special attention because alopecia (hair loss) is common. The nurse recommends mild protein shampoos and avoidance of harsh treatments, such as permanents or frostings, until the hair regrows during remission.

DISCHARGE PLANNING

HOME CARE PREPARATION

Discharge planning for the client with lupus is similar to that for clients with rheumatoid arthritis. The client is generally treated at home but may need repeated hospitalizations during exacerbations of disease. Usually, however, the client does not need rehabilitation or a long-term care facility because severe joint deformity and prolonged immobility are not common.

HEALTH TEACHING

Two major differences exist between systemic lupus (SLE) and rheumatoid arthritis in terms of education of the client and family or significant others. First, the nurse teaches the client with SLE how to protect the skin (Chart 23–11). Second, body temperature is monitored carefully in SLE. Fever is the major sign of an exacerbation, during which the client can be-

CHART 23–11

Education Guide ◆ Skin Protection and Care for Clients with Lupus Erythematosus

- Cleanse your skin with a mild soap like Ivory.
- Dry your skin thoroughly by patting rather than rubbing.
- Apply lotion liberally to dry skin areas.
- Avoid powder and other drying agents, such as rubbing alcohol.
- Use cosmetics that contain moisturizers.
- Avoid direct sunlight and any other type of ultraviolet lighting (including tanning beds).
- Wear a large-brimmed hat, long sleeves, and long pants when in the sun.
- Use a sun-blocking agent with at least a sunburn protection factor (SPF) of 30.
- Inspect your skin daily for open areas and rashes.

come seriously ill. The nurse teaches the client to report any other unusual or new clinical manifestation to the physician immediately.

PSYCHOSOCIAL PREPARATION

Many clients become frustrated that family members, significant others, and the lay public do not have a good understanding of lupus. When lupus is in complete remission, the client appears to be healthy. However, an exacerbation can necessitate rapid admission to a critical care unit. This unpredictability disrupts the client's life and can cause fear and anxiety. The nurse helps the client identify coping strategies and support systems that can help the client function in the community. Chapter 7 covers stress management and coping in detail.

HEALTH CARE RESOURCES

Although The Arthritis Foundation is a general resource for all clients with connective tissue disease, the Lupus Foundation is a national organization, with chapters in every state, that provides information and assistance for clients with lupus. Local support groups and services are offered without charge to the client.

Progressive Systemic Sclerosis

OVERVIEW

Progressive systemic sclerosis (PSS), one of a family of diseases, is often referred to as systemic scleroderma. "Scleroderma" means hardening of the skin, which is only one clinical manifestation of PSS. As the name implies, PSS is a systemic disease. It is less common than systemic lupus erythematosus (SLE) but is associated with a higher mortality rate. Chart 23-10 shows a comparison of the clinical manifestations of these two diseases.

PSS is a chronic connective tissue disease that is characterized by inflammation, fibrosis, and sclerosis of the skin and vital organs. The inflammatory process is so similar to that of lupus that clients are often diagnosed as having probable SLE until the disease progresses. The inflamed tissue undergoes fibrotic and then sclerotic changes. The most obvious tissue affected is the skin, but renal involvement is the leading cause of death. Unfortunately, clients with PSS do not respond well to steroids and immunosuppressants that are used for lupus, and the mortality rate is therefore higher.

The prognosis seems to be worse when the client presents with a group of manifestations that occur at the same time—the CREST syndrome:

- *c*alcinosis (calcium deposits)
- *R*aynaud's phenomenon
- *e*sophageal dysmotility
- *s*clerodactyly (scleroderma of the digits)
- *t*elangiectasia (spider-like hemangiomas)

The disease tends to progress rapidly, but spontaneous remissions and exacerbations can occur.

Little is known about the cause of PSS, but autoimmunity is suspected. The occurrence of more than one case per family is uncommon, although other connective tissue diseases may be noted in the family history.

Progressive systemic sclerosis has been described in people of all races and in all geographic areas. Women are affected three to four times more often than men. The onset of the disease is usually between the ages of 30 and 50 years. The incidence is higher in coal miners, who have a high incidence of silicosis —which may be a predisposing or contributing factor to PSS.

COLLABORATVE MANAGEMENT

ASSESSMENT

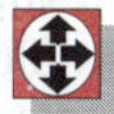

MUSCULOSKELETAL MANIFESTATIONS

Arthralgia (joint pain) and stiffness are common manifestations that the nurse can elicit during the musculoskeletal examination. The acute inflammation that occurs in people with rheumatoid arthritis is not common, and deformities are rare.

SKIN MANIFESTATIONS

Findings on inspection of the skin depend on the stage of the scleroderma (Fig. 23-10). Typically, there is a painless, symmetric, pitting edema of the hands and fingers, which may progress to include the entire upper and/or lower extremities and face. In this edematous phase, the fingers are described as sausage-like. The skin is taut, shiny, and free from wrin-

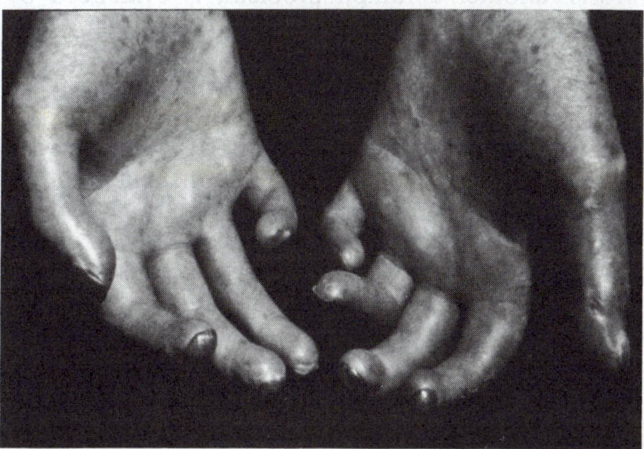

FIGURE 23-10 ◆ Late-stage skin changes seen in clients with progressive systemic sclerosis. (From the Arthritis Teaching Slide Collection, copyright 1980. Used by permission of the Arthritis Foundation.)

kles. If diffuse scleroderma occurs, swelling is replaced by tightening, hardening, and thickening of skin tissue; this phase is sometimes called the *indurative phase*. The skin loses its elasticity, and range of motion is markedly decreased; ulcerations may occur. Joint contractures may develop, and the client may be unable to perform activities of daily living independently.

SYSTEMIC MANIFESTATIONS

Major organ damage is likely to develop in clients with diffuse scleroderma, specifically affecting:

- The gastrointestinal tract
- The cardiovascular system
- The pulmonary system
- The renal system

Gastrointestinal tract involvement, particularly of the esophagus, is common. The esophagus loses its motility, and dysphagia and esophageal reflux result. A small, sliding hiatal hernia may be present, and swallowing may be difficult. Reflux of gastric contents can cause esophagitis and subsequent ulceration, particularly in the lower two thirds of the esophagus. Intestinal changes are similar to those of the esophagus. Peristalsis is diminished, which causes clinical manifestations similar to a partial bowel obstruction; malabsorption is a frequent complication.

In addition to assessing problems of the digestive tract, the nurse observes for *cardiovascular* manifestations. Raynaud's phenomenon occurs in various degrees in most clients with progressive systemic sclerosis. On exposure to cold or emotional stress, the small arterioles in the digits of both hands and feet rapidly constrict, which causes decreased blood flow. In severe cases, the client experiences digit necrosis, excruciating pain, and autoamputation of distal digits (the tips of digits fall off spontaneously). (See Chapter 35 for a complete discussion of this disorder.) The nurse notes vasculitic lesions, often around the nail beds (periungual lesions), in many clients. Myocardial fibrosis, another common problem, is evidenced by electrocardiographic changes (ECG), cardiac dysrhythmias, and chest pain.

Lung involvement in the client with PSS may go undetected until autopsy. Fibrosis of the alveoli and interstitial tissues is present in almost all clients with the disease, but clinical manifestations may not be present.

Renal involvement is an important aspect of the overall disease process and frequently causes malignant hypertension and death. The nurse assesses for signs of impending organ failure, such as changes in urinary output.

LABORATORY ASSESSMENT

The laboratory findings in a client with progressive systemic sclerosis (PSS) are similar to those in a client with systemic lupus. Clinical findings and the client's response to drug therapy help the physician differentiate the two diseases. Additional tests ordered for the client depend on which organs seem to be affected. Upper and lower gastrointestinal series are commonly performed because of the frequency of gastrointestinal clinical manifestations.

INTERVENTIONS

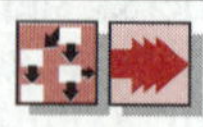

The aim of medical management of PSS is to force the disease into remission and thus slow disease progression. The physician uses drug therapy primarily for this purpose, but it is often unsuccessful. Systemic steroids and immunosuppressants are used in large doses and often in combination.

Local skin protective measures can help to maintain the client's skin integrity. The nurse pays special attention to skin care by having the client use mild soap and lotions and gentle cleaning techniques. The nurse inspects the skin daily for further changes or open lesions. Skin ulcers are treated according to their type and location.

In addition to drug therapy to control the overall disease process, specific measures can provide comfort. The client with PSS not only experiences chronic joint pain but also has severe, acute pain during episodes of Raynaud's phenomenon. A bed cradle and footboard keep bedcovers away from the skin in severe cases. The nurse adjusts the room temperature to prevent chilling, which can precipitate digit vasospasm. If clients can tolerate touching of the affected areas, they can wear gloves and socks to increase warmth. Because cigarette smoking and extreme emotional stress can also cause recurrence of symptoms, the client should try to avoid or minimize these factors as much as possible.

The client with esophageal involvement may need small, frequent meals rather than the traditional three meals daily. Clients should minimize the intake of foods and liquids that stimulate gastric secretion, for example, spicy foods, caffeine, and alcohol. The nurse instructs the client to keep his or her head elevated for 1 to 2 hours after meals. Some clients may need to be in this position continuously. Histamine antagonists and antacids help to reduce and neutralize gastric acid. To help the client avoid choking, the nurse collaborates with the dietitian for dietary changes (Chart 23-12).

Nursing care for the client with joint pain and decreased mobility is very similar to that for the client with rheumatoid arthritis (see Rheumatoid Arthritis earlier in this chapter).

DISCHARGE PLANNING

Discharge planning for the client with progressive systemic sclerosis is similar to that for the client with lupus. The client is treated at home, but the client may need frequent hospitalizations if major organ involvement occurs during exacerbations.

CHART 23-12

Nursing Care Highlight ◆ The Client with Progressive Systemic Sclerosis and Esophagitis

- Keep the client's head elevated at least 60 degrees during meals and for at least 1 hour after each meal.
- Provide small, frequent meals rather than three large meals each day.
- Give the client small amounts of food for each bite, and explain the importance of chewing each bite carefully before swallowing.
- Provide semisoft foods, such as mashed potatoes and pudding or custard; liquids are most likely to cause choking.
- Collaborate with the dietitian about the client's diet.
- Teach the client to avoid foods that increase gastric secretion, for instance, caffeine, pepper, and other spices.
- Give antacids if the physician prescribes them.

Gout

OVERVIEW

Gout, or gouty arthritis, is a systemic disease in which urate crystals deposit in joints and other body tissues, causing inflammation. The cause and treatment of gout have been firmly established. The classic case of well-advanced disease is seldom seen today unless the client does not comply with the therapeutic regimen.

There are two major types of gout: primary and secondary.

Primary gout is the most common type and results from one of several inborn errors of purine metabolism. An end-product of purine metabolism is uric acid, which is usually excreted by the kidneys. In primary gout, uric acid production exceeds the excretion capability of the kidneys and sodium urate is deposited in synovium and other tissues, which results in inflammation. Primary gout is inherited as an X-linked trait; males are affected through female carriers. About 25% of clients have a family history of gout. Primary gout affects middle-aged and older men (85% to 90% of clients with gout) and postmenopausal women. The peak time of onset is during a person's 30s and 40s.

Secondary gout involves hyperuricemia (excessive uric acid in the blood) that is caused by another disease. Secondary gout affects people of all ages. Renal insufficiency, diuretic therapy, and certain chemotherapeutic agents decrease the normal excretion of waste products, including uric acid. Disorders such as multiple myeloma and certain carcinomas bring about increased uric acid production because of greater turnover of cellular nucleic acids. Treatment involves management of the underlying disorder.

There are four phases of the primary disease process:

- Asymptomatic hyperuricemic
- Acute
- Intercritical (intercurrent)
- Chronic

The client is usually unaware of the asymptomatic hyperuricemic phase unless he or she has had a serum uric acid level determination. The client's serum level is elevated, but no overt signs of the disease are present.

The first "attack" of gouty arthritis begins the acute phase. The client experiences excruciating pain and inflammation in one or more small joints, usually the metatarsophalangeal joint of the great toe. Of all clients with gout, 75% have inflammation of this joint (podagra) as the initial manifestation.

Months or perhaps years can pass before additional attacks occur—this is the intercritical, or intercurrent, phase of the disease. The client is asymptomatic, and no abnormalities are found on examination of the joints.

After repeated episodes of acute gout, deposits of urate crystals develop under the person's skin and within major organs, particularly in the renal system. The client is then classified as having chronic tophaceous gout. Urate kidney stone formation is more common than renal insufficiency in chronic gout.

COLLABORATIVE MANAGEMENT

ASSESSMENT

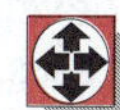

The historical data that the nurse collects include age, sex, and a family history of gout. Gout affects men, particularly those who have relatives with gout. A complete medical history is needed to determine whether gout has been caused by another problem. In women, especially, there is a tendency to overuse diuretics, which can lead to secondary gout.

ACUTE GOUT

Overt manifestations are present in the acute and chronic phases of gout. The nurse encounters a client with acute gout most often because chronic gout is not common today in the United States. Joint inflammation is the most frequent finding and is usually so painful that the client seeks medical care. The nurse uses inspection skills only; the inflamed area is usually too painful and swollen to be touched or moved.

CHRONIC GOUT

When the client has chronic gout, the nurse inspects the skin for tophi, or deposits of sodium urate crystals (Fig. 23-11). Common sites for tophi are the

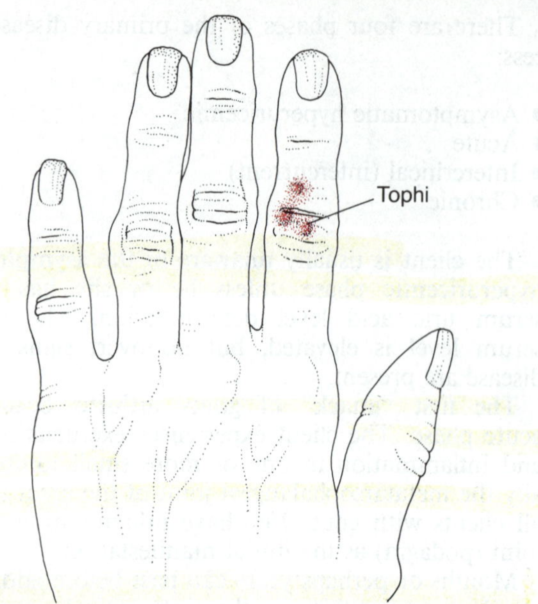

FIGURE 23-11 ◆ Typical appearance of tophi, which are common in chronic gout, on an index finger.

ear, arms, and fingers near joints. The tophi are hard on palpation and are irregular in shape. When the skin over the tophi is irritated, it may break open and a yellow, gritty substance is discharged. Infection may result. Although tophi may occur anywhere, they commonly appear on the outer ear.

Other manifestations of chronic gout include signs of renal calculi (stones) or renal dysfunction. Stones develop in about 20% of clients with gout. In some cases, urate kidney stones occur before the arthritis is present.

The physician orders determinations of serum uric acid levels to validate hyperuricemia. Because the serum uric acid level can be altered by food intake, serial measurements are usually taken. A consistent level of more than 8 mg/100 mL is generally considered abnormal. Urinary uric acid levels are also measured; an overproduction of uric acid is confirmed by an excretion of more than 600 mg per 24 hours after a 5-day restriction of purine intake.

The physician orders renal function tests, such as blood urea nitrogen (BUN) and serum creatinine level, to monitor possible kidney involvement. A definitive diagnostic test for the disease is synovial fluid aspiration (arthrocentesis) to detect the needle-like crystals that are characteristic of the disorder (See Other Diagnostic Assessment under Rheumatoid Arthritis.)

INTERVENTIONS

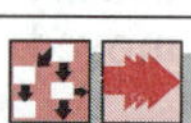

Gout is one of the easiest diseases for the physician to diagnose and treat in its early phases. If the client receives treatment and complies with drug therapy, the client should experience no further symptoms and no change in body image or lifestyle. The client with gout is usually treated on an outpatient basis.

Drug Therapy Drug therapy is the primary component of management for clients with gout. In acute gouty "attacks," the inflammation subsides spontaneously within 3 to 5 days, but most clients cannot tolerate the pain for that long. The drugs used in acute gout are different from those used in chronic gout. The physician typically prescribes a combination of colchicine (Colsalide, Novocolchicine✱) and a nonsteroidal anti-inflammatory drug, such as indomethacin (Indocin, Novomethacin✱) or ibuprofen (Motrin, Amersol✱), for *acute* gout. The client takes these medications until the inflammation subsides, usually for 4 to 7 days, or until severe diarrhea occurs (a side effect of colchicine).

For clients with chronic gout, the physician prescribes drugs to promote uric acid excretion or to reduce its production on a continuous, maintenance basis. Allopurinol (Zyloprim) is the drug of choice. As a xanthine oxidase inhibitor, it prevents the conversion of xanthine to uric acid. Probenecid (Benemid, Benuryl✱) is also effective as a uricosuric drug in gout (it promotes excretion of excess uric acid). Combination drugs, such as ColBENEMID, that contain probenecid and colchicine are also available. The physician and nurse monitor serum uric acid levels to determine the effectiveness of these medications.

Diet Therapy Whether to recommend special dietary restrictions for clients with gout is controversial. Some physicians advocate a strict low-purine diet, advising the client to avoid such foods as organ meats, shellfish, and oily fish with bones, such as sardines. Some physicians believe that limiting protein foods, especially red and organ meats, is sufficient. Still others do not believe that diet restrictions affect treatment. It is well known, however, that excessive alcohol intake and fad "starvation" diets can cause a gouty attack. The nurse helps the client determine which foods may precipitate a gout attack.

In addition to food and beverage restrictions, clients with gout should avoid all forms of aspirin and diuretics because they may precipitate an attack. Likewise, excessive physical or emotional stress can exacerbate the disease. The nurse may need to teach stress management techniques (see Chap. 7).

Having the client drink more fluids is one of the best measures to prevent urinary stone formation. Such a measure helps to dilute the urine and prevent sediment formation. Uric acid is less likely to form urinary stones in urine that has a high pH because it is more soluble in that environment. The client's urinary pH can be increased by intake of alkaline ash foods, such as citrus fruits and juices, and milk and certain dairy products. However, the value of adhering to a strict diet that is rich in these foods is questionable.

The client with a diagnosis of gout is seldom hospitalized unless renal complications develop. If clients follow the prescribed interventions, chronic tophaceous gout should not develop.

OTHER CONNECTIVE TISSUE DISEASES

The care of clients with connective tissue diseases (CTDs) is often similar regardless of the specific diagnosis. This part of the chapter describes other fairly common diseases that are classified as CTDs.

Polymyositis/Dermatomyositis

Polymyositis is a diffuse, inflammatory disease of striated muscle that causes symmetric weakness and atrophy. When a rash accompanies polymyositis, the disease is called dermatomyositis. Both diseases vary in their mode of onset and progression and are characterized by spontaneous remissions and exacerbations. Women are affected twice as often as men, and 30- to 60-year-olds are the most susceptible to either disease.

In addition to proximal muscle and possible skin involvement, the client typically has polyarthritis, polyarthralgia (pain around multiple joints), and Raynaud's phenomenon (see Chap. 35). Clients with dermatomyositis have the characteristic heliotrope (lilac) rash and periorbital edema. Malignant neoplasms occur more frequently in these clients than in the rest of the population, with as many as 30% of clients older than age 55 having internal malignancies. Many clients have difficulty in swallowing and/or talking because of severe muscle weakness.

Clients are treated with high-dose steroids, immunosuppressive agents, and supportive care, with particular attention to nutrition.

Systemic Necrotizing Vasculitis

Necrotizing vasculitis is a term for a group of diseases whose primary manifestation is arteritis (inflammation of arterial walls), which causes ischemia in tissues usually supplied by the involved vessels.

Polyarteritis nodosa affects middle-aged men and involves every body system. Treatment is similar to that for people with systemic lupus, but the prognosis is not as promising. Renal disorders and cardiac involvement are the most frequent causes of death.

Hypersensitivity vasculitis is the most common form of vasculitis and primarily causes skin lesions as an allergic response to drugs, infections, or tumors.

Takayasu's arteritis, or the aortic arch syndrome, is also called the "pulseless" disease. Women in their 20s, particularly those of Japanese descent, are affected most often. Cerebral ischemia is manifested by visual changes, syncope, and vertigo.

The drug of choice for most types of vasculitis is steroids.

Polymyalgia Rheumatica

Polymyalgia rheumatica (PMR) is a clinical syndrome characterized by stiffness, weakness, and aching of the proximal musculature, that is, the shoulder and pelvic girdles. Systemic manifestations, such as fever, arthralgias (pain around joints), and weight loss, occur in the majority of cases. The disease commonly occurs in women older than 50 years of age and typically responds to steroid therapy in 3 to 5 days.

Giant cell (temporal) arteritis is frequently associated with polymyalgia rheumatica. The branches of the aorta are vasculitic, which causes headaches and changes in vision. This disorder is easy to miss because most clients with PMR are elderly women who complain of declining vision (also an age-related change). Corticosteroids are highly effective in controlling giant cell arteritis.

Ankylosing Spondylitis

Ankylosing spondylitis is also known as Marie-Strumpell disease and, more recently, as rheumatoid spondylitis. As shown in Figure 23–12, the disease affects the vertebral column and causes spinal deformities. Although this disorder is present in both sexes

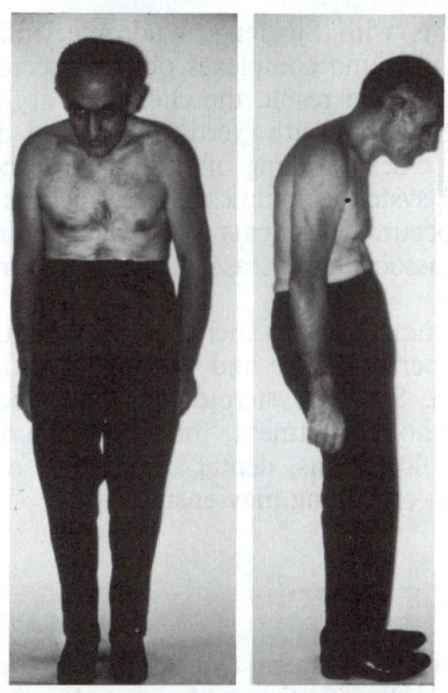

FIGURE 23–12 ◆ Spinal deformity and posture that are often seen in clients with advanced spondylitis. (From the Arthritis Teaching Slide Collection, copyright 1980. Used by permission of the Arthritis Foundation.)

at any age in adulthood, young Caucasian males under age 40 are most commonly affected. Other features include iritis (inflammation of the iris), arthritis or arthralgia, and nonspecific systemic manifestations, such as malaise and weight loss.

Although the exact cause is unknown, ankylosing spondylitis is associated with the HLA-B27 antigen. Compromised respiratory function caused by a rigid chest wall is the major threat to health. Most clients function normally but live with chronic discomfort. Anti-inflammatory drugs and physical therapy are key components of management.

Reiter's Syndrome

Like ankylosing spondylitis, Reiter's syndrome is associated with the HLA-B27 antigen. The disease most often affects young Caucasian males. The complete syndrome is a triad of arthritis, conjunctivitis, and urethritis (inflammation of the urethra) resulting from exposure to sexually transmitted disease or dysentery (infectious diarrhea). Urethritis is often the first clinical manifestation.

Although the disease is characterized by this triad of manifestations, other conditions, such as circinate balanitis (ring-like inflammation of the glans penis) and skin lesions, are equally significant for confirmation of the diagnosis.

Management is symptomatic and may be complex if there is organ involvement. Nonsteroidal anti-inflammatory drugs and physical therapy are generally prescribed.

Sjögren's Syndrome

In clients with Sjögren's syndrome, inflammatory cells and immune complexes obstruct secretory ducts and glands. As a result, the client has dry eyes (sicca syndrome), dry mouth (xerostomia), and dry vagina. In severe cases, swelling of the parotid and lacrimal areas and systemic manifestations, such as fever and fatigue, occur. Of clients with the syndrome 50% have an associated disease, such as rheumatoid arthritis.

Local management includes meticulous mouth, eye, and perineal care and the use of artificial tears and saliva. Systemic steroids may also be administered. Without treatment, the client can lose vision and oral ulcerations, dental caries, and difficulty in swallowing or talking may ensue.

Infectious Arthritis

Any infectious agent can invade the joint space and cause inflammation and tissue destruction. Certain pathogens, such as *Staphylococcus aureus,* destroy tissue rapidly; others, especially viruses, do not cause irreversible damage. The cornerstone of management is local and/or systemic antibiotic therapy.

CHART 23-13

Health Promotion Guide ◆ Prevention and Early Detection of Lyme Disease

- Avoid heavily wooded areas or areas with thick underbrush.
- Use an insect repellent on your skin and clothes when you are in an area where ticks are likely to be found.
- Wear long-sleeved tops and long pants.
- Wear closed shoes and a hat or cap.
- Bathe immediately after being in an infested area, and inspect your body for ticks (about the size of a pinhead), paying special attention to your arms, legs, and hairline.
- Gently remove with tweezers or fingers any tick that you find. Dispose of the tick by flushing it down the toilet (burning a tick could spread infection).
- Wait 4 to 6 weeks after being bitten by a tick before being tested for Lyme disease (testing before this time is not reliable).
- Report symptoms, such as a rash or influenza-like illness, to your physician.

Lyme Disease

Lyme disease has recently been added to the list of connective tissue diseases (CTDs). Unlike many CTDs, however, the cause has been identified. The infected deer tick *(Ixodes dammini)* transmits a bacterium (a spirochete) that causes a circular rash, malaise, fever, headache, and muscle or joint aches.

If Lyme disease is not diagnosed and treated, later complications, such as arthritis, enlarged lymph nodes, and neurologic and cardiac problems, can result. Prompt treatment with antibiotics, such as tetracycline, is usually effective. Chart 23-13 lists ways to avoid Lyme disease.

Pseudogout

Pseudogout is a disease that mimics the clinical manifestations of gout. The crystals that deposit in joints, however, are calcium pyrophosphate, not sodium urate. Most often, these crystals migrate to cartilage, but they can also deposit in tendons, ligaments, and synovium.

The client most susceptible to pseudogout is an elderly male who is hospitalized. Although the cause is not certain, the incidence is highest in men who have metastatic cancer or endocrine imbalances, such as hypothyroidism. Nonsteroidal anti-inflammatory drugs usually control the manifestations of the disease.

Disease-Associated Arthritis

A number of diseases can cause secondary arthritis. Tuberculosis, Crohn's disease, ulcerative colitis, hemophilia, psoriasis, and sickle cell anemia are typical examples. To manage joint involvement, the primary disease is treated. For example, when a client with Crohn's disease has a remission, joint manifestations also subside. Conditions in which joint involvement can occur are presented in Table 23–3.

Fibrositis

The term fibrositis, or fibromyalgia, describes a syndrome characterized by trunk, extremity, and/or facial pain and tenderness without other objective findings. The primary manifestations are pain, muscle stiffness and spasm, sensory changes, and exhaustion, which may be attributable to severe sleep disturbances. Tender areas, known as *trigger points,* typically can be palpated to elicit pain in a predictable, reproducible pattern. Physical therapy, nonsteroidal anti-inflammatory drugs, and muscle relaxants usually provide temporary relief.

In most clients, fibrositis is the result of deep sleep deprivation. Clients may need hypnotics and other sleep-inducing methods to overcome this sleep disturbance. Antidepressive agents, such as amitriptyline (Elavil, Apo-Amitriptyline✱) or nortriptyline (Pamelor), may promote sleep and reduce muscle spasm. These drugs should be used with caution in the elderly because they can cause confusion and orthostatic hypotension. Trazadone (Desyrel) is the preferred drug for this population. The nurse observes the client for side effects and monitors for postural blood pressure changes.

Secondary fibrosis syndromes can accompany any connective tissue disease, particularly lupus and rheumatoid disease, and may not necessarily be related to sleep patterns.

TABLE 23–3 Disorders Associated with Arthritis

- Crohn's disease
- Ulcerative colitis
- Tuberculosis
- Hemophilia
- Whipple's disease
- Intestinal bypass surgery
- Hyperparathyroidism
- Hyperthyroidism
- Diabetes mellitus
- Sickle cell anemia crisis
- Psoriasis
- Infection

Local Inflammatory Disorders

Two of the most common inflammatory conditions are localized to specific connective tissues: *bursitis* and *tendinitis.* Both usually occur in the shoulder and are caused by aging, irritation, and/or trauma. During middle age, the tendons become frayed, irregular, and calcified, which causes inflammation of tendons and adjacent bursae. This syndrome, which may be acute or chronic, occurs most often in women. The dominant arm is usually involved. Intra-articular steroid injections and systemic anti-inflammatory drugs are administered.

Mixed Connective Tissue Disease

When a client presents with clinical manifestations that are not typical of any one connective tissue disease, a diagnosis of mixed CTD is made. Approximately 10% of clients with CTDs are classified as having mixed disease. Some of these are *overlap syndromes,* in which two or more diseases occur at the same time. Common examples are systemic lupus erythematosus (SLE) plus progressive systemic sclerosis (PSS) and rheumatoid arthritis (RA) plus SLE.

Management depends of the clinical manifestations, but often the client is treated as having SLE.

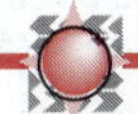

IMPLICATIONS FOR NURSING RESEARCH

Because many connective tissue diseases result in chronic pain and impaired mobility, the nursing profession should address the following research questions:

- What are the most appropriate pain relief measures for chronic joint pain?
- What is the best method to accurately assess the client's level of mobility?
- What are the best nursing interventions to help the client cope with fatigue?
- When are cold and heat applications best applied for maximum effectiveness in a client with joint involvement?
- What are the best ways for nurses to assist with body image disturbance in a client with severe joint deformity or skin lesions?

SELECTED BIBLIOGRAPHY

*Aglietti, P., Rinonapoli, E., Stringa, G., & Taviani, A. (1983). Tibial osteotomy for the varus osteoarthritic knee. *Clinical Orthopaedics and Related Research, 176,* 239–251.

*American Nurses' Association and Arthritis Health Professionals Association Nursing Task Force. (1983). *Outcome* *standards for rheumatology nursing practice.* Kansas City: American Nurses' Association.

Bailey, J. M., & Nielson, B. I. (1993). Uncertainty and appraisal in women with rheumatoid arthritis. *Orthopaedic Nursing, 12*(2), 63–67.

*Blake, S. A. (1985). Noncemented femoral prosthesis: Intraoperative focus. *Orthopaedic Nursing, 4*(1), 40–42.

Blalock, S. J., DeVellis, B. M., DeVellis, R. F., et al. (1992). Psychological well-being among people recently diagnosed with rheumatoid arthritis: Do self-perceptions of abilities make a difference? *Arthritis and Rheumatism, 35,* 1267–1272.

*Boggs, J. (1982). *Arthritis, living and loving: Information about sex.* Atlanta: The Arthritis Foundation.

*Bradley, L. A. (1985). Psychological aspects of arthritis. *Bulletin on the Rheumatic Diseases, 35,* 1–12.

*Brassell, M. P. (1988). Pharmacologic management of rheumatic diseases. *Orthopaedic Nursing, 7*(2), 43–51.

*Brinkley, L. B. (1989). Predeposit autologous blood for elective orthopaedic surgery. *Orthopaedic Nursing, 8*(1), 25–28.

Calkins, E. (1991). Arthritis in the elderly. *Bulletin on the Rheumatic Diseases, 40*(1), 1–9.

Clough, D. H. (1991). The effects of cognitive distortion and depression on disability in rheumatoid arthritis. *Research in Nursing and Health, 14,* 439–446.

Cornwell, C. J., et al. (1990). Perceived health status, self-esteem and body image in women with rheumatoid arthritis and systemic lupus erythematosus. *Research in Nursing and Health, 13*(2), 99–107.

Crosby, L. (1991). Factors which contribute to fatigue associated with rheumatoid arthritis. *Journal of Advanced Nursing, 16,* 974–981.

*Doheney, M. O. (1985). Porous coated prosthesis: Concepts and care considerations. *Orthopaedic Nursing, 4*(5), 43–45.

*Dunajcik, L. M. (1989, April). The hip: When the joint must be replaced. *RN,* 62–71.

*Fessel, W. J. (1988). Epidemiology of systemic lupus erythematosus. *Rheumatic Disease Clinics of North America, 14,* 15–23.

Fife, R. Z. (1993). Methotrexate use in juvenile rheumatoid arthritis. *Orthopaedic Nursing, 12*(1), 32–36.

*Follman, D. A. (1988). Nursing care concerns in total shoulder replacement. *Orthopaedic Nursing, 7*(3), 29–31.

Fries, J. F., Williams, C. A., Ramey, D., & Bloch, D. A. (1993). The relative toxicity of disease-modifying antirheumatic drugs. *Arthritis and Rheumatism, 36,* 297–306.

Gavula, D. (1990). Lyme disease. *Topics in Emergency Medicine, 12*(3), 15–22.

Giger, J. N., & Davidhizar, R. E. (1991). Transcultural nursing: Assessment and intervention. St. Louis: Mosby Year Book.

*Guccione, A. A. (1989). Understanding arthritis in the elderly. *Topics in Geriatric Care and Rehabilitation, 3*(5), 1–8.

Hahn, B. H. (1990). Lupus nephritis: Therapeutic decisions. *Hospital Practice, 25*(3A), 89–93, 96–97, 103–104.

Hardin, J. G. (1992). Complications of cervical arthritis. *Postgraduate Medicine, 91,* 309–315, 318.

Hynes, D. (1992). Oral NSAIDs: The best choice in practice. *Practitioner, 236,* 328–330.

*Ignatavicius, D. D. (1987). Meeting the psychosocial needs of patients with rheumatoid arthritis. *Orthopaedic Nursing, 6*(3), 16–20.

Kaplan, D., Ginzler, E. M., & Feldman, J. (1992). Arthritis and hypertension in patients with systemic lupus erythematosus. *Arthritis and Rheumatism, 35,* 423–428.

*Koerner, M. E., & Dickinson, G. R. (1983). Adult arthritis: A look at some of its forms. *American Journal of Nursing, 83,* 255–262.

Lambert, V. A. (1991). Arthritis. *Annual Review of Nursing Research, 9,* 3–18.

*Lee, B. C. (1989, April). Be ready for Lyme disease in your own back yard. *RN,* 26–31.

*Malek, C. J., & Brower, S. A. (1984). Rheumatoid arthritis: How does it influence sexuality? *Rehabilitation Nursing, 9,* 26–28.

*Maly, B. J., Turk, M. A., & Kinney, C. L. (1988). Rehabilitation in joint and connective tissue diseases. *Archives of Physical Medicine and Rehabilitation, 69*(Suppl.), S71–S112.

Manne, S. L., & Zautra, A. J. (1993). Coping with arthritis: Current status and critique. *Arthritis and Rheumatism, 35,* 1273–1280.

McInnes, J. (1992). A controlled evaluation of continuous passive motion in patients undergoing total knee replacement. *Journal of the American Medical Association, 268,* 1423–1428.

Mirabelli, L. (1990). Caring for patients with rheumatoid arthritis. *Nursing, 20*(9), 67–68, 70, 72.

*Mooney, N. E. (1983). Coping with chronic pain in rheumatoid arthritis: Patient behaviors and nursing interventions. *Rehabilitation Nursing, 8,* 20–21, 24–25.

*Moskowitz, R. W. (1982). Management of osteoarthritis. *Bulletin on the Rheumatic Diseases, 31,* 31–34.

*Navarro, A. H. (1983). Physical therapy in the management of rheumatoid arthritis. *Clinical Rheumatology in Practice, 1,* 125–130.

Peeters, W. (1992). Effect of rheumatoid arthritis upon other members of the family. *Clinical Rheumatology, 11*(2), 185–188.

*Pigg, J. S., Driscoll, P. W., & Caniff, R. (1985). *Rheumatology nursing: A problem-oriented approach.* New York: Wiley.

*Riggs, G. K., & Gall, E. P. (1984). *Rheumatic diseases: Rehabilitation and management.* Boston: Butterworth.

*Rothfield, N. F. (1989). The diagnostic pictures of systemic lupus erythematosus. *Hospital Practice, 24,* 37–46.

*Salmond, S. W. (1989). Stress and stressors in rheumatoid arthritis. *Journal of Advanced Nursing, 1*(4), 35–43.

*Salvati, E. A. (Ed.). (1988). Long term results of cemented joint replacement: Is cement obsolete? *Orthopedic Clinics of North America, 19,* 467–668.

*Schumacher, H. R., Jr. (1988). *Primer on the rheumatic diseases.* Atlanta: The Arthritis Foundation.

*Simpson, C. F. (1983). Heat, cold, or both. *American Journal of Nursing, 83,* 270–272.

*Smeltzer, K. J. (1987). Fibromyalgia: The frustration of diagnosis and treatment. *Orthopaedic Nursing, 6*(3), 28–31.

*Strand, C. V., & Clark, S. R. (1983). Adult arthritis: Drugs and remedies. *American Journal of Nursing, 83,* 266–270.

*Sutton, J. D. (1984). The hospitalized patient with arthritis. *Nursing Clinics of North America, 19,* 617–625.

Wallace, D. J. (1990). Managing arthritis in the elderly. *AORN, 51,* 1074, 1076–1077, 1080.

*Walsh, C. R., & Wirth, C. R. (1985). Total knee arthroplasty: Biomechanical and nursing considerations. *Orthopaedic Nursing, 4*(2), 29–34.

Ward, M. M., & Leigh, J. P. (1993). Marital status and progression of functional disability in patients with rheumatoid arthritis. *Arthritis and Rheumatism, 36*, 581–588.

Weinblatt, M., Polisson, R., Blotner, S. D., et al. (1993). The effects of drug therapy on radiographic progression of rheumatoid arthritis. *Arthritis and Rheumatism, 36*, 613–619.

*Whitney, R. (1989). Unlock the mystery of lupus. *Today's OR Nurse, 11*(3), 10–12, 30–32.

*Wilske, K. R., & Healey, L. A. (1985). Polymyalgia rheumatica and giant cell arteritis. *Postgraduate Medicine, 77*, 243–248.

*Zeigler, G. C. (1984). Systemic lupus erythematosus and systemic sclerosis. *Nursing Clinics of North America, 19*, 673–695.

SUGGESTED READINGS

Bailey, J. M., & Nielson, B. I. (1993). Uncertainty and appraisal of uncertainty in women with rheumatoid arthritis. *Orthopaedic Nursing, 12*(2), 63–67.

This study examined the relationships between degree of uncertainty, appraisal of uncertainty, and length of illness among 23 women with rheumatoid arthritis. The authors' findings suggested that nurses who work with clients with rheumatoid arthritis should be aware that high levels of uncertainty can lead to distress, anxiety, and coping problems.

Blalock, S. J., DeVellis, B. M., DeVellis, R. F., (1992). Psychological well-being among people recently diagnosed with rheumatoid arthritis: Do self-perceptions of abilities make a difference? *Arthritis and Rheumatism, 35*, 1267–1272.

This study examined the effect of satisfaction with abilities on psychological well-being. The higher the satisfaction, the lower the psychological distress, and vice versa.

Fife, R. Z. (1993). Methotrexate use in juvenile rheumatoid arthritis. *Orthopaedic Nursing, 12*(1), 32–36.

Although this article discussed the use of methotrexate (MTX) in children with arthritis, it presents an excellent overview of this drug. The author begins with a history, then discusses action, side effects, and toxicity associated with MTX.

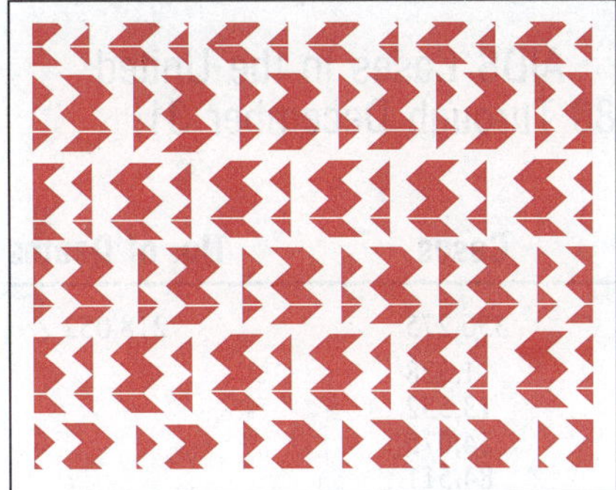

CHAPTER 24

Interventions for Clients with Immunologic Disorders

CHAPTER HIGHLIGHTS

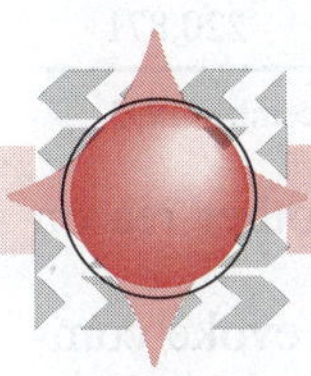

The immune system protects the body from disease through constant surveillance and destruction of foreign invaders. Occasionally, however, the immune system malfunctions. This malfunction may take the form of *inadequate* function, *excess* function, or *inappropriate* function. Clients who have inadequate immune function are at increased risk for infection and cancer. Clients who have excessive or inappropriate immune function are at increased risk for tissue damage. For some clients, malfunction of the immune system is the cause of disease; for others, it is the result.

This chapter presents categories of immune disorders:

- Immunodeficiencies
- Hypersensitivities
- Autoimmunities
- Gammopathies

IMMUNODEFICIENCIES

A deficient response of the immune system that is due to a missing or damaged immune component is an immunodeficiency. The immunodeficient person cannot defend adequately against potentially harmful substances that an immunocompetent person can normally combat. An immunodeficient person's immune system cannot recognize or eliminate antigens normally, and the person is therefore susceptible to infection, malignancy, and other disease.

In some newborns, a specific substance or function that is essential to normal immune activity may be absent; these newborns are said to have a congenital or primary immunodeficiency. Other people at birth have a normally functioning immune system but later, as a consequence of another disease, injury, or unknown cause, *acquired* (secondary) immunodeficiency develops; these people are referred to as *immunocompromised* because their immune systems have been compromised, resulting in an impaired ability to neutralize, destroy or eliminate antigens (see Chap. 22).

The client who has an immunodeficiency manifests clinical symptoms that vary in severity and occur in multiple systems of the body. For many immunodeficiencies, the cause is unknown or uncontrollable, the pathophysiology is not well understood, and effective treatment may not be available. The complications, but not the actual immune defect, can be treated. Most immunodeficiencies are chronic conditions, and periods of wellness are interspersed with the occurrence of clinical problems.

The immunodeficient person constantly faces the possibility that the next infection might be fatal. Normal environmental exposures to people, objects, and microorganisms may pose significant danger. Nurses are instrumental in teaching the immunodeficient person how to avoid infection and which signs and symptoms to monitor if an infection occurs. The nurse assesses the client for subtle changes related to early infection and treats the client quickly according to physician's orders. Supporting the client and family is an essential part of nursing care.

TABLE 24–1 AIDS Cases in the United States from 1980 Through December 31, 1993

Age	Cases	No. of Deaths
Adult/Adolescent	356,275	218,052
13–19	1,528	
20–24	13,552	
25–29	54,075	
30–34	84,511	
35–39	80,397	
40–44	55,186	
45–49	30,515	
50–54	16,507	
55–59	9,563	
60–64	5,475	
65+	4,963	
Male	252,363	
Female	32,477	
Pediatric	5,229	2,819
<5	4,187	
5–12	1,042	
Total	361,504	220,871

Data from Centers for Disease Control and Prevention, December 1993.

ACQUIRED IMMUNODEFICIENCIES

Acquired Immunodeficiency Syndrome

OVERVIEW

Acquired immunodeficiency syndrome (AIDS) is the late stage of a continuum of symptoms that result from infection with the human immunodeficiency virus (HIV). AIDS is not the same as HIV infection, and not everyone infected with HIV has AIDS. Persons with AIDS are profoundly immunosuppressed and usually have lived with HIV for several years before AIDS develops. The nurse provides education, physical care, and psychologic support for the person living with AIDS.

AIDS is a serious, debilitating, and eventually fatal disease. To date, 84% of those with AIDS have been between the ages of 25 and 49 (Table 24–1). To be diagnosed as having AIDS, a person must be infected with HIV, have a clinical disease that indicates a cellular immunodeficiency, and have no other reason to be cellularly immunodeficient.

The care of the person with AIDS can evoke complex personal issues for the nurse. Nurses must acknowledge their own fear of acquiring HIV and any negative attitudes regarding possible client lifestyles contributing to HIV infection, such as intravenous (IV) drug use or homosexual behaviors. Knowledge and practice of appropriate infection control techniques can reduce the nurse's fears about becoming infected through client care. To provide competent, compassionate nursing care to the person with AIDS, nurses must be willing to suspend judgment.

PATHOPHYSIOLOGY

The Centers for Disease Control and Prevention (CDC) classification scheme for HIV infection is based on the pathophysiology of the disease as immune function progressively worsens (Table 24–2). The classification begins with acute infection and spans a continuum that culminates with AIDS. *The person with HIV can transmit the virus to others at all stages of disease.*

Acute infection (CDC group I) can occur within 1 to 8 weeks after infection with HIV and is characterized by a flu-like syndrome that resolves completely. The next stage is asymptomatic infection (CDC group II), in which the infected person has no signs or symptoms of the disease. The first symptomatic stage occurs with the appearance of persistent generalized lymphadenopathy (lymph node enlargement lasting more than 3 months) (CDC group III).

The next stage includes constitutional disease, which can include persistent fever or diarrhea (more

TABLE 24–2 Centers for Disease Control (CDC) Classification of Human Immunodeficiency Virus (HIV)

Class	Criteria
Group I	• Acute infection with HIV • Flu-like symptoms, resolve completely • HIV antibody-negative
HIV Asymptomatic	
Group II	• HIV antibody-positive • No laboratory or clinical indicators of immune deficiency
HIV Symptomatic	
Group III	• HIV antibody-positive • Persistent generalized lymphadenopathy

Group IV-A	• HIV antibody-positive
	• Constitutional disease
	  • Persistent fever or diarrhea
	  • Weight loss >10% normal body weight

Group IV-B	• Same as group IV-A, plus
	• Neurologic disease
	  • Dementia
	  • Neuropathy
	  • Myelopathy

Group IV-C	• Same as group IV-B, plus • CD_4 T-cell count <200/mm^3 • Opportunistic infection
Group IV-D	• Same as group IV-C, plus • Pulmonary tuberculosis, invasive cervical cancer, or other malignancy

Data from Centers for Disease Control and Prevention, March 1993.

than 1 month), or involuntary loss of more than 10% of body weight (CDC group IV-A). Neurologic disease, including dementia, neuropathy and myelopathy are indicators for CDC group IV-B classification. CDC groups IV-C and IV-D include a CD_4 T-lymphocyte (see Chap. 22) count below 200 mm^3 and such clinical conditions as opportunistic infections, recurrent pneumonia, invasive cervical cancer, pulmonary tuberculosis, or other cancers.

The time from initial HIV infection to development of AIDS ranges from 18 months to more than 10 years. The range differs among people, depending on the way in which HIV was acquired and a variety of personal factors. For people who have direct blood contact through transfusion of HIV-contaminated blood, AIDS develops more quickly; for people who become HIV-positive as a result of a single sexual encounter, there is a longer latency period before the condition progresses to AIDS. Other personal factors that may influence how rapidly a person's HIV-positive status progresses to AIDS includes:

- Frequency of re-exposures to HIV
- The presence of other sexually transmitted diseases (syphilis, herpes simplex virus)
- Nutritional status
- Pregnancy
- Stress

ETIOLOGY

The cause of the acquired immunodeficiency syndrome (AIDS) is the profound suppression of immune responses that results from infection with the human immunodeficiency virus (HIV). Two subtypes of the virus have been identified: type 1 (HIV-1) and type 2 (HIV-2). Type 1 is the form of the virus most frequently isolated from infected persons in the Western hemisphere, Europe, and Asia. Type 2 is endemic to West Africa. Although they differ in the viral surface molecules, both HIV subtypes can cause AIDS.

The HIV belongs to a special class of viruses known as retroviruses. Retroviruses differ from ordinary viruses in their efficiency of cellular infection. Retroviruses have only ribonucleic acid (RNA) as their genetic material. The most important difference between retroviruses and ordinary viruses is the presence of a special complex of enzymes within the retrovirus, called reverse transcriptase. This enzyme complex increases the efficiency of viral replication once the retrovirus enters a human cell.

Once a retrovirus gains entry into the body and infects a human cell, the reverse transcriptase enzymes force the human cell's deoxyribonucleic acid (DNA) synthesis machinery to use the viral RNA as a pattern and make a piece of human DNA complementary to the viral RNA. This new piece of DNA is then incorporated successfully into the person's cellular DNA, where it can remain for a long time. When this new DNA is actively transcribed or replicated, the result is the synthesis of huge numbers of viral particles.

After many rounds of replication, in which hundreds to thousands of new viruses or viral particles are produced, these viruses and viral particles leave the human cell (Fig. 24–1). Once the particles are in the host's body fluids, they can infect other cells and continue the viral replication process.

The HIV retrovirus attaches to, infects, and ultimately destroys immune system cells with a CD4 surface receptor. These cells include T4 lymphocytes (CD_4 cells) and macrophages (see Fig. 22–3). The T4 lymphocyte, also called the helper or inducer lymphocyte, regulates the activity of all immune system cells (see Chap. 22). When infected by HIV, the T4 cell does not function normally, causing general malfunction of the whole immune system. The results of HIV infection are:

- Lymphocytopenia with selective T4 cell depletion
- Abnormal T cell function
- Increased production of incomplete and nonfunctional antibodies
- Abnormally functioning macrophages

As a result of these immune dysfunctions, the client with HIV is susceptible to *opportunistic* infections (infection by organisms that take advantage of a defective immune system) and cancer. Macrophages

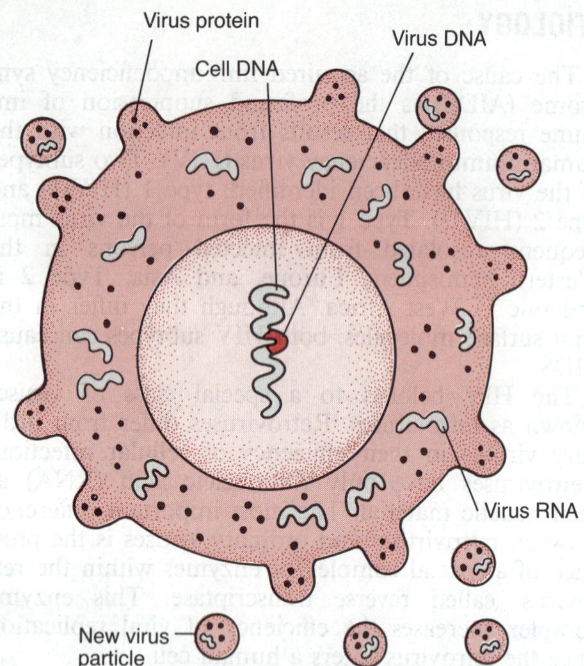

FIGURE 24–1 ◆ A T-lymphocyte infected with human immunodeficiency virus (HIV). The virus can be seen budding from the infected T cell.

that are infected by HIV are not destroyed by infection; they act as a reservoir for the virus.

INCIDENCE/PREVALENCE

The incidence of AIDS in the United States has grown exponentially from its initial occurrence in the early 1980s. In 1981, 291 new cases of AIDS were reported; in 1991, 45,506 new cases were reported (MMWR, 1992). The Public Health Service (PHS) estimates that 1 million persons in the United States are infected with HIV. It has been projected that by the end of 1993, 390,000 to 500,000 people in North America will have AIDS and that 285,000 to 340,000 persons will have died from the disease. The case fatality rate for all reported cases of AIDS is 66% (Centers for Disease Control, 1992).

Epidemiologic and demographic data have shown that most people with AIDS in the United States are (1) men who have had homosexual and bisexual contact (57%) or (2) persons of both sexes who have used intravenous drugs (22%) (Table 24–3). However, the demographics of the disease are rapidly changing. In 1991, the incidence of AIDS increased 3.6% for males and 15% for females. A disproportionate number of cases of AIDS have occurred in racial and ethnic minority groups. Approximately 46% of all AIDS cases in North America have occurred in African-Americans and Hispanics, who constitute only 18.5% of the population. The rates for women and minority groups are reflected in changes in AIDS rates by exposure categories, with a 0.4% decrease in those exposed through male homosexual and bisexual contact and a 9.8% increase in those exposed through IV drug use (Table 24–4).

TABLE 24–3 Distribution of Adult AIDS Cases in the United States by Exposure Category from 1980 Through December 31, 1993

Category	Cases
Male homosexual contact	193,162
Intravenous drug use	86,961
Male homosexual contact and intravenous drug use	23,483
Hemophilia/coagulation disorder	3,134
Heterosexual contact	23,038
Transfusion	6,304
Undetermined	20,193

Data from Centers for Disease Control and Prevention, December 1993.

AIDS is a disease with high mortality. The overall case fatality rate is about 65% for adults and 54% for children; that is, more than 50% of all people who have been diagnosed with AIDS have died (Centers for Disease Control, 1992). To date, there have been no reports of a cure or of a reversal of the immune defect.

Transcultural Considerations. AIDS has been reported in 162 countries and in each state of the United States (World Health Organization, 1991). Reporting of AIDS cases to the World Health Organization is generally incomplete. However, in 1991, a total of 418,403 cases were reported (World Health Organization, 1991). The pattern of HIV infection and the manifestations of AIDS differ in countries such as West Africa, where HIV-2 is the predominant viral strain.

The main difference in the pattern of HIV-2 infection is that it occurs primarily in the heterosexual population, with equal numbers of men and women infected. The modes of transmission are the same as that of HIV-1. The large number of infected females results in a high rate of perinatal transmission and large numbers of HIV-infected children.

Women are the fastest-growing group with HIV

TABLE 24–4 Distribution of AIDS Cases by Race and Ethnic Group in the United States (1980 Through December 31, 1993)

Category	No. of Cases
White, not Hispanic	181,358
Black, not Hispanic	114,959
Hispanic	61,337
Asian/Pacific Islander	2,399
American Indian/Alaskan Native	794
Unknown	662
Total	361,509

Data from Centers for Disease Control and Prevention, December 1993.

infection and AIDS (Kelly & Holman, 1993; Smeltzer & Whipple, 1991). Women who have HIV appear to have a poorer outcome with shorter survival. This outcome may be the result of late diagnosis and social and economic factors that reduce access to medical care rather than the result of viral pathology.

Gynecologic symptoms, particularly persistent vaginal candidiasis, may be the first signs of HIV in women (Kelly & Holman, 1993). Additional symptoms associated with HIV in women include genital herpes, pelvic inflammatory disease, and neoplasia of the genital tract. Because the current CDC classification for HIV does not include these symptoms, diagnosis in women is often delayed.

Most women with HIV are of childbearing age. The effect of pregnancy on the course of HIV infection is not known. There is conflicting evidence that it may or may not speed up the progression of disease.

COLLABORATIVE MANAGEMENT

ASSESSMENT

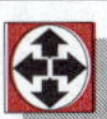

Continuous, careful, and comprehensive assessment of the client who has AIDS is crucial. The client with AIDS may have signs and symptoms related to disease in multiple organ systems. Subtle changes must be assessed so that infections and other clinical problems can be found early and treated effectively.

HISTORY

Information relevant to HIV and AIDS from the general history includes biographic data such as age, sex, occupation, and residence. The nurse thoroughly assesses the current complaint or current illness, including its nature, when it started, severity of symptoms, associated problems, and any interventions to date. The nurse questions the client about when the diagnosis of AIDS was made and what clinical symptom led to that diagnosis. The nurse asks the client to give a chronology of infections and clinical problems since the diagnosis. The nurse assesses past health history, including whether the client received a blood transfusion between 1978 and 1985.

The client is questioned about sexual practices and history of sexually transmitted diseases. The nurse should elicit a history of major diseases, including tuberculosis and hepatitis. If the person is a hemophiliac, the nurse asks about treatment with clotting factors. The client is asked about past or present drug use, including needle exposure and sharing. The nurse assesses the client's level of knowledge regarding the diagnosis, symptom management, diagnostic tests, treatments, community resources, and modes of transmission of the virus. The nurse also assesses the client's familiarity with and use of safer sex practices, and his or her understanding of correct methods.

PHYSICAL ASSESSMENT/CLINICAL MANIFESTATIONS

The nurse looks for many possible signs and symptoms. These include shortness of breath or cough, fevers, night sweats, fatigue, nausea and vomiting, weight loss, lymphadenopathy, diarrhea, visual changes, headache, memory loss, confusion, seizures, personality changes, dry skin, rashes, skin lesions, pain, and discomfort (Chart 24–1).

OPPORTUNISTIC INFECTIONS Opportunistic infections with a variety of organisms occur because of the profound immune suppression of the person with AIDS (see Chart 24–1). They may result from primary infection or the reactivation of a latent infection. Opportunistic infections account for most of the clinical manifestations observed in AIDS. These infections can be protozoan, fungal, bacterial or viral. The nurse may note the presence of more than one infection in a client with AIDS.

Protozoal Infections

Pneumocystis carinii *Pneumonia* *Pneumocystis carinii* pneumonia (PCP) is the most common opportunistic infection and occurs in 75% to 80% of persons with HIV (Henry & Holzemer, 1992). The nurse notes dyspnea on exertion, tachypnea, a persistent dry cough, and fever. The client with PCP complains of fatigue and weight loss. On auscultation of the lungs, the nurse notes crackles.

Toxoplasmosis Toxoplasmosis encephalitis, caused by *Toxoplasma gondii,* is acquired through contact with contaminated cat feces or the ingesting of infected, undercooked meat. The client may experience subtle changes in mental status, neurologic deficits, headaches and fever. Other symptoms include difficulties with speech, gait, and vision, seizures, lethargy, and confusion. The nurse performs a comprehensive baseline mental status examination and monitors the client to detect subtle changes.

Cryptosporidiosis Cryptosporidiosis is a gastroenteritis caused by *Cryptosporidium.* In AIDS this illness ranges from a mild diarrhea to a cholera-like syndrome with wasting and electrolyte imbalance. The nurse notes voluminous diarrhea with a volume loss of up to 15 to 20 L/day.

Fungal Infections

Candida albicans *Infection* *Candida albicans* is part of the natural flora of the gastrointestinal tract. In the person with AIDS, candidiasis occurs because the regulatory mechanisms of the immune system are no longer able to control fungal overgrowth. *Candida* stomatitis or esophagitis is a frequent finding in AIDS. A client with a candidal infection complains of food tasting "funny," mouth pain, difficulty in swallowing, and retrosternal pain (pain behind the ribs). On examination of the mouth and the back of

CHART 24-1

Key Features of AIDS

Immunologic Manifestations
- Low white blood cell counts:
  - T_4:T_8 ratio <2
  - T_4 count <200/mm^3
- Hypergammaglobulinemia
- Opportunistic infections
- Lymphadenopathy
- Fatigue

Integumentary Manifestations
- Dry skin
- Poor wound healing
- Skin lesions
- Night sweats

Respiratory Manifestations
- Cough
- Shortness of breath

Gastrointestinal Manifestations
- Diarrhea
- Weight loss
- Nausea & vomiting

Central Nervous System Manifestations
- Confusion
- Dementia
- Headache
- Fever
- Visual changes
- Memory loss
- Personality changes
- Pain
- Seizures

Opportunistic Infections
- Protozoal Infections
  - *Pneumocystis carinii* pneumonia
  - Toxoplasmosis
  - Cryptosporidiosis
  - Isosporiasis
  - Microsporidiosis
  - Strongyloidiasis
  - Giardiasis
- Fungal Infections
  - Candidiasis
  - Cryptococcosis
  - Histoplasmosis
  - Coccidiomycosis
- Bacterial Infections
  - *Mycobacterium avium* complex infection
  - Tuberculosis
  - Nocardiosis
- Viral Infections
  - Cytomegalovirus infection
  - Herpes simplex virus infection
  - Varicella-zoster virus infection

Malignancies
- Kaposi's sarcoma
- Non-Hodgkin's lymphoma
- Hodgkin's lymphoma
- Invasive cervical carcinoma

the throat, the nurse sees the characteristic "cottage cheese"-like, yellow-white plaques and inflammation. Esophagitis is diagnosed by endoscopic biopsy and culture. Women who have AIDS may have vaginal candidiasis, characterized by severe pruritus (itching), perineal irritation, and vaginal discharge.

Cryptococcosis Cryptococcosis is a severe, debilitating meningitis and occasionally a disseminated disease in AIDS. It is caused by *Cryptococcus neoformans.* Clinical manifestations of meningitis include fever, headache, blurred vision, nausea and vomiting, nuchal rigidity (stiff neck), mild confusion, and other mental status changes. The client sometimes experiences seizures and other focal neurologic abnormalities. Some clients present with mild symptoms and may complain only of malaise and fever with or without headaches.

Histoplasmosis Histoplasmosis, caused by *Histoplasma capsulatum,* begins as a respiratory infection and progresses to disseminated infection in persons with AIDS. The nurse may note dyspnea, fever, cough and weight loss. The client's spleen, liver and lymph nodes may be enlarged.

Bacterial Infections

Mycobacterium avium *Complex Infection* The most common bacterial infection associated with AIDS is *Mycobacterium avium* complex (MAC). This complex is caused by *Mycobacterium intracellulare* or *Mycobacterium avium,* which infects the respiratory or gastrointestinal tract. MAC is a disseminated infection. Positive cultures may be obtained from lymph nodes, bone marrow, and blood. Clinical manifestations include fever, debility, weight loss, malaise, and sometimes lymphadenopathy or organ disease.

Tuberculosis Tuberculosis, caused by *Mycobacterium tuberculosis,* occurs in 2% to 10% of persons with AIDS. People with HIV are at an increased risk for active tuberculosis. More than 50% of all clients who have AIDS and tuberculosis have extrapulmonary sites of disease that can include the central nervous system, bones, liver, spleen, skin and gastrointestinal tract. The client's systemic symptoms include fever, chills, night sweats, weight loss, and anorexia. Pulmonary involvement causes symptoms of cough, dyspnea and chest pain. Symptoms of extrapulmonary infection vary with the site. The person with tuberculosis and a CD4 count below 200 mm^3 may not have a positive purified protein derivative (PPD) skin test because of their inability to mount an immune response to the antigen. Therefore, other diagnostic measures should include chest x-ray, an acid-fast sputum smear, and sputum culture.

The nurse who delivers aerosol treatments that induce coughing, such as pentamidine isethionate prophylaxis, to clients with AIDS should be screened with a PPD skin test every 6 months.

Viral Infections

Cytomegalovirus Infection Cytomegalovirus (CMV) can infect multiple sites in people with AIDS. These include the eye (CMV retinitis), respiratory and gastrointestinal tracts, and central nervous system. CMV infection can also result in many nonspecific symptoms associated with AIDS, such as fever, malaise, weight loss, fatigue, and lymphadenopathy. CMV retinitis causes visual impairment ranging from slight to total bilateral blindness (see Chap. 46).

Cytomegalovirus infection is also responsible for colitis, with diarrhea, abdominal bloating and discomfort, and weight loss. In addition, CMV can cause encephalitis, pneumonitis, adrenalitis, hepatitis, or disseminated infection.

Herpes Simplex Virus Infection Herpes simplex virus (HSV) infections in people with AIDS occurs in the perirectal area and in the oral or genital areas. Clients describe numbness or tingling at the site of infection up to 24 hours before vesicle formation. Vesicular lesions are painful. Chronic ulcerative lesions form following vesicle rupture. The nurse notes fever, pain, bleeding and lymph node enlargement in the affected area. Systemic symptoms include headache, myalgia and malaise.

Varicella-Zoster Virus Infection Varicella-zoster virus (VZV) infection usually does not represent a new infection for people with AIDS. This virus causes chickenpox, and it is present in many nerve ganglia of people who have had chickenpox. When these people are immunocompromised, the VZV leave the nerve ganglia, enter body fluids and other tissue areas, causing *shingles.* Symptoms begin with pain and burning along dermatome nerve tracts. Large fluid-filled vesicles form and eventually crust over. Systemic symptoms include headache and low-grade fever.

MALIGNANCIES The altered immunocompetence associated with AIDS increases the risk for cancer in this group. Cancers associated with AIDS include Kaposi's sarcoma (KS), Hodgkin's lymphoma, and non-Hodgkin's lymphoma.

Kaposi's Sarcoma The most common malignancy associated with AIDS is Kaposi's sarcoma, which occurs in 1% to 21% of clients with AIDS. Hemophiliacs with HIV have the lowest incidence of KS, but men who became infected through homosexual contact have the highest.

KS presents as small, purplish-brown, palpable discrete lesions that are usually not painful or pruritic; they can occur anywhere on the person's body. Most clients with KS present with mucocutaneous (skin or mucous membrane) lesions. In some, extracutaneous lesions develop, especially in the lymph nodes, gastrointestinal tract, or lungs. The nurse assesses the KS lesions for number, size, and location and monitors their progression over time. KS is diagnosed by biopsy and histologic examination of the lesion.

Malignant Lymphomas Malignant lymphomas associated with AIDS are primarily non-Hodgkin's B-cell lymphomas. Systemic symptoms include weight loss, fever, and night sweats. (See Chapter 39 on the clinical course and nurse care issues relevant to malignant lymphomas.)

OTHER CLINICAL MANIFESTATIONS

AIDS Dementia Complex HIV-associated dementia complex, or AIDS dementia complex (ADC), refers to the signs and symptoms that indicate central nervous system involvement in the person with AIDS. ADC occurs in up to 70% of persons with AIDS. It is probably the result of direct infection of cells within the central nervous system by HIV. The three components that characterize ADC are cognitive, motor, and behavioral impairments (Chart 24–2). Symptoms range from subclinical to severe dementia.

CHART 24–2

Key Features of AIDS Dementia Complex

Cognitive Impairment

- Slowed thinking
- Slowed reaction time to external stimuli
- Loss of concentration while thinking or speaking
- Memory loss
- Forgetfulness
- Wandering attention

Motor Impairment

- Loss of coordination
- Loss of balance
- Increased minor accidents such as tripping, bumping into things, or dropping things
- Slowed motor performance
- Leg weakness

Behavioral Impairment

- Apathy
- Withdrawal
  or
- Irritability
- Hyperactivity

Other neurologic complications of HIV infection include peripheral neuropathies and myopathies. Symptoms of peripheral neuropathies include paresthesias and burning sensations, pain, and gait changes. Myopathies are accompanied by leg weakness, ataxia, and muscle pain.

Slim Disease Slim disease, or wasting syndrome, is not due to any single factor. It may be the result of altered metabolism from malignancy or opportunistic infection. Diarrhea, malabsorption, anorexia, and oral and esophageal lesions can all contribute to weight loss. Weight loss is persistent and sometimes extreme, and the client may appear to be quite thin or emaciated.

Integumentary Changes Many clients complain of dry, itchy, irritated skin and, sometimes, diffuse rashes. The nurse may observe eczema or psoriasis. The nurse also may note petechiae, or bleeding gums as a result of a low number of platelets.

PSYCHOSOCIAL ASSESSMENT

Psychosocial data collection for a client with AIDS is extremely important. The nurse asks about the client's social support system, including family, significant others, and friends. To protect the client's confidentiality, the nurse assesses who in this support system is aware of the client's diagnosis so that the nurse does not inadvertently mention it. Some clients, because of real or threatened discrimination, are quite selective about whom they tell about their diagnosis. Nurses should respect the client's choices as much as possible without compromising care. The nurse can offer resources to help the client with disclosure to sexual partners or significant others.

The client may be closest to a lover or a friend who is not legally recognized as next of kin. The nurse obtains the name and phone number of that person and learns whether a durable power of attorney document has been executed.

The nurse elicits information about the client's activities of daily living as well as any changes that may have occurred since diagnosis. The nurse assesses the client's employment status and occupation, social activities and hobbies, living arrangements, and financial resources, including health insurance.

To plan care and monitor changes, the nurse assesses the client's anxiety level, mood, and cognitive ability. The nurse asks the client about any experiences with discrimination and how they were handled. After the nurse assesses the client's level of self-esteem and changes in body image, together the nurse and client identify the client's strengths and coping strategies. The nurse gathers information about any suicidal ideation, depression, or other psychologic problems. The nurse also obtains information about the client's involvement with support groups or other community resources.

LABORATORY ASSESSMENT

LYMPHOCYTE COUNTS A lymphocyte count is generally performed as part of a complete blood count (CBC) with differential (see Chap. 22). The normal white blood cell count (WBC) is between 4500 and 11,000 cells/mm^3, with a differential of approximately 30% to 40% lymphocytes (an absolute number of 1500 to 4500). Clients with AIDS are often leukopenic, having a white blood cell count of less than 3500 cells/mm^3) and usually lymphopenic (having less than 1500 cells/mm^3).

T4:T8 RATIO As an important part of an immune profile, the percentage and number of T4 and T8 cells are determined. People with HIV infection usually have a lower than normal number of T4 cells. Some clients with AIDS have fewer than 100 cells/mm^3 (normal range is between 800 and 1200 cells/mm^3). At the same time, the number of T8 cells is usually normal. The normal ratio of T4 to T8 cells is approximately 2:1. In AIDS, because of a low number of T4 cells, this ratio is low. Low T4 cell counts and a low T4:T8 ratio are associated with increased clinical manifestations of disease.

ANTIBODY TESTS Tests to determine whether a person is infected with HIV include methods designed to detect antibody to the virus or viral products. HIV antibody can be measured by means of an enzyme-linked immunosorbent assay (ELISA) and a Western blot analysis. Following infection with the virus, it usually takes from 3 weeks to 3 months for a person to test positive for HIV antibodies. However, in some infected people, it can take up to 36 months for antibodies to be detectable (Imagawa, 1989). False-negative results (incorrectly indicating the absence of HIV infection) have been reported:

- Early in the infection
- In people with cancer
- In people on long-term immunosuppressive therapies

ELISA The client's serum is mixed with HIV that was grown in culture. If the client has antibodies to HIV, they will bind to the HIV antigens and can be detected. If antibodies are present, the test is positive. Two considerations in HIV antibody testing are sensitivity and specificity. False-positive test results (incorrectly indicating the presence of HIV infection) occur in approximately 0.1% of those tested with the ELISA. False-positive results (McMahon, 1988) have been reported:

- In multiparous or pregnant women
- In intravenous drug users
- In people with a history of malaria
- In clients with lymphomas
- In those with reactivity to the HLA-DR4 leukocyte antigen

Western Blot If the results of an ELISA are positive, they are confirmed by Western blot analysis. This test is not as widely available as ELISA because of its cost and complexity. The Western blot analysis is a more specific test that can detect the presence of the client's serum antibodies to four specific major HIV antigens. A positive Western blot is based on the presence of antibodies to two of the major HIV antigens.

The result is considered indeterminate if two of the major antibodies are not detected but other antibodies to HIV are present in the client's serum. If the result is indeterminate, the person should be retested. In people whose tests are positive, conversion from an indeterminate to a positive Western blot usually occurs within 6 months. If a person has a positive test result for antibody to HIV, it does not mean that he or she has AIDS but that there has been infection with the virus.

VIRAL CULTURE Virus culture techniques are available to determine the presence of HIV. One method involves placing the infected client's blood cells in a culture medium and measuring the amount of reverse transcriptase activity over a 28-day period. The more reverse transcriptase present, the more actively the virus is thought to be replicating.

ANTIGEN ASSAY

p24 Antigen Assay The p24 antigen assay is used to quantify the amount of p24 (HIV viral core protein) present in the client's serum. Antibodies to p24 are mixed with the serum and can detect even low levels of viral antigen present in serum. However, the assay is not as sensitive as antibody tests. The p24 test is sometimes used to chart a client's disease progression.

Polymerase Chain Reaction The polymerase chain reaction (PCR) technique detects the presence of HIV genetic material in the client's cells. A process of amplifying or copying of a specific gene sequence is used. Even if only a few infected cells are present in a serum sample, minute amounts of HIV products are amplified by the PCR in sufficient quantities to be detected. This test is useful in diagnosing HIV infection in people who have no other indication of infection.

OTHER LABORATORY TESTS Other laboratory tests are essential to establish and monitor the overall condition of the client and to detect or diagnose any infections or secondary clinical processes. Standard tests that are done include blood chemistries, complete blood count (CBC) with differential and platelets, prothrombin time and partial thromboplastin time, serologic test for syphilis (STS), hepatitis B surface antigen, and immunoglobulin levels. Tests that are sometimes done to further evaluate the immune profile of a client include skin testing for delayed hypersensitivity and bone marrow aspiration with biopsy and cultures.

OTHER DIAGNOSTIC ASSESSMENT

On the basis of the clinical symptoms with which the client presents, other diagnostic tests are chosen. Frequently included are:

- Tests of stool for ova and parasites
- Biopsies of skin, lymph nodes, lungs, liver, gastrointestinal tract, or brain
- Chest x-ray
- Gallium scans
- Bronchoscopy, endoscopy, or colonoscopy
- Liver and spleen scans
- Computed tomography scans
- Pulmonary function tests
- Assays for arterial blood gases

ANALYSIS

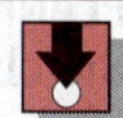

COMMON NURSING DIAGNOSES

The priorities for nursing diagnoses when caring for a client with AIDS are:

1. Impaired Gas Exchange related to anemia, respiratory infection or malignancy (*Pneumocystis carinii* pneumonia, cytomegalovirus pneumonitis, pulmonary Kaposi's sarcoma, and/or *Mycobacteria* infection), anemia, fatigue or pain
2. Altered Nutrition: Less than Body Requirements related to high metabolic need, nausea/vomiting, diarrhea, difficulty chewing or swallowing, anorexia
3. Diarrhea related to infection, food intolerance, medications
4. Impaired Skin Integrity related to KS, infection, altered nutritional state, incontinence, immobility, hyperthermia, malignancy
5. High Risk for Infection related to immune deficiency
6. Altered Thought Processes related to AIDS dementia complex, central nervous system infection, or malignancy
7. Self-Esteem Disturbance related to changes in body image changes, decreased self-esteem, and helplessness
8. Social Isolation related to stigma, transmissibility of the virus, infection control practices, and fear

ADDITIONAL NURSING DIAGNOSES

Clients who have AIDS may present with one or more of the following additional diagnoses:

- Activity Intolerance related to fatigue, discomfort, central nervous system defect, weakness, or anemia
- High Risk for Injury related to central nervous system deficit, mental status changes, depression, and/or thrombocytopenia
- Pain related to neuropathy, myelopathy, malignancy or infection

- Sensory/Perceptual Alterations (Visual) related to CMV retinitis and blindness
- Sleep Pattern Disturbance related to pain, discomfort, anxiety or depression
- Ineffective Individual Coping related to the diagnosis of AIDS
- Ineffective Family/Significant Other Coping related to the diagnosis of AIDS
- Anticipatory Grieving related to potential loss of role and function, and impending death of self

PLANNING AND IMPLEMENTATION

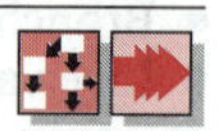

IMPAIRED GAS EXCHANGE

PLANNING: CLIENT GOALS The major goals are that the client will:

- Maintain adequate oxygenation and perfusion
- Experience minimal dyspnea and discomfort

INTERVENTIONS Interventions include drug therapy, respiratory support and maintenance, comfort, and rest (Client Care Plan).

Drug Therapy Appropriate drug therapy is initiated according to identification of an infectious or neoplastic cause for respiratory difficulty (Chart 24–3). One of the two treatments of choice for *Pneumocystis carinii* pneumonia (PCP) is trimethoprim-sulfamethoxazole (Apo-sulfatrim♣, Bactrim, Protrin♣, Septra). It can be given intravenously or orally, depending on the severity of infection. A high percentage of clients with AIDS experience adverse reactions to this medication, including nausea, vomiting, hyponatremia, rashes, fever, leukopenia, thrombocytopenia, and hepatitis.

The second drug of choice is pentamidine isethionate (Lomidine♣, PenTam), usually given intravenously or intramuscularly. Aerosolized pentamidine isethionate is used prophylactically in those with T4 counts below 200 and in those who have already had PCP.

Respiratory Support and Maintenance In addition to drug therapy, the client needs appropriate nursing care to maintain respiratory function and to avoid complications. The nurse assesses the client's respiratory rate, rhythm, depth and breath sounds, and vital signs, and monitors for cyanosis at least every 8 hours. The nurse applies and maintains oxygen therapy and room humidification, as ordered. In addition, the nurse monitors mechanical ventilation, performs suctioning and chest physical therapy as needed, and evaluates blood gas results.

Comfort The nurse assesses the client's comfort. Clients with respiratory difficulties often are more comfortable with the head of the bed elevated. The nurse helps the client pace activities to minimize

CHART 24–3

Drug Therapy for AIDS-Related Opportunistic Infections and Malignancies

Drug	Indication	Usual Dosage	Nursing Interventions	Rationale
Trimethoprim (TMP) and sulfamethoxazole (SMX) (Apo-sulfatrim♣, Bactrim, Protrin♣, Septra)	• *Pneumocystis carinii* pneumonia	• PO 160 mg TMP and 800 mg SMX every 12 hours	• Monitor input and output (I&O) • Encourage fluids	• Input and output are monitored because TMP-SMX is nephrotoxic
			• Monitor CBC, urinalysis, bilirubin, creatinine, alkaline phosphatase	• These values are monitored because TMP-SMX suppresses the immune system
			• Assess for sore throat, pallor, purpura, jaundice, weakness	• These signs are assessed for because TMP-SMX is hepatotoxic
Pentamidine isethionate (Lomidine♣, Pentam)	• *P. carinii* pneumonia	• IM or IV 4 mg/kg once daily for 14–21 days	• Monitor blood pressure, heart rate and rhythm • Administer with client lying down	• BP and heart rate are monitored because pentamidine causes hypotension when administered rapidly
			• Monitor for hypoglycemia • Administer IV over 1 hour	• Monitoring is necessary because pentamidine causes severe hy-

CHART 24-3

Drug Therapy for AIDS-Related Opportunistic Infections and Malignancies *Continued*

Drug	Indication	Usual Dosage	Nursing Interventions	Rationale
				poglycemia that may be fatal
			• Monitor liver function, CBC	• Liver function and CBC are monitored because pentamidine is hepatotoxic and immunosuppressive
Pentamidine isethionate (Pentam)	• *P. carinii* pneumonia	• Inhalant 300 mg every 4 weeks via nebulizer	• See above	• See above
Pyrimethamine (with sulfadiazine) (Daraprim)	• Toxoplasmosis	• PO 50–75 mg/day for 1–3 weeks, then 25 mg/day for 4–5 weeks	• Administer with food or milk • Monitor CBC and platelets	• Pyrimethamine irritates the GI tract • The CBC and platelets are monitored because pyrimethamine suppresses bone marrow activity
Sulfadiazine	• Toxoplasmosis • Nocardiasis	• PO 500–2000 mg daily every 6 hours for 3–4 weeks	• Monitor urine output, CBC	• Urine output and the CBC are monitored because sulfadiazine causes renal toxicity
			• Encourage fluids	• Fluids are necessary because sulfadiazine suppresses bone marrow activity
			• Advise client to avoid sun • Assess for sore throat, pallor, purpura, jaundice, weakness	• Clients should avoid the sun because sulfadiazine increases photosensitivity
Dapsone (Avlosulfon✱, DDS)	• Toxoplasmosis	• PO 50–100 mg daily	• Monitor CBC • Assess for fever, sore throat, purpura, jaundice	• The CBC is monitored because dapsone suppresses bone marrow activity
Metronidazole (Flagyl)	• Cryptosporidiosis • Giardiasis	• PO 7.5 mg/kg every 6 hours, IV 15 mg/kg initial dose, then 7.5 mg/kg every 6 hours	• Administer with food or milk	• Food or milk is recommended because metronidazole irritates the GI tract
			• Teach client to avoid alcohol during treatment • Assess for dry mouth, dizziness, fungal infection	• Alcohol causes formation of acetaldehyde and headache, nausea, vomiting, and diarrhea
Ketoconazole (Nizoral)	• Candidiasis • Coccidioidomycosis • Histoplasmosis	• PO 200–400 mg/day, single dose	• Administer with food or milk • Avoid antacids for 2 hours	• Ketoconazole irritates the GI tract • Gastric acid is needed to activate drug
			• Teach client to avoid sun and al-	• Ketoconazole increases photosensi-

Chart continued on following page

CHART 24-3

Drug Therapy for AIDS-Related Opportunistic Infections and Malignancies *Continued*

Drug	Indication	Usual Dosage	Nursing Interventions	Rationale
			cohol during treatment	tivity
			• Monitor hepatic function	• Hepatic function is monitored because ketoconazole is hepatotoxic
Fluconazole (Diflucan)	• Candidiasis • Cryptococcal meningitis	• PO, IV 200–400 mg initially, then 100–200 mg daily for 2–4 weeks	• Monitor hepatic function • Assess for abdominal pain, fever, diarrhea	• Hepatic function is monitored because fluconazole is hepatotoxic
Rifampin (Rifadin, Rofact✱)	• *Mycobacterium avium* complex • Tuberculosis	• PO 10 mg/kg/day	• Assess breath sounds, sputum	• Assessment of breath sounds and sputum determines treatment effectiveness
			• Monitor hepatic function, CBC • May turn body secretions orange	• Rifampin is hepatotoxic
Ethambutol (Myambutol, Etibi✱)	• *Mycobacterium avium* complex • Tuberculosis	• PO 15 mg/kg 2–3 times a week	• Assess vision changes	• Vision changes are assessed because ethambutol causes retrobulbar neuritis and decreased visual acuity (reversible)
			• Assess hepatic and renal function, CBC, urinalysis	• This assessment is necessary because ethambutol increases uric acid concentrations • Ethambutol suppresses bone marrow activity
Amphotericin B (Fungizone)	• Candidiasis • Other fungal infections	• IV 0.3–1 mg/kg/day	• Assess renal function	• Renal function is assessed because amphotericin B is nephrotoxic
			• Assess infusion site	• Amphotericin B causes thrombophlebitis
			• Assess CBC	• The CBC is checked because amphotericin B suppresses bone marrow activity • Amphotericin B is *very* toxic
Ciprofloxacin (Cipro)	• *Mycobacterium avium* complex • Urinary tract infections	• PO 250–750 mg every 12 hours, IV 200–400 mg every 12 hours	• Monitor I&O • Encourage fluids	
			• Administer on empty stomach (1 hour before or 2 hours after meals) if tolerated	• An empty stomach is recommended for best absorption
			• Teach client to avoid sun • Assess for dizzi-	• Clients should avoid the sun because ciprofloxacin

CHART 24-3

Drug Therapy for AIDS-Related Opportunistic Infections and Malignancies *Continued*

Drug	Indication	Usual Dosage	Nursing Interventions	Rationale
			ness, fungal infection • Infuse over 1 hour	increases photosensitivity
Clofazimine (Lamprene)	• *Mycobacterium avium* complex	• PO 50–100 mg every day	• Assess vision changes, dizziness, drowsiness	• Vision changes and dizziness are assessed because clofazimine increases sedation
			• Instruct client to avoid sun	• Clofazimine increases photosensitivity (especially of eyes)
			• Use lotions for dry skin • Monitor hepatic and renal function	• Clients should use lotions because clofazimine causes dry, scaly skin
Pyrazinamide (Tebrazid✱)	• Tuberculosis	• PO 20–30 mg/kg/day	• Monitor hepatic function, uric acid	• Pyrazinamide is hepatotoxic and increases uric acid concentration
			• Assess temperature every 4 hours	• The client's temperature is assessed because pyrazinamide stimulates fever
Isoniazid (Laniazid, Isotamine✱)	• Tuberculosis	• PO, IM 5–10 mg/kg/day or 15 mg 2–3 times a week	• Administer on empty stomach	• Taking isoniazid on an empty stomach enhances absorption
			• Monitor hepatic function	• Isoniazid is hepatotoxic
			• Assess for vision changes	• Vision changes are assessed because isoniazid is neurotoxic
			• Instruct client to avoid alcohol and tyramine containing foods	• Isoniazid is an MAO inhibitor
Ganciclovir	• Cytomegalovirus retinitis	• IV 5 mg/kg every 12 hours for 14–21 days	• Monitor neutrophil and platelet count • Infuse over 1 hour	• Neutrophil and platelet counts are monitored because ganciclovir suppresses bone marrow activity
Acyclovir (Zovirax)	• Herpes simplex • Herpes zoster • Varicella zoster	• PO 200–800 mg 5 times a day, IV 5–10 mg/kg every 8 hours for 7–10 days	• Monitor renal function • Encourage fluids • Rotate infusion site	• Acyclovir is nephrotoxic • Various infusion sites are used because acyclovir is a blood vessel irritant
Zidovudine (Retrovir)	• HIV seropositivity	• PO 200 mg every 4 hours	• Must be administered around the clock	• Zidovudine is given around the clock for maximum antiviral effect

Chart continued on following page

CHART 24-3

Drug Therapy for AIDS-Related Opportunistic Infections and Malignancies *Continued*

Drug	Indication	Usual Dosage	Nursing Interventions	Rationale
			• Assess for dizziness	• Dizziness is assessed because zidovudine crosses the blood-brain barrier
			• Monitor CBC, hepatic and renal function	• Zidovudine suppresses bone marrow activity • Hepatotoxic • Nephrotoxic
Didanosine (Videx)	• HIV seropositivity	• PO 125–300 mg every 12 hours	• Administer on empty stomach • Instruct client to chew tablet, or crush	• Taking didanosine on an empty stomach enhances absorption
			• Monitor for dizziness, neuropathy, pancreatitis	• Didanosine crosses the blood-brain barrier
Interferon alfa-2b	• Kaposi's sarcoma	• IM, SC 30 million IU/m^2 three times weekly	• Monitor vital signs, cardiac status	• Vital signs and cardiac status are monitored because interferon alfa-2b poses a danger of hyperviscosity
			• Assess for bleeding, low-grade fever, malaise, muscle aches, headache, chills, infection, nausea	• Interferon alfa-2b causes malaise and flu-like symptoms

AIDS = acquired immunodeficiency syndrome; I&O = input and output; HIV = human immunodeficiency virus; CBC = complete blood count; MAO = monoamine oxidase; GI = gastrointestinal

shortness of breath and exhaustion. The nurse provides the patient with psychologic support during periods of respiratory distress.

Rest and Activity The nurse consults with the client to pace client activities to conserve energy. The nurse guides and assists the client in active and passive range of motion exercises. Activities such as bathing and range of motion exercises are scheduled so that the client is not fatigued at meal time.

ALTERED NUTRITION: LESS THAN BODY REQUIREMENTS

Many clients with AIDS have difficulty maintaining their weight and nutritional status. This problem may be associated with fatigue, anorexia, nausea and vomiting, difficult or painful swallowing, diarrhea, or a wasting syndrome.

PLANNING: CLIENT GOALS The major goal is that the client will achieve or maintain optimum weight through adequate nutrition and hydration.

INTERVENTIONS Because there are multiple factors for alterations in nutrition in AIDS, the proper diagnostic procedures are undertaken to determine the cause. Once the cause is determined, appropriate therapy is initiated. For example, in the client who has candidal esophagitis, nutrition is affected because of the client's difficulty in swallowing.

Drug Therapy Therapy can include ketoconazole (Nizoral) or fluconazole (Diflucan) orally or intravenous amphotericin B (Fungizone). The nurse administers the medication as ordered and monitors the client. Medication can cause nausea and vomiting, which further compromise nutritional status. The nurse provides mouth care and ice chips and keeps unpleasant odors out of the client's environment. Antiemetics are used as ordered.

Diet Therapy The nurse monitors the client's weight, intake and output, and calorie count. The nurse assesses the client's food preferences and any dietary cultural or religious practices. The nurse instructs the client in a high-calorie, high-protein, low-microbial, nutritionally sound diet (see Chap. 39). In collaboration with the dietitian, the nurse provides an appropriate diet for the client. Small, frequent meals are better tolerated than large meals. The use of supplemental vitamins and fluids is indicated in some cases. For the client who cannot achieve adequate nutrition through food, tube feedings or total parenteral nutrition may be needed.

Mouth Care For clients who are susceptible to oral ulceration or infection, the nurse provides meticulous mouth care. Rinses of sodium bicarbonate with normal saline every 2 hours or several times a day are helpful. The client is given a soft toothbrush and advised to drink plenty of fluids. For oral pain that interferes with the client's ability to eat, analgesics or viscous lidocaine may be necessary.

DIARRHEA

Clients with AIDS frequently suffer from diarrhea. Sometimes an infectious cause (e.g., *Giardia* or *Amoeba*) can be determined and treated. Sometimes an infection is the etiologic factor, but no effective therapy is available, as in the case of cryptosporidiosis or cytomegalovirus colitis. In some cases, clients with AIDS have diarrhea and no infectious etiology can be identified.

PLANNING: CLIENT GOALS The major goals are that the client will:

- Experience decreased diarrhea
- Maintain fluid, electrolyte, and nutritional status
- Minimize incontinence

INTERVENTIONS For most clients with AIDS and diarrhea, symptomatic management is all that is available. Antidiarrheals, such as diphenoxylate hydrochloride (Diarsed♣, Lomotil), given on a regular schedule, provide the client with some degree of relief. In collaboration with the dietitian, the nurse offers dietary counseling and helps to provide appropriate foods. Recommended dietary changes include less roughage and less fatty, spicy, or sweet food. Clients should avoid alcohol and caffeine. Some clients experience symptomatic relief if they eliminate dairy products from the diet. Clients are assisted to eat smaller amounts of food more often and to drink plenty of fluids, especially between meals.

The nurse provides the client with a bedside commode or a bedpan if needed. Some clients cannot reach the bathroom in time because of immobility or anal sphincter weakness, others because of the urgency to defecate. The nurse provides privacy, support, and understanding.

IMPAIRED SKIN INTEGRITY

The most common skin lesion occurring in AIDS is Kaposi's sarcoma (KS). Cutaneous involvement may be localized or disseminated. Large lesions can cause pain, and restrict movement or ambulation. They can impede circulation, causing open, weeping, painful lesions. Another cause of impaired skin integrity is herpes simplex virus infection.

PLANNING: CLIENT GOALS The major goals are that the client will:

- Experience healing of any existing lesions
- Avoid increased skin breakdown or secondary infection

INTERVENTIONS Kaposi's sarcoma can be treated locally with radiotherapy, intralesional chemotherapy, or cryotherapy. KS is responsive to local radiation therapy, but this treatment is only transiently effective.

Systemic therapy is used in clients with rapidly progressive disease or with significant involvement of the gastrointestinal tract, lungs, or other organs. These therapies include chemotherapy (single-agent or combination), alpha interferon, and alpha interferon–zidovudine combinations.

Treatment of painful KS lesions includes the use of analgesics and comfort measures. KS lesions that are open and weeping must be kept clean and dressed to minimize the risk of secondary infection. Some clients with cutaneous KS are concerned about their appearance and the risk of being identified by others as having HIV. The use of make-up if open lesions are not present, long-sleeved shirts, and hats may help the client maintain a normal appearance.

For the client with a herpes simplex virus abscess, the nurse provides meticulous skin care. The nurse cleans the abscess regularly with a diluted solution of povidone-iodine (Betadine) and leaves it open to the air or exposed to a heat lamp to help it dry. This infection can be painful and necessitates the use of analgesics, assistance with position, and other comfort measures. For some clients with this type of abscess, Domeboro soaks help to promote healing. Herpes simplex virus infection is treated with acyclovir (Zovirax) given intravenously or by mouth and, in some cases, topically, depending on the severity of the infection.

HIGH RISK FOR INFECTION

The client with AIDS is susceptible to opportunistic infections because of immunodeficiency secondary to HIV infection.

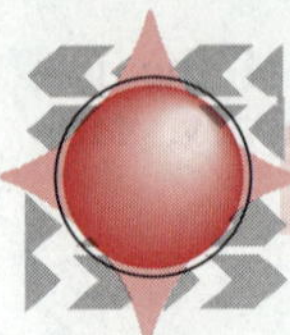

CLIENT CARE PLAN

The Client with AIDS

Nursing Diagnosis No. 1: Ineffective Breathing Pattern related to *Pneumocystis*, cytomegalovirus, Kaposi's sarcoma, or *Mycobacterium avium* infection

Expected Outcomes	Nursing Interventions	Rationale
The client will experience minimal or no dyspnea or discomfort.	◆ Use fluids, oxygen therapy, and elevation of the head of the bed.	◆ These measures minimize dyspnea.
◆ Has a respiratory rate and depth within normal limits for activity level	◆ Assess respiratory status; vital signs; level of consciousness; rate, depth, and rhythm of respirations; and breath sounds.	◆ Changes should be monitored.
The client will experience adequate oxygenation or perfusion.	◆ Monitor arterial blood gas levels.	◆ These levels indicate oxygenation of the blood.
◆ Has PaO_2 >80 mmHg	◆ Administer medication as ordered and watch for side effects.	◆ Medication side effects are common.
The client will maintain a patent airway.	◆ Ensure room humidification.	◆ Most clients have a dry cough.
◆ Has no adventitious breath sounds on auscultation	◆ Use ventilation, suction, and chest physical therapy as ordered.	
The client will be able to perform activities of daily living (ADL) and other activities.	◆ Ensure activity moderation/pacing.	◆ Moderation and assistance minimize shortness of breath and exhaustion.
	◆ Assist with activities of daily living.	
	◆ Use antipyretics for fever.	◆ Reduction of fever lowers the metabolic rate and conserves energy resources.
	◆ Support the client.	◆ Providing supportive care as needed reduces the client's physical and emotional energy demands and conserves energy resources for other functions.

Nursing Diagnosis No. 2: Altered Nutrition: Less than Body Requirements related to high metabolic need, nausea, vomiting, diarrhea, difficulty chewing or swallowing, and anorexia

Expected Outcomes	Nursing Interventions	Rationale
The client will maintain appropriate weight for height and body build.	◆ Monitor intake and output and calorie count.	◆ These measures indicate fluid balance and adequacy of calorie intake.
◆ Shows no weight loss	◆ Provide meals and snacks with high protein, high calorie, and high nutritional value.	◆ Proper intake provides calories and improves nutrition.
◆ Shows weight increase in proportion to height and body build	◆ Offer high-calorie supplements (e.g., Ensure, Sustacal).	◆ Supplements provide many calories and nutrients in an easy-to-use can.
	◆ Give enteral or parenteral feedings if needed.	◆ Clients who cannot get adequate calories orally need other types of feedings.
	◆ Offer low microbial food.	◆ Some foods bring microorganisms into the client's internal environment, increasing the risk for infection.
The client will maintain adequate nutrition and hydration.	◆ Supplement with fluids and vitamins.	◆ Supplements ensure adequate fluid and vitamin levels.

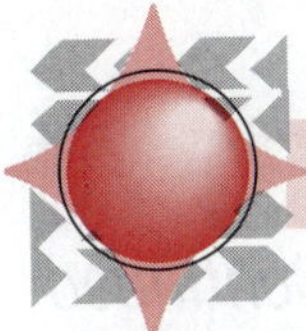

CLIENT CARE PLAN

The Client with AIDS *Continued*

Nursing Diagnosis No. 2: Altered Nutrition: Less than Body Requirements related to high metabolic need, nausea, vomiting, diarrhea, difficulty chewing or swallowing, and anorexia

Expected Outcomes	Nursing Interventions	Rationale
◆ Fluid intake equal to the amount of fluid lost plus 100 mL ◆ Ingests a minimum of 2500 kcal/d ◆ Evidences no loss of weight from baseline		
The client will identify foods tolerated. ◆ Lists 25 preferred foods that do not cause discomfort	◆ Provide small, frequent meals.	◆ Smaller meals are usually better tolerated.
	◆ Use antiemetics, if needed. ◆ Provide a soft or bland diet.	◆ Antiemetics minimize nausea. ◆ Foods that are easy to eat or digest will help if the client has mouth sores or abdominal pain.
	◆ Provide meticulous mouth care.	◆ Mouth care minimizes mouth soreness and infection.

Nursing Diagnosis No. 3: Diarrhea related to infection, food intolerance, and medications

Expected Outcomes	Nursing Interventions	Rationale
The client will experience decreased diarrhea and stable fluid, electrolyte, and nutritional status. ◆ Has no weight fluctuation >1 pound/day ◆ Maintains serum sodium, potassium, calcium, and chloride values within normal ranges	◆ Provide dietary counseling: ◆ Less roughage, alcohol, spicy foods, sweets, fatty foods, and dairy products ◆ Smaller amounts of food more frequently ◆ Adequate amounts of fluids, especially between meals	◆ Dietary changes aid in decreasing diarrhea.
	◆ Administer antidiarrheals routinely, as ordered.	◆ Antidiarrheals such as diphenoxylate hydrochloride (Lomotil) or tincture of opium may be necessary on a routine basis.
The client will experience minimal or no incontinence.	◆ Provide a commode or bedpan.	◆ Sometimes the client cannot reach the bathroom.
◆ Eliminates all wastes on a bedpan or commode.	◆ Support the client and allow privacy.	◆ Incontinence can be embarrassing.

Nursing Diagnosis No. 4: Impaired Skin Integrity related to Kaposi's sarcoma, infection, altered nutritional state, incontinence, immobility, hyperthermia, and malignancy

Expected Outcomes	Nursing Interventions	Rationale
The client will not experience increased skin breakdown or secondary infection.	◆ Monitor the progress of lesions.	◆ Monitoring allows institution of early treatment.

Continued on following page

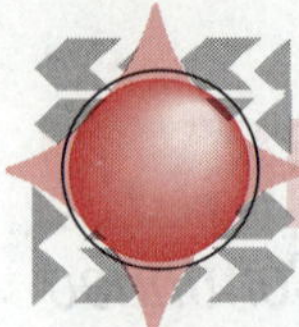

CLIENT CARE PLAN

The Client with AIDS *Continued*

Nursing Diagnosis No. 4: Impaired Skin Integrity related to Kaposi's sarcoma, infection, altered nutritional state, incontinence, immobility, hyperthermia, and malignancy

Expected Outcomes	Nursing Interventions	Rationale
♦ Develops no new skin lesions	♦ Avoid pressure (use eggcrate, air, or water mattresses).	♦ Pressure increases the possibility of skin breakdown.
The client will experience healing of existing lesions. ♦ Has decreased lesion size and number from baseline ♦ Evidences no redness or drainage from the lesion sites ♦ Has re-epithelialization over all lesion sites	♦ Use careful hygienic measures.	♦ Some clients have perirectal abscesses and massive diarrhea.
The client will remain comfortable. ♦ Expresses comfort	♦ Provide skin care.	♦ Skin care allows maintenance of cleanliness and skin integrity.
	♦ Give analgesics, if needed.	♦ Some skin lesions (e.g., herpes simplex virus lesions) are painful.
	♦ Use lotions and emollients for dry skin.	♦ Dry skin is more susceptible to break down.
	♦ Use Universal Precautions.	♦ Virus is shed from the wound.

Nursing Diagnosis No. 5: High Risk for Infection related to immune deficiency

Expected Outcomes	Nursing Interventions	Rationale
The client will remain free from cross-contamination–induced infection. ♦ Limits close contact with other people ♦ Maintains a core body temperature of <100°F (38°C) ♦ Does not have pathogenic organisms in cultures of blood, urine, and wound drainage	♦ Initiate protective isolation procedures according to institutional policy (e.g., thorough hand washing between seeing clients, reverse isolation, private room, wearing masks).	♦ Protective isolation reduces the number of vector-transmissible microorganisms.
	♦ Keep supplies for the client (e.g., paper cups, straws, dressing materials, gloves) separate from supplies for other clients.	♦ Keeping separate supplies limits the potential for cross-contamination infection.
	♦ Limit the number of care personnel entering the client's room.	♦ Limiting care personnel decreases the client's exposure to nonself microorganisms.
	♦ Have the client maintained in a private room.	♦ A private room reduces traffic and exposure to nonself microorganisms.
	♦ Allow healthy adult visitors only.	♦ Allowing only healthy adult visitors prevents transmission of microorganisms by small children, who may incubate microorganisms and inadvertently transmit them to the client by not adhering to infection control procedures.

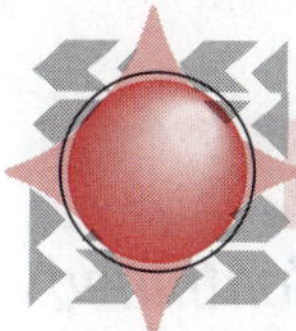

CLIENT CARE PLAN

The Client with Aids *Continued*

Nursing Diagnosis No. 5: High Risk for Infection related to immune deficiency

Expected Outcomes	Nursing Interventions	Rationale
	◆ Reduce exposure to environmental microorganisms by having the client avoid raw fruits and vegetables and by not having standing water in the client's room (e.g., remove vases, humidifiers, and water games).	◆ Reducing exposure to environmental microorganisms prevents contact with potentially harmful microorganisms.
	◆ Clean the client's room at least once per day.	◆ Daily cleaning inhibits proliferation of environmental microorganisms.
The client will remain free from autocontamination-induced infection. ◆ Complies with prescribed hygiene measures ◆ Maintains a core body temperature of <100°F (38°C) ◆ Does not have pathogenic organisms in cultures of blood, urine, and wound drainage	◆ Instruct or assist the client with daily bathing using antimicrobial soap.	◆ Daily bathing reduces microorganisms on skin surfaces.
	◆ Touch the client gently to avoid injuring the skin.	◆ Touching the client gently prevents new portals of entry for microorganisms.
	◆ Instruct and assist the client to perform oral hygiene every 4 hours including the use of antimicrobial rinses, mouth swabs, and moisturizing rinses.	◆ Oral hygiene reduces the number of oral tract microorganisms.
	◆ Change IV tubing every 48 hours.	◆ Regular IV changes reduce the risk of contamination.
	◆ Prevent rectal trauma by initiating a bowel program, administering stool softeners and laxatives, and promoting the use of sitz baths.	◆ These measures reduce intestinal stasis and bacterial overgrowth.
	◆ Change wound dressings daily, teaching the client or performing central venous catheter site care according to institutional protocols.	◆ Daily dressing changes reduce the number of colony-forming microorganisms at the site of a portal of entry and allow inspection of the site for signs and symptoms of infection.
	◆ Teach the client to identify signs and symptoms of infections and instruct him or her to inform a health care professional should any new symptom occur.	◆ Often the client is more in touch with subtle changes that occur. Involving the client can assist with early detection of infection.
	◆ Avoid invasive procedures, such as injections, rectal temperatures, and urinary catheterization.	◆ Invasive procedures and trauma can disrupt mucosal linings and skin, resulting in a portal of entry for infectious organisms.
	◆ Encourage the client to cough and deep breathe; counsel the client about smoking cessation.	◆ These measures help prevent respiratory infections.

Continued on following page

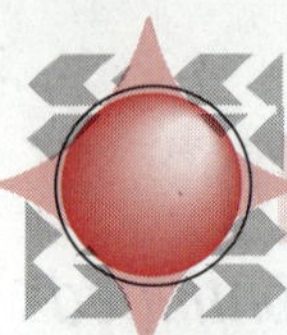

CLIENT CARE PLAN

The Client with Aids *Continued*

Nursing Diagnosis No. 5: High Risk for Infection related to immune deficiency

Expected Outcomes	Nursing Interventions	Rationale
The client will not experience septicemia. ♦ Does not experience a "left shift" in white blood cell (WBC) populations ♦ Maintains a core body temperature of <100°F (38°C) ♦ Does not have pathogenic organisms in cultures of blood, urine, and wound drainage ♦ Maintains a pulse rate and blood pressure (BP) within normal limits	♦ Assess the client for signs and symptoms of infection: ♦ Measure oral temperature q 4 hours. ♦ Inspect wound areas for redness, swelling, or drainage q 8 hours. ♦ Auscultate the client's lungs q 8 hours. ♦ Check the client's urine for odor and cloudiness. ♦ Monitor the client's pulse and BP q 4 hours.	♦ These assessments identify infectious processes early.
	♦ Monitor the differential WBC, especially the ANC.	♦ These values determine the client's risk for infection and indicate a return of immune function.
	♦ If symptoms of infection are present, notify the physician immediately and be prepared to:	♦ Institute appropriate treatment.
	♦ Obtain specimens of blood for culture through the venous access device and the peripheral vein before antibiotic therapy is initiated.	♦ Blood cultures help to determine whether microorganisms are present in the blood and whether the venous access device is the source of contamination.
	♦ Obtain specimens for culture of open lesions, urine, and sputum.	♦ These cultures help determine the origin of the infection and to identify the infecting organism.
	♦ Administer prescribed antibiotic, antifungal, or antiviral therapy.	♦ These agents limit proliferation of microorganisms within the client and prevent progression to sepsis.

Nursing Diagnosis No. 6: Altered Thought Processes related to AIDS dementia complex, CNS infection, or malignancy

Expected Outcomes	Nursing Interventions	Rationale
The client will maintain orientation and level of consciousness. ♦ States the correct date and location ♦ Correctly identifies known visitors and health care providers	♦ Assess the client's mental status and neurovital signs. ♦ Reorient the client, and use clocks, calendars, windows, and so on.	♦ Neurologic status should be followed. ♦ Use of these aids helps to reorient the client.
The client and others will remain safe. ♦ Incurs no injuries ♦ Experiences no seizure activity	♦ Provide a safe environment. ♦ Use seizure precautions. ♦ Organize and pace the client's activities.	♦ The environment can pose hazards. ♦ Use of standard seizure precautions and organized activities promotes safety.

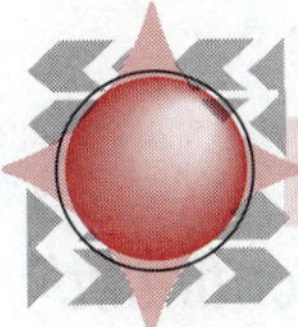

CLIENT CARE PLAN

The Client with AIDS *Continued*

Nursing Diagnosis No. 6: Altered Thought Processes related to AIDS dementia complex, CNS infection, or malignancy

Expected Outcomes	Nursing Interventions	Rationale
	♦ Use anticonvulsants as necessary.	♦ Some clients also need corticosteroids to reduce intracranial pressure.
The client will trust the nurse. ♦ Initiates open communication with the nurse	♦ Structure and assist with activities of daily living.	♦ These actions help to develop client comfort and trust.
	♦ Offer emotional support to the client and significant others.	♦ Neurologic problems are difficult to accept.

Nursing Diagnosis No. 7: Self Esteem Disturbance related to body image changes, decreased self-esteem, and helplessness

Expected Outcomes	Nursing Interventions	Rationale
The client will maintain normalcy and accept himself or herself. ♦ Expresses positive feelings about himself or herself. ♦ Verbalizes positive approaches to assist in the adjustment process before and after discharge.	♦ Provide a climate of acceptance.	♦ The client's self-acceptance is enhanced if others accept him or her.
	♦ Allow for privacy.	♦ Providing privacy shows respect for the person.
	♦ Offer a safe environment.	♦ A safe environment allows for the expression of fears and anxiety.
	♦ Encourage self-care, independence, control, and decision making.	♦ These actions are normal.
	♦ Help formulate attainable short-term goals.	♦ Achieving goals enhances self-esteem.
	♦ Be honest with your feelings.	♦ Honesty from others shows respect for the dignity of the person.

Nursing Diagnosis No. 8: Social Isolation related to stigma, transmissibility of the virus, infection control practices, and fear

Expected Outcomes	Nursing Interventions	Rationale
The client will identify behaviors that lead to social isolation.	♦ Do not place the client in isolation.	♦ Transmission of HIV does not occur by casual contact.
	♦ Teach the client and significant others the modes of human immunodeficiency virus (HIV) transmission.	♦ Teaching reduces the fear of transmission.
	♦ Touch the client frequently.	♦ Touching the client and avoidance of unnecessary protective clothing allow the client to know you are not afraid of contracting AIDS from him or her.

Continued on following page

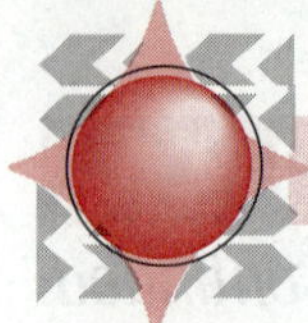

CLIENT CARE PLAN

The Client with AIDS *Continued*

Nursing Diagnosis No. 8: Social Isolation related to stigma, transmissibility of the virus, infection control practices, and fear

Expected Outcomes	Nursing Interventions	Rationale
	♦ Do not wear protective gloves, masks, or other protective clothing when not coming into contact with the client's body fluids.	♦ Transmission of HIV does not occur through casual contact.
	♦ Listen to the client.	♦ Listening helps you to identify client fears.
	♦ Ask the client to list his or her support people.	♦ Enlisting support people increases social interactions.

PLANNING: CLIENT GOALS The major goal is the prevention of opportunistic diseases.

INTERVENTIONS Several strategies can help the client to minimize the chances of acquiring an infection. These strategies are investigational and include drug therapy as well as approaches to enhance immune function.

Drug Therapy Chart 24–3 lists treatments for opportunistic infections and neoplasms. Several experimental medications have demonstrated antiretroviral effects in vitro and in animal studies.

Zidovudine, or AZT (Retrovir), is an antiviral medication that was approved by the United States Food and Drug Administration in mid-1987 for use in people with AIDS who have recently had *Pneumocystis carinii* pneumonia or for those who have HIV infection and a T4 cell count lower than 500/mm^3. AZT can be given orally or intravenously; the usual dose is 200 mg orally every 4 hours. Side effects include a potentially severe macrocytic anemia that often necessitates regular transfusions. Clients also complain of mild headache, nausea, abdominal pain and diarrhea; and, less commonly, changes in white blood cell count or liver function tests. Didanosine or ddI (Videx) is an antiviral used for persons who are unable to tolerate zidovudine or who have had continued loss of immune function despite AZT therapy.

Immune Enhancement Research is also being conducted to evaluate modalities that may enhance or reconstitute the immune system of clients who are made immunodeficient by HIV infection. Some of these methods include bone marrow transplantation, lymphocyte transfusion, and the administration of lymphokines and other biologic response modifiers.

The human immunodeficiency virus (HIV) can remain latent inside a cell for long periods and can cause an active infection when the cell is stimulated. The specific signals for the cell to become activated are not known, but concurrent viral or parasitic infections are suspected. The nurse teaches the client to avoid exposure to infection.

ALTERED THOUGHT PROCESSES

Neurologic changes and alterations in thought processes are major areas of concern for clients with AIDS. These changes may be due to the psychologic stressors that accompany the disease or to organic disorders caused by opportunistic infections, cancer, or HIV encephalitis.

PLANNING: CLIENT GOALS The major goals are that the client will:

- Demonstrate improved mental status
- Sustain no injury

INTERVENTIONS Clients with AIDS suffer from enormous loss and psychologic stress, which complicate the assessment of any changes in behavior or affect. The nurse establishes baseline neurologic and mental status by using neurologic assessment tools (see Chap. 40). All changes can then be compared with this baseline. Subtle changes in memory, ability to concentrate, affect, and behavior are evaluated. Differential diagnosis is important to determine whether the cause of the neurologic changes is treatable.

Orientation The nurse reorients the confused client to person, time, and place as needed. The nurse reminds the client of the nurse's identity and explains what is to be done at any given time. Using calendars, clocks, and radios and putting the bed close to a window all may help to keep the client oriented. The nurse gives simple directions and uses short, uncomplicated sentences. The nurse explains activities in simple language and involves the client in planning the daily schedule. Relatives or significant others are asked to bring in familiar items from home for the client's room. Items in the client's environment are arranged in the same location as at home for consistency.

Drug Therapy Chart 24–3 lists agents appropriate for different conditions contributing to altered thought processes in the person who has AIDS.

Safety Measures Attention to safety is crucial to the well-being of the neurologically impaired client with AIDS. The client may not be aware of activities or surroundings. The client may need assistance with bathing, dressing, eating, ambulating, and other activities of daily living. The environment, whether it is the hospital room, long-term care facility, or home, is made safe and comfortable. Some clients are prone to seizures. The nurse institutes seizure precautions, including padded side rails and the availability of an airway. Anticonvulsants may be added to the client's medications.

The nurse assesses the client with neurologic disease for signs and symptoms of increased intracranial pressure. The nurse should immediately report any changes in level of consciousness, vital signs, pupil size or reactivity, or limb strength to the physician for appropriate intervention. Some clients are given corticosteroids to reduce intracranial pressure.

Support The nurse works closely with the family and significant others of the neurologically impaired client. There is great trauma in seeing a loved one who cannot provide self-care or who is demonstrating unusual or child-like behaviors. The nurse answers questions honestly and sensitively and teaches the family and significant others how to reorient the client. They are encouraged to continue to provide the client with news of family happenings or current events. The nurse identifies community resources for the client and family.

SELF ESTEEM DISTURBANCE

The client with AIDS is susceptible to changes in self-esteem and self-concept. Contributing to this are real and often dramatic changes in appearance that alter the person's body image. In addition, many clients experience significant changes in their relationships with others and in day-to-day activities, often including a job or other productive activity. All of these abrupt changes disrupt the client's self-concept.

PLANNING: CLIENT GOALS The major goals are that the client will:

- Identify positive aspects of oneself
- Accept oneself

INTERVENTIONS The nurse and other members of the health care team provide a climate of acceptance for clients with AIDS. The nurse promotes a trusting relationship and assists clients in expressing feelings and identifying positive aspects of themselves. The nurse allows for the client's privacy but does not avoid or isolate the client. The nurse encourages the client's self-care, independence, control, and decision-making. The nurse helps the client formulate short-term attainable goals and offers encouragement and praise when they are achieved.

SOCIAL ISOLATION

Many clients with AIDS experience discrimination, rejection, and isolation from others (Research Applications for Nursing). Friends or health care workers sometimes avoid or refuse to have anything to do

RESEARCH APPLICATIONS FOR NURSING

People with AIDS May Be at Risk for Depression and Suicide

Longo, M. B., Spross, J. A., & Locke, A. (1990). Identifying major concerns of persons with acquired immunodeficiency syndrome: A replication. *Clinical Nurse Specialist, 4*(1), 21–26.

The purpose of this descriptive study was to determine what the major concerns are of people who are diagnosed with AIDS. The investigators stated that if the major concerns were identified, health care professionals could use this information to identify appropriate support resources and to obtain a better understanding of what the person with AIDS must experience on a day-to-day basis. The study design was exploratory descriptive, using a semi-structured interview instrument to answer the question: "What are the major physical and psychological concerns of persons with AIDS?" Thirty-four subjects were interviewed. Most subjects were young, Caucasian, homosexual men. Five major themes were identified as major concerns of persons with AIDS: uncertainty of the future, desire to maintain health, social unacceptability, fatigue, and weight loss.

Critique. Content validity for the instrument was based on an extensive review of relevant literature; however, reliability was not established at the time of data collection. Even though the interview was semi-structured, incoming information was of a qualitative nature because of the use of open-ended questions. Tape recording the subjects' responses rather than having the interviewer write them on the interview tool could have strengthened the study. The results cannot be generalized to women or heterosexuals with AIDS.

Possible Nursing Implications. The five themes revealed by the results of this study are associated with client depression and suicide ideation. Nurses caring for people who have AIDS should gather assessment data relevant to these five themes. Such information may help identify clients at risk for depression and/or suicide at a time when supportive interventions may be effective.

with these clients. Misunderstanding and fear lead to misuse of proper infection control procedures so that clients are inappropriately isolated in hospitals.

PLANNING: CLIENT GOALS The major goals are that the client will:

- Identify behaviors that cause social isolation
- Demonstrate behaviors that reduce social isolation

INTERVENTIONS Interventions for social isolation are focused on activities to promote social interactions and on education to reduce fear of AIDS transmission.

Promotion of Social Interaction The nurse does not isolate the client but establishes a therapeutic nurse-client relationship. The nurse shows understanding and concern while helping the client to find ways to minimize feelings of rejection and isolation. The nurse reduces barriers to social contact for the client. Client social support resources are assessed. Family and significant others are taught about mode of HIV transmission and how to take Universal Precautions to reduce anxiety and increase contact with the client (see Chap. 27).

The nurse encourages the client to verbalize feelings about self, coping skills, and sense of ability to control the situation. The nurse helps the client to identify support systems, including those already in place and those that need to be arranged.

Education for Prevention of AIDS Transmission The most important aspect for prevention of HIV transmission is education. All people, regardless of age, sex, ethnicity, or sexual orientation, are susceptible to HIV infection. Because of the mode of viral transmission and the fragile nature of the virus, AIDS is a preventable disease.

The human immunodeficiency virus (HIV) has been isolated from multiple body secretions and tissues, including blood, semen, vaginal secretions, breast milk, amniotic fluid, urine, feces, saliva, tears, cerebrospinal fluid, lymph nodes, cervical cells, Langerhans cells, corneal tissue, and brain tissue of infected persons. HIV is primarily transmitted in three ways:

- *Sexual:* Genital, anal or oral sexual contact with exposure of mucous membranes to infected semen or vaginal secretions
- *Parenteral:* Sharing of needles contaminated with infected blood or receiving contaminated blood or blood products
- *Perinatal:* From the placenta, from contact with maternal blood and body fluids during birth, or from breast milk from an infected mother to child

HIV infection is not usually transmitted by casual contact in the home, school, or workplace. Studies of persons sharing household utensils, towels and linens, and toilet facilities in crowded households showed no evidence of HIV transmission (Friedland, et al., 1990). Transmission by insect vectors is "highly improbable" (Gershon et al., 1990).

SEXUAL TRANSMISSION Abstinence and mutually monogamous sex with a noninfected partner are the only absolutely safe methods of preventing the transmission of HIV infection through sexual contact. However, this may not be reasonable for a number of personal, cultural, and economic factors.

Safer sex practices are those that reduce the risk of nonintact skin or mucous membranes coming in contact with potentially infected body fluids and blood (Chart 24–4). Such practices include:

- The use of a latex condom and a spermicide containing nonoxynol-9 for genital and anal intercourse
- The use of a condom or latex barrier (dental dam) over the genitals or anus during oral-genital or oral-anal sexual contact
- The use of latex gloves for finger or hand contact with the vagina or rectum

CHART 24–4

Health Promotion Guide ◆ Condom Use to Prevent Sexually Transmitted Diseases

- Use latex condoms rather than natural membrane condoms.
- Store condoms in a cool, dry place.
- Do not use condoms that were in damaged packages or those that show signs of age, such as those that are brittle, sticky, or discolored.
- Handle condoms carefully to avoid puncturing them.
- Put a condom on before making any genital contact. Hold the tip of the condom and unroll it onto the erect penis, making sure that no air is trapped in the tip. Leave space at the tip to collect semen.
- Use adequate lubrication. Use water-based lubricants only. Petroleum or oil-based lubricants such as petroleum jelly, cooking oil, shortening, and lotions can damage the condom.
- Using a spermicide lubricated condom, or additional spermicide can provide additional protection against sexually transmitted diseases.
- Replace a broken condom immediately. If ejaculation occurs after the condom breaks, there may be some protection in the immediate use of a spermicide.
- After ejaculation, the condom must remain on until the penis is withdrawn. While the penis is still erect, hold the condom against the base of the penis while withdrawing.
- Never reuse condoms.

From Centers for Disease Control. (1988). Condoms for prevention of sexually transmitted diseases. *Morbidity and Mortality Weekly Report, 37*(9), 133–137.

PARENTERAL TRANSMISSION Preventive practices to reduce the risk of parenteral transmission among intravenous drug users include the use of proper cleaning of "works" (needles, syringes and other drug paraphernalia). Clients are instructed to clean drug paraphernalia by using a solution of 1 part chlorine (ordinary household) bleach to 10 parts water. The solution is aspirated through the needle into the syringe twice before the "works" are shared. Drug users are advised to carry a small container with this solution whenever they might be sharing needles. Another option is a needle exchange program, in which needles and syringes are used only once and exchanged for clean ones.

The risk of AIDS transmission through blood and blood products has been reduced to an national average of 0.02% (Durham & Cohen, 1991). Several measures have been implemented to protect the nation's blood supply. All donated blood in North America is screened for the HIV antibody. Blood that reacts positively is discarded. However, current tests detect the antibody rather than the virus itself. Because of time lag in antibody production (seroconversion) after exposure to the HIV, infected blood can test negative for HIV antibodies. In addition, there is the possibility of false-negative results. The small but real possibility of transmission of HIV through blood and blood products has resulted in the use of more stringent indications for transfusion and an increase in the use of autologous transfusion.

PERINATAL TRANSMISSION The risk of perinatal transmission is 20% to 50% for each pregnancy, and it increases to 65% for women having previously infected a child (Smeltzer & Whipple, 1991). It is not known whether transmission occurs transplacentally in utero or during exposure to blood and vaginal secretions during birth. Women with HIV infection should delay pregnancy until more information regarding perinatal transmission is available.

TRANSMISSION AND HEALTH CARE WORKERS Needlestick injuries are the primary means of exposure to HIV infection for health care workers. In addition, transmission to health care workers occurs through exposure of nonintact skin and mucous membranes to blood and body fluids. Because there is a time lag between the time of infection with HIV and the production of serum antibodies (seroconversion), infected people can test negative for HIV yet still transmit the virus to others. Therefore, the best prevention for health care providers is the scrupulous and consistent application of universal precautions for *all* clients as recommended by the Centers for Disease Control and Prevention (CDC) (see Chap. 27).

As a result of the report of possible HIV transmission by a dentist during invasive dental procedures, the public has become concerned about transmission of HIV to clients by health care workers. It is recommended that HIV-infected health care workers wear gloves when they are in contact with clients' nonintact skin or mucous membranes. Infected workers with weeping dermatitis or exudative lesions should not perform direct care activities. The Centers for Disease Control (1991b) also has issued recommendations for preventing HIV transmission by health care workers during exposure-prone invasive procedures. These include any procedure where there is a risk of percutaneous injury to the health care worker in which the worker's blood is likely to make contact with the patient's body cavity, subcutaneous tissues, or mucous membranes. These recommendations are intended to reduce the risk of HIV transmission to clients (Table 24–5).

TABLE 24–5 Recommendations for Preventing Human Immunodeficiency Virus by Health Care Workers

- Workers should adhere to Universal Precautions.
- Workers with exudative lesions or weeping dermatitis should not perform direct patient care or handle patient care equipment and devices used in invasive procedures.
- Workers must follow guidelines for disinfection and sterilization of reusable equipment used in invasive procedures.
- Workers infected with HIV are not restricted from practice of non-exposure–prone procedures, provided that they comply with Universal Precautions and sterilization/disinfection recommendations.
- Workers should identify exposure-prone procedures by institutions where they are performed.
- Workers who perform exposure-prone procedures should know their HIV antibody status.
- Workers who are infected with HIV should seek advice from an expert review panel before performing exposure-prone procedures to determine under what circumstances they may continue to practice these procedures. These circumstances would include notification of prospective clients of HIV positivity.

Adapted from Centers for Disease Control (1991b). Recommendations for preventing transmission of human immunodeficiency virus and hepatitis B virus to patients during exposure-prone invasive procedures. *Morbidity and Mortality Weekly Report, 40*(RR-8), 1–9.

TESTING Testing plays a role in prevention because those who test positive can be educated and encouraged to modify their behaviors to prevent transmission to others. The CDC has issued recommendations describing who should be advised to seek HIV antibody testing (Chart 24–5). Pre-test and post-test counseling must be performed by appropriately trained personnel. Counseling is necessary for the client to make an informed decision about testing, and it provides an opportunity to teach the client risk-reduction behaviors. Post-test counseling is needed to interpret the results, discuss risk reduction, and provide psychologic support and health promotion information for the client with a positive test result.

Recommendations for people who have had positive test results for antibody to HIV are presented in Chart 24–6. People who test positive should also be counseled on how to inform sexual partners and those with whom they have shared needles.

CHART 24–5

Health Promotion Guide ◆ CDC Recommendations for Human Immunodeficiency Virus (HIV) Testing

You should be tested for AIDS if you fall within one or more of the following groups:

- People with sexually transmitted disease
- Intravenous drug abusers
- People who consider themselves at risk
- Women of childbearing age with identifiable risks, including:
  - Having used IV drugs
  - Having engaged in prostitution
  - Having had sexual partners who were infected or at risk
  - Having had contact with countries with high HIV prevalence
  - Having received a transfusion between 1978 and 1985
- People planning to get married
- People undergoing medical evaluation or treatment for signs and symptoms that may be HIV-related
- People admitted to hospitals
- People in correctional institutions such as jails and prisons
- Prostitutes and their customers

Modified from Centers for Disease Control (1987). Public Health Service guidelines for counseling and antibody testing to prevent HIV infection and AIDS. *Morbidity and Mortality Weekly Report, 36*(31), 509–515.

DISCHARGE PLANNING

The usual course of illness is one of intermittent acute infections interspersed with periods of relative wellness over months or years and, ultimately, a chronic, progressive debilitation. Because of the fluctuating nature of HIV infection, the client often spends long periods at home between hospital admissions or clinic visits. In some instances, especially as the illness becomes more severe, the client may need referral to a long-term care facility, home health care agency, or hospice for care outside of the hospital.

The nurse, in collaboration with the social worker, dietitian, and other available resources, works with clients to plan what will be needed and how they will manage at home with self-care and activities of daily living.

HOME CARE PREPARATION

If the client is discharged to home, the nurse carefully assesses the client's status, ability to function, and actual or potential needs for care. Some clients do not need care but do need to maintain a link with the physician or primary care providers. Others need help or care in the home. Home care can range from assistance with activities of daily living for someone with weakness, debility, or limited function, to round-the-clock nursing care, medications, and nutritional support for someone who is severely or terminally ill. The nurse assesses available resources, including family members and significant others who are willing and able to function as caregivers. The nurse helps to make arrangements for outside caregivers or respite care, if needed. Clients may need referrals or help in planning housing, finances, insurance, legal services, funeral arrangements, and spiritual counseling.

HEALTH TEACHING

Educating the client, family, and significant others is a high priority, especially when the nurse is preparating the client for discharge. The nurse instructs client about modes of transmission of the virus and about what behaviors prevent transmission, (safer sex guidelines, not sharing toothbrushes, razors, and other potentially blood-contaminated articles). Caregivers need instruction about infection control precautions to prevent transmission of the virus while caring for the client in the home (Chart 24–7). The nurse also teaches the caregiver nursing techniques

CHART 24–6

Education Guide ◆ Recommendations for HIV-Positive People

- Seek regular medical evaluation and follow-up.
- Either avoid sexual activity or inform your prospective partner of your antibody test results and protect him or her from contact with your body fluids during sex. "Body fluids" includes blood, semen, urine, feces, saliva, and women's genital secretions. Use a condom and avoid practices that may injure body tissues (for example, anal intercourse). Avoid oral-genital contact and open mouthed, intimate kissing.
- Inform your present and previous sex partners, and any persons with whom needles may have been shared, of their potential exposure to HIV and encourage them to seek counseling and antibody testing from their physicians or at appropriate health clinics.
- Don't share toothbrushes, razors, or other items that could become contaminated with blood.
- If you use drugs, enroll in a drug treatment program. Needles and other drug equipment must never be shared.
- Don't donate blood, plasma, body organs, other body tissue, or sperm.
- Clean blood or other body fluid spills on household or other surfaces with freshly diluted household bleach—1 part bleach to 10 parts water. (Do not use bleach on wounds.)
- Inform your doctor, dentist, and eye doctor of your positive HIV status so that proper precautions can be taken to protect you and others.
- Women with a positive antibody test should avoid pregnancy until more is known about the risks of transmitting HIV from mother to infant.

CHART 24–7

Education Guide ♦ Infection Control for Home Care of the Person with AIDS

Direct Care

- Follow Universal Precautions and good hand-washing techniques.
- Do not share razors or toothbrushes.

Housekeeping

- Wipe up feces, vomitus, sputum, urine, blood or other body fluids and the area with soap and water. Dispose of solid wastes and solutions used for cleaning by flushing them down the toilet. Disinfect the area by wiping with a 1:10 solution of household bleach (one part bleach to ten parts water). Wear gloves during cleaning.
- Soak rags, mops, and sponges used for cleaning in a 1:10 bleach solution for 5 minutes to disinfect them.
- Wash dishes and eating utensils in hot water and dishwashing soap or detergent.
- Clean bathroom surfaces with regular household cleaners, then disinfect them with a 1:10 solution of household bleach.

Laundry

- Rinse clothes, towels, or bedclothes if they become soiled with feces, vomitus, sputum, urine, or blood. Then dispose of the soiled water by flushing it down the toilet. Launder these clothes with hot water and detergent with one cup of bleach added per load of laundry.
- Keep soiled clothes in a plastic bag.

Waste Disposal

- Dispose of needles and other "sharps" in a labeled puncture-proof container such as a coffee can with a lid, using Universal Precautions to avoid needlestick injuries. Decontaminate full containers by adding a 1:10 bleach solution. Then seal the container with tape and place it in a paper bag. Dispose of the container in the regular trash.
- Remove solid waste from contaminated trash such as paper towels or tissues, dressings, disposable incontinence pads, and disposable gloves, then flush the waste down the toilet. Place these items in tied plastic bags and dispose of them in the regular trash.

for use in the home and coping and support strategies.

The nurse teaches the client, family, and significant others how to protect the client from infection. They are taught to identify signs and symptoms of potential infections and what to do if these appear. The nurse instructs the client about the importance of self-care strategies, such as good hygiene, balanced rest and exercise, skin care, mouth care, and safe administration of any ordered medications (including potential side effects). Dietary teaching stresses:

- Good nutrition
- The avoidance of raw or rare fish, fowl or meat
- Thorough washing of fruits and vegetables
- Proper food handling
- Refrigeration practices

The nurse also teaches the client about preventing infections by avoiding large crowds, especially in enclosed areas, not traveling to countries with poor sanitation, and not cleaning pet litter boxes.

PSYCHOSOCIAL PREPARATION

Clients with AIDS who are discharged to home or another care facility are often concerned about the possible social stigma and rejection that they may experience. The nurse is aware that this fear is realistic and helps the client to identify ways to avoid problems as well as coping strategies for difficult situations. Family and significant others are supported in efforts to help clients and protect them from discrimination.

The nurse encourages the client to continue as many usual activities as possible. Except when clients are too ill or too weak, they can continue to work and participate in most social activities. Because of potential stigma and discrimination, clients are supported in their selection of friends and relatives with whom to discuss the diagnosis. Sexual partners and care providers should be informed; beyond that, it is up to the client. Some clients experience severe depression or anxiety about the future (Longo, et al., 1990). Almost all feel the burden of having a fatal disease that is widely considered to be unacceptable and thus feel compelled to maintain some secrecy about the illness. Referrals to community resources, mental health professionals, and support groups can help the client verbalize fears and frustrations and cope with the illness.

HEALTH CARE RESOURCES

In many cities, community organizations have been set up to assist the person with AIDS. These organizations are often composed of volunteers, and they offer excellent services to the community. The types and number of services vary by agency and city, but many include HIV testing and counseling, clinic services, buddy systems, support groups, respite care, education and outreach, referral services, and even residences. Clients may also need referrals to other local resources, such as home care agencies, companies that provide home intravenous therapy, community mental health agencies, Meals on Wheels, and others.

EVALUATION

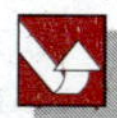

The overall goals are to:

- Maintain the maximum possible level of function for as long as possible

- Minimize infections
- Maintain quality of life and dignity during the course of progressive illness

On the basis of the identified nursing diagnoses, the nurse evaluates care for the client with AIDS. Expected outcomes for this client population are that the client will:

- Demonstrate adequate respiratory function
- Attain adequate weight and nutritional and fluid status
- Maintain skin integrity
- Not develop opportunistic infections
- Remain oriented and/or in a safe environment
- Maintain self-esteem
- Maintain a support system and involvement with others
- Comply with the appropriate and available therapy

Nutrition-Related Deficiencies

Adequate and balanced nutrition is necessary for the proper functioning of the immune system. For example, lymphocytes are highly active metabolic cells that constantly shed surface components (such as immunoglobulin and marker antigens) and need appropriate nutrients for resynthesis of these components. Immunodeficiency that is related to nutrition is considered to be an acquired abnormality and results from multiple factors—biologic, political, economic, and cultural. Acquired immunodeficiencies from inadequate or inappropriate nutrition are potentially preventable and treatable.

Malnutrition is a major cause of immunodeficiencies in the world. It is seen with the greatest frequency in developing countries, in the urban and rural poor of developed countries, and in the chronically ill. An important group at high risk for malnutrition are hospitalized adult medical-surgical clients. Four points should be kept in mind:

- Anorexia that is associated with chronic disease, acute infection, or treatment often leads to a reduced oral intake.
- Absorption, assimilation, or utilization of nutrients is sometimes impaired because of gastrointestinal diseases or absorption problems.
- Host defense mechanisms, which are mobilized in infection, result in increased demand for nutrients, and these demands are met at the expense of the body's stores.
- Hospitalized clients are often treated with a semistarvation regimen with many hours of nothing by mouth because of procedures that will be performed, or with many hours of administration of intravenous fluids that lack essential nutrients.

Malnutrition can impair any or all aspects of the immune system; the degree of impairment is related to the severity of the malnutrition. An excess of nutrients, especially fats and certain carbohydrates, can also have a detrimental effect on immune function. Nutritional problems are almost never simple; they are a complex of deficiency or excess of one or multiple nutrients.

PROTEIN-CALORIE MALNUTRITION

Protein-calorie malnutrition (PCM) affects all aspects of the immune system. The greatest impairment is noted in cell-mediated immunity, with a decreased number of T lymphocytes, reduced delayed hypersensitivity, and thymic changes. The result is *anergy* (no cutaneous delayed hypersensitivity response to common antigens) and an increased incidence of infection in the malnourished host. The incidence of PCM is unknown, but estimates range from 25% to 50% of hospitalized adult medical-surgical clients. PCM causes a deficiency in energy and protein synthesis, which necessitates the use of other body stores (if available).

The usual manifestations of PCM in adults include:

- Leanness and cachexia
- Decreased effort tolerance
- Lethargy
- Intolerance to cold
- Ankle edema
- Dry, flaking skin and various types of dermatitis
- Poor wound healing
- A higher than usual incidence of postoperative infection

The management strategy for clients with PCM is to treat the precipitating event and to supply protein and calories, sometimes with supplements of other specific nutrients. In clients with severe PCM, first any infections are treated and fluid and electrolyte imbalances are corrected. Then a gradual but steady repletion of protein and energy is undertaken. Often this refeeding begins parenterally because a severely malnourished gut undergoes atrophy of the mucosa and depletion of gastric enzymes, which result in an inability to tolerate food. Replenishment of protein and calories is accompanied by vitamin supplementation as appropriate, nutrition education, psychosocial stimulation, and a progressive increase in physical activity.

Protein-calorie malnutrition is easier to prevent than it is to treat. The nurse is aware of hospitalized clients who are at risk for PCM. To reduce this risk, the nurse:

- Measures height and weight when the client is admitted to the agency and reweighs the client at least weekly
- Monitors the client's ability to eat the ordered diet and the amounts eaten
- Obtains dietary consultation when needed
- Evaluates whether nutrients consumed are sufficient to meet basal and stress-related energy needs
- Avoids prolonged use of standard intravenous fluids that provide less than 200 calories/L.

- Assesses and monitors laboratory values for serum albumin and leukocyte counts
- Schedules tests and procedures so that the client spends minimal time fasting

IMMUNODEFICIENCIES RELATED TO OBESITY

The incidence and severity of infectious disease increase among obese people. Impaired cell-mediated immunity and decreased intracellular killing by neutrophils are associated with obesity, which makes obese people more susceptible to infection. Excess dietary fats have a generalized suppressive action on all aspects of immune function. Although more research is needed regarding the interaction between obesity and specific immune functions, appropriate nutrition is an important factor in maintaining or improving host immunologic defenses.

CONGENITAL IMMUNODEFICIENCIES: ANTIBODY-MEDIATED IMMUNODEFICIENCIES

Congenital, or primary, immunodeficiencies are disorders in which the immunodeficient person is born with a defect in the development or function of one of the immune components. As a result, the immune response does not adequately protect the client from infection, cancer, or other disease. Fortunately, most congenital immunodeficiencies are rare.

Some congenital immunodeficiencies are inherited as an X-linked trait (such as Bruton's disease or Wiskott-Aldrich syndrome), and some are autosomal recessive (such as immunodeficiency with ataxia-telangiectasia). For many congenital immunodeficiencies, however, the genetic defect and inheritance pattern have not been clearly identified. Examples of congenital immunodeficiencies are listed in Table 24-6.

TABLE 24–6 Congenital Immunodeficiencies

Antibody-Mediated Immunodeficiencies
- X-linked agammaglobulinemia (Bruton's)
- Acquired hypogammaglobulinemia (common variable immunodeficiency)
- Selective IgA deficiency

Cell-Mediated Immunodeficiencies
- Congenital thymic aplasia (DiGeorge's syndrome)
- Chronic mucocutaneous candidiasis

Combined Immunodeficiencies
- Severe combined immunodeficiencies (SCID)
- Wiskott-Aldrich syndrome
- Immunodeficiency with ataxia-telangiectasia
- Nezelof's syndrome

Congenital immunodeficiencies are classified according to the type of immune function that is impaired:

- Antibody-mediated
- Cell-mediated
- Combined

Because cell-mediated and combined immunodeficiencies are so severe that the affected person usually does not survive infancy, only the antibody-mediated immunodeficiencies (seen in adults) are discussed in this chapter.

Bruton's Agammaglobulinemia

OVERVIEW

A prototypic congenital antibody-mediated immunodeficiency is Bruton's or X-linked agammaglobulinemia. Boys born with this disease present at about 6 months of age, after the loss of maternal antibodies, with recurrent sinusitis, pneumonia, otitis, furunculosis, meningitis, and septicemia with extracellular pyogenic organisms, such as *Pneumococcus, Streptococcus,* and *Haemophilus.* Laboratory evaluation of the client with Bruton's agammaglobulinemia reveals an absence of circulating immunoglobulin.

COLLABORATIVE MANAGEMENT

Except for clients with poliomyelitis, chronic echovirus infection, or a lymphoreticular malignancy, the overall prognosis is fairly good if antibody replacement is begun early in life. Intravenous or intramuscular immune serum globulin is given to these clients on a regular basis, usually about 100 to 400 mg/kg every 3 to 4 weeks (Chart 24–8). The dosage and schedule are individualized. Intermittent courses of antibiotics are used for specific infections. Long-term prophylactic antibiotic therapy may also be used. Despite therapy, severe sinopulmonary disease later develops in some clients.

Common Variable Immunodeficiency

OVERVIEW

Common variable immunodeficiency, or acquired hypogammaglobulinemia, is characterized by recurrent bacterial infections similar to those seen in clients with Bruton's disease. The client has low levels of circulating immunoglobulins of all classes.

Acquired hypogammaglobulinemia differs from Bruton's disease in that it first appears later in life (usually in adolescents or young adults), occurs almost equally in males and females, and is associated with a less severe susceptibility to infection. Frequent complications include giardiasis (intestinal infection

CHART 24-8

Nursing Care Highlights ◆ Administration of Intravenous Immune Serum Globulin

Indications	Dosage	Interventions	Rationale
B cell or humoral immunodeficiencies Bruton's hypogammaglobulinemia Common variable immunodeficiency Combined immunodeficiencies: severe combined immunodeficiencies Pediatric AIDS	• Gamimune, 100–200 mg/kg or 2–4 mL/kg, IV once monthly *or* • Sandoglobulin, 0.2–0.3 g/kg, IV once monthly	• Observe client closely and monitor vital signs during infusion and for 30–60 min thereafter.	• Monitoring detects signs of anaphylaxis and routine side effects. Side effects occur in 10% of clients and include skeletal pain, back pain, nausea, chills, headache, chest tightness, and abdominal cramps.
		• Slow the rate of infusion or stop it temporarily if side effects occur.	• Side effects appear to be related to the rate of infusion.

with the protozoon *Giardia lamblia*), bronchiectasis, gastric carcinoma, lymphoreticular malignancy, and cholelithiasis (gallbladder stones).

COLLABORATIVE MANAGEMENT

Treatment for common variable hypogammaglobulinemia is similar to that for Bruton's disease. Regular administration of intravenous or intramuscular immune serum globulin and the regular or intermittent use of antibiotics protect the affected person against infection.

Selective Immunoglobulin A Deficiency

OVERVIEW

Selective immunoglobulin A (IgA) deficiency is the most common congenital immunodeficiency, occurring in 1 per 600 to 800 population (Workman, et al., 1993). The client may be asymptomatic or may have chronic recurrent respiratory tract infections, atopic diseases, and/or collagen-vascular diseases. Usually, clients with selective immunoglobulin A deficiency have a normal life span. Because IgA is the major immunoglobulin in secretions, bacterial infections are seen primarily in the respiratory, gastrointestinal, and urogenital tracts. Some adults with IgA deficiency also have a malabsorption syndrome.

COLLABORATIVE MANAGEMENT

Therapy for selective IgA deficiency is limited to appropriate and vigorous treatment of infections. Unlike other immunoglobulin deficiencies, selective IgA deficiency should never be treated with administration of exogenous immune globulin for two reasons. First, exogenous immune globulin contains very little IgA. Second, because clients who have selective IgA deficiency do make normal amounts of all other classes of immunoglobulins, they are at high risk for severe allergic reactions to exogenous immune globulin. If malabsorption syndrome accompanies the selective IgA deficiency, the client will need nutritional supplementation (such as total parenteral nutrition).

SECONDARY IMMUNODEFICIENCIES

Specific immunodeficiencies may be "secondary" to other disease states that cause the loss of immunoglobulins or destruction of lymphocytes (T and B cells). For example, severe malabsorption states, such as protein-losing enteropathy, can cause the loss of albumin and immunoglobulins through the intestinal tract. Loss of serum proteins through extensive burns, renal problems, eczema, or other skin diseases can also cause depletion of immunoglobulins. Increased catabolism of immunoglobulin resulting in hypogammaglobulinemia can occur in nephrotic syndrome or multiple myeloma. Many diseases, such as Hodgkin's lymphoma, cause a cell-mediated (or T-cell) deficiency.

The most common cause of secondary immunodeficiency is *iatrogenesis.* An iatrogenic immunodeficiency is an immunodeficiency or immunosuppressive state that is induced in a person by medical therapies or procedures. Many of the drugs and other treatment modalities used for various diseases can cause immunosuppression. Sometimes this is a desired effect, as in the case of organ transplantation or the treatment of certain autoimmune disorders. At other times, immunosuppression is an undesirable, complicating side effect of therapy that is used for another intent, such as cancer chemotherapy, and may even necessitate an alteration in the therapeutic regimen. Various therapies cause different types and degrees of immunosuppression. The challenge is deriving maximal therapeutic effect without leaving the client overly immunosuppressed and therefore susceptible to potentially serious complications.

Drug-Induced Immunodeficiencies

Several classes of drugs have powerful and significant immunosuppressive effects. Some induce a general immunosuppression; others are more specific and affect one part of the immune system more than another.

Immunodeficiencies Caused by Cytotoxic Drugs

Cytotoxic drugs are usually not selective but interfere with all rapidly proliferating cells. White blood cells, including immunocompetent lymphocytes and phagocytes, are rapidly proliferating and therefore susceptible to this type of destruction (see Chaps. 22 and 26). The result is a decrease in the number of lymphocytes and phagocytic cells. Cytotoxic agents also interfere with the ability of lymphocytes to synthesize and release their products (such as lymphokines and antibodies), thereby causing a general immunosuppression. Most cytotoxic drugs are used in the treatment of cancer (see Chap. 22).

Immunodeficiencies Caused by Corticosteroids

Corticosteroids are adrenocortical hormones used in the treatment of many immunologically mediated diseases, neoplasms, and several neurologic and endocrine disorders. Corticosteroids have both anti-inflammatory and immunosuppressive effects. They inhibit inflammation by stabilizing the vascular membrane, decreasing permeability, thereby blocking the migration and mobilization of neutrophils and monocytes. In addition, corticosteroids disrupt the synthesis of arachidonic acid, the main precursor for a variety of vasoactive amines.

Corticosteroids sequester T cells in the bone marrow, reducing the number of circulating T cells and resulting in lymphopenia and suppressed cell-mediated immunity.

Corticosteroids appear to interfere with IgG synthesis and the binding of immunoglobulin to antigen. These drugs have many physiologic and immunologic effects, which can alter disease activity. Numerous side effects are also associated with corticosteroid therapy, including:

- Central nervous system changes, such as euphoria, insomnia, or psychosis
- Cardiovascular changes, such as hypertension and edema
- Gastrointestinal tract effects, such as gastric irritation, ulcers, and increased appetite (with weight gain)
- Other changes, such as cataracts, hyperglycemia and glucose intolerance, muscle weakness, osteoporosis, delayed wound healing, redistribution of body fat

Immunodeficiencies Caused by Cyclosporine

Cyclosporine (Sandimmune) is a specific immunosuppressant that selectively suppresses the helper subset of T lymphocytes by blocking proliferation and development (see Chap. 22). Cyclosporine has been used primarily to prevent organ transplant rejection and graft-versus-host disease (see Chaps. 39 and 72). The drug is undergoing clinical trials for use in other disorders, such as uveitis, rheumatoid arthritis, and other autoimmune diseases.

Radiation-Induced Immunodeficiencies

Radiation is cytotoxic to proliferating and resting cells. Because most lymphocytes are sensitive to radiation, exposure can induce a profound lymphopenia in lymphoid organs and in the circulation, thereby causing a general immunosuppression. Whether or not immunodeficiency occurs after radiation therapy depends on the location and dose of radiation received. Exposure to the iliac and femur in adults can cause generalized immunosuppression because the medullary areas of these bones are the primary blood cell–producing sites in adults. Total nodal irradiation is used in certain diseases, such as Hodgkin's disease, to induce immunosuppression. This treatment results in a lymphopenia and a decreased T-cell function.

HYPERSENSITIVITIES

Hypersensitivity is a state of altered reactivity in which a previously sensitized immune system reacts in an excessive or inappropriate way with resultant tissue damage and pathology. The primary function of the immune system is to protect the host from harm. However, the same protective mechanisms, if prolonged or excessive, have a deleterious effect and may produce tissue damage (Workman, 1993).

Immune mechanisms that result in tissue damage to the host are classified into four basic types of hypersensitivity:

- Type I (immediate) hypersensitivity (anaphylactic) reactions
- Type II (cytotoxic) reactions
- Type III (immune complex–mediated) reactions
- Type IV (delayed) hypersensitivity reactions (Table 24–7).

TABLE 24–7 Mechanisms and Examples of Types of Hypersensitivities

Mechanism	Clinical Examples
Type I: Immediate	
Reaction of IgE antibody on mast cells with antigen, which results in release of mediators	• Hay fever • Allergic asthma • Anaphylaxis
Type II: Cytotoxic	
Reaction of IgG with host cell membrane or antigen adsorbed by host cell membrane	• Autoimmune hemolytic anemia • Goodpasture's syndrome • Myasthenia gravis
Type III: Immune Complex–Mediated	
Formation of immune complex of antigen and antibody, which deposits in walls of blood vessels and results in complement release and inflammation	• Serum sickness • Vasculitis • Systemic lupus erythematosus • Rheumatoid arthritis
Type IV: Delayed	
Reaction of sensitized T cells with antigen and release of lymphokines, which activate macrophages and induce inflammation	• Poison ivy • Graft rejection • Tuberculosis • Sarcoidosis

Clinical manifestations may be the consequence of one or any combination of these mechanisms of tissue injury.

TYPE I: IMMEDIATE HYPERSENSITIVITY REACTIONS

Type I, or immediate, hypersensitivity occurs when IgE responds to an otherwise harmless antigen, such as pollen, and causes the release of histamine and other vasoactive amines from basophils, eosinophils and mast cells (see Chap. 22). This response results in an acute inflammatory reaction and symptoms such as bronchospasm, wheezing, and rhinorrhea.

On first exposure to an allergen (an antigen that provokes allergic sensitization with IgE), the host responds by making antigen-specific IgE. This antigen-specific IgE then binds to the surface of basophils and mast cells. These cells have large numbers of granules that contain vasoactive amines (including histamine) that are released when stimulated (see Chap. 22). Once the antigen-specific IgE is formed, the host is sensitized to that allergen.

In a type I hypersensitivity reaction, the previously sensitized person is re-exposed to the provoking allergen. The allergen binds to two adjacent IgE molecules on the surface of a basophil or mast cell and causes distortion of the cell membrane. This distortion initiates a series of biochemical events that cause the granules in the cell to swell, migrate, and fuse with the cell membrane. The granular contents (vasoactive amines) are then expelled and released into the extravascular space. This process is called *degranulation.*

The most important mediator is *histamine,* a short-acting vasoactive amine. Histamine causes increased capillary permeability, mucous secretion (both nasal and bronchial), smooth muscle contractions (especially of bronchioles and small blood vessels), and an itching sensation (pruritus), sometimes accompanied by redness. These symptoms last for approximately 10 minutes, with the maximum reaction occurring 1 to 2 minutes after the histamine is released.

Clinical examples of type I reactions include systemic anaphylaxis, allergic asthma, and atopic (genetic tendency to have allergies) allergies such as hay fever, allergic rhinitis, and allergies to specific allergens. Allergens can be:

- Inhaled (e.g., plant pollens, fungal spores, animal dander, house dust, grass, ragweed)
- Ingested (e.g., foods, food additives, drugs)
- Injected (e.g., bee venom, drugs, biologic substances such as contrast dyes and adrenocorticotropic hormone)
- Contacted (e.g., pollens, foods)

Chapter 66 describes methods of allergy testing.

Anaphylaxis

OVERVIEW

Anaphylaxis, the most dramatic example of a type I hypersensitivity reaction, is a rapid, systemic, simultaneous occurrence after reactions in multiple organs. It generally occurs within seconds to minutes of exposure to an allergen. Anaphylaxis is not common, but it can be fatal.

Many substances can trigger anaphylaxis in a susceptible person. The most common allergens are:

- Drugs, especially antibiotics such as penicillin, the cephalosporins, vancomycin, and amphotericin B
- Foreign proteins that are used as therapeutic agents, such as adrenocorticotropic hormone (ACTH), insulin, vaccines, allergen extracts, and muscle relaxants
- Insect venom, especially from bees, wasps, hornets, and fire ants
- Certain foods, such as shellfish, berries, chocolate, eggs, and nuts

There are many other potential triggers of anaphylaxis (Table 24–8).

TABLE 24–8 Common Agents That Cause Anaphylaxis

Drugs/Foreign Proteins

- Antibiotics (penicillin, cephalosporins, tetracycline, sulfonamides, streptomycin, vancomycin, chloramphenicol, amphotericin B, others)
- Adrenocorticotropic hormone, insulin, vasopressin, protamine*
- Allergen extracts, muscle relaxants, hydrocortisone, vaccines, local anesthetics (lidocaine, procaine)*
- Whole blood, cryoprecipitate, immune serum globulin*
- Radiocontrast media*
- Opiates

Foods

- Shellfish
- Eggs
- Legumes, nuts
- Grains
- Berries
- Preservatives

Insects/Animals

- Hymenoptera: bees, wasps, hornets
- Fire ants
- Snake venom

Other Agents

- Pollens
- Exercise
- Heat/cold
- Other

* Anaphylaxis that is caused by these substances is probably a result of direct mast cell degranulation, rather than an IgE-mediated hypersensitivity event.

COLLABORATIVE MANAGEMENT

ASSESSMENT

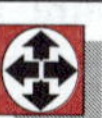

Typically, a client who is experiencing an anaphylactic reaction first complains of a feeling of uneasiness, apprehension, weakness, and a feeling of impending doom. The nurse notes that the client is anxious and frightened. These feelings are followed, often quickly, by a generalized pruritus and urticaria. The nurse sees erythema and sometimes angioedema of the eyes, lips, or tongue. Frequently, discrete cutaneous wheals or urticarial eruptions appear that are intensely pruritic and sometimes merge together and give a red, blotchy appearance over a large area.

Histamine and other chemical mediators cause bronchoconstriction, mucosal edema, and excess mucus. On respiratory assessment, the nurse notes congestion, rhinorrhea, dyspnea, and increasing respiratory distress with audible wheezing.

On auscultation, the nurse detects crackles, wheezing, and diminished breath sounds. Clients may experience laryngeal edema as a feeling of having a "lump in the throat," hoarseness, and stridor (a crowing sound). Distress increases as the tongue and larynx become more edematous and excess mucous secretion continues. The nurse may note increasing stridor and anxiety as the airway begins to close. Respiratory failure may follow quickly as a complication of laryngeal edema and suffocation or lower airway bronchoconstriction causing hypoxemia (insufficient oxygenation of blood) and hypercapnia (increased carbon dioxide in blood).

In performing the cardiovascular assessment, the nurse usually finds hypotension and a rapid, weak, possibly irregular pulse. These findings are due to chemical mediators, which cause vasodilation and increased capillary permeability with resultant leakage of intravascular fluids. The client may be syncopal (faint) and diaphoretic. The nurse notes increasing anxiety, confusion, and eventual loss of consciousness if the client is not treated immediately. Dysrhythmias, shock, and cardiac arrest may occur within minutes as intravascular volume is lost. Less often, the client may complain of abdominal cramping, may have diarrhea, or may vomit. Death can be caused by respiratory failure (70% of deaths) and/or by shock and cardiac dysrhythmias.

INTERVENTIONS

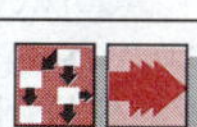

EMERGENCY RESPIRATORY MANAGEMENT

Emergency respiratory management is critical for the client having an anaphylactic reaction because the severity of the reaction and the gravity of the consequences increase with time. An airway must be established and/or stabilized immediately. The nurse may need to initiate cardiopulmonary resuscitation. Epinephrine (1:1000), 0.2 to 0.5 mL, should be given subcutaneously as soon as possible after a person displays symptoms of systemic anaphylaxis. This agent constricts blood vessels, increases myocardial contraction, and dilates the bronchioles. The same dose may be repeated every 15 to 20 minutes if needed. Other drugs commonly administered during anaphylaxis are listed in Chart 24–9.

Antihistamines, such as diphenhydramine (Allerdryl✱, Benadryl), 25 to 100 mg, are usually given intravenously, intramuscularly, or orally to treat angioedema and urticaria. This agent blocks the histamine receptor site (H_1) in vascular and bronchiolar smooth muscle. If the extent of upper airway narrowing requires it, the physician may insert a small endotracheal tube or perform an emergency tracheostomy.

If the client can breathe independently, the nurse administers oxygen, as ordered, to minimize hypoxemia. Oxygen should be started via nasal cannula at 5 to 10 L/minute or via face mask at 40% to 60% before arterial blood gas results are obtained. The nurse monitors tissue oxygen saturation using pulse oximetry. Arterial blood gas concentrations are monitored to determine the adequacy of the oxygenation, with the PO_2 maintained between 80 and 100 mmHg. The nurse uses suction to remove excess mucous se-

CHART 24-9

Drug Therapy for Anaphylaxis

Drug	Mechanism	Side Effects
Sympathomimetics		
• Epinephrine (Adrenalin)	• Rapidly stimulates alpha- and beta-adrenergic receptors of autonomic nervous system (alpha: vasoconstriction; beta: bronchodilation)	• Pallor, tachycardia and palpitations, nervousness, muscle twitching, sweating, anxiety, insomnia, hypertension, headache, hyperglycemia
• Isoproterenol (Isuprel)	• Stimulated beta-adrenergic receptors, relaxing bronchial muscle and dilating vessels	• Same as for epinephrine.
• Ephedrine sulfate (Vatronol)	• Similar to isoproterenol, but with longer duration of action	• Same as for epinephrine.
Antihistamines		
• Diphenhydramine HCl (Allerdryl✱, Benadryl)	• Competes with histamine for H_1 receptors on effector cells, thus blocking effects of histamine on bronchioles, gastrointestinal tract, and blood vessels	• Drowsiness, confusion, insomnia, headache, vertigo, photosensitivity, diplopia, nausea, vomiting, dry mouth
Corticosteroids		
• Prednisone (PO) • Hydrocortisone sodium succinate (Solu-Cortef) (IV/IM) • Methylprednisolone sodium succinate (Solu-Medrol) (IV/IM) • Beclomethasone (inhalant)	• Anti-inflammatory; inhibits mast cell degranulation	• Fluid and sodium retention, hypertension, Cushingoid state, gastric distress, adrenal suppression, psychosis, osteoporosis, susceptibility to infection
Methlyxanthines		
• Aminophylline (Aminophyllin, Palaron✱)	• Relaxes bronchial smooth muscle	• Restlessness, dizziness, palpitations, tachycardia, nausea, vomiting, epigastric distress, headache, convulsions
Vasopressors		
• Norepinephrine (Levophed)	• Raises blood pressure and cardiac output in severely decompensated states	• Headache, tachycardia, fibrillation, decreased urinary output, hypertension, metabolic acidosis
• Dopamine (Intropin)		• Arrhythmias, tachycardia, hypertension, dyspnea, nausea and vomiting, azotemia, headache
Inhaled Beta-Adrenergic Agonists		
• Metaproterenol (Alupent, Metaprel)	• Rapidly stimulates beta-2 receptor sites in pulmonary smooth muscle, causing bronchodilation	• Palpitations, tachycardia, dysrhythmias, hypokalemia
• Albuterol (Proventil, Ventolin)	• Same as for metaproterenol	• Same as for metaproterenol, plus painful urination, flushing of the face

cretions, if indicated, and closely assesses and records the client's rate, rhythm, and depth of respirations as well as the presence of bronchospasm and abnormal breath sounds. The nurse elevates the client's bed to 45 degrees unless this is contraindicated because of hypotension.

For severe bronchospasm, the client is given aminophylline (Aminophyllin, Palaron✱), 6 mg/kg intravenously, over 20 to 30 minutes. If the client is taking aminophylline regularly, no more than 3 mg/kg is given. Maintenance aminophylline (0.3 to 0.5 mg/kg/hour) is initiated. The client may be given an inhaled beta-adrenergic agonist such as metaproterenol (Alupent) or albuterol (Proventil) every 2 to 4 hours. For persistent symptoms (after 1 to 2 hours), corticosteroids are added to prevent the late recurrence of symptoms.

The nurse's primary role of caring for the client with anaphylaxis is assessment to detect changes in any body system and monitoring for adverse effects of drug therapy. For severe anaphylaxis, the client is admitted to a critical care unit for cardiac, pulmonary arterial, and capillary wedge pressure monitoring. The nurse carefully observes the client for fluid overload from the rapid administration of medications and intravenous fluids, and reports changes to the physician immediately. The client may be discharged from the hospital when respiratory and cardiovascular systems have returned to baseline functioning.

PREVENTION

Because of the rapid onset of life-threatening symptoms and the potential for a fatal outcome, sometimes even with appropriate medical intervention, the prevention of anaphylaxis is of paramount importance. The nurse teaches the client with a history of allergic reactions to avoid allergens whenever possible, to wear a medical alert (Medic-Alert) bracelet, and to alert health care personnel about their specific allergies. Some clients must carry an emergency anaphylaxis kit, such as a bee sting kit with injectable epinephrine, or an epinephrine injector, such as EpiPen Auto-Injector (Center Laboratories). The EpiPen device is an easy-to-use, spring-loaded injector that delivers 0.3 mg of epinephrine per dose (in 2 mL).

The medical record of a client with a history of anaphylactic symptoms should prominently display the list of allergens to which the client is sensitive. A careful history is taken before *any* drug or therapeutic agent is given. Skin tests should be performed before the administration of substances with a highly associated incidence of anaphylactic reactions, such as allergenic extract or horse serums. Physicians and nurses should be aware of common cross-reacting agents. For example, a client with a history of sensitivity to penicillin is also likely to react to cephalosporins because both have a similar biochemical structure.

If an agent must be used despite a history of allergenic reactions, precautionary measures should be taken. An intravenous solution should be started and intubation equipment and a tracheostomy set put at the bedside. The substance should be given first intradermally, and then subcutaneously, and then intramuscularly in increasing doses at 20- to 30-minute intervals so that the initial dose by the next route does not exceed the final dose by the previous route. When carefully done, this procedure is fairly safe.

Atopic Allergy

Atopic reactions are allergic manifestations that occur in people who are genetically predisposed to respond to a variety of environmental allergens by forming immunoglobulin E (IgE). Once the person has sensitized IgE, allergic symptoms occur on re-exposure to the allergen via degranulation of mast cells (see type I hypersensitivity earlier). Conditions such as allergic asthma, allergic rhinitis, urticaria, and eczematous dermatitis are manifested alone or in combination. Urticaria and asthma are described here because they are noted most frequently in a medical-surgical setting.

Urticaria

OVERVIEW

Uricaria ("hives") is characterized by local wheals and erythema of the skin. Urticaria is essentially anaphylaxis that is limited to the skin. Urticaria can be due to exposure to drugs, transfusions, insect stings, desensitization injections, and certain foods, especially eggs, shellfish, nuts, and berries. Urticaria can also be associated with a viral infection, such as hepatitis, infectious mononucleosis, or rubella, or with physical stimuli, such as cold, sunlight, heat, vibration, or exercise. In chronic urticaria, the offending agent is often unknown.

COLLABORATIVE MANAGEMENT

The client experiencing urticaria initially reports pruritis (itching), followed by the appearance of wheals. The nurse notes pink, raised, edematous, and pruritic areas that vary in size and shape; these areas are commonly called hives (Fig. 24-2). Sometimes, larger wheals clear in the center and appear as rings of erythema. The nurse observes that crops of hives appear, usually last a few hours, and then disappear as new ones appear in a different location. In some

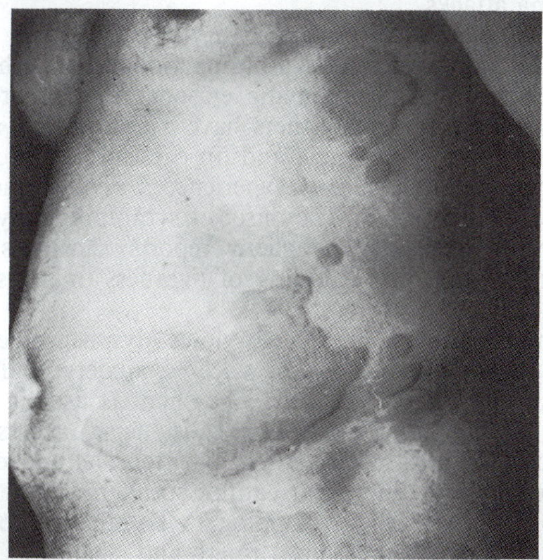

FIGURE 24-2 ◆ Urticaria (hives). (From Moschella, S. L., & Hurley, H. J. [1992]. *Dermatology* [3rd ed., p. 287]. Philadelphia: W. B. Saunders).

cases, urticaria is associated with angioedema, particularly of the hands, eyelids, lips, and genitalia.

Urticaria is self-limiting and will disappear within 7 to 10 days. Treatment during this time is symptomatic and usually includes an oral antihistamine, such as diphenhydramine (Allerdryl♣, Benadryl), 25 to 50 mg every 4 to 6 hours, cyproheptadine hydrochloride (Periactin, Vimicon♣), 4 to 8 mg three times a day, or hydroxyzine (Atarax, Vistaril), 25 to 50 mg three times a day. For a more severe reaction, especially urticaria with angioedema, corticosteroids (usually prednisone [Apo-prednisone♣]) may be used.

The nurse helps the client identify the allergen that caused the urticaria and explains strategies for avoiding exposure to that allergen. Nurses help clients suffering from chronic urticaria, for whom the allergen is often not known, to reduce stress in their lives. Nurses also teach clients to avoid caffeine, tobacco, alcohol, and aspirin, all of which tend to exacerbate symptoms. Chronic urticaria undergoes spontaneous remission within 2 years in approximately 50% of cases.

Allergic Asthma

OVERVIEW

Approximately 10% to 20% of the adult asthmatic population suffer from extrinsic/asthma, i.e., asthma that is caused by allergenic exposure (e.g., to pollens, molds, dust, or animal dander). Extrinsic asthma results in bronchoconstriction, edema, and increased mucus production. Approximately 50% of adult asthmatics have intrinsic asthma, which is precipitated by nonallergenic factors, such as viral infection, exercise, cold, cigarette smoke, changes in temperature or humidity, gasoline fumes, and paint fumes. Emotional stress seems to exacerbate an attack but may not have a primary etiologic role. In some adults, both allergenic and nonallergenic factors may trigger asthma attacks.

Adult clients with asthma vary greatly in the frequency and severity of symptoms. Some people have only occasional symptomatic episodes that are relatively mild and brief. Others have a mild cough and wheeze most of the time, and on exposure to known allergens or other factors experience a severe exacerbation of symptoms. The onset of symptoms may be acute or gradual. The client reports shortness of breath, cough, and a feeling of tightness or pressure in the chest.

On assessment, the nurse notes dyspnea, tachypnea, nonproductive cough, wheezes, anxiety, and increasing respiratory distress. The client is usually sitting or even leaning forward, is using accessory muscles for breathing, is often hypertensive, and may be dehydrated. The client cannot speak more than a couple words without stopping to breathe. Respirations become increasingly rapid and shallow. The client then experiences fatigue and becomes cyanotic, confused, and lethargic as the PO_2 drops and PCO_2 rises. Pulmonary function test results are abnormal and arterial blood gas tests indicate hypoxemia (decreased arterial oxygen) and hypercapnia (increased arterial carbon dioxide).

COLLABORATIVE MANAGEMENT

Treatment of asthma centers on control of causative factors, treatment of acute episodes, and maintenance drug therapy. An asthma attack is treated as an emergency, and the nurse intervenes promptly to interrupt symptoms. At the same time, the nurse acts calmly and confidently to reassure and support an anxious client.

Medications used to treat an acute attack include:

- Beta-adrenergic agents (e.g., epinephrine, isoproterenol, ephedrine), which relax bronchial smooth muscle and inhibit mediator release
- Theophylline and derivatives, which act in a similar fashion
- Corticosteroids, in some cases

Oxygen is administered to maintain a PO_2 value higher than 60 mmHg. The nurse monitors fluid intake and output and electrolytes and administers intravenous fluids to replace loss. Asthmatic clients are usually given maintenance therapy with theophylline and bronchodilators or cromolyn sodium.

(For a more detailed discussion of asthma, see Chapter 30 under Chronic Airflow Limitation [CAL]).

TYPE II: CYTOTOXIC REACTIONS

In a type II (cytotoxic) reaction, the body makes special autoantibodies directed against self cells or tissues that have some form of foreign protein attached to them. The autoantibody binds to the self cell and forms an antigen-antibody complex, or immune complex. The self cell is then destroyed by complement-mediated lysis (see Chap. 22). Clinical examples of type II reactions include Coombs'-positive hemolytic anemias, thrombocytopenic purpura, hemolytic transfusion reactions, hemolytic disease of the newborn, Goodpasture's syndrome, and drug-induced hemolytic anemia.

An interesting variant of a type II reaction occurs when the autoantibody is made to a receptor. For example, in Graves disease, the antibody known as long-acting thyroid stimulator (LATS) is made to the thyroid-stimulating hormone receptor on the thyroid gland. LATS binds with the receptor and stimulates it, which results in the production of abnormally high levels of thyroxine.

Another clinical example involving an antireceptor antibody is myasthenia gravis. An autoantibody is made to the acetylcholine receptor on muscle. The antibody binds to the receptor at the neuromuscular junction, which blocks acetylcholine and thus prevents transmission of the impulse from the nerve that would stimulate the muscle. The result is profound muscular weakness.

Hemolytic Blood Transfusion Reaction

OVERVIEW

A hemolytic transfusion reaction occurs when a person is given ABO-incompatible blood. Early in a person's life, natural antibodies (agglutinins) to ABO antigens, which are found on erythrocyte cell membranes, develop. If a client is transfused with incompatible blood, the antibodies bind to the antigens on the donor's erythrocytes and coat them, and the cells agglutinate, or clump together. Agglutination of cells results in blockage of small blood vessels and capillaries. The immune complex activates complement, which results in destruction of the erythrocytes. Through this destruction, hemoglobin is released and, ultimately, the renal tubules are blocked and acute renal failure results.

The most common causes of hemolytic transfusion reaction are mistakes in labeling of blood and transfusion of blood to the wrong client. Nurses can help prevent this type of reaction by ensuring that the client who is receiving blood has recently been typed and crossmatched and by double-checking the blood before use (see Chap. 39).

COLLABORATIVE MANAGEMENT

When the first symptom of a hemolytic reaction appears, the nurse stops the transfusion but continues intravenous administration of normal saline through new tubing. The nurse notifies the physician immediately. The nurse monitors the client's vital signs and urinary output every 15 to 30 minutes. If symptoms of shock develop, appropriate intervention is initiated with epinephrine, intravenous fluids, and oxygen. Samples of blood from the client are taken and sent to the blood bank, and urine is sent to the laboratory for determination of hemoglobin. The nurse remains calm and reassures the client that appropriate actions are being taken. If there is evidence of renal involvement, a potent diuretic, such as mannitol (Osmitrol✱), is given.

Drug-Induced Hemolytic Anemia

OVERVIEW

Certain drugs precipitate a type II reaction to erythrocytes. This occurs by two main mechanisms:

- Drugs such as penicillin and the sulfonamides form bonds with the erythrocyte membrane. Antibodies are made, and the antigen-antibody reaction leads to clumping and destruction of erythrocytes.
- Methyldopa (Aldomet, Dopamet✱) and some other drugs alter the erythrocyte surface chemically, thereby exposing an antigen that stimulates and reacts with an autoantibody, and leads to destruction of the cells.

COLLABORATIVE MANAGEMENT

Treatment of drug-induced hemolytic anemia starts with discontinuation of the offending drug. Otherwise, treatment is symptomatic. Complications such as hemolytic crisis and renal failure can be life-threatening.

TYPE III: IMMUNE COMPLEX REACTIONS

OVERVIEW

In a type III reaction, soluble immune complexes are formed, usually in the setting of antigen excess (Fig. 24–3). These circulating immune complexes are then deposited in the vessel wall, usually of small vessels. Common sites include the kidneys, skin, joints, and other small blood vessels. The deposited immune complex activates complement, and tissue or vessel damage results.

There are many immune complex disorders in which the type III reaction is the major mechanism of clinical manifestations. Many of these are known as connective tissue disorders. For example, the clinical manifestations of rheumatoid arthritis are caused by immune complexes that lodge in joint spaces followed by destruction of tissue, and later scarring and fibrous changes. In a similar fashion, the clinical manifestations of systemic lupus erythematosus result from immune complex deposition in the vessels (vasculitis), the glomeruli (nephritis), the joints (arthralgia/arthritis), and other organs and tissues. In this disorder, the immune complex is composed of cellular DNA and anti-DNA antibodies. (For a detailed discussion of these and other connective tissue disorders, see Chapter 23.)

Serum sickness is a complex of symptoms that occurs after the administration of foreign serum or certain drugs. It is caused by collection of immune complexes in the walls of vessels in the skin, joints, and the glomeruli of the kidney. The most common causes of serum sickness today are penicillin and related drugs and some horse serum antitoxins. Serum sickness used to be quite common when vaccines were made with horse or rabbit serum, but now most vaccines are made with human serum or antigen fragments. Relatively new agents that can cause serum sickness are antilymphocyte globulin and antithymocyte globulin, used to suppress the immune response in organ transplantation.

The client experiencing serum sickness has symptoms of fever, arthralgia (achy joints), rash, lymphadenopathy (enlarged lymph nodes), malaise, and possibly polyarthritis and nephritis, usually about 7 to 12

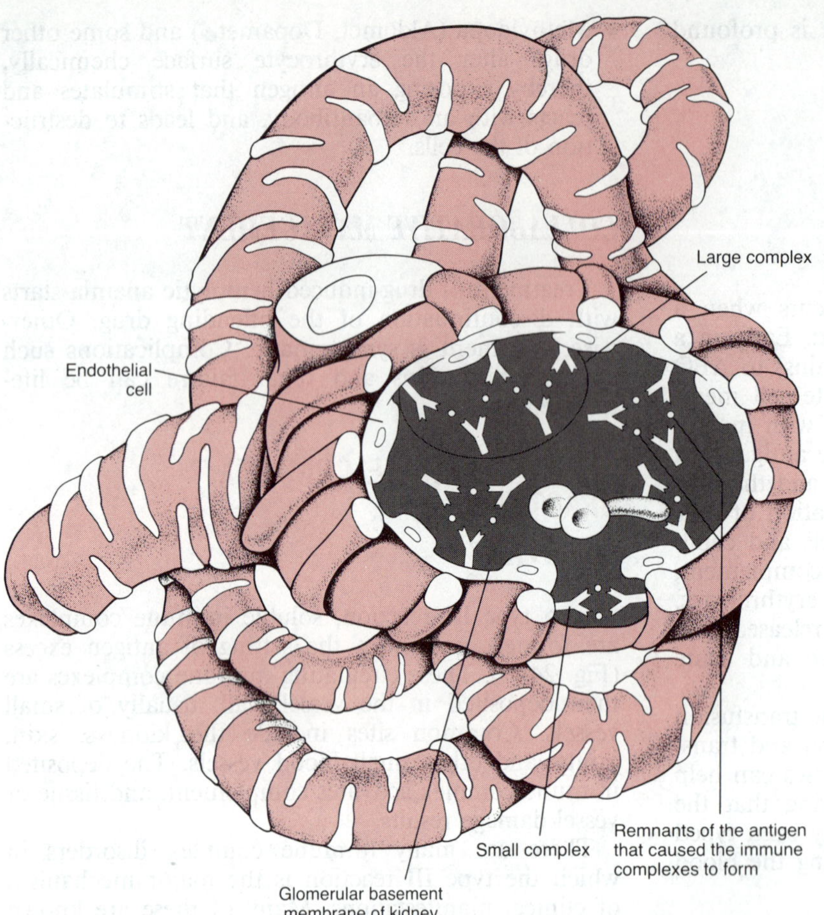

FIGURE 24-3 ◆ An immune complex in a type III hypersensitivity reaction.

days after administration of the causative agent. The nurse alerts the client to the possibility of serum sickness and what symptoms to look for. When administering a foreign serum to a client, the nurse is also prepared for the possibility of a type I anaphylactic reaction and has emergency equipment and medications close at hand.

COLLABORATIVE MANAGEMENT

Serum sickness is usually self-limiting, and symptoms subside after several days. Treatment is usually symptomatic, with antihistamines given for pruritus and aspirin for arthralgias. Prednisone is given if symptoms are severe.

TYPE IV: DELAYED HYPERSENSITIVITY REACTIONS

In a type IV reaction, the important cell is the T lymphocyte. Antibodies and complement are not involved. Sensitized T lymphocytes (from a previous exposure) respond to an antigen by producing and releasing certain lymphokines (chemical mediators). These lymphokines act to recruit, retain, and activate macrophages that help to destroy the antigen. A type IV response typically occurs hours to days after exposure rather than immediately, as in a type I hypersensitivity reaction. A type IV reaction is characterized by an accumulation of lymphocytes and macrophages. These events cause edema, ischemia, and tissue destruction at the site of response.

An example of a type IV reaction is a positive purified protein derivative (PPD) test. In a client who had previously been exposed to tuberculosis, an intradermal injection of this agent causes sensitized T cells to accumulate at the injection site, release lymphokines, and recruit and activate macrophages. Induration and erythema at the site of the injection appear approximately 24 to 48 hours later.

Clinical examples of type IV hypersensitivity reactions include contact dermatitis, poison ivy skin rashes, local response to insect stings, allograft (tissue transplant) rejections, and granulomatous diseases in which the antigen is unknown (e.g., sarcoidosis).

AUTOIMMUNITIES

OVERVIEW

Autoimmunity is a process whereby a host develops and expresses immunologic reactivity, especially in the form of antibodies, against self components.

For unknown reasons, certain cells or tissues of the body are recognized as nonself or no longer tolerated as self, and immune reactions to them occur. The responses, both antibody and cell mediated, are similar to normal immune responses against nonself, although they are inappropriate and sometimes excessive. Although the reasons for alterations in self-tolerance are not known, there are multiple theories.

Much research is ongoing in the area of autoimmunity, but there are still few confirmed, established data. Not only is the etiology of autoimmunity uncertain; there is also a lack of consensus as to which diseases are truly autoimmune. Diseases that are generally believed to be autoimmune include systemic lupus erythematosus, polyarteritis nodosa, rheumatoid arthritis, autoimmune hemolytic anemia, rheumatic fever, and Hashimoto's thyroiditis (Table 24–9).

Connective tissue disorders, also sometimes referred to as collagen disorders, are characterized by changes in connective tissue. Many of these diseases are considered to be autoimmune, and for most, autoantibodies have been detected. Connective tissue disorders include systemic lupus erythematosus, rheumatoid arthritis, scleroderma, and polyarteritis nodosa. Most of the connective tissue disorders are characterized as organ-nonspecific autoimmunities, which means that the autoantibodies and the tissue damage are not limited to a specific organ. These disorders can be differentiated from organ-specific autoimmunities in which tissue damage occurs in a specific organ (see Chap. 23).

COLLABORATIVE MANAGEMENT

Treatment of autoimmunities depends on the organ or organs affected. Common to most autoimmunities, however, is the use of anti-inflammatory drugs and immunosuppressive drugs.

TABLE 24–9 Autoimmune Disorders*

Disorder	Autoantigen	Comments
Systemic or Non–Organ-Specific		
Systemic lupus erythematosus	• DNA, DNA proteins	• Autoantibodies to a number of entities; immune complex-mediated damage
Rheumatoid arthritis	• IgG	• Immune complex-mediated damage in joints (arthritis, fibrosis)
Progressive systemic sclerosis	• DNA proteins	• Autoantibodies against nuclear materials; sclerosis
Mixed connective tissue disease	• DNA proteins	• Autoantibodies to ribonucleoprotein
Organ-Specific		
Autoimmune hemolytic anemia	• Erythrocytes	• Killing of antibody-coated erythrocytes
Autoimmune thrombocytopenic purpura	• Platelets	• Killing of antibody-coated platelets or innocent bystander effect
Myasthenia gravis	• Acetylcholine receptor	• Blocking of impulse transmission by autoantibody to acetylcholine receptor on muscle
Graves' disease	• Thyroid-stimulating hormone receptor	• Stimulation by autoantibody to thyroid-stimulating hormone receptor
Rheumatic fever	• Myocardial cells	• Cross-reaction of antibody with myocardial cells
Idiopathic Addison's disease	• Adrenal cell	• Antibody- and cell-mediated adrenal cytotoxicity
Hashimoto's thyroiditis	• Thyroid cell surface	• Antibody and cell-mediated thyroid cytotoxicity
Pernicious anemia	• Intrinsic factor/parietal cell	• Autoantibodies to intrinsic factor, intrinsic factor/B_{12} complexes, and parietal canalicula cells
Goodpasture's syndrome	• Basement membrane	• Anti-glomerular basement membrane antibodies, which also cross-react with pulmonary basement membrane
Glomerulonephritis	• Glomerular basement membrane	• Autoantibodies and/or immune complex-mediated damage
Uveitis	• Uvea	• ? Cell-mediated and humoral damage
Vasculitis	• Unknown	• Probably primarily immune complex-mediated damage

* Other inflammatory, granulomatous, degenerative, and atrophic disorders are thought to be autoimmune because there is no more reasonable alternative explanation.

GAMMOPATHIES: MULTIPLE MYELOMA

OVERVIEW

Gammopathies are relatively rare disorders that involve abnormal reproduction of the lymphoid cells that produce immunoglobulins. More specifically, gammopathies are associated with increased production of an abnormal clone of immunoglobulin-secreting plasma cells, which are derived from B lymphocytes (see Chap. 22). Several terms other than gammopathies are used to describe this group of diseases: monoclonal gammopathies, plasma cell dyscrasias, paraproteinemias, dysproteinemias, and immunoglobulinopathies.

The most common example of disease in this group is multiple myeloma. Other gammopathies are plasmacytoma, Waldenström's macroglobulinemia, heavy chain disease, and histiocytoses.

Multiple myeloma is a malignant condition in which a clone of transformed plasma cells multiplies in bone marrow. The result is disruption of normal bone marrow function and eventual invasion and destruction of adjacent bone. In addition, the ability of the plasma cells to make functional antibodies decreases, leaving the client immunocompromised. The cause of multiple myeloma is unknown, but genetic predisposition, oncogenic viruses, inflammatory stimuli, and chronic antigenic stimulation have all been identified as possible etiologic factors.

Essentially, an excess number of abnormal plasma cells invade the bone marrow, develop into tumors, and ultimately destroy bone. They then invade lymph nodes, liver, spleen, and kidneys. These plasma cells produce an abnormal antibody, which is often referred to as a myeloma protein, or the *Bence Jones protein,* and is found in the blood and urine of people with multiple myeloma. Multiple myeloma occurs in middle-aged and elderly clients and in men more often than in women.

The onset of multiple myeloma is insidious, and most people remain asymptomatic until the disease is advanced. Some people are diagnosed without symptoms by the presence of Bence Jones proteinuria and an elevated total serum protein level. The major complaint is usually skeletal pain, especially in the pelvis, spine, and ribs. Clients also experience weakness, fatigue, and recurrent infection. Other clinical manifestations include osteoporosis (bone loss) and hypercalcemia (increased serum calcium) related to destruction of bone. If there is vertebral involvement and destruction, spinal cord compression and paraplegia may occur. Pathologic fractures are also common.

Anemia is a major problem for these clients. Anemia is due to invasion of the bone marrow by plasma cells and, therefore, a failure of normal marrow function. Thrombocytopenia (decreased serum platelets) and granulocytopenia (decreased serum granulocytes) also occur. Renal failure occurs in approximately 20% of clients and is due to increased calcium levels, severe proteinuria, and hyperuricemia (increased serum uric acid).

COLLABORATIVE MANAGEMENT

The diagnostic work-up shows pancytopenia (a decrease of all serum blood cells), a high total serum protein level, hyperuricemia, hypercalcemia, an elevated serum creatinine level, and Bence Jones proteinuria. Radiograph and isotope scans show the extent of bony destruction. X-rays show bones with multiple dark lesions that give the bone a "Swiss cheese" appearance.

Treatment includes systemic chemotherapy and supportive care of complications. The chemotherapeutic agent most commonly used is melphalan (Alkeran), which is often given with corticosteroids and cyclophosphamide (Cytoxan). Supportive care is important for control of symptoms and prevention of complications, especially bone fractures, renal failure, and infections.

Clients need fluids (approximately 3 to 4 L/day) to offset the potential problems of hypercalcemia and proteinuria. (Additional interventions for reducing the serum calcium level are presented in Chapters 16 and 26.)

The nurse is alert for back pain and the development of neurologic symptoms in the lower extremities. These symptoms may indicate impending spinal cord compression and should be diagnosed and treated (with surgery or radiation) as soon as possible to prevent paraplegia. The nurse teaches the client to recognize signs and symptoms of infection so that infections can be diagnosed and treated early and efficiently. Blood transfusions are often required for anemia. Pain control is essential. Analgesics, orthopedic supports, local radiation, and relaxation techniques are all helpful.

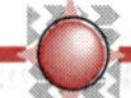

IMPLICATIONS FOR NURSING RESEARCH

Nursing research is needed in all areas of physiological and psychological care of clients with immune disorders. Potential nursing research questions include:

- What interventions can improve client coping skills and management of immune disorders?
- What are the psychosocial needs of persons with HIV and their significant others at different stages of disease? Are these needs different based on gender, age, and culture?
- What educational strategies are most effective in modifying behaviors that will reduce HIV trans-

mission? How should health information be modified for different genders, age groups and cultures?

- What is the relationship of stress and other psychosocial variables to HIV and autoimmune diseases?
- What is the extent of health care worker compliance with universal precautions and how can this be increased?

SELECTED BIBLIOGRAPHY

Abbas, A., Lichtman, A., & Pober, J. (1991). *Cellular and molecular immunology.* Philadelphia: W. B. Saunders.

Bird, K. D. (1991). The use of spermicide containing nonoxynol-9 in the prevention of HIV infection. *AIDS, 5,* 791–796.

Brettle, R. P., & Leen, C. L. S. (1991). The natural history of HIV and AIDS in women. *AIDS, 5,* 1283–1292.

Centers for Disease Control. (1992). Update: Acquired immunodeficiency syndrome—United States, 1991. *Mortality and Morbidity Weekly Report, 41*(26), 463–468.

Centers for Disease Control. (1987). Public Health Service guidelines for counseling and antibody testing to prevent HIV infection and AIDS. *Morbidity and Mortality Weekly Report, 36*(31), 509–515.

Centers for Disease Control. (1991a). Statistics from the Centers for Disease Control. *AIDS, 5,* 1545–1547.

Centers for Disease Control. (1991b). Recommendations for preventing transmission of human immunodeficiency virus and hepatitis B virus to patients during exposure-prone invasive procedures. *Morbidity and Mortality Weekly Review, 40*(RR-8), 1-9.

Cotran, R., Kumar, V., & Robbins, S. (1989). *Robbins pathologic basis of disease* (4th ed). Philadelphia: W. B. Saunders.

Cox, P. H., Martin, M. A., Styer, C. M. & Beall, G. N. (1990). Outcomes of treatment with AZT of patients with AIDS and symptomatic infection. *Nurse Practitioner, 15*(5), 36–44.

Durham, J. D., & Cohen, F. L. (1991). *The person with AIDS: Nursing perspectives* (2nd ed.). New York: Springer.

Frey, A. (1991). Intravenous administration of immune globulin. *Journal of Intravenous Nursing, 14,* 396–405.

Friedland, G., Kahl, P., Saltzman, B., Rogers, M., Feiner, C., Mayers, M., Schable, C. & Klein, R. S. (1990). Additional evidence for lack of transmission of HIV infection by close interpersonal (casual) contact. *AIDS, 4,* 639–644.

Gawlikowski, J. (1992). White cells at war. *American Journal of Nursing, 92*(3), 44–51.

Gershon, R. R. M., Vlahov, D., & Nelson, K. E. (1990). The risk of transmission of HIV-1 through non-percutaneous, non-sexual modes—a review. *AIDS, 4,* 645–650.

Groer, M. (1991). Psychoneuroimmunology. *American Journal of Nursing, 91*(8), 33–38.

Guyton, A. C. (1991). *Textbook of medical physiology* (8th ed.). Philadelphia: W. B. Saunders.

Henry, S. B., & Holzemer, W. L. (1992). Critical care management of the patient with HIV infection who has *Pneumocystis carinii* pneumonia. *Heart and Lung, 21*(3), 243–249.

Howard, B. A. (1994). Guiding allergy sufferers through the medication maze. *RN, 56*(4), 26–30.

Huston, C. (1991). What's wrong with this patient? Deficiency of immunoglobulin A. *RN, 54*(9), 47–48, 50.

Imagawa, D. T., Lee, M. H., Wolinsky, S. M., Sano, K., Morales, F., Kwok, S., Shinsky, J. J., Nishanian, P. G., Giorgi, J., Fahey, J. L., Dudley, J., Visscher, B. R., & Detels, R. (1989). Human immunodeficiency virus type 1 infection in homosexual men who remain seronegative for prolonged periods. *New England Journal of Medicine, 320*(22), 1458–1489.

Kelly, P., & Holman, S. (1993). The new face of AIDS. *American Journal of Nursing, 93*(3), 26–32.

Kulwicki, A., & Cass, P. (1994). An assessment of Arab American knowledge, attitudes, and beliefs about AIDS. *Image, 26*(1), 13–17.

Kyle, R. (1992). Diagnostic criteria of multiple myeloma. *Hematology/Oncology Clinics of North America, 6*(2), 347–358.

Larson, E., & Ropka, M. E. (1991). An update on nursing research and HIV infection. *Image, 23* (1), 4–12.

Levy, J. A. (1990). Changing concepts in HIV infection: Challenges for the 1990s. *AIDS, 4,* 1051–1058.

Longo, M. B., Spross, J. A., & Locke, A. (1990). Identifying major concerns of persons with acquired immunodeficiency syndrome: A replication. *Clinical Nurse Specialist, 4*(1), 21–26.

McMahon, K. (1988). The integration of HIV testing and counseling into nursing practice. *Nursing Clinics of North America, 23*(4), 803–821.

Meisenhelder, J. B. (1994). Contributing factors to fear of HIV contagion in registered nurses. *Image, 26*(1), 65–69.

Meyer, C. (1991). Nursing and AIDS: A decade of caring. *American Journal of Nursing, 91*(12), 26–30.

Moeser, L. (1991). Anaphylaxis: a preventable complication of home infusion therapy. *Journal of Intravenous Nursing, 14*(2), 108–112.

O'Neill, S. (1990). Critical difference: Anaphylactic shock. *American Journal of Nursing, 90*(12), 40.

Parsons, L., & Klopovich, P. (1990). Immune globulin therapy. *Seminars in Oncology Nursing, 6*(2), 136–139.

Patton, B., & Holt, J. (1992). When your patient is allergic. *American Journal of Nursing, 92*(9), 58–61.

Pillon, L. (1991). Cyclosporine: A nursing focus on immunosuppressive therapy. *Dimensions in Critical Care Nursing, 10*(32), 68–73.

Sande, M. A., & Volberding, P. A. (1992). *The medical management of AIDS* (3rd ed.). Philadelphia: W. B. Saunders.

Schenkein, D. (1992). Intravenous IgG for treatment of autoimmune disease. *Hospital Practice, 27*(10A), 29–36, 39–40, 42.

Scherer, P. (1990). How AIDS attacks the brain. *American Journal of Nursing, 90*(1), 44–52.

Smeltzer, S. C., & Whipple, B. (1991). Women and HIV infection. *Image, 23*(4), 249–256.

Swanson, B., Cronin-Stubbs, D., & Coletti, M. A. (1990). Dementia and depression in persons with AIDS: Causes and care. *Journal of Psychosocial Nursing, 28*(10), 33–39.

Timmerman, P. (1993). Intravenous immunoglobulin in oncology nursing practice. *Oncology Nursing Forum, 20*(1), 69–75.

Verma, I. (1990). Gene therapy. *Scientific American, 263*(5), 68–72.

Vickers, P. (1990). SCID syndrome. *Nursing90, 4*(2), 32–33.

Weinstein, R. (1992). Bone involvement in multiple myeloma. *American Journal of Medicine, 93*(6), 591–594.

Wilson, R. (1992). *Critical care manual: Applied physiology and principles of therapy* (2nd ed.). Philadelphia: F. A. Davis.

Workman, M. L. (1993). The immune system: Your defensive partner and offensive foe. *AACN Clinical Issues in Critical Care, 4*(3), 568–593.

Workman, M. Ellerhorst-Ryan, J., & Koertge, V. (1993). *Nursing care of the immunocompromised patient.* Philadelphia: W. B. Saunders.

World Health Organization. (1991). Statistics from the World Health Organization and the Centers for Disease Control. *AIDS, 5,* 1399–1403.

SUGGESTED READINGS

Cox, P. H., Martin, M. A., Styer, C. M. & Beall, G. N. (1990). Outcomes of treatment with AZT of patients with AIDS and symptomatic infection. *Nurse Practitioner, 15*(5), 36–44.

This article describes the effects of azidothymidine, or zidovudine (AZT) treatment over 5 to 87 weeks. The indications for dose reduction and treatment of toxicities are discussed.

Kelly, P., & Holman, S. (1993). The new face of AIDS. *American Journal of Nursing, 93*(3), 26–32.

This article attempts to alert the nurse that AIDS is on the rise among heterosexual women. Helpful suggestions regarding sexual history taking are presented, as are the early clinical manifestations specific to women with AIDS. Self-assessment questions are included at the end of the chapter.

Kulwicki, A., & Cass, P. (1994). An assessment of Arab American knowledge, attitudes, and beliefs about AIDS. *Image, 26*(1), 13–17.

The focus of this research article was to determine the knowledge levels, attitudes, and beliefs about AIDS among young, male Arab immigrants to the United States. The results indicated that this population is at risk for becoming infected with HIV because of extensive misconceptions about the transmission of the virus.

Larson, E., & Ropka, M. E. (1991). An update on nursing research and HIV infection. *Image, 23*(1), 4–12.

This review surveys the nursing literature between 1987 and 1990 and identifies major HIV-related topics researched. The authors also identify gaps in the literature.

Swanson, B., Cronin-Stubbs, D., & Coletti, M. A. (1990). Dementia and depression in persons with AIDS: Causes and care. *Journal of Psychosocial Nursing, 28*(10), 33–39.

This article focuses on the need to differentiate dementia from depression in persons with AIDS by assessing neuropsychologic function. The authors outline nursing strategies to promote safety and humanistic care.

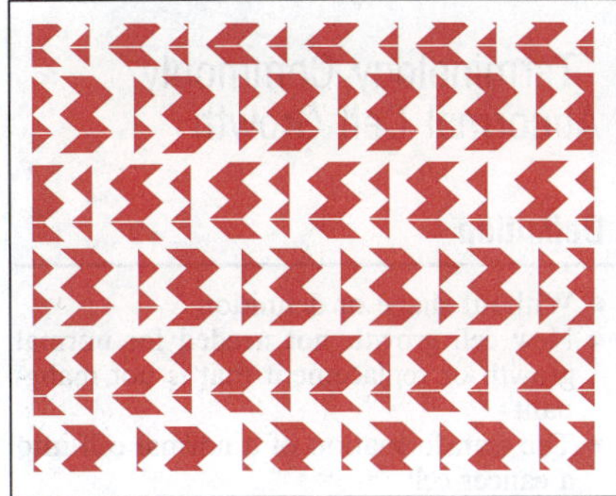

CHAPTER 25

Altered Cell Development and Growth

CHAPTER HIGHLIGHTS

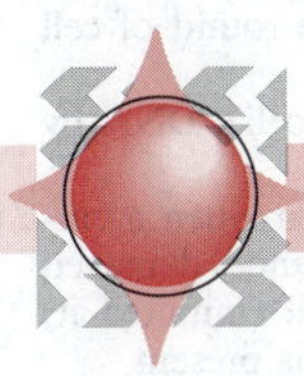

Altered cell growth occurs to some degree in all people. Many types of altered cell growth are harmless (benign) and do not require intervention. The most serious and harmful type of altered cell growth is cancer, or malignant cell growth. Without intervention, cancer usually leads to the death of the person. Cancer is a common problem: approximately 1.3 million people in the United States and Canada are newly diagnosed with cancer each year (American Cancer Society, 1994). Cancer has serious consequences, requires extensive and expensive intervention, and is responsible for much of the health care services provided in acute care settings. Nurses, therefore, must understand the causes, consequences, and treatments of cancer.

HISTORICAL PERSPECTIVE

Cancer is not a new disorder. There is evidence that even prehistoric humans experienced cancer. Some types of cancer are more prevalent today, especially among industrialized societies, than in centuries past. Two primary reasons for this increase are the increasing longevity and the increased exposure to substances within the environment that stimulate cancer development.

More than 5 million Americans are alive today who have a history of cancer, nearly 3 million of whom can be considered cured (American Cancer Society, 1994). Cancer will occur in approximately one of every three people currently living in North America (American Cancer Society, 1994), although cancer risk differs for each person. Factors influencing cancer development are discussed later in this chapter. The terminology for the concepts of abnormal cell growth and cancer is presented in Table 25-1.

OVERVIEW

Although the continuous growth of cells and tissues is expected during infancy and childhood, many human body cells continue to "grow" by cell division (mitosis) long after development and maturation are complete. Such cells are located in tissues where constant damage or wear is likely to occur and where continued cell growth is necessary to replace dead or damaged tissues. Body cells that retain the ability to divide throughout a person's life span are the cells of the skin, hair, mucous membranes, bone marrow, linings of glandular organs (lungs, stomach, intestines, bladder, uterus), and support cells of the brain (glial cells), among others. The growth of these cells is well regulated so that only the right number of cells is always present in any tissue or organ.

Some tissues and organs do not continue to grow by cell division after development is complete. For example, heart muscle cells no longer divide after fetal life. Therefore, the number of heart muscle cells a person has is fixed at birth. The size of the heart increases as the person grows because each of the cells gets larger, but the number of muscle cells in the heart does not increase. Growth that causes an organ or tissue to increase in size by having the individual cells become larger is called *hypertrophy.* Growth that causes an organ or tissue to increase in size by having the number of cells increase is called *hyperplasia* (Fig. 25-1).

Any new or continued cell growth not needed for normal development or for replacement of dead and damaged tissues is referred to as *neoplasia,* and neoplasia is always abnormal. Whether the new cells are benign or malignant, neoplastic cells develop from normal cells (parent tissues or cells). Thus, cancer cells or any neoplastic cells were once normal cells that were damaged or changed so that they no longer look, grow, or function in the normal way. The strict control mechanisms regulating normal growth and function have been lost or suppressed. To understand how cancer cells disrupt physiologic processes, it is first necessary to understand the regulation and function of normal cells.

Biology of Normal Cells

Normal cells function interactively to make the whole person function at an optimal level. To

TABLE 25-1 Terminology Commonly Associated with Abnormal Cell Growth

Term	Definition
Anaplastic	• Without shape or definition
Benign	• New cell growth not needed for normal growth or replacement that is not malignant
Carcinogenesis	• The transformation of a normal cell into a cancer cell
Doubling time	• The amount of time it takes for a tumor to double in size by mitotic cell divisions
Fibronectin	• A large, extracellular, transformation-sensitive cell-surface protein present on normal cells that allows normal cells to adhere tightly together
Gene expression	• The activation, or "turning on," of a specific gene to the extent that it synthesizes a specific protein that influences the activity of a cell or group of cells
Gene repression	• The deactivation, or "turning off," of a specific gene so that it is silent and does not synthesize a protein
Generation time	• The period of time necessary for one cell to enter and complete one round of cell division by mitosis
Initiation	• The damage of a normal cell's DNA by a carcinogen
Latency	• The period of time between when a carcinogenic agent or substance damaged the DNA of a normal cell (initiated it) and when an overt cancer is present
Malignant	• Cancerous, new growth of cells by invasion that is not needed for normal development or tissue replacement
Metastasis	• Invasive growth of cancer cells from the original tumor into distant areas
Mitosis	• Cell division by exact duplication
Morphology	• Appearance or shape
Multipotent	• An undifferentiated cell that has multiple potentials for maturation and differentiation (also called totipotent and pluripotent)
Neoplasia	• New cell growth not needed for normal body growth or replacement of dead or missing tissue
Oncogene	• Developmental gene (proto-oncogene) expressed at an inappropriate time, capable of transforming a normal cell into a cancer cell
Ploidy	• The chromosome content of a cell
Aneuploid	• Chromosome content of a cell that is greater or lesser than the normal chromosomal number for the species
Diploid	• Normal chromosome content of a cell for the species (for example, human cells have 46 chromosomes [23 pairs] per cell)
Primary tumor	• A tumor formed in a specific tissue as a result of a carcinogenic agent or event
Promotion	• Enhancement of cell division in a cell initiated by a carcinogen
Proto-oncogene	• A developmental gene expressed during early embryonic development
Secondary tumor	• A tumor formed as a result of breaking off from a primary tumor and spreading to distant sites (metastasis)
Transformation	• The changing of a normal cell into a cancer cell by a carcinogenic agent or event

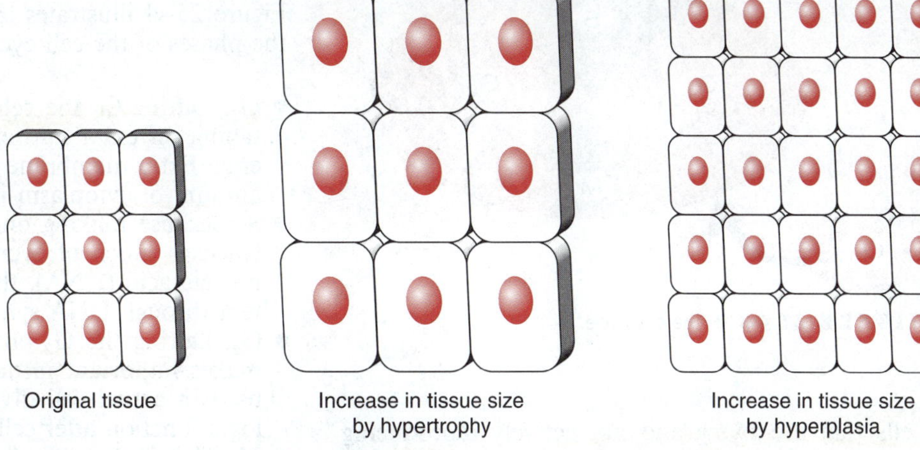

FIGURE 25-1 ◆ Tissue growth by hypertrophy and hyperplasia.

achieve this optimal function, each individual cell performs in a predictable manner.

CHARACTERISTICS OF NORMAL CELLS

HAVE LIMITED CELL DIVISION

Normal cells divide (undergo mitosis) only for one of two reasons: (1) to develop normal tissues or (2) to replace lost or damaged normal tissues. Even when capable of mitosis, normal cells do not divide when all cell surfaces are in contact with other cells (contact inhibition of cell division).

SHOW SPECIFIC MORPHOLOGY

Each normal cell type has a distinct and recognizable appearance, size, and shape. Figure 25–2 shows the distinctive appearances of some normal cells.

HAVE A SMALL NUCLEAR-TO-CYTOPLASMIC RATIO

As shown in Figure 25–2, the space that the nucleus occupies inside a normal cell is small compared with the size of the rest of the cell. As a result, the nuclear space is small in proportion to the cytoplasmic space.

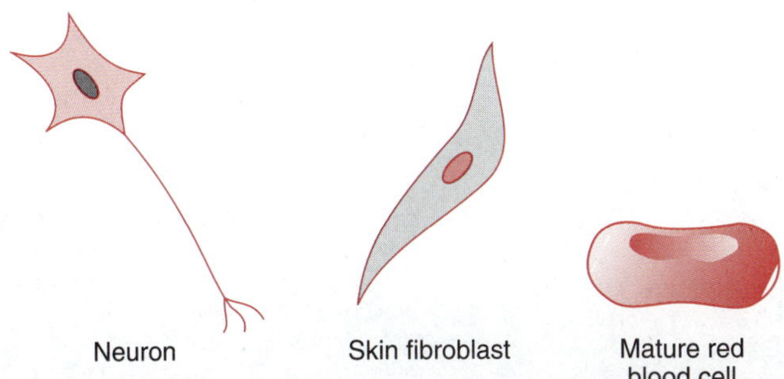

FIGURE 25–2 ◆ Distinctive morphology of some normal cells.

PERFORM SPECIFIC DIFFERENTIATED FUNCTIONS

Every normal cell must perform at least one function to contribute to whole-body homeostasis. For example, skin cells make keratin, liver cells make bile, cardiac muscle cells contract rhythmically, nerve cells generate and conduct impulses, and red blood cells make and carry hemoglobin.

ADHERE TIGHTLY TOGETHER

Normal cells make and secrete cell-surface proteins that protrude from the cell surface, allowing cells to bind closely and tightly together. One protein that makes normal cells tightly adherent is fibronectin. In the presence of fibronectin, normal cells composing any normal tissue are bound tightly to each other.

ARE NONMIGRATORY

Because normal cells are tightly bound together and respect tissue borders, they do not wander from one tissue to the next (with the exception of erythrocytes and leukocytes).

GROW IN AN ORDERLY AND WELL-REGULATED MANNER

Normal cells capable of mitosis do not divide unless conditions are optimal for cell division. These conditions include the need for more cells, adequate space, and the presence of sufficient nutrients and other resources. Cell division, occurring in a well-recognized pattern, is described by the cell cycle. Figure 25-3 shows the phases of the cell cycle.

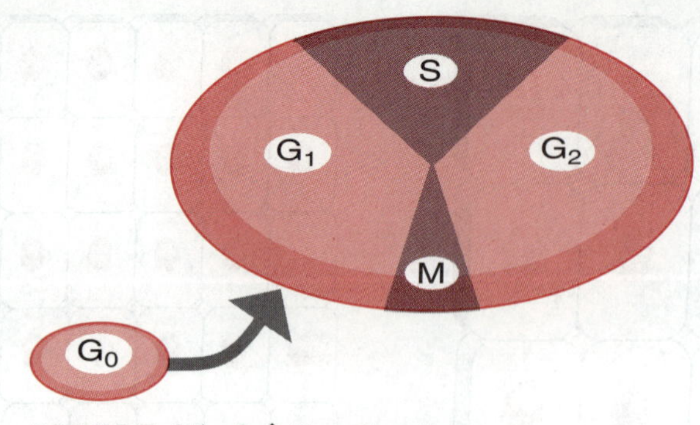

FIGURE 25-3 ◆ The cell cycle.

Cells that are living and not actively reproducing are not in the cell cycle but in a reproductive resting state termed G_0. During this period, cells actively carry out their specific functions but do not divide. Most normal cells spend most of their existence in the G_0 state.

Mitotic cell division makes one cell divide and become two cells. These two cells are identical not only to each other but also to the original cell that started the mitotic cell division. The processes of entering and completing the cell cycle are rigidly controlled. Figure 25-4 illustrates the activities occurring during the phases of the cell cycle:

- G_1. During G_1 the cell is preparing for division by taking on extra nutrients and generating more energy. Extra membrane is made at this time, and the amount of cytoplasm increases.
- S. Because making one cell into two cells requires twice as much of everything, including deoxyribonucleic acid (DNA), the cell doubles its DNA content through DNA synthesis at this time.
- G_2. During the G_2 phase of the cell cycle, the cell makes important intracellular proteins that will be used in actual cell division and in normal physiologic function after cell division is complete.
- M. The single cell splits apart into two cells during mitosis, or the M phase.

The concept of each normal, mature cell having a specific structure and function is interesting, considering that all mature human beings started life as a single cell. The function and behavior of that first single cell and its daughter cells for several generations are quite different from normal differentiated

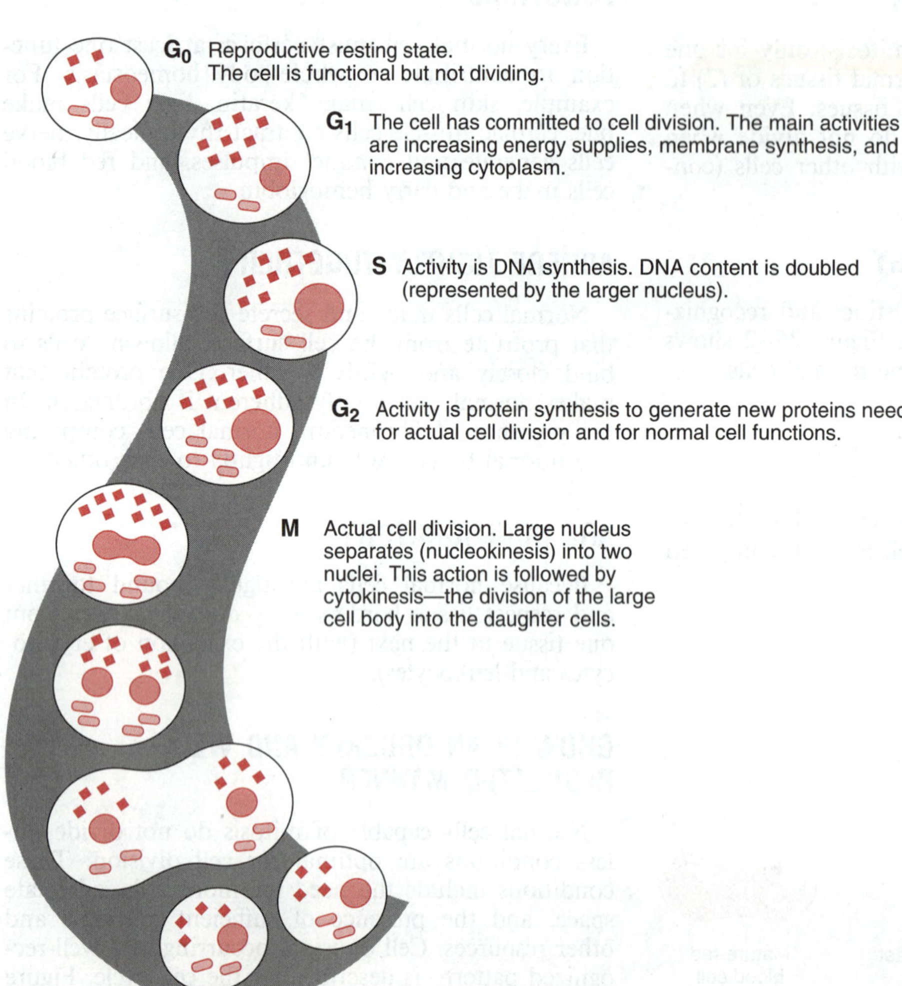

FIGURE 25-4 ◆ Cellular events during mitotic cell division.

human cells. Some of their differences and mechanisms of regulation have helped in the understanding of cancer development.

CHARACTERISTICS OF NORMAL EARLY EMBRYONIC CELLS

DEMONSTRATE RAPID AND CONTINUOUS CELL DIVISION

Early embryonic cells (from conception to the eighth day after conception) spend most of their time within the cell cycle, actively reproducing. The generation time for these cells ranges from 2 to 8 hours.

SHOW ANAPLASTIC MORPHOLOGY

Anaplasia means without structural shape or differentiation. Early embryonic cells do not look like the mature cells they will eventually become; instead, they all have the same anaplastic appearance. They are small and round (Fig. 25-5).

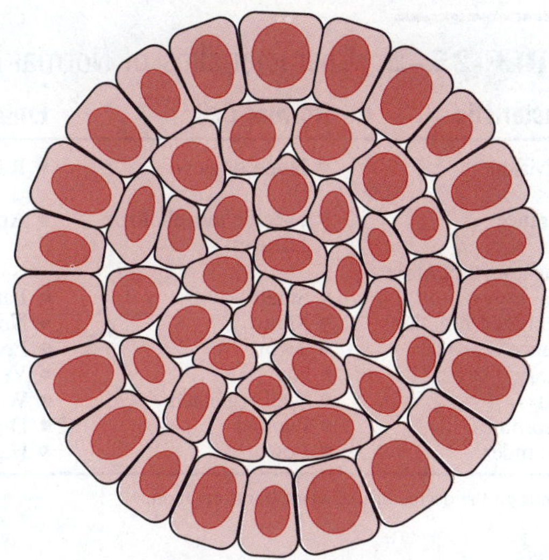

FIGURE 25-5 ◆ Early embryonic cells at about 5 days after conception.

HAVE A LARGE NUCLEAR-TO-CYTOPLASMIC RATIO

The nucleus of an early embryonic cell takes up most of the space inside of the cell. The ratio of nuclear space to cytoplasmic space is larger than that of a normal differentiated cell.

PERFORM NO DIFFERENTIATED FUNCTIONS

In the early embryonic period, cells do not have any differentiated functions. They have not committed to a specific maturity at this time. Each early embryonic cell is totally flexible and can mature to become any body cell. This flexibility is called pluripotency, multipotency, or totipotency because each cell has an unlimited maturational potential.

ADHERE LOOSELY TOGETHER

Early embryonic cells do not make fibronectin and are not tightly bound together.

ARE ABLE TO MIGRATE

Because early embryonic cells are not tightly bound together, they do not remain in one place within the embryo. Instead, they migrate throughout the early embryo.

Commitment

At some point in early embryonic development, the cells initiate the steps to become differentiated. In response to an unknown signal or signals, each cell commits itself to a specific differentiated maturational outcome. At the time of commitment, the cell has not taken on any differentiated features or functions, but positions itself within a group that will eventually take on specific morphologic features and functional behavior.

Commitment involves turning off specific early embryonic genes that regulated the early rapid growth. These early embryonic regulatory genes, called *proto-oncogenes,* are not needed again throughout the person's life.

After the early embryonic regulatory genes are "turned off" (repressed), other specific genes that control the expression of specific differentiated functions must be "turned on" (expressed) selectively in different cell types. For example, the gene for insulin is actively expressed only in the fetal pancreatic beta cells and is repressed in all other cells. It is the selective expression of different genes that directs the normal growth and differentiation of specific body cells.

Biology of Abnormal Cells

Because body cells do not exist in isolation but are subjected to personal and environmental changes, events can alter how the cells grow or function. When either cell growth or cell function is changed, the cells are considered abnormal. Table 25-2 compares the characteristics of normal cells, embryonic cells, benign tumor cells, and cancer cells.

CHARACTERISTICS OF BENIGN TUMOR CELLS

Benign tumor cells are normal cells that are growing in the wrong place, at the wrong time, or at the wrong rate.

TABLE 25–2 Characteristics of Normal and Abnormal Cells

Characteristic	Normal Cell	Embryonic Cell	Benign Tumor Cell	Malignant Cell
Cell division	• None or slow	• Rapid, continuous	• Continuous or inappropriate	• Rapid or continuous
Appearance	• Specific morphologic features	• Anaplastic	• Specific morphologic features	• Anaplastic
Nuclear-to-cytoplasmic ratio	• Small	• Large	• Small	• Large
Differentiated functions	• Many	• None	• Many	• Some–none
Adherence	• Tight	• Loose	• Tight	• Loose
Migratory	• No	• Yes	• No	• Yes
Growth	• Well regulated	• Well regulated	• Expansion	• Invasion
Chromosomes	• Diploid	• Diploid	• Diploid	• Aneuploid*
Mitotic index	• Low	• High	• Low	• High*

* Depends on the degree of malignant transformation.

DEMONSTRATE CONTINUOUS OR INAPPROPRIATE CELL GROWTH

Benign tumors are tissues that are not necessary for normal structure or function. Moles and polyps are two examples of benign tumors.

SHOW SPECIFIC MORPHOLOGY

Benign tumors strongly resemble, and sometimes exactly resemble, the parent tissues from which they arose. They retain the specific morphologic features of the parent tissue.

HAVE A SMALL NUCLEAR-TO-CYTOPLASMIC RATIO

Just like completely normal cells, benign tumor cells have a small nucleus compared with the size of the rest of the cell.

PERFORM DIFFERENTIATED FUNCTIONS

Not only do benign tumors look like their parent tissues; they also perform the same differentiated functions as those of the parent tissue. For example, one type of benign tumor is endometriosis. In this condition, the normal lining of the uterus (endometrium) grows in an abnormal place (such as on an ovary, on the peritoneum, or, occasionally, even on the nasal septum). The displaced endometrium acts just like normal endometrium by exhibiting increased vascularity and tissue thickness each month under the influence of estrogen and progesterone. When these hormone levels drop and the normal endometrium sheds from the uterus, the displaced endometrium—wherever it is—also sheds.

ADHERE TIGHTLY TOGETHER

Benign tumor cells make and secrete fibronectin. As a result, benign tumor cells bind tightly to one another. In addition, many benign tissues are "encapsulated," or surrounded with fibrous connective tissue, which assists in holding the benign tissue together.

ARE NONMIGRATORY

A major feature of benign tissues is that they do not wander. They remain tightly bound together and do not invade other body tissues.

GROW IN AN ORDERLY MANNER

Benign tumor cells follow normal cell growth patterns. Growth may continue beyond an appropriate time, but the rate of growth is usually what is normal for the parent tissue. The benign tumor grows by hyperplastic expansion.

CHARACTERISTICS OF MALIGNANT CELLS

Most cancer cells (malignant cells) no longer look like or function like the tissue from which they arose. The following characteristics are commonly found among malignant tumors.

DEMONSTRATE RAPID OR CONTINUOUS CELL DIVISION

Some cancer cells have a short generation time (2 to 4 hours); others have a generation time even longer than that of normal cells. Most cancer cells have a generation time that is the same as the generation time of the parent tissue from which they arose.

A major distinction between normal cells and cancer cells is that cancer cells divide nearly continuously. Almost as soon as mitosis is complete, the daughter cells begin a new round of mitosis. In addition, cancer cells continue to divide even when contacted on all surface areas by other cells; thus, their growth is not contact inhibited. The persistence of cancer cell division, even under adverse conditions, is one factor that makes the disease so difficult to control.

SHOW ANAPLASTIC MORPHOLOGY

Cancer cells lose the specific shape and appearance of their parent cells, becoming anaplastic in appearance. As a cancer cell progresses in its malignant path, it becomes smaller and rounder in appearance. This lack of a specific morphologic appearance can make the diagnosis of cancer type difficult because many types of malignant cells look very much alike.

HAVE A LARGE NUCLEAR-TO-CYTOPLASMIC RATIO

The nucleus of a cancer cell is larger than that of a normal cell, and the cancer cell is small. The nucleus occupies much of the space within the cancer cell, which creates a large nuclear-to-cytoplasmic ratio.

LOSE SOME OR ALL DIFFERENTIATED FUNCTIONS

Along with losing the appearance of the parent cell, cancer cells lose some of the differentiated functions that the parent tissue performed.

ADHERE LOOSELY TOGETHER

Cancer cells make little, if any, fibronectin. As a result, they adhere poorly to each other and little pressure is needed to allow some cancer cells to break off from the primary tumor.

ARE ABLE TO MIGRATE

Because cancer cells do not bind tightly together and because they have many enzymes on their cell surfaces, they are able to slip through blood vessels and tissues and spread from the original site of the tumor to many other body sites. This ability to spread (metastasize) is a key characteristic of cancer cells.

GROW BY INVASION

Cancer cells expand and extend into other tissues, both those close by and those more remote from the original tumor, by invasion. This form of tissue spreading is called metastasis. Together with persistent growth, metastasis makes untreated cancer a deadly disease.

CANCER DEVELOPMENT

Carcinogenesis/Oncogenesis

The terms *carcinogenesis* and *oncogenesis* are synonyms for the beginning or development of cancer. Table 25–3 summarizes important concepts related to cancer development. The process of changing a cell that expresses normal appearance and function into a cell that expresses malignant characteristics is called malignant transformation. Malignant transformation occurs through the steps of initiation, promotion, progression, and metastasis (McMillan, 1992).

INITIATION

The first step in changing a normal cell to a cancer cell (carcinogenesis) is initiation. Normal cells can become cancer cells if their proto-oncogenes are turned back on at an inappropriate time (any time after early embryonic development is complete). Anything that can penetrate a cell, gain access to the nucleus, and damage the DNA can damage the genes, turning on genes that should remain repressed and turning off normal genes (Yarbro, 1992). Substances that can change the expression of a cell's genes to the extent that the cell expresses malignant characteristics are called carcinogens. Carcinogens may be chemicals, physical agents, or viruses. Table 25–4 lists some common carcinogens and the resultant cancers. (Carcinogenic/oncogenic mechanisms are described

TABLE 25–3 Key Concepts Related to Cancer Development

- Neoplastic cells originate from normal body cells.
- Transformation of a normal cell into a cancer cell involves mutation of the genes (DNA) of the normal cell.
- Early embryonic genes activated at an inappropriate time can cause a cell to develop into a tumor.
- Only one cell has to undergo malignant transformation for cancer to begin.
- Benign tumors grow by expansion, whereas malignant tumors grow by invasion.
- Most tumors arise from cells that are capable of cell division.
- Primary prevention of cancer involves avoiding exposure to known causes of cancer.
- Secondary prevention of cancer involves screening for early detection.
- Tobacco use is a causative or permissive factor in 30% of all malignant neoplasms.
- Tumors that metastasize from the primary site into another organ are still designated as tumors of the originating tissue.

TABLE 25–4 Common Environmental Carcinogens

Carcinogen	Cancer Site or Associated Neoplasm
Alcoholic beverages	• Liver, esophagus, mouth, pharynx, larynx
Alkylating agents (melphalan, cyclophosphamide, chlorambucil, nitrosoureas)	• Acute myelocytic leukemia, bladder (cyclophosphamide)
Androgenic steroids	• Liver
Aromatic amines	• Bladder
Arsenic (inorganic)	• Lung, skin
Asbestos	• Lung, pleura, peritoneum, pericardium
Benzene	• Acute myelocytic leukemia
bis-Chloromethyl ether	• Lung
Chromium	• Lung
Chronic hepatitis B infection	• Liver
Cyclosporine	• Non-Hodgkin's lymphoma
Diethylstilbestrol (prenatal exposure)	• Vagina (adenocarcinoma)
Human T-cell lymphotropic virus type I (HTLV-I)	• Adult T-cell leukemia/lymphoma
Immunosuppressive drugs (azathioprine, cyclosporine)	• Non-Hodgkin's lymphoma
Ionizing radiation	• Almost all organs
Isopropyl alcohol production	• Nasal sinuses
Mustard gas	• Lung, larynx, nasal sinuses
Nickel dust	• Lung, nasal sinuses
Phenacetin	• Renal pelvis, bladder
Polycyclic hydrocarbons	• Lung, scrotum, skin (squamous carcinoma)
Sunlight (ultraviolet)	• Skin, intraocular melanoma
Synthetic estrogens	• Endometrium
Tobacco	• Lung, mouth, pharynx, larynx, esophagus, pancreas, bladder, kidney, renal pelvis
Vinyl chloride	• Liver (angiosarcoma)
Wood dust	• Nasal sinuses

From Li, F. P. (1989). Cancer epidemiology and prevention. In E. Rubenstein & D. D. Federman (Eds.), *Scientific American Medicine*, Section 12, Subsection 1.

later in this chapter. Chapters presenting the care of clients with specific cancers discuss the role of specific carcinogens (when known) in the development of the malignant neoplasm under the heading "Etiology.")

Pure carcinogens initiate mutational changes in a cell's genes and are thus called *initiators.* Initiation is an irreversible event that can lead to cancer development if it does not interfere with the cell's ability to reproduce.

Once a cell has been initiated, it can become a cancer cell if the cellular changes induced during initiation are enhanced by the process of promotion. One cancer cell is not significant, however, unless it has the ability to reproduce. If the cancer cell cannot reproduce, it cannot form a tumor. *If growth conditions are right, however, widespread metastatic disease can develop from just one cancer cell.*

PROMOTION

Once a normal cell has been initiated by a carcinogen and can express cancer cell characteristics, it can become a tumor if its growth is enhanced. The time between a cell's initiation and the development of an overt tumor is called the latency period. The latency period ranges from months to years and depends on the type of cell initiated and the presence of promoters.

Promoters are substances that promote or enhance the growth of initiated cells (Pitot, 1986). They can also shorten the latency period. Some substances identified as promoters are hormones, drugs, and a wide variety of industrial chemicals.

PROGRESSION

After cancer cells have grown to the point that a detectable tumor is formed (a 1-cm tumor has at least 1 billion cells in it), other events must occur for this tumor to become a significant health problem for the client. First, the tumor must establish its own blood supply. In the early stages, the center cells of the tumor can receive nutrition by diffusion from the surrounding fluids. However, after the tumor reaches 1 cm, diffusion is not efficient and the center cells start to die. To continue to grow and survive, the tumor makes a substance called tumor angiogenesis factor (TAF). TAF stimulates capillaries and other blood vessels in the area to grow new branches into the tumor (Pitot, 1986). These blood vessels ensure the continued nourishment of the tumor.

As the tumor cells continue to divide, some of the new cells change from the original initiated cancer cell. Actual colonies or subpopulations within the tumor begin to appear, and these subpopulations differ in some ways from the original cancer cell. Some of the differences provide certain subpopulations with advantages that enable them to survive no matter how the environmental conditions around them change. These advantages are thus called "selection advantages" (Fidler & Hart, 1982). The changes that a tumor undergoes at this time allow it to progress in its malignant expression. Over time the tumor cells come to have fewer and fewer normal cell characteristics.

The original tumor formed from the transformed normal cells is called the *primary* tumor. It is usually identified by the tissue from which it arose (parent tissue), such as in breast cancer or lung cancer. When primary tumors are located in vital organs, such as the brain or the lungs, they can grow to such an extent that they either lethally damage the vital organ or "crowd out" healthy organ tissue and interfere with the ability of the organ to perform its vital function. Other times, the primary tumor is located in a soft-tissue compartment that can expand without damage as the tumor grows. One such site is the breast. The breast is not a vital organ, and even if it had a large tumor in it, the presence of the primary tumor would not cause the client's death. It is when the tumor spreads from the original site into vital areas that life functions can be disrupted.

METASTASIS

In the process of metastasis, cancer cells move from their original location by severing connections with the original group and establish colonies at remote sites. These additional tumors are called metastatic tumors or secondary tumors. Even though the tumor is now in another organ, it is still a cancer from the original altered tissue. For example, when breast cancer spreads to the lung and the bone, it is a breast cancer in the lung and in the bone. It is not lung cancer and it is not bone cancer. Metastasis occurs through several progressive steps depicted in Figure 25–6 (Nicolson, 1979).

EXTENSION INTO SURROUNDING TISSUES

Tumors secrete enzymes that open up areas of surrounding tissue. Mechanical pressure, created as the tumor increases in size, forces tumor cells to invade new territory.

PENETRATION INTO BLOOD VESSELS

The same enzymes that open up areas of surrounding tissue make large pores in the blood vessels of the client. This allows tumor cells to enter the blood vessels.

RELEASE OF TUMOR CELLS

Because tumor cells are loosely held together, clumps of cells break off the primary tumor in the blood vessels and are transported to remote sites.

INVASION OF TISSUE AT SITE OF ARREST

Tumor cells circulate through the blood and enter tissues at remote sites. When conditions in the remote site are appropriate for the tumor, the cells arrest and invade the surrounding tissues, creating secondary tumors. Table 25–5 lists the common sites of metastasis for specific tumor types. Three routes are responsible for metastatic spread:

- Local seeding
- Blood-borne metastasis
- Lymphatic spread

LOCAL SEEDING

Local seeding is a form of metastatic spread that involves distribution of shed cancer cells in the local area of the primary tumor. In ovarian cancer, for example, cells often spill from the primary tumor into the peritoneal cavity and set up multiple seeding sites there.

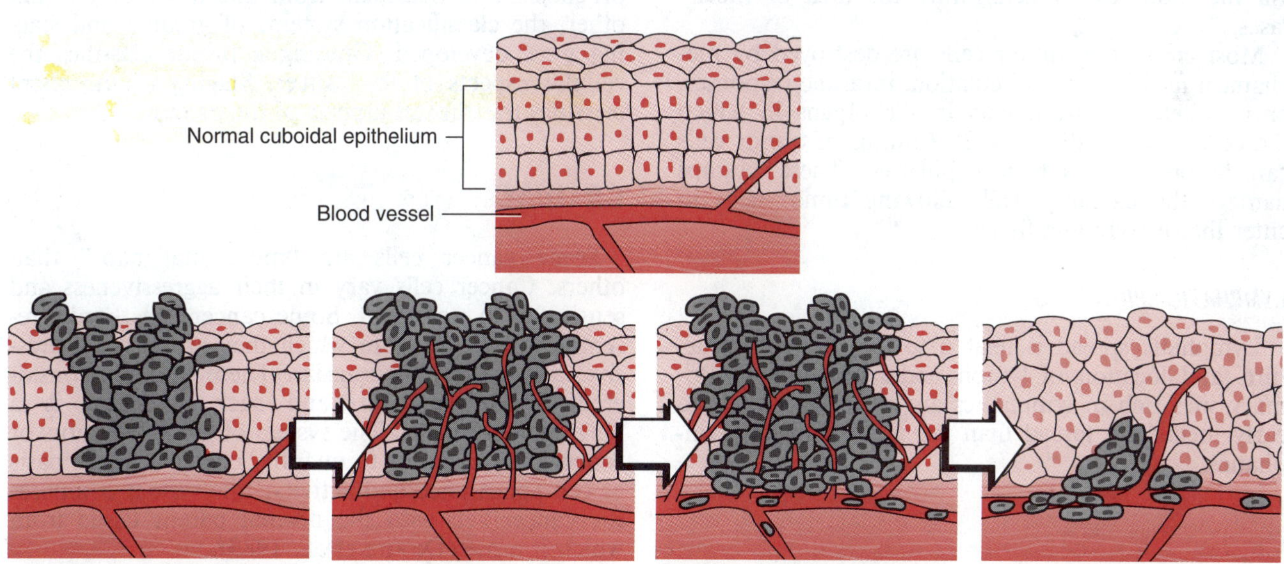

Malignant transformation
Some normal cuboidal cells have undergone malignant transformation and have divided enough times to form a tumorous area within the cuboidal epithelium.

Tumor vascularization
Cancer cells secrete tumor angiogenesis factor (TAF), stimulating the blood vessels to bud and form new channels growing into the tumor.

Blood vessel penetration
Cancer cells have broken off from the main tumor. Enzymes on the surface of the tumor cells make holes in the blood vessels, allowing cancer cells to enter blood vessels and travel around the body.

Arrest and invasion
Cancer cells clump up in blood vessel walls and invade new tissue areas. If the new tissue areas have the right conditions to support continued growth of cancer cells, new tumors (metastatic tumors) will form at this site.

FIGURE 25–6 ◆ The steps of metastasis.

TABLE 25–5 Common Sites of Metastasis for Different Cancer Types

Cancer Type	Sites of Metastasis
Breast cancer	• Bone* • Lung* • Liver • Brain
Lung cancer	• Brain* • Bone • Liver • Lymph nodes • Pancreas
Colorectal cancer	• Liver* • Lymph nodes • Adjacent structures
Prostate cancer	• Bone (especially spine and legs)* • Pelvic nodes
Melanoma	• Gastrointestinal tract • Lymph nodes • Lung • Brain
Primary brain cancer	• Central nervous system

* Most common site of metastasis for the specific malignant neoplasm.

BLOOD-BORNE METASTASIS

Blood-borne metastasis through release of tumor cells into the blood is the most common cause of cancer spread. Combined with seeding, distribution via the bloodstream determines the area of metastases.

Most circulating tumor cells are destroyed by mechanical factors in the circulation, immune responses, or unsuitable environments in the organs in which the cells stop (Dudjak, 1992). Clumps of tumor cells can become trapped in capillaries. These clumps damage the capillary wall, allowing tumor cells to enter the surrounding tissue.

LYMPHATIC SPREAD

Lymphatic spread is related to the number, structure, and location of lymph nodes and vessels. Primary sites rich in lymphatics are more susceptible to early metastatic spread than are areas with few lymphatics.

Cancer Classification

Terminology for neoplasia describes the tissue of origin for neoplastic cells and classifies the tumor as benign or malignant. Prefixes include *fibro-* (originating from fibrous or connective tissues), *adeno-* (originating from glandular tissues), and *lipo-* (originating from fat cells).

Benign tumor names are derived from these prefixes and the suffix -oma. Cancer terminology incorporates the roots *sarc-* and *carcino-*. Sarcomas are cancers of connective tissues, bone, muscle, and cartilage. Carcinomas are cancers of the epithelial tissues, glands, and ducts. Other terms and characteristics describe the tumor's biologic behavior, anatomic site, and degree of differentiation.

One biologic feature used to further categorize cancer cells is the number and appearance of the chromosomes. Normal human cells have 46 chromosomes (23 pairs); the normal diploid number. When malignant transformation occurs, changes in the genes and chromosomes also occur. Some tumor cells gain or lose whole chromosomes and may have structural abnormalities of the remaining chromosomes. When a tumor cell has more or less than the normal diploid number of chromosomes, it is said to be aneuploid. The degree of aneuploidy generally increases with the degree of malignant transformation.

Approximately 100 different types of cancer arise from various tissues or organs. Figure 25–7 compares cancer distribution by site and sex. Cancers are divided into two major categories: solid and hematologic.

Solid tumors are associated with the organs from which they develop, for example, breast cancer and lung cancer. Hematologic cancers (e.g., leukemias and lymphomas) originate from blood cell–forming tissues, which communicate with all organs.

Cancer Grade and Stage

To ensure standardization of cancer diagnosis, prognosis, and treatment from one institution to another, the classification systems of grading and staging were developed. Grading a tumor classifies the cellular aspects of the cancer. Staging of the client classifies the clinical aspects of the cancer.

GRADING

Some cancer cells are "more malignant" than others. Cancer cells vary in their aggressiveness and sensitivity to treatment. Some cancer cells hardly resemble the tissue from which they arose, are aggressive, and rapidly metastasize. These cells are considered more malignant, and such a tumor is a "high-grade tumor." The system of grading tumors or cancer cells attempts to quantify cancer. On the basis of cell appearance and activity, this system compares the cancer cell with the normal parent tissue from which it arose (DeVita et al., 1989).

Many groups have established grading systems for different kinds of cancer cells. Although each system is slightly different, overall they resemble the standard system listed in Table 25–6. This standard rates tumor cells from lowest to highest; the lowest rating is given to those tumors that closely resemble normal cells, and the highest rating is given to those tumors that have little resemblance to normal cells.

Grading the cancer cells is the first step in con-

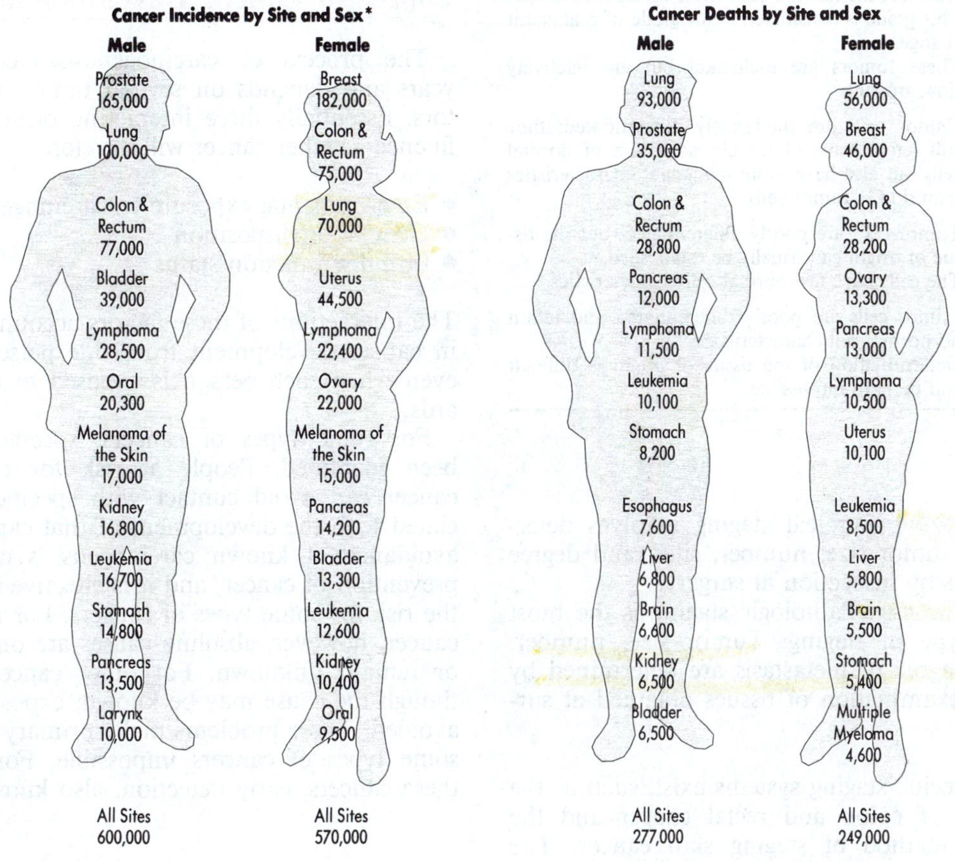

FIGURE 25–7 ◆ Cancer incidence and death by site and sex. (Redrawn from American Cancer Society [1993]. *Cancer facts and figures 1993* (p. 12]. Atlanta: American Cancer Society, Inc.).

firming the presence of a malignant neoplasm. Grading provides one means of evaluating the client with cancer for prognosis and appropriate therapy. This step also allows health care professionals to evaluate the results of management and to compare statistics reported from local, regional, national, and international sources.

STAGING

Staging determines the exact location of the cancer and the degree of metastasis present at the time of diagnosis. Staging is important because, for most cancers, the smaller the tumor is at diagnosis and the less it has spread, the greater the chances are that treatment will result in a cure. The stage of a tumor influences what type of therapy is appropriate. Staging is done in three different ways:

1. *Clinical Staging.* Clinical staging is accomplished by assessing the client's clinical manifestations and evaluating clinical signs for the tumor size and degree of metastasis. Clinical tests are used, and tumor cells may be obtained for biopsy, but clinical staging does not include major surgery.

TABLE 25–6 Grading of Malignant Tumors

Grade	Cellular Characteristics
GX	• Grade cannot be determined.
G1	• Tumor cells are well differentiated and closely resemble the normal cells from which they arose. • This grade is considered a low grade of malignant change. • These tumors are malignant but are relatively slow growing.
G2	• Tumor cells are moderately differentiated; they still retain some of the characteristics of normal cells but also have more malignant characteristics than do G1 tumor cells.
G3	• Tumor cells are poorly differentiated, but the tissue of origin can usually be established. • The cells have few normal cell characteristics.
G4	• Tumor cells are poorly differentiated and retain no normal cell characteristics. • Determination of the tissue of origin is difficult and perhaps impossible.

2. *Surgical Staging.* Surgical staging involves determining the tumor size, number, sites, and degree of metastasis by inspection at surgery.
3. *Pathologic Staging.* Pathologic staging is the most definitive type of staging. Tumor size, number, sites, and degree of metastasis are determined by pathologic examination of tissues obtained at surgery.

Some site-specific staging systems exist, such as the Dukes staging of colon and rectal cancer and the Clark's levels method of staging skin cancer. The American Joint Committee on Cancer (AJCC) developed the TNM (tumor, node, metastasis) system to describe the anatomic extent of cancers. The stages guide treatment and are useful for prognosis and comparison of the end results of treatment. The TNM staging system is based on the concept that similar cancers share similar patterns of growth and extension. TNM staging systems are specific to each solid tumor site. Table 25–7 gives basic definitions for the specific staging systems. TNM staging is not applicable to several types of cancers, however, particularly those that arise in the bone marrow or lymphoid tissues. Staging for these cancers is discussed in Chapter 39.

The growth of tumors is discussed in terms of doubling time, the amount of time it takes for a tumor to double in size, and the mitotic index, the percentage of cells within a tumor that are actively dividing at any point. The smallest tumor likely to be detected by a physical examination or diagnostic test is 1 cm in diameter. At this size, a tumor contains 1 billion cells. To reach this size, a tumor will have undergone at least 30 doublings (Cooper, 1992). A tumor with a mitotic index of less than 10% is a relatively slow-growing tumor, whereas a tumor with a mitotic index of 85% is a fast-growing tumor. Tumors have a wide range of growth rates. Fast-growing tumors, such as lymphomas, may double in 4 weeks; an adenocarcinoma of the lung may double in 21 to 40 weeks (DeVita et al., 1993).

Causes of Cancer Development

The process of carcinogenesis/oncogenesis takes years and depends on several tumor and client factors. Essentially three interacting primary factors influence whether cancer will develop:

- Environmental exposure to carcinogens
- Genetic predisposition
- Immune function status

The interactions of these factors account for variation in cancer development from one person to another, even when each person is exposed to the same hazards.

For some types of cancers, specific causes have been identified. People at risk for these types of cancer can avoid contact with specific agents associated with the development of that cancer type. The avoidance of known carcinogens is called primary prevention of cancer, and it is effective in minimizing the risk for some types of cancers. For many types of cancer, however, absolute causes are only speculative or remain unknown. For other cancer types, even though the cause may be known, exposure cannot be avoided. These problems make primary prevention of some types of cancers impossible. For people with these cancers, early detection, also known as second-

TABLE 25–7 Staging of Cancer—TNM Classification

	Primary Tumor (T)
TX	• Primary tumor cannot be assessed
T0	• No evidence of primary tumor
Tis	• Carcinoma in situ
T1, T2, T3, T4	• Increasing size and/or local extent of the primary tumor
	Regional Lymph Nodes (N)
NX	• Regional lymph nodes cannot be assessed
N0	• No regional lymph node metastasis
N1, N2, N3	• Increasing involvement of regional lymph nodes
	Distant Metastasis (M)
MX	• Presence of distant metastasis cannot be assessed
M0	• No distant metastasis
M1	• Distant metastasis

Modified from American Joint Committee on Cancer. (1988). O. H. Beahrs, D. E. Henson, R. V. Hutter, & M. H. Myers (Eds.), *Manual for staging of cancer* (3rd ed., p. 7). Philadelphia: J. B. Lippincott.

ary prevention, can be helpful because treatment outcome is usually better with diagnosis of small tumors that have not metastasized (Appendix 4).

ONCOGENE ACTIVATION

Regardless of the specific cause, the mechanism of carcinogenesis appears to be the same—the activation of proto-oncogenes into oncogenes. When a normal cell is exposed to any carcinogen (initiator), the normal cell's DNA can be damaged or mutated. The mutations can cause the early embryonic genes (proto-oncogenes), which should be repressed forever, to be turned on again at an inappropriate time (Yarbro, 1992). When these genes are activated or turned on, they are called oncogenes and can cause the cell to change from normal to malignant (Bishop, 1982).

About 50 different proto-oncogenes that can be activated into oncogenes have been identified so far, and scientists estimate that at least 50 more exist (Cooper, 1990; Yarbro, 1992). *These oncogenes are not abnormal genes.* They are all part of every cell's normal make-up and were critically important in early development. Oncogenes become a problem only if they are activated (derepressed), after development is complete, as a result of exposure to carcinogenic agents or events. Activation of some specific oncogenes causes specific cancers. For example, activation of the *cMYC* oncogene, located on chromosome 8, can cause Burkitt's lymphoma. Extrinsic and intrinsic factors are associated with the activation of oncogenes.

EXTRINSIC FACTORS INFLUENCING CANCER DEVELOPMENT

Up to 80% of cancer in North America may be the result of environmental, or extrinsic, factors (Cooper, 1992). Environmental carcinogens are chemical, physical, or viral agents that cause cancer. Table 25–4 lists established environmental causes of human cancer.

CHEMICAL CARCINOGENESIS

Many chemicals capable of causing malignant transformation appear to have similar chemical structures. The study of chemical carcinogenesis began with epidemiologic findings of the high incidence of certain cancers among people who were chronically exposed to large amounts of some chemicals, especially coal tar, aromatic amines, and chemicals used in leather tanning. More than 20 organic and inorganic industrial chemicals, drugs, and other products used in everyday life are carcinogenic to humans, and hundreds of additional chemicals are suspected of being carcinogenic.

Some chemicals are complete carcinogens that can both initiate and promote cancer. Others are pure initiating agents, or incomplete carcinogens. Still others are only promoting agents. Some substances appear to be only mildly carcinogenic, so that it takes chronic exposure to large amounts of the substance before a cancer develops. Two such substances are tobacco and alcohol. However, these two substances can act as co-carcinogens; when taken together, they enhance the carcinogenic activity of each other or other carcinogens.

Cells are not equally susceptible to chemically induced malignant transformation. Normal cells that retain the capacity for mitotic cell division are at greater risk for cancer development than are normal cells not capable of cell division. The fact is borne out by looking at the tissues that most commonly develop cancer. Cancers commonly arise in bone marrow cells, skin cells, the lining of the gastrointestinal tract, the ductal cells of the breast, and the lining of the lungs. All of these cells normally undergo mitotic cell division. Cancers of nerve tissue, cardiac muscle, and skeletal muscle are rare. These cells do not normally undergo mitotic cell division.

Approximately 30% of cancers diagnosed in North America are related to tobacco use (Cooper, 1992). It is the single most important source of preventable chemical carcinogenesis. Tobacco contains many different chemical compounds, including complete carcinogens and co-carcinogens. Thus, tobacco use or ingestion can initiate and promote cancer.

The risk of a person who uses tobacco for cancer depends on his or her immune function, amount of exposure, depth and mode of exposure, and tar content of the tobacco. The type of cancer that develops depends on the susceptibility of specific sites to various concentrations of tobacco and its metabolites.

The tissues associated with the greatest risk for cancer are those that have direct contact with the tobacco smoke. Cigarette smoking is a major cause of cancer of the lungs, larynx, oral cavity, and esophagus, and it contributes to the development of bladder, pancreas, and kidney cancer. There is also a link between smoking and cancers of the breast, stomach, and uterine cervix (American Cancer Society, 1994). Table 25–8 summarizes cancer deaths attributable to tobacco use.

PHYSICAL CARCINOGENESIS

Physical agents or events may cause cancer by the same mechanism as for chemical carcinogens, that is, by induction of DNA damage. Two types of physical agents suspected of causing cancer are radiation and chronic irritation (Pitot, 1986).

RADIATION

Radiation is a physical agent that is capable of carcinogenesis. Even small doses of radiation affect cells. Some effects are temporary and reparable; other effects are irreversible and may be lethal to the damaged cell. The two types of radiation associated with carcinogenesis are ionizing and ultraviolet. Both ion-

TABLE 25–8 Cancer Mortality and Morbidity Attributable to Tobacco Use

Cancer Site	Men		Women		Total SAM
	Deaths/yr	*SAM*	*Deaths/yr*	*SAM*	
Lip, oral cavity, pharynx	5,754	3,958	2,689	1,110	5,068
Esophagus	6,310	3,717	2,345	1,257	4,974
Stomach	8,463	1,455	5,772	1,467	2,922
Pancreas	11,513	3,459	11,634	1,653	5,112
Larynx	2,959	2,385	664	274	2,660
Trachea, lung, bronchus	82,459	65,659	36,227	27,170	92,829
Cervix uteri	0	0	4,562	1,685	1,685
Urinary bladder	6,597	2,447	3,114	853	3,299
Kidney, other urinary site	5,424	1,319	3,403	403	1,722

From Centers for Disease Control. (1987). Smoking-attributable mortality and years of potential life lost—United States. *Morbidity and Mortality Weekly Report, 30,* 42.

SAM = smoking-attributable mortality; sums may not equal total because of rounding.

izing radiation and ultraviolet radiation produce gene mutations and chromosomal damage. Although radiation exposure induces cancers more frequently among cells that can divide, it can cause cancer among nondividing cells as well.

IONIZING RADIATION Ionizing radiation can induce all types of human cancers, depending on the intensity and duration of cellular absorption. Ionizing radiation occurs naturally in the environment in such minerals as radon, uranium, and radium. Most rocks and soil contain various concentrations of uranium and radium. The decay of radium results in the release of radon into the air and water. It is thought that decay of radium in the bricks, foundations, and soil surrounding many homes may be a major source of exposure to radon for the general population.

The two most important routes of entry for ionizing radiation are ingestion and inhalation. Ingestion is most likely to occur with contaminated foods or water. Inhaled radioactive particles can be deposited in any compartment of the respiratory tract. Inhalation of radioactive particles may also exert toxic effects on other structures, including the pulmonary lymph nodes, gastrointestinal tract, blood, and tissue compartments such as skeleton, liver, and kidneys.

Other sources of ionizing radiation include diagnostic and therapeutic x-rays and cosmic radiation. Even though the carcinogenic risk is low, there is concern about the risk of exposure to diagnostic and therapeutic x-rays. Emphasis is now placed on careful selection of clients for diagnostic x-rays, proper shielding of noninvolved body areas, and limitation of routine diagnostic procedures for which the risk might outweigh the benefit.

ULTRAVIOLET RADIATION Ultraviolet (UV) radiation is the most common type of solar radiation. UV rays do not penetrate deeply, and the most common type of cancer associated with UV exposure is skin cancer. People at risk are those with fair complexions and outdoor occupations. The degree of risk also increases with lower latitudes, higher altitudes, and less cloud cover.

Sources of UV radiation include the sun, tanning parlors, and such industrial equipment as welding arcs and germicidal lights. Cell-damaging effects of UV radiation are cumulative, and multiple exposures to large doses are necessary for carcinogenesis.

CHRONIC IRRITATION

Chronic irritation and tissue trauma have been suspected as predisposing physical agents to cancer development; however, this theory has not yet been supported directly. The incidence of skin cancer is higher in people with burn scars and other tissues that have sustained severe injury. Chronically irritated tissues may undergo frequent mitosis and, thus, are at an increased risk for spontaneous DNA mutations (Pitot, 1986).

VIRAL CARCINOGENESIS

Relatively few viruses have proved to be carcinogenic to humans. Evidence of viral carcinogenesis has been found that relates hepatitis B virus (HBV) to liver cancer, Epstein-Barr virus (EBV) to Burkitt's lymphoma, human T-cell lymphotropic virus (HTLV) to adult T-cell leukemia and lymphoma, and human papillomavirus (HPV) to cervical carcinoma. When viruses infect body cells, they break the DNA chain and insert their own genetic material into the human DNA chain. Breaking of the DNA along with viral gene insertion mutates the normal cell's DNA and can activate an oncogene. Viruses capable of causing cancer are known as oncoviruses.

DIETARY FACTORS RELATED TO CARCINOGENESIS

Epidemiologic data relate cancer development to many dietary practices or combinations of dietary practices and environmental exposures. However, the

CHART 25-1

Health Promotion Guide ◆ Dietary Habits to Reduce Cancer Risk

- Avoid the excessive intake of animal fat.
- Avoid nitrites (found in prepared lunch meats, sausage, bacon).
- Minimize your intake of red meat.
- Keep your alcohol consumption to no more than one or two drinks per day.
- Eat more bran.
- Eat more cruciferous vegetables, such as broccoli, cauliflower, Brussels sprouts, and cabbage.
- Eat foods high in vitamin A (such as apricots, carrots, and leafy green and yellow vegetables) and vitamin C (such as fresh fruits and vegetables, especially citrus fruits).

relationship of diet to carcinogenesis is poorly understood. Because dietary considerations are rarely independent of other possible carcinogenic agents, evidence of dietary contributions to the development of cancer is clouded. Dietary factors suspected of being related to cancer development include low crude fiber intake, high intake of red meat, and high intake of animal fat. Preservatives, contaminants, preparation methods, and additives (dyes, flavorings, and sweeteners) are being assessed for possible carcinogenic effects.

Certain foods and other nutrients, such as green vegetables, fruits, vitamins (A, C, D, and E), calcium, and selenium, may be protective against cancer development (Cooper, 1992). Chart 25-1 identifies foods considered to have high carcinogenic potential and foods that may have a protective effect.

INTRINSIC FACTORS INFLUENCING CANCER DEVELOPMENT

In addition to a person's expression of oncogenes, other intrinsic factors affect whether that person is likely to develop cancer. Intrinsic factors include:

- Immune system function
- Age
- Genetic predisposition

IMMUNOCOMPETENCE

The function of the immune system is to protect the body from foreign invaders and nonself cells (see Chap. 22). Nonself cells include cells that are made in the body but that are no longer normal, such as cancer cells. The part of the immune system responsible for protection against cancer is cell-mediated immunity. Natural killer (NK) cells together with the helper T cells are most important for immune surveillance (Applebaum, 1992).

The instrumental role of the immune system in protecting the body from cancer is supported by cancer incidence statistics in immunosuppressed people. Children younger than 2 years of age and adults older than 60 years have immune systems that function at less than optimal level. These populations also have a higher incidence of cancer compared with that of the general population. Organ transplant recipients who are taking immunosuppressive drugs to reduce the risk of organ rejection also have a higher incidence of cancer. In clients with acquired immunodeficiency syndrome, the incidence of cancer may be as high as 70% (Cooper, 1992; Pitot, 1986).

AGE

Advancing age is probably the single most significant risk factor related to the development of cancer (American Cancer Society, 1991b). Of all cancers, 50% occur in people older than 65 years (American Cancer Society, 1994). The higher cancer incidence in this age group may reflect lifelong accumulation of DNA mutations that result in cell transformation and cancer. The body may no longer be able to repair these mutations as it did in the early years. The effectiveness of the immune system, especially cell-mediated immunity, is also reduced in the elderly population. This reduction results in a limited ability to recognize and eliminate altered self cells. Cancer assessment considerations for the elderly are given in Chart 25-2 (see p. 558).

Manifestations of a cancer in elderly clients may be overlooked and attributed to changes that coincide with normal aging. It is essential that elders be aware of and report symptoms, such as the seven warning signs of cancer (Table 25-9), to health care providers. Health care providers must treat these reports with respect and thoroughly investigate all manifestations suggestive of disease.

GENETIC PREDISPOSITION

As previously discussed, oncogenes are primarily intrinsic factors related to carcinogenesis. Proto-onco-

TABLE 25-9 The Seven Warning Signs of Cancer

- C Changes in bowel or bladder habits
- A A sore that does not heal
- U Unusual bleeding or discharge
- T Thickening or lump in the breast or elsewhere
- I Indigestion or difficulty swallowing
- O Obvious change in a wart or mole
- N Nagging cough or hoarseness

CHART 25-2

Nursing Focus on the Elderly ◆ Cancer Assessment Considerations

Cancer Type	Assessment Consideration
Colorectal cancer	• Ask the client whether bowel habits have changed over the past year, for example, in consistency, frequency, or color. • Is there any obvious blood in the stool? • Test at least one stool specimen for the presence of occult blood during the client's hospitalization. • Encourage the client to have a baseline colonoscopy. • Encourage the client to reduce dietary intake of animal fats, red meat, and smoked meats. • Encourage the client to increase dietary intake of bran, vegetables, and fruit.
Bladder cancer	• Ask the client about the presence of: Pain on urination Blood in the urine Cloudy urine Increased frequency or urgency
Prostate cancer	• Ask the client about: Hesitancy Change in the size of the urine stream Pain in back or legs History of urinary tract infections
Skin cancer	• Examine skin areas for moles or warts. • Ask the client about changes in moles, for example, color, edges, or sensation.
Leukemia	• Observe the skin for color, the presence of petechiae, or ecchymosis. • Ask the client about: Fatigue Bruising Bleeding tendency History of infections and illnesses Night sweats Unexplained fevers
Lung cancer	• Observe the skin and mucous membranes for color. • How many words can the client say between breaths? • Ask the client about: Cough Hoarseness Smoking history Exposure to inhalation irritants Shortness of breath Activity tolerance Frothy or bloody sputum Pain in the arms or chest Difficulty swallowing

genes, precursors of oncogenes, are passed on from generation to generation. The development of cancer, however, depends on more than the presence of such genes. For a cancer to develop, the proto-oncogene needs to be damaged or altered to allow expression of the oncogene. In some people, the location of specific proto-oncogenes is different and may allow them to be activated to oncogenes more easily (Cooper, 1990). These variations in gene location are inheritable.

Patterns of genetic predisposition for cancer other than oncogenes have also been identified, including:

- Inherited predisposition for specific cancers
- Inherited conditions associated cancer
- Familial clustering
- Chromosomal aberrations

Table 25-10 lists different conditions associated with a genetic predisposition for cancer development.

Transcultural Considerations The incidence of cancer varies among races. American Cancer Society (1992) data show that African-Americans have a higher incidence of cancer than Caucasians do, and the death rate is higher for African-Americans. The overall incidence among African-Americans has increased 27% since 1960; in that same period, it increased 12% for Caucasians (American Cancer Society, 1991a). Cancer sites and cancer-related mortality

TABLE 25-10 Conditions Associated with a Genetic Predisposition for Cancer

Condition	Specific Cancer Type
Inherited cancers*	• Retinoblastoma • Wilms' tumor
Familial clustering	• Breast cancer • Melanoma
Bloom's syndrome	• Leukemia
Familial polyposis	• Colorectal cancer
Chromosomal aberrations	
Down syndrome (47 chromosomes)	• Leukemia
Klinefelter's syndrome (47, XXY)	• Breast cancer
Turner's syndrome (45, XO)	• Leukemia • Gonadal carcinoma • Meningioma • Colorectal cancer

* Not all retinoblastomas or Wilms' tumors are inherited.

TABLE 25–11 Racial Differences in Cancer Development

Race	Common Cancer Types
Caucasian	1. Lung 2. Breast 3. Colorectal 4. Prostate
African-American	1. Lung 2. Prostate 3. Breast 4. Colorectal 5. Uterine
Asian	1. Breast 2. Colorectal 3. Prostate 4. Lung 5. Stomach
Hispanic	1. Prostate 2. Breast 3. Colorectal 4. Lung

Data from American Cancer Society. (1994). *Cancer facts and figures—1994.* Atlanta: American Cancer Society, Inc.

rizes the major cancers commonly occurring among Caucasian, African-American, Asian, and Hispanic populations.

When risks for the development of cancer are assessed, however, race and genetic predisposition cannot be considered in a vacuum. Behavior that is related to culture or ethnic group, geographic location, diet, and socioeconomic factors must also be assessed. The American Cancer Society (1991a) has reported that cancer incidence and survival are often related to socioeconomic factors, such as the availability of health care services or the belief that seeking early health care has a positive effect on the outcome of cancer diagnosis (see the accompanying Research Applications for Nursing).

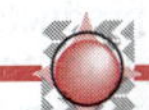

IMPLICATIONS FOR NURSING RESEARCH

Nurses can play a major role in educating people about cancer prevention for those cancers that have a known, avoidable cause. In addition, by increasing the public awareness of cancer screening and early detection methods, nurses may help reduce the mortality rate from those cancers for which causes remain unidentified. The following questions are amenable to nursing research:

- What methods are most effective in motivating clients to avoid the use of tobacco products?
- What methods are most effective in teaching clients dietary habits that lower cancer risks?
- Are nurse-managed cancer screening programs effective for secondary prevention of cancer?

RESEARCH APPLICATIONS FOR NURSING

African-American Women May Be More Likely to Seek Medical Attention for Possible Breast Cancer Than Caucasian Women

Lauver, D. (1992). Psychosocial variables, race, and intention to seek care for breast cancer symptoms. *Nursing Research, 41*(4), 236–241.

Many people equate a diagnosis of cancer with a death sentence. When such people have one or more symptoms associated with cancer, they often either ignore the symptom or delay seeking medical attention that would confirm or rule out a diagnosis of cancer. If the client does have cancer, this delay in seeking medical attention can adversely affect the outcome because earlier intervention is more likely to result in cure or long-term survival than is either late intervention or no intervention.

Although African-American women have a lower incidence of breast cancer than do Caucasian women, their overall chances of surviving the disease are lower. Lauver sought to determine whether race was a major factor influencing a woman's intention to seek medical attention if she should develop one or more symptoms of breast cancer. This research used a comparative, test-retest design that measured the subject's responses to a hypothetical question. In this way, the investigators measured *intention to act* rather than actual *action* of the subjects to a given situation. The results of the study showed African-American women to have slightly greater intentions to seek medical attention for symptoms of breast cancer than did Caucasian women. The greater intentions were also associated with a stronger view that seeking medical attention would be useful.

Critique The investigators statistically controlled for differences in education and socioeconomic levels between the two age groups. The number of subjects was adequate (96), and the instruments used were valid and reliable. Measuring intention versus action limits the generalizability of the results.

Possible nursing implications The intention to seek medical assistance was positively related to how useful that behavior was viewed by the subjects. Therefore, one way nurses may be able to encourage clients to seek medical assistance when cancer symptoms first appear (or even before they appear) is to stress how valuable early interventions are in curing cancer and prolonging life.

- Are there cultural barriers to public education about cancer risk education?

SELECTED BIBLIOGRAPHY

American Cancer Society. (1991a). *Cancer facts and figures for minority Americans.* Atlanta: American Cancer Society, Inc. (91–75M–No. 5623)

American Cancer Society. (1991b). *Proceedings of the national workshop on cancer control and the older person.* Atlanta: American Cancer Society, Inc. (91-3M-No. 3043)

American Cancer Society. (1994). *Cancer facts & figures—1994.* Atlanta: American Cancer Society, Inc. (93-400M-No. 5008.93.)

Applebaum, J. (1992). The role of the immune system in the pathogenesis of cancer. *Seminars in Oncology Nursing, 8*(1), 51-62.

Baird, S., McCorkle, R., & Grant, M. (1991). *Cancer nursing: A comprehensive textbook.* Philadelphia: W. B. Saunders.

*Bishop, J. (1982). Oncogenes. *Scientific American, 246*(3), 80-92.

Boring, C., Squires, T., & Heath, C. (1992). *Cancer statistics for African Americans.* Atlanta: American Cancer Society, Inc. (Professional Education Publication 3034-PE)

Cartmel, B., Loescher, L., & Villar-Werstler, P. (1992). Professional and consumer concerns about the environment, lifestyle, and cancer. *Seminars in Oncology Nursing, 8*(1), 20-29.

Cooper, G. (1990). *Oncogenes.* Boston: Jones & Bartlett Publishers.

Cooper, G. (1992). *Elements of human cancer.* Boston: Jones & Bartlett Publishers.

Dangle, R. (1992). Cancer epidemiology. In J. Clark & R. McGee (Eds.), *Core curriculum for oncology nursing* (2nd ed)., pp. 289-299). Philadelphia: W. B. Saunders.

*DeVita, V., Hellman, S., & Rosenberg, S. (Eds.). (1993). *Cancer: Principles and practice of oncology* (4th ed.). Philadelphia: J. B. Lippincott.

Dudjak, L. (1992). Cancer metastasis. *Seminars in Oncology Nursing, 8*(1), 40-50.

*Fidler, I., & Hart, I. (1982). Biologic diversity in metastatic neoplasia: Origins and implications. *Science, 217*(4564), 998.

Frank-Stromberg, M. (1991). Evaluating cancer risk. In S. Baird, R. McCorkle, & M. Grant (Eds.), *Cancer nursing: A comprehensive textbook* (pp. 155-189). Philadelphia: W. B. Saunders.

Frank-Stromberg, M., & Olsen, S. (1993). *Cancer prevention in minority populations: Cultural implications for health care professionals.* St. Louis: C. V. Mosby.

*Fraser, M., & Tucker, M. (1989). Second malignancies following cancer therapy. *Seminars in Oncology Nursing, 5*(1), 43.

Gallucci, B. (1991). Cancer biology: Molecular and cellular aspects. In S. Baird, R. McCorkle, & M. Grant (Eds.), *Cancer nursing: A comprehensive textbook* (pp. 115-129). Philadelphia: W. B. Saunders.

*Gullatte, M. (1989). Cancer prevention and early detection in Black Americans: Colon and rectum. *Journal of the National Black Nurses' Association, 3*(2), 49-56.

Heusinkveld, K. (1991). Preventive oncology. In S. Baird, R. McCorkle, & M. Grant (Eds.), *Cancer nursing: A comprehensive textbook* (pp. 143-154). Philadelphia: W. B. Saunders.

Hubbard, S., & Liotta, L. (1991). The biology of metastasis. In S. Baird, R. McCorkle, & M. Grant (Eds.), *Cancer nursing: A comprehensive textbook* (pp. 130-142). Philadelphia: W. B. Saunders.

Jenkins, J. (1992). Biology of cancer: Current issues and future prospects. *Seminars in Oncology Nursing, 8*(1), 63-69.

Jenkins, C., McPhee, S., Bird, J., & Bonilla, N. (1990). Cancer risks and prevention practices among Vietnam refugees. *Western Journal of Medicine, 153*(1), 34-39.

Lauver, D. (1992). Psychosocial variables, race, and intention to seek care for breast cancer symptoms. *Nursing Research, 41*(4), 236-241.

Lind, J. (1992). Tumor cell growth and cell kinetics. *Seminars in Oncology Nursing, 8*(1), 3-9.

Mack, E., McGrath, T., Pendleton, D., & Zieber, N. (1993). Reaching poor populations with cancer prevention and early detection programs. *Cancer Practice, 1*(1), 35-39.

McMillan, S. (1992). Carcinogenesis. *Seminars in Oncology Nursing, 8*(1), 10-19.

Mettlin, C., & Mirand, A. (1991). The causes of cancer. In S. Baird, R. McCorkle, & M. Grant (Eds.), *Cancer nursing: A comprehensive textbook* (pp. 104-114). Philadelphia: W. B. Saunders.

*Nicolson, G. (1979). Cancer metastasis. *Scientific American, 240*, 66.

Olsen, S., & Frank-Stromborg, M. (1994). Cancer prevention and screening activities reported by African American nurses. *Oncology Nursing Forum, 21*(3), 487-494.

Olsen, S., & Frank-Stromborg, M. (1991). Cancer screening and early detection. In S. Baird, R. McCorkle, & M. Grant (Eds.), *Cancer nursing: A comprehensive textbook* (pp. 190-218). Philadelphia: W. B. Saunders.

*Orleans, C., Strecher, V., Schoenbach, V., Salmon, M., & Blackmon, C. (1989). Smoking cessation initiatives for Black Americans: Recommendations for research and intervention. *Health Education Research, 4*(1), 13-25.

Palos, G. (1994). Cultural heritage: Cancer screening and early detection. *Seminars in Oncology Nursing, 10*(2), 104-113.

*Pitot, H. (1986). *Fundamentals of Oncology* (2nd ed.). New York: Marcel Dekker.

Yarbro, J. (1992). Oncogenes and cancer suppressor genes. *Seminars in Oncology Nursing, 8*(1) 30-39.

SUGGESTED READINGS

Cartmel, B., Loescher, L., & Villar-Werstler, P. (1992). Professional and consumer concerns about the environment, lifestyle, and cancer. *Seminars in Oncology Nursing, 8*(1), 20-29.

The authors identify known and potential environmental risk factors for cancer development. The article assists the reader to be an educated consumer of potentially damaging products, procedures, or lifestyles. The information presented in the article can help students and practicing nurses educate clients about choices and changes that reduce cancer risk.

Olsen, S., & Frank-Stromborg, M. (1991). Cancer screening and early detection. In S. Baird, R. McCorkle, & M. Grant (Eds.), *Cancer Nursing: A comprehensive textbook* (pp. 190-218). Philadelphia: W. B. Saunders.

This chapter clearly describes the various methods for cancer screening and early detection. The authors present the advantages and disadvantages of each method as well as the role of the nurse in educating clients about risks and benefits.

Yarbro, J. (1992). Oncogenes and cancer suppressor genes. *Seminars in Oncology Nursing, 8*(1), 30-39.

This up-to-date article presents background information on the existence and purposes of specific gene types important in cancer development. Explanations are clear, and the use of scientific jargon is avoided. The article provides a link between cancer biology information available in the usual nursing literature and the basic science literature. Reading level is appropriate for advanced undergraduate nursing students.

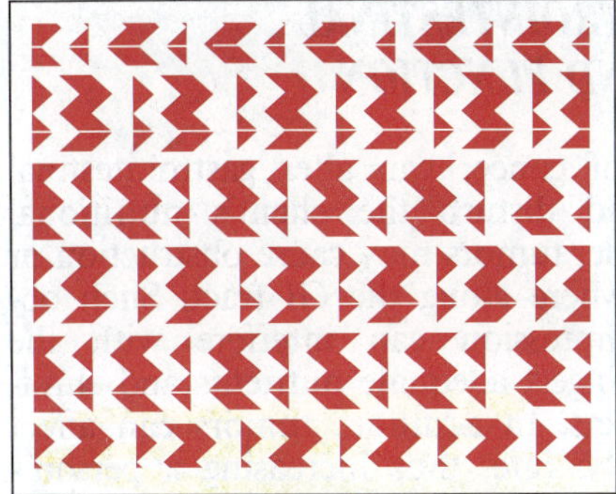

CHAPTER 26

Interventions for Clients with Cancer

CHAPTER HIGHLIGHTS

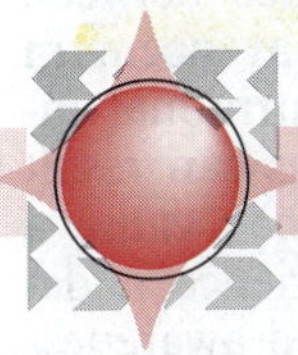

Cancer is a disease that affects many body systems at the same time. Although many cancers can be cured or controlled, cancer is one of the diseases that clients fear most. A diagnosis of cancer elicits psychologic and emotional responses and is a threat to human relationships, financial security, and role responsibilities. The family and friends of people who have cancer are also affected (Jassak, 1992).

Nursing care of clients with cancer incorporates traditional and nontraditional methods. This chapter addresses common issues associated with cancer development, diagnosis, treatment, and survival. Table 26-1 lists key concepts associated with cancer treatment and care. Specific issues regarding diagnosis, treatment, and nursing care for clients with specific cancers are presented in the chapters associated with the system in which the cancer has developed.

GENERAL DISEASE-RELATED CONSEQUENCES OF CANCER

Cancer can develop in any organ or tissue (Cooper, 1992). Cancer destroys normal tissue, resulting in decreased function in that tissue or organ. Even when cancers occur in nonvital tissues or organs, they can cause a person's death by metastasizing (spreading) into vital organs and disrupting critical physiologic

TABLE 26–1 Key Points Concerning Clients Undergoing Cancer Treatment

- With multiapproach to cancer treatment, 50% of clients with cancer can be cured of their disease.
- Surgery is most effective for cancer therapy when tumors are small and well localized.
- Radiation therapy is only effective on the tissues directly within the radiation path.
- Side effects of radiation therapy are confined to the tissues within the radiation path.
- The most common side effects of radiation therapy are skin irritation, fatigue, and altered taste sensation.
- Chemotherapy is systemic therapy for cancer and affects all body tissues.
- The most common side effects of chemotherapy are alopecia, nausea and vomiting, mucositis, skin changes, and bone marrow suppression.
- The most life-threatening side effect of chemotherapy is bone marrow suppression.

processes (see Chap. 25). Cancers can produce serious health problems, especially when they cause obstruction, pressure, hemorrhage, infection, or ulceration in vital tissues or organs.

Cancer development and metastasis commonly lead to:

- Impaired immune and hematopoietic (blood-producing) function
- Altered gastrointestinal (GI) tract structure and function
- Motor and sensory deficits
- Decreased respiratory function

Not only do these impairments cause great physical and emotional distress to the client; without intervention, persistent cancer invasion of normal tissues leads to death.

IMPAIRED IMMUNE AND HEMATOPOIETIC FUNCTION

Impaired immune and hematopoietic function occurs most often in clients who have leukemia and lymphoma, but such impairment can occur with any cancer that invades the bone marrow (Gallucci, 1991). Tumor cells enter the bone marrow, causing decreased production of healthy white blood cells, which are needed for normal immune function (see Chap. 22). Thus, clients who have cancer, especially leukemia, are at an increased risk for infection.

When cancer invades the bone marrow, clients also have a decreased number of red blood cells and platelets. These abnormalities may be caused by the cancer itself, such as in leukemia, or by cancer treatment. In either case, the client becomes anemic and has an increased tendency to bleed. (For a more complete discussion of cancer's effects on the hematologic system, see Chapter 39.)

ALTERED GASTROINTESTINAL STRUCTURE AND FUNCTION

The presence of cancer can alter gastrointestinal (GI) function and disturb the client's nutritional status. For example, tumors may cause obstruction or compression anywhere along the GI tract. Such obstruction or compression can interfere with the client's ability to ingest adequate nutrients and eliminate waste products. In addition, tumors can affect the basal metabolic rate, thus increasing a person's requirements for protein, carbohydrates, and fat at the same time the person has less energy available to prepare food and eat.

Many tumors metastasize to the liver, causing profound damage to liver tissues. The liver has many important metabolic functions and participates in the digestion and utilization of proteins and fats. Diminished liver function contributes to malnutrition and death among clients with cancer.

The anorexia experienced by clients with cancer often interferes with the client's ability to meet energy requirements. Cachexia (extreme body wasting and malnutrition) develops from the imbalance between food intake and energy use. Cachexia may occur in spite of what appears to be adequate nutritional intake. Changes in a client's taste sensations can result from the cancer or the treatment and may cause a decrease in appetite. Clients often experience a decreased ability to taste sweets, an increased awareness of bitterness, and an aversion to red meat. A complete list of cancer-related factors that can contribute to malnutrition is presented in Table 26–2.

The role of nutritional support for the client with cancer, especially the client undergoing cancer therapy, is complex and controversial. Often a diet high in protein and carbohydrates is ordered to assist the client to maintain his or her weight and to provide nutrients needed for energy and cellular repair. However, some scientists believe that excessive intake of protein, carbohydrates, and vitamins increases the nutrition of the cancer cells and contributes to cancer progression. Some vitamins, when taken in large amounts, counteract the effect of some chemotherapeutic agents. In addition to these controversial issues, clients often believe that by eating more food, especially a diet that is low in fat and high in fiber, grains, fruit and vegetables, their cancer can be cured more easily. Clients' tolerance for different types of food may change during cancer treatment. At present, no one nutritional plan meets the needs of all clients with cancer.

MOTOR AND SENSORY DEFICITS

Motor (movement) and sensory deficits can occur when cancers invade bone or compress nerves. In most clients with bone metastases, the primary cancer is in the prostate, breast, or lung. Bone sites most affected include the vertebrae, ribs, pelvis, and femur. The humerus, scapula, sternum, skull, and clavicle

TABLE 26–2 Causes of Malnutrition in Clients with Cancer

Anorexia
- Local causes
  - Pelvic or abdominal tumors
  - Hepatic metastases
  - Intestinal compression or obstruction
  - Others
- Remote causes
  - Food aversions
  - Early satiety
- Treatment-related causes
  - Postsurgical small stomach or stasis
  - Drugs, including chemotherapy
  - Radiation—local and systemic effects
- Systemic illness
  - Infection
  - Hepatitis or pancreatitis
  - Endocrinopathies
- Taste disorders
  - Drugs (e.g., metronidazole)
  - Remote effects of neoplasm and its treatment
  - Local disease and its treatment (e.g., stomatitis, nasopharyngeal tumor, radiation, and surgery)
  - Nausea and vomiting
- Psychogenic causes
  - Depression
  - Anxiety
  - Conditioned aversions
- Intolerance of institutional food

Difficulty in Eating
- Head and neck tumors and their treatment
- Xerostomia
- Stomatitis
- Loss of teeth and dental problems
- Dysphagia and odynophagia

Maldigestion or Malabsorption
- Pancreatitic insufficiency
- Bile salt deficiency
- Hypersecretory states
  - Zollinger-Ellison syndrome
  - Pancreatic cholera
  - Bowel infiltration
  - Diffuse invasion (e.g., lymphoma)
  - Local blockage
  - Fistula
- Postsurgical causes
  - Esophageal surgery (with vagotomy, gastric stasis diarrhea, and steatorrhea)
  - Gastrectomy—dumping, achlorhydria, or afferent loop syndrome
  - Small intestine resections
- Postirradiation causes
  - Enteritis (may occur as late sequela)
  - Fistula
  - Stenosis
  - Obstruction

Protein-Losing Enteropathy

Malutilization
- Cancer cachexia
- Steroids
  - Nitrogen wasting
  - Hyperglycemia
  - Calcium loss

are also common metastatic sites. Bone metastases can cause fractures, spinal cord compression, and hypercalcemia. Each of these problems causes decreased mobility for the client.

The client may also experience sensory changes if the spinal cord is damaged by tumor compression or if nerve ganglia are compressed. In addition, many malignant tumors metastasize to the brain and disrupt both sensory and motor functions.

Pain is another sensory change that the client with cancer may experience. Pain does not always accompany cancer, but it can be a significant problem for clients with terminal cancer. Table 26–3 lists common causes of pain in clients with cancer. The most common approach to pain management is pharmacologic. However, nonpharmacologic interventions may also be effective (Research Applications for Nursing). (Chapter 8 provides an in-depth discussion of pain etiology and management.)

DECREASED RESPIRATORY FUNCTION

Cancer can disrupt a client's respiratory function in several ways and often results in death. Tumors involving the airways can cause airway obstruction. If lung tissue is involved, lung capacity is decreased. Tumor growth can also press on vascular and lymphatic structures in the chest, blocking blood flow through the chest and lungs, resulting in pulmonary edema and dyspnea. Tumors also can thicken the alveolar membrane and damage pulmonary blood vessels, reducing the effectiveness of gas exchange.

TREATMENT-RELATED CONSEQUENCES OF CANCER

The purpose of any treatment for cancer is to prolong the client's survival time or improve the client's quality of life. Although some spontaneous regressions of malignant tumors have been reported, the vast majority of clients who have cancer would die within months of diagnosis without appropriate cancer therapy.

Therapies for cancer include the following:

- Surgery
- Radiation
- Chemotherapy
- Hormonal manipulation
- Immunotherapy

These therapies may be used individually or in combination to kill tumor cells. What type and

TABLE 26–3 Causes of Pain in Clients with Cancer

Effects of Cancer

- Bone infiltration by primary or metastatic tumor (most common cause of pain)
- Nerve infiltration involving peripheral nerves, nerve plexus, or spinal cord
- Nerve compression
- Soft-tissue infiltration
- Visceral involvement
- Muscle spasm
- Lymphedema
- Increased intracranial pressure
- Myopathy

Treatment

- Surgery, especially thoracotomy, mastectomy, radical neck dissection; phantom limb
- Chemotherapy
  - Peripheral neuropathy
  - Postherpetic neuralgia
  - Extravasation
  - Dysesthesias
  - Aseptic necrosis of the humeral head
- Nerve block
- Postoperative adhesions
- Postirradiation fibrosis, especially when fields include plexus
- Postirradiation myopathy
- Mucositis

Debility or Immobility

- Constipation
- Capsulitis of shoulder
- Pressure ulcer
- Pulmonary embolus
- Penile spasm or urinary catheterization

Concurrent Disorders

- Musculoskeletal disease
  - Myofascial
  - Lumbar disk disease
  - Osteoporosis
  - Osteoarthritis
  - Others
- Migraine
- Miscellaneous

Data from Foley, K. M. (1984). A review of pain syndrome in patients with cancer. *The management of cancer pain symposium.* Nutley, NJ: Roche Laboratories; and Twycross, R. G. (1988). The management of pain in cancer: A guide to drugs and dosages. *Oncology, 2*(4), 35–44.

RESEARCH APPLICATIONS FOR NURSING RESEARCH

Music Therapy May Help Reduce Pain Perception in Clients with Cancer

Beck, S. (1991). The therapeutic use of music for cancer-related pain. *Oncology Nursing Forum, 18*(8), 1327–1337.

This article describes the results of a crossover, experimental study undertaken to evaluate the effectiveness of music therapy as a form of non-pharmacologic intervention for pain reduction. The subjects were clients with cancer who were receiving analgesics on schedule rather than on demand. Experimental subjects listened to relaxing music of their choice for 45 minutes a day for 3 days in a row. Control subjects listened to 45 minutes of sound (low-frequency 60-hertz hum) for 45 minutes each day for 3 days in a row. Halfway through the study, subjects were crossed over into the opposite treatment group. Subjects rated their pain using the McGill Pain Questionnaire and their mood using a Mood Visual Analogue Scale. Data were analyzed using ANOVA. Results indicated that pain was perceived to be significantly less for subjects listening to relaxing music. Music had no significant effect on mood.

Critique Even though the number of subjects in the study was low (15) and the type of cancer was not controlled for, homogeneity of other variables within the group and the fact that the design was random crossover strengthen the study. Because the study was small, however, results cannot be generalized to other groups of clients with cancer.

Possible nursing implications Despite the limitations in this study, its results are of clinical significance to nurses caring for clients with cancer experiencing pain. Thus, use of a noninvasive and nonpharmacologic approach combined with other modalities may assist in reducing the perception of pain and increasing the quality of life for the client with cancer.

amount of therapy a client with cancer receives is determined by:

- The specific type of cancer present
- The extent of the disease
- The overall health of the client

For most types of cancer, one or more regimens of therapy (protocols) have been established, based on experiments with cancer cells, animals, and other clients with cancer.

Surgery

RATIONALE FOR SURGERY AS A CANCER THERAPY

Surgery for cancer involves the removal of diseased tissue. If cancer is confined to the tissue removed, surgery alone can result in "cure" for that cancer. Although many cancers have spread too far at the time of diagnosis for surgery alone to be curative, surgery may still be a useful part of the diagnosis,

TABLE 26–4 Diagnostic/Biopsy Surgeries for Cancer

Biopsy Type	Description	Problem/Limitations
Needle	• Aspiration of cells in a fluid or in very soft tissue • Bore a "core" of solid tissue by using a long needle, or making a punch, scrape, or bite.	• Sample error—may biopsy only non-cancerous cells in a tissue or organ • Sample size may not be adequate for accurate testing. • Procedure may spread cancer by seeding it into surrounding tissues. • Procedure may damage healthy tissue.
Incisional	• Wedge of suspected tissue is removed from a larger tissue mass, leaving some tumor cells remaining in the tissue.	• Sample error • Tumor seeding • Damage to healthy tissue
Excisional	• Complete removal of an entire lesion without removing any adjacent normal tissues	• Tumor seeding • Leaving micrometastasis • Damage to healthy tissue
Staging	• Multiple needle or incisional biopsies in tissues where metastasis is suspected or likely	• Tumor seeding • Sample error • Damage to healthy tissue

treatment, follow-up, and rehabilitation (Harvard & Topping, 1991).

MECHANISM OF ACTION

Surgery is the oldest form of cancer treatment and the first method that was used to cure cancer. Surgery may be prescribed for the client with cancer for one or more of the following purposes:

- Prophylaxis
- Diagnosis
- Cure
- Control
- Palliation
- Determination of therapy effectiveness
- Reconstruction

PROPHYLAXIS

Prophylactic surgery is performed when a client has either an existing "premalignant" condition or a known family history that strongly predisposes the person to the subsequent development of cancer. With this type of surgery, an attempt is made to remove the tissue or organ "at risk" and thus prevent the development of cancer. An example of prophylactic surgery for a premalignant condition is removal of a benign mole from a location where it would receive continuous irritation or exposure to sunlight.

DIAGNOSIS (BIOPSY)

Diagnostic surgery can provide histologic proof of malignancy. Usually, all or part of a suspected lesion is removed for microscopic examination and testing. Specific types of biopsies are summarized in Table 26–4.

CURE

Surgery for cure is a treatment that can, without additional therapy, result in a cure rate of 25% to 30%. With this type of surgery, all gross and microscopic tumor is either removed or destroyed. Types of curative surgeries are described in Table 26–5.

CONTROL (CYTOREDUCTIVE SURGERY)

Cancer control, or cytoreductive surgery, is a "debulking" procedure that consists of removing part of the tumor while *known* gross tumor is left. This type of surgery alone cannot result in a cure, but it does

TABLE 26–5 Curative Surgeries for Cancer

Surgery Type	Description	Purpose/Use
Local excision	• Removal of all identifiable tumor along with a small margin of normal tissues	• Small, localized tumors
Wide local excision (radical)	• Removal of identifiable tumor plus immediate tissue or adjacent tissue	• Small tumors with only local tissue invasion
Wide excision	• Removal of tumor, surrounding tissue, adjacent structures, and usual lymph channels draining the area	• Small to moderate size tumors with known local invasion
Extended radical excision	• Removal of tumor, lymphatics, adjacent organs and all tissues in the region	• Tumor infiltrate in a wide area but with no known distant metastasis

decrease the number of cancer cells present and may increase the effectiveness of other therapies.

PALLIATION

The aim of palliative surgery is not to cure (or even increase survival time in many instances) but to improve the client's quality of life during the survival time. The surgeon removes tumor tissue that is causing the client such distressing symptoms as pain, intestinal obstruction, or difficulty in swallowing. What is done specifically during palliative surgery depends on what is causing a problem to the client.

DETERMINATION OF THERAPY EFFECTIVENESS ("SECOND-LOOK" SURGERY)

Second-look surgery is essentially a "rediagnosis" after treatment. The purpose is to assess the disease status in clients who have been treated and who have no symptoms of remaining or recurrent tumor. The results of this surgery serve as a basis for discontinuing or continuing specific therapy.

RECONSTRUCTIVE OR REHABILITATIVE SURGERY

Reconstructive-rehabilitative surgery for clients who have cancer is relatively new; this means that people with cancer are surviving long enough to need reconstruction. This type of surgery is indicated to increase function, enhance cosmetic appearance, or both. Examples include breast reconstruction after mastectomy, replacement of the esophagus after radiation damage, bowel reconstruction, revision of scars, release of contractures, and placement of penile implants.

SIDE EFFECTS OF SURGICAL THERAPY FOR CANCER

Unlike surgery performed for many other reasons, cancer surgery often involves the loss of a specific body part or loss of function of a body part. Sometimes whole organs are removed, such as the kidney, lung, breast, testes, arm, or tongue. Any organ loss results in diminished functional capacity. How much function is lost and how the loss physically affects the client depend on the location and extent of the surgery. Some surgical procedures for cancer also may result in significant scarring or disfigurement. In addition to actual loss of a body part and anxiety about the chances of surviving the disease, clients may be grieving about a loss of body image or a change in lifestyle imposed by the cancer or its treatment.

NURSING CARE OF CLIENTS UNDERGOING SURGERY

Nursing care associated with surgery for cancer is not vastly different from that related to surgery for other reasons (see Chaps. 19 to 21). The nurse considers all the physical and psychosocial factors related to the client's ability (or the ability of family and significant others) to cope with the uncertainty of cancer and its treatment along with changes in body image and role. For example, surgery involving the genitals, urinary tract, colon, and rectum may cause permanent damage to these organs. Surgical procedures that create a urinary or fecal diversion (such as a colostomy) may disturb innervation, causing erectile impotence and ejaculatory dysfunction in men and painful intercourse (dyspareunia) in women.

Radiation

RATIONALE FOR RADIATION AS A CANCER THERAPY

The purpose of all types of radiation therapy for cancer is to destroy malignant cells with minimal exposure of the normal cells to the cell-damaging actions of the radiation. The effects of radiation are localized only to those tissues in the path of radiation. Some effects are apparent within days or weeks after radiation treatment; other effects may not be apparent for months to years after radiation therapy is completed.

MECHANISM OF ACTION

Most of the radiation used for treatment of malignant tumors is *ionizing* radiation. When cells are exposed to this type of radiation, source of the atoms within the cell are "kicked out" of orbit, resulting in a tremendous release of intracellular energy. Ionizing radiation is naturally given off by some substances, such as radium and cobalt, and it also can be generated by machines called linear accelerators. Naturally occurring radiation is called *gamma* radiation; radiation generated by machine is called *roentgen* radiation. Their effect on cells is exactly the same.

Cells damaged by radiation either die outright or become unable to divide. Cellular damage, caused by a combination of intracellular oxidation and the tight binding together of the deoxyribonucleic acid (DNA) strands, inhibits the capacity of the cell to divide.

Radiation damage can occur any time a cell is exposed to radiation; it is not confined to cells that are actively in the cell cycle (Iwamoto, 1991). However, cells in the cell cycle experience more damage when they are exposed to radiation than do nondividing cells. Radiation damage is not cell cycle phase–specific, although some phases are more sensi-

TABLE 26–6 Characteristics of Different Types of Gamma Radiation

Type of Ray	Characteristics
Gamma	• Gamma rays are very light with a low energy transfer potential and travel very rapidly (at the speed of light), allowing them to be concentrated and penetrate deeply into tissues. • This is the most common type of radiation used for the treatment of cancer. • This type of radiation can also cause serious, irreversible harm to tissues. • Exposure to this type of radiation must be avoided or severely limited.
Beta	• Beta rays are heavier with moderate to high speed. They have a high linear energy transfer potential, and do not penetrate tissues or other substances well. • Some beta rays are used inside the body for specific radiation therapy. • Beta rays are used in some diagnostic tests. • Beta rays do pose some health hazards to humans exposed to them but exposure must be considerable for damage to occur.
Alpha	• Alpha rays are very heavy and slow. They easily transfer energy to surroundings and quickly lose their ability to penetrate tissues (0.04 mm into tissue). • Currently, alpha rays are used in laboratory tests rather than as treatment for cancer. • This type of radiation is harmful to humans only if it is ingested chronically.

tive than others. The cell cycle phase sensitivity to radiation in descending order is M, G2, G1, and S. (Chapter 25 reviews the different phases of the cell cycle.)

Three different types of energy, or rays, are produced as a result of gamma radiation: gamma, beta, and alpha rays (Hilderley & Dow, 1991). These rays vary in their ability to penetrate tissues and damage cells. Table 26–6 summarizes the features of these three types of gamma radiation, and Figure 26–1 depicts the penetrating ability of each.

The intensity of the radiation emitted decreases with the inverse square of the distance from the radiation source (Fig. 26–2). In practice this means that the dose of radiation received at a distance of 2 inches from the radiation source is only 25% of the dose received at a distance of 1 inch from the radiation source; the dose of radiation received at 3 inches from the source is only one-ninth the dose received at a distance of 1 inch from the source (Hassey, 1987).

The amount of radiation aimed at or delivered to a tissue is called *exposure*, and how much of this exposure is absorbed by the recipient tissue is called the *dose*. Therefore, the dose is always some fraction or percentage of the exposure and depends on the:

- Energy level
- Absorption type
- Intensity
- Proximity
- Duration of exposure

KILLING EFFECTS OF RADIATION

If the absorbed dose of radiation is high enough, all cells will be killed immediately. However, this is not what usually happens with therapeutic radiation. Instead, radiation damage to the DNA is not usually apparent until the cell attempts to divide (Strohl, 1990). In a population of tumor cells treated with a single exposure of radiation, all cells within the tumor absorb the radiation slightly differently; thus, their overall response to the radiation is slightly different. A few cells die immediately on exposure, and more die within the next 24 hours as they attempt to divide. Some cells are sterile as a result of this single treatment; still others repair the radiation-induced damage and continue to reproduce for many cell generations.

Because of the varying responses of all the cancer cells within a given tumor, radiation for cancer therapy is administered as a series of divided doses. Small doses are delivered on a daily basis for a set period of time. Giving radiation treatment in a series rather than as a single dose presents multiple opportunities to catch and destroy cancer cells that survived the initial hit of radiation.

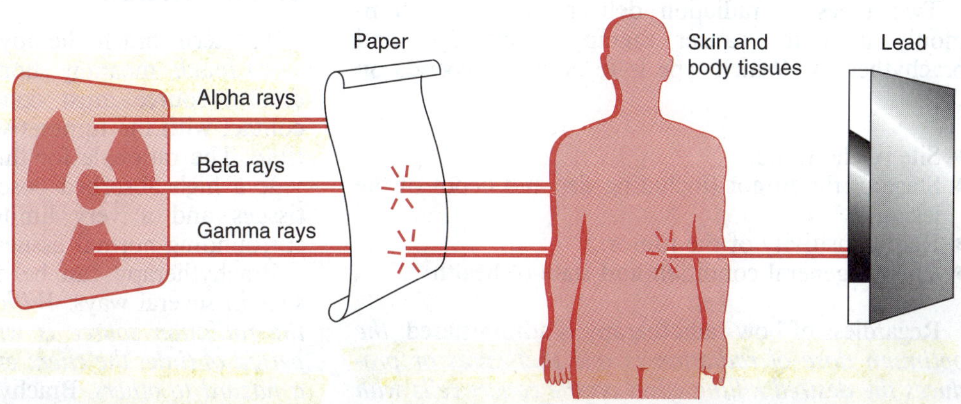

FIGURE 26–1 ◆ Penetrating capacity of different types of radiation.

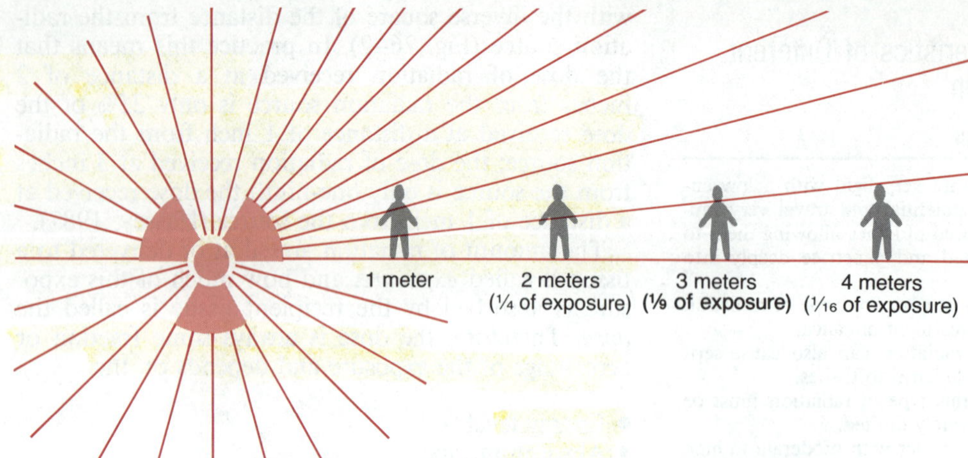

FIGURE 26-2 ◆ The inverse square law of radiation exposure. (From Sedholm, L. N., & Yann, M. I. Y. [1985]. Radiation therapy and nurses' fears of radiation exposure. *Cancer Nursing, 8,* 129–134.)

The total therapeutic dose of radiation to a tumor varies according to the:

- Tumor's size
- Tumor's location
- Tumor's degree of radiation sensitivity
- Radiation sensitivity of the surrounding normal tissues

Some normal tissues are more sensitive to radiation than other normal tissues. For example, a total dose of 1200 rad might be prescribed for a primary liver tumor, but a total dose of 5000 to 6000 rad might be prescribed for a breast carcinoma (delivered over 25 to 30 separate days). If a 6000-rad dose were delivered to the liver, such extensive damage would occur to the liver tissue that the client would experience liver failure and die even if the tumor were eradicated.

Dividing the dose of radiation over many days is called *fractionation.* Standard radiotherapy is usually fractionated between 180 and 250 rad/day, multiplied by as many days as necessary to achieve the optimum prescribed dosage with the least amount of acute and late effects to normal tissues.

Two types of radiation delivery are most commonly used for cancer therapy: teletherapy and brachytherapy. Which type is to be used depends on the:

- Site of the tumor
- Stage of the tumor (including size and depth of the lesion)
- Radiosensitivity of the tumor
- Client's general condition and state of health

Regardless of how radiotherapy is administered, *the optimum dose of radiation is one that cures or produces the desired killing effect on the cancer cells with an acceptable level of damage to normal tissues* (some damage to normal tissues cannot be avoided).

TELETHERAPY

The term teletherapy is derived from the Greek prefix *tele,* meaning far or distant. With teletherapy, the actual radiation source is external to the client and remote from the tumor site. Because the source is external, the client never emits radiation and poses no hazard to anyone else. This type of therapy is also called "beam" radiation.

To increase the accuracy of radiation delivery to the cancer cells, exact localization of the tumor is determined before teletherapy begins. Once the pattern of radiation delivery has been established, the client must always be in exactly the same position for all treatments. The nurse should make sure that the client can get into and maintain this position with relative ease. Position-fixing devices and markings, either on the client's body or on the position-fixing devices, are used to ensure that the client assumes the proper position each day of the treatment.

BRACHYTHERAPY

The term brachytherapy is derived from the Greek word *brach,* meaning short. In brachytherapy, the radiation source must come into direct, continuous contact with the tumor tissues for a specific period of time. The rationale for this treatment plan is to provide a high absorbed dose of radiation in the tumor tissues and a very limited absorbed low dose in surrounding normal tissues (Strohl, 1990).

Brachytherapy can be delivered to the tumor tissues in several ways. *With all types of brachytherapy, the radiation source is within the client; thus, for a period of time, the client emits radiation and can pose a hazard to others.* Brachytherapy involves the use of radioactive isotopes, which can be either in solid form or may be soluble in body fluids. Radiation is delivered to the body surface, interstitial tissues, and body cavities.

UNSEALED RADIATION SOURCES

Soluble isotopes are unsealed radioactive sources. They are administered orally, intravenously, or as an intracavitary instillation. Because the isotopes are unsealed, they are not completely confined to any one area of the body, although they may concentrate more in some specific body tissues than in others. These soluble isotopes enter body fluids, and eventually they are eliminated from the body in various excreta (waste products). *These excreta are radioactive and can be harmful to other people.*

An example of brachytherapy with soluble isotopes is the ingestion or injection of the radionuclide iodine-131 (an iodine base with a half-life of 8.05 days) to treat hyperthyroidism and some thyroid malignancies. The radioactive iodine becomes sequestered in the thyroid gland. The radioactivity of the iodine-131 destroys the thyroid cancer cells. Most of this isotope is eliminated from the body within 48 hours. Once the isotope is eliminated, neither the client nor the excreta are radioactive.

SEALED RADIATION SOURCES

The solid forms of brachytherapy involve the use of sealed radiation sources implanted either within or close to the tumor target tissues. These implants may be temporary or permanent. Most of the implants emit lower energy radiation continuously to the tumor tissues. Some devices, such as seeds or needles, can be placed into the tissues and will stay in place alone. Other solid isotope devices must be held in place within the tissue or cavity by other pieces of equipment. The needles and seeds are radioactive at the time of insertion or implantation, and they have already been preloaded with the radioactive isotope. This type of procedure is called "hot implantation." Some of these devices are so small and the half-life of the isotope so short that the device is permanently left in place (most often for clients with prostate cancer). Other devices are removed from the client and are reused in other clients.

In the technique of afterloading, the implant, without the radioactive isotope, is placed within the cavity, with special devices (applicators) that hold it in position. When placement has been ascertained and the client is in the proper environment, the implants are loaded with the radioisotope. After the prescribed dose has been delivered, the implant, radioisotopes, and position-holding devices are removed. *With solid implants, the client emits radiation while the implant is in place, but the excreta are not radioactive* (Chart 26–1).

The radiation delivered by brachytherapy is ionizing and has the same tissue effects and limitations as ionizing radiation delivered by external sources. Most commonly, brachytherapy is used in conjunction with teletherapy for maximum tumor kill (Strohl, 1990).

CHART 26–1

Nursing Care Highlight ◆ Care of the Client with Sealed Implants of Radioactive Sources

- Assign the client to a private room with a private bath.
- Place a "Caution: Radioactive Material" sign on the door of the client's room
- Wear a dosimeter film badge at all times while caring for clients with radioactive implants. The badge offers no protection, but measures an individual's exposure to radiation and should be used by only one individual.
- Pregnant nurses should not care for these clients; do not allow children under 16 years of age or pregnant women to visit.
- Limit each visitor to one-half hour per day. Be sure visitors are at least 6 ft from the source.
- Never touch the radioactive source with bare hands. In the rare instance that it is dislodged, use a longhandled forceps to retrieve it. Deposit the radioactive source in the lead container kept in the client's room.
- Save all dressings and bed linens until after the radioactive source is removed. After the source is removed, dispose of dressings and linens in the usual manner. Other equipment can be removed from the room at any time.

SIDE EFFECTS OF RADIATION THERAPY FOR CANCER

Because the immediate and long-term side effects for all types of radiation are limited to the tissues exposed to the radiation, side effects vary according to the site. Skin changes and hair loss (alopecia) are local but are likely to be permanent, depending on total absorbed dose (Hilderley & Dow, 1991; Sitton, 1992a, 1992b).

Depending on the dose, altered taste sensations and fatigue are two systemic side effects often noted in clients receiving external beam radiation, regardless of the site of radiation. The changes in taste sensation are attributed to the metabolites that are rapidly released and absorbed systemically from dead and dying cells. In particular, many clients experience an aversion to the taste of red meats. The symptom of fatigue may be related to the hypermetabolism and increased energy demands needed to repair radiation-damaged cells (Hilderley & Dow, 1991).

Radiation damage to normal tissues during cancer therapy can initiate inflammatory responses that cause tissue fibrosis and scarring. The effects of these processes may not be apparent for many years after radiation treatment. For example, women who receive high-dose radiation therapy for uterine cancer may experience radiation-induced changes in the colon years later, resulting in constipation and obstruction. Because radiation treatment can also cause mutation of normal cells, normal tissues in the radiation path are at an increased risk for undergoing malignant changes any time after therapy is completed (Fraser and Tucker, 1989).

NURSING CARE OF CLIENTS UNDERGOING RADIATION THERAPY

Most clients are anxious about the use of radiation. The nurse should be knowledgeable about the nature of radiation and should be able to explain its purpose and side effects to clients and families.

Chart 26–2 summarizes skin care and precautions for clients during radiation therapy. The nurse instructs the client not to remove the markings when cleaning the skin until the entire course of radiation therapy is completed. Skin in the path of radiation becomes very dry and may break down. The nurse instructs the client not to use lotions or ointments in these areas unless the radiologist prescribes them. Because skin in the radiation path is more sensitive to sun damage, the nurse advises clients to avoid direct skin exposure to the sun.

CHART 26–2

Education Guide ◆ Radiation Therapy for Cancer

- Wash the irradiated area gently each day with either water alone, or a mild soap and water.
- Use your hand rather than a washcloth to be more gentle.
- Rinse soap thoroughly from your skin.
- Take care not to remove the markings that indicate exactly where the beam of radiation is to be focused.
- Dry the irradiated area with patting motions rather than rubbing motions, using a clean, soft towel or cloth.
- Use no powders, ointments, lotions or creams on your skin at the radiation site unless they are prescribed by your *radiologist.*
- Wear soft clothing over the skin at the radiation site.
- Avoid wearing belts, buckles, straps, or any type of clothing that binds or rubs the skin at the radiation site.
- Keep the irradiated area from being exposed to the sun.
- Avoid heat exposure.

Normal tissues most sensitive to external radiation are hematopoietic (blood-producing), epithelial (including skin, mucous membranes, and hair follicles), and gonadal (reproductive) tissues. Some changes caused by radiation are permanent. Long-term problems experienced by clients vary with the location and dose of radiation administered. For example, radiation to the throat and upper chest can cause the client to have difficulty in swallowing. Head and neck radiation may damage the salivary glands and cause the client to have a dry mouth. The nurse teaches the client what types of symptoms might be expected from the location and dose of radiation he or she is receiving.

Chemotherapy

Chemotherapy, the treatment of disease through the use of chemical agents, has assumed a major role in the management of clients with cancer. Chemotherapy as a cancer treatment is used to cure, to increase mean survival time, and to decrease the chance of specific life-threatening complications.

RATIONALE FOR CHEMOTHERAPY AS A CANCER THERAPY

A characteristic of cancer growth is the ability of cancer cells to separate from the original tumor, spread to new areas, and establish new cancers at distant sites; this process is called metastasis (Cooper, 1992). It is clear that clients with metastatic disease will die of their cancers unless treatment focuses on the metastatic cancer cells as well as the original cancer cells (Fraser & Tucker, 1989). Chemotherapy is instrumental in the treatment of cancer because the effects of chemotherapy are exerted systemically and thus provide the opportunity to kill metastatic cancer cells that may have escaped local treatment. Table 26–7 indicates the general responsiveness of chemotherapy for specific cancers.

MECHANISM OF ACTION

Chemotherapy can be a successful form of cancer treatment because it has some demonstrated selectivity for cancer cells over normal cells. The killing effect of chemotherapy on cancer cells appears to be related to its ability to damage deoxyribonucleic acid (DNA) and interfere with successful cell division. Because of this mechanism of action, the tumors most sensitive to chemotherapy are those that have rapid growth.

Unfortunately, chemotherapeutic agents usually are administered systemically and exert their cytotoxic (cell-damaging) effects against both healthy and cancerous cells. The normal cells most profoundly affected by systemic chemotherapy are those that undergo frequent cell division. These tissues include

TABLE 26–7 General Tumor Responsiveness to Standard Chemotherapy

Malignancies Usually Very Responsive to Chemotherapy

- Acute lymphocytic leukemia (ALL)
- Chronic lymphocytic leukemia (CLL)
- Lymphoma (Hodgkin's)
- Choriocarcinoma
- Small cell lung cancer

Malignancies Often Responsive to Chemotherapy

- Breast carcinoma
- Testicular carcinoma
- Prostatic carcinoma
- Head and neck carcinoma
- Acute myelocytic leukemia (AML)
- Chronic myelocytic leukemia (CML)

Malignancies Occasionally Responsive to Chemotherapy

- Colo-rectal carcinomas
- Central nervous system tumors
- Multiple myeloma
- Ovarian carcinoma
- Uterine carcinoma

Malignancies Usually Non-responsive to Chemotherapy

- Renal cell carcinoma
- Pancreatic carcinoma
- Bladder carcinoma
- Liver carcinoma (primary)
- Non-small cell carcinomas of the lung

Data from: Guy, J. (1991). Medical oncology—the agents. In S. Baird, R. McCorkle, & M. Grant (Eds.), *Cancer nursing: a comprehensive textbook* (pp. 266–290). Philadelphia: W.B. Saunders.

skin, hair, epithelial lining of the gastrointestinal tract, spermatocytes, and hematopoietic cells (Tenenbaum, 1989).

Chemotherapy encompasses a broad classification of drugs or chemical compounds that are effective in killing cancer cells. Agents used for chemotherapy are classified by:

- The specific types of biologic action they exert in the cancer cell
- The specific period in the life of a cell during which the chemotherapeutic agent is most likely to succeed in disrupting vital cell processes

Table 26–8 lists categories and specific chemotherapeutic agents.

ANTIMETABOLITES

Antimetabolites are chemicals that have structures similar to normal metabolites that play essential roles in critical enzymatic cell processes. Most enzymatic reactions require "cofactors" in order to begin or to continue the reaction. Many cofactors are vitamins. Antimetabolites closely resemble these cofactors and literally fool the cancer cells into using the antimetabolites in critical physiologic reactions rather than the real cofactors. Because antimetabolites cannot function as proper cofactors, their presence interferes with some critical cell processes needed for successful cell division and cell division is either impaired or prevented. Most antimetabolites are structurally similar to vitamins, coenzymes, and nucleotides (purines and pyrimidines).

ANTITUMOR ANTIBIOTICS

Antitumor antibiotics make up a class of antineoplastic drugs that were initially developed to combat standard bacterial infections. The mechanism of action is to inflict significant damage on the cell's DNA, thus interrupting DNA or ribonucleic acid (RNA) synthesis (and sometimes both). Exactly how the interruptions occur varies with each antibiotic.

ALKYLATING AGENTS

All alkylating agents cause cross-linking of DNA by various means. Whatever the mechanism, the double strands of DNA become more tightly bound together (usually in intermittent areas rather than continuously down the whole strand). This tight binding causes some areas of the DNA to be misread or not read at all during DNA and RNA synthesis, thus resulting in inhibition of cell division.

ANTIMITOTIC AGENTS

Antimitotic agents are alkaloids derived from specific plants. The vinca alkaloids are derived from the periwinkle plant. Their primary mechanism of action is to interfere with the proper formation of microtubules so that cells cannot complete mitosis during cell division. As a result, either the cell does not divide at all, or it divides only once, resulting in two daughter cells that have unequal amounts of DNA and thus cannot continue to divide.

MISCELLANEOUS CHEMOTHERAPEUTIC AGENTS

The actions of other chemotherapeutic agents do not fit any of the broad categories of chemotherapeutic agents. Because the number of such agents is small, they are described here.

PROCARBAZINE

Procarbazine (Matulane, Natulanar) is an enzyme inhibitor that appears to have several effects on DNA. Although the mechanism of action is not well understood, the agent inhibits both DNA and RNA synthesis and causes the double strands of DNA to "fall apart."

DACARBAZINE

Although the exact mechanism of action is not known, dacarbazine (DTIC) exerts some cross-linking

TABLE 26–8 Categories of Chemotherapeutic Agents

Generic Name	Trade Name	Usual Dose	Nadir
	Antimetabolites		
• Methotrexate	• Amethopterin, MTX, Mexate, Folex	• 3.3 mg/m²	• 10–14 days
• 6 Mercaptopurine	• Purinethol	• 80–100 mg/m²	• 5–40 days
• 6 Thioguanine	• 6-TG	• 2–3 mg/kg	• 1–4 weeks
• 5 Fluorouracil	• 5-FU, Adrucil, Efudex, Fluoroplex	• 300–750 mg/m²	• 9–14 days
• FUDR	• Floxuridine	• 0.1–0.6 mg/kg	• 4–7 days
• Cytosine arabinoside	• Cytosar, Ara-C, Cytarabine	• 100–200 mg/m²	• 4–7 days
	Antibiotics		
• Bleomycin	• Blenoxane	• 10–20 U/m²	• 7–14 days
• Dactinomycin	• Actinomycin-D, Cosmegen	• 1–2 mg/m²	• 14–21 days
• Doxorubicin	• Adriamycin, Rubex	• 50–80 mg/m²	• 10–15 days
• Daunorubicin	• Cerubidine	• 30–60 mg/m²	• 10–14 days
• Mithramycin	• Mithracin, Plicamycin	• 0.8–1.6 mg/m²	• 10–12 days
• Mitomycin-C	• Mutamycin	• 10–20 mg/m²	• 21–50 days
• Mitoxantrone	• Novantrone	• 14 mg/m²	• 7–10 days
	Alkylating Agents		
• Cyclophosphamide	• Cytoxan, Proytox🍁	• 50–500 mg/m²	• 7–14 days
• Cisplatin	• Platinol, Abiplatin🍁	• 25–120 mg/m²	• 10–20 days
• Mechlorethamine	• Nitrogen mustard, Mustargen	• 1.6 mg/m²	• 10–14 days
• Busulfan	• Myleran	• 1–8 mg/m²	• 14–21 days
• Chlorambucil	• Leukeran	• 1–4 mg/m²	• >28 days
• Melphalan	• Alkeran	• 1–6 mg/m²	• 14–21 days
• Carmustine	• BCNU	• 200–250 mg/m²	• 4–6 weeks
• Lomustine	• CCNU, CecNU	• 130 mg/m²	• 4–6 weeks
• Triethylene thiophosphoramide	• Thiotepa	• 10–30 mg/m²	• 15–30 days
• Streptozocin	• Zanosar	• 500–1500 mg/m²	• 14 days
	Antimitotics		
• Vincristine	• Oncovin, Vinerex	• 0.5–2.0 mg/m²	• 7 days
• Vinblastine	• Velban, Velbe🍁, VLB	• 5–10 mg/m²	• 5–11 days
• Vindesine	• DAVA, Eldesine	• 2 mg/m²	• 2–7 days
• Etoposide	• VP16, VePeside	• 50–100 mg/m²	• 8–10 days
• Taxol	• Paclitaxel	• 100–250 mg/m²	• 8–11 days
	Other Agents		
• Procarbazine	• Matulane, Natulanar	• 100–300 mg	• 14–28 days
• Dacarbazine	• DTIC	• 75–250 mg/m²	• 10–14 days
• Hydroxyurea	• Hydrea	• 25 mg/kg	• 4–7 days
• Asparaginase	• Elspar, Kidrolase🍁	• 200–1000 IU/kg	• 4–10 days

or alkylating of nucleotide effects on DNA and, to a more limited extent, on RNA. Thus, it is sometimes classified as an alkylating agent, although it is more than that.

HYDROXYUREA

Hydroxyurea (Hydrea) interferes with DNA synthesis in much the same way that antimetabolites do, although it is not similar to any known metabolite.

ASPARAGINASE

Asparaginase (Elspar, Kidrolase🍁) is an enzyme that degrades the amino acid asparagine. Some tumor cells, as with most normal cells, require this amino acid in order to survive and divide. Normal cells, however, have an additional "survival pathway" that converts other asparagine precursors into asparagine in the cell, whereas some tumor cells cannot accomplish this.

COMBINATION CHEMOTHERAPY

Chemotherapy for cancer usually involves the timed administration of more than one specific antineoplastic drug, or combination chemotherapy. Using more than one drug is much more effective in killing cancer cells than using a single agent. Unfortunately, the damage caused to normal tissues is increased with combination chemotherapy.

Table 26–9 presents a standard protocol of combination chemotherapy for Hodgkin's lymphoma. The selection of drugs is based on known tumor sensitivity to the drugs and the degree of side effects expected to result. For example, most chemothera-

TABLE 26–9 Typical Combination Chemotherapy Schedule for Clients with Hodgkin's Lymphoma

MOPP

M = Mechlorethamine (nitrogen mustard)
6 mg IV/m^2 on days 1 and 8
O = Oncovin (vincristine)
2.0 mg IV/m^2 on days 1 and 8
P = Procarbazine (Matulane)
100 mg PO/m^2 continuously days 1 through 14
P = Prednisone (APO-prednisone✱)
40 mg PO/m^2 continuously days 1 through 14 (only during cycles 1 and 4)

These drugs are given together as a "cycle." The cycle is administered for the first 2 weeks followed by a resting or recovery period of 2 weeks. After the recovery period, the ABVD regimen is administered (on one day) followed by a 2-week recovery period.

ABVD

A = Adriamycin (doxorubicin)
25 mg IV/m^2
B = Bleomycin (Blenoxane)
10 units IV/m^2
V = Vinblastine (Velban,Velbe✱)
6 mg IV/m^2
D = Dacarbazine (DTIC)
375 mg IV/m^2

peutic drugs suppress bone marrow activity and immune function to some degree, and some agents have a more profound effect than others. The following agents are considered profoundly immunosuppressive: busulfan, cyclophosphamide, etoposide, dactinomycin, doxorubicin, and mechlorethamine. In addition to variation in the degree to which chemotherapeutic agents suppress immune function, there is also variation in the timing of drug-induced immunosuppression.

The time during which bone marrow activity and peripheral white blood cell counts are at their lowest levels after chemotherapy is the *nadir*. The nadir occurs at different times for different chemotherapeutic agents (see Table 26–8). For instance, the expected nadir after cytosine arabinoside administration is 5 to 7 days; after methotrexate, 10 to 14 days, and after mitomycin-C, about 4 weeks. Combination chemotherapy is planned to avoid prescribing different drugs with nadirs at or near the same time in order to minimize immunosuppression.

DRUG DOSAGE

Doses of most chemotherapeutic agents are calculated according to the type of cancer present and the client's size. A few drug dosages are calculated in terms of milligrams per kilogram (mg/kg) of body weight. More frequently, calculations are based on milligrams per square meter (mg/meter^2) of total body surface area (TBSA). This parameter takes into account the client's height and weight and is calculated as follows: Multiply the height of the client (in centimeters) by the weight of the client (in kilograms), and divide the result by 10,000 (moving the decimal point four spaces to the left). As an example, a woman who is 68 inches tall (173 cm) and weighs 143 pounds (65 kg) would have a TBSA of 11,245 cm^2, or 1.12 m^2.

DRUG SCHEDULE

Chemotherapeutic agents are administered on a regular basis, timed to maximize cancer cell kill and to minimize complications caused by damage to normal cells. The schedule may vary somewhat to accommodate individual client responses to therapy, but usually chemotherapy is scheduled every 3 to 4 weeks for a specified number of times (on an average, 6 to 12 times). The entire planned schedule is the *course* of chemotherapy; the individual days of administration are the *rounds*.

DRUG ADMINISTRATION

Most chemotherapeutic drugs are administered intravenously, although other routes may be used for specific cancers (Table 26–10). Techniques and nursing care considerations for routes other than intravenous (IV) are described with the specific cancer type most commonly associated with the special administration route.

The intravenous route is the one most preferred for chemotherapy because the therapeutic effects of the drugs are rapidly available and many of these agents are irritating or damaging to tissues. A major complication of IV administration is extravasation, or movement of the IV needle so that the drug leaks into the surrounding skin and subcutaneous tissues.

TABLE 26–10 Routes of Chemotherapy Administration

Route	Typical Cancer
Oral	• Hodgkin's lymphoma • Leukemia (maintenance phase) • Small cell lung cancer
Intravenous	• Most solid tumors, leukemias • Lymphomas
Intra-arterial	• Hepatic tumors (primary and metastatic) • Head and neck cancers

Isolated limb perfusion	• Cancers confined to a limb
	  • Osteogenic sarcoma
	  • Ewing's sarcoma
	  • Rhabdomyosarcoma
	  • Regional melanoma

Intracavitary	
• Intraperitoneal	• Ovarian cancer
• Intraventricular	• Brain tumors
• Intrathecal	• Brain tumors • Prophylaxis for acute lymphocytic leukemia

The results of extravasation when the administered agents are vesicants (chemicals that cause tissue damage on direct contact) can include pain, infection, and tissue loss, sometimes necessitating surgical intervention. (See Table 15–7 for chemotherapeutic agents that are known vesicants.)

The most important nursing intervention for extravasation is prevention (Wood & Gullo, 1993). (See also Chapter 15 and Chart 15–9.) Most extravasations resolve without extensive treatment if less than 0.5 mL of the irritating drug has infiltrated into the tissues. If a larger amount has infused into the tissues, however, extensive tissue damage occurs and surgical intervention may be necessary (Barton-Burke et al., 1991). Immediate treatment depends on the specific agent extravasated. With some agents, cold compresses to the area are appropriate; for others, warm compresses are recommended. Antidotes may be injected into the site of extravasation. The nurse consults with the oncologist and pharmacist to determine the specific antidote needed for the agent extravasated.

Most chemotherapeutic agents are readily absorbed through the skin and mucous membranes. As a result, health care workers, especially nurses and pharmacists, who prepare and/or administer chemotherapeutic agents are at risk for absorbing these agents during occupational exposure. Even at low doses, chronic exposure to chemotherapeutic agents can seriously affect health. Therefore, nurses and other health care professionals must use extreme caution and wear protective clothing whenever preparing, administering, or disposing of chemotherapeutic agents. The Occupational Safety and Health Administration (OSHA) and the Oncology Nursing Society have established practice guidelines and protective standards.

SIDE EFFECTS OF CHEMOTHERAPY FOR CANCER

Clients experience distress as a result of specific serious side effects associated with aggressive chemotherapy. These side effects include alopecia (hair loss), nausea and vomiting, the development of open sores on mucous membranes (mucositis), and various skin changes. Common side effects of chemotherapy on the hematopoietic (blood-producing) system can be life-threatening and are the most frequent reason for altering the dosage or the schedule of chemotherapy. Chemotoxic effects on the blood-forming cells of the bone marrow also produce specific side effects, including immunosuppression, anemia, and thrombocytopenia (decreased numbers of platelets).

NURSING CARE OF CLIENTS UNDERGOING CHEMOTHERAPY

The major nursing care issue during chemotherapy for cancer is management of the client's distressing symptoms associated with the therapy. For some clients, the symptoms are so disagreeable that they decide not to remain in treatment.

ALOPECIA

OVERVIEW

Clients receiving chemotherapy for cancer frequently experience whole body hair loss. Some drugs, such as methotrexate and cytoxan, may cause only some thinning of scalp hair. Others, such as doxorubicin, vincristine, and cisplatin, cause a more complete hair loss.

COLLABORATIVE MANAGEMENT

The nurse reassures the client that hair loss is temporary. Usually, hair regrowth begins about 1 month after chemotherapy is completed. The nurse cautions the client that the new hair may differ from the client's original hair in color, texture, and thickness.

No known treatment totally prevents alopecia. Techniques to reduce the amount of chemotherapeutic agents that reaches the hair follicles during treatment have been somewhat effective in reducing scalp hair loss. These techniques include applying ice packs and caps to the scalp and/or applying a scalp tourniquet during chemotherapy administration and for a few hours immediately afterward. These techniques are not endorsed by oncologists or oncology nurses because it is believed that some circulating cancer cells escape chemotherapy, resulting in a less favorable treatment outcome.

Nurses can assist clients in selecting a type of head covering that suits the client's financial means and lifestyle. High-quality wigs are expensive but can look very much like the client's own hair. Many local units of the American Cancer Society offer wigs that other clients have used temporarily and have donated to be lent to other clients with cancer.

Clients can disguise hair loss relatively inexpensively by the creative use of scarves and turbans. Both are available in many fabrics, styles, and prices. Many clients wear caps while alopecia is present.

NAUSEA AND VOMITING

OVERVIEW

Nausea and vomiting are caused by chemotherapy-induced stimulation of chemoreceptor trigger zones in the brain. Most chemotherapeutic agents are emetogenic (vomiting-inducing) to some degree, depending on the dose, but the agents that produce the most severe nausea and vomiting include cisplatin, doxorubicin, mithramycin, nitrogen mustard, vinblastine, and etoposide. Most of these agents induce nausea and vomiting during drug administration and for 1 to 2 days afterward. Cisplatin induces delayed nausea and vomiting that can continue as long as 5 to 7 days after administration.

COLLABORATIVE MANAGEMENT

A multitude of oral and parenteral antiemetics (agents that alleviate nausea and vomiting) are available, including the phenothiazine derivatives, benzodiazepines, and serotonin antagonists. These agents vary in their effectiveness in controlling chemotherapy-induced nausea and vomiting. Many antiemetics are central nervous system (CNS) depressants and may induce drowsiness and/or confusion in clients. Usually, one or more antiemetics are administered before the chemotherapy as well as afterward. Other drugs used in combination with the antiemetics are corticosteroids. A new class of antiemetics that seem to act at the chemoreceptor trigger zone is the serotonin antagonists. One of these, ondansetron (Zofran), has been very beneficial for clients with previously resistant chemotherapy-induced nausea and vomiting (Egan et al., 1992).

The nurse assists the client with chemotherapy-induced nausea and vomiting to achieve comfort through nonpharmacologic means. Progressive muscle relaxation and guided imagery may help reduce anxiety and relieve some nausea and vomiting. The nurse also assesses the client for complications associated with excessive vomiting, such as dehydration and electrolyte imbalances.

Some facilities have created clinical pathways for clients with nausea, vomiting, and dehydration related to cancer and its treatment. For an example, see page 576.

CHART 26–3

Nursing Care Highlights ◆ Mouth Care for Clients with Mucositis

- Examine the client's mouth (including under the roof and tongue and between the teeth and cheek) every 4 hours.
- Document the location, size, and character of fissures, blisters, sores, or drainage.
- Get an order to obtain specimens of sores or drainage for culture.
- Brush the teeth and tongue with a soft-bristled brush or sponges every 8 hours.
- Rinse the mouth with solution of ½ peroxide and ½ normal saline every 12 hours.
- Avoid use of alcohol or glycerin-based mouthwashes.
- Administer antimicrobial medications as prescribed.
- Administer topical analgesic medications as prescribed or as needed.
- Help the conscious client to "swish and spit" room-temperature tap water or normal saline as needed.
- Apply petrolatum jelly to the client's lips after each episode of mouth care and as needed.
- Assist the client in using "artificial saliva" as needed, if ordered.
- Assist the client in menu choices to avoid spicy or hard food.
- Offer complete mouth care before and after every meal.

MUCOSITIS

OVERVIEW

Mucositis is the presence of sores in mucous membranes. Clients undergoing chemotherapy for cancer frequently have mucositis of the entire gastrointestinal (GI) tract, especially in the mouth (stomatitis). Normally, the mucous membrane of the GI tract undergoes rapid cell division and replaces dead or damaged cells quickly. Under the influence of chemotherapy, mucous membrane cells are killed more rapidly than they are replaced, resulting in the formation of sores. Mouth sores are painful and interfere with the client's desire and ability to eat. (Chart 26–3 lists nursing care highlights for people with mucositis.)

COLLABORATIVE MANAGEMENT

A major component in the management of oral mucositis is oral hygiene. The nurse stresses the importance of good and frequent oral hygiene, which includes tooth cleaning and mouth rinsing. Because most clients with chemotherapy-induced mucositis also have bone marrow suppression, clients must take care to avoid traumatizing the oral mucosa. The nurse instructs the client to use a soft-bristled toothbrush or disposable mouth sponges. Clients should avoid using dental floss and water pressure gum cleaners (such as a water pick) at this time. The nurse encourages the client to rinse the mouth at least every hour with plain water or saline. The nurse warns the client about use of commercial mouthwashes that contain alcohol or other drying agents that may further irritate the mucosa.

It is very important for clients to keep oral hygiene equipment clean. The nurse should remind clients not to share toothbrushes with anyone. Clients can clean toothbrushes daily by running them through a home dishwasher or rinsing them with either a concentrated solution of liquid bleach or hydrogen peroxide.

Many compounds are available for pain relief from stomatitis or mucositis. Many hospitals offer their own special mixture that can be used as a "swish and spit" topical medication. These mixtures usually contain a local anesthetic combined with anti-inflammatory agents. The nurse stresses that these mixtures are not to be swallowed.

BONE MARROW SUPPRESSION

OVERVIEW

Bone marrow suppression results in decreased numbers of circulating leukocytes, erythrocytes, and platelets. Decreased leukocyte numbers cause immu-

1 - 7-3
2 - 3-11
3 - 11-7

LAST ☐ Chemotherapy Date ______
☐ Radiation Date ______

CARE NEED	DAY 1 ADMIT DAY date ______	DAY 2 date ______	DAY 3 date ______	Day 4 date ______
ASSESSMENTS/ TREATMENTS	Postural BP on admission & prn Weight documented I&O Baseline vital signs documented Vital signs q shift and prn Review old chart Previous admit for n/v/d date: ____ Safety/fall assessment	AM weight I&O Vital signs q shift - stable Evaluate lab results	AM weight I&O Vital signs ONLY 7-3 and 3-11 if stable	
FLUIDS/ NUTRITIONS	Start IV hydration @ admit 1000cc D_5 ½NS 20 KCL @ 100 IV antiemetics Adjust IV fluids based on lab results within 8° of admit Clear liquids as tolerated	IV fluids continue Start PO or PR antiemetics q 6° around-the-clock Cont. IV antiemetics for BREAKTHROUGH Clear liquids-intake: 7-3 500; 3-11 400; 11-7 100 Advance to full liquid dinner or as tolerated	DC or HL IV by noon Antiemetics AC and HS PO only Advance to regular diet for lunch Fluid intake: 7-3 600; 3-11 500; 11-7 100	
LAB/ DIAGNOSTICS	CBC-if not available from MD office SMA 20-SMA 7 stat	SMA-7		
ACTIVITY	Up to BR Ambulate in room 1x day/evenings	Up to BR Ambulate ½ length of hallway TID	Ambulate full length of hallway TID	
SELF-CARE	Mouth care Face/hand washing Feeding	Mouth care Self bath @ bedside Feeding	Mouth care Shower	
DISCHARGE PLANNING	Evaluate home care support Refer to Social Services if: Social Work intervention needed	Document discharge plan: Social Services or Nursing	Finalize home care needs	Discharge by 11:00 AM
TEACHING	____ Assess current knowledge of antiemetics; document on kardex	____ Medication instruction ____ Dietary consult evaluate need for diet counseling	____ Review/reinforce med instruction ____ Review/reinforce diet instruction	____ Verbalizes understanding of meds for home care and diet
	RN ____ D ____ E ____ N	RN ____ D ____ E ____ N	RN ____ D ____ E ____ N	RN ____ D ____ E ____ N

Initial	Signature	Initial	Signature	Initial	Signature	Initial	Signature

Good Samaritan Hospital
A division of Good Samaritan Community Healthcare
407-14th Ave. SE, PO Box 1247, Puyallup, WA 98371-0192 (206) 848-6661

Oncology
Clinical Pathway
Nausea/Vomiting/Dehydration

Clinical Pathway: Nausea, vomiting, and dehydration in clients with cancer. (Karen Graybeal, MS, RN; Cynthia Marion, RN, OCN; Margaret Brown, MN, RN, OCN; Patty Patch, RN, OCN; Deanna Kruckenberg, RN, OCN; courtesy of Good Samaritan Hospital, Puyallup, WA.)

CP

nosuppression. Decreased erythrocytes and platelets cause hypoxia, fatigue, and increased bleeding tendency.

Immunosuppression, which places the client at extreme risk for infection, is the major dose-limiting side effect of chemotherapy for cancer. Most chemotherapeutic agents suppress bone marrow function to some degree. The agents associated with severe bone marrow suppression include busulfan, cyclophosphamide, cytosine arabinoside, dactinomycin, doxorubicin, daunorubicin, etoposide, mitomycin-C, nitrogen mustard, and triethylenethiophosphoramide. Suppression of immune function is the most life-threatening side effect for the client and presents the nurse with a most serious challenge—to provide the client with the understanding, environment, and support to withstand this potentially devastating complication.

The clinical problems associated with the immediate effects of cancer treatment on immune function are related primarily to a transient loss or impairment of inflammatory responses to tissue injury or invasion by microorganisms. The severity and duration of the impairment are related directly to the dosage of specific chemotherapeutic agents. Although this impairment is usually temporary, with good recovery of inflammatory responses evident within weeks or months of therapy completion, the seriousness of the potential infection complications makes this problem a major treatment concern. The infectious processes most commonly observed during this period include those of fungal origin, yeast, some residual viral breakthrough, and a wide variety of bacteria.

Decreased numbers of circulating erythrocytes (anemia) and platelets (thrombocytopenia) result from the generalized bone marrow suppression caused by some chemotherapeutic agents. The anemia causes the client to feel fatigued, and some tissues must operate under hypoxic conditions. The cardiac and respiratory systems may be overtaxed in their effort to maintain adequate oxygenation. Thrombocytopenia increases the risk for uncontrolled bleeding. When the client's platelets are less than $50,000/mm^3$, any small trauma can lead to episodes of prolonged bleeding. When the number of platelets is less than $20,000/mm^3$, the client may experience spontaneous and uncontrollable bleeding, which necessitates extensive transfusion therapy and other interventions to resolve.

CHART 26–4

Nursing Care Highlight ◆ Care of the Client with Immunosuppression

- Place the client in a private room whenever possible.
- Use good hand-washing technique before touching the client or any of the client's belongings.
- Ensure that the client's room and bathroom are cleaned at least once each day.
- Do not use supplies from common areas for immunosuppressed clients. For example, keep a sleeve or box of paper cups in the client's room and do not share this box with any other client. Other articles include drinking straws, plastic knives and forks, dressing materials, gloves, and bandages.
- Limit the number of care personnel entering the client's room.
- Monitor vital signs every 4 hours; note minor temperature elevation, which may suggest early sepsis.
- Inspect the client's mouth at least every 8 hours.
- Inspect the client's skin and mucous membranes (especially the anal area) for the presence of fissures and abscesses at least every 8 hours.
- Inspect open areas, such as IV sites, every 4 hours for manifestations of infection.
- Change wound dressings daily.
- Obtain specimens of all suspicious areas for culture, and promptly notify physician.
- Assist the client in performing coughing and deep breathing exercises.
- Encourage activity at appropriate level for the client's current health status
- Change IV tubing daily.
- Keep frequently used equipment in the room for use by the client only (e.g., blood pressure cuff, stethoscope, thermometer).
- Limit visitors to healthy adults.
- Wear a mask when entering the room.
- Use strict aseptic technique for all invasive procedures.
- Monitor the white blood cell count, especially the absolute neutrophil count (ANC), daily.
- Avoid the use of indwelling urinary catheters.
- Keep fresh flowers and potted plants out of the client's room.
- Teach the client to eat a low-bacteria diet (see Chart 26–5).

COLLABORATIVE MANAGEMENT

The nurse works closely with the client and other health care professionals to provide safe care to clients at risk for infection. Chart 26–4 lists specific nursing care actions to prevent infection among immunosuppressed clients. Good hand washing by the nurse before contact with the client is the cornerstone for prevention of infection. The nurse should practice asepsis (prevention of contact with microorganisms) when any invasive technique or procedure must be done.

Many clients remain at home during periods of immunosuppression. The nurse teaches the client and family precautions to take to reduce the client's chances of developing an infection (Chart 26–5).

The nurse provides a safe hospital environment for the client with thrombocytopenia and teaches the client how to avoid excessive bleeding when he or she is discharged from the hospital before the platelet count has returned to normal. Chart 26–6 lists nursing actions to reduce the client's risk for bleeding

CHART 26–5

Education Guide ♦ Prevention of Infection

- Avoid crowds and other large gatherings of people who might be ill.
- Do not share personal toilet articles, such as toothbrushes, toothpaste, washcloths, or deodorant sticks, with others.
- If possible, bathe daily.
- Wash the armpits, groin, genitals, and anal area at least twice a day with an antimicrobial soap.
- Clean your toothbrush daily by either running it through the dishwasher or rinsing it in liquid laundry bleach.
- Wash your hands thoroughly with an antimicrobial soap before you eat or drink, after touching a pet, after shaking hands with anyone, as soon as you come home from any outing, and after using the toilet.
- Eat a low-bacteria diet, and avoid salads, raw fruit and vegetables, undercooked meat, pepper, and paprika.
- Wash dishes between use with hot, sudsy water or use a dishwasher.
- Do not drink water that has been standing for longer than 15 minutes.
- Do not reuse cups and glasses without washing.
- Do not change pet litter boxes.
- Take your temperature at least once a day.
- Report any of the following signs or symptoms of infection to your physician immediately:
  - Temperature over 100° F (38°C)
  - Persistent cough (with or without sputum)
  - Pus or foul-smelling drainage from any open skin area or normal body opening
  - Presence of a boil or abscess
  - Urine that is cloudy or foul-smelling or that causes burning on urination
- Take all prescribed medications as the doctor ordered.
- Do not dig in the garden or work with houseplants.

during hospitalization. The nurse teaches the client practices to prevent bleeding and what to do if bleeding should occur after the client is discharged (Chart 26–7).

Hormonal Manipulation

RATIONALE FOR HORMONAL MANIPULATION AS CANCER THERAPY

Hormones are naturally occurring special chemicals secreted by endocrine (ductless) glands and picked up by capillaries. Once in the bloodstream, hormones circulate to all body areas but exert their effects only on specific target tissues (this is different for each hormone). Some hormones make hormone-sensitive tumors grow more rapidly. Some tumors actually require the presence of specific hormones in order to divide. Therefore, altering the availability of these hormones to hormonally sensitive tumors can directly alter the growth rate of the tumor.

MECHANISM OF ACTION

HORMONES

Hormonal manipulation can help to control some types of cancer for many years; however, this therapy does not lead to cure. The endocrine system usually keeps hormones within narrow ranges, and a balance is maintained. When a large amount of one hormone is administered, it upsets the balance and disturbs the uptake of some other hormones. If a tumor depends on hormone A for growth and a large quantity of hormone B (structurally but not functionally related to A) is given to the client, hormone B will interfere with the tumor's uptake of hormone A or will limit

CHART 26–6

Nursing Care Highlight ♦ Care of the Client with Thrombocytopenia

- Handle the client gently.
- Use a lift sheet when moving and positioning the client in bed.
- Avoid intramuscular injections and venipunctures.
- When injections or venipunctures are necessary, use the smallest-gauge needle for the task.
- Apply firm pressure to the needlestick site for 10 minutes or until site no longer oozes blood.
- Apply ice to areas of trauma.
- Test all urine and stool for the presence of occult blood.
- Observe IV sites every 2 hours for bleeding.
- Avoid trauma to rectal tissues:
  - Do not take temperatures rectally.
  - Do not administer enemas.
  - Administer well-lubricated suppositories and with caution.
  - Advise the client not to have anal intercourse.
- Measure the client's abdominal girth daily.
- Use an electric razor.
- Teach the client to avoid mouth trauma by:
  - Using soft-bristled toothbrush or tooth sponges
  - Not flossing
  - Avoiding dental work, especially extractions
  - Avoiding hard foods
  - Making certain that dentures fit and do not rub
- Encourage the client not to blow the nose or insert objects into the nose.
- Instruct the client to avoid contact sports.
- Advise the client to wear shoes with firm soles whenever he or she is ambulating.

CHART 26-7

Education Guide ◆ The Client at Risk for Bleeding

- Use an electric razor.
- Use a soft-bristled toothbrush, and do not floss.
- Do not have dental work done without consulting your doctor.
- Do not take aspirin or any aspirin-containing products. Read the label to be sure that the product does not contain aspirin or salicylates.
- Do not participate in contact sports or engage in any activity that is likely to result in you being bumped, scratched, or scraped.
- If you are bumped, apply ice to the site for at least 1 hour.
- Notify your doctor if you:
  - Experience an injury and persistent bleeding results.
  - Have excessive menstrual bleeding.
  - See blood in your urine or bowel movement.
- Avoid anal intercourse.
- Take a stool softener to prevent straining during a bowel movement.
- Do not use enemas or rectal suppositories.
- Avoid bending over at the waist.
- Do not wear clothing or shoes that are tight or that rub.
- Avoid blowing your nose or placing objects in your nose. If you must blow your nose, do so gently without blocking either nasal passage.

the amount of hormone A that is produced (through competition or feedback inhibition) so that the tumor growth is slowed. Thus, hormonal therapy may increase survival time. Table 26-11 lists drugs commonly used in hormonal manipulation for cancer therapy.

HORMONE ANTAGONISTS

Hormone antagonists, which are competitors for the hormones at the receptor sites, often are antibodies that are specific for the receptor. When hormone antagonists are administered, they bind to the specific hormone receptor of the tumor cell and prevent the hormone from binding to the receptor. Therefore, if a tumor requires the presence of a certain hormone to grow and the hormone can enter the cell only through a receptor, the use of hormone antagonists can slow down tumor growth.

SIDE EFFECTS OF HORMONAL MANIPULATION FOR CANCER

In women, androgens and the antiestrogen receptor drugs cause masculinizing manifestations. Chest and facial hair may develop. Menses (menstrual periods) stop, and breast tissue shrinks. Women usually experience some fluid retention. For men and women who are receiving androgens, acne may develop, hypercalcemia is common, and liver dysfunction may occur when therapy is prolonged. Women receiving estrogens or progestins have irregular but heavy menses, fluid retention, and breast tenderness. Male and female clients taking estrogen or progestins are at an increased risk for thrombus formation.

When men take estrogens, progestins, or antiandrogen receptor drugs, usually some feminine clinical manifestations develop over time. Facial hair diminishes or disappears, and the man's facial skin becomes smoother. There is a redistribution of body fat and gynecomastia (breast development in men) can occur. Testicular and penile atrophy occurs to some degree. Although sexual function may continue, achieving and maintaining an erection are much more difficult.

Immunotherapy—Biologic Response Modifiers

Biologic response modifiers (BRMs) are defined as agents or approaches that modify the client's biologic responses to tumor cells with a beneficial result (Clark & Longo, 1986). The BRMs in current use or under investigation for use as cancer therapy are cytokines. Cytokines are small, protein hormones synthesized by the various leukocytes. Cytokines that are synthesized by the mononuclear phagocytes (macrophages, neutrophils, eosinophils, and monocytes) are monokines; the cytokines produced by lymphocytes (especially the T lymphocytes) are lymphokines. Essentially, cytokines make the immune system work better (see Chap. 22 and especially Table 22-5).

TABLE 26-11 Common Agents Used for Hormonal Manipulation of Cancer

Type of Agent	Example
Hormones	
Estrogens	• Estradiol • Diethylstilbestrol • Estrace • Premarin
Androgens	• Halotestin • Fluoxymesterone
Progestins	• Megace • Provera • Depo-Provera • Amen
Hormone Antagonists	
Antiestrogen	• Tamoxifen
Antiandrogen	• Flutamide
Antiadrenal	• Lysodrene

RATIONALE FOR BIOLOGIC RESPONSE MODIFIERS AS A CANCER THERAPY

Cytokines enhance the effectiveness of the immune system. Immune function plays an important role in cancer prevention (see Chaps. 22 and 25). Therefore, cytokines and other biologic response modifiers (BRMs) have the potential to be therapeutic as a cancer treatment by stimulating the client's immune system to recognize transformed self cells (cancer cells) and to mount actions to eliminate and/or destroy them. In addition, some BRMs may be useful by playing a supporting role. Other BRMs (colony-stimulating factors) stimulate faster recovery of bone marrow function after treatment-induced suppression.

MECHANISM OF ACTION

Cytokine activity is similar to the action of any other kind of peptide hormone, in that one cell produces and secretes a cytokine—which then exerts its effects on other cells of the immune system (Guyton, 1991). The cells responding to the cytokine may be right next to the cytokine-secreting cell or quite remote from it. The cells that change their activity in response to the cytokine are "responder" cells. For a responder cell to be able to respond to the presence of a cytokine, the membrane of the responder cell must have a specific receptor for the cytokine to bind to and initiate changes in the responder cell's activity.

BIOLOGIC RESPONSE MODIFIERS FOR CANCER THERAPY

Two categories of biologic response modifiers are being used as cytotoxic therapy for cancer: interleukins and interferons. These agents can stimulate some immune system cells to attack and destroy cancer cells.

INTERLEUKINS

Eight interleukins have been identified (see Table 22–5). Many are now synthetically produced through recombinant DNA technology. Interleukins help different immune system cells recognize and destroy body cells that are no longer normal. In particular, interleukins 1, 2, and 6 appear to "charge up" the immune system and enhance attacks on cancer cells by macrophages, natural killer (NK) cells, lymphokine-activated killer (LAK) cells, and tumor-infiltrating lymphocytes. At present, cancer treatment with interleukins is experimental. The best responses have occurred in clients with renal cell carcinoma, colorectal cancer, and melanoma.

INTERFERONS

In 1957, interferons were discovered as a substance produced by cells that had been exposed to viruses. These substances can protect noninfected cells from viral infection and replication. There are many types of interferons, and although they all have similar functions, each type has properties and functions that are unique.

The interferon that has been most completely characterized is interferon alfa-2b. Although different body cells can produce interferon, leukocytes produce the most interferon. Today, interferons are mass-produced synthetically by recombinant DNA technology. Cancer-related functions of interferon include the ability to:

- Slow down the cell division of tumor cells
- Stimulate the proliferation and activation of natural killer cells
- Help cancer cells resume a more normal appearance and revert to their previous characteristics
- Inhibit expression of oncogenes

Although interferons are approved for use as a treatment for hairy cell leukemia only, they have been effective to some degree in the treatment of renal cell carcinoma, ovarian cancer, and cutaneous T-cell lymphoma.

BIOLOGIC RESPONSE MODIFIERS FOR CANCER SUPPORT

The biologic response modifiers (BRMs) approved for use as supportive therapy during cancer treatment are the colony-stimulating factors (Table 26–12). Essentially, the colony-stimulating factors are used to induce more rapid recovery of the bone marrow after suppression by chemotherapy.

The therapeutic value of this effect may be twofold. First, when bone marrow suppression is less severe and/or of shorter duration, clients are less at risk for life-threatening infections and anemia. Second, because the colony-stimulating factors allow more rapid recovery of the bone marrow, clients can receive their chemotherapy on time and may even be able to tolerate higher doses. These effects have the potential for improving the curative outcome of chemotherapy.

SIDE EFFECTS OF BIOLOGIC RESPONSE MODIFIER THERAPY FOR CANCER

Clients receiving interleukins at therapeutic doses experience generalized and severe inflammatory reactions. Fluid shifts and capillary leak are widespread. Tissue swelling affects the function of all major organs and can be life-threatening. Clients receiving such therapy should be cared for in intensive care and monitoring units. These effects are limited to the period of acute drug administration and resolve spontaneously when treatment is completed.

Many of the biologic response modifiers (BRMs) induce general symptoms of mild inflammatory reactions during and immediately after administration.

TABLE 26–12 Colony-Stimulating Factors

Factor	Granulocyte/Macrophage Colony-Stimulating Factor (GM-CSF)	Granulocyte Colony-Stimulating Factor (G-CSF)	Erythropoietin (EPO)
Generic Name	• Sargramostim	• Filgrastim	• Epoetin alfa
Brand Name	• Leukine (Immunex) • Prokine (Hoechst/Roussel)	• Neupogen (Amgen)	• Epogen (Amgen) • Procrit (Ortho Biotech)
Source	• T-cells (lymphokine)	• Monocytes • Fibroblasts • Endothelial epithelial cells	• Renal
Cell Type Affected	• All granulocytes • Neutrophils • Eosinophils • Monocytes/macrophages	• Neutrophil	• Red blood cells
Indications	• To accelerate myeloid recovery in patients with non-Hodgkin's lymphoma, ALL, and Hodgkin's disease who are undergoing autologous bone marrow transplantation	• To decrease the incidence of infection, manifested by febrile neutropenia, in patients with non-myeloid malignancies receiving myelosuppressive anticancer drugs associated with a significant incidence of severe neutropenia with fever	• Anemia of chronic renal failure patients • Anemia in AZT-treated HIV patients
Dosage	• 250 mcg/m²/day × 21 days as a 2-hour IV infusion beginning 2 to 4 hours after autologous bone marrow transplantation and not less than 24 hours after the last dose of chemotherapy and 12 hours after the last dose of radiotherapy	• 5 mcg/kg/day, SC or IV, as a single daily injection not less than 24 hours after cytotoxic chemotherapy or in the 24 hours preceding chemotherapy • Give for up to two weeks, until the absolute neutrophil count has reached 10,000 mm³ following the expected chemotherapy-induced neutrophil nadir.	• Starting dose 50–100 μ/kg T.I.W. • IV for dialysis patients • IV or SQ for non-dialysis CRF patients • Individualize dose to reach the HCT target range of 30–33%.

These symptoms include fever, chills, rigors, and flu-like general malaise. Symptoms are worse when higher doses are given and seem to become less severe over time. Fever is treated with acetaminophena. Clients with rigors, if severe, are managed with meperidine (Demerol, pethidine✱).

ONCOLOGIC EMERGENCIES

Cancer is considered a chronic disease; however, a number of acute conditions associated with cancer and/or its treatment can occur. These conditions, or complications, often require immediate medical intervention and are thus *oncologic emergencies.* Early diagnosis is essential to avoid life-threatening situations.

Sepsis and Disseminated Intravascular Coagulation

OVERVIEW

Sepsis, or septicemia, is a condition in which microorganisms enter the bloodstream. Septic shock is a life-threatening result of sepsis and a frequent cause of death in clients with cancer. These clients are at increased risk for infection and sepsis because their white blood cell counts are often low and their immune function is usually impaired. (Chapter 36 describes the pathophysiology of sepsis and septic shock.)

Disseminated intravascular coagulation (DIC) is a condition indicating a problem with a person's blood clotting process. DIC is triggered by many severe illnesses, including cancer. In clients with cancer, DIC is caused by sepsis (usually gram-negative infection), by release of thrombin or thromboplastin (clotting factors) from cancer cells, or by blood transfusions. DIC is most often associated with leukemia and with adenocarcinomas of the lung, pancreas, stomach, and prostate.

In clients with DIC, extensive, abnormal clot formation occurs throughout small blood vessels. The widespread clotting consumes all circulating clotting factors and platelets. This process is followed by extensive bleeding. Bleeding from many sites is the most common problem and ranges from minimal to fatal hemorrhage. Blockage of blood vessels from clots decreases blood flow to major body organs and results in pain, stroke-like signs and symptoms, dyspnea, tachycardia, oliguria (decreased urine output), and bowel necrosis (tissue death). (Chapter 36 describes the pathophysiology of DIC and the collaborative management of sepsis-induced DIC.)

COLLABORATIVE MANAGEMENT

Disseminated intravascular coagulation (DIC) is a life-threatening problem. The mortality rate is 70% even when appropriate therapies are instituted. Therefore, the best treatment plan for sepsis and DIC is prevention. The nurse identifies those clients at greatest risk for development of sepsis and DIC. Strict adherence to aseptic technique is practiced during invasive procedures and during manipulation of non-intact skin and mucous membranes in clients who are immunocompromised. The nurse teaches the client and family members the early clinical manifestations of infection and sepsis and when to seek medical assistance.

When sepsis is present and DIC is likely, treatment is focused on reducing the infection and halting the DIC process. Appropriate intravenous antibiotic therapy is initiated. During the early phase of DIC, anticoagulants (especially heparin) are administered to limit unnecessary clotting and prevent the rapid consumption of circulating clotting factors. When DIC has progressed to the later phase, when hemorrhage is the problem, cryoprecipitated clotting factors are administered.

Syndrome of Inappropriate Antidiuretic Hormone

OVERVIEW

In healthy people, antidiuretic hormone (ADH) is secreted by the posterior pituitary gland only when more fluid (water) is needed in the body, such as when plasma volume is decreased (see Chapter 14). In people with certain health problems, however, ADH is secreted when it is *not* needed by the body, or it is secreted inappropriately.

Cancer is the most common cause of the syndrome of inappropriate ADH (SIADH). The type of cancer most frequently associated with this complication is carcinoma of the lung (especially small cell lung cancer), but SIADH may occur in other types of cancer as well, especially when tumors are present in the brain. Some tumors actually make and secrete ADH, and other tumors stimulate the brain to synthesize and secrete ADH. In addition, certain drugs frequently used in the care of clients with cancer can cause the problem (most notably morphine sulfate and cyclophosphamide).

In SIADH, excessive amounts of water are reabsorbed by the kidney and put into systemic circulation. The increased water causes hyponatremia (decreased serum sodium levels) and some degree of fluid retention. Mild symptoms, including weakness, muscle cramps, loss of appetite, and fatigue, occur, with serum sodium levels ranging from 115 to 120 mEq/L (normal range is 135 to 145 mEq/L). More serious signs and symptoms are related to water intoxication; these include weight gain, nervous system changes (especially personality changes), confusion, and extreme muscle weakness. As the sodium level approaches 110 mEq/L, seizures, coma, and eventually death may follow unless the condition is rapidly treated.

COLLABORATIVE MANAGEMENT

Management of the syndrome of inappropriate antidiuretic hormone (SIADH) is accomplished in two ways: treating the condition and treating the cause.

First, the condition itself is treated. Treatment regimens for SIADH usually include fluid restriction (sometimes total fluid intake is reduced to 1 L/day), increased sodium intake, and drug therapy. A drug commonly used for this condition is demeclocycline, a form of tetracycline antibiotic. Clients take this drug orally. The mechanism of action appears to be antagonistic to ADH. Because hypernatremia can develop suddenly, serum sodium levels should be monitored closely with this regimen.

The second method for treating clients with cancer-induced SIADH is to reduce or eliminate the underlying cause. The immediate institution of appropriate cancer therapy, usually either radiation or chemotherapy, can cause such tumor regression that ADH synthesis and release processes return to normal.

Spinal Cord Compression

OVERVIEW

Spinal cord compression (damage from pressure) occurs when a tumor directly enters the spinal cord or when the vertebral column collapses from tumor entry. Tumors may begin in the spinal cord but more commonly spread to the spinal cord from other areas of the body, such as the lung, prostate, breast, and colon. Spinal cord compression causes back pain, usually before neurologic changes occur. Neurologic deficits are related to the spinal level of compression and include numbness, tingling, loss of urethral, vaginal, and rectal sensation, and muscle weakness. If paralysis occurs, it is usually permanent.

COLLABORATIVE MANAGEMENT

Nurses who manage the care of clients with spinal cord compression must recognize the condition early. The nurse assesses the client for neurologic changes consistent with spinal cord compression. The nurse also teaches the client and family to recognize symptoms of early spinal cord compression and to seek medical assistance as soon as symptoms are apparent.

Treatment is largely palliative. Usually, high-dose

radiation is administered in an effort to reduce tumor in the area and to relieve the compression. Radiation may be given in conjunction with chemotherapy to treat the total disease. Occasionally, surgery is performed to remove the tumor from the area and rearrange the bony tissue so that less pressure is placed on the spinal cord. External back or neck braces may be prescribed for the client to reduce the weight borne by the spinal column and to reduce pressure on the spinal cord or spinal nerves.

Hypercalcemia

OVERVIEW

Hypercalcemia (an increased serum calcium level) occurs most often in clients who have bone metastasis. It is a late manifestation of extensive malignancy. The presence of cancer in bone causes the bone to release calcium into the bloodstream. In clients with cancer in other parts of the body, especially the lung, head and neck, kidney, or lymph nodes, the tumor secretes parathyroid hormone (parathormone), which causes bone to release calcium (Baird et al., 1991). Decreased physical mobility also contributes to or worsens hypercalcemia.

Early signs and symptoms of hypercalcemia include fatigue, loss of appetite, nausea, vomiting, constipation, and polyuria (increased urine output). More serious signs and symptoms include severe muscle weakness, diminished deep tendon reflexes, paralytic ileus, dehydration, and electrocardiographic (ECG) changes. The severity of signs and symptoms depends on how high the serum calcium level is and how quickly it developed (see also Chapter 16).

COLLABORATIVE MANAGEMENT

For many clients in whom hypercalcemia develops as a consequence of cancer, the process takes place very slowly over time, which allows the body time to adapt to this electrolyte change. As a result, the symptoms of hypercalcemia in these clients may not be evident until the serum calcium level is greatly elevated. Because adaptation does occur, treatment of hypercalcemia associated with cancer is instituted only when clinical manifestations are present.

Conservative management may be enough to reduce the serum calcium to an acceptable level. Oral hydration alone can be effective. When parenteral hydration is needed, normal saline is the fluid of choice.

Many drugs lower serum calcium levels, some quite dramatically (e.g., oral glucocorticoids, calcitonin, diphosphonate, gallium nitrate, mithramycin). These agents do not cure hypercalcemia, but reduce the serum calcium levels temporarily (Hawthorne, et al., 1992). In addition, when cancer-induced hypercalcemia is life-threatening or is accompanied by renal impairment, dialysis can temporarily reduce serum calcium levels.

Superior Vena Cava Syndrome

OVERVIEW

Superior vena cava (SVC) syndrome occurs when the superior vena cava is compressed or obstructed by tumor growth (Fig. 26–3). Compression of the SVC can lead to a painful and life-threatening emergency. The problem occurs most often in clients with lymphomas and bronchogenic carcinoma, but clients with cancer of the breast, esophagus, colon, and testes may also be affected.

The signs and symptoms associated with superior vena cava syndrome result from blockage of blood flow in the venous system of the head, neck, and upper trunk. Early signs and symptoms generally occur in the early morning and include edema of the face, especially around the eyes (periorbital edema), and tightness of the shirt or blouse collar (Stokes' sign). As the compression worsens, the client typically experiences edema in the arms and hands, dyspnea, erythema of the upper body, and epistaxis (nosebleeds). Late life-threatening signs and symptoms include hemorrhage, cyanosis, mental status changes from lack of blood to the brain, decreased cardiac output, and hypotension (low blood pressure). Death can result if compression is not relieved.

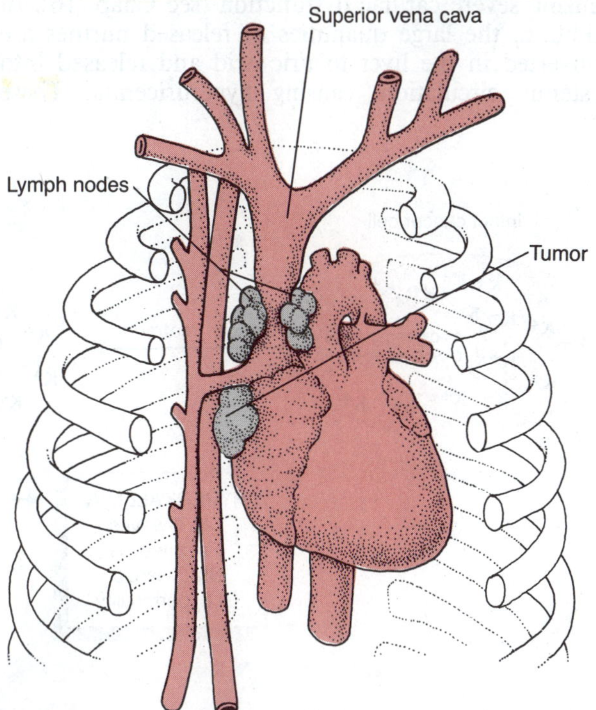

FIGURE 26–3 ◆ Compression of the superior vena cava in SVC syndrome. (From Varricchio, C. [1985]. Clinical management of superior vena cava syndrome. *Heart and Lung*, *14*, 411.)

COLLABORATIVE MANAGEMENT

Superior vena cava (SVC) syndrome is often a late-stage manifestation, with tumor usually being widespread. High-dose radiation therapy to the mediastinal area is most frequently the treatment of choice and can provide temporary relief in about 70% of clients with cancer-induced SVC syndrome (Glover & Glick, 1991). Surgery is *not* performed for this condition because the tumor may have increased the intrathoracic pressure to such an extent it may not be possible to close the chest after the procedure.

The best therapeutic and palliative results occur when SVC syndrome is in the early stages. The nurse assesses each client for the signs and symptoms of SVC syndrome and notifies the physician.

Tumor Lysis Syndrome

OVERVIEW

In the tumor lysis syndrome (TLS), large quantities of tumor cells are destroyed rapidly; their intracellular contents, including potassium and purines (DNA components), are released into the bloodstream faster than the body's homeostatic mechanisms can handle them (Fig. 26–4). Unlike the other oncologic emergencies, tumor lysis syndrome is a positive sign that cancer treatment is effective (Hawthorne et al., 1992). However, if TLS is severe or left untreated, it can cause severe tissue damage and death. Serum potassium levels can increase to the point of hyperkalemia, causing severe cardiac dysfunction (see Chap. 16). In addition, the large quantities of released purines are converted in the liver to uric acid and released into systemic circulation, causing hyperuricemia. These uric acid molecules precipitate in the kidney, forming a sludge in the kidney tubules, blocking them, and leading to acute renal failure.

The tumor lysis syndrome is most commonly seen in clients receiving radiation and/or cancer drug therapy for cancers that are very sensitive to the therapies. Such cancers include leukemia, lymphoma, small cell lung cancer, and multiple myeloma.

COLLABORATIVE MANAGEMENT

The best management for tumor lysis syndrome is prevention through hydration. Hydration alone can dilute the serum potassium level and increases the glomerular filtration rate. As a result, urine flows through the kidney at a greatly increased rate, preventing precipitation of uric acid crystals, enhancing renal excretion of potassium, and mechanically flushing out any sludge in the renal tubule.

For clients with tumors that are known to be very sensitive to cancer therapy, the nurse instructs the client to drink at least 3000 mL (5000 mL is more desirable) of fluid each day on the day before the treatment, the day of the treatment, and for 3 days after the treatment. Some fluids should be alkaline in nature because this helps to prevent crystallization of uric acid. The nurse stresses to the client the importance of keeping the fluid intake relatively consistent throughout the 24-hour day and helps the client by drawing up a schedule of fluid intake.

Because some clients experience nausea and vomiting after cancer therapy and therefore may not feel like taking oral fluids, the nurse stresses the importance of following the antiemetic regimen. The nurse also instructs the client to contact the physician or cancer clinic immediately if nausea and vomiting

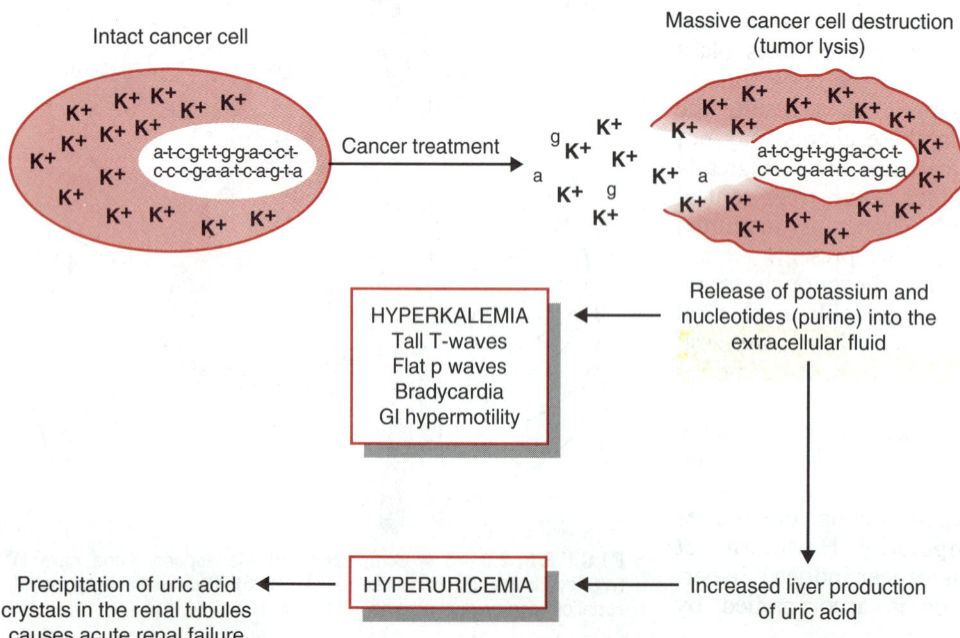

FIGURE 26–4 ◆ Pathology of tumor lysis syndrome.

prevent adequate fluid intake so that the client can be started on parenteral fluids.

For clients who become hyperkalemic and/or hyperuricemic, treatment becomes more aggressive. In addition to increased fluid intake (oral or parenteral), diuretics (especially osmotic types) are given to increase urine flow through the kidney. These are administered with caution because it is crucial that the client avoid becoming dehydrated. Drugs that increase the excretion of purines, such as allopurinol (Alloprin✱, Zyloprim), are administered. To reduce serum potassium levels, clients may be given intravenous infusions containing glucose and insulin. When hyperkalemia and hyperuricemia are more severe and persistent, the client may require dialysis.

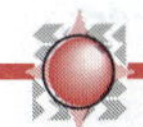

IMPLICATIONS FOR NURSING RESEARCH

Cancer is a major health problem among industrialized societies. Nurses involved in the care of clients with cancer have focused on aspects of symptom management and protection. A new role for nurses in prevention of cancer is emerging as nurses become more involved in public education and cancer screening programs. Some questions to be explored to enhance the effectiveness of nursing interventions in cancer prevention and quality of life for clients with cancer are as follows:

- What methods are most effective in motivating clients to avoid the use of tobacco products?
- What methods are most effective in teaching clients dietary habits that lower cancer risks?
- Are nurse-managed cancer screening programs effective for secondary prevention of cancer?
- What nursing interventions are most effective for preventing infection in neutropenic clients?
- Which mouth care protocols are most effective in preventing or ameliorating stomatitis?
- How effective are nonpharmacologic interventions in reducing pain perception in clients with cancer?
- How effective are nonpharmacologic interventions in reducing nausea and vomiting in clients with cancer?

SELECTED BIBLIOGRAPHY

American Cancer Society (1994). Cancer facts and figures—1994. Atlanta: American Cancer Society.

American Cancer Society (1991). *Proceedings of the national workshop on cancer control and the older person.* Atlanta: American Cancer Society.

Baird, S., Donehower, M., Stalsbroten, V., & Ades, T. (Eds.). (1991).*A cancer source book for nurses* (6th ed.). Atlanta: American Cancer Society.

Baird, S., McCorkle, R., & Grant, M. (Eds.). (1991). *Cancer nursing: A comprehensive textbook.* Philadelphia: W. B. Saunders.

Barton-Burke, M., Wilkes, G., Berg, D., Bean, C., & Ingwersen, K. (1991). *Cancer chemotherapy: A nursing process approach.* Boston: Jones and Bartlett.

Beck, S. (1991). The therapeutic use of music for cancer-related pain. *Oncology Nursing Forum, 18*(8), 1327–1337.

Belcher, A. (1992). *Cancer nursing.* St. Louis: Mosby Year Book.

Bryce, J. (1994). S.I.A.D.H. *Nursing94, 24*(4), 33.

Cheson, B. (1991). Clinical trials program. *Seminars in Oncology Nursing, 7*(4), 235–242.

*Clark, J., & Longo, D. (1986). Biologic response modifiers. *Mediguide to Oncology, 6,* 1–10.

Cooper, G. (1992). *Elements of human cancer.* Boston: Jones & Bartlett.

Davis, K., & Attie, M. (1991). Management of severe hypercalcemia. *Critical Care Clinics, 7*(1), 175–190.

Dillon, P. (1994). Ovarian cancer: Confronting the silent killer. *Nursing94, 24*(5), 66–68.

DiStasio, S. (1993). Zofran makes chemo bearable. *RN, 56*(5), 56–59.

Doane, L., Fisher, L., & McDonald, T. (1990). How to give peritoneal chemotherapy. *American Journal of Nursing, 90*(4), 58–65.

Dudjak, L., & Fleck, A. (1991). BRMs: New drug therapy comes of age. *RN, 54*(10), 41–48.

Egan, A., Taggart, J., & Bender, C. (1992). Management of chemotherapy-related nausea and vomiting using a serotonin antagonist. *Oncology Nursing Forum, 19*(5), 791–800.

Ersek, M. (1991). Biological response modifiers. In S. Baird, M. Donehower, V. Stalsbroten, & T. Ades (Eds.), *A cancer source book for nurses* (6th ed., pp. 83–90). Atlanta: American Cancer Society.

Flyge, H. (1993). Meeting the challenge of neutropenia. *Nursing93, 23*(7),60–64.

*Fraser, M., & Tucker, M. (1989). Second malignancies following cancer therapy. *Seminars in Oncology Nursing, 5*(1), 43.

Gallucci, B. (1991). Cancer biology: Molecular and cellular aspects. In S. Baird, R. McCorkle, & M. Grant (Eds.), *Cancer nursing: A comprehensive textbook* (pp. 115–129). Philadelphia: W. B. Saunders.

Glover, D., & Glick, J. (1991). Oncologic emergencies. In A. Holleb, D. Fink, & G. Murphy (Eds.), *American Cancer Society textbook of clinical oncology* (pp. 513–532). Atlanta: American Cancer Society.

Goodman, M. (1991). Delivery of cancer chemotherapy. In S. Baird, R. McCorkle, & M. Grant (Eds.), *Cancer nursing: A comprehensive textbook* (pp. 291–320). Philadelphia: W. B. Saunders.

Groenwald, S., Frogge, M., Goodman, M., & Yarbro, C. (1992). *The care of individuals with cancer.* Boston: Jones and Bartlett.

Guy, J. (1991). Medical oncology—the agents. In S. Baird, R. McCorkle, & M. Grant (Eds.), *Cancer nursing: A comprehensive textbook* (pp. 266–290). Philadelphia: W. B. Saunders.

*Hassey, K. (1987). Principles of radiation therapy and protection. *Seminars in Oncology Nursing, 3,* 23–29.

Havard, C., & Topping, A. (1991). Surgical oncology. In S. Baird, R. McCorkle, & M. Grant (Eds.), *Cancer nursing: A comprehensive textbook* (pp. 235–245). Philadelphia: W. B. Saunders.

Hawthorne, J., Schneider, S., & Workman, M. (1992). Common electrolyte imbalances associated with malignancy. *AACN Clinical Issues in Critical Care, 3*(3), 714–723.

Hilderley, L., & Dow, K. (1991). Radiation oncology. In S.

Baird, R. McCorkle, & M. Grant (Eds.), *Cancer nursing: A comprehensive textbook* (pp. 246–265). Philadelphia: W. B. Saunders.

Holleb, A., Fink, D., & Murphy, G. (Eds.). (1991). *American Cancer Society textbook of clinical oncology.* Atlanta: American Cancer Society.

Hood, L., & Abernathy, E. (1991). Biological response modifiers. In S. Baird, R. McCorkle, & M. Grant (Eds.), *Cancer nursing: A comprehensive textbook* (pp. 321–343). Philadelphia: W. B. Saunders.

Iwamoto, R. (1991). Radiation therapy. In S. Baird, M. Donehower, V. Stalsbroten, & T. Ades (Eds.), *A cancer source book for nurses* (6th ed., pp. 63–72). Atlanta: American Cancer Society.

Jassak, P. (1992). Families: An essential element in the care of the patient with cancer. *Oncology Nursing Forum, 19*(6), 871–882.

*Jassak, P., & Sticklin, L. (1986). Interleukin-2: An overview. *Oncology Nursing Forum, 13*(6), 17.

*Maddock, P. (1987). Brachytherapy sources and applicators. *Seminars in Oncology Nursing, 3*(1), 15.

Miaskowski, C. (1991). Oncologic emergencies. In S. Baird, R. McCorkle, & M. Grant (Eds.), *Cancer nursing: A comprehensive textbook* (pp. 885–893). Philadelphia: W. B. Saunders.

Peterson, J. (1991). Chemotherapy. In S. Baird, M. Donehower, V. Stalsbroten, & T. Ades (Eds.), *A cancer source book for nurses* (6th ed., pp. 73–82). Atlanta: American Cancer Society.

Russell, S. (1994). Septic shock: Can you recognize the clues? *Nursing94, 24*(4), 40–48.

Schneider, S. Clinical implications for the administration of colony stimulating factors. *Journal of Orthopaedic Nursing.* In press.

Sitton, E. (1992a). Early and late radiation-induced skin alterations. Part I: Mechanisms of skin changes. *Oncology Nursing Forum, 19*(5), 801–807.

Sitton, E. (1992b). Early and late radiation-induced skin alterations. Part II: Nursing care of irradiated skin. *Oncology Nursing Forum, 19*(6), 907–912.

Skalla, K., & Lacasse, C. (1992). Patient education for fatigue. *Oncology Nursing Forum, 19*(1), 1537–1541.

Strohl, R. (1992). Implications of diagnosis and staging on treatment goals and strategies. In J. Clark & R. McGee (Eds.), *Core curriculum for oncology nursing* (2nd ed., pp. 303–308). Philadelphia: W. B. Saunders.

Strohl, R. (1992). The elderly patient receiving radiation treatment: Sequelae and nursing care. *Geriatric Nursing, 13*(3), 152–156.

Szopa, T. (1992). Implications of surgical treatment for nursing. In J. Clark & R. McGee (Eds.), *Core curriculum for oncology nursing* (2nd ed., pp. 309–318). Philadelphia: W. B. Saunders.

Tenenbaum, L. (1989). *Cancer chemotherapy: A reference guide.* Philadelphia: W. B. Saunders.

Wood, L., & Gullo, S. (1993). IV vesicants: How to avoid extravasation. *American Journal of Nursing, 93*(4), 42–46.

Workman, M., Ellerhorst-Ryan, J., & Koertge, V. (1993). *Nursing care of the immunocompromised patient.* Philadelphia: W. B. Saunders.

Yasko. J., & Rust, D. (1989). Trends in chemotherapy administration. *Seminars in Oncology Nursing, 5*(2), 3.

Zwingler, R. (1994). Cancer update 94. *Nursing94, 24*(4), 59.

SUGGESTED READINGS

Cheson, B. (1991). Clinical trials program. *Seminars in Oncology Nursing, 7*(4), 235–242.

Many clients with cancer who are treated at major medical centers are asked to participate in "clinical trials" for new cancer therapy regimens. This article provides background information on what clinical trials are and how participation would or would not benefit individual clients. Nurses can use this information to allow clients to make an informed decision on whether or not to participate in a clinical trial.

Dudjak, L., & Fleck, A. (1991). BRMs: New drug therapy comes of age. *RN, 54*(10), 41–48.

This article concisely, yet simply, explains the purpose and mechanism of action for the most common biologic response modifiers (BRMs). The authors include a brief review of the immune system. Nursing responsibilities are categorized in relation to administration of the BRMs and collaborative management of the side effects. A self-assessment test is included at the end of the article.

Jassak, P. (1992). Families: An essential element in the care of the patient with cancer. *Oncology Nursing Forum, 19*(6), 871–882.

This excellent article describes the important role family members play in assisting the person with cancer to live life to its fullest. Because cancer treatment is a prolonged process and cancer is now considered a chronic illness, clients with cancer experience a long period of interaction with health care delivery systems. Most of these systems focus specifically on the client with cancer and offer very limited support or assistance to family members. This article provides information for nurses to use in assessing the needs of the entire family when one member has cancer. The author presents nursing diagnoses with a family focus as well as the major psychosocial problems that most clients and families with cancer experience.

Skalla, K., & Lacasse, C. (1992). Patient education for fatigue. *Oncology Nursing Forum, 19*(1), 1537–1541.

Most clients with cancer experience some degree of fatigue. The causes of fatigue are related to the disease process, side effects of treatment (especially radiation therapy), and poor nutrition. This distressing manifestation interferes with a client's activities of daily living and quality of life. Clients often believe that the manifestation of fatigue is a personal weakness and that they are abnormal. This article provides information for the nurse to assure and reassure clients that fatigue is a normal physiologic response to cancer and that it will resolve.

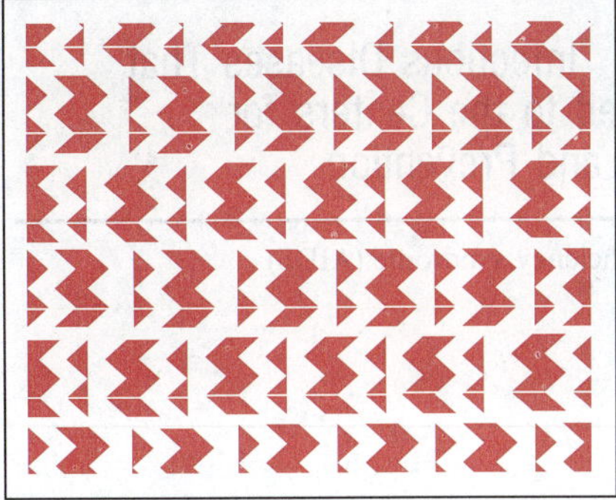

CHAPTER 27

Interventions for Clients with Infection

CHAPTER HIGHLIGHTS

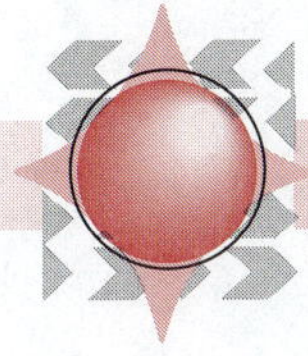

An infection is caused by the invasion of the body by microorganisms. Infections can be communicable (e.g., hepatitis and influenza) or noncommunicable (e.g., pancreatitis and cellulitis).

New microorganisms continue to emerge as causes of human disease. However, vaccines and more effective antibiotics have made many infections and infectious diseases among the most easily preventable and treatable illnesses. In addition, as people live longer and as medical technology improves, more invasive procedures are being performed and more immunosuppressive therapies are being used. Thus, microorganisms that previously caused no harm can gain access to the body and cause infection. The nurse's understanding of the infectious process can help prevent or minimize the effects of infection.

OVERVIEW

THE INFECTIOUS PROCESS

DEFINITIONS

The process of infection requires a pathogen, or causative agent, and a susceptible host, or recipient of infection. A pathogen is any microorganism capable of producing disease in a person. People are surrounded by countless microorganisms with differing degrees of pathogenicity (ability to cause disease).

Virulence is often used as a synonym for *pathogenicity*. However, virulence is related more to the frequency with which a pathogen causes disease in exposed people (degree of communicability) and its ability to invade and damage a host. Virulence can also indicate the severity of the disease. Another important characteristic is invasiveness, the ability of pathogens to spread and grow in the tissues of a host after entrance.

Most microorganisms commonly live in or on the human host without causing disease. Some microbes are actually beneficial. For example, each body location harbors its own characteristic bacteria, or normal flora. One important function of normal flora is to compete with and prevent infection by unfamiliar microorganisms attempting to invade a body site. In some instances, microorganisms may be present in the tissues of the host yet not cause symptomatic disease; this process is called colonization.

In many instances, microorganisms behave as parasites; that is, the microorganisms live at the expense of their human hosts. In this interaction with its host, the microbe gains some advantage and infection occurs. Infection is the establishment of a host-parasite interaction.

Subclinical infection causes no apparent reaction in the host and thus elicits no detectable symptoms. Most often, subclinical infection can be identified only by the immune response of the host. This is demonstrated by a rise in the titer of antibody directed against the infecting agent. Clinically apparent infection in which the host-parasite interaction causes obvious injury is accompanied by one or more clinical manifestations and is known as infectious disease. Disease caused by an infectious agent may range from mild to fatal.

The Centers for Disease Control and Prevention (formerly the Centers for Disease Control [CDC]) collects information about the occurrence and nature of infectious diseases. The CDC then makes recommendations to health care agencies for infection control and prevention. Certain diseases must be reported to the CDC (Table 27–1).

TABLE 27–1 Infectious Diseases That Must Be Reported to the Centers for Disease Control and Prevention

- Acquired immunodeficiency syndrome (AIDS)
- Amebiasis
- Anthrax
- Aseptic meningitis
- Botulism
- Brucellosis
- Cholera
- Diphtheria
- Encephalitis, primary infections
- Encephalitis, postinfectious
- Gonorrhea
- Hepatitis A
- Hepatitis B
- Hepatitis, non-A, non-B
- Hepatitis, unspecified
- Legionellosis
- Leprosy
- Leptospirosis
- Malaria
- Measles (rubeola)
- Meningococcal infections
- Mumps
- Pertussis
- Plague
- Poliomyelitis, paralytic
- Psittacosis
- Rabies, human
- Rheumatic fever
- Rubella (German measles)
- Rubella congenital syndrome
- Salmonellosis
- Shigellosis
- Syphilis, primary and secondary
- Tetanus
- Toxic shock syndrome
- Trichinosis
- Tuberculosis
- Tularemia
- Typhoid fever
- Typhus fever (Rocky Mountain spotted fever)
- Varicella (chickenpox)

CHAIN OF INFECTION

The development of an infectious disease depends on the chain of infection (Fig. 27–1). Transmission of infection requires the following factors:

- Reservoir
- Pathogen
- Susceptible host
- Portal of entry
- Mode of transmission
- Portal of exit

Preventing the spread of infection depends on breaking the chain of infection at any point. Eliminating the microorganism, providing the host with immunity, or, most often, interrupting the mode of transmission breaks the chain of infection. In the health care setting, nurses and other personnel interrupt the pathogen's transmission by scrupulous hand washing, implementing barrier precautions, and using antimicrobial agents.

RESERVOIR

Reservoirs, or sources of infectious agents, are numerous. A reservoir is any place where the pathogen is found; it can be animate (living) or inanimate (not living). Animate reservoirs include people, animals, and insects. Inanimate reservoirs include soil, water, other environmental sources, and medical equipment, such as intravenous (IV) solutions and urine collection devices. The host's own body can be a reservoir; pathogens can colonize in skin and body substances, such as feces, sputum, saliva, and wound drainage. A person with an active infection or an asymptomatic carrier (a person who does not have a disease but harbors the infectious agent) can be a reservoir. A

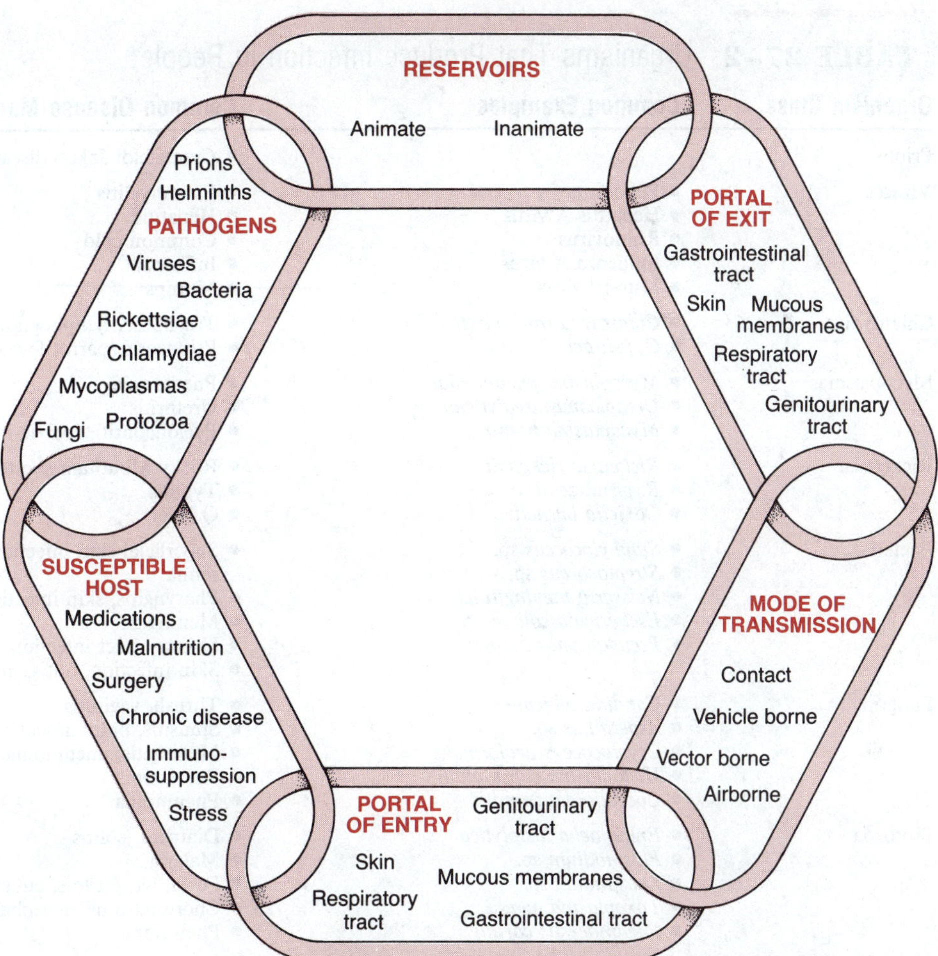

FIGURE 27-1 ♦ The chain of infection—the process by which pathogens are transmitted from the environment to a host, invade the host, and cause infection.

carrier can be incubating the pathogen before signs and symptoms develop, have a subclinical infection, be convalescing from an infection, or be a chronic carrier of the pathogen. Examples of community reservoirs are sewage or stagnant water and certain improperly cooked foods.

PATHOGEN

Several different classes of microorganisms produce infection (Table 27–2). Survival and continued multiplication of a pathogen are often accompanied by the production of toxins. Toxins are protein molecules released by bacteria to affect host cells at a distant site. Exotoxins are produced and released by certain bacteria into the surrounding environment. Botulism, tetanus, and diphtheria are attributed to exotoxins. Endotoxins are produced in the cell walls of certain bacteria and released only with cell lysis. Typhoid and meningococcal diseases are caused by endotoxins.

HOST

Several host factors influence the development of infection (Table 27–3). The human body has an efficient system for self-protection against pathogens known as host defense (see later discussion). Breakdown of any of these defense mechanisms may increase the susceptibility of the host to infection.

The client's immune status plays the largest role in determining his or her risk for infection. Congenital abnormalities as well as acquired health problems, such as acquired immunodeficiency syndrome (AIDS), can result in numerous immunologic deficiencies. Such depression of the immune system may render the host particularly susceptible to infection or cripple the host's ability to combat organisms that have gained entry.

NATURAL IMMUNITY Natural immunity is resistance to infection that occurs without previous exposure to an infecting organism. Several host factors influence natural immunity. *Age* has frequently been cited as a risk factor for the development of infection. Elderly clients are clearly at increased risk for infection, probably because of their decreased ability to produce an adequate immune response. Immunity declines in the elderly, as evidenced by decreasing T-cell and primary antibody responses (also see Chap. 22).

Transcultural Considerations Ethnicity may influence host susceptibility to infection. For example,

TABLE 27–2 Organisms That Produce Infection in People*

Organism Class	Common Examples	Common Disease Manifestations
Prions		• Creutzfeldt-Jakob disease
Viruses	• Poliovirus	• Poliomyelitis
	• Hepatitis A virus	• Hepatitis
	• Rhinovirus	• Common cold
	• Influenza A virus	• Influenza
	• Mumps virus	• Mumps
Chlamydiae	• *Chlamydia trachomatis*	• Trachoma, lymphogranuloma venereum, conjunctivitis
	• *C. psittaci*	• Psittacosis (parrot fever)
Mycoplasmas	• *Mycoplasma pneumoniae*	• Pneumonia
	• *Ureaplasma urealyticum*	• Urethritis
	• *Mycoplasma hominis*	• Pyelonephritis, pelvic inflammatory disease
Rickettsiae	• *Rickettsia rickettsii*	• Rocky Mountain spotted fever
	• *R. prowazekii*	• Typhus
	• *Coxiella burnetii*	• Q fever
Bacteria	• *Staphylococcus* sp.	• Superficial skin infections, osteomyelitis, pneumonia, bacteremia
	• *Streptococcus* sp.	• Pharyngitis, skin infections, pneumonia
	• *Neisseria meningitidis*	• Meningitis
	• *Escherichia coli*	• Urinary tract infection
	• *Pseudomonas aeruginosa*	• Skin infection, otitis, urinary tract infection
Fungi	• *Candida albicans*	• Thrush, vaginitis
	• *Aspergillus* sp.	• Sinusitis, brain abscess
	• *Cryptococcus neoformans*	• Meningitis, pneumonia
	• *Histoplasma capsulatum*	• Pneumonia
	• *Coccidioides immitis*	• Pneumonia
Protozoa	• *Entamoeba histolytica*	• Diarrhea, colitis
	• *Plasmodium* sp.	• Malaria
	• *Leishmania* sp.	• Fever, weight loss, cutaneous lesions
	• *Toxoplasma gondii*	• Chorioretinitis, encephalitis
	• *Pneumocystis carinii*	• Pneumonia
Helminths	• *Ancylostoma duodenale* (hookworm)	• Anemia
	• *Ascaris lumbricoides* (roundworm)	• Intestinal obstruction
	• *Enterobius vermicularis* (pinworm)	• Anal pruritus
	• *Schistosoma* sp. (blood flukes)	• Hydronephrosis
	• *Taenia solium* (pork tapeworm)	• Epilepsy from cysticercosis

* Organisms are presented in order of increasing complexity.

the incidence of tuberculosis in Native Americans, Mexican-Americans, and Soviet-Americans is higher than that in Caucasians (Giger & Davidhizar, 1991). Whether genetic differences influence disease resistance or whether apparent differences in immunity are due to other factors, such as nutrition or living conditions, is still unclear.

OTHER FACTORS Hormonal factors play a role in the incidence and mortality rate of many infectious diseases. People with diabetes mellitus and adrenal insufficiency experience increased numbers of acute and chronic bacterial infections.

Certain environmental factors may influence a person's immune status and thus his or her susceptibility to or ability to fight infection. Examples include alcohol consumption, inhalation of toxic chemicals that may suppress bone marrow function, and certain vitamin deficiencies. Malnutrition, especially protein-calorie malnutrition (which may result from chronic illnesses, such as end-stage renal disease, hepatic or gastrointestinal disease, or alcoholism), places a client at increased risk for infection.

Finally, certain types of medical interventions may suppress or impair the normal immune response. Corticosteroid therapy, chemotherapy for malignant neoplasms, and cytotoxic therapy specifically intended to suppress the immune response (e.g., cyclophosphamide for lupus nephritis and cyclosporine in organ transplant recipients) increase the client's risk for infection. Medical devices, such as percutaneous intravascular catheters, urethral catheters, and endotracheal tubes, also impair or violate normal host defense mechanisms.

PORTAL OF ENTRY

Microorganisms may enter the body in a variety of ways (Table 27–4).

RESPIRATORY TRACT A number of pathogens enter the body through the respiratory tract. Microbes in

TABLE 27-3 Host Factors that Influence Risk of Infection

Host Factor	Increased Risk of Infection
Natural immunity	• Congenital or acquired immunodeficiencies
Normal flora	• Alteration of normal flora by antibiotic therapy
Age	• Infants and elderly clients
Hormonal factors	• Pregnancy, diabetes, corticosteroid therapy, and adrenal insufficiency
Phagocytosis	• Defective phagocytic function, circulatory disturbances, and neutropenia
Skin/mucous membranes/normal excretory secretions	• Break in skin or mucous membrane integrity; interference with flow of urine, tears, or saliva; interference with cough reflex or ciliary action; changes in gastric secretions
Nutrition	• Malnutrition
Environmental factors	• Smoking, alcohol consumption, and inhalation of toxic chemicals
Medical interventions	• Invasive therapy, chemotherapy, radiation therapy, and steroid therapy; surgery

contaminated droplets are sprayed into the air when people with infected oral, nasal, or throat tissues talk, cough, or sneeze. These droplets are then inhaled by a susceptible host and either localize in the lung or are distributed via the lymphatic system or the bloodstream to other areas of the body. Microorganisms that enter the body by the respiratory tract but produce distant infection include *Mycobacterium tuberculosis,* influenza virus, and *Neisseria meningitidis* (the organism most commonly responsible for epidemic meningitis).

GASTROINTESTINAL TRACT Some pathogens enter the body through the gastrointestinal (GI) tract. Of these, some stay in the GI tract and produce disease (e.g., enteroviruses, *Giardia,* and the organisms that cause self-limited food poisoning). Others invade the GI tract to produce local and then distant infection (e.g., *Salmonella enteritidis*). Still others produce limited GI symptoms, causing either a systemic infection (e.g., *Salmonella typhi*) or profound involvement of another organ (e.g., hepatitis A virus). *Clostridium difficile* can cause diarrhea, especially in the elderly, and occurs when antibiotic therapy destroys the normal flora of the bowel. When diarrhea subsides, stool culture may still be positive for the microbe.

TABLE 27-4 Portals of Entry of Selected Disease-Producing Organisms

Portal of Entry	Infecting Organisms	Resultant Diseases
Respiratory tract	• *Neisseria meningitidis*	• Meningococcal pneumonia, meningococcal meningitis, meningococcemia
	• *Cryptococcus neoformans*	• Cryptococcal meningitis, cryptococcal pneumonia
	• *Mycobacterium tuberculosis*	• Tuberculosis
	• Influenza A virus	• Influenza
	• *Streptococcus pneumoniae*	• Pneumococcal pneumonia
	• Measles virus (rubeola)	• Measles
	• *Legionella pneumophila*	• Legionnaires' disease
	• Varicella-zoster virus	• Chickenpox
Gastrointestinal tract	• *Salmonella enteritidis*	• Gastroenteritis
	• *Salmonella typhi*	• Typhoid fever
	• *Giardia lamblia*	• Diarrhea
	• *Clostridium botulinum*	• Botulism
	• Poliovirus	• Poliomyelitis
	• Hepatitis A virus	• Hepatitis A
Genitourinary tract	• *Neisseria gonorrhoeae*	• Gonorrhea
	• *Chlamydia trachomatis*	• Lymphogranuloma venereum, cervicitis, urethritis, endometritis
	• Enterobacteriaceae (*Escherichia coli, Klebsiella* sp., *Serratia* sp., *Proteus* sp.)	• Urinary tract infections
Intact skin or mucous membranes	• Rhinovirus	• Common cold
	• Respiratory syncytial virus	• Pneumonia, bronchiolitis, tracheobronchitis
	• *Schistosoma* sp.	• Schistososome dermatitis (swimmer's disease)
	• Herpes simplex virus	• Oral or genital herpes
Bloodstream	• Hepatitis B virus	• Hepatitis B
	• *Plasmodium*	• Malaria
	• *Clostridium tetani*	• Tetanus
	• Human immunodeficiency virus (HIV)	• AIDS

GENITOURINARY TRACT A third portal of entry for microorganisms is the genitourinary tract. Urinary tract infection is one of the most common infectious diseases treated each year. Microorganisms (often normal colonic bacterial flora) colonize the perineal area, the urethral meatus, and the bladder, especially in a woman with a short urethra. The elderly woman is at an even greater risk because of decreased resistance to infection, stress incontinence, or, possibly, inability to practice proper hygiene.

SKIN/MUCOUS MEMBRANES Some pathogens, such as *Treponema pallidum,* can enter the body through intact skin or mucous membranes. Most enter through breaks in these normally effective surface barriers. Sometimes a medical procedure creates a break in the normal cutaneous (skin) or mucocutaneous (mucous membrane) barriers, as in surgical wound infections and catheter-acquired bacteremia (bacteria in the bloodstream).

BLOODSTREAM Microorganisms can gain direct access to the bloodstream. Insects can inject organisms into the bloodstream by biting the host, causing such infections as malaria, Lyme disease, and Rocky Mountain spotted fever.

MODE OF TRANSMISSION

For infection to be transmitted, a mechanism must transport the invading organism from the infected source to a susceptible host. Microorganisms are transmitted by several routes, and the same microorganism may be transmitted by more than one route. The four common routes are:

- Contact transmission
- Airborne transmission
- Vehicle transmission
- Vector-borne transmission

CONTACT TRANSMISSION Many infections are spread by contact, which may be direct or indirect. With *direct* contact, the source and host come into physical contact; microorganisms are transferred directly, usually through skin to skin or mucous membrane to mucous membrane. Often called person-to-person transmission, direct contact is best illustrated by the sexual spread of venereal disease.

Indirect contact leading to transmission of infectious agents involves transfer of microorganisms from a source to a host by passive transfer from an inanimate (not living) intermediate object (also called a fomite). Contaminated articles, especially those that may contact nonintact skin or mucous membranes, may serve as sources of infection. One example of transmission through indirect contact is transfer of hepatitis B virus from a contaminated source to a susceptible host by a device for capillary blood sampling.

Another method of indirect contact, *droplet spread,* involves transmission of infection through contact with infective secretions. Droplets are relatively large, usually greater than 5 μm in size. These droplets are most often produced when a person talks or sneezes, and they travel through the air only a short distance (usually less than 3 feet, or 1 meter). Susceptible hosts may acquire infection by contact with droplets deposited on the membranes of the nose, mouth, or conjunctivae. A common example of droplet-spread infection is measles. Susceptible people who are closest to the infected source have the highest risk for infection with a droplet-spread organism.

Oral-fecal transmission is another example of indirect contact for the spread of infection. Ingestion of enteric pathogens (e.g., eating food prepared by a person with hepatitis A infection who does not wash his or her hands) can cause transmission of the virus.

AIRBORNE TRANSMISSION Airborne transmission occurs when small, airborne, infected particles leave the infected source and travel farther than 3 feet (approximately 1 meter) in the air. These particles are usually contained in droplet nuclei or dust; they are most often propelled from the respiratory tract by coughing or sneezing. A susceptible person then inhales the particles directly into the respiratory tract. Tuberculosis, legionnaires' disease, and chickenpox are transmitted by the airborne route.

VEHICLE TRANSMISSION Vehicle transmission occurs when infectious agents are transmitted through a common source, such as contaminated food, water, or intravenous fluid. Salmonellosis is an example of a vehicle-transmitted disease.

VECTOR-BORNE TRANSMISSION Vector-borne transmission of infection involves insects and animals that act as intermediaries between two or more hosts. For example, ticks can transmit Rocky Mountain spotted fever and mosquitoes can spread malaria.

PORTAL OF EXIT

The portal of exit completes the chain of infection. An infecting organism exits from the once-susceptible person who has become a reservoir for infection. Exit from the host most often occurs through the portal of entry. An organism, such as *Mycobacterium tuberculosis,* enters the susceptible client's respiratory tract and exits the respiratory tract as the infected host coughs into the air. However, some organisms may exit from the infected host by several routes. For example, varicella-zoster virus can spread through direct contact with infective fluid in the chickenpox vesicles and by droplet contact.

DEFENSE AGAINST INFECTION

Several host factors influence the development of infection. Strong and intact host defenses can prevent a microbe from entering the body, or they can destroy a pathogen that has gained entry. Conversely, impaired host defenses may be unable to defend against microbial invasion, allowing entry of microorganisms that can destroy host cells and cause infection.

Host defense mechanisms may be classified as nonspecific or specific.

NONSPECIFIC DEFENSES

Nonspecific mechanisms, most often representing the first encounter an invading pathogen has with its human host, include:

- Body tissues, such as the skin and mucous membranes
- Phagocytosis
- Inflammation

BODY TISSUES Intact skin forms the first and most important physical barrier to the entry of microorganisms into the body. In addition to providing a mechanical barrier, the skin's slightly acidic pH (resulting from the breakdown of lipids into fatty acids), together with the normal skin flora, creates an unfriendly environment for pathogenic bacteria.

Mucous membranes, by their mucociliary action, provide some mechanical protection against pathogenic invasion. More important, however, mucous membranes are bathed in secretions that inactivate many microorganisms. Lysozymes, which are enzymes that dissolve the cell walls of some bacteria, are present in large quantities in many body secretions, particularly in nasal mucus and tears.

Other body systems provide natural barriers to infection. The respiratory tract can clear about 90% of all inhaled material by filtration in the upper airways, humidification, mucociliary transport, and expulsion by coughing. Peristaltic action mechanically empties the gastrointestinal tract of pathogenic organisms. In addition, the acid pH of the stomach, intestinal secretions, pancreatic enzymes, and bile, together with the competition from normal bowel flora, provides an environment that protects the gastrointestinal tract from invasion by harmful organisms. In the genitourinary tract, the flushing action of urine eliminates pathogenic organisms. The low pH of urine also maintains a sterile environment, although certain microorganisms, like *Escherichia coli,* can thrive in an acid medium. Table 27-5 summarizes the action of body tissues in defending a host.

PHAGOCYTOSIS Phagocytosis occurs when a foreign substance evades the first-line mechanical barriers and enters the body. Various types of leukocytes function differently in the immune reaction, but neutrophils bear the primary responsibility for phagocytosis. This process of engulfing, ingesting, killing, and disposing of an invading organism is an essential mechanism in host defense. Phagocytic dysfunction dramatically increases a client's risk for infection and recurrent infections.

TABLE 27-5 Nonspecific Defense Mechanisms

Body Tissue	Type of Action	Defense Action
Intact skin	• Physical • Chemical	• Provides a barrier • Normal flora and acid pH create a hostile environment
Mucous membranes	• Mechanical	• Mucociliary action clears bacteria
	• Chemical	• Lysosomes dissolve bacterial wall
Respiratory tract	• Mechanical	• Mucociliary action • Cough
	• Chemical	• Lysosome action • Humidification
Gastrointestinal tract	• Mechanical • Chemical	• Peristalsis • Enzymes • Acid pH • Normal bowel flora
Genitourinary tract	• Mechanical • Chemical	• Flushing action of urine • Acid pH

INFLAMMATION Inflammation is another important nonspecific defense mechanism in preventing the spread of infection. Inflammation occurs when tissue becomes damaged. The damaged cells release enzymes, and polymorphonuclear leukocytes are attracted to the infected site from the bloodstream. One important enzyme, histamine, increases the permeability of the capillaries in the inflamed tissues, thus allowing fluid, proteins, and white blood cells to enter the inflamed area. Still other enzymes activate fibrinogen, which causes the leaked fluid to clot and prevents its flow away from the damaged site into unaffected tissue, essentially "walling off" the inflamed tissue. The process of phagocytosis then disposes of the invading microorganism and often the dead tissue. If the inflammation is caused by infection, the end products of inflammation form the substance commonly known as pus, which is subsequently absorbed or exits the body through a break in the skin. (See also Chapter 22 for a discussion of the inflammatory response.)

SPECIFIC DEFENSES

Specific defenses against infection, that is, specific responses to specific microorganisms, are provided by the antibody-mediated and cell-mediated immune systems. The antibody-mediated immune system produces antibodies directed against certain pathogens. These antibodies inactivate or destroy the invading microorganism as well as protect against future infection with that microorganism. Resistance to other microorganisms is mediated by the action of specifically sensitized T lymphocytes and is called cell-mediated immunity. The components of the immune system work both independently and together to protect against infection (see Chap. 22).

INFECTION CONTROL IN HEALTH CARE FACILITIES

Infection acquired in the hospital, nursing home, or other inpatient setting (not present or incubating at the time of admission) is termed *nosocomial.* Nosocomial infections can be endogenous (from the client's own flora) or exogenous (from outside the client, usually from the health care facility environment or the hands of health care workers). The hospital stay of 5 to 10 days required for treatment of nosocomial infections costs approximately $4 billion annually. The costs associated with the additional morbidity and mortality cannot be measured. Infection control within a health care facility is designed to reduce the risk of nosocomial infection and thus reduce morbidity and mortality and their associated costs. A program for infection control includes infection control policies and procedures (usually found in a designated manual), surveillance, and client and staff education. The program is coordinated and implemented by an infection control practitioner who is usually a nurse certified in infection control (CIC).

Infection or the spread of infection can be prevented or controlled in health care facilities in at least five ways:

- Hand washing
- Hygiene
- Sanitation
- Disinfection/sterilization
- Barriers (such as gloves)

Every health care facility employee who comes in contact with clients or client care areas is involved in some aspect of the infection control program of the health care facility.

HAND WASHING Hand washing is the *single most effective* mechanism for preventing the spread of infection. Effective hand washing consists of wetting, soaping, lathering, applying friction, rinsing, and drying adequately. Friction may be supplied by soft brushes or simply by rubbing the skin surfaces together. Friction is essential to emulsify the oils on the skin and to disperse transient bacteria and soil from the skin surface. To avoid chapped or cracked skin, nurses should rinse and dry their hands thoroughly.

Health care personnel should always wash their hands before and after direct contact with a client and immediately after contact with blood, secretions, or excretions. The use of gloves does not eliminate the need for hand washing. The Centers for Disease Control and Prevention (CDC) recommends the use of antiseptic solutions, such as chlorhexidine or povidone-iodine, for hand washing in the care of clients who are at high risk (e.g., immunocompromised clients). The use of these solutions is widely accepted in caring for clients who are colonized or infected with virulent or multiply-resistant organisms.

OTHER INFECTION CONTROL MEASURES Proper *hygiene,* including bathing and grooming, is important in preventing infection for both the client and the health care personnel. Strict attention to *sanitation* in a health care facility is also especially important, because proper procedures for infectious waste (e.g., soiled dressings) disposal and incineration must be followed in keeping with CDC guidelines. *Sterilization* and *disinfection* procedures keep equipment and the physical environment (like hospital rooms) clean, with no or minimal microorganisms that harm clients. For example, the housekeeping staff uses strong but safe cleaning chemicals that disinfect or destroy most microbes.

In addition to these measures, the nurse must try to keep clients with infections from clients who are highly susceptible to infection, such as a new postoperative or immunocompromised client. This helps prevent transmission of infection from client to client.

Barriers are items placed between the client and the health care provider. Gloves, masks, and gowns are examples (see the next paragraph).

BARRIER PRECAUTIONS

Meticulous hand washing is essential within any health care facility. In some instances, however, hand washing alone may not be sufficient for infection control. Barrier precautions, also called isolation precautions, are designed to prevent the spread of infection in these circumstances. These precautions have changed dramatically over the past 20 years as transmission of infections has become better understood and new infections have emerged.

In 1983, the Centers for Disease Control (CDC) issued its initial guidelines for isolation precautions for use in health care facilities. However, these recommendations are based entirely on information that was available in 1983 regarding the transmission of infectious organisms. Additional guidelines from the CDC continue to be distributed periodically to health care facilities. The latest guidelines are reviewed by each health care facility's infection control committee and then tailored to meet the specific needs of that facility. Each health care facility develops its own policies and procedures for barrier precautions, but the principles are similar.

HISTORY OF CDC GUIDELINES The CDC isolation guidelines of 1983 describe two alternative systems:

- Category-specific isolation precautions
- Disease-specific isolation precautions

Both systems are designed to prevent an infection from being spread from one client to another.

Category-Specific Isolation Precautions Category-specific precautions group isolation procedures into seven distinct categories on the basis of the disease's mode of transmission. In this system, category-specific isolation instruction cards are usually posted outside the client's room. Although not all categories are used today in most health care facilities, each category is described briefly in Table 27–6.

Category-specific isolation is associated with several advantages. The system is relatively simple, convenient, and familiar in most health care institutions. However, because many diseases are grouped into a few broad categories, unnecessary techniques are used for some infections. Thus, overisolation may occur. To avoid this problem, the CDC recommended an alternative system, or disease-specific isolation.

Disease-Specific Isolation Precautions Disease-specific isolation involves the use of a single instruction card for all clients with a transmissible infection. This instruction card lists all possible isolation specifications (e.g., masks, gowns, gloves, and private room) and requires that a health care professional indicate which are appropriate for a specific disease. Use of only those particular precautions needed to interrupt the transmission of a specific disease eliminates overisolation and the costs of unnecessary precautions. However, the disease-specific system requires more training and attention on the part of health care personnel.

UNIVERSAL PRECAUTIONS

Guidelines In 1987, the CDC published Universal Precautions guidelines. Although infection control practitioners believed all clients' blood and body fluids to be potentially infectious, this concept was not widely accepted by health care personnel until the 1987 guidelines were published. The CDC issued the guidelines in response to concern about the transmission of human immunodeficiency virus (HIV), which causes acquired immunodeficiency syndrome (AIDS). Hepatitis B virus (HBV) is also a commonly transmitted blood-borne disease that affects health care workers more often than HIV infection does. About 200 health care workers die from HBV complications each year (Weber et al., 1991; Yassi & McGill, 1991).

Unlike the category-specific isolation precautions for the protection of clients in health care facilities, Universal Precautions protect health care workers who come into contact with clients. All clients are considered potentially infected with a blood-borne disease.

Table 27–7 outlines the guidelines for Universal Precautions. Since these guidelines were published, the CDC has specified which body fluids are the highest risk for transmission of any blood-borne disease and which ones are not. For example, exposure to saliva is less of a risk than is exposure to blood in a person's stool (Table 27–8).

Problems with Universal Precautions Two areas of concern about Universal Precautions are being addressed: needlestick injuries and glove quality.

Even though the CDC requires that needles no longer be recapped and that sharps containers for needle disposal be available, a number of needlestick injuries still occur each year, most often to nurses (Haiduven et al., 1992). Several manufacturers have developed needleless systems or needle protection systems to prevent needlestick injuries.

Research has shown that latex gloves are superior to vinyl gloves, but virus leakage may occur with either type. To help resolve this problem, newer gloves are being double-dipped and protected with

TABLE 27–6 Category-Specific Isolation Precautions

Isolation Category	Private Room*	Masks	Gowns	Gloves	Common Diseases Placed into Isolation Category
Strict isolation	• Always	• Always	• Always	• Always	• Varicella-zoster (chickenpox); pharyngeal diphtheria; shingles (zoster), localized in an immunocompromised client or disseminated
Contact isolation	• Always	• For close contact	• If soiling with infective material is likely	• If contact with infective material is likely	• Acute respiratory tract infection in infants and young children; disseminated herpes simplex; methicillin-resistant *Staphylococcus aureus;* pediculosis; scabies
Respiratory isolation	• Always	• For close contact	• No	• No	• Measles; meningococcal meningitis, pneumonia, or meningococcemia; mumps; pertussis
Acid-fast bacteria isolation	• Always	• Yes	• Only to prevent gross contamination	• No	• Tuberculosis (primary pulmonary or pharyngeal)
Enteric precautions	• Only if the client's hygiene is poor	• No	• If soiling with infective material is likely	• If contact with infective material is likely	• Enteroviral infection, including meningitis; infectious gastroenteritis (e.g., giardiasis, salmonellosis, shigellosis); hepatitis A, *Clostridium difficile* enterocolitis
Drainage and secretion precautions	• No	• No	• If soiling with infective material is likely	• If contact with infective material is likely	• Minor or limited abscess, wound, burn, or skin infection; conjunctivitis
Blood and body fluid precautions	• Only if the client's hygiene is poor	• If contact with blood or body fluids is likely	• If contact with splashes of blood or body fluids is likely	• If contact with blood or body fluids is likely	• AIDS; hepatitis B; non-A, non-B hepatitis; malaria

* In most instances when a private room is required, clients infected with the same organism may share a room.

TABLE 27–7 Universal Precautions

These precautions are to be used with all clients to protect health care providers from blood-borne communicable diseases.

- *Gloves* should be worn for contact with blood and body fluids, nonintact skin, and mucous membranes of all clients; for handling surfaces or items soiled with blood and body fluids; and for performing venipuncture and other vascular access procedures. Gloves should be changed after each client contact.
- *Masks or protective goggles* should be worn during procedures that are likely to cause splashes of blood or body fluids.
- *Gowns or aprons* should be worn during procedures that are likely to result in splashes of blood or body fluids.
- *Hand washing* should be done immediately on contact with blood or other body fluids. One should wash hands as soon as gloves are removed.
- *Needles and sharp instruments* should be placed in puncture-resistant containers for disposal to prevent injuries from needles or other sharp items. Needles should not be recapped, bent, or removed from the syringe.
- *Mouth-to-mouth resuscitation* should be performed with use of mouthpieces or other ventilation devices.

Data from Centers for Disease Control. (1987). Recommendations for prevention of HIV transmission in health-care settings. *Morbidity and Mortality Weekly Report, 36*(2S), 3–17.

special chemicals that kill pathogens on contact (Korniewicz, 1992).

BODY SUBSTANCE PRECAUTIONS Universal Precautions have been expanded by infection control experts to include other materials from the body besides blood and body fluids; this isolation category is called body substance precautions or body substance isolation (BSI). With the increased occurrence of gastrointestinal microorganisms, like *Clostridium difficile,* any client's feces is considered a potential source of infection. Therefore, *in addition* to wearing barriers for protection from blood and certain body fluids, the nurse and other health care personnel should always wear gloves when coming in contact with feces or anything contaminated with feces, like soiled linen and underpads. Gowns may also be necessary to protect the staff's uniform.

By using body substance precautions, several categories under the category-specific isolation system can be eliminated (e.g., enteric precautions, drainage and secretion precautions, and blood and body fluid precautions). As a result, many infection control programs have condensed their categories for isolation into five (or fewer) groups: body substance, strict, respiratory, acid-fast and contact precautions.

Another trend in infection control practice discourages the term *isolation,* which implies that the client is removed from everyone else. Nonprofessional health care facility employees are often afraid of isolation and fear that they will "catch" an infection from the isolated client. The terms *barrier* and *precautions* are preferred.

Whichever system for precautions is used, the nurse must be careful to prevent the client's solitude and to promote quality care. In some cases, initiating barrier precautions may be associated with untoward psychosocial effects. For the few clients who must be confined to their rooms, the constant environment of the hospital room may be difficult to tolerate. Family members may also express fear or anxiety because the client is isolated. Clients in strict isolation, visited only by persons wearing masks, gowns, and gloves, may actually experience sensory deprivation (see Chap. 9).

TABLE 27–8 Categories of Body Fluids for Universal Precautions

Body Fluids to Which Universal Precautions Apply

- Blood and other body fluids containing visible blood
- Semen and vaginal/cervical secretions
- Tissues
- Cerebrospinal fluid
- Amniotic fluid
- Synovial fluid
- Pleural fluid
- Peritoneal fluid
- Pericardial fluid

Body Fluids to Which Universal Precautions Do Not Apply Unless They Contain Visible Blood

- Feces
- Nasal secretions
- Sputum
- Vomitus
- Sweat
- Tears
- Urine
- Breast milk
- Saliva, except in dentistry

OCCUPATIONAL EXPOSURE TO SOURCES OF INFECTION

The Occupational Safety and Health Administration (OSHA) is a federal agency that protects all workers from injury or illness at their place of employment. Unlike the guidelines developed by the Centers for Disease Control, OSHA regulations are law. Employers can be disciplined for noncompliance with OSHA regulations.

In 1991, Congress passed the Bloodborne Pathogens Standard prepared by OSHA (Table 27–9). Effective as of March 6, 1992, this legislation eliminates or minimizes occupational exposure to hepatitis B virus (HBV), human immunodeficiency virus (HIV), and other blood-borne pathogens. The standard does not specify the type of workplace but defines whether an employee is at risk for occupational exposure to blood or body fluids.

In addition to standards protecting workers from blood-borne diseases, OSHA is developing regulations that address protection from the newer resistant strains of tuberculosis. Some states in the United States have already implemented legislation for this purpose. As for occupational exposure, each facility

TABLE 27–9 OSHA Standard for Blood-Borne Pathogens

- Employers whose workers are at risk of "occupational exposure" must establish a written exposure control plan that is updated annually. This plan must be available to all employees.
- Employers must implement and enforce procedures that reduce the risk of occupational exposure, including, but not limited to, Universal Precautions, hand washing, and providing supplies for avoidance of blood or other infectious materials.
- Employers must provide and launder protective garments and other equipment, such as gloves, gowns, masks, face shields, goggles, and ventilation devices. Gloves must be hypoallergenic or powderless for those employees who are allergic to glove material.
- Employers must provide the hepatitis B vaccine to all employees at no cost to the employee within 10 days of employment. If the employee refuses the vaccine, the employer must obtain a signed statement indicating this refusal.
- Employers must provide postexposure evaluation for all employees who are exposed to blood or other infectious material.
- Employers must train employees about the hazards of blood and other infectious materials, and the Bloodborne Pathogens Standard; this training must be done annually.

Adapted from the Occupational Safety and Health Administration. (1991).

will be required to provide employee education and counseling, tuberculosis screening, specially designed client isolation rooms, and special masks that protect the health care worker.

COMPLICATIONS OF INFECTION

Most complications of infection relate to inadequate treatment. This may range from an incorrect choice of antibiotics to poor compliance by clients. Perhaps the most obvious complication of inadequate treatment is relapse. Relapse may be serious because:

1. Some infections may become active again in a more subtle fashion. Thus, the client may think that the infection is getting slowly better on its own, but the infection is not under control.
2. Noncompliance with the drug regimen (e.g., taking the medication when the client feels like it) prevents contact of the harmful microorganism with sufficient concentrations of the antibiotic.

LOCAL COMPLICATIONS

Serious complications of infection may result from incomplete antibiotic therapy. Local infections that could be cured without complications, such as cellulitis and pneumonia, may progress to abscess formation if appropriate drug therapy is not continued. Although adequate antibiotic therapy does not always prevent abscess, early therapy may prevent or at least limit the size of an abscess.

SYSTEMIC COMPLICATIONS

In addition to abscess formation, systemic complications may develop as a result of inadequate therapy. If a client's infection is not completely resolved or if it is being treated with drugs that are not effective against the offending microorganism, the pathogen may enter the bloodstream. Systemic sepsis or septicemia results. Even small local infections, if left untreated or treated inadequately, may spread locally or via the bloodstream to produce significant complications, such as leukocytosis (increased white blood cell count) or leukopenia (decreased white blood cell count) and disseminated intravascular coagulation (DIC) (see Chap. 26). After pathogens invade the bloodstream, virtually no site is protected from invasion.

Clients with sepsis may progress to sepsis-induced distributive shock, also known as septic shock. In septic shock, insufficient cardiac output is compounded by hypovolemia; inadequate blood supply to vital organs leads to hypoxia (lack of oxygen) and metabolic failure (see Chap. 36).

COLLABORATIVE MANAGEMENT

ASSESSMENT

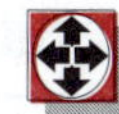

HISTORY

Careful attention to the history of a client with a possible infectious disease helps the nurse determine risk factors for infection. The age of a client, history of cigarette smoking or alcohol use, current illness or disease (such as diabetes), past and current medication use, familial predisposition, and poor nutritional status may place the client at increased risk for a number of infectious diseases.

The nurse also determines whether the client has been exposed to infectious agents. A history of recent exposure to someone with similar clinical symptoms or to contaminated food or water, as well as the time of exposure, assists in identifying a possible source for infection. Nurses may find this information helpful for determining the incubation period for the disease and thus for providing a clue to its cause.

Contact with animals, including pets, may facilitate exposure to infection. The nurse asks the client about recent contact with animals at home, at work, or in the course of leisure activities, such as hunting. The nurse also asks the client about recent contact with insects.

The nurse obtains a travel history from the client. Travel to areas both within and outside the client's home country may expose a susceptible client to infectious organisms not encountered in the local community.

A thorough sexual history may reveal sexual behavior associated with increased risk of sexually transmitted diseases. The nurse should obtain a history of intravenous drug use and a transfusion history to assess the client's risk for hepatitis B, hepatitis C, and human immunodeficiency virus (HIV) infections.

Ascertaining the type and location of symptoms may provide a key to the affected organ system. The order of onset of symptoms may also provide clues to the client's specific problem.

PHYSICAL ASSESSMENT/CLINICAL MANIFESTATIONS

Disorders caused by pathogens vary, depending on the cause and the site of infection. Common clinical manifestations are associated with specific sites of infection (Chart 27-1). Symptoms of local infection at any site include pain, swelling, heat, redness, and pus. The nurse carefully inspects the skin for these symptoms.

Fever (generally a body temperature above 38° C [101° F]), chills, and malaise are primary indicators of a systemic infection. Fever may also accompany other noninfectious disorders, and infection *can* be present without fever. The elderly client whose normal body temperature may be 1° to 2° lower than in younger adults may manifest fever at 37° C (99° F). The nurse assesses the client for these symptoms and carefully questions the client about the history and patterns of symptoms.

Lymphadenopathy, photophobia, pharyngitis, and gastrointestinal disturbance (usually diarrhea or vomiting) are often associated with infection. The nurse palpates the cervical and axillary lymph nodes to detect enlargement and examines the throat for redness. Other lymph nodes are also palpated for enlargement. In the elderly, a change in mental status may be the first, if not the only, presenting symptom. The nurse determines the client's baseline mental status for comparison. The client typically becomes increasingly confused and disoriented (Chart 27-2).

CHART 27-1

Key Features of Infection of Specific Sites

Gastrointestinal Infections
- Fever
- Nausea and vomiting
- Diarrhea
- Abdominal distention

Genitourinary Infections
- Dysuria
- Frequency
- Urgency
- Hematuria
- Fever
- Purulent discharge
- Pelvic or flank pain

Respiratory Infections
- Cough
- Congestion
- Rhinitis
- Sore throat
- Sputum
- Fever
- Chest pain

Skin Infections
- Redness
- Warmth
- Swelling
- Drainage
- Pain

Generalized Infections
- Fever
- Malaise
- Fatigue
- Muscle aches
- Joint pain

CHART 27-2

Nursing Focus on the Elderly ◆ Infection

- Assess for atypical clinical manifestations of infection, such as confusion and unusual behavior. Typical manifestations, such as fever and pain, may not be present.
- Monitor renal function carefully when the client receives antibiotic therapy, especially aminoglycosides.
- Observe for and report adverse effects of antibiotic therapy because they may cause serious complications or death in an elderly client.
- Monitor for diarrhea from *Clostridium difficile* infection; obtain a specimen for culture if diarrhea occurs.
- Keep the client well hydrated because the elderly client is at high risk for dehydration.

PSYCHOSOCIAL ASSESSMENT

The client with an infectious disease often has psychosocial concerns. Typically, several diagnostic tests must be performed, and definitive identification of the microorganism responsible for the client's symptoms may be prolonged. This delay produces frustration and anxiety for the client. The nurse assesses the client's level of understanding about various diagnostic procedures and the time that may be required to obtain accurate results.

Frequently noted symptoms of infection are prolonged feelings of malaise and fatigue. The nurse assesses the client's psychologic and sociologic adjustment to a decreased energy level. The nurse evaluates the client's current level of activity and the impact of these symptoms on usual family, occupational, and recreational activities.

An additional stress associated with the diagnosis of an infection is the potential spread of infection to others. The client may curtail family and social interactions for fear of spreading the illness. The nurse assesses the client's and family's levels of understanding of the infection, its mode of transmission, and mechanisms that may limit or prevent transmission. The nurse assesses the effects of the client's illness on usual interpersonal interactions.

Finally, a number of transmissible infectious diseases, especially those associated with socially unacceptable lifestyles (such as intravenous drug abuse), are associated with some degree of social labeling. The client may feel socially isolated and may experience guilt related to behavior that increases the risk for infection. The nurse observes carefully for signs of the client's reaction to social labels and how these feelings further affect socialization.

LABORATORY ASSESSMENT

The definitive diagnosis of an infectious disease requires identification of a microorganism in the tissues of an infected client. Direct examination of blood, body fluids, and tissues under a microscope in the laboratory may not yield positive identification of an organism. However, laboratory assessment usually provides helpful information about the microorganism, such as its shape, motility, and reaction to various staining agents. Even when direct microscopy does not prove diagnostic, enough information is often gathered for initiating appropriate antibiotic therapy.

CULTURE AND SENSITIVITY The most definitive procedure for identification of a microorganism is *culture,* or isolation of the pathogen by cultivation in tissue cultures or various artificial media. Specimens for culture may be obtained from almost any body fluid or tissue. The physician usually decides when and where the specimen for culture is taken. The nurse often obtains the specimen when ordered.

Proper collection and handling of specimens for culture are essential for obtaining accurate results. The specimen collected by the nurse must be appropriate for the suspected infection. Material must be in sufficient quantity, freshly obtained, and placed in a sterile container that adequately preserves the specimen and microorganism to be examined. Chart 27–3 suggests techniques for collecting specimens for culture. The nurse always checks with the laboratory or laboratory manual for the specific procedure to be followed in a particular facility.

After isolation of a microorganism in culture, antibiotic sensitivity testing is usually performed to determine the effects of various antibiotics on that particular microorganism. A microorganism that is killed by acceptable levels of an antibiotic is considered *sensitive* to that drug. An organism that is not killed by tolerable levels of an antibiotic is considered *resistant* to that drug. If sensitivity testing is desired, the nurse ensures that the laboratory slip is marked for a "C & S," indicating that both culture and sensitivity testing are to be performed on the specimen. Preliminary results are usually available in 24 to 48 hours, but the final results generally take 72 hours.

SEROLOGY A less specific laboratory test for determining the presence of an infectious microorganism is a serologic test—a blood test to look for antibodies that react with a certain antigen. Serologic tests are available for virtually all classes of microorganisms. Examples of diseases for which serologic studies commonly aid diagnosis include syphilis, mononucleosis, Rocky Mountain spotted fever, and cryptococcosis.

A positive serologic result does not necessarily indicate active infection but merely signifies that the client has had previous exposure to the antigen in question. Two serum specimens are typically obtained from a client—the first during the acute phase of illness, and the second 7 to 10 days later. A fourfold or greater rise in antibody titer in the second specimen indicates a recent infection.

COMPLETE BLOOD COUNT A complete blood count (CBC) is nearly always performed on the client with a suspected infectious disease. Five types of leukocytes (white blood cells) have been identified: neutrophils, lymphocytes, monocytes, eosinophils, and basophils. In most active infections, especially those caused by bacteria, the total leukocyte count is elevated. Various diseases are characterized by changes in the percentages of the different types of leukocytes. The differential count most often shows an increased number of immature neutrophils, or a shift to the left. A few infectious diseases, however, are associated with neutropenia, (decreased neutrophils), such as malaria and infectious mononucleosis.

ERYTHROCYTE SEDIMENTATION RATE The erythrocyte sedimentation rate (ESR) measures the rate at which red blood cells fall through plasma. This rate is most significantly affected by an increased number of acute-phase reactants, which occurs with inflammation. Thus, an elevated ESR (>20 mm/hr) indicates inflammation or infection somewhere in the body. Chronic infection, most notably osteomyelitis, and chronic abscesses are commonly associated with an elevated ESR. The effectiveness of therapy is often monitored by a fall in this value.

RADIOGRAPHIC ASSESSMENT

X-rays are often obtained to determine activity or destruction by an infectious microorganism. Radiologic studies (such as chest films, sinus films, joint films, gastrointestinal studies, and renal films) are typically obtained for diagnosis of infection in a specific body site.

A more sophisticated technique for diagnosis of an infection is computed tomography. This method is particularly helpful in assessing the presence and location of abscesses.

OTHER DIAGNOSTIC ASSESSMENT

Another diagnostic tool for the evaluation of a client with an infectious disease is *ultrasonography.* This noninvasive procedure is particularly helpful in detecting infection that has affected the heart valves.

CHART 27–3

Nursing Care Highlight ◆ Collection Techniques for Commonly Cultured Specimens

Specimen	Collection Method	Comments
Blood	1. Decontaminate the skin with 70% alcohol followed by 2% tincture of iodine, allowed to dry. 2. Perform venipuncture and collect 10 mL of blood (2 mL in infants). 3. Inject into sterile culture bottles—usually one vented and one unvented for anaerobic culture.	Three separate specimens are usually collected over a 24-hr period to ensure isolation of the causative organism.
Urine		
Clean void	1. Clean the urethral meatus with tincture of iodine or other antiseptic solution. 2. Have the client void small amount and then collect approximately 2 mL of midstream urine specimen into a sterile container.	The specimen may be refrigerated. If not, the specimen must be delivered to the laboratory within 30 min to be useful for quantitative studies.
Indwelling catheter	1. Clean the aspiration site on catheter drainage tubing with iodine. 2. Collect a 2-mL specimen into a sterile container.	
Wound	1. Decontaminate the skin with 70% alcohol. 2. Swab an active margin of the wound with a sterile swab and place the swab into a sterile tube.	
Throat	1. Swab an inflamed area of the throat, especially areas of exudate. 2. Place the swab into sterile medium for transport.	Inform the laboratory of any suspected organism other than group A streptococcus.
Sputum	1. Collect first morning expectorated sputum into a sterile container.	Production of an adequate specimen may be aided by saline aerosol administration or by postural drainage. Sputum specimens may also be collected via tracheal or transtracheal aspiration.
Pus (abscesses)	1. Decontaminate the skin with alcohol. 2. Coat a sterile swab rapidly with pus. 3. Insert the swab immediately into a specially prepared anaerobic transport tube.	Deliver the specimen to the laboratory immediately.
Vagina	1. Wipe the vagina clean of secretions with dry gauze. 2. Swab the exudate with a sterile swab. 3. Insert into a sterile container or into specially prepared medium.	If trichomoniasis is suspected, place the swab in a small amount of sterile saline and send to the laboratory immediately.
Rectal swab	1. Insert the swab into the rectum approximately 1 in and rotate once. 2. Place into transport medium.	The specimen is usually sent on 3 consecutive days. The swab should show obvious soiling.
Stool	1. Collect stool in a clean waxed cardboard container.	Deliver to the laboratory immediately. The specimen is often collected on 3 consecutive days
Intravenous catheters	1. Clean the catheter insertion site with alcohol. 2. Withdraw the catheter and cut off approximately a 5-cm tip with sterile scissors. 3. Place into a sterile container.	In general, catheter tips that are contaminated during removal will grow only a few colonies, whereas infected catheters usually show heavy growth.

Scanning techniques using radioactive substances, such as gallium, can determine the presence of inflammation. Inflammatory tissue is identified by its increased uptake of the injected radioactive material.

To obtain tissue for culture, biopsy of the infected site may be necessary. Biopsy sites may include the liver, bone marrow, skin, pleura, lymph nodes, kidney, bone, or even the brain. To obtain specimens for examination, invasive procedures (such as bronchoscopy or endoscopy) or even surgery (such as open lung biopsy or laparotomy) may be necessary. These procedures are described in detail elsewhere in this text.

ANALYSIS

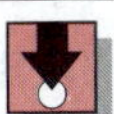

COMMON NURSING DIAGNOSES

The most common nursing diagnoses for clients with an infection or infectious disease include:

1. Hyperthermia related to increased metabolic state
2. Fatigue related to increased metabolic energy production
3. Social Isolation related to effects of illness

ADDITIONAL NURSING DIAGNOSES

The inclusion of other nursing diagnoses depends on the type and extent of the infection. For example, a client with pneumonia might experience Ineffective Airway Clearance; a client with a sexually transmitted disease may have Altered Sexuality Patterns.

PLANNING AND IMPLEMENTATION

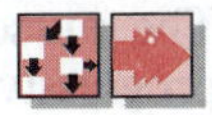

HYPERTHERMIA

PLANNING: CLIENT GOALS The primary goal is that the client's body temperature will return to normal.

INTERVENTIONS Fever (hyperthermia) is one way in which the body attempts to destroy pathogens. The primary concern is to provide measures to eliminate the underlying cause of hyperthermia—to destroy the causative microorganism. Interventions are implemented to reduce fever, such as:

- Antibiotic therapy
- Antipyretic therapy
- External cooling
- Fluid administration

Antibiotic Therapy The cornerstone of therapy for infectious diseases is antibiotic drug therapy, also called antimicrobial or anti-infective therapy. The sulfonamides, the first antibiotic group, were used in the mid-1930s. Shortly thereafter, in the 1940s, penicillin became the first antibiotic used systemically. Since these early days, a wide variety of antimicrobial drugs have been developed for treatment as well as prevention of infection associated with virtually every class of microorganism. Effective antibiotics are available to treat nearly all bacterial infections. However, fewer effective antifungal agents have been developed, and these drugs generally exhibit more toxicity than do antibacterial agents. Few effective chemotherapeutic agents are currently available for treatment of infections caused by viruses.

Effective antibiotic therapy requires:

- Delivery of the appropriate agent
- Sufficient dosage
- Proper route of administration
- Sufficient duration of therapy

Fulfilling these four requirements ensures that a concentration of drug is delivered in excess of that needed to inhibit or kill the infecting microorganism. The physician, often in consultation with the pharmacist, decides about each requirement. The nurse needs to know the drug actions, side effects, and toxic effects as well as teach them to the client.

Antibiotics act on susceptible pathogens by:

- Inhibiting cell wall synthesis (penicillins and cephalosporins)
- Injuring the cytoplasmic membrane (antifungal agents)
- Inhibiting biosynthesis (reproduction) (erythromycin, tetracycline, and gentamicin)
- Inhibiting nucleic acid synthesis (actinomycin)

The nurse observes and reports side effects and toxic effects, which vary according to the specific classification of the drug. Most antibiotics can cause nausea, vomiting, and rashes along with a long list of other problems. The nurse ensures that the prescribed drug is not one to which the client is allergic. The nurse must obtain an accurate allergy history before drug therapy begins.

Antipyretic Therapy The physician prescribes antipyretic drugs, such as aspirin (Ancasal✱) and acetaminophen (Tylenol, Ace-Tabs✱), to reduce hyperthermia. However, because antipyretics mask fever, monitoring the course of the client's disease may be difficult. Therefore, unless the client is extremely uncomfortable or if hyperthermia presents a significant risk (e.g., in clients with heart failure, febrile seizures, or head injury), antipyretics are not usually ordered.

The nurse must be alert for waves of sweating after each dose. Sweating may be accompanied by a fall in blood pressure and subsequent return of fever. These unpleasant side effects of antipyretic therapy can often be alleviated by liberal administration of fluids and by regular scheduling of drug administration.

External Cooling Cooling or hypothermia blankets, or ice bags and packs, are highly effective external mechanisms for reducing fever. For convenience, cooling blankets are used extensively in the hospital setting, yet there are no universal guidelines for their use. Caruso et al. (1992) found that warmer blanket temperatures provide rates of cooling similar to those of colder temperatures and are more comfortable for the client (Research Applications for Nursing).

Alternatives to cooling blankets may be used, particularly in settings other than hospitals. The nurse may sponge the client's body with tepid water or saline solution or apply cool compresses to the skin and pulse points to reduce body temperature. The nurse observes the client for shivering during any form of external cooling. Shivering indicates that the client is possibly being cooled too quickly.

Fluid Administration In clients with fever, there is increased fluid volume loss from rapid evaporation of body fluids as well as increased perspiration. As body temperature increases, fluid volume loss increases. The nurse carefully monitors for signs of dehydration, such as increased thirst, decreased skin turgor, and dry mucous membranes. The nurse encourages increased oral fluid intake and administers intravenous fluids as prescribed by the physician (see Chap. 15 for additional information on fluid volume deficit).

RESEARCH APPLICATIONS FOR NURSING

Higher Temperatures in Cooling Blankets May Be As Effective As Lower Temperatures—But More Comfortable for Clients

Caruso, C. C., Hadley, B. J., Shukla, R., Frame, P., & Khoury, J. (1992). Cooling effects and comfort of four cooling blanket temperatures in humans with fever. *Nursing Research, 41*(2), 68–72.

Cooling blanket temperatures vary tremendously from 3.3° C (38° F) to 36.7° C (98° F). The study attempted to determine which temperature was the best for reducing fever as well as promoting comfort. The occurrence of shivering was also measured.

The 89 adult clients who completed the study were evenly distributed among four treatment groups for sex, race, cause of fever, and initial body temperature. Infection was the most common cause of fever. Each group used a cooling blanket having a different temperature.

There was no difference in the subjects' fever reduction or shivering. However, subjects with the warmer cooling blankets were more comfortable. Clients using the blankets for a shorter time were more comfortable than those using the blankets for a longer time.

Critique The sample was fairly large, and individual variables were controlled by stratified randomization. The researchers used several measures, in addition to fever reduction, to determine which blanket temperature might be best.

Possible nursing implications This study supports other findings that warmer blanket temperatures are just as effective for fever reduction as colder blanket temperatures and are more comfortable for the client. Nurses should work with their facilities to ensure that warmer blankets are used to reduce fever.

FATIGUE

PLANNING: CLIENT GOALS The primary goal is that the client will progress to the previous level of activity.

INTERVENTIONS Whether a client achieves the goal depends on recognition and correction of factors that contribute to activity intolerance. Malaise and easy fatigability are classic clinical manifestations of an infectious process. Fever accelerates many metabolic processes, which accentuates weight loss and nitrogen wasting. The heart rate increases, and water loss may be excessive; both factors contribute to a feeling of general malaise.

Nutrition The nurse observes the client for causative factors of malaise and easy fatigability, such as nutritional deficiencies or fluid and electrolyte imbalances. The nurse collaborates with the client and dietitian to establish a dietary program that is tolerable for the client and meets calorie and protein requirements.

Activity Management The nurse encourages bed rest during the acute phase of the client's illness while treatment for the underlying infection is initiated. The nurse works closely with the client to develop a progressive program for return to his or her normal level of activity. The program depends on the client's response to antibiotic therapy, as evidenced by diminished clinical manifestations of infection. Frequent rest periods are encouraged. Throughout the course of the client's illness, the nurse encourages the client to verbalize feelings of frustration and discouragement related to chronic fatigue and decreased ability to perform activities of daily living.

SOCIAL ISOLATION

PLANNING: CLIENT GOALS The primary goal is that the client will not experience feelings of social isolation.

INTERVENTIONS Education is the major intervention for meeting this goal. The nurse develops an educational program to instruct the client and the family about the mode of transmission of infection and mechanisms that prevent its spread to others. The nurse also initiates appropriate barrier precautions.

The nurse ensures that the client and family understand the client's disease process and its cause. The nurse specifically explains the mode of transmission of the infecting microorganism, the risk for transmission to others, and mechanisms that may prevent transmission. If necessary, the nurse ensures that the client and family can state specific ways in which precautions will be instituted in the home after discharge from the hospital.

Because the client requiring precautions may feel secluded, the nurse encourages health care personnel as well as family members and friends to maintain contact with the client. The nurse reminds all personnel caring for the client that the *disease*—not the client—requires isolation. The nurse encourages family members and friends to visit the client, and to use the appropriate barrier precautions when necessary. Communication by telephone is often effective for continuing contact with loved ones. Television and radio help bring the outside world into the lives of clients confined to their rooms. (For other suggestions for the care of a client experiencing sensory deprivation, see Chap. 9).

DISCHARGE PLANNING

HOME CARE PREPARATION

The client with an infectious disease who is discharged from the hospital to home may require continued, long-term antibiotic therapy. The nurse emphasizes the importance of a clean home environment, especially for the client who continues to be immunocompromised or who is uniquely susceptible to superinfection (i.e., reinfection or second infection of the same kind) because of antimicrobial drug therapy. Medications often need to be refrigerated. The nurse ensures that the client has access to proper storage facilities and instructs the client to check for signs of improper storage, such as discoloration of the medication.

The nurse questions the client to be sure that hand washing facilities are available in the home. The nurse provides supplies and instructions as needed and reviews other measures to prevent transmission of infection with the client and family or significant other.

HEALTH TEACHING

The teaching plan for the client with an infectious disease addresses several important issues.

- The nurse explains the disease and makes certain that the client understands what is causing the illness.
- The nurse explains whether the pathogen causing the client's infection can be spread to family members, social contacts, or other community contacts.
- If the client has an infectious disease caused by a transmissible agent, the nurse explains how the pathogen causing the client's infection is transmitted.
- If the client has an infectious disease that is potentially transmissible, the nurse teaches the client, family, or home caregivers the precautions for preventing transmission of infection.

General household cleaning measures are often sufficient (e.g., a dishwasher for dishes, a washer and dryer for laundry). If these are not available, dishes can be sanitized with weak bleach solution (100 parts per million [ppm] available chlorine) attained by adding 30 mL (1 ounce) of bleach to 4 gallons of water. Clothing soiled with blood or other body fluids can be washed with bleach or disinfectant (e.g., Lysol). Recommended cleaning measures should be based on actual available equipment or facilities.

For clients who are discharged to the home setting to complete a course of antibiotic therapy, the nurse also explains the importance of compliance with the planned drug regimen. The nurse emphasizes the importance of both the timing of doses and the completion of the planned number of days of therapy. The nurse also teaches the client how the agents should be taken (e.g., before meals, with meals, and without other agents). The nurse explains to the client and family about the side effects of medications to be taken at home. Side effects include those that are expected (such as gastric distress after the oral administration of erythromycin) as well as more severe adverse reactions (such as rash, fever, or other systemic signs and symptoms of an acute adverse drug reaction). The nurse also teaches the client about allergic manifestations (Table 27–10). The nurse emphasizes the need for the client and family or significant other to notify the physician if adverse or allergic reactions occur.

In the past, many clients who had a severe infection were hospitalized for several weeks or more simply to receive intravenous (IV) antibiotic therapy. Since the implementation of the DRG (diagnosis-related groups) prospective payment system in hospitals, many clients have been discharged with an IV device in place and continue to receive IV antibiotics at home. The client, a family member, or a home care nurse administers the drugs. When a client is discharged with an indwelling intravascular device in place, the nurse teaches the client or family members who are assisting the client how to care for it. The

TABLE 27–10 Allergic Reactions to Antibiotic Therapy

- Flushing
- Wheezing
- Sneezing
- Pruritus
- Urticaria
- Rashes
- Maculopapular to exfoliative dermatitis
- Vascular eruptions
- Erythema multiforme (Stevens-Johnson syndrome)
- Angioneurotic edema
- Serum sickness (headache, fever, chills, hives, malaise, and conjunctivitis)
- Anaphylaxis (laryngeal edema, bronchospasm, hypotension, vascular collapse, and cardiac arrest)
- Death

nurse also instructs the client to be alert for malfunction of the device as well as for signs of inflammation resulting from infection at the catheter insertion site (e.g., redness, heat, pain, swelling, and purulent discharge).

PSYCHOSOCIAL PREPARATION

The client with an infection is often anxious and fearful that the infection will be transmitted to family members or friends. The nurse allays these fears by teaching the client and the family ways of preventing the spread of disease. Careful attention is paid to the client's concerns. The nurse makes concrete suggestions (e.g., "Your wife can wear gloves when changing your dressing") to address specific concerns.

The client with an infectious disease associated with lifestyle behaviors, such as sexual activity or intravenous drug abuse, may experience guilt related to the disease. The nurse encourages the client to verbalize feelings associated with the illness. The nurse assists the client in locating support systems that may help alleviate these problems. Supportive family members, friends, or groups can help in easing the client's adjustment to illness.

HEALTH CARE RESOURCES

In unusual instances, a client who has been hospitalized for an infectious disease may not be able to return to the home setting immediately. In such circumstances, temporary placement in a long-term care facility may be advantageous. The staff nurse carefully notes the client's care requirements, medication schedules, and personal needs and preferences on the transfer documents. When possible, the staff nurse communicates directly with a nurse at the receiving facility to facilitate a smooth transition from the hospital to the intermediate care setting.

Because of the early discharge trend from hospitals, clients with severe or chronic infections may be discharged to home before completing long-term antibiotic therapy. Clients may continue to receive intravenous antibiotic therapy at home. Ambulatory clients may be asked to return to an outpatient facility every third day to have a new peripheral venous catheter placed for use as a heparin lock. Implanted ports may be used for convenience and to decrease the chance of infection at the skin site. The client's primary nurse communicates with the outpatient facility staff to effect a smooth transition from the hospital to the outpatient setting.

A home health care service may be used to ensure appropriate administration of antibiotics at the client's home. These home care services have proved efficient, effective, and much less expensive than hospitalization or intermediate care facilities. Occasional visits from a home care nurse may also facilitate detection of early antimicrobial failures, toxic reactions, or other side effects of therapy.

EVALUATION

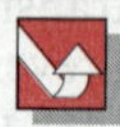

On the basis of the identified common nursing diagnoses, the nurse evaluates the care of the client with an infectious disease. Expected outcomes for the client with an infection include that the client:

- Describes and complies with the antibiotic regimen as ordered
- Maintains normal body temperature
- Returns to his or her usual level of activity
- Describes and implements precautions so that infection is not transmitted to others
- Exhibits no clinical manifestations of recurrence, relapse, or reinfection

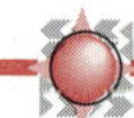

IMPLICATIONS FOR NURSING RESEARCH

Many issues relating to the care and management of clients with infections or infectious diseases remain unresolved and are appropriate topics for nursing research. Possible research questions include:

- ◆ How can elderly clients be better protected from nosocomial infections while in a health care facility?
- ◆ What would make health care personnel more compliant with hand washing?
- ◆ What are the psychosocial effects of universal precautions on clients who are in health care facilities?
- ◆ What is the most ideal temperature for cooling blankets?

SELECTED BIBLIOGRAPHY

American Nurses' Association. (1991). *ANA position statement on post-exposure programs in the event of occupational exposure to HIV/HBV*. Washington, D.C.: Author.

* Brown, R. B. (1988). Prescribing antibiotics in home health care: Problems and prospects. *Geriatrics, 43*(12), 43–49.

Bryant, J., & Lewicki, L. J. (1992). Infection control. In G. M. Bulachek & J. C. McCloskey (Eds.), *Nursing interventions: Essential nursing treatments* (2nd ed., pp. 247–253). Philadelphia: W. B. Saunders.

Caruso, C. C., Hadley, B. J., Shukla, R., Frame, P., & Khoury, J. (1992). Cooling effects and comfort of four cooling blanket temperatures in humans with fever. *Nursing Research, 41*(2), 68–72.

* Centers for Disease Control. (1987). Recommendations for prevention of HIV transmission in health-care settings. *Morbidity and Mortality Weekly Report, 36*(2S), 3–17.

* Coleman, D. (1987). The when and how of isolation. *RN, 50*(10), 5–8.

Cuzzell, J. Z. (1993). The right way to culture a wound. *American Journal of Nursing, 93*(5), 48–50.

* Farber, B. (1988). The multi-lumen catheter: Proposed guidelines for its use. *Infection Control and Hospital Epidemiology, 9,* 206–208.

* Garner, J. S., & Faverno, M. S. (1985). *Guidelines for handwashing and hospital environmental control. Hospital infections program.* Atlanta: Centers for Disease Control.

Giger, J. N., & Davidhizar, R. E. (1991). *Transcultural nursing: Assessment and intervention.* St. Louis: Mosby Year Book.

* Griffin, J. P. (1986). Nursing care of the immunosuppressed patient in an intensive care unit. *Heart & Lung, 15,* 179–186.

* Gurevich, I., & Tafuro, P. (1985). Nursing measures for the prevention of infection in the compromised host. *Nursing Clinics of North America, 20,* 257–260.

Haiduven, D. J., DeMaio, T. M., & Stevens, D. A. (1992). A five-year study of needlestick injuries: Significant reduction associated with communication, education, and convenient placement of sharps containers. *Infection Control and Hospital Epidemiology, 13,* 265–271.

Kolodner, D. E. (1993). The new federal bloodborne pathogens standard: Significance to the health care worker. *MEDSURG Nursing, 2*(1), 59–61.

Korniewicz, D. M. (1992). Effectiveness of glove barriers used in clinical settings. *MEDSURG Nursing, 1*(1), 29–32.

Korniewicz, D., Kirwin, M., Cresci, K., Markut, C., & Larson, E. (1992). In-use comparison of latex gloves in two high-risk units: Surgical intensive care and acquired immunodeficiency syndrome. *Heart & Lung, 21,* 81–84.

Korniewicz, D., Kirwin, M., & Larson, E. (1991). Do your gloves fit the task? *American Journal of Nursing, 23,* 38–40.

* Larson, E. (1988). Guidelines for use of antimicrobial agents. *American Journal of Infection Control, 16,* 253–263.

Larson, E., McGreer, A., Quaraishi, A., Krenzischek, D., Parsons, B. J., Holdford, J., & Hierholzer, W. J. (1991). Effect of an automated sink on handwashing practices and attitudes in high-risk units. *Infection Control and Hospital Epidemiology, 12,* 422–428.

* Larson, E. L. (Ed.). (1984). *Clinical microbiology and infection control.* Boston: Blackwell Scientific.

Lehne, R. A. (1990). *Pharmacology for nursing care.* Philadelphia: W. B. Saunders.

* Mermel, L., & Maki, D. (1988). Epidemic bloodstream infections from hemodynamic pressure monitoring: Sign of the times. *Infection Control and Hospital Epidemiology, 10,* 47–53.

Much, J. K., & Cotteta, T. A. (1993). Stress of occupational exposure to blood or body fluids: Managing the response. *MEDSURG Nursing, 2*(1), 49–56.

Occupational Safety and Health Administration. (1991). Occupational exposure to bloodborne pathogens: Final rule. *Federal Register,* 29CFR part 1910 subpart 2 (amended) 1919. 1030 (d) (2) (i).

* Pritchard, V. (1988). Preventing and treating geriatric infections. *RN, 51*(3), 36–38.

Weber, D., Hoffman, K. K., & Rutala, W. (1991). Management of the healthcare worker infected with human immunodeficiency virus: Lessons from nosocomial transmission of hepatitis B Virus. *Infection Control and Hospital Epidemiology, 12,* 625–629.

* Wenzel, R. P. (1987). *Prevention and control of nosocomial infections.* Baltimore: Williams & Wilkins.

Yassi, A., & McGill, M. (1991). Determinants of blood and body fluid exposure in a large teaching hospital: Hazards of the intermittent intravenous procedure. *American Journal of Infection Control, 19*(3), 129–134.

SUGGESTED READINGS

Cuzzell, J. Z. (1993). The right way to culture a wound. *American Journal of Nursing, 93*(5), 48–50.

This article describes the correct way to obtain specimens for culture from various types of wounds. The author provides several tips to ensure an accurate culture result, such as irrigating with saline before culture if the wound has copious drainage.

Haiduven, D. J., DeMaio, T. M., & Stevens, D. A. (1992). A five-year study of needlestick injuries: Significant reduction associated with communication, education, and convenient placement of sharps containers. *Infection Control and Hospital Epidemiology, 13,* 265–271.

This study was conducted at the Santa Clara Valley Medical Center in San Jose, California, in an effort to reduce the number of needlesticks in high-risk areas such as critical care. The researchers were able to decrease needlestick injuries by 60% over a 4-year period by repeated in-service education sessions, communication with staff, and placement of sharps containers in every client's room and other convenient locations.

Korniewicz, D. M. (1992). Effectiveness of glove barriers used in clinical settings. *MEDSURG Nursing, 1*(1), 29–32.

This article discusses the importance of nurses' involvement in the selection of gloves used in the clinical setting. Latex gloves are safer than vinyl gloves; however, other factors, such as improved chemical and physical protection and glove fit, need to be evaluated. The author lists questions to use in glove evaluation.

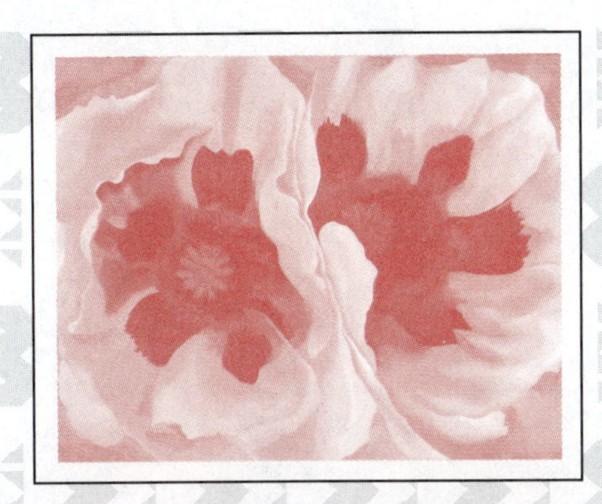

UNIT

Problems of Oxygenation: Management of Clients with Problems of the Respiratory Tract

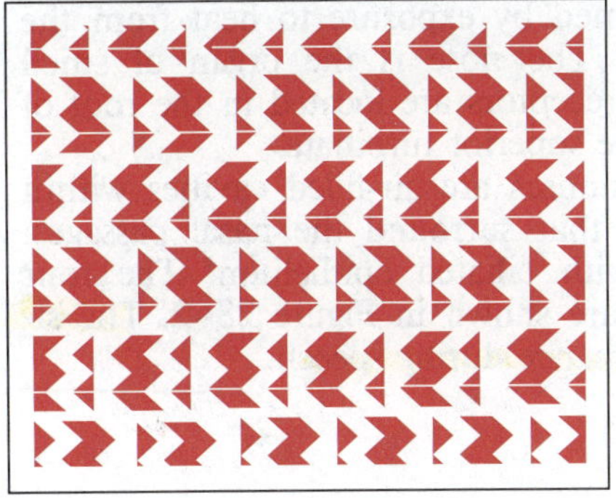

CHAPTER 28

Assessment of the Respiratory System

CHAPTER HIGHLIGHTS

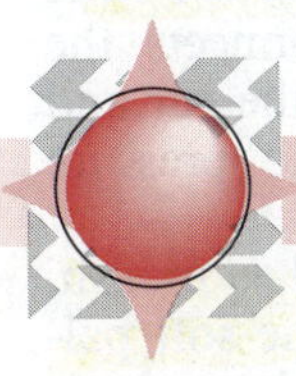

Respiratory disease currently ranks as the sixth leading cause of death in the United States (Boring, et. al., 1994). As clients with chronic respiratory impairments live longer because of advances in diagnosis, treatment, and management, the nurse is confronted with planning and implementing care for increasing numbers of clients with various respiratory disorders. The nurse needs an adequate knowledge base regarding the anatomy, physiology, and pathophysiology of the respiratory system to meet this challenge.

ANATOMY AND PHYSIOLOGY REVIEW

The two major purposes of the respiratory system are to provide oxygen for metabolism in the tissues and to remove carbon dioxide, the waste product of metabolism. The respiratory system performs several secondary functions, such as:

- Maintaining acid-base balance
- Producing speech
- Facilitating the sense of smell
- Maintaining body water levels
- Ensuring heat balance

Upper Respiratory Tract

The upper airways consist of the nose, the sinuses, the pharynx, and the larynx (Fig. 28–1).

NOSE AND SINUSES

The nose, a rigid structure that is bony in the upper one third and cartilaginous in the lower two thirds, contains two passages that are separated in the middle by the septum. The septum and the interior walls of the nasal cavity are lined with mucous membranes, as is the rest of the respiratory tract. The nostrils (anterior nares), or external openings into the nasal cavities, are lined with skin and hair follicles (vibrissae). Vibrissae are the first defense mechanisms of the respiratory system. They defend against foreign particles or organisms from entering the lungs. The posterior nares are openings from the nasal cavity into the nasopharynx.

Three major bony projections called *turbinates,* or conchae, arise from the lateral walls of the internal portion of the nose (see Fig. 28–1). Turbinates increase the total surface area for filtering, heating, and humidifying inspired air before it passes into the nasopharynx. Thus, inspired air entering the nose is filtered first by vibrissae in the nares. Particles that are not filtered out in the nares are trapped in the mucous layer of the turbinates. These particles are passed posteriorly by cilia (hair-like projections) to the oropharynx, where they are swallowed. Inspired air is humidified by contact with the mucous membrane and is warmed by exposure to heat from the vascular network. The nose is the organ of smell because olfactory receptors are located in the roof of the nose and in the superior turbinate.

The paranasal sinuses are air-filled cavities within the hollow bones that surround the nasal passages. They are lined with ciliated epithelium. The four paranasal sinuses are shown in Figure 28–2. The sinuses provide resonance during speech.

PHARYNX

The pharynx, or throat, is located behind the oral and nasal cavities. It is divided into the nasopharynx, the oropharynx, and the laryngopharynx (see Fig. 28–1). The pharynx is a passageway for both the respiratory and digestive tracts.

Located behind the nose, the nasopharynx lies above the soft palate and contains the adenoids and the eustachian tube. The adenoids (pharyngeal tonsils) are located in the back of the throat in the roof of the nasopharynx. They act as an important defense mechanism by trapping organisms entering the nose and the mouth. The eustachian tube connects the nasopharynx with the middle chamber of the ear and opens during swallowing to equalize the pressure within the middle ear.

The oropharynx is located behind the mouth, below the nasopharynx. It extends from the soft palate to the base of the tongue. The palatine tonsils (also known as faucial tonsils) are located on the anterolateral borders of the oropharynx. The tonsils

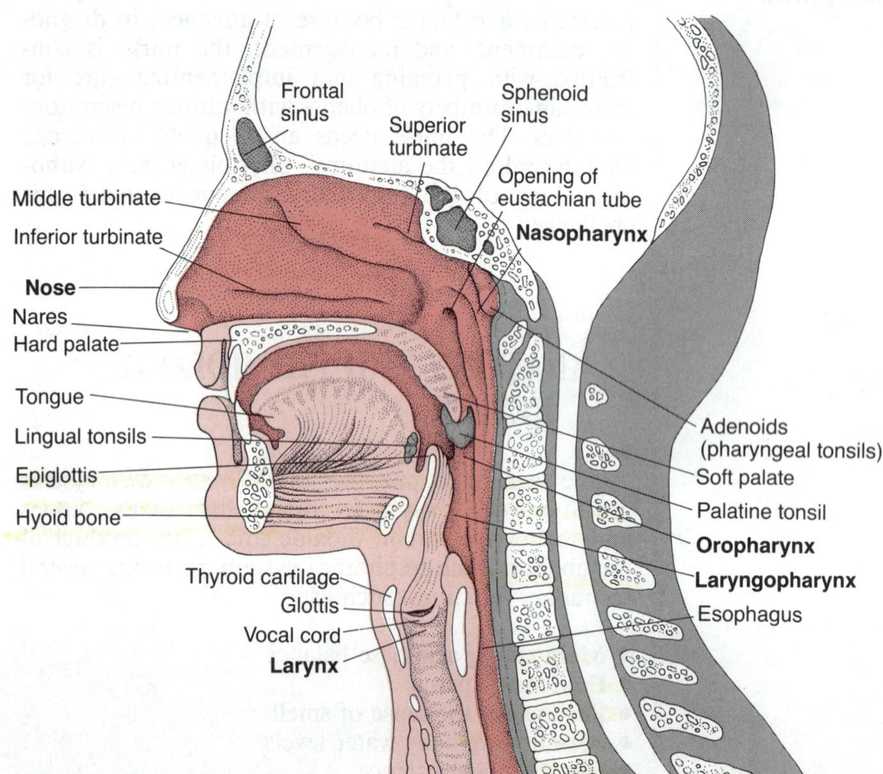

FIGURE 28–1 ◆ Structures of the upper respiratory tract.

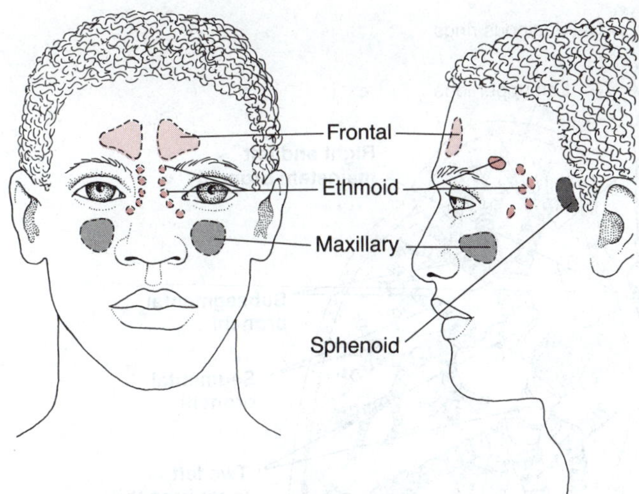

FIGURE 28-2 ◆ The paranasal sinuses.

also guard the body against invading organisms entering the nose and throat. Normally, when food is propelled through the oropharynx into the esophagus, the larynx closes off for swallowing. This mechanism prevents the aspiration of food into the lower airways.

Located behind the larynx, the laryngopharynx extends from the base of the tongue to the esophagus. The laryngopharynx is the critical dividing point where solid foods and fluids are separated from air. At this point, the passageway bifurcates into the larynx and the esophagus.

LARYNX

The larynx is located above the trachea, just below the pharynx at the root of the tongue. It is innervated by the recurrent laryngeal nerves. The larynx, commonly called the *voice box,* is composed of several cartilages (Fig. 28-3). The thyroid cartilage is the largest and is commonly referred to as the Adam's apple. The cricoid cartilage, which contains the vocal cords, lies below the thyroid cartilage. The cricoid cartilage is the only complete ring of cartilage in the airway. The cricothyroid membrane is below the level of the vocal cords and joins the thyroid and cricoid cartilages. This site is used in an emergency for access to the lower airways. The procedure, a cricothyroidotomy (an opening made between the thyroid and cricoid cartilage), is also called a cricothyrotomy and results in a tracheostomy. The two arytenoid cartilages, to which the posterior ends of the vocal cords are attached, are used together with the thyroid cartilage in vocal cord movement.

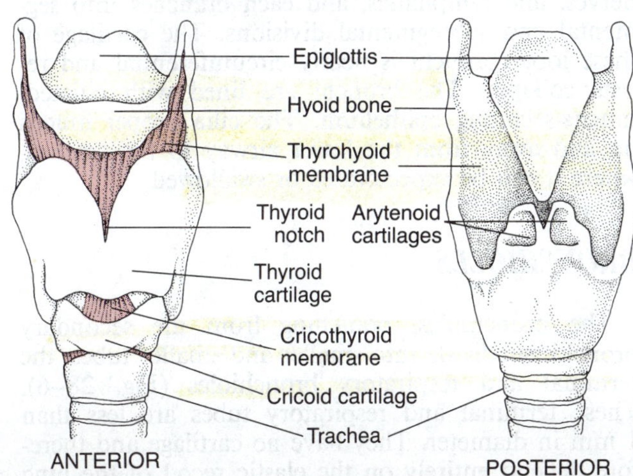

FIGURE 28-3 ◆ Structures of the larynx.

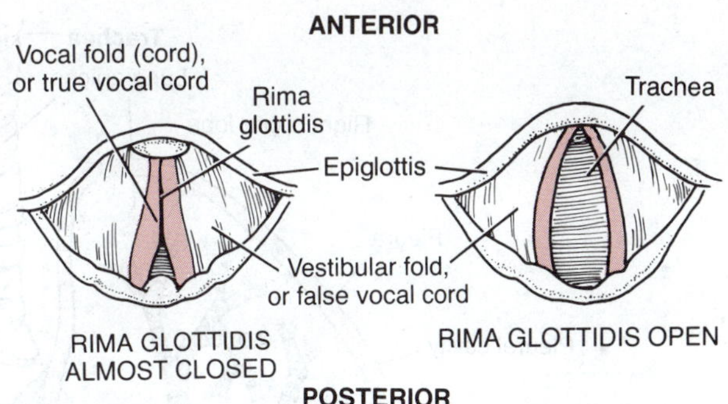

FIGURE 28-4 ◆ Detail of the vocal cords and glottis.

Inside the larynx are two pairs of vocal cords, the false and true cords. The opening between the true vocal cords is the *glottis* (Fig. 28-4). The glottis plays an important role in coughing, which is the most fundamental defense mechanism of the lungs. The *epiglottis* is a leaf-shaped, elastic structure that is attached along one edge to the top of the larynx. Its hinge-like action prevents food from entering the tracheobronchial tree by closing over the glottis during swallowing.

Lower Respiratory Tract

The lower airways consist of the trachea; two mainstem bronchi; lobar, segmental, and subsegmental bronchi; bronchioles; alveolar ducts; and alveoli (Fig. 28-5). The tracheobronchial tree is an inverted tree-like structure consisting of muscular, cartilaginous, and elastic tissues. This system of bifurcating tubes, which decrease in size from the trachea to the respiratory bronchioles, allows the passage of gases to and from the pulmonary parenchyma. Gas exchange takes place in the pulmonary parenchyma between the alveoli and the pulmonary capillaries.

TRACHEA

The trachea, commonly termed the windpipe, is located in front of (anterior to) the esophagus. It begins at the lower border of the cricoid cartilage of the larynx and extends to the level of the fourth or fifth thoracic vertebra. The trachea branches into the

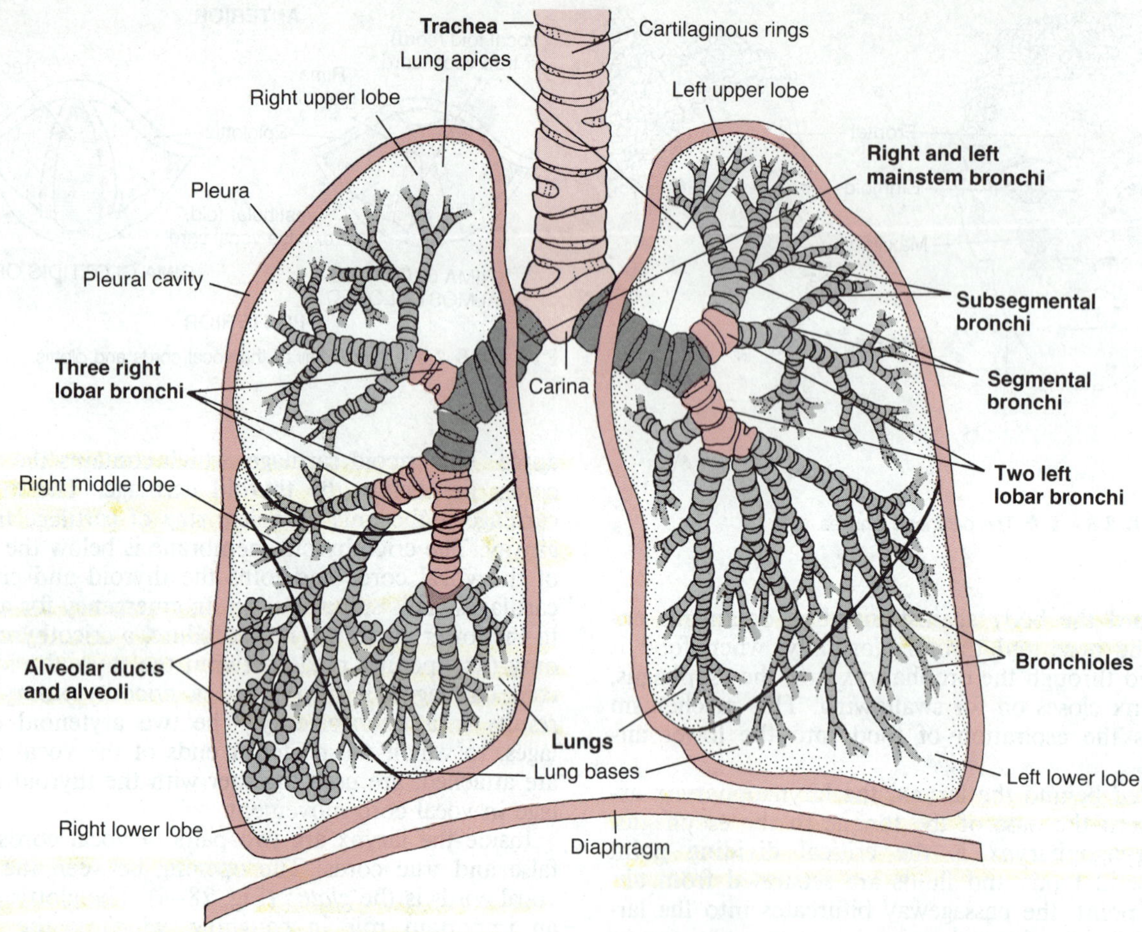

FIGURE 28-5 ◆ Structures of the lower respiratory tract (structural size and proportions not drawn to scale.)

right and left mainstem bronchi at the carina. The carina is located at the sternal angle where the manubrium joins the sternum.

The trachea is composed of six to ten C-shaped cartilaginous rings. The open portion of the "C" is the back (posterior) portion of the trachea; it contains smooth muscle that is shared with the esophagus. Low pressure must be maintained in endotracheal and tracheostomy tube cuffs so as not to cause erosion of this posterior wall and create a tracheoesophageal fistula.

MAINSTEM BRONCHI

The mainstem, or primary, bronchi begin at the carina. The structure of a bronchus resembles that of the trachea. The right bronchus is slightly wider, shorter, and more vertical than the left bronchus. Because of the more vertical line of the right bronchus, accidental intubation of the right bronchus is possible when an endotracheal tube is passed. Also, if a foreign object is aspirated from the pharynx, it most likely enters the right bronchus.

LOBAR, SEGMENTAL, AND SUBSEGMENTAL BRONCHI

The mainstem bronchi further divide into the five secondary, or lobar, bronchi that enter each of the five lobes of the lung. Each lobar bronchus is surrounded by connective tissue, blood vessels, nerves, and lymphatics, and each branches into segmental and subsegmental divisions. The cartilage of these lobar bronchi is nearly circumferential and resists collapse. The bronchi are lined with ciliated, mucus-secreting epithelium. The cilia propel mucus up and away from the lower airway to the trachea, where it can be expectorated or swallowed.

BRONCHIOLES

The bronchioles, branching from the secondary bronchi, subdivide into smaller and smaller tubes, the terminal and respiratory bronchioles (Fig. 28-6). These terminal and respiratory tubes are less than 1 mm in diameter. They have no cartilage and therefore depend entirely on the elastic recoil of the lung for patency. The terminal bronchioles contain no cilia and do not participate in gas exchange.

ALVEOLAR DUCTS AND ALVEOLI

Alveolar ducts, which resemble a bunch of grapes, branch from the respiratory bronchioles. Alveolar sacs arise from these ducts. The alveolar sacs contain clusters of alveoli, which are the basic units of gas exchange (see Fig. 28-6). It is estimated that the lungs contain about 300 million alveoli, surrounded by pulmonary capillaries. Because these microscopic alveoli are so numerous and share common walls, the surface area for gas exchange in the lungs is extensive. In a healthy adult, this surface area is approximately the size of a tennis court. *Acinus* is a term used to indicate all structures distal to the terminal bronchiole (e.g., respiratory bronchiole, alveolar duct, and alveolar sac).

Certain cells located in the walls of the alveoli secrete *surfactant,* a phospholipid protein that reduces the surface tension in the alveoli. Without sufficient surfactant, atelectasis (collapse of the alveoli) ultimately occurs. In atelectasis, gas exchange is less than optimal because the surface area is reduced.

LUNGS

The lungs are solid, sponge-like, elastic, cone-shaped organs located in the pleural cavity in the thorax. They extend from just above the clavicles to the diaphragm (the major muscle of inspiration). The lungs are composed of millions of alveoli and their related ducts, bronchioles, and bronchi. The right lung, which is larger than the left, is divided into three lobes: upper, middle, and lower. The left lung, which is somewhat narrower than the right lung to accommodate the heart, is divided into two lobes.

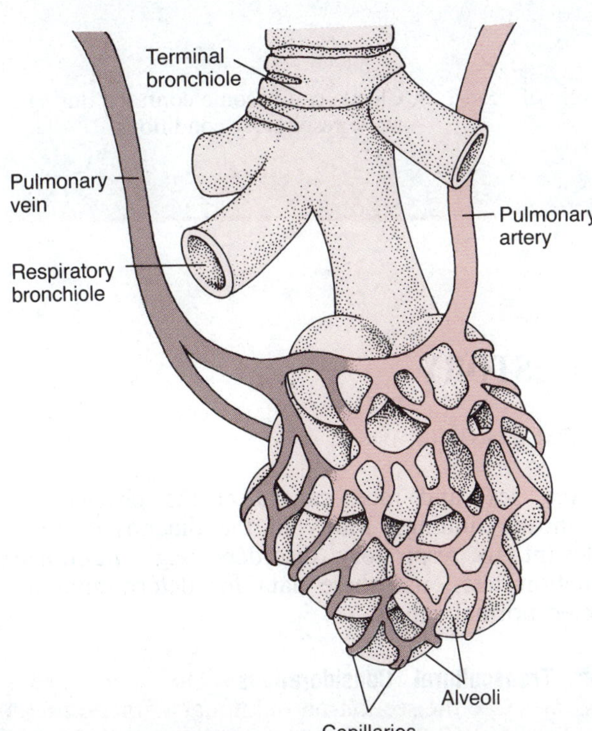

FIGURE 28-6 ◆ The terminal and respiratory bronchioles.

The hilum is the point at which the primary bronchus, pulmonary blood vessels, nerves, and lymphatics enter each lung. Innervation of the respiratory structures is accomplished by the phrenic nerve (diaphragm), vagus nerve (thorax), and thoracic nerves (intercostal muscles).

Composed of two surfaces, the pleura, a continuous smooth membrane, totally encloses the lung. The parietal pleura lines the inside of the thoracic cavity, including the upper surface of the diaphragm. The visceral pleura covers the pulmonary surfaces, including the major fissures between the lobes. A thin fluid layer, which is produced by the cells lining the pleura, lubricates these two surfaces, thereby allowing them to glide smoothly and painlessly during respirations.

Blood flow through the lungs occurs via two separate systems: the pulmonary system and the bronchial system. The bronchial arteries, arising from the thoracic aorta, are part of the systemic circulation and do not participate in gas exchange. This system carries the blood necessary to meet the metabolic demands of the lungs. The pulmonary circulation is composed of a highly vascular capillary network. Oxygen-depleted blood travels from the right ventricle of the heart into the pulmonary artery, which eventually branches into arterioles and venules that form the capillary networks. The capillaries are enmeshed around and through the alveoli, the site of gas exchange (see Fig. 28-6). Freshly oxygenated blood then travels through the pulmonary venous circulation to the left atrium, where it is pumped throughout the systemic circulation.

Accessory Muscles of Respiration

Accessory muscles of respiration include the scalene muscles, which elevate the first two ribs; the sternocleidomastoid muscles, which raise the sternum; and the trapezius and pectoralis muscles, which fix the shoulders. Additionally, various back and abdominal muscles are used in disease states.

Respiratory Changes Associated with Aging

Respiratory changes that occur with aging are described in Chart 28-1. Many changes associated with elderly clients are due to a lifetime of exposure to environmental stimuli (e.g., cigarette smoke, air pol-

CHART 28-1

Nursing Focus on the Elderly ◆ Changes in the Respiratory System Related to Aging

Physiologic Change	Nursing Implications	Rationale
Chest Wall		
Anteroposterior diameter increases. Slope changes. Progressive kyphoscoliosis occurs. Decreased mobility occurs. Osteoporosis is possible.	• Discuss the normal changes of aging. • Discuss the need for increased rest periods during exercise. • Encourage adequate calcium intake (especially during a woman's premenopause phase).	• Clients may be anxious because they must work harder to breathe. • Older clients have less tolerance for exercise. • Calcium intake helps prevent osteoporosis by building bone in younger clients.
Alveoli		
Alveolar membranes thicken. Diffusion capacity decreases. Elastic recoil decreases. Dilation of bronchioles and alveolar ducts occurs. Ability to cough decreases.	• Encourage vigorous pulmonary hygiene (i.e., encourage the client to turn, cough, and deep breathe), especially if the client is confined to bed or has had surgery.	• There is increased potential for mechanical or infectious respiratory complications in these situations.
Lungs		
Residual volume increases. Decreased capacity results in less efficient oxygen and carbon dioxide exchange. Elasticity decreases.	• Include inspection, palpation, percussion, and auscultation in lung assessments. • Assess the client's respirations for abnormal breathing patterns. • Encourage frequent oral hygiene.	• Inspection, palpation, percussion, and auscultation are needed to detect normal age-related changes. • Periodic breathing patterns (e.g., Cheyne-Stokes) can occur. • Oral hygiene aids in the removal of secretions.
Pharynx and Larynx		
Muscles atrophy. Vocal cords become slack. Laryngeal muscles lose elasticity and cartilage.	• Have face-to-face conversations with clients when possible.	• Voices of clients may be soft and difficult to understand.
Pulmonary Artery		
Increased vascular resistance to blood flow through pulmonary vascular system occurs. Risk of hypoxia increases.	• Assess the client's level of consciousness.	• Clients can become confused during acute respiratory conditions.

lutants, and industrial fumes and irritants) and heredity. Respiratory disease is a major cause of acute illness and chronic disability in elderly clients. Although respiratory function normally declines with increasing age, there is usually little difficulty with the demands of ordinary activity. However, the sedentary elderly client often reports feeling breathless during exercise.

It is difficult to differentiate the normal changes related to aging from the pathologic changes associated with respiratory disease or exposure to pollutants. In addition, disorders of the neuromuscular and cardiovascular systems that occur with aging may cause abnormal respiration even if the lungs are normal. Adequate functioning of both of these systems is essential for the respiratory system to perform its various functions.

HISTORY

Demographic Data

Age, sex, and race, can affect the physical and diagnostic findings. Many of the diagnostic studies relevant to respiratory disorders (e.g., pulmonary function tests) use these data for determining predicted normal values.

Transcultural Considerations The largest chest volumes (see the section on pulmonary function tests) are found in Caucasians and the smallest volumes are found in Native Americans. The chest volumes of African-Americans are significantly larger than those of Asian-Americans, but not as large as those of Caucasians (Jarvis, 1992).

Personal and Family History

PAST MEDICAL HISTORY

The nurse questions clients about their past respiratory history (Table 28–1). The circumstances of some chest injuries and surgeries may suggest that the present illness is related. For example, a foreign body lodged in the lung may cause recurrent coughing or a pulmonary abscess.

SMOKING HISTORY

The nurse asks about smoking in a comprehensive respiratory assessment. The nurse questions the client about the use of cigarettes, cigars, pipe tobacco, and marijuana and other controlled substances. Information on the client's association with smokers on a daily basis (passive smoking) is also important. If the client smokes, the nurse asks how long the client has smoked and how many packs a day, and if the client has quit, how long ago he or she stopped smoking. The smoking history is documented in pack-years (number of packs smoked per day multiplied by number of years). The nurse assumes a nonjudgmental attitude when questioning the client about smoking because the client may harbor guilt and denial about this habit.

TABLE 28–1 Important Aspects to Assess in a Respiratory System History

- Childhood illnesses:
  - Asthma
  - Pneumonia
  - Communicable diseases
  - Hay fever
  - Allergies
  - Eczema
  - Frequent colds
  - Croup
- Adult illnesses:
  - Pneumonia
  - Sinusitis
  - Tuberculosis
  - Diabetes
  - Hypertension
  - Heart disease
- Immunizations: influenza and pneumococcal (Pneumovax) vaccine
- Surgeries of the upper or lower respiratory system
- Injuries to the upper or lower respiratory system
- Hospitalizations
- Date of last chest x-ray, pulmonary function test, tuberculin test, or other diagnostic tests, and results
- Recent weight loss
- Night sweats

CURRENT AND PAST MEDICATION USE

The nurse questions the client about medications taken for breathing problems and also about drugs taken for other conditions. The nurse determines which over-the-counter medications, such as cough syrups, antihistamines, decongestants, inhalants, and nasal sprays, the client is using. The nurse also assesses home remedies. The nurse asks about past medication use and why it was discontinued. For example, a client may have used numerous bronchodilator metered-dose inhalers but may prefer one particular drug for relieving shortness of breath.

ALLERGIES

Data about allergies are extremely important and relevant to the respiratory history. The nurse determines whether the client has any known allergies to foods, dust, molds, pollen, bee stings, trees, grass, animal dander and saliva, or medications. The nurse asks the client to explain his or her specific allergic response. For example, does he or she wheeze, have trouble breathing, cough, sneeze, or experience rhinitis after exposure to the allergen? Has the client ever been treated for an allergic response? If the client has received treatment, the nurse asks about the circumstances regarding, and the type of, the allergic treatment.

TRAVEL AND AREA OF RESIDENCE

Travel and area of residence may be relevant for a history of exposure to certain diseases. For example, histoplasmosis, a fungal disease caused by inhalation of contaminated dust, is found in the central United States, the Mississippi and Missouri river valleys, and Central America. Coccidioidomycosis, another fungal disease, is found predominantly in the western and southwestern United States, Mexico, and portions of Central America.

FAMILY HISTORY

The nurse obtains a family history to rule out respiratory disorders with a genetic component. Some of the conditions the nurse asks about are cystic fibrosis, asthma, allergies, kyphoscoliosis, emphysema, and lung cancer. The nurse assesses for a family history of infectious disease such as tuberculosis because of the possibility of the client's exposure.

Diet History

An evaluation of the client's diet history may reveal allergic reactions after ingestion of foods containing certain preservatives, such as various benzoic acid derivatives. These include tartrazine (a component of FD & C Yellow No. 5), which is used as a coloring agent in foods and beverages (Tse, 1982). Preservatives such as sulfites are widely used to maintain the freshness of vegetables in restaurant salads, to prevent discoloration of dried fruit and uncooked potatoes, and to preserve processed fruits, vegetables, and juices. These preservatives are also used in the production of wine and beer. Signs and symptoms range from rhinitis, chest tightness, weakness, shortness of breath, urticaria, and severe wheezing to loss of consciousness.

Socioeconomic Status

A thorough occupational history is particularly relevant. The incidence of occupational pulmonary disease continues to increase annually. Occupational pulmonary diseases include pneumoconiosis (resulting from the inhalation of dust such as coal dust, stone dust, and silicone dust), toxic lung injury, and hypersensitivity disease. The occupational history includes exact dates of employment and a brief job description. Exposure to industrial dusts (both organic and inorganic) or noxious chemicals found in smoke and fumes may cause respiratory disease. Some of the most susceptible clients include coal miners, stonemasons, cotton handlers, welders, potters, plastic and rubber manufacturers, printers, farm workers, and steel foundry workers.

The nurse obtains information about the client's home and living conditions, such as the type of heat used (e.g., gas heater, woodburning stove, fireplace, and kerosene heater) and exposure to environmental irritants (e.g., noxious fumes, chemicals, animals, birds, and air pollutants). The nurse considers the home, community, and workplace for environmental factors possibly causing or contributing to the client's lung disease.

The nurse also asks about the client's hobbies and leisure activities. Pastimes such as painting, working with ceramics, model airplane building, furniture refinishing, or woodworking may have exposed the client to harmful chemical irritants.

Current Health Problem

The chief complaint is a brief statement, in the client's own words, describing the client's reason for seeking help. If there are several problems, they are listed in order of the client's priorities. Whether the pulmonary problem is acute or chronic, the client's chief complaint is likely to include cough, sputum production, chest pain, and shortness of breath at rest or on exertion.

While discussing the client's chief complaint, the nurse also explores the history of the present illness. This analysis includes the following:

- Onset
- Duration
- Location
- Frequency
- Progressing and radiating patterns
- Quality and number of symptoms
- Aggravating and relieving factors
- Associated signs and symptoms
- Treatment

COUGH

Cough is the cardinal sign of respiratory disease. The nurse asks the client how long the cough has persisted (e.g., 1 week, 3 months). The nurse also asks whether it occurs at a specific time of day (e.g., on awakening in the morning) or in relation to any physical activity. The nurse determines whether the cough is productive or nonproductive, congested, dry, tickling, or hacking.

SPUTUM PRODUCTION

An important symptom that is associated with coughing is sputum production. The nurse notes the color, consistency, odor, and amount of sputum, because these characteristics suggest the underlying pathologic process. Sputum may be clear, white, tan, gray, or if infection is present, yellow or green. Voluminous, pink, frothy sputum is characteristic of pulmonary edema. Pneumococcal pneumonia is often associated with rust-colored sputum, and foul-smelling sputum is often found in anaerobic infections such as lung abscess. The presence of blood in the sputum may be noted as streaks in clients with an acute respiratory tract infection; clients with tuberculosis, pulmonary infarction, or tumors may expectorate grossly bloody sputum (hemoptysis).

Sputum can be quantified by describing its production in terms of measurements such as teaspoon, tablespoon, ½ cup, and cup. Normally, the tracheobronchial tree can produce up to 3 ounces (90 mL) of sputum per day. The nurse determines whether sputum production is increasing, which may result from external stimuli (such as an irritant in the work setting) or from an internal cause (such as chronic bronchitis or a pulmonary abscess).

CHEST PAIN

A detailed description of chest pain helps the nurse differentiate pleural, musculoskeletal, cardiac, and gastrointestinal pain. The lungs have no pain-sensitive nerves, but the ribs, muscles, parietal pleura, and tracheobronchial tree do. Because perception of pain is purely subjective, the nurse analyzes pain in relation to the characteristics described in the history of the present illness. Coughing, deep breathing, or swallowing usually makes pulmonary pain worse (Green, 1992). (Chapter 8 discusses pain in detail.)

DYSPNEA

The perception of shortness of breath (breathlessness) or difficulty breathing is subjective and varies among clients. A client's perception may not be consistent with the severity of the presenting problem. For that reason, the nurse determines the type of onset (slow or abrupt), the duration (number of hours, time of day), relieving factors (changes of position, medication use, activity cessation), and evidence of audible sounds (wheezing, crackles, stridor).

The nurse tries to quantify dyspnea by determining whether this symptom interferes with activities of daily living (ADL) and, if so, how severely. For example, is the client short of breath while dressing, showering, shaving, or eating? Does dyspnea on exertion occur after the client walks one block or after climbs one flight of stairs? Table 28-2 correlates dyspnea classifications with ADL performance. The nurse also may use a dyspnea assessment scale to assess dyspnea (see Chap. 30).

The nurse inquires about paroxysmal nocturnal dyspnea (PND) and orthopnea, which are commonly associated with chronic pulmonary disease and left ventricular failure. In PND, the client has a sudden onset of difficulty breathing that is severe enough to awaken him or her from sleep. The term *orthopnea* is used when the client needs to be in an upright position to have easier breathing.

TABLE 28-2 Correlation of Dyspnea Classification with Performance of Activities of Daily Living

Classification	Activities of Daily Living Key
Class I: No significant restrictions in normal activity. Employable. Dyspnea occurs only on more than normal or strenuous exertion.	• *4:* No breathlessness, normal.
Class II: Independent in essential ADL but restricted in some other activities. Dyspneic on climbing stairs or on walking on an incline but not on level walking. Employable for only sedentary job or under special circumstances.	• *3:* Satisfactory, mild breathlessness. Complete performance is possible without pause or assistance, but not entirely normal.
Class III: Dyspnea commonly occurs during usual activities, such as showering or dressing, but the client can manage without assistance from others. Not dyspneic at rest; can walk for more than a city block at own pace but cannot keep up with others of own age. May stop to catch breath partway up a flight of stairs. Is probably not employable in any occupation.	• *2:* Fair, moderate breathlessness. Must stop during activity. Complete performance is possible without assistance, but performance may be too debilitating or time-consuming.
Class IV: Dyspnea produces dependence on help in some essential ADL such as dressing and bathing. Not usually dyspneic at rest. Dyspneic on minimal exertion; must pause on climbing one flight, walking more than 100 yards, or dressing. Often restricted to home if lives alone. Has minimal or no activities out of home.	• *1:* Poor, marked breathlessness. Incomplete performance; assistance is necessary.
Class V: Entirely restricted to home and often limited to bed or chair. Dyspneic at rest. Dependent on help for most needs.	• *0:* Performance not indicated or recommended; too difficult.

PHYSICAL ASSESSMENT

Nose and Sinuses

The nurse inspects and palpates the nose and the sinuses. The nurse inspects the client's external nose for deformities or tumors and the nostrils for symmetry of size and shape. Nasal flaring may indicate increased respiratory effort.

For the nurse to observe the interior nose easily, the client tilts his or her head back. The nurse may use a nasal speculum and nasopharyngeal mirror for a more thorough examination of the nasal cavity; usually, a penlight is sufficient.

Using the penlight, the nurse inspects the internal mucous membranes, the nasal septum, and the inferior and middle turbinates for color, swelling, drainage, and bleeding. The mucous membrane of the nose normally appears redder than the oral mucosa, but it may appear pale, engorged, and bluish gray in clients with allergic rhinitis. The nurse checks the nasal septum for evidence of bleeding, perforation, or deviation. Some degree of septal deviation is common in most adults and appears as an S shape, inclining toward one side or the other. A perforated septum is noted if the light shines through the perforation into the opposite nostril; it is often found in cocaine users. Nasal polyps, a frequent cause of obstruction, appear as pale, shiny, gelatinous structures attached to the turbinates (see also Chap. 29).

The nurse palpates the nose and the paranasal sinuses to detect tenderness or swelling. Only the frontal and maxillary sinuses are readily accessible to clinical examination because the ethmoid and sphenoid sinuses lie deep within the skull (see Fig. 28-2). Using the thumbs, the nurse checks for sinus tenderness by pressing upward on the frontal and maxillary areas; both sides are assessed simultaneously. Tenderness in these areas suggests inflammation or acute sinusitis.

The nurse may use transillumination of the sinuses to detect sinusitis. A darkened room and a penlight are needed for this procedure. Normally, the nurse sees a faint glow of light through the bone outlining the sinus. Transillumination is absent or decreased in sinusitis. Computed tomographic (CT) scans and x-rays of the sinuses are more definitive tools for detecting inflammation or sinusitis.

Pharynx, Trachea, and Larynx

Examination of the mouth and the pharynx begins with inspection of the external structures of the mouth. Chapter 52 describes a complete physical assessment of the oral cavity, and Chapter 53 discusses disorders of the oral cavity.

Using a tongue depressor, the nurse presses down one side of the tongue at a time (to avoid stimulating the client's gag reflex) to visualize the structures of the posterior pharynx. As the client says "ah," the nurse notes the rise and fall of the soft palate and uvula and observes for color and symmetry, evidence of mucopurulent discharge (postnasal drainage), edema or ulceration, and tonsillar enlargement.

The nurse inspects the neck and trachea for symmetry, alignment, masses, swelling, bruises, and the use of accessory neck muscles in breathing. The nurse palpates lymph nodes for size, shape, mobility, consistency, and tenderness. Tender nodes are usually movable and suggest inflammation. Malignant nodes are often hard and fixed to the surrounding tissue.

The nurse palpates the trachea for deviation, tenderness and masses. The nurse palpates the trachea by gently placing the fingers because firm palpation may elicit coughing or gagging. The trachea is located near the sternal notch. The spaces between each side of the trachea and the ends of the notch should be equal. Many pulmonary disorders cause the trachea to deviate from the midline. Masses push the trachea away from the affected area, whereas atelectasis causes a pull toward the affected area.

The larynx is usually examined by a specialist with a laryngoscope. The nurse may observe an abnormal voice, especially hoarseness, when there are abnormalities of the larynx.

Lungs and Thorax

Before examining the thorax, the nurse becomes familiar with anatomic landmarks. Identifying the location of physical assessment findings depends on accurate numbering of the ribs, intercostal spaces, and vertebrae and on accurate use of imaginary lines drawn on the chest (Fig. 28–7).

INSPECTION

Inspection of the chest begins with assessment of the posterior thorax, with the client in a sitting position if possible. The client should be undressed to the waist and draped for privacy and warmth. The chest is observed by comparing one side with the other. The nurse works from the top (apex) and moves downward toward the base. The nurse inspects the posterior thorax for skin color and condition, scars, lesions, masses, and spinal deformities such as kyphosis, scoliosis (see Chap. 50), and lordosis (see also Fig. 49–3).

The nurse notes the rate, rhythm, and depth of inspirations, as well as symmetry of chest movement. The nurse observes the type of breathing, such as

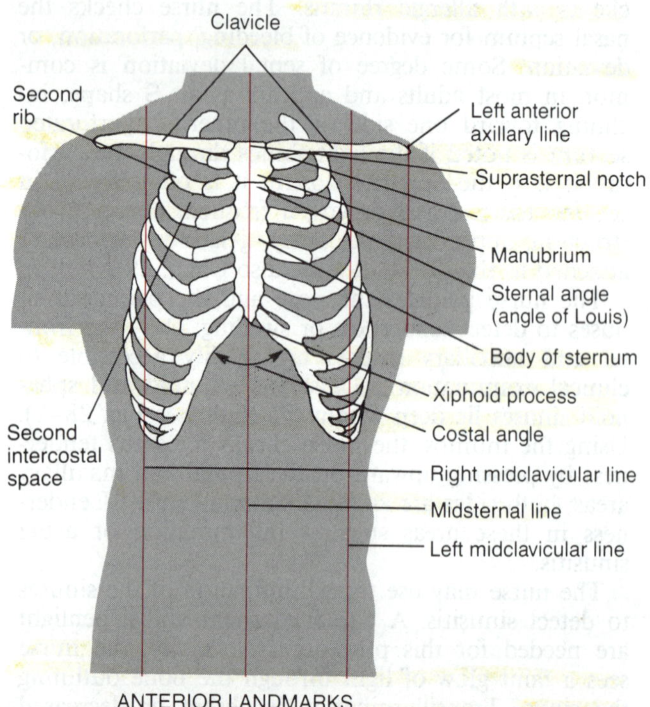

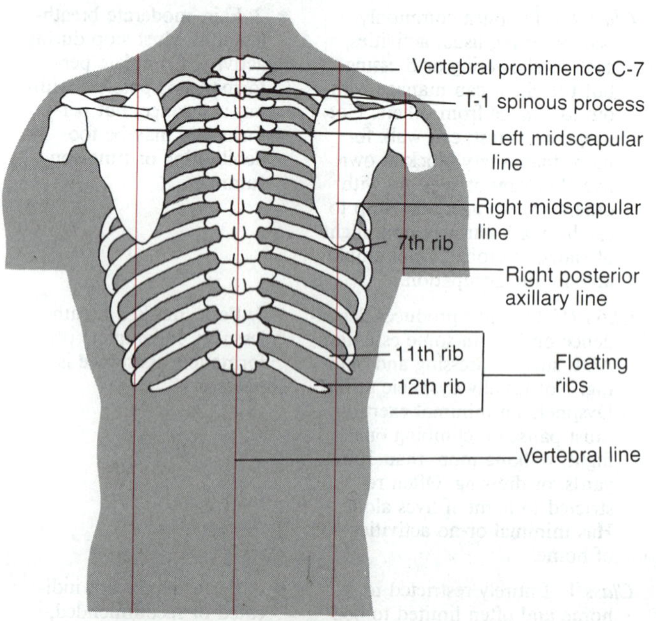

FIGURE 28–7 ♦ Anterior and posterior thoracic landmarks.

pursed-lip or diaphragmatic breathing, and the use of accessory muscles. In observing respiration, the nurse notes the duration of the inspiratory (I) and expiratory (E) phases. The ratio of these phases *(the I/E ratio)* is normally 1:2. A prolonged expiratory phase indicates obstruction of air outflow and is frequently seen in clients with chronic airflow limitation (CAL).

The nurse notes the client's chest configuration and compares the anteroposterior (AP) diameter with the lateral diameter. This ratio normally ranges from 1:2 to about 5:7, depending on the client's body build. The ratio approximates 1:1 in the client with emphysema, thus giving the client the typical barrel chest appearance (see Fig. 30–5).

The nurse observes for normal upward and outward symmetric movement of the chest on inspiration. An impaired movement or unequal expansion may indicate underlying disease of the lung or the pleura. Normally, the ribs slope downward. However, clients with air trapping in the lungs caused by chronic asthma or emphysema have little or no slope to the ribs (i.e., the ribs are more horizontal).

The nurse also checks for abnormal retractions of the intercostal spaces during inspiration, which indicate airflow obstruction. These retractions may be due to fibrosis of the underlying lung, severe acute asthma, emphysema, or tracheal or laryngeal obstruction. Abnormal bulging of the interspaces on expiration results from forced prolonged expiration, as in asthma and emphysema, or it may result from a loss of thoracic structure, as with multiple rib fractures.

PALPATION

After inspecting the chest, the nurse palpates the chest. Palpation enables the nurse to assess symmetry of respiratory movement and observable abnormalities, to identify areas of tenderness, and to elicit vocal or tactile fremitus (vibration).

In palpation, the nurse places his or her thumbs posteriorly on the spine at the level of the ninth ribs; the fingers are extended laterally around the rib cage. As the client inhales, both sides of the chest should move upward and outward together in one symmetric movement; the nurse's thumbs thus move apart. On exhalation, the thumbs should come back together as they return to the midline. Splinting or decreased movement on one side (unilateral expansion) may be due to pleuritic pain, trauma, or pneumothorax (air in the pleural cavity). Respiratory lag or impairment of thoracic movement may also indicate the presence of a pulmonary mass, pleural fibrosis, atelectasis, pneumonia, or a lung abscess.

The nurse palpates the thorax for any abnormalities found on inspection (e.g., masses, lesions, bruises, and swelling). The nurse also palpates for tenderness, particularly if the client has reported pain. *Crepitus,* or subcutaneous emphysema, is a crackling sensation felt beneath the fingertips and should be noted, especially around a wound site. Crepitus indicates that air is trapped within the tissues.

Vocal fremitus is a vibration of the chest wall that is produced when the client speaks; when perceived by palpation, it is termed *tactile fremitus.* To elicit tactile fremitus, the nurse places the palm or the base of the fingers against the client's chest wall and instructs the client to say "ninety-nine." The nurse compares vibrations (with the same hand) from one side of the chest with those from the other side, moving from the apices to the bases of the lung. Palpable vibrations are transmitted from the tracheobronchial tree, along the solid surface of chest wall, to the nurse's hand.

The nurse notes symmetry of the vibrations and areas of enhanced, diminished, or absent fremitus. Fremitus is decreased if the transmission of sound waves from the larynx to the chest wall is slowed. This situation can occur when the pleural space is filled with air (pneumothorax), fluid (pleural effusion), or solid tissue (pleural thickening). Fremitus is increased over large bronchi because of their proximity to the chest wall. Disease processes such as pneumonia and pulmonary abscesses decrease the distance that vibrations must travel to reach the chest wall, also resulting in increased tactile fremitus.

PERCUSSION

The nurse uses percussion to assess for pulmonary resonance, the boundaries of organs, and diaphragmatic excursion. Percussion involves tapping the chest wall, which sets the underlying tissues into motion and produces audible sounds. The nurse places the distal joint of the middle finger of the less dominant hand firmly on the surface to be percussed. No other part of the nurse's hand touches the client's chest wall because it dampens the vibrations. The plexor (in this case, the tapping finger of the dominant hand) is used to deliver quick, sharp strikes to the distal joint of the positioned finger (Fig. 28–8). The nurse maintains a loose, relaxed wrist while delivering the taps with the tip of the plexor or middle finger, not the finger pad. The nurse repeats this technique two or three times and listens to the intensity, pitch, quality, and duration of the sound produced.

Percussion produces five distinguishable notes. These sounds assist the nurse in determining the density of the underlying structures (i.e., whether the lung tissue contains air or fluid or is solid). The five percussion notes elicited are described in Table 28–3. Percussion of the thorax is performed over the rib intercostal spaces because percussing the sternum, ribs, or scapulae yields sound indicating the solid bone. Percussion penetrates only 2 to 3 inches (5 to 7 cm), so deeper lesions are not detected with this technique.

The percussion technique begins with the client sitting in an upright position; the nurse assesses the posterior thorax first. The nurse proceeds systematically, beginning at the apex and working toward the base. The apex of the lung rises about ¾ to 1½ inches

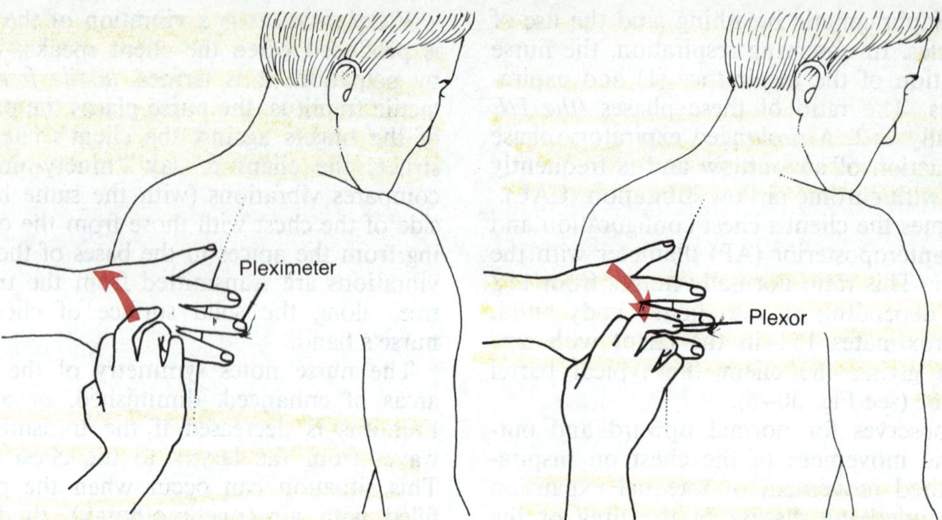

FIGURE 28–8 ◆ Percussion technique.

(2 to 4 cm) above the clavicle anteriorly. Posteriorly, there is approximately a 2-inch (5-cm) width of lung tissue at the apex.

While percussing the posterior chest, the nurse assesses the client's diaphragmatic excursion: the distance the diaphragm moves during inspiration and expiration. Diaphragmatic excursion may be measured by noting the difference in the level of dullness percussed at rest from that percussed at full inspiration. The nurse instructs the client to "take a deep breath and hold it" while the nurse percusses downward until dullness is noted at the lower border of the lung. Normal resonance of the lung stops at the diaphragm, where the sound becomes dull, and this site is marked. The nurse repeats the process after instructing the client to "let out all your breath and hold." The difference between the two markings or sounds is the diaphragmatic excursion, which may range from 1 to 2 inches (3 to 5 cm) (Finesilver, 1992). The diaphragm is normally higher on the right because of the location of the liver. Diaphragmatic excursion may be decreased in clients with pleurisy or emphysema.

The nurse continues assessment of the thorax with percussion of the anterior and lateral chest. The boundaries of organs such as the heart and the liver can be percussed anteriorly by noting the change in percussion notes. The percussion note changes from resonance of the normal lung to dullness at the borders of the heart and the liver. If a dull percussion note is found over lung tissue, the nurse expects that fluid or solid material (as in pneumonia, pleural effusion, fibrosis, atelectasis, and tumor) is replacing the normal air-containing lung.

AUSCULTATION

Auscultation is the most reliable assessment technique and includes listening for normal breath sounds, adventitious (abnormal) sounds, and voice sounds. Auscultation provides information about the

TABLE 28–3 Characteristic Features of the Five Percussion Notes

Note	Pitch	Intensity	Quality	Duration	Findings
Resonance	• Low	• Moderate to loud	• Hollow	• Long	• Resonance is characteristic of normal lung tissue.
Hyperresonance	• Higher than resonance	• Very loud	• Booming	• Longer than resonance	• Hyperresonance indicates the presence of trapped air, so it is commonly heard over an emphysematous or asthmatic lung and occasionally over a pneumothorax.
Flatness	• High	• Soft	• Extreme dullness	• Short	• An example location is the sternum. Flatness percussed over the lung fields may indicate a massive pleural effusion.
Dullness	• Medium	• Medium	• Thud-like	• Medium	• An example location is over the liver and the kidneys. Dullness can be percussed over atelectatic lung or consolidated lung.
Tympany	• High	• Loud	• Musical, drum-like	• Short	• Examples are the cheek filled with air and the abdomen distended with air. Over the lung, a tympanic note usually indicates a large pneumothorax.

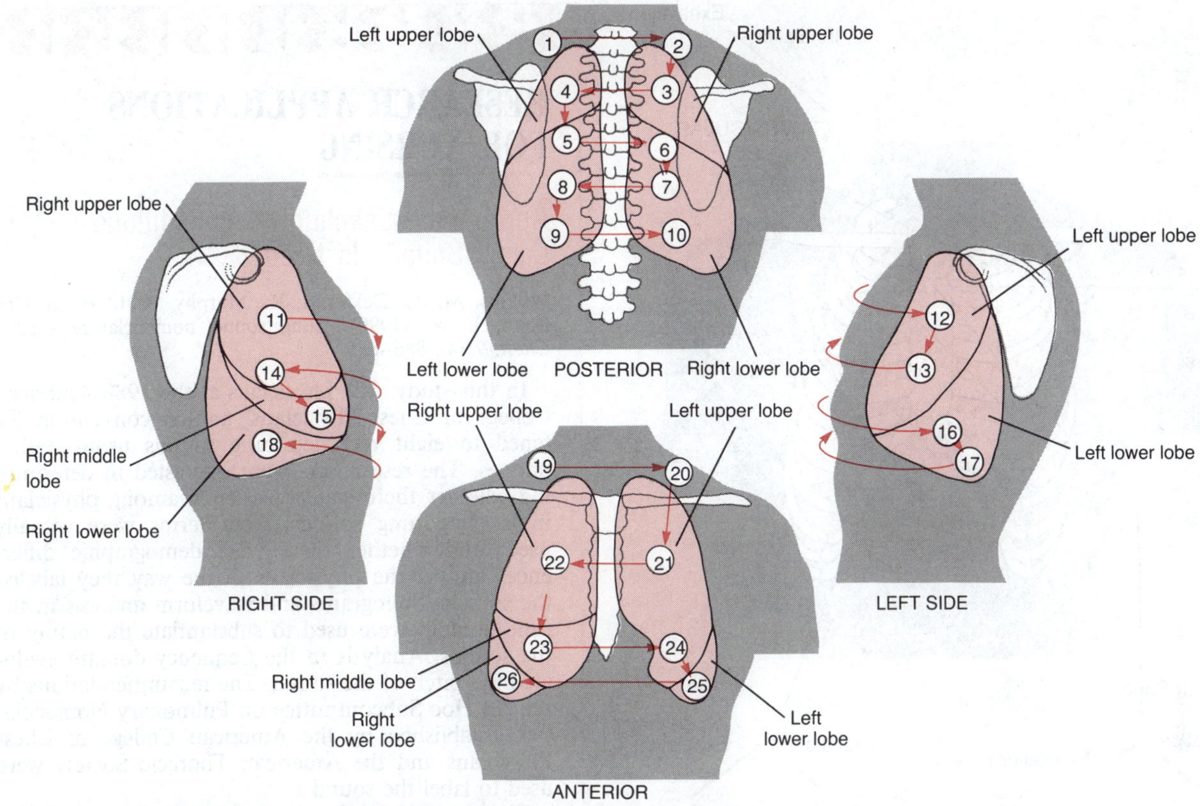

FIGURE 28-9 ◆ Sequence for percussion and auscultation.

flow of air through the tracheobronchial tree. It enables the nurse to identify the presence of fluid, mucus, or obstruction in the respiratory system. The nurse uses the diaphragm of the stethoscope for auscultation because it is designed to detect high-pitched sounds.

The auscultation procedure begins with the client sitting in an upright position. The nurse uses a systematic approach and works from the apices of the lungs to the basal segments (Fig. 28-9). Auscultation is performed on the posterior, anterior, and lateral thorax. With the stethoscope pressed firmly against the chest wall (clothing can distort or muffle sounds), the nurse instructs the client to breathe slowly and deeply with an open mouth. The nurse listens to a full respiratory cycle and notes the quality and intensity of the breath sounds. The nurse then listens for adventitious sounds and their locations. The nurse observes the client for signs of lightheadedness or dizziness caused by hyperventilation during auscultation. The nurse allows the client to breathe normally for a few minutes if these symptoms occur.

NORMAL BREATH SOUNDS

Normal breath sounds are produced as air vibrates while passing through the respiratory passages from the larynx to the alveoli. Breath sounds are identified by their location, intensity, pitch, and duration within the respiratory cycle (e.g., early or late inspiration and expiration). Normal breath sounds are known as vesicular, bronchovesicular, and bronchial (or tubular). Figure 28-10 illustrates normal breath sounds and their location. The nurse describes these sounds as normal, decreased, diminished, or absent.

VESICULAR BREATH SOUNDS

Vesicular breath sounds are low-pitched, soft, breezy sounds resembling wind blowing through the trees. The inspiratory phase is longer and more audible than the expiratory phase; expiration is heard as a puff. There is no perceptible pause between inspiration and expiration. Vesicular sounds are normal breath sounds. They are heard over most of the peripheral lung fields, with the exception of the area between the scapulae posteriorly or above the sternum anteriorly.

BRONCHOVESICULAR BREATH SOUNDS

Bronchovesicular breath sounds are a mixture of vesicular and bronchial sounds. The sound is harsh and moderate in pitch and intensity; inspiration is equal to expiration in duration. These sounds are heard over the thorax where the bronchi are closest to the chest wall (i.e., anteriorly near the mainstem bronchi at the level of the first and second intercostal spaces and in the intrascapular region posteriorly). Bronchovesicular breath sounds, when audible elsewhere, may indicate normal aging or an abnormality

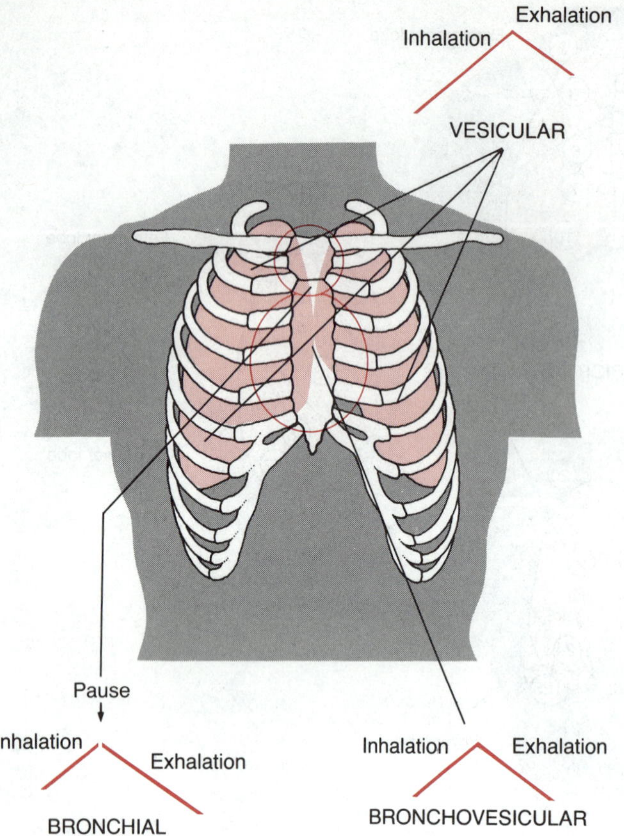

FIGURE 28–10 ◆ Location of normal breath sounds. I, inspiration; E, expiration.

such as pulmonary consolidation and chronic airway disease.

BRONCHIAL BREATH SOUNDS

Bronchial breath sounds are also called tubular sounds because they resemble the sound produced by wind going through a long tube. The bronchial breath sound is loud, harsh, or coarse, with a blowing, hollow quality. The expiratory phase is prolonged and longer than the inspiratory phase, and there is a noticeable pause between the two phases. Bronchial breath sounds are normally heard over the trachea. When these sounds are heard peripherally, they are abnormal. Peripheral bronchial breath sounds are due to transmission of centrally generated bronchial sounds to an area of increased density such as in clients with atelectasis, tumor, or pneumonia.

ADVENTITIOUS BREATH SOUNDS

Adventitious sounds are abnormal breath sounds superimposed on normal sounds and indicate pathologic changes in the tracheobronchial tree. Table 28–4 classifies and describes the adventitious sounds: crackle, wheeze, rhonchus, and pleural friction rub (American College of Chest Physicians and the

RESEARCH APPLICATIONS FOR NURSING

Appropriate Labeling of Adventitious Lungs Sounds Is Needed

Wilkins, M. A., Dexter, J. R., Murphy, R. L. H., & Del-Bono, E. A. (1990). Lung sound nomenclature survey. *Chest, 98*(4), 886–889.

In this study, 277 physicians at the 1988 American College of Chest Physicians' annual convention listened to eight recorded lung sounds using stethophones. The researchers were interested in determining whether there was consistency among physicians in labeling lung sounds, what terms were actually used, and whether there were demographic differences among the physicians in the way they labeled the sounds. Sonograms and waveform analysis in the time domain were used to substantiate the nature of the sounds. Analysis in the frequency domain evaluated the pitch of the sound. The recommendations by the Ad Hoc Subcommittee on Pulmonary Nomenclature established by the American College of Chest Physicians and the American Thoracic Society were used to label the sound.

The researchers found that the terms "crackles" and "rales" were used with equal frequency to describe discontinuous sounds but not at all to describe continuous sounds. Crackles is the recommended term, but the researchers suggested that the terms are synonymous. Most of the physicians used the term "stridor" or "wheeze" to correctly describe continuous lung sounds. The researchers, however, believed that more participants in the study should have labeled the sound of laryngeal obstruction as stridor.

The term "rhonchi" was used incorrectly to describe both continuous and discontinuous lung sounds. Because of confusion, the recommendation has been for the term rhonchi to be used to describe low-pitched continuous sounds. The researchers suggested that the term needs clarification among practitioners. They also noted that a rhonchus might not be easily recognized because it lacks distinctive sound characteristics.

Additional findings included that the majority of the participants were not able to recognize a pleural friction rub, and that no demographic differences among the physicians were found in sound labeling.

Critique The survey took place in an exhibit hall, but the process was not described. Because of the setting, the concentration ability and motivation of the physician being surveyed could be questioned. In addition, the hearing ability of participants was not addressed. The absence of a clinical situation may account for some of the results noted.

Possible nursing implications Nurses should recognize the difficulties in accurately describing lung sounds and work to improve their own ability to do so on the basis of the recommended nomenclature, rather than physicians' descriptions. This is especially true for rhonchi and the pleural friction rub.

American Thoracic Society Joint Committee on Pulmonary Nomenclature, 1975). Various subclassifications of these categories exist. Adventitious sounds vary in pitch, intensity, and duration and the phase of the respiratory cycle in which they occur. The terms for adventitious sounds vary among respiratory care practitioners (Research Applications for Nursing). The nurse is encouraged to document exactly what is heard on auscultation instead of relying on numerous labels.

VOICE SOUNDS

If the nurse discovers abnormalities during the physical assessment of the lungs and thorax, the client is assessed for vocal resonance. Auscultation of voice sounds through the normally air-filled lung produces a muffled, unclear sound because sound vibrations travel poorly through air. Vocal resonance is increased when the sound must travel through a solid or liquid medium as in clients with a consolidated area of the lung, pneumonia, atelectasis, pleural effusion, tumor, or abscess.

BRONCHOPHONY

Bronchophony is the abnormally loud transmission of voice sounds through an area of increased density. For assessment of bronchophony, the client repeats the number "ninety-nine" while the nurse systematically auscultates the thorax.

WHISPERED PECTORILOQUY

Whispered pectoriloquy is much more sensitive than bronchophony and is perceived by having the client whisper the number sequence "one, two, three." Normally, whispered words sound faint and indistinct; if they are heard loudly and distinctly, the nurse suspects consolidation of lung tissue and correlates this finding with other physical assessment findings.

EGOPHONY

Egophony is another form of abnormal vocal resonance and has a high-pitched, bleating, nasal quality. The nurse instructs the client to repeat the letter "E" and auscultates the thorax. Egophony exists when this

TABLE 28–4 Characteristic Features of Adventitious Breath Sounds

Adventitious Sound	Occurrence in the Respiratory Cycle	Character	Association
Discontinuous			
Fine crackle	• Either phase; more commonly heard on inspiration	• Popping, discontinuous sounds caused by air passing through moisture in alveoli or bronchioles. Sounds like hair being rolled between fingers near the ear.	Atelectasis Interstitial fibrosis Pulmonary edema Bronchitis Pneumonia Tuberculosis
Coarse crackle	• More prominent on expiration	• Lower pitched, coarse, discontinuous rattling sounds caused by fluid or secretions in large airways. Likely to change with coughing or suctioning.	Chronic bronchitis Pneumonia Tumors Chronic pulmonary diseases
Continuous			
Wheeze	• Audible during both inspiration and expiration	• Squeaky, musical, continuous sounds associated with air rushing through narrowed airways. May be heard without a stethoscope.	Inflammation Bronchospasm Edema Tumors Secretions Obstruction by foreign body Pulmonary vessel engorgement (as in cardiac "asthma")
Rhonchus	• Audible during both inspiration and expiration	• Lower-pitched, coarse, continuous snoring sounds.	Thick tenacious secretions Sputum production
Pleural friction rub	• Heard during both inspiration and expiration	• Rough, grating, scratching sounds caused by the inflamed surfaces of the pleura rubbing together. Often associated with pain on deep inspirations.	Pleurisy Tuberculosis Pulmonary infarction Pneumonia Lung cancer

CHART 28–2

Lab Profile ◆ Respiratory Assessment

Test	Normal Range for Adults	Significance of Abnormal Findings
Blood Studies		
Complete Blood Count		
Red blood cells	• Females: 4.2–5.4 million/mm^3 • Males: 4.7–6.1 million/mm^3	• *Elevated levels* (polycythemia) may be due to the excessive production of erythropoietin that occurs in response to a hypoxic stimulus, as in CAL and from living at high altitude. • *Decreased levels* indicate possible anemia, hemorrhage, or hemolysis.
Hemoglobin	• Females: 12–16 g/dL or 7.4–9.9 mmol/L • Males: 14–18 g/dL or 8.7–11.2 mmol/L • **Elderly:** values slightly decreased	• Same as for red blood cells
Hematocrit	• Females: 37%–47% • Males: 42%–52% • **Elderly:** values may be slightly decreased	• Same as for red blood cells
White blood cells, total	• 5000–10,000/mm^3	• *Elevations* indicate possible acute infections or inflammations, pneumonia, meningitis, tonsillitis, or emphysema. • *Decreased levels* may indicate an overwhelming infection or an autoimmune disorder.
Differential White Blood Cell (Leukocyte) Count		
Neutrophils	• 55%–70% of total	• *Elevations* indicate possible acute infection (influenza, pneumonia) or CAL. • *Decreased levels* indicate possible viral disease.
Eosinophils	• 0–450/mm^3 or 1%–4% of total	• *Elevations* indicate possible CAL, asthma, or allergies.
Basophils	• 0.5%–1% of total	• *Elevations* indicate possible inflammation. • *Decreased levels* may be seen in an acute allergic reaction.
Lymphocytes	• 20%–40% of total	• *Elevations* indicate possible viral infection, pertussis, and infectious mononucleosis. • *Decreased levels* may be seen during corticosteroid therapy.

letter is heard as a flat, nasal sound of "A" through the stethoscope. This abnormal sound indicates an area of consolidation, pleural effusion, or abscess.

PSYCHOSOCIAL ASSESSMENT

The nurse assesses aspects of the client's lifestyle that may significantly affect respiratory function. Some respiratory conditions may be exacerbated by stress. The nurse questions the client about present life stresses and the coping patterns used to reduce stress.

Chronic respiratory illnesses may cause changes in family roles and relationships, social isolation, financial problems, and unemployment or disability. By discussing coping mechanisms, the nurse assesses the client's reaction to these psychosocial stressors and discovers strengths as well as ineffective behaviors. For example, the client may react to stress with dependence on family members, withdrawal, or noncompliance with interventions. After completing the psychosocial assessment, the nurse assists the client in determining the support systems available to help the client cope with respiratory impairment.

DIAGNOSTIC ASSESSMENT

Laboratory Tests

BLOOD TESTS

Several laboratory tests (Chart 28–2) are relevant to the care of clients with respiratory disorders. A red blood cell count provides data regarding the transport of oxygen to the lungs. A hemoglobin deficiency directly affects tissue oxygenation because hemoglobin

CHART 28–2

Lab Profile ◆ Respiratory Assessment *Continued*

Test	Normal Range for Adults	Significance of Abnormal Findings
Monocytes	• 2%–8% of total	• *Elevations*—see Lymphocytes entry; also may indicate tuberculosis. • *Decreased levels*—see Lymphocytes entry.
Arterial Blood Gases		
PaO_2	• 80–100 mmHg • **Elderly:** values may be lower	• *Elevations* indicate possible excessive oxygen administration. • *Decreased levels* indicate possible CAL, chronic bronchitis, cancer of the bronchi and lungs, cystic fibrosis, respiratory distress syndrome, anemias, atelectasis, or any other cause of hypoxia.
$PaCO_2$	• 35–45 mmHg	• *Elevations* indicate possible CAL, pneumonia, anesthesia effects, or use of opioids (respiratory acidosis). • *Decreased levels* indicate hyperventilation/respiratory alkalosis.
pH	• 7.35–7.45	• *Elevations* indicate metabolic or respiratory alkalosis. • *Decreased levels* indicate metabolic or respiratory acidosis.
HCO_3^-	• 21–28 mEq/L	• *Elevations* indicate possible respiratory acidosis as compensation for a primary metabolic alkalosis. • *Decreased levels* indicate possible respiratory alkalosis as compensation for a primary metabolic acidosis.
SaO_2 (oxygen saturation)	• 95%–100% • **Elderly:** values may be slightly lower	• *Decreased levels* indicate possible impaired ability of hemoglobin to release oxygen to tissues.
Sputum Studies		
Gram's stain	• Negative	• Presence of gram-positive or gram-negative bacteria indicates the type of microorganism that is causing the respiratory infection.
Culture and sensitivity	• Negative	• Presence of microorganisms indicates possible respiratory infections (e.g., pneumonia or bronchitis).
Acid-fast stain	• No acid-fast bacilli	• Presence of bacilli indicates possible tuberculosis.
Cytologic tests	• Negative	• Presence of abnormal cells indicates possible malignancy.

CAL, chronic airflow limitation. (formerly referred to as COPD, chronic obstructive pulmonary disease)

transports oxygen to the cells and could cause hypoxemia.

Arterial blood gas (ABG) analysis assesses oxygenation (arterial oxygen pressure [PaO_2]), alveolar ventilation (arterial carbon dioxide pressure [$PaCO_2$]), and acid-base balance. Blood gas studies provide valuable information for monitoring treatment results, adjusting oxygen therapy, and evaluating the client's responses to treatment and therapy such as during weaning from mechanical ventilation.

SPUTUM TESTS

Sputum specimens obtained by expectoration or tracheal suctioning assist in the identification of pathogenic organisms or abnormal cells such as in a malignancy or a hypersensitivity state. Sputum culture and sensitivity analyses identify bacterial infection with either gram-negative or gram-positive organisms and determine the vulnerability to specific antibiotics. Cytologic examination is performed on sputum to help diagnose and specify malignant lesions by identifying cancer cells. Benign conditions, such as a hypersensitivity state, may also be identified by cytologic testing. Eosinophils and Curschmann's spirals (a mucus form) are often found by cytologic study in clients with allergic asthma.

The nurse correlates the laboratory results with the history and assessment findings to form nursing diagnoses, formulate care plans, and implement client teaching. Chapter 17 has more detail regarding the assessment of acid-base balance and Chapter 38 has more information on the complete blood count.

Radiographic Examinations

STANDARD RADIOGRAPHY

Chest x-rays are taken for clients with respiratory tract disorders to evaluate the present status of the chest and to provide a baseline for comparison with future changes. The diagnostic intent of the test helps to determine the type that is ordered. Types of chest x-rays include:

- Anteroposterior (AP): front to back
- Posteroanterior (PA): back to front
- Right lateral (RL) or left lateral (LL) views

Chest x-rays can be used to assess pathologic changes in the lung such as those occurring in clients with pneumonia, atelectasis, pneumothorax, and tumor. The presence of pleural fluid and the position and placement of an endotracheal tube or other invasive lines and catheters also can be detected by chest radiography. However, these films have limitations; they may appear normal even in a severe form of certain diseases, such as chronic bronchitis, asthma, and emphysema.

Sinus and facial x-rays are taken to assess the fluid levels in the sinus cavities to assist in the diagnosis of acute or chronic sinusitis.

BRONCHOGRAPHY

Bronchography is performed to diagnose abnormalities of the bronchi, such as narrowing, dilation, and obstruction.

CLIENT PREPARATION To prepare the client, the nurse ensures that he or she has nothing by mouth for several hours before the test to prevent aspiration. The protective laryngeal reflex and swallowing mechanism will be impaired because of sedation and the local anesthesia.

Because the dye used could cause an allergic reaction, the nurse assesses the client for allergies to iodine, shellfish, and contrast media. The nurse also assesses for allergy to any local anesthetic agent.

The nurse assesses the client for anxiety, fears, concerns, and lack of knowledge. Clients are often anxious about not being able to breathe during the procedure. The nurse offers support and reassurance as indicated and provides any additional information that is appropriate.

PROCEDURE In bronchography, the physician instills a liquid contrast medium into the trachea, and then takes x-rays of the bronchial tree. The client's chest is tilted at various angles to assist the flow of the contrast medium.

FOLLOW-UP CARE After the procedure, the nurse assesses the client's vital signs frequently for 24 hours and monitors the client for dyspnea or bleeding. A slight temperature elevation may be normal. The nurse does not allow the client to have anything by mouth until the gag reflex returns. To promote expectoration of secretions and facilitate removal of the dye, the nurse encourages coughing and deep breathing, along with fluid intake after the client is permitted to have fluids by mouth.

TOMOGRAPHY

Tomography is valuable in the assessment of the client with a respiratory disorder because pulmonary densities, tumors, and lesions can be seen. Positron emission tomography (PET) is useful for studying ventilation-perfusion relationships in the lung. Computed tomography (CT) provides cross-sectional views of the thorax and produces a three-dimensional assessment of the lungs and the thorax. CT can be used with or without an intravenously (IV) injected contrast agent. Nursing interventions for clients undergoing CT include education about the procedure and determination of the client's sensitivity to the contrast medium.

VENTILATION-PERFUSION SCANNING

A ventilation-perfusion scan (also known as a V/Q scan) visualizes the distribution of pulmonary blood flow and patterns of ventilation after the injection of IV contrast media or the inhalation of a radiopaque agent. Comparison of ventilation and perfusion scans helps confirm diagnoses such as pulmonary embolism, pneumonia, tumor, and fibrosis. The report may read "high probability" or "low probability" (of a certain condition).

Other Diagnostic Tests

MAGNETIC RESONANCE IMAGING

Magnetic resonance imaging (MRI) assists in the diagnosis of respiratory system disorders by providing information about the type and condition of the tissues being imaged along any plane inside the body: vertically, horizontally, and diagonally. This noninvasive procedure requires little client preparation other than the removal of all metal objects. Clients with pacemakers, aneurysm clips, inner-ear implants, cardiac valves, or metallic foreign objects in the body are not candidates for MRI. The nurse informs the client of possible claustrophobia and discomfort from lying inside the magnet's small cylinder on a hard, cool table. The nurse instructs the client in the use of relaxation techniques and imagery to help decrease these feelings. In addition, the nurse informs the client that the noises heard during the examination are the natural, rhythmic sounds of radio frequency pulses, which may range from barely audible to noticeable.

ENDOSCOPIC EXAMINATIONS

Endoscopic diagnostic studies to assess respiratory disorders include bronchoscopy, laryngoscopy, and mediastinoscopy. These procedures are summarized in Table 28-5.

TABLE 28–5 Care of the Client Undergoing Endoscopic Tests for Respiratory Disorders

Procedure	Purpose and Description	Nursing Interventions	Rationale
Bronchoscopy	• To assess airway anatomy for tumors, obstruction, and atelectasis • To assist in the diagnosis of tuberculosis or cancer by biopsy of lesions • To remove thick secretions, mucous plugs, or foreign bodies • A flexible fiberoptic bronchoscope is inserted through the mouth, nose, endotracheal tube, or tracheostomy tube. The procedure may be done in the operating room or the radiology department. Oxygen administration and cardiac monitoring are usually used.	• Allow the client nothing by mouth for several hours before the test. • Assess for allergies to iodine or local anesthetics. • Administer pretest medications (atropine, diazepam) as ordered. • Prepare the client for topical anesthetic administration into the oropharynx. • Remove the client's dentures if present. • After the procedure, monitor the client's vital signs for 15 min until stable. • After the procedure, allow the client nothing by mouth until the gag reflex returns. • Discourage smoking, talking, and coughing for several hours.	• The client may aspirate gastric contents if vomiting occurs. • A knowledge of allergies helps prevent allergic reactions. • Pretest medications help decrease secretions and reduce anxiety. • Explanations about the effects of the anesthetic agent (numbness and gagging) help to decrease anxiety. • Injury may occur if dentures are left in place. • Assessing vital signs helps the nurse to detect respiratory distress and signs of complications related to the procedure. • Allowing the client nothing by mouth reduces the possibility of aspiration. • Throat irritation is decreased by avoiding certain activities.
Transbronchial needle aspiration	• Used with flexible bronchoscopy to perform biopsy of areas of the lung and surrounding lymph nodes	• Same as for bronchoscopy	• Same as for bronchoscopy
Laryngoscopy	• *Direct:* To detect or remove lesions or foreign bodies in the larynx or to diagnose cancer by removing tissue for biopsy or samples for culture. A fiberoptic laryngoscope is used. • *Indirect:* To assess the function of the vocal cords or to obtain tissue for biopsy. Observations are made during rest and phonation by using a laryngeal mirror, head mirror, and light source.	• Allow the client nothing by mouth for several hours before the test. • Assess the client for allergies to iodine, contrast media, or local anesthetics. • Administer pretest medications (atropine, diazepam) as ordered. • Assess the client for fears concerning the procedure. Assure the client that he or she will be monitored for any respiratory problems. • For indirect laryngoscopy, assist the client to sit in an upright position and encourage normal breathing. • After the procedure, allow the client nothing by mouth until the gag reflex returns. • Encourage coughing and fluid intake. • Assess vital signs frequently for 24 hr. Assess the client for bleeding. • After the procedure, administer lozenges or gargles as ordered.	• Aspiration is possible if vomiting occurs. • A knowledge of allergies helps prevent allergic reactions. • Pretest medications help decrease secretions and reduce anxiety. • Reassurance helps decrease fears about not being able to breathe during the procedure. • An upright sitting position facilitates the passage of the laryngeal mirror into the mouth. • The client may aspirate gastric contents if vomiting occurs. • Hydration and coughing promote the expectoration of secretions. • Frequent monitoring of vital signs enables the nurse to detect changes such as dyspnea. • Lozenges and gargles help to relieve sore throat.
Mediastinoscopy	• To inspect and remove samples for biopsy of lymph nodes that drain the lung • To detect metastasis of lung cancer • To obtain tissue for biopsy for diagnosis of tuberculosis or sarcoidosis • The procedure is done in the operating room with the client given local or general anesthesia; a suprasternal incision is used.	• Explain preoperative measures and the procedure to the client. • Postoperatively, assess the client for bleeding, pneumothorax, and vocal cord paralysis. • Assess the client for pain, and administer analgesics as ordered.	• Explanations about the anticipated procedure help to decrease anxiety. • Ongoing assessment for complications helps to ensure prompt treatment. • Medication decreases discomfort associated with the procedure.

PULMONARY FUNCTION TESTS

Pulmonary function tests (PFTs) evaluate the ability of the lungs to maintain ventilation and the effects of ventilation and oxygenation on the cardiopulmonary circulatory system. The overall evaluation of the lungs requires multiple pulmonary function studies that vary in complexity and sophistication. Such studies measure lung volumes and capacities, flow rates, diffusion capacity, gas exchange, airway resistance, and distribution of ventilation. The physician interprets the results by comparing the client's results with normal results, which are predicted according to age, sex, height, and weight.

PFTs are useful in screening clients for pulmonary disease even before the onset of signs or symptoms. Serial testing gives objective data that may be used as a guide to treatment (e.g., changes in pulmonary function can support a decision to continue or discontinue a specific therapy). Preoperative evaluation of clients with pulmonary function tests may identify clients at risk for postoperative pulmonary complications. One of the most common reasons for performing such tests is to determine the cause of breathlessness. When performed while the client exercises, pulmonary function tests help to determine whether dyspnea is caused by a pulmonary or a cardiac dysfunction or by muscle deconditioning. These tests are also useful for determining the effect of the client's occupation on pulmonary function and evaluating any related disability for legal purposes.

CLIENT PREPARATION The nurse prepares the client for PFTs by explaining the purpose and value of the tests for planning the client's care. The client is advised not to smoke for 6 to 8 hours before testing. According to institutional policy and procedure, the nurse withholds bronchodilator medication for 4 to 6 hours before the test. Many clients with respiratory impairment fear further breathlessness and are usually anxious before these so-called breathing tests. The nurse helps to alleviate apprehension by explaining to the client what the client will experience during and after the testing.

PROCEDURE PFTs can be performed at the client's bedside or in the respiratory laboratory. The client is asked to breathe through the mouth only. A nose clip may be used to prevent air from escaping. The client is asked to perform different breathing maneuvers while measurements are obtained. Table 28–6 describes the most frequently used PFTs and their purpose.

FOLLOW-UP CARE Because numerous breathing maneuvers are performed during pulmonary function tests, the nurse observes the client for increased dyspnea or bronchospasm after such studies. The nurse notes whether bronchodilator medication was administered during testing and alters the client's medication schedule as indicated.

TABLE 28–6 Characteristics and Purposes of Pulmonary Function Tests

Test	Purpose
FVC (forced vital capacity) records the maximal amount of air that can be exhaled after maximal inspiration.	• FVC gives an indication of respiratory muscle strength and ventilatory reserve. FVC is often reduced in chronic airway disease because of air trapping.
FEV_1 (forced expiratory volume in 1 sec) records the maximal amount of air that can be exhaled in the first second of expiration.	• FEV_1 is effort dependent and declines normally with age. This measure provides an estimate of the amount of obstruction of the client's breathing.
FEV_1/FVC is the ratio of expiratory volume in 1 sec to FVC.	• This ratio provides a much more sensitive indication of obstruction to airflow. This ratio is the hallmark of obstructive pulmonary disease.
$FEF_{25\%-75\%}$ records the forced expiratory flow over the 25%–75% volume (middle half) of the FVC.	• This measure provides a more sensitive index of obstruction in the smaller airways.
FRC (functional residual capacity) records the amount of air remaining in the lungs after normal expiration. FRC is an anatomic measurement of the lung compartment and requires use of the helium dilution technique.	• Increased FRC indicates hyperinflation or air trapping, which may result from obstructive pulmonary disease. FRC is normal or decreased in restrictive pulmonary diseases.
TLC (total lung capacity) records the amount of air in the lungs at the end of maximal inhalation.	• Increased TLC indicates air trapping associated with obstructive pulmonary disease. Decreased TLC indicates restrictive disease.
RV(residual volume) records the amount of air remaining in the lungs at the end of a full, forced exhalation.	• RV is increased in obstructive pulmonary disease such as emphysema.
DLCO (diffusion capacity for carbon monoxide) is a comparison of the amount of carbon monoxide (milliliters per minute) exhaled with the amount inhaled.	• This measure reflects the movement of gas across the alveolar capillary membrane into the alveolar blood. DLCO is reduced whenever the alveolar-capillary membrane is diminished, as occurs in emphysema, pulmonary hypertension, and pulmonary fibrosis. It is increased with exercise and in conditions such as polycythemia and congestive heart disease.

THORACENTESIS

Thoracentesis is the aspiration of pleural fluid or air from the pleural space. This procedure is used for diagnosis or treatment. Pleural fluid may be drained to relieve pulmonary compression and the resultant respiratory distress caused by cancer, empyema, pleurisy, or tuberculosis. Aspiration of the pleural fluid and subsequent bacteriologic examination can assist in the diagnosis of respiratory disease. To assist in further assessment of the parietal pleura, thoracentesis is usually followed by a pleural biopsy. Thoracentesis also allows the instillation of medications into the pleural space, which may be necessary to prevent further fluid formation in certain cases of pleural effusion caused by lung cancer.

CLIENT PREPARATION Adequate client preparation is essential before thoracentesis to ensure the client's cooperation during the procedure and to prevent

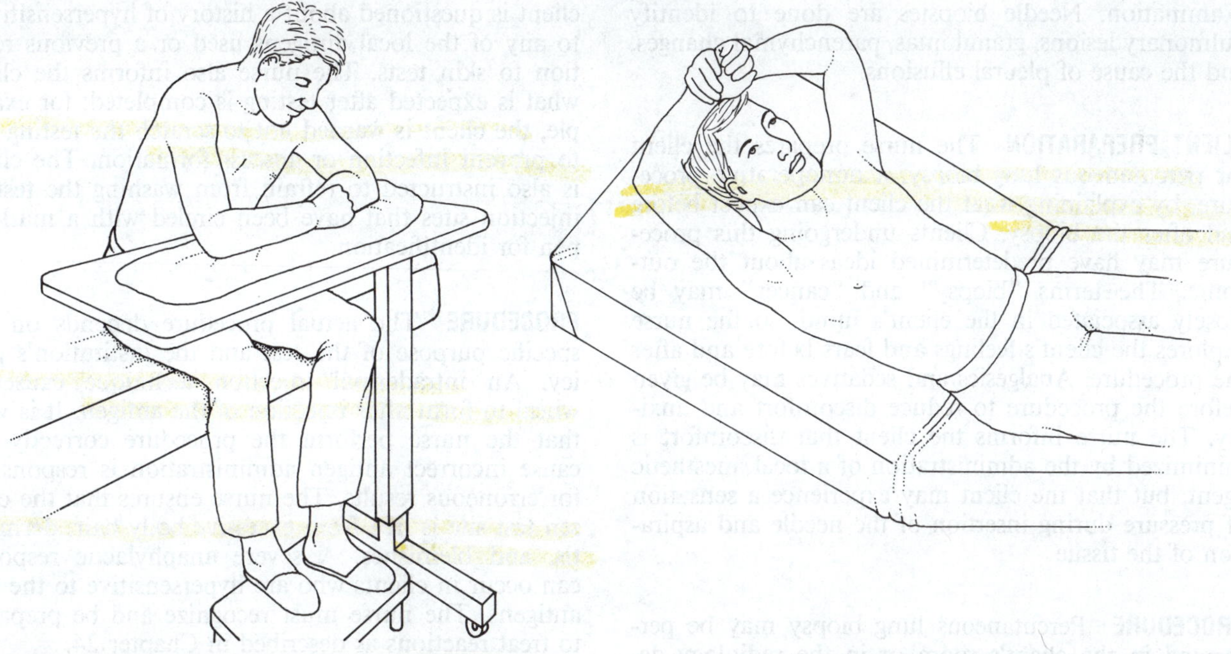

Sitting on the edge of a bed with the feet supported. The arms and shoulders are elevated, and the head is resting on the overbed table, which is padded with pillows or bath blankets.

Sitting in bed in semi-Fowler's position with the arm on the side on which the procedure will be performed raised above the head.

FIGURE 28–11 ◆ Positions for thoracentesis.

complications. The nurse tells the client to expect a stinging sensation from the local anesthetic agent and a feeling of pressure when the needle is inserted. The nurse reinforces the importance of the client's remaining immobile (avoiding coughing, deep breathing, or sudden movement) during the procedure to avoid puncture of the visceral pleura or lung.

Figure 28–11 illustrates appropriate positions for thoracentesis. These positions widen the intercostal spaces and permit the physician to have easy access to the pleural cavity. The nurse properly positions and physically supports the client. Pillows are used to make the client comfortable and to provide physical support.

Before the procedure, the nurse checks the client's history for hypersensitivity to local anesthetic agents. The entire chest or back is exposed, and the aspiration site is shaved if necessary. The actual site depends on the volume and location of the effusion, which is determined by radiography and physical examination procedures such as percussion.

PROCEDURE Thoracentesis is usually done at the bedside. After draping the client and cleaning the skin with a germicidal solution, the physician uses an aseptic technique and injects a local anesthetic agent into the selected intercostal space. The nurse keeps the client informed of the procedure while observing for shock, pain, nausea, pallor, diaphoresis, cyanosis, tachypnea, and dyspnea. The physician advances the thoracentesis needle with a syringe attached into the pleural space. Gentle suction is applied as the fluid in the pleural space is slowly aspirated. A vacuum collection bottle is sometimes necessary to remove larger volumes of fluid. To prevent hypovolemic shock and circulatory collapse, no more than 1200 mL of fluid is removed at one time. After the physician withdraws the needle, pressure is applied to the puncture site, followed by the application of a small sterile dressing.

FOLLOW-UP CARE After thoracentesis, the physician orders a chest x-ray to rule out possible pneumothorax and subsequent mediastinal shift. The nurse monitors the client's vital signs and auscultates breath sounds while noting absent or diminished sounds on the affected side. The nurse observes the puncture site and dressing for leakage or bleeding. The nurse also assesses for other complications after thoracentesis, such as reaccumulation of fluid in the pleural space, subcutaneous emphysema, pyrogenic infection, and tension pneumothorax. The client is encouraged to breathe deeply to promote re-expansion of the lung. The nurse documents the procedure in the client's chart and notes the client's tolerance, the volume and character of the fluid removed, any specimens sent to the laboratory, the location of the puncture site, and respiratory assessment findings before, during, and after the procedure.

PERCUTANEOUS LUNG BIOPSY

A percutaneous lung biopsy is performed to obtain tissue for pathogenic analysis by culture or cytologic examination. Needle biopsies are done to identify pulmonary lesions, granulomas, parenchymal changes, and the cause of pleural effusions.

CLIENT PREPARATION The nurse prepares the client for percutaneous lung biopsy, a nonoperative procedure, by explaining what the client can expect before and after the biopsy. Clients undergoing this procedure may have predetermined ideas about the outcome. The terms "biopsy" and "cancer" may be closely associated in the client's mind, so the nurse explores the client's feelings and fears before and after the procedure. Analgesics and sedatives may be given before the procedure to reduce discomfort and anxiety. The nurse informs the client that discomfort is minimized by the administration of a local anesthetic agent, but that the client may experience a sensation of pressure during insertion of the needle and aspiration of the tissue.

PROCEDURE Percutaneous lung biopsy may be performed in the client's room or in the radiology department with fluoroscopic monitoring. The positioning of the client for percutaneous needle biopsy is similar to that for thoracentesis. After the physician cleans the skin with an antibacterial agent, he or she administers a local anesthetic agent. Under sterile conditions, the physician inserts a spinal-type needle through the skin into the pleural space, aspirates fluid, and obtains tissue for microscopic examination. The nurse then applies a dressing.

FOLLOW-UP CARE The nurse monitors the client's vital signs and breath sounds every 4 hours for 24 hours. Signs of respiratory distress (e.g., dyspnea, pallor, diaphoresis, and tachypnea) are reported. Pneumothorax is the major complication after needle biopsy, so the physician may order a chest x-ray after the procedure. The nurse has the necessary equipment available for continuous chest drainage, if needed.

SKIN TESTS

Skin tests are used in combination with other diagnostic data to diagnose various infectious diseases (such as tuberculosis), viral diseases (such as mononucleosis and mumps), and fungal diseases (such as coccidioidomycosis and histoplasmosis). The presence of allergic hypersensitivity and the status of the immune system can be demonstrated through skin testing. Exposure to the allergen or organism used in testing produces a specific reaction (delayed hypersensitivity reaction) of the client's immune system. (For further discussion, see Chapters 22 and 24.)

CLIENT PREPARATION The nurse explains the purpose of skin testing and the procedure to the client to ensure cooperation and to alleviate anxiety. The client is questioned about a history of hypersensitivity to any of the local antigens used or a previous reaction to skin tests. The nurse also informs the client what is expected after testing is completed; for example, the client is warned not to scratch the testing site to prevent infection or abscess formation. The client is also instructed to refrain from washing the test or injection sites that have been circled with a marking pen for identification.

PROCEDURE The actual procedure depends on the specific purpose of the test and the institution's policy. An intradermal injection technique causes a wheal to form after injection of the antigen. It is vital that the nurse perform the procedure correctly because incorrect antigen administration is responsible for erroneous results. The nurse ensures that the chosen test site is free from excessive body hair, dermatitis, and blemishes. A severe anaphylactic response can occur in clients who are hypersensitive to the test antigens. The nurse must recognize and be prepared to treat reactions as described in Chapter 24.

FOLLOW-UP CARE The reaction at injection sites is interpreted 24 to 72 hours after administration of the test antigen. If the testing is done as an outpatient procedure, the nurse instructs the client when to return to have the results read. The nurse documents the amount of induration (hard swelling) in millimeters and the presence of erythema and vesiculation (formation of small blister-like elevations).

PULSE OXIMETRY

Pulse oximetry is a noninvasive test that registers how saturated the client's hemoglobin is with oxygen. This arterial oxygen saturation (SaO_2) is recorded as a percentage, with ideal normal values being 95% to 100%. The oxygen saturation of elderly clients may be a little lower. After a hypoxic client uses up his or her readily available oxygen (measured as the arterial oxygen pressure [PaO_2] on arterial blood gas [ABG] testing), the reserve oxygen, that attached to the hemoglobin (SaO_2), is drawn on to provide oxygen to the tissues.

The pulse oximeter uses a wave of infrared light and a sensor placed on the client's finger, toe, nose, earlobe, or forehead to measure oxygen saturation, which is then displayed on a monitor. Although pulse oximetry does not replace ABG analysis, it is more convenient, less expensive, and less uncomfortable than ABG studies. A pulse oximeter reading can alert the nurse to hypoxemia before clinical signs occur (e.g., dusky skin and nail beds).

The nurse may consider results lower than 91% (and certainly below 86%) an emergency, necessitating immediate treatment. If the SaO_2 is below 85%, the body's tissues have a difficult time becoming oxygenated. An SaO_2 of less than 70% is life-threatening (Sonnesso, 1991).

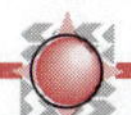

IMPLICATIONS FOR NURSING RESEARCH

Some of the questions that nurses could study with regard to assessment of the respiratory system include:

- Can more information about a client's coughing be obtained? For example, could a coughing assessment scale be developed? What is the effect of coughing on a client's coping mechanisms? What behaviors are observed in addition to coughing?
- What characteristics of chest pain are most frequently assessed?
- How reliable are the current methods of assessing dyspnea?
- What is the most effective way for nurses to learn to identify abnormal breath sounds?
- How can nurses reach consensus on the labeling of adventitious breath sounds?
- How effective is prediagnostic teaching?
- What do clients perceive as the nurse's role before and after undergoing a diagnostic test?

SELECTED BIBLIOGRAPHY

*American College of Chest Physicians and the American Thoracic Society Joint Committee on Pulmonary Nomenclature (1975). Pulmonary terms and symbols. *Chest, 67,* 583–593.

Bates, B. (1991). *A guide to physical examination and history taking* (5th ed.). Philadelphia: J. B. Lippincott.

Boring, C. C., Squires, T. S., Tong, T., & Montgomery, S. (1994). Cancer statistics, 1994. *CA-A Cancer Journal for Clinicians, 44*(1), 7–26.

Carrieri-Kohlman, V., Douglas, M., Gormley, J., & Stulborg, M. (1993). Desensitization and guided mastery: Treatment approaches for the management of dyspnea. *Heart & Lung, 22*(3), 226–234.

*Clemente, C. D. (Ed.). (1985). *Gray's anatomy of the human body* (30th ed.). Philadelphia: Lea & Febiger.

Davis, D., & Scarpa, N. (1991). Transbronchial needle aspiration. *Gastroenterology Nursing, 14*(2), 80–84.

*Davis, N. (1988). Danger signs—pleural friction rub. *Nursing88, 18*(1), 70–71.

Ehrhardt, B. S., & Graham, M. (1990). Pulse oximetry: An easy way to check oxygen saturation. *Nursing90, 20*(3), 50–54.

Finesilver, C. (1992). Respiratory assessment. *RN, 55*(2), 22–30.

Ganong, W. F. (1993). *Review of medical physiology* (16th ed.). Los Altos, CA: Appleton & Lange Medical.

Gift, A. G. (1990). Dyspnea. *Nursing Clinics of North America, 25*(4), 955–965.

Green, E. (1992). Solving the puzzle of chest pain. *American Journal of Nursing, 93*(1), 32–40.

Guyton, A. C. (1991). *Textbook of medical physiology* (8th ed.). Philadelphia: W. B. Saunders.

Jarvis, C. (1992). *Physical examination and health assessment.* Philadelphia: W. B. Saunders.

Kernicki, J. G. (1993). Differentiating chest pain: Advanced assessment techniques. *Dimensions of Critical Care Nursing, 12*(2), 66–76.

*Kersten, L. D. (1989). *Comprehensive respiratory nursing: A decision making approach.* Philadelphia: W. B. Saunders.

Kuhn, J. K., & McGovern, M. (1992). Respiratory assessment of the elderly. *Journal of Gerontological Nursing, 18*(5), 40–43.

Lehrer, S. (1993). *Understanding lung sounds* (2nd ed.). Philadelphia: W. B. Saunders.

Nield, M., & Kim, M. J. (1991). The reliability of magnitude estimation for dyspnea measurement. *Nursing Research, 40*(1), 17–19.

Pagana, K. D., & Pagana, T. J. (1992). *Mosby's diagnostic and laboratory test reference.* St. Louis: Mosby Year Book.

*Report of the American College of Chest Physicians and the American Thoracic Society Ad Hoc Subcommittee on Pulmonary Nomenclature. (1977). *ATS News, 3,* 5–6.

Roberts, A. (1991). The respiratory system, part 1. *Nursing Times, 87*(2), 53–56.

Roberts, A. (1991). The respiratory system, part 2. *Nursing Times, 87*(7), 53–56.

Sonnesso, G. (1991). Are you ready for pulse oximetry? *Nursing91, 21*(8), 60–64.

Spyr, J., & Preach, M. A. (1990). Pulse oximetry: Understanding the concept, knowing the limits. *RN, 53*(5), 38–45.

*Stevens, S. A., & Becker, K. L. (1988). How to perform a picture perfect respiratory assessment. *Nursing88, 18*(1), 57–63.

Stiesmeyer, J. K. (1993). A four-step approach to pulmonary assessment. *American Journal of Nursing, 93*(8), 22–28, 31.

*Tse, C. S. T. (1982). Food products containing tartrazine. *New England Journal of Medicine, 306,* 681–682.

Wilkins, M. A., Dexter, J. R., Murphy, R. L. H., & Del-Bono, E. A. (1990). Lung sound nomenclature survey. *Chest, 98*(4), 886–889.

*Wilkins, R., Hodghin, J., & Lopez, B. (1988). *Lung sounds: A practical approach.* St. Louis: C. V. Mosby.

*Williams, T. F. (Ed.). (1984). *Rehabilitation in the aging.* New York: Raven.

SUGGESTED READINGS

Gift, A. G. (1990). Dyspnea. *Nursing Clinics of North America, 25*(4), 955–965.

This article discusses the nurse's role in the management of symptoms of dyspnea. A model of dyspnea is discussed as well as various standardized tools used in the assessment of dyspnea. Treatment, including oxygen therapy, pharmacologic therapy, and psychologic and physical techniques, is presented, and the efficacy of each treatment method is discussed.

Spyr, J., & Preach, M. A. (1990). Pulse oximetry: Understanding the concept, knowing the limits. *RN, 53*(5), 38–45.

The article begins by laying a solid foundation for understanding pulse oximetry readings. Basic principles of oxygen transport, the role of hemoglobin, the arterial oxygen saturation measurement, and the oxyhemoglobin dissociation curve are discussed. Difficulties in obtaining accurate readings are considered, including information on how the nurse can overcome these difficulties. The article concludes by comparing 11 brands of pulse oximeters in a chart form.

Finesilver, C. (1992). Respiratory assessment. *RN, 55*(2), 22–30.

This comprehensive article begins with a discussion of aspects of a client's history that are important in an assessment of the respiratory system and then considers each phase of physical assessment related to the respiratory system. The figures and photographs are explicit. A continuing education test is included.

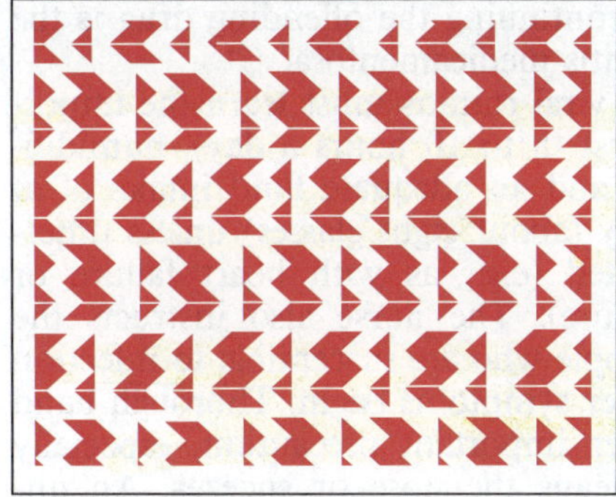

CHAPTER 29

Interventions for Clients with Upper Airway Problems

CHAPTER HIGHLIGHTS

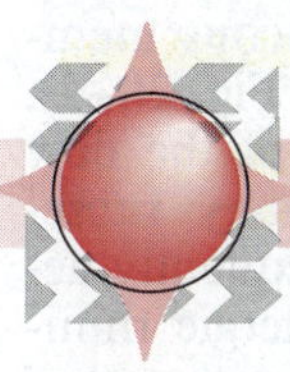

Disorders of the upper respiratory tract are common. The nurse encounters clients with diseases of the upper respiratory system in homes, clinics, primary care practitioners' offices, emergency departments, and hospitals and nursing homes. These diseases may be acute, chronic, emergent, self-limiting, or terminal. A major nursing priority for the client with disorders of the upper airway is to maintain a patent and functioning airway.

DISORDERS OF THE NOSE AND SINUSES

Rhinitis

OVERVIEW

Rhinitis is an inflammation of the nasal mucosa and is the most common disorder to affect the nose and sinuses of adults. The etiology of rhinitis often involves an interplay of viruses, bacteria, and allergens.

Acute rhinitis may be caused by allergens, bacteria, or a virus. *Allergic rhinitis,* frequently called "hay fever" or "allergies," is commonly initiated by sensitivity reactions to allergens, especially plant pollens and molds. Acute episodes tend to be seasonal; that is, they disappear after a few weeks and recur at the same time the following year. *Chronic,* or *perennial, rhinitis* presents intermittently or continuously when a person is exposed to certain allergens, such as dust, animal dander, wool, and foods (e.g., seafood). Rhinitis also can occur after excessive use of nose drops or sprays (rhinitis medicamentosa) as a rebound effect causing nasal congestion or after nasal inhalation of cocaine.

Acute viral rhinitis (*coryza,* or the common cold) is caused by one of more than 30 viruses. It usually spreads from one person to another via droplet nuclei from sneezing or coughing and is most contagious in the first 2 to 3 days after symptoms appear. The condition is self-limiting unless a complication, such as otitis media, sinusitis, bronchitis, or pneumonia, occurs. These complications are most likely seen in the young, elderly, or immunosuppressed people, especially if they live or work in crowded conditions or in group settings, such as a long-term care facility.

COLLABORATIVE MANAGEMENT

ASSESSMENT

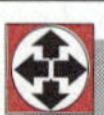

In both acute and chronic allergic rhinitis, the offending substance causes a release of vasoactive mediators (e.g., histamine, serotonin, bradykinin, and prostaglandin), which induces vasodilation and increased capillary permeability. Edema and swelling of the nasal mucosa result, and the client complains of headache, nasal irritation, sneezing, nasal congestion, *rhinorrhea* (watery drainage from the nose), and itchy, watery eyes. Chapter 24 further describes the physiologic mechanisms that occur in allergic reactions of the hypersensitivity type.

In addition to the clinical manifestations observed in clients with allergic rhinitis, clients with viral infections often present with fatigue, a sore, dry throat, and, at times, a low-grade fever with chills.

INTERVENTIONS

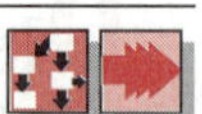

Management of the client with any type of rhinitis includes symptomatic relief and client education. The physician prescribes appropriate drug therapy, and the nurse instructs the client as indicated. Drugs, including antihistamines and decongestants, are commonly given but must be used with caution in the elderly because of side effects such as vertigo, hypertension, urinary retention, and insomnia. These medications work by causing vasoconstriction and, subsequently, by decreasing edema. Antipyretics are administered if fever is present in the client with viral rhinitis. Antibiotic therapy is usually not prescribed to prevent primary or secondary bacterial infection because these agents do not kill the offending virus. Decreasing or discontinuing the offending drug is the treatment for rhinitis medicamentosa.

The client with viral rhinitis must learn the importance of proper rest (8 to 10 hours a day), humidification of the air, and an adequate fluid intake of at least 2000 mL/day (about eight glasses) unless otherwise contraindicated (e.g., as with heart failure or chronic renal failure). The nurse also instructs the client to avoid people who are susceptible to infection for 2 to 3 days after symptoms begin. Thorough hand washing is another important precaution, especially after the client cleans the nose or sneezes. An uncomplicated cold typically subsides within 7 days.

The client with recurrent allergic rhinitis can undergo allergy testing to determine the cause, and desensitization may help to prevent future episodes. The client may be able to avoid the offending substance. Chapter 24 further discusses allergies.

Sinusitis

OVERVIEW

Sinusitis is an inflammation of the mucous membranes of one or more of the sinuses (see Fig. 28–2). *Acute sinusitis* results in the obstruction of the flow of secretions from the sinuses, which may subsequently become infected. The disorder frequently accompanies or follows acute or chronic allergic rhinitis. It can also occur in conjunction with other influencing factors, including a deviated nasal septum, polyps, tumors, chronically inhaled air pollutants or cocaine, facial trauma, nasotracheal intubation, or cystic fibrosis. In *chronic sinusitis,* the mucous membrane becomes permanently thickened from prolonged or repeated inflammation or infection.

The causative organism in sinus infection is usually *Streptococcus pneumoniae, Haemophilus influenzae, Diplococcus,* or *Bacteroides.* Anaerobic infections can also cause sinusitis. Sinusitis most often develops in the maxillary and frontal sinuses.

COLLABORATIVE MANAGEMENT

ASSESSMENT

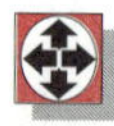

The clinical manifestations of sinusitis include nasal swelling and congestion, headache, facial pressure, and pain (usually aggravated by movement of the head to a dependent position), tenderness on percussion over the involved area, low-grade fever, and purulent or bloody nasal drainage.

INTERVENTIONS

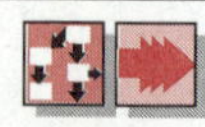

Nonsurgical Management The treatment for sinusitis includes the use of broad-spectrum antibiotics, analgesics for pain and fever (e.g., acetaminophen [Tylenol, Ace-Tabs♣]), decongestants (e.g., phenylephrine [Neo-Synephrine], terfenadine [Seldane], astemizole [Hismanal]), steam humidification, and nasal saline irrigations. The nurse instructs the client to increase free water intake to more than ten glasses of water or juice per day unless medically contraindicated. When this treatment plan is not successful, the physician orders additional evaluations with sinus films and computed tomography. Surgical intervention may be necessary.

Surgical Management

Antral Irrigation Antral irrigation, also known as maxillary antral puncture and lavage, is an outpatient surgical procedure. Following local anesthesia, a large-gauge needle is inserted under the inferior turbinate of the nose and into the maxillary sinus on the affected side. Fluid or purulent material from the sinus is withdrawn. The sinus is then irrigated with saline solution, an antibiotic solution, or both.

Other Surgical Procedures If antral irrigation is not successful, other surgical procedures may be used to open the sinus cavities in clients with chronic sinusitis. In the *Caldwell-Luc procedure,* the surgeon makes an incision in the anterior wall of the maxillary sinus under the upper lip. The infected mucosa in the maxillary sinus is removed. With the *nasal antral window procedure,* the surgeon creates an opening in the anterior portion of the inferior turbinate to allow for unobstructed drainage through the nares. With either procedure, the client may have difficulty eating for a few days postoperatively because of pain and swelling. Chart 29–1 covers nursing care for clients undergoing these procedures.

When the ethmoid sinuses need to be opened, the surgeon uses an external approach for better visualization and preservation of structures. The surgical incision is made along the side of the nose from the middle of the eyebrow (Webber-Ferguson incision).

The surgical procedure for frontal sinusitis differs from that for the other areas, in that the diseased tissue of the frontal sinus can be completely removed and the sinus obliterated. An osteoplastic flap, with a coronal or "hairline" incision requires the replacement of the sinus mucosal lining with subcutaneous fat obtained from the client's abdomen. Postoperatively, the client usually experiences both sinus and incisional pain, and the abdominal donor site may be tender for several days.

Endoscopic Sinus Surgery Endoscopic sinus surgery has become a revolutionary method of diagnosing and treating sinus disorders. Direct inspection of the sinuses by the use of a sinus endoscope is an improved surgical procedure for refractory sinus disorders. Completed with the client under general anesthesia in an outpatient surgical center, the procedure takes only minutes. The client goes home the same day and can return to work in approximately 5 days. Nasal mucosa may take up to 4 to 6 weeks to heal. The nurse instructs the client in frequent use of saline nasal sprays to prevent intranasal and sinus crusting and promote healing.

CHART 29–1

Nursing Care Highlight ◆ Postoperative Care for Clients with Sinus Surgery

- Position the client in the semi-Fowler's position to promote drainage and prevent swelling.
- Perform gentle oral hygiene to promote healing and prevent injury to the surgical incision.
- Use ice compresses as ordered for 24 hours.
- Change the "moustache" dressing under the nose as needed, and record the type and amount of drainage.
- Instruct the client to eat soft foods and increase fluid intake.
- Instruct the client to limit the Valsalva maneuver (no coughing, blowing the nose, or straining at stool) for at least 2 weeks postoperatively to prevent bleeding and tissue damage.

Fracture of the Nose

OVERVIEW

Nasal fractures commonly occur from injuries that are received during falls, during participation in sports, or from trauma related to violence or motor vehicle accidents. If the bone or cartilage is not displaced, usually no serious complications result from the fracture and treatment may not be necessary. Displacement, however, can cause airway obstruction or cosmetic deformity and is a potential source of infection.

COLLABORATIVE MANAGEMENT

ASSESSMENT

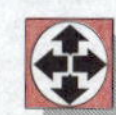

During the initial assessment, the nurse notes and documents nasal deviation, a malaligned nasal bridge, a change in nasal breathing, crepitus on palpation, midface ecchymosis, and pain. Blood or clear (cerebrospinal) fluid rarely drains from one or both nares, but such drainage could indicate a skull fracture. Radiographic examination is not always useful in nasal fractures but is very important in evaluating the patient for other concurrent facial fractures.

INTERVENTIONS

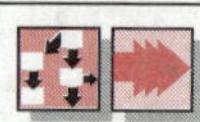

The physician performs a simple closed reduction of the fracture using local or general anesthesia within the first 24 hours after injury. After 24 hours, the fracture is more difficult to reduce because of edema and scar formation. Simple closed fractures need not be surgically treated; treatment focuses on pain relief and local cold compresses to decrease swelling.

Rhinoplasty For severe fractures or those that do not heal properly, a closed or open reduction with or without rhinoplasty is required. Rhinoplasty is a surgical reconstruction of the nose for cosmetic purposes and for functional improvement of airflow. The client returns from surgery with packing in both nostrils to prevent bleeding and to provide a *stent* (object that provides support and structure) for the reconstructed nose. The ½-inch gauze packing is typically treated with an antibiotic ointment, such as bacitracin (Bacitin✱) to reduce the risk of infection. The client typically has a "moustache" dressing, or drip pad, usually a folded 2 × 2 gauze pad, placed under the nose. A splint or cast may cover the nose for additional alignment and protection (Fig. 29–1). The nurse or client changes the drip pad as necessary.

Postoperatively, the nurse observes the client for edema and bleeding and takes vital signs every 4 hours until discharge. The nurse assesses how often the client swallows. Repeated swallowing may indicate posterior nasal bleeding. The nurse checks the pharynx with a penlight for bleeding, and, if present, notifies the physician.

The nurse places the client in semi-Fowler's position and instructs him or her to move slowly and to rest as much as possible. The nurse applies cool compresses to the nose, eyes, or face to reduce swelling and prevent excessive discoloration. Once the effects of anesthesia are eliminated and the physician has so ordered, the nurse allows the client to select soft foods and encourages an increased fluid intake. To prevent bleeding, the nurse also instructs the client to limit the Valsalva maneuver, such as forceful coughing or straining at stool, for the first few days after removal of the nasal packing. Laxatives or stool softeners may be appropriate to facilitate defecation. The client avoids aspirin and non-steroidal anti-inflammatory drugs during this time to prevent the possibility of bleeding. The physician may order prophylactic antibiotics to prevent postoperative infection and pain medication to relieve discomfort. The nurse explains to the client that edema and discoloration usually last for several weeks and that the final surgical result will be evident in 6 to 12 months.

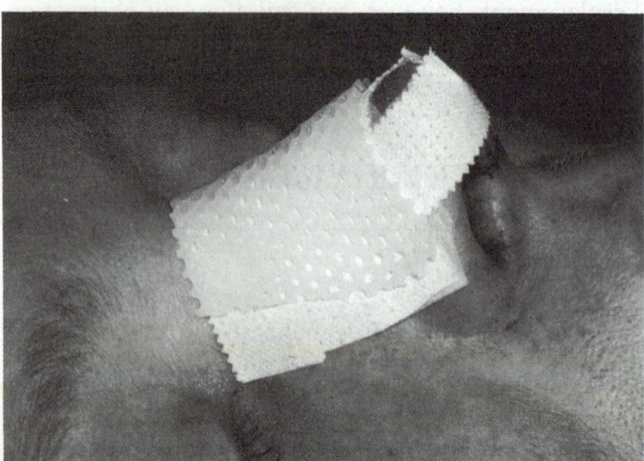

FIGURE 29–1 ◆ A basic rhinoplasty dressing, including an Aquaplast cast. (From Johnson, C. M., Jr., & Toriumi, D. M. [1990]. *Open structure rhinoplasty.* Philadelphia: W. B. Saunders.)

Nasoseptoplasty Nasoseptoplasty, or submucous resection (SMR), may be necessary to straighten a deviated septum when chronic symptoms (e.g., a "stuffy" nose) or discomfort occurs. A slight deviation of the nasal septum is present in most adults and causes no symptoms. Major deviations may obstruct the nasal passages or interfere with airflow and sinus drainage. The surgeon removes the deviated section of the cartilage and bone. The amount resected depends on the type and degree of deformity present.

Nursing care is similar to that for the client with a rhinoplasty. Nasoseptoplasty is often an ambulatory surgery procedure; the nurse reviews written instructions with the client on discharge.

Epistaxis

OVERVIEW

Epistaxis (nosebleed) is a common problem because of the rich capillary network within the nose. Nosebleeds may occur as a result of trauma, hypertension (especially in the elderly), blood dyscrasia (e.g., leukemias), inflammation, tumor, decreased humidity, excessive nose blowing, and nose picking. Men are usually affected more than women, and the elderly tend to bleed most often from the posterior portion of the nose.

COLLABORATIVE MANAGEMENT

ASSESSMENT

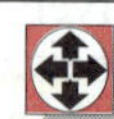

The client may be holding a tissue or gauze pad up to the nares while explaining to the nurse what happened. Often the client will report that the bleeding started after sneezing or blowing the nose. The nurse notes the amount and color of the blood and takes a set of vital signs. The nurse also assesses and documents the number, duration, and causes of previous bleeding episodes.

INTERVENTIONS

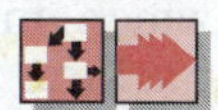

Chart 29-2 summarizes emergency first aid interventions for the client with a nosebleed. If the nosebleed does not respond to the described interventions, medical attention is needed. The physician cauterizes the affected capillaries with silver nitrate or electrocautery, then follows with anterior packing. Anterior packing is most commonly used and is very effective in controlling bleeding from the anterior nasal cavity.

When bleeding originates in the posterior nasal region, the physician uses a posterior pack to stop the bleeding. A string is attached to a large gauze pack and then threaded through the nose and out the mouth. The physician positions the pack in the posterior nasal cavity above the pharynx, then tapes the string to the client's cheek to prevent movement of the pack. This procedure is uncomfortable and may cause airway obstruction if the pack slips.

The nurse observes the client for respiratory distress and for tolerance of the packing. The physician may prescribe humidification and oxygen as well as bed rest and antibiotics. To maintain gag and cough reflexes and optimal level of consciousness, the client should not receive any sedatives and only limited pain medication. The nurse provides oral care and ensures adequate hydration, which is important because of mouth breathing. The nurse uses pulse oximetry, a cardiac monitor, or both, as ordered, to observe for hypoxemia and hypercapnia. After the physician removes the packing, the nurse may apply petroleum jelly to the nares for lubrication and comfort. Nasal saline solution and humidification may be helpful for added moisture and to prevent crusting and rebleeding.

CHART 29-2

Nursing Care Highlight ◆ Emergency Care of a Nosebleed

1. Position the client in an upright position, leaning forward, to prevent blood from entering the stomach and possible aspiration.
2. Reassure the client and attempt to keep him or her quiet to reduce anxiety and blood pressure.
3. Apply direct lateral pressure to the nose for 5 minutes, and apply ice or cool compresses to the nose and face if possible.
4. Maintain universal or body substance precautions.
5. If nasal packing is necessary, loosely pack both nares with gauze or nasal tampons.
6. To prevent rebleeding from dislodging clots, instruct the client not to blow the nose for several hours after the bleeding stops.
7. Seek medical assistance if these measures are ineffective or if the bleeding occurs frequently.

Cancer of the Nose and Sinuses

OVERVIEW

Tumors of the nasal cavities and sinuses are relatively uncommon and may be benign or malignant. Malignant lesions of these areas can occur at all ages, but the peak incidence is 40 to 45 years in males and 60 to 65 years in females. There is a higher incidence of nasopharyngeal cancer in Asian-Americans. The cause is believed to be environmental.

COLLABORATIVE MANAGEMENT

ASSESSMENT

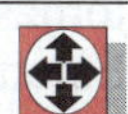

The onset of sinus malignancies is insidious, and symptoms are frequently interpreted by clients as representing sinusitis. Therefore, clients may have relatively advanced disease when they are first diagnosed. Detection and diagnosis are often delayed because the symptoms mimic those of common upper respiratory tract illnesses. Persistent nasal obstruction, drainage, bloody discharge, and pain that does not improve after treatment of sinusitis suggest nasal or sinus malignancy. Cervical lymph node enlargement usually occurs on the side most burdened with tumor mass.

INTERVENTIONS

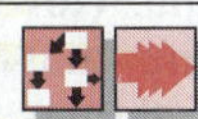

Radiation therapy is the primary treatment for nasopharyngeal cancers. Surgical resection may be indicated in radiation therapy failures. Chemotherapy has not proved to be effective. The specific surgical procedure performed depends on the amount of tumor, its anatomic location, and tissue invasion. The primary deficit is change in body image, speech, and alteration in nutrition, especially when the maxilla and floor of the nose are involved in the resection.

The nurse provides general postoperative care (see Chap. 21), including maintenance of a patent airway, wound care, strict attention to nutrition, and tracheostomy care (if present). (Tracheostomy care is covered later in this chapter.) The nurse provides meticulous mouth and maxillary cavity care for the client with saline irrigations using a water pick (e.g., Water Pik) or a syringe. The nurse also assesses for alterations in comfort and for infection. Optimal nutrition is essential during the perioperative period for adequate healing.

Nasal Polyps

Nasal polyps are benign, grape-like clusters of mucous membrane and loose connective tissue. Polyps typically occur bilaterally and are often caused by irritation to the nasal mucosa or sinuses, allergies, or infection (chronic sinusitis). If polyps become too large, airway obstruction may result.

Benign nasal polyps are treated medically with nasally inhaled steroids in conjunction with removal of the polyps. Surgical removal (polypectomy) can be accomplished with either local or general anesthesia. The nurse observes the client for postoperative bleeding. The nostrils are usually packed with gauze for 24 hours postoperatively. Nasal polyps tend to recur if not completely resected.

Inverting papilloma is a rare, histologically benign condition, consisting of a space-occupying lesion that erodes nasal and maxillary skeletal structures. Often initially diagnosed as benign polyps, inverting papillomas grow by pressure into other adjacent structures. Extensive sinus and nasal surgery is necessary for complete removal. If these papillomas are completely resected, they do not recur.

FACIAL TRAUMA

OVERVIEW

Facial trauma is defined by the specific bones (i.e., mandibular, maxillary, zygomatic, orbital, or nasal fractures) and the side of the face involved. Mandibular (lower jaw) fractures can occur at any location of the mandible and make up the majority of facial fractures. Le Fort I is a nasoethmoid complex fracture. Le Fort II is a transverse maxillary *and* nasoethmoid complex fracture. Le Fort III is a combination of I and II plus an orbital-zygoma fracture, often called "craniofacial dysjunction" because it leaves the midface with no connection to the skull. Nasal fractures have been discussed earlier in this chapter. Because the face is very vascular, there is often much bleeding with facial trauma.

COLLABORATIVE MANAGEMENT

ASSESSMENT

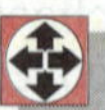

The first priority in the management of facial trauma is assessment for a patent airway. Signs and symptoms of an upper airway obstruction include stridor, shortness of breath, dyspnea, anxiety, restlessness, hypoxia, hypercarbia, decreased oxygen saturation, cyanosis, and loss of consciousness (see also upper airway obstruction later in this chapter). After establishing the airway, the nurse assesses the amount and site of soft-tissue trauma, bleeding, and palpable fractures. Additional findings on assessment include edema of soft tissue, asymmetry, pain, or leakage of cerebrospinal fluid through the ears and/or nose, which may indicate temporal bone or basilar skull fracture. Because orbital and maxillary fractures can entrap the globe, the nurse assesses vision and extraocular movement (EOM) and also observes for neurologic changes (see Chap. 40). Because spinal cord trauma and skull fractures often occur in conjunction with facial trauma, cranial computed tomography, facial series, and cervical spine films are then obtained.

INTERVENTIONS

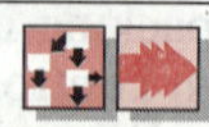

The nurse's first intervention is to establish and maintain a patent airway. The nurse must anticipate the need for emergent intubation, tracheotomy, or cricothyroidotomy. When the client arrives at a trauma center, key personnel have specific duties, including controlling hemorrhage, establishing an airway, and assessing for the extent of injury. If the signs and symptoms of shock are present (see Chap. 36), fluid resuscitation and identification of bleeding sites must be initiated immediately.

In head and neck trauma, the nurse should be astute in the areas of trauma and critical care nursing. Time is paramount in stabilizing the client. Early treatment and response of the appropriate services, including the trauma team, maxillofacial surgeon, general surgeon, otolaryngologist, plastic surgeon, and dentist, optimize the client's post-trauma recovery period. (Consult a specialized trauma book for more information about trauma care.)

Stabilization of the fractured segment of a *mandibular fracture* allows the teeth to heal in proper alignment or occlusion. The client remains in fixed centric occlusion for 6 to 10 weeks. Antibiotic therapy may be prescribed because of oral wound contamination. Delay in treatment, infection of the adjacent tooth, or poor oral care may result in infection in the mandibular segment. The client may then require surgical debridement, intravenous antibiotic therapy, and an extended period in fixation.

Inner maxillary fixation (IMF) is a common method of securing a mandibular fracture. The physician can repair nondisplaced alligned fractures in a clinic or office using local dental anesthesia. General anesthesia is used for repair of displaced or complex fractures or fractures that occur with other facial bone fractures.

If the mandibular fracture is repaired with titanium plates, the nurse teaches the client oral care, soft-diet restrictions, and follow-up care with a dentist. The plates are permanent and do not interfere with magnetic resonance imaging (MRI) studies.

Postoperatively, the nurse teaches oral care with a water-irrigating device, such as a Water Pik. If the client is in inner maxillary fixation, the nurse teaches self-care with wires in place, including a dental liquid diet. The nurse also explains the proper method of cutting the wires if emesis occurs. The client keeps wire cutters with him or her at all times for this emergency. The nurse instructs the client to return to the physician for rewiring as soon as possible to reinstitute fixation.

Nutrition is important for any client with fractures. Because of oral fixation, pain, and surgery, clients may not attend to their nutritional needs. Dietary consultations are important for teaching and support.

DISORDERS OF THE ORAL PHARYNX AND TONSILS

Pharyngitis

OVERVIEW

Pharyngitis is an inflammation of the mucous membranes of the pharynx. It may precede, or occur simultaneously with, acute rhinitis or sinusitis.

Acute pharyngitis has multiple causes (Table 29–1). The most common bacterial organism causing pharyngitis is group A beta-hemolytic *Streptococcus,* but most adult cases are caused by a virus. The incidence of streptococcal infection rises between late fall and spring, especially in the colder climates.

TABLE 29–1 Causes of Pharyngitis

Bacterial Causes
- *Streptococcus*
- *Staphylococcus*
- *Haemophilus influenzae*
- Pneumococcus
- *Corynebacterium diphtheriae*
- *Neisseria gonorrhoeae*

Viral Causes
- Adenovirus
- Rhinovirus
- Epstein-Barr virus
- Cytomegalovirus (CMV)
- Influenza virus
- Parainfluenza virus
- Herpesvirus
- Coxsackievirus A
- Echovirus

Other Causes
- *Chlamydia*
- *Mycoplasma pneumoniae*
- *Candida*
- Physical and chemical causes
  - Alcohol
  - Tobacco
  - Heat
  - Irritants
  - Dehydration
  - Trauma

COLLABORATIVE MANAGEMENT

ASSESSMENT

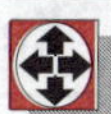

Pharyngitis is characterized by soreness and dryness in the throat, pain, pain on swallowing (odynophagia), difficulty in swallowing (dysphagia), and fever. Viral and bacterial pharyngitis is often difficult to differentiate on physical assessment. When inspecting the mucous membranes of a throat infected with either virus or bacteria, the nurse may note a mild to severe hyperemia (redness) with or without enlarged erythematous tonsils and with or without exudate. The nurse asks about nasal discharge, which can vary from thin and watery to thick and purulent. Cervical lymphadenopathy may be present in either viral or bacterial pharyngitis. With a parapharyngeal (or tonsillar) abscess, the client may have a characteristic "hot potato" voice—a thickened voice of poor quality.

Clinical studies indicate that streptococcal or other bacterial infections are more often associated with enlarged erythematous tonsils with exudate, purulent nasal discharge, and cervical lymphadenopathy. Chart 29–3 (see p. 640) outlines the clinical manifestations of viral versus bacterial pharyngitis. Viral pharyngitis is communicable for 2 to 3 days, and symptoms usually subside within 3 to 10 days after onset. It is usually a self-limiting disease.

Bacterial pharyngitis, such as group A streptococcal infection, however, can lead to dangerous medical complications (Table 29–2). The two most serious complications, acute glomerulonephritis (see Chap. 71) and rheumatic fever (see Chap. 34), occur in 1% to 3% of cases. Acute glomerulonephritis generally occurs 7 to 10 days after the acute infection, and rheumatic fever may develop 3 to 5 weeks after an acute streptococcal infection.

Throat cultures are important to differentiate viral from group A beta-hemolytic streptococcal infection. To obtain a specimen, the nurse or physician rubs a cotton swab over each tonsillar area and the posterior

TABLE 29–2 Complications of Group A Streptococcal Infection

- Rheumatic fever
- Acute glomerulonephritis
- Peritonsillar abscess
- Retropharyngeal abscess
- Otitis media
- Sinusitis
- Mastoiditis
- Bronchitis
- Pneumonia
- Scarlet fever

CHART 29–3

Key Features of Acute Viral and Bacterial Pharyngitis

Feature	Viral Pharyngitis	Bacterial Pharyngitis
Temperature	• Low-grade or no fever	• High fever (above 101° F [38° C], and usually 102°–104° F [38.5°–40° C])
Ear manifestations	• Retracted and/or dull tympanic membrane	• Retracted and/or dull tympanic membrane
Throat manifestations	• Scant or no tonsillar exudate	• Severe hyperemia of pharyngeal mucosa, tonsils, and uvula
	• Slight erythema of pharynx and tonsils	• Erythema of tonsils with yellow exudate
Neck manifestations	• Possible lymphadenopathy	• Anterior cervical lymphadenopathy and tenderness
Skin manifestations	• No rash	• Possible scarlatiniform rash • Possible petechiae on chest and/or abdomen
Dysphagia, odynophagia	• Present	• Present
Other symptoms	• Cough	• No cough
	• Rhinitis	
	• Mild Hoarseness	• Voice characterized by pain on voicing and slurred speech
	• Headache	• Arthralgia • Myalgia
Laboratory data	• Complete blood count usually normal	• Complete blood count abnormal
	• White blood cell count usually lower than 10,000/mm³	• White blood cell count usually higher than 12,000/mm³
	• Negative throat culture results	• Throat culture results positive for beta-hemolytic streptococcus
Onset	• Gradual	• Abrupt

pharynx. The cotton swab is then streaked on a blood agar plate (Fig. 29–2), which is incubated for 24 hours.

An easier and faster method for determining the type of infection is a test using latex agglutination for group A streptococcal antigen; results are ready in 10 minutes. With immediate results and rapid initiation of treatment, the incidence of sequelae of streptococcal infection should decrease. Throat culture results are not entirely accurate; both false-negative and false-positive results occur.

A complete blood count is performed when the client's condition is severe or not improving. The client may exhibit extremely high fevers, lethargy, or signs and symptoms of complications. A complete blood count may indicate other causes of pharyngitis.

When taking a history, the nurse inquires about the client's recent contacts (within the last 10 days) with people who have been ill. Of particular importance is whether the client has been ill with symptoms of a cold or upper respiratory tract infection recently or in the past. Documenting previous streptococcal infections is essential. The nurse also notes a history of rheumatic fever, valvular heart disease, streptococcal infections, or penicillin allergy. Because diphtheria (*Corynebacterium diphtheriae* infection) can cause pharyngitis, the nurse documents whether the client has had a diphtheria immunization.

INTERVENTIONS

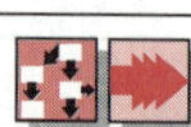

Most sore throats in adults are viral and do not warrant the use of antibiotics. The treatment plan includes rest, increased fluid intake, humidification of the air, analgesics for pain, warm saline throat gargles, and throat lozenges containing mild anesthetics.

The management of bacterial pharyngitis involves the use of antibiotics and the same supportive care provided for viral pharyngitis. For streptococcal infection, the physician typically prescribes penicillin V (Pen-Vee K, Apo-Pen-VK✱), 250 mg orally every 6 hours for 10 days. If the client is allergic to penicillin, erythromycin is the alternative. The nurse counsels the client on the importance of completing the entire 10-day dosage of antibiotics, even if symptoms subside. If the client cannot tolerate the medication, the nurse notifies the physician so that a change in the antibiotic regimen can be made. If compliance is a concern or the client cannot swallow pills, long-acting benzathine penicillin, 1.2 million units, can be administered intramuscularly in a single dose to eradicate the organism. The client should be re-evaluated if there is no improvement in 3 days or if the symptoms are still present after completion of the antibiotic course.

The nurse instructs the client in the proper proce-

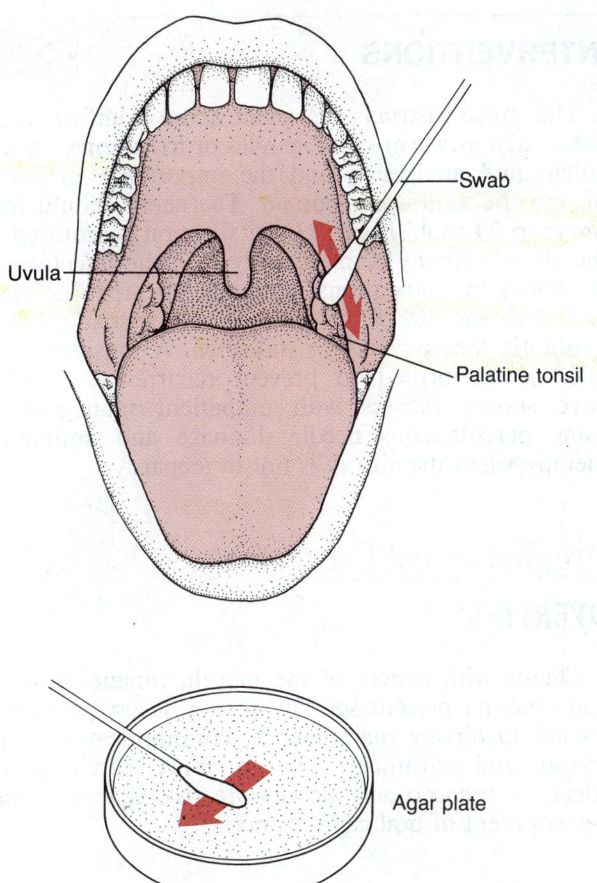

FIGURE 29–2 ◆ Throat culture technique.

dure for taking an oral temperature reading. This reading is taken in the morning and in the evening until convalescence is complete. The client is not contagious after 24 hours of antibiotic treatment. Family members or significant others who experience a sore throat should be evaluated, and a throat culture may be indicated.

Tonsillitis

OVERVIEW

Tonsillitis is an inflammation and infection of the tonsils and the lymphatic tissue located on each lateral side of the oropharynx (where the palatine, or faucial tonsils, are located). The tonsils consist of lymphatic tissue that is shaped like a small almond. Each tonsil is covered by a mucous membrane. These lymphatic tissues filter microorganisms, thus functioning as a protective mechanism for the respiratory and gastrointestinal tracts.

Tonsillitis is a contagious, airborne infection. Acute or chronic tonsillitis can occur in any age group, but 5- to 10-year-old children are affected most often. The infection is usually more severe when it occurs in adolescents or adults.

The acute form usually lasts 7 to 10 days and is most often caused by a bacterial organism. The most common organism is *Streptococcus*. Other bacterial pathogens include *Staphylococcus aureus, Haemophilus influenzae,* and *Pneumococcus*. Viruses may also cause tonsillitis. Chronic tonsillitis usually results either from an acute infection that did not resolve or from recurrent infections.

COLLABORATIVE MANAGEMENT

ASSESSMENT

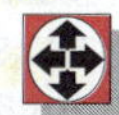

Chart 29–4 summarizes the signs and symptoms of acute tonsillitis. Diagnostic studies are performed to rule out other causes of the sore throat and fever (such as acute pharyngitis). The following diagnostic studies may be ordered for a client with suspected tonsillitis: complete blood count, throat culture and sensitivity (C&S) studies, Monospot test, and chest x-ray if respiratory symptoms are present. In bacterial infections, the white blood cell count is elevated. Throat culture and sensitivity studies identify the causative bacterial organism and direct the choice of regimen.

INTERVENTIONS

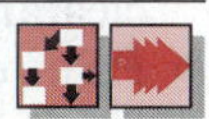

The physician orders systemic antibiotics (usually penicillin or erythromycin) for 7 to 10 days. Warm saline throat gargles, analgesics, antipyretics, and lozenges with topical anesthetic ingredients may provide symptomatic relief.

CHART 29–4

Key Features of Acute Tonsillitis

- Sudden onset of a mild to severe sore throat
- Fever
- Muscle aches
- Chills
- Dysphagia, odynophagia (painful swallowing of food)
- Pain in the ears
- Headache
- Anorexia
- Malaise
- "Hot potato" voice (thickened voice of poor quality)
- Tonsils visually swollen and red with pus
- Tonsils may be covered with a white or yellow exudate
- Purulent drainage may be expressed upon pressing a tonsil
- Uvula visually edematous or inflamed
- Cervical lymph nodes usually tender and enlarged

Indications for surgical intervention include:

- Recurrent acute infections or chronic infections that have not responded to antibiotic therapy
- Peritonsillar abscess
- Infected hypertrophy of the tonsils or adenoids that obstructs the airway
- Diphtheria carriage, because the tonsils are the source of infection

The indication for surgery becomes stronger in the presence of evidence of *repeated* group A beta-hemolytic streptococcal infections. Surgery is generally not indicated if the client is experiencing an acute tonsillar infection (except with an acute peritonsillar abscess) or has a blood dyscrasia, such as aplastic anemia, hemophilia, or leukemia.

The most common surgical procedure for removing the tonsils is dissection and snare. The adenoids are removed with an adenoid curette or adenotome. A tonsillectomy and adenoidectomy (T&A) is usually performed with the client under general anesthesia, but this procedure is performed infrequently in adults. Postoperatively, the nurse focuses care on the following nursing diagnoses:

- High Risk for Injury related to ineffective airway clearance
- Pain related to surgery and edema
- Fluid Volume Deficit related to bleeding

Peritonsillar Abscess

OVERVIEW

Peritonsillar abscess (PTA), or *quinsy,* is a complication of acute tonsillitis. The acute infection spreads from the tonsil to the surrounding peritonsillar tissue, which forms an abscess. It is one of the most common abscesses of the head and neck area. The common cause of PTA is group A beta-hemolytic streptococcus. Anaerobic organisms may also be the etiologic agent.

COLLABORATIVE MANAGEMENT

ASSESSMENT

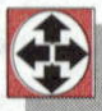

At physical examination, signs of infection are pronounced. Pus forms behind the tonsil and causes a marked asymmetric swelling and deviation of the uvula. Because of the swelling, the client may experience drooling, severe throat pain that may radiate to the ear, a voice change, and difficulty in swallowing. The client may also exhibit a tonic contraction of the muscles of mastication (trismus) and may complain of difficult breathing.

INTERVENTIONS

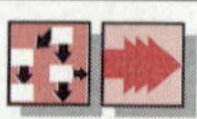

The nurse instructs the client about comfort measures such as warm saline gargles or irrigations, an ice collar, and analgesics, and the importance of completing the antibiotic regimen. The client should improve in 24 to 48 hours. Hospitalization is required if the client's airway is in jeopardy or if the infection is refractory to conventional antibiotic therapy. Incision and drainage (I&D) of the abscess plus additional antibiotic therapy may be indicated. A tonsillectomy may be performed to prevent recurrence. Studies have shown success with outpatient management using percutaneous needle drainage and antibiotic therapy when the airway is not in jeopardy.

Oropharyngeal Cancer

OVERVIEW

Clients with cancer of the mouth, tongue, tonsils, and pharynx present special nursing needs, primarily related to airway maintenance, communication, nutrition, and self-image. The combined carcinogenic effects of tobacco and alcohol are risk factors in the development of oral cavity cancers.

COLLABORATIVE MANAGEMENT

ASSESSMENT

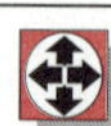

Signs and symptoms of oropharyngeal cancer are described under the heading Head and Neck Cancer later in this chapter and in Chapter 53.

INTERVENTIONS

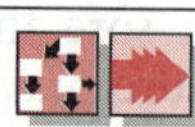

For small tumors, the physician prescribes either radiation or surgery. A combination of surgery plus radiation is indicated for larger, more aggressive tumors. Chemotherapy is still experimental, used in combination with other modalities, but shows promise in controlling disease. Surgical resection depends on location, size, and tumor type. The primary deficits following surgical resection are speech and swallowing and changes in appearance.

Management of clients with head and neck cancer requiring extensive surgery is complex and involves close collaboration with other health care professionals. Each member of the multidisciplinary team (speech therapist, nutritionist, dentist, psychologist, discharge planner, physical therapist, nurse, and physician) assists the client in adjusting to the numerous changes imposed by the diagnosis of cancer and the treatment regimen. (See Discharge Planning for the client with head and neck cancer for additional information about psychosocial preparation, home care preparation, health teaching, and health care resources.)

DISORDERS OF THE LARYNX

Laryngitis

OVERVIEW

Laryngitis is an inflammation of the mucous membranes lining the larynx and may or may not include edema of the vocal cords. It is commonly associated with upper respiratory tract infections and can be an entity itself or a symptom of a related disease process. Etiologic factors include exposure to irritating inhalants and pollutants, including chemical agents, tobacco, alcohol, and smoke; overuse of the voice; inhalation of volatile gases, such as glue, paint thinner, and butane; or intubation.

COLLABORATIVE MANAGEMENT

ASSESSMENT

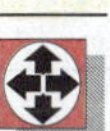

The nurse assesses the client for acute hoarseness, dry cough, and dysphagia. Complete but temporary voice loss *(aphonia)* also may occur. The physician performs a laryngeal examination to assist in the diagnosis. A laryngeal mirror is used to visualize the larynx and to differentiate inflammation, polyps, edema, and tumor. The physician may further order radiography and computed tomography (CT) of the neck and fiberoptic laryngoscopic examination. Most clients are referred to an ear, nose, and throat (ENT) specialist (also called an otolaryngologist) for any suspected disorder other than acute laryngitis.

INTERVENTIONS

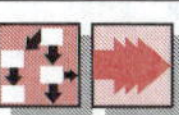

Nursing management is aimed toward relief of presenting symptoms and the introduction of further preventive measures. Treatment consists of voice rest, steam inhalations, increased fluid intake, and use of topical throat lozenges. The physician may order antibiotic therapy and bronchodilators when sinusitis, bronchitis, or a bacterial upper respiratory infection is also present. The nurse informs the client and family about immediate acute care therapies, infection prevention, and avoidance of alcohol, tobacco, and pollutants.

Preventive therapy is aimed toward increasing the client and family's awareness of the hazards of tobacco and alcohol use. The nurse also emphasizes the activities that place an added strain on the larynx, such as singing, cheering, public speaking, heavy lifting, and whispering. Speech therapy is often the treatment of choice for vocal cord injuries and should be implemented for any voice disorder. For recurrent bouts of laryngitis, further medical and speech therapy evaluation are necessary.

Vocal Cord Paralysis

OVERVIEW

Vocal fold (cord) paralysis may result from injury, trauma, or a disease process affecting the larynx, the laryngeal nerves, or the vagus nerve. Prolonged intubation with an endotracheal (ET) tube may cause temporary or, rarely, permanent paralysis. Laryngeal paralysis may occur in clients with central neurologic disorders. Damage to the vagus nerve (by chest injury) or medulla (part of the brain stem) may lead to innervation dysfunction. The superior and recurrent laryngeal nerve may be damaged in disorders or trauma involving the chest, esophagus, or thyroid. Paralysis of both vocal cords may result from a direct traumatic injury or a bilateral cerebrovascular accident (CVA), especially involving the brain stem, or following total thyroidectomy.

COLLABORATIVE MANAGEMENT

ASSESSMENT

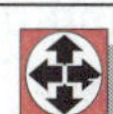

Vocal fold paralysis may be unilateral or bilateral. When only one vocal cord is involved, as is commonly the case, the airway remains patent but voice use may be affected. Symptoms of *abducted* bilateral vocal cord paralysis include hoarseness; a breathy, weak voice; and aspiration of food. *Adducted* vocal cord paralysis presents with airway obstruction and dyspnea and may be considered a medical emergency if the symptoms are severe and the client is unable to compensate. Stridor is the prime presenting symptom. Clients with vocal cord dysfunction are at risk for aspiration because of their inability to protect their airway by normal vocal cord closure.

INTERVENTIONS

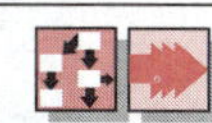

The nurse assesses for airway compromise, as evidenced by signs and symptoms of upper airway obstruction. Securing a patent airway is the primary intervention. The nurse positions the client in a high Fowler's position to protect the airway. Dyspnea with stridor indicates an inadequate airway, and the nurse immediately notifies the physician. Emergent endotracheal intubation, cricothyroidotomy, or tracheostomy may be necessary.

Many surgical procedures have been used to improve the voice. In one procedure, polytef (Teflon) is injected into the affected cord so that it will enlarge

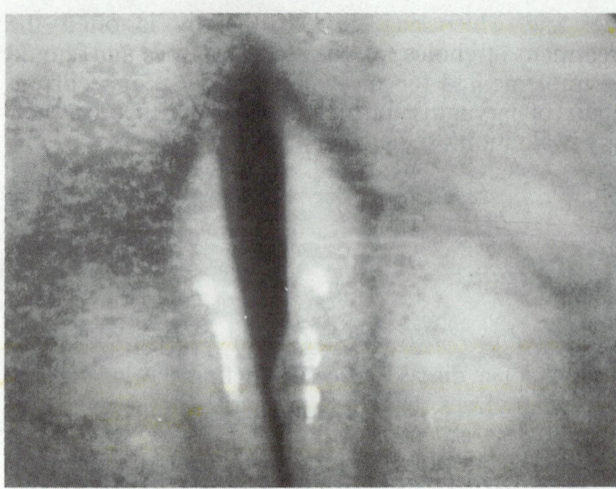

FIGURE 29-3 ◆ Unilateral left vocal cord nodule caused by contact and voice abuse, often seen following viral illnesses. Differential diagnosis includes cancer and trauma. The origin of the nodule may be scar tissue, bacterial, or viral.

toward the unaffected cord, which in turn leads to improved approximation.

Additional nursing interventions include teaching clients to hold their breath during swallowing. This intervention may allow the larynx to elevate, close, and divert the food stream posteriorly into the esophagus during swallowing. The nurse evaluates the client for aspiration of liquids and saliva related to vocal cord dysfunction. Signs and symptoms include immediate coughing on swallowing of liquids, a "wet"-sounding voice, and fever. Chest x-rays and chest auscultation are also useful to diagnose aspiration pneumonia.

Nodules and Polyps of the Vocal Cords

OVERVIEW

Nodules often appear at the point where the vocal cords touch during voicing. Nodules are hypertrophied fibrous tissue (Fig. 29-3) that may result from overuse of the voice and may appear after an infectious process. The populations most affected are teachers, coaches, sports fans, singers, and people who use their voices in noisy environments.

Vocal cord polyps (Color Fig. 29-1) are chronic edematous masses. Polyps occur most commonly in adults who smoke, who have many allergies, and who live in dry climates. Vocal cysts also may occur.

COLLABORATIVE MANAGEMENT

ASSESSMENT

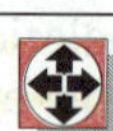

Both nodules and polyps are painless, but they produce hoarseness because of the loss of coordinated approximation of the vocal cords (Fig. 29-4).

INTERVENTIONS

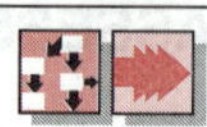

Nursing management of the client with vocal cord nodules or polyps is aimed at client and family education. The nurse teaches the client about the hazards of tobacco use, smoking cessation programs (see Chart 31-4), and the importance of voice rest. Conservative treatment includes not whispering, and avoiding heavy lifting.

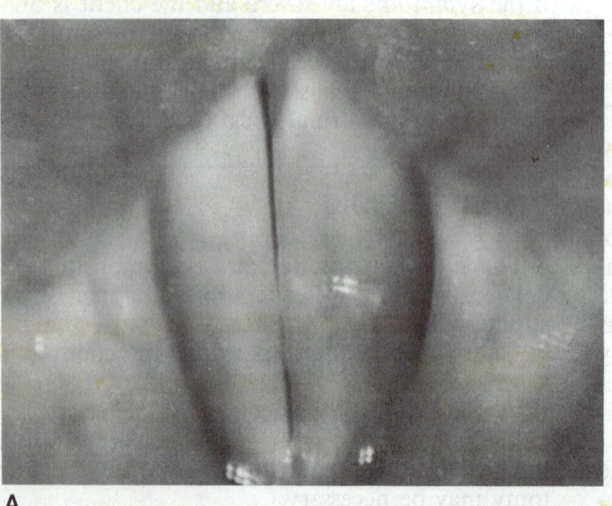

A

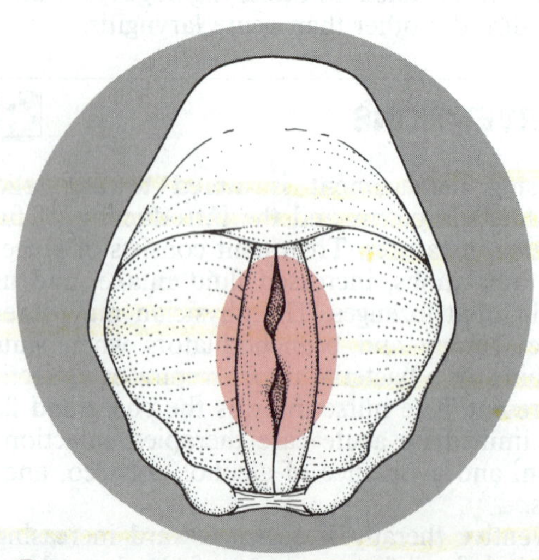

B

FIGURE 29-4 ◆ *A*, Close-up picture of normal vocal folds in phonation. Saying the word "E" in a high pitch allows the examiner to evaluate the total movement of the cords in all pitch ranges and evaluate membrane contact. *B*, Vocal cord nodules and polyps prevent approximation of the vocal cords. Hoarseness results.

Humidification and specialized speech therapy help to reduce the intensity of speech. Speech therapy is a primary treatment for behavioral voice changes. A conservative approach using speech therapy may make surgery unnecessary.

If hoarseness or the presenting voice disturbance is not relieved, the physician may excise the nodules or polyps under direct laryngoscopy. Laser is used to excise or strip the mucous membrane of the affected cord. (Direct laryngoscopy is described in Table 28–5.) If both cords are involved, one cord is usually allowed to heal before surgery is performed on the other cord.

After surgery, the client will need about 14 days of complete voice rest to promote healing. The client can use alternative methods of communication, such as a slate board, pen and paper, "magic slate," or alphabet board. The nurse places a sign on the client's door, over the bed, and on the intercom system to help implement this important nursing intervention. Because these procedures are often done with the client ambulatory, proper education is imperative *before* the operation and before the client returns home.

Laryngeal Trauma

OVERVIEW

Laryngeal trauma is a result of crushing or direct blow injury, fracture, or intrinsic injury. Intrinsic injuries are caused by prolonged endotracheal intubations.

COLLABORATIVE MANAGEMENT

ASSESSMENT

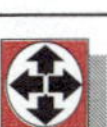

Symptoms of trauma to the larynx include dyspnea, aphonia, hoarseness, and subcutaneous emphysema. Bleeding from the airway (hemoptysis) may occur, depending on the location of the trauma. The physician performs a direct visual examination of the larynx to determine the exact nature of the injury.

INTERVENTIONS

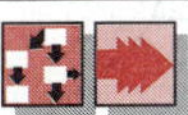

Management of clients with laryngeal injuries consists of assessing and frequent monitoring of vital signs (every 15 to 30 minutes), including respiratory status and pulse oximetry. The nursing priority is to maintain a patent airway. The nurse places oxygen and humidification as ordered to maintain adequate oxygen saturation. If the client has respiratory difficulty, as evidenced by signs such as increasing tachypnea, anxiety, sternal retraction, shortness of breath, dyspnea, restlessness, decreased oxygen saturation, decreased level of consciousness, nasal flaring, and stridor, the nurse stays with the client and instructs other trauma team members to prepare for emergent cricothyroidotomy (cricothyrotomy) or tracheostomy.

For lacerations of the mucous membranes, cartilage exposure, and paralysis of the cords, surgical intervention is necessary. Repair of the larynx is performed as soon as possible to prevent laryngeal stenosis and to cover any exposed cartilage. An artificial airway may be indicated. Maintenance of a patent airway is of the utmost priority.

UPPER AIRWAY OBSTRUCTION

OVERVIEW

Upper airway obstruction is a life-threatening emergency. It is defined as any significant interruption in airflow through the nose, mouth, pharynx, or larynx. Early recognition is essential to prevent further complications, including respiratory arrest. Some potential causes of upper airway obstruction are:

- Tongue edema (surgery, trauma)
- Occlusion by the tongue (e.g., with loss of protective reflexes, loss of pharyngeal muscle tone, unconsciousness and coma)
- Laryngeal edema
- Peritonsillar and pharyngeal abscess
- Head and neck carcinoma
- Thick secretions in the airway
- Cerebral disorders (i.e., cerebrovascular accident)
- Smoke inhalation edema
- Facial, tracheal, and/or laryngeal trauma
- Foreign body aspiration
- Burns of the head and/or neck area
- Anaphylaxis

COLLABORATIVE MANAGEMENT

ASSESSMENT

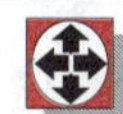

Prompt nursing and medical care are essential to prevent a partial airway obstruction from progressing to a complete obstruction. A client with a partial obstruction (e.g., caused by limited edema or a small foreign body) may have few symptoms. Unexplained or persistent recurrent symptoms warrant evaluation even though the symptoms are vague. The physician orders diagnostic procedures, such as chest x-ray, lateral neck films, direct laryngoscopic examination, and computed tomography to rule out any potentially life-threatening condition, such as a tumor, foreign body, or infection. Upper airway obstruction can be a frightening experience for the client and family.

The nurse observes for signs of hypoxia and hypercapnea, restlessness, increasing anxiety, sternal retractions, "seesawing" chest, abdominal movements, or a feeling of impending doom related to actual air hunger. The nurse performs pulse oximetry for the ongoing monitoring of oxygen saturation and assesses for stridor, cyanosis, and changes in level of consciousness.

INTERVENTIONS

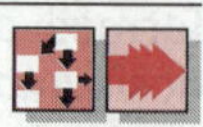

The nurse assesses for the cause of the obstruction. When obstruction is due to the tongue falling back or to the accumulation of secretions, the nurse places the client's head and neck in a slightly extended position, inserts an oral airway, and may use suction to remove obstructing secretions. If the airway obstruction results from a foreign body, the nurse performs abdominal thrusts (Fig. 29-5).

Upper airway obstruction may necessitate emergent procedures, such as a cricothyroidotomy, endotracheal intubation, or tracheostomy. These procedures are often preceded or followed by direct laryngoscopy to evaluate the cause of obstruction. The physician uses direct laryngoscopy in a controlled situation as the treatment of choice for removal of foreign bodies.

Cricothyroidotomy Cricothyroidotomy is a life-saving emergency procedure and is usually performed outside the hospital by emergency medical personnel or in the emergency department by a physician. A cricothyroidotomy is a stab wound at the cricothyroid membrane between the thyroid cartilage and the cricoid cartilage ring (see Fig. 28-3). Any hollow tube —but preferably a tracheostomy tube—can be placed through this opening to keep the new airway open until a formal tracheotomy can be performed. This procedure is warranted when it is the *only* way to secure an airway for the client. Alternatively, the physician can make an incision by inserting a 14-gauge needle immediately into the cricoid space to allow air into and out of the lungs, thus bypassing the obstruction.

Endotracheal Intubation To accomplish endotracheal intubation, a tube is inserted into the trachea via the nose (nasotracheal) or mouth (orotracheal) by a physician, a nurse anesthetist, or another specially trained nurse. Nursing care related to endotracheal tubes is discussed in Chapter 31.

Tracheostomy Tracheostomy is usually an elective procedure that takes approximately 10 minutes to perform. The procedure takes place in the operating room (preferably) with the client under local or general anesthesia, or it can be done at the bedside. An emergency tracheostomy is reserved for the client who cannot be immediately intubated with an oral or

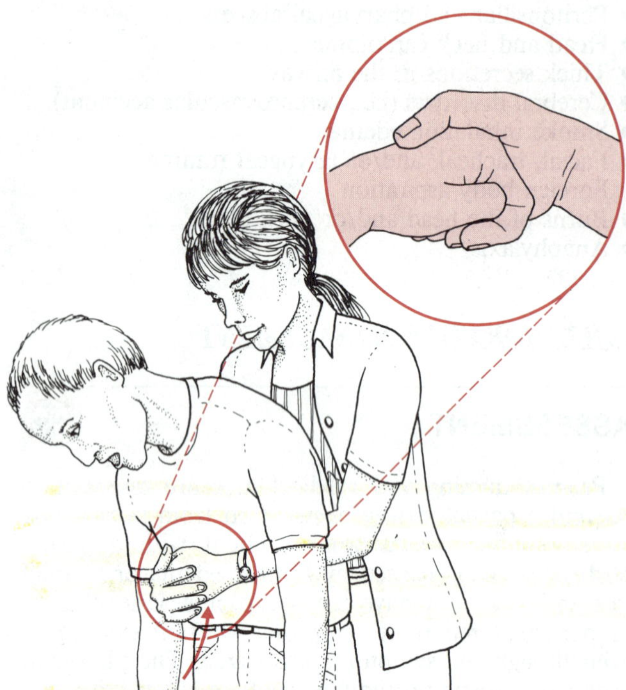

With the **conscious victim standing or sitting,** place your fist between the victim's lower rib cage and navel. Wrap the palm of your other hand around your fist. A quick inward, upward thrust expels the air remaining in the victim's lungs and with it the foreign body. If the first thrust is unsuccessful, repeat several thrusts in rapid succession until the foreign body is expelled or until the victim loses consciousness.

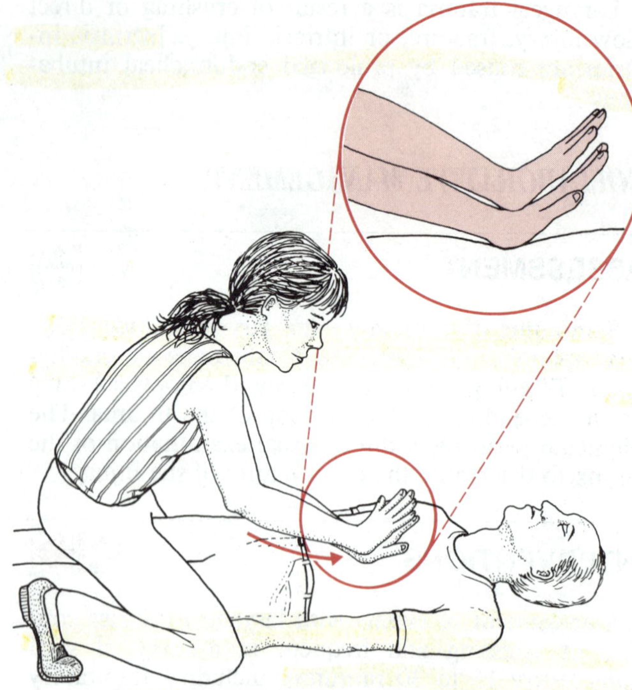

With the **unconscious victim lying supine,** straddle the victim's thighs. Place your hands one over the other as shown, with the heel of the bottom hand just above the victim's navel. Quickly thrust inward and upward, toward the victim's head.

FIGURE 29-5 ◆ The abdominal thrust maneuver (formerly referred to as the Heimlich maneuver) for relief of upper airway obstruction caused by a foreign body.

nasal endotracheal tube. The airway can be established in less than 2 minutes in an emergent situation. Care of the client with a tracheostomy is discussed in detail later in this chapter. Clients who have been placed on mechanical ventilation as part of the treatment for upper airway obstruction or respiratory failure may require elective tracheostomy after 7 or more days of continuous oral or nasal intubation.

NECK TRAUMA

OVERVIEW

Injuries to the neck are most often caused by a knife, gun, or traumatic accident. Clients with neck trauma may have multiple injuries, including cardiovascular, respiratory, gastrointestinal, and neurologic damage. The final outcome of this type of injury depends on the initial assessment and management. (Consult a critical care or emergency textbook as well as Chapter 42 for more in-depth information. Advanced Cardiac Life Support courses are also valuable.)

COLLABORATIVE MANAGEMENT

ASSESSMENT

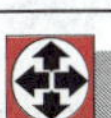

The first priority in the management of neck trauma is assessment for a patent airway. (Signs and symptoms of an upper airway obstruction are discussed earlier in this chapter.) The nurse then assesses the cardiovascular system for signs of internal or external bleeding, or impending shock.

The nurse performs a baseline neurologic assessment for mental status, sensory level, and motor function. Injury to the carotid artery may result in stroke or paralysis related to interruption of blood to the brain. The physician may order a carotid angiogram (see Chap. 32) to rule out vascular injuries.

Injuries involving the esophagus also may occur with neck trauma. The nurse assesses for chest pain and tenderness, oral bleeding, and crepitus. The physician may order a barium or meglumine diatrizoate (Gastrografin) swallow to rule out esophageal perforation injury.

INTERVENTIONS

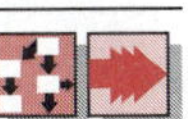

Cervical spine injuries often occur at the same time as a neck injury (see Chap. 42). The nurse and emergency personnel must take great care not to exacerbate these injuries by causing neck movement while establishing the airway. The nurse prepares to assist in emergency intubation, cricothyrotomy, or tracheostomy to establish a patent airway. Interventions for clients in shock are detailed in Chapter 36.

HEAD AND NECK CANCER

OVERVIEW

Head and neck cancer interferes with breathing, eating, facial appearance, self-image, speech, and communication. This form of cancer can be a devastating disease even if it is successfully treated. The role of the nurse is challenging in caring for clients with these complex problems. The client can receive appropriate care only through accurate identification of the location and size of the original tumor. A interdisciplinary health care team approach is essential to address the entire spectrum of needs of these clients.

Head and neck cancer can be a curable disease when discovered early. The prognosis for those who present with more advanced disease depends on the extent and location of the tumor. Untreated cancer of the head and neck is inevitably a fatal disease, and untreated clients usually die within 2 years of diagnosis.

PATHOPHYSIOLOGY

Most head and neck cancers (80%) are squamous cell (mucosal epithelial) carcinomas (Fig. 29-6) and pathogenesis of these tumors is usually related to tobacco and alcohol use. Many head and neck tumors present as malignant ulcerations with underlying infiltration.

The development of malignancy in the mucosa is a process requiring several years and takes place in a step-like manner, similar to that seen in the bronchial epithelium. When mucosa is subjected to an irritating substance, it responds by transforming itself into a

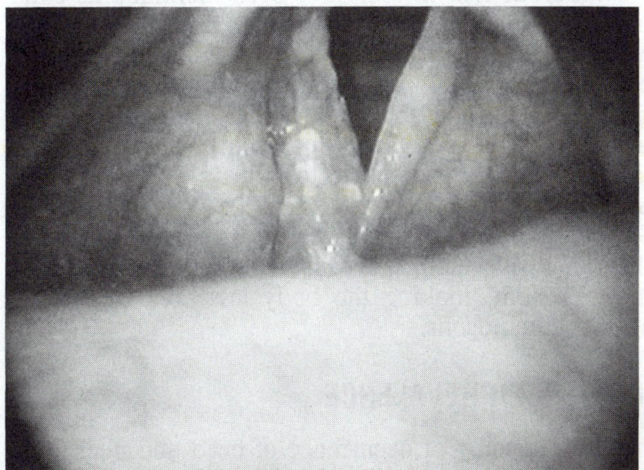

FIGURE 29-6 ◆ Laryngeal cancer is frequently caused by the combination of alcohol and tobacco. This illustration shows a squamous cell cancer of the true vocal cords, involving primarily the entire surface of the right true vocal cord.

tougher mucosa (squamous metaplasia), by increasing the mucosal thickness (acanthosis or hyperplasia), or by developing a keratin layer (keratosis).

When the irritating substance contains a carcinogen, these benign protective changes may be accompanied by epithelial atypia or dysplasia. These atypical lesions may then take the form of white, patchy lesions or red, velvety patches. Head and neck carcinoma is often diagnosed on the basis of white, patchy mucosal lesions called leukoplakia, or red patches called erythroplasia.

Growth and spread of the carcinoma depend on the site of the primary tumor. Spread is predominantly to adjacent anatomic areas like mucosa, muscle, and bone, although cartilage and bone may act as barriers in the early stages. Anatomic barriers of the larynx and surrounding structures are present in the glottic area, but fewer barriers exist in the subglottic and supraglottic areas. Few anatomic barriers exist in the oropharynx. Oral cancers are discussed further in Chapter 53.

Systemic dissemination through the lymphatic system may also occur, although the lymph system often contains the tumor in the head and neck region for some time before dissemination. When metastasis occurs, it is most commonly to the lungs or liver. Metastasis to the head and neck *from* other primary sites is rare.

The histologic description of squamous cell cancers includes carcinoma in situ, well-differentiated carcinoma, moderately differentiated carcinoma, or poorly differentiated carcinoma. Most head and neck cancers are of squamous origin, but they also can be of salivary gland or thyroid (papillary or follicular) origin. They can also be epidermoid, adenoid cystic, malignant melanoma, or adenocarcinoma. These tumors are treated by various methods directed by the type of tumor and its known response to therapies.

ETIOLOGY

Numerous risk factors have been identified as contributing to the development of head and neck cancer. The two most important risk factors are tobacco and alcohol use, and especially the combination of the two. Other risk factors include chewing tobacco, pipe smoking, marijuana, voice abuse, chronic laryngitis, exposure to industrial chemicals or hardwood dust, and complete neglect of oral hygiene. Steroid use has been implicated in association with the other risk factors because steroids alter the immune system, making the body less able to defend against carcinogens.

INCIDENCE/PREVALENCE

The frequency of occurrence of head and neck carcinoma is increasing. The National Cancer Institute (NCI) estimates 42,100 newly diagnosed cases of *oral* and *laryngeal* cancers per year, accounting for more than 4% of all carcinomas and more than 11,000 deaths per year.

In the United States in 1994, the NCI projected 12,500 total cases of *laryngeal* cancer, 9800 of those in males (Boring, 1994). In females, laryngeal cancer usually appears in the 50s or 60s; in males, the incidence peaks in the 60s and 70s. In 1994, the NCI estimated 3800 deaths from laryngeal cancer.

Laryngeal cancer represents 2.3% of all malignant tumors in males and 0.4% of all malignant tumors in females, excluding basal and squamous cell carcinomas of the skin. Most clients with laryngeal cancers are diagnosed when the tumor is limited to the larynx. Tumor locations within the larynx are shown in Figure 29–7.

Transcultural Considerations The rate of death for men of all races due to cancer of the larynx has not shown any changes over three decades, but there has been a 110% increase in the non-Caucasian population, up from 2.3 to 4.9 cases. Death rates for women with oral or laryngeal cancers have increased for all races over the past three decades. Oral cancer death rates are up from 1.5 to 1.8 for women of all races, and up from 1.7 to 2.3 for non-Caucasians. Deaths due to cancer of the larynx is up from 0.2 to 0.5 for women of all races and are up from 0.3 to 0.8 for non-Caucasian women (Boring, et al, 1992).

COLLABORATIVE MANAGEMENT

ASSESSMENT

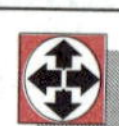

HISTORY

The client with head and neck cancer may have difficulty speaking because of hoarseness, shortness of

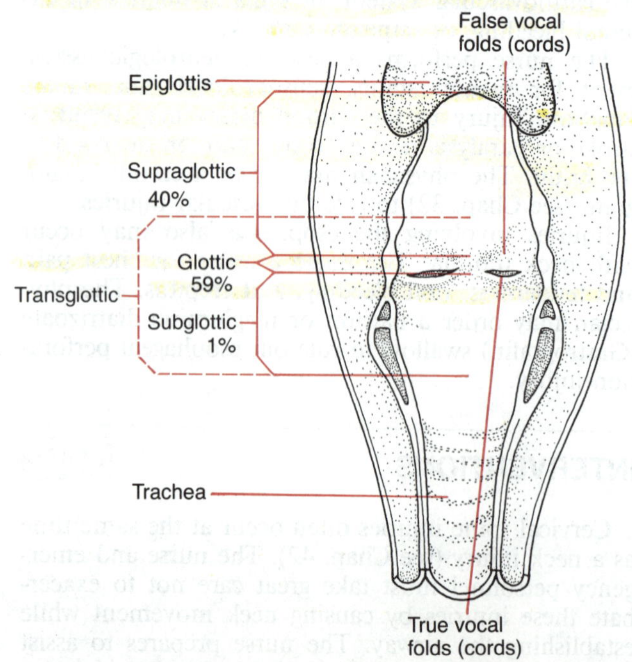

FIGURE 29–7 ◆ Sites and incidence of primary laryngeal tumors.

breath, tumor bulk, and pain. The nurse should be sensitive to these difficulties during the interview.

The nurse questions the client about tobacco and alcohol use, history of recurrent acute or chronic laryngitis or pharyngitis, oral sores, and lumps in the neck. The nurse calculates the client's smoking history in terms of pack-years. The nurse asks about alcohol intake, that is, how many drinks per day and for how many years. Questions of this nature may be uncomfortable for both the client and the nurse but are an important part of the history. The nurse also ascertains whether the client has been exposed to any environmental pollutants.

The nurse assesses problems related to risk factors. For example, nutrition may be poor because of alcohol intake, with subsequent impairment of liver function. The nurse assesses dietary habits and any reported weight loss. The nurse notes a history of chronic lung disease, which has an impact on the client's breathing pattern and is an important operative risk factor.

PHYSICAL ASSESSMENT/CLINICAL MANIFESTATIONS

Table 29–3 summarizes the warning signs of head and neck cancer. With *laryngeal* cancer, hoarseness may occur because of tumor bulk and a lack of ability to approximate vocal cords in a normal fashion during phonation. Lesions of the true vocal cords are the earliest form of laryngeal cancer. A careful evaluation is important for anyone who has a history of hoarseness, sores in the mouth, or a lump in the neck for a period of 3 to 4 weeks or longer.

The techniques of inspection and palpation of the head and neck are an important part of the physical examination. A nurse who is specially trained may perform a laryngeal examination, which includes the use of the laryngeal mirror or fiberoptic laryngoscope. Lesions may be visualized by direct inspection, and the nurse palpates the neck for tumor nodal involvement. A cranial nerve assessment (see Chapter 40) is also valuable because some tumors have an affinity for dissemination along these nerves.

PSYCHOSOCIAL ASSESSMENT

The typical client with head and neck carcinoma is a man with a long-standing history of cigarette and/or alcohol use. The client or family may experience denial, guilt, blame, or shame once the diagnosis is suspected. The nurse assesses the availability and adequacy of support systems and coping mechanisms. Because clients frequently require extensive assistance at home following treatment, assessment and documentation of social and family support are essential. The nurse consults the social worker for assistance as needed. The nurse also evaluates cognitive functioning (see Chapter 40), level of education, and literacy of the client and family because of the importance of preoperative and postoperative teaching.

The nurse notes any family history of cancer as well as the client's age, sex, occupation, interests, and ability to perform the activities of daily living. The nurse investigates whether the client's occupation requires continual oral communication, whether the client will need retraining in other vocational areas, or whether he or she will be able to resume the same job after surgery, radiation, or combined therapy.

TABLE 29–3 Warning Signs of Head and Neck Cancer

- Pain
- A lump in the mouth, throat, or neck
- Difficulty in swallowing
- Color changes in the mouth or tongue to red, white, gray, dark brown, or black
- An oral lesion or sore that does not heal in 2 weeks
- Persistent or unexplained oral bleeding
- Numbness of the mouth, lips, or face
- Change in the fit of dentures
- Burning sensation when drinking citrus juices or hot liquids
- Persistent, unilateral ear pain
- Hoarseness or change in voice quality
- Persistent or recurrent sore throat
- Shortness of breath
- Anorexia and weight loss

LABORATORY ASSESSMENT

The routine diagnostic laboratory tests include a complete blood count, bleeding times, urinalysis, and SMA-20. The nurse is alert to a decrease in hemoglobin and hematocrit values and an increase in alkaline phosphatase levels. Protein and albumin levels indicate protein stores and define nutritional risks often seen in clients with alcoholism. The changes may indicate, but are not specific for, malignancies and nutritional deficits. Renal and liver function tests are usually performed to rule out metastatic disease and to evaluate the client's ability to metabolize medications and chemotherapeutic agents.

RADIOGRAPHIC ASSESSMENT

Many types of radiographic studies are useful diagnostic tools. X-ray of the skull, sinuses, neck, and chest may identify possible metastases, second primary tumors, or the extent of tumor invasion. Computed tomography (CT) of the head and neck helps evaluate the tumor's exact location. CT may or may not include the use of a contrast medium.

OTHER DIAGNOSTIC ASSESSMENT

Magnetic resonance imaging (MRI) is a diagnostic test that can differentiate normal from diseased tissue. MRI is more sensitive than CT in defining the extent of soft-tissue invasion.

The brain, bone, and liver may also be evaluated with nuclear imaging, bone scans, and SPECT (single-photon emission computerized technology). These tests help to locate additional tumor sites.

Other diagnostic tests include direct and indirect laryngoscopy, tumor mapping, and biopsy. Panendoscopy is a procedure performed with general anesthesia to define the extent of the tumor. This procedure includes laryngoscopy, nasopharyngoscopy, esophagoscopy, and bronchoscopy. Anatomic tumor mapping uses biopsy to outline and identify tumor location. At the time of the panendoscopy, the biopsy confirms the diagnosis and determines the tumor type, histologic presentation, and defined location. Tumor staging according to the TNM Classification (see Chapter 25 and Table 25-7) is done at this time.

ANALYSIS

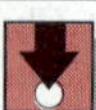

COMMON NURSING DIAGNOSES

Four nursing diagnoses are common in most clients with head and neck carcinomas:

1. Ineffective Airway Clearance related to impaired airway from the disease process (i.e., tumor invasion or obstruction, edema, and chronic lung disease)
2. High Risk for Aspiration related to anatomic changes and alteration of protective reflexes in oropharyngeal cancer
3. Anxiety related to fear of the unknown
4. Body Image Disturbance related to tumor and treatment modalities

ADDITIONAL NURSING DIAGNOSES

In addition to the most common diagnoses, the client may present with one or more of the following diagnoses:

- Pain related to tumor invasion of tissues and nerves and surgical intervention
- Altered Nutrition: Less than Body Requirements related to dysphagia, anxiety, or tumor process; surgical resection; or chronic alcohol intake
- Impaired Verbal Communication related to tumor invasion, associated aphonia, hoarseness, pain, and/or surgical resection
- Altered Cerebral Tissue Perfusion related to wound breakdown, recurrent tumor, and resultant interruption of arterial blood flow from carotid rupture
- Impaired Tissue Integrity and Impaired Skin Integrity related to altered circulation, nutritional deficit, tumor invasion, radiation, chemical factors (body secretions or substances), or surgical wound
- Ineffective Individual Coping related to altered body image, communication method, and/or ineffective social network support
- Impaired Social Interaction related to body image disturbance and lifestyle practices
- Impaired Adjustment related to self-care of the tracheostomy and nasogastric tubes, alternative communication methods, and body image disturbance
- Knowledge Deficit related to treatment regimen and unfamiliarity with information resources

PLANNING AND IMPLEMENTATION

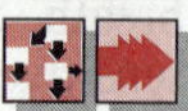

INEFFECTIVE AIRWAY CLEARANCE

PLANNING: CLIENT GOALS The major goal is that the client will attain and/or maintain a patent airway.

INTERVENTIONS The primary goal of treatment is removal or eradication of the cancer with preservation of as much normal function as possible. The physician presents available treatment options to the client. Modalities may be used alone or in combination. When planning treatment options, the physician considers general physical condition, nutritional status, age, effects of the tumor on body function, and, most importantly, the client's personal choice. The physician considers the client's ability to manage his or her own care postoperatively before recommending extensive surgery.

The treatment of laryngeal cancer may range from radiation therapy for a small specific area or tumor, to total laryngopharyngectomy, with bilateral neck dissections followed by radiation therapy. The specific treatment depends on the extent and location of the lesion. Voice conservation procedures are elected only if they can be accomplished without risking incomplete removal of the tumor. The nurse, as a member of the collaborative team, focuses on the client's total needs, including preoperative preparation, competent in-hospital care, discharge planning and teaching, and extensive outpatient rehabilitation.

Nonsurgical Management The nurse monitors the client's respiratory system by assessing respiratory rate, breath sounds, pulse oximetry results, arterial blood gas values, and results of pulmonary function tests. Signs of respiratory distress may indicate narrowing of the airway related to tumor growth, edema, or both. The nurse positions the client to obtain optimal air exchange. The nurse educates the client and family about the use of Fowler's and semi-Fowler's positions. Clients may find that by sitting upright in a reclining chair they can be supported and therefore breathe more comfortably. Texts on hospice care can provide additional information on palliation and pain control for those clients who elect no therapy and for those whose therapy has not been effective.

Radiation Therapy Treatment of small cancers in specific locations with radiation offers a cure rate of 80% and above. Treatment of larger cancers offers a lower cure rate when radiation is used as a single-modality therapy. Standard therapy uses 5000 to 7500 rad, usually over 6 weeks. The physician may recommend radiation alone, before or after surgery, or in combination with surgery. Because radiation therapy causes alterations in tissue healing, it might *not* be recommended preoperatively. Radiation therapy is commonly an outpatient procedure (see Chap. 26).

The nurse monitors for major side effects at the site of the radiation, including dysphagia, pain, and skin and mucous membrane irritation. Systemic lethargy is not uncommon. Adequate nutrition and hydration can lessen the side effects of radiation therapy.

Chemotherapy Chemotherapy is not usually used alone for cancers of the head and neck. It remains under experimental clinical investigation for these cancers. At times, it is an adjuvant to surgery or radiation. The most commonly used chemotherapeutic agents for cancer of the neck include methotrexate (Mexate), vincristine sulfate (Oncovin), bleomycin sulfate (Blenoxane), and cisplatin (Platinol). Methotrexate often is used for patients who cannot undergo rigorous surgery, radiation, or chemotherapy. Often, terminal patients receive methotrexate for control (not cure) of the disease, and for assistance in pain control. Chapter 26 includes a detailed discussion of the care of clients receiving chemotherapy.

Surgical Management Tumor size and location (TNM Classification) defines the extent of surgical intervention for cancer of the head and neck. The method of reconstruction is also determined by the tumor size and amount of tissue to be resected and reconstructed. Surgical procedures for head and neck cancers include laryngectomy (total and partial), tracheostomy, and oropharyngeal cancer resections.

Laryngectomy and Related Surgical Procedures The major types of resections for laryngeal cancer include cordal stripping, *cordectomy* (excision of a vocal cord), partial laryngectomy, and total laryngectomy. If neck lymph nodes are involved or if the tumor carries with it a known high rate of nodal spread, the surgeon performs a nodal neck dissection in conjunction with removal of the primary tumor. A pathologist evaluates the resected lymph nodes for tumor invasion.

PREOPERATIVE CARE As the client advocate, the nurse educates the client and family about the tumor. The physician explains the surgical procedure and obtains the client's informed consent. The nurse discusses and interprets the implications of such consent.

The nurse explains about self-care of the airway, compensatory methods of communication, suctioning, pain control methods, the critical care environment (including ventilators and critical care routines), nutritional support, feeding tubes, and outcome goals for discharge. The client will need to learn new methods of speech postoperatively. The nurse prepares the client for this change through preoperative teaching. The nurse establishes with the client an alternative form of communication (e.g., pen and pencil, "magic slate," picture or alphabet board) before surgery.

The explanations of routines and outcomes of care are very important because these discussions are used to plan the hospitalization and rehabilitation. Multidisciplinary teams of speech pathologists, social workers, dietitians, and occupational and physical therapists along with the nurses and physicians are vitally important in the preoperative evaluation and preparation of clients with cancer. Chapter 19 describes general preoperative assessment and education in detail.

OPERATIVE PROCEDURES Hemilaryngectomy (vertical or horizontal) and supraglottic laryngectomy are types of partial voice conservation laryngectomies. Table 29–4 presents more specific information on the various surgical procedures.

A tracheostomy (discussed later) is often performed with a partial laryngectomy to protect the airway. The tracheostomy can be either a temporary or a permanent airway. With a total laryngectomy, the upper airway is diverted and separated from the pharynx and esophagus, and the trachea is brought out through the skin in the neck and sutured in place, thus creating a permanent stoma. This airway

TABLE 29–4 Surgical Procedures for Laryngeal Cancer and Their Effect on Voice Quality

Procedure	Description	Resulting Voice Quality
Laser surgery	• Tumor reduced or destroyed by laser beam through laryngoscope	• Normal/hoarse
Transoral cordectomy	• Tumor (early lesion) resected through laryngoscope	• Normal (high cure rate)/hoarse
Laryngofissure	• No cord removed (early lesion)	• Normal (high cure rate)
Supraglottic partial laryngectomy	• Hyoid bone, false cords, and epiglottis removed • Neck dissection on affected side performed if nodes involved	• Normal/hoarse
Hemilaryngectomy or vertical laryngectomy	• One true cord, one false cord, and one-half of thyroid cartilage removed	• Hoarse voice
Total laryngectomy	• Entire larynx, hyoid bone, strap muscles, one or two tracheal rings removed • Nodal neck dissection if nodes involved	• No natural voice

opening is *always* permanent and is referred to as a laryngectomy stoma.

Neck dissection includes removal of the lymph nodes of the neck involved in the tumor, the sternocleidomastoid muscle, the jugular vein, the 11th cranial nerve, and surrounding involved soft tissue. Because the 11th cranial nerve—the spinal accessory nerve—is resected during the nodal dissection, shoulder drop will be present postoperatively. Physical therapy exercises are imperative and help the client to ease the shoulder drop by increasing the use of other muscle groups.

POSTOPERATIVE CARE Head and neck surgical procedures often last longer than 8 hours. The client may spend the immediate postoperative period in the surgical intensive care unit because of the duration of anesthesia and the amount of resection and reconstruction. The nurse monitors the client's airway patency, vital signs, hemodynamic status, and level of comfort. The nurse is also alert to the possibility of postoperative hemorrhage and other general complications of anesthesia and surgery (see Chap. 21). The nurse monitors vital signs every hour for the first 24 hours, then every 2 hours until the client is stable. After the client is transferred from the critical care unit, vital signs can be monitored every 4 hours or according to agency policy. The nurse is attentive to dependent areas of the body and prevents pressure sores by movement every 2 hours. The client is generally out of bed by the second postoperative day.

Complications after a head and neck cancer resection can include airway obstruction, hemorrhage, wound breakdown, and tumor recurrence. The priorities in postoperative head and neck cancer care include airway maintenance and ventilation; wound, flap, and reconstructive tissue care (Client Care Plan); pain management; nutrition; and psychological adjustment, including speech therapy.

Airway Maintenance and Ventilation. In the immediate postoperative period, the client may need ventilatory assistance because of a long-term smoking history, chronic lung disease, and long duration of anesthesia. Although many clients also have chronic lung disease, weaning usually is not difficult because (1) the thoracic and abdominal cavities are not entered during the surgical procedure and (2) the cough mechanism is intact. When weaned from the ventilator, the client typically uses a tracheostomy collar (over the artificial airway or open stoma) with oxygen and humidification to help mobilize mucus secretions. Secretions may remain blood-tinged for 1 to 2 days. The nurse maintains body substance precautions and reports any increase in bleeding to the physician. Humidification helps to remove crusts and prevent obstruction of the tube with secretions. Sterile saline instillation of 5 to 10 mL every 2 hours or as needed may also be ordered.

Clients who have had a *total laryngectomy* and need an appliance to prevent scar tissue contracture at the skin tracheal border use a laryngectomy tube. This tube is similar to a conventional tracheostomy tube but is shorter and fatter with a larger lumen and

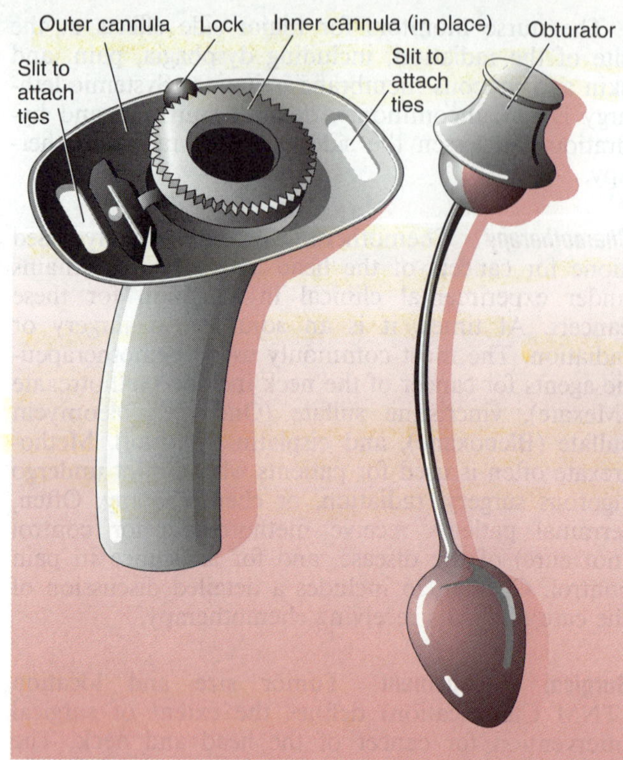

FIGURE 29-8 ◆ A laryngectomy tube. Note that the outer cannula is shorter and has a diameter wider than that of a tracheostomy tube.

a more acute angle (Fig. 29-8). Laryngectomy tube care is similar to tracheostomy tube care (see later in this chapter), except that the client can change the laryngectomy tube on a daily or an as-needed basis. A laryngectomy button is similar to a laryngectomy tube but is made of a silicone-like substance (Silastic), has a single lumen, and is very short. A button is very comfortable for the laryngectomy patient, is easily removed for cleaning, and is available in various sizes and lengths for custom fit. The nurse provides a "magic slate" or paper and pencil for communication because the client has no oral communication capabilities.

Coughing, deep breathing, and saline instillation are often totally effective in clearing secretions. The lack of surgical interruption in the thoracic cavity or abdomen improves the ability to cough. The nurse instructs the client in the proper techniques for coughing and deep breathing (see Chap. 19) to clear secretions.

Oral secretions can be suctioned with a Yankauer or tonsillar suction. The nurse teaches clients to suction away from the side of an oral cavity cancer resection to preserve continuity of the wounds immediately after surgery. The nurse teaches clients self-care by providing this catheter for suctioning oral airway secretions. Using a table mirror for visualization, clients can participate in their own care. The nurse provides a clean environment for the catheter.

Stoma care following total laryngectomy is a combination of wound care and airway care. Careful inspection of the stoma with a flashlight is routine. The nurse cleans the suture line with half-strength hydro-

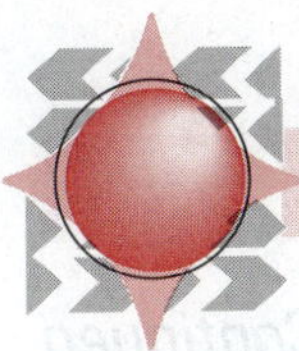

CLIENT CARE PLAN

The Client Who Has Had Head and Neck Surgery

Nursing Diagnosis No. 1: Ineffective Airway Clearance related to impaired airway from disease process (i.e., tumor invasion/obstruction, edema, chronic lung disease) and surgical intervention

Expected Outcomes	Nursing Interventions	Rationale
The client will attain and/or maintain a patent airway.	◆ Monitor airway patency. ◆ Assess for signs and symptoms of respiratory distress.	◆ Ongoing assessment promotes early detection and treatment of complications.
	◆ Place client in semi-Fowler's or Fowler's position as soon as possible postoperatively.	◆ Positioning makes breathing easier and facilitates oxygenation, secretion removal, and airway patency.
	◆ Suction client via the artificial airway frequently postoperatively (q 30–60 minutes and advance to q 2 hr and as needed).	◆ Suctioning and tube (if present) care promote removal of secretions that could obstruct airway.
Lung sounds will be maintained at the client's baseline or improved.	◆ Suction oral cavity as ordered using a Yankauer tonsillar tip catheter.	◆ A laryngectomy tube prevents scar tissue contracture and maintains airway.
	◆ Inspect and clean laryngectomy stoma q 2 hr and as needed. Use cotton-tipped applicators with peroxide and saline.	◆ Peroxide removes crusts and secretions.
	◆ Perform laryngectomy tube care q 4 hr, and advance to q shift, as needed, if ordered.	◆ Suction and cleaning procedures help to prevent obstruction and infection and promote healing.
	◆ Have the client cough and deep breathe; if ordered, instill saline as needed.	◆ Pulmonary hygiene exercises prevent pooling of secretions and promotes oxygenation and ventilation.
Breathing efforts will be without distress.	◆ Place an appropriate-sized laryngectomy set at bedside.	◆ Having duplicate equipment readily available enables prompt response in the event of distress or if urgent replacement of the tube is required (i.e., if the tube accidentally comes out).
	◆ Document assessment findings and the client's response to interventions.	◆ Documentation provides an ongoing, permanent record of the client's progress and care requirements.

Nursing Diagnosis No. 2: Impaired Tissue Integrity and Impaired Skin Integrity related to the surgical wound

Expected Outcomes	Nursing Interventions	Rationale
The client's surgical wound area will remain intact and will heal without complications.	◆ Assess wound integrity, capillary refill, and color q 1–2 hr for 48 hrs.	◆ Ongoing assessment promotes early detection and treatment of complications.
	◆ Strip surgical drains q 1–2 hr to ensure correct functioning. ◆ Record each drain amount separately at least q shift.	◆ An accumulation of drainage beneath the skin or reconstructive flaps impairs tissue nutrition, resulting in vascular insufficiency and tissue breakdown.

Continued on following page

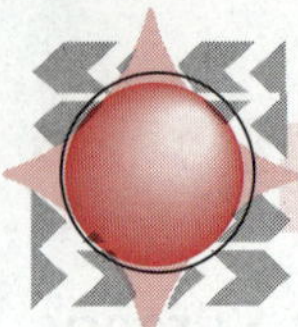

CLIENT CARE PLAN

The Client Who Has Had Head and Neck Surgery *Continued*

Nursing Diagnosis No. 2: Impaired Tissue Integrity and Impaired Skin Integrity related to the surgical wound

Expected Outcomes	Nursing Interventions	Rationale
	◆ Avoid constricting dressings, ties, or oxygen tubing around the suture lines or reconstructive flaps.	◆ Pressure on altered or operated skin and tissue causes alteration in circulation.
	◆ Keep wound clean and dry; perform routine wound care as ordered.	◆ Appropriate wound care promotes healing and prevents complications.
	◆ Ensure adequate nutrition by the enteral or parenteral feeding method.	◆ Nutrition is imperative for tissue nutrition and healing.
	◆ Document assessment findings and the client's response to interventions.	◆ Documentation provides an ongoing, permanent record of care.

Nursing Diagnosis No. 3: High Risk for Impaired Tissue Integrity and Impaired Skin Integrity related to tumor resection, wound breakdown, altered circulation, nutritional deficit, and chemical factors (body secretions or substances)

Expected Outcomes	Nursing Interventions	Rationale
The client's wound will remain intact without complications of infection, bleeding, dehiscence, or fistula.	◆ Monitor for signs of infection (e.g., redness, pus, suture line separation, increasing white blood cell count, fever, malaise).	◆ Ongoing assessment promotes early detection and treatment of complications.
	◆ Assess for saliva or refluxed enteral feeding in wound secretions.	◆ Feedings or saliva in the wound represents a pharyngocutaneous fistula and wound infection.
	◆ Provide wound care, as ordered, q 2–4 hr.	◆ Aggressive nursing care keeps the wounds clean and free of cellular debris and promotes granulation tissue formation and healing.
	◆ Maintain adequate nutrition via enteral or parenteral route, as ordered.	◆ Adequate nutrition helps to prevent wound breakdown and promotes healing.

Nursing Diagnosis No. 4: High Risk for Altered (Cerebral) Tissue Perfusion related to wound breakdown, recurrent tumor, and resultant interruption of arterial blood flow from carotid rupture

Expected Outcomes	Nursing Interventions	Rationale
The client's carotid artery will remain intact without bleeding complications. If bleeding occurs, the client will suffer minimal or no re-	◆ Maintain carotid precautions if the carotid artery is exposed:	
	◆ Keep the carotid artery and dressing wet with *sterile* saline	◆ Keeping the carotid dressing clean and moist prevents drying

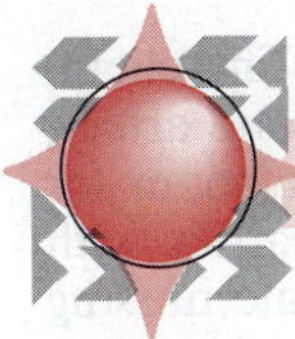

CLIENT CARE PLAN

The Client Who Has Had Head and Neck Surgery *Continued*

Nursing Diagnosis No. 4: High Risk for Altered (Cerebral) Tissue Perfusion related to wound breakdown, recurrent tumor, and resultant interruption of arterial blood flow from carotid rupture

Expected Outcomes	Nursing Interventions	Rationale
sidual complications (i.e., stroke, cerebral insufficiency, cardiac damage).	at all times, as ordered by the physician.	and infection, which could cause bleeding, and promotes granulation of tissue over the carotid artery.
	◆ Change dressings q 2 hr to maintain a wet-to-wet dressing.	
	◆ Move client to room closest to the nursing station or to the intensive care unit.	◆ Being prepared for a carotid bleed may result in a more positive outcome.
	◆ Place two large-gauge IV lines, as ordered.	
	◆ Keep dressing supplies, sterile saline, gloves, and IV solution (lactated Ringer's) at the bedside.	
	◆ Be sure client has had a type and cross-match for blood ordered.	
	◆ Alert operating room of any client receiving carotid precautions.	
	◆ Monitor for and report any bleeding to the physician.	◆ Ongoing assessment promotes early detection and treatment of complications. ◆ A small amount of bright red bleeding that stops spontaneously may herald a true carotid bleed.
	◆ Discuss with client and family the potential for carotid rupture along with prevention, precautions, preparations, and goals of care.	◆ Client and family education helps promotes understanding, acceptance, and participation in the plan of care.
	◆ If carotid bleeding occurs:	
	◆ Apply immediate direct pressure to the artery and ***do not remove pressure.***	◆ Direct pressure applied to the arterial bleeding site prevents rapid blood loss.
	◆ Call for assistance!	◆ Assistance will be needed for this emergency situation.
	◆ Direct another nurse to call the physician ***immediately.***	
	◆ Secure the client's airway.	◆ A patent airway will help to ensure oxygenation.
	◆ Institute intravenous hydration as per standing order.	
	◆ If possible, talk to the client during emergency care.	◆ Talking to the client provides reassurance.
	◆ Transport to the operating room and ***do not remove pressure*** during transport.	

gen peroxide to prevent secretions from forming crusts and obstructing the airway. Suture line care is performed every 1 to 2 hours initially, advancing to every 4 hours by the fifth postoperative day. The mucosa of the stoma and trachea should be bright and shiny without crusts, similar to the appearance of the buccal mucosa.

Wound, Flap, and Reconstructive Tissue Care. Commonly used reconstructive flaps are pectoralis major myocutaneous flaps, island flaps, rotation flaps, trapezius flaps, split-thickness skin grafts (STSGs), and free flaps with microvascular anastomosis. These flaps may be used for reconstruction after any type of head and neck resection. After neck dissection, the surgeon places an STSG over the exposed carotid artery before covering it with skin flaps or reconstructive flaps.

The first 24 hours are critical. The nurse evaluates all flaps every hour for the first 72 hours, monitoring capillary refill, color, and Doppler activity of the major feeding vessel. The nurse reports any changes immediately because surgical intervention may be indicated. The nurse positions the client to protect the native or reconstructed vascular supply of the reconstructed flaps.

Hemorrhage. Hemorrhage is a possible postoperative complication for all clients undergoing surgery, but it is not common in clients who have had composite resections (see later) or laryngectomy. The physician often places a closed surgical drain (see Chap. 21) in the neck area to collect blood and drainage for approximately 72 hours postoperatively. The drain also helps to seat the reconstructed skin flaps. Any obstruction of the drains, or equipment malfunction, may cause a buildup of blood or serum under the flaps. This accumulation jeopardizes the vascular supply of the flaps by interfering with both arterial supply and venous drainage. Malfunction of the drains may necessitate a surgical procedure to remove accumulated clots.

Wound Breakdown. Wound breakdown is a frequent complication because of the common presentation of poor nutrition in these clients and because of wound contamination from oral contaminants. Often the tumor has also affected the client's ability to eat, causing significant weight loss. A history of alcohol use further complicates the nutritional status.

The nurse treats such wound breakdown with packing and local care as ordered to keep the wound clean and stimulate the growth of healthy granulation tissue. Wounds may be extensive, and the carotid artery may be exposed underneath the dehisced wounds. At the initial surgical resection, split-thickness skin grafts are placed over the carotid for protection in the event of such a wound dehiscence. As the wound heals, granulation tissue covers the artery and prevents rupture. If granulation is slow and the carotid artery is at risk, another surgical flap may be raised to cover the carotid artery and close the wound.

If the carotid artery ruptures because of drying or infection, the nurse places *immediate constant pressure* over the site and secures the airway. The client, still with direct manual pressure on the carotid artery, is *immediately* transported to the operating room for carotid resection. Carotid artery rupture carries with it a high risk of stroke and death. Immediate nursing response can save the client's life.

Pain Management. Following cancer surgery, the client's pain should be controlled and the client should still be able to participate in care. Morphine (Statex✱) often is given by intravenous (IV) bolus and continuously for the first days after surgery. As the client progresses, acetaminophen with codeine, then acetaminophen alone can be given, all by feeding tube. Oral medications for pain and discomfort are started only after the client can tolerate oral nutrition. After discharge, clients still require pain medication, especially if they are receiving radiation therapy. An adjunct to the pain regimen may be liquid nonsteroidal anti-inflammatory drugs (NSAIDs); these drugs provide excellent pain relief and can be used in conjunction with opioid analgesics (see also Chap. 8).

Nutrition. A nasogastric, gastrostomy, or jejunostomy tube is placed intraoperatively for nutritional support while the aerodigestive tract heals. Initially, however, the client receives IV fluids (see Chap. 15) or parenteral nutrition (see Chap. 61) until the gastrointestinal tract has recovered from the effects of anesthesia. After that, nutrients may be administered via the feeding tube (see Chart 55-5 and Table 61-9). The nutritional support team or dietitian assesses the client preoperatively and is available for consultations after surgery. A standard postoperative therapeutic goal is 35 to 40 kcal/kg of body weight. Protein and insensible water loss must also be very carefully calculated.

The nasogastric tube (the most commonly used tube type) usually remains in place for about 10 days after surgery. Before removing the tube, the nurse assesses the client's ability to swallow if the client is to receive nutrition by mouth. A client *cannot* aspirate following an uncomplicated total laryngectomy because the airway and esophagus are separated completely. The nurse reassures the client that he or she will not aspirate and stays with the client during the first few swallowing attempts. The nurse anticipates that swallowing may be uncomfortable at first and may administer analgesics as ordered.

Speech Rehabilitation. Because the client's voice and speech can be expected to be altered after surgery, the speech pathologist and nurse discuss the principles of speech therapy with the client and family early in the course of the treatment plan. The differences will depend on the type of surgical resection (see Table 29-4). Speech production varies with client practice, amount of resection, and radiation effects, but the client's speech can be very understandable.

The speech rehabilitation plan for clients undergoing total laryngectomy consists initially of writing, then using an artificial larynx, then learning esophageal speech. The client needs support and encouragement from the speech pathologist, hospital team, and family while relearning to speak. This process can be time-consuming and necessitates concentration each time the client speaks. Having a laryngectomee from one of the local self-help organizations visit the client and family is quite beneficial. The International Association of Laryngectomees is very active and supportive, as is the American Cancer Society Visitor Program.

Mechanical Devices. Clients who cannot attain esophageal speech can use mechanical devices called electro-larynges. Most contain a battery-powered device that is placed against the side of the neck or cheek. The air inside the mouth and pharynx is vibrated, and the client articulates as usual. Another external device (Cooper Rand), also battery-powered, consists of a plastic tube, placed within the client's mouth, that vibrates on articulation.

Esophageal Speech. Most total laryngectomees can attempt esophageal speech. Clients produce esophageal speech by the eructation of air swallowed or injected through the pharyngoesophageal (P-E) segment and articulate words in the mouth. The voice produced is a monotone; it cannot be raised or lowered and carries no pitch. Clients must have adequate hearing, or esophageal speech will be difficult because they use the mouth to shape the words as they hear them. Hearing-impaired clients may require hearing aids. In the English language, the vocal cords are necessary for 15 consonants; the remaining ten consonants can be formed by shaping the mouth.

Initially, gastrointestinal bloating occurs as a result of swallowing air for esophageal speech. Antacids may help to diminish bloating sensations. Esophageal speech also helps to strengthen the respiratory and abdominal musculature, which aids the client in expectorating secretions and in breathing.

Tracheoesophageal Fistula. A tracheoesophageal fistula (TEF) may be used if esophageal speech is insufficient for communication and if the client meets strict criteria. A surgical fistula is created between the trachea and the esophagus either at the time of the laryngectomy or in the postoperative period (Fig. 29–9). The surgeon places a catheter into the laryngectomy stoma and surgically creates a fistula into the esophagus. Usually, the catheter is then sutured to the neck to prevent accidental dislodgment. After the fistula heals, a silicone prosthesis, such as the Blom-Singer prosthesis (Fig. 29–10), is inserted in place of the catheter. The client covers the stoma and the opening of the prosthesis with a finger or opens and closes the opening with a special valve to divert air from the lungs, through the trachea, into the esophagus, and out of the mouth. Lip and tongue movement, not the prosthesis itself, produces speech.

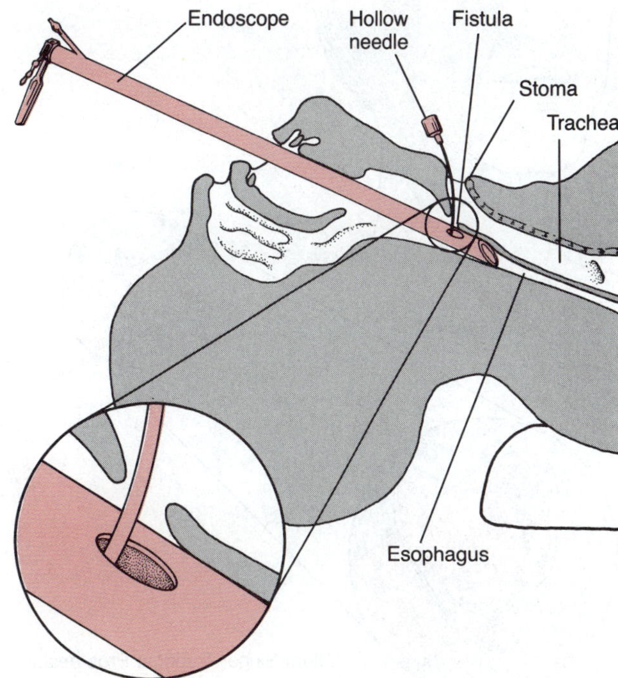

FIGURE 29–9 ◆ One method of creating a tracheoesophageal fistula (TEF).

Surgical Procedures for Other Head and Neck Cancers

The major types of resections, defined by the tumor location of the *oropharyngeal cancer,* are called composite resections. Composite resections are a combination of surgical procedures that include partial or total glossectomies, partial mandibulectomies, and, if required, nodal neck dissections. Tracheostomy may be planned to provide an adequate airway. More information on oral cancer is found in Chapter 53.

The major types of resections for *nasopharyngeal cancer* include maxillectomies and palatectomies.

Base of skull cancers involving the interface of the cranium and the facial structures are defined by tumor location in the anterior, middle, and posterior cranial fossae. Base of skull cancers are resected by a combination of otolaryngologic, neurosurgical, and neurovascular physicians and by skilled nursing staff.

Tracheostomy A tracheostomy can be performed as an emergency procedure or as a scheduled surgical procedure. A tracheotomy is a surgical incision into the trachea for the purpose of establishing an airway. Tracheostomy is the (tracheal) stoma, or opening, that results from the tracheotomy. Indications for tracheostomy, other than to attain or maintain a patent airway for clients with head and neck cancer, are listed in Table 29–5. The tracheostomy can be temporary or permanent.

PREOPERATIVE CARE The preoperative care for the client undergoing a tracheostomy is similar to that for a client scheduled for a laryngectomy. The nurse focuses on the client's knowledge deficits through teaching and discusses tracheostomy care, communication, and speech.

OPERATIVE PROCEDURES Initially, the anesthesiologist or nurse anesthetist extends the neck and places an endotracheal tube in order to maintain the airway.

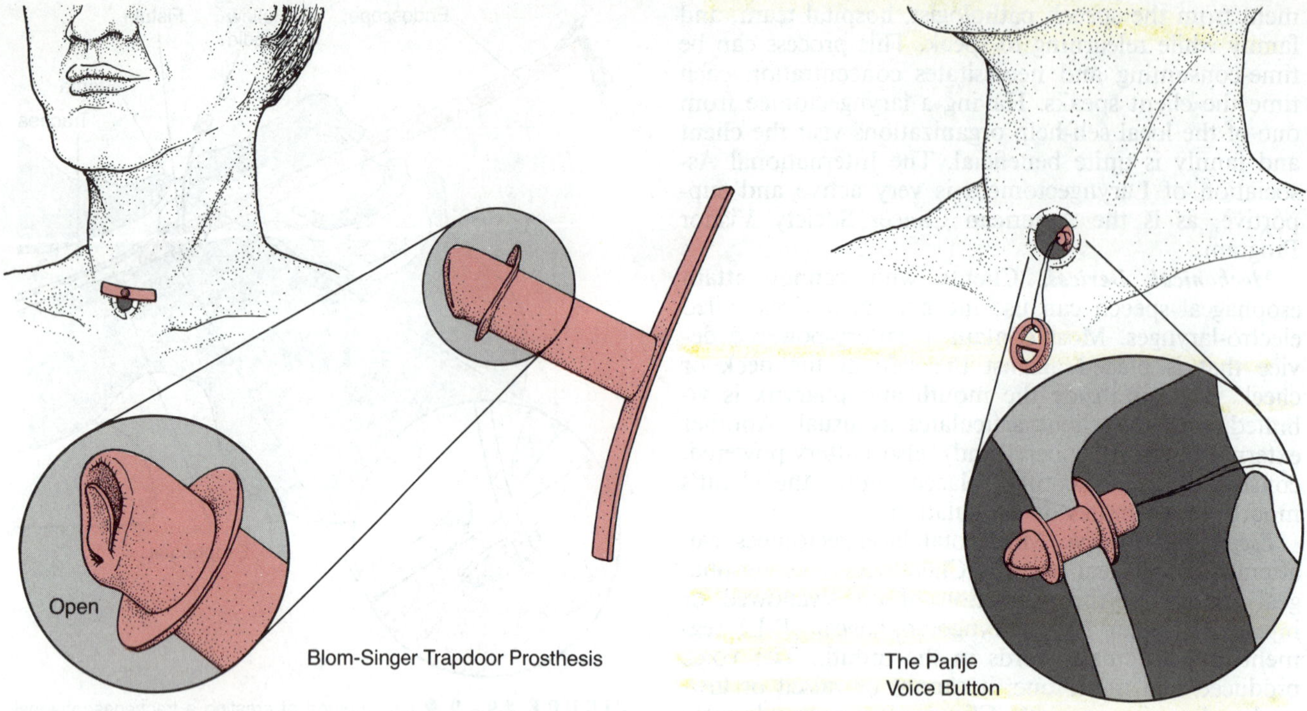

FIGURE 29-10 ♦ Examples of tracheoesophageal prostheses.

The surgeon then makes an incision through the anterior skin of the neck, dissects the subcutaneous tissue for exposure, separates the thyroid, and identifies the thyroid artery and tracheal rings. Another incision is made through the second and third or third and fourth tracheal rings to enter the trachea (Fig. 29-11). The types of incisions and specific techniques vary, depending on the surgeon's preference and the reason for the surgery.

After the surgeon enters the trachea, the endotracheal tube is very carefully removed while the tracheostomy tube is inserted. The surgeon secures the tracheostomy tube in place with sutures and tracheostomy ties and orders a chest x-ray to ensure proper placement of the tube. In clients who cannot be intubated, tracheostomy can be done with the client awake and with local anesthesia.

TABLE 29-5 Indications for a Tracheostomy

- Prolonged intubation or need for mechanical ventilation
- Acute airway obstruction when oral or nasal intubation is not feasible
- Obstructive sleep apnea refractory to conventional therapy
- Control of pulmonary secretions refractory to conventional methods
- Decreased airway dead space in combination with other indicators
- Airway protection (e.g., following head and neck cancer surgery)
- Airway reconstruction following laryngeal trauma or laryngeal cancer surgery

POSTOPERATIVE CARE Immediate postoperative nursing care focuses on ensuring a patent airway, confirming the presence of bilateral breath sounds, recovering the client from anesthesia, and assessing for complications from the procedure.

Complications. Six major complications may arise in the postoperative period:

- Tube obstruction with secretions
- Tube dislodgment or accidental decannulation

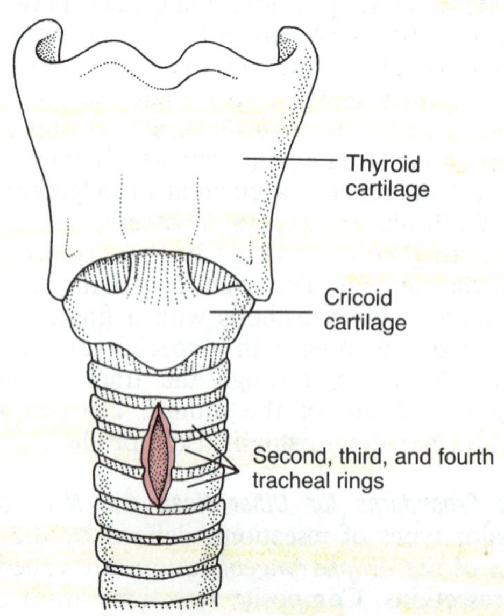

FIGURE 29-11 ♦ A vertical tracheal incision for a tracheostomy.

- Pneumothorax
- Subcutaneous emphysema
- Bleeding
- Infection

Refer to Table 29–6 for signs and symptoms, management, and prevention of other serious complications of tracheostomy.

Tube Obstruction. The nurse prevents obstruction from secretions through humidification and suctioning, by helping the client with coughing and deep breathing, providing inner cannula care, and instilling saline, as ordered. If tube obstruction occurs as a result of prolapse of the cuff over the end of the tracheostomy tube, the physician repositions or replaces the tube. Specific signs and symptoms of obstruction include difficulty in breathing; noisy respirations from the tracheostomy; difficulty in inserting the suction catheter; thick, dry secretions; and unexplained peak pressures if a mechanical ventilator is in use.

Tube Dislodgment or Accidental Decannulation. The nurse prevents tube dislodgment and decannulation by securing the tube in place, thus minimizing manipulation and traction of the tube from oxygen or ventilator tubing or accidental pulling by the client. Tube dislodgment in the first 72 hours after surgery is a medical emergency because the tracheostomy tract has not matured and tissue planes are not well defined. If unable to immediately replace the airway, the nurse calls the resuscitation team for help. Attempts at replacement of a fresh tracheostomy can lead to cannulation of subcutaneous tissue planes instead of the trachea itself. Securing the tube in the proper manner initially almost always prevents this problem.

TABLE 29–6 Complications of Tracheostomy

Complications and Description	Signs and Symptoms	Management	Prevention
Tracheomalacia: Constant pressure exerted by the cuff causes tracheal dilation and erosion of cartilage.	• An increased amount of air is required in the cuff to maintain the seal. • A larger tracheostomy tube is required to prevent an air leak at the stoma. • Food particles are seen in tracheal secretions. • The client does not receive tidal volume on the ventilator.	• No special management is needed unless bleeding occurs.	• Use an uncuffed tube as soon as possible. • Monitor cuff pressure and air volumes closely and detect changes.
Tracheal stenosis: Narrowed tracheal lumen is due to scar formation from irritation of tracheal mucosa by the cuff.	• Stenosis usually seen after the cuff is deflated or the tracheostomy tube is removed. • The client has increased coughing; inability to expectorate secretions; or difficulty in breathing or talking.	• Tracheal dilation or surgical intervention is used.	• Prevent pulling of and traction on the tracheostomy tube. • Properly secure the tube in the midline position. • Maintain proper cuff pressure. • Minimize oronasal intubation time.
Tracheoesophageal fistula (TEF): Excessive cuff pressure causes erosion of the posterior wall of the trachea. A hole is created between the trachea and the anterior esophagus. The client at highest risk also has a nasogastric tube present.	• Similar to tracheomalacia: • Food particles are seen in tracheal secretions. • Increased air in cuff is needed to achieve a seal. • The client has increased coughing and choking while eating. • The client does not receive the set tidal volume on the ventilator.	• Oxygen is given manually by mask to the client to prevent hypoxemia. • A small soft tube feeding is used instead of a nasogastric tube for tube feedings. A gastrostomy or jejunostomy may be performed. • The client with a nasogastric tube is monitored closely, and assessment is done for tracheoesophageal fistula and aspiration.	• Maintain cuff pressure. • Monitor the amount of air needed for inflation and detect changes. • Progress to deflated cuff or cuffless tube as soon as possible.
Trachea-innominate artery fistula: A malpositioned tube causes its distal tip to push against the lateral wall of the tracheostomy. Continued pressure causes necrosis and erosion of the innominate artery. ***This is a medical emergency.***	• The tracheostomy tube pulsates in synchrony with the heart beat. • There is exsanguination from the stoma. • This is a life-threatening complication.	• The tracheostomy tube is removed immediately. • Direct pressure is applied to the innominate artery at the stoma site. • Emergency surgery is done for repair.	• Correct the tube size, length, and midline position. • Prevent pulling or tugging on the tracheostomy tube. • Immediately notify the physician of pulsating tube.

TABLE 29–7 Types of Tracheostomy Tubes

Type	Description
Double-lumen tube	• The double-lumen tube has three major parts: • *Outer cannula*—fits into the stoma and keeps the airway open. The face plate indicates the size and type of tube and has small holes on both sides for securing the tube with tracheostomy ties. • *Inner cannula*—fits snugly into the outer cannula and locks into place. Provides the universal adapter for use with the ventilator and other respiratory therapy equipment. Some may be removed, cleaned, and reused; others are disposable. • *Obturator*—is a stylet with a blunt end used to facilitate direction of the tube when inserting or changing a tracheostomy tube. It is removed immediately after tube placement and is always kept with the client and at the bedside in case of accidental decannulation.
Single-lumen tube	• The single-lumen tube is a long tube used for clients with long or extra thick necks. Often called a "bull neck trach" because of the long distance from the skin to the trachea or the longer length of the trachea in large people. More intensive nursing care is required with this tube because there is no inner cannula to ensure a patent lumen.
Cuffed tube	• A cuff, when inflated, seals the airway. Used with mechanical ventilation, in preventing aspiration of oral or gastric secretions, or for tube feeding. A pilot balloon attached to the outside of the tube may indicate the presence or absence of air in the cuff.
Cuffless tube	• The cuffless tube is a plastic, silicone-like (Silastic), or metal tube, usually double lumen. Used for long-term airway management in those clients who require a tracheostomy and who can protect themselves from aspiration and who do not require mechanical ventilation. Many people can speak with this tube in place.
Fenestrated tube	• The fenestrated tube has a pre-cut opening (fenestration) in the upper posterior wall of the outer cannula. It is used to wean the client from a tracheostomy by ensuring that the client can tolerate breathing through his or her natural airway before the entire tube is removed. This tube allows the client to speak.
Cuffed fenestrated tube	• The cuffed fenestrated tube facilitates mechanical ventilation and speech. It is often used for clients with spinal cord paralysis or neuromuscular disease who do not require ventilation all the time. When not on the ventilator, the client can have the cuff deflated and the tube capped for speech. A cuffed fenestrated tube is never used in weaning from a tracheostomy because the cuff, even fully deflated, may partially obstruct the airway.
Metal tracheostomy tube	• The metal tracheostomy tube is used for permanent tracheostomy. It is a cuffless double-lumen tube and can be cleaned and reused indefinitely. A special adapter attaches a manual resuscitation bag. Popular types are the Jackson and Holinger tubes.
Talking tracheostomy tube	• The talking tracheostomy tube provides a means of communication for the client who is using a ventilator on a long-term basis. An extra air channel allows air to flow up through the vocal cords so that the client can speak with the cuff inflated. The air can cause drying of the vocal cords from constant dry airflow. Examples are the Pitt Trach Speaking Tube (National Catheter Corporation) and Communitrach (Implant Technologies, Inc.).

The nurse ensures that a tracheostomy tube of the same type (including an obturator) and size (or one size smaller) is at the client's bedside *at all times,* along with a tracheostomy insertion tray. After 72 hours, if decannulation occurs, the nurse extends the client's neck and opens the tissues of the stoma to secure the airway. With the obturator inserted into the tracheostomy tube, the nurse quickly and gently replaces the tube and removes the obturator. The nurse checks for airflow through the tube and for bilateral breath sounds. If unable to secure the airway, the nurse notifies a more experienced nurse or physician for assistance. The nurse attempts to ventilate via a bag-valve mask. If the client is in distress and further attempts to secure the airway fail, the nurse calls the resuscitation team, including an anesthesiologist, for assistance.

Pneumothorax. Pneumothorax (air in the chest cavity) can develop during the tracheostomy procedure if the thoracic cavity is accidentally entered. When pneumothorax occurs, it does so medially and superiorly at the apex of the lung. Chest x-ray after placement is used to assess for pneumothorax.

Subcutaneous Emphysema. When there is an opening (rent) in the trachea, air escapes into fresh tissue planes of the neck, causing subcutaneous emphysema. It can progress throughout the chest and axilla and into the face. The nurse inspects and palpates for air under the skin of a client with a new tracheostomy.

Bleeding. A small amount of bleeding from the tracheostomy incision can be expected for the first few days, but constant oozing warrants surgical intervention, cauterization, or ligation of vessels. With a physician order, the nurse initially wraps a petroleum (Vaseline) gauze around the tube and packs it gently into the wound to apply pressure to the bleeding sites.

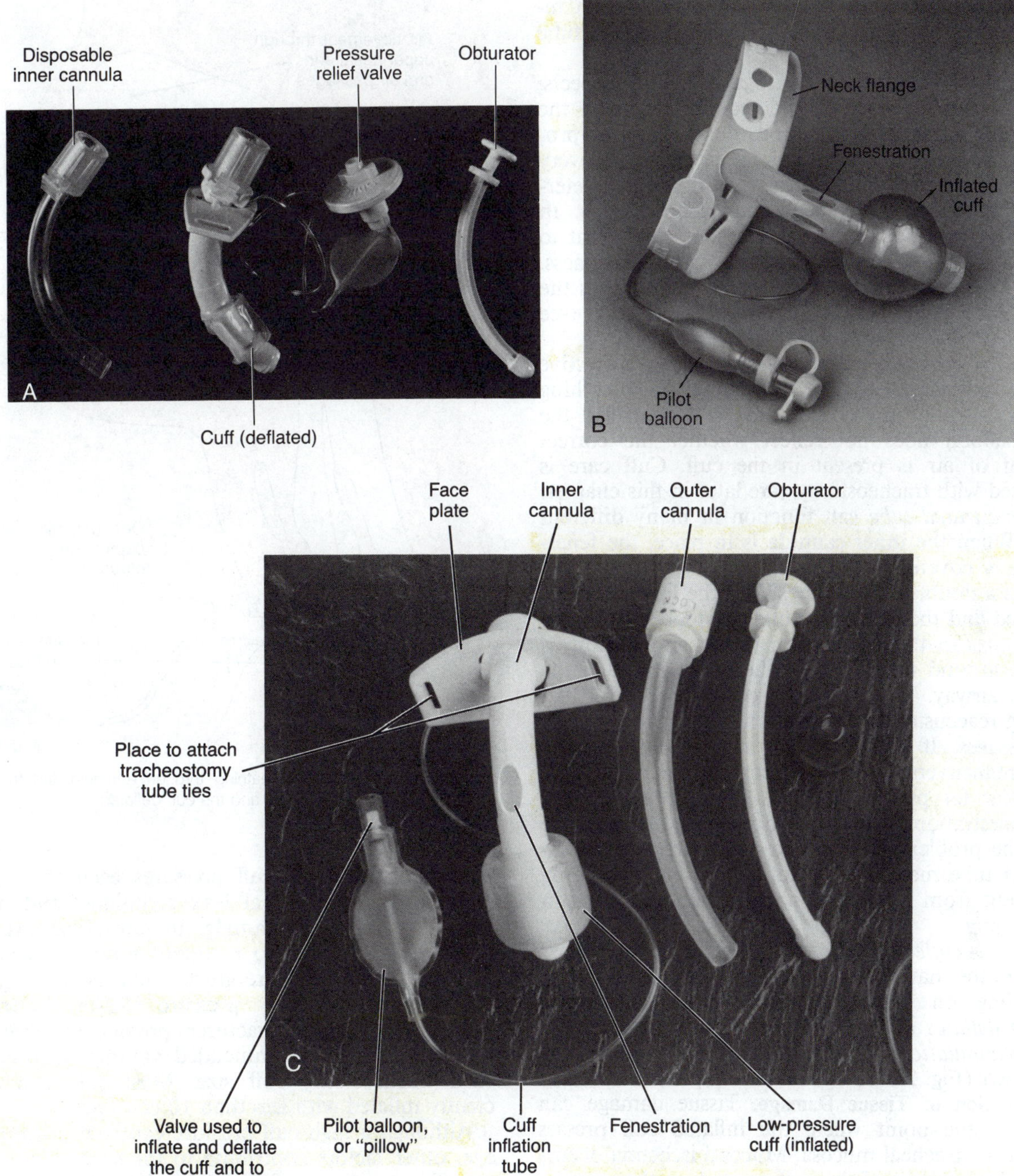

FIGURE 29-12 ◆ Tracheostomy tubes. *A*, Double-lumen tracheostomy tube. (Courtesy of Mallinckrodt Medical, Shiley Tracheostomy Products, Irvine, CA.) *B*, Single-lumen tracheostomy tube. (Courtesy of Concord Portex, Keene, NH.) *C*, The Shiley fenestrated low-pressure cuffed tracheostomy tube. (Courtesy of Mallinckrodt Medical, Shiley Tracheostomy Products, Irvine, CA.)

Infection. The nurse uses sterile technique to prevent infection during suctioning and tracheostomy care and assesses the stoma site for purulent drainage, redness, pain, swelling, or cellulitis. Tracheostomy dressings may be used to keep the stoma clean and dry; moist dressings provide an excellent medium for bacterial growth. Prevention and early detection of a local infection are therefore important. Diligent wound care prevents most local infections.

Tracheostomy Tubes. A variety of tracheostomy tubes are available (Table 29-7 and Fig. 29-12). The one chosen depends on the specific needs of the client. Tracheostomy tubes are available in numerous sizes and are made of various types of materials, such as plastic or metal. The tubes may be disposable or reusable. A tracheostomy tube may or may not have a cuff. It may also have an inner cannula that can be either disposable or reusable. A cuffed tube is used in acute care settings for clients receiving mechanical ventilation. A non-cuffed tube is used for airway maintenance when mechanical ventilation is not required or for the client being discharged with a tube in place.

For *tubes* with an *inner cannula,* the nurse inspects, suctions, and cleans the inner cannula. During the immediate postoperative period, the nurse may provide cannula care frequently as needed, perhaps every 30 to 60 minutes. Thereafter, care is usually determined by the client's needs and agency policy. In planning for self-care, the nurse teaches the client to remove the inner cannula and check for cleanliness. As the teaching progresses, the nurse also teaches the client suctioning and tracheostomy cleaning (see later).

A *cuffed tube* may not always be entirely protective against aspiration because movement of breathing and swallowing moves the tube. Additionally, the pilot balloon does not reflect whether the correct amount of air is present in the cuff. Cuff care is discussed with tracheostomy care later in this chapter.

A *fenestrated tube* can function in many different ways. When the inner cannula is in place, the fenestration is covered over (closed) and the tube functions as a double-lumen tube. With the inner cannula removed and the red decannulation stopper locked in place, air can then pass through the fenestration as well as around the tube. Air then flows through the natural airway. The client can cough and speak, becoming reaccustomed to breathing through the upper air passages. If the client has trouble with any of these maneuvers, the nurse and physician evaluate the client for proper tube placement, patency, size, and fenestration. The nurse does not cap the tube until the problem is identified and corrected. A fenestrated tube may or may not have a cuff. Weaning the client from a tracheostomy is discussed later in this chapter.

With a *cuffed fenestrated tube,* some air flows through the natural airway when the client is not depending on mechanical ventilation. The nurse *always deflates the cuff before capping the tube with the decannulation cannula; otherwise, the client has no airway* (Fig. 29–13).

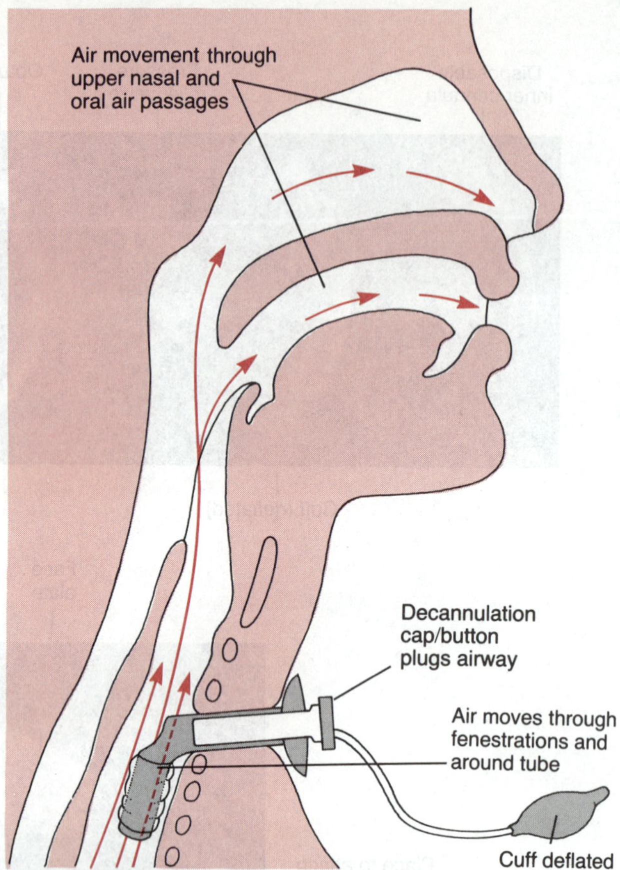

FIGURE 29–13 ◆ Breathing through a fenestrated tracheostomy tube with a cap in place and the cuff deflated.

Prevention of Tissue Damage. Tissue damage can occur at the point where the inflated cuff presses against the tracheal mucosa. Mucosal ischemia occurs when the pressure of the cuff exerted on the mucosa exceeds the capillary perfusion pressure. Arterial capillary perfusion pressure is 30 mmHg, venous capillary perfusion pressure is 18 mmHg, and lymphatic perfusion pressure is 5 mmHg. Therefore, the nurse ensures a cuff pressure between 14 and 20 mmHg to reduce the incidence of tracheal damage.

Most cuffs are designed to use a high volume of air while maintaining a low pressure on the tracheal mucosa. The nurse inflates the cuff to provide an adequate seal between the trachea and the cuff while creating the least amount of pressure. There are two methods of cuff inflation: the "minimal leak technique" (for cuffs without pressure relief valves), and the "occlusive technique" (for cuffs with pressure relief valves).

The nurse checks cuff pressures each shift, especially with the minimal leak technique, and maintains it at 14 to 20 mmHg. In rare situations, cuff pressure is increased to maintain ventilator volumes when peak pressures are greater than 50 mmHg and positive end-expiratory pressure (PEEP) is greater than 10 mmHg. Manufacturers provide guidelines for the approximate recommended volumes allowed for each tracheostomy cuff size. Most cuffs are sufficiently inflated with less than 10 cc of air.

Although a high cuff pressure causes tracheal damage, other factors contribute to the severity of damage. The condition of the client determines, to a degree, the susceptibility to tissue damage. The client who is malnourished, hypotensive, dehydrated, hypoxic, or receiving corticosteroids is unable to promote adequate tissue healing and is vulnerable to further tissue damage. Duration of intubation, extent and technique of suctioning, and stabilization of the tube against friction and movement are important factors that determine the extent of tracheal mucosa damage. The nurse minimizes local airway damage through the maintenance of proper cuff pressures, proper stabilization of the tube, judicious suctioning, and the prevention and treatment of malnutrition, hemodynamic instability, or hypoxia.

Humidification and Warming of Air. Humidification and warming of air are essential for any client with an artificial airway. The tube bypasses the upper air passages of the nose and mouth, which normally humidify, warm, and filter the air before it reaches the lower part of the respiratory tract. If humidification and warming are not adequate, tracheal damage can result from extremes in humidity and air temperature. In addition, thick, dried secretions form, which can occlude the proximal and distal airway.

To prevent these complications, the nurse provides a humidification source, as ordered. The nurse then assesses, on an ongoing basis, for a fine mist emerging from the tracheostomy collar or T-piece during inspiration and expiration. To increase the amount of humidification delivered, the respiratory therapist attaches a warming device to the humidification source. At the same time, a temperature probe is placed in the tubing circuit. Temperature is constantly monitored and is generally maintained between 37° and 38° C (98.6° to 100.4° F), but no greater than 40° C (104° F). The nurse monitors the client's temperature by feeling the tubing during client care and by checking the temperature probe. In addition, the nurse ensures adequate hydration, which also helps to liquify secretions.

Suctioning. Suctioning (Chart 29-5) maintains a patent airway and promotes gas exchange by removing secretions from clients who cannot adequately cough. The nurse assesses the client's need for suction, indicated by audible or noisy secretions, crackles or rhonchi on auscultation, restlessness, increased pulse and/or respiratory rates, the presence of mucus in the artificial airway, client requests for suctioning, and/or an increase in the peak airway pressure on the ventilator.

Suctioning is most often through an artificial airway (Fig. 29-14) but can be accomplished either through the nose or mouth. Suctioning of both routes is considered routine for clients with retained secretions.

The technique of suctioning *through the nose* holds similar complications as suctioning through an artificial airway. Entry through the nasal vault into the nasopharynx can be painful for the client. Slow, careful placement of the catheter, with a good understanding of the nasopharyngeal anatomy, can make the procedure less traumatic. The nurse may place a nasopharyngeal airway through which to suction to prevent trauma to the nasal mucosa. The nurse advances the catheter through the nasopharynx and into the laryngopharynx while at the same time giving the client oxygen by mask or nasal cannula. Once the catheter enters the larynx, the client may cough. On inhalation, the nurse inserts the catheter through the vocal cords and into the trachea. Occasionally, the catheter can be disconnected from suction and attached to an oxygen source, with the client receiving oxygen via the catheter.

Suctioning is associated with several complications:

- Hypoxia
- Tissue (mucosal) trauma
- Infection
- Vagal stimulation
- Bronchospasm

CHART 29-5

Nursing Care Highlight ◆ Suctioning the Artificial Airway

1. Assess the need for suctioning (routine unnecessary suctioning causes mucosal damage, bleeding, and bronchospasm).
2. Wash hands. Don protective eyewear. Maintain universal or body substance precautions.
3. Explain to the client that sensations such as shortness of breath and coughing are to be expected but that any discomfort will be very short in duration.
4. Check the suction source. Occlude the suction source, and adjust the pressure dial to between 80 and 120 mmHg to prevent hypoxemia and trauma to the mucosa.
5. Set up a sterile field.
6. Preoxygenate the client with 100% oxygen for 30 seconds to 3 minutes (at least three hyperinflations) to prevent hypoxemia. Keep hyperinflations synchronized with inhalation.
7. Quickly insert the suction catheter until resistance is met. Do not apply suction during insertion.
8. Withdraw the catheter 0.4 to 0.8 inch (1 to 2 cm), and begin to apply suction. Use intermittent suction and a twirling motion of the catheter during withdrawal. Never suction longer than 10 to 15 seconds.
9. Hyperoxygenate for 1 to 5 minutes or until the client's baseline heart rate and oxygen saturation are within normal limits.
10. Repeat as needed for up to three total suction passes.
11. Suction mouth as needed, and provide mouth care.
12. Describe secretions, and document client's responses.

Hypoxia. The causes of hypoxia include:

- Ineffective oxygenation before, during, and after suctioning
- Use of a catheter that is too large for the artificial airway
- Prolonged suctioning time
- Excessive suction pressure
- Too-frequent suctioning.

The nurse prevents hypoxia by hyperoxygenating the client with 100% oxygen from an oxygen-delivery device (Ambu bag attached to an oxygen source). Suctioning can be done by a one- or two-person technique. If the client is able to take deep breaths, the nurse instructs the client to do so three or four times before suctioning, using the existing oxygen delivery system. If possible, simultaneous monitoring of

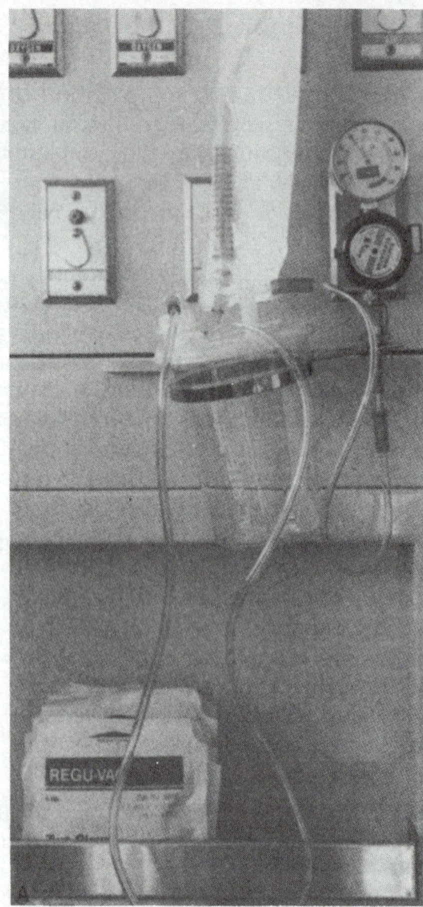

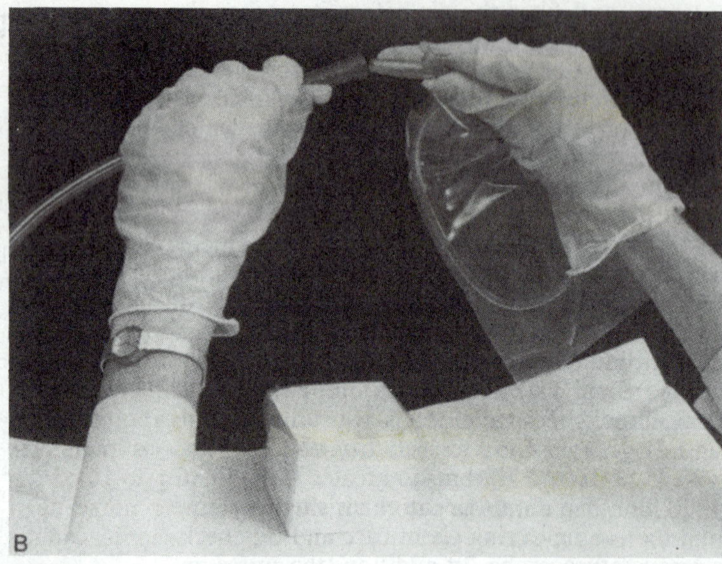

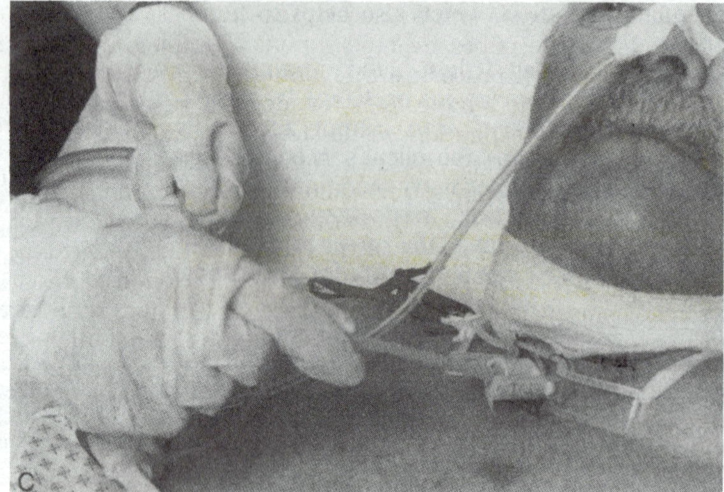

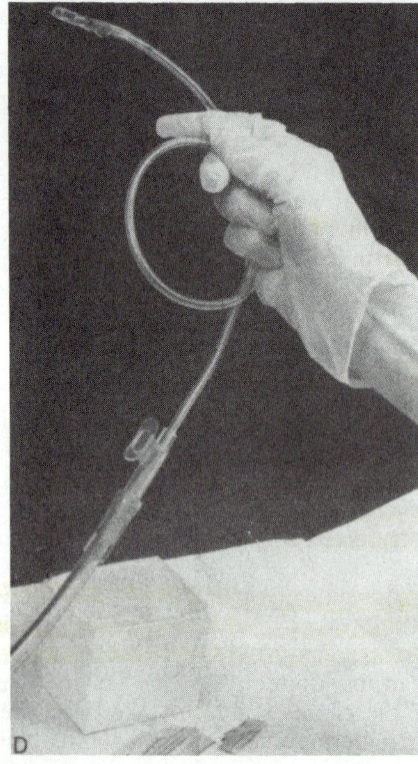

FIGURE 29-14 ◆ Sterile technique for suctioning. *A*, Bedside suction canister, tubing, and tonsil tip (also called Yankauer's pharyngeal suction tip) attached to wall vacuum. *B*, Attaching a suction catheter to the suction source. *C*, Suctioning by passing a catheter through a tracheostomy tube. *D*, Holding the catheter with one hand away from the client to prevent possible contamination between suctioning passes (From Kersten, L. D. [1989]. *Comprehensive respiratory nursing: A decision making approach.* Philadelphia: W. B. Saunders.)

heart rate or use of a pulse oximeter is helpful in assessing tolerance of the suctioning procedure. The nurse assesses the client for signs and symptoms of hypoxia (e.g., increased heart rate and blood pressure, oxygen desaturation, cyanosis, restlessness, anxiety, and cardiac dysrhythmias). Oxygen desaturation below 90% as determined by pulse oximetry indicates hypoxemia. If hypoxia occurs, the nurse terminates the suctioning procedure. Using the 100% oxygen-delivery system, the nurse reoxygenates the client until baseline parameters are achieved.

The nurse prevents hypoxia by using a catheter of the correct size. The size should not exceed half of the size of the tracheal lumen. In adults, the standard catheter size is 12 or 14 French (Fr.). Adequate catheter size facilitates efficient removal of secretions without causing hypoxemia.

Tissue Trauma. The mucosa of the respiratory tract is extremely fragile, and frequent suctioning, prolonged suctioning time, excessive suction pressure, and nonrotation of the catheter cause damage.

The nurse prevents tissue trauma by suctioning only when indicated. The nurse lubricates the catheter with sterile water or saline before insertion and suctions only during the withdrawal of the catheter. Use of a twirling motion during withdrawal prevents excessive grabbing of the mucosa. In addition, the nurse applies suction intermittently for only 10 to 15 seconds. The nurse can estimate this time frame by holding his or her own breath and counting to 10 or 15 during suctioning. At the end of the 15 seconds, the suctioning procedure is finished. Fifteen seconds does not seem long to a healthy person, but most clients requiring suctioning have respiratory compromise and cannot tolerate more than 15 seconds of suctioning.

Infection. Each catheter pass introduces bacteria into the trachea. In the hospital, the nurse uses sterile technique for suctioning and for all suctioning equipment, including suction catheters, gloves, and saline or water. After suctioning the artificial airway, the nurse then suctions the mouth. Oral suction equipment is never used for suctioning an artificial airway. This is because the mouth is contaminated with bacteria, necessary for digestion, which could be introduced into the lungs. Home suctioning procedures emphasize clean technique because of the lower number of virulent organisms in the home environment compared with that in the hospital.

Vagal Stimulation and Bronchospasm. Vagal stimulation results in severe bradycardia, hypotension, heart block, ventricular tachycardia, or asystole. If vagal stimulation occurs, the nurse stops suctioning immediately and oxygenates the client manually with 100% oxygen. Bronchospasm sometimes occurs when the catheter passes into the airway. The client may require a bronchodilator to relieve the bronchospasm and respiratory distress.

Tracheostomy Care. Tracheostomy care (Chart 29–6) keeps the tracheostomy tube free of obstructing secretions, maintains a patent airway, and provides wound care. This procedure is performed whether or not the client is able to clear secretions. The nurse performs tracheostomy care according to agency policy, usually every shift and as needed.

CHART 29–6

Nursing Care Highlight ◆ Tracheostomy Care

1. Assemble the necessary equipment.
2. Wash your hands. Maintain universal or body substance precautions.
3. Suction the tracheostomy tube if necessary.
4. Remove old dressings and excess secretions.
5. Set up a sterile field.
6. Remove and clean the inner cannula. Use half-strength hydrogen peroxide to clean the cannula, and sterile saline to rinse it. If the inner cannula is disposable, remove the cannula and replace it with a new one.
7. Clean the stoma site and then the tracheostomy plate with half-strength hydrogen peroxide followed by sterile saline. Ensure that none of the solutions enters the tracheostomy.
8. Change tracheostomy ties if they are soiled. Secure new ties in place before removing soiled ones to prevent accidental decannulation. If a knot is needed, tie a *square* knot that is visible on the side of the neck. One or two fingers should be able to be placed between the tie tape and the neck.
9. Document the type and amount of secretions and the general condition of the stoma and surrounding skin. Document the client's response to the procedure and any teaching or learning that occurred.

The extent of both suctioning and tracheostomy care depends entirely on the needs of the client. The need for suctioning and tracheostomy care are determined by the amount and consistency of secretions, the medical diagnosis (specifically pulmonary diseases), the ability of the client to cough and deep breathe, the need for mechanical ventilation, and wound care required. The nurse inspects the inner lumen of a single-lumen tube with a flashlight or penlight to assess for the presence of secretions.

The nurse changes tracheostomy ties once a day to keep them clean and not act as a medium for infection. A properly secured tie allows space for only one or two fingers to be placed between the tie and the neck. Tube movement causes irritation and coughing, which in turn may cause decannulation. *It is imperative to keep the tube secure while changing the ties to prevent accidental decannulation.* One way to accomplish this safely is to keep the old ties on the tube when changing ties. However, a secure hand on the tube is the most reliable method of tube stabilization. The nurse includes the client in this process as a step toward self-care. Figure 29–15 demonstrates a correct technique for applying a tracheostomy dressing.

Bronchial and Oral Hygiene. *Bronchial hygiene* measures promote a patent airway, prevent pulmonary infections, and stimulate the pulmonary system. The nurse turns and repositions the client every 1 to 2

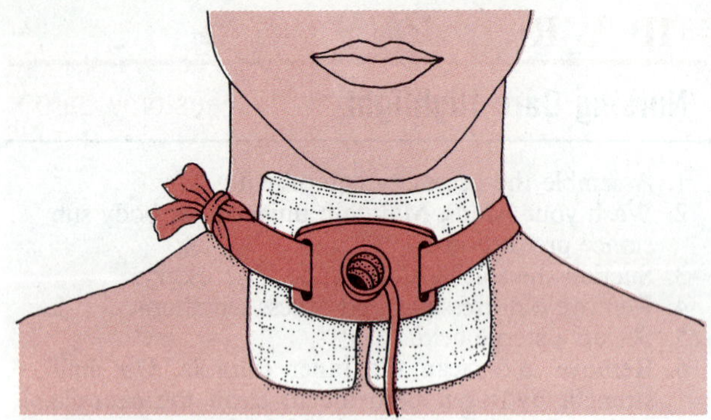

FIGURE 29-15 ◆ Placement of pre-cut gauze and tie around a tracheostomy tube.

hours, supports out-of-bed activities, and encourages ambulation. These interventions promote lung expansion and gas exchange and facilitate the mobilization of secretions. Coughing and deep breathing, combined with the *chest physical therapy* techniques of percussion, vibration, and postural drainage, are powerful measures in promoting pulmonary care (see Chap. 30).

Frequent *oral hygiene* is important not only to ensure a patent airway but also to prevent bacterial overgrowth and dental caries and to promote client comfort. The nurse maintains universal or body substance precautions during the procedure. Cleansing the mouth with glycerine swabs and mouthwash, which contains significant amounts of alcohol, are contraindicated because these interventions dry the oral mucosa, change its pH, and promote bacterial growth. The nurse instead uses a toothette or soft-bristle brush moistened in water for mouth care. Hydrogen peroxide solutions can help to remove crusted materials but may break down granulating tissue and are used only with a physician's order.

During oral care, the nurse examines the mouth for any alterations in mucosal integrity, dental abnormalities, and alterations in tissue integrity. Ulcers (aphthous or herpes simplex), bacterial or fungal *(Candida)* growth, or other infections are treated medically. Application of lip balms or water-soluble jelly can prevent cracked lips and further skin breakdown and can help keep the client comfortable. Providing mouth care is a simple but very effective method of promoting oral health, comfort, and esthetic appearance. Offering an opportunity for the client or family member to perform mouth care encourages participation in care and increases the client's self-esteem.

Speech and Communication. The client will be able to speak when there is a cuffless tube, when a fenestrated tracheostomy tube is in place, and when the fenestrated tube is capped or covered. Until one of the methods for natural vocalization is feasible, the nurse establishes a means of communication that is easy for the client to use. A writing tablet, "magic slate," communication board with pictures and letters, hand signals, or a computer, as well as a call light within reach, is essential to promote communication and decrease the client's frustration from not being able to speak or be understood. The nurse moves the client closer to the nurses' station and marks the central call light system with indicators to indicate that the client cannot speak. Questions phrased for "yes" or "no" answers help the client respond efficiently.

The inability to talk is a major stressor for the client. Every effort to facilitate communication and speech is important. When the client can tolerate cuff deflation, he or she places a finger over the tracheostomy tube on exhalation. This forces air up through the larynx, vocal cords, and mouth and allows for articulation. During the process of decannulation, when the fenestrated tube is "capped," the client experiences a very positive but secondary benefit of speech without the need to cover the tube.

Emotional Care. Addressing psychologic concerns is an important aspect of nursing care of clients recovering from a tracheostomy. While providing physical care to the client, the nurse keeps in mind the emotional impact of an artificial airway. Acknowledging the client's frustration in communication and allowing sufficient time for communication are critically important. When speaking to the client, the nurse uses a normal tone of voice. The tracheostomy tube has not altered the client's ability to hear or understand.

Weaning. Weaning the client from a tracheostomy tube entails a gradual decrease in the tube size and ultimate removal of the tube. The nurse carefully monitors this process, especially after each change. The physician or a specially trained nurse performs the steps in the process.

First, the cuff is deflated as soon as the client can manage secretions and does not require mechanical ventilation. This change allows the client to breathe through the tube and also through the upper airway. Next, the tube is changed to an uncuffed tube; then the size of the tube is gradually decreased. When a small fenestrated tube is placed (a No. 4 or No. 6, depending on the size of the airway) the tube is capped so that all air passes through the upper airway and the fenestra, with none passing through the tube. The tube is removed after the client tolerates more than 24 hours of capping. The nurse places a dry dressing over the stoma, which then gradually heals on its own. A small scar remains.

Another device used for the transition from tracheostomy to natural breathing is a tracheostomy button. The button maintains patency of the stoma and facilitates spontaneous breathing. The Kistner tracheostomy tube and Olympic tracheostomy button are examples of this type of device. To function, they must fit properly. A disadvantage of these buttons is the possibility of decannulation: The tube dislodges from the trachea but remains in the anterior subcutaneous tissues of the neck.

HIGH RISK FOR ASPIRATION

PLANNING: CLIENT GOALS The major goal is for the client not to aspirate food, gastrointestinal contents, or oral secretions into the lungs.

INTERVENTIONS Depending on tumor size and location or type of tumor resection, the client may aspirate during eating. This incident can result in life-threatening pneumonia, weight loss, further hospitalization, and increased costs.

Because of anatomic or surgical changes in the upper respiratory tract and altered swallowing mechanisms, the client with head and neck cancer is at risk for aspiration. The presence of a nasogastric (NG) feeding tube may further increase the potential for aspiration because of the incompetent LES (lower esophageal sphincter). The one exception is the client who has had a total laryngectomy; such a person is *not* at risk because the airway is separated from the esophagus, making aspiration impossible.

A Dynamic Swallow Study evaluates a client's ability to protect the airway from aspiration and helps to determine the appropriate method of swallow rehabilitation. Bedside clinical assessment of swallowing is important but carries with it a high rate of inaccuracy. In many cases, the physician must institute enteral feedings either because the client cannot swallow or because of continued aspiration potential.

When an NG tube is in place, the nurse helps to prevent aspiration through routine reflux precautions, including elevating the head of the bed and strictly adhering to tube feeding regimens, including no bolus feedings at night. The nurse checks residual feeding amounts before each bolus feeding (or every 4 to 6 hours with continuous feeding) and evaluates the client's tolerance of the tube feeding. If the residual volume is too high (above 100 mL), the nurse withholds the feeding and notifies the physician. The nurse adds food coloring to the tube feeding and observes tracheal secretions. If aspiration occurs, secretions may be the color of the food coloring. Methylene blue is not used today as an additive to tube feedings because it is systemically excreted through the lungs and can appear in pulmonary secretions. See Chapters 55 and 61 for other interventions related to NG tubes and tube feedings.

Swallowing can be a major problem for the client with a tracheostomy tube in place. In a normal swallow, the larynx elevates and moves forward to protect itself from the passing stream of food and saliva. Laryngeal elevation also assists in the opening of the cricopharyngeal muscle, the upper esophageal sphincter. The tracheostomy tube sometimes tethers the larynx in place, rendering it unable to execute this motion efficiently. The result is difficulty in swallowing. Likewise, when the tracheostomy tube cuff is inflated, it can balloon posteriorly and interfere with the passage of food through the esophagus. The common wall of the posterior trachea (trachealis muscle) and the anterior esophagus is very thin, allowing this pushing phenomenon.

Provided that the tracheostomy tube is not capped, the nurse usually inflates the cuff during feeding to prevent aspiration. The nurse then instructs the client to keep the head of the bed elevated for at least 30 minutes after feeding and keeps the cuff inflated for the same time period. Clients with head and neck cancer who are cognitively intact, however, may adapt to eating normal food when the tracheostomy tube is small and the cuff is not inflated.

If the client has had a subtotal, vertical, or supraglottic laryngectomy, he or she *must* be observed for aspiration. It is imperative that the nurse and the speech and language pathologist teach the client the procedure for alternate methods of swallowing without aspirating. Especially effective after partial laryngectomy or base-of-tongue resection is the "supraglottic method" of swallowing (Chart 29–7). To reinforce teaching and learning, the nurse places a chart in the client's room detailing the steps. A Dynamic Swallow Study is performed to evaluate the client's ability to protect the airway and to guide rehabilitation therapy for swallowing.

ANXIETY

PLANNING: CLIENT GOALS The major goal is that the client will verbalize decreased anxiety through increased knowledge and understanding about the specific, individualized treatment plan.

INTERVENTIONS The client may benefit from multidisciplinary conferences with the physician, clinical nurse specialist, dietitian, speech-language pathologist, physical therapist, psychologist, social worker, discharge planning nurse, as well as the general nursing staff. The nurse explores with the client the reason for anxiety (e.g., fear of the unknown, lack of preoperative teaching, fear of pain, fear of airway compromise, fear of hospitalization, and loss of control). Many times the client and family can benefit from further information. Before the client is scheduled for surgery and while the client is still at home, home care nurses or community-sponsored associations, such as the American Cancer Society, may be able to alleviate the fears of the client and family about the disease process and surgical interventions.

The nurse administers antianxiety agents, such as diazepam (Valium, Meval✱), with caution because of

CHART 29–7

Education Guide ◆ The Supraglottic Method of Swallowing

1. Position yourself in an upright, preferably out-of-bed, position.
2. Clear your throat.
3. Take a deep breath.
4. Place ½ to 1 teaspoon of food into your mouth.
5. Hold your breath, or "bear down" (Valsalva maneuver).
6. Swallow twice.
7. Release your breath, and clear your throat.
8. Swallow twice again.
9. Breathe normally.

* *Note:* This method exaggerates the normal protective mechanisms of cessation of respiration during the swallow. The double swallow attempts to clear food that may be pooling in the pharynx, vallecula, and piriform sinuses. This method is used only after a dynamic radiographic swallow study has demonstrated that it is appropriate and safe for the client.

the possibility of hypercarbia and hypoxia in an already compromised client. The location of the tumor and any other concurrent lung disease may be causing some degree of airway obstruction. For anxiety in these clients, the physician prescribes drug therapy judiciously.

BODY IMAGE DISTURBANCE

PLANNING: CLIENT GOALS The goal is for the client to state that he or she understands and, in time, accepts body image changes and returns to the previous lifestyle within the limits of the disease.

INTERVENTIONS The client with head and neck cancer experiences a permanent change in body image because of deformity, the presence of a stoma or artificial airway, speech changes, and a change in the method of eating. The client may be aphonic (unable to speak) or may have permanent hoarseness or speech deficits. The nurse helps the client to set realistic goals, starting with involvement in self-care. The nurse teaches alternative communication methods so that the client can functionally communicate in the hospital and after discharge.

The nurse and family must make all attempts to ease the client into a more normal social environment. The nurse provides encouragement and positive reinforcement while demonstrating acceptance and caring behaviors. The family may benefit from counseling sessions that the nurse initiates in the hospital.

After surgery, the client may feel reserved and socially isolated because of the change in voice and facial appearance. To cover the laryngectomy stoma, the tracheostomy tube, and postoperative changes related to surgery, the client can wear loose-fitting, high-collar shirts or sweaters (e.g., turtleneck), scarves, and jewelry. Cosmetics may aid in covering any disfigurement. Most surgeons try to place the surgical incisions in the client's natural skin fold lines if doing so does not pose a risk for cancer recurrence. (See Chapter 10 for a detailed discussion of body image, including additional nursing interventions.)

DISCHARGE PLANNING

HOME CARE PREPARATION

The client is usually ready to be discharged from the hospital within 2 weeks if no complications occur. By this time, the client should be able to provide his or her own care, which may include some or all of the following:

- Tracheostomy or stoma care
- Oral, nasogastric, or gastrostomy feedings
- Wound care
- Methods of communication

The client should feel safe and secure with the extended plan of care.

The client and family may feel more secure about discharge if they receive a referral to a community health agency familiar with the care of clients recovering from head and neck cancer. The multidisciplinary team assesses the client's specific discharge needs and makes the appropriate referrals to home care agencies, including such professionals as nutritionists, nurses, physical therapists, speech pathologists, and social workers. The nurse coordinates the scheduling for chemotherapy or radiation therapy with the client and family.

HEALTH TEACHING

Although education begins during preoperative teaching sessions, most self-care is taught in the hospital. The nurse teaches the client and family how to care for the stoma or tracheostomy or laryngectomy tube, depending on the type of surgery performed. The nurse reviews incision and airway care, including cleaning and inspecting for signs of infection. The nurse teaches clean suction technique and reviews the client's plan of care.

The nurse instructs the client to use a shower shield over the tracheostomy tube or laryngectomy stoma when bathing to prevent water from entering the airway. To shield the airway during the day, the client may wear a protective cover, or stoma guard.

For clients with permanent stomas following laryngectomy or for those with permanent tracheostomies, covering the permanent opening has a double benefit: filtering the air entering the stoma and keeping humidity in the airway as well as enhancing esthetic appearance. To protect the airway and increase humidity, the nurse instructs the client to cover the airway with cotton or foam. Attractive coverings are available in the form of cotton scarves, crocheted bibs, and jewelry. Using colored seam binding for tracheostomy ties after the stoma has matured may enhance the client's overall body image. The client's shirt or dress color can be matched or coordinated with seam bindings of various colors. The nurse also teaches the client how to increase humidity in the home. The nurse may teach the client to instill normal saline into the artificial airway 10 to 15 times a day as ordered.

The client continues the selected method of alternative communication that began in the hospital. The client wears a medical alert (Medic Alert) bracelet and carries a special identification card (Fig. 29–16). For clients who have had a laryngectomy, these cards are available from their local chapters of the International Association of Laryngectomees. They instruct the reader in providing an emergency airway or resuscitating the client who has a stoma.

Chart 29–8 summarizes the highlights of self-care for the client being discharged after laryngeal cancer surgery. Many of the highlights are also applicable to someone being discharged following any resection for head and neck cancer.

PSYCHOSOCIAL PREPARATION

The client who goes home with a permanent stoma, tracheostomy tube, nasogastric tube, and wounds experiences an alteration in body image. The

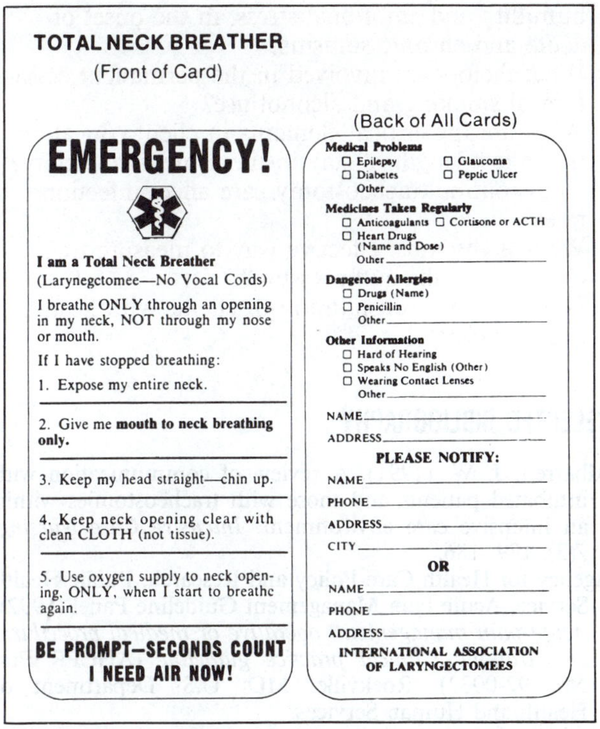

TOTAL NECK BREATHER
(Front of Card)

EMERGENCY!

I am a Total Neck Breather
(Laryngectomee—No Vocal Cords)

I breathe ONLY through an opening in my neck, NOT through my nose or mouth.

If I have stopped breathing:

1. Expose my entire neck.
2. Give me **mouth to neck breathing only.**
3. Keep my head straight—chin up.
4. Keep neck opening clear with clean CLOTH (not tissue).
5. Use oxygen supply to neck opening. ONLY, when I start to breathe again.

BE PROMPT—SECONDS COUNT
I NEED AIR NOW!

(Back of All Cards)

Medical Problems
☐ Epilepsy ☐ Glaucoma
☐ Diabetes ☐ Peptic Ulcer
Other ______

Medicines Taken Regularly
☐ Anticoagulants ☐ Cortisone or ACTH
☐ Heart Drugs (Name and Dose)
Other ______

Dangerous Allergies
☐ Drugs (Name)
☐ Penicillin
Other ______

Other Information
☐ Hard of Hearing
☐ Speaks No English (Other)
☐ Wearing Contact Lenses
Other ______

NAME ______
ADDRESS ______

PLEASE NOTIFY:

NAME ______
PHONE ______
ADDRESS ______
CITY ______

OR

NAME ______
PHONE ______
ADDRESS ______

INTERNATIONAL ASSOCIATION OF LARYNGECTOMEES

FIGURE 29-16 ◆ Emergency wallet card for identification of laryngectomees.

nurse stresses the importance of returning to a normal lifestyle as much as possible. About half of these clients return to full-time employment. The remainder work part time or apply for disability income. Most clients can resume many of their usual activities within 4 to 6 weeks after surgery or longer after a combination of radiation therapy and surgery. The client may be frustrated at times while trying to adjust to changes in smell, taste, and communication during this time.

The client with a total laryngectomy cannot produce audible sounds during laughing and crying, and excess mucous secretions may appear unexpectedly when these emotions or coughing or sneezing occurs. This expectoration can be embarrassing, and the client must always be prepared to cover the stoma with a handkerchief or gauze. The client who has undergone composite resections will have difficulty with both speech *and* swallowing. These clients may have tracheostomies and feeding tubes to deal with in public places.

The nurse tries to prepare the client for these changes, but another client who has adjusted to these changes is usually more effective in preparing the client for discharge. Counseling by other health care

CHART 29-8

Education Guide ◆ Home Laryngectomy Care

- Avoid swimming, and use care when showering or shaving.
- Lean slightly forward and cover the stoma when coughing or sneezing.
- Wear a stoma guard or loose clothing to cover the stoma.
- Clean the stoma with mild soap and water. Lubricate the stoma with non-oil-based ointment as needed.
- Increase humidity by using saline in the stoma as instructed, a bedside humidifier, pans of water, and houseplants.
- Obtain and wear a Medic-Alert bracelet and emergency card for life-threatening situations.

RESEARCH APPLICATIONS FOR NURSING

Social Support Promotes Optimal Rehabilitation Outcomes after Head and Neck Cancer

Baker, C. A. (1992). Factors associated with rehabilitation in head and neck cancer. *Cancer Nursing, 15*(6), 395–400.

In this study of 51 head and neck cancer survivors, perceived social support, perceived severity of dysfunction, and degree of disfigurement were examined in relation to rehabilitation outcomes.

Outcomes were measured using a self-scored instrument that elicited data on 12 functional areas of daily living. Areas scored, for example, included ambulation, mobility, social interaction, alertness, sleep and rest, work, recreation, and home management. A facial disfigurement severity scale was used to assess the degree of disfigurement. The subjects used a ladder scale to identify extremes in problem areas, such as shoulder function, swallowing, taste, and speech. Perceived social support was measured on a 25-item Likert-type scale that measures worth, intimacy, social interaction, nurturance, and assistance.

Results indicated that facial disfigurement was not significantly associated with rehabilitation outcomes, but perceived social support and degree of dysfunction were significantly correlated with rehabilitation.

Critique In this well-designed study, the researcher collected and analyzed the data appropriately, using previously tested tools. Further research, as the author states, should focus on interventions that would strengthen social support as well as limit physical dysfunction.

Possible nursing implications This study emphasizes the importance of social support in relation to positive rehabilitation outcomes. The nurse needs to incorporate psychosocial assessment, intervention, and evaluation into the plan of care for head and neck clients at the earliest possible time. Resources for clients will need to be identified as well.

The nurse should continue to focus on teaching and promoting functional activities, such as swallowing, shoulder movement, and speech. The plan of care should include the prevention of complications that, if they were to occur, could result in more physical dysfunction.

professionals can also offer valuable support. One important nursing study looked at various factors associated with rehabilitation outcomes. The results are reviewed in Research Applications for Nursing.

HEALTH CARE RESOURCES

Clinic or physician follow-up visits occur early after discharge. Very often, a home care nurse is involved with the client's care after discharge and becomes a very important resource for the client and family. The home care or hospital nurse informs the client and family of community organizations, such as the American Cancer Society, and local laryngectomee clubs, which can offer support, accurate information, and friendships. When the client has problems paying for health care services, equipment supply and prescriptions, a visiting nurse agency may be helpful in directing the client to available resources.

EVALUATION

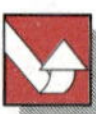

On the basis of the identified nursing diagnoses, the nurse evaluates the entire plan of care for the client with head and neck cancer. The expected outcomes are that the client:

- Maintains a patent airway
- Attains or maintains clear lung sounds in all lung fields
- Demonstrates an understanding of head and neck cancer and its treatment
- Performs self-care of the artificial airway and wound
- Performs the activities of daily living (ADLs) independently or with minimal assistance
- States that levels of anxiety are reduced
- Resumes as normal a lifestyle as possible through rehabilitation
- States understanding of and adapts to body image changes
- Attains or maintains adequate nutrition
- Does not aspirate gastric contents or food
- Complies with smoking and alcohol cessation programs

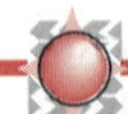

IMPLICATIONS FOR NURSING RESEARCH

Many factors contribute to the development of upper airway diseases. There are several possible questions for nursing research:

- ♦ What role does emotional stress play in the onset of the common cold?
- ♦ How can the nurse be most effective in helping a client with a total laryngectomy accept the accompanying changes in body image?
- ♦ What is the role of stressors, such as changes in humidity and emotional stress, in the onset of acute and chronic sinusitis?
- ♦ What factors are involved in the permanent cessation of smoking and alcohol use?
- ♦ What are the critical elements in client education that affect length of stay in the acute care facility?
- ♦ Does routine tracheostomy care affect infection rates?
- ♦ What is the most effective way to measure tracheostomy tube cuff pressure?
- ♦ How frequent is aspiration in clients with head and neck cancers?

SELECTED BIBLIOGRAPHY

Albarren, J. W. (1991). A review of communication with intubated patients and those with tracheostomies within an intensive care environment. *Intensive Care Nursing, 7*(3), 179–186.

Agency for Health Care Policy and Research, Public Health Service, Acute Pain Management Guideline Panel (1992). *Acute pain management: operative or medical procedures and trauma: Clinical practice guideline* (AHCPR Pub No. 92-0032). Rockville, MD: U.S. Department of Health and Human Services.

American Cancer Society (1990). Cancer of the larynx. *Ca: A Cancer Journal for Clinicians, 40*(3), 133–183.

American Cancer Society (1991). *Cancer facts and figures.* New York: Author.

American Joint Committee on Cancer (AJCC) (1992). *Manual for staging of cancer* (4th ed.). Philadelphia: J. B. Lippincott.

Badhwar, A. K., & Druce, H. M. (1992). Allergic rhinitis. *Medical Clinics of North America, 76*(4), 789–804.

Baker, C. A. (1992). Factors associated with rehabilitation in head and neck cancer. *Cancer Nursing, 15*(6), 395–400.

Barkett, P. A. (1991). Obstructed airway with wired jaws: How to respond when a patient with wired jaws vomits. *Nursing91, 21*(12), 33.

Bartkiw, T. P., & Pynn, B. R. (1993). Close-up on mandible fracture. Nursing 93, *23*(12), 45.

Boring, C. C., Squires, T. S., & Heath, C. W. (1992). Cancer statistics for African Americans. *CA: A Cancer Journal for Clinicians, 42*(1), 7–17.

Boring, C. C., Squires, T. S., Tong, T, & Montgomery, S. (1994). Cancer statistics, 1994. *CA: A Cancer Journal for Clinicians, 44*(1), 7–26.

De Lorenzo, R. A., & Mayer, D. (1991). Laryngeal trauma: Uncovering the hidden injury. *Journal of Medical Emergency Services, 16*(9), 77–83.

*Dropkin, M. J. (1989). Coping with disfigurement and dysfunction after head and neck cancer surgery: A conceptual framework. *Seminars in Oncology Nursing, 5*(3), 213–219.

Droughton, M. L., & Krech, R. L. (1992). Head and neck cancer resection and reconstruction: From past to present. *Today's OR Nurse, 14*(9), 25–34.

Foster, J. (1992). Intensive care of the patient with cancer after reconstructive surgery. *Focus on Critical Care, 19*(2), 122–127.

Gantz, N. M., & Sogg, A. J. (1992). An update on sinusitis. *Patient Care, 26*(8), 141–143, 147–148, 157–163.

*Grant, M., Rhiner, M., & Padilla, G. (1989). Nutritional management in the head and neck cancer patient. *Seminars in Oncology Nursing, 5*(3), 195–204.

*Hancher, K. (1988). Social adjustment of laryngectomy

patients. *Journal: Society of Otorhinolaryngology Head-Neck Nurses, 6*(2), 4–8.

Howard, B. A. (1994). Guiding allergy sufferers through the medication maze. *RN, 57*(4), 26–30.

Hudak, M. (1993). Implementing case management for a head and neck unit. *ORL–Head and Neck Nursing, 11*(2), 16–20.

*Janzen, V. D. (1987). Rhinological disorders in the elderly. *Journal of Otolaryngology, 15,* 228–230.

Keithley, J., & Kohn, C. (1992). Advances in nutritional care of medical-surgical patients. *MEDSURG Nursing, 1*(1), 13-21.

*Kersten, L. D. (1989). *Comprehensive respiratory nursing: A decision making approach.* Philadelphia: W. B. Saunders.

*Knapp, B. A. (1989). Nursing management of the patient requiring head and neck reconstructive surgery. In W. R. Panje (Ed.), *Musculocutaneous flap reconstruction of the head and neck.* New York: Raven Press.

Kryger, M. H. (Ed.) (1990). *Introduction to respiratory medicine* (2nd ed.). New York: Churchill Livingstone.

LaMuraglia, M. V., Meister, M., & Di Bona, N. (1991). Tracheal resection and reconstruction: Indications, surgical procedure, and postoperative care. *Heart & Lung, 20*(3), 245–254.

Lockhart, J. S., Troff, J. L., & Artim, L. S. (1992). Total laryngectomy and radical neck dissection: A case study. *AORN Journal, 55*(2), 458–459, 462–464, 466, 468–469, 471–473, 475–476, 478–479.

*Lockhart, J. S., & Griffin, C. (1986). Action stat! Epistaxis. *Nursing86, 16*(11), 33.

Maas, A. (1991). A model for quality of life after laryngectomy. *Social Science and Medicine, 33*(12), 1373–1377.

*Mapp, C. (1988). Trach care: Are you aware of all the dangers? *Nursing88, 18*(7), 34–43.

McCall, M. (1993). It killed George, or managing the peritonsillar abscess patient effectively. *ORL–Head and Neck Nursing, 11*(1), 10–12.

*Montanari, J., & Spearing, C. (1986). The fine art of measuring tracheal cuff pressure. *Nursing86, 16*(7), 46–49.

Norman, P. S. (1991). Allergic rhinitis: Combined therapy improves control. *Consultant, 31*(8), 25–29.

Pasterkamp, H., & Sanchez, I. (1992). Tracheal sounds in upper airway obstruction. *Chest, 102*(3), 963–965.

Pattern, B. C., & Holt, J. (1992). When your patient is allergic. *American Journal of Nursing, 92*(9), 58–61.

*Richardson, J. L., Graham, J. W., & Shelton, D. R. (1989, November). Social environment and adjustment after laryngectomy. *Health and Social Work,* 283–292.

Robbins, K. T. (1991). *Neck dissection classification and TNM staging of head and neck cancer.* American Academy of Otolaryngology–Head and Neck Surgery Foundation, Inc.

Saber, S. K. (1991). Nutritional management of intermaxillary fixation patients. *Advances in Clinical Care, 6*(5), 24–25.

Servodidio, C. A., Abramson, D. H., & Romanella, A. (1991). Self-assessment quiz . . . ethmoid sinus fracture. *Journal of Ophthalmic Nursing Technology, 10*(6), 273, 282.

Sievers, A. E. (1991). Decannulation of the patient with a tracheostomy. *Colleagues in Caring.* Irvine, CA: Shiley, Inc.

*Sievers, A. E. (1984). Nursing care. In P. J. Donald (Ed.), *Head and neck cancer: Management of the difficult case.* Philadelphia: W. B. Saunders.

*Sievers, A. E. (1984). Nutritional care. In P. J. Donald (Ed.), *Head and neck cancer: Management of the difficult case.* Philadelphia: W. B. Saunders.

Sievers, A. E., Leonard, R., & McKenzie, S. (1992). The safe use of an adaptive early feeding device for impaired patients. *ORL–Head and Neck Nursing, 10*(3), 17–19.

Sicola, V. R. (1992). Hat and me. *ORL–Head and Neck Nursing, 10*(2), 8–9.

Slavin, R. G. (1991). Management of sinusitis. *Journal of the American Geriatrics Society, 39*(2), 212–217.

Stam, H. J., Koopmans, J. P., & Mathieson, C. M. (1991). The psychosocial impact of a laryngectomy: A comprehensive assessment. *Journal of Psychosocial Oncology, 9*(3), 37–58.

Steuer, K. (1991). Facial fractures: Diagnosis to discharge. *AORN Journal, 54*(4), 773–777, 780–784, 786–787, 789–792.

*Thawley, S. E., Panje, W. R., Batsakis, J. G., & Lindberg, R. D. (1987). *Comprehensive management of head and neck tumors.* Philadelphia: W. B. Saunders.

Weber, M., & Reimer, M. (1993). Laryngectomy: Grieving disfigurement and dysfunction. *The Canadian Nurse, 89*(3), 31–34.

Weimert, T. A. (1992). Common ENT emergencies: The acute nose and throat, part 2. *Emergency Medicine, 24*(6), 26–28, 31–32, 34–36.

SUGGESTED READINGS

Hudak, M. (1993). Implementing case management for a head and neck unit. *ORL–Head and Neck Nursing, 11*(2), 16–20.

This valuable article reviews the process of case management by organizing the work process according to the case type and delivering the outlined care within a specified time frame. Using the client with laryngeal cancer and undergoing a total laryngectomy as an example, Hudak develops a critical pathway. This pathway targets elements of care over a defined period of time. This coordination of care ensures system knowledge of each client's progress and defines outcome goals.

LaMuraglia, M. V., et al. (1991). Tracheal resection and reconstruction: Indications, surgical procedure, and postoperative care. *Heart & Lung, 20*(3), 245–254.

The article discusses pathophysiology of tracheal conditions that might necessitate a tracheal resection and reconstruction. Preoperative diagnostic tests and preoperative teaching are reviewed. The detailed surgical procedure is described, as is the guardian suture, which secures the neck in a chin-to-chest position to reduce stress on the anastomosis. A comprehensive nursing care plan and a continuing education test are included.

Lockhart, J. S., et al. (1992). Total laryngectomy and radical neck dissection: A case study. *AORN Journal, 55*(2), 458–466+.

This comprehensive article covers statistics on laryngeal cancer, the various anatomic locations of tumors, diagnostic testing and staging. Much of the article follows Mr. Y., diagnosed with T4 N2 M0 Stage IV laryngeal cancer, from diagnosis through surgery and discharge. The surgery is described in a step-by-step fashion and includes intraoperative nursing roles. Specific nursing diagnoses for each phase of the case, along with description of the tracheoesophageal puncture to restore speech after total laryngectomy, are presented.

Steuer, K. (1991). Facial fractures: Diagnosis to discharge. *AORN Journal, 54*(4), 773–787+.

Initially, the article reviews the anatomy of the facial skeleton, then common fractures of the nasal bones, zygoma, mandible, maxilla (including Le Fort fractures), and the orbital rim. Various surgical procedures (tracheostomy, intramaxillary fixation, fracture elevation, intraosseous wiring, bone grafting) are described. Numerous figures are included.

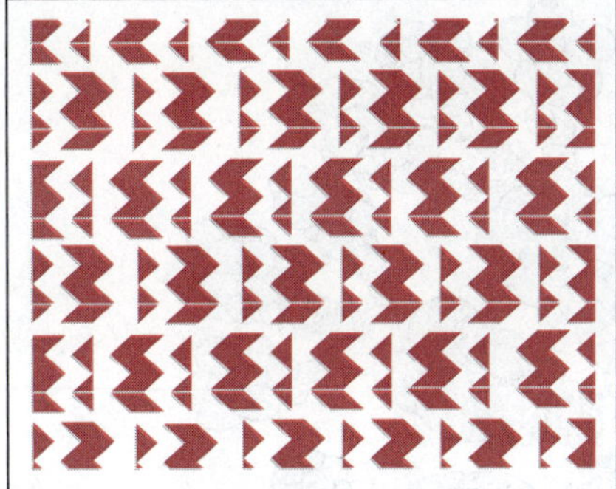

CHAPTER 30

Interventions for Clients with Lower Airway Problems

CHAPTER HIGHLIGHTS

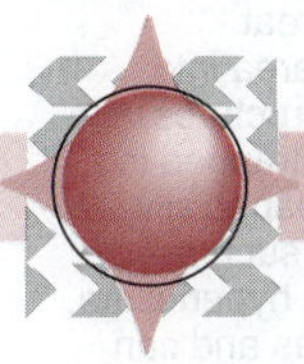

Disorders of the lower airways are common in adults. Some disorders may be aggravated by environmental irritants; others have a familial tendency. The major nursing diagnoses include Impaired Gas Exchange, Ineffective Breathing Pattern, and Ineffective Airway Clearance. For the elderly client with a respiratory disorder, some general nursing considerations are listed in Chart 30-1.

CHRONIC AIRFLOW LIMITATION

OVERVIEW

Chronic airflow limitation is the term for a group of chronic lung diseases including pulmonary emphysema, chronic bronchitis, and bronchial asthma. The previously used terms chronic obstructive pulmonary disease (COPD) and chronic obstructive lung disease (COLD) are becoming outdated. Experts have argued that these diseases are not truly "obstructive" and that chronic airflow limitation (CAL) is a more accurate descriptor.

PATHOPHYSIOLOGY

Even though most clients with respiratory problems present with two or more diseases (e.g., emphysema

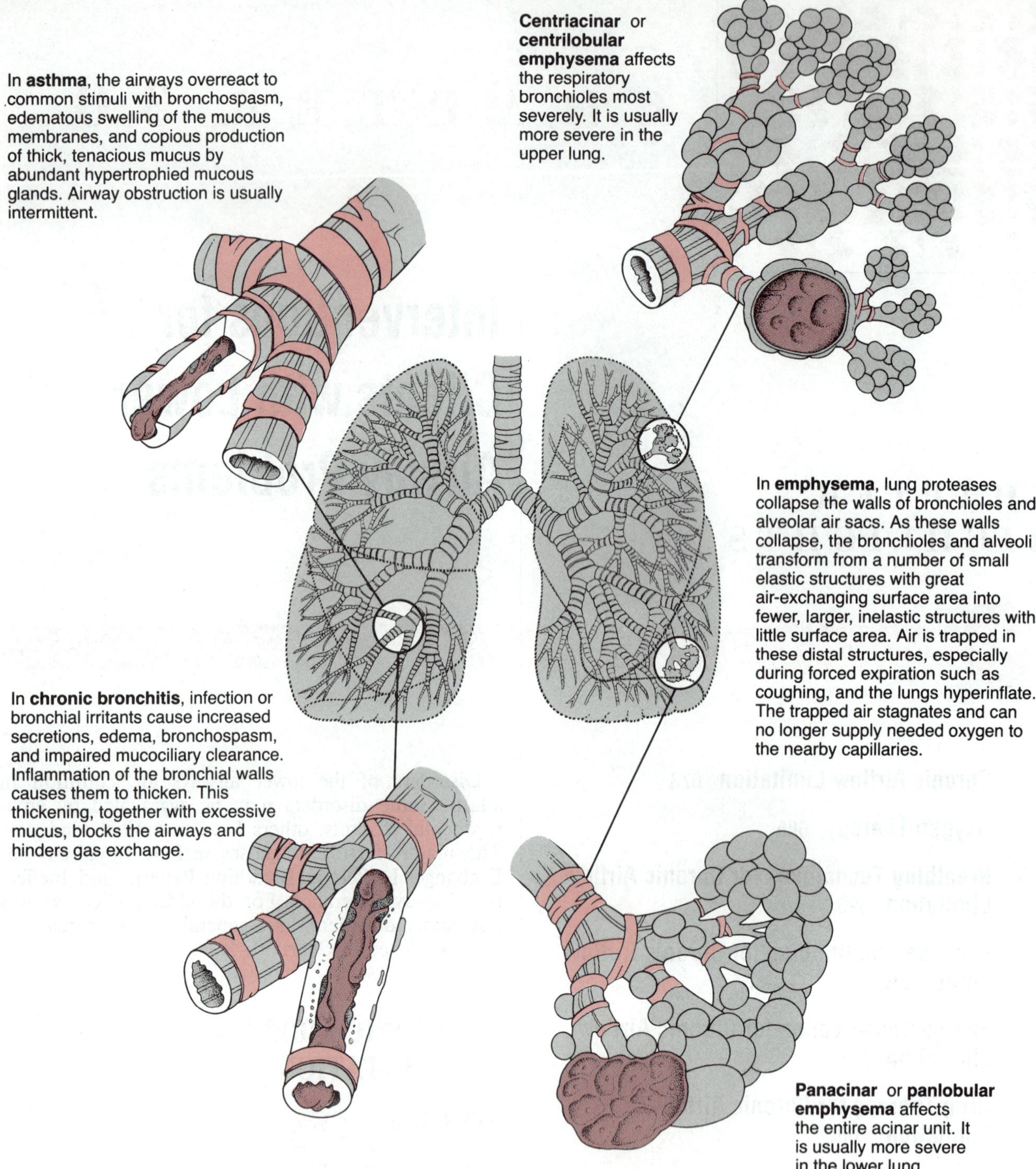

FIGURE 30–1 ♦ The pathophysiology of chronic airflow limitation.

and chronic bronchitis) at the same time, the pathophysiologic process of each disease is described separately (Fig. 30–1).

PULMONARY EMPHYSEMA

Pulmonary emphysema is characterized by the destruction of alveoli, the narrowing of small airways (bronchioles), and the trapping of air.

SPECIFIC PATHOLOGIC CHANGES Four pathologic changes occur in the client (see Fig. 30–1):

- Loss of lung elasticity. Proteases (lung enzymes) alter or destroy the alveoli and the small airways by breaking down elastin. As a result, the alveolar sacs lose their elasticity, and the small airways col-

CHART 30–1

Nursing Focus on the Elderly ◆ Respiratory Disorders

- Provide rest periods between such activities as bathing, meals, and ambulation.
- Place the client in an upright position for meals to prevent aspiration.
- Encourage nutritional fluid intake after the meal to promote increased calorie intake.
- Schedule medications around routine activities to increase medication compliance.
- Arrange chairs in strategic locations to allow the client with dyspnea to walk and rest as needed.
- Encourage prompt access to a health care facility for any sign or symptom of infection.
- Ensure that the client has received the pneumococcal vaccine.
- Encourage the client to have an annual flu vaccination.

lapse or narrow. Some alveoli are destroyed, whereas others remain enlarged.

- Hyperinflation of the lung. The enlarged alveoli prevent the lung from returning to its normal resting state during expiration.
- Formation of bullae. The alveolar walls deteriorate and connect to form bullae (air-filled spaces) that can be seen on x-ray examination.
- Small airway collapse and air trapping. As the client attempts to forcibly exhale air trapped in the enlarged alveoli, positive intrathoracic pressures collapse the small airways.

EFFECTS OF PATHOLOGIC CHANGES ON BREATHING Emphysema, like other CAL diseases, increases the work of breathing. In moderate to severe emphysema, the work of breathing is increased because the hyperinflated lung causes the diaphragm to flatten (Fig. 30–2). The flattened diaphragm requires the use of accessory respiratory muscles, such as the neck and abdominal muscles, during expiration when the diaphragm must rise against gravity. A healthy person uses about 65% of the diaphragm and 35% of the accessory muscles to breathe; clients with emphysema use about 30% of the diaphragm and 70% of the accessory muscles to breathe. Increased use of the accessory muscles for breathing increases the client's need for oxygen and may give the sensation of "air hunger." The client usually reacts by starting inspiration before expiration has been completed. The result is a dyspneic client with an inefficient and uncoordinated pattern of breathing.

EFFECTS OF PATHOLOGIC CHANGES ON GAS EXCHANGE In addition to air hunger, the increased work of breathing may affect gas exchange, which alters arterial blood gas (ABG) values. Arterial blood gases are not changed in the client with early or mild disease. However, clients with advanced disease often produce carbon dioxide faster than their ability to eliminate it; this situation causes carbon dioxide retention and chronic respiratory acidosis (see Chap. 18). In addition, the client with late-stage emphysema has a low arterial blood oxygen concentration (PaO_2) because it is difficult for oxygen to move from diseased lung tissue into the bloodstream.

CLASSIFICATION OF EMPHYSEMA Emphysema is classified according to the pattern of destruction and dilation of the gas-exchanging units, or acini, of the

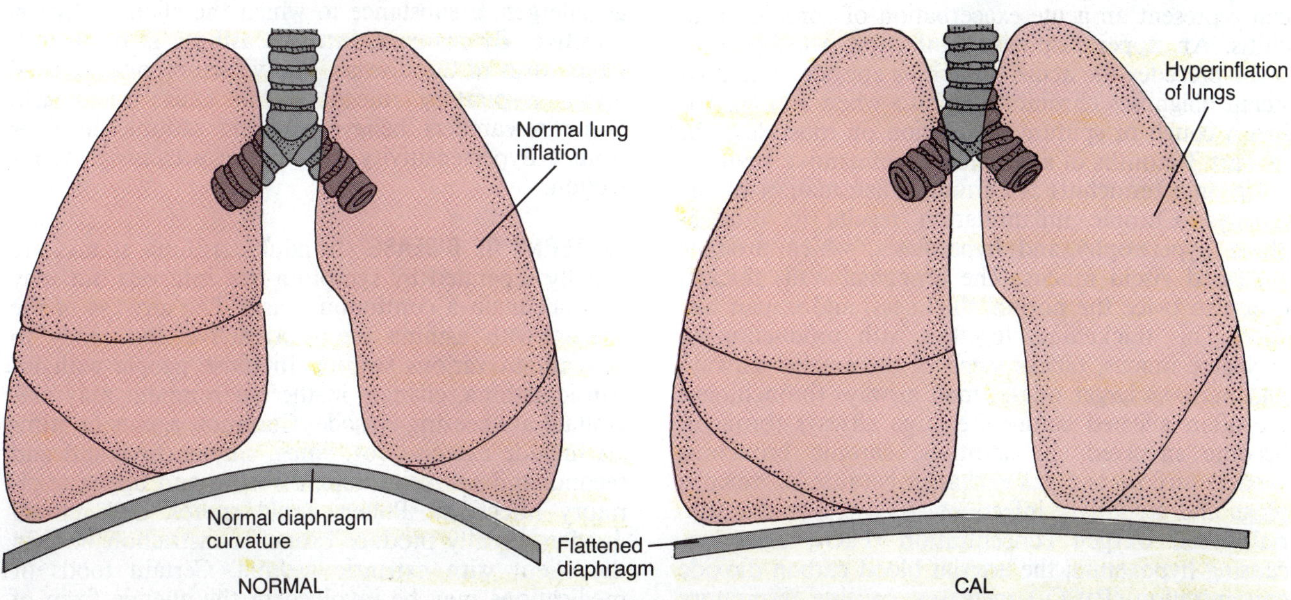

FIGURE 30–2 ◆ Comparison of diaphragm shape and lung inflation in the normal client and in the client with chronic airflow limitation.

lung. The patterns of emphysema may exist alone or in combination in the same lung. Emphysema can be divided into three types (see Fig. 30-1):

- Panlobular
- Centrilobular
- Paraseptal

Panlobular (panacinar) *emphysema* (PLE) involves destruction of the alveoli in the pulmonary acinus until only a few strands of tissue and blood vessels remain. Panacinar emphysema is a diffuse disease that is usually more severe in the lower lung area.

In *centrilobular* (centriacinar) *emphysema* (CLE), openings selectively develop in respiratory bronchioles and allow spaces to develop as tissue walls disintegrate. Although centrilobular emphysema is a diffuse disease process that commonly affects the upper portions of the lung most severely, damage to the acini varies greatly within the same lung segment.

In *paraseptal emphysema,* the disease is confined to the distal portion of the acinus; only alveolar ducts and alveoli are involved. This disease type tends to be localized and is associated with the formation of bullae. Spontaneous pneumothorax, with the formation of blebs, can result in the diseased lung area. Spontaneous pneumothorax is a collapse of a portion of the lung because of an opening from the lung side into the pleural space. A bleb is a collection of air within the pleura that is generally less than 1 to 2 cm.

ACUTE AND CHRONIC BRONCHITIS

Bronchitis results from exposure to infectious or noninfectious irritants, especially tobacco smoke. The irritant produces an inflammatory response, which causes vasodilation, congestion, mucosal edema, and bronchospasm. Unlike emphysema, bronchitis affects the small and large airways rather than the alveoli. Airflow may or may not be limited.

Acute bronchitis can occur as a single episode or can represent an acute exacerbation of chronic bronchitis. An upper respiratory infection, usually viral, often precedes the acute bronchitis episode. The physician diagnoses chronic bronchitis when a client has had a cough or sputum production on most days for at least 3 months of a year for 2 consecutive years.

Chronic bronchitis is chronic inflammation of the airways. Chronic inflammation results in mucous gland hypertrophy and hyperplasia, which produce increased viscid mucus. The bronchial walls thicken (often to twice the normal thickness) and impair airflow. This thickening, together with production of excessive mucus, blocks some of the smaller airways and narrows larger ones. Small airways (bronchioles) are often affected before the large airways (bronchi) become involved. In addition, chronic bronchitis hinders airflow and gas exchange because of mucous plugs and secondary infections. As a result, the arterial blood oxygen concentration (PaO_2) decreases, causing hypoxemia; the arterial blood carbon dioxide concentration ($PaCO_2$) increases, causing respiratory acidosis.

BRONCHIAL ASTHMA

Bronchial asthma is characterized by reversible airflow obstruction. It is primarily a disease of inflammation that precipitates bronchospasm. Asthma, like bronchitis, affects the airways, not the alveoli. Therefore, asthma does not typically lead to emphysema; however, asthma may coexist with emphysema and bronchitis.

Bronchial hyperresponsiveness is a cardinal feature of asthma. Once the client is exposed to the stimulus, chemical mediators are immediately released. Within minutes of being exposed, the client experiences:

- Dyspnea
- Wheezing and cough due to inflammation
- Increased mucus production
- Bronchospasm

This acute-phase reaction may subside quickly and be followed by a secondary decline in lung function called the late-phase response. Onset of the late phase is associated with inflammation. Airway obstruction lasts longer, the obstruction is less responsive to bronchodilator therapy, and airway reactivity increases.

Because inflammation plays the key role in asthma, anti-inflammatory therapy is the cornerstone for the control of asthma. Beta-agonists and other bronchodilator medications help control symptoms but have no effect on the underlying disease and do not alter inflammation or bronchial hyperreactivity (National Institute of Health, 1991). Asthma is a chronic disease that affects people of all ages and races. It not only is a disabling disease but can be fatal.

TYPES OF ASTHMA Asthma can be divided into extrinsic and intrinsic types. Extrinsic asthma (IgE-mediated), the allergic form of bronchial asthma, is seen more in children than in adults. The client experiences an asthma attack as a response to exposure to an allergen, a substance to which the client is hypersensitive. By contrast, intrinsic asthma is the nonallergic form of the disease. Many factors, often a viral upper respiratory infection, can cause an attack. Some researchers believe intrinsic asthma develops from a hypersensitivity to the viruses causing the infection.

PATTERNS OF DISEASE In adults, asthma attacks are usually separated by symptom-free intervals but may also occur on a continuous basis. The airways of the person with asthma are overreactive and ready to respond to various stimuli. In those people with intrinsic asthma, changes in the environment may precipitate a wheezing episode. Common agents or stimuli include exercise, fog, smog, smoke (firsthand and secondhand smoke), odors, aerosols, and upper respiratory infections. Pollen, mold spores, and animal danders usually produce bronchoconstriction only in the client with extrinsic asthma. Certain foods or medications may be involved in the allergic form of asthma as well (Chart 30-2). Emotional excitement,

CHART 30–2

Education Guide ◆ Asthma

- Avoid potential environmental asthma triggers, such as smoke, fireplaces, dust, mold, and weather changes (especially warm to cold, or sudden barometric changes).
- Avoid medications that could trigger asthma, for example, aspirin, nonsteroidal anti-inflammatory drugs (NSAIDs), and beta-blockers.
- Avoid food that has been prepared with monosodium glutamate (MSG) or metabisulfite.
- If you experience symptoms of exercise-induced asthma, use your bronchodilator inhaler 30 minutes before exercise to prevent or reduce bronchospasm.
- Be sure you know the proper technique and correct sequence when you use metered-dose inhalers.
- Be sure to get adequate rest and sleep.
- Reduce stress and anxiety; learn relaxation techniques; adopt coping mechanisms that have worked for you in the past.
- Wash all bedding with *hot* water to destroy the dust mite.
- Monitor your peak expiratory flow rates as you were instructed.
- Seek immediate emergency care if you experience any of the following:
  - Gray or blue fingertips or lips
  - Difficulty breathing, walking, or talking
  - Retractions of the neck, chest, or ribs
  - Nasal flaring
  - Failure of medications to control worsening symptoms
  - Peak expiratory flow rates declining steadily after treatment, or a flow rate 50% below your usual flow rate

anxiety, hormonal changes, and fatigue are not causes of asthma but may aggravate, initiate, or accompany an episode of wheezing or dyspnea (Gift & Cahill, 1990).

PATHOLOGY OF BRONCHOCONSTRICTION Inhaled agents stimulate the contraction of airway smooth muscle by different mechanisms. After being inhaled, the agent comes in contact with several different cells within the airway lumen before it reaches the airway smooth muscle. Some agents cause bronchoconstriction by *directly* stimulating the smooth muscle. The direct effects of many environmental stimuli disappear within a short distance of the airway lumen. These agents, then, are more likely to cause smooth muscle contraction indirectly by affecting *neural* pathways. Three neural pathways have been studied in environmentally produced bronchoconstriction: muscarinic, alpha-adrenergic, and neuropeptide.

The non-neural mechanisms of bronchoconstriction involve humoral cells: macrophages, eosinophils, and mast cells. Macrophages are present throughout the tracheobronchial tree. Eosinophils are the principal inflammatory cell in the pathophysiologic process of asthma. The extent of eosinophils in the sputum, peripheral circulation, and airway tissues correlates with severity of the disease. Mast cells in the lung release histamine and slow-reacting substance of anaphylaxis during allergic reactions, especially those caused by pollen.

COMPLICATIONS OF CHRONIC AIRFLOW LIMITATION

HYPOXEMIA Hypoxemia is defined as a PaO_2 of 55 mmHg or less, with an oxygen saturation of 85% or less. The client will experience subtle changes as hypoxemia ensues. Initially, the client may experience mood changes, be unable to concentrate, and be forgetful. Cyanosis is a late sign of hypoxemia.

RESPIRATORY ACIDOSIS Rising carbon dioxide levels in the arterial blood ($PaCO_2$) result in respiratory acidosis. Common signs of carbon dioxide retention (hypercapnia) include:

- Headache
- Fatigue
- Increased drowsiness and lethargy
- Dizziness
- Tachypnea/hyperventilation

RESPIRATORY INFECTIONS The client with chronic airflow limitation (CAL) is susceptible to respiratory infections. Acute respiratory infections cause increased production of mucus, increased irritability of bronchial smooth muscle, and edema of the involved mucosa. Airflow is limited, the work of breathing increases, and dyspnea results. A bacterial cause cannot be identified in most acute respiratory illnesses. However, severely compromised and debilitated clients with CAL are treated with antibiotics even when an organism has not been isolated. Some physicians prescribe antibiotics on an as-needed basis; the client self-administers the antibiotic according to changes in sputum appearance, which may indicate infection.

CARDIAC FAILURE Cardiac failure, especially cor pulmonale (right ventricular heart failure caused by pulmonary disease), must be considered in a client with worsening dyspnea. This complication is most frequently associated with chronic bronchitis, but clients with advanced emphysema are also likely to develop this problem. Detection of cor pulmonale (also called pulmonary heart disease) is difficult because its clinical signs are generally masked by those of the underlying lung disease. Signs and symptoms are listed in Chart 30-3.

Chronic airflow limitation (CAL) places a heavy workload on the heart, especially the right side of the heart, which is responsible for pumping blood into the lungs. As the disease progresses, the amount of oxygen in the blood decreases, which causes major blood vessels in the lung to constrict. To pump blood through these narrowed vessels, the right side of the heart must generate high pressures. In response to

CHART 30-3

Key Features of Cor Pulmonale (Pulmonary Heart Disease)

- Hypoxia and hypoxemia
- Increasing dyspnea
- Fatigue
- Weakness
- Enlarged and tender liver
- Warm cyanotic extremities with bounding pulses
- Cyanotic lips
- Distended neck veins
- Right ventricular enlargement (hypertrophy)
- Lower sternal or epigastric pulsations
- Gastrointestinal disturbances, such as nausea or anorexia
- Dependent edema
- Metabolic and respiratory acidosis
- Pulmonary hypertension

this heavy workload, the right chambers of the heart enlarge and thicken, which causes right-sided heart failure, or cor pulmonale. Heart failure is frequently a cause of death in clients with CAL. (Treatment for right-sided heart failure is discussed in Chapter 34.)

CARDIAC DYSRHYTHMIAS Clients with CAL frequently experience cardiac dysrhythmias. These dysrhythmias may be a result of hypoxemia (from decreased oxygen to the heart muscle), other cardiac disease, the effect of drugs, or respiratory acidosis (see Chap. 34). Treatment for dysrhythmias is described in Chapter 33.

STATUS ASTHMATICUS Status asthmaticus is a major complication associated with bronchial asthma. It is a severe, potentially life-threatening acute episode of airway obstruction that tends to intensify once it begins and often does not respond to common therapy. The client arrives in the emergency department of the hospital with extremely labored breathing and wheezing. Use of accessory muscles for breathing and distention of neck veins are commonly noted. If the condition is not reversed, the client can experience cor pulmonale, pneumothorax and eventually cardiac or respiratory arrest. Intravenous fluids, potent bronchodilators, steroids (to decrease inflammation), epinephrine, and oxygen are administered immediately in an attempt to reverse the acute condition. The nurse also prepares for emergency intubation. When wheezing diminishes, management is similar to that for any client with chronic airflow limitation.

ETIOLOGY

CIGARETTE SMOKING

Smoking is the most important risk factor for chronic airflow limitation (CAL). The client with 8 pack-years usually has obstructive lung changes but no signs and symptoms of disease. The client with 20 or more pack-years typically has CAL (Kersten, 1989).

Transcultural Considerations The prevalence of smoking remains higher among African-Americans, blue-collar workers, and less educated people than in the overall population of the United States. Approximations of smoking prevalence range from 37% among the least educated people to 14% among the most educated. Smoking prevalence is highest among Northern Plains Native Americans (42% to 70%) and Alaskan Natives (56%). The overall prevalence of smoking for both men and women has decreased over the past two decades, but the decrease for women has been proportionately less than that for men. The prevalence of smoking is approximately 28% for men and 23% for women (National Center for Health Statistics, 1993).

The harmful effects of tobacco result in part because inhaled smoke stimulates excess release of the enzyme elastase protease from cells that are normally found in the lung. The elastase protease breaks down elastin, the major component in alveoli. By impairing the action of cilia, smoking also inhibits the cilia from clearing the tracheobronchial tree of mucus, cellular debris, and fluid.

In addition to the increased risk of chronic airflow limitation from active smoking, much attention has been given to passive smoking, or secondhand smoke. Although a person may not smoke, exposure to smoke, particularly in a small or confined space, may contribute to the development of upper and lower respiratory problems, including CAL. As a result of this finding, there has been a movement in the United States to designate smoking and nonsmoking areas and to create smoke-free environments.

FAMILY HISTORY

Emphysema and chronic bronchitis occur in families more often than would be expected by chance. This may be related to family smoking habits. However, in some people, a genetic defect results in decreased levels of the substance $alpha_1$-antitrypsin. $Alpha_1$-antitrypsin normally works to inhibit or prevent proteases from breaking down the elastic tissue (alveoli) of the lungs. When the amount of $alpha_1$-antitrypsin is decreased, more damage can be done by the proteases.

The client with $alpha_1$-antitrypsin deficiency emphysema is frequently young, has rapidly progressive pulmonary disease, and may have the disease in the absence of smoking. Panlobular emphysema is typically seen in clients with $alpha_1$-antitrypsin deficiency. The physician prescribes prolastin, an emzyme replacement.

Other CAL diseases also have a strong familial association:

- Asthma, especially extrinsic asthma, tends to occur in families. Intrinsic asthma may occur in clients with a family or personal history of allergies.

- Cystic fibrosis, an inherited autosomal recessive disease, is often discussed in relation to CAL.

Although cystic fibrosis involves many organs besides the lungs (sweat glands and the pancreas), it is the main cause of chronic lung disease in children. These clients are now being diagnosed earlier and are living into their 30s and even 40s. Cystic fibrosis is no longer just a disease of children. Treatment is aimed at clearing secretions, preventing airway obstruction, and preventing and treating infection. More information on cystic fibrosis can be found in current pediatric textbooks.

AIR POLLUTION

It appears at present that the effect of air pollution is additive to tobacco exposure. Air pollution alone plays only a relatively small role in clients with emphysema and chronic bronchitis. For the client with asthma, however, increased air pollution can cause an asthma attack.

INCIDENCE/PREVALENCE

The prevalence of chronic bronchitis and emphysema has been estimated around 13.5 million and 2 million, respectively, in the United States. Another 12 million suffer from asthma, and 10 million have acute bronchitis (Benson and Marano, 1994). Since 1979, the number of people who suffer from these conditions has doubled. More than 30,000 children and young adults are affected by cystic fibrosis.

Chronic airflow limitation (CAL) is responsible for a greater restriction of activity than is any other major disease category. For example, nearly 20% of people with asthma have some limitation in their daily activities.

The prevalence of smoking among various groups was discussed under Etiology, and the relationship between smoking and CAL has already been addressed. Although CAL is seen more in men, the incidence among women is increasing. CAL typically affects the middle-aged and elderly adult. Asthma is seen in the young adult as well. In 1990, more than 86,000 deaths occurred in the United States from chronic pulmonary disease (National Center for Health Statistics, 1993).

COLLABORATIVE MANAGEMENT

ASSESSMENT

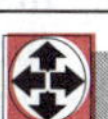

HISTORY

DEMOGRAPHIC FACTORS The nurse considers age, sex, and ethnic/cultural background when taking a history from a client who has, or is suspected of having, chronic airflow limitation (CAL). Each of these factors can place the client at risk for CAL. For example, CAL is seen more often in the elderly male client. The nurse also reviews family history because certain types of CAL diseases, especially extrinsic asthma and panlobular emphysema, occur in families.

The nurse obtains a thorough smoking history, if appropriate. Cigarette smoking tends to be the most harmful, but the effects of cigarette smoking vary from person to person. The nurse takes a careful smoking history, which includes:

- The length of time the client has smoked
- The number of packs or amount of tobacco smoked daily
- The type of cigarette or other tobacco smoked (for tar and nicotine content)

The nurse then quantifies this information into pack-years (for cigarette smokers) as follows:

$$\text{years of smoking} \times \text{packs smoked per day} = \text{pack-years}$$

NATURE OF DISEASE PRESENTATION The nurse asks the client to discuss his or her chief complaint and pays particular attention to the client's ability to answer questions. Can the client give clear answers and state them in complete sentences? Or is breathlessness so severe that the client gives one- or two-word answers to the questions?

Cough, dyspnea, and wheezing are the three classic signs and symptoms of CAL, although they occur in various combinations and intensity. The nurse questions the client about each of these symptoms. Early signs and symptoms of CAL include mild shortness of breath, especially on exertion (also known as dyspnea on exertion, or DOE), and a slight cough in the morning. A long-term cough is associated most often with chronic bronchitis. The nurse determines the coughing pattern by asking the client:

- When, if ever, are you troubled by coughing?
- How does the cough sound? Dry? Hacking? Loose?
- Is the cough worse in the morning or at night?
- Is the cough worse after you smoke or are exposed to irritants?

The client's cough may be productive or nonproductive of sputum. If the cough is productive, the nurse asks whether sputum is clear or colored and how much is expectorated each day. The sputum should be clear. The nurse also asks the client to recall the time of day when most sputum is expectorated. Smokers typically have a productive cough when they get up in the morning, nonsmokers generally do not. The nurse asks whether sputum production has increased or changed.

Shortness of breath and coughing may be much worse when the client with CAL experiences an acute respiratory tract infection. The sputum usually turns from clear to yellowish or greenish as a result of the infection, and wheezing is likely to occur. Wheezing is more commonly associated with asthma.

The nurse determines how long any of the signs and symptoms have been present, whether they are intermittent or continuous, and whether they have become progressively worse over time. The accompanying Research Applications for Nursing addresses the client's perception of the severity of his or her symptoms. Clients with asthma describe their signs and symptoms as intermittent; clients with chronic bronchitis and emphysema describe their signs and symptoms as continuous and getting worse.

In addition to determining the onset, duration, and severity of the classic symptoms of CAL, the nurse always asks the client about the relationship between activity tolerance and dyspnea. The client is asked to compare his or her activity level and shortness of breath with those of a month ago and a year ago. Likewise, the nurse asks about any difficulty with eating and sleeping. Many clients sleep in a semisitting position because breathlessness prevents them from lying down (orthopnea).

The nurse weighs the client at admission and compares this weight with previous weights. Clients with CAL have increased metabolic requirements associated with the increased work of breathing. The increased metabolic requirements plus bothersome dyspnea often result in poor food intake and inadequate nutrition. The nurse asks the client to recall a typical day's meals and fluid intake. The nurse determines whether the client uses any breathing exercises (such as pursed-lip breathing) during dyspneic episodes to help make eating easier and asks for a demonstration. The nurse obtains additional information about the client's usual daily activities and any difficulty with sleeping, bathing, dressing, or sexual activities.

PHYSICAL ASSESSMENT/CLINICAL MANIFESTATIONS

Regardless of the client's specific chronic airflow limitation (CAL) disease, the nurse inspects the chest to determine the breathing rate and pattern. Clients with respiratory muscle fatigue typically breathe with rapid, shallow respirations. The respiratory rate could be as high as 40 to 50 breaths per minute. The nurse observes the client's breathing to determine the use of accessory muscles (abdominal and neck) and abnormal retractions. Three breathing patterns are commonly seen in clients with respiratory muscle fatigue (Table 30–1):

- Abdominal paradox
- Respiratory alternans
- Asynchronous breathing

The nurse systematically palpates the client's anterior chest, feeling for areas of tenderness and abnormal retractions or moves and feeling for symmetric chest expansion. In the client with emphysema, the nurse expects to find limited excursion (movement) of the diaphragm because it is typically flattened and below its usual resting state. In palpating the posterior chest for tactile fremitus (vibrations felt while the

RESEARCH APPLICATIONS FOR NURSING

Subjective Assessments of Asthmatic Symptoms May Be Accurate

Janson-Bjerklie, S., Ferketich, S., Benner, P., & Becker, G. (1992). Clinical markers of asthma severity and risk: Importance of subjective as well as objective markers. *Heart & Lung, 21*(3), 265–272.

In addition to experiencing severe anxiety associated with life-threatening stressors, clients with asthma may be subjected to the condescending attitudes of health care professionals.

Because emotions are thought to aggravate the severity of an asthma attack, some health care providers might assume that emotions also cause the acute symptoms of asthma. Such unfounded beliefs interfere with the accuracy of the health assessment, leading the health care professional to ignore the client's subjective judgment of the severity and risk of symptoms.

These investigators observed the course of 95 asthmatic adults who kept an asthma symptoms diary and measured their peak expiratory flow rates twice daily with a peak flowmeter. The study showed that the subjective assessments clients with asthma make about the severity and risk of their symptoms are accurate, closely matching objective clinical measures of the risk and severity of asthma attacks. Nineteen subjects visited the emergency department a total of 29 times with what they judged to be severe asthma attacks, and nine visits were severe enough to result in hospital admission. Because these clients had reported previously negative experiences with the attitudes of the emergency department health care providers, they saw coming to the emergency department as a last resort and a major concession to their illness. Instead, they tried a wide range of self-care strategies, such as drinking hot liquids, taking medication, self-massage, and self-talk, before deciding on an emergency department visit.

Critique There were many variables in this study, and the reliability and validity of some of the instruments were not clearly discussed. There could have been more discussion about those who visited the emergency department versus those who did not as well as about those clients who visited the emergency department but were not admitted to the hospital.

Possible nursing implications Because the nurse is often the first health care professional to assess the client in asthmatic distress who comes to the emergency department, the nurse should remember that first impressions have a lasting impact. The nurse should take the subjective statements of the client with asthma seriously and incorporate the client's symptoms and behavioral cues into the nursing assessment. Not only will the accuracy of the assessment improve, but the quality and effectiveness of nursing interventions are likely to be enhanced as well.

TABLE 30–1 Three Breathing Patterns Commonly Seen in Clients with Respiratory Muscle Fatigue

- Abdominal paradox: the diaphragm is nonfunctional; inspiration is accomplished by the intercostal and abdominal accessory muscles
- Respiratory alternans: diaphragmatic breathing alternates with abdominal paradox; may serve to rest the diaphragm
- Asynchronous breathing: the chest wall motion is unorganized; reflects the uncoordinated activity of fatigued muscles

client speaks), the nurse notes decreased fremitus when the client says "ninety-nine" because vibrations are not transmitted through obstructed airways.

The nurse percusses the chest, anteriorly and posteriorly, for hyperresonance in the client with emphysema related to trapped air in the alveoli. On percussion of the anterior chest, hyperresonance is often easily identified over the area of usual cardiac dullness.

The nurse then auscultates the chest to determine the depth of inspiration and to listen for adventitious breath sounds. Crackles are associated with emphysema and chronic bronchitis; wheezes are most commonly heard in a client with asthma. The nurse notes the pitch and location of the sound as well as where in the respiratory cycle the sound is heard. A silent chest may indicate airflow obstruction or pneumothorax.

In addition to assessing breathing patterns and breath sounds, the nurse assesses for signs and symptoms of CAL complications. The nurse can detect early signs of hypoxemia by assessing the client's level of consciousness every 8 hours. With a concurrent respiratory infection, the client may have fever and sputum changes. Because cardiac complications are likely, the nurse determines heart rate and rhythm. The nurse assesses for swelling of the feet and ankles (dependent edema) or other signs and symptoms of right-sided heart failure (see Chart 30–1 and Chap. 34).

The nurse also assesses for signs and symptoms of the following specific CAL diseases.

EMPHYSEMA The most common clinical manifestation experienced by the client with emphysema is dyspnea. As the disease progresses, dyspnea worsens. Although the focus of discussions among health care professionals about dyspnea is varied, most agree there is both a subjective and an objective component to dyspnea. The nurse assesses the degree of dyspnea by questioning the client, but this may aggravate the problem. Another approach the nurse can use is an assessment tool called a Visual Analog Dyspnea Scale (VADS). The VADS is a straight line with verbal anchors at the beginning and end of a 100-mm line. The nurse asks the client to place a mark on the line to indicate his or her breathing difficulty. The Modified Borg Scale, a 10-point scale that rates breathlessness from nothing at all to maximal, is also used to rate perceived breathlessness. Figure 30–3 illustrates an assessment guide that combines subjective and objective assessments. The nurse uses these scales to assess dyspnea, determine the effectiveness of bronchodilator and other therapy, and pace the client's activities.

In advanced disease, the client becomes orthopneic, that is, the client must be in a sitting position, often leaning forward with his or her arms over several pillows or an overbed table (Fig. 30–4) to breathe easier. The nurse observes for orthopnea.

The nurse also assesses for cough, which may produce only minimal sputum, and examines the client's chest, which usually has an altered shape known as a barrel chest (Fig. 30–5). In a client with a barrel chest, the ratio between the anteroposterior (AP) diameter of the chest and its lateral (transverse) diameter is 2:2 rather than the normal ratio of 1:2. This change in shape results from hyperinflation of alveoli and flattening of the diaphragm, which are typical of emphysema.

Dyspnea Assessment Guide

Direct Measure of Dyspnea

Indicate the amount of shortness of breath you are having at this time by marking the line.

shortness of breath as bad as can be

no shortness of breath

Subjective Symptoms

On a scale of 0–4 with 0 indicating no distress and 4 indicating much distress, how much are you presently distressed by: *(circle answer).*

poor appetite	0	1	2	3	4
worn out or weak	0	1	2	3	4
suffocation	0	1	2	3	4
tightness	0	1	2	3	4
congestion	0	1	2	3	4
a feeling of panic or anxiety	0	1	2	3	4

Objective Sign

Rise of the clavicle during inspiration:
ABSENT = not detected
MILD = seen but not pronounced
SEVERE = pronounced

FIGURE 30–3 ◆ An example of a dyspnea assessment tool. (Redrawn from Gift, A. G. [1989]. A dyspnea assessment guide. *Critical Care Nurse, 9*[8], 79.)

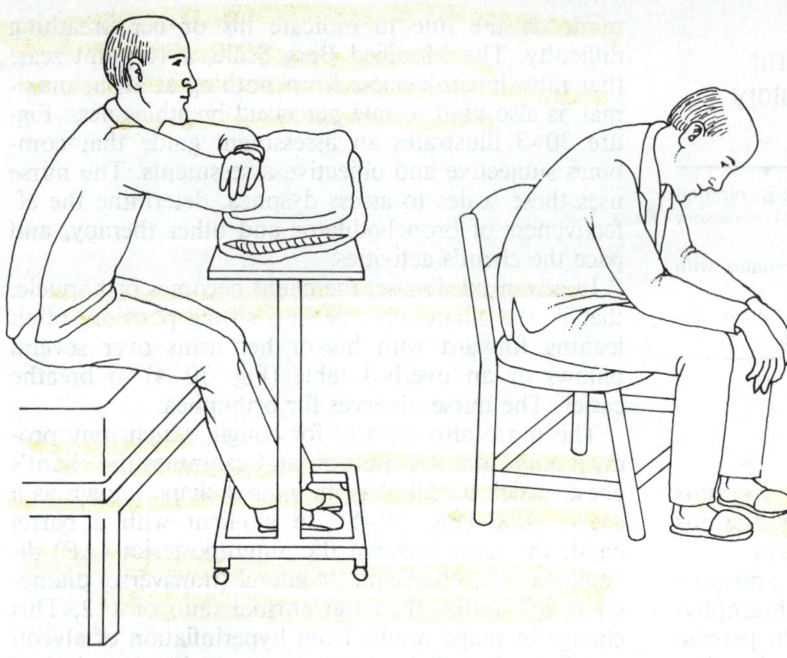

Sitting on the edge of a bed with the arms folded and placed on two or three pillows positioned over a nightstand.

Sitting in a chair with the feet spread a shoulder-width apart and leaning forward with the elbows on the knees. Arms and hands are relaxed.

FIGURE 30-4 ◆ Orthopnea positions that clients with chronic airflow limitation can assume to ease the work of breathing.

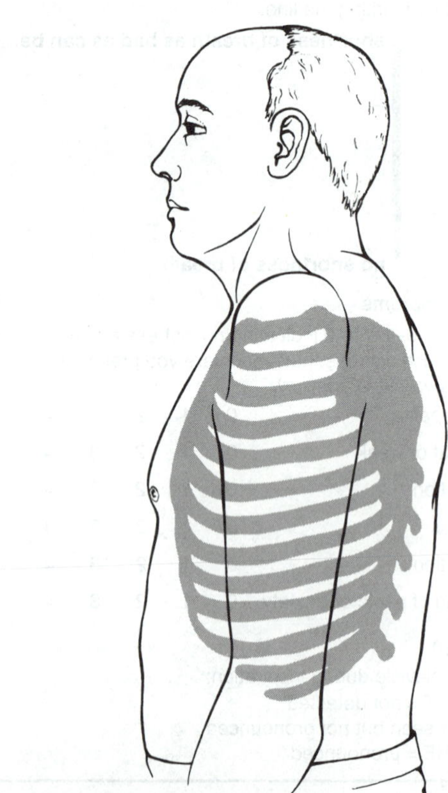

FIGURE 30-5 ◆ Typical barrel chest in a client with chronic airflow limitation.

The client with emphysema may be referred to as a "pink puffer." Because arterial oxygen levels do not change remarkably until the terminal stage, the client is not usually cyanotic until then. Instead, the nurse observes a pinkish skin color (most easily observed if the client has light-colored skin). The pink puffer also appears cachectic, is typically malnourished, and complains of a chronic cough and worsening dyspnea.

Inadequate nutrition in clients with CAL, particularly elderly clients with emphysema, has been documented since the early 1960s. Malnutrition in the elderly client with CAL is a vicious cycle. The dyspnea, fatigue, abdominal bloating, and sputum production prevent the client from wanting to prepare or eat a meal. However, in malnutrition, lung tissue and respiratory muscle further deteriorate, which makes breathing even more difficult.

In addition to promoting structural changes, malnutrition impairs the immune system. The client is then more likely to develop a respiratory infection that can be life threatening in the presence of CAL. This problem is particularly critical for the elderly client, who typically has a compromised immune system as a normal change associated with aging.

CHRONIC BRONCHITIS The client with chronic bronchitis is often a "blue bloater." The bronchitic client typically has a cyanotic, or blue-tinged, dusky appearance and complains of excessive sputum production. The nurse observes the client for cyanosis, delayed capillary refill, and clubbing of the fingers (Fig.

30–6), which indicate chronically decreased arterial oxygen levels. Clubbing is most often associated with a compensatory polycythemia.

BRONCHIAL ASTHMA During an asthma attack, the nurse assesses the client for dyspnea, wheezing, and coughing. The cough is usually productive if the client also has an upper respiratory tract infection. The client complains of chest tightness and a feeling of suffocation. Between attacks, the client's signs and symptoms usually disappear.

PSYCHOSOCIAL ASSESSMENT

Like any chronic disease, chronic airflow limitation (CAL) affects all aspects of a person's life: social, economic, and psychologic.

SOCIAL ASPECTS CAL can affect socialization in two ways:

1. Friends may avoid the client because of annoying coughs, excessive sputum, or dyspnea.
2. The client may choose to be isolated because dyspnea interferes with his or her ability to socialize with friends.

The nurse questions the client about interests and hobbies but cautions the client to avoid exposure to irritants, such as aerosols, smoke, and the harsh chemicals used to build or refinish furniture.

The client is also questioned about home conditions. The nurse determines whether the client lives near a constant source of air pollution, such as a chemical factory or a freeway. Crowded living conditions promote the transmission of communicable respiratory diseases. Exposure to such animals as cats, dogs, and hamsters may cause allergic responses or asthma attacks.

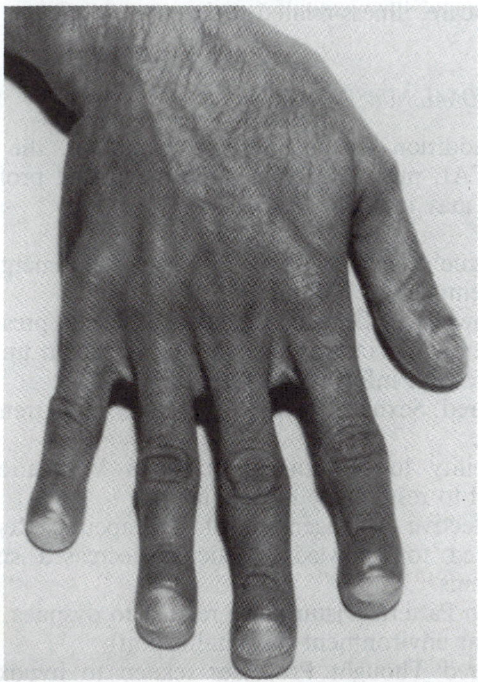

FIGURE 30–6 ◆ Clubbing. (From Hinshaw, H., & Murray, J. [1980]. *Diseases of the chest* [4th ed]. Philadelphia: W. B. Saunders.)

ECONOMIC ASPECTS The client's economic status may be affected by the disease. Both income and health insurance coverage are concerns for the client. If the client is the head of the household, severe CAL may require a role reversal with the spouse or mate. This change may have a negative impact on the client's self-image. When the client is employed, the nurse questions him or her about on-the-job exposure to cigarette smoke or to other substances that may irritate the respiratory system.

PSYCHOLOGIC ASPECTS The nurse assesses the psychologic impact of CAL and the client's ability to cope with chronic disease. Anxiety and fear related to episodes of dyspnea and feelings of breathlessness directly influence the client's ability to participate in a full life. Work, family, social, and sexual roles can be affected. The nurse asks whether the client is aware of support groups sponsored by the American Lung Association (ALA). Various hospitals and physicians' offices also offer group support.

LABORATORY ASSESSMENT

Arterial blood gas (ABG) values identify abnormalities of oxygenation, ventilation, and acid-base status. The nurse compares serial, or repeated, ABG values to assess changes in the client's status over time. In general, as CAL progresses, the amount of oxygen in the blood decreases (hypoxemia), and the amount of carbon dioxide in the blood increases (hypercarbia). Chronic respiratory acidosis (increased $PaCO_2$) then results, with metabolic alkalosis (increased arterial bicarbonate) occurring as compensation. Not all clients with CAL are carbon dioxide retainers, even when hypoxemia is present. Carbon dioxide is more easily diffused across the alveolar membrane than oxygen is.

Sputum samples are collected for culture from clients who exhibit signs of an acute respiratory tract infection. A bacterial cause cannot be identified in most acute respiratory illnesses. A white blood cell count may help identify leukocytosis.

Other blood tests that may be indicated in clients with CAL include hemoglobin, hematocrit, and red blood cell count to determine polycythemia (a compensatory increase in red blood cells in the chronically hypoxic client). The eosinophil count on the white blood cell differential is often increased in the client with extrinsic (allergic) asthma.

RADIOGRAPHIC ASSESSMENT

The physician orders routine chest x-rays to rule out other chest diseases and to determine the progress of clients with respiratory tract infections and chronic disease. In a client with advanced emphysema, chest x-rays usually show marked overinflation and a flattened diaphragm. Chest x-rays may not be helpful in the diagnosis of early or moderate disease, however.

OTHER DIAGNOSTIC ASSESSMENT

CAL is classified from mild to severe on the basis of results of pulmonary function tests (PFTs). Airflow rates and lung volume measurements help distinguish airway disease from restrictive patterns that are typical of interstitial lung disease. The three major components of PFTs are measurements that determine lung volumes, flow volume curves, and diffusion capacity. Each test is performed before and after the client inhales a bronchodilator agent. In the client with asthma, an improvement in abnormal results is usually observed after inhalation of a bronchodilator. If no reversibility is seen after bronchodilator treatment, however, the diagnosis of asthma cannot be excluded.

Three lung volume measurements most relevant to CAL are:

- Vital capacity (VC)
- Residual volume (RV)
- Total lung capacity (TLC)

Although most of the measured lung volumes or capacities change to some degree with chronic lung disease, residual volume usually increases markedly. This increase reflects the trapped, stagnant air remaining in the lungs.

Flow volume curves measure the client's ability to move air into and out of the lung. The rate of airflow out of the lungs during a rapid, forceful, and complete expiration from total lung capacity to residual volume (forced expiratory volume, or FEV) indirectly measures the flow-resistive properties of the lung. A diagnosis of chronic lung disease is based primarily on the FEV_1 (the FEV in the first second of expiration). FEV_1 can also be expressed as a percentage of the forced vital capacity (FVC). As the disease progresses, the ratio of FEV_1 to FVC becomes smaller.

The third part of pulmonary function testing is diffusion, formerly called the "diffusing" capacity of the lung. This test measures how well a test gas (carbon monoxide) diffuses across the alveolar-capillary membrane and combines with the hemoglobin of red blood cells. In emphysema, the decrease in diffusion ability results from the destruction of alveolar walls, which leads to a significant decrease in surface area for diffusion of gas into the blood. In asthma and bronchitis, even though lung volumes are increased, the diffusion capacity is usually normal.

Pulmonary function tests are further discussed in Chapter 28 and outlined in Table 28–6. Typical pulmonary function findings in CAL are given in Table 30–2.

Clients with CAL may have a decreased oxygen saturation, often as low as 91%. Pulse oximetry results lower than 91% (and certainly below 86%) may be considered an emergency necessitating immediate treatment. Chapter 28 contains more information on pulse oximetry.

ANALYSIS

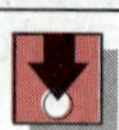

COMMON NURSING DIAGNOSES

The most common nursing diagnoses for clients with chronic airflow limitation (CAL) are:

1. Impaired Gas Exchange related to alveolar membrane changes, airflow limitation, respiratory muscle fatigue, excess mucus production
2. Ineffective Breathing Pattern related to airflow obstruction (narrowed airways), fatigue, and decreased energy
3. Ineffective Airway Clearance related to excessive secretions, fatigue and decreased energy, ineffective cough
4. Altered Nutrition: Less than Body Requirements related to dyspnea, excessive secretions, anorexia, and fatigue
5. Anxiety related to loss of control during dyspneic episodes or asthma attacks, dyspnea, change in health status, and situational crisis
6. Activity Intolerance related to fatigue, dyspnea, and an imbalance between oxygen supply and demand
7. High Risk for Infection related to retained secretions, ineffective airway clearance
8. Powerlessness related to difficulty in performing self-care, illness-related regimen

ADDITIONAL NURSING DIAGNOSES

In addition to the common diagnoses, the client with CAL may also have other associated problems, which may include:

- Fatigue related to change in metabolic energy, hypoxemia
- Knowledge Deficit (disease process, prescribed treatments, activity limitations) related to unfamiliarity with information resources
- Altered Sexuality Patterns related to extreme fatigue
- Inability to Sustain Spontaneous Ventilation related to respiratory muscle fatigue
- Ineffective Management of Therapeutic Regimen related to knowledge deficits, decreased support systems
- Sleep Pattern Disturbance related to dyspnea, unfamiliar environment (hospitalization)
- Altered Thought Processes related to hypoxemia, sleep deprivation

TABLE 30–2 Pulmonary Function Findings in Chronic Airflow Limitation

Test	Findings
Residual volume (RV): the volume of gas remaining in the lungs after a maximal expiration	• Loss of elastic recoil causes RV to be increased in emphysema and chronic bronchitis because of the narrowing and obstruction of airways.
Total lung capacity (TLC): the total amount of gas in the lungs at the end of a maximal inspiration	• TLC is increased in emphysematous clients because of loss of elastic recoil. TLC is normal in clients with chronic bronchitis.
Vital capacity (VC): the maximal amount of gas that can be expired after a maximal inspiration	• VC may be normal or decreased in the client with CAL.
Forced vital capacity (FVC): VC that is produced from a maximal forced expiratory effort	• FVC is often increased in CAL clients secondary to air trapping.
Forced expiratory volume (FEV_1, FEV_2): volume of air that is exhaled during a specified time (in seconds) while measuring FVC	• FEV mainly reflects resistance in large airways and is usually reduced in the client with CAL.
Functional residual capacity (FRC): the amount of gas remaining in the lungs at the end of a tidal expiration	• FRC is increased in clients with chronic bronchitis if obstruction is severe.
Diffusion: measure of carbon monoxide uptake across the alveolar capillary membrane	• The diffusion value is decreased in severe emphysema. Chronic bronchitis has little effect on diffusion.

PLANNING AND IMPLEMENTATION

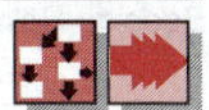

IMPAIRED GAS EXCHANGE

PLANNING: CLIENT GOALS The primary goal is for the client to attain and maintain PaO_2 (or oxygen saturation) and $PaCO_2$ levels within normal ranges. The minimum goal for most clients is a PaO_2 of 55 to 60 mmHg and an oxygen saturation between 91% and 95%, but this goal varies according to the client's age, attitude, and disease process.

Other goals include that the client will:

- Demonstrate a decrease in tachycardia and confusion (from the hypoxemia)
- State that fatigue is reduced
- Demonstrate techniques and methods that support improved oxygenation without carbon dioxide retention

Some facilities have created clinical pathways to guide the planning of care for the client with asthma. For an example, see pages 686 and 687.

INTERVENTIONS The nurse assesses the client at frequent intervals (every 2 to 4 hours), especially during the acute phase of the illness. The nurse provides the prescribed oxygen, assesses the client's response to treatment, and intervenes to prevent complications. Additional interventions can be found in the Client Care Plan.

If the client's condition continues to deteriorate despite treatment, more aggressive therapy is required. Intubation and mechanical ventilation may be necessary for clients in respiratory failure, such as those who are unable to sustain spontaneous ventilation. Chapter 31 discusses mechanical ventilation in detail.

Maintaining Airway Patency The nurse's first intervention to improve gas exchange is to maintain a patent airway. The nurse maintains the client's head and neck in alignment, assists the client in liquefying secretions, and clears the airway of secretions. (More information on airway obstruction can be found in Chapter 29.)

Oxygen Therapy Oxygen (O_2) is a potent drug prescribed by the physician for relief of symptoms of hypoxia (inability to get sufficient oxygen into the lungs) and its resultant hypoxemia (decreased tissue oxygenation). Arterial blood gas (ABG) analysis is the best tool for determining the need for oxygen therapy and for evaluating its effects. Oxygen need can also be determined by noninvasive monitoring, such as pulse oximetry.

The average client requires an oxygen flow of 2 to 4 L/minute via nasal cannula or up to 40% via Venturi mask. The client who is hypoxemic and also has chronic hypercarbia requires lower levels of oxygen delivery, usually 1 to 2 L/minute via nasal cannula. A low arterial oxygen level is this client's primary drive for breathing.

INDICATIONS FOR OXYGEN THERAPY Oxygen is used for both acute and chronic respiratory conditions associated with decreased PaO_2 levels. The goal of oxygen therapy is to use the lowest fraction of inspired oxygen (FIO_2) to produce the most acceptable oxygenation without causing the development of harmful side effects. Although oxygen improves the PaO_2 level, it does not cure the condition or stop the disease process.

Oxygen therapy is indicated in other conditions that may be associated with the respiratory problem or complicating the hypoxemia, for example, increased oxygen demand, decreased blood oxygen-carrying capability, and decreased cardiac ouptut.

Conditions that increase oxygen demand include sepsis, fever, and the increased workload of dyspnea. Insufficient amounts of hemoglobin or altered hemoglobin quality result in the inability of the hemoglobin to carry enough oxygen to the tissues.

HAZARDS OF OXYGEN THERAPY Oxygen therapy is associated with several hazards. The nurse understands these hazards to detect early signs and symptoms.

Combustion. Oxygen itself does not burn, but it supports combustion. Therefore, a fire burns more

University Hospitals of Cleveland

Care Path Name: Asthma
DRG: 97 ELOS: 4.7 days
Expected Disposition: Home

Collaborative Problem List

1. Ineffective breathing R/T asthma
2. Probable alteration in health maintenance R/T deficit in knowledge to: control of asthma

FOCUS	Emergency Room	DAY 1	DAY 2	DAY 3	DAY 4
Laboratory/Tests/ Procedures	CXR-PA/LAT EKG CBC/diff SMA7 Pulse Ox ABG Theo level Peak flows-baseline & after 3rd aerosol	Peak flow q4h ABG—see criteria SMA7 qd Theo level qd Bedside Spirometry	Electrolytes qam Peak flow qs Theo level Bedside Spirometry	Peak flow qom CXR Room Air ABG PFT's	
Consults		Resp			
Physical Assessment	VS q20 min ×3 Chest Assessment q20 min ×3		VS q4h & PRN Chest Assessment q4h	VS qs Chest Assessment qs	
Activity	As Tolerated	As Tolerated			
Treatments	Oxygen 2L NC IV Hep Lock	Oxygen 2L NC Admission weight VS q4h Chest Assessment q4h		DC Oxygen?	
Diet	As Tolerated				
Medications	Albuterol Aerosol q 20 min ×3 Solu-Medrol 60 mg IV ×1 Aminophylline Load & Drip—see protocol for dosage	Albuterol Aerosol q2 × 6 then q3 × 4 Solu-Medrol 60 mg q6h Amino Drip	Albuterol Aerosols qhr Assess Continuation of Solu-Medrol & Amino Drip	PO Inhalers with spacers q4h Prednisone Theo-Dur	
Discharge Planning		Social Service Consult PRN	Social Service Consult F/U Plan in progress		
Teaching		Begin Med Teaching			
Date					
Variance					
RN Signature Days					
RN Signature Evenings					
RN Signature Nights					

Discharge Outcome:	Met	Not Met	Comments	Date/Initials
1. Respiratory status normal for patient as evidenced by a. asymptomatic b. peak flow 60% predicted c. absence of pulsus paradoxus d. no use of accessory muscles e. RR less than 20 f. absence of or decrease in wheezing 2. Adequate health maintenance as evidenced by control of asthma by knowledge re: a. proper use of inhalers b. demonstrate use of peak flow meter c. recognize signs of drug toxicity d. able to modify ADL's to meet needs e. state early warning signs of asthma exacerbation f. able to seek appropriate medical care when necessary.				
Discharge Assessment Questions	**Yes**	**No**	**Comments**	**Date/Initials**
1. Are you wheezing? a. at rest b. with activity				
2. Are you short of breath? a. at rest b. with activity				
3. Can you walk across the room without getting SOB?				
4. Can you speak in a full sentence without getting SOB?				
5. Do you cough? a. at rest b. with activity c. after your peak flow				
6. Do you feel you are ready to go home?				
7. Could you go back to your usual activities now?				

Clinical Pathway: Asthma. (Courtesy of University Hospitals of Cleveland.)

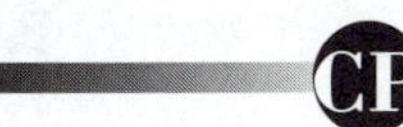

readily in the presence of oxygen. The nurse takes special precautions during the administration of oxygen, including posting a sign on the door of the client's room. Smoking is prohibited in the client's room, and all electrical equipment must be grounded (three prongs). Grounded outlets are usually designated with a green or red dot on the plate. Frayed cords must be repaired because they can cause a spark that can ignite a flame. Any type of flammable solution containing alcohol or oil is prohibited from the room when oxygen is in use.

Oxygen-Induced Hypoventilation. Oxygen-induced hypoventilation is seen in the client whose principal respiratory drive is hypoxia (hypoxic drive), that is, the client with chronic airflow limitation (CAL) who also has hypercarbia.

In the client with CAL, the arterial carbon dioxide level ($PaCO_2$) gradually rises over time. The central chemoreceptors in the brain (medulla) are normally sensitive to *high carbon dioxide levels, which stimulate breathing*. When the $PaCO_2$ increases above 60 to 65 mmHg, however, this normal mechanism shuts off. At that point, peripheral chemoreceptors found in the carotid and aortic arch bodies become the major stimulus for breathing. These peripheral receptors are sensitive to low PaO_2 levels. When PaO_2 drops below 55 to 60 mmHg, these receptors signal the brain to increase the respiratory rate or depth, which results in a *hypoxic drive to breathe* (Fig. 30–7).

The hypoxic drive occurs only in the presence of severely elevated $PaCO_2$ levels (i.e., in the client who has hypoxemia *and* hypercarbia). When the client with PaO_2 levels less than 55 to 60 mmHg (*and* $PaCO_2$ levels greater than 60 to 65 mmHg) receives oxygen therapy, the PaO_2 level increases; but the hypoxic drive, the *only* stimulation for breathing, is eliminated. As a result, the client experiences respiratory depression that could lead to apnea or respiratory arrest.

Oxygen therapy is given at the lowest liter flow (usually 1 to 2 L/minute) necessary to treat the hypoxemia without raising the $PaCO_2$. A system that delivers precise oxygen concentrations in low

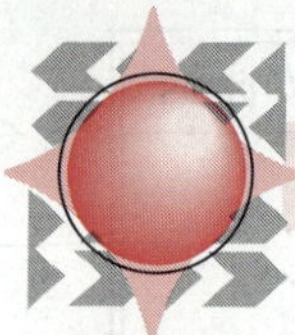

CLIENT CARE PLAN

The Client with Chronic Airflow Limitation

Nursing Diagnosis No. 1: Impaired Gas Exchange related to alveolar membrane changes, airflow limitation, respiratory muscle fatigue, excess production of mucus, and intrapulmonary shunting

Expected Outcomes	Nursing Interventions	Rationale
The client demonstrates correct use of techniques and methods that support improved oxygenation.	♦ Assess oxygenation of the client, including: a. Level of consciousness b. Pulse oximetry c. Breathing pattern, rate, and depth; chest expansion; dyspnea; nasal flaring; pursed-lip breathing; prolonged expiratory phase; and use of accessory muscles d. Peak expiratory flow rate	♦ Information will provide answers to questions of hypoxemia.
	♦ Instruct client and monitor proper placement of oxygen devices (e.g., nasal cannula).	♦ Clients with hypoxemia will desaturate rapidly once oxygen is removed.
	♦ Teach energy conservation techniques: a. Encourage sitting for most activities, such as peeling potatoes or talking on the phone. b. Teach the client never to hold his or her breath while performing activities. c. Be aware that activities involving the arms may increase dyspnea. d. Plan rest between periods of activity.	♦ Increased activity and work of breathing will increase oxygen consumption. These techniques assist the client in oxygen conservation.
	♦ Instruct the client in the following: a. Pursed-lip breathing b. Diaphragmatic breathing c. Relaxation therapy d. Controlled cough techniques	♦ These techniques assist the client with better ventilation.
	♦ Formulate a plan with the client and family for pacing activities of daily living.	♦ Planned activities are better controlled and provide better data for evaluation.
The client demonstrates correct technique to normalize $PaCO_2$.	♦ Assess the quality and quantity of sputum: color, consistency, amount, and odor.	♦ Increased mucus and inflammation can cause airflow limitation.
	♦ Maximize the effect of medical interventions by proper sequence of respiratory treatments and by judicious use of bronchodilators and steroids.	♦ These interventions result in decreased airflow limitation.
	♦ Instruct and monitor client's technique with metered-dose inhalers.	♦ Correct technique, sequence, and use are key to effective treatment.

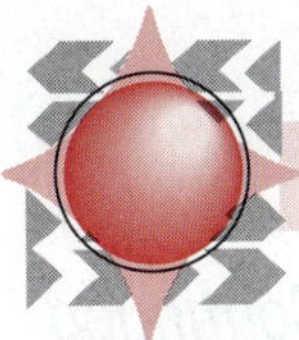

CLIENT CARE PLAN

The Client with Chronic Airflow Limitation *Continued*

Nursing Diagnosis No. 1: Impaired Gas Exchange related to alveolar membrane changes, airflow limitation, respiratory muscle fatigue, excess production of mucus, and intrapulmonary shunting

Expected Outcomes	Nursing Interventions	Rationale
	◆ Teach potential hazard of excessive inspired oxygen to clients and family.	◆ Clients with chronic hypercapnia have blunted CO_2 drives to breathe.
	◆ Teach signs and symptoms of hypercapnia: a. Headache b. Confusion	◆ Acute hypercapnia can result in respiratory failure.

Nursing Diagnosis No. 2: Ineffective Breathing Pattern related to airflow obstruction (narrowed airways), fatigue, and decreased energy from respiratory muscle fatigue

Expected Outcomes	Nursing Interventions	Rationale
The client will demonstrate a breathing pattern that decreases the work of breathing.	◆ Assess respiratory rate, depth, and rhythm at least every shift.	◆ Assessment provides the nurse with baseline information.
	◆ Assist the client in maintaining proper positioning during dyspneic episodes: a. Sitting up and leaning on over-bed table b. Sitting up and resting with elbows on knees c. Standing and leaning against the wall	◆ These positions can decrease the work of breathing.
	◆ Teach pursed-lip and diaphragmatic breathing techniques.	◆ These breathing techniques facilitate increased expiratory flow.
	◆ Teach energy conservation techniques.	◆ Respiratory muscles fatigue easily in CAL clients.
	◆ Initiate respiratory muscle training, if appropriate.	◆ Inspiratory muscle training can assist in strengthening the diaphragm.
	◆ Identify in writing various factors that elicit an anxious response.	◆ This process gives the client control of his or her situation.
	◆ Help the client to formulate a plan for coping with dyspneic and wheezing episodes.	◆ A plan prepares the client for episodes of anxiety.
	◆ Allow the client to verbalize feelings.	◆ Verbalization tends to prevent or decrease anxiety.
	◆ Teach the client various interventions for anxiety: a. Relaxation techniques b. Biofeedback	◆ Interventions decrease stress.
	◆ Refer the client for professional counseling if necessary.	◆ Counseling assists the client with self-analysis and coping techniques.

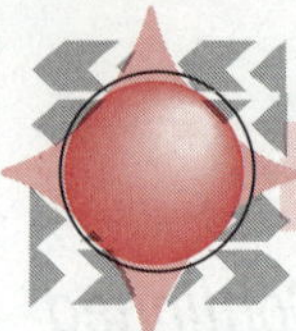

CLIENT CARE PLAN

The Client with Chronic Airflow Limitation *Continued*

Nursing Diagnosis No. 3: Ineffective Airway Clearance related to excessive secretions, fatigue and decreased energy, and ineffective cough

Expected Outcomes	Interventions	Rationales
The client will demonstrate effective airway clearance techniques. The client will attain optimal lung sounds.	◆ Assess sputum for color, amount, consistency, and odor.	◆ Secretions can obstruct airways.
	◆ Assess the client's ability to expectorate sputum with ease.	◆ Observe the client's cough efforts to determine best technique.
	◆ Assess breath sounds at least every 8 hours.	◆ Assessment provides vital information of respiratory status.
	◆ Monitor fluid intake daily.	◆ Dehydration impairs ciliary action.
	◆ Position the client to prevent aspiration.	◆ Aspiration is the leading cause of pneumonia in the elderly.
	◆ Teach a method of controlled cough.	◆ This technique will produce the best results with the least effort.
	◆ Suction as necessary to remove secretions.	◆ Suctioning is based on breath sound assessment.
	◆ Teach postural drainage and chest physiotherapy techniques, if ordered: a. Assess level of consciousness. b. Observe for hypoxemia. c. Assess breath sounds for wheezes caused by bronchospasm.	◆ Chest physiotherapy can cause hypoxemia and bronchospasm.

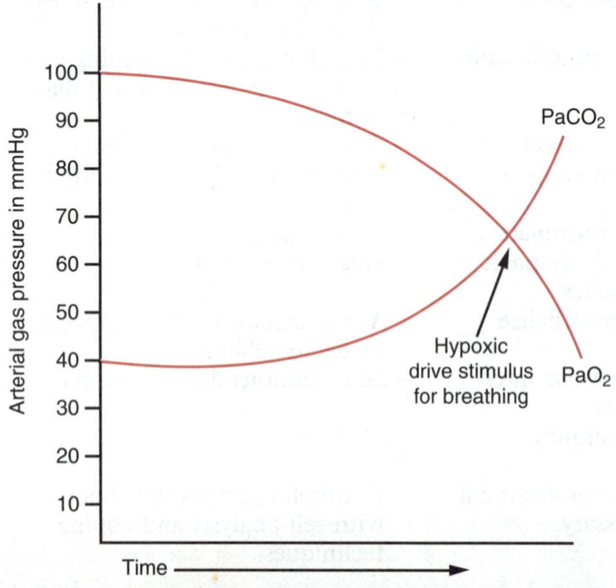

FIGURE 30–7 ◆ Arterial gas changes in chronic lung disease, showing the point when the hypoxic drive becomes the stimulus for breathing.

amounts, such as a nasal cannula or Venturi mask, is preferred for any client with CAL. The nurse closely monitors the respiratory rate and depth of a client with CAL who receives oxygen. This monitoring is especially important when it is the first time the client has received oxygen or when the $PaCO_2$ levels are not known. Signs and symptoms of hypoventilation are seen during the first 30 minutes of oxygen administration; the client's color improves ("pinking up") related to an increase in the PaO_2 level before the apnea or respiratory arrest occurs from the loss of the hypoxic drive.

Oxygen Toxicity. Oxygen toxicity is related to:

- The concentration of oxygen delivered
- The duration of oxygen therapy
- The degree of lung disease present before oxygen therapy is started

In general, an oxygen concentration greater than 50% administered continuously for more than 24 to 48 hours may damage the lungs.

The pathophysiologic mechanism and clinical manifestations of lung injury associated with oxygen toxicity are the same as those for adult respiratory distress syndrome (ARDS) (see Chap. 31). The nurse observes for initial symptoms, which include nonproductive cough, substernal chest pain, gastrointestinal upset, and dyspnea. As exposure to high concentrations of oxygen continues, the symptoms become more severe and are accompanied by decreased vital capacity, decreased vital compliance (which results in more dyspnea), crackles, and hypoxemia. Prolonged exposure to high concentrations of oxygen cause structural damage to the lungs. Atelectasis, pulmonary edema, pulmonary hemorrhages, and hyaline membrane formation result. Mortality depends on the ability of the health care team to correct the underlying disease process and to decrease the oxygen amount delivered.

The toxic effects of oxygen are difficult to treat; hence, the physician orders the lowest concentrations of oxygen required by the client. The nurse closely monitors arterial blood gases during oxygen administration and notifies the physician of PaO_2 levels greater than 100 mmHg. The nurse also monitors the prescribed oxygen concentration and length of time of administration to identify the client at higher risk. High concentrations of oxygen are avoided unless absolutely necessary. The addition of continuous positive airway pressure (CPAP) with an oxygen mask, Bilevel positive airway pressure (Bi-Pap) (Fig. 30–8) or positive end-expiratory pressure (PEEP) on the mechanical ventilator (see Chap. 31) may reduce the amount of oxygen needed. As soon as the client's clinical condition allows, the physician decreases the prescribed amount of oxygen.

Absorption Atelectasis. Nitrogen normally plays a large role in the maintenance of patent airways and alveoli. When high concentrations of oxygen are delivered

- Nitrogen is washed out
- The oxygen diffuses from the alveoli into the pulmonary circulation
- The alveoli collapse

Collapsed alveoli cause atelectasis, called absorption atelectasis, which the nurse detects by auscultation. The nurse monitors the client closely for crackles and/or decreased breath sounds every 1 to 2 hours when the client is initially placed on oxygen therapy and frequently thereafter.

OXYGEN DELIVERY SYSTEMS Oxygen can be delivered by numerous systems. The nurse understands the rationale for the type of oxygen delivery system used for a particular client and uses the equipment properly. The type of delivery system depends on the following:

- The concentration of oxygen required by the client
- The concentration of oxygen achieved by a delivery system
- The importance of accuracy and control of the oxygen concentration

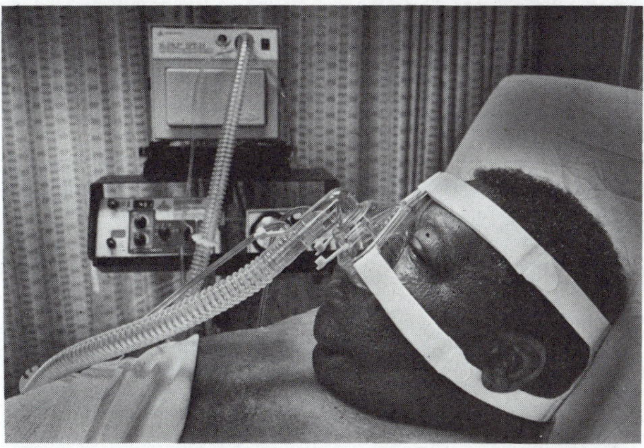

FIGURE 30–8 ◆ The client breathes comfortably on bilevel positive airway pressure (Bi-PAP), which combines the effects of continuous positive airway pressure (CPAP) (applied with exhalation) with the principles of pressure support ventilation (applied with inspiration). Bi-PAP or CPAP is commonly used during sleep to prevent sleep apnea.

- The client's comfort
- Expense to the client
- The importance of humidity
- The client's mobility

Oxygen delivery systems are classified according to the rate at which oxygen is delivered. There are two systems: low-flow systems and high-flow systems. Low-flow systems do not provide enough oxygen to meet the total inspiratory effort of the client. Part of the tidal volume is supplied by the client's inspiring room air. The total concentration of oxygen received depends on respiratory rate and tidal volume. In contrast, high-flow systems provide a flow rate that is adequate to meet the entire inspiratory effort and tidal volume of the client regardless of the respiratory pattern. High-flow systems are used for critically ill clients.

Low-Flow Oxygen Delivery Systems. Low-flow delivery systems include (Table 30–3):

- Nasal cannula
- Simple face mask
- Partial rebreather mask
- Non-rebreather mask

These systems are inexpensive, easy to use, and fairly comfortable for the client. A major disadvantage is that the actual amount of oxygen obtained per liter is variable and depends on the client's breathing pattern. The oxygen delivered by the system is diluted with room air (21%), which lowers the amount of oxygen the client actually receives.

Nasal Cannula. The nasal cannula, or nasal prongs (Fig. 30–9), is used at flow rates of 1 to 6 L/minute. Approximate oxygen concentrations of 24% (at 1 L/minute) to 44% (at 6 L/minute) can be achieved. Flow rates higher than 6 L/minute do not significantly increase oxygenation because the anatomic reserve or dead space (oral and nasal cavities) is full. In

TABLE 30–3 Comparison of Low-Flow Oxygen Delivery Systems

System	FIO_2 Delivered	Nursing Interventions	Rationale
Nasal cannula	• 24%–40% FIO_2 at 1–6 L/min • ≈24% at 1 L/min • ≈28% at 2 L/min • ≈32% at 3 L/min • ≈36% at 4 L/min • ≈40% at 5 L/min • ≈44% at 6 L/min	• Ensure that prongs are in the nares properly.	• A poorly fitting nasal cannula leads to hypoxemia and skin breakdown.
		• Provide water-soluble jelly to nares PRN.	• This substance prevents mucosal irritation related to the drying effect of oxygen; promotes comfort.
		• Assess the patency of the nostrils.	• Congestion or a deviated septum prevents effective delivery of oxygen through the nares.
		• Assess the client for changes in respiratory rate or depth.	• The respiratory pattern affects the amount of oxygen delivered. A different delivery system may be needed.
Simple face mask	• 40%–60% FIO_2 at 5–10 L/min; flow rate must be set at least 5 L/min to flush mask of carbon dioxide • ≈40% at 5 L/min • ≈45%–50% at 6 L/min • ≈55%–60% at 8 L/min	• Be sure mask fits securely over nose and mouth.	• A poorly fitting mask reduces the FIO_2 delivered.
		• Assess skin and provide skin care to the area covered by the mask.	• Pressure and moisture under the bag may cause skin breakdown.
		• Monitor the client closely for risk of aspiration.	• The mask limits the client's ability to clear the mouth, especially if vomiting occurs.
		• Provide emotional support to the client who feels claustrophobic.	• Emotional support decreases anxiety, which contributes to a claustrophobic feeling.
		• Suggest to physician to switch the client from a mask to the nasal cannula during eating.	• Use of the cannula prevents hypoxemia during eating.
Partial rebreather mask	• 70–90% at 6–15 L/min, a liter flow rate high enough to maintain bag two-thirds full during inspiration	• Make sure that the reservoir does not twist or kink, which results in a deflated bag.	• Deflation results in decreased oxygen delivered and rebreathing of exhaled air.
		• Adjust the flow rate to keep the reservoir bag inflated (two-thirds full during inspiration).	• The flow rate is adjusted to meet the pattern of the client.
Non-rebreather mask	• 60%–100% FIO_2 at liter flow to maintain bag two-thirds full	• Interventions as for partial rebreather mask; this client requires close monitoring.	• Rationales are for partial rebreather mask. • Monitoring ensures proper functioning and prevents harm.
		• Make sure that valves and rubber flaps are patent, functional, and not stuck. Remove mucus or saliva.	• Valves should open during expiration and close during inhalation to prevent dramatic decrease in FIO_2. Suffocation can occur if the reservoir bag kinks or if the oxygen source disconnects.
		• Closely assess the client on increased FIO_2 via non-rebreather mask. Intubation is the only way to provide more precise FIO_2.	• The client may require intubation.

addition, high flow rates increase mucosal irritation. With the use of a nasal cannula, an effective oxygen concentration can be delivered to both nose breathers and mouth breathers.

The nasal cannula is frequently used for the client with chronic airflow limitation (CAL) and for long-term maintenance of clients with other illnesses. The CAL client who retains carbon dioxide should *never* receive oxygen at a rate higher than 2 to 3 L/minute unless he or she is on a mechanical ventilator because of the concern of apnea or respiratory arrest. The nurse places the nasal prongs in the nostrils, with the openings facing the client. When a flow rate higher than 2 L/minute is needed, the nurse adds humidification upon order (Fig. 30–10). The nurse checks the water level and charges the humidifier as needed.

Simple Face Mask. A simple face mask is used to deliver oxygen concentrations of 40% to 60% for

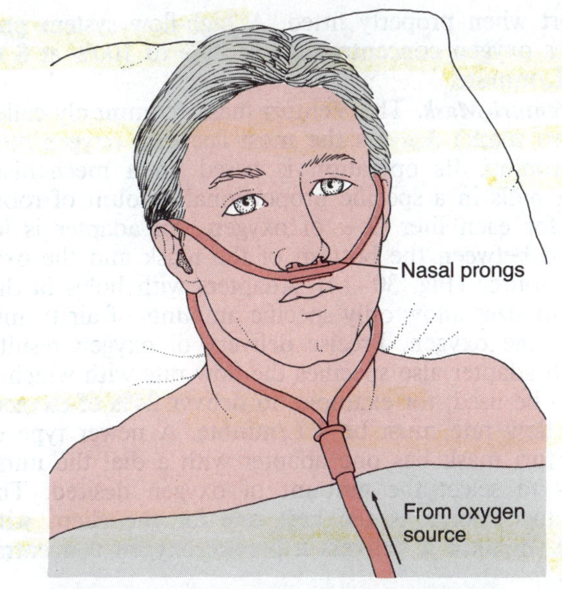

FIGURE 30–9 ◆ A nasal cannula (prongs).

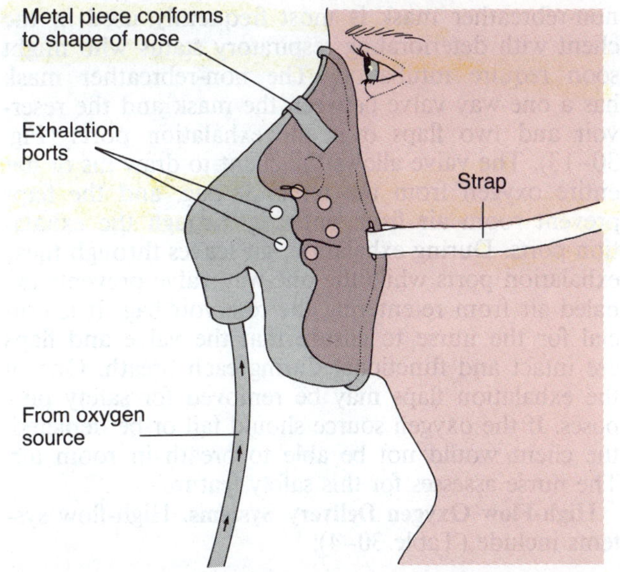

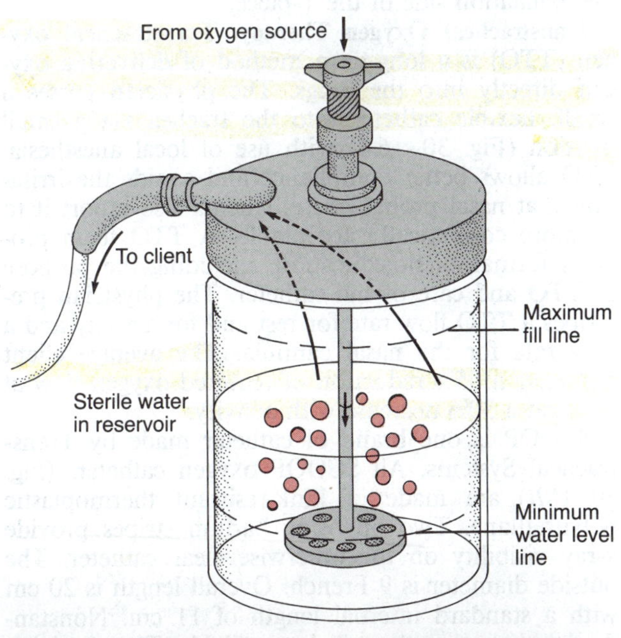

FIGURE 30–10 ◆ A bubble humidifier bottle used with oxygen therapy.

short-term oxygen therapy or in an emergency (Fig. 30–11). A minimal flow rate of 5 L/minute is needed to prevent the rebreathing of exhaled air. The nurse gives special attention to skin care and to the proper fitting of the mask so that inspired oxygen concentration is maintained.

Partial Rebreather Mask. A partial rebreather mask provides oxygen concentration of 70% to 90%, with flow rates of 6 to 15 L/minute. It consists of a mask with a reservoir bag but no flaps (Fig. 30–12). The client first rebreathes one-third of the exhaled tidal volume, which is high in oxygen, thus providing a high FIO_2. The nurse ensures that the bag remains

FIGURE 30–11 ◆ A simple face mask used to deliver oxygen.

slightly inflated at the end of inspiration; otherwise, the client will not be getting the desired oxygen prescription. If needed, the nurse calls the respiratory therapist for assistance.

Non-rebreather Mask. A non-rebreather mask provides the highest concentration of the low-flow systems and can deliver an FIO_2 greater than 90%, depending on the client's ventilatory pattern. The

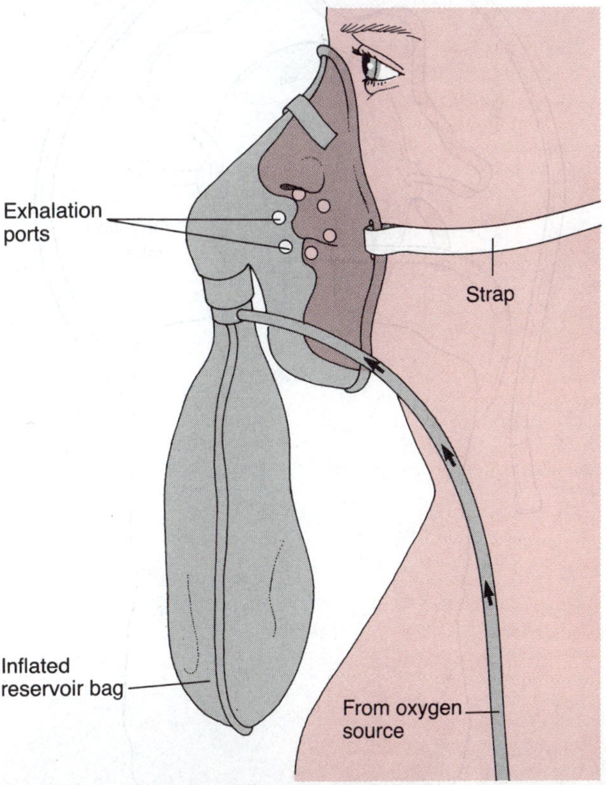

FIGURE 30–12 ◆ A partial rebreather mask.

non-rebreather mask is most frequently used in the client with deteriorating respiratory status who might soon require intubation. The non-rebreather mask has a one-way valve between the mask and the reservoir and two flaps over the exhalation ports (Fig. 30–13). The valve allows the client to draw his or her entire oxygen from the reservoir bag, and the flaps prevent room air from entering through the exhalation ports. During exhalation, air leaves through these exhalation ports while the one-way valve prevents exhaled air from re-entering the reservoir bag. It is crucial for the nurse to ensure that the valve and flaps are intact and functional during each breath. One of the exhalation flaps may be removed for safety purposes. If the oxygen source should fail or be depleted, the client would not be able to breath in room air. The nurse assesses for this safety feature.

High-Flow Oxygen Delivery Systems. High-flow systems include (Table 30–4):

- Venturi mask
- Aerosol mask
- Face tent
- Tracheostomy collar
- T-piece

These devices deliver a consistent and accurate oxygen concentration that meets the client's inspiratory effort when properly fitted. A high-flow system provides oxygen concentrations of 24% to 100% at 8 to 15 L/minute.

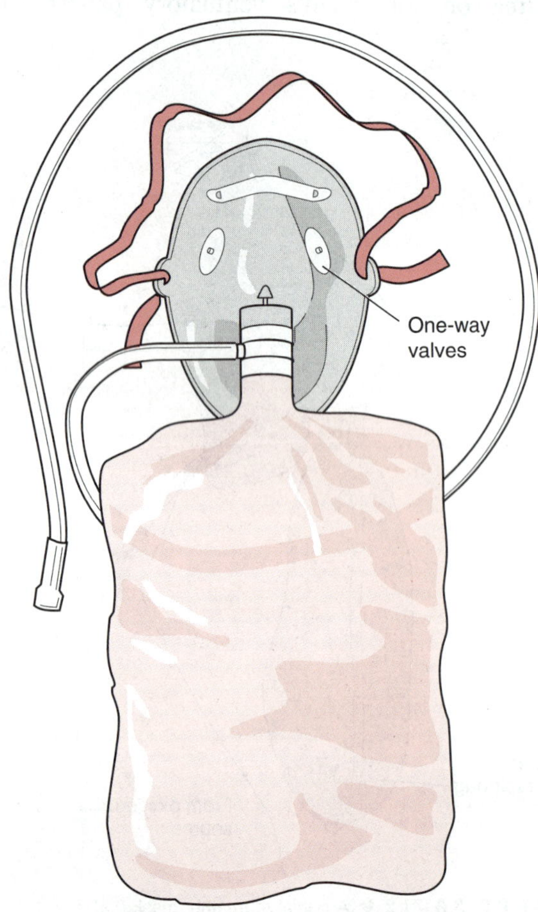

FIGURE 30–13 ◆ A non-rebreather mask.

Venturi Mask. The Venturi mask (commonly called Venti mask) delivers the most accurate oxygen concentration. Its operation is based on a mechanism that pulls in a specific proportional amount of room air for each liter flow of oxygen. An adapter is located between the bottom of the mask and the oxygen source (Fig. 30–14). Adapters with holes of different sizes allow only specific amounts of air to mix with the oxygen. Precise delivery of oxygen results. Each adapter also specifies the flow rate with which it is to be used; for example, to deliver 24% of oxygen, the flow rate must be 4 L/minute. A newer type of Venturi mask has one adapter with a dial the nurse uses to select the amount of oxygen desired. The Venturi system is the best one for the client with CAL because it delivers a precise oxygen concentration.

Other High-Flow Systems. The face tent, aerosol mask, tracheostomy collar, and T-piece are often used to administer high humidity. A dial on the humidification source regulates the oxygen concentration being delivered. A *face tent* fits over the client's chin, with the top extending halfway across the face. The oxygen concentration varies, but the face tent is useful instead of a tight-fitting mask for the client who has facial trauma and burns. An *aerosol mask* is used for the client who requires high humidity after extubation or upper airway surgery or for the client who has thick secretions. The *tracheostomy collar* can be used to deliver high humidity and the desired oxygen to the client with a tracheostomy. A special adapter, called the *T-piece,* can be used to deliver any desired FIO_2 to the client with a tracheostomy, laryngectomy, or endotracheal tube (Fig. 30–15). The flow rate is regulated so that the aerosol does not disappear on the exhalation side of the T-piece.

Transtracheal Oxygen Therapy. Transtracheal oxygen (TTO) is a long-term method of delivering oxygen directly into the lungs. The physician passes a small, flexible catheter into the trachea via a small incision (Fig. 30–16*A*) with use of local anesthesia. TTO allows better compliance and avoids the irritation that nasal prongs cause. Clients also report it to be more cosmetically acceptable. A TTO team provides formal client education, including the purpose of TTO and care of the catheter. The physician prescribes a TTO flow rate for rest and for activity and a flow rate for the nasal cannula. The average client will have a 55% reduction of required oxygen flow at rest and a 30% decrease with activity.

SCOOP is one brand of catheter made by Transtracheal Systems. All SCOOP oxygen catheters (Fig. 30–16*B*) are made of kink-resistant thermoplastic polyurethane. Two opposing barium stripes provide x-ray visibility on the otherwise clear catheter. The outside diameter is 9 French. Overall length is 20 cm with a standard internal length of 11 cm. Nonstandard catheter lengths are also available. The physician determines proper length after viewing the post-procedure x-ray with an 11-cm Pre SCOOP stent in

TABLE 30–4 Comparison of High-Flow Oxygen Delivery Systems

System	FIO_2 Delivered	Nursing Interventions	Rationale
Venturi mask (Venti mask)	• 24%–55% FIO_2 with flow rates of 4–10 L/min; provides high humidity	• Perform constant surveillance to ensure accurate flow rate for specific FIO_2.	• An accurate flow rate ensures FIO_2 delivery.
		• Keep the orifice for the Venturi adapter open and uncovered.	• If the Venturi orifice is covered, the adapter does not function and oxygen delivery varies.
		• Provide a mask that fits snugly and tubing that is free of kinks.	• FIO_2 is altered if kinking occurs or if the mask fits poorly.
		• Assess the client for dry mucous membranes.	• Humidity or aerosol can be added to the system to prevent the drying effect of oxygen.
		• Change to a nasal cannula during mealtimes.	• Oxygen is a drug that needs to be given continuously.
Aerosol mask, face tent, tracheostomy collar	• 24%–100% FIO_2 with flow rates of at least 10 L/min; provides high humidity	• Assess that aerosol mist escapes from the vents of the delivery system during inspiration and expiration.	• Humidification should be delivered to the client.
		• Empty condensation from the tubing.	• Emptying prevents the client from being lavaged with water and promotes an adequate flow rate.
		• Change the aerosol water container as needed.	• Adequate humidification is ensured only when there is sufficient water in the canister.
T-piece	• 24%–100% FIO_2 with flow rates of at least 10 L/min; provides high humidity	• Empty condensation from the tubing.	• Condensation interferes with flow rate and may drain into the tracheostomy if not emptied.
		• Keep the exhalation port open and uncovered.	• If the port is occluded, the client can suffocate.
		• Position the T-piece so that it does not pull on the tracheostomy or endotracheal tube.	• The weight of the T-piece pulls on the tracheostomy and causes pain or erosion of skin at the insertion site.
		• Make sure the humidifier creates enough mist. A mist should be seen during inspiration and expiration.	• An adequate flow rate is needed to meet the inspiratory effort of the client. If not, FIO_2 is decreased.

place. Oxygen is attached to the catheter using a SCOOP oxygen hose with a Luer taper connection. Catheters are sterilely packaged individually or in pairs and contain a cleaning rod(s), lubricating jelly, physician and client instructions and a registration card.

NURSING MANAGEMENT OF CLIENTS RECEIVING OXYGEN
Regardless of the type of oxygen delivery system used, the nurse understands the indications, advantages, and disadvantages of each. The nurse also ensures the proper use and maintenance of the oxygen delivery equipment.

If humidification is needed, the nurse ensures that a constant mist of humidification escapes from the vents of the delivery system during inspiration and expiration. A sufficient amount of sterile water must be in the humidification container, and an adequate flow rate must be maintained so that proper humidification is delivered to the client (see Fig. 30–10). Condensation often forms in the tubing and is removed as needed by disconnecting the tubing and emptying the water into an appropriate receptacle. For prevention of bacterial contamination, the fluid should never be drained back into the humidification bottle.

If the client requires a mask but is able to eat, the nurse requests an order for a nasal cannula at an appropriate liter flow for mealtimes only. The nurse replaces the mask after the meal is completed. To increase the client's mobility, up to 50 feet of connecting tubing can be used with proper connecting pieces. Chart 30–4 and also Tables 30–3 and 30–4 discuss other nursing interventions for the client receiving oxygen.

INEFFECTIVE BREATHING PATTERN

PLANNING: CLIENT GOALS The major goal is that the client will achieve an effective breathing pattern that

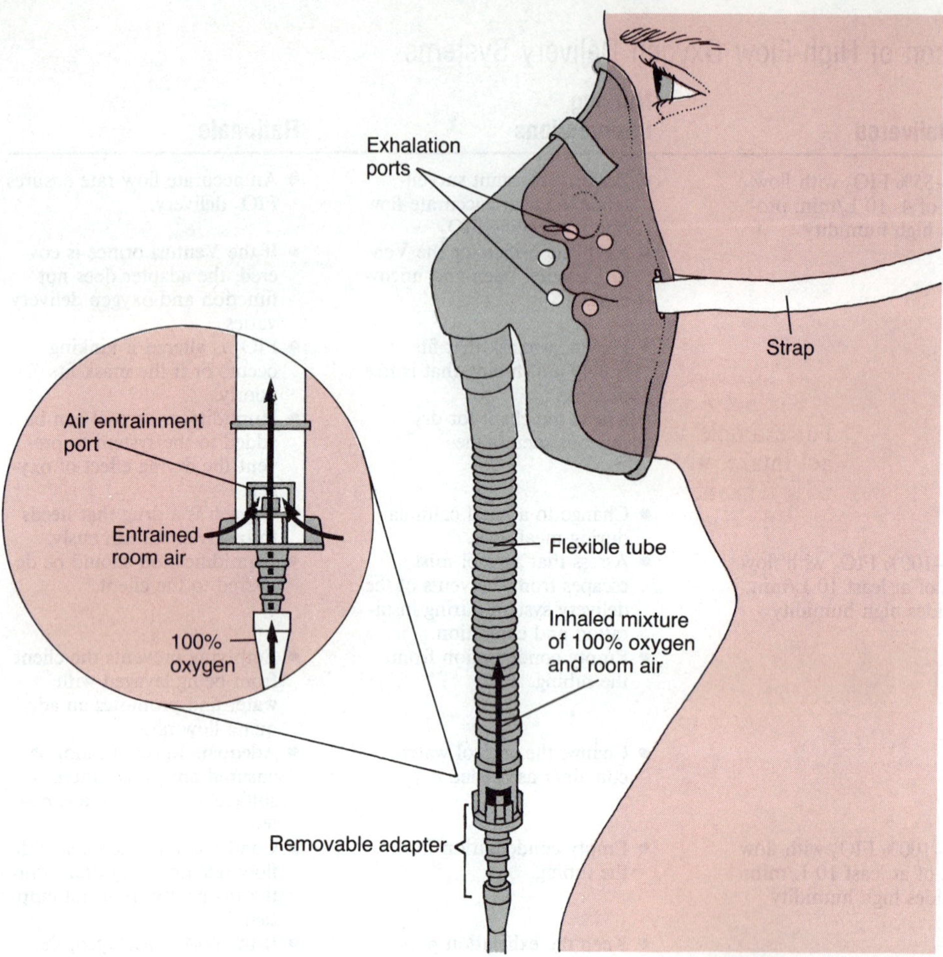

FIGURE 30–14 ◆ A Venturi mask for precise oxygen delivery.

decreases the work of breathing. Specific goals may be for the client to have:

- A respiratory rate, depth, and timing within normal limits
- A respiratory rhythm within normal limits for his or her age
- Synchronous thoracoabdominal movement
- Use of accessory muscles appropriate to activity level

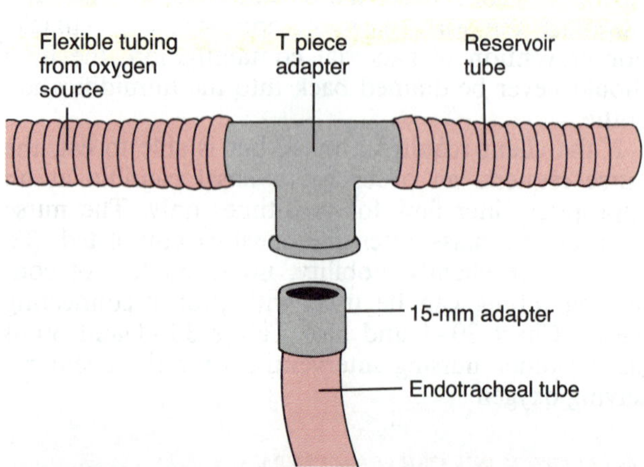

FIGURE 30–15 ◆ A T-piece apparatus for attachment to an endotracheal or tracheostomy tube.

INTERVENTIONS Before any interventions can be implemented, the nurse, physician, and respiratory therapist assess the client to determine his or her breathing pattern, especially the rate, rhythm, depth, and use of accessory muscles. The client with chronic airflow limitation (CAL) relies more on accessory muscles than on the diaphragm for ventilation. However, these muscles are less efficient than the diaphragm, and consequently the client experiences increased work of breathing. The nurse determines whether there are any contributing factors to the increased work of breathing, such as respiratory tract infection. Interventions are aimed at improving the client's breathing efforts and decreasing the work of breathing (see Client Care Plan).

Breathing Techniques Diaphragmatic or abdominal and pursed-lip breathing maneuvers may be beneficial interventions for managing dyspneic episodes. The client uses these techniques, shown in Chart 30–5, during all activities. The amount of stagnant air in the lung is minimized, and the client gains confidence and control in managing dyspnea.

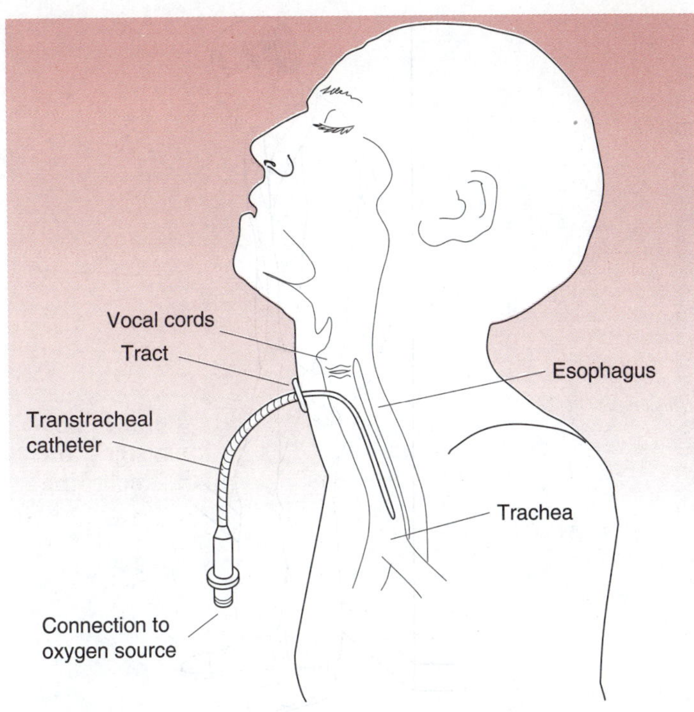

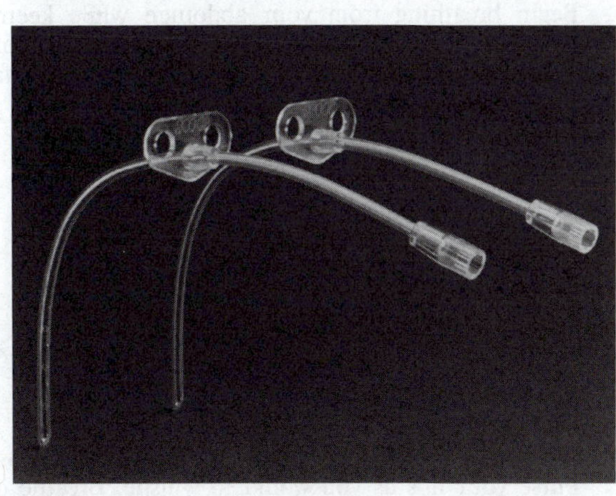

FIGURE 30–16 ◆ *A*, Example of transtracheal oxygen delivery. *B*, The SCOOP brand transtracheal oxygen catheter.

CHART 30–4

Nursing Care Highlight ◆ The Client Receiving Oxygen Therapy

- Check the physician's order with the type of delivery system and liter flow or percentage of oxygen actually in use.
- Obtain an order for humidification if oxygen is being delivered at 2 L/minute or more.
- Be sure the oxygen and humidification equipment is functioning properly.
- Check the skin around the client's ears, back of the neck, and face every 4 to 8 hours for pressure points and signs of irritation.
- Pad the elastic band and change its position frequently to prevent skin breakdown.
- Lubricate the client's nostrils and face with water-soluble jelly to relieve the drying effects of oxygen.
- Position the tubing so it does not pull on the client's face, nose, or artificial airway.
- Ensure that there is no smoking and no candles or matches are lit in the immediate area.
- Assess and document the client's response to oxygen therapy.
- Provide the client with ongoing teaching and reassurance to enhance the client's compliance with oxygen therapy.

DIAPHRAGMATIC OR ABDOMINAL BREATHING In diaphragmatic breathing, the client attempts to consciously increase diaphragmatic movement. Lying on the back allows the abdomen to relax.

PURSED-LIP BREATHING The technique of pursed-lip breathing uses the mild resistance of partially opposed lips to prolong exhalation and to increase airway pressure, thereby delaying dynamic compression of airways and minimizing the effects of air trapping. Many clients with CAL learn this technique on their own. Pursed-lip breathing can be used during diaphragmatic or abdominal breathing. The nurse teaches both of these breathing techniques when the client is free from dyspnea.

Positioning The nurse assists the client to an upright position with the head of the bed elevated to promote easier breathing patterns. The client uses various positions to assist in alleviating dyspnea (see Fig. 30–4). In one position, the client sits on the edge of the bed with the arms resting on two or three pillows on an overbed table. If extra pillows are not available, the client may lean on a table or rest on the elbows. These positions promote increased chest expansion, relax the chest muscles, and place the diaphragm in the proper position to contract while conserving energy by supporting the client's arms and upper body. The client may also find this position particularly helpful during an acute attack when he or she is tired but too short of breath to lie back.

The client uses the standing position (Fig. 30–17) when there is no place to sit. Clients with CAL use a

CHART 30–5

Education Guide ◆ Breathing Exercises

Diaphragmatic or Abdominal Breathing

Lie on your back with your knees bent.

Place your hands or a book on your abdomen to create resistance.

Begin breathing from your abdomen while keeping your chest still. You can tell if you are breathing correctly if your hands or the book rises and falls accordingly.

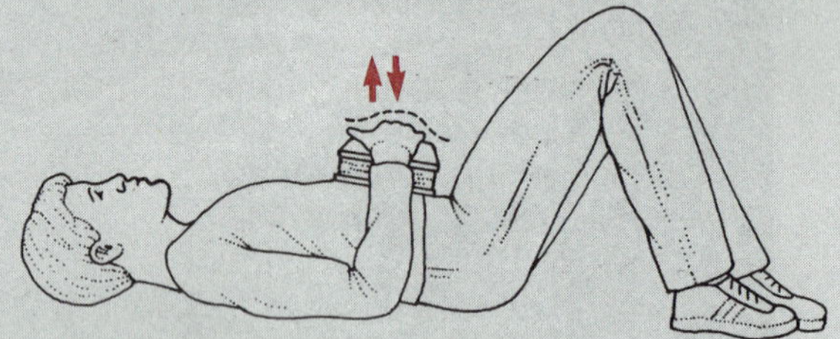

Pursed-Lip Breathing

Close your mouth and breathe in through your nose.

Purse your lips as you would to whistle. Breathe out slowly through your mouth, without puffing your cheeks. Spend at least twice the amount of time it took you to breathe in. Use your abdominal muscles to squeeze out every bit of air you can.

Remember to use pursed-lip breathing during any physical activity. Always inhale before beginning the activity and exhale while performing the activity. Never hold your breath.

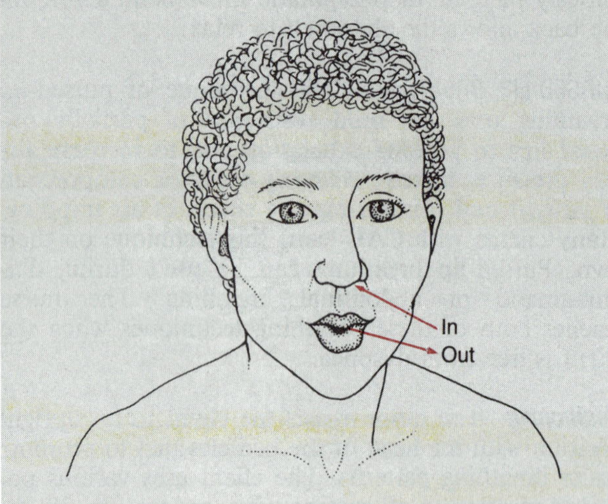

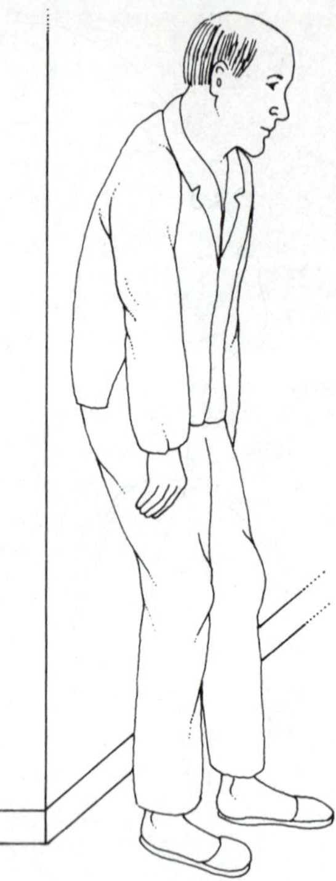

FIGURE 30–17 ◆ The standing position that is used to help clients with chronic airflow limitation to breathe. The client stands with his or her back and hips against a wall and with the feet about 30 cm (12 inches) from the wall. The shoulders are relaxed and bent slightly forward.

greater proportion of their accessory muscles for breathing. Supporting the thorax, therefore, allows these muscles to work better.

Exercise Conditioning Clients suffering from exercise-induced shortness of breath respond to dyspnea by limiting their activity, even basic activities of daily living. Over time, the muscles of respiration and the general large muscle groups weaken, becoming less efficient in their use of oxygen. The end result is increased dyspnea with lower activity levels. (Table 28–2 summarizes the relationship between dyspnea and the performance of daily activities.)

Exercise conditioning is part of a complete pulmonary rehabilitation program. Conditioning of the large muscle groups (indirect) or retraining of the respiratory muscles (direct) can be done. The indirect approach is accomplished through any general exercise program.

Two direct techniques currently used are isocapneic hyperventilation and resistive breathing. Isocapneic hyperventilation is designed to increase endurance. The client hyperventilates into a machine that controls the concentrations of oxygen and carbon dioxide. In resistive breathing, the client breathes against a set resistance. Resistive breathing theoretically trains respiratory muscles for both strength and endurance. Retraining of the respiratory muscles is currently done predominantly in research settings.

Energy Conservation Energy conservation is the planning and placing of activities for maximal tolerance by the client and minimal discomfort of the client. The nurse or therapist (physical or occupational) begins by asking the client to describe a typical daily schedule. Then, each activity is divided into its smaller parts to determine whether that task can be performed in a different way or at a different time of the day. The nurse assists the client in planning and pacing activities for the day. Rest periods are paced between activities. It is helpful for the nurse and the client to develop a chart outlining the day's activities and planned rest periods. Once a day, the nurse and client review the previous day's plan and make adjustments as indicated to promote energy conservation yet provide activity.

The nurse reminds the client to avoid working with his or her arms raised. Activities involving the arms decrease exercise tolerance because the accessory muscles of respiration are then used to stabilize the shoulders. Many activities involving the arms can be done sitting at a table leaning on the elbows.

The nurse reminds the client to adjust work heights. Improper working height causes back strain and fatigue. The best work height for a table top is 5 cm (2 inches) below the bent elbow. Rapid, jerky arm motions cause shortness of breath and fatigue and put an extra strain on the heart. Clients should be reminded to keep arm motions smooth and flowing. Long-handled dustpans, sponges, and feather dusters minimize bending and reaching.

The nurse gives suggestions to the client about the organization of work spaces so that items used most often are within easy reach. Measures like dividing laundry or groceries into small parcels that can be handled easily, using disposable plates to save washing time, and letting dishes dry in the rack also conserve energy. The nurse suggests that clients straighten bed covers before getting out of bed for easier bed making. Talking requires energy and use of the lungs; therefore, the nurse instructs the client not to talk when engaged in other activities that require energy, for example, walking. In addition, the nurse instructs the client that the key to any activity is to remember to avoid holding his or her breath and to always exhale while performing any activity.

INEFFECTIVE AIRWAY CLEARANCE

PLANNING: CLIENT GOALS The major goal is that the client will attain optimal lung sounds. Additional goals include that the client will:

- Maintain a patent airway
- Demonstrate an effective cough
- Remain free from aspiration

INTERVENTIONS The client with chronic bronchitis and advanced emphysema often has difficulty with removal of secretions, which results in compromised breathing and inadequate oxygenation. In addition to impairing breathing, excessive mucus predisposes the client to respiratory infections. The nurse auscultates breath sounds routinely as part of physical assessment but also before and after interventions as part of the evaluation for this nursing diagnosis. Careful use of drugs combined with controlled coughing, hydration, and postural drainage may help in airway clearance. If these measures fail, a tracheostomy may be required on a temporary or permanent basis.

Drug Therapy The physician uses five main classes of drugs in the management of chronic airflow limitation (CAL):

- Bronchodilators
- Anticholinergics
- Corticosteroids
- Cromolyn sodium
- Mucolytics

Chart 30–6 summarizes these drugs.

BRONCHODILATORS The technique preferred for the administration of the bronchodilators is via the metered-dose inhaler (MDI) because it delivers the drug directly to the lung. Side effects are reduced because only a limited amount of the drug gets into the general circulation. The bronchodilators are divided into sympathomimetics and methylxanthines.

Sympathomimetics. The sympathomimetic drugs, or adrenergic bronchodilators, are drugs that mimic, or act like, the sympathetic nervous system. These drugs cause bronchodilation through activation of the enzyme adenylate cyclase, which converts adenosine triphosphate (ATP) to cAMP. These drugs are rapidly metabolized and, hence, are short acting. In choosing the specific drug, the physician considers the beta-adrenergic activity of each drug. Beta$_1$-receptors are located in the heart, whereas beta$_2$-receptors are located in the lung. The more selective beta$_2$-adrenergic drugs (e.g., metaproterenol [Alupent], albuterol [Proventil, Ventolin], and terbutaline [Brethine]) generally do not stimulate the heart directly, have a faster onset of action, and are longer in duration. Many of the sympathomimetics can be administered in an inhaled form (Chart 30–7).

Methylxanthines. Methylxanthines act to increase the levels of adenosine 3′,5′-cyclic monophosphate (cAMP), the body's own natural bronchodilator. Other major actions include antagonism of adenosine and prostaglandins, which are natural bronchoconstrictors.

Aminophylline. In an acute flare-up of asthma or severe bronchospasm caused by any type of CAL, the physician typically prescribes a loading dose of intravenous aminophylline. The maintenance dose is 0.5 mg/kg/hr in otherwise healthy, nonsmoking adults. Doses up to 1.2 mg/kg/hr may be required for heavy smokers.

Theophylline. Theophylline is useful in managing severe bronchospasms and is usually given orally in immediate- or sustained-release preparations. The drug is well absorbed orally, with peak serum concentrations occurring in 1 to 2 hours. Achieving a therapeutic level can be challenging because various conditions influence the serum concentrations (Table 30–5). Recommended therapeutic serum levels for theophylline range from 10 to 20 μg/mL, but many clients do well at levels of 5 to 10 μg/mL. The nurse monitors for side and toxic effects of theophylline and reports them immediately to the physician. The physician makes adjustments in dosage based on the client's clinical response to therapy. Both the physician and the nurse carefully monitor serum levels of the drug to prevent toxic levels.

Over-the-Counter Bronchodilators. The Food and Drug Administration believes people should have ready access to certain bronchodilator drug products. A potential for abuse exists, however, particularly

CHART 30–6

Drug Therapy for Chronic Airflow Limitation (CAL)

Drug	Usual Dosage	Nursing Interventions	Rationale
Bronchodilators			
Sympathomimetics (adrenergics; beta stimulants)			
Metaproterenol (Metaprel, Alupent)	• MDI: 2–4 puffs q4–6h • PO: 20 mg tid • Aerosol: 0.2–0.3 mL q4–6h	• Instruct the client to use the bronchodilator inhaler before the steroid inhaler (if ordered). • Teach the client the correct method of using the inhaler and observe the client's technique.	• Use of the beta$_2$ agent inhaler first opens the airways and facilitates deeper penetration of the steroid. • Correct technique ensures proper inhalation. Sequencing the steps in using an inhaler can be tricky for children and the elderly. Two critical variables are the speed of inhalation and the duration of breath holding.
Albuterol (salbutamol, Proventil, Ventolin)	• MDI: 2–4 puffs q4–6h • PO: 2–4 mg q6–8h • Aerosol: 0.5 mL q4–6h	• Observe the client for fine finger tremors.	• The nurse observes the client to detect side effects of this selective beta$_2$ agent.
Pirbuterol (Maxair)	• MDI: 1–2 puffs q4–6h	• Observe the client for tremors, nervousness, insomnia, headache, tachycardia, and palpitations.	• The nurse observes the client to detect side effects. The drug stimulates beta-adrenergic receptors in the heart and lungs.
Isoetharine (Bronkosol)	• MDI: 2–4 puffs q3–6h • Nebulizer: 0.5 mL diluted 1:3 with saline	• Observe the client for tachycardia, palpitations, headache, and blood pressure alterations.	• Same as for pirbuterol.
Epinephrine (Adrenalin, Primatene Mist, Bronkaid Mistometer,🍁 Dysne-Inhal🍁)	• MDI: 2–3 puffs q2–4h • SC or IM: 0.2–0.5 mL of 1:1000 solution; may repeat in 10–15 min • IV: 0.1–0.25 mL of 1:1000 solution	• Observe the client for anxiety, tremors, and palpitations. • Assess the client for a history of hypertension, hyperthyroidism, and ischemic heart disease.	• The nurse observes the client to detect side effects. The drug is fast acting, with an onset of about 20 min. • The nurse observes the client to detect possible contraindications.
Isoproterenol (Isuprel, Medihaler-Iso)	• MDI: 2–3 puffs 4–6 times/day	• Monitor the client for palpitations.	• The nurse monitors the client to detect severe cardiac dysrhythmias, especially with IV administration.
Terbutaline (Brethine, Brethaire, Bricanyl)	• MDI: 2–4 puffs q4–8h • PO: 5 mg q8h • SC: 0.25 mg, not to exceed 0.5 mg q4h	• Monitor the client for palpitations and tachycardia.	• The nurse monitors the client to detect these infrequent side effects. The drug has a more selective beta$_2$ action, a slower onset, and a longer duration than do other sympathomimetics.
Methylxanthines			
Aminophylline (contains 80% theophylline; Corophyllin🍁)	• IV loading dose: 5–7 mg/kg over 20–40 min • IV maintenance dose: 0.5–1.2 mg/kg/hr	• Monitor drug levels.	• Monitoring blood levels detects possible toxicity. The drug has a narrow therapeutic range of 10–20 μg/mL.

CHART 30–6

Drug Therapy for Chronic Airflow Limitation (CAL) *Continued*

Drug	Usual Dosage	Nursing Interventions	Rationale
		• Observe the client for nausea and vomiting, diarrhea, tachycardia, palpitations, dizziness, and restlessness.	• The nurse observes the client to detect side effects and potential toxic effects.
		• Space doses equally throughout a 24-h period.	• Spacing of doses ensures even coverage throughout the day.
		• Give in saline by an infusion pump.	• Infusion is constant, steady, and controlled.
		• Avoid caffeine intake.	• Avoidance of caffeine reduces other sources of sympathetic stimulation.
Theophylline (Slo-Phyllin, Theo-Dur, Theobid, Uniphyl, Slo-bid gyrocaps, Acet-Am✱)	• PO: Initially: 10–12 mg/kg/day, increased by 25% at 3-day intervals until a maximal oral dose of 13 mg/kg/day in 2–4 divided doses (usually 400–800 mg/day) is reached	• Same as for aminophylline.	
		• Administer with food, such as milk and crackers.	• Taking the drug with food prevents gastrointestinal irritation.
		• Instruct the client to take medication even when feeling good.	• A therapeutic blood level is maintained.
		• Know whether the medication is the immediate-release form or the timed-release form.	• Sustained-release preparations give better coverage than do regular preparations, which makes them ideal for clients who awaken at night with shortness of breath.
Anticholinergics			
Ipratropium bromide (Atrovent)	• MDI: 2 puffs qid	• Instruct the client to close eyes while activating inhaler if not using spacer.	• Medication in the eyes will cause temporary blurring of vision.
		• Monitor the client for cough, dry mouth, blurred vision, palpitations.	• The nurse monitors the client to detect side effects.
Atropine	• Aerosol: 0.2% (1 mg) 0.5% (2.5 mg) 5–10 mg q6–8h (long-term maintenance) 2.5–5 mg q4–6h (acute severe asthma)	• Monitor for troublesome anticholinergic side effects (i.e., drying of mucous secretions, decreased mucociliary transport, tachycardia).	• The nurse monitors the client to detect side effects.
Corticosteroids			
Prednisone (Deltasone, Apo-Prednisone✱, Winpred✱) Methylprednisolone (Solu-Medrol, Medrol✱)	• PO, IV: Dosage varies	• Instruct the client about the side effects of long-term steroid use, such as: a. Hyperglycemia b. Osteoporosis c. Increased fat production and weight gain d. Immunologic impairment e. Reduced inflammatory response f. Increased gastric acidity	• The nurse warns the client of possible side effects, many of which are irreversible but must be treated.

Chart continued on following page

CHART 30–6

Drug Therapy for Chronic Airflow Limitation (CAL) *Continued*

Drug	Usual Dosage	Nursing Interventions	Rationale
		• Monitor serum potassium levels for hypokalemia.	• Systemic steroids cause potassium loss with sodium and water retention.
		• Instruct the client to take medication with food.	• Food minimizes gastric irritation.
		• Instruct the client never to discontinue steroid use suddenly.	• Sudden discontinuation of steroids precipitates adrenal crisis and shock.
Beclomethasone (Vanceril, Beclovent, Rotacaps✱)	• MDI: 2–4 puffs tid–qid	• Observe the client's mouth daily for oral candidiasis.	• Oral candidiasis is a complication of inhaled steroids.
		• Instruct the client in the proper sequencing of sympathomimetic and steroid inhalers, if appropriate, and observe the client's technique.	• Proper sequencing and technique promote optimal distribution of the steroid.
		• Instruct the client to drink 8 ounces of water after inhaling steroids or gargle and rinse mouth after use.	• Drinking water washes away excess medication from the back of the throat and thus minimizes the growth of *Candida.*
		• Provide reservoir spacer.	• A spacer decreases oropharyngeal deposition of the drug.
Triamcinolone (Azmacort)	• MDI: 2–6 puffs tid–qid	Same as for beclomethasone.	
Flunisolide (AeroBid)	• MDI: 2–4 puffs bid	Same as for beclomethasone.	
Cromolyn sodium			
(Intal, Rynacrom✱)	• MDI: 1 or 2 puffs qid	• Observe the client for maculopapular rash and urticaria.	• The nurse observes the client to detect rare side effects.
		• Instruct the client that cromolyn is a prophylactic drug.	• Encourage the client to seek other treatment during an acute attack.
		• Inform the client that an optimal response may not occur before 2 months of daily use.	• Continued use is promoted until the drug takes effect.
Mucolytics			
Acetylcysteine (Mucomyst, Airbron✱)	• Aerosol (nebulizer): 3–5 mL (20%) 3–4 times daily; 6–10 mL (10%) 3–4 times daily	• Observe the client for nausea and bronchospasm.	• The nurse observes the client to detect common side effects.
Iodinated glycerol (Organidin)	• PO: 60 mg qid	• Instruct the client to have T_3 and T_4 tests done before starting therapy and then at the 3-month follow-up examination.	• The iodine content can cause hypothyroidism.
Saturated solution of potassium iodide (SSKI)	• PO: 300 mg in liquid (500 mg/ml) q4–6h	• Same as for iodinated glycerol.	
		• Observe the client for hypersensitivity and dermatologic reactions.	• The nurse observes the client to detect side effects.

MDI = metered-dose inhaler.

CHART 30–7

Education Guide ◆ How to Use an Inhaler Correctly

Without a Spacer (Preferred Technique)

1. Before each use, remove the cap and shake the inhaler according to the instructions in the package insert.
2. Tilt your head back slightly and breathe out fully.
3. Open your mouth and place the mouthpiece 1 to 2 inches away.
4. As you begin to breathe in deeply through your mouth, press down firmly on the canister of the inhaler to release one dose of medication.
5. Continue to breathe in slowly and deeply (usually over 3 to 5 seconds).
6. Hold your breath for at least 10 seconds to allow the medication to reach deep into the lungs, then breathe out slowly.
7. Wait at least 1 minute between puffs.
8. Replace the cap on the inhaler.
9. At least once a day, remove the canister and clean the plastic case and cap of the inhaler by thoroughly rinsing in warm, running tap water.

Without a Spacer (Alternative Method)

1. Follow steps 1 and 2 above.
2. Place the mouthpiece into your mouth, over your tongue, and seal your lips tightly around it.
3. Follow steps 4 to 9 above.

With a Spacer

1. Before each use, remove the caps from the inhaler and the spacer.
2. Insert the mouthpiece of the inhaler into the non-mouthpiece end of the spacer.
3. Shake the whole unit vigorously 3 or 4 times.
4. Place the mouthpiece into your mouth, over your tongue, and seal your lips tightly around it.
5. Press down firmly on the canister of the inhaler to release one dose of medication into the spacer.
6. Breathe in slowly and deeply. If the spacer makes a whistling sound, you are breathing in too rapidly.
7. Remove the mouthpiece from your mouth and, keeping your lips closed, hold your breath for at least 10 seconds, then breathe out slowly.
8. Wait at least 1 minute between puffs.
9. Replace the caps on the inhaler and the spacer.
10. At least once a day, clean the plastic case and cap of the inhaler by thoroughly rinsing in warm, running tap water; at least once a week, clean the spacer in the same manner.

when these preparations are taken with prescription drugs. The nurse teaches clients that over-the-counter (OTC) preparations contain active ingredients and are to be respected. The three principal ingredients in most nonprescription bronchodilator products are epinephrine, ephedrine, and theophylline, along with other additives. The nurse asks whether the client routinely uses over-the-counter preparations and cautions the client about the potential for their abuse.

ANTICHOLINERGICS Most of the autonomic nerves in the airways are branches of the vagus nerve. They are predominantly located in the large and medium-sized airways. Release of acetylcholine at these sites results in smooth muscle contraction. An anticholinergic agent, then, acts as a bronchodilator.

CORTICOSTEROIDS Steroid preparations reduce inflammation in the throat and lungs but also act to stimulate cAMP production and cause bronchodilation. Steroids may be given by the intravenous, oral, or inhalation route. The physician prescribes systemic steroids with great care. Side effects are usually related to long-term use; adrenal suppression is potentially the most hazardous. When long-term use is necessary, alternate-day therapy minimizes adrenal suppression as well as other side effects. A 2-day dose of the steroid is given every other day. (See Chapter 63 for more information on steroids and steroid side effects.)

Some steroid drugs may be administered via aerosol. If the client requires 30 mg or less of a steroid, it can often be administered via the aerosol route or in combination with the oral form to decrease oral steroid needs. The major advantage of the aerosol route is equivalent or greater bronchodilation and protec-

TABLE 30–5 Factors that Influence Theophylline Clearance

Factors that Decrease Clearance (Resulting in Increased Drug Levels)	Factors that Increase Clearance (Resulting in Decreased Drug Levels)
Diseases	
• Renal failure	• Hyperthyroidism
• Cirrhosis or other liver abnormalities	
• Congestive heart failure	
• Alcoholism	
• Upper respiratory tract infections	
• Hypothyroidism	
Drugs	
• Caffeine	• Isoproterenol (Isuprel)
• Allopurinol (Zyloprim)	• Rifampin (Rifadin, Rofact✽)
• Erythromycin (E-Mycin, Apo-Erythro✽)	• Phenobarbital (Luminal✽)
• Cimetidine (Tagamet)	• Phenytoin (Dilantin)
• Oral contraceptives	
• Ciprofloxacin (Cipro)	
• Calcium channel blockers	
Other factors	
• Older age, elderly	• Cigarette smoking

tion with fewer systemic side effects. A possible side effect of steroid aerosols and inhalers is *Candida* infection of the oropharynx. The nurse assesses for a bright, fire red or cherry red color of the mouth. Whitish plaques may also be present.

If the physician has prescribed both an inhaled bronchodilator and an inhaled steroid for administration at the same time, the nurse instructs the client to use the bronchodilator first. With dilation of the large airways, a greater portion of the steroid preparation reaches the peripheral airways.

CROMOLYN SODIUM Cromolyn sodium (Intal) can be used prophylactically in clients with asthma whose symptoms are not controlled adequately by bronchodilators or as a first-line treatment before bronchodilators are given. It is not useful during acute attacks. The desired effects of cromolyn are to reduce the severity and frequency of asthma attacks and to reduce the need for bronchodilators and steroids. Cromolyn probably acts by strengthening the mast cell membrane to prevent release of histamine and thereby decreases bronchospasm in the allergic asthmatic. Cromolyn is administered via metered-dose inhaler or as solution in a nebulizer, usually four times a day.

MUCOLYTICS The physician orders mucolytic agents for clients with thick, tenacious (sticky) mucous secretions. Nebulizer treatments with normal saline or with a mucolytic agent like acetylcysteine (Mucomyst) and normal saline help to thin secretions and facilitate expectoration. Most expectorants (e.g., iodinated glycerol [Organidin]) contain alcohol and must be used carefully in the elderly debilitated client who may be at risk for falls.

Controlled Coughing Because clients with chronic airflow limitation (CAL) produce more mucus than healthy people do, they may benefit from specific coughing at certain times of the day. The nurse teaches the client to cough on arising early in the morning to get rid of mucus that collected during the night. Coughing to expectorate mucus before mealtimes may facilitate a more pleasant meal, and coughing before bedtime may ensure clear lungs for an uninterrupted night's sleep.

To cough effectively, the client sits in a chair or on the side of a bed with feet placed firmly on the floor. The nurse instructs the client to turn his or her shoulders inward and to bend the head slightly downward, hugging a pillow against the stomach. The pillow helps decrease chest discomfort.

The nurse then instructs the client to take a few diaphragmatic breaths (see Charts 19–4 and 30–5). After the third to fifth deep breath (in through the nose, out through pursed lips), the nurse instructs the client to slowly bend forward while producing two or three strong coughs from the same breath. The first cough moves the secretions; the second and third coughs facilitate expectoration. The nurse notes the color, consistency, odor, and amount of secretions. As the client returns to a sitting position, he or she takes a comfortable deep breath. The entire coughing procedure is repeated at least twice. After coughing exercises, the nurse allows the client to rest and then assists the client in providing mouth care.

Chest Physiotherapy and Postural Drainage Chest physiotherapy (PT) with postural drainage (Fig. 30–18) is a technique that assists in mobilizing secretions from peripheral to central airways, in re-expanding lung tissue, and in promoting efficient use of the respiratory muscles. Chest PT combines chest percussion with vibration to loosen secretions. Postural drainage uses specific positions and gravity to assist in removing bronchial secretions. Postural drainage with chest PT may be helpful for select CAL patients with excessive secretions and airway clearance problems but should not be used routinely on all CAL clients (Eid et al., 1991).

Suctioning Suctioning is based on the auscultation of adventitious breath sounds and not performed on a routine schedule. For the client with a weak cough and weak pulmonary musculature unable to expectorate effectively, the nurse performs nasotracheal suctioning. The nurse assesses the client for dyspnea and tachycardia or other dysrhythmias during the suctioning procedure and for improved breath sounds afterward. (Chapter 29 discusses suctioning in detail.)

Positioning When the client can tolerate sitting in a chair, the nurse assists him or her out of bed for 1-hour periods, two to three times a day. This intervention helps mobilize secretions and also places the diaphragm in a position to provide more effective ventilation of the lungs.

Hydration Unless hydration is medically contraindicated, the nurse teaches clients with CAL to drink 2 to 3 L/day to maintain adequate hydration, which helps liquefy secretions. Humidifiers may be useful for clients living in a dry climate or who complain of dry heat during the winter. The nurse instructs the client to clean the humidifier daily to prevent the growth of mold spores.

ALTERED NUTRITION: LESS THAN BODY REQUIREMENTS

PLANNING: CLIENT GOALS The goal is for the client to achieve and then maintain a body weight within 10% of ideal.

INTERVENTIONS Clients with acute or chronic lung disease often complain of food intolerance, nausea, early satiety, loss of appetite, and meal-related dyspnea. In addition, the increased work of breathing raises calorie and protein requirements. These situations lead to protein-calorie malnutrition for many clients with chronic airflow limitation (CAL). Malnourished clients lose total body mass, respiratory muscle mass, respiratory muscle strength, lung elasticity, and alveolar capillary surface area, which contributes to an ineffective breathing pattern.

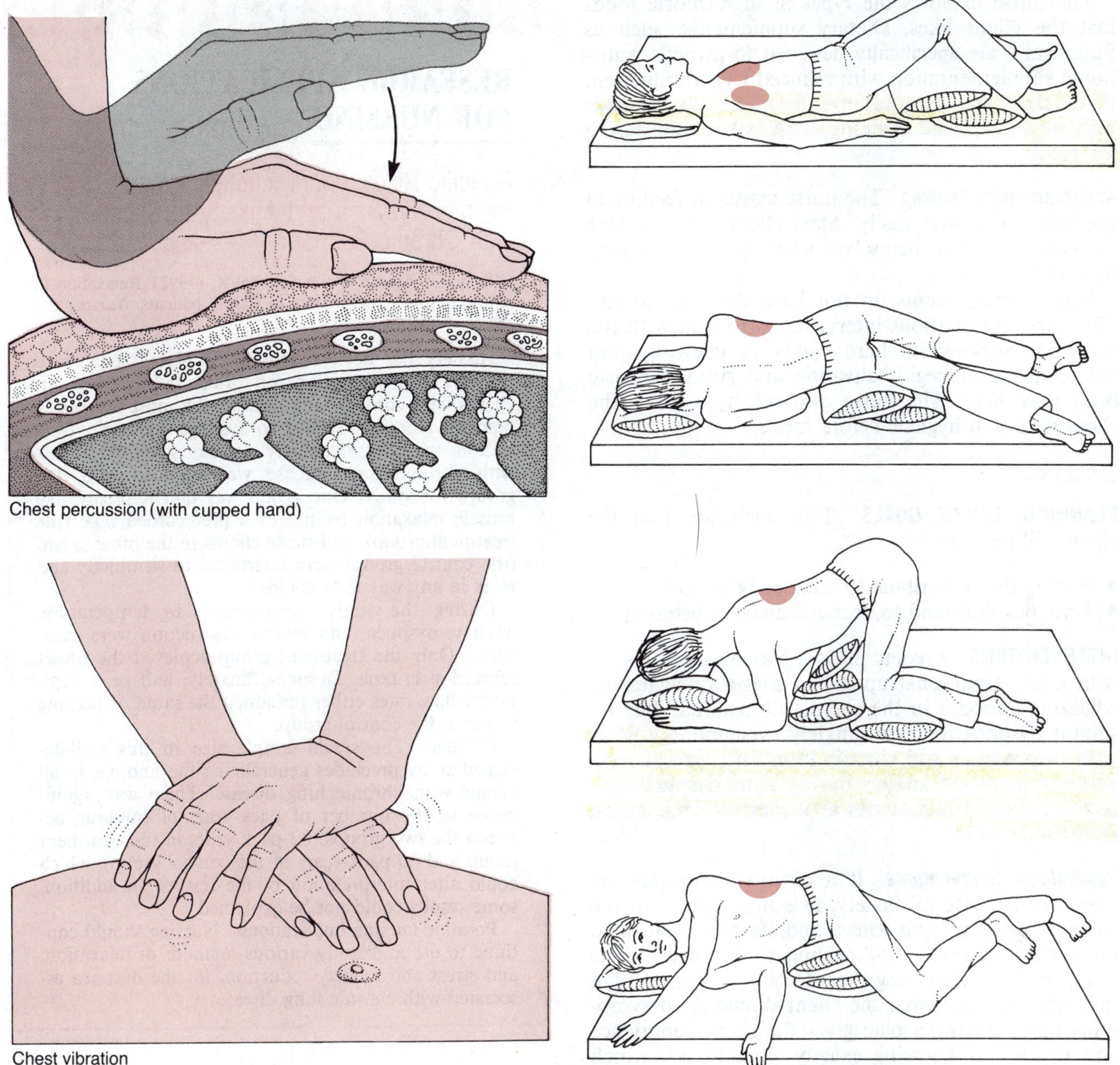

FIGURE 30–18 ♦ Chest physiotherapy (chest PT) and postural drainage. *A*, percussion and vibration techniques. The nurse may use one or two hands with vibration, which is performed when the client exhales or coughs. *B*, Position for postural drainage of respiratory secretions.

The nurse identifies clients at risk or those experiencing this complication and initiates dietary consultation. The nurse and dietitian monitor the client's weight and other indicators of nutrition, such as skin condition and serum albumin levels.

Dyspnea Management Shortness of breath is the most common complaint of clients related to eating. The nurse teaches the client that shortness of breath during mealtimes can be minimized by resting before meals. The client plans the biggest meal of the day for the time when he or she is most hungry. Four to six small meals a day may be preferred. The nurse suggests the use of pursed-lip breathing and abdominal breathing to alleviate the dyspnea. A bronchodilator used 30 minutes before the meal may be helpful if the meal-related dyspnea is due to bronchospasm or secretions.

Food Selection Abdominal bloating and a feeling of fullness often prevent the client from eating a complete meal. In the acute care setting, clients may need assistance in choosing menus; the nurse reminds them to choose foods that are easy to chew and not gas forming. Dry foods stimulate coughing, and foods like milk and chocolate increase the thickness of saliva and secretions. The nurse advises avoidance of these foods in the symptomatic client. The nurse also teaches the client to avoid caffeinated beverages; they promote diuresis and contribute to dehydration.

The nurse explores the types of high-calorie foods that the client likes. Dietary supplements, such as Pulmocare, are specifically designed to provide nutritional supplementation with reduced CO_2 production. If the client has early satiety, the nurse recommends that the client avoid drinking fluids before and during the meal.

Assistance with Feeding The nurse assists in feeding of the client who tires easily. Most clients do not have the energy to feed themselves when they are working hard to breathe.

Many times, clients do not have the urge to eat. The nurse tries various interventions to deal with the anorexia. Sucking on hard candy or chewing gum before meals to begin salivation and stimulate taste buds may help. The nurse also offers to assist the client with oral hygiene before meals.

ANXIETY

PLANNING: CLIENT GOALS Two goals are that the client will identify

- Factors that contribute to anxious behaviors
- Activities that tend to decrease anxious behaviors

INTERVENTIONS Anxiety plays a major role in clients with CAL. Emotional upset can trigger or aggravate wheezing episodes in the client with asthma. The resultant dyspnea increases anxiety even more. Clients with emphysema and chronic bronchitis typically experience increased anxiety during acute dyspneic episodes, especially if they feel as if they are choking on excess secretions.

Psychologic Interventions If a client's symptoms are worsened because of anxiety, it is important that the client understand this effect and have a clear plan prepared in advance for dealing with anxiety. The nurse and the client together develop a written plan that states exactly what the client should do if symptoms flare. Having a plan gives the client confidence and control in knowing exactly what to do, which often helps reduce anxiety.

The nurse helps clients to think of themselves, for example, not as asthmatics, but as people who have asthma. The client is encouraged to discuss his or her feelings and concerns with the nursing staff and other members of the health care team. The nurse explores other alternative psychologic approaches to help the client control dyspneic episodes and panic attacks. Examples include relaxation techniques (see Chap. 7), hypnosis therapy, and biofeedback. An example of the successful use of relaxation is described in the Research Applications for Nursing. Biofeedback helps the client determine the impact of various stimuli on symptoms. The client ultimately learns to relax and control these stimuli to avoid the aggravating symptoms.

The client uses pursed-lip and diaphragmatic breathing techniques in conjunction with relaxation therapy. The nurse instructs the client in the various techniques and assesses the client's understanding and performance of the techniques. The client practices the techniques daily and uses the techniques during panic attacks or episodes of dyspnea.

Professional counseling, if recommended, should be viewed by the client as a positive suggestion; in no way should the client view this need as a failure to cope. The nurse helps the client believe that talking with a professional counselor can make a big difference in the course of the disease.

Drug Therapy Some clients may benefit from drugs that reduce anxiety. These drugs are particularly helpful for some clients with asthma during an attack.

RESEARCH APPLICATIONS FOR NURSING

Specific Relaxation Techniques May Reduce Dyspnea and Anxiety in Clients with Chronic Pulmonary Disease

Gift, A. G., Moore, T., & Soeken, K. (1992). Relaxation to reduce dyspnea and anxiety in COPD patients. *Nursing Research, 41*(4), 242–246.

Anxiety has been shown to be closely related to dyspnea, the sensation of difficult breathing. In clients with chronic lung disease, the most frequently reported emotions related to dyspnea are panic, frustration, worry, and anxiety. In this study 26 clients with chronic lung disease were divided into two groups for study. One group was taught progressive muscle relaxation by use of a prerecorded tape (the treatment group), and those clients in the other group (the control group) were instructed to sit quietly and relax in any way they could.

During the study, peripheral skin temperature, anxiety, dyspnea, and airway obstruction were measured. Only the treatment group achieved the preset relaxation criteria. Dyspnea, anxiety, and peak expiratory flow rates either remained the same or became worse in the control group.

Critique The small sample size in this well-designed study precludes generalizing the findings to all clients with chronic lung disease. There was significance to the number of pack-years of smoking between the two groups (82 pack-years in the treatment group and 50 pack-years in the control group), which could alter interpretation of the results. In addition, some results could not be explained.

Possible nursing implications Nursing should continue to use and study various methods of relaxation, and stress and anxiety reduction, for the dyspnea associated with chronic lung disease.

ACTIVITY INTOLERANCE

PLANNING: CLIENT GOALS The goals are for the client to:

- Perform activities of daily living without assistance or with limited assistance

- Adjust his or her daily schedule, making minimal changes in usual routine or lifestyle
- Perform activities, including walking for short distances, without experiencing dyspnea or tachycardia

INTERVENTIONS The client with emphysema and chronic bronchitis typically experiences chronic fatigue. While in the acute phases of the illness, the client may require extensive assistance with activities of daily living, like bathing and grooming. As the client's acute episode resolves, the nurse encourages the client to pace activities and provide as much self-care as possible. The nurse instructs the client not to rush through morning activities because rushing is likely to increase hypoxemia, dyspnea, and fatigue. As the client gradually increases his or her level of activity, the nurse continually assesses the physiologic response by noting skin color changes, pulse rate and regularity, and blood pressure. If the physician has ordered supplemental oxygen, it should be used continually, particularly during such periods of increased energy use as bathing or walking for short periods. Other interventions, such as energy conservation, are discussed under the nursing diagnosis of Ineffective Breathing Pattern.

HIGH RISK FOR INFECTION

PLANNING: CLIENT GOALS The goals are that the client will:

- Not experience secondary respiratory infection
- Recognize early signs and symptoms of infection and seek prompt treatment

INTERVENTIONS Clients who have excessive secretions or have artificial airways are at increased risk for respiratory infections. The risk is greatly increased in an elderly person. The nurse teaches the client to avoid large crowds of people, such as in a shopping center. The nurse also teaches the client the importance of having influenza injections ("flu shots") and pneumococcal vaccinations to prevent these potentially deadly diseases. The highest mortality from these diseases is in elderly clients with CAL.

POWERLESSNESS

PLANNING: CLIENT GOALS The goals are that the client will:

- Identify aspects of life that he or she can control
- Identify personal strengths

INTERVENTIONS The client who has a feeling of powerlessness may be depressed, angry, apathetic, or withdrawn. The nurse assesses each client's reaction to powerlessness through observation and exploration with the client. The nurse asks the client to describe how he or she feels, specifically related to the impact of the disease on lifestyle and daily routines. The nurse helps the client identify strengths and discourages a focus on limitations.

The nurse also assists the client in identifying resources and support systems, such as the family, significant others, and clergy. In her nursing research, Reed (1991) found that family, clergy, and friends were identified by hospitalized clients more frequently than nurses as spiritual resource persons. The client may also wish to talk with other clients who have the same disease or choose to confer with a counselor. The nurse makes the necessary arrangements at the client's request.

DISCHARGE PLANNING

HOME CARE PREPARATION

The client with chronic airflow limitation (CAL) is usually discharged from the hospital to his or her previous home setting. For clients with advanced disease, however, 24-hour care may be needed for activities of daily living and to monitor the client for acute episodes or progression of the illness. The client may not be able to enjoy work or recreational activities because he or she spends all available energy on the work of breathing. If arrangements for home care are not possible, the client may need to be transferred to a long-term care setting.

Most clients can benefit from a structured pulmonary rehabilitation program (Table 30–6). Pulmonary rehabilitation programs vary, but the overall goal of these multidisciplinary programs is to increase a person's ability to compensate for and live with CAL. In collaboration with the physician, the nurse refers clients with CAL to a pulmonary rehabilitation program before illness becomes severe. Clients with the least severe functional abnormality benefit the most.

The nurse works with the hospital discharge planning nurse to obtain the necessary equipment for care at home. Possible needs include oxygen therapy, including transportable oxygen for out-of-home use, a hospital-type bed, and a nebulizer.

HEALTH TEACHING

Clients with a chronic, disabling disease like CAL need to know as much about the disease as possible so that they can better manage it and themselves. Specifically, the client and family members or significant others should be able to discuss medications,

TABLE 30–6 Areas of Focus in a Pulmonary Rehabilitation Program

- Education
- Exercise conditioning
- Energy conservation
- Breathing retraining
- Bronchial hygiene
- Dietary counseling
- Vocational training
- Psychologic counseling

diet therapy regimen, and activity progression. They need to identify and avoid stressors that can exacerbate the disease. The nurse stresses the importance of communication between the client and family. Spouses or family members frequently avoid any communication they believe will upset the client. Family therapy may be needed to facilitate communication techniques.

The nurse instructs the client in techniques of breathing that include:

- Pursed-lip breathing
- Diaphragmatic breathing
- Positioning
- Relaxation therapy
- Coughing and deep breathing
- Energy conservation

Figure 30–19 is a sample CAL client education checklist used for discharge teaching. Education related to specific interventions has been discussed under the various nursing diagnoses. Two factors may interfere with teaching the hospitalized client: the shortened length of stay coupled with a multitude of topics to discuss, and the client's level of tolerance and dyspnea. It may be unrealistic to cover all of the topics in the education checklist during a single hospitalization. The primary nurse or case manager will coordinate teaching with the home health or clinic staff.

Hypoxemic clients can benefit from long-term use of oxygen at home. As with other therapies, the physician's decision to prescribe home oxygen is made with calculated analysis. The physician may prescribe oxygen only during periods of exercise or while sleeping if hypoxemia occurs only during these times. Continuous, long-term administration of oxygen can reverse tissue hypoxia and decreased pulmonary vascular resistance; it can also improve cognitive ability and well-being.

CRITERIA FOR HOME OXYGEN THERAPY The client must be clinically stable and optimally treated before the need for home oxygen is considered. For Medicare to cover the cost of continuous oxygen therapy, the client must have severe hypoxemia. Severe hypoxemia is defined as a PaO_2 level of less than 55 mmHg or an arterial oxygen saturation of less than 85% on room air and at rest. A variation of this criterion is a PaO_2 value of 56 to 59 mmHg or an arterial oxygen saturation value of 86% to 89% with a secondary diagnosis of symptomatic congestive heart failure, cor pulmonale as seen on an electrocardiogram, or erythrocytosis with a hematocrit of 56%. Specific criteria are also established for coverage of nocturnal oxygen and portable oxygen therapy. Medicare guidelines are continually changing; therefore, it is important for the nurse to be aware of these criteria and the documentation required to meet the standards.

TEACHING ABOUT HOME OXYGEN THERAPY After the need for home oxygen therapy is verified, the nurse begins a teaching plan about oxygen therapy. The client, with the nurse's assistance, selects a durable medical equipment (DME) company to deliver oxygen equipment and a community health nursing agency for follow-up care in the home. The physician re-evaluates the client's need for oxygen therapy approximately 6 months after discharge from the health care facility and yearly thereafter.

While providing discharge planning and teaching, the nurse is sensitive to the client's psychologic adjustment to oxygen therapy. The nurse encourages the client to share feelings and concerns. The client may be concerned about social acceptance by and misconceptions of friends. The nurse helps the client realize that compliance with oxygen therapy is important so that normal activities of daily living and events that bring enjoyment can be continued.

EQUIPMENT FOR HOME OXYGEN THERAPY The nurse or respiratory therapist teaches the client about the equipment needed for home oxygen therapy:

- The oxygen source
- The oxygen delivery device
- The humidification source
- Safety aspects of using and maintaining the equipment

Home oxygen is provided in one of three ways:

- Compressed gas in a tank or a cylinder
- Liquid oxygen in a reservoir
- An oxygen concentrator

Compressed gas in an oxygen tank (green) is the most common type of oxygen source. The large H cylinder is used as a stationary source; the small E tank is available for transporting the client (Fig. 30–20). Even smaller (and lighter) D or C cylinders are available for the client to carry. An oxygen tank is economical, and pure oxygen can be delivered at a wide range of flow rates.

The second type of home oxygen, liquid oxygen, is oxygen gas that has been liquefied by cooling to −300° F (−147° C); thus, a concentrated amount of oxygen is available in a lightweight and easy-to-carry container similar to a thermos bottle (Fig. 30–21). This type of oxygen lasts longer than oxygen in a conventional tank of the same size; however, it is expensive, and the oxygen evaporates if it is not used continuously.

The last type of home oxygen source is the oxygen concentrator (Fig. 30–22), which is an electric machine that removes nitrogen, water vapor, and hydrocarbons from room air. Oxygen is concentrated from room air and is delivered at more than 90%. The concentrator is the least expensive of the systems but is not portable and is often noisy.

Humidification is rarely needed for any of these

Checklist for CAL Client Education

The Client Has Received the Following Education:	Date	Signature
A. Basic anatomy and physiology of the respiratory system 1. Structures composing the respiratory system 2. Functions of the respiratory passageways	______	______
B. Pathophysiology related to condition 1. Name of lung disease 2. Generalized physiologic effects 3. Generalized psychosocial effects	______	______
C. Medications 1. Medication safety 2. Name of each medication 3. Action of each medication 4. Dosage 5. How to take each medication 6. How to use a metered dose inhaler with or without a "spacer" 7. Recognition of side effects 8. Importance of carrying a medication list and a medical alert (Medic Alert) bracelet or card	______	______
D. Respiratory therapy interventions and bronchial hygiene 1. Proper care and cleaning of home equipment, i.e., oxygen, cannulas, nebulizers 2. Sequence of treatments 3. Adequate hydration 4. Postural drainage and chest physiotherapy (optional and only with excessive secretions) 5. Prevention of respiratory tract infection: a. Avoid exposure to crowds and people with respiratory tract infections b. Signs and symptoms of respiratory tract infection c. Use of prescribed antibiotics with as needed (prn) schedule d. Influenza immunization; pneumococcal immunization e. Use of measures to promote oronasal hygiene	______	______
E. Management of dyspnea 1. Controlled cough maneuver 2. Pursed-lip breathing 3. Diaphragmatic breathing 4. Positioning techniques 5. Stress management and relaxation techniques	______	______
F. Adaptation of a daily routine 1. Daily schedule of graded exercises 2. Walking exercise on level ground 3. Stair climbing 4. Activities of daily living: adjust activities according to individual fatigue patterns	______	______
G. Nutrition 1. Type of diet prescribed 2. Balanced diet: meat, dairy, grain, fruit and vegetables: 2:2:4:4 ratio 3. Low salt intake	______	______
H. Control of environment 1. Environmental problems related to pulmonary disease 2. Ways to make the environment conducive to living with pulmonary disease a. Avoid irritants and use air purification system b. Use mask when exposed to dusts and cold air c. Stay indoors with air conditioning operating when air quality is poor d. Check air quality telephone recording	______	______
I. Smoking 1. Rationale for smoking cessation 2. Suggest ways to stop smoking	______	______
J. Body image and human sexuality 1. Alterations in self-esteem and body image related to pulmonary disease 2. Communication in human relationships. 3. Alterations in sexual relationships related to pulmonary disease	______	______
K. Available community resources 1. Discharge planning; referral to home care professionals 2. Available community services: Meals on Wheels; American Lung Association; American Heart Association; American Cancer Society	______	______

FIGURE 30–19 ◆ A checklist for education of the client with chronic airflow limitation.

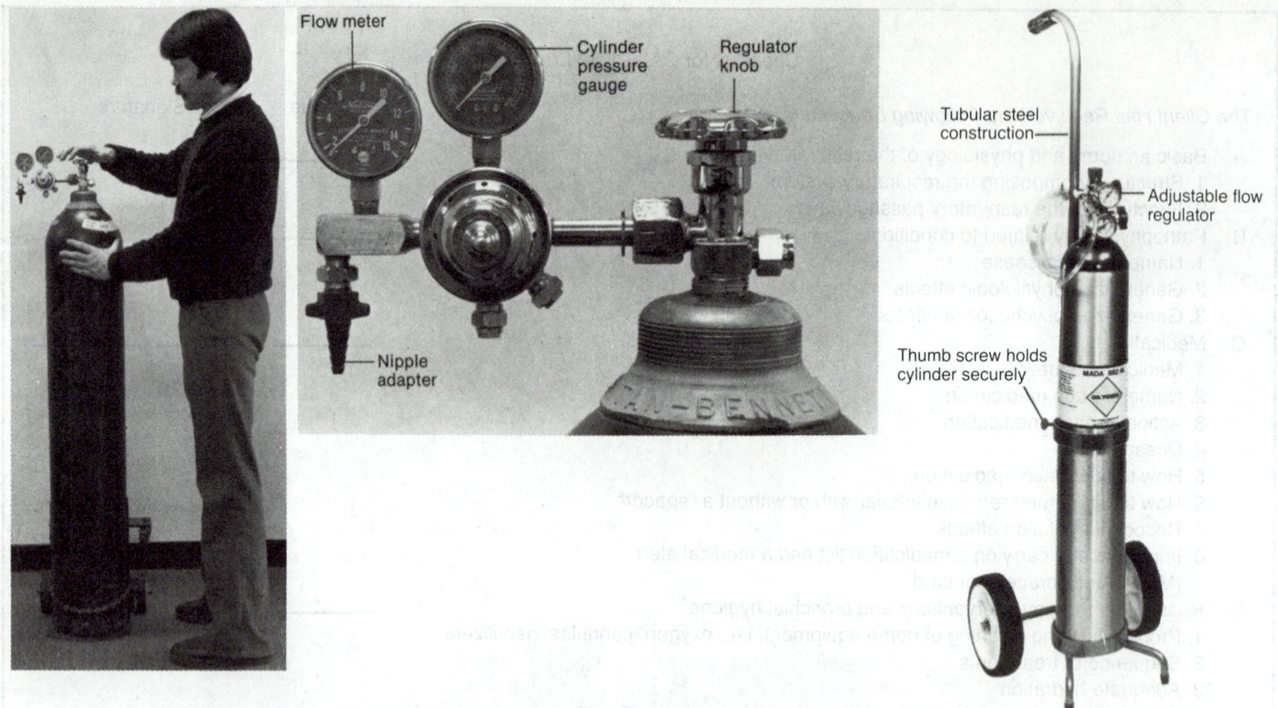

FIGURE 30–20 ◆ Comparison of a large H oxygen cylinder (*left* and *center*), with a stand, regulator, and flowmeter, and a small E cylinder (right). (Left and center photographs, From Kersten, L. D. [1989]. *Comprehensive respiratory nursing: A decision making approach.* Philadelphia: W. B. Saunders; right photograph, Courtesy of Mada Medical Products, Inc., Carlstadt, NJ.)

oxygen systems. Nevertheless, humidification may help when the physician prescribes a flow rate higher than 2 L/minute.

PSYCHOSOCIAL PREPARATION

The client with chronic airflow limitation (CAL) faces a lifelong disease with remissions and exacerbations. The nurse explains to both the client and the family that the client may experience periods of anxiety, depression, and ineffective coping. The client may also have self-directed anger, particularly if he or she was a smoker and recognizes that smoking contributed to the disease.

Financial concerns often increase the client's anxiety and interfere with disease management. The client's condition may worsen to the point that he or she cannot work. Disability benefits through Social Security or private disability insurance plans can help ease the financial burden. Medicare or other health insurers may assist with payment for home oxygen therapy and nebulizer treatments. The nurse collaborates closely with the social worker or discharge planning nurse to help the client make the necessary arrangements.

HEALTH CARE RESOURCES

The nurse provides appropriate referrals as necessary. Home care visits may be warranted, particularly if the client must use home oxygen therapy for the

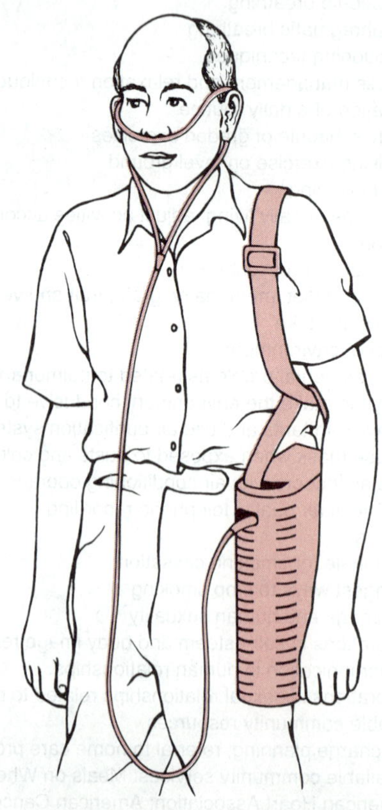

FIGURE 30–21 ◆ Liquid oxygen.

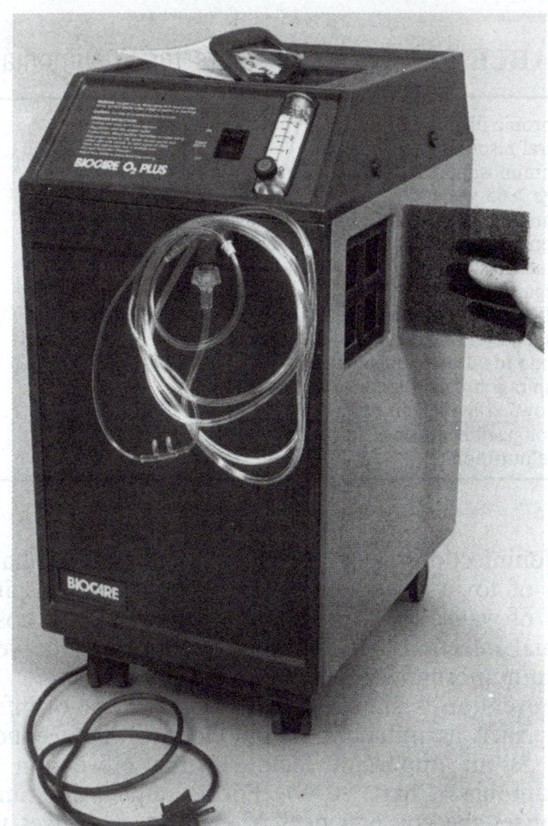

FIGURE 30–22 ◆ An oxygen concentrator for long-term oxygen delivery. (From Kersten, L. D. [1989]. *Comprehensive respiratory nursing: A decision making approach.* Philadelphia: W. B. Saunders.)

first time. Referral to assistance programs, such as Meals on Wheels, can be extremely helpful. The nurse provides the client with a list of various support groups and Better Breathing groups sponsored by the American Lung Association. If the client is having difficulty with smoking cessation and indicates the need for assistance, the nurse makes the appropriate referrals.

EVALUATION

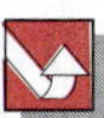

The nurse evaluates the care of the client with chronic airflow limitation on the basis of the identified nursing diagnoses. The expected outcomes are that the client:

- Attains and maintains ventilation parameters (PaO_2, $PaCO_2$) within the normal range for the client
- Demonstrates lung sounds optimal for the client
- Demonstrates breathing techniques of pursed-lip breathing and abdominal or diaphragmatic breathing
- Demonstrates positioning techniques to use during dyspneic episodes
- Identifies various methods of conserving energy
- Maintains a patent airway by removing excessive secretions
- Demonstrates controlled coughing
- Increases or maintains fluid intake
- Attains and maintains body weight within 10% of ideal
- States methods of reducing anxiety
- Identifies personal strengths rather than focusing on limitations
- Performs self-care independently or with minimal assistance for as long as possible
- States the need to avoid irritants and sources of infection

RESPIRATORY INFECTIONS

Pneumonia

OVERVIEW

Pneumonia is an inflammatory process that results in edema of the interstitial lung tissue and extravasation of fluid into the alveoli, thus causing hypoxemia. Although pneumonia was once a major cause of death, antibiotics have reduced mortality significantly.

PATHOPHYSIOLOGY

Pneumonia results from an infection of the pulmonary tissue, including the interstitial spaces, the alveoli, and often the bronchioles. The pneumonic process begins when pathogens successfully penetrate the airway mucus and multiply in the alveolar spaces. To do this, they must survive the lung's many defenses against microbial invasion. As the pathogenic organisms multiply, edematous fluid forms, and other evidence of inflammation becomes apparent. White blood cells migrate into the alveoli and cause thickening of the alveolar wall. Fluid fills the alveoli, which protects the organisms from phagocytosis and facilitates the movement of organisms to other alveoli. In this way, the infection spreads. If the invading organisms obtain access to the bloodstream, septicemia results. Chapter 27 discusses the infectious process in detail.

The edema of inflammation stiffens the lung, thus causing decreased lung compliance and a decline in the vital capacity (VC) of the lung. Decreased production of surfactant further reduces compliance and leads to atelectasis. Some of the venous blood coming into the lungs passes through the underventilated area. This unoxygenated blood then travels to the left side of the heart. As a result, arterial oxygen tension falls, causing hypoxemia (insufficient oxygen in the blood).

Fever is the systemic response to the infection. The client may develop shaking chills in an attempt to increase heat production and raise the metabolic rate. An increase in metabolic demand causes secondary tachypnea with tachycardia. Blood pressure may fall because of peripheral vasodilation and decreased circulating blood volume secondary to dehydration. Cardiac function may be compromised by hypoxemia and enhanced metabolism. Congestive heart failure or shock may result; cardiac irritability may be enhanced because of inadequate tissue oxygenation, thus causing dysrhythmias.

The extent of pulmonary involvement after the microbial invasion depends on the defenses of the host. In an immunocompromised host, bacteria can multiply. Tissue necrosis results when multiplying anaerobic organisms form an abscess that perforates the bronchial wall. Pneumonia may occur as diffuse patches throughout both lungs (bronchopneumonia), or it may cause consolidation (solidification, lack of air spaces) in one lobe.

Pneumonias are classified as community-acquired or nosocomial (hospital-acquired). Common organisms are listed in Table 30–7. A third group of pneumonias is associated with the immunocompromised client who is susceptible to both community-acquired and nosocomial infections. *Pneumocystis carinii,* a protozoan, is the most frequent cause of pneumonia in the immunocompromised client. *Pneumocystis* pneumonia is the most life-threatening infection in the client with AIDS.

ETIOLOGY

In general, pneumonia develops when a person's defense mechanisms cannot combat the virulence of the invading organisms. Risk factors are given in Table 30–8. Several types of organisms cause pneumonia, including bacteria, viruses, mycoplasmas, fungi, rickettsiae, protozoa, and helminths (worms). The incidence of fungal pneumonias is increasing in critically ill and immunosuppressed clients; these pneumonias are not communicable. Examples of fungal and viral agents that could cause pneumonia are listed in Table 30–9.

TABLE 30–7 Common Organisms Causing Community and Nosocomial Pneumonias

Community-Acquired Pneumonias

- *Mycoplasma pneumoniae*
- *Streptococcus pneumoniae*
- *Haemophilus influenzae*
- *Legionella pneumophila*

Nosocomial Pneumonias

- *Staphylococcus aureus*
- *Klebsiella pneumoniae*
- *Pseudomonas aeruginosa*
- Fungi (various types)

TABLE 30–8 Risk Factors for Pneumonia

- Chronic illness
- Viral respiratory infections
- Immunosuppression/neutropenia
- Age >65 years
- Impaired gag, cough, or swallow reflex
- Depressed cerebral function (altered level of consciousness)
- Tracheostomy or endotracheal tube
- Organ transplants
- AIDS
- Exposure to noxious gas (e.g., cigarette smoke, air pollution)
- Abdominal or thoracic surgery
- Aspiration of upper airway organisms
- Crowded living conditions
- Prolonged bed rest or immobility
- Malnutrition

Noninfectious causes of pneumonia include inhalation of toxic gases, chemicals, or smoke and aspiration of water, food, fluid, or vomitus. Because nosocomial infections are prevalent in facilities, the very ill, immunosuppressed client is at high risk.

Prevention is aimed at reducing the cause of infection, such as influenza in the elderly. Client education is an important factor in the prevention of pneumonia (Chart 30–8). For example, the nurse discusses the consequences of smoking and gives the client information on local support groups for smoking cessation, if desired.

In the hospital setting and in all facilities, the nurse follows strict hand washing techniques to avoid the spread of nosocomial infection. In addition, respiratory therapy equipment is well maintained and decontaminated or changed as recommended by the respiratory therapy personnel.

The nurse identifies clients at risk for aspiration and, thus, aspiration pneumonia. These at-risk clients include those with a feeding tube, impaired swallowing or coughing mechanisms, an altered level of con-

TABLE 30–9 Viral and Fungal Agents that Could Cause Pneumonia

Viruses

- Influenza A virus
- Adenovirus
- Varicella-zoster virus
- Togavirus (rubella)
- Paramyxovirus
- Herpes simplex virus
- Cytomegalovirus (CMV)
- Epstein-Barr virus

Fungi

- *Candida*
- *Histoplasma*
- *Coccidioides*
- *Blastomyces*
- *Cryptococcus*
- *Aspergillus*

CHART 30-8

Health Promotion Guide ◆ Preventing Pneumonia

- Know whether you are at risk for pneumonia.
- Have the annual influenza vaccine after discussing appropriate timing of the vaccination with your primary health care provider.
- Discuss the once-in-a-lifetime pneumococcal vaccine with your primary health care provider and have the vaccination as recommended.
- Avoid crowded public areas during flu and holiday seasons.
- Cough, turn, move about, and do deep-breathing exercises as directed by your nurse or other health care professional.
- If you are using respiratory equipment at home, clean the equipment as you have been taught.
- Avoid indoor pollutants, such as dust, second-hand (passive) smoke, and aerosols.
- If you don't smoke, don't start.
- If you smoke, seek professional help on how to stop, or at least decrease, your habit.
- Be sure to get enough rest and sleep on a daily basis.
- Eat a healthy, balanced diet and take in a sufficient amount of nonalcoholic fluids each day.

sciousness, or decreased mobility and the elderly. Specific interventions to prevent aspiration are discussed in Chapter 29.

INCIDENCE/PREVALENCE

Pneumonia and influenza remain a leading cause of death, ranking fifth in the United States. Pneumonia accounts for up to 20% of all nosocomial infections and is a prevalent condition affecting the elderly. Pneumonia is the most frequent cause of death by infection among clients 65 years old or older; and it is the third leading cause of death for clients older than 85 years. Risk factors for pneumonia in the elderly are summarized in Table 30-10. Mortality is highest in clients who develop complications of

TABLE 30-10 Predisposing Factors for Pneumonia in the Elderly

- Chronic airflow limitation
- Congestive heart failure
- Influenza
- Alcoholism
- Immobility
- Reduced cellular immunity
- Loss of ciliary action
- Decreased chest wall compliance
- Decreased muscle strength
- Poor nutritional status

TABLE 30-11 Common Complications of Pneumonia

Hypoxemia	• Arterial oxygen <55 mmHg
Ventilatory failure	• Lungs unable to mechanically move gas in and out of lungs, resulting in hypoxemia and hypercapnia
Atelectasis	• Collapse of the affected lobes of the lungs
Pleural effusion	• Collection of fluid in the pleural space (usually sterile fluid that resolves)
Pleurisy	• Pain caused by friction between layers of pleura

pneumonia (Table 30-11). During late fall and winter, a higher incidence of pneumonia is likely because this illness frequently follows viral infection.

COLLABORATIVE MANAGEMENT

ASSESSMENT

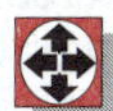

HISTORY

In preparing to take the history from the client who may have pneumonia, the nurse considers risk factors consistent with infection (see Table 30-8). The nurse collects essential data from the client or from a family member if the client is too dyspneic. The nurse documents the following:

- Age
- Living, work, or school environment
- Diet, exercise, and sleep routines
- Tobacco and alcohol use
- Past and current use of medications
- Previous history of drug addiction or intravenous drug use

The nurse lists the client's past illnesses, particularly those with a respiratory origin, and determines whether the client has been exposed to influenza or pneumonia or has experienced a recent viral episode. In addition, the nurse notes a history of any rashes, insect bites, or exposure to animals.

If the client has chronic respiratory problems, the nurse asks whether respiratory equipment is used in the home. It is essential to determine whether the client's cleaning regimen is adequate to prevent infection. The nurse also notes previous inoculations with influenza or pneumococcal vaccine.

PHYSICAL ASSESSMENT/CLINICAL MANIFESTATIONS

The nurse first observes the general appearance of the client. He or she may have flushed cheeks, bright eyes, and an anxious expression. The client may have chest or pleuritic pain or discomfort, myalgia, headache, chills, fever, cough, dyspnea, tachypnea, or sputum production. Severe chest muscle weakness may also be present from sustained coughing.

In assessing the elderly, the nurse is aware of risk and predisposing factors (see Tables 30–8 and 30–10). The elderly often have weakness, fatigue, lethargy, confusion, and poor appetite. Fever and cough may be absent. Hypoxemia, however, is generally present.

The nurse observes the client's breathing pattern, position, and use of accessory muscles. The acutely compromised client is uncomfortable in a lying position and sits upright, balancing with the hands. The nurse assesses the client's cough and the amount, color, consistency, and odor of sputum produced because these characteristics offer diagnostic clues about the offending pathogen.

On auscultation, the nurse hears crackles when there is fluid in interstitial and alveolar areas. Wheezing may be heard as a result of inflammation and exudate in the airways. Bronchial breath sounds are heard over areas of density or consolidation. Tactile fremitus is increased over areas of pneumonia, and percussion is dulled in these areas. Chest expansion may be diminished or unequal on inspiration. Chapter 28 discusses respiratory assessment in more detail.

In evaluating vital signs, the nurse compares the results with baseline values. The client who has pneumonia is likely to be hypotensive with orthostatic changes. A rapid, weak pulse may indicate hypoxemia, dehydration, or impending shock.

The nurse also inspects the skin of the client for a rash, which may occur with *Mycoplasma* infection, cytomegalovirus (CMV) infection, or Rocky Mountain spotted fever. The pathophysiology of selected clinical manifestations of pneumonia is summarized in Table 30–12.

TABLE 30–12 Pathophysiology of Selected Clinical Manifestations of Pneumonia

Clinical Manifestation	Pathophysiology
Increased respiratory rate/dyspnea	• Stimulation of chemoreceptors • Increased work of breathing due to decreased lung compliance • Stimulation of J receptors • Anxiety • Pain
Hypoxemia	• Alveolar consolidation • Capillary shunting
Cough	• Fluid accumulation in the subepithelial mechanoreceptors in the trachea, bronchi, and bronchioles
Sputum	• Purulent, blood-tinged, or rusty in color • A result of the inflammatory process in which fluid from the pulmonary capillaries and red blood cells moves into the alveoli
Fever	• Phagocytes release endogenous pyrogens that cause the hypothalamus to increase body temperature
Pleuritic chest discomfort	• Inflammation of the parietal pleura causes pain on inspiration

PSYCHOSOCIAL ASSESSMENT

The client with pneumonia experiences pain, fatigue, and dyspnea, which promote anxiety. The nurse assesses anxiety by looking at the client's facial expression and general tenseness of facial and shoulder muscles. The nurse listens to the client carefully and uses a calm, slow approach to assessment. The client with dyspnea speaks in broken sentences because of airway obstruction and muscle fatigue. The nurse gauges the length of the interview on the degree of dyspnea or breathing discomfort the client experiences.

LABORATORY ASSESSMENT

Sputum is obtained from the client and examined by Gram stain, culture, and sensitivity testing. A sputum sample is obtained easily from the client who can cough into a specimen container. Extremely ill clients may require nasotracheal suctioning by the nurse or suctioning via a tracheostomy or endotracheal tube. The nurse obtains a sputum specimen from these clients by using a sputum trap (Fig. 30–23) while suctioning.

A complete blood count (CBC) is obtained to determine leukocytosis, which is a common finding except in the elderly. Blood cultures may be performed to determine whether the organism has invaded the bloodstream. Urine may be examined for hematuria, pyuria, or the presence of protein in the septic client with pneumonia.

Arterial blood gases (ABGs) determine baseline arterial oxygen and carbon dioxide levels and help identify a need for supplemental oxygen. Serum electrolyte, blood urea nitrogen, and creatinine levels are also assessed. The client may develop an increased blood urea nitrogen level as a result of increased catabolism and a diminished glomerular filtration rate. Electrolyte changes occur with dehydration, a result of fever and malaise.

RADIOGRAPHIC ASSESSMENT

In general, pneumonia appears on chest x-ray as an area of increased density. It may involve a lung segment, a lobe, one lung, or both lungs. The chest x-ray is essential for early diagnosis of pneumonia in elderly clients because their symptoms are often vague.

OTHER DIAGNOSTIC ASSESSMENT

The nurse obtains oxygen saturation values by using pulse oximetry. This noninvasive test (see Chap. 28) helps detect hypoxemia.

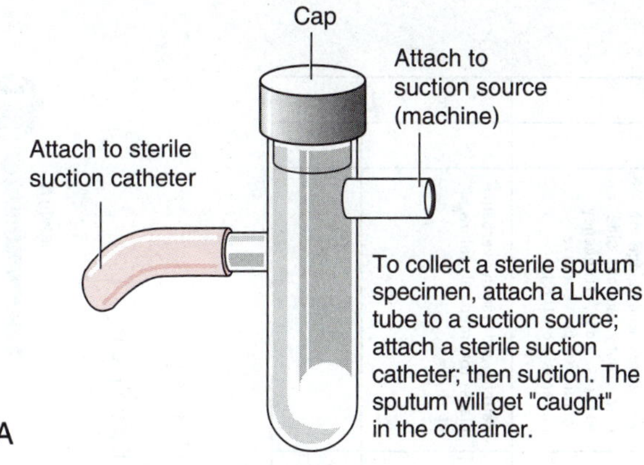

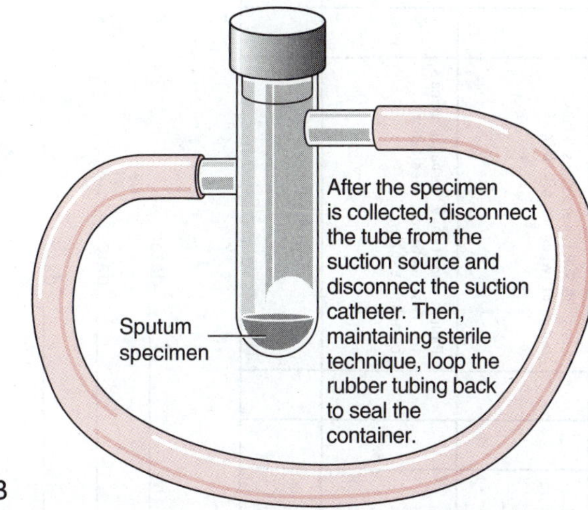

FIGURE 30–23 ◆ Method of collecting a sterile sputum specimen using a Lukens tube.

ANALYSIS

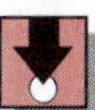

COMMON NURSING DIAGNOSES

Two of the nursing diagnoses commonly identified for the client with pneumonia are:

1. Impaired Gas Exchange related to effects of alveolar-capillary membrane changes
2. Ineffective Airway Clearance related to effects of infection, excessive tracheobronchial secretions, fatigue and decreased energy, chest discomfort, and muscle weakness

ADDITIONAL NURSING DIAGNOSES

In addition to the common diagnoses, the client may have associated problems, which may include those listed for the client with chronic airflow limitation (CAL) and:

- Pain related to effects of inflammation of the parietal pleura, coughing
- Hyperthermia related to an increased metabolic rate, dehydration
- Fluid Volume Deficit related to fever, infection, increased metabolic rate
- Ineffective Breathing Pattern related to fatigue, decreased energy, pain, the inflammatory process, and anxiety
- Sleep Pattern Disturbance related to pain, dyspnea, unfamiliar environment (e.g., hospitalization)

PLANNING AND IMPLEMENTATION

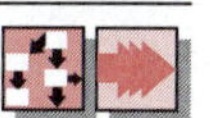

IMPAIRED GAS EXCHANGE

PLANNING: CLIENT GOALS The major goal is that the client will attain and maintain PaO_2 and $PaCO_2$ levels within baseline ranges. Other goals are similar to those for the client with CAL and have been listed previously.

Some facilities have created clinical pathways to plan care for the client with pneumonia. An example of such a pathway is found on page 716.

INTERVENTIONS Interventions for treatment and management of impaired gas exchange for the client with pneumonia are similar to those discussed earlier for the client with CAL. The gas exchange affected most in pneumonia is that of oxygen; therefore, hypoxemia is the primary problem. Carbon dioxide retention is not as common in pneumonia as it is, for example, in chronic emphysema.

Incentive spirometry, also referred to as sustained maximal inspiration, is a type of bronchial hygiene therapy used in pneumonia. The objective is to improve inspiratory muscle performance and to prevent or reverse atelectasis. The nurse obtains an incentive spirometer and instructs the client to exhale fully, then place the mouthpiece in the mouth and take a long, slow, deep breath for 3 to 5 seconds. The nurse evaluates the client's technique and records the volume of air inspired. The client performs 5 to 10 breaths per session every hour while awake. Chapter 19 has more information on incentive spirometry.

INEFFECTIVE AIRWAY CLEARANCE

PLANNING: CLIENT GOALS The major goal is that the client will have optimal breath sounds. The goal may be to have clear lungs in all lobes on auscultation or to have, minimally, improved breath sounds. Other goals are similar to those for the client with CAL and have been listed previously.

INTERVENTIONS Interventions for the treatment and management of ineffective airway clearance for the client with pneumonia are similar to those discussed earlier for the client with CAL. The client with pneumonia often has difficulty clearing secretions because of fatigue, muscle weakness, chest discomfort, and

HARBOR HOSPITAL CENTER

CLINICAL PATHWAY

Pneumonia LOS 5.4 DRG 090

	DAY 1	O	C	DAY 2	O	C	DAY 3	O	C	DAY 4	O	C
Special Orders Tests (Consults)	CBC, SMAC20, PT, PTT, STS, CXR, UA Sputum - Gram stain, C&S, SA02			CBC, SMA7			CXR					
Treatment	IV fluids, IV antibiotics after gram stain report. Protective cough - CPT/or suction Reactive airways - Bronchodilators 02 via NC to maintain SA02 > 92%, I&O.			IV fluids. IV antibiotics. Respiratory Rx as ordered. 02 to maintain SA02 > 92%, I&O			IV fluids. IV antibiotics. Respiratory Rx as ordered. 02 to maintain SA02 > 92%, I&O			IV fluids (if needed). IV antibiotics. I&O's.		
Nutrition	Diet as ordered, encourage fluids.			As tolerated, encourage fluids.			As tolerated, encourage fluids.			Diet as tolerated, encourage fluids.		
Activity	Bed rest with BRP.			OOB as tolerated.			Ambulate with assistance.			Ambulatory.		
Teaching	Verbalize rationale for: coughing and deep breathing, no smoking, increase fluid intake. Demonstrates - proper use of MDI (if indicated).			Identifies risk factors for U.R.I. Demonstrate competency in use of MDI.			Lists S&S R.I. verbalizes knowledge of when to call MD.			Verbalizes knowledge of medications: action, side effects, dose, frequency. Identifies preventative methods for U.R.I.		
Discharge Planning	Assess support system and resources. Assess need for Smoking Cessation program.			Evaluate need for Home Health for medication monitoring, need for home 02.			Patient and family verbalize need for rest, nutrition, medication compliance after D/C.			Patient and family verbalize plans for medical follow-up.		
Variance												

EXPECTED OUTCOMES

1. The patient will ______________________________ date
2. The patient will ______________________________ date
3. The patient will ______________________________ date

O = Ordered

C = Completed

(CP007)

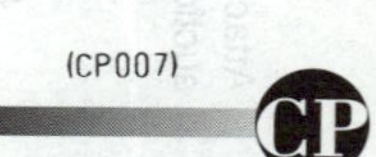

excessive secretions. The nurse assists the client to cough and deep breathe at least every 2 hours. The alert client may use an incentive spirometer to facilitate deep breathing and stimulate coughing. Chest physiotherapy (CPT or chest PT), which was once thought to be useful for clearing secretions in the client with pneumonia, is no longer recommended in uncomplicated pneumonia. Whereas dehydration should be avoided, there is no evidence that hydration helps clear secretions. Adequate hydration may help in thinning secretions, which makes them easier to remove. The nurse monitors the client's intake and output to ensure adequate hydration when fever and tachypnea are present.

It is common for clients with pneumonia to be treated with antibiotics on an outpatient basis. The key to the effective treatment of pneumonia is identification of the organism causing the pneumonia. A sputum culture identifies the organism, and a sensitivity study identifies the antibiotic most effective in treating the organism. Antibiotics are given for all types of pneumonias except viral pneumonias (Table 30–13). Aerosolized pentamidine may be used if *Pneumocystis carinii* pneumonia (PCP) is diagnosed. Pentamidine has antiprotozoal activity and is administered via a specialized nebulizer (Respirgard II), which nebulizes the medication into particles small enough to be delivered to the alveoli. Pentamidine is used in the treatment and prevention of *Pneumocystis* pneumonia.

The physician prescribes bronchodilators, especially $beta_2$-agonists (see Chart 30–6), when bronchospasm is part of the disease process. They are usually administered initially by aerosol nebulizer and then by metered-dose inhaler (see Chart 30–7). The use of mucolytic agents and expectorants has been found to be of marginal value in the treatment of pneumonia. Inhaled steroid preparations are generally not used with acute pneumonia except when the client also has bronchial asthma or respiratory failure.

TABLE 30–13 Drug Therapy for Various Types of Pneumonia

Type of Pneumonia	Drug Therapy
Community-acquired pneumonias	
Streptococcus pneumoniae (gram +)	• Penicillins
Haemophilus influenzae (gram −)	• First- and second-generation cephalosporins • Tetracyclines • Quinolones • Trimethoprim/sulfamethoxazole
Mycoplasma pneumoniae *Legionella pneumophila* (gram −)	• Macrolide antibiotics (such as Erythromycin)
Viruses	• No specific drug for viruses
Nosocomial pneumonias	
Staphylococcus aureus (gram +)	• Broad-spectrum penicillins
Klebsiella pneumoniae (gram −)	
Pseudomonas aeruginosa (gram −)	• Penicillins with a beta-lactamase-inhibitor added • Second- and third-generation cephalosporins • Aminoglycosides • Quinolones • Macrolide antibiotics • Trimethoprim/sulfamethoxazole • Vancomycin
Fungi	• Antifungals (such as Amphotericin B or fluconazole [Diflucan])
Other pneumonias	
Pneumocystis carinii pneumonia	• Trimethoprim/sulfamethoxazole • Pentamidine
Aspiration pneumonia (usually anaerobes such as *Bacteroides*)	• Clindamycin (Cleocin, Dalacin C✱) • Second-generation cephalosporins

DISCHARGE PLANNING

HOME CARE PREPARATION

No special structural changes are needed in the home. If the home consists of more than one story, the client may prefer to stay on the first floor for a few weeks because stair climbing may increase fatigue and dyspnea. Bath and hygiene needs may be met by using a bedside commode if a bathroom is not located on the first level. Home care needs depend on the client's level of fatigue, dyspnea, and family and social support.

HEALTH TEACHING

The nurse's most important health teaching for the client and family is educating them to avoid upper respiratory tract infections and viruses. The client must:

- Avoid crowds, especially in the fall and winter when viruses are prevalent
- Avoid people who have a cold or flu
- Avoid exposure to irritants, such as smoke

The influenza vaccine is recommended annually and the pneumococcal vaccine currently once in a lifetime. A balanced diet and adequate fluid intake are essential. The nurse reviews all medications with the client and family and emphasizes that antibiotic therapy must be completed. The nurse instructs the client to notify the physician if chills, fever, persistent cough, dyspnea, hemoptysis, chest discomfort, or increasing fatigue recurs or if symptoms fail to resolve.

The client is instructed to get plenty of rest and gradually increase exercise.

PSYCHOSOCIAL PREPARATION

The prolonged convalescent phase of pneumonia, particularly in the elderly client, can be frustrating and perhaps depressing. Fatigue, weakness, and a residual cough can last for weeks. The client may fear that he or she will never return to a "normal" level of functioning. It is important that the nurse prepare the client for the course of the disease and offer reassurance so that complete recovery will occur. The client may benefit from a home health nurse assessment initially after discharge.

HEALTH CARE RESOURCES

Clients who smoke are taught that smoking is a risk factor for pneumonia. The nurse provides information on smoking cessation classes through the American Lung Association (ALA) and American Cancer Society. The physician may prescribe nicotine patches. The physician and nurse warn the client of the danger of myocardial infarction if he or she continues to smoke while using the patches. It is recommended that the client be enrolled in a smoking cessation program in conjunction with use of the nicotine patches to assist in the nicotine withdrawal process. The nurse can also give the client information booklets on pneumonia provided by the ALA. If the client has not already been vaccinated against influenza or pneumococcal pneumonia, he or she should be encouraged to take this preventive measure.

EVALUATION

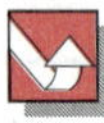

On the basis of the identified nursing diagnoses, the nurse evaluates the care of the client with pneumonia. The expected outcomes are that the client:

- Attains and maintains acceptable PaO_2, $PaCO_2$, and oxygen saturation values
- Is able to think clearly without confusion
- Maintains a patent airway and has an effective cough
- Has improved breath sounds
- Controls dyspnea
- Performs self-care and other daily activities independently
- Walks for short distances without experiencing dyspnea or tachycardia
- Describes and complies with the medication regimen
- States risk factors associated with pneumonia
- States interventions to prevent pneumonia

Pulmonary Tuberculosis

OVERVIEW

In 1900, tuberculosis (TB) was the leading cause of death in the United States and Europe. After significant reduction in its incidence, TB is currently on the rise, especially in clients with HIV and acquired immunodeficiency syndrome (AIDS). Continuous assessment and intervention to prevent the spread of the disease must continue. Increasing numbers of the homeless, people with AIDS, and resistant strains of the TB organism present new challenges to the control and eradication of TB.

PATHOPHYSIOLOGY

Tuberculosis is a highly communicable disease caused by *Mycobacterium tuberculosis.* The tubercle bacillus is transmitted via aerosolization, that is, an airborne route. When an infected person coughs, laughs, sneezes, or sings, droplet nuclei are produced and may be inhaled by others. When the tubercle bacillus reaches a susceptible site (bronchi or alveoli), it multiplies freely. An exudative response causes a nonspecific pneumonitis. With the development of acquired immunity, further multiplication of bacilli is controlled in the majority of initial lesions. The lesions typically resolve and leave little or no residual. However, a small percentage of people who are initially infected will develop the disease (5% to 15%).

Cell-mediated, or type IV, immunity develops 2 to 10 weeks after infection and is manifested by a significant reaction to a tuberculin test, that is, inflammation and necrosis. A primary infection may be microscopic in size and may never appear on an x-ray. The process of infection occurs in the following way:

- The granulomatous inflammation created by the tubercle bacillus in the lung becomes surrounded by collagen, fibroblasts, and lymphocytes.
- Caseation necrosis (necrotic tissue being turned into a granular mass) occurs in the center of the lesion. If this area becomes evident on x-ray, it is called Ghon's tubercle, or the primary lesion.

Areas of caseation then undergo resorption, hyaline degeneration, and fibrosis. These necrotic areas may calcify (calcification) or may liquefy (liquefaction). If liquefaction occurs, the liquid material then empties into a bronchus, and the evacuated area becomes a cavity (cavitation). Bacilli continue to proliferate in the necrotic cavity wall. The evacuated material leads to endobronchial spread of disease into new areas of the lung; this process can be a recurring one.

A lesion may also progress by direct extension if bacilli multiply rapidly and there is a marked exudative response to the inflammation. These lesions may extend through the pleura, which results in tuberculous pleural effusion with a small number of organisms. Pericardial effusions may also occur.

Miliary tuberculosis, or hematogenous tuberculosis, occurs when a large number of organisms enter the bloodstream and the disease becomes disseminated. Many tiny, discrete nodules scattered throughout the lung are typically seen on chest x-ray. The brain, meninges, liver, kidney (see Chap. 71), and bone marrow are commonly involved as a result of dissemination.

Initial infection is seen more often in the middle or lower lobes of the lung. The regional lymph nodes, particularly the hilar and paratracheal nodes, are commonly involved. There is usually an asymptomatic interval after infection that lasts for years, or less commonly decades, before clinical symptoms develop. The upper lobes are the most common site of reinfection. The TB classification adopted and revised by the American Lung Association is shown in Table 30–14.

ETIOLOGY

The organism *Mycobacterium tuberculosis* is a nonmotile, nonsporulating, acid-fast rod that secretes niacin. The tubercle bacillus is transmitted via aerosolization.

People who are most commonly infected are those having repeated close contact with an infected person who has not yet been diagnosed with TB. After the infected person has received medication for 2 to 3 weeks, the risk of transmission is greatly reduced.

INCIDENCE/PREVALENCE

Figures for 1981 reveal that TB accounted for only 0.8% of deaths in the United States and that the incidence of TB was declining steadily. From 1985 on, though, the number of new TB cases has increased to more than 20,000 annually. Ten million persons are estimated to be infected in the United States. The World Health Organization estimates that there are 10 million new cases each year, with 2 to 3 million deaths per year worldwide.

TABLE 30–14 American Lung Association Classification of Tuberculosis (TB)

0	No TB exposure, not infected
1	TB exposure, no evidence of infection
2	TB infection, no disease
3	TB: clinically active (clients with completed diagnostic evidence of TB: both a significant reaction to tuberculin skin test and clinical or x-ray evidence of TB)
4	TB: not clinically active (clients with previous history of TB or with abnormal chest x-ray but no significant tuberculin skin test reaction or clinical evidence)
5	TB: suspect (diagnosis pending) (used during diagnostic testing of suspect clients, for no longer than a 3-month period)

The highest at-risk populations currently include:

- Those in constant, frequent contact with an untreated individual
- Those with immune dysfunction or HIV
- Those living in crowded areas, such as long-term care facilities, prisons, and mental health facilities
- The elderly, the homeless, and minorities
- Those from a lower socioeconomic group

Transcultural Considerations Groups known to have higher incidence of tuberculosis include African-Americans, Asians and Pacific Islanders, Native Americans and Alaskan Natives or Inuits, Hispanics, current or past prison inmates, alcoholics, intravenous drug users, the elderly, and foreign-born people from Asia, Africa, the Caribbean, and Latin America (Centers for Disease Control [CDC], 1990). The risk of progression from infection to active disease increases markedly for clients with HIV infection.

COLLABORATIVE MANAGEMENT

ASSESSMENT

Early detection of TB depends on subjective findings rather than the presentation of symptoms. TB has an insidious onset, and many clients are not aware of symptoms until the disease is well advanced. A diagnosis of tuberculosis should be considered for any client with a persistent cough or other symptoms compatible with TB, such as weight loss, anorexia, fatigue, night sweats, or fever.

HISTORY

A thorough history includes assessment of past exposure to TB. The nurse inquires about the client's country of origin and travel to foreign countries in which there is a high incidence of TB. The nurse must note whether the client has had previous tests for TB and what the results were. In addition, the nurse asks whether the client has had bacille Calmette-Guérin (BCG) vaccine, a vaccine containing attenuated tubercle bacilli that is given routinely in many foreign countries to produce increased resistance to TB. Anyone who has received BCG will have a positive skin test and should be evaluated for TB with a chest x-ray.

PHYSICAL ASSESSMENT/CLINICAL MANIFESTATIONS

The client with TB typically has progressive fatigue, lethargy, nausea, anorexia, weight loss, irregular menses, and a low-grade fever, which may have been present for weeks or months. Fever may also be accompanied by night sweats. The client finally notices a cough and the production of mucoid and mucopurulent sputum, which is occasionally streaked with blood. Chest tightness and a dull, aching chest pain may accompany the cough. The physical examination of the chest does not provide conclusive evidence of tuberculosis. The nurse may hear dullness with percussion over involved parenchymal areas, bronchial breath sounds, crackles, and increased transmission of spoken or whispered sounds. Partial obstruction of a bronchus because of endobronchial disease or compression by lymph nodes may produce localized wheezing.

OTHER DIAGNOSTIC ASSESSMENT

Sputum culture of *Mycobacterium tuberculosis* confirms the diagnosis. Three samples are usually obtained for an acid-fast smear. After medications are started, sputum samples are obtained again to determine the effectiveness of therapy. Most clients have negative cultures after 3 months.

In the future, we can expect to see polymerase chain reaction (PCR) assays performed for rapid identification of the mycobacterium. This process allows amplification of mycobacterial DNA and identification of the mycobacteria within hours instead of days to weeks. This will allow earlier diagnosis and treatment of the client with TB (Brisson-Noel et al., 1991).

The tuberculin test (Mantoux test) result is the most reliable determinant of infection with TB. A small amount (0.1 mL) of intermediate-strength purified protein derivative (PPD) containing 5 tuberculin units is given intradermally in the forearm. An area of induration measuring 10 mm or more in diameter 48 to 72 hours after injection indicates the person has been exposed to TB. A positive reaction does not mean that active disease is present but indicates exposure to TB or the presence of inactive (dormant) disease. For persons with HIV infection, a reaction of 5 mm or greater is considered positive. A negative skin test result does not rule out tuberculosis disease or infection. People with HIV infection are more likely to have false-negative results (CDC, 1990).

Once a person's skin test is positive, chest x-ray is essential to rule out clinically active TB or to detect old, healed lesions. Caseation and inflammation may be seen on the x-ray if the disease is active.

Routine skin tests and chest x-rays are no longer recommended in these clients. They should be instructed to seek medical attention if they experience symptoms suggestive of TB (American Thoracic Society, 1992). The radiographic presentation in HIV-infected clients, however, may be unusual. Such clients may have infiltrates in any lung zone, often associated with hilar adenopathy, or may have a normal chest x-ray (CDC, 1990).

INTERVENTIONS

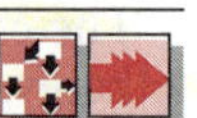

Chemotherapy is the most effective method of treating the disease and preventing transmission. Active TB is treated with a combination of drugs to which the organism is susceptible. Therapy is continued until the disease is under control. The use of multiple-drug regimens destroys organisms as quickly as possible and minimizes the emergence of drug-resistant organisms. Current therapy (Chart 30–9) uses isoniazid (INH) and rifampin throughout the therapy; pyrazinamide is added for the first 2 months. This permits shortening of the therapy from 6 to 12 months to 6 months for most clients. Ethambutol and streptomycin may be added to the treatment.

The nurse's major role is teaching clients about drug therapy. The nurse recognizes that the client who is anxious may not absorb information well. The nurse repeats the information and obtains the assistance of family members if they are available. In instructing, the nurse uses teaching aids, such as those available through the ALA. The client should be able to describe his or her treatment regimen and major side effects for which to call the health care agency and physician.

TB is frequently treated outside the acute care setting, so the client convalesces in the home setting. In this setting, respiratory isolation is not necessary because family members have already been exposed. However, the nurse instructs the client to cover his or her mouth and nose when coughing or sneezing, to confine used tissues to plastic bags, and to wear a mask when in contact with crowds until medication is effective in suppressing the infection.

The nurse informs the client that examinations of sputum are needed every 2 to 4 weeks once drug therapy is initiated. When results of two sputum cultures are negative, the client is no longer considered infectious and can usually return to former employment. The nurse reminds the client to avoid excessive exposure to silicone or dust because these substances can cause further lung damage.

The nurse places a hospitalized client with active TB in respiratory isolation precautions (see Chap. 27) in a well-ventilated room. The room should have at least six exchanges of fresh air per minute and should be ventilated to the outside if possible. The nurse wears a HEPA respirator (Fig. 30–24) when caring for the client and a gown when there is the possibility of contamination of clothing. Hands are always thoroughly washed before and after caring for the client. Isolation is discontinued when the client is no longer considered infectious.

Clients may prevent nausea related to the medications by taking the daily dose at bedtime. Antinausea drugs may also prevent this symptom. The nurse instructs the client about the need for adequate nutrition and a well-balanced diet to promote healing. The nurse recommends an increased intake of foods rich in iron, protein, and vitamin C. The nurse consults the nutritionist for specialized needs. The nurse should know the patient's ideal body weight so that progress toward the goal can be evaluated. (See Chapter 61 for further discussion of nutrition.)

The client with tuberculosis notices changes in physical stamina, which may be frightening. The client also faces concerns about the prognosis of the disease. The nurse is realistic in offering a positive outlook for the client as long as he or she complies with the medication regimen and suggests that fatigue

CHART 30-9

Drug Therapy for Tuberculosis

Drug	Usual Dosage	Nursing Interventions	Drug Action/Rationale for Use
Isoniazid (INH)	• 5 mg/kg PO, IM (max 300 mg) daily; 15 mg/kg (max 900 mg) biweekly	• Observe for drug interactions. It may inhibit drug metabolism of phenytoin, carbamazepine, primidone, and warfarin. • Instruct the client to take on empty stomach and avoid antacids. • Monitor for signs of hepatitis and neurotoxicity effects.	• Isoniazid inhibits synthesis of mycolic acids and acts to kill actively growing organisms in the extracellular environment and inhibits growth of dormant organisms in the macrophages and caseating granulomas.
Rifampin (RIF)	• 10 mg/kg PO (max 600 mg) daily or biweekly	• Instruct the client that secretions will be orange in color and will permanently discolor soft contact lenses. • Observe for drug interactions. It may enhance elimination of theophylline, steroids, opioids, oral hypoglycemics, warfarin, and occasionally vitamin D. • Observe for hepatotoxic effects. • RIF decreases effectiveness of oral contraceptives.	• Rifampin has the unique ability to kill slower growing organisms that reside in the caseating granuloma and macrophage.
Pyrazinamide (PZA)	• 15–30 mg/kg PO (max 2000 mg) daily; 50 mg/kg biweekly	• Observe for hepatotoxic effects.	• Pyrazinamide is the most active drug at killing mycobacteria present in macrophages. The acidic environment in the macrophage inhibits most agents.
Ethambutol (EMB)	• 15 mg/kg daily PO; 50 mg/kg biweekly	• Obtain baseline visual acuity and color discrimination, especially to the color green. Repeat testing q 1–2 months.	• Ethambutol inhibits bacterial RNA synthesis. It is slow acting and must be used in combination with other bactericidal agents.
Streptomycin (SM)	• 1000 mg IM, or IV over 1 hr, daily for 2 months followed by biweekly injections until treatment is completed	• Obtain baseline audiometric test q 1–2 months. It can impair the 8th cranial nerve. Elderly clients are especially susceptible.	• Streptomycin is an aminoglycoside antibiotic that is active against extracellular organisms only.
Amikacin	• 15 mg/kg daily IM, IV (usual dose 1 g)	• Ensure adequate hydration, monitor renal function, and hearing. Amikacin can lead to renal toxicity and ototoxicity.	• Amikacin is an aminoglycoside antibiotic that can be used if streptomycin is not available.

Current treatment recommendations:

INH + RIF + PZA + EMB or SM (induction phase)—2 months. Daily dosing. Ethambutol or streptomycin is included in the initial phase until drug susceptibility is determined.

INH + RIF (continuation phase)—4 months. Daily or 2–3 times/week dosing.

Continue treatment for at least 6 months, and 3 months beyond the time when the result of sputum culture converts to negative.

Clients with a drug resistance, coexisting HIV infection, or inability to take certain antituberculosis drugs require longer duration of therapy, i.e., 9 total months, and at least 6 months after culture conversion.

Current treatment information and data from the official ATS statement. A joint statement of the ATS, American Academy of Pediatrics, The Centers for Disease Control, and the Infectious Disease Society of America. (1992). Control of Tuberculosis in the United States. *American Review of Respiratory Disease, 146*(6), 1623–1633; U. S. Department of Health and Human Services, Recommendations of the Advisory Council for the Elimination of Tuberculosis. (1993). Initial therapy for tuberculosis in the era of multidrug resistance. *Morbidity and Mortality Weekly Report, 42*(RR-7), 1–8.

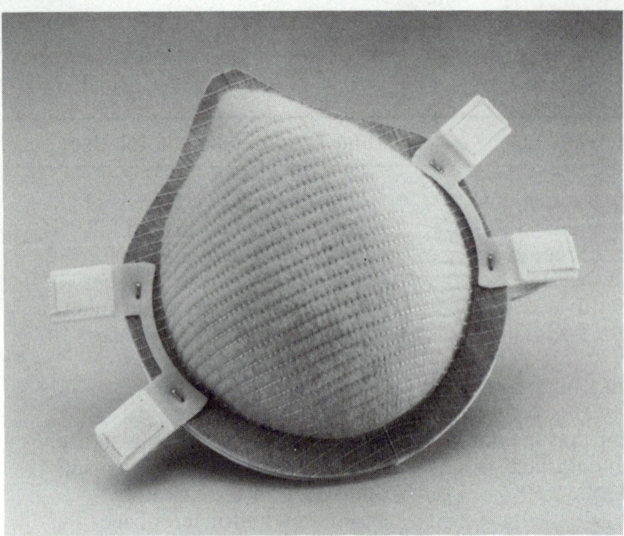

FIGURE 30-24 ◆ A HEPA respirator used in the care of clients with active or "rule out" tuberculosis. (Courtesy of Uvex Safety, Smithfield, RI.)

will diminish as the treatment progresses. With current resistant strains of TB, however, the nurse must also emphasize that noncompliance regarding medication could lead to an infection that is difficult to treat or that has total drug resistance. The nurse listens carefully to the client's concerns throughout the treatment and responds in a supportive manner. The client's return to work and usual daily routines is likely to reduce anxiety.

DISCHARGE PLANNING

HOME CARE PREPARATION

Most clients with tuberculosis are treated outside the hospital. However, clients may be diagnosed with TB while in the hospital if pneumonia is suspected or other possible complications exist. Discharge may be delayed if the living situation is considered to lead to high risk or if the client is likely to be noncompliant. The nurse may consult with the social service worker in the hospital or the community health nursing agency to ensure the client's discharge to the appropriate environment with continued supervision. The home health nurse follows up on potentially infected people in the home environment. It would be futile to treat the client and then return him or her to the same environment only to become reinfected.

HEALTH TEACHING

The client is instructed to follow the drug regimen exactly as prescribed and always to have a supply of the medication on hand. The nurse stresses side effects and ways of minimizing them to ensure compliance. The nurse reminds the client with TB that the disease is usually no longer communicable after medication has been taken for 2 to 3 consecutive weeks. However, the client must continue with the prescribed medication for 6 months or longer as ordered.

If the client has experienced weight loss and severe lethargy, he or she should gradually resume usual activities. The client must maintain proper nutrition to prevent recurrence of infection. The nurse instructs the client that rifampin will discolor the urine and other body fluids and may permanently stain contact lenses.

A key to preventing the transmission of TB is the identification of those in close contact with the infected person so that they can be tested and treated as necessary. Public health professionals have an important role in this aspect of care. When contacts have been identified, these people are assessed with a tuberculin test and chest x-ray to determine infection with TB. Multidrug therapy may be indicated. In addition, certain high-risk clients receive prophylactic therapy.

PSYCHOSOCIAL PREPARATION

The nurse provides the client with information about tuberculosis. This information will help the client who may encounter others with concerns about the contagious aspect of the infection. The nurse reassures the client that after 2 weeks of drug therapy, it is unlikely that the client will infect anyone.

HEALTH CARE RESOURCES

The nurse instructs the client to receive follow-up care by a physician for at least 1 year during active treatment. In addition, the ALA, an organization that uses volunteers, can provide free information to the client about the disease and its treatment. Alcoholics Anonymous and other health care resources for clients with alcoholism are available as well, if needed. The nurse assists the client who uses illegal drugs to locate an appropriate drug treatment program.

EVALUATION

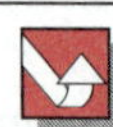

The nurse evaluates the care for a client with tuberculosis on the basis of the identified nursing diagnoses. The expected outcomes are that the client:

- Complies with the treatment regimen and follow-up care
- Maintains body weight through adequate nutritional intake
- States that anxiety about disease and treatment has been reduced
- Returns to the usual level of activity before treatment is discontinued (within 1 year)

Lung Abscess

OVERVIEW

A lung abscess is a localized area of lung destruction caused by liquefaction necrosis, which is usually related to pyogenic bacteria. Clients who have this problem often have a history of pneumonia, possibly complicated by aspiration of oropharyngeal contents or proximal obstruction due to tumor or foreign body. Other causes of aspiration leading to abscess include alcoholism that causes loss of consciousness, seizure disorders or other neurologic deficits, and swallowing disorders. An obstruction of a bronchus may cause a necrotizing process in the distal lung that eventually becomes an abscess. Multiple abscesses and cavities commonly form in clients with TB or fungal infections of the lung. Immunosuppressed clients, such as those receiving chemotherapy or those with a disease like leukemia or AIDS, are particularly susceptible to fungal infections. Most common organisms are anaerobic bacteria, *Staphylococcus* or other gram-positive organisms, or gram-negative or opportunistic infections such as fungi.

COLLABORATIVE MANAGEMENT

ASSESSMENT

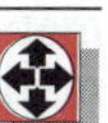

The nurse notes a client's recent history of influenza, pneumonia, febrile illness, cough, and foul-smelling sputum production. In addition, the nurse inquires about the sputum color and odor and about any pleuritic chest pain (a stabbing pain, especially when taking a deep breath). The client is often febrile, pale, fatigued, and cachectic. The nurse may note decreased breath sounds on auscultation and dullness on percussion in the involved area. Bronchial breath sounds and crackles are frequently heard over the site of the lesion. The physician orders a chest x-ray and sputum samples to assist in the diagnosis.

INTERVENTIONS

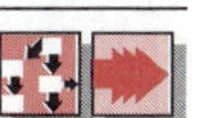

Nursing diagnoses and interventions identified for the client with pneumonia also apply to the client with a lung abscess. Medical treatment is directed toward drainage of the abscess and antibiotics. The physician may prescribe more than one antibiotic. The nurse, then, provides frequent mouth care and observes for oral overgrowth of *Candida albicans.*

Pulmonary Empyema

OVERVIEW

Empyema refers to a collection of pus in the pleural space. The most common cause of empyema is pulmonary infection, lung abscess, or infected pleural effusion. Pneumonia or lung abscess can spread across the pleura; or obstruction of lymph nodes can cause a retrograde flood of infected lymph into the pleural space. In addition, an intrahepatic or subphrenic abscess can spread through the diaphragm's lymphatic system. Thoracic surgery and chest trauma are common predisposing conditions in which bacteria are introduced directly into the pleural space. Blood from trauma may accumulate in the pleural space. Incomplete evacuation of this blood presents a culture medium for bacterial growth.

COLLABORATIVE MANAGEMENT

ASSESSMENT

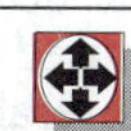

Important history findings include recent febrile illness (including pneumonia), chest pain, dyspnea, cough, and trauma. The nurse notes the characteristics of the sputum. On physical assessment, the nurse may observe diminished chest wall motion. If a pleural effusion is present, the nurse notes decreased or absent fremitus on palpation, a flat percussion note on percussion, and decreased breath sounds on auscultation. With compression of lung tissue adjacent to the effusion, the nurse auscultates bronchial breath sounds, egophony, and whispered pectoriloquy.

Some clients have fever, chills, night sweats, and weight loss. If there is cardiorespiratory compromise, the client may be hypotensive. The nurse may note a displacement of the PMI (point of maximal impulse) on auscultation of the heart because of a mediastinal deviation.

The physician orders a chest x-ray and obtains a sample of the pleural fluid via thoracentesis (see Chap. 28) for help in making the diagnosis. Empyema fluid is thick, opaque, exudative, and intensely foul smelling. The pleural fluid is sent to the laboratory and is analyzed for color, red blood cell count, white blood cell count and differential, glucose and protein levels, lactate dehydrogenase (LDH), and pH. Gram and acid-fast stains of the smears and cytology studies are also done. A protein concentration higher than 3 g/100 mL of pleural fluid indicates an exudative process.

INTERVENTIONS

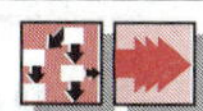

Therapy for empyema focuses on emptying the empyema cavity, re-expanding the lung, and controlling the infection. The physician usually treats the client with antibiotics appropriate for the isolated pathogen. In addition, closed chest drainage is used to promote lung expansion. The physician places one or more chest tubes in the inferior parts of the empyema sac. Underwater seal drainage is used without suction initially, but negative pressure may be added if the lung fails to expand. The physician removes the tube when the lung is fully expanded and the infectious process is under control (see also Chapter 31). Open thoracotomy and decortication (removal) of a portion of the pleura may be needed for thick pus or marked pleural thickening. Nursing considerations are the same as those for clients with a pleural effusion, pneumothorax, or infection.

Influenza

Influenza, or "flu," is an acute viral respiratory infection that can occur in adults of all ages. Because influenza is highly contagious, epidemics are common and can lead to complications like pneumonia or death, especially in elderly and immunocompromised clients. Influenza may be caused by one of several viruses, usually referred to as A, B, and C. The client with this disorder typically complains of severe headache, muscle aches, fever, chills, fatigue, weakness, and anorexia. Clinical manifestations associated with the respiratory system, such as a sore throat, cough, and rhinorrhea (watery discharge from the nose), generally follow the initial symptoms for a week or more. Most clients continue to complain of general malaise for 1 to 2 weeks after the acute episode has resolved.

Treatment of influenza is symptomatic because antibiotics are ineffective against viral infections. The nurse recommends that the client remain in bed for several days and drink copious amounts of fluids unless contraindicated by some other physical condition, such as chronic renal failure or congestive heart failure. Saline gargles may ease sore throat pain; when ordered, antihistamines may reduce rhinorrhea. Other palliative measures are the same as those for clients with acute rhinitis (see Chap. 29).

During the past two decades, vaccinations for the prevention of influenza have been developed and widely administered. With advanced refinement of the vaccine, allergic reaction is rare. The vaccine is altered every year on the basis of specific viral strains that are likely to pose a problem during the influenza season, that is, late fall and winter. It is highly recommended that clients older than 65 years and those with chronic illness or immune compromise receive the vaccine each year, typically during October or November.

SARCOIDOSIS

OVERVIEW

Sarcoidosis is one of a group of diseases within a broader classification of pulmonary diseases called interstitial lung disease. Interstitial lung disease is used interchangeably with the term *fibrotic lung disease.* The hallmark of sarcoidosis is noncaseating granuloma. The granulomas of sarcoidosis can occur in almost any organ or tissue of the body, but most frequently affected are the lung, liver, spleen, lymph nodes, eyes, small bones of the hands and feet, and skin.

Pulmonary sarcoidosis is a chronic disorder of the alveolar structure that develops over time in a stepwise manner. Growths called granulomas characterize the disease. Granulomas are composed of lymphocytes, macrophages, epithelioid cells, and giant cells.

It is currently believed that the development of pulmonary sarcoidosis involves the activation of T lymphocytes; the stimulus for this activation is unknown. The stimulus causes normal resident immune cells (the T lymphocytes) to recruit additional immune cells, probably by releasing chemotactic factor. Monocytes are then attracted to the T lymphocytes. Monocytes are precursors of macrophages, epithelioid cells, and the multinucleated giant cells that compose the granuloma. Alveolitis is the term that describes this process of accumulation of inflammatory immune cells in the alveoli.

The presence of T lymphocytes and macrophages and of the substances they secrete leads to disorder of the cellular arrangement in the lung. Individual cell shapes are also altered. It is believed that the T lymphocytes are primarily responsible for granuloma formation and that the activated macrophages are primarily responsible for interstitial fibrosis (because of their ability to recruit and increase the number of fibroblasts). The fibrosis results in a loss of lung compliance (elasticity) and a loss of functional ability to exchange gases. Cor pulmonale (right-sided cardiac failure) is often present because the heart can no longer pump against the noncompliant, fibrotic lung.

The development of the fiberoptic bronchoscope (see Chap. 28) has allowed researchers to sample the epithelial fluid of the lower respiratory tract to investigate the alveolitis of clients with active disease. This test confirms that pulmonary sarcoidosis is a disease associated with an intense cellular immune response in the alveolar structure.

Transcultural Considerations In the United States, sarcoidosis affects African-Americans ten times more frequently than Caucasians. The overall prevalence is similar in women and men, but it is twice as common in women of childbearing age as in women of other ages. A distinctive feature of sarcoidosis is its age distribution: most cases develop in people who are between 20 and 40 years old.

COLLABORATIVE MANAGEMENT

Indications for treatment vary. If the client is asymptomatic and has no abnormalities of pulmonary function, no treatment is given. If pulmonary function is reduced and there are pulmonary infiltrates, corticosteroids (e.g., prednisone) are administered. A daily maintenance dose of 10 to 15 mg may be needed. After the symptoms resolve, the maintenance dose may be reduced and eventually withdrawn, but relapses may occur. The nurse focuses on psychosocial issues involving the younger adult with a chronic, potentially debilitating illness and intervenes as indicated. The nurse also teaches about side effects of steroid therapy and other aspects of the client's physical care as indicated and appropriate.

OCCUPATIONAL PULMONARY DISEASE

OVERVIEW

Exposure to occupational or environmental toxic dust and particulate matter may cause a variety of respiratory disorders. Depending on the degree and intensity of exposure, the smoking history, and underlying pulmonary disease, clients may experience acute reversible effects or chronic pulmonary disease. *Pneumoconiosis* is chronic respiratory disease related to the inhalation of dust.

ACUTE OCCUPATIONAL DISEASES

In many people, asthma results from occupational exposures. These clients usually have no childhood or family history of the disease. In some cases, symptoms may develop after several years of exposure. *Occupational asthma* may be difficult to recognize because the client may continue to experience respiratory distress when away from the work setting. The most easily recognized signs of occupational asthma consist of wheezing and dyspnea, which occur within minutes of exposure to the offending agent.

With the rapid development of the chemical industry, it has been found that large numbers of inorganic and organic substances can cause asthma by direct bronchial irritation. Aside from chemical irritants, enzymes used in the food processing, detergent, and pharmaceutical industries may be asthma-inducing agents. Plant- and animal-derived materials may also be sources of irritation.

Byssinosis is an occupational pulmonary disease of textile workers caused by excessive inhalation of certain vegetable fiber dusts. Chest tightness, coughing, wheezing, and dyspnea are characteristic and especially prominent on the first day back to work after a break in exposure, such as a holiday or a weekend. Evidence suggests that chronic pulmonary damage results from prolonged exposure. However, the chest tightness, dyspnea, and decline in expiratory flow are completely reversible in many people.

Acute symptoms may be caused by working with the dusts of a variety of cereal grains. Acute conjunctivitis, rhinitis, and pharyngitis, as well as a *hypersensitivity pneumonitis,* may be the presenting symptoms. Workers who complain of cough and dyspnea often show no pulmonary function abnormalities. It is believed that symptoms result from a relatively benign hypersecretory condition of the bronchial mucosa without a high risk of disability.

Excessive exposure to irritant gases like ammonia, sulfur dioxide, chlorine, ozone, and nitrogen dioxide may produce an acute respiratory illness called *toxic pneumonitis.* Exposure may cause inflammation or edema of any portion of the respiratory tract. This condition may be fatal if not treated immediately.

Both transient pleural effusions and recurrent attacks of pleurisy are recognized with increased frequency among workers exposed to asbestos. In addition, asbestos exposure may cause exudative or hemorrhagic effusions. Exposure to talc and zeolite dusts is associated with benign pleural effusions.

CHRONIC OCCUPATIONAL DISEASES

Silicosis, a chronic fibrosing disease of the lungs, is produced by excessive inhalation of free crystalline silica dust. Mining and quarrying are associated with a high incidence of silicosis. Hazardous exposure to silica dust also occurs in foundry work, tunneling, sandblasting, pottery making, stone masonry, and the manufacture of glass, tile, and bricks. The finely ground silica used in soaps, polishes, and filters is especially dangerous.

Chronic silicosis results from exposure to low concentrations of silica dust for 20 years or more. The formation of selective nodules in the pulmonary parenchyma is characteristic. This process may be accompanied by progressive massive fibrosis.

Uncomplicated, or simple, silicosis is often entirely asymptomatic and causes only mild ventilating restriction and evidence of fibrosis on an x-ray. Clients with chronic complicated disease experience significant dyspnea on exertion, marked reduction in lung volume, and massive fibrosis causing obstructive problems. Malaise, anorexia, and weight loss may be present with an outcome of respiratory failure.

Asbestosis refers to diffuse interstitial fibrosis caused by exposure to asbestos. There is generally a considerable latency period between the initial exposure and the onset of clinical manifestations of fibrosis, often 10 to 20 years. People who are at risk for asbestosis are asbestos miners and millers and those employed in the building trade and shipyards, such as loggers, insulation workers, pipe fitters, steamfitters, sheet metal workers, and welders. Asbestos causes a diffuse pleural thickening with diaphragmatic calcification. Pulmonary function abnormalities usually indicate a restrictive ventilatory defect. Removal of the worker from exposure does not necessarily prevent the effects of the disease. The chances of arresting the disease are best in its early stages. Clients with this disease frequently have respiratory infections.

Talcosis is a pulmonary fibrosis that occurs after years of exposure to high concentrations of talc dust. Significant exposures can occur during the manufacture of paints, ceramics, asphalt, roofing materials, cosmetics, and rubber goods. The clinical picture of the client closely resembles that of asbestosis.

Two different respiratory diseases can develop from chronic excessive inhalation of coal dust: *coal workers' pneumoconiosis* and *chronic bronchitis.* The clinical picture of these illnesses is similar to that of silicosis.

Berylliosis is sarcoidosis with a defined cause, that is, exposure or sensitivity to beryllium. The typical exposure history includes involvement in an operation in which metals are heated to fumes (e.g., welding, burning, or casting) or are machined to dust. Clients with berylliosis are more likely to progress to advanced irreversible disease than are those with sarcoidosis of unknown etiology.

COLLABORATIVE MANAGEMENT

Prevention is extremely important for avoiding pulmonary disability caused by dust-related disease. The nurse or other public health advocate stresses the importance of using masks and ensuring adequate ventilation when working in potentially harmful environments. When assessing the client who has respiratory distress, the nurse ascertains whether symptoms are acute or chronic. If the client is having an allergic reaction, avoidance of the allergen is stressed.

Nursing interventions for clients experiencing occupational pulmonary disorders are based on the fact that restrictive pulmonary disease is present, that is, there are deficits in chest wall compliance, vital capacity, and total lung volume. These deficits are related to the fibrotic process, which restricts lung expansion. Most nursing diagnoses appropriate for clients with chronic airflow limitation (CAL), as delineated earlier in this chapter, apply to these clients. Hypoxemic clients require supplemental oxygen. In addition, respiratory therapies to promote sputum clearance are essential.

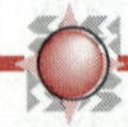

IMPLICATIONS FOR NURSING RESEARCH

Research is needed to develop methods for assessment and management of symptoms in the chronically ill adult with pulmonary impairment. Research ideas and questions that nurses could address include:

- How effective are specific strategies for reducing dyspnea, such as relaxation, exercise, symptom monitoring, breathing strategies, coping, and self-care strategies?
- What standardized methods of measurement for dyspnea are applicable to both critically ill and chronically ill clients?
- What strategies are the most effective for relieving dyspnea?
- How can the nurse be most effective in reducing anxiety and fear in the client experiencing dyspnea?
- What are the optimal techniques for preventing infection in the immunocompromised client?
- How can the nurse help decrease mortality associated with asthma?

SELECTED BIBLIOGRAPHY

American Association of Respiratory Care. (1991a). Clinical practice guideline: Oxygen therapy in the acute care hospital. *Respiratory Care, 36*(12), 1410–1413.

American Association of Respiratory Care. (1991b). Guidelines: Pulse oximetry. *Respiratory Care, 36*(12), 1407–1409.

* American Thoracic Society. (1987). Standards for the diagnosis of patients with chronic obstructive pulmonary disease (COPD) and asthma. *American Review of Respiratory Disease, 136*, (1), 225–244.

American Thoracic Society. (1990a). Diagnostic standards and classification of tuberculosis. *American Review of Respiratory Disease, 142*(3), 725–735.

American Thoracic Society. (1990b). Research priorities in respiratory nursing. *American Review of Respiratory Disease, 142*(6), 1459–1464.

American Thoracic Society. (1991). Standards of nursing care for adult patients with pulmonary dysfunction. *American Review of Respiratory Disease, 144*(1), 231–236.

American Thoracic Society. (1992). Control of tuberculosis in the United States (the official ATS statement). *American Review of Respiratory Disease, 146*(6), 1623–1633.

Benson, V., & Marano, M. A. (1994). *Current estimates from the National Health Interview Survey.* DHHS Pub. No. (PHS) 94-1517. Hyattsville, MD: National Center for Health Statistics.

Bolgiano, C. S., Bunting, K., & Shoenberger, M. M. (1990). Administering oxygen therapy: What you need to know. *Nursing90, 20*(6), 47–51.

Boutotte, J. (1993). T.B. the second time around. *Nursing93, 23*(5), 42–50.

Brisson-Noel, A., Aznar, C., Chureau, C., Nguyen, S., Pierre, C., Bartoli, M., Bonete, R., Pialoux, G., Gicquel, B., & Garrigue, G. (1991). Diagnosis of tuberculosis by DNA amplification in clinical practice evaluation. *Lancet, 338*(8763), 364–366.

Brock, E. T. & Shucard, D. W. (1994). Sleep apnea. *American Family Physician,* 49(2), 385–394.

Brown, R. (1991). Pneumonia and lower respiratory tract infections. *Hospital Practice, 26*(Suppl. 5), 37–42.

Busse, W. W., Lemanske, R. F., & Dick, E. C. (1992). The relationship of viral respiratory infections and asthma. *Chest 101*(6), 385s–388s.

* Carrieri, V. K., & Janson-Bjerklie, S. (1986). Dyspnea. In Carrieri, V. K., Lindsey, A. M., & West, C. M. (1993). *Pathophysiological phenomena in nursing: Human responses to illness* (pp. 191–218). Philadelphia: W.B. Saunders.

Carrieri-Kohlman, V., Douglas, M. K., Gormley, J. M., & Stulbarg, M. S. (1993). Desensitization and guided mastery: Treatment approaches for the management of dyspnea. *Heart & Lung, 22*(3), 226–234.

* Carroll, P. F. (1989). Good nursing gets COPD patients out of hospitals. *RN, 52*(7), 24–28.

Carter, R. (1990). Restoring functional capacity. *The Journal of Respiratory Care Practitioners,* Oct./Nov., 12–18, 49.

Caruthers, D. (1990). Infectious pneumonia in the elderly. *American Journal of Nursing, 90*(2), 56–60.

Centers for Disease Control. (1990). Guidelines for preventing the transmission of tuberculosis in health-care settings, with special focus on HIV-related issues. *Morbidity and Mortality Weekly Report, 39*(RR–17), 1–26.

DeLetter, M. C. (1991). Nutritional implications for

chronic airflow limitation patients. *Journal of Gerontological Nursing, 17*(5), 21–26.

DesJardins, T. (1990). *Clinical manifestations of respiratory disease* (2nd ed.). St. Louis: C.V. Mosby.

Dunston, J. (1990). How managed care can work for you. *Nursing90, 20*(10), 56–59.

* Egglund, E. (1987). Teaching the ABC's of C.O.P.D. *Nursing87, 17*(1), 60–64.

Eid, N., Buchheit, J., Neuling, M., & Phelps, H. (1991). Chest physiotherapy in review. *Respiratory Care, 36*(4), 270–282.

Elpern, E. H., & Girzadas, A. M. (1993). Tuberculosis update: New challenges of an old disease. *MEDSURG Nursing, 2*(3), 176–183.

Faryniarz, K., & Mahler, D. (1990). Writing an exercise prescription for patients with COPD. *The Journal of Respiratory Diseases, 11*(7), 638–648.

Fedson, D. (1992). Clinical practice and public policy for influenza and pneumococcal vaccination of the elderly. *Clinics in Geriatric Medicine, 8*(1), 183–199.

Gianaris, P. G., & Golish, J. A. (1994). Changing strategies in the management of asthma. *Postgraduate Medicine, 95*(5), 105–110.

* Gift, A. (1989). Clinical measurement of dyspnea. *Dimensions of Critical Care Nursing, 8*(4), 210–216.

Gift, A. G., & Cahill, C. (1990). Psychophysiologic aspects of dyspnea in chronic obstructive pulmonary disease: A pilot study. *Heart & Lung, 19*(3), 252–257.

Gift, A. G., Moore, T., & Soeken, K. (1992). Relaxation to reduce dyspnea and anxiety in COPD patients. *Nursing Research, 41*(4), 242–246.

Gross, N. (1990). Chronic obstructive pulmonary disease: Current concepts and therapeutic approaches. *Chest, 97*(2), 19s–23s.

Haas, F., & Axen, K. (1991). *Pulmonary therapy and rehabilitation: Principles and practice* (2nd ed.). Baltimore: Williams & Wilkins.

* Hahn, K. (1989). Sexuality and COPD. *Rehabilitation Nursing, 14*(4), 191–195.

* Howard, J., Davis, J., & Roghmann, K. (1987). Respiratory teaching of patients: How effective is it? *Journal of Advanced Nursing, 12*(2), 207–214.

Janelli, L. M., Scherer, Y. K., & Schmieder, L. E. (1991). Can a pulmonary health teaching program alter patients' ability to cope with COPD? *Rehabilitation Nursing, 16*(4), 199–202.

Janson-Bjerklie, S., Ferketich, S., Benner, P., & Becker, G. (1992). Clinical markers of asthma severity and risk: Importance of subjective as well as objective markers. *Heart & Lung, 21*(3), 265–272.

Jess, L. W. (1992a). Chronic bronchitis and emphysema: Airing the differences. *Nursing92, 22*(3), 34–41.

Jess, L. W. (1992b). When your patient has asthma. *Nursing92, 22*(4), 48–51.

* Johnson, A. P. (1988). The elderly and COPD. *Journal of Gerontological Nursing, 14*(12), 20–24, 35–36.

Kacmarek, R. M., Mack, C. W., & Dimas, S. (1990). *The essentials of respiratory care* (3rd ed.). St. Louis: Mosby Year Book.

Kaufman, J., Fox, R., & Swearengen, P. (1990). How a support group can help your chronically ill patient. *Nursing90, 20*(10), 65–66.

* Kersten, L. D. (1989). *Comprehensive respiratory nursing: A decision making approach.* Philadelphia: W. B. Saunders.

Kronenberg, R. S., & Griffith, D. E. (1993). Chronic bronchitis: Key points in evaluation. *Postgraduate Medicine, 94*(8), 93–100.

Lareau, S. C. (1993). Respiratory problems. In D. L. Carnevali & M. Patrick (Eds.), *Nursing management for the elderly* (3rd ed., pp. 625–657). Philadelphia: J. B. Lippincott.

Lordi, G. M., & Reichman, L. B. (1993). Pulmonary complications of asbestos exposure. *American Family Physician, 48*(8), 1471–1477.

Make, B. (1991). COPD: Management and rehabilitation. *American Family Physician, 43*(4), 1315–1324.

McCue, J. D. (1993). Pneumonia in the elderly. *Postgraduate Medicine, 94*(95), 39–40, 43–48, 51.

McDowell, K. (1993). Drugs for acute bronchitis: An up-to-date guide. *Nursing93, 23*(5), 32I–32L.

National Center for Health Statistics. (1993). *Health United States, 1992 and healthy people 2000 review.* DHHS Pub. No. (PHS) 93–1232. Hyattsville, MD: Public Health Service.

National Institute of Health. (1991). Guidelines for the diagnosis and management of asthma. *National asthma education program: Expert panel report* (91–3042). Bethesda: U.S. Department of Health and Human Services.

Nelson, D. M. (1992). Interventions related to respiratory care. *The Nursing Clinics of North America, 27*(2), 301–323.

O'Brien, L. M., & Bartlett, K. A. (1992). TB plus HIV spells trouble. *American Journal of Nursing, 92*(5), 28–34.

O'Donnell, D. E., Webb, K. A., & McGuire, M. A. (1993). COPD: Benefits of exercise training. *Geriatrics, 48*(1), 59–69.

* Openbrier, D. R., Fuoss, C., & Mall, C. (1988). What patients on home oxygen therapy want to know. *American Journal of Nursing, 88*(2), 198–202.

* Openbrier, D. R., Hoffman, L., & Wesmiller, S. (1988). Home oxygen therapy. *American Journal of Nursing, 88*(2), 192–197.

Petty, T. (1990). *Treatment of asthma in the 1990's.* Princeton: Excerpta Medica.

Piirila, P. (1992). Changes in crackle characteristics during the clinical course of pneumonia. *Chest, 102*(1), 176–183.

Reed, P. G. (1991). Preferences for spiritually related nursing interventions among terminally ill and nonterminally ill hospitalized adults and well adults. *Applied Nursing Research, 4*(3), 122–128.

Reinke, L. F., & Hoffman, L. A. (1992). Breathing space: How to teach asthma co-management. *American Journal of Nursing, 92*(10), 40–51.

Ruben, F. L. (1993). Viral pneumonias: The increasing importance of a high index of suspicion. *Postgraduate Medicine, 93*(7), 57–60, 63–64.

Sexton, D. L. (1990). *Nursing care of the respiratory patient.* Norwalk, CT: Appleton & Lange.

Strolley, J. M., & Buckwalter, K. C. (1991). Iatrogenesis in the elderly. Nosocomial infections. *Journal of Gerontological Nursing, 17*(9), 30–34.

Swearingen, P., & Keen, J. (1991). *Manual of critical care* (2nd ed.). St. Louis: C. V. Mosby.

U. S. Department of Health and Human Services. (1993). Recommendations of the Advisory Council for the elimination of tuberculosis: Initial therapy for tuberculosis in the era of multidrug resistance. *Morbidity and Mortality Weekly Report, 42*(RR-7), 1–8.

Vork, K. L., & Olson, D. K. (1990). Asbestos review and update. *American Association of Occupational Health Nurses, 38*(4), 160–164.

Weaver, T. E., & Narsavage, G. L. (1992). Physiological and psychological variables related to functional status in chronic obstructive pulmonary disease. *Nursing Research, 41*(5), 286–291.

Webster, J. R., & Kadah, H. (1991). Unique aspects of respiratory disease in the aged. *Geriatrics, 46*(7), 31–43.

Wilson, S. F., & Thompson, J. M. (1990). *Respiratory disorders.* St. Louis: Mosby Year Book.

Wisinger, D. (1993). Bacterial pneumonia: *S. pneumoniae* and *H. influenzae* are the villains. *Postgraduate Medicine, 93*(7), 43–46, 49–50, 52.

Yeaw, E. M. J. (1992). Good lung down? *American Journal of Nursing, 92*(3), 27–32.

Yoshikawa, T. T. (1992). Tuberculosis in aging adults. *Journal of the American Geriatrics Society, 40*(2), 178–187.

SUGGESTED READINGS

Boutotte, J. (1993). T.B. the second time around. *Nursing93, 23*(5), 42–50.

The article discusses the recent rise in tuberculosis (TB) and the populations particularly affected. Transmission, screening, diagnosis, and prevention are detailed. Nursing considerations and interventions are addressed throughout. The drugs used to treat TB are presented in an organized, informative chart. A continuing education test is included.

Carrieri-Kohlman, V., Douglas, M. K., Gormley, J. M., & Stulbarg, M. S. (1993). Desensitization and guided mastery: Treatment approaches for the management of dyspnea. *Heart & Lung, 22*(3), 226–234.

The article begins by reviewing previous research related to desensitization and guided mastery for decreasing various phobias and symptoms, including dyspnea. Other authors have reported that a greater intensity of dyspnea can be tolerated when clients are in a safe (monitored, supervised) environment.

These authors present two treatment approaches to clients with dyspnea, one for desensitization and one for guided mastery. Both treatments were used with the client exercising on a treadmill. Specific findings are not presented as a research study; rather, the treatments are suggested as a conceptual model for the management of dyspnea. A 77-item reference list is included.

Nelson, D. M. (1992). Interventions related to respiratory care. *Nursing Clinics of North America, 27*(2), 301–323.

This article selected for study 11 labels from the Iowa Intervention Project Group related to respiratory care. A total of 182 nursing activities are included in the study. Nurses who work with respiratory clients in an intensive care setting were asked to indicate to what extent each nursing activity was characteristic of the corresponding nursing intervention label. Results are listed under each label.

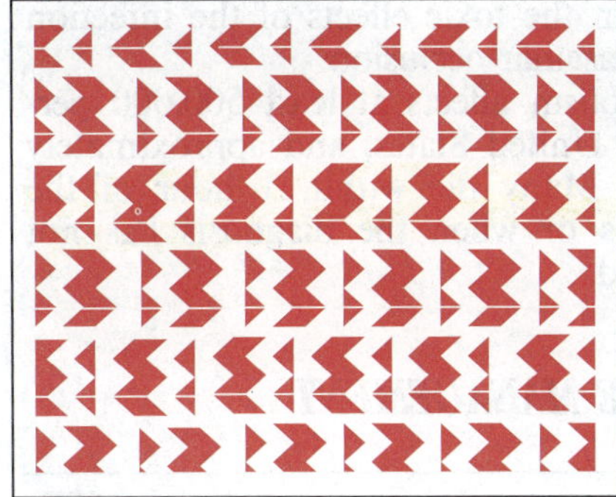

CHAPTER 31

Interventions for Critically Ill Clients with Respiratory Problems

CHAPTER HIGHLIGHTS

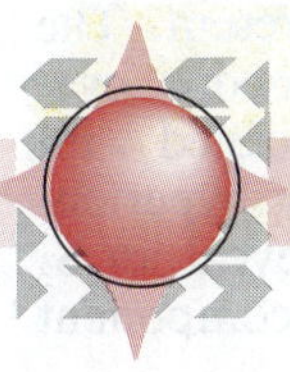

The client with a disorder of the lower respiratory tract can be extremely ill from an acute or chronic problem. With a growing elderly population, critical respiratory conditions are increasing in frequency. Even with prompt treatment, these often lead to death. The nurse must be familiar with the numerous modalities for sustaining breathing or lessening the work of breathing. The nurse must be prepared to handle respiratory emergencies and complications while allaying the client's anxiety and fear.

Pulmonary Embolism

OVERVIEW

The release or entry of solid, liquid, or gaseous particles into the venous system is characteristic of embolism. The particulate matter is then transported to the lungs by the venous blood. The larger matter lodges into the pulmonary capillary bed as an embolus and obstructs circulation. Any substance can cause an embolism, but a blood clot is the most common.

The most common acute pulmonary disease in hospitalized clients is pulmonary embolism (PE). In most people with a PE, a blood clot from a deep venous thrombosis (DVT) breaks loose from one of the veins in the lower extremities or the pelvis. The thrombus detaches, travels through the vena cava and right side of the heart, and then lodges at a bifurcation or in a capillary of the pulmonary artery. Platelets accumulate behind the embolus, triggering the release of serotonin and thromboxane A_2, which causes vasoconstriction. Widespread pulmonary vasoconstriction and pulmonary hypertension impair ventilation and perfusion. Deoxygenated blood shunts into the arterial circulation to produce hypoxemia. Approximately 12% of clients with PE do *not* have hypoxemia, however.

Major risk factors for DVT include:

- Prolonged immobilization
- Surgery
- Obesity
- Advancing age
- Hypercoagulability
- Previous history of thromboembolism

In addition, smoking, pregnancy, estrogen therapy, congestive heart failure, stroke, malignant neoplasms (particularly of the lung or prostate), Trousseau's syndrome, or major trauma increases a client's risk for DVT.

Nursing interventions that help prevent pulmonary embolism are those that also prevent venous stasis and DVT. These interventions include:

- Initiating passive and active range-of-motion exercises for the extremities of immobilized and postoperative clients
- Ambulating postoperative clients soon after surgery
- Using antiembolism and pneumatic compression stockings and devices postoperatively
- Avoiding the use of tight garters, girdles, and constricting clothing
- Preventing pressure under the popliteal space (such as with a pillow)

The physician may order small doses of prophylactic heparin administered subcutaneously every 8 hours. Heparin prevents hypercoagulability in clients immobilized for a prolonged period after surgery or restricted to bed rest. Adequate fluid intake and the avoidance of oral contraceptives are also preventive. (Further information on the prevention of DVT is found in Chapter 19).

Fat, oil, air, tumor cells, amniotic fluid, foreign objects like broken intravenous (IV) catheters, injected particles, and infected fibrin clots or pus can gain access to the venous system and cause pulmonary emobolism. Fat emboli from fracture of a long bone and oil emboli from lymphangiography do not impede blood flow; rather, they result in vascular injury and an adult respiratory distress syndrome (ARDS) (see later in this chapter). Amniotic fluid embolus is associated with a mortality rate of 80% to 90%; it occurs in 1 per 20,000 to 30,000 deliveries and can be a complication of abortion or amniocentesis. Septic emboli commonly arise from a pelvic abscess, an infected intravenous line, and the nonsterile injections of illegal drugs. The problem with septic emboli lies in the toxic effects of the infection more than in the vascular occlusion.

Pulmonary embolism affects at least 500,000 persons a year in the United States, and approximately 10% of these die. Many die within 1 hour of the onset of symptoms or when the diagnosis has not even been suspected.

COLLABORATIVE MANAGEMENT

ASSESSMENT

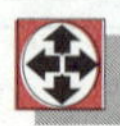

Chart 31-1 outlines the key features of pulmonary embolism. The nurse assesses the client for dyspnea accompanied by tachypnea, tachycardia, and pleuritic chest pain (sharp, stabbing-type pain on inspiration). These symptoms are found in 80% of clients diagnosed with PE. Because the onset of symptoms is usually abrupt, the client generally is extremely anxious and fearful. Breath sounds may be normal, but crackles occur in 50% of clients with PE. The nurse typically notes a dry cough that may result in hemoptysis. A low-grade fever may be present. The nurse assesses for distended neck veins, syncope, cyanosis, and hypotension. Hypotension associated with massive emboli indicates acute pulmonary hypertension. Auscultation of heart sounds may reveal an S_3 or S_4 sound with an altered pulmonic component of S_2.

The hyperventilation from hypoxia and pain initially leads to respiratory alkalosis, which the nurse confirms with low $PaCO_2$ values on arterial blood gas (ABG) analysis. As blood continues to be shunted without picking up oxygen from the lungs, the $PaCO_2$ level will start to rise. This leads to respiratory acidosis. Later, metabolic acidosis results from tissue hypoxia.

ABG studies and pulse oximetry may reveal hypoxemia but these results alone are not sufficient for

CHART 31–1

Key Features of Pulmonary Embolism

Symptoms

- Dyspnea
- Pleuritic chest pain
- Apprehension
- Cough
- Hemoptysis

Signs

- Tachypnea
- Crackles
- Tachycardia
- S_3 or S_4 heart sound
- Diaphoresis
- Fever

the diagnosis of PE. A client with a small embolus may not be hypoxemic, and PE is not the only cause of hypoxemia. The chest x-ray is typically normal.

One of the most important studies to determine PE is the ventilation-perfusion lung scan (V/Q scan). A negative perfusion scan rules out PE. If the V/Q scan is inconclusive, pulmonary angiography, the most definitive and specific test for PE, may be done. Electrocardiogram findings are abnormal, nonspecific, and transient. T wave changes and ST segment abnormalities develop in almost 50% of clients, but left axis and right axis deviations occur with equal frequency.

In a few clients, the physician performs thoracentesis (see Chap. 28) or transesophageal echocardiography (TEE; see Chap. 32) for help in detecting PE. The physician often orders Doppler ultrasound studies or impedance plethysmography (IPG) to document the presence of DVT and to support a diagnosis of PE.

INTERVENTIONS

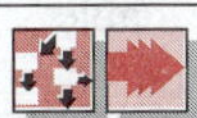

When a client complains of the acute onset of dyspnea with associated pleuritic chest pain, the nurse notifies the physician immediately. The nurse attempts to reassure the client and assists him or her to a position of comfort with the head of the bed elevated. The nurse prepares for oxygen administration and blood gas analysis while continuing to monitor and assess the client for additional signs and symptoms.

Oxygen Therapy Oxygen therapy (see Chap. 30) is important for the client with pulmonary embolism (PE). The severely hypoxemic client may be placed on a mechanical ventilator and monitored closely with ABGs. In less severe cases, oxygen may be administered by nasal cannula or mask. Pulse oximetry may be useful in monitoring arterial oxygen saturation, which reflects the degree of hypoxemia.

The nurse assesses the client on an ongoing basis for any changes in status. The nurse assesses vital signs, lung sounds, and cardiac and respiratory status at least every 1 to 2 hours. The nurse notes increasing dyspnea, dysrhythmias, distended neck veins, and pedal or sacral edema. The nurse also notes the presence of crackles and adventitious sounds on auscultation of the lungs along with any cyanosis of the lips, conjunctiva, oral mucous membranes, or nail beds.

Anticoagulation Therapy The physician usually orders anticoagulation to keep the embolus from enlarging and prevent the formation of new clots. Active bleeding, stroke, and recent trauma are some possible contraindications to use of anticoagulants. Before proceeding, the physician evaluates each client for risks and determines the risk versus the benefit of therapy. Heparin is commonly used unless the PE is massive or accompanied by hemodynamic instability. A thrombolytic enzyme agent may then be used to break up the existing clot. The physician and nurse review the client's partial thromboplastin time (aPTT, also called PTT) before therapy is initiated, every 4 hours when therapy is initiated, and then usually daily thereafter. Therapeutic PTT values usually range between 2 and 2½ times the control value.

Heparin therapy usually continues for 7 to 10 days. The physician starts most clients on oral anticoagulants, such as warfarin (Coumadin, Warfilone✱), on the third day of heparin use. Therapy with both heparin and warfarin continues until the prothrombin time (PT) reaches 1½ times normal, usually 3 to 5 days. Heparin is then discontinued. The nurse and physician monitor the client's PT daily. Therapeutic PT values usually range between 1½ and 2 times the control value. The physician usually continues warfarin for 3 to 6 weeks, but particular clients at high risk may take warfarin indefinitely. Charts 31-2 and 31-3 further discuss the drugs used and laboratory tests monitored. (Chapter 35 also discusses anticoagulants and associated nursing care.)

When thrombolytic enzyme therapy is contraindicated in a client with massive or multiple large pulmonary emboli with shock, surgical embolectomy may be necessary. Embolectomy involves removal of the embolus or emboli from the pulmonary arteries.

The physician considers placing a vena cava filter as a lifesaving measure for some clients, including:

- Clients with an absolute contraindication to anticoagulation
- Clients with recurrent or major bleeding while receiving anticoagulants
- Clients with septic PE
- Clients undergoing pulmonary embolectomy

The physician orders a pulmonry angiogram before placing the filter. (Placement of a vena caval filter is detailed in Chapter 35.)

Lung Cancer

OVERVIEW

Lung cancer is the leading cause of cancer-related mortality worldwide. The prognosis remains poor. Cancer of the lung is essentially incurable unless surgical resection can be accomplished. The overall 5-year survival rate for all clients with lung cancer is 13%. Metastatic disease is often present, and only 16% of clients have localized disease at the time of diagnosis (Boring et al., 1994). Because of metastasis, treatment of lung cancer is often aimed toward relieving symptoms (palliation) rather than cure. It has been estimated that 85% of lung cancers might be prevented through the elimination of cigarette smoking. (Chapter 25 further discusses causes of cancer development.) Therefore, the nurse plays a major role in public education to prevent the *initiation* of smoking. The nurse also uses interventions that improve the quality of life for clients with lung cancer.

CHART 31-2

Drug Therapy for Pumlonary Embolism

Drug	Usual Dosage	Nursing Interventions	Rationale
Heparin sodium (Hepalean✱)	• 5000–15,000 units IVP initially; then dose adjustment is based on PTT, usually 4000–5000 units IVP q4h, 700–1200 units/hr on continuous drip or, less preferably, intermittent infusion	• Monitor PTT.	• Ongoing assessment helps detect side effects and prevent complications.
		• Know expected therapeutic PTT range for each client.	
		• Report PTT results.	• Reporting enables the physician to begin early treatment of a prolonged PTT.
		• Monitor client for bleeding or bruising.	
		• Do not use with salicylates.	• An increased anticoagulation effect can occur with salicylates.
		• Monitor platelets for thrombocytopenia.	• White clot syndrome, a type of arterial thrombosis, can occur.
		• Have the antidote, protamine sulfate, available.	• Being prepared for an emergency helps prevent further complications.
		• Apply pressure to venipuncture and IM injection sites.	• Pressure at puncture sites helps promote clotting.
		• Avoid use of firm toothbrushes, straight razors, and rectal thermometers.	• Safety measures help prevent bleeding.
Warfarin sodium (Coumadin, Warfilone sodium✱)	• 10–15 mg PO for 3 days initially; then dose adjustment is based on PT, usually 2–10 mg PO daily	• Monitor PT.	• Ongoing assessment helps detect side effects and prevent complications.
		• Know expected therapeutic PT range for each client.	
		• Report PT results.	• Reporting enables the physician to begin early treatment of a prolonged PT.
		• Monitor the client for bleeding or bruising.	
		• Monitor for fever and skin rash.	• Adverse drug reaction can occur.
		• Consult the pharmacist about potential drug interactions.	• There are many drug interactions with warfarin.
		• Have the antidote, vitamin K, available.	• Being prepared for an emergency helps prevent further complications.
		• Apply pressure to venipuncture and IM injection sites.	• Pressure at puncture sites helps promote clotting.
		• Avoid use of firm toothbrushes, straight razors, and rectal thermometers.	• Safety measures help prevent bleeding.
		• Teach the client which foods are high in vitamin K.	• Food sources of vitamin K will alter PT.
Alteplase (tissue plasminogen activator, recombinant; tPA; Activase)	• 100 mg IV infusion over 2 hr	• Assess for internal and external bleeding.	• Bleeding is the most common adverse effect.
		• Reconstitute with sterile water without preservative immediately before use.	• Recommended preparation ensures drug stability.
		• Administer with caution to clients who had	• Other drugs with anticoagulation effects in-

CHART 31-2

Drug Therapy for Pulmonary Embolism *Continued*

Drug	Usual Dosage	Nursing Interventions	Rationale
		been receiving aspirin, dipyridamole, heparin, or other anticoagulants.	crease the risk of bleeding.
Streptokinase	• 250,000 IU by IV infusion over 30 min as loading dose, then 100,000 IU/hr over 24–72 hr via continuous IV infusion pump	• Draw blood samples for PTT and PT before starting infusion. • Reconstitute and further dilute with sterile normal saline; roll to mix—do not shake. • Monitor the client for internal and external bleeding. • Avoid IM injections, venipunctures, other invasive procedures, or excessive handling of the client during therapy.	• The rate of infusion depends on blood studies. • Recommended preparation ensures drug stability. • Bleeding is a common adverse effect. • Safety measures help prevent bleeding. • Bruising is common.
Urokinase	• 4400 IU/kg by IV infusion as a priming dose, then 4400 IU/kg/hr for 12–24 hr via continuous IV infusion pump	• Reconstitute with sterile water, then further dilute; total volume should not exceed 200 mL. • Monitor the client for internal and external bleeding. • Avoid IM injections, venipunctures, other invasive procedures, or excessive handling of the client during therapy.	• Recommended preparation ensures drug stability. • Bleeding is a common adverse effect. • Safety measures help prevent bleeding. • Bruising is common.

IVP = intravenous push, or bolus; PTT = partial thromboplastin time; PT = prothrombin time; IU = international units.

PATHOPHYSIOLOGY

More than 90% of all primary lung cancers arise from the bronchial epithelium. These cancers are collectively called bronchogenic carcinomas. Lung cancers are classified according to their histologic cell type as:

- Small cell or oat cell
- Epidermoid or squamous cell
- Adenocarcinoma
- Large cell

The last three types are often referred to as non–small cell lung cancers. Tumor cell types are summarized in Table 31-1.

METASTASIS

Lung cancers metastasize (spread) by direct extension, lymphatic invasion, and blood-borne avenues. Bronchial tumors can spread by direct invasion and grow to occlude the bronchus partially or completely. Invasion of the bronchial wall and encircling or obstruction of the airway can also occur. Pulmonary spread can compress lung structures other than the airway, including the alveoli, nerves, blood vessels, or lymph vessels.

The patterns of metastasis depend on the type of tumor cell and the anatomic location of the tumor. Lymphatic spread is usually associated with embolization and invasion by tumor. The mediastinal, paratracheal, and central hilar lymph nodes are most commonly involved. Lower lobe tumors tend to metastasize diffusely more often by lymph channels than do tumors located in other portions of the lung.

Hematogenous (blood-borne) metastasis of lung cancer is due to invasion of the pulmonary venous system. Tumor emboli spread to other distant areas of the body. Distant sites of metastasis include the lower thoracic and upper lumbar vertebrae, long bones, adrenal glands, central nervous system, and liver.

Additional pathophysiologic manifestations, known

CHART 31–3

Lab Profile ◆ Blood Tests Used to Monitor Anticoagulation Therapy

Test	Normal Range for Adults	Significance of Abnormal Findings
Partial thromboplastin time (PTT, aPTT [APTT])	• Normal values for each local laboratory may vary. • When activator reagents are used by the laboratory, the normal clotting time is shortened. • Common normal ranges are 20–30 sec in some laboratories, or 30–40 sec in others. • Therapeutic range for PE is 2–2.5 times the normal value (e.g., if normal is 20–30 sec, then therapeutic range is 40–75 sec).	*Subtherapeutic times* may signify that the client is not receiving enough heparin to prevent extension of the blood clot. An increase in the dosage or rate of infusion is usually indicated. *Therapeutic times* mean that the clotting time is increased from normal, but this increase is indicated in the case of PE. *Prolonged times* in clients with PE (i.e., >75 sec) indicate that the client is at risk of serious spontaneous bleeding. Heparin is usually held or decreased until the PTT drops back into the therapeutic range.
Prothrombin time (protime, PT)	• 11–12.5 sec • Therapeutic range for anticoagulant therapy in PE is 1.5–2 times the normal or control value in seconds. • Control values can vary day to day because reagents used may vary. • If INR values are reported with the PT, therapeutic range for PE is 2.5–3.0, or 3.0–4.5 for recurrent PE.	*Subtherapeutic values* may signify that the client is not receiving enough warfarin. An increase in the dosage is usually indicated. *Therapeutic values* mean that the protime is increased from normal, but this increase is indicated in the case of PE. *Prolonged values* in the treatment of PE indicate that the client is at risk for bleeding. The warfarin dose is usually decreased or held, the client is instructed to eat foods high in vitamin K, or an injection of vitamin K may be given.

PE = pulmonary embolism; INR = International normalized ratio; apTT or APTT = activated partial thromboplastin time.

as paraneoplastic syndromes, complicate certain lung cancers. The paraneoplastic syndromes are caused by various hormones, antigens, or enzymes. Small cell carcinomas are most commonly associated with paraneoplastic syndromes. Tables 31–2 and 31–3 list the endocrine and nonendocrine paraneoplastic syndromes that may be associated with lung cancer.

STAGING

The staging of lung cancer is based on the TNM system (T, primary *t*umor; N, regional lymph *n*odes; M, distant *m*etastasis). The TNM staging system determines the anatomic extent of the disease and predicts prognosis. The TMN System is further described in Chapter 25.

Staging groups are used clinically because of the significant relationship between the extent of the disease and survival rates. Table 31–4 describes stage grouping for lung cancers. Figure 31–1 shows the various anatomic stages of lung cancer (Mountain et al., 1991).

ETIOLOGY

EXPOSURE

Lung cancers have been associated with repeated exposure to substances that cause chronic tissue irritation or inflammation. Cigarette smoking is the major risk factor and is responsible for 80% to 90% of all lung cancers. The risk for development of lung cancer is ten times greater for men and five times greater for women who smoke (Faber, 1991).

Increased risk for lung cancer is directly related to:

- Total exposure to cigarette smoke as determined by the number of years of smoking
- The number of cigarettes smoked per day
- The depth of inhalation
- The tar and nicotine content of cigarettes

Pipe and cigar smoking also increase the risk. The incidence of lung cancer decreases when smoking stops and, after 15 years of smoking cessation, approaches that of those who have never smoked (Faber, 1991).

Studies demonstrate that nonsmoking spouses and children of a smoker have a higher risk for lung cancer from inhalation of "passive" smoke. Passive smoke, also referred to as sidestream smoke, contains many of the carcinogens found in actively inhaled tobacco smoke. Others at risk from passive smoking include those heavily exposed to passive smoke in the work place, such as people who work in bars and restaurants.

Other risk factors include occupational exposure to

TABLE 31–1 Differential Features of the Major Types of Lung Cancer

Type	Approximate Incidence	Characteristics	Treatment
Small-Cell (oat cell)	• 20%	• Centrally located tumors (80%), rapidly growing, most malignant type • High rate of metastasis via the lymph and circulatory systems with early extrathoracic involvement • Associated with paraneoplastic syndromes • Prognosis poor; survival usually not more than 2 yr with treatment	• Combination chemotherapy is the initial treatment of choice • Surgical resectability poor • Palliative endobronchial laser therapy to relieve obstruction • Radiation not recommended for metastatic disease
Non–Small-Cell			
Epidermoid (squamous cell)	• 30%	• Frequently originates in a central or hilar location and at the bifurcation points of segmental bronchi • In a peripheral location, cavities may form in lung tissue • Strong association with cigarette smoking • Slower growing, less invasive; metastasis often limited to the thorax, including regional nodes, pleura, and chest wall • Commonly associated with obstructive symptoms and pneumonias; client presents with chest pain, cough, dyspnea, and hemoptysis	• Surgical resectability good if stage I or stage II • Chemotherapy and radiation therapy may be used to palliate symptoms
Adenocarcinoma	• 30%–35%	• Tumors are located peripherally • Slow growing • Hematogenous spread occurs frequently and usually early in the course of the disease • High frequency of metastasis to brain; other sites include: adrenals, liver, bone, and kidneys • Predominant type in nonsmokers; most frequent type of lung cancer found in women • Often arises in previously scarred or fibrotic lungs	• Surgical resectability good if stage I or stage II • Moderately good response to chemotherapy • Radiation therapy used to palliate pulmonary and metastatic disease
Large-cell	• 11%	• Peripheral, subpleural lesions with necrotic surfaces or cavities • Often form larger tumor masses than adenocarcinoma • Slow growing • Metastasis is similar to that for adenocarcinoma with addition of gastrointestinal tract • Prognosis poor	• Surgical resectability good if stage I or stage II • Chemotherapy has limited benefit • Palliative radiation therapy

asbestos, beryllium, chromium, coal distillates, cobalt, iron oxide, mustard gas, petroleum distillates, radiation, tar, nickel, and uranium. Atmospheric and industrial pollution that contains benzopyrenes and hydrocarbons has also been associated with an increased incidence of lung cancer.

TABLE 31–2 Endocrine Paraneoplastic Syndromes Associated with Lung Cancer

Ectopic Hormone	Manifestation
Adrenocorticotropic hormone (ACTH)	• Cushing's syndrome
Antidiuretic hormone	• Syndrome of inappropriate antidiuretic hormone (SIADH)
Follicle-stimulating hormone (FSH)	• Gynecomastia
Parathyroid hormone	• Hypercalcemia
Ectopic insulin	• Hypoglycemia

OTHER ETIOLOGIC FACTORS

Some hereditary conditions predispose to cancer, although they are not strongly linked to bronchogenic carcinoma. However, evidence for adenocarcinoma and alveolar cell carcinoma suggests familial factors. These factors do not seem to be related to smoking and are found in families with other tumors, acquired immunodeficency syndrome (AIDS), or inheritable disorders of the lung. Clients with chronic respiratory diseases are also at higher risk for lung cancer. Research has shown a possible link between vitamin A deficiency in the diet and the development of lung cancer (Faber, 1991). A person who smokes *and* has one or more of the predisposing factors is at the greatest risk for the disease (Elpern, 1992).

PREVENTION

Primary prevention for lung cancer is directed at reducing the number of new and existing cases of tobacco smoking. Extensive educational strategies

TABLE 31–3 Nonendocrine Paraneoplastic Syndromes Associated with Lung Cancer

Tissue/System	Manifestation
Connective tissue	• Arthralgia • Digital clubbing
Hematologic system	• Anemia • Leukocytosis • Thrombocytopenia purpura • Polycythemia • Thrombocytosis
Neuromuscular system	• Peripheral neuropathy • Carcinomatous myopathy • Cortical cerebellar degeneration • Seizure • Polymyositis • Myasthenia-like syndrome
Integumentary system	• Dermatomyositis • Scleroderma • Acanthosis nigricans
Vascular system	• Thrombophlebitis • Nonbacterial endocarditis
Renal system	• Arterial thrombosis • Nephrotic syndrome • Proteinuria

start with elementary school children to discourage them from beginning to smoke. Nurses are actively involved in encouraging nonsmokers not to begin to smoke, in promoting smoking cessation programs, and in establishing a smoke-free environment. Nurses from the Canadian Cancer Society's Industrial Education Program visit places of employment to enducate workers about the dangers of smoking. This avenue of education has also been successfully used in the United States (Frank-Stromborg & Rohan, 1992). Smoking cessation programs for assisting those who smoke are available in most geographic areas. Chart 31–4 reviews interventions to help ,a person stop smoking. The nurse encourages nonsmokers to avoid sidestream smoking by avoiding environmental exposure. Smoke-free environments or areas have been established in most public places.

The nurse also educates workers about safety precautions, such as wearing specialized masks and protective clothing to reduce occupational hazards. The nurse encourages people who are at high risk through smoking history, occupational hazards, or possible genetic background to seek frequent health examinations.

TABLE 31–4 TMN Stage Grouping for Lung Cancer

Occult carcinoma	TX	N0	M0
Stage 0	Tis	Carcinoma in situ	
Stage I	T1	N0	M0
	T2	N0	M0
Stage II	T1	N1	M0
	T2	N1	M0
Stage III-a	T3	N0	M0
	T3	N1	M0
	T1–3	N2	M0
Stage III-b	Any T	N3	M0
	T4	Any N	M0
Stage IV	Any T	Any N	M1

From Mountain, C. F., Greenberg, M. D., & Fraire, A. E. (1991). Tumor stages in non–small cell carcinoma of the lung. *Chest, 99*(5), 1258.

INCIDENCE/PREVALENCE

Lung cancer is a major health problem throughout the world. Estimates for 1993 were approximately 170,000 new cases of lung cancer and 149,000 deaths from this disease in the United States. Lung cancer represents 17% of new cancers in men and 12% of new cancers in women. Deaths from lung cancer account for 34% of cancer deaths in men and 22% of cancer deaths in women (Boring et al., 1993). Beginning in 1986, deaths from lung cancer in women exceeded deaths from all other cancers, including breast cancer.

Transcultural Considerations Lung cancer occurs more frequently and with higher mortality in non-Caucasians. Lung cancer is the most common newly diagnosed cancer in African-Americans (Boring et al., 1992).

The impact of industrial factors on the geographic variation in lung cancer rates is pronounced. Mortality rates are higher in countries with significant paper and petroleum industries.

COLLABORATIVE MANAGEMENT

ASSESSMENT

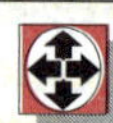

HISTORY

RISK FACTORS The nurse extensively questions the client about risk factors, including smoking and occupational hazards in the workplace, and warning signals (Table 31–5). A detailed history of the duration, frequency, and intensity of exposure is elicited. Cigarette smoking history is described in "pack-years." To calculate this value, the number of packs smoked per day is multiplied by the number of years the person has smoked. For example, a person who has smoked two packs per day for 22 years has a 44 pack-year smoking history.

HOARSENESS AND COUGH When obtaining the history, the nurse notes vague but persistent subjective complaints. Hoarseness is an early sign of lung cancer caused by laryngeal nerve invasion. In addition, the

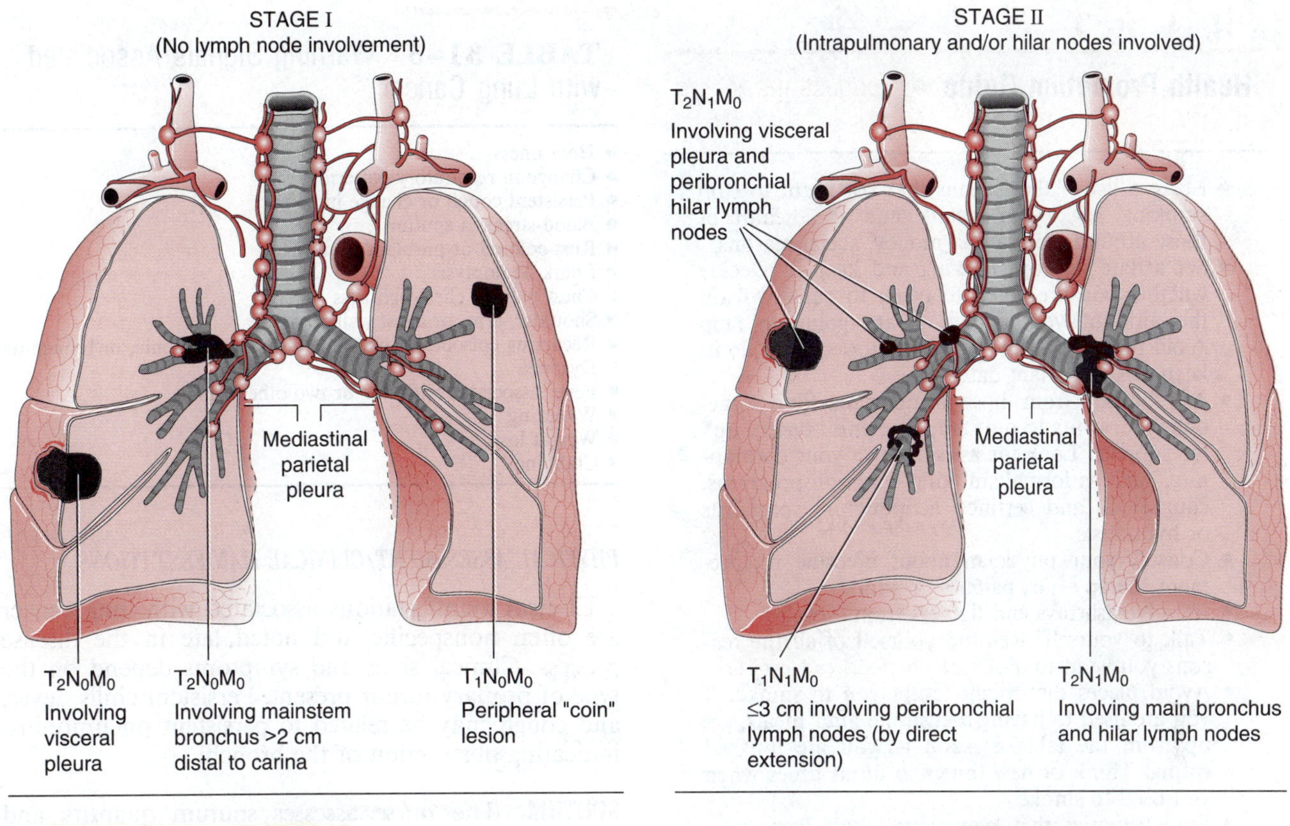

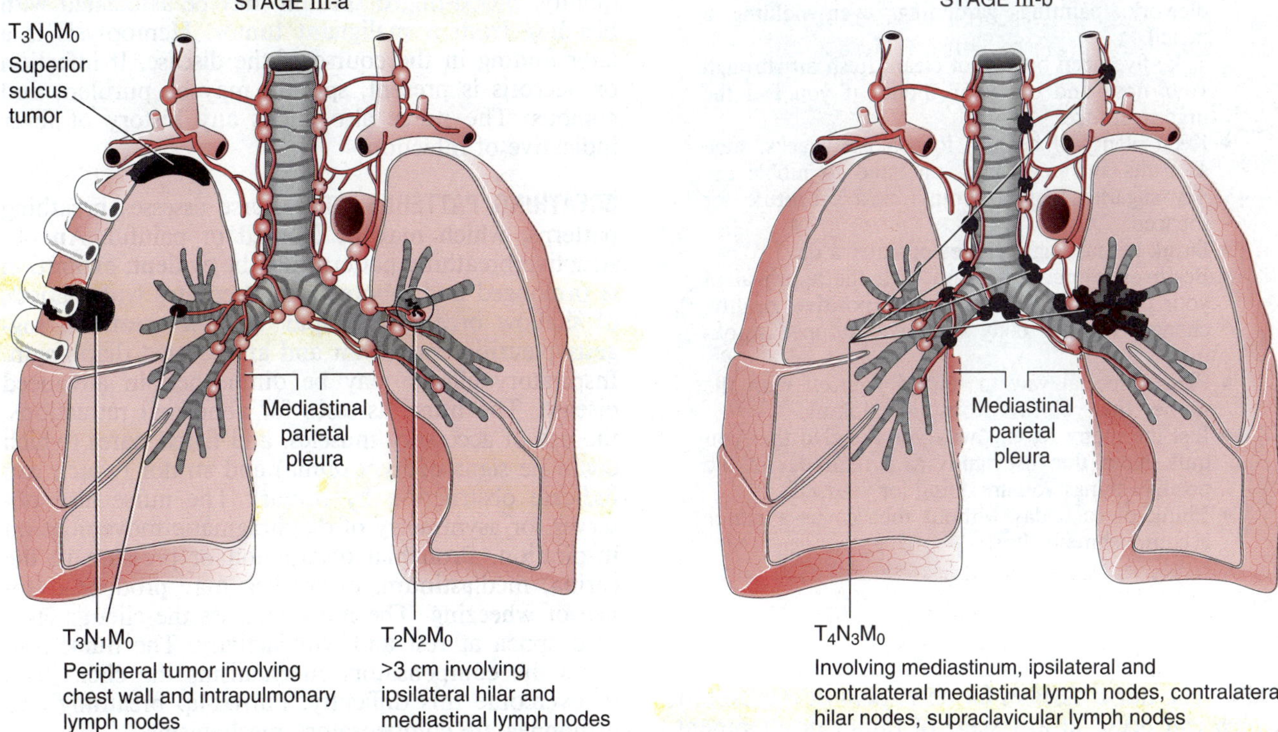

FIGURE 31–1 ◆ Anatomic staging of lung cancer. (Redrawn from Mountain, C. F., Greenberg, M. D., & Fraire, A. E. [1991]. Tumor stages in non-small cell carcinoma of the lung. *Chest*, *99*[5], 1258.)

nurse asks whether changes in position affect hoarseness, because a recumbent position often exacerbates (worsens) this sign. The nurse questions the client about a persistent cough or change in cough and whether the cough is productive of sputum. The nurse also notes a history of any change in respiratory pattern, shortness of breath, or hemoptysis (blood in the sputum).

CHART 31–4

Health Promotion Guide ◆ Suggestions to Help You Stop Smoking

- Make a list of the reasons that you want to stop smoking, e.g., your health and the health of those around you, saving money, social reasons.
- Set a date to stop smoking and keep it. Decide whether you are going to begin to cut down on the amount you smoke or are going to stop "cold turkey." Whatever way you decide to do it, keep this important date!
- Ask for help from those around you. Find someone who wants to quit smoking and "buddy up" for support. Look for assistance in your community, such as formal smoking cessation programs, counselors, and certified acupuncture specialists or hypnotists.
- Consult your physician about nicotine replacement therapy (i.e., patches or gum).
- Remove ashtrays and lighters from view.
- Talk to yourself! Remind yourself of all the reasons you want to quit.
- Avoid places that might tempt you to smoke. If you are used to having a cigarette after meals, get up from the table as soon as you are finished eating. Think of new things to do at times when you used to smoke.
- Find activities that keep your hands busy: needlework, painting, gardening, even holding a pencil.
- Take five deep breaths of clean, fresh air through your nose and out your mouth if you feel the urge to smoke.
- Keep plenty of healthy, low-calorie snacks, such as fruits and vegetables, on hand to nibble on. Try sugarless gum or mints as a substitute for tobacco.
- Drink at least eight glasses of water a day.
- Begin an exercise program with the approval of your physician. Be aware of the positive, healthy changes in your body since you stopped smoking.
- Plan a special way to reward yourself with the money that you save from not smoking.
- List the many reasons why you are glad that you quit. Keep that list handy as a reminder of the positive things you are doing for yourself.
- Think of each day without tobacco as a major accomplishment. It is!

PAIN The nurse assesses for chest pain or discomfort, which can occur at any stage of tumor development. Chest pain may be localized or unilateral and can range from mild to severe. The nurse assesses for any vague sensation of fullness, tightness, or pressure in the chest, which may suggest obstruction. A piercing chest pain or pleuritic pain may accompany inspiration. Subscapular pain radiating to the arm commonly results from tumor invasion in advanced disease.

TABLE 31–5 Warning Signals Associated with Lung Cancer

- Hoarseness
- Change in respiratory pattern
- Persistent cough or change in cough
- Blood-streaked sputum
- Rust-colored or purulent sputum
- Frank hemoptysis
- Chest pain or chest tightness
- Shoulder, arm, or chest wall pain
- Recurring episodes of pleural effusion, pneumonia, or bronchitis
- Dyspnea
- Fever associated with one or two other signs
- Wheezing
- Weight loss
- Clubbing

PHYSICAL ASSESSMENT/CLINICAL MANIFESTATIONS

Clinical manifestations associated with lung cancer are often nonspecific and noted late in the disease process. Clinical signs and symptoms depend on the type of primary tumor present. Persistent chills, fever, and cough may be related to persistent pneumonitis, indicating obstruction of the bronchi.

SPUTUM The nurse assesses sputum quantity and quality. Blood-tinged sputum may be associated with bleeding from a malignant tumor. Hemoptysis is a later finding in the course of the disease. If infection or necrosis is present, sputum may be purulent and copious. The nurse also elicits any history of fever indicative of infection.

BREATHING PATTERNS The nurse assesses breathing patterns, which may be labored or painful. An obstructive breathing pattern may be evident; expiration is prolonged and labored and alternates with periods of shallow breathing. Rapid, shallow breathing suggests pleuritic chest pain and an elevated diaphragm. Inspiratory efforts may be diminished in advanced disease. The nurse assesses for abnormal retractions, the use of accessory muscles, and flared nares (which could be signs of hypoxemia) and stridor (which can indicate obstruction by tumor). The nurse also observes for asymmetry of diaphragmatic movement on inspiration. Bronchial obstruction or pressure in the carina, mediastinum, or trachea may produce dyspnea or wheezing. The nurse assesses the client's level of dyspnea at rest and with activity. The nurse also notes the compensatory mechanisms the client uses to overcome this difficulty. Pursed-lip breathing and orthopnea are compensatory mechanisms.

FREMITUS On palpation of the chest wall, the nurse may find areas of tenderness or masses. Changes in tactile fremitus (vibrations felt on the chest wall) indicate areas of consolidation (the process whereby air spaces in the lung are replaced with solid material, such as tumor or fluid). Fremitus is decreased or absent when the bronchus is obstructed or the pleural space is occupied by a tumor. Palpation of the trachea may reveal deviation from midline or "shifting" related to a thoracic mass.

MASSES By percussion of the chest wall the nurse examines for areas of dullness or obvious masses. With diaphragmatic excursion, resonance usually occurs around the tenth rib. In the presence of a pleural effusion, the nurse may detect an unusually high diaphragmatic level (Epps, 1992).

BREATH SOUNDS The nurse auscultates the chest to determine changes in breath sounds directly related to the presence of a tumor. Wheezes indicate partial obstruction of airflow in passages narrowed by tumors. Decreased or absent breath sounds is an ominous sign. Absent breath sounds indicate impairment of air passages from obstruction by a tumor or replacement of lung tissue with a solid tumor or fluid. Auscultation of vocal fremitus (i.e., bronchophony, perctoriloquy, and egophony [see chap. 28]) reveals changes in the sound normally heard. Increased loudness or sound intensity indicates consolidation or compression of the pleural tissue by tumor. Auscultation of a pleural friction rub suggests an inflammatory response to an invading tumor.

CARDIAC STATUS The nurse notes distant heart sounds, which may indicate cardiac tamponade related to an extended tumor. Dysrhythmias may be present as a result of hypoxemia. The nurse may also observe cyanosis of the lips and fingertips, or clubbing (see Fig. 30–6).

LATE SIGNS AND SYMPTOMS Late manifestations of lung cancer may include nonspecific systemic symptoms, such as fatigue, recent weight loss, anorexia, dysphagia, and nausea and vomiting. Superior vena cava syndrome may result from intrathoracic spread of the malignant tumor; this syndrome constitutes an emergency (see Chap. 26). Lethargy and somnolence may develop; therefore, the nurse performs a baseline neurologic assessment. Bowel and bladder tone and function may be affected by tumor spread to the spine and spinal cord.

PSYCHOSOCIAL ASSESSMENT

To complete the psychosocial assessment of the client with lung cancer, the nurse evaluates various parameters, including:

- Age
- Occupation
- Previous experience with illness
- Marital status
- Dependents
- Support systems
- Usual coping mechanisms

Symptoms associated with lung cancer, especially dyspnea, often add to the client's feelings of fear and anxiety. Clients with a history of cigarette smoking may experience feelings of guilt and shame. The nurse conveys acceptance of the client and interacts in a nonjudgmental way.

Societal awareness of the poor prognosis of lung cancer poses many challenges for the client and family. Few clients with the diagnosis of lung cancer are candidates for curative therapy. Most clients with lung cancer are given palliative treatment that is limited to relief of symptoms. Overall survival time is only moderately lengthened. Fear of abandonment and separation is commonly noted in clients with lung cancer (Houston & Kendall, 1992).

The client and family will undergo a rapid course of changes in activities of daily living and associated adjustments. Progression of lung cancer increases dependency, decreases tolerance for activity, and decreases self-esteem. Clients and their families daily confront anticipatory grief related to loss of role functions and ultimately the loss of life. With sensitivity to this situation, the nurse:

- Supports the client and family through the diagnosis and treatment phases
- Assesses the client's emotional response to the diagnosis of lung cancer
- Listens carefully to the client's and family's concerns

Family members play an important role in the physical and psychosocial care of the client. Family members and significant others can help alleviate the client's anxiety level, anticipate needs, and act as a liasion between the staff and the client. The nurse recognizes that the family and significant others also have unmet psychosocial needs and assists them in expressing their needs and concerns.

The nurse identifies resources to assist the client and family in the treatment phase, through the progression of illness, and during anticipatory and actual bereavement. The nurse assesses the grief response as the client and family react to their situation and adjusts care accordingly. (Chapter 12 covers grief and loss in detail.)

LABORATORY ASSESSMENT

A definitive diagnosis of lung cancer is made by isolation of malignant cells. Cytologic examination of early morning sputum specimens may identify tumor cells. However, even with a lung tumor, malignant cells may not be obtained in sputum. With pleural effusion, thoracentesis may enable fluid to be obtained for cytologic examination.

RADIOGRAPHIC ASSESSMENT

Pulmonary lesions are frequently seen on chest x-ray, but tomograms and computed tomography (CT) scans are used to clearly visualize the lesions. CT scan identifies and localizes the extent of masses in the chest, including mediastinal and lymph node involvement.

OTHER DIAGNOSTIC ASSESSMENT

Fiberoptic bronchoscopy is extremely important in the diagnosis of lung cancer. It provides direct visualization of the tracheobronchial tree. Specimens and "bronchial brushings" can thus be obtained, especially when lesions are located endobronchially or are close to an airway. Transthoracic and transbronchial needle biopsy may also be used in an attempt to obtain malignant cells.

To identify metastasis in mediastinal lymph nodes, the physician may perform mediastinoscopy by inserting a scope through a small anterior chest incision at the suprasternal notch. Mediastinoscopy is an important staging tool for determining the extent of the lung cancer and formulating a treatment plan. If scalene (near the first rib) or supraclavicular lymph nodes are palpable, biopsy of these nodes may also be done.

To determine a definitive diagnosis and assess overall pulmonary status, other diagnostic studies may be needed, including percutaneous needle biopsy, direct surgical biopsy, and thoracentesis with pleural biopsy. A magnetic resonance imaging (MRI) study may be ordered to identify possible invasion or compression of vascular structures by tumor. Radionuclide scans of the liver, spleen, brain, and bone may be used to assess metastasis of lung cancer. Pulmonary function studies and arterial blood gas analysis may be included to determine the client's overall respiratory status.

ANALYSIS

COMMON NURSING DIAGNOSES

Three nursing diagnoses are common in clients with lung cancer:

1. Impaired Gas Exchange related to decreased lung capacity secondary to tissue destruction
2. Ineffective Airway Clearance related to tumor obstruction and increased tracheobronchial secretions
3. Pain related to tumor pressure on surrounding tissues and erosion of tissues

ADDITIONAL NURSING DIAGNOSES

In addition to the common diagnoses, the client may present with one or more of the following diagnoses:

- Ineffective Breathing Pattern related to decreased energy, fatigue, pain, tracheobronchial obstruction, anxiety
- Activity Intolerance related to imbalance between oxygen supply and demand, dyspnea, fatigue, generalized weakness, weight loss, malnourishment, pain, depression
- Fluid Volume Excess related to compromised antidiuretic hormone regulating mechanism
- High Risk for Injury related to metabolic imbalances, e.g. hypercalcemia
- Fatigue related to increased metabolic energy production, overwhelming emotional demands, states of discomfort, altered body chemistry (e.g., chemotherapy)
- High Risk for Trauma related to weakness
- Altered Nutrition, Less than Body Requirements related to the active disease process (increased metabolism), anorexia, nausea, vomiting
- Decreased Cardiac Output related to electrical malfunction secondary to hypoxic dysrhythmias
- Impaired Physical Mobility related to decreased strength and endurance, fatigue, intolerance to activity, dyspnea
- Anticipatory Grieving related to actual or potential loss of health status
- Anxiety related to change in health status, situational crisis, threat of death, loss of control
- Fear related to pain, threat of death, effects of loss of body part or function
- Altered Role Performance related to change in health status, role loss
- Ineffective Family Coping, Disabling or Compromised, related to effects of major life events, effects of impending death of family member, temporary family disorganization and role changes, effects of acute or chronic illness
- Ineffective Individual Coping related to effects of acute or chronic illness, loss of control over body part or function, major changes in lifestyle, situational crisis, knowledge deficit regarding therapeutic regimen/disease process/prognosis

PLANNING AND IMPLEMENTATION

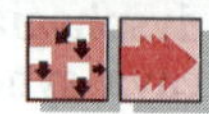

IMPAIRED GAS EXCHANGE

PLANNING: CLIENT GOALS The major goal is that the client will be adequately oxygenated, as evidenced by decreased symptoms of hypoxia (such as dyspnea) and decreased signs of hypoxemia (i.e., acceptable blood gas or pulse oximetry results).

INTERVENTIONS The nurse evaluates the hypoxemic client's respiratory status as often as indicated by his or her condition, perhaps every 2 to 4 hours. Color of the skin, lips, ear lobes, and nail beds is noted. The nurse also assesses for signs of respiratory distress, such as dyspnea and use of accessory muscles for breathing. The client in obvious distress is further evaluated by pulse oximetry and arterial blood gas studies.

Nonsurgical Management

Oxygen Therapy If the client is hypoxemic, the nurse provides supplemental oxygen via mask or nasal cannula as ordered. Even if the client is not overtly hypoxemic, the physician may order oxygen as needed to relieve dyspnea (difficulty breathing) and anxiety in the lung cancer client. (See also Oxygen Therapy in Chapter 30 for associated nursing care.)

Drug Therapy If the client is experiencing bronchospasm, the physician may prescribe bronchodilators (as for clients with asthma) and corticosteroids to decrease bronchospasm, inflammation, and edema (see Chap. 30).

CHEMOTHERAPY Chemotherapy is frequently the treatment of choice for lung cancers, especially small-cell lung cancer, because of metastasis. Chemotherapy may also be used in conjunction with surgical treatment modalities. Chemotherapy agents commonly administered for the treatment of lung cancer include combinations such as:

- Cyclophosphamide, doxorubicin, methotrexate, and procarbazine
- Etoposide and cisplatin
- Mitomycin, vinblastine, and cisplatin

The nurse understands the mode of action of each chemotherapeutic agent and takes measures to control common side effects (Table 31–6). The nurse supports the client and family throughout the course of chemotherapy. The nurse educates the client and family about this treatment modality and how to prevent and manage potential side effects. (See Chapter 26 for further discussion of chemotherapeutic agents and associated nursing care.)

IMMUNOTHERAPY Many clients with lung cancer are immunocompromised (unable to adequately defend against potentially harmful substances). Treatment is directed at enhancing an effective immune response, which favorably affects the course of the disease. Immunotherapeutic agents (cytokines) that are "growth factors" are most commonly administered. Cytokines decrease the time that the client is neutropenic (has a low white blood cell count) and allow continuation of chemotherapy (see also Chaps. 22 and 26).

Radiation Therapy Radiation therapy can be an effective primary treatment for localized, unresectable, intrathoracic lung tumors. Radiotherapy can also be helpful for palliation of hemoptysis, obstruction of the bronchi and great veins (superior vena cava syndrome), dysphagia related to esophageal compression, and pain due to bone metastasis. Preoperative irradiation may be attempted to shrink a tumor and promote resectability. After surgical resection of primary tumors, radiation has successfully reduced re-

TABLE 31–6 Side Effects of Chemotherapeutic Agents Used in the Treatment of Lung Cancer

	Side Effects				
Drug	Alopecia	Nausea and Vomiting	Bone Marrow Suppression	Diarrhea	**Specific Toxic Effects**
Cisplatin (Platinol)	+	++++	+++	–	• Constipation • Nephrotoxic effects • Ototoxic effects • Hypophosphatemia
Cyclophosphamide (Cytoxan, Procytox✱)	++	++	++	+	• Hemorrhagic cystitis • Syndrome of inappropriate antidiuretic hormone (SIADH) • Hyperpigmentation
Doxorubicin (Adriamycin)	+++	++	+++	+	• Tissue vesicant • Cardiotoxic effects • Mucositis • Hyperpigmentation
Etoposide VP-16, Vepesid)	+++	+++	++++	–	• Constipation • Postural hypotension
Methotrexate (MTX)	+	++	+++	+	• Mucositis
Mitomycin-C (Mutamycin)	+++	++	+++	+	• Tissue vesicant • Pulmonary injury
Procarbazine (Matulane)	+	+++	+++	+++	• Postural hypotension • Myalgia • Arthralgia
Vinblastine (VLB, Velban)	+	+++	+	–	• Tissue vesicant • Pain at tumor site • Jaw pain • Neurotoxic effects • Loss of deep tendon reflexes

– no symptoms; + mild; ++ moderate; +++ severe; ++++ profound.

sidual pleural or mediastinal disease. Because of the high frequency of brain metastasis with small-cell carcinoma and adenocarcinoma, prophylatic brain radiation may be recommended for clients with these types of lung cancer.

Laser Therapy Neodymium-YAG lasers and (rarely) carbon dioxide lasers have been used for palliation of endobronchial obstruction in clients with benign or malignant tumors that are accessible by bronchoscopy. The surgeon debulks the obstructive portion of the tumor, and the airway is reopened. Laser therapy does not produce systemic or toxic effects and is well tolerated by most clients.

Thoracentesis and Pleurodesis Pleural effusions can be a common problem for clients with lung cancer. Effusions can be caused by involvement of the visceral or parietal pleura by tumor and also by mediastinal lymphatic obstruction or obstructive pneumonitis. The goal of treatment is to remove pleural fluid and prevent its accumulation. Thoracentesis (see Chap. 28) removes fluid from the intrapleural space and relieves immediate signs and symptoms of hypoxia.

The physician performs thoracentesis by inserting a specialized needle into the intercostal space at the level of fluid accumulation. The physician then aspirates pleural fluid with a syringe; alternatively, tubing can be connected to the needle and attached to sterile vacuum collection bottles. After accessible fluid is aspirated, the physician removes the needle and applies a bandage over the site. A chest x-ray after the tap documents the presence or absence of pneumothorax, a potential complication of the procedure.

The nurse offers reassurance throughout the procedure and assesses the client's breathing pattern at the same time. After the procedure, the nurse:

- Continues to assess respiratory status
- Monitors vital signs
- Assesses the puncture site for bleeding, redness, swelling, and discomfort

Fluid can rapidly reaccumulate in the pleural space, and the client may again experience respiratory compromise within a few days. Repeated thoracentesis can create pain and anxiety and place the client at risk for further complications. As an alternative to repeated thoracentesis, the physician inserts a chest tube to drain the fluid and instills a sclerosing agent. A sclerosing agent is an irritant that causes inflammation and results in fibrosis of tissue. Doxycycline, thiotepa, bleomycin, nitrogen mustard, and 5-fluorouracil as well as talc have been used for this treatment. The aim of thoracentesis and intrapleural administration of one of these agents is to create a *pleurodesis,* which causes adherence of the pleura to the chest wall. Thus, the potential space is eliminated, and reaccumulation of effusion is prevented.

Before pleurodesis, the nurse medicates the client with an analgesic and/or sedative, as ordered. The physician anesthetizes the pleural surfaces by injecting 1% lidocaine through the chest tube. The physician instills the sclerosing agent; then the nurse or physician clamps the chest tube to prevent drainage of the agent. The physician may order that the client be rotated through various positions at 15- to 30-minute intervals. However, this repositioning process has been eliminated at some medical centers because limited research has demonstrated that dispersion of the sclerosing agent is not enhanced by rotation of the client's position (Lorch, et al., 1988). Chart 31-5 reviews nursing care of the client undergoing pleurodesis.

Surgical Management Surgery is the treatment of choice for stage I and stage II non-small cell lung cancer (see Fig. 31-1). Total resection of a non-small cell primary bronchogenic tumor is undertaken in hope of achieving a cure. If complete resectability is not possible, the surgeon removes the bulk of the tumor and decreases the possibility of metastatic extension. The choice of surgical procedure depends on the findings of the staging process and the client's overall health and functional status.

CHART 31-5

Nursing Care Highlight ♦ The Client Undergoing Pleurodesis

- Reinforce explanation of the pleurodesis and inform the client that medication will be provided to promote comfort before the procedure. (The physician may administer IV analgesia/sedation immediately before the procedure.)
- Ensure that the chest tube is clamped after instillation of the sclerosing agent.
- Monitor vital signs and respiratory status at the completion of the procedure and then at least every 30 min until the effects of the IV medication have dissipated.
- Thereafter, monitor vital signs every 4 hr for 24 hr. (The client may experience a low-grade fever. Pleurodesis creates pleuritis between the visceral and parietal layers, thus preventing reaccumulation of fluid.)
- If a rotation schedule is ordered, assist the client to the correct position for appropriate time frames and provide reassurance.
- Unclamp the chest tube after completion of the rotation schedule or at the specified time ordered by the physician.
- Assess chest tube drainage and document the amount and character of the drainage.
- Perform a complete respiratory assessment every 8 hr and observe for signs and symptoms of distress, including those of pneumothorax.
- Analgesics may be administered as needed to promote the client's comfort.
- When drainage has decreased (<150 mL in 12–24 hr), the physician may remove the chest tube. Maintain an occlusive dressing at the insertion site for a minimum of 48 hr.

Thoracotomy A thoracotomy is an opening into the thoracic cavity to locate tumors, perform a biopsy, or identify sites of bleeding or injury. Thoracotomy is most often performed to remove all or a portion of the lung.

PREOPERATIVE CARE The goals of preoperative care are to relieve anxiety and promote the client's participation. The nurse employs interventions to relieve the client's anxiety related to the diagnosis of lung cancer, postoperative management, and loss of a portion or all of a lung. The nurse encourages the client to express fears and concerns, reinforces the physician's explanation of the surgical procedure, and provides education related to the postoperative course. The nurse teaches the client the following:

- Anticipated location of the surgical incision, if known
- Shoulder exercises
- Chest tube and drainage system (except after pneumonectomy)
- Other routines (see Chap. 19)

OPERATIVE PROCEDURES Three types of incisions can be made:

- Posterolateral thoracotomy
- Anterolateral thoracotomy
- Median sternotomy

A posterolateral thoracotomy incision begins in the submammary fold of the anterior chest, is drawn down below the scapular tip and along the course of the ribs, and then curves posteriorly and upward as far as the spine of the scapula.

An anterolateral thoracotomy involves an incision below the breast and above the costal margins. This incision extends from the anterior axillary line and then turns downward to avoid the axillary apex.

A median sternotomy is a straight incision from the suprasternal notch to below the xyphoid process. The sternum must be transected with an electric or air-driven saw.

POSTOPERATIVE CARE General care of the client after thoracotomy is reviewed in the Client Care Plan. Postoperative management of clients who have undergone thoracotomy requires closed-chest drainage to drain air and blood that may accumulate in the pleural space. A chest tube is a drain placed in the pleural space to restore intrapleural pressure, allowing re-expansion of the lung. The chest tube also prevents air and fluid from returning to the chest. The drainage system consists of:

- One or more chest tubes or drains
- A collection container placed below the chest level
- A water seal to keep air from entering the chest

The tip of the tube used to drain air is usually placed anteriorly near the lung apex. The tube that drains liquid is placed laterally near the base of the lung. After lung resection, two tubes, anterior and posterior, are used. The puncture wounds are covered with airtight dressings.

The chest tube is connected to approximately 6 feet of tubing that leads to a collection device placed several feet below the chest. The tubing allows the client to turn and move easily. The position of the collection device below the chest uses gravity and allows drainage of the pleural space. When two chest tubes are inserted, they are usually joined by a Y connector near the client's body; the 6 feet of tubing is attached to the Y connector.

The separate water seal mechanism of the chest drainage system acts as a one-way valve. In setting up current chest drainage systems, the nurse adds a specified amount of sterile saline to the water seal chamber. In older systems, the end of the tubing was placed beneath the surface of a sterile saline solution to create the water seal. The water seal closes the open end of the system (or the end of the tubing) from the atmosphere. When the positive pressure in the lungs during exhalation pushes air out of the pleural space through the tubing, the air bubbles into saline and cannot re-enter the chest.

Earlier chest drainage systems consisted of one-, two-, and three-bottle systems. Technology has greatly improved these bulky glass bottle systems through the availability of one-piece disposable chest drainage systems. The Pleur-evac system, one of the most widely distributed systems, uses a one-piece disposable, molded plastic unit with three chambers. This system duplicates the formerly used three-bottle system. From right to left, the system contains chambers for drainage, a water seal, and suction control (Fig. 31–2). The plastic devices reduce the risk of breakage or contamination of the drainage system and allow the client increased mobility. All systems are vented so that incoming pleural air cannot build up, and further air entry into the chest is prevented. Suction may be added, as ordered.

In one of the newer drainage systems, a knob on the collection device can be set to the ordered amount of suction. The wall suction source dial is then turned until a small orange floater valve appears in a certain window (Fig. 31–3). When the orange valve is in the window, the right amount of suction has been applied. With this system, the nurse notes the absence of bubbling in the chamber, which is normal for this so-called dry suction system.

The nurse routinely checks to ensure the sterility and patency of the system. The nurse tapes the tubing junctions to prevent accidental disconnections and maintains an occlusive dressing at the chest tube insertion site. Sterile gauze is kept at the bedside to cover the insertion site immediately in the event that the chest tube becomes accidentally dislodged. The nurse keeps heavy padded clamps at the bedside for use if the drainage system is inadvertently interrupted or to facilitate changing of the drainage system when necessary. The nurse carefully positions the drainage tubing to prevent kinks and large loops of tubing,

Text continued on page 748

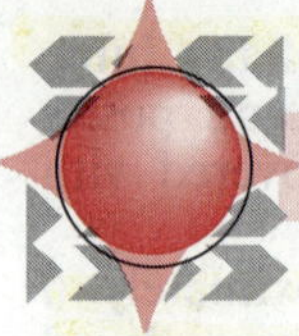

CLIENT CARE PLAN

The Client Who Has Had a Thoracotomy for Lung Cancer

Nursing Diagnosis No. 1: Impaired Gas Exchange related to ventilation-perfusion imbalance secondary to removal of all or part of a lung and ineffective airway clearance

Expected Outcomes	Nursing Interventions	Rationale
The client will have adequate lung expansion and mobilization of secretions. The client's blood gases and pulse oximetry will be within his or her normal range.	◆ Perform complete respiratory assessment every 2 hr. Assess: breath sounds; rate, depth, and pattern of respirations; signs and symptoms of hypoxia, including restlessness and irritability; and position of mediastinum.	◆ Ongoing astute assessments alert the nurse to subtle and early signs and symptoms of changes in respiratory status.
	◆ Monitor vital signs, pulse oximetry, and arterial blood gases as ordered. Report abnormalities to the physician.	◆ Prompt reporting of abnormalities enable the physician to institute early treatment and prevent further complications.
	◆ Administer oxygen therapy as ordered.	◆ Supplemental oxygen will help correct hypoxemia.
	◆ Maintain patency and integrity of the chest tube and drainage system, if present.	◆ A properly functioning chest drainage system promotes adequate drainage of blood and air that may accumulate in the pleural space, allowing re-expansion of the lung.
	◆ Assess for and report signs and symptoms of air leak from the chest tube or hemorrhage.	◆ Prompt reporting of abnormalities help prevent further complications.
	◆ Perform pain assessment and administer analgesics as ordered. (Observe for signs and symptoms of respiratory depression related to opioids.)	◆ Effective pain management promotes the client's participation in deep breathing and mobility, thus fostering optimal respiratory effort.
	◆ Reposition the client every 2 hr. Check order for positioning carefully and seek clarification if necessary (Do not place the client on the operative side after pneumonectomy.)	◆ Repositioning promotes lung expansion.
	◆ Encourage the client to perform deep-breathing exercises every 2 hr and to use incentive spirometry devices as soon as he or she is physically able.	◆ Breathing exercises promote lung expansion and help prevent atelectasis and pneumonia.
	◆ Coach in effective coughing technique if secretions are present. Assist to high-Fowler's position with knees bent and feet flat on bed. Instruct the client to obtain maximal inspiration and to hold the breath for 2 sec; follow by having the client cough twice with the mouth open, pause, and then inhale through the nose and rest.	◆ Effective coughing improves airway clearance and prevents stasis of secretions.

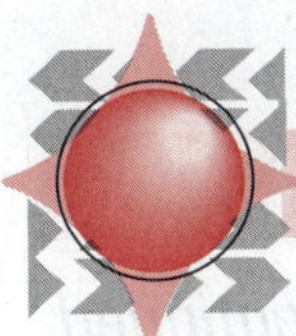

CLIENT CARE PLAN

The Client Who Has Had a Thoracotomy for Lung Cancer *Continued*

Nursing Diagnosis No. 1: Impaired Gas Exchange related to ventilation-perfusion imbalance secondary to removal of all or part of a lung and ineffective airway clearance

Expected Outcomes	Nursing Interventions	Rationale
	◆ Assist the client to remove and properly dispose of secretions.	◆ Proper disposal of secretions is required for infection control purposes.
	◆ Assist the client to sit in a chair, when ordered, and monitor tolerance.	◆ Lung expansion is enhanced when the client is able to be out of bed.

Nursing Diagnosis No. 2: Pain related to tissue trauma as a result of surgery, inflammation of incised muscles, and presence of chest tubes

Expected Outcomes	Nursing Interventions	Rationale
The client will be as pain-free and alert as possible.	◆ Perform a complete pain assessment using designed pain level scale (i.e., 0 = no pain, 5 = severe pain).	◆ Obtain the baseline pain assessment rating and use it for comparison with the routine pain assessment score to determine the effectiveness of pain management interventions.
	◆ Assist with incisional splinting during deep-breathing exercises, with turning, and in anticipation of cough stimulation.	◆ Splinting promotes the client's comfort and participation in measures that promote respiratory function.
	◆ Secure the chest tube to prevent excessive discomfort resulting from movement of the tube. ◆ Promote optimal comfort through proper positioning, hygiene, gentle massage, and relaxation techniques.	◆ Nonpharmacologic nursing interventions are instrumental in helping the client to achieve optimal comfort.
	◆ Administer analgesics as ordered. Plan activities to coincide with peak of analgesic effectiveness. Observe for signs and symptoms of respiratory depression associated with opioids. ◆ Use diversional activities as appropriate.	◆ The client's participation in respiratory excursion activities will be increased with effective pain management.
	◆ Document the client's response to the pain control regimen and seek adjustment as needed.	◆ Ongoing assessment and evaluation of the effectiveness of the pain control regimen are essential to the client's optimal comfort.
The client will maintain normal arm and shoulder movement and	◆ Educate the client about the possible complication and pre-	◆ The client is more likely to actively participate in preventive

Continued on following page

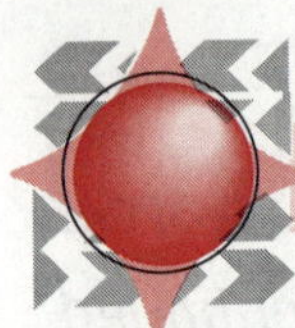

CLIENT CARE PLAN

The Client Who Has Had a Thoracotomy for Lung Cancer *Continued*

Nursing Diagnosis No. 3: Activity Intolerance related to restricted arm and shoulder movement

Expected Outcomes	Nursing Interventions	Rationale
function as evidenced by the ability to perform range-of-motion exercises on the operative side.	vention of "frozen shoulder syndrome."	measures when he or she is knowledgeable about this potential postoperative complication.
	◆ Monitor and report restricted arm and shoulder movement postoperatively.	◆ Ongoing assessments help detect early signs of complications.
	◆ Perform passive range-of-motion exercises to the affected arm and shoulder 2 times every 4 hr during the first 24 hr postoperatively, and then 10 times every 2 hr.	◆ Exercising maintains strength, facilitates mobility, and prevents fixation.
	◆ Instruct the client in active range-of-motion exercises beginning the second day after surgery.	◆ Active participation by the client promotes well-being, autonomy, and independence.
	◆ Encourage the client to use the affected arm for activities of daily living and place frequently used items on the same side of the bed as the operative side to facilitate reaching and gentle stretching.	
	◆ Administer analgesic as needed to promote active participation in exercises.	◆ Effective levels of analgesia allow the client to perform prescribed exercises and prevent complications.
	◆ Offer encouragement and support for the client's progress.	◆ Positive reinforcement enables the client to continue the rehabilitation process.

Nursing Diagnosis No. 4: Body Image Disturbance related to actual change in body structure and function

Expected Outcomes	Nursing Interventions	Rationale
The client will verbalize feelings about loss of all or part of a lung and identify ways in which to compensate for altered lung capacity.	◆ Establish a therapeutic nurse/client relationship by building trust and confidence.	◆ Sincere behaviors that display concern and caring enable the client to feel comfortable and at ease with the nurse.
	◆ Encourage expression of feelings and concerns related to lung cancer diagnosis, grief about loss of lung, and effects on lifestyle.	◆ Ventilation of feelings and concerns can serve as an effective coping strategy and assist the client to express needs.
	◆ Support a realistic hope of regaining aspects of usual activities.	◆ Hope is a universal coping mechanism and can enable the client to attain activity potential within the present physical limitations.

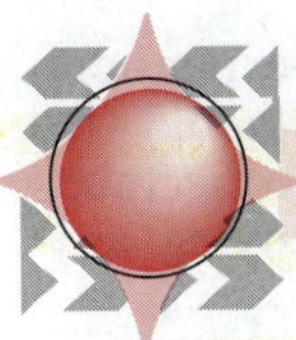

CLIENT CARE PLAN

The Client Who Has Had a Thoracotomy for Lung Cancer *Continued*

Nursing Diagnosis No. 4: Body Image Disturbance related to actual change in body structure and function

Expected Outcomes	Nursing Interventions	Rationale
	◆ Assist the client to identify activities that can be performed with present lung capacity.	◆ Identification of activities that can be performed by the client encourages independence and increased self-esteem.
	◆ Identify measures to promote increased endurance and participation in activities (i.e., carefully schedule activities, ensure rest periods and proper nutrition).	◆ Energy conservation and health promotion activities assist the client to achieve optimal physical activity.
	◆ Provide support for accomplishments and encourage the concept of slow progression without compromising respiratory status.	◆ Positive reinforcement of achievements enhances body image and self-esteem.

Nursing Diagnosis No. 5: Knowledge Deficit related to care after hospitalization

Expected Outcomes	Nursing Interventions	Rationale
The client will verbalize follow-up care and signs and symptoms to report to the primary care provider.	◆ Review the discharge instructions with the client, including: follow-up visit, medications, permitted activities, and arm and shoulder exercises.	◆ Ensuring that the client understands required information before discharge promotes the client's participation in the treatment plan and minimizes anxiety after discharge.
	◆ Instruct the client to report signs and symptoms of fever, cough and sputum production, increased discomfort, or dyspnea to the primary care provider (physician or nurse).	◆ Early detection and treatment of possible respiratory infection or other respiratory complications can reduce the extent of the complication.
	◆ Encourage the client to pace tolerable activities and rest periods. ◆ Reinforce that heavy lifting is to be avoided for 6 months and to stop any activity that provokes excessive dyspnea or discomfort.	◆ When the client understands how to balance and limit activities, complications can be prevented.
	◆ Review and educate the client about additional proposed treatment as indicated (chemotherapy, radiation therapy).	◆ Education related to further treatment modalities fosters the client's understanding of and compliance with the treatment plan and can reduce anxiety and possible misconceptions.
	◆ Refer the client to appropriate community resources, if indicated (e.g., home health agency, American Cancer Society, American Lung Association).	◆ Community resources are an additional avenue for information and support.

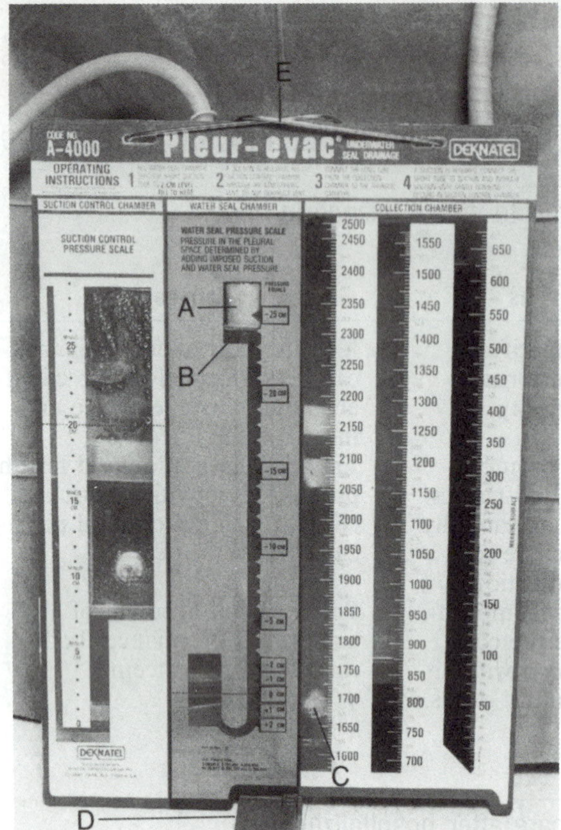

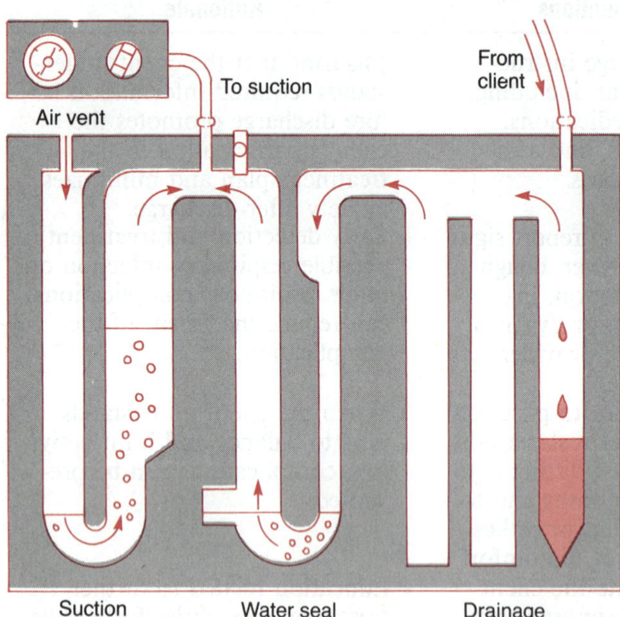

FIGURE 31-2 ◆ The Pleur-evac drainage system, a commercial three-bottle chest drainage device. *Top,* Float valve (A); well indicator (B); self-sealing diaphragm for drainage sampling (C); floor stand (D); and hooks from which to hang the unit (E). (From Kersten, L. D. [1989]. *Comprehensive respiratory nursing: A decision making approach.* Philadelphia: W. B. Saunders.) *Bottom,* Schematic of the drainage device.

which can impede drainage and lung re-expansion. Vigorous stripping of the chest tube should be avoided (Teplitz, 1991). Gentle milking of the tube, however, may prevent obstruction by moving any blood clots.

The nurse assesses the client's respiratory status and notes the amount and type of drainage. Immediately after surgery, the nurse hourly records the amount of drainage. Drainage of more than 100 mL/hr is considered excessive, and the physician is notified. After the first 24 hours, the nurse usually assesses drainage and the drainage system minimally every 8 hours.

The nurse checks the water seal chamber for unexpected bubbling created by an air leak in the system. During forceful expiration or coughing, bubbling is anticipated because air in the chest is being expelled. Continuous bubbling indicates that an air leak is present, and efforts must be made to identify its source. On the physician's order, the nurse gently applies a padded clamp on the drainage tubing close to the occlusive dressing. If the bubbling stops, the air leak can be at the chest tube insertion site or within the chest. Further assessment of the insertion site and chest tube position is necessary, and the nurse consults the physician for identified problems. Air bubbling that does not cease when the nurse applies a padded clamp indicates that the air leak is between the clamp and the drainage system. For ensuring patency and sterility of the system, this tubing and drainage device should be replaced, as ordered.

The nurse also checks for rising and falling of fluid in the water seal as the client breathes in and out. These fluctuations act like a manometer by representing the pressure changes in the pleural space and reliably indicate overall respiratory effort. Fluctuations of 5 to 10 cm (2 to 4 inches) during normal breathing are common. The absence of fluctuations could mean that the tubing is obstructed by a kink, the client is lying on the tubing, or dependent fluid has filled a loop of tubing. Expanded lung tissue can also block the chest tube eyelets during expiration. Another explanation is that no more air is leaking into the pleural space.

Suction can be added to current collection systems on the physician's order. Suction enhances the pressure difference between the pleural space and the drainage system. This causes the pressure to drop inside the system by 15 to 20 cm. In some systems, the ordered amount of suction, often a negative 20 cm, is determined by the height of the saline in the water seal chamber. When suction is added, air is pulled down into the water seal chamber. When the depth of the saline solution is 20 cm, the amount of negative pressure required to pull air to the bottom of the chamber where it bubbles out into the solution is 20 cm of water. While suction is applied, the nurse notes gentle bubbling in the chamber. The depth of the saline determines the maximal suction level on the system. Increasing the suction source causes more bubbling, but it cannot increase the effective suction because the outside air offsets any further air re-

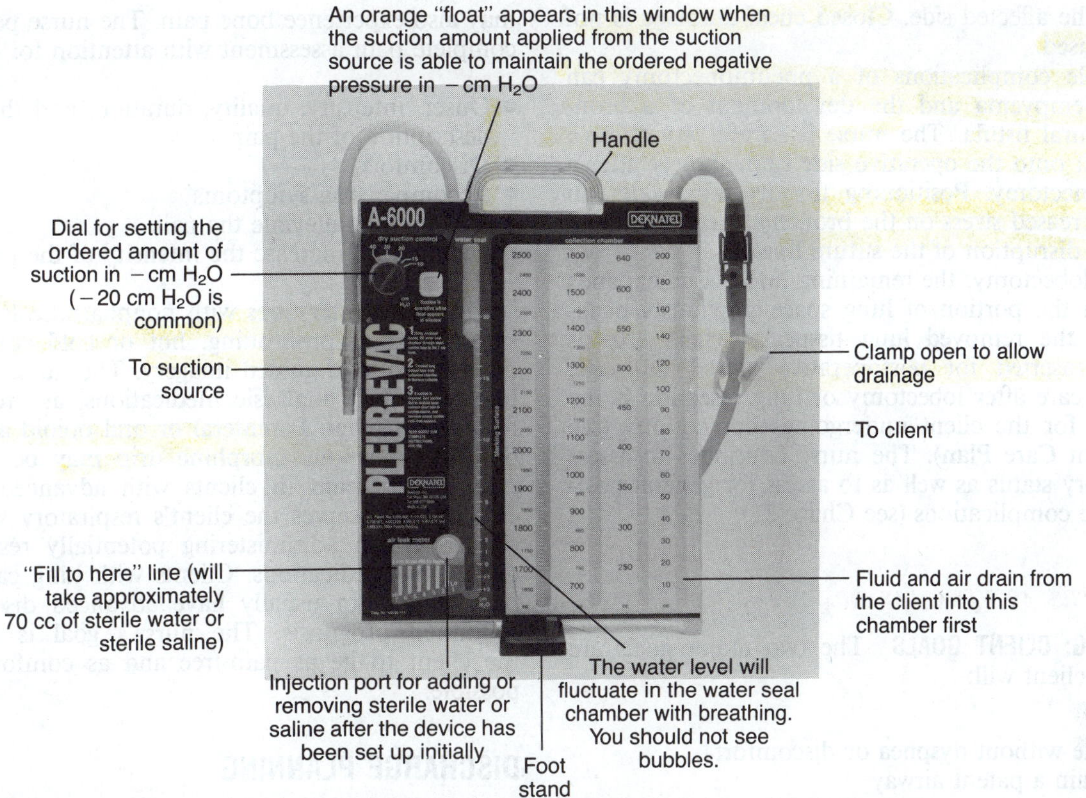

FIGURE 31–3 ◆ The A-6000 dry suction control Pleur-evac chest drainage system. (Courtesy of Deknatel, Inc., Fall River, MA.)

moval. When vigorous bubbling is noted, an air leak may be present. Bubbling also enhances evaporation, and the nurse adds more sterile saline in the chamber as needed.

Other Procedures

PREOPERATIVE CARE The preoperative care for the client undergoing these surgical procedures is the same as for the client having a thoracotomy.

OPERATIVE PROCEDURES

Pneumonectomy. Pneumonectomy, removal of an entire lung, is required for:

- Large, centrally located bronchogenic tumors
- Involvement of a main stem bronchus
- Invasion of the main pulmonary artery

Less frequent indications for this type of surgery include extensive unilateral tuberculosis (TB), extensive bronchiectasis, multiple lung abscesses, and rare varieties of malignant tumors. When a pneumonectomy is performed, the mainstem bronchus is severed and sutured at its bifurcation. The pulmonary artery and veins are also ligated.

Lobectomy. The resection of a single pulmonary lobe, called a lobectomy, can be curative for many carcinomas that develop within a single lobe. It is the usual surgical procedure for most stage I and stage II lung cancers.

When the tumor is confined to a single lobe and easily resectable, the procedure is known as a *simple* lobectomy. Resection is extended to the mainstem bronchus and is followed by a bronchial anastomosis.

When carcinomas are within or compress a lobar bronchus, they are removed by using a *sleeve* lobectomy (bilobectomy), which includes the adjacent lobe.

Resection. A limited pulmonary resection is any surgical resection of the lung that does not involve a complete lobectomy. A *limited* surgical resection is considered only when the lung tumor is in stage I, the tumor size is 3 cm or less, and the client's pulmonary status is compromised. A lung resection may be used if the client cannot tolerate a lobectomy or pneumonectomy.

A *segmental* resection (segmentectomy) is a pulmonary resection that includes the bronchus, pulmonary artery and vein, and lung parenchyma of the involved lung segment or segments, which are divisions of lobes.

A *wedge* resection is removal of the peripheral portion of small localized areas of disease.

POSTOPERATIVE CARE After pneumonectomy, the pleural cavity on the affected side is an empty space. The physician sometimes inserts a clamped chest tube for only a day. This is because it is helpful for serous fluid to accumulate in the empty space and create adhesions, which reduce mediastinal shift toward the affected side. Closed chest drainage is not usually used.

Possible complications of a pneumonectomy can include empyema and the development of a bronchial-pleural fistula. The nurse is careful *not* to turn the client onto the operative side immediately after a pneumonectomy. Positioning the operative side can place increased stress on the bronchial stump incision and risk disruption of the suture line.

After lobectomy, the remaining lung tissue expands to fill in the portion of lung space previously occupied by the removed lung tissue. A chest tube is usually inserted for postoperative closed drainage. Nursing care after lobectomy or lung resection is the same as for the client undergoing thoracotomy (see the Client Care Plan). The nurse continues to assess respiratory status as well as to assess for general postoperative complications (see Chap. 21).

INEFFECTIVE AIRWAY CLEARANCE

PLANNING: CLIENT GOALS The two major goals are that the client will:

- Breathe without dyspnea or discomfort
- Maintain a patent airway

INTERVENTIONS The client who produces copious secretions may benefit from the use of a humidifier and a vaporizer, which provide moisture to loosen the secretions. The nurse suctions the client, as indicated and as ordered, to clear secretions from the airway. If the client also has an underlying chronic lung disease, beta-agonists and inhaled steroids may relieve symptoms. In moderately advanced disease, postural drainage and chest physiotherapy may help.

The client with lung cancer fatigues easily and is often most comfortable resting in a semi-Fowler's position. Dyspnea can be reduced with supplemental oxygen, use of a morphine drip, and positioning for comfort and to facilitate drainage of secretions. The severely dyspneic client may be most comfortable sitting in a lounge or a reclining chair. The nurse monitors the amount of blood loss in the client with hemoptysis. Because blood is an excellent medium for bacterial growth, the nurse is alert for signs and symptoms of infection. The nurse and physician work closely together to provide a regimen that is effective in relieving pain, discomfort, and dyspnea.

PAIN

PLANNING: CLIENT GOALS The major goal is that the client will experience relief or reduction of pain and discomfort.

INTERVENTIONS The client with lung cancer may experience chest pain and possibly subscapular pain radiating to the arm. With bone metastasis, the client may also experience bone pain. The nurse performs a complete pain assessment with attention to:

- Onset, intensity, quality, duration, and the client's description of the pain
- Discomfort
- Accompanying symptoms
- Factors that alleviate the pain
- Factors that increase the intensity of the pain

The nurse intervenes with nonpharmacologic measures, such as positioning, hot or cold compresses, distractions, and guided imagery. The nurse administers prescribed analgesic medications, as ordered, to foster pain relief. Parenteral or oral opioid analgesics or an intravenous morphine drip may be used for more severe pain in clients with advanced disease. The nurse observes the client's respiratory status for changes when administering potentially respiratory-depressing medications. Clients with lung cancer experiencing pain usually have advanced disease and a limited prognosis. The nurse's goal is to assist the client to be as pain-free and as comfortable as possible.

DISCHARGE PLANNING

HOME CARE PREPARATION

Clients and their families usually have significant needs upon the client's discharge from the acute care setting. The nurse works with the client and family before discharge to determine what they perceive their needs will be. Appropriate referrals are made to community agencies, including home health nursing or hospice programs as indicated. The nurse coordinates arrangements for oxygen and other respiratory therapy to be available if needed by the client at home.

HEALTH TEACHING

The nurse reviews with the client and family any limitations of physical activity and prescribes an acceptable activity level. Nurses provide instruction on dealing with dyspnea and explain positions that facilitate easier breathing, such as leaning forward and sitting in a chair. The nurse emphasizes the need to prevent exposure to others with infections and outlines which signs and symptoms should be reported to health care professionals. The nurse instructs the family to call the physician when the prescribed pain medications or respiratory therapy is not providing comfort to the client and when the client is not receiving adequate relief from dyspnea. The nurse also provides specific information about medications as well as safety precautions for the use of oxygen.

PSYCHOSOCIAL PREPARATION

Psychosocial interventions differ, depending on the prognosis. The client with resectable carcinoma of the lung can be encouraged to have an optimistic outlook and to gradually resume normal activities. The nurse continues to help the client and family with their fear of death and anxiety related to the cancer diagnosis as well as the client's uncertain future health status.

The client whose prognosis is poor is one who, with the family, is facing death. The nurse helps by facilitating the expression of fears and concerns. The nurse encourages the client and family to maintain open lines of communication and stresses the importance of quality of life issues as defined by the client. The nurse's continued support and understanding can help the client and family through this difficult time. The nurse or social worker makes referrals to community hospice and home care agencies as indicated. (Chapter 12 presents nursing interventions for people experiencing loss and grief.)

HEALTH CARE RESOURCES

For the client in the terminal phase of lung cancer, a referral to a hospice program can be beneficial. The discharge planning nurse or social worker can assist in making these arrangements. Hospice programs provide support to the terminally ill client and the family by meeting physical and psychosocial needs, adjusting the palliative care regimen as needed, making home visits, and providing volunteers for errands and respite care. The American Cancer Society may also be able to provide assistance through support groups for clients and families or through the use of equipment, such as a hospital bed.

EVALUATION

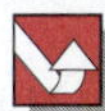

In evaluating the care of the client with lung cancer, the nurse expects that the client will:

- Maintain a patent airway
- State that pain or discomfort is reduced or alleviated
- Breathe without severe dyspnea
- Maintain acceptable arterial blood gases
- Resolve the reality of the diagnosis and prognosis
- State an understanding of the treatment plan
- Experience no major complications from radiation therapy, chemotherapy, or surgery

Acute Respiratory Failure

OVERVIEW

PATHOPHYSIOLOGY

Acute respiratory failure can be classified as:

- Ventilatory failure
- Oxygenation failure
- A combination of both ventilatory and oxygenation failure

Whatever the underlying disorder, the client in acute respiratory failure is always hypoxemic.

With normal respiration, oxygen diffuses into the capillaries, and carbon dioxide diffuses out of the capillaries. Ventilatory failure (hypoventilation) occurs when the client cannot eliminate carbon dioxide from the alveoli. Carbon dioxide retention also results in hypoxemia. Oxygen reaches the alveoli but cannot be absorbed or used properly.

Ventilatory failure is usually the result of one or more of the following three mechanisms:

- A mechanical abnormality of the lungs or chest wall
- A defect in the respiratory control center in the brain
- An impairment in the function of the respiratory muscles

Ventilatory failure is usually defined by a $PaCO_2$ level above 45 mmHg in clients who have otherwise healthy lungs. The most common cause of ventilatory failure is a problem with the lung itself, particularly chronic airflow limitation.

In oxygenation failure, the lungs can move air sufficiently but cannot oxygenate the pulmonary blood properly. Causes include the following:

- Impaired diffusion of oxygen at the alveolar level
- Right to left shunting of blood in the pulmonary vessels
- Ventilation-perfusion mismatching
- Breathing air with too low a concentration of oxygen
- Abnormal hemoglobin, which fails to absorb the oxygen

ETIOLOGY

There are numerous diseases and conditions that can result in *ventilatory failure.* Disorders that impair the respiratory muscles include:

- Neuromuscular disorders, such as multiple sclerosis, myasthenia gravis, Guillain-Barré syndrome, or poliomyelitis
- Spinal cord injuries that affect the nerves that supply the intercostal muscles

Any central nervous system lesion or infection can impair the central respiratory mechanism in the brain, such as:

- Cerebral vascular accident (CVA, or stroke)
- Cerebral edema
- Increased intracranial pressure
- Meningitis

Overdosage of some drugs, such as opioid analgesics and sedatives, may lead to hypoventilation. Other conditions that can result in ventilatory failure include:

- Massive obesity
- Sleep apnea
- Upper airway obstruction, including obstruction of an endotracheal tube with secretions or tubing kinks

Many diseases and disorders of the lung can cause *oxygenation failure.* In right-to-left shunting of the blood, areas of the lungs are still being perfused but gas exchange is not able to occur (which leads to hypoxemia), such as in pneumonia, atelectasis, and lung tumors. A client at high altitudes or who inhales a toxic chemical, gas, or smoke (as in mine work, from automotive exhaust [carbon monoxide], or in a fire) is breathing air with decreased oxygen. Other conditions that can result in oxygenation failure include adult respiratory distress syndrome (ARDS), near-drowning, and aspiration of any other liquid.

The third cause of acute respiratory failure is a *combination* of ventilatory failure and oxygenation failure. This type occurs in clients who have abnormal lungs, as in all forms of chronic airflow limitation (CAL, i.e., chronic bronchitis, emphysema, and asthma). The bronchioles and alveoli are diseased (oxygenation failure), and the work of breathing increases until the respiratory muscles are not able to continue (ventilatory failure). Acute respiratory failure results.

COLLABORATIVE MANAGEMENT

ASSESSMENT

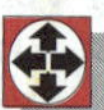

The nurse assesses for dyspnea, the hallmark of respiratory failure. With use of a dyspnea assessment guide (see Fig. 30–3), if one is available, the nurse objectively evaluates the client's dyspnea. The client may or may not perceive his or her dyspnea, depending on the process, nature, and course of the underlying condition. In addition, the client needs to be alert enough to be aware of the sensation of difficult breathing. Dyspnea tends to be more intense when it develops rapidly. Slowly progressive respiratory failure may first manifest as dyspnea on exertion (DOE) or when lying down. The client notes it is easier to breathe in an upright position (orthopnea). In the client with chronic airflow limitation, a minor increase in dyspnea from the baseline condition may represent severe gas exchange abnormalities.

In addition to dyspnea, the nurse assesses for a change in the client's respiratory rate or pattern, a change in lung sounds, and the signs and symptoms of hypoxemia and hypercapnia (see Chap. 30). Pulse oximetry may indicate decreased oxygen saturation, but the physician will also order arterial blood gas (ABG) analysis. The nurse and physician review the ABG studies to identify the degree of hypercapnia and hypoxemia.

INTERVENTIONS

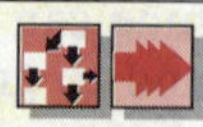

The physician orders oxygen therapy for the client with acute respiratory failure to keep the PaO_2 level above 60 mmHg while treating the underlying cause of the respiratory failure. (Oxygen therapy is discussed in detail in Chapter 30.) If supplemental oxygen cannot maintain acceptable PaO_2 levels, the physician may order mechanical ventilation (discussed later in this chapter).

The nurse assists the client to find a position of comfort that allows easier breathing. The nurse assists the client with interventions such as relaxation and diversion to decrease the anxiety commonly associated with dyspnea. Energy-conserving measures are instituted. The physician may order pulmonary medications administered systemically or by metered-dose inhaler (MDI) to open the bronchioles and promote gas exchange. The nurse instructs the client on the use of the inhaler and about the medications. Deep breathing and other breathing exercises are encouraged. (See Chapter 30 for further discussion of interventions for dyspnea and hypoxemia.)

Adult Respiratory Distress Syndrome

OVERVIEW

Adult respiratory distress syndrome (ARDS) is a form of acute respiratory failure characterized by:

- Hypoxemia
- Decreased pulmonary compliance
- Dyspnea
- Noncardiac bilateral pulmonary edema
- Dense pulmonary infiltrates

ARDS usually occurs after an acute catastrophic event in people with no previous pulmonary disease. The mortality rate is approximately 50%. Terminology for ARDS includes the current term *noncardiac pulmonary edema* and the former term *shock lung.*

Despite diverse causes leading to injury of the lung in ARDS, no common pathway has been found in its development, but the principal clinical manifestations are similar. In some forms of ARDS, the pathophysiologic mechanism is understood; in many others, it is not. The *major* site of injury in the lung is the alveolar capillary membrane, which is normally permeable to only small molecules. The interstitium of the lung normally remains relatively dry, but in clients with ARDS, there is increased extravascular lung fluid containing a high concentration of proteins.

Other significant changes occur in the alveoli and respiratory bronchioles. The type II pneumocyte is responsible for producing surfactant, a substance that maintains the elasticity of lung tissue. Surfactant activity is reduced in ARDS either because of destruction of the type II pneumocyte or inactivation or dilution of surfactant. Consequently, the alveoli become unstable and tend to collapse unless they are filled with fluid from the interstitial space. These alveoli can no longer participate in gas exchange. As a result, interstitial edema forms around terminal airways, which are compressed and obliterated. Lung volume is thus further reduced, and there is even less compliance (elasticity). As the leak expands, fluid, protein, and blood cells collect in the interstitium and alveoli. Lymph channels are compressed and ineffective. Poorly ventilated alveoli receive blood. Thus, the shunt fraction increases, and hypoxemia and ventilation-perfusion mismatching result.

ARDS is associated with a number of causative factors. Some major causes include:

- Shock
- Trauma
- Serious nervous system injury
- Pancreatitis
- Fat and amniotic fluid emboli
- Pulmonary infections
- Sepsis
- Inhalation of toxic gases (smoke, oxygen)
- Pulmonary aspiration
- Drug ingestion (e.g., heroin, opioids, aspirin)
- Hemolytic disorders
- Multiple blood transfusions

Serious nervous system injury, such as trauma, cerebrovascular accidents, tumors, and sudden increases in cerebrospinal fluid pressure, may cause massive sympathetic discharge. Systemic vasoconstriction with redistribution of large volumes of blood into the pulmonary circuit results. The marked elevation of hydrostatic pressure, then, probably causes lung injury. Processes that produce cerebral hypoxia, such as shock and ascent to high altitudes, may operate by a similar mechanism.

Some factors produce ARDS by direct injury to the lung. For example, aspiration of gastric contents leads to mechanical obstruction or produces an acid burn to the airway when the pH of the gastric contents is less than 2.5. In such a direct injury, rapid necrosis of the alveolar type I pneumocyte occurs. The injured capillary endothelium allows protein and cellular elements to escape from the intravascular space. Radiation, near-drowning, and inhalation of toxic gases similarly injure the alveolar and capillary endothelium. In addition, trauma, sepsis, drowning, and burns cause the release of thromboplastins, which form fibrin clots in the peripheral blood. The clots, together with platelets and leukocytes, are filtered out in the lung. In many cases of ARDS, especially after trauma, production of plasminogen activation inhibitors by the liver is enhanced. Fibrinolysis is prevented, and microemboli remain in the lung. Disseminated intravascular coagulation (DIC) plays a role in some clients.

The incidence of ARDS is unknown. It was estimated in 1980 that 150,000 cases of ARDS occurred in the United States per year. It is likely that the incidence has increased because of the improved treatment of other forms of catastrophic illness.

A major goal in the prevention of ARDS is early recognition of the client who is at high risk for the syndrome. Because clients with aspiration of gastric contents are at great risk, the nurse closely assesses and monitors elderly clients receiving tube feeding and clients with neurologic deficits and altered swallowing and gag reflexes. The nurse meticulously follows all infection control guidelines, including handwashing, invasive line and wound care, and body substance precautions. In addition, the nurse carefully observes clients who are being treated for any of the diseases or disorders associated with ARDS.

COLLABORATIVE MANAGEMENT

ASSESSMENT

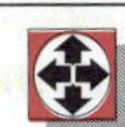

The nurse assesses the client's respirations and notes whether increased work of breathing is evident, as indicated by hyperpnea, grunting respiration, cyanosis, pallor, and retraction intercostally (between the ribs) or suprasternally (above the ribs). The nurse notes the presence of diaphoresis and any change in mental status. The nurse finds no abnormal lung sounds on auscultation because the edema of ARDS occurs first in the interstitial spaces and not in the airways. The nurse monitors vital signs frequently to assess for hypotension, tachycardia, and dysrhythmias.

The primary laboratory study for establishing the diagnosis of ARDS is a lowered arterial PaO_2 value, which is determined by arterial blood gas (ABG) measurements. The client with ARDS is poorly responsive to high concentrations of oxygen. Because a widening alveolar oxygen gradient (increased FIO_2 does not yield corresponding increased PaO_2 levels) develops with increased shunting of blood, the client has a progressive need for higher concentrations of oxygen. A large difference between the predicted and actual alveolar oxygen tension indicates shunting. The physician orders sputum cultures to isolate any organisms causing an infection that must be treated. Because decreased mortality depends on aggressive therapy, sputum may be obtained through bronchoscopy with protective brushings and by transtracheal aspiration.

The chest x-ray shows the diagnostic diffuse haziness or "whited-out" appearance of the lung. An electrocardiogram rules out cardiac abnormalities and usually reveals no specific changes. The placement of a Swan-Ganz hemodynamic monitoring catheter is a diagnostic tool: in the client with ARDS, the pulmonary capillary wedge pressure is usually normal. This pressure differs from the client with cardiogenic pulmonary edema in whom the pulmonary capillary wedge pressure is higher than 15 mmHg.

INTERVENTIONS

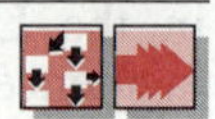

Clients with adult respiratory distress syndrome (ARDS) usually require endotracheal intubation and mechanical ventilation with positive end-expiratory pressure (PEEP) and continuous positive airway pressure (CPAP). Sedation may be necessary for adequate ventilation and for reducing the work of breathing. Because one of the side effects of PEEP is tension pneumothorax, the nurse assesses lung sounds frequently and maintains a patent airway with suctioning. Intubation and mechanical ventilation are discussed later. Positioning may be important in promoting gas exchange. The Research Applications for Nursing explains the semiprone position.

Corticosteroids are seldom used in the treatment of ARDS, although they may impair neutrophil mobilization and stabilize the capillary membrane. Their efficacy, however, has not been determined. Antibiotics are used to treat infections with organisms identified by culture.

The optimal type of fluid therapy for the client with ARDS remains unknown. A colloidal solution may be effective for intravascular volume expansion. However, the value of colloid therapy is unknown. Fluid volume should be titrated to maintain adequate cardiac output and tissue perfusion. Judicious diuresis may help decrease extravascular *lung* fluid, but care should be taken to prevent overall dehydration and hypotension.

Clients with ARDS are at risk for malnutrition, which further compromises the respiratory system. An altered immune response as well as an altered ventilatory response to hypoxemia may occur with undernourished clients. Diaphragmatic functioning is also altered. Therefore, enteral nutrition in the form of tube feeding or parenteral nutrition in the form of hyperalimentation is instituted.

The Client Requiring Mechanical Ventilation

OVERVIEW

Through the use of mechanical ventilation, clients who have severe derangements of gas exchange may be supported until the underlying process has resolved or has been adequately treated. Thus, mechanical ventilation is nearly always a temporary life-support technique. In some instances, however, the need for ventilatory support may not be temporary but lifelong. This is especially true for clients with chronic, progressive neuromuscular diseases that preclude effective spontaneous ventilation.

Mechanical ventilation is most commonly used for clients with hypoxemia and progressive alveolar hypoventilation with respiratory acidosis. The hypoxemia is usually due to intrapulmonary shunting of blood when external devices cannot provide sufficiently high FIO_2. Mechanical ventilation is also indicated:

- For clients who need respiratory support after cardiac, thoracic, or upper abdominal surgery
- For clients who are barely maintaining adequate gas exchange at the cost of expending energy with high work of breathing
- For clients who require general anesthesia or heavy sedation to allow diagnostic or therapeutic interventions

RESEARCH APPLICATIONS FOR NURSING

Consider the Semi-Prone Position for Clients with ARDS

Schmitz, T. M. (1991). The semi-prone position in ARDS: Five case studies. *Critical Care Nurse, 11*(5), 22–23.

In mechanically ventilated clients with adult respiratory distress syndrome (ARDS), optimal tissue oxygenation is primarily promoted by large increases in both the client's fraction of inspired oxygen (FIO_2) and the use of positive end-expiratory pressure (PEEP). In this pilot study, the researcher capitalizes on a traditional nursing intervention—that of positioning—and applies it to the problem of ventilation-perfusion mismatching in five clients who have adult respiratory distress syndrome. On the basis of previous preliminary studies using the prone position in adult respiratory distress syndrome, Schmitz compares the effects of the supine position and the right and left semiprone positions on arterial oxygen tension, heart rate, ventilatory peak inspiratory pressure, and arterial blood pressure. Three clients demonstrated the best oxygenation in the right semiprone position and improved their arterial oxygen tension an average of 30 mmHg. In six of ten instances, the semiprone position was related to improved oxygenation. The semiprone position was associated with a decrease in arterial oxygen tension four times.

Critique The sample size was too small for definite conclusions to be drawn. Baseline blood studies and continuous pulse oximetry may assist the data analysis process in future studies. However, the study provided important preliminary information that may help in the design of future studies.

Possible nursing implications Improvement in arterial oxygen tension ranged from 15 to 50 mmHg in clients turned from the supine to the semiprone position. In many clients with adult respiratory distress syndrome, these increases would allow adjusting down the amount of FIO_2 and PEEP necessary for adequate gas exchange. With evaluation of changes in the client's respiratory status, including arterial oxygen saturation or arterial oxygen tension, the semiprone position should be considered an alternative to the lateral and supine positions in clients with adult respiratory distress syndrome.

COLLABORATIVE MANAGEMENT

ASSESSMENT

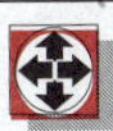

The nurse assesses the client about to undergo intubation in the same way as for other clients with respiratory problems. Once mechanical ventilation has been initiated, the nurse assesses the respiratory system on an ongoing basis. The nurse monitors and assesses for complications related to the artificial airway or ventilator as well as for those related to mechanical ventilation (see the Interventions text).

INTERVENTIONS

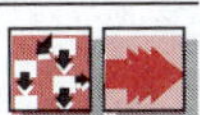

Endotracheal Intubation Clients who need mechanical ventilation require an artificial airway. The most common type of artificial airway for establishing and maintaining the airway on a *short-term* basis is the endotracheal tube (ET tube). If the client requires an artificial airway for longer than a specified period, usually longer than 10 to 14 days, the physician considers a tracheostomy (see Chap. 29) to avoid mucosal and vocal cord damage.

The goals of intubation include:

- Maintaining a patent airway
- Reducing the work of breathing
- Providing a means to remove secretions
- Providing ventilation and oxygen

Major indications for intubation are listed in Table 31–7.

THE ENDOTRACHEAL TUBE An ET tube is a long polyvinyl chloride tube that is passed through the mouth or nose and into the trachea (Fig. 31–4). When properly positioned, the tip of the endotracheal tube rests approximately 2 to 3 cm (0.8 to 1.2 inches) *above* the carina (where the trachea divides into the right and left mainstem bronchi). The technique for oral intubation is the easiest and quickest method for establishment of an airway; therefore, it is also performed as an emergency procedure. The nasal route is reserved for elective intubation, for some facial or oral traumas and surgeries, or when oral intubation is not possible. An experienced, specially trained professional, such as an anesthesiologist, nurse anesthetist, or pulmonologist (MD), performs the intubation.

TABLE 31–7 Indications for Intubation

- Airway protection when the client loses reflexes because of anesthesia, medications, disease, or decreased level of consciousness
- A need for mechanical ventilation
- Suctioning of secretions when the client cannot handle secretions (as in diseases of chronic airflow limitation)
- Airway obstruction

An ET tube has several parts (Fig. 31–4). The shaft of the tube contains a radiopaque vertical line for the length of the tube that permits demonstration of correct placement by chest x-ray. Short horizontal lines (depth markings) are used to designate the correct placement of the tube at the nares or mouth (at the incisor tooth) and to identify how far the tube has been inserted.

The cuff at the distal end of the tube, with proper inflation, produces a seal between the trachea and the cuff. The seal prevents aspiration and ensures delivery of a set tidal volume when mechanical ventilation is used. When the cuff is inflated, no air can pass through the cuff to the vocal cords, nose, or mouth; therefore, the client is not able to talk when the cuff is inflated.

The pilot balloon with a one-way valve permits air to be inserted into the cuff, yet prevents air from escaping. This balloon is used as a general guideline for determining the absence or presence of air in the cuff; it will not tell how much or how little air is present.

The universal adapter, which is 15 mm in diameter, enables attachment to ventilator tubing or other types of oxygen delivery systems. The size of the tube is indicated on the adapter or the shaft of the tube. Adult tube sizes range from 5 to 10 mm. Size 8.5 or 9.0 is commonly used for men; size 7.5 or 8.0 (smaller sizes) is commonly used for women.

PREPARING FOR INTUBATION The nurse knows the proper procedure for summoning intubation personnel to the bedside in an emergency situation. The nurse explains the procedure to the client as clearly as possible under the circumstances. Basic life-support measures, such as the establishment of a patent airway and the administration of 100% oxygen via a resuscitation (Ambu) bag with a face mask, are crucial to the client's survival until help arrives. The coordination for resuscitation with a bag and mask device can be cumbersome; therefore, practice is necessary.

In an emergency, the nurse brings the code (or "crash") cart, respiratory equipment box, and suction equipment (which is often already on the code cart) to the bedside. The nurse maintains a patent airway through positioning and the insertion of an oral airway until the client is intubated. During intubation, the nurse continuously monitors for changes in the client's vital signs, signs of hypoxia or hypoxemia, dysrhythmias, and aspiration. The nurse also ensures that each intubation attempt lasts no longer than 30 seconds. After 30 seconds, oxygen via mask and manual resuscitation bag is provided to prevent hypoxia and potential cardiac arrest. The nurse suctions as necessary.

VERIFYING TUBE PLACEMENT Immediately after an ET tube is inserted, its placement must be verified. To do this, the nurse assesses for bilateral equal breath sounds, bilateral equal chest excursion, and air emerging from the ET tube. If breath sounds and

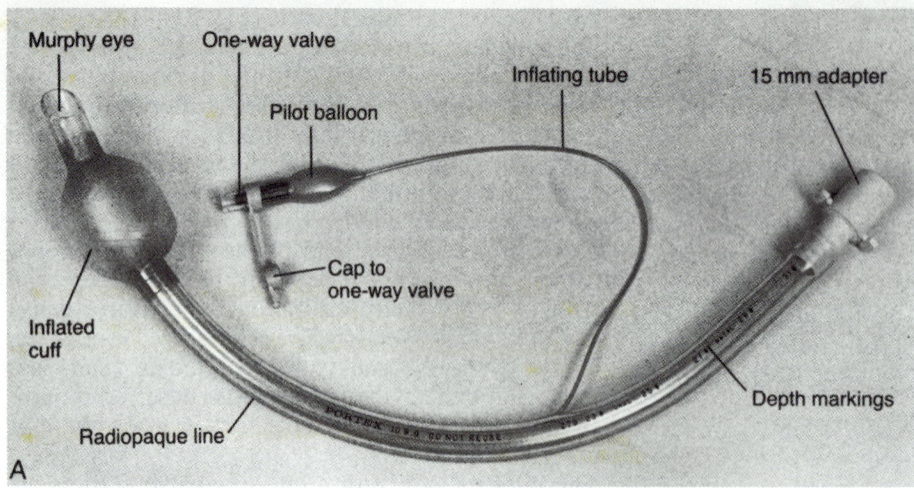

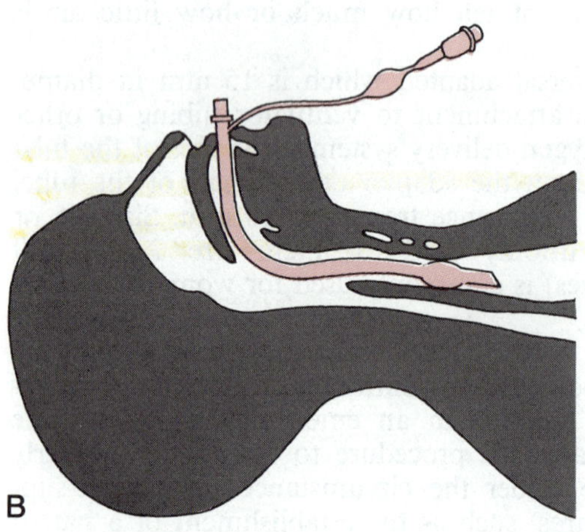

FIGURE 31-4 ◆ *A,* Components of an endotracheal tube (From Kersten, L. D. [1989]. *Comprehensive respiratory nursing: A decision making approach.* Philadelphia: W. B. Saunders.) *B,* Correct placement of an oral endotracheal tube.

chest wall movement are absent on the left side, the tube may be in the right mainstem bronchus. The person intubating the client should be able to reposition the tube without repeating the entire intubation procedure.

The nurse auscultates over the stomach to rule out esophageal intubation. If the tube is in the stomach, the nurse hears louder breath sounds over the stomach than over the chest and notes abdominal distention. The absence of bilateral equal breath sounds requires reintubation. The nurse continuously monitors chest wall movement and breath sounds until tube placement is verified by chest x-ray.

STABILIZING THE TUBE The nurse, respiratory therapist, or anesthesia personnel stabilize the ET tube at the mouth or nose. The tube is marked at the level at which it touches the incisor tooth, lip, or naris. Two persons working together use a head halter technique to secure the tube. Chart 31-6 outlines the steps in the procedure. An oral airway may also need to be inserted to keep the client from biting an oral tube. Ongoing nursing care requires an oral tube to be moved to the opposite side of the mouth daily. This maneuver helps prevent pressure and necrosis of the lip and mouth area, prevent nerve damage, and facilitate a thorough inspection and cleaning of the mouth. One person stabilizes the tube at the correct position and prevents head movement while a second person applies the tape. After the procedure is completed, the nurse verifies the presence of bilateral and equal breath sounds.

NURSING CARE The nurse assesses tube placement, breath sounds, and chest wall movement regularly. The nurse prevents pulling or tugging on the tube by the client to prevent dislodgment or "slipping" of the tube and checks the pilot balloon to ensure the cuff is inflated. Suctioning, coughing, and speaking attempts by the client place extra stress on the tube and also can cause dislodgment. Head flexion moves the tube away from the carina; head extension moves the tube closer to the carina. Rotation of the head also causes the tube to move. Mouth secretions and tongue manipulations can loosen the tape and allow malposition of the tube. The nurse applies soft wrist re-

CHART 31–6

Nursing Care Highlight ♦ Taping an Oral Endotracheal Tube

1. If the client is alert, instruct her or him not to move and to keep the head in the midline position while you tape the tube. Provide reassurance as follows:
   a. State that taping the tube takes about 5 min.
   b. Emphasize that the procedure will not interfere with breathing or cause pain.
2. To make a halter, cut two strips of tape, one 65 cm (26 in) long and the other 15–20 cm (6–8 in) long.
3. Lay the 65-cm (26-in) length flat with the adhesive side up. Place the 15-cm (6-in) length sticky side down in the middle of the longer strip. The sticky sides of the tape are apposed so that the hair bordering the client's posterior neck area does not stick to the halter.

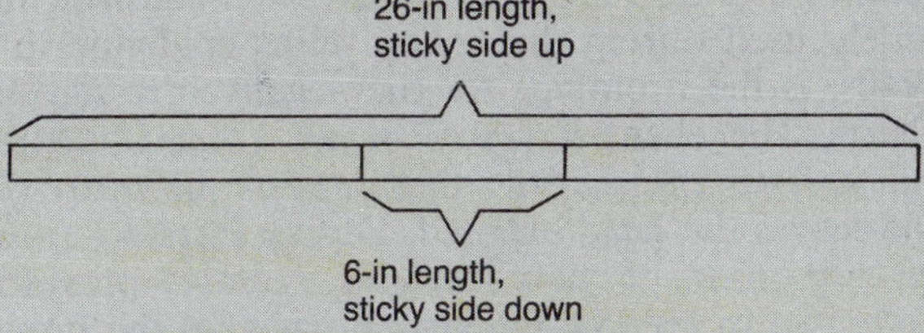

4. Place the halter under the client's neck.

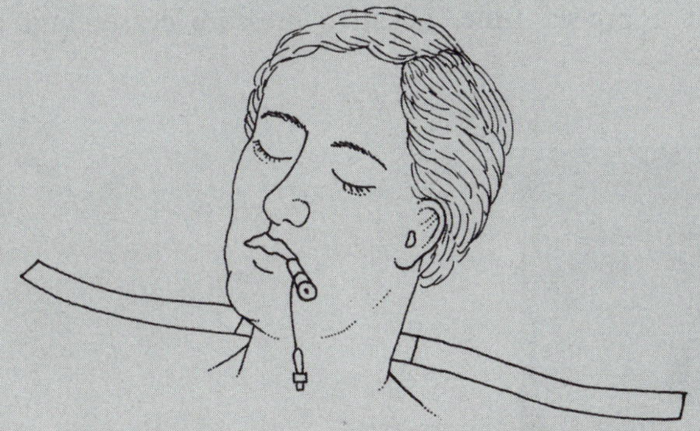

5. Split or tear each tape end lengthwise to the point at which the endotracheal tube exits from the mouth.
   a. Be careful not to tear the tape too far. The halter will not fit if the tape is torn to a point beyond the mouth.
   b. Trim excess tape with scissors, as needed.

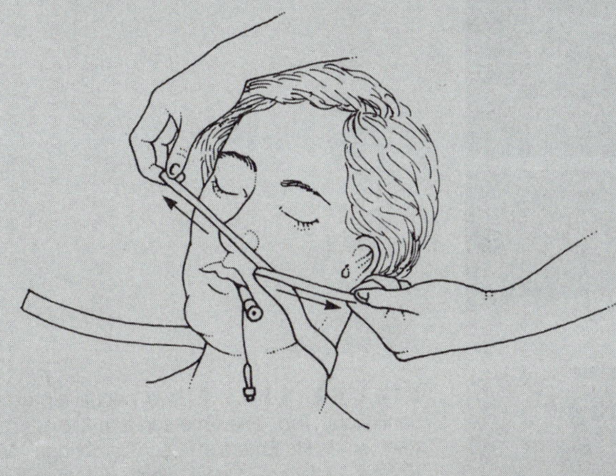

6. Prepare the skin by applying tincture of benzoin to the face and tube where tape contact is anticipated. Properly prepared skin surfaces are vital for tape adhesion and adequate tube stabilization. Whenever possible:
   a. Allow at least 1 min for the benzoin to dry before tape application. Do not "fan" dry.
   b. Test that benzoin is dry before applying tape. (When benzoin dries, it is slightly "sticky" to the touch).
   c. For diaphoretic skin, wash with soap and water and dry before benzoin application.
7. To tape one side of the face:
   a. Wrap the top split end beneath the nose and across the opposite cheek.

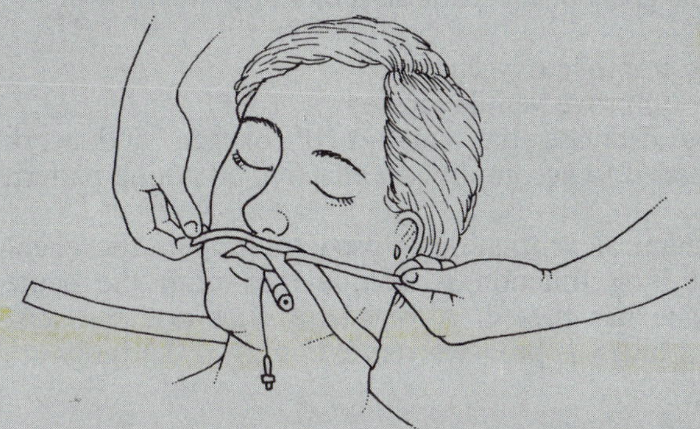

   b. Wrap the bottom split end around the tube.

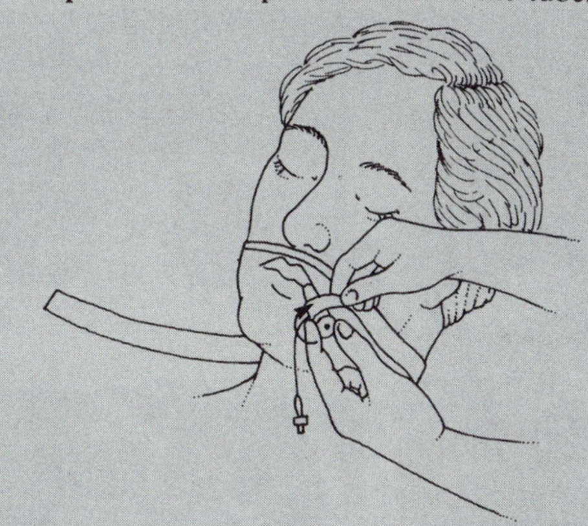

8. Repeat step 7 with the other end of the tape wrapping the bottom split end beneath the bottom lip and wrapping the top split end around the tube.
9. When you are finished wrapping the tube, fold a ¼-in end of tape back on itself to make a pull tab. This pull tab facilitates later tape removal.

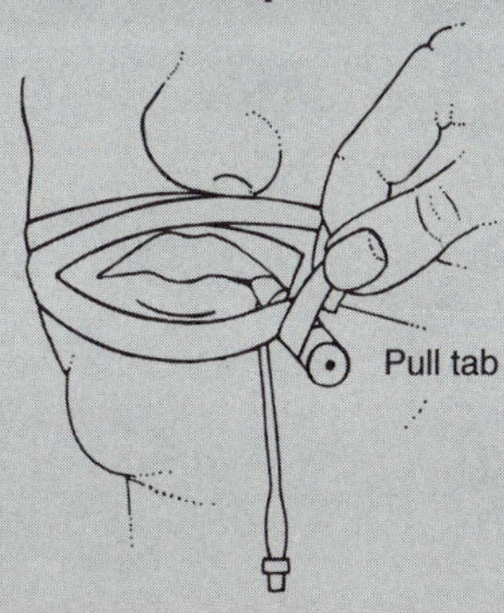

Modified from Kersten, L. D. (1989). *Comprehensive respiratory nursing: A decision making approach.* Philadelphia: W. B. Saunders.

straints, as ordered, when the client is voluntarily or involuntarily pulling on the tube. Without restraints, accidental extubation can result. The nurse obtains permission for restraints from the client or family after explaining the rationale. More information on management of the artificial airway is found in Chapter 29 (tracheostomy, suctioning), Chapter 30 (oxygen therapy), and later in this chapter (mechanical ventilation).

Mechanical Ventilation Mechanical ventilation to support and maintain a client's respiratory function is widely used on medical-surgical units, in nursing homes, and in the home setting as well as in critical care units. The nurse plays a pivotal role in the coordination of care and the prevention of complications.

The goals of mechanical ventilation are:

- To improve oxygenation
- To improve ventilation
- To decrease the amount of oxygen and work needed to accomplish an effective breathing pattern

Mechanical ventilation is used to support the client until lung function is adequate or until the acute episode has passed. A ventilator does not cure diseased lungs; it provides ventilation until the lungs are able to resume the process of breathing. Therefore, the nurse must remember why the client is using the ventilator so that aggressive attempts to correct the underlying cause of the respiratory failure are always at the forefront of the management plan. If normal oxygenation, ventilation, and respiratory muscle strength are achieved, mechanical ventilation can be discontinued.

TYPES OF VENTILATORS A wide variety of ventilators are available. The ventilator selected depends on the severity of the disease process and the length of time that ventilator support is required. Two major types of ventilators are: negative-pressure and positive-pressure.

Negative-Pressure Ventilators. The negative-pressure ventilator (Fig. 31–5) is noninvasive. The iron lung, widely used during the poliomyelitis epidemic in the 1940s, is the prototype for the negative-pressure ventilator. The client is placed in an airtight apparatus that surrounds either the chest area or the entire body and leaves the head exposed. During inspiration, with the expansion of the chest wall, negative pressure is generated in the chest cavity. Because of the pressure gradient created, air rushes from the atmosphere (high pressure) into the thoracic cavity (low pressure). At a pre-set time, negative pressure ceases and ex-

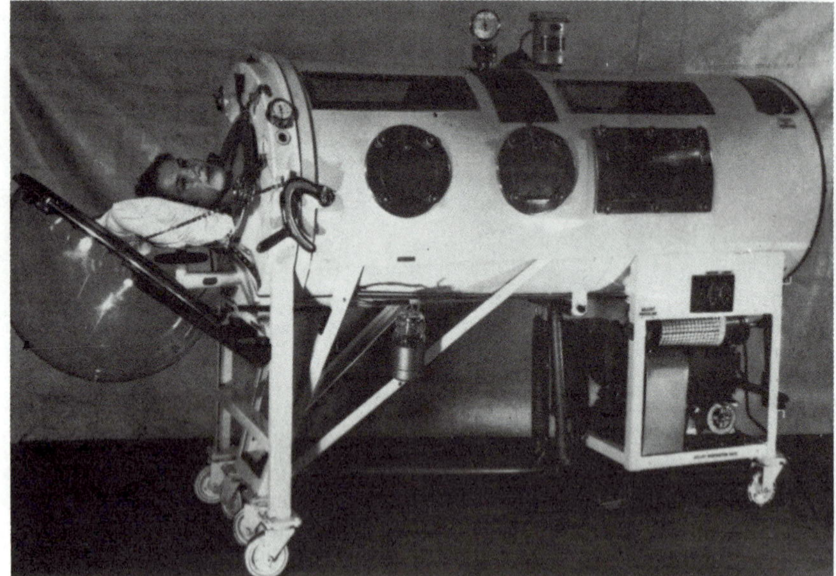

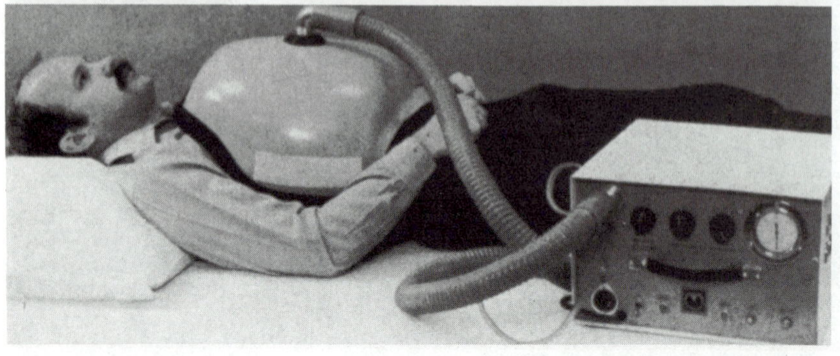

FIGURE 31–5 ♦ Two negative-pressure ventilators. *Top,* The Emerson Iron Lung. (Courtesy of J. H. Emerson Co., Cambridge, MA.) *Bottom,* Lifecare Chest Shell. (From Hill, N. [1986]. Clinical application of body ventilators. *Chest, 90*[6], 900.)

piration occurs. This negative-pressure ventilator creates pressure gradients that mimic normal physiologic ventilation.

Newer negative-pressure ventilators include the cuirass, poncho, and body wrap. These ventilators are used for clients with neuromuscular disease, central nervous system disorders, spinal cord injuries, and chronic airflow limitation (CAL). Clients may use negative-pressure ventilation for home nighttime ventilatory support so that their muscles can rest. Advantages are that an artificial airway is not required, and the newer models are lightweight and easy to use. The enclosing ventilator makes some direct nursing care more difficult. In addition, the client must be able to clear oral secretions and must have compliant (elastic) lungs to benefit from this mode of ventilation.

Positive-Pressure Ventilators. The positive-pressure ventilator is the most widely used type in the acute care setting. During inspiration, pressure is generated that *pushes* air into the lungs and expands the chest. In most instances, an endotracheal tube or tracheostomy is needed. Positive-pressure ventilators are classified according to the mechanism that ends inspiration and starts expiration. Inspiration is terminated or cycled in three major ways:

- Pressure-cycled
- Time-cycled
- Volume-cycled

Pressure-Cycled Ventilators. The pressure-cycled ventilator pushes air into the lungs until a pre-set airway pressure is reached. Tidal volumes and inspiratory time are variable. Pressure-cycled ventilators are often used for short periods, such as in the postanesthesia care unit and for respiratory therapy. The most common examples are the Puritan-Bennett PR-2 (Fig. 31–6) and the Bird Mark 7 and 8.

Time-Cycled Ventilators. The time-cycled ventilator pushes air into the lungs until a preset time has elapsed. Tidal volume and pressure are variable, depending on the characteristics of the client and the ventilator. The time-cycled ventilator is used primarily in pediatric and neonatal populations. Some examples are the Bird Babybird and the Monaghan 225.

Volume-Cycled Ventilators. The volume-cycled ventilator pushes gas into the lungs until a preset volume is delivered. A constant tidal volume is delivered regardless of the pressure needed to deliver the tidal volume. However, a pressure limit is set to prevent excessive pressure from being exerted on the lungs. The advantage of the volume-cycled ventilator is that a constant tidal volume is delivered regardless of the changing compliance of the lungs and chest wall or the airway resistance found in the client or ventilator. Examples include the Bear I, II (Fig. 31–7), and III; Puritan-Bennett MA-1, MA-2, and MA-3; and Monaghan 225/SIMV.

Microprocessor Ventilators. The microprocessor ventilators are the most sophisticated of the positive-pressure ventilators. A computer or microprocessor is built into the ventilator to allow ongoing monitoring of ventilatory functions, alarms, and client parameters. The ventilator often has components of volume-, time-, and pressure-cycled ventilators. The microprocessor ventilator is more responsive to clients who have severe lung disease, who require prolonged weaning trials, and who may not be able to be ventilated on older volume-cycled ventilators. Examples include the Bear IV and V, Puritan-Bennett 7200, Erisa, and Siemens Servo C and Servo D.

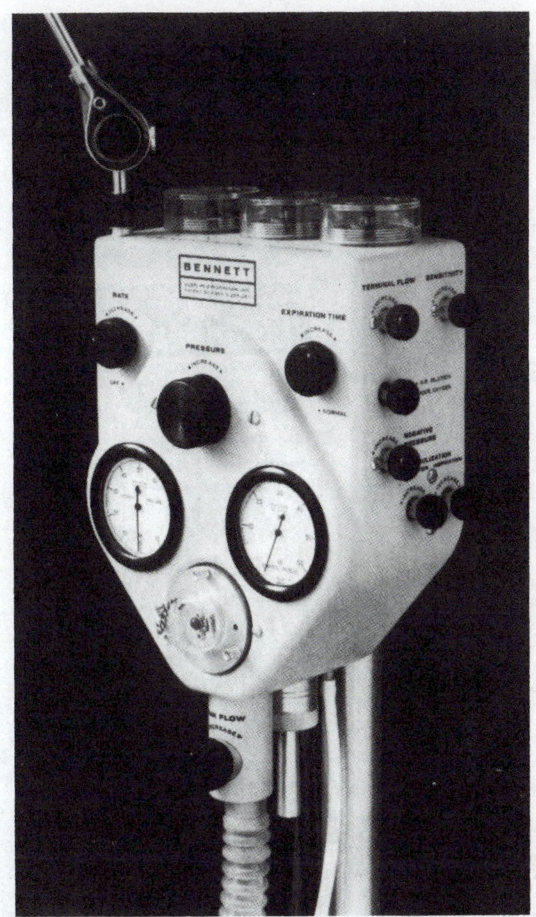

FIGURE 31–6 ◆ Puritan-Bennett PR-2 pressure-cycled ventilator. (Courtesy of Puritan-Bennett Corp., Overland Park, KS.)

MODES OF VENTILATION The "mode" of ventilation describes the way in which the client receives breaths from the ventilator.

Controlled Ventilation. Controlled ventilation is the least used mode. The client receives a set tidal volume at a set rate. This mode may be used for clients who cannot initiate respiratory effort, for example, those with polio or Guillain-Barré syndrome. It may be used for clients who are "paralyzed" as part of their medical management, such as those in status epilepticus or those with severely elevated intracranial pressure. If a client on controlled ventilation attempts to initiate a breath, the efforts are blocked by the ventilator. This maneuver results in the client's "fighting" the ventilator.

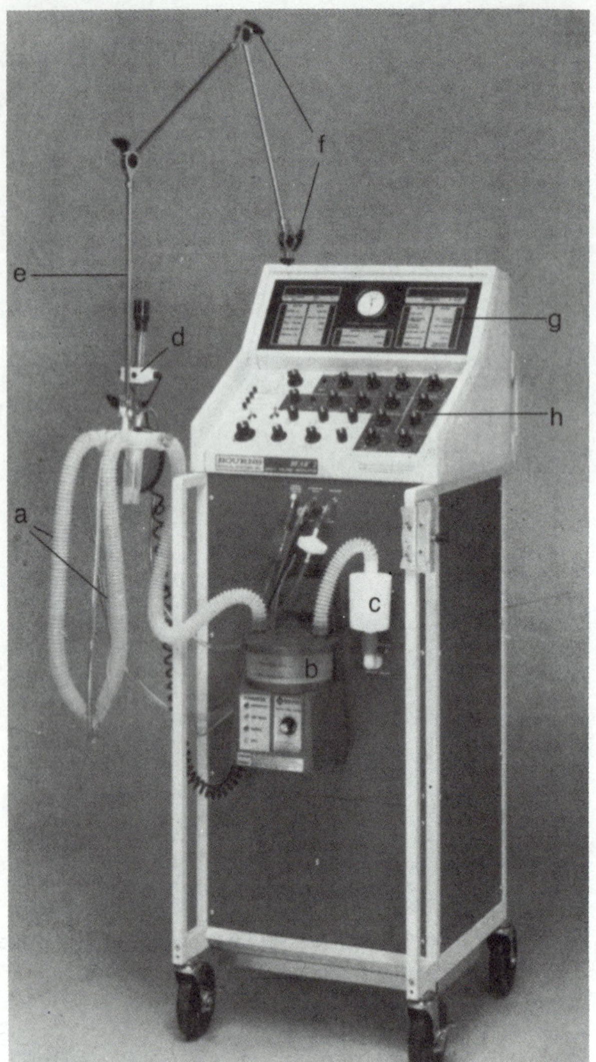

FIGURE 31-7 ◆ Bear II Adult Volume Ventilator. (Courtesy of Bear Medical Systems, Inc., Riverside, CA.)

Assist-Control Ventilation. Assist-control (AC) ventilation is the most commonly used mode. It is used mainly as a resting mode. The ventilator takes over the work of breathing for the client. Tidal volume and ventilatory rate are preset on the ventilator. If the client does not trigger spontaneous breaths, a minimal ventilatory pattern is established. The ventilator is also programmed to respond to the client's inspiratory effort if the client does initiate a breath. In this case, the ventilator delivers the pre-set tidal volume while allowing the client to control the rate of breathing.

One disadvantage of the AC mode is that if the client's spontaneous ventilatory rate increases, the ventilator continues to deliver a pre-set tidal volume with each breath. The client may then hyperventilate, and respiratory alkalosis occurs. Causes of hyperventilation, such as pain, anxiety, or acid-base imbalances, must be corrected.

Synchronized Intermittent Mandatory Ventilation. Synchronized intermittent mandatory ventilation (SIMV) is similar to AC ventilation in that tidal volume and ventilatory rate are pre-set on the ventilator. Therefore, if the client does not breathe, a minimal ventilatory pattern is established. In contrast to the AC mode, SIMV allows the client to breathe spontaneously at his or her own rate and tidal volume between the ventilator breaths. SIMV can be used as a primary ventilatory mode or as a weaning modality. When SIMV is used as a weaning mode, the number of mechanical breaths (SIMV breaths) is gradually decreased (i.e., from 12 to 2), and the client gradually resumes spontaneous breathing. The mandatory ventilator breaths are delivered when the client is ready to inspire, which promotes synchrony between the ventilator and the client.

Other Modes of Ventilation. Newer modes of ventilation, such as pressure support and continuous flow (flow-by), are available only in microprocessor ventilators. Both modalities decrease the work of breathing and are often used for weaning clients from mechanical ventilation. Another mode is maximum mandatory ventilation (MMV).

VENTILATOR CONTROLS AND SETTINGS The volume-cycled ventilator is the most widely used ventilator in the acute care setting. Regardless of the type of volume-cycled ventilator used, the controls and types of settings are universal (Fig. 31-8). The physician prescribes the ventilator settings, and usually the ventilator is readied or "set up" by the respiratory department. The nurse assists in connecting the client to the ventilator. The nurse understands and monitors the ventilator settings as part of the nursing care for the client.

Tidal Volume. Tidal volume (V_T) is the volume of air that the client receives with each breath; it can be measured on either inspiration or expiration. The average prescribed tidal volume ranges between 7 and 15 mL/kg of body weight. Adding a zero to the weight of clients in kilograms gives an estimate of tidal volume.

Rate, or Breaths per Minute. Rate, or breaths per minute (BPM), is the number of ventilator breaths delivered per minute. It is usually set between 10 and 14 breaths per minute.

Fraction of Inspired Oxygen. The fraction of inspired oxygen (FIO_2) is the oxygen concentration delivered to the client. The prescribed FIO_2 is determined by the arterial blood gas value and the client's condition. Ventilators can provide 21% to 100% oxygen, depending on the client's needs.

The oxygen delivered to the client is warmed to body temperature (37° C [98.6° F]) and humidified to 100%. Humidification and warming are necessary because the upper air passages of the respiratory tree that normally warm, humidify, and filter air are bypassed by the endotracheal tube or tracheostomy tube. Humidification and warming are needed to prevent mucosal damage and to facilitate clearance of secretions.

Sighs. Sighs may be used to prevent atelectasis in special circumstances. Sighs are volumes of air that are 1½ to 2 times the set tidal volume, delivered 6 to 10 times per hour.

Peak Airway (Inspiratory) Pressure. Peak airway (in-

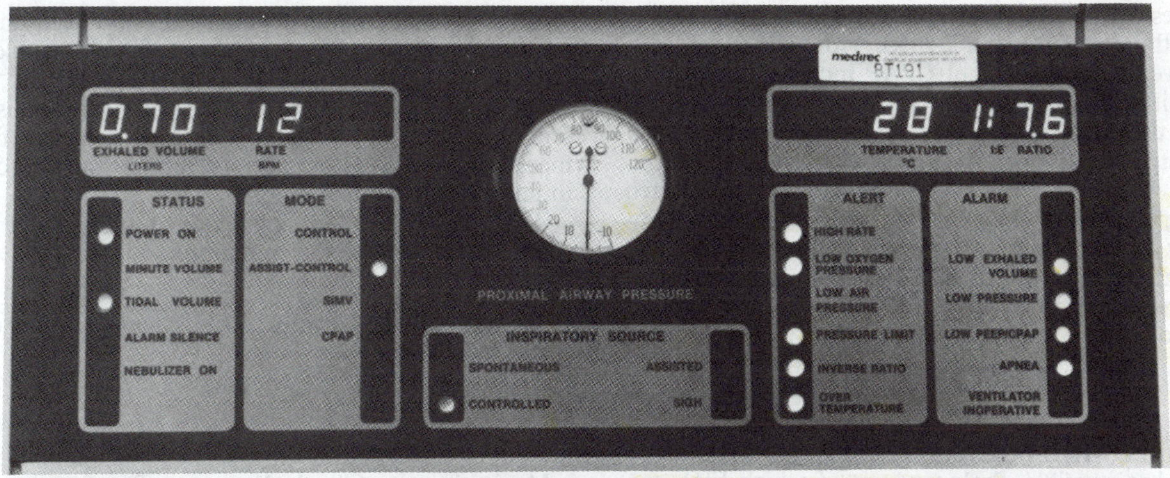

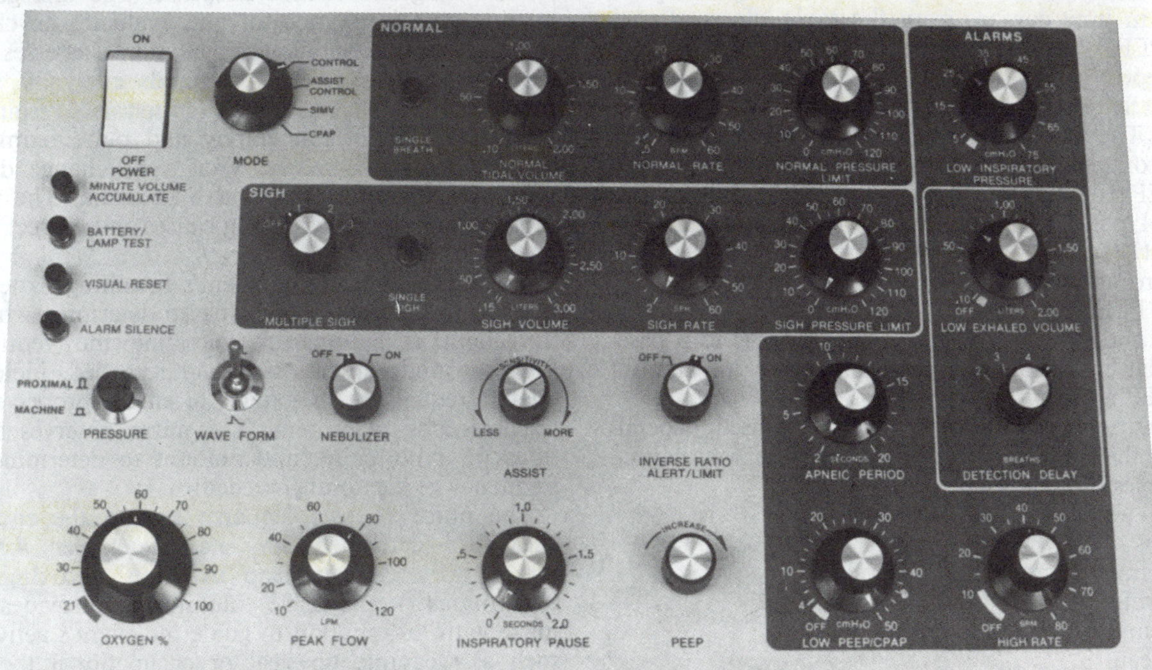

FIGURE 31-8 ◆ Display signals and alarms *(top)* and control panel *(bottom)* of a typical volume-cycled ventilator. (From Kersten, L. D. [1989]. *Comprehensive respiratory nursing: A decision making approach.* Philadelphia: W. B. Saunders.)

spiratory) pressure (PIP) indicates the pressure needed by the ventilator to deliver a set tidal volume at a given dynamic compliance. The peak airway pressure measurement appears on the digital readout or display on the front or top of the ventilator (labeled proximal airway pressure in Fig. 31–8). Peak pressure is the highest pressure indicated during inspiration. Monitoring trends in PIP reflect changes in compliance (elasticity) of the lungs and resistance in the ventilator or client. An increased PIP reading means increased airway resistance (bronchospasm), increased amount of secretions, pulmonary edema, or decreased pulmonary compliance (the lungs or chest wall are "stiffer," or harder to inflate). An upper pressure limit is set on the ventilator to prevent barotrauma (lung damage from excessive pressure). When the limit is reached, the high-pressure alarm sounds, and the remaining volume is not given.

Continuous Positive Airway Pressure. Continuous positive airway pressure (CPAP) is the application of positive airway pressure throughout the entire respiratory cycle for spontaneously breathing clients. Sedating medications should be given cautiously or not at all when a client is receiving CPAP so that respiratory effort is not suppressed. CPAP keeps the alveoli open during inspiration and prevents alveolar collapse during expiration. This process results in increased functional residual capacity (FRC), improved gas exchange, and improved oxygenation. CPAP is used primarily as a weaning modality. During CPAP, no ventilator breaths are delivered; the ventilator delivers oxygen and provides monitoring and an alarm system. The respiratory pattern is determined by the client's efforts. Normal levels of CPAP are 5 to 15 cm H_2O, adjusted to promote adequate oxygenation. If no pressure is set on the ventilator, the client receives no positive pressure. The client is essentially using the ventilator as a T-piece with alarms.

Newer modifications of CPAP include nasal CPAP and BiPAP) (see Chap. 30 and Fig. 30–8). The physician uses these modifications for select indications.

Positive End-Expiratory Pressure. Positive end-expiratory pressure (PEEP) is positive pressure exerted during the expiratory phase of ventilation. PEEP improves oxygenation by enhancing gas exchange and preventing atelectasis. It is indicated for the treatment of persistent hypoxemia that does not improve with an acceptable oxygen concentration. PEEP is often added when the arterial PaO_2 value remains low with an FIO_2 of 50% to 70% or greater.

The need for PEEP indicates a severe gas exchange disturbance. It is important to lower the FIO_2 delivered when possible. Prolonged use of a high FIO_2 can result in lung damage from the toxic effects of oxygen. PEEP prevents alveoli from collapsing; the lungs are kept partially inflated so that alveolar capillary gas exchange is facilitated throughout the ventilatory cycle. The effect should be an increase in arterial blood oxygenation so that the F_IO_2 can be decreased.

PEEP is "dialed in" with the PEEP dial on the control panel. The amount of PEEP is often 3 or 5 cm H_2O and is read (monitored) on the peak airway pressure dial, the same dial used to read the PIP. When PEEP is added, the dial does not return to zero at the end of exhalation; rather, it returns to a baseline that has been increased from zero by the amount of PEEP applied.

Other Settings. Other settings may be used, depending on the type of ventilator and mode of ventilation. Examples of additional settings include:

- Flow
- Inspiratory and expiratory cycle
- Waveform
- Expiratory resistance
- Plateau

NURSING MANAGEMENT The institution of mechanical ventilation for a client involves a complex decision-making process for both the family and the health-care professionals. Both physical and psychologic concerns of the client and family must be addressed. The mechanical ventilator frequently causes anxiety for the client and family. Therefore, the nurse carefully explains the purpose of the ventilator and that some different sensations might be felt. The client and family are encouraged to express their concerns. The nurse acts as the coach who both physically and psychologically helps and supports the client and family through this experience. In emergency situations, these explanations may not be accomplished until the emergency has been controlled.

When caring for a ventilated client, the nurse's responsibility is to the client first and the ventilator second. It is vital that the nurse understand the reason for which the client requires mechanical ventilation. Such causes as excessive amounts of secretions, sepsis, and trauma require different interventions to facilitate ventilator independence. In addition, an appreciation of the client's chronic health problems, particularly chronic airflow limitation (CAL), left-sided heart failure, anemia, and malnutrition, is essential. These problems may impede weaning from mechanical ventilation and therefore warrant close monitoring and intervention.

There are three nursing goals in caring for the client with mechanical ventilation:

- To monitor and evaluate the client's response to the ventilator
- To safely manage the ventilator system
- To prevent complications

Monitoring the Client's Response. The first goal of nursing care is to monitor and evaluate the client's response to the ventilator. The nurse assesses vital signs and listens to breath sounds every 30 to 60 minutes initially, monitors noninvasive respiratory parameters (e.g., capnography and pulse oximetry), and checks ABG values. Vital signs change during episodes of hypercapnea and hypoxemia. The nurse should note any precipitating causes and correct them promptly.

The nurse assesses the client's breathing pattern in relation to the ventilatory cycle to determine whether the client is fighting or tolerating the ventilator. Breath sounds are assessed and recorded, including bilateral equal breath sounds, to ensure proper endotracheal tube placement. The nurse observes secretions for type, color, and amount to determine the frequency of suctioning needed.

The nurse assesses the area around the endotracheal tube or tracheostomy site at least every 4 hours for color, tenderness, skin irritation, and drainage. Continuous noninvasive monitoring provides the nurse with information to guide the client's activities, such as weaning, physical or occupational therapy, and self-care. These activities can be paced so that oxygenation and ventilation are adequate. The nurse interprets ABG values to evaluate ventilation and suggest ventilator settings that help the client.

Because the nurse spends the most time with the client, the nurse is most likely to be the first person to recognize slight changes in the vital signs, fatigue or distress in the client, or changes in the ABG values. The nurse then promptly confers with the physician and implements the appropriate interventions.

While monitoring and evaluating the client's clinical status, the nurse also serves as an excellent resource for addressing the psychologic needs of the client and family. Anxiety can play a major role in the client's tolerance of mechanical ventilation. Therefore, skilled and sensitive nursing care promotes psychologic well-being and facilitates synchrony with the ventilator. Communication can be frustrating and anxiety-producing because the client cannot speak. The client and family may panic because they prematurely believe the client has lost his or her voice.

They must be reassured that the endotracheal tube prevents speech but that it is temporary.

Alternative, creative methods of communication must be individualized to meet the client's needs. Magic slates, writing paper, computers, and tracheostomy tubes that permit talking are potential means of facilitating communication. Finding a successful means for communication is important because the client often experiences feelings of isolation related to the inability to speak. Anticipation of the client's needs, easy access to frequently used belongings, and a nursing call light within reach are effective ways of giving the client a sense of control over the environment. In addition, the client is not isolated from participation in self-care.

Managing the Ventilator System. The second goal of nursing care is directed toward safe management of the ventilator system. Ventilator settings are ordered by the physician and include the following:

- Tidal volume
- Respiratory rate
- FIO_2
- Mode of ventilation (assist-control, synchronized intermittent mandatory ventilation)
- Any adjunctive modes, such as positive end-expiratory pressure (PEEP), pressure support, or continuous flow

Nurses perform and document ventilator checks according to the standards of the unit or facility and respond promptly to emergency situations as indicated by alarms. During a ventilator check, the nurse compares the ventilator settings ordered by the physician with the actual settings. The nurse checks the level of water in the humidifier and the temperature of the humidification system to ensure that they are within normal limits. Extremes in temperature cause damage to the mucosa of the airways. Any condensation in the ventilator tubing is removed by draining water into drainage collection receptacles, which should be emptied frequently. For prevention of bacterial contamination, moisture and water from the tubings are never allowed to enter the humidifier.

Mechanical ventilators have alarm systems that warn the nurse of a problem with either the client or the ventilator. Alarm systems must be activated and functional at all times. It is crucial for the nurse to recognize an emergency and to intervene promptly so that complications are prevented. If the cause of the alarm cannot be determined, the nurse ventilates the client manually with a resuscitation bag until the problem is corrected by a second nurse, the respiratory therapist, or a physician. The two major alarms on a ventilator indicate either a high pressure or a low exhaled volume. Table 31-8 presents nursing interventions for various causes of ventilator alarms.

Ensuring proper functioning of the ventilator also includes care of the endotracheal tube or tracheostomy tube. A patent airway is maintained through suctioning only as needed. Indications for suctioning in the ventilated client include:

- The presence of secretions
- Increased PIP
- The presence of rhonchi
- Decreased breath sounds

Careful maintenance of the endotracheal tube or tracheostomy tube also ensures a patent airway. The nurse frequently assesses the tube's position, especially for the client whose airway is attached to heavy ventilator tubing that may pull on the tracheostomy or endotracheal tube. The nurse positions the ventilator tubing in such a way that the client can move, yet will avoid pulling on the endotracheal or tracheostomy tube. The endotracheal tube can move and slip into the right mainstem bronchus. To detect minimal changes in the tube's position, the nurse marks the level at which the tube touches the client's mouth or nose. The nurse gives mouth care frequently to promote adequate oral hygiene and to prevent loosening of the tape that holds the tube.

Preventing Complications. The third goal in providing nursing care of the client receiving mechanical ventilation is to prevent complications. Most of these complications are due to the positive pressure from the ventilator. Nearly every body system is affected.

Cardiac Complications. Cardiac complications of mechanical ventilation include hypotension and fluid retention. Hypotension is caused by the application of positive pressure, which increases intrathoracic pressure and inhibits blood return to the heart. The decreased venous return to the right side of the heart decreases cardiac output and is clinically reflected as hypotension. Hypotension is most frequently seen in the client who is dehydrated or requires high peak airway (inspiratory) pressure (PIP) to be ventilated. The nurse instructs the client to avoid a Valsalva maneuver and puts a plan of care into effect to prevent constipation, which could result in a Valsalva maneuver. Fluid is retained because of decreased cardiac output. The kidneys receive less blood flow and stimulate the renin-angiotensin-aldosterone system to retain fluid. In addition, humidified air via the ventilator system can contribute to fluid retention. The nurse monitors the client's fluid intake and output, weight, and hydration, and signs of hypovolemia.

Lung Complications. The lungs experience barotrauma (damage to the lungs by positive pressure) and acid-base abnormalities. *Barotrauma* includes pneumothorax, subcutaneous emphysema, and pneumomediastinum. Clients at risk for barotrauma have diseases of chronic airflow limitation (CAL), have blebs, are on PEEP, have dynamic hyperinflation, or require high pressures to ventilate the lungs (decreased compliance or "stiff" lungs, as seen in ARDS). Blood gas abnormalities, another pulmonary complication of mechanical ventilation, can be corrected by appropriate ventilator changes and adjustment of fluid and electrolyte imbalances.

Gastrointestinal and Nutritional Complications. Gastrointestinal alterations result from the stress of mechanical ventilation. Stress ulcers occur in approximately 25% of clients receiving mechanical venti-

TABLE 31–8 Nursing Interventions for Various Causes of Ventilator Alarms

Cause	Interventions
High Pressure Alarm (Sounds when peak inspiratory pressure reaches the set alarm limit [usually set 10–20 mmHg above the client's baseline PIP])	
There is an increased amount of secretions in the airways or a mucous plug	• Suction as needed.
The client coughs, gags, or bites on the oral ET.	• Insert oral airway to prevent biting on the ET tube.
The client is anxious or fights the ventilator	• Provide emotional support to decrease anxiety. • Explain all procedures to the client. • Provide sedation or paralyzing agent per the physician's order.
Airway size decreases related to wheezing or bronchospasm	• Auscultate breath sounds. • Consult with the physician for management of bronchospasm.
Pneumothorax occurs	• Auscultate breath sounds. • Consult with the physician about a new onset of decreased breath sounds or unequal chest excursion, which may be due to pneumothorax.
The artificial airway is displaced; the ET tube may have slipped into the right mainstem bronchus	• Assess the chest for unequal breath sounds and chest excursion. • Obtain a chest x-ray as ordered to evaluate the position of the ET tube. • After the proper position is verified, tape the tube securely in place.
Obstruction in tubing occurs because the client is lying on the tubing or there is water or a kink in the tubing	• Assess the system, moving from the artificial airway toward the ventilator. • Empty water from the ventilator tubing and remove any kinks.
There is increased PIP associated with deliverance of a sigh	• Consult with respiratory therapist or physician to adjust the pressure alarm.
Decreased compliance of the lung is noted; a trend of gradually increasing PIP is noted over several hours or a day	• Evaluate the reasons for the decreased compliance of the lungs. Increased PIP occurs in ARDS.
Low Exhaled Volume (or Low-Pressure Alarm) (Sounds when there is a disconnection or leak in the ventilator circuit or a leak in the client's artificial airway cuff)	
A leak in the ventilator circuit prevents breath from being delivered	• Assess all connections and all ventilator tubings for disconnection.
The client stops spontaneous breathing in the SIMV or CPAP mode or on pressure support ventilation	• Evaluate the client's tolerance of the mode.
A cuff leak occurs in the ET or tracheostomy tube	• Evaluate the client for a cuff leak. A cuff leak is suspected when the client is able to talk (air escapes from the mouth) or when the pilot balloon on the artificial airway is flat (see section on tracheostomy tubes in Chap. 29).
The exhalation valve on Bear I or II is wet	• Keep exhalation valve and flow tube horizontal. • Unsnap and check the membrane for dampness. If the sensor is wet, gently dab dry and resnap.

PIP = peak inspiratory pressure; ET = endotracheal; ARDS = adult respiratory distress syndrome; CPAP = continuous positive airway pressure; SIMV = synchronized intermittent mandatory ventilation.

lation. Prophylactic antacids, sucralfate (Carafate, Sulcrate✱), and the histamine blockers cimetidine (Tagamet) and ranitidine (Zantac) are often instituted as soon as the client is intubated. The nurse administers these medications as well as suggests therapeutic strategies for stress management (see Chap. 7).

Malnutrition is a prevalent problem in clients receiving mechanical ventilation. Because many other acute or life-threatening events are occurring simultaneously, nutrition is often neglected. Malnutrition is an extreme problem for these clients and a major reason that clients cannot be weaned from the ventilator. In clients with malnutrition, the respiratory muscles lose their mass and strength. The diaphragm, which is the major organ of inspiration, is affected early in this process. When the diaphragm and other muscles of respiration are weakened, an ineffective breathing pattern emerges, fatigue occurs, and the client cannot be weaned from the ventilator.

A balanced diet via the parenteral or enteral route is essential whenever a ventilator is used. Furthermore, nutrition for the client with CAL requires that special attention be given to the percentage of carbohydrates in the client's diet. During metabolism, carbohydrates are broken down to glucose to produce energy (ATP), carbon dioxide, and water. Excessive carbohydrate loads increase carbon dioxide production, which the CAL client may be unable to exhale. Hypercapnic respiratory failure results. Enteral and parenteral formulas with a higher fat content (e.g., Pulmocare, Nutrivent, Intralipids) can be an alternative source of calories to combat this problem.

Another important aspect of nutritional support is electrolyte replacement. Electrolytes also have a major impact on the efficiency of respiratory muscle function. Specifically, the nurse and physician closely monitor potassium, calcium, magnesium, and phosphate levels, and the nurse replenishes deficiencies as ordered. All four electrolytes are important in respiratory muscle contraction and function and can easily be added to the nutritional regimen.

Infection. Infections are always a potential threat for the client requiring a ventilator. The endotracheal or tracheostomy tube bypasses the body's normal process of filtering and warming air and provides bacteria direct access to the lower parts of the respiratory system. Within 48 hours, the artificial airway is usually colonized with bacteria. An environment is established in which pneumonia can develop. In addition, aspiration of colonized fluid from the mouth or the stomach can occur and be a source of pathogens. Pneumonic infections are associated with prolonged hospitalization and increased morbidity. Therefore, the focus must be on prevention of infections through strict adherence to infection control standards, especially hand washing, during suctioning, and care of the tracheostomy or endotracheal tube. The nurse implements ongoing oral care and pulmonary hygiene, including chest physiotherapy, postural drainage, and turning and positioning, to prevent pneumonia. More information on pneumonia can be found in Chapter 30.

Muscular Complications. Overall muscle deconditioning can occur because of immobility. Getting out of bed, ambulating with assistance, and performing exercises with the nurse, physical therapist, and occupational therapist not only improve muscle tone and strength but also boost the client's morale, facilitate gas exchange, and promote oxygen delivery to all muscles.

Chart 31–7 reviews nursing care of the client on mechanical ventilation.

Ventilator Dependence. The final complication of mechanical ventilation is ventilator dependence, or inability to wean. Ventilator dependence can be psychologic or physiologic but more often has a physiologic basis. The older client, especially one who has smoked or who has an underlying lung dysfunction like CAL, is at risk for ventilator dependence. The longer a client uses a ventilator, the more difficult the weaning process. The respiratory muscles fatigue and cannot assume breathing. The health care team attempts to optimize all major body systems and to exhaust every method of weaning before a client is declared unweanable. The nursing diagnosis of Dysfunctional Ventilatory Weaning Responses (DVWR)

CHART 31–7

Nursing Care Highlight ◆ The Client on Mechanical Ventilation

- At least once every shift check to be sure the ventilator settings are set as ordered.
- Check to be sure alarms are set (especially low pressure and low exhaled volume).
- Observe the exhaled volume digital display to be sure the client is receiving the prescribed tidal volume.
- Empty ventilator tubings when moisture collects. Never empty fluid in the tubing back into the cascade.
- If the client is on PEEP, observe the peak airway pressure dial to determine the proper level of PEEP.
- Assess the client's respiratory status each shift and as needed:
  a. Observe the client's color (especially lips and nail beds).
  b. Observe the client's chest for bilateral expansion.
  c. Auscultate the lungs for rales, rhonchi, wheezes, equal breath sounds, and decreased or absent breath sounds.
  d. Obtain pulse oximetry reading.
  e. Evaluate ABGs as ordered.
- Take vital signs at least every 4 hr.
- Be sure the tracheostomy cuff (or the endotracheal cuff) is adequately inflated to ensure tidal volume.
- Administer mouth care *at least* twice per shift.
- Observe the client's need for tracheal/oral/nasal suctioning every 2 hr. Provide adequate suctioning every 4 hr and as needed. Provide tracheostomy care every shift.
- Change tracheostomy tape or endotracheal tube tape as needed. Observe the client's mouth around the endotracheal tube for pressure sores.
- Move the oral endotracheal tube to the opposite side of the mouth once every 24 hr to prevent ulcers.
- Maintain accurate intake and output records to monitor fluid balance.
- Turn the client at least every 2 hr and get the client out of bed as ordered to promote pulmonary hygiene and prevent complications of immobility.
- Schedule treatments and nursing care at intervals to provide rest.
- Explain all procedures and treatments; provide access to a call bell; visit the client frequently.
- Include the client and his or her family in care whenever possible (especially suctioning and tracheostomy care).
- Provide a letter board or pencil and paper for communication. Request consultation with a speech therapist for assistance, if necessary.
- Observe ventilated clients for gastrointestinal distress (diarrhea, constipation, tarry stools).
- Document pertinent observations in the client's medical record (chart).

Courtesy of Our Lady of Lourdes Medical Center, Camden, NJ.

TABLE 31–9 Weaning Methods

Synchronous Intermittent Mandatory Ventilation

- The client breathes between the machine's preset breaths per minute rate.
- The client is initially set on a synchronized intermittent mandatory ventilation (SIMV) rate of 12, meaning the client receives a minimum of 12 breaths per minute by the ventilator.
- The client's respiratory rate will be a combination of ventilator breaths and spontaneous breaths.
- As the weaning process ensues, the physician orders gradual decreases in the SIMV rate, usually at a decrease of 1 to 2 breaths per minute.

T-Piece Technique

- The client is taken off the ventilator for short periods (initially 5 to 10 min) and allowed to breathe spontaneously.
- The ventilator is replaced with a T-piece (see Chap. 30) or CPAP, which delivers humidified oxygen.
- The ordered FIO_2 may be higher for the client on the T-piece than on the ventilator.
- Weaning progresses as the client is able to tolerate progressively longer periods off the ventilator.
- Nighttime weaning is not usually attempted until the client is able to maintain spontaneous respirations most of the day.

Pressure Support Ventilation

- Pressure support ventilation (PSV) allows the client's respiratory effort to be augmented by a predetermined pressure assist from the ventilator (Henneman, 1991).
- As the weaning process ensues, the amount of pressure applied to inspiration is gradually decreased.
- Another method of weaning with PSV is to maintain the pressure but gradually decrease the ventilator's preset breaths per minute rate.

would be applicable during the weaning attempts (Jenny & Logan, 1994). The physician and nurse, often with a social worker or psychologist and a member of the clergy, discuss with the family and the client, as able, the client's quality of life, goals, and values. In accordance with this discussion, arrangements are made for home ventilation, nursing home placement, or withdrawal of life support (in terminal cases).

WEANING Weaning is the process of going from ventilatory dependence to spontaneous breathing. The weaning process can be prolonged if complications develop. Many of these complications can be avoided by skillful nursing care. For example, turning and positioning the client not only promote comfort and prevent skin breakdown but also facilitate gas exchange and prevent pulmonary complications, such as pneumonia and atelectasis. Table 31–9 summarizes various weaning techniques.

EXTUBATION Removal of the endotracheal (ET) tube is termed extubation. The tube is removed when the indication for intubation has been resolved. Before removal, the nurse explains the procedure to the client. The nurse or respiratory therapist sets up the prescribed oxygen delivery system at the bedside and brings in the equipment for emergency reintubation. The nurse or respiratory therapist hyperoxygenates the client and thoroughly suctions the ET tube as well as the oral cavity. The cuff of the ET tube is then rapidly deflated, and the tube is removed at peak inspiration. The nurse instructs the client to take deep breaths and to cough. It is normal for large amounts of oral secretions to have accumulated in the back of the throat. The nurse or respiratory therapist administers oxygen, usually ordered to be by face mask or nasal cannula. The FIO_2 is usually ordered at 10% higher than the level that was maintained while the ET tube was in place.

Monitoring after extubation is essential. The nurse monitors the client's vital signs every hour initially, assesses the client's ventilatory pattern, and assesses for any signs or symptoms of respiratory distress. It is common for the client to experience hoarseness and a sore throat for a few days after extubation. The nurse instructs the client to:

- Sit in a semi-Fowler's position
- Take deep breaths every ½ hour
- Use an incentive spirometer (see Chap. 19) every 2 hours
- Limit speaking in the immediate period after extubation

These measures facilitate gas exchange and decrease laryngeal edema and vocal cord irritation. The nurse also closely observes the client for signs or symptoms of upper airway obstruction (see Chap. 29). Early signs are mild dyspnea, coughing, and the inability to expectorate secretions. With the onset of these signs, the nurse notifies the physician, who evaluates the need for reintubation. The nurse is especially concerned if the client develops stridor, which is a late sign of a narrowed airway. Stridor is a high-pitched, crowing noise during inspiration caused by laryngospasm or edema above or below the glottis. Racemic epinephrine, a topical aerosol vasoconstrictor, is given, and reintubation is performed.

CHEST TRAUMA

Thoracic injuries are directly responsible for approximately 25% of all civilian traumatic deaths; 50% of the injured succumb before arriving at health care facilities. Only 5% to 15% of all thoracic injuries require thoracotomy. The remainder can be treated with basic resuscitation, intubation, or chest tube placement. Emergency personnel's basic and initial approach to all chest injuries is ABC (airway, breathing, circulation) followed by rapid assessment and treatment of potentially life-threatening conditions.

Pulmonary Contusion

Pulmonary contusion, a potentially lethal injury, is the most common chest injury seen in the United States. After a contusion, respiratory failure can develop over time rather than instantaneously. This condition most frequently follows injuries caused by rapid deceleration during vehicular accidents. Interstitial hemorrhage, which is almost invariably associated with intra-alveolar hemorrhage, is characteristic of pulmonary contusion. The resultant interstitial edema causes a decrease in pulmonary compliance and a decreased area for gas exchange. The client usually becomes hypoxemic and dyspneic. The bronchial mucosa becomes irritated, and the client has increased bronchial secretions.

Clients who may initially be asymptomatic can develop respiratory failure. The client presents with hemoptysis, decreased breath sounds, crackles, and wheezes. The chest x-ray of pulmonary contusion may show a hazy opacity in the lobes or parenchyma. If there is no disruption of the parenchyma, resorption of the lesion often occurs without treatment.

Treatment includes maintenance of ventilation and oxygenation. Central venous pressure is monitored closely, and fluid intake is restricted accordingly. The client in obvious respiratory distress may require mechanical ventilation with use of positive end-expiratory pressure (PEEP) to inflate the lungs and provide positive-pressure ventilation. A vicious circle occurs in which more muscle effort is required for ventilation, and the client becomes progressively hypoxemic. When the client attempts to compensate, he or she tires easily, becomes less efficient in breathing, and becomes more fatigued and hypoxemic. Flail chest may also be associated with a pulmonary contusion accompanied by parenchymal damage. The sequela to this situation is the probable development of ARDS.

Rib Fracture

After chest wall contusion, rib fractures are the next most common injury to the chest wall. Rib fractures most frequently result from direct blunt trauma to the chest, usually with involvement of the fifth through ninth ribs. Direct force applied to the ribs tends to fracture them and drive the bone ends into the thorax. Thus, there is a potential for intrathoracic injury, such as pneumothorax or pulmonary contusion. Pneumothorax is almost invariably present if ribs one through four are fractured.

The client usually experiences pain with movement and splints the chest defensively. Thoracic splinting results in impaired ventilation and inadequate clearance of tracheobronchial secretions. If the client has pre-existing pulmonary disease, the likelihood of atelectasis and pneumonia related to the rib fracture is increased. Clients with injuries to the first or second ribs, flail chest, seven or more fractured ribs, or expired volumes less than 15 mL/kg have a poor prognosis; intrathoracic injury occurs in 50% of these cases.

Treatment for uncomplicated rib fractures is nonspecific because the fractured ribs unite spontaneously. The chest is usually not splinted by tape or other materials. The primary consideration for the client is to decrease pain so that adequate ventilatory status is maintained. Intercostal nerve block may be used if pain is severe. Potent analgesia that causes respiratory depression is avoided.

Flail Chest

OVERVIEW

Flail chest is frequently associated with high-speed vehicular accidents. It is more common in older clients because their declining agility predisposes them to vehicular accidents, pedestrian accidents, and falls. It is associated with a high mortality rate (40%) and is one of the most critical chest injuries.

Flail chest (paradoxic respiration) is the inward movement of the thorax during inspiration, with outward movement during expiration. It usually involves one hemithorax (one side of the chest) and results from multiple rib fractures due to blunt chest trauma. Flail chest occurs when a loose segment of chest wall is left because of a fracture of two or more adjacent ribs. The movement of this segment becomes paradoxic to the expansion and contraction of the rest of the chest wall. Flail chest can also occur from bilateral fracture of multiple costochondral junctions (without rib fracture) anteriorly. There may be associated injury to the lung tissue under the flail segment. Gas exchange is significantly impaired, as is the ability to cough and clear secretions. Defensive splinting because of the rib fracture further reduces the client's ability to exert the extra effort required for breathing.

COLLABORATIVE MANAGEMENT

ASSESSMENT

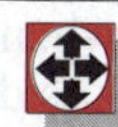

The nurse assesses the client with a flail chest for:

- Paradoxic chest movement
- Dyspnea
- Cyanosis
- Tachycardia
- Hypotension

Anxiety is usually associated with the experience of pain and dyspnea.

INTERVENTIONS

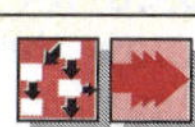

Interventions for flail chest include:

- The administration of humidified oxygen
- Pain management
- Promotion of lung expansion through deep breathing and positioning
- Secretion clearance by coughing and tracheal aspiration.

The nurse gives psychosocial support to this extremely anxious client by explaining all procedures, talking slowly, and allowing the client time to verbalize feelings and concerns.

The client with a flail chest may be treated conservatively with vigilant respiratory care. The physician may prescribe mechanical ventilation if such complications as respiratory failure or shock ensue. The physician and the nurse monitor ABG values closely along with vital capacity. With severe hypoxemia and hypercapnia, the client is intubated and placed on a ventilator with PEEP. If there is a pulmonary contusion or an underlying pulmonary disease, the potential for respiratory failure increases. Flail chest is best stabilized by positive-pressure ventilation rather than surgical intervention. Operative stabilization is reserved for extreme cases of flail chest.

The nurse monitors the client's vital signs and fluid and electrolyte balance closely so that hypovolemia or shock can be treated immediately. If the client has a pulmonary contusion, the nurse monitors central venous pressure and administers fluids as ordered. The nurse assesses the client for pain and intervenes to relieve the client's pain. The physician may order analgesic medication by the intravenous, epidural, or nerve block routes.

Pneumothorax

Any thoracic injury that allows accumulation of *atmospheric air* in the pleural space results in a rise in intrathoracic pressure and a reduction in vital capacity, depending on the amount of pulmonary collapse produced. Pneumothorax is often caused by blunt chest trauma and is associated with some degree of hemothorax. The pneumothorax can be open (when the pleural cavity has become exposed to the outside air, as through an open wound in the chest wall) or closed.

Assessment findings include:

- Diminished breath sounds on auscultation
- Hyperresonance on percussion
- Prominence of the involved hemithorax, which moves poorly with respirations

In addition, the client may have pleuritic pain, tachypnea, and subcutaneous emphysema (air under the skin in the subcutaneous tissues). A chest x-ray is used for diagnosis. Chest tubes may be indicated to allow the air to escape and the lung segment to reinflate.

Tension Pneumothorax

OVERVIEW

Tension pneumothorax, one of the most rapidly developing and life-threatening complications of blunt chest trauma, results from an air leak in the lung or chest wall. Air that is forced into the thoracic cavity causes complete collapse of the affected lung. The air that enters the pleural space during expiration does not exit during inspiration. As a result, air progressively accumulates under pressure, compresses the mediastinal vessels, and interferes with venous return. Because this process leads to decreased diastolic filling of the heart, cardiac output is compromised. If not promptly detected and treated, tension pneumothorax is quickly fatal. Typical causes of tension pneumothorax are:

- Blunt chest trauma in which the parenchymal injury has failed to seal
- Mechanical ventilation with PEEP
- Closed chest drainage (chest tubes)
- Insertion of central venous access lines

COLLABORATIVE MANAGEMENT

ASSESSMENT

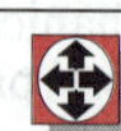

Assessment findings with tension pneumothorax include:

- Tracheal deviation to the unaffected side
- Respiratory distress
- Unilateral absence of breath sounds
- Distended neck veins
- Cyanosis

On percussion, there is a hypertympanic sound over the affected hemithorax. Pneumothorax is detectable on a chest x-ray. ABG assays demonstrate hypoxia and respiratory alkalosis.

INTERVENTIONS

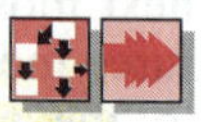

The physician inserts a large-bore needle into the second intercostal space in the midclavicular line of the affected side as initial treatment for tension pneumothorax. After this lifesaving measure is completed, the physician places a chest tube into the fourth intercostal space of the midaxillary line and attaches the tube to a water seal drainage system until the lung reinflates.

Hemothorax

OVERVIEW

Hemothorax is one of the most common problems encountered after blunt chest trauma or penetrating injuries. A *simple* hemothorax is a blood loss of less than 1500 mL into the thoracic cavity; a *massive* hemothorax is a blood loss of more than 1500 mL.

Bleeding is frequently caused by injuries to the

lung parenchyma, such as pulmonary contusions or lacerations, which are often associated with rib and sternal fractures. Massive intrathoracic bleeding in blunt chest trauma generally stems from the heart, great vessels, or major systemic arteries, such as the intercostal arteries.

COLLABORATIVE MANAGEMENT

ASSESSMENT

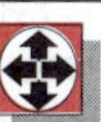

Physical assessment findings vary with the size of the hemothorax. If the hemothorax is small, the client may be asymptomatic. If the hemothorax is larger, the client experiences respiratory distress. In addition, breath sounds are diminished on auscultation. The percussion note on the involved side is dull. Blood in the pleural space is visualized by a chest x-ray and confirmed by diagnostic thoracentesis.

INTERVENTIONS

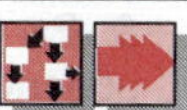

Interventions are aimed at evacuating the blood in the pleural space to normalize pulmonary function and to prevent infection related to blood accumulation. The physician inserts anterior and posterolateral chest tubes to evacuate the pleural space and to reduce the rush of clotted blood. The physician and the nurse carefully monitor the chest tube drainage, and chest x-rays are evaluated serially.

The physician considers open thoracotomy when there is initial evacuation of 1500 to 2000 mL of blood or when there is persistent bleeding at the rate of 200 mL/hr over 3 hours. The nurse:

- Monitors the client's vital signs, blood loss, and overall intake and output
- Assesses the client's response to the chest tubes
- Administers intravenous fluids and blood as ordered

Autotransfusion of the blood lost through chest drainage should be considered.

Tracheobronchial Trauma

Most tears of the tracheobronchial tree result from severe blunt trauma primarily involving the mainstem bronchi. Injuries to the cervical trachea usually occur at the junction of the trachea and cricoid cartilage. These injuries are frequently caused by striking the anterior neck against the dashboard or steering wheel during a vehicular accident. Clients with lacerations of the trachea develop massive air leaks, which produce pneumomediastinum (air in the mediastinum) and extensive subcutaneous emphysema. Upper airway obstruction may also occur and produce severe respiratory distress and inspiratory stridor. Major cervical tears are managed by cricothyroidotomy or tracheostomy below the level of injury.

The nurse assesses the client for hypoxemia by ABG assays. On the physician's order, the nurse administers oxygen appropriately. Depending on the degree of injury, the client may require mechanical ventilation. Frequent assessment of vital signs is essential because the client is likely to be hypotensive and in shock. The nurse continues to assess for subcutaneous emphysema and auscultates lungs to assess for further complications every 1 to 2 hours initially. Decreased breath sounds or wheezing may indicate further obstruction, atelectasis, or pneumothorax. Care of the client with a tracheostomy is discussed in Chapter 29. Mechanical ventilation is discussed earlier in this chapter.

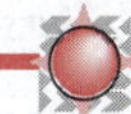

IMPLICATIONS FOR NURSING RESEARCH

Although many technologic advances have been made in the area of mechanical ventilation, only a few vaccines are available to prevent the multiple respiratory infections in clients of all ages. Diseases that cause immunosuppression increase the susceptibility to infections and associated complications (e.g., TB and pneumonia). Research needs to focus on this area as well as on the area of lung cancer and pulmonary diseases.

Questions that nursing needs to address include:

♦ What is the effect of teaching about risk factors and warning signs of lung cancer on the morbidity and mortality of the disease?
♦ What factors are most important in successful weaning from the ventilator?
♦ How can the nurse be most effective in reducing dyspnea in the client with a lower respiratory tract disorder?
♦ How can the nurse be most effective in reducing anxiety and fear in the client experiencing dyspnea?

SELECTED BIBLIOGRAPHY

American Cancer Society. (1993). *Cancer facts and figures—1993.* Atlanta: American Cancer Society.

Arbour, R. (1993). Weaning a patient from a ventilator. *Nursing93, 23*(2), 52–56.

Belcher, A. (1992). *Cancer nursing* (pp. 55–67). St. Louis: Mosby Year Book.

Berckman, K. L., & Austin, J. K. (1993). Casual attribution, perceived control, and adjustment in patients with lung cancer. *Oncology Nursing Forum, 20*(1), 23–30.

Boring, C. C., Squires, T. S., & Heath, C. W. (1992). Cancer statistics for African Americans. *CA: A Cancer Journal for Clinicians, 42*(1), 7–17.

Boring, C. C., Squires, T. S., Tong, T., & Montgomery, S. (1994). Cancer statistics, 1994. *CA: A Cancer Journal for Clinicians, 44*(1), 7–26.

Burns, S. M. (1991). Preventing diaphragm fatigue in the ventilated patient. *Dimensions of Critical Care Nursing, 10*(1), 13–20.

Burns, S. M. (Ed.). (1991). Weaning from long-term mechanical ventilation. *AACN Clinical Issues in Critical Care Nursing, 2*(3), 359–472.

Carroll, P. (1991). What's new in chest-tube management. *RN, 54*(5), 34–40.

Carroll, P. (1992). Nursing the thoracotomy patient. *RN, 55*(6), 34–41.

Cheever, K. H. (1993). Assisting with chest tube insertion. *Nursing93, 23*(1), 32C, 32F.

Connolly, M. A., & Shekleton, M. E. (1991). Communicating with ventilator dependent patients. *Dimensions of Critical Care Nursing, 10*(2), 115–121.

Curry, K., & Casday, L. (1992). Managing spontaneous pneumothorax. *The Nursing Spectrum, 1*(7), 12–13.

Dettenmeier, P. A., & Johnson, T. M. (1991). The art and science of mechanical ventilator adjustments. *Critical Care Nursing Clinics of North America, 3*(4), 575–583.

Do's and don'ts of anticoagulation therapy. (1993). *Nursing93, 23*(5), 32X.

Elpern, E. H. (1992). Lung cancer. In S. L. Groenwald, M. H. Frogge, M. Goodman, & C. H. Yarbro, et al. (Eds.), *Cancer nursing principles and practice* (2nd ed., pp. 952–973). Boston: Jones and Bartlett.

Epps, M. E. (1992). Diagnostic testing for patients with lung cancer. *Nursing Clinics of North America, 27*(3), 615–630.

Faber, L. P. (1991). Lung cancer. In A. Holleb, et al. (Eds.), *American cancer society textbook of clinical oncology* (pp. 194–211). Atlanta: American Cancer Society.

Finesilver, C. (1992). Perfecting the art: Respiratory assessment. *RN, 55*(2), 22–29.

Finkelmeier, B. A., & Garolis, S. (1993). Readers comment on response to chest tube instillation question [Letter]. *Critical Care Nurse, 13*(1), 17–18.

Frank-Stromborg, M., & Rohan, K. (1992). Nursing's involvement in primary and secondary prevention of cancer: Nationally and internationally. *Cancer Nursing, 15*(2), 79–108.

Fraser, R., & Paré, J. A. (1991). *Diagnosis of disease of the chest* (3rd ed.). Philadelphia: W. B. Saunders.

Garfinkel, L., & Silverberg, E. (1991). Lung cancer and smoking trends in the United States over the past 25 years. *CA: A Cancer Journal for Clinicians, 41*(3), 137–145.

Glover, J., & Miaskowski, C. (1994). Small cell lung cancer: Pathophysiologic mechanisms and nursing implications. *Oncology Nursing Forum, 21*(1), 87–97.

Hamlin, W., Schnobel, L. & Smith, B. (1991). The patient with noncardiac pulmonary edema. *Journal of Post Anesthesia Nursing, 6*(1), 43–49.

Harley, N. H., & Harley, J. H. (1990). Potential lung cancer risk from indoor radon exposure. *CA: A Cancer Journal for Clinicians, 40*(5), 265–275.

Heffner, J. E., & Unruh, L. C. (1992). Tetracycline pleurodesis: Adios, farewell, adieu [Editorial]. *Chest, 101*(1), 5–6.

Henneman, E. A. (1991). The art and science of weaning from mechanical ventilation. *Focus on Critical Care, 18*(6), 490–501.

Hess, D. (1991). Noninvasive respiratory monitoring during ventilatory support. *Critical Care Nursing Clinics of North America, 3*(4), 565–574.

Hinson, J. A., & Perry, M. C. (1993). Small cell lung cancer. *CA: A Cancer Journal for Clinicians, 43*(4), 216–225.

Hirsh, J., Dalen, J. E., Deykin, D., & Poller, L. (1992). Heparin: Mechanism of action, pharmacokinetics, dosing considerations, monitoring, efficacy, and safety. *Chest, 102*(Suppl. 4), 3375–3455.

Houston, S. J., & Kendall, J. A. (1992). Psychosocial implications of lung cancer. *Nursing Clinics of North America, 27*(3), 681–690.

Hunter, F. C., & Mitchell, S. (1993). Managing ARDS. *RN, 56*(7), 52–58.

Jassak, P. (1992). Families: An essential element in the care of the patient with cancer. *Oncology Nursing Forum, 19*(6), 871–882.

Jenny, J., & Logan, J. (1994). Promoting ventilator independence: A grounded theory perspective. *Dimensions of Critical Care Nursing, 13*(1), 29–37.

Kelleghan, S. I., Salemi, C., & Padilla, S., et al. (1993). An effective continuous quality improvement approach to the prevention of ventilator-associated pneumonia. *American Journal of Infection Control, 21*(6), 322–330.

* Kersten, L. D. (1989). *Comprehensive respiratory nursing: A decision making approach.* Philadelphia: W. B. Saunders.

Krebel, A. (1991). Weaning from a mechanical ventilator: Current controversies. *Heart & Lung, 20*(4), 321–331.

Larson, P. J., Lindsey, A. M., Dodd, M. J., Brecht, M., & Packer, A. (1993). Influence of age on problems experienced by patients with lung cancer undergoing radiation therapy. *Oncology Nursing Forum, 20*(3), 473–480.

* Lorch, D. G., Gordon, L., Wooten, S., et al. (1988). Effect of patient positioning on distribution of tetracycline in the pleural space during pleurodesis. *Chest, 93*(3), 527–529.

* Lush, M. T., Janson-Bjerklie, S, Carrieri, V. K., & Lovejoy, N. (1988). Dyspnea in the ventilator-assisted patient. *Heart & Lung, 17*(5), 528–535.

Macey, B. A., & Landstrom, L. L. (1993). Replacing a chest-tube drainage-collection device. *American Journal of Nursing, 93*(3) 95–96.

Martini, N. (1993). Operable lung cancer *CA: A Cancer Journal for Clinicians, 43*(4), 201–214.

Mason, S. G. (1992). When a ventilator patient is going home. *RN, 55*(10), 60–64.

McGuire, D. B., & Shiedler, V. R. (1992). Pain. In S. L. Groenwald, M. H. Frogge, M. Goodman, & C. H. Yarbro, et al. (Eds.), *Cancer nursing principles and practice* (2nd ed., pp. 385–433). Boston: Jones and Bartlett.

Mills, J., & Luce, J. M. (1992). Pulmonary emergencies. In C. E. Saunders & M. T. Ho (Eds.), *Current emergency diagnosis and treatment* (4th ed., pp. 451–467). Norwalk, CT: Appleton & Lange.

Moldowan, C. (1992). Improved outcome for post-thoracotomy patients using intermittent bupivacaine with epinephrine by the CADD-Plus Ambulatory Infusion Pump. *Journal of Intravenous Nursing, 15*(6), 333–337.

Mountain, C. F., Greenberg, S. D., & Fraire, A. E. (1991). Tumor stage in non–small cell carcinoma of the lung. *Chest, 99*(5), 1258–1259.

Nathanson, L. K., Shimi, S. M., Wood, R. A. B., & Cuschieri, A. (1991). Videothorascopic ligation of bulla and pleurectomy for spontaneous pneumothorax. *Annals of Thoracic Surgery, 52*(2), 316–319.

Noll, M. L. (Ed.). (1990). Respiratory care in adults. *AACN Clinical Issues in Critical Care Nursing, 1*(2), 237–326.

Olsen, G. N. (1991). Stair climbing as an exercise to predict the postoperative complications of lung resection: Two years' experience. *Chest, 99*(3), 587–590.

Penny, S. L., & Shell, J. A. (1991). Lung cancer. In S. E.

Otto (Ed.), *Oncology nursing* (pp. 439–495). St. Louis: Mosby–Year Book.

Pierce, J. D., Wiggins, S. A., Plaskon, C., & Glass, C. (1993). Pressure support ventilation: reducing the work of breathing during weaning. *Dimensions of Critical Care Nursing, 12*(6), 282–290.

Rose, M. A. (1991). Intervention strategies for smoking cessation: The role of oncology nursing. *Cancer Nursing, 14*(5), 225–231.

Sabiston, D. C. (1990). Carcinoma of the lung. In D. C. Sabiston & F. C. Spencer (Eds.), *Surgery of the chest* (5th ed., pp. 554–577). Philadelphia: W. B. Saunders.

Sarna, L., Lindsey, A. M., Dean, H., Brecht, M., & McCorkle, R. (1993). Nutritional intake, weight change, symptom distress, and functional status over time in adults with lung cancer. *Oncology Nursing Forum, 20*(3), 481–489.

Saul, L. (Ed.). (1991). *Activase therapy in acute myocardial infarction and acute massive pulmonary embolism.* Califon, NJ: Gardiner-Caldwell SynerMed.

Schmitz, T. M. (1991). The semi-prone position in ARDS: Five case studies. *Critical Care Nurse, 11*(5), 22–33.

Sheppard, K. C. (1993). The relationships among nursing diagnoses in discharge planning for patients with lung cancer. *Nursing Diagnosis, 4*(4), 148–155.

Sonnesso, G. (1990). Negative pressure ventilation: New uses for an old technique. *AACN Clinical Issues in Critical Care Nursing, 1*(2), 313–317.

Stiesmeyer, J. K. (1992). Care of the elderly mechanically ventilated patient: Preserving the fragile environment. *AACN Clinical Issues in Critical Care Nursing, 3*(1), 129–136.

Superior vena cava syndrome. *American Journal of Nursing, 93*(2), 52.

Taggart, J. A., & Lind, M. A. (1994). Evaluating unplanned endotracheal extubations. *Dimensions of Critical Care Nursing, 13*(3), 114–122.

Tampinco-Golos, I. (1993). Endoscopic thoracotomy. *Nursing93, 23*(8), 62–64.

Tampinco-Golos, I. (1992). Endoscopic thoracotomy: A new approach to thoracic surgery. *AORN Journal, 55*(5), 1167, 1169–1172, 1174–1177, 1180.

Teplitz, L. (1991). Update: Are milking and stripping chest tubes necessary? *Focus on Critical Care, 18*(6), 506–511.

Thelan, L. A., Davie, J. K., & Urden, L. D. (1990). *Textbook of critical care nursing: Diagnosis and management* (pp. 467–469). St. Louis: C. V. Mosby.

Thompson, K. S., Caddick, K., Mathie, J., Newlon, B., & Abraham, T. (1991). Building a critical path for ventilator dependency. *American Journal of Nursing, 91*(7), 28–31.

Turner, J. A. T. (1992). Nursing care of the terminal lung cancer patient. *Nursing Clinics of North America, 27*(3), 691–702.

Underwood, S. M. (1991). African-American men: Perceptual determinants of early cancer detection and cancer risk reduction. *Cancer Nursing, 14*(6), 281–288.

Watson, P. G. (1992). The optimal functioning plan: A key element in cancer rehabilitation. *Cancer Nursing, 15*(4), 254–263.

Wilson, D. J. (1993). Chronic ventilator-dependent patients. In J. M. Clochesy, C. Breu, S. Cardin, E. Rudy, & A. Whittaker (Eds.), *Critical care nursing* (pp. 623–640). Philadelphia: W. B. Saunders.

Wilson, S. F., & Thompson, J. M. (1990). *Respiratory disorders.* St. Louis: Mosby–Year Book.

Wright, J., Doyle, P., & Yoshihara, G. (1993). Advances in mechanical ventilation. In J. Clochesy, C. Breu, S. Cardin, E. Rudy, & A. Whittaker (Eds.), *Critical care nursing* (pp. 602–622). Philadelphia: W. B. Saunders.

SUGGESTED READINGS

Hirsh, J., Dalen, J. E., Deykin, D., & Poller, L. (1992). Heparin: Mechanism of action, pharmacokinetics, dosing considerations, monitoring, efficacy, and safety. *Chest, 102*(Suppl. 4), 337S–345S.

Heparin is considered in great detail in this article. Chemical structure, mechanism of action, administration, pharmacokinetics, and pharmacodynamics are discussed. A review of laboratory monitoring of the anticoagulant effect by activated partial thromboplastin time (APTT) and associated therapeutic ranges is included. The side effects of bleeding, osteoporosis, thrombocytopenia, and skin lesions are addressed. The article concludes by discussing the low-molecular-weight heparins, a new class of anticoagulants.

Stiesmeyer, J. K. (1992). Care of the elderly mechanically ventilated patient: Preserving the fragile environment. *AACN Clinical Issues in Critical Care Nursing, 3*(1), 129–136.

The article begins by reviewing normal aging changes in the pulmonary structures. A summary of various modes of ventilation follows. Complications to which the elderly mechanically ventilated client is susceptible are discussed, including pneumonia, malnutrition, and pneumothorax. The author suggests methods to prevent, identify, and treat the complications. The article concludes with a discussion about weaning the elderly client from the ventilator. Criteria for readiness to wean and ability to wean as well as indicators of failure to wean are discussed. A 36-term reference list is included.

Thompson, K. S., Caddick, K., Mathie, J., Newlon, B., & Abraham, T. (1991). Building a critical path for ventilator dependency. *American Journal of Nursing, 91*(7), 28–31.

In this article, one hospital presents its approach to weaning ventilator-dependent clients. A special care unit is used, and a nurse case manager collaborates and coordinates care. A 30-day critical pathway developed in collaboration is presented.

Turner, J. A. T. (1992). Nursing care of the terminal lung cancer patient. *Nursing Clinics of North America, 27*(3), 691–702.

Lung cancer is viewed on a continuum of care spanning curative treatment and palliative care. Terminal care is described as the time when treatment goals are aimed toward control of symptoms and quality of life. The author outlines palliative care, as well as ethical issues faced by the client and nurse, and emphasizes active participation of the client in decision-making for as long as possible.

Watson, P. G. (1992). The optimal functioning plan: A key element in cancer rehabilitation. *Cancer Nursing, 15*(4), 254–263.

This important article addresses the rehabilitation needs of clients with cancer throughout the trajectory of disease—diagnosis, treatment, and post-treatment periods. Watson describes an Optimal Functioning Plan (OFP), developed to achieve optimal client status in physical functioning, nutrition, self-care, psychosocial support, and management of cancer signs and symptoms. This proactive model provides guidelines and strategies to promote independence of and empowerment for the client based on individual goals, regardless of prognosis.

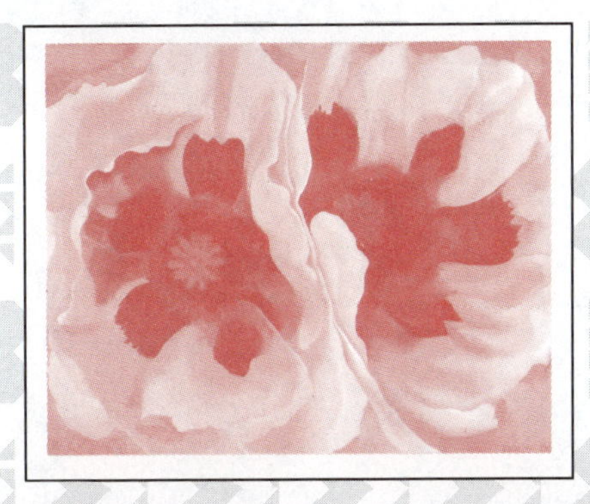

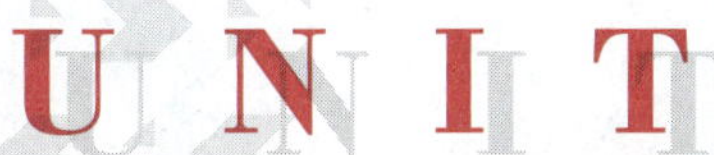

UNIT

7

Problems of Cardiac Output and Tissue Perfusion: Management of Clients with Problems of the Cardiovascular System

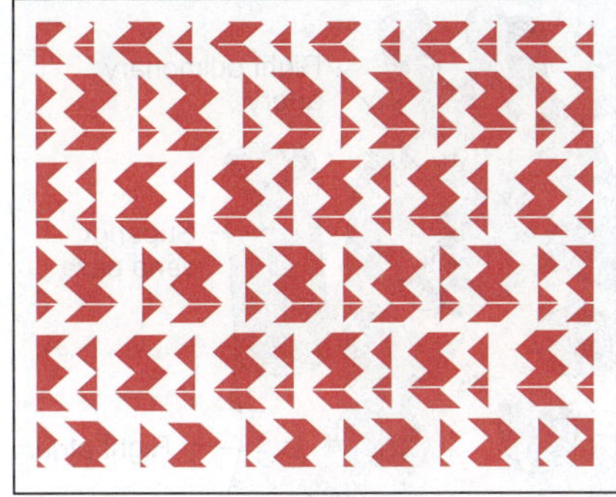

CHAPTER 32

Assessment of the Cardiovascular System

CHAPTER HIGHLIGHTS

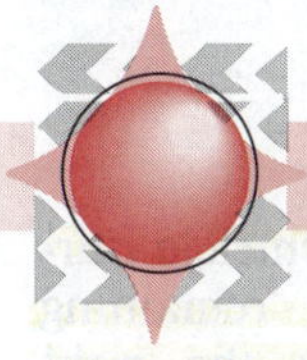

Since 1979, there has been a 23.4% decline in the death rate from cardiovascular disease in the United States. Despite this dramatic reduction, cardiovascular disease remains the major cause of mortality, resulting in the deaths of nearly 1 million people each year in the United States. Additionally, the American Heart Association (AHA) estimates that approximately one in four people has experienced, and is living with, some form of cardiovascular disease (AHA, 1992).

ANATOMY AND PHYSIOLOGY REVIEW

Heart

STRUCTURE

The human heart is a cone-shaped, hollow, muscular organ located between the lungs (Fig. 32–1). It is approximately the size of an adult fist. The heart rests on the diaphragm, tilting forward and to the left in the client's chest. The apex of the heart is rotated anteriorly. This small organ must pump continuously. Each beat of the heart pumps approximately 60 mL of blood, which is about 5 L/minute. During strenuous physical activity, the heart can double the

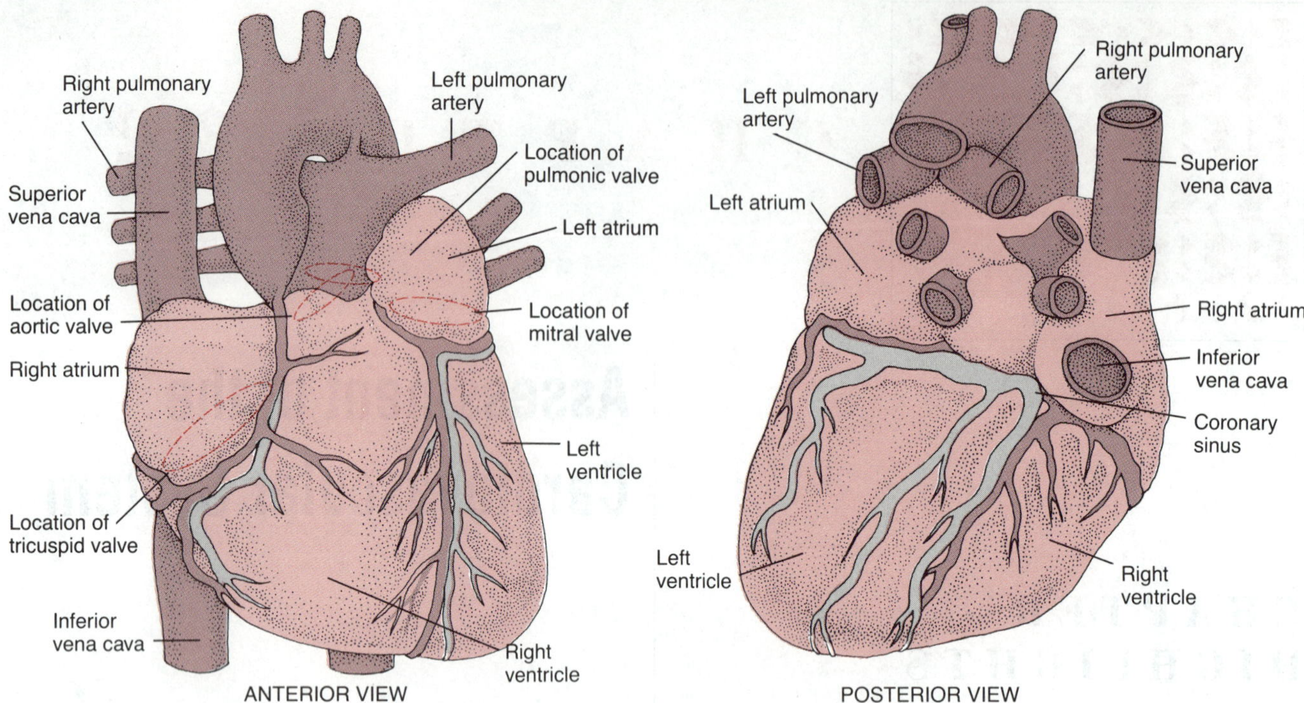

FIGURE 32–1 ◆ Surface anatomy of the heart.

amount of blood pumped to meet the increased oxygen needs of the peripheral tissues.

The heart is encapsulated by a protective covering called the *pericardium* (Fig. 32–2). The cardiac muscle tissue is composed of three layers:

- The epicardium
- The myocardium
- The endocardium

The epicardium, the outer surface, is a thin transparent tissue. The myocardium, the middle layer, is composed of striated muscle fibers interlaced into bundles. This layer is responsible for the heart's contractile force. The innermost layer, the endocardium, is composed of endothelial tissue. This tissue lines the inside of the chambers of the heart and covers the four heart valves.

CHAMBERS OF THE HEART

A muscular wall, known as the septum, separates the heart into two halves: right and left. Each half has an upper chamber called an *atrium* and a lower chamber called a *ventricle* (Fig. 32–3).

RIGHT SIDE OF THE HEART

The right atrium is a thin-walled structure that receives deoxygenated venous blood (venous return) from all the peripheral tissues by way of the superior and inferior venae cavae and from the heart muscle by way of the coronary sinus. Most of this venous return flows passively from the right atrium through the opened tricuspid valve to the right ventricle during ventricular diastole, or filling. The remaining venous return is actively propelled by the right atrium into the right ventricle during atrial systole, or contraction.

The right ventricle is a flat muscular pump located behind the sternum. The right ventricle generates enough pressure (about 25 mmHg) to close the tricuspid valve, to open the pulmonic valve, and to propel blood into the pulmonary artery and the lungs. The workload of the right ventricle is light compared with that of the left ventricle because the pulmonary system is a low-pressure system, which imposes less resistance to flow.

LEFT SIDE OF THE HEART

After blood is reoxygenated in the lungs, it flows freely from the four pulmonary veins into the left atrium. Blood then flows through an opened mitral valve into the left ventricle during ventricular diastole. When the left ventricle is almost full, the left atrium contracts, pumping the remaining blood volume into the left ventricle. Finally, with systolic contraction, the left ventricle generates enough pressure (about 120 mmHg) to close the mitral valve and open the aortic valve. Blood is propelled into the aorta and into the systemic arterial circulation. Blood flow through the heart is shown in Figure 32–2.

The left ventricle is ellipsoid and is the largest and most muscular chamber of the heart. Its wall is two to three times the thickness of the right ventricular wall. The left ventricle must generate a higher pressure than the right ventricle because it must contract

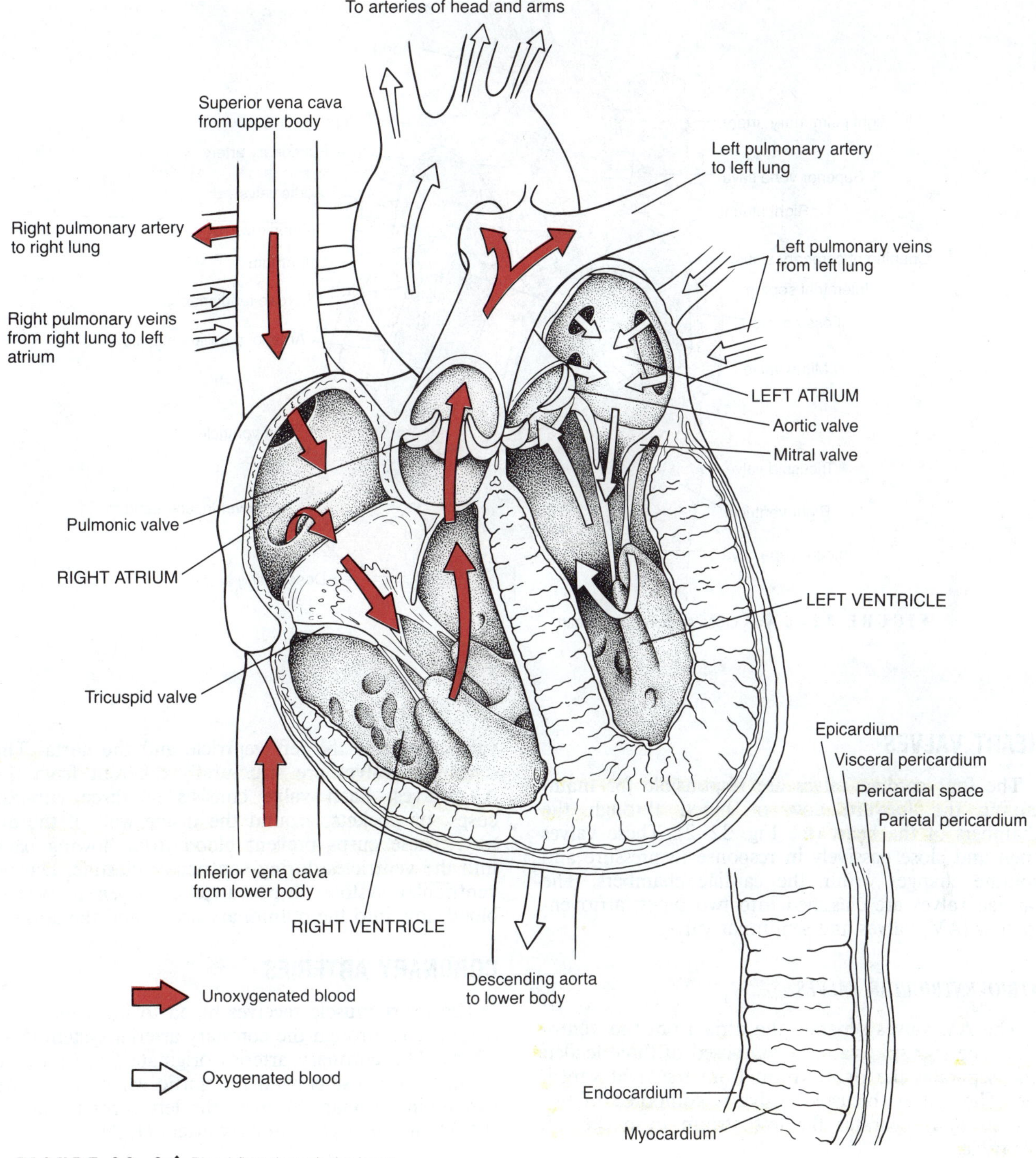

FIGURE 32-2 ◆ Blood flow through the heart.

against a high-pressure systemic circulation, which imposes a greater resistance to flow. If pressure rises in the circulatory system (as with hypertension), there is greater resistance. Thus, the left ventricle must generate a higher pressure to open the aortic valve and empty its contents, increasing left ventricular workload.

Blood is propelled from the aorta throughout the systemic circulation to the various tissues of the body; it returns to the right atrium because of pressure differences. The pressure of blood in the aorta in a young adult averages about 100 to 120 mmHg, whereas the pressure of blood in the right atrium averages about 0 to 5 mmHg. These differences in pressure produce a pressure gradient, whereby blood flows from an area of higher pressure to an area of lower pressure. The heart and vascular structures are responsible for maintaining these pressures.

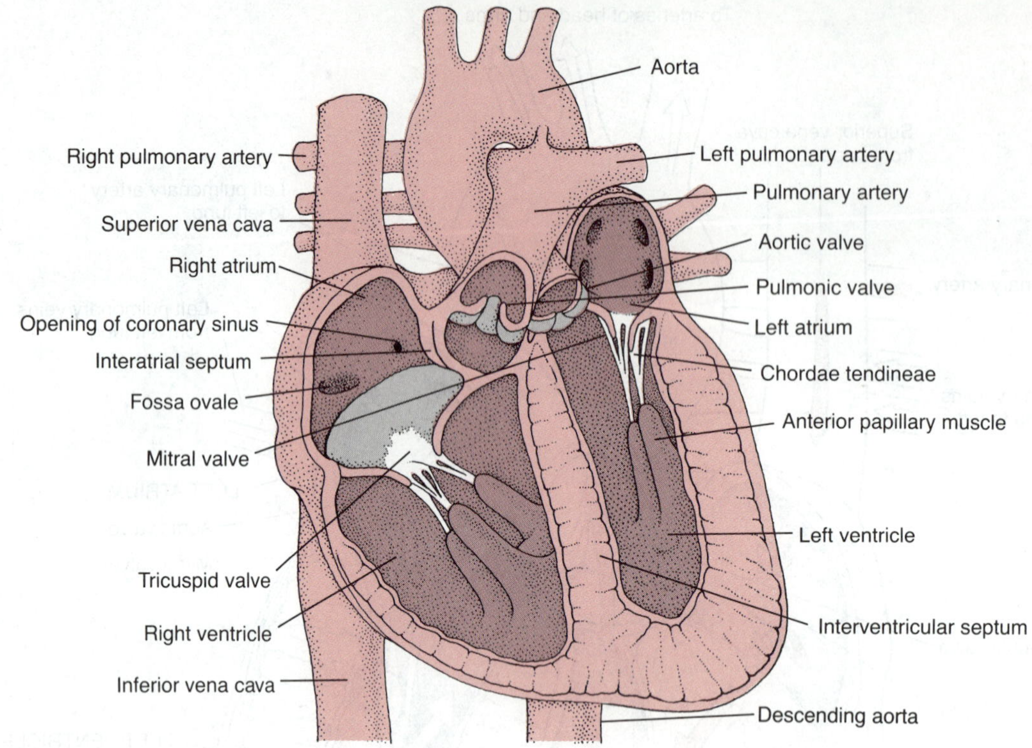

FIGURE 32–3 ◆ A cross-section of the heart.

HEART VALVES

The four cardiac valves are responsible for maintaining the forward flow of blood through the chambers of the heart (see Fig. 32–2). These valves open and close passively in response to pressure and volume changes within the cardiac chambers. The cardiac valves are classified into two types: atrioventricular (AV) valves and semilunar valves.

ATRIOVENTRICULAR VALVES

The AV valves separate the atria from the ventricles. The tricuspid valve is composed of three leaflets and separates the right atrium from the right ventricle. The mitral (bicuspid) valve is composed of two leaflets and separates the left atrium from the left ventricle.

During ventricular diastole, the valves act as funnels, facilitating the flow of blood from the atria to the ventricles. There is some overlapping of the valve leaflets during closure to prevent the backflow (regurgitation) of blood into the atria.

SEMILUNAR VALVES

There are two semilunar valves: the pulmonic and the aortic valve. Each is named for the arteries in which it is located. The pulmonic valve separates the right ventricle and the pulmonary artery. The aortic valve separates the left ventricle and the aorta. The semilunar valves are structurally different from the AV valves. Each valve consists of three cup-like cusps, or pockets, around the inside wall of the artery. These cusps prevent blood from flowing back into the ventricles during ventricular diastole. During ventricular systole, these valves are open to permit blood flow into the pulmonary artery and the aorta.

CORONARY ARTERIES

The heart muscle receives blood to meet its metabolic needs through the coronary arterial system (Fig. 32–4). The coronary arteries originate from an area on the aorta just beyond the aortic valve. There are two main coronary arteries: the left coronary artery (LCA) and the right coronary artery (RCA).

LEFT CORONARY ARTERY

The LCA divides into two branches: the left anterior descending (LAD) and the circumflex coronary artery (CCA). The LAD branch descends toward the anterior wall and the apex of the left ventricle. It supplies blood to the anterior wall of the left ventricle, the anterior ventricular septum, the anterior papillary muscle, and portions of the right ventricle. In addition, the LAD branch usually supplies the anterior apex of the left ventricle and portions of the posterior apex.

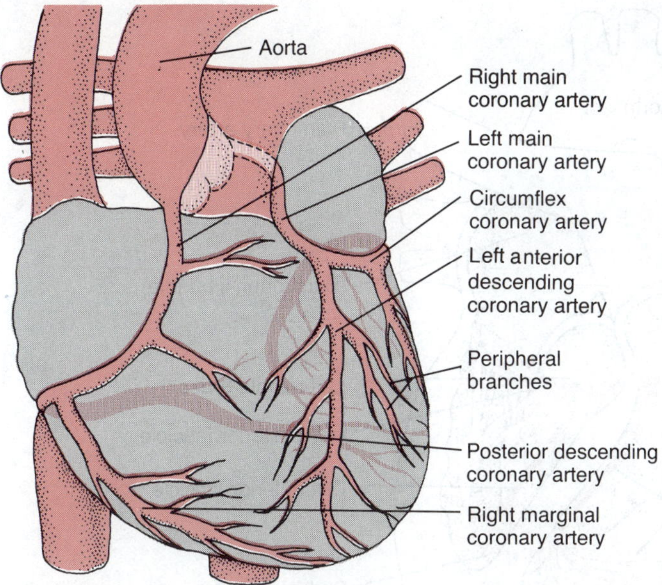

FIGURE 32-4 ◆ The coronary arterial system.

The CCA descends toward the lateral wall of the left ventricle and apex. It supplies blood to the left atrium, the lateral and posterior surfaces of the left ventricle, and sometimes the posterior interventricular septum. In some people, the CCA supplies the sinoatrial (SA) node and the AV node. Peripheral branches (diagonal and obtuse marginal) arise from the LAD and the CCA and form an abundant network of vessels throughout the entire myocardium. Sometimes, these peripheral branches anastomose. Anastomosis maintains blood supply to a region, even if the main blood vessel supplying the area becomes blocked.

RIGHT CORONARY ARTERY

The RCA originates from the right sinus of Valsalva; encircles the heart, passing through the right AV groove (the junction between the right atrium and the right ventricle); and descends toward the apex of the right ventricle. The RCA supplies the right atrium, the right ventricle, and the inferior portion of the left ventricle. The posterior descending branch of the RCA supplies the posterior wall of the septum and the posterior left papillary muscle. In many people (more than 50%), the RCA supplies the SA node and the AV node. Considerable variation in the branching pattern of the coronary arteries exists among individuals.

Coronary artery blood flow to the myocardium occurs primarily during diastole, when coronary vascular resistance is minimized. To maintain adequate blood flow through the coronary arteries, the diastolic blood pressure must be at least 60 mmHg, or autoregulatory mechanisms are activated to maintain blood flow to the myocardium.

FUNCTION

ELECTROPHYSIOLOGIC PROPERTIES OF THE HEART

The electrophysiologic properties of heart muscle are responsible for regulating heart rate and rhythm. Cardiac muscle cells are unique and possess the following special properties:

- Automaticity
- Excitability
- Conductivity
- Contractility
- Refractoriness

Automaticity refers to the ability of all cardiac cells to initiate an impulse spontaneously and repetitively. Excitability is the ability of the cells to respond to a stimulus by initiating an impulse (depolarization). Conductivity means that cardiac cells transmit the electrical impulses they receive. Because the cells possess the property of contractility, they also contract in response to an impulse. Refractoriness means that cardiac cells are unable to respond to stimuli because they have not yet repolarized from an earlier stimulus. These properties are more completely described in Chapter 33.

CONDUCTION SYSTEM OF THE HEART

The cardiac conduction system is composed of specialized tissue capable of rhythmic electrical impulse formation (Fig. 32-5). It can conduct impulses much more rapidly than other cells located in the myocardium. The SA node, located at the junction of the right atrium and the superior vena cava, is considered the main regulator of heart rate. The SA node is composed of pacemaker cells, which spontaneously initiate impulses at a rate of 60 to 100 per minute, and myocardial working cells, which transmit the impulses to surrounding atrial muscle.

An impulse from the SA node initiates the process of depolarization and hence the activation of all myocardial cells. Depolarization occurs in the right atrium first, followed by the left atrium. Activation of the atria occurs normally in 0.11 second or less.

The atrioventricular (AV) node contained in the junctional area is located on the right side of the interatrial septum in front of the coronary sinus. After the impulse reaches the AV node from the SA node, conduction of the impulse is delayed 0.07 to 0.1 second. This delay allows the atria to contract completely before the ventricles are stimulated to contract.

The bundle of His is a continuation of the AV node and runs in the inferior border of the interventricular septum. It then divides into the right and left bundle branches.

The bundle branches extend downward through the ventricular septum and fuse with the Purkinje fiber

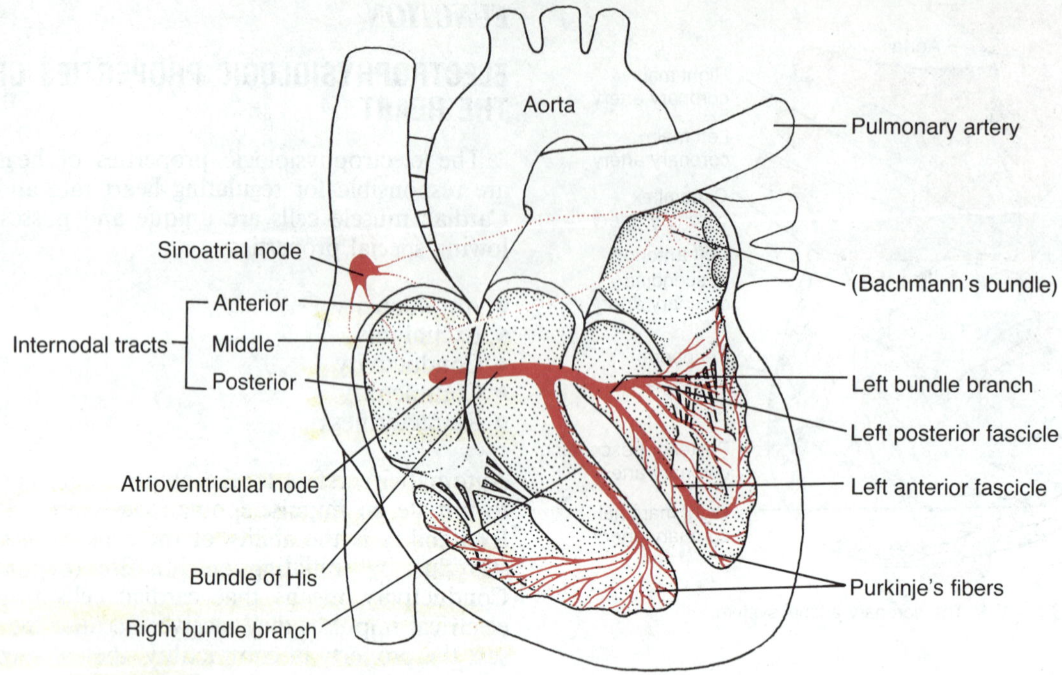

FIGURE 32–5 ♦ The conduction system of the heart.

system. The Purkinje fibers are the terminal branches of the conduction system and are responsible for carrying the wave of depolarization to both ventricular walls. The Purkinje fibers can act as an intrinsic pacemaker, but their discharge rate is only 20 to 40 beats per minute. Thus, these intrinsic pacemakers seldom initiate an electrical impulse.

SEQUENCE OF EVENTS DURING THE CARDIAC CYCLE

The phases of the cardiac cycle are generally described in relation to changes in pressure and volume in the left ventricle during filling (diastole) and ventricular contraction (systole) (Fig. 32–6). Diastole, normally about two thirds of the cardiac cycle, consists of relaxation and filling of the atria and ventricles, whereas systole consists of the contraction and emptying of the atria and ventricles.

Cardiac muscle contraction results from the release of large numbers of calcium ions from the sarcoplasmic reticulum, which diffuse into the myofibril sarcomere (the basic contractile unit of the myocardial cell). Calcium ions promote the interaction of actin and myosin protein filaments, causing a linking and overlapping of these filaments. As the protein filaments slide over or overlap each other, cross-bridges, or linkages, are formed. These cross-bridges act as force-generating sites. The sliding of these protein filaments of multiple myofibril sarcomeres causes shortening of the sarcomeres, producing myocardial contraction.

Relaxation of the cardiac muscle occurs when calcium ions are pumped back into the sarcoplasmic reticulum, causing a decrease in the number of calcium ions around the myofibrils. This reduced number of ions causes the protein filaments to disengage or dissociate, the sarcomere to lengthen, and the muscle to relax.

MECHANICAL PROPERTIES OF THE HEART

The electrical and mechanical properties of cardiac muscle determine the function of the cardiovascular system. The heart is able to adapt to various pathophysiologic conditions (e.g., stress, infections, and hemorrhage) to maintain adequate blood flow to the various body tissues. Blood flow to the tissues is measured clinically as the cardiac output (CO), the amount of blood pumped from the left ventricle each minute. Cardiac output is the basic determinant of heart function. Cardiac output depends on the relationship between heart rate (HR) and stroke volume (SV); it is the product of these two variables.

$$\text{cardiac output} = \text{heart rate} \times \text{stroke volume}$$

CARDIAC OUTPUT AND CARDIAC INDEX

Cardiac output is the volume of blood in liters ejected by the heart each minute. Normally, cardiac output in the adult ranges from 4 to 7 L/minute (Wilson, 1992). Because cardiac output requirements vary according to a person's body size, the cardiac index is calculated to adjust for size differences. The cardiac index can be determined by dividing the cardiac output by the body surface area. It is based on the assumption that cardiac output is more proportional to body surface area than to body mass.

$$\text{cardiac index} = \frac{\text{cardiac output}}{\text{body surface area}}$$

The normal range of cardiac index is 2.7 to 3.2 L/minute/m² of body surface area, thus adjusting for the client's body size and variability in cardiac function (Wilson, 1992).

HEART RATE

Heart rate refers to the number of times the ventricles contract per minute. The normal resting heart rate for an adult is between 60 and 100 beats per minute (AHA, 1992). Increases in heart rate increase myocardial oxygen demand. Rate is extrinsically controlled by the autonomic nervous system. This allows for the rapid adjustments in rate necessary to regulate cardiac output. The parasympathetic system slows the heart rate, whereas sympathetic stimulation has an excitatory effect. Circulating endogenous catecholamines such as epinephrine and norepinephrine also affect the heart rate. An increase in catecholamine levels usually causes an increase in heart rate, and vice versa.

Other factors, such as the central nervous system (CNS) and baroreceptor (pressoreceptor) reflexes, influence the effects of the autonomic nervous system on the heart rate. Pain, fear, and anxiety can cause an increase in heart rate. When the baroreceptors are stimulated, reflex changes can influence heart rate. The baroreceptor reflex acts as a negative-feedback system. Sensors in the aortic arch recognize pressure in the arteries and regulate the resistance of blood vessels in the periphery. If a client experiences hypotension, the baroreceptors in the aortic arch sense a lessened pressure in the blood vessels. A signal is relayed to the parasympathetic system to have less inhibitory effect on the sinoatrial (SA) node, which results in a reflex increase in heart rate.

Additional factors can affect the heart rate. Examples are body temperature, medications, hormonal influence, arterial blood gas tensions, and electrolyte concentrations.

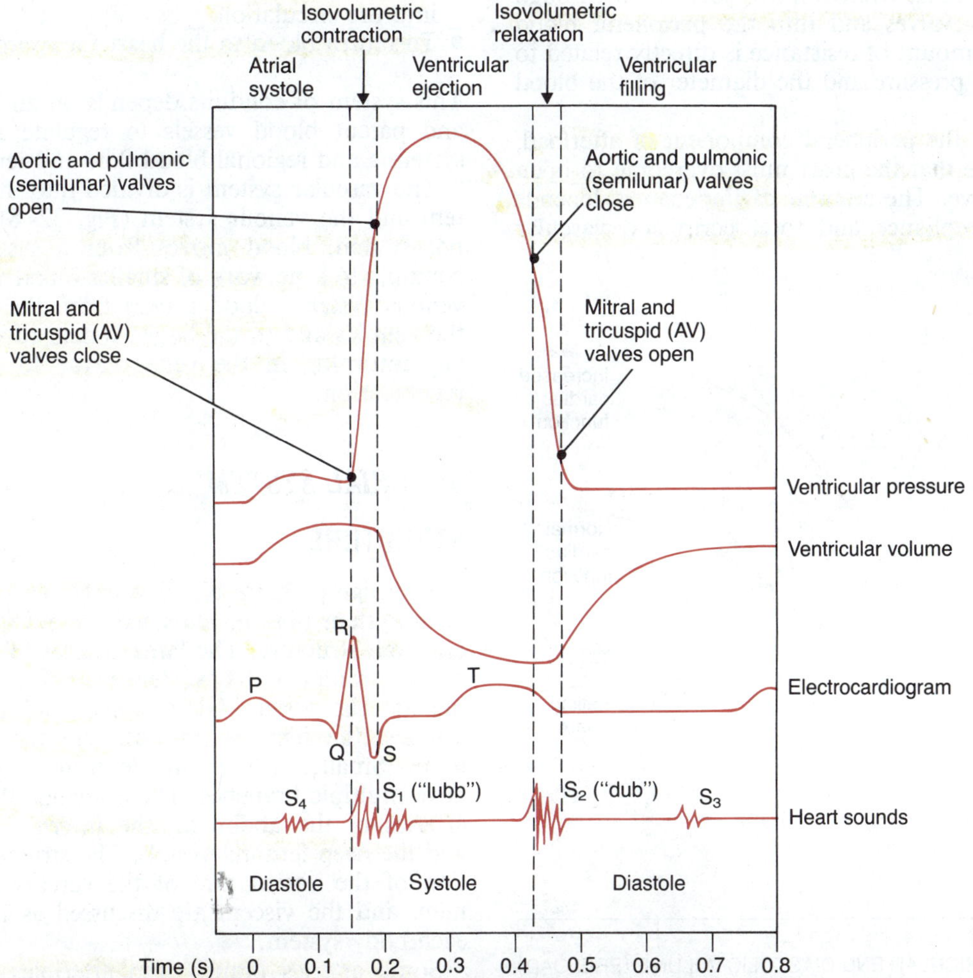

FIGURE 32-6 ◆ The events of the cardiac cycle.

STROKE VOLUME

Stroke volume is the amount of blood ejected by the left ventricle during each systole. Several variables influence stroke volume and, ultimately, cardiac output. These variables include heart rate, preload, afterload, and contractility. Heart rate was discussed earlier.

PRELOAD Preload refers to the degree of myocardial fiber stretch at the end of diastole just before contraction. The stretch imposed on the muscle fibers results from the volume contained within the ventricle at the end of diastole. Preload is determined by left ventricular end-diastolic (LVED) volume.

An increase in ventricular volume increases muscle fiber length and tension, thereby enhancing contraction and improving stroke volume. This statement is derived from Starling's law of the heart, which can be summarized as follows: the more the heart is filled during diastole (within limits), the more forcefully it contracts. However, *excessive* filling of the ventricles results in excessive LVED volume and pressure and decreased cardiac output (Fig. 32–7).

AFTERLOAD Another determinant of stroke volume is afterload. Afterload is the pressure or resistance that the ventricles must overcome to eject blood through the semilunar valves and into the peripheral blood vessels. The amount of resistance is directly related to arterial blood pressure and the diameter of the blood vessels.

Impedance, the peripheral component of afterload, is the pressure that the heart must overcome to open the aortic valve. The amount of impedance depends on aortic compliance and total peripheral vascular resistance, a combination of blood viscosity and arteriolar constriction. A decrease in stroke volume can result from an increase in afterload without the benefit of compensatory mechanisms.

CONTRACTILITY Contractility also affects stroke volume and cardiac output. Myocardial contractility occurs independently of preload and refers to the force of contractions generated by the myocardium. The myocardium has an inherent ability to alter its contractile force and velocity. Contractility is increased by such factors as sympathetic stimulation and calcium release. Increases in myocardial contractility cause increases in myocardial oxygen consumption. Factors such as hypoxia and acidemia decrease contractility.

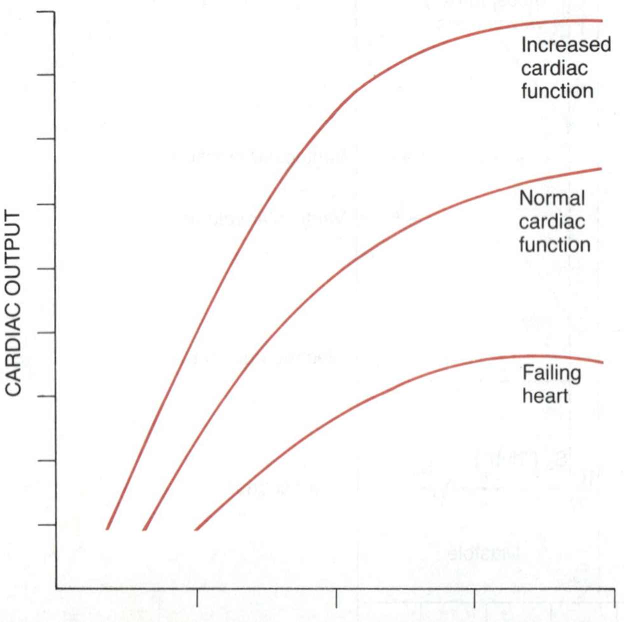

FIGURE 32–7 ◆ Length-tension ventricular function curves.

Vascular System

The purpose of the vascular system is:

- To provide conduits for blood to travel from the heart to nourish the various tissues of the body
- To carry away cellular wastes to the excretory organs
- To allow lymphatic flow to drain tissue fluid back into the circulation
- To return blood to the heart for recirculation

This system of conduits depends on an efficient heart and patent blood vessels to regulate and maintain systemic and regional blood flow and temperature.

The vascular system is divided into the arterial system and the venous system (Fig. 32–8). In the arterial system, blood moves from a system of larger conduits to a network of smaller blood vessels. In the venous system, blood travels from the capillaries to the venules and to the larger system of veins, eventually returning in the venae cavae to the heart for recirculation.

ARTERIAL SYSTEM

STRUCTURE

The high-pressure blood vessels of the arterial vascular system may be classified according to their size and wall structure. The large arteries follow relatively straight routes and have few branches. Such arteries include the aorta, the common and external ileac arteries, the femoral arteries, and the popliteal arteries. Smaller arteries divide from larger ones and have multiple branches. These include the mesenteric arteries of the abdomen, the internal iliac arteries, and the deep femoral vessels. The structure and function of the vasculature of the cerebrum, the abdomen, and the viscera are discussed as they relate to each body system.

Some arteries branch into arterioles, which measure less than 0.5 mm in diameter, whereas some

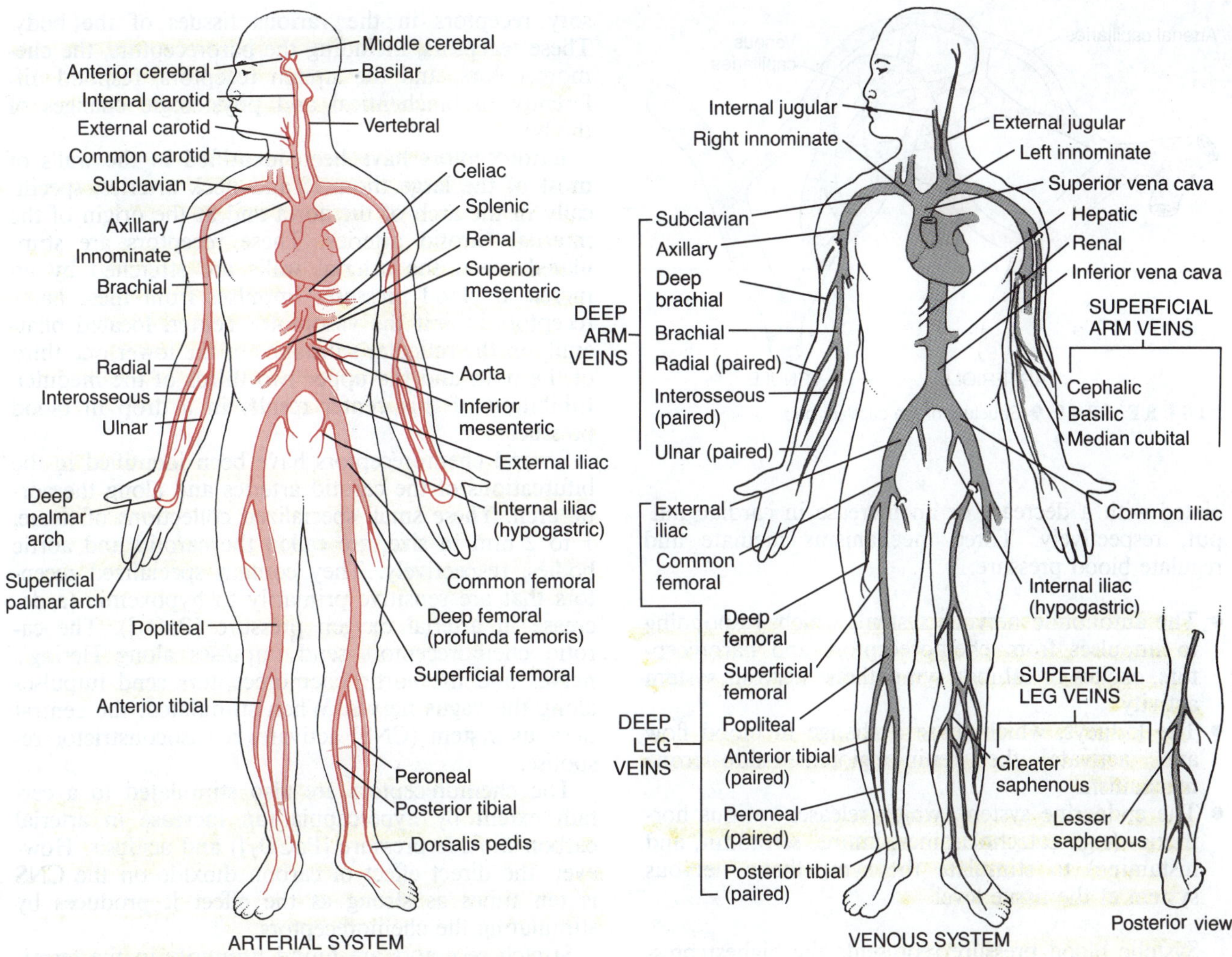

FIGURE 32–8 ◆ Anatomy of the arterial and venous systems.

arteries anastomose with other arteries. The arterioles branch into terminal arterioles, which join with the capillary or capillaries and ultimately join with venules, forming the capillary network (Fig. 32–9). The exchange of nutrients across the capillary membrane occurs primarily by three processes: osmosis, filtration, and diffusion. (See Chapter 14 for detailed discussions of osmosis, filtration, and diffusion.)

FUNCTION

The arterial system delivers blood to various tissues for nourishment. At the tissue level, nutrients, chemicals, and body defense substances are distributed and exchanged for cellular waste products, depending on the needs of the particular tissue. The arteries transport the cellular wastes to the excretory organs, such as the kidneys, the liver, and the lungs, to be reprocessed or removed. The arteries also contribute to the tissue's temperature regulation. Blood can be either directed toward the skin to promote heat loss or diverted away from the skin to conserve heat.

BLOOD PRESSURE

Blood pressure is the force of blood exerted against the vessel walls. Pressure in the larger blood vessels is greater (about 80 to 100 mmHg) and decreases as blood flow reaches the capillaries (about 25 mmHg). By the time blood enters the right atrium, blood pressure is approximately 0 to 5 mmHg.

INDIRECT MEASUREMENT OF BLOOD PRESSURE

The blood pressure in the arterial system is determined primarily by the quantity of blood flow or cardiac output and the resistance in the arterioles.

$$\text{blood pressure} = \text{cardiac output} \times \text{peripheral vascular resistance}$$

Therefore, any factor that increases cardiac output or total peripheral vascular resistance increases blood pressure. In general, blood pressure is maintained at a relatively constant level so that an increase or decrease in total peripheral vascular resistance is asso-

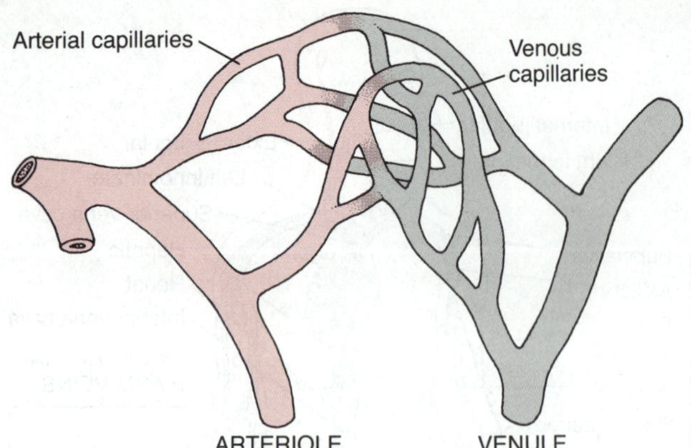

FIGURE 32-9 ◆ Structure of the capillary bed.

ciated with a decrease or an increase in cardiac output, respectively. Three mechanisms mediate and regulate blood pressure:

- The autonomic nervous system, which, responding to impulses from chemoreceptors and baroreceptors, excites or inhibits sympathetic nervous system activity
- The kidneys, which sense a change in blood flow and activate the renin-angiotensin-aldosterone mechanism
- The endocrine system, which releases various hormones (e.g., catecholamines, kinins, serotonin, and histamine) to stimulate the sympathetic nervous system at the tissue level

Systolic blood pressure represents the highest pressure occurring in an artery with each contraction of the heart; diastolic blood pressure represents the lowest pressure during the relaxation phase of the heart. In the adult, systolic pressure is normally 90 to 140 mmHg and diastolic pressure is normally 60 to 90 mmHg (AHA, 1992). Blood pressure is expressed as a fraction: systolic/diastolic.

Systolic pressure is affected by a number of factors, including cardiac output. When cardiac output decreases, systolic pressure also decreases. Diastolic pressure is primarily determined by the amount of vasoconstriction in the periphery. An increase in peripheral vascular resistance increases diastolic pressure.

REGULATION OF BLOOD PRESSURE

The autonomic nervous system (ANS) and the renal system are primarily responsible for regulating blood pressure, although external factors can also affect a person's blood pressure.

AUTONOMIC NERVOUS SYSTEM Blood pressure is regulated by balancing the sympathetic and parasympathetic nervous systems of the autonomic nervous system. Changes in sympathetic and parasympathetic activities are responses to messages sent by the sensory receptors in the various tissues of the body. These receptors, including the baroreceptors, the chemoreceptors, and the stretch receptors, respond differently to biochemical and physiologic changes of the body.

Baroreceptors have been identified in the walls of most of the large thoracic and neck arteries, specifically in the arch of the aorta and at the origin of the internal carotid arteries. These receptors are stimulated when the arterial walls are stretched by an increased blood pressure. Impulses from these baroreceptors inhibit the vasomotor center, located bilaterally in the reticular substance of the lower one third of the pons and the upper two thirds of the medulla. Inhibition of this center results in a drop in blood pressure.

Several chemoreceptors have been identified in the bifurcations of the carotid arteries and along the aortic arch. These small specialized collections of tissue, 1 to 2 mm in size, are called the carotid and aortic bodies, respectively. They contain specialized receptors that are sensitive primarily to hypoxemia (a decrease in arterial oxygen pressure [PaO_2]). The carotid chemoreceptors send impulses along Hering's nerves and the aortic chemoreceptors send impulses along the vagus nerves. When stimulated, the central nervous system (CNS) activates a vasoconstrictor response.

The chemoreceptors are also stimulated to a certain extent by hypercapnia (an increase in arterial carbon dioxide pressure [$PaCO_2$]) and acidosis. However, the direct effect of carbon dioxide on the CNS is ten times as strong as the effect it produces by stimulating the chemoreceptors.

Stretch receptors are found primarily in the terminal portions of the venae cavae and the right atrium. These receptors are sensitive to pressure or volume changes. When a client is hypovolemic, the stretch receptors in the blood vessels sense a reduced volume or pressure and elicit fewer impulses to the CNS. This reaction stimulates the sympathetic nervous system to increase heart rate and to constrict the peripheral blood vessels.

RENAL SYSTEM The renal system also helps to regulate cardiovascular activity. When renal blood flow or pressure decreases, the kidneys tend to retain sodium and water. Blood pressure tends to rise because of fluid retention and because of activation of the renin-angiotensin-aldosterone mechanism. Vascular volume is also regulated by the release of antidiuretic hormone (vasopressin) from the posterior pituitary gland (see Chap. 14).

EXTERNAL FACTORS Other factors can influence the activity of the cardiovascular system. For example, emotional behaviors, such as excitement, pain, and anger, stimulate the sympathetic nervous system to increase blood pressure. Increased physical activity such as exercise increases blood pressure and pulse rate as well. Body temperature can affect the metabolic needs of the tissues, thereby influencing the delivery of blood. In hypothermia, tissues require fewer nutrients and blood pressure falls. In hyperthermia, the metabolic requirement of the tissues is greater, and blood pressure rises.

VENOUS SYSTEM

STRUCTURE

The venous system is composed of a series of veins that are located adjacent to the arterial system. In addition, a second venous circulation is superficial and runs parallel to the subcutaneous tissue of the extremity. These two venous systems are connected by communicating veins, which provide a means for blood to travel from the superficial veins to the deep veins. Blood flow is directed toward the deep venous circulation.

The venules collect blood from the capillaries and the terminal arterioles. Venules also serve as a location where white blood cells enter into and exit from the body tissues.

Venules branch into veins, which are low-pressure blood vessels. Veins have the ability to accommodate large shifts in volume with minimal changes in venous pressure. This flexibility allows the venous system to accommodate the administration of intravenous (IV) fluids and blood transfusions, blood loss, and dehydration. In both the superficial and deep venous systems, all veins, except for the smallest and the largest veins, have valves directing blood flow back to the heart, preventing retrograde flow (backflow).

FUNCTION

The primary function of the venous system is to provide for the return of blood from the capillaries to the right side of the heart for circulation. It also acts as a reservoir for a large portion of the blood volume. In contrast to the arterial system, which consists of a high-pressure, continuous flow system through relatively rigid conduits, the venous system consists of a low-pressure, intermittent flow system through collapsible tubes working against the effects of gravity.

Gravity exerts an increase in hydrostatic pressure (capillary blood pressure) when the client is in an upright position, which delays venous return. When the client is lying down, the hydrostatic pressure is lessened, and thus there is less hindrance of venous return to the heart.

Cardiovascular Changes Associated with Aging

A number of physiologic changes in the cardiovascular system occur with advancing age (Chart 32–1). Many of these changes result in loss of cardiac reserve. Thus, these changes may not be evident when the older adult is resting. They become apparent only when the person is physically or emotionally stressed and the heart cannot meet the demands of the body.

HISTORY

The nurse obtains a thorough history, which includes demographic data, personal and family history, diet, socioeconomic status, and a functional assessment. Information relative to risk factors and symptoms of cardiovascular disease is the focus of the history.

Demographic Data

Demographic data include the client's age, sex, and ethnic origin. The incidence of conditions such as coronary artery disease (CAD) and valvular disease increases with age (Braunwald, 1992; Eliopoulos, 1991). The incidence of CAD also varies with the client's sex (Braunwald, 1992). Women who are premenopausal have a lower incidence of CAD than do men.

Transcultural Considerations Information about the client's ethnic or cultural background is important because some disease conditions may be more prevalent in specific ethnic groups. For example, high blood pressure is particularly prevalent in African-American women. African-Americans, Puerto Ricans, Cubans, and Mexican-Americans have a higher incidence of hypertension than do Caucasians (Jarvis, 1992).

Age, sex, and ethnic background, as well as a family history of cardiovascular disease, are considered nonmodifiable or uncontrollable risk factors for cardiovascular disease (Braunwald, 1992). Modifiable risk factors (e.g., high blood pressure and excessive blood cholesterol level) are risk factors that, if controlled, can reduce the risk of heart disease. These factors are discussed in detail later under Socioeconomic Status and in Chapter 37.

Personal and Family History

The nurse notes a history of major illnesses, such as diabetes mellitus, renal disease, anemia, high blood pressure, stroke, bleeding disorders, connective tissue diseases, chronic pulmonary diseases, heart disease, and thrombophlebitis. These conditions can influence the client's cardiovascular status.

The nurse also asks about previous experiences with the health care system. For example, previous hospitalizations may have included treatment for injuries, surgeries, and diagnostic testing (e.g., electrocardiography and cardiac catheterization) in either an inpatient or an outpatient (ambulatory) setting. It is important for the nurse to ask specifically about

CHART 32-1

Nursing Focus on the Elderly ◆ Changes in the Cardiovascular System Related to Aging

Structure/Function	Change	Nursing Implications*	Rationale
Cardiac valves	• Calcification and mucoid degeneration occur, especially in the mitral valve.	• Assess heart sounds for murmurs. • Question clients about dyspnea.	• Murmurs may be detected before other symptoms.
Conduction system	• Pacemaker cells decrease in number. Fibrous tissue and fat in the SA node increase. • Few muscle fibers remain in the atrial myocardium and bundle of His.	• Assess the ECG and heart rhythm for dysrhythmias or a heart rate less than 60 beats per minute	• The SA node may lose its inherent rhythm. • Dysrhythmias (both atrial and ventricular) tend to be more common in older adults.
Left ventricle	• The size of the left ventricle increases. • The left ventricle becomes stiff and less distensible. • The ejection phase becomes longer and there is a delay in early diastolic filling to compensate for the stiff ventricle, allowing the heart to "empty" more effectively.	• Assess the ECG for a widening QRS complex and a longer QT interval. • Assess for activity intolerance. • Assess the heart rate at rest and with activity.	• Conduction time increases. • Ventricular changes result in decreased stroke volume, ejection fraction, and cardiac output; the heart is less able to meet increased oxygen demands. • Maximal heart rate with exercise is decreased.
Blood flow in coronary vessels	• The distribution of blood flow changes, with more blood flowing to venous vessels and sinusoids and less flowing to the coronary arteries.	• Assess for activity intolerance.	• The heart is less able to meet increased oxygen demands.
Aorta and other large arteries	• The aorta and other large arteries thicken and become stiffer and less distensible. Systolic blood pressure increases to compensate for the stiff arteries. • Systemic vascular resistance increases as a result of less distensible arteries, so the left ventricle pumps against greater resistance, contributing to left ventricular hypertrophy.	• Assess blood pressure. • Note increases in systolic, diastolic, and pulse pressures. • Assess for activity intolerance and shortness of breath. • Assess the peripheral pulses.	• Hypertension may occur, which must be treated to avoid target organ damage. • Left ventricular hypertrophy decreases cardiac output and may lead to congestive heart failure.
Baroreceptors	• Baroreceptors become less sensitive.	• Assess the client's blood pressure with the client lying, then sitting or standing. • Assess for dizziness when the client changes from a lying to a sitting or standing position. • Teach clients to change positions slowly.	• Orthostatic (postural) changes occur because of ineffective baroreceptors. Changes may include drops in blood pressure of 10 mmHg or more, dizziness, and fainting.

* ECG, electrocardiogram.

streptococcal infections and rheumatic fever because these conditions may lead to valvular abnormalities of the heart. In addition, the nurse inquires about any known congenital heart defects.

The nurse questions clients about any known sensitivity to penicillin or any drugs that may be needed in an emergency, such as lidocaine (Xylocaine). A thorough assessment of all prescription drugs and over-the-counter drugs that the client is taking is imperative. The nurse specifically asks clients if they have recently used cocaine or any IV "street" drugs, because they may be associated with chest pain or endocarditis. The nurse also asks female clients if they are taking oral contraceptives. There is an increased incidence of myocardial infarction (MI) and cerebrovascular accident in older women who take oral contraceptives, but only if they smoke, have diabetes, or have hypertension (Mishell, 1989).

A family history includes information about the age and health status, as well as deaths, of immediate family members (i.e., parents, siblings, spouse, and children). The nurse may also ask about the extended family, including grandparents and grandchildren. The nurse can record this information in a narrative outline or as a diagram with the client's history.

Diet History

A diet history might include the client's recall of food and fluid intake during a 24-hour period, self-imposed or medically prescribed dietary restrictions or supplementations, and the amount and type of alcohol consumption. The nurse and the dietitian examine the type of foods selected by the client for the amount of sodium, sugar, cholesterol, and fat. These elements have been associated with coronary artery disease and high blood pressure. A diet history also examines the client's attitudes toward food, knowledge level of essential and nonessential dietary elements, and willingness to make changes in the diet. Cultural beliefs and economic status can influence the client's choice of food items and must be reviewed. Family members or significant others who are responsible for shopping and cooking are included in the discussion.

Socioeconomic Status

Social history includes information about the client's domestic situation, such as marital status, number of children, household members, living environment, and occupation. The nurse also identifies the client's support systems. It is especially important for the nurse to explore the possibility that the client might have difficulty paying for medications or treatment.

The nurse asks about the client's occupation, including the type of work performed and the requirements of the specific job. For instance, does the job involve lifting of heavy objects? Is the job emotionally stressful? What does a day's work entail? Does the client's job require him or her to be outside in extremes of weather?

Lifestyle habits that are specific risk factors for heart disease include cigarette smoking, physical inactivity, obesity, and type A behavior. These factors are considered modifiable or controllable risk factors.

CIGARETTE SMOKING

Cigarette smoking is a major risk factor for cardiovascular disease, specifically coronary artery disease (CAD) and peripheral vascular disease (PVD) (AHA, 1992). According to the U. S. Department of Health and Human Services (DHHS), cigarette smoking is directly responsible for 21% of all deaths from CAD (DHHS, 1990). Three compounds in cigarette smoke (tar, nicotine, and carbon monoxide) have been implicated in the development of CAD.

The smoking history should include the number of cigarettes smoked daily, the duration of the smoking habit, the age of the client when smoking started, and the pattern of inhaling. Typically, the nurse records the smoking history in pack-years, which is the number of packs per day multiplied by the number of years that the client smoked. The nurse should also inquire about the client's desire to quit, past attempts to quit, and the methods used.

The risks to the cardiovascular system from cigarette smoking appear to be noncumulative and transient. Three to four years after a client has stopped smoking, his or her cardiovascular risk appears to be similar to that of a person who has never smoked. The nurse asks clients who do not currently smoke if they have ever smoked and when they quit.

PHYSICAL INACTIVITY

Physical inactivity is also considered a significant risk factor in the development of heart disease. Regular physical activity promotes cardiovascular fitness and produces beneficial changes in blood pressure and levels of blood lipids and clotting factors. Unfortunately, few people in the United States engage in the recommended 30 minutes daily of light-to-moderate exercise, equivalent to a 30-minute brisk walk. According to DHHS (1990), only 22% of Americans engage in this much exercise 5 times a week and only 10% engage in vigorous physical activity, enough to promote cardiopulmonary fitness, 3 times a week. This puts more people at risk for CAD owing to physical inactivity than any other factor. The nurse questions clients concerning the type of exercise in which they engage, how long they have participated in the exercise, and the frequency and the intensity of the exercise.

OBESITY

Obesity affects about 26% of the United States population (DHHS, 1990). It is particularly a problem for poor and minority populations, such as Hispanic-American and African-American women (Jarvis, 1992). Obesity is associated with hypertension, hyperlipidemia, and diabetes; all are known contributors to cardiovascular disease. The nurse examines the client for his or her pattern of obesity, also known as waist/hip ratio. Clients with abdominal obesity (greater waist than hip circumference) are more likely to develop cardiovascular disease than are clients with fat distributed in their buttocks, hips, and thighs (greater hip than waist circumference).

The nurse reviews the client's patterns of dieting and weight loss to identify any patterns of weight loss and regain. Clients with patterns of weight loss and regain have higher cardiovascular morbidity and mortality than do clients with stable weights. It is also important to identify the age of onset of obesity. Clients with an early onset of obesity (during adolescence) with an elevated waist/hip ratio appear to be at especially high risk for cardiovascular disease (Weigle, 1992).

TYPE A PERSONALITY

Researchers have identified people with type A personalities as being more vulnerable to the development of heart disease (Braunwald, 1992). Type A personalities are highly competitive, are overly concerned about meeting deadlines, and are often hostile and angry. Although there is a positive correlation between people identified as having type A personalities and heart disease, conclusive proof remains elusive.

Current Health Problems

Inquiring about the client's major concerns helps the nurse to establish priorities in nursing care and management. The nurse asks the client to describe his or her concerns. Then the nurse expands on the client's description by obtaining information about their onset, duration, chronology and frequency, location, quality, intensity, associated symptoms, and precipitating or aggravating and relieving factors. Major symptoms identified by clients with cardiovascular disease include:

- Chest pain or discomfort
- Dyspnea
- Fatigue
- Palpitations
- Weight gain
- Syncope
- Extremity pain

CHEST PAIN

Chest pain or discomfort, a cardinal symptom of heart disease, can result from ischemic heart disease, pericarditis, and aortic dissection. Chest pain can also be due to noncardiac conditions, such as pleurisy, pulmonary embolus, hiatal hernia, and anxiety. Nurses must thoroughly evaluate the nature and characteristics of the client's chest pain. Because chest pain resulting from myocardial ischemia is life-threatening and can lead to serious complications, the cause of chest pain should be considered ischemic (reduced or obstructed blood flow to the myocardium) until proven otherwise.

In many health care settings, the nurse may be the first health care professional to evaluate the client with chest pain. Nursing research by Bonnono et al. (1992) found that nurses accurately assessed clients for potential myocardial infarctions when compared with physician assessments (Research Applications for Nursing).

When assessing for chest pain, the nurse uses alternative terms such as "discomfort," "heaviness," and "indigestion." Often, clients deny a true pain in the chest but admit to discomfort or a feeling of indigestion. The client may also use other descriptors, such as aching, choking, strangling, tingling, squeezing, constricting, and vise-like.

The nurse asks the client to identify when the pain was first noticed (onset). Did the pain begin suddenly or develop gradually (what was its manner of onset)? How long did the pain last (what was its duration)? If the client has repeated chest pain episodes, the nurse assesses how long the pain usually lasts (its chronol-

RESEARCH APPLICATIONS FOR NURSING

In Emergency Services, Nurses and Physicians Tend to Have the Same Clinical Impressions of Clients with Chest Pain

Bonnono, C., Hedges, J. R., Peterson, C., & Collings, J. L. (1992). Initial nursing impression in patients with chest discomfort. *Journal of Emergency Nursing, 18*(1), 28–32.

This study examines the ability of nurses and physicians to evaluate accurately clients with chest pain who entered the emergency department of one hospital. The study subjects were all older than 30 years of age and reported angina. Of 148 clients, 39 (26%) had evidence of myocardial ischemia.

The researchers found that there was a statistically significant agreement between the nurse's and the physician's clinical impressions, on the basis of diagnosis, hospital admission, and admission to the coronary care unit.

Critique This study shows the importance of the nurse in accurately evaluating the cause or the source of chest pain. Several methods were used to measure the dependent variable—the likelihood of nurse-physician agreement.

Possible nursing implications This study supports the contribution of nurses in guiding the physician's initial clinical impression of chest pain in people who have nondiagnostic electrocardiographic changes. Further studies are needed to evaluate how communication of findings by primary nurses to physicians can be improved.

TABLE 32–1 Assessment of Chest Pain: How Various Types of Chest Pain Differ

Source	Onset	Quality and Severity	Location and Radiation	Duration and Relieving Factors
Angina	• Sudden, usually in response to exertion	• Squeezing vise-like pain	• Substernal, may spread across the chest and the back and/or down the arms	• Usually lasts 15 min, relieved with rest, nitroglycerin administration, or oxygen therapy
Myocardial infarction	• Sudden, without precipitating factors	• Intense stabbing vise-like pain or pressure, severe	• Substernal, may spread throughout the anterior chest and to the arms, the jaw, the back, or the neck	• Usually lasts 30 min or longer or is relieved with opioids
Pericarditis	• Sudden	• Sharp stabbing, moderate to severe	• Substernal, usually spreads to the left side or the back	• Intermittent, relieved with sitting upright, analgesia, or, the administration of anti-inflammatory agents
Pleuropulmonary	• Variable	• Moderate ache, worse on inspiration	• Lung fields	• Continuous until the underlying condition is treated or the client has rested
Esophageal/gastric	• Variable	• Squeezing, heartburn, variable severity	• Substernal, may spread to the shoulders or the abdomen	• Variable, may be relieved with antacid administration or food intake
Anxiety	• Variable, may be in response to stress or fatigue	• Dull ache to sharp stabbing, may be associated with numbness in fingers	• Usually the left side of chest without radiation	• Usually lasts a few minutes

ogy and frequency). Is this pain different from any other episodes of pain? The nurse asks the client to describe what activities he or she was doing at the time it first occurred (e.g., sleeping, watching television, arguing, and running) (precipitating factors). The client can be asked to point to the area where the chest pain occurred (its location). Did the pain stay in one specific area or did it move (what was its radiation)?

In addition, the client describes how the pain feels and whether it is sharp or dull (its quality). To understand how severe the pain is, the nurse asks the client to grade the pain from zero to ten, with zero indicating the absence of pain and ten indicating severe pain (intensity). The client may also report other signs and symptoms that occur at the same time (associated symptoms), such as dyspnea, diaphoresis, nausea, and vomiting. Other factors that need to be addressed are those that may have made the chest pain worse (aggravating factors) or made the pain less intense (relieving factors). Chest pain may arise from a variety of sources (Table 32–1). The nurse must address these areas to find the origin of the client's chest pain.

DYSPNEA

Dyspnea is a symptom that can occur from both heart and pulmonary disease. Dyspnea is objectively described as difficult or labored breathing and is subjectively experienced as uncomfortable breathing, or shortness of breath. When obtaining the client's history, the nurse ascertains what factors precipitate and relieve dyspnea, what level of activity produces dyspnea, and what the assumed body position was when dyspnea first occurred.

There are several types of dyspnea. Dyspnea that is associated with exertional activity, such as climbing stairs, is referred to as dyspnea on exertion (DOE). This is usually an early symptom of heart failure.

The client with advanced heart disease may develop orthopnea, in which dyspnea appears as soon as the client assumes the lateral recumbent position. The client may use several pillows at night to elevate the head or sleep in a recliner to prevent nighttime breathlessness. The severity of orthopnea is measured by the number of pillows or the amount of head elevation needed to provide restful sleep. Orthopnea is usually relieved within a matter of minutes by sitting up or standing.

Paroxysmal nocturnal dyspnea occurs after the client has been recumbent for several hours. When the client is in a lateral recumbent position, blood from the splanchnic beds and lower extremities is redistributed to the venous system, thereby increasing venous return. This increase in blood volume returning to the heart elevates pulmonary venous and pulmonary arterial pressures. A diseased heart is unable to compensate for the increased intravascular volume and is ineffective in pumping the additional fluid into the circulatory system. Therefore, pulmonary congestion results. Clients awaken abruptly, often with a feeling of suffocation and panic. They usually sit upright with their legs dangled over the bedside to relieve the dyspnea. It may take as long as 20 minutes before the client obtains relief, which can be quite distressing.

FATIGUE

Fatigue may be described as the inability to complete routine activities of daily living (ADL). The client may indicate that a certain activity takes longer to complete. Fatigue in itself is not diagnostic of heart disease. Nevertheless, in clients with heart disease, fatigue may result from nocturia, insomnia, and exertional and nocturnal dyspnea. Fatigue that occurs after mild activity and exertion usually indicates an inadequate cardiac output (low stroke volume). The nurse questions the client to determine when he or she has experienced fatigue as well as what activities can be performed. The nurse asks if he or she can perform the same activities as a year ago or the same activities as others of the same age. Often, clients limit their activities in response to fatigue without being aware how much less active they have become.

PALPITATIONS

A feeling of fluttering in the chest or an unpleasant awareness of the heartbeat is referred to as palpitations. Palpitations may result from a change in heart rate or rhythm or from an increase in the force of heart contractions. Rhythm disturbances that may cause palpitations include paroxysmal atrial tachycardia, premature contractions, and sinus tachycardia. Palpitations that occur during or after strenuous physical activity, such as running and swimming, may indicate overexertion or possibly heart disease. Some noncardiac factors that may precipitate palpitations include anxiety, stress, fatigue, insomnia, and the ingestion of caffeine, nicotine, or alcohol.

WEIGHT GAIN

A sudden increase in weight of 2.2 pounds (1 kg) can be the result of an accumulation of excessive fluid (1 L) in the interstitial spaces, commonly known as *edema.* It is possible, however, for weight gains of up to 10 to 15 pounds (4.5 to 6.8 kg, or 4 to 7 L of fluid) to occur before any associated edema occurs. The nurse should inquire whether the client has experienced a tightness of shoes, noted indentations from socks, or noted tightness of rings. Generalized edema is referred to as *anasarca.*

SYNCOPE

Syncope refers to a transient loss of consciousness. The most common cause is decreased perfusion to the brain. Any condition that suddenly reduces the cardiac output, resulting in decreased cerebral blood flow, could potentiate a syncopal episode. Conditions such as cardiac rhythm disturbances (ventricular dysrhythmias or Stokes-Adams attack) and valvular disorders (aortic stenosis) may potentiate this symptom.

Syncope in the aging client may result from hypersensitivity of the carotid sinus bodies, located in the neck arteries. Pressure applied to the carotid arteries (e.g., during turning the head, shrugging the shoulders, shaving, or buttoning a shirt) stimulates a vagal response. A decrease in blood pressure and heart rate usually results, but an exaggerated response may produce syncope. Syncope in the older adult may also result from orthostatic (postural) hypotension due to an age-affected baroreceptor response.

Near-syncope refers to dizziness with an inability to remain in an upright position. The nurse explores the circumstances that lead to dizziness or syncope.

EXTREMITY PAIN

Extremity pain may result from two conditions: ischemia from atherosclerosis and venous insufficiency of the peripheral blood vessels. Clients who report a moderate-to-severe cramping sensation in their legs or buttocks associated with an activity such as walking have *intermittent claudication* related to reduced arterial tissue perfusion. Claudication pain is usually relieved by resting or lowering the affected extremity to decrease tissue demands or to enhance arterial blood flow. Leg pain that results from prolonged standing or sitting is related to venous insufficiency from either incompetent valves or venous obstruction. This pain may be relieved by elevating the extremity.

Functional History

After obtaining the history of the client's cardiac status, the client may be classified according to the New York Heart Association's Functional Classification (Table 32–2). The four classifications (I, II, III, and IV) depend on the degree to which ordinary physical activities (routine activities of daily living [ADL]) are affected by heart disease.

PHYSICAL ASSESSMENT

A thorough physical assessment is the foundation for the nursing data base and the formation of nursing diagnoses. Any changes noted during the client's hospital course can be compared with this initial data base. The nurse evaluates vital signs (blood pressure, pulse rate, and respiration rate) when the client is admitted to the hospital and at least every 4 hours until the client's condition improves.

TABLE 32–2 New York Heart Association Functional Classification of Cardiovascular Disability

Class I

- Clients with cardiac disease but without resulting limitations of physical activity
- Ordinary physical activity does not cause undue fatigue, palpitation, dyspnea, or anginal pain.

Class II

- Clients with cardiac disease resulting in slight limitation of physical activity
- They are comfortable at rest.
- Ordinary physical activity results in fatigue, palpitation, dyspnea, or anginal pain.

Class III

- Clients with cardiac disease resulting in marked limitation of physical activity
- They are comfortable at rest.
- Less than ordinary physical activity causes fatigue, palpitation, dyspnea, or anginal pain.

Class IV

- Clients with cardiac disease resulting in inability to carry on any physical activity without discomfort
- Symptoms of cardiac insufficiency or of the anginal syndrome may be present even at rest.
- If any physical activity is undertaken, discomfort is increased.

Excerpted from *Diseases of the heart and blood vessels—nomenclature and criteria for diagnosis,* 6th edition, Boston, Little, Brown and Company, copyright 1964 by the New York Heart Association, Inc.

General Appearance

Physical assessment begins with the client's general appearance. The nurse assesses the following areas: the general build and appearance of the client, as well as skin color; distress level; level of consciousness; presence of shortness of breath; position; and verbal responses.

Clients with chronic heart failure may appear malnourished, thin, and cachectic. Latent signs of severe heart failure are ascites, jaundice, and anasarca as a result of prolonged congestion of the liver. Heart failure may cause fluid retention, and clients may have engorged neck veins and generalized dependent edema.

Coronary artery disease is suspected in clients with yellow lipid-filled plaques on the upper eyelids (xanthelasma) or earlobe creases. Clients with poor cardiac output and decreased cerebral perfusion may have mental confusion, memory loss, and slowed verbal responses.

Integumentary System

Assessment and evaluation of the integumentary system is determined primarily by the color and temperature of the skin. The best areas for the nurse to assess circulation include the nail beds, the mucous membranes, and the conjunctival mucosa, because small blood vessels are located near the surface of the skin.

SKIN COLOR

If there is normal blood flow or adequate perfusion of a given area in light-colored skin, it appears pink, perhaps rosy in color, and warm to touch. Decreased flow is depicted as cool, pale-looking, and moist skin. Pallor is characteristic of anemia and can be seen in areas such as the nail beds, the palms, and the conjunctival mucous membranes.

A bluish or darkened discoloration of the skin and mucous membranes is referred to as *cyanosis.* Cyanosis results from an increased amount of deoxygenated hemoglobin.

In central cyanosis, there is decreased oxygenation of the arterial blood in the lungs, which manifests as a bluish tinge of the conjunctivae and the mucous membranes of the mouth and tongue. Central cyanosis may indicate impaired lung function or a right-to-left shunt found in congenital heart conditions.

Because of impaired circulation, there is a marked desaturation of hemoglobin in the peripheral tissues, which produces a bluish or darkened discoloration of the nail beds, the earlobes, the lips, and the toes. Peripheral cyanosis occurs in severe heart disease when blood flow to the peripheral vessels is decreased by peripheral vasoconstriction. The clamping down of the peripheral blood vessels is the result of a low cardiac output or an increased extraction of oxygen from the peripheral tissues. Peripheral cyanosis localized in an extremity is usually a result of arterial or venous obstruction.

SKIN TEMPERATURE

The temperature of the skin can be assessed for symmetry by touching different areas of the client's body (e.g., arms, hands, legs, and feet) with the dorsal surface of the hand or fingers. Decreased blood flow results in decreased skin temperature. The skin temperature is lowered in several clinical conditions, including heart failure, peripheral vascular disease, and shock.

Extremities

The nurse assesses the client's hands, arms, feet, and legs for skin changes, vascular changes, clubbing, capillary filling, and edema. Skin mobility and turgor are affected by the fluid status of the client. Dehydration and aging reduce skin turgor, and edema decreases skin mobility. Vascular changes of an affected extremity may include paresthesia, muscle fatigue and discomfort, numbness, pain, coolness, and loss of hair distribution from a reduced blood supply. Clubbing of the fingers and toes results from chronic oxygen deprivation in these tissue beds. Clubbing is characteristic in clients with advanced chronic pulmonary disease, congenital heart defects, and cor pulmonale. Clubbing can be identified by assessing the angle of the nail bed. The angle of the normal nail bed is 160 degrees; with clubbing, the angle of the nail bed increases to greater than 180 degrees and the base of the nail becomes spongy. Figure 32–10 describes the assessment of clubbing using the Schamrath method.

Capillary filling of the fingers and the toes is an indicator of peripheral circulation. Pressing or blanching the nail bed of a finger or a toe produces a whitening effect; when pressure is released, a brisk return of color should occur in the nail bed. If color returns within 3 seconds, peripheral circulation is considered intact. If the capillary refill time exceeds 3 seconds, the lack of circulation may be due to arterial insufficiency from atherosclerosis or spasm. Rubor (dusky redness) that replaces pallor in a dependent foot suggests arterial insufficiency.

Peripheral edema is a common finding in clients with cardiovascular problems. The location of edema helps the nurse to determine its potential cause. Bilateral edema of the legs may be seen in clients with heart failure or with chronic venous insufficiency. Abdominal and leg edema can be seen in clients with heart disease and cirrhosis of the liver. Localized edema in one extremity may be the result of venous obstruction (thrombosis) or lymphatic blockage of the extremity (lymphedema). Edema may also be noted in dependent areas, such as the sacrum, when a client is confined to bed.

The nurse documents the location of edema as precisely as possible (e.g., mid-tibial or sacral) and the number of centimeters from an anatomic landmark. Although some health care practitioners attempt to grade edema as mild, moderate, and severe, or 1+, 2+, 3+, or 4+, no universal scale is used. In addition, these values are not precise and are subjective. Instead of using a grading scale, the nurse determines whether the edema is pitting (the skin can be indented) or nonpitting, how deep the pit is (in millimeters), and how long the pit lasts (in seconds).

Blood Pressure Measurement

The indirect measurement of arterial blood pressure is done by sphygmomanometry (Chart 32–2). This technique of measurement is described in greater detail in nursing skills books.

The normal blood pressure in adults older than 45 years of age ranges from 90 to 140 mmHg for systolic pressure and 60 to 90 mmHg for diastolic pressure (AHA, 1989). A blood pressure that exceeds 140/90 mmHg increases the workload of the left ventricle and oxygen consumption. A blood pressure less than 90/60 mmHg may be inadequate in providing proper and sufficient nutrition to the cells of the body.

In certain circumstances, such as shock, the Korotkoff sounds are less audible or absent. In such circumstances, the nurse might palpate the blood pressure, use an ultrasonic device (Doppler device), or obtain a direct measurement by arterial catheter. When a blood pressure is palpated, the diastolic pressure is usually not obtainable. More information on direct measurement of arterial pressure is available under Hemodynamic Monitoring in this chapter.

POSTURAL BLOOD PRESSURE

Clients may report dizziness or lightheadedness when they move from a flat supine position to a sitting or a standing position at the edge of the bed. Normally, these symptoms are transient and pass

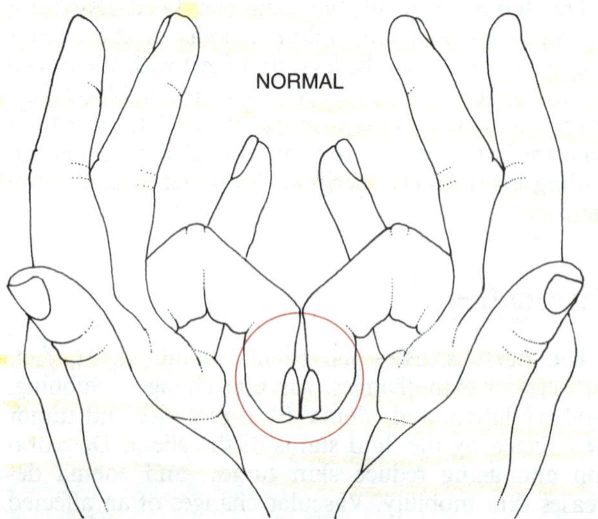

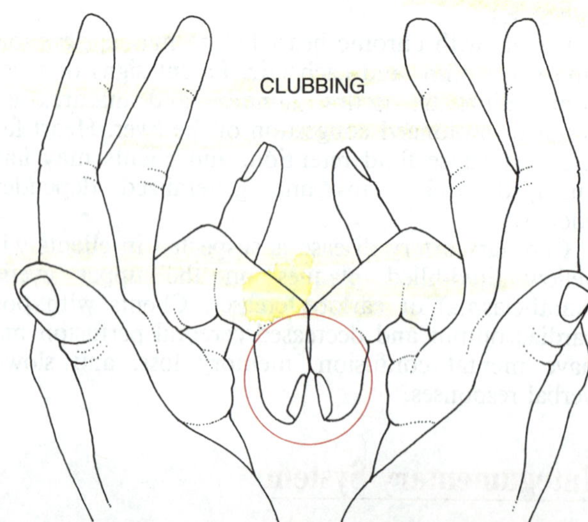

FIGURE 32–10 ◆ Assessment of clubbing by the Schamrath method. The client places the fingernails of the ring fingers together and holds them up to a light. If the examiner can see a diamond shape between the nails, there is no clubbing. Clubbing is identified by the absence of the diamond shape.

CHART 32–2

Nursing Care Highlight ◆ Tips for Accurate Blood Pressure Measurement

- Select the proper cuff size:
  - Adult cuff size is 12- to 14-cm wide and 30-cm long.
  - Pediatric cuff size is 8- to 10-cm wide and 26-cm long.
  - Larger adult cuff size is 18- to 20-cm wide.
- Ensure that equipment is properly assembled and calibrated:
  - The cuff bladder should be intact inside the cuff.
  - The sphygmomanometer should be calibrated to 0 mmHg every few months to ensure reliability.
  - The cuff must be placed above the area to be auscultated (e.g., if the right arm is used, the cuff is placed above the brachial artery).
- Follow these steps to ensure correct blood pressure measurement and recording:
  - After palpating the brachial or radial pulse, inflate the cuff 30 mmHg above the level at which those pulses disappear. Release the cuff slowly to palpate the systolic pressure. Reinflate the cuff, and auscultate the systolic and diastolic pressures. The auscultated pulses are referred to as the Korotkoff sounds.
  - Record measurements on both arms to rule out dissecting aortic aneurysm, coarctation of the aorta, vascular obstruction, and possibly errors in measurement. Perform subsequent readings on the extremity with the highest pressure.
  - If the client's arms are inaccessible (after amputation or mastectomy) you can obtain readings using the client's thigh or calf. Auscultate the popliteal artery or the posterior tibial artery, respectively.
  - Obtain and record the client's blood pressure with the client in different positions, including supine, sitting, and standing positions.
  - Record the position of the client and the site used to obtain the blood pressure.

quickly; however, when these symptoms become pronounced, they may be due to orthostatic (postural) hypotension. Postural hypotension occurs when the client's blood pressure is not adequately maintained when moving from a lying to a sitting or standing position. It is defined as a blood pressure fall of more than 10 to 15 mmHg of the systolic pressure or a fall of more than 10 mmHg of the diastolic pressure *and* a 10% to 20% increase in heart rate (Bates, 1991). The causes of postural hypotension include medications, depletion of blood volume, prolonged bed rest, and age-related changes or disorders of the autonomic nervous system.

To detect orthostatic changes in blood pressure, the nurse first takes the client's blood pressure when the client is supine. After remaining supine for at least 3 minutes, the client changes position to sitting or standing. Normally, as the client rises, systolic pressure drops slightly or remains unchanged while diastolic pressure rises slightly. After the client's change in position, a time delay of 1 to 3 minutes should be permitted before auscultating a blood pressure and palpating the radial pulse. The cuff should remain in the proper position on the client's arm. The nurse observes and records any signs or symptoms of distress in the client. If the client is unable to tolerate the position change, he or she is returned to the previous position of comfort.

As a person ages, the autonomic nervous system may lose the ability to compensate rapidly for the gravitational effects of position change and therefore cause postural hypotension. With autonomic insufficiency, there is no increase in heart rate when the client moves to an upright position. Autonomic insufficiency can also occur from the effects of some cardiac drugs, including digoxin, calcium channel blockers, and beta-adrenergic blockers, that inhibit increases in heart rate. Antiparkinsonian drugs, such as levodopa (Dopar), can cause severe postural hypotension as well.

PARADOXICAL BLOOD PRESSURE

Paradoxical blood pressure is defined as an exaggerated decrease in systolic pressure by more than 10 mmHg (normal is 3 to 10 mmHg) during the inspiratory phase of the respiratory cycle (Braunwald, 1992). It is sometimes referred to as pulsus paradoxus. Certain clinical conditions, including pericardial tamponade, constrictive pericarditis, and pulmonary hypertension, that potentially alter the filling pressures in the right and left ventricles, may produce a paradoxical blood pressure. During inspiration, the filling pressures normally decrease slightly. But with decreased fluid volume in the ventricles because of these pathologic conditions, there is an exaggerated or marked reduction in cardiac output. The procedure for assessing a paradoxical blood pressure is found in Chart 34–10 of Chapter 34.

PULSE PRESSURE

The difference between the systolic and diastolic values is referred to as pulse pressure. A normal pulse pressure for an adult is 30 to 40 mmHg. This value can be used as an indirect measure of the client's cardiac output. An increased pulse pressure may be seen in clients with slow heart rates, aortic regurgitation, atherosclerosis, hypertension, and aging. Decreased pulse pressure is rarely normal and results from increased peripheral vascular resistance or decreased stroke volume in clients with heart failure or cardiogenic shock. Decreased pulse pressure can also be seen in clients who are hypovolemic or who have mitral stenosis or regurgitation.

CHART 32-3

Nursing Care Highlight ◆ Assessment of Jugular Venous Pressure and Central Venous Pressure

1. Place the client in a supine position.
2. Raise the head of the bed to approximately 30 to 45 degrees.
3. Shine a light across the client's neck (tangential lighting) to highlight the pulsations of the internal jugular vein.
4. To differentiate the internal jugular vein from the carotid artery, occlude the internal jugular vein with a fingertip at its base, then release. This maneuver easily eliminates the pulse wave in the internal jugular vein.

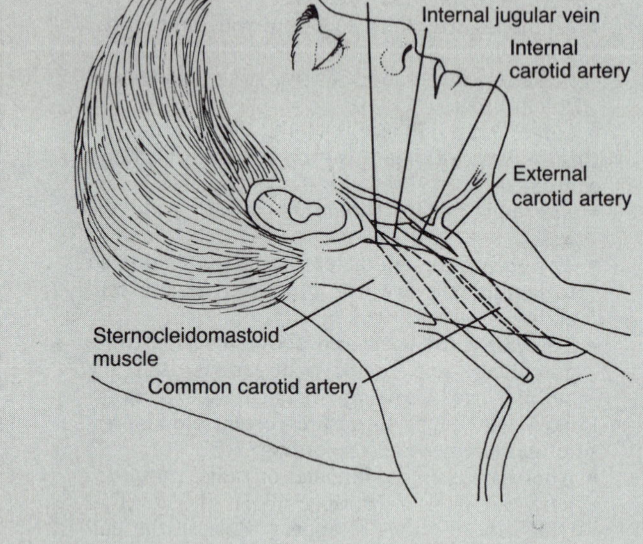

5. Locate the meniscus (the highest point at which pulsations of the internal jugular vein can be seen).
6. Locate the sternal angle (angle of Louis), which can be felt as a notch at the top of the sternum. It is roughly 4 cm above the right atrium.
7. With a centimeter rule, measure the vertical distance from the sternal angle to the meniscus of the internal jugular vein. The reading in centimeters equals the JVP, which generally does not exceed 4 cm.
8. To calculate CVP, add 4 cm to JVP.

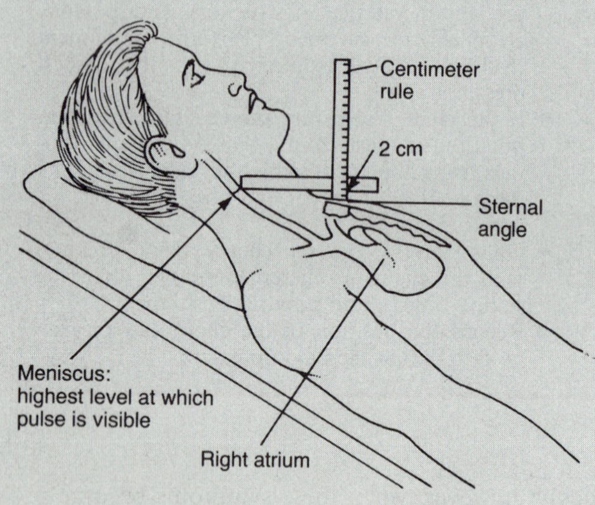

Venous and Arterial Pulsations

VENOUS PULSATIONS

The nurse observes the venous pulsations in the neck to assess the adequacy of blood volume and central venous pressure (CVP). The nurse can assess jugular venous pressure (JVP) to estimate the filling volume and pressure on the right side of the heart (Chart 32-3). The right internal jugular vein is usually used to estimate JVP, because this vessel contains fewer valves than the left.

JVP is normally 3 to 10 cm (Bates, 1991). Increases in JVP are usually caused by right ventricular failure. Other causes include tricuspid regurgitation or stenosis, pulmonary hypertension, cardiac tamponade, constrictive pericarditis, hypervolemia, and superior vena cava obstruction.

The nurse determines hepatojugular reflux by positioning the client with the head of the bed elevated to

45 degrees and locating the internal jugular vein. The nurse compresses the right upper abdomen for 30 to 40 seconds. Sudden distention of the neck veins after abdominal compression is usually indicative of right-sided heart failure.

ARTERIAL PULSATIONS

Assessment of arterial pulsations gives the nurse information about vascular integrity and circulation. All major peripheral pulses, including the temporal, carotid, brachial, radial, ulnar, femoral, popliteal, posterior tibial, and dorsalis pedis pulses, need to be assessed for presence or absence, amplitude, contour, rhythm, rate, and equality. The nurse examines the peripheral arteries in a head-to-toe approach with a side-to-side comparison (Fig. 32-11).

A hypokinetic pulse is a weak pulsation indicative of a narrow pulse pressure. It is seen in clients with hypovolemia, aortic stenosis, and decreased cardiac output.

A hyperkinetic pulse is a large, "bounding" pulse caused by an increased ejection of blood. It is seen in clients with a high cardiac output (with exercise or thyrotoxicosis) or with increased sympathetic system activity (with pain, fever, or anxiety).

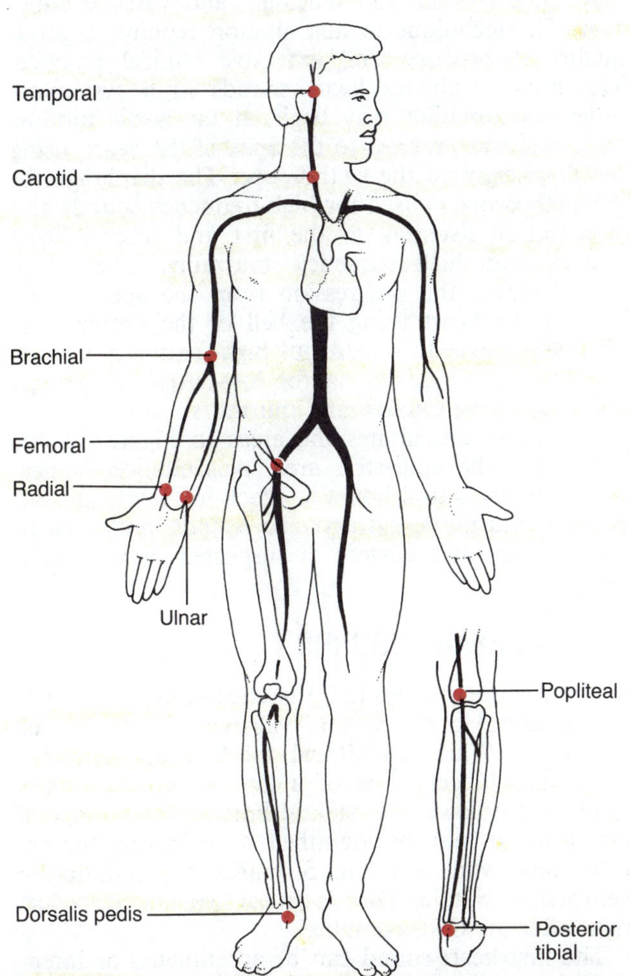

FIGURE 32-11 ◆ Pulse points for assessment of arterial pulses.

In pulsus alternans, a weak pulse alternates with a strong pulse, despite a regular heart rhythm. It is seen in clients with severely depressed cardiac function. Clients may be asked to hold their breath to exclude any false readings. The nurse may palpate the brachial or radial arteries to assess this condition, but it is more accurately assessed by auscultation of blood pressure.

Auscultation of the carotid arteries is necessary to assess for bruits. Bruits are swishing sounds that may develop over narrowed carotid arteries. Using the bell of the stethoscope over the skin of the carotid artery with the client holding his or her breath, the nurse can assess for the absence or presence of sounds. Normally, there are no sounds if the carotid artery has uninterrupted blood flow. A bruit may develop when the internal diameter of the vessel is narrowed by 50% or more. A bruit does not indicate the severity of disease in the carotid arteries. The severity of disease is determined by Doppler flow studies and arteriography.

Precordium

Assessment of the precordium (the area over the heart) is done by inspection, palpation, percussion, and auscultation. The nurse places the client in a supine position, with the head of the bed slightly elevated for the client's comfort. Some clients may require greater elevation of the head of the bed (to 45 degrees) for ease and comfort in breathing.

INSPECTION

Cardiac examination is usually done in a systematic order, beginning with inspection. The nurse inspects the chest from the side, at a right angle, and downward over areas of the precordium where vibrations are visible. Cardiac motion is of low amplitude, and sometimes the inward movements are more easily detected by the naked eye.

The nurse can examine seven precordial areas (Fig. 32-12), noting any prominent precordial pulsations. Movement over the aortic, pulmonic, and tricuspid areas is abnormal. Pulsations in the mitral area (the apex of the heart) are considered normal and are referred to as the apical impulse, or the point of maximal impulse (PMI). The PMI should be located at the left fifth intercostal space (ICS) medial to the mid-clavicular line. If the apical impulse appears in more than one intercostal space and has shifted lateral to the mid-clavicular line, it may indicate left ventricular hypertrophy.

PALPATION

The nurse palpates with the fingers and the most sensitive part of the palm of the hand to detect pre-

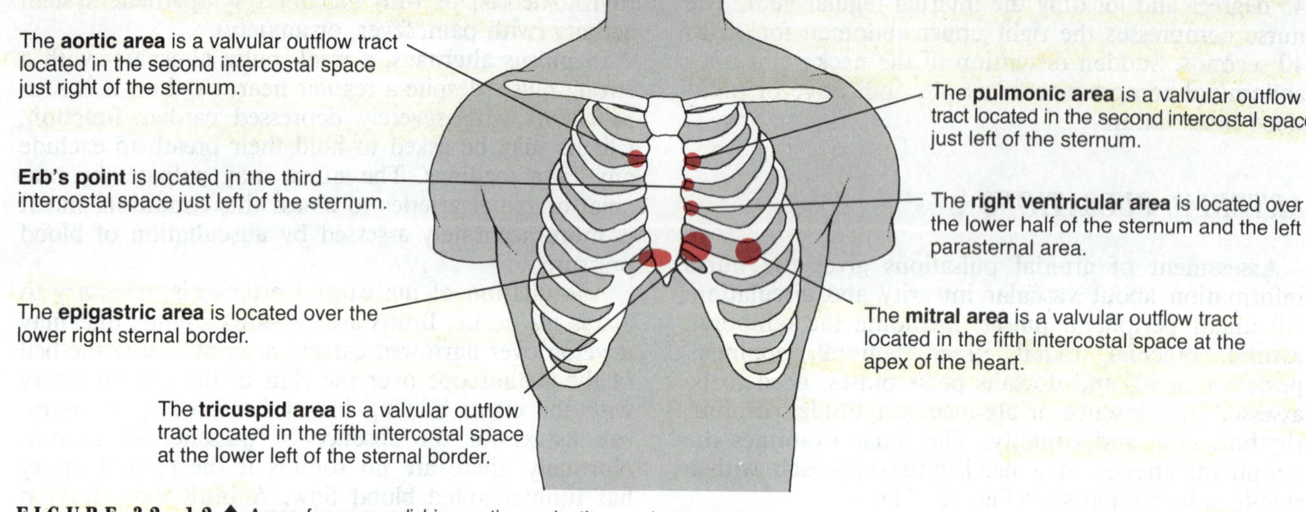

FIGURE 32-12 ◆ Areas for myocardial inspection, palpation, and auscultation.

cordial motion and thrills, respectively. The nurse palpates the seven precordial areas, starting with the aortic area. Turning the client on his or her left side brings the heart closer to the surface of the chest. This may be helpful for the nurse to achieve maximal tactile sensitivity.

An abnormal forceful thrust accompanied by a sustaining outward movement felt over the left anterior chest usually indicates left ventricular enlargement. An outward systolic lift along the left sternal border extending from the fourth to the fifth intercostal space represents right ventricular enlargement.

Heaves and lifts are terms found with pulsations associated with valvular diseases or pulmonary hypertension. Thrills are vibrations that are associated with abnormal heart valve function (mitral regurgitation, tricuspid regurgitation, and pulmonic stenosis). When palpating for heaves or thrills, the nurse should consider several factors, including the location, the amplitude, the duration, the distribution, and the timing in relation to the cardiac cycle.

PERCUSSION

Cardiac size is usually determined most accurately by chest x-ray. The nurse can perform percussion to estimate the size of the heart.

With the client in the supine position, the nurse begins percussion at the left anterior axillary line in the fifth intercostal space on the chest using the middle fingers of both hands. By striking one finger against the other on the surface of the chest, sounds are produced. Sounds produced by percussion over specific anatomic regions include dullness (heart and liver), tympany (stomach and intestine), flatness (muscle), resonance (normal lung), and hyperresonance (abnormal lung, such as in emphysema).

AUSCULTATION

Auscultation evaluates heart rate and rhythm, cardiac cycle (systole and diastole), and valvular function. The technique of auscultation requires a good-quality stethoscope and extensive clinical practice. The nurse evaluates heart sounds in a systematic order; examination may begin at the aortic outflow tract area and progress to the apex of the heart, using the diaphragm of the stethoscope. The diaphragm of the stethoscope is used for high-frequency sounds and is useful in listening to the first and second heart sounds and high-frequency murmurs. The nurse should repeat the progression from the apex to the base of the heart using the bell of the stethoscope. The bell is able to screen out high-frequency sounds and is useful in listening for low-frequency gallops (diastolic filling sounds) and murmurs.

The nurse auscultates the areas in Figure 32-12, except for the epigastric area. Auscultation is performed every 4 to 8 hours to check for heart rate and rhythm, murmurs, extrasystolic sounds, and rubs in the presence of a current or suspected cardiac problem.

NORMAL HEART SOUNDS

The first heart sound (S_1) is created by the closure of the mitral and tricuspid valves (AV valves) (see Fig. 32-6). When auscultated, the first heart sound is softer and longer; it is of a low pitch and is best heard at the lower left sternal border or the apex of the heart. It may be identified by palpating the carotid pulse while listening. S_1 marks the beginning of ventricular systole. On electrocardiogram, it occurs right after the QRS complex.

The first heart sound can be accentuated or intensified in conditions such as exercise, hyperthyroidism, and mitral stenosis. A decrease in sound intensity occurs in clients with mitral regurgitation and heart failure.

The second heart sound (S_2) is caused mainly by the closing of the aortic and pulmonic valves (semilunar valves) (see Fig. 32–6). S_2 is characteristically shorter. It is higher pitched and is heard best at the base of the heart at the end of ventricular systole.

Splitting of heart sounds is often difficult to differentiate from diastolic filling sounds (gallops). A splitting of S_1 (closure of the mitral valve followed by closure of the tricuspid valve) occurs physiologically because left ventricular contraction occurs slightly before right ventricular contraction. However, closure of the mitral valve is louder than closure of the tricuspid valve, so that splitting is often not heard. Normal splitting of S_2 occurs because of the longer systolic phase of the right ventricle. Splitting of S_1 and S_2 can be accentuated by inspiration (increased venous return) and narrows during expiration.

ABNORMAL HEART SOUNDS

PARADOXICAL SPLITTING

Abnormal splitting of S_2 is referred to as paradoxical splitting, which is characteristic of a wider split heard on expiration. Paradoxical splitting of S_2 is heard in clients with severe myocardial depression causing early closure of the pulmonic valve or a delay in aortic valve closure. Such conditions include myocardial infarction, left bundle branch block, aortic stenosis, aortic regurgitation, and right ventricular pacing (Braunwald, 1992).

GALLOPS AND MURMURS

Gallops and murmurs are common abnormal heart sounds, which may occur when heart disease is present.

GALLOPS Diastolic filling sounds (S_3) and (S_4) are produced when blood enters a noncompliant chamber during rapid ventricular filling. The third heart sound (S_3) is produced during the rapid filling phase of ventricular diastole when blood flows from the atrium to a noncompliant ventricle. The sound arises from vibrations of the valves and supporting structures. The fourth heart sound (S_4) occurs as blood enters the ventricles at the end of ventricular diastole.

S_3 is termed *ventricular gallop*, and S_4 is referred to as *atrial gallop*. These sounds can be caused by decreased compliance of either or both ventricles. The nurse can best hear left ventricular diastolic filling sounds with the client on his or her left side, using the bell of the stethoscope at the apex and the left lower sternal border during expiration.

An S_3 heart sound is probably a normal finding in children or young adults up to 30 years of age. An S_3 gallop in clients older than 40 years of age is considered abnormal and represents a decrease in left ventricular compliance. S_3 can be detected as an early sign of heart failure, ventricular septal defect, or ruptured papillary muscle.

An atrial gallop (S_4) may be heard in clients with hypertension, anemia, ventricular hypertrophy, myocardial infarction, aortic or pulmonic stenosis, and pulmonary emboli. It may also be heard with advancing age because of a stiffened ventricle.

The auscultation of both S_3 and S_4, called a *summation,* or *quadruple gallop,* is an indication of severe heart failure. If the quadruple rhythm is present, it is sometimes difficult to delineate the four heart sounds because the client is tachycardiac (has shortened diastolic filling time). The two sounds actually fuse, producing a rhythm that sounds like a horse galloping.

MURMURS Murmurs reflect turbulent blood flow through normal or abnormal valves. They are classified according to their timing in the cardiac cycle: systolic murmurs (such as aortic stenosis and mitral regurgitation) occur between S_1 and S_2, whereas diastolic murmurs (such as in mitral stenosis and aortic regurgitation) occur between S_2 and S_1. Murmurs can occur during presystole, midsystole, or late systole or diastole or last throughout both phases of the cardiac cycle. Murmurs are also graded according to their intensity, depending on their level of loudness (Table 32–3).

The nurse describes the location of a murmur by where it is best heard on auscultation. Some murmurs may transmit or radiate from their loudest point to other areas, including the neck, the back, and the axilla. The configuration of a murmur is described as crescendo (increases in intensity) or decrescendo (decreases in intensity). The quality of murmurs can be further characterized as harsh, blowing, whistling, rumbling, or squeaking. The murmur is also described by its pitch, usually high or low.

PERICARDIAL FRICTION RUB

A pericardial friction rub originates from the pericardial sac and occurs with the movements of the heart during the cardiac cycle. Rubs are usually transient and are a sign of inflammation, infection, or

TABLE 32–3 Grading of Heart Murmurs

• Grade I	Very faint
• Grade II	Faint, but recognizable
• Grade III	Loud, but moderate in intensity
• Grade IV	Loud and accompanied by a palpable thrill
• Grade V	Very loud, accompanied by a palpable thrill, and audible with the stethoscope partially off the client's chest
• Grade VI	Extremely loud, may be heard with the stethoscope slightly above the client's chest

infiltration. Pericardial friction rubs may be heard in clients with pericarditis resulting from myocardial infarction and cardiac tamponade.

The three phases of cardiac movement—atrial systole, ventricular diastole, and ventricular systole—can produce three components of a rub. Usually, only one or two components can be heard. With each movement, a short, high-pitched scratchy sound is produced; the loudest component is heard in systole. The nurse may be most able to auscultate the rubs when the client sits, leans forward, and exhales. The pericardial friction rub is better heard with the diaphragm of the stethoscope.

PSYCHOSOCIAL ASSESSMENT

To many people, the heart is the symbol of their existence and longevity. A client with a heart-related illness, whether acute or chronic, usually perceives it as a major life crisis. Clients and families and significant others confront not only the possibility of death, but also fears about pain, disability, lack of self-esteem, physical dependence, and changes in family role dynamics. The nurse may assess the meaning of the illness to the client and family members by asking, "What do you understand about what happened to you (or the client)?" and "What does that mean to you?" When the client or family members perceive the stressor as overwhelming, formerly adequate support systems may no longer be effective. In these circumstances, clients and families attempt to cope to regain a sense or feeling of control.

Coping behaviors vary from client to client. Clients who feel helpless to meet the demands of the situation may exhibit behaviors such as disorganization, fear, and anxiety. The nurse may ask the client or family members, "Have you ever encountered such a situation before?" "How did you manage that situation?" and "Who can you turn to for help?" The answers to these questions often reassure the client that he or she has encountered difficult situations in the past and has the ability and resources to cope with them.

A common and normal response is *denial,* which is a defense mechanism to enable clients to cope with threatening circumstances. The client may deny that he or she has the current cardiovascular condition, may state that it was present but is now absent, or may be excessively cheerful. Denial of the seriousness of the illness while following the treatment regimen is a protective response. Denial becomes maladaptive only when the client is noncompliant with significant portions of medical and nursing care (see Chapter 7 on coping).

Family members and significant others of the client with heart disease may be more anxious than the client. Often, they recall all the events of the illness, are unprotected by denial, and are afraid of recurrence. Disagreements may occur between the client and family members over compliance with appropriate follow-up care.

DIAGNOSTIC ASSESSMENT

Laboratory Tests

Assessment of the client with cardiac dysfunction includes examination of the blood for abnormalities. This is done to establish a diagnosis, to detect concurrent disease, to assess risk factors, and to monitor response to treatment. Normal values for serum cardiac enzymes and serum lipids are listed in Chart 32–4.

SERUM CARDIAC ENZYMES

Events leading to cellular injury cause a release of enzymes from intracellular storage, and circulating levels of these enzymes are dramatically elevated. Acute myocardial infarction (MI) can be confirmed by abnormally high levels of enzymes or isoenzymes in the serum.

CREATINE KINASE

Creatine kinase (CK) is an enzyme specific to cells of the brain, the myocardium, and skeletal muscle. The appearance of CK in the blood indicates tissue necrosis or injury, and CK levels follow a predictable rise and fall during a specified period of time. Cardiac specificity must be determined by measuring isoenzyme activity. There are three isoenzymes of CK: CK-MM is the predominant isoenzyme of skeletal muscle; CK-MB is found in myocardial muscle; and CK-BB occurs in the brain. CK-MB activity is most specific for MI and shows a predictable rise and fall during 3 days, with a peak level occurring approximately 24 hours after the onset of chest pain.

LACTATE DEHYDROGENASE

Lactate dehydrogenase (LDH) is widely distributed in the body and is found in the heart, the liver, the kidney, the brain, and the erythrocytes. LDH elevation starts within 12 to 24 hours after an MI, reaches a peak between 48 and 72 hours, and falls to normal in 7 days. Because LDH is not specific to the myocardial cell, assessment of isoenzymes and patterns of elevation is necessary for confirmation of MI. There are five isoenzymes for LDH, of which LDH_1 and LDH_2 are found in the heart. If the serum level of LDH_1 is higher than the concentration of LDH_2, the pattern is said to have flipped, signifying myocardial damage.

CHART 32-4

Lab Profile ◆ Cardiovascular Assessment

Test	Normal Range for Adults	Significance of Abnormal Findings*
Serum Cardiac Enzymes		
Creatine kinase	• Females: 10–55 U/mL, or 30–135 U/L • Males: 12–70 U/mL, or 55–70 U/L (values higher after exercise)	• *Elevations* indicate possible brain, myocardial, and skeletal muscle necrosis or injury.
CK–MM (CK_3)	• 95%–100% of total CK	• *Elevations* occur with muscle injury.
CK–MB (CK_2)	• 0%–5% of total CK	• *Elevations* occur with myocardial injury or after percutaneous transluminal angioplasty and intracoronary streptokinase infusion.
CK–BB (CK_1)	• 0%	• *Elevations* occur with brain tissue injury.
Lactate dehydrogenase	• 45–90 U/L, or 0.4–1.7 mmol/L	• *Elevation* occurs with injury to heart, liver, kidney, brain, and erythrocytes.
LDH_1	• 17%–27% of total LDH	• *Elevation* occurs higher than LDH_2 with myocardial damage.
LDH_2	• 27%–37% of total LDH	
LDH_1/LDH_2 ratio	• <1	• *Elevation* occurs with myocardial damage.
Serum Lipids		
Total lipids	• 400–1000 mg/dL	• *Elevation* indicates increased risk of CAD.
Cholesterol	• 150–200 mg/dL, or 3.9–6.5 mmol/L • **Elderly:** range increases with age	• *Elevation* indicates increased risk of CAD.
Triglycerides	• Females: 35–135 mg/dL, or 0.35–1.35 g/L • Males: 40–60 mg/dL, or 0.4–1.6 g/L • **Elderly:** range increases with age	• *Elevation* indicates increased risk of CAD
Plasma high-density lipoproteins	• Females: mean of 55–60 mg/dL • Males: mean of 45–50 mg/dL • **Elderly:** range increases with age	• *Elevations* may protect against CAD.
Plasma low-density lipoproteins	• 60–180 mg/dL • **Elderly:** range increases with age	• *Elevation* indicates increased risk of CAD.
HDL/LDL ratio	• 3:1	• *Elevated ratios* may protect against CAD.

* CAD, coronary artery disease.

ASPARTATE AMINOTRANSFERASE

Another enzyme that may be assessed to monitor the presence and the progression of an acute cardiovascular event is aspartate aminotransferase (AST; previously known as serum glutamic-oxaloacetic transaminase [SGOT]). Like LDH, it is not specific to cardiac muscle tissue.

SERUM LIPIDS

Elevated lipid levels are considered a coronary artery disease (CAD) risk factor. Cholesterol, triglycerides, and the protein components of high-density lipoproteins (HDL) and low-density lipoproteins (LDL) are evaluated to assess a client's degree of risk for CAD. A serum cholesterol level greater than 260 mg/dL gives a client a three times greater risk of CAD than a serum level of 200 mg/dL.

Each of the lipoproteins contains varying proportions of cholesterol, triglyceride, protein, and phospholipid. HDL contains mainly protein and 20% cholesterol, whereas LDL is predominantly cholesterol. Elevated LDL levels are positively correlated with CAD, whereas elevated HDL levels are negatively correlated and may be a protective factor. HDL converts cholesterol to a less active form.

A nonfasting blood sample for the measurement of serum cholesterol levels is acceptable. However, if triglycerides are to be evaluated, the physician obtains the specimen after a 12-hour fast.

BLOOD COAGULATION TESTS

Blood coagulation tests evaluate the ability of the blood to clot and are important in clients with a greater tendency to form thrombi (e.g., clients with atrial fibrillation, prosthetic valves, or infective endocarditis). They are also important for clients receiving anticoagulant therapy (e.g., during cardiac surgery, after thrombolytic therapy, and during treatment of an established thrombus).

PROTHROMBIN TIME

Prothrombin time (PT) is used when initiating and maintaining therapy with oral anticoagulants, such as sodium warfarin (Coumadin, Warfilone✱). It measures the activity of prothrombin, fibrinogen, and factors V, VII, and X.

PARTIAL THROMBOPLASTIN TIME

Partial thromboplastin time (PTT) is assessed in clients receiving heparin (Hepalean✱). It measures deficiencies in all coagulation factors, except factors VII and XIII.

ARTERIAL BLOOD GASES

Arterial blood gas (ABG) determinations are frequently obtained in the client with cardiovascular disease. Determination of tissue oxygenation, carbon dioxide removal, and the acid-base status is essential to appropriate intervention and treatment. Complete discussion of ABGs can be found in Chapter 17.

SERUM ELECTROLYTES

Fluid and electrolyte balance is essential for normal cardiovascular performance. Cardiac manifestations often occur when there is an imbalance in either fluids or electrolytes in the body. For example, the cardiac effects of hypokalemia (high serum potassium level) include increased electrical instability, ventricular dysrhythmias, the appearance of U waves on the electrocardiogram, and an increased risk of digitalis toxicity. The effects of hyperkalemia on the myocardium include slowed ventricular conduction and contraction, followed by asystole (cardiac standstill).

Cardiac manifestations of hypocalcemia are ventricular dysrhythmias, prolonged QT interval, and cardiac arrest. Hypercalcemia shortens the QT interval and causes AV block, digitalis hypersensitivity, and cardiac arrest.

Serum sodium values reflect fluid balance and may be decreased, indicating a fluid excess in clients with heart failure.

Because magnesium regulates some aspects of myocardial electrical activity, hypomagnesemia has been implicated in some forms of rapid ventricular dysrhythmias. Another manifestation of hypomagnesemia is hypokalemia that is unresponsive to potassium replacement.

COMPLETE BLOOD COUNT

The erythrocyte count is usually decreased in rheumatic fever and subacute infective endocarditis. It is increased in heart diseases characterized by inadequate tissue oxygenation.

Decreased hematocrit and hemoglobin levels (e.g., caused by hemorrhage or hemolysis from prosthetic valves) indicate anemia and can manifest as angina or aggravate heart failure. Vascular volume depletion with hemoconcentration (e.g., hypovolemic shock and excessive diuresis) results in an elevated hematocrit.

The leukocyte count is typically elevated after MI and in the various infectious and inflammatory diseases of the heart (e.g., infective endocarditis and pericarditis). Chapter 38 discusses the complete blood count in detail.

Radiographic Examinations

CHEST RADIOGRAPHY

Routinely, posteroanterior and left lateral x-ray views of the chest are taken to determine the size, silhouette, and position of the heart. In acutely ill clients, a simple anteroposterior view is taken at the bedside. Cardiac enlargement, pulmonary congestion, cardiac calcifications, and placement of central venous catheters, endotracheal tubes, and hemodynamic monitoring devices are all assessed by x-ray.

CARDIAC FLUOROSCOPY

Fluoroscopy is a simple x-ray examination that reveals the action of the heart. Continuous visual observation of the heart, the lungs, and vessel movement on a luminescent x-ray screen in a darkened room is provided. Fluoroscopy is used to place and position intracardiac catheters and IV pacemaker wires and can be helpful in identifying abnormal structures, calcifications, and tumors of the heart. In critically ill clients, fluoroscopy can be performed at the bedside for the placement of intracardiac catheters of IV pacemaker wires. The client preparation and follow-up depend on the procedure. Commonly, fluoroscopy is used in conjunction with cardiac catheterization, and the client is taken to a special cardiac catheterization room (see later discussion of cardiac catheterization).

ANGIOGRAPHY

Angiography of arterial vessels, or arteriography, is an invasive diagnostic procedure that involves fluoroscopy and x-ray studies. This procedure is performed when an arterial obstruction, narrowing, or aneurysm is suspected. The radiologist performs selective arteriography to evaluate specific areas of the arterial system. For example, coronary arteriography, which is performed during left-sided cardiac catheterization, assesses arterial circulation within the heart (see later in this chapter). Angiography can also be performed on arteries in the extremities, the mesentery, or the cerebrum.

CLIENT PREPARATION The radiologist explains the procedure and the risks to the client before the client or the designated responsible party signs a consent form. Because this procedure involves injection of contrast medium (sometimes called a dye) into the arterial system, the risks are serious. They include allergic reaction, hemorrhage, thrombosis, embolism, and death. The client is told to expect a warm sensation when dye is injected during the procedure. The nurse assesses the client for any allergies to contrast medium, iodine-containing substances such as seafood, or local anesthetics. The nurse also shaves and scrubs the area that will be catheterized with an antiseptic skin preparation per the health care agency's policy and procedure. Most often, the femoral artery in a groin area is used. The nurse documents vital signs and marks and describes pedal pulses in the client's medical record.

PROCEDURE The radiologist or the technician places the client in a supine position on an x-ray table in the radiology department. A radiologist usually performs this procedure and begins by injecting a local anesthetic into the tissue surrounding the artery being catheterized. Contrast medium is injected via this catheter, and fluoroscopy and x-ray studies are done.

FOLLOW-UP CARE After the procedure, the client is typically restricted to bed rest in the supine position for 8 to 12 hours. The nurse ensures that the extremity that was catheterized is not flexed during this time. A pressure dressing or bandage is kept in place over the injection site; there may be a sandbag over the dressing.

The nurse assesses the insertion site for bloody drainage or hematoma formation, assesses distal pulses, and compares skin temperature in the affected extremity with that in the opposite extremity. Vital signs are assessed at the time of every dressing, pulse, and temperature check, the first measurement being obtained immediately after the client is transferred from the radiology department. These assessments usually continue every 15 minutes for 1 hour, then every 30 minutes for 2 hours, followed by every 4 hours or as necessary per the health care agency's protocol. The nurse notifies the radiologist immediately if bleeding, loss of pulses, or changes in vital signs occur. The nurse carefully administers the prescribed IV or oral fluids after the procedure, because the contrast medium may be toxic to the kidneys.

CARDIAC CATHETERIZATION

The most definitive, but most invasive, test in the diagnosis of heart disease is cardiac catheterization. Cardiac catheterization may include studies of the right and/or left side of the heart and the coronary arteries. Some of the most common indications for cardiac catheterization are listed in Table 32–4.

CLIENT PREPARATION Many clients express a great deal of anxiety and fear regarding cardiac catheterization. The nurse assesses the client's physical and psychosocial readiness and knowledge level.

The nurse reviews the purpose of the procedure. The nurse informs the client how long the procedure usually takes, states who will be present while it is going on, and describes the appearance of the catheterization laboratory. The client is also informed about the sensations that may be experienced during the procedure, such as palpitations (as the catheter is passed up to the left ventricle); a feeling of heat or hot flash (as the dye is injected into either side of the heart); and a desire to cough (as the dye is injected into the right side of the heart). The nurse may use written, illustrated materials or videotapes, if available, to assist the client's understanding.

The risks of cardiac catheterization are usually explained by the cardiologist. The risks vary with the procedures to be performed and the client's physical status (Table 32–5). Right-sided heart catheterization is less risky than left-sided catheterization. Several complications may follow coronary arteriography, such as:

- Myocardial infarction (MI)
- Cerebrovascular accident (CVA)
- Arterial bleeding
- Thromboembolism
- Lethal dysrhythmias
- Death

TABLE 32–4 Indications for Cardiac Catheterization

- To confirm suspected heart disease, including coronary artery disease, myocardial disease, valvular disease, and valvular dysfunction
- To determine the location and extent of the disease process
- To assess:
  - Stable, severe angina unresponsive to medical management
  - Unstable angina pectoris
  - Uncontrolled heart failure, ventricular dysrhythmias, or cardiogenic shock associated with acute myocardial infarction, papillary muscle dysfunction, ventricular aneurysm, or septal perforation
  - Whether cardiac surgery is necessary
- To evaluate:
  - Effects of medical treatment on cardiovascular function
  - Percutaneous transluminal coronary angioplasty or coronary artery bypass graft patency

TABLE 32–5 Complications of Cardiac Catheterization

Right-Sided Heart Catheterization

- Thrombophlebitis
- Pulmonary embolism
- Vagal response

Left-Sided Heart Catheterization and Coronary Arteriography

- Myocardial infarction
- Cerebrovascular accident
- Arterial bleeding or thromboembolism
- Dysrhythmias

Right- or Left-Sided Heart Catheterization*

- Cardiac tamponade
- Hypovolemia
- Pulmonary edema
- Hematoma or blood loss at insertion site
- Reaction to contrast medium

* In addition to those cited for each procedure.

The cardiologist or the radiologist obtains a written informed consent from the client or the responsible party.

The client may be admitted to the hospital before the catheterization procedure. Standard preoperative tests are performed, which usually include chest x-ray, complete blood count, urinalysis, and 12-lead electrocardiogram. The client receives nothing by mouth after midnight or has only a liquid breakfast if the catheterization is to take place in the afternoon. The nurse shaves the catheterization site and antiseptically prepares the skin according to the hospital's policy.

Nursing assessment before the procedure includes measurement of the client's vital signs, auscultation of the heart and the lungs, and evaluation of peripheral pulses. The nurse questions the client as to any prior history of allergy to iodine-containing substances (e.g., seafood and contrast agents). An antihistamine may be given to a client with a positive history. A mild sedative is given before the procedure. Digitalis preparations and diuretics are usually not given on the day of catheterization.

PROCEDURE The client is taken to the cardiac catheterization laboratory (sometimes referred to as the "cath lab") and is placed supine on an x-ray table. The client is securely strapped to the table. The nurse informs the client that this precaution is necessary because the table turns like a cradle during the procedure. The physician injects a local anesthetic at the insertion site. The nurse in the catheterization laboratory instructs the client to report any angina or chest pain or other symptoms to the staff. During the procedure, the client may experience discomfort and pain at the insertion site if the anesthetic wears off.

Right-Sided Heart Catheterization The right side of the heart is catheterized first and may be the only side examined. The cardiologist inserts a catheter through the femoral vein to the inferior vena cava or through the basilic vein to the superior vena cava. The catheter is advanced through either the inferior or the superior vena cava and, guided by fluoroscopy, is advanced through the right atrium, through the right ventricle, and at times, into the pulmonary artery (Fig. 32–13). Intracardiac pressures (right atrial, right ventricular, pulmonary artery, and pulmonary artery wedge pressures) are obtained, and blood samples are withdrawn. Contrast dye or medium is usually injected to detect any cardiac shunts or regurgitation from the pulmonic or tricuspid valves.

Left-Sided Heart Catheterization The left-sided heart catheterization is more risky than the right-sided heart catheterization. The cardiologist passes the catheter in a retrograde direction to reach the heart. This technique is accomplished by advancing the catheter from the femoral or brachial artery up the aorta, across the aortic valve, and into the left ventricle (Fig. 32–14). The cardiologist may pass the cath-

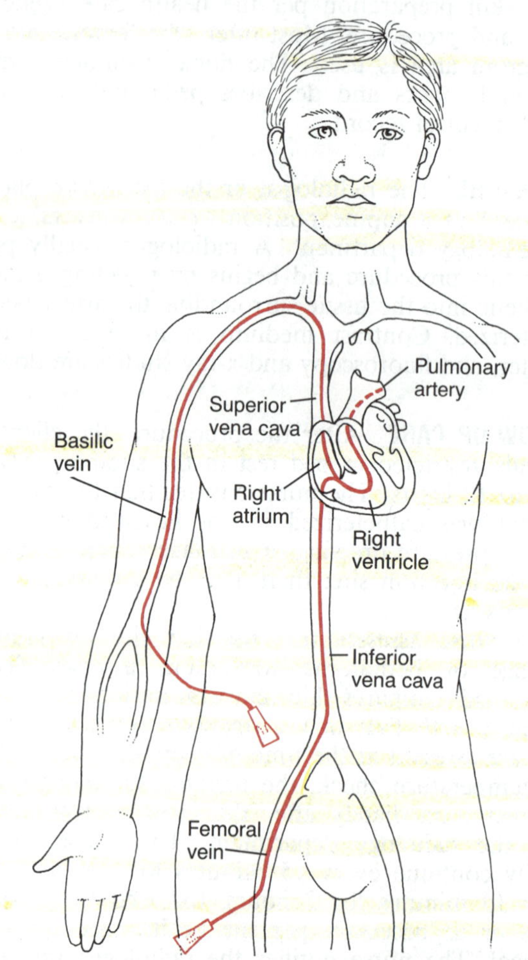

FIGURE 32–13 ◆ Right-sided heart catheterization. The catheter is inserted into the femoral vein and advanced through the inferior vena cava (or, if into an antecubital or basilic vein, through the superior vena cava), right atrium, and right ventricle and into the pulmonary artery.

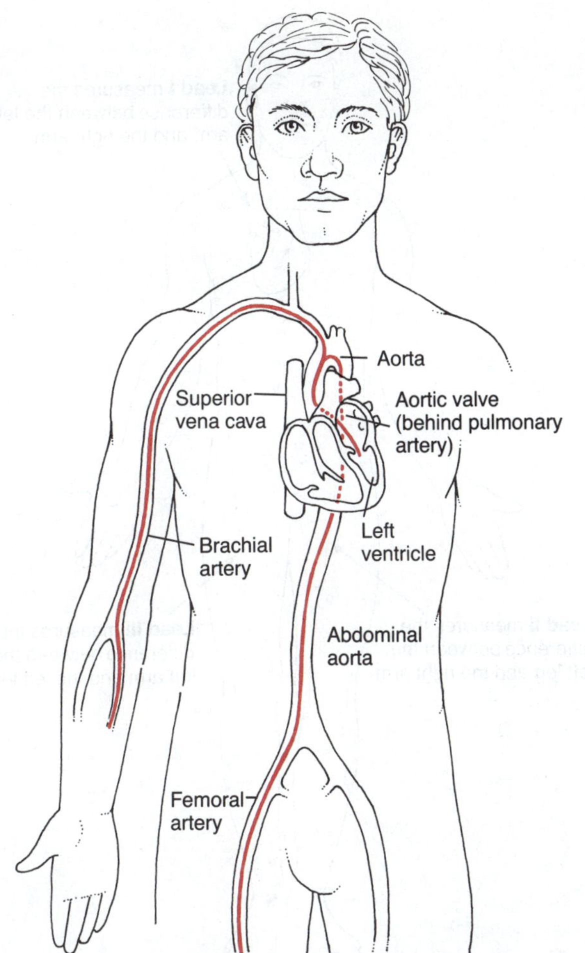

FIGURE 32-14 ◆ Left-sided heart catheterization. The catheter is inserted into the femoral artery or the antecubital artery. The catheter is passed through the ascending aorta, through the aortic valve, and into the left ventricle.

eter from the right side of the heart through the atrial septum, using a special needle to puncture the septum. Intracardiac pressures and blood samples are obtained. The pressures of the left atrium, the left ventricle, and the aorta and mitral and aortic valve status are evaluated. In addition, the cardiologist injects contrast dye into the ventricle; cineangiograms (rapidly changing films) evaluate left ventricular motion. Calculations are made of end-systolic volume, end-diastolic volume, stroke volume, and ejection fraction.

Coronary Arteriography The technique for coronary arteriography is the same as that for left-sided heart catheterization. The catheter is advanced into the aortic arch and positioned selectively in the right or the left coronary artery. Injection of contrast medium permits visualization of the coronary arteries. By assessing the flow of dye through the coronary arteries, information about the site and severity of coronary lesions is obtained.

FOLLOW-UP CARE After the cardiac catheterization, the client is typically restricted to bed rest for 8 to 12 hours; the client is supine, with the insertion site extremity straight. A pressure dressing or bandage may be placed over the insertion site. A 5- or 10-pound sandbag or a C clamp may be applied over the insertion site to ensure hemostasis. The nurse has many postcatheterization responsibilities. First, the nurse monitors vital signs every 15 minutes for 1 hour, then every 30 minutes for 2 hours or until vital signs are stable, and then every 4 hours or according to the hospital's policy. The nurse observes the insertion site for bloody drainage or hematoma formation when taking vital signs. Peripheral pulses in the affected extremity, as well as skin temperature and color, are monitored with every vital signs check.

The nurse must be constantly vigilant for complications of cardiac catheterization (see Table 32–5). The nurse assesses the client's reports of pain and discomfort at the insertion site, chest pain, nausea, or feelings of lightheadedness. By carefully monitoring the client's heart rhythm and pulse rate and auscultating heart sounds, the nurse may detect dysrhythmias. Because the contrast medium acts as an osmotic diuretic, the nurse notes any changes in blood pressure or pulse indicative of hypovolemia and monitors urinary output. The nurse also ensures that the client receives sufficient oral and IV fluids for adequate excretion of the dye. The nurse may administer pain medication for insertion site discomfort, as ordered.

If the client experiences chest pain, dysrhythmias, bleeding, hematoma formation, or a dramatic change in peripheral pulses in the affected extremity, the nurse reports these findings to the physician immediately and provides prompt intervention. The nurse is also alert for neurologic changes such as visual disturbances, slurred speech, difficulty in swallowing, and extremity weakness.

DIGITAL SUBTRACTION ANGIOGRAPHY

Digital subtraction angiography (DSA) combines x-ray detection methods and a computerized subtraction technique with fluoroscopy for visualization of the cardiovascular system. There is no interference from adjacent structures, such as bone and soft tissue.

CLIENT PREPARATION DSA involves the injection of dye into the venous system. Therefore, before the procedure, the nurse assesses the client for a history of allergies to contrast medium (dye), iodine, or seafood.

PROCEDURE For a DSA, the radiologist injects dye into the venous system via the superior vena cava. As the contrast medium circulates through the heart and the arterial system, a fluoroscopic image intensifier displays the vessels and focuses the image. A computer then converts the images to numbers. The first image obtained before the injection of the dye is subtracted from the postinjection images.

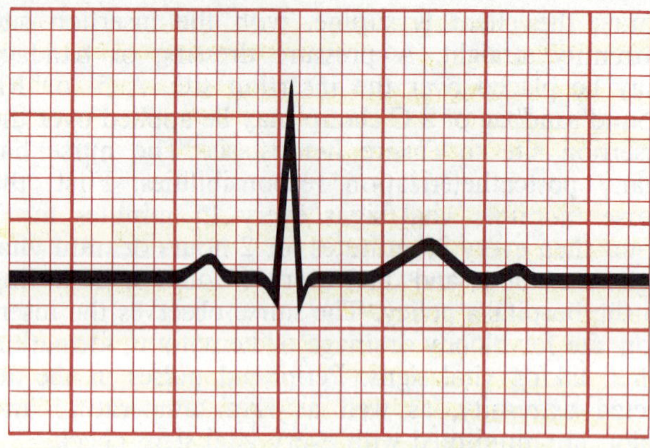

FIGURE 32–15 ◆ A normal ECG pattern.

FOLLOW-UP CARE Because DSA does not involve an arterial puncture and because little contrast dye is used, nursing care after the procedure is not as extensive as that after cardiac catheterization. The nurse monitors the client for vital signs and assesses the injection site for bleeding or discomfort.

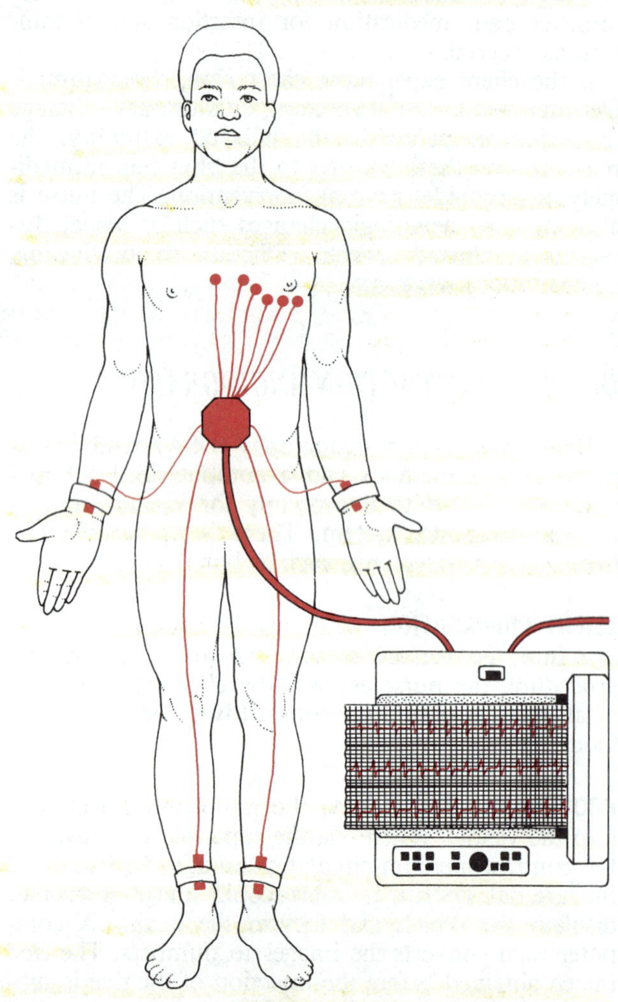

FIGURE 32–16 ◆ Electrode placement for a 12-lead ECG.

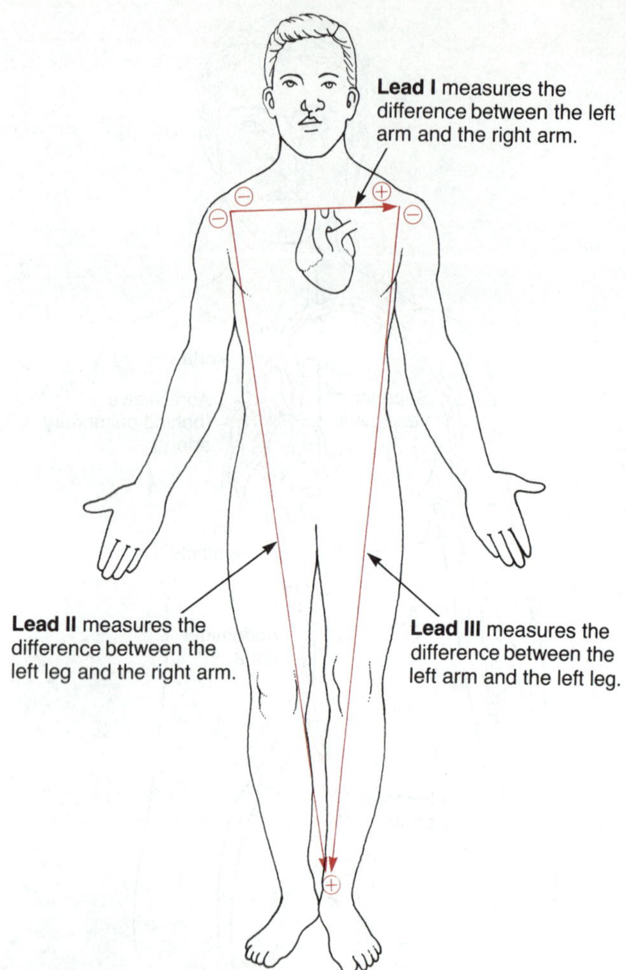

FIGURE 32–17 ◆ Standard ECG limb leads.

Other Diagnostic Tests

ELECTROCARDIOGRAPHY

The electrocardiogram (ECG) is a routine part of every cardiovascular evaluation and is one of the most valuable diagnostic tests. Various forms are available: resting ECG, continuous ambulatory ECG (Holter monitoring), and exercise ECG (stress test). The resting ECG provides information about cardiac dysrhythmias, myocardial ischemia, the site and extent of myocardial infarction, cardiac hypertrophy, electrolyte imbalances, and the effectiveness of cardiac drugs. The normal ECG pattern of one cardiac cycle is illustrated in Figure 32–15. Further discussion of the interpretation and evaluation of normal and abnormal patterns is found in Chapter 33.

RESTING ELECTROCARDIOGRAPHY

The ECG graphically records electrical current generated by the heart. This current is measured by electrodes placed on the skin and connected to an amplifier and strip chart recorder (Fig. 32–16). In the stan-

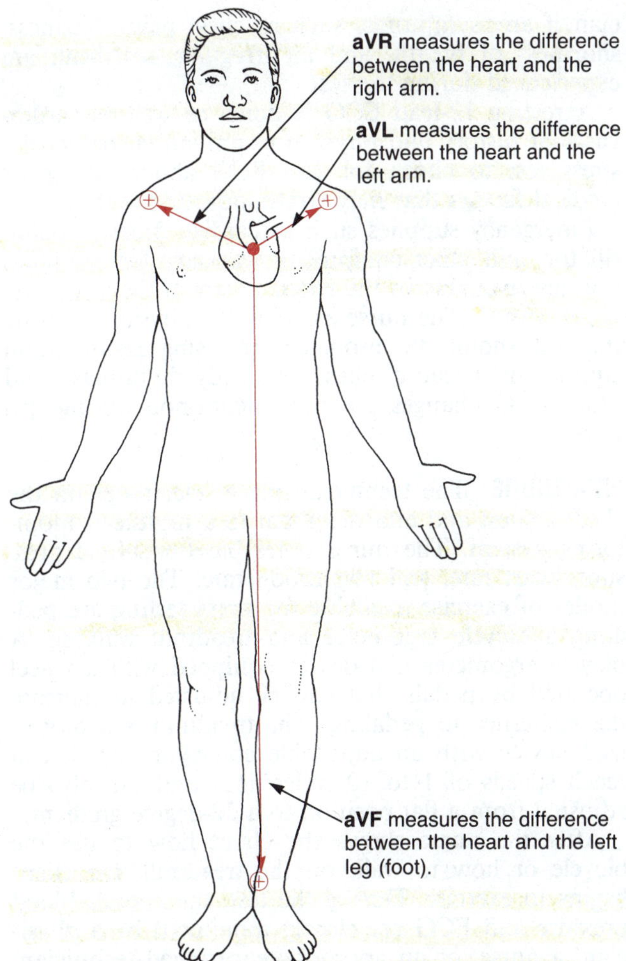

FIGURE 32-18 ◆ Unipolar augmented ECG leads.

dard 12-lead ECG, five electrodes attached to the arms, legs, and chest measure current from 12 different views or leads—three bipolar limb leads (Fig. 32-17), three unipolar augmented leads (Fig. 32-18), and six unipolar precordial leads (Fig. 32-19). Placement of the leads allows the physician to view myocardial electrical conduction from different axes or positions, identifying sections of the heart in which electrical conduction is abnormal.

CLIENT PREPARATION The nurse explains the purpose and procedure of the resting ECG and informs the client that the test is safe and painless. Some clients may fear that they will be electrocuted by the machine. The nurse reassures them that the machine does not emit electricity but rather measures the electrical activity of the heart. The nurse reminds the client to lie as still as possible during the test.

PROCEDURE The ECG is performed with the client in a supine position with the chest exposed. Before applying the electrodes, the nurse or the technician washes the skin to reduce skin oils and to improve electrode contact. Electrode paste, gel, or saline pads are applied to the electrode sites if metal plates or suction cups are used. To ensure good contact between the skin and the electrodes for the limb leads, the electrodes should be placed on a flat surface above the wrists and the ankles. A total of ten electrodes are used for a standard ECG and are attached to lead wires that connect to the ECG machine. The 12-lead ECG reading is obtained by selecting the indicators on the machine.

FOLLOW-UP CARE No specific follow-up care is warranted. The nurse washes off any gel or paste used.

AMBULATORY ELECTROCARDIOGRAPHY

Ambulatory ECG (also called Holter monitoring) allows continuous recording of cardiac activity during an extended period (usually 24 hours) while the client is performing the usual activities of daily living. The ambulatory ECG allows assessment and correlation of dyspnea, chest pain, central nervous system symp-

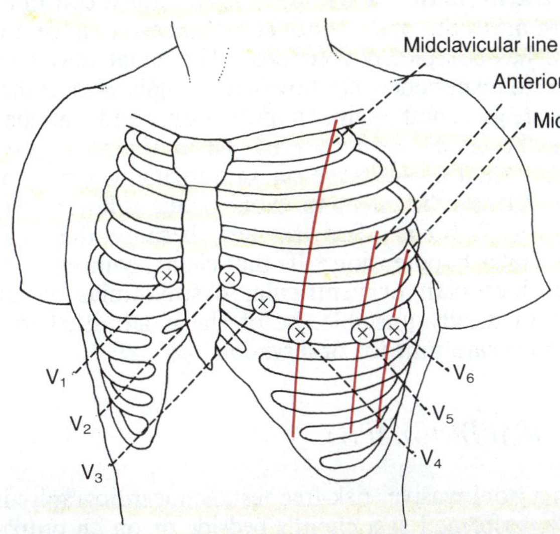

V_1 measures horizontally at the fourth intercostal space at the right sternal border.
V_2 measures horizontally at the fourth intercostal space at the left sternal border.
V_3 measures horizontally midway between V_2 and V_4.
V_4 measures horizontally at the fifth intercostal space at the midclavicular line.
V_5 measures horizontally at the fifth intercostal space at the anterior axillary line.
V_6 measures horizontally at the fifth intercostal space at the midaxillary line.

FIGURE 32-19 ◆ Unipolar precordial ECG leads.

toms (such as lightheadedness and syncope), and palpitations with actual cardiac events and the client's activities.

CLIENT PREPARATION The nurse encourages the client to maintain a normal day's schedule. He or she is instructed to keep a diary, or log, in which to note the time of activities, such as eating, sleeping, walking, and working, and to record any symptoms, such as chest pain, lightheadedness, fainting, and palpitations. The nurse instructs the client to avoid operating heavy machinery, using electric shavers and hair dryers, and bathing or showering. These activities may interfere with the ECG recorder. If the client is hospitalized, the nurse may need to make the entries for the log.

PROCEDURE The ECG technician places the electrodes on the client's chest and attaches them to the Holter monitor. The monitor is a small portable ECG tape recorder about the size of a transistor radio. The monitor is worn in a sling or holder around the client's chest or waist. After the prescribed monitoring period, the technician removes the electrodes and the monitor system. The ECG tape is analyzed by a microcomputer to allow correlation of the ECG findings with activities noted in the client's diary.

FOLLOW-UP CARE No specific follow-up care is needed.

EXERCISE ELECTROCARDIOGRAPHY (STRESS TEST)

The exercise ECG test (also known as the exercise tolerance, or stress, test) assesses the cardiovascular response to an increased workload. The stress test helps to determine the heart's functional capacity and screens for asymptomatic coronary artery disease. Dysrhythmias that develop during exercise may be identified, and the effectiveness of antidysrhythmic drugs can be evaluated.

CLIENT PREPARATION Because risks are associated with exercising, the client must be adequately informed about the purpose, the procedure, and the risks involved. A written consent must be obtained. Anxiety and fear are common before stress testing. The nurse assures the client that the procedure is performed in a controlled environment with prompt nursing and medical attention available. The nurse instructs the client to get plenty of rest the night before the procedure. The client should not eat anything after going to bed, or at least not within 2 hours before the test. The client should not smoke or drink alcohol or caffeine-containing beverages on the day of the test. The physician decides whether the client should stop the administration of any cardiac medications. The client is advised to wear comfortable, loose clothing and rubber-soled, supportive shoes. The nurse instructs the client to tell the physician if any symptoms, such as chest pain, dizziness, shortness of breath, and an irregular heartbeat, are experienced during the test.

A resting 12-lead ECG is done, as well as cardiovascular history and physical examination, before the stress test to check for any ECG abnormalities or medical factors that may contraindicate the test.

Emergency supplies such as cardiac drugs, a defibrillator, and other equipment necessary for resuscitation are available in the room in which the stress test is performed. The nurse assisting the physician during the test should be proficient in using resuscitation equipment because chest pain, dysrhythmias, and other ECG changes are not uncommon during this test.

PROCEDURE The technician places electrodes on the client's chest and attaches them to a multilead monitoring system. The nurse notes baseline blood pressure, heart rate, and respiration rate. The two major modes of exercise available for stress testing are pedaling a bicycle ergometer and treadmill walking. A bicycle ergometer is a device equipped with a wheel operated by pedals that can be adjusted to increase the resistance to pedaling. The treadmill is a motorized device with an adjustable conveyor belt; it can reach speeds of 1 to 10 miles/hour and can also be adjusted from a flat position to a 22-degree gradient.

After the nurse shows the client how to use the bicycle or how to walk on the treadmill, the client begins to exercise. During the test, the client's blood pressure and ECG are closely monitored by a physician, a nurse, or an appropriately trained technician. The client exercises until one of the following occurs:

- A predetermined heart rate is reached and maintained.
- Signs and symptoms, such as chest pain, fatigue, extreme dyspnea, vertigo, hypotension, and ventricular dysrhythmias, appear.
- Significant ST segment depression occurs.

FOLLOW-UP CARE After the test, the nurse continues to monitor the ECG and blood pressure until the client has completely recovered. The client may continue to experience cardiovascular signs and symptoms (e.g., chest pain, hypotension, and fatigue). After the client has recovered, he or she can return home if the test was done on an outpatient basis. The nurse advises the client to avoid taking a hot shower for 1 to 2 hours after the test, because this may precipitate hypotension. If the client continues to have chest pain or ventricular dysrhythmias or appears medically unstable, he or she is admitted to a coronary care unit for observation.

ECHOCARDIOGRAPHY

As a noninvasive, risk-free test, echocardiography is easily performed at a client's bedside or on an outpatient basis. Echocardiography uses ultrasound to assess the cardiac structure and mobility, particularly of the valves. Echocardiograms help to assess and diagnose cardiomyopathy, valvular disorders, pericardial effusion, left ventricular function, ventricular aneurysms, and cardiac tumors.

CLIENT PREPARATION There is no special preparation for echocardiography. The nurse informs the client that the test is painless and takes 30 to 60 minutes to complete. The nurse instructs the client to lie quietly during the test. The nurse assists the client to lie slightly on his or her left side with the head of the client elevated 15 to 20 degrees.

PROCEDURE During an echocardiogram, a small transducer lubricated with gel to facilitate movement and conduction is placed on the client's chest at the level of the third or fourth intercostal space near the left sternal border. The transducer transmits high-frequency sound waves and receives them back from the client as they are reflected from different structures. These echoes are usually videotaped simultaneously with the client's ECG and can be recorded on graph paper for a permanent copy.

Figure 32–20 is a representation of how echocardiograms examine the heart. After the images are taped, cardiac measurements that require several images can be obtained. Some routine measurements are chamber size, ejection fraction, and flow gradient across the valves.

Echocardiograms may also be performed transesophageally. Transesophageal echocardiography examines cardiac structure and function with an ultrasound transducer placed immediately behind the heart in the esophagus or the stomach. The transducer provides especially detailed views of such posterior cardiac structures as the left atrium, the mitral valve, and the aortic arch. Preparation and follow-up are similar to those for the client having an upper gastrointestinal endoscopic examination (see Chap. 52).

FOLLOW-UP CARE There is no specific follow-up care for a client having an echocardiogram.

PHONOCARDIOGRAPHY

Phonocardiography is the graphic recording of heart sounds during auscultation. It can be helpful in determining the exact timing and characteristics of extra heart sounds and murmurs.

A phonocardiography machine simultaneously records the pulse wave, ECG, and heart sounds. A pressure-sensitive transducer is applied to the selected pulse (e.g., apical or carotid artery), and the ECG is

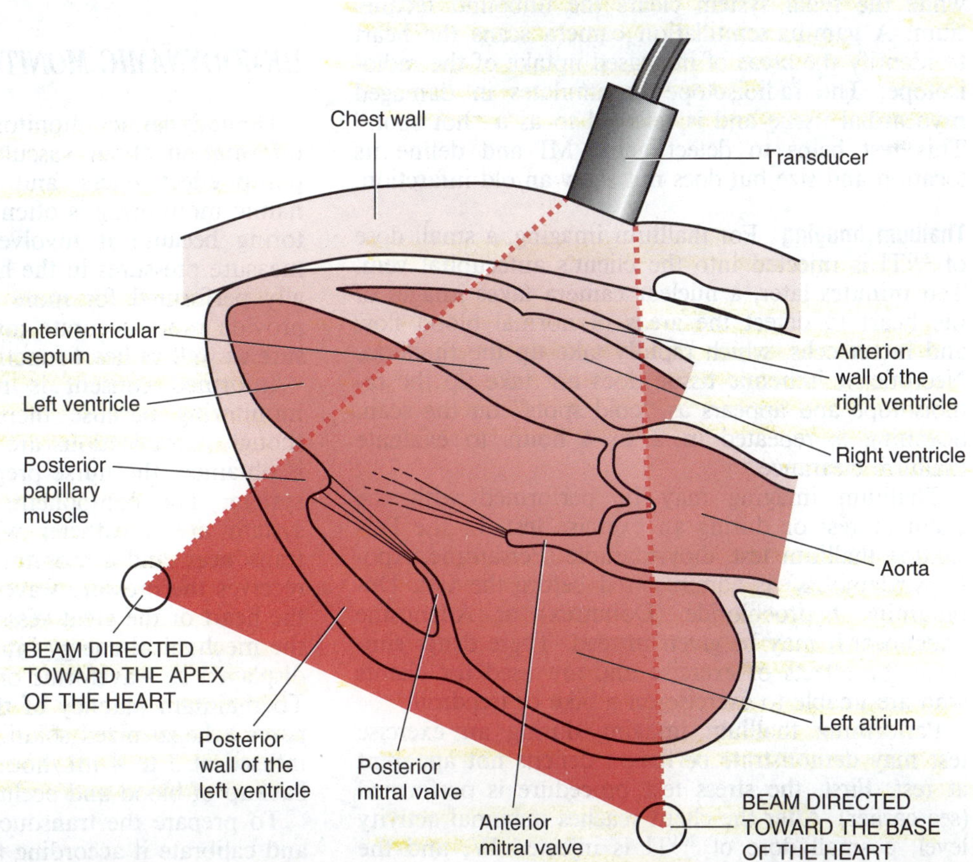

FIGURE 32–20 ◆ Echocardiographic imaging of the heart.

obtained through standard limb leads. A special microphone, used in the same manner as a stethoscope, is applied to the various areas for auscultation on the client's chest. Client preparation and follow-up care are similar to those for echocardiography (see earlier).

NUCLEAR CARDIOGRAPHY

The use of radionuclide techniques in cardiovascular assessment is called nuclear cardiology. Using radioactive tracer substances, cardiovascular abnormalities can be viewed, recorded, and evaluated. These studies are useful for detecting myocardial infarction (MI) and decreased myocardial blood flow and for evaluating left ventricular ejection.

CLIENT PREPARATION The nurse tells the client that the tests are relatively noninvasive and that the radiation exposure and risks are minimal. The client is informed that the test involves the IV injection of small amounts of radioisotope. The client or responsible party must give written consent.

PROCEDURE The most common tests in nuclear cardiology include technetium (^{99m}Tc) pyrophosphate scanning, thallium imaging, and multigated cardiac blood pool imaging.

Technetium Pyrophosphate Scanning A small dose of ^{99m}Tc pyrophosphate is injected into the client's antecubital vein. The client then waits at least 2 hours while the renal system clears the unbound technetium. A gamma-scintillation camera scans the heart to identify the areas of increased uptake of the radioisotope. The radioisotope accumulates in damaged myocardial tissue and is referred to as a "hot spot." This test helps to detect acute MI and define its location and size but does not show an old infarction.

Thallium Imaging For thallium imaging, a small dose of ^{201}Tl is injected into the client's antecubital vein. Ten minutes later, a nuclear camera takes images of the heart to detect the areas of normal blood flow and intact cells, which rapidly take up the thallium. Necrotic or ischemic tissue does not take up the radioisotope and appears as "cold spots" on the scan. Scanning is repeated in 2 to 4 hours to evaluate thallium clearance.

Thallium imaging may be performed with the client at rest or during an exercise test. In the Persantine thallium test, dipyridamole (Persantine, Apo-Dipyridamole✱) is administered before the test. Dobutamine hydrochloride (Dobutrex) or Adenosine (Adenocard) may be given instead. These drugs simulate the effects of exercise and are used for clients who are unable to exercise on a bike or treadmill.

Performing thallium imaging during an exercise test may demonstrate perfusion deficits not apparent at rest. First, the stress test procedure is performed (see earlier). After the client reaches maximal activity level, a small dose of ^{201}Tl is injected IV, and the client continues to exercise for approximately 1 to 2 minutes. The scanning is then done.

Thallium imaging is used to assess myocardial scarring and perfusion, to detect the location and extent of an acute or chronic MI, to evaluate graft patency after coronary bypass surgery, and to evaluate antianginal therapy, thrombolytic therapy, or balloon angioplasty.

Multigated Cardiac Blood Pool Scanning A multigated cardiac blood pool, or multigated angiogram (MUGA) scan utilizes a computer to analyze ventricular function. ECG leads are attached to the client. The ECG is synchronized with a computer and a gamma-scintillation camera. The technician injects a small amount of ^{99m}Tc intravenously (attached to either human serum albumin or autologous red blood cells). After 3 to 5 minutes, the scanning begins. The computer constructs an average cardiac cycle that represents the summation of several hundred heartbeats.

From this information, the computer calculates the ejection fraction (the amount of blood the left ventricle ejects with each contraction) and the ejection velocity. Areas of decreased, absent, or paradoxical movement of the left ventricle may be identified.

FOLLOW-UP CARE The client may complain of fatigue, depending on which test is performed, or discomfort at the antecubital injection site. If a stress test was paired with the ^{201}Tl study, the nurse needs to be aware of the same follow-up care as for the stress test (see earlier).

HEMODYNAMIC MONITORING

Hemodynamic monitoring provides quantitative information about vascular capacity, blood volume, pump effectiveness, and tissue perfusion. Hemodynamic monitoring is often referred to as direct monitoring because it involves procedures that directly measure pressures in the heart and great vessels. Usually performed for more seriously ill clients, it can provide more accurate measurements of blood pressure as well as heart function and volume status.

Informed consent is required for hemodynamic monitoring because there are significant risks, although complications are uncommon. After consent is obtained, the nurse prepares a pressure-monitoring system. The components of a pressure-monitoring system are a catheter with an infusion system, a transducer, and a monitor (Fig. 32–21). The catheter receives the pressure waves (mechanical energy) from the heart or the great vessels. The transducer converts the mechanical energy into electrical energy, which is displayed as waveforms or numbers on the monitor. To maintain patency of the catheter, the nurse prepares a heparinized solution. This solution is usually infused at 3 to 4 mL/hour under pressure to prevent backup of blood and occlusion of the catheter.

To prepare the transducer, the nurse must balance and calibrate it according to the equipment manufac-

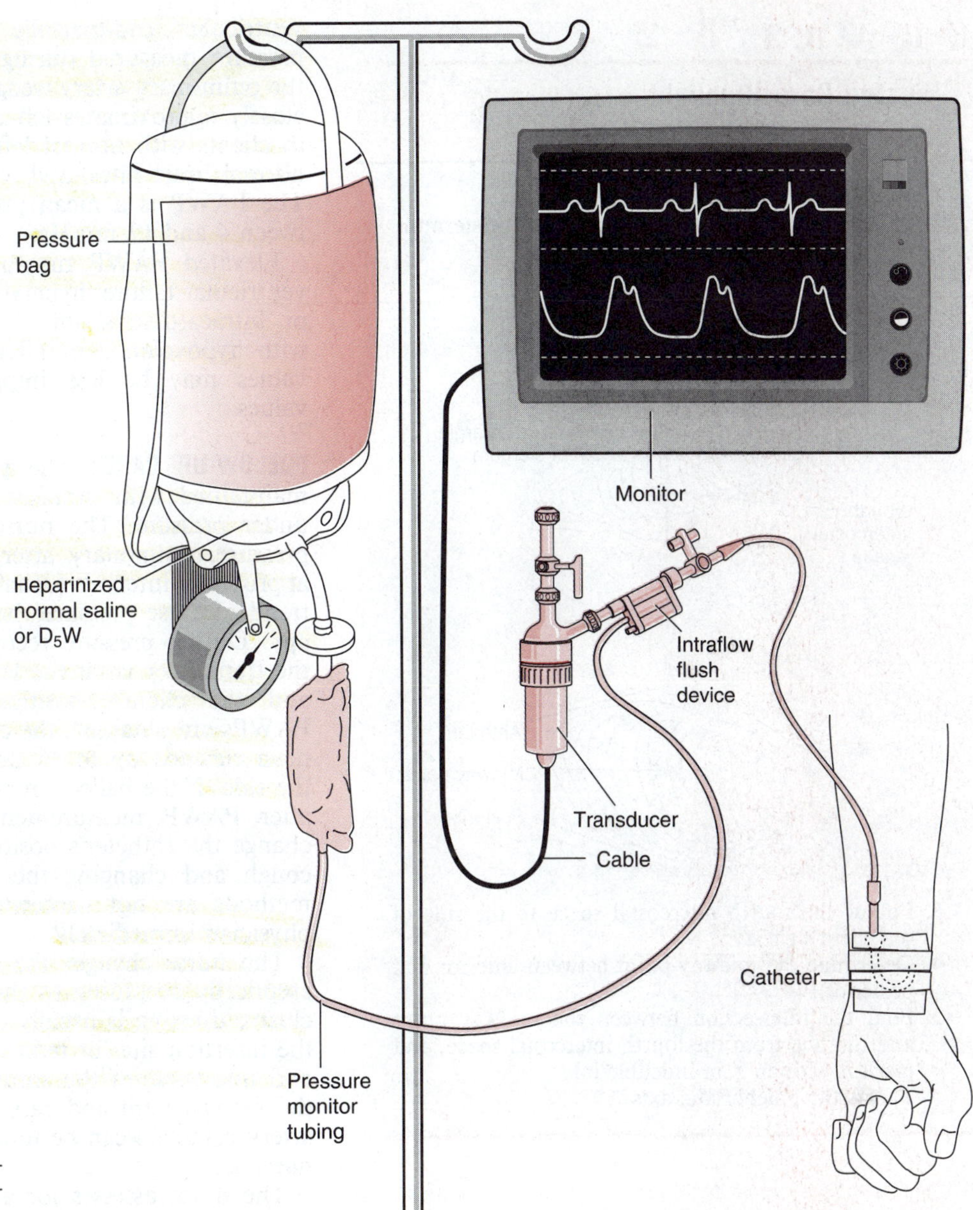

FIGURE 32–21 ◆ The components of a hemodynamic monitoring system.

turer's specifications and the hospital's policy. Finally, the nurse must identify the phlebostatic axis (Chart 32–5) and level the transducer to it. When the monitoring system is prepared, the physician inserts the catheter.

RIGHT ATRIAL, PULMONARY ARTERY, AND PULMONARY WEDGE PRESSURES

A pulmonary artery catheter is a triple-lumen or quadruple-lumen catheter with the capacity to measure right atrial and indirect left atrial pressures or pulmonary artery wedge pressure (PAWP). A cardiac output may also be obtained from the catheter.

CLIENT PREPARATION The physician explains the procedure and advises the client and family members or the significant other of the risks. Then the physician obtains a written consent for the procedure. The client and the family should understand that the hemodynamic monitoring system represents an assessment tool, and although it is used to guide therapy, it is not itself a treatment. The nurse asks the client to remain still and supine for the insertion of the catheter.

PROCEDURE The physician inserts a balloon-tipped catheter percutaneously through a large vein and directs it to the right atrium (RA). When the catheter tip reaches the RA, the physician inflates the balloon and the catheter advances with the flow of blood through the tricuspid valve, into the right ventricle, past the pulmonic valve, and into a branch of the pulmonary artery. The balloon is deflated after the

CHART 32–5

Nursing Care Highlight ◆ Identification of the Phlebostatic Axis

1. Position the client supine.
2. Palpate the fourth intercostal space at the sternum.

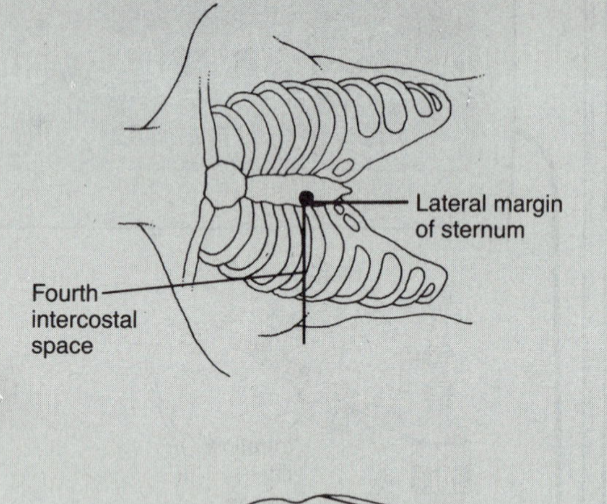

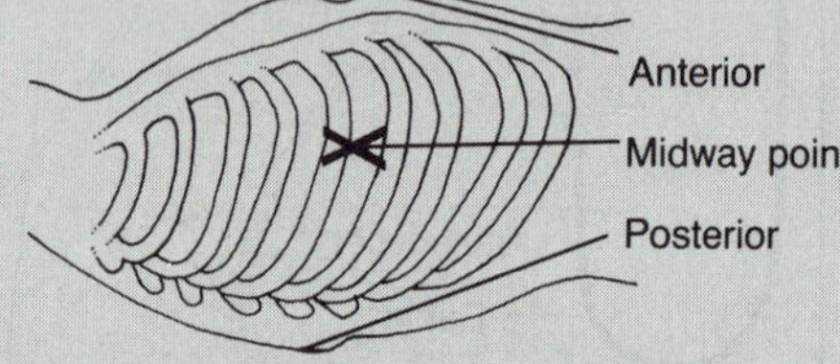

3. Follow the fourth intercostal space to the side of the client's chest.
4. Determine the midway point between anterior and posterior.
5. Find the intersection between the midway point and the line from the fourth intercostal space, and mark it with an X in indelible ink.
   This is the phlebostatic axis.

catheter tip reaches the pulmonary artery. Waveforms visualized on the oscilloscope as the pulmonary artery catheter is advanced (Fig. 32–22) and fluoroscopy are used to determine the location of the catheter.

RA pressure is measured by a pressure sensor on the catheter inside the right atrium. Normal RA pressure ranges between 1 and 8 mmHg (Daily & Kenner, 1992). Increased RA pressures may occur with right ventricular failure, whereas low RA pressures are usually indicative of hypovolemia.

Normal pulmonary artery pressure (PAP) is 15 to 28 mmHg/5 to 16 mmHg, with a mean of 15 (Daily & Kenner, 1992) and may be constantly visible on the monitor. When the balloon is inflated, the catheter wedges into a branch of the pulmonary artery. The tip of the catheter is able to sense pressures transmitted from the left atrium, which reflects left ventricular end-diastolic pressure (LVEDP). The pressure measured during balloon inflation is called the pulmonary artery wedge pressure (PAWP). PAWP closely approximates left atrial pressure and LVEDP in clients with normal left ventricular function, with normal heart rates, and without mitral valve disease. The PAWP is a mean pressure and is normally between 4 and 12 mmHg.

Elevated PAWP measurements may indicate left ventricular failure, hypervolemia, mitral regurgitation, or intracardiac shunt. A decreased PAWP is seen with hypovolemia or afterload reduction. Individual values may be less important than the trend in values.

FOLLOW-UP CARE The patency of the catheter is maintained with infusion of a heparinized solution under pressure. The nurse obtains and records RA pressure, pulmonary artery pressure, and PAWP at appropriate intervals (usually every 1 to 4 hours). The trend of these pressures helps to guide medical therapy. During pressure recording, it is important that the transducer be at the level of the phlebostatic axis and the client's position be appropriate. While PAWPs are obtained, the client is usually supine with head elevated up to 45 degrees or turned slightly to the side. If the balloon remains in the wedge position after PAWP measurement, the nurse attempts to change the catheter's position by asking the client to cough and changing the client's position. If these methods are not successful, the nurse notifies the physician immediately.

The nurse changes the dressing over the catheter aseptically according to the hospital's policy. An occlusive dressing is usually applied. The nurse inspects the insertion site for redness, heat, swelling, drainage, and intactness of the sutures. Detailed discussion of the management and care of clients with pulmonary artery catheters can be found in texts on critical care nursing.

The nurse assesses for a number of complications associated with pulmonary artery catheters. For example, pulmonary infarction or pulmonary rupture may occur if the catheter remains in the wedge position. Air embolism is possible if the balloon has ruptured and repeated attempts are made to inflate it. Ventricular dysrhythmias may occur if the catheter tip slips back into the right ventricle and irritates the myocardium. Thrombus and embolus formation may occur at the catheter site. Infection may result and bleeding may be pronounced if the infusion system becomes disconnected.

CARDIAC OUTPUT

The measurement of cardiac output using the thermodilution method can also be obtained with the pulmonary artery catheter. The nurse injects a specified amount (5 or 10 mL) of iced or room-temperature IV solution (normal saline or dextrose in water) into the proximal port of the catheter. The solution

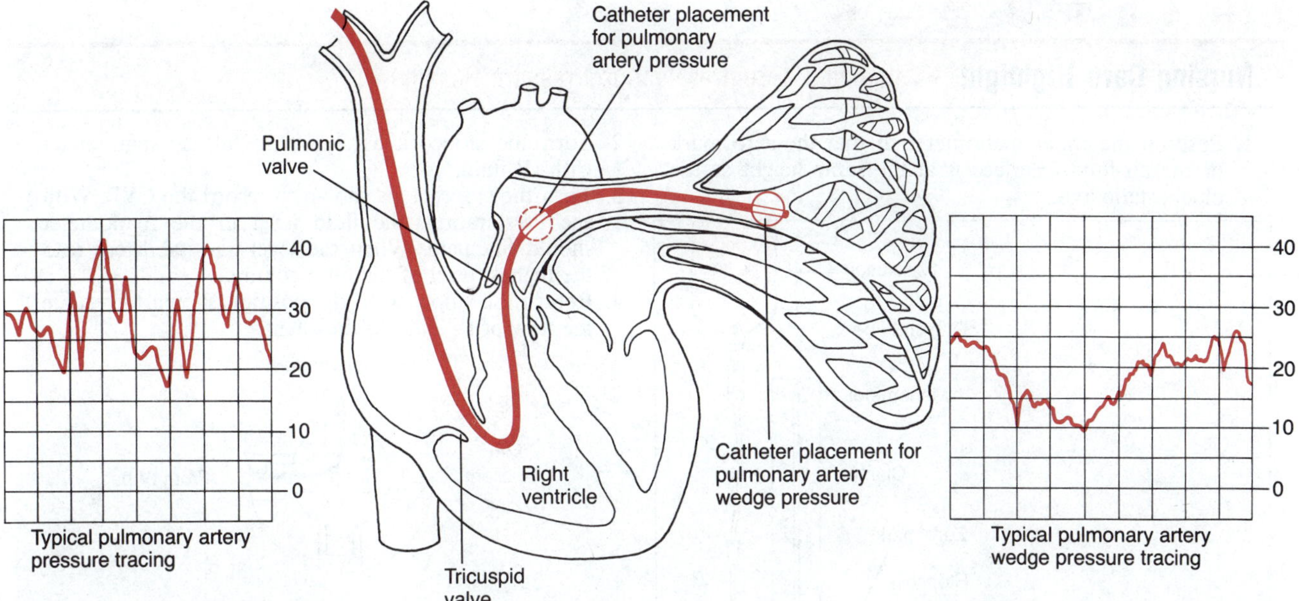

FIGURE 32–22 ◆ Cardiac pressure waveforms can be visualized on the oscilloscope.

mixes with the blood in the right atrium and travels with the flow of blood through the heart. A temperature-sensitive device located on the tip of the catheter in the pulmonary artery registers and senses the change in temperature of the blood. The information is transmitted to a cardiac output computer, which displays a digital value. The normal range of cardiac output in the adult client is 4 to 7 L/minute (Wilson, 1992). The cardiac index, the cardiac output adjusted for the person's size, may also be calculated. The normal range of cardiac output is 2.5 to 4.5 L/minute/mm^2.

CENTRAL VENOUS PRESSURE MONITORING

If the physician desires measurement of pressures from the right atrium or central veins but a pulmonary artery catheter and pressure-monitoring system are not appropriate, pressures may be obtained with a water manometer attached to a conventional IV system. Central venous pressures (CVPs) are similar to right atrial pressures, but CVPs are measured in centimeters of water rather than millimeters of mercury. A normal CVP is 3 to 8 cm H_20.

The physician inserts a catheter through the venous system into the right atrium. A chest x-ray is taken to assess placement. The nurse levels the manometer with the phlebostatic axis to ensure accurate pressure measurement (Chart 32–6).

Elevated CVPs may indicate right ventricular failure. Low CVPs may indicate hypovolemia. Caution must be used in predicting the function of the left side of the heart from a CVP reading.

Care of the site is similar to care of the pulmonary artery catheter site. Complications include pneumothorax during insertion, hemorrhage, infection, and catheter occlusion.

SYSTEMIC INTRA-ARTERIAL MONITORING

Direct measurement of arterial blood pressure is by invasive arterial catheter in critically ill clients. The physician usually inserts an intra-arterial catheter into the radial artery, but the femoral, brachial, or dorsalis pedis arteries may also be used. After the physician has inserted the catheter, the catheter is attached to pressure tubing and a heparinized solution is infused constantly under pressure to maintain the integrity of the system. A transducer attached to the tubing allows continuous direct monitoring of the arterial blood pressure. Direct measurements of blood pressure are usually 10 to 15 mmHg greater than indirect measurements. The arterial catheter may also be used to obtain blood samples for arterial blood gas values and other blood tests.

Because the arterial vasculature is a high-pressure system, frequent assessment of the arterial site and infusion system are essential. The nurse notes any bleeding around the intra-arterial catheter or any loose connections and corrects the situation immediately. Collateral circulation is assessed by Doppler or Allen's tests before and during the time when an arterial catheter is in place. Color, pulse, and temperature at the insertion site should be scrupulously monitored for any early signs of circulatory compromise or venous thrombosis. Complications of systemic intra-arterial monitoring may include pain, in-

CHART 32–6

Nursing Care Highlight ◆ Obtaining a Central Venous Pressure Reading

1. Position the water manometer so that the zero mark or the air-fluid interface is at the same height as the phlebostatic axis.

IV solution
Drip chamber
Manometer
Clamp
Zero mark
Stopcock
Phlebostatic axis
Right atrium
0

2. Turn the stopcock as shown to fill the manometer with IV fluid.
3. Turn the stopcock as shown to record the CVP. With each respiration, the fluid level in the manometer should fluctuate. When the level has stabilized, read the highest level of the fluid column.
4. Return the stopcock to the position shown to resume the flow of IV fluid to the client.

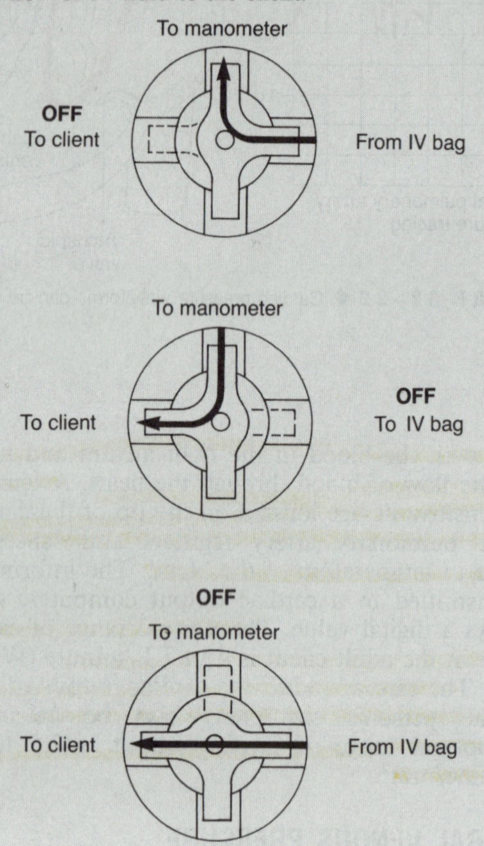

fection, arteriospasm, obstruction at the site with potential for distal infarction, air embolism, and hemorrhage.

ELECTROPHYSIOLOGIC STUDIES

An electrophysiologic study (EPS) is an invasive procedure during which programmed electrical stimulation of the heart is used to induce and evaluate lethal dysrhythmias and conduction abnormalities. Clients who have survived cardiac arrest, have recurrent tachydysrhythmias, or experience unexplained syncopal episodes may be referred for EPS. Induction of the dysrhythmia during EPS permits accurate diagnosis of the dysrhythmia and aids in the search for an effective treatment. These procedures hold risks similar to those for cardiac catheterization and are performed in a special catheterization laboratory, where conditions are strictly controlled and immediate treatment is available for any adverse effects.

CLIENT PREPARATION The preparation of clients for EPS studies parallels preparation of the client undergoing cardiac catheterization (see earlier). Clients may express fear or anxiety, because attempts are made to induce lethal dysrhythmias similar to those that led to the clients' initial hospitalization or resuscitation. The nurse reassures the client that EPS is a planned, controlled event and immediate treatment will be available for any dysrhythmia induced during the studies. An electrophysiologist (a physician who specializes in these studies) usually explains the purpose of the studies; describes the procedure, including benefits and risks; and obtains a written consent.

PROCEDURE The client is taken to a cardiac catheterization laboratory or a similar laboratory where he or she is asked to assume a supine position on an x-ray table. Limb lead electrodes and chest leads are attached for continuous ECG monitoring. Defibrillation pads are placed on the client's chest and back. The nurse or the technician prepares the insertion site according to the hospital's policy. The electrophysiologist injects a local anesthetic into the selected site. A multipolar electrode catheter is then inserted into the femoral vein. The catheter is advanced, guided by fluoroscopy, until one electrode rests in the high right atrium, one electrode is adjacent to the bundle of His, and one electrode is in the right ventricle. Additional electrodes may be placed for endocardial mapping.

During EPS, baseline conduction times can be measured: the AH interval (conduction time from the low right atrium through the His bundle) and the HV interval (conduction time from the proximal His bundle to the ventricular myocardium). The catheter may be programmed to pace at varying rates to determine SA and AV node function or it may be programmed to deliver premature paced stimuli in an effort to initiate and evaluate the client's tachydysrhythmia.

If the dysrhythmia is induced, it may terminate spontaneously or be treated by the physician. The physician might elect to use properly timed stimuli, rapid pacing, medications, or countershock to terminate the dysrhythmia.

The client needs to be advised to tell the staff of any symptoms that he or she is experiencing. During rapid pacing, the client may be aware of the rapid heartbeat and state that he or she is experiencing palpitations. Clients may also experience chest pain or loss of consciousness if they become hypotensive. Clients often experience back discomfort during the procedure, because they must remain supine for 2 to 6 hours. Pain may develop at the insertion site as the anesthetic wears off.

FOLLOW-UP CARE The follow-up care is the same as that for the client who has undergone cardiac catheterization. The nurse may provide comfort measures to alleviate back discomfort, including massage and position changes. If the client lost consciousness during the procedure and received electrical cardioversion or defibrillation, the client may complain of chest discomfort over the area where the electrical current was applied. The nurse assesses the skin for any signs of redness, swelling, or burns. In addition, the client might describe a loss of memory of the events during the procedure, and the nurse needs to provide reassurance and explain the events of the procedure in careful detail.

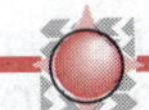

IMPLICATIONS FOR NURSING RESEARCH

During the past few years, nurses have become more proficient in assessing the cardiovascular system. However, a number of questions remain unanswered:

- ◆ How can the nurse best assess chest pain and differentiate the type that a client experiences?
- ◆ Because some nurses do not take blood pressures using the AHA procedure (even if they know how), how can nurses be convinced to use the recommended procedure?
- ◆ How can nurses best emotionally support the client experiencing cardiovascular problems?
- ◆ What is the best way to help a client change lifestyle habits to prevent or to reduce his or her risk of cardiovascular disease?

SELECTED BIBLIOGRAPHY

American Heart Association. (1992). *Heart and stroke facts* (pp. 1–3). Dallas: Author.

*American Nurses' Association Division on Medical-Surgical Nursing Practice and American Heart Association Council on Cardiovascular Nursing. (1981). *Standards of cardiovascular nursing practice.* Kansas City: American Nurses' Association.

Bates, B. (1991). *A guide to physical examination and history taking* (5th ed.). Philadelphia: J. B. Lippincott.

Beattie, S., Billiard, S. J., & Meinhardt, S. L. (1990). The use of cardiac catheterization data to design nursing care plans. *Critical Care Nurse, 10*(6), 43–52.

*Berne, R. M., & Levy, M. N. (1986). *Cardiovascular physiology* (5th ed.). St. Louis: C. V. Mosby.

Bonnono, C., Hedges, J. R., Peterson, C., & Collings, J. L. (1992). Initial nursing impression in patients with chest discomfort. *Journal of Emergency Nursing, 18*(1), 28–32.

Braunwald, E. (Ed.). (1992). *Heart disease: A textbook of cardiovascular medicine* (4th ed.). Philadelphia: W. B. Saunders.

Chassie M. B., & Bradley D. H. (1992). Psychosocial intervention for the critically ill adult. In B. M. Dossey, C. E. Guzzetta, & C. V. Kenner (Eds.), *Critical care nursing* (3rd ed., pp. 101–122). Philadelphia: J. B. Lippincott.

*Clark, S. (1988). Ineffective coping: Patient and family. In L. S. Kern (Ed.), *Cardiac critical care nursing.* Rockville, MD: Aspen Publishers.

Conn, V., Taylor, S., & Abele, P. (1991). Myocardial infarction survivors: Age and gender differences in physical health, psychosocial state and regimen adherence. *Journal of Advanced Nursing, 16,* 1026–1034.

Daily, E. K., & Kenner, C. V. (1992). Hemodynamic monitoring. In B. M. Dossey, C. E. Guzzetta, & C. V. Kenner (Eds.), *Critical care nursing* (3rd ed., pp. 231–258). Philadelphia: J. B. Lippincott.

Department of Health and Human Services. (1990). *Healthy people 2000: National health promotion and disease prevention objectives.* Washington D. C.: U. S. Government Printing Office.

Di Lucente, L., & Gorcsan, J. (1991). Transesophageal

echocardiography: Application to the postoperative cardiac surgery patient. *Dimensions of Critical Care Nursing, 10*(2), 74–80.

Eliopoulos, C. (1991). *Gerontological nursing.* Philadelphia: J. B. Lippincott.

*Fahey, V. A. (1988). *Vascular nursing.* Philadelphia: W. B. Saunders.

*Fitzgerald, S. T. (1989). Occupational outcomes after treatment for coronary heart disease: A review of the literature. *Cardiovascular Nursing, 25*(1), 1–6.

*Froelicher, E. S. (1989). Exercise testing. In S. L. Underhill, S. L. Woods, E. Froelicher, & C. J. Halpenny (Eds.), *Cardiac nursing* (2nd ed., pp. 418–430). Philadelphia: J. B. Lippincott.

Gawlinski, A., & Jensen, G. (1991). The complications of cardiovascular aging. *American Journal of Nursing, 91*(11), 26–30.

Guzzetta C. E., & Casey P. E. (1992). Cardiovascular assessment. In B. M. Dossey, C. E. Guzzetta, & C. V. Kenner (Eds.), *Critical care nursing.* (3rd ed., pp. 397–411). Philadelphia: J. B. Lippincott.

Havens, L. L., & Weaver, J. W. (1992). Cardiovascular system. In M. O. Hogstel (Ed.), *Clinical manual of gerontological nursing* (pp. 70–90). St. Louis: Mosby Year Book.

Hayden, R. (1992). What keeps oxygenation on track? *American Journal of Nursing, 92*(12), 32–43.

Hochrein, M., & Sohl, L. (1992). Heart smart: A guide to cardiac tests. *American Journal of Nursing, 92*(12), 22–25.

Jarvis, C. (1992). *Physical examination and health assessment.* Philadelphia: W. B. Saunders.

*Kennedy, G. (1988). Clinical cardiac assessment. In L. S. Kern (Ed.), *Cardiac critical care nursing* (pp. 1–31). Rockville, MD: Aspen Publishers.

*Kirkendall, W. M., Feinleib, M. D., & Fries, E. D. (1988). *Recommendations for human blood pressure determination by sphygmomanometers.* Dallas: American Heart Association.

*Lane, L. D., & Winslow, E. H. (1987). Oxygen consumption, cardiovascular response, and perceived exertion in healthy adults during rest, occupied bedmaking, and unoccupied bedmaking activity. *Cardiovascular Nursing, 23*(6), 31–36.

McCauley, K. M. (1992). Cognitive strategies for emotional distress after myocardial infarction. *Med–Surg Nursing Quarterly, 1*(2), 56–70.

Mishell, D. R. (1989). Correcting misconceptions about oral contraceptives. *American Journal of Obstetrics and Gynecology, 161,* 1385–1389.

*New York Heart Association Criteria Committee. (1964). *Diseases of the heart and blood vessels: Nomenclature and criteria for diagnosis* (6th ed.). Boston: Little, Brown.

Swearingen, R. L., & Keen, J. L. (1991). *Manual of critical care.* (2nd ed.). St. Louis: Mosby Year Book.

*Tilkian, A. G., & Daily, E. K. (1986). *Cardiovascular procedures: Diagnostic techniques and therapeutic procedures.* St. Louis: C. V. Mosby.

*Tortora, G. (1989). *Principles of human anatomy* (5th ed.). New York: Harper & Row.

Van Bushirk, M. C., & Gradman, A. H. (1993). Monitoring blood pressure in ambulatory patients. *American Journal of Nursing, 93*(6), 44–47.

Weigle, D. S. (1992). The pathophysiology of obesity: Implications for treatment. *Clinician Reviews, 2*(5), 81–102.

Wilson, R. F. (1992). *Critical care manual.* Philadelphia: F. A. Davis.

Wingate, S. (1991). Women and coronary heart disease: Implications for the clinical setting. *Focus on Critical Care, 18*(3), 212–218.

SUGGESTED READINGS

Conn, V., Taylor, S., & Abele, P. (1991). Myocardial infarction survivors: Age and gender differences in physical health, psychosocial state and regimen adherence. *Journal of Advanced Nursing, 16,* 1026–1034.

This article examines the physical and psychosocial status of people who had a myocardial infarction (MI), particularly in relationship to age and gender. The compliance rate with the post–MI regimen was also evaluated.

McCauley, K. M. (1992). Cognitive strategies for emotional distress after myocardial infarction. *Med-Surg Nursing Quarterly, 1*(2), 56–70.

This article discusses the emotional reactions that clients with MIs have, especially denial, anxiety, and depression. The author also provides ideas for interventions to help these clients cope with their health problem.

Van Bushirk, M. C., & Gradman, A. H. (1993). Monitoring blood pressure in ambulatory patients. *American Journal of Nursing, 93*(6), 44–47.

This article describes ambulatory blood pressure monitoring (ABPM), including how it works, how it is analyzed, and what costs associated with the system are. A list of ABPM manufacturers is also provided.

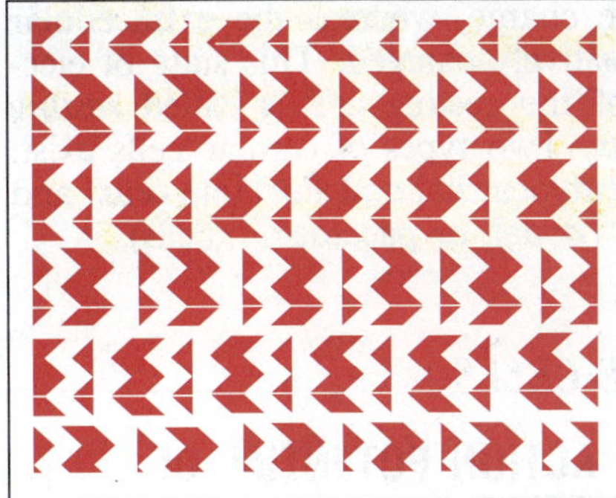

CHAPTER 33

Interventions for Clients with Dysrhythmias

CHAPTER HIGHLIGHTS

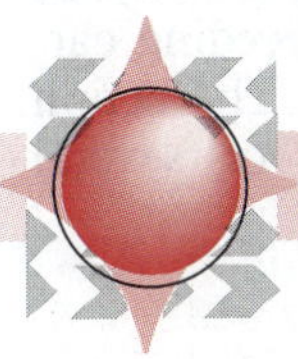

Cardiac dysrhythmias are disturbances of cardiac electrical impulse formation, conduction, or both. Many diseases can affect the electrical activity of the heart, causing dysrhythmias. Many dysrhythmias are benign. Some dysrhythmias affect the pumping efficiency of the heart, leading to hemodynamic instability. A few dysrhythmias result in cardiac arrest. To understand dysrhythmias thoroughly and to interpret these disturbances correctly, the nurse must understand cardiac electrophysiology, the conduction system of the heart, and the principles of electrocardiography.

REVIEW OF CARDIAC ELECTROPHYSIOLOGY

Electrophysiologic Properties

The electrophysiologic properties of cardiac cells regulate heart rate and rhythm. Specialized cardiac muscle cells possess unique properties: automaticity, excitability, conductivity, and contractility.

AUTOMATICITY

Automaticity (spontaneous depolarization) is the ability of cardiac cells to generate an electrical impulse spontaneously and repetitively without external neurohormonal influence. The movement of electrolytes into the cells changes the electrical balance. Normally, only primary pacemaker cells possess this property. Under certain conditions, such as myocardial ischemia and infarction, electrolyte imbalances, and drug therapy, any cardiac cell may exhibit this property, generating electrical impulses independently and creating dysrhythmias.

EXCITABILITY

Excitability is the ability of nonpacemaker cardiac cells to respond to an electrical impulse generated from pacemaker cells and to depolarize. Depolarization occurs when the normally negatively charged cells develop a positive charge. This is accomplished through the inward movement of sodium resulting from the excitation process. Myocardial cells and Purkinje cells exhibit excitability.

CONDUCTIVITY

Conductivity is the ability to transmit an electrical stimulus from cell membrane to cell membrane. Consequently, excitable cells depolarize in rapid succession from cell to cell until all cells have depolarized. This wave of depolarization gives rise to the deflections of the ECG waveforms that are recognized as the P wave and the QRS complex.

CONTRACTILITY

Contractility is the ability of cardiac muscle cells to shorten their fiber length in response to electrical stimulation, generating sufficient pressure to propel blood forward. This is the mechanical activity of the heart. The atria contract and pump blood into the ventricles. The ventricles contract and eject blood out into the great vessels, producing the cardiac output.

Action Potential

The cardiac cell membrane (sarcolemma) exhibits selective permeability to ions. This creates an electrical imbalance, known as an action potential, across the cell membrane. Channels and gates selectively promote and restrict ionic movement across the membrane. Cardiac muscle cells are interconnected by specialized junctions called intercalated disks. Electrical impulses are transmitted through these junctions, which are low-resistance pathways, to adjacent cells until all cells have been stimulated. The heart's intricate interconnecting network allows it to function as though it were a single muscle fiber.

The intracellular environment of the cardiac cell at rest has a negative charge, whereas the extracellular environment is positively charged. This state of electrical imbalance of the resting cell is called *resting membrane potential.* Two types of cardiac cells exist: fast-response cells (myocardial and Purkinje cells) and slow-response cells (nodal, or pacemaker, cells).

FAST-RESPONSE CELLS

PHASES OF THE ACTION POTENTIAL OF FAST-RESPONSE CELLS

When myocardial and Purkinje cells are at rest, their cellular membrane is permeable to potassium but relatively impermeable to sodium. Therefore, potassium freely diffuses out of cells (efflux), following its concentration gradient, because there is more potassium inside the cells than outside. Because potassium is a positive ion (cation), this diffusion leaves the cells negatively charged relative to the outside environment, which becomes positively charged. The electrical difference is approximately −90 millivolts (mV) in ventricular cells during resting membrane potential at the end of phase 4 of the preceding cardiac cycle. The cells are ready for action. The action potential of fast-response cells consists of several phases (Fig. 33–1).

PHASE 0

Phase 0 is the phase of rapid depolarization. A stimulus from an impulse generated from pacemaker cells reaches the excitable myocardial and Purkinje cells. The stimulus causes a sudden increase in cell membrane permeability to sodium, initiating depolarization, or electrical stimulation of cells. As sodium, a cation, diffuses into the cells (influx), the cells become less negatively charged, allowing the membrane voltage to reach threshold, at approximately −60 mV. At threshold, fast sodium channels open, allowing sodium to diffuse rapidly into the cells, following its concentration gradient. The internal environment of the cells becomes positive, at approximately +20 mV. Depolarization is complete. As depolarization occurs from cell to cell, a wave of positive current is created. The ECG lead system senses this current and inscribes a P wave during atrial depolarization or a QRS complex during ventricular depolarization.

PHASE 1

Phase 1 is the phase of early rapid repolarization. Sodium channels are inactivated, and there is a small efflux of potassium and a small influx of chloride across the cell membrane. As the positive potassium ions leave the cells and the negative chloride ions enter the cells, myocardial and Purkinje cells have a decreased positive charge until they are nearly electrically equal with the extracellular environment.

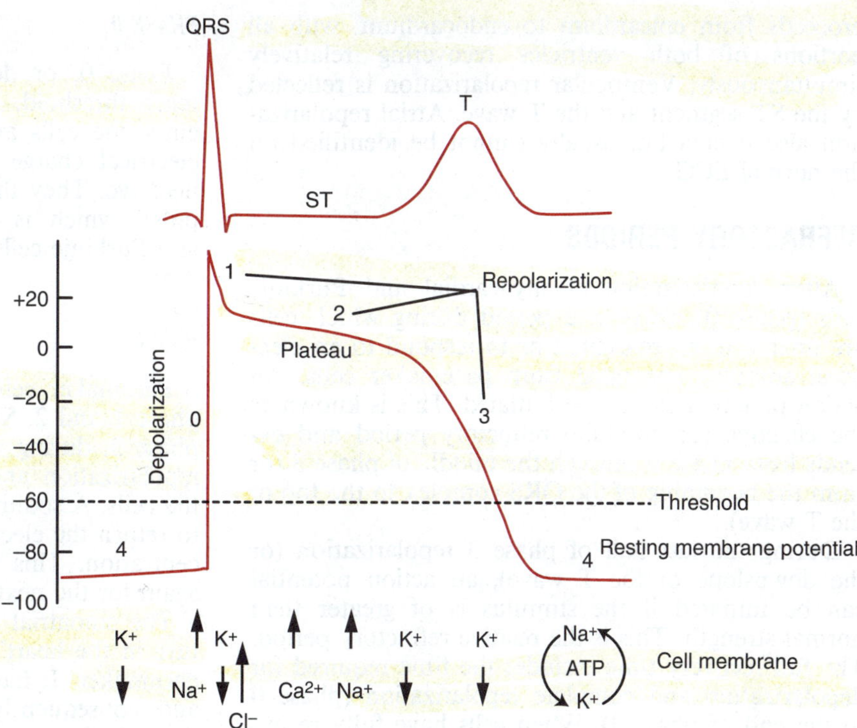

FIGURE 33-1 ◆ Action potential of a fast-response cell (muscle cell). Exchange of ions across the cell membrane occurs at different points of the action potential. At rest, the inside of the cardiac cell is more negatively charged than the outside of the cell and the cell membrane is more permeable to potassium (K^+) than to sodium (Na^+) ions. With a sufficient electrical stimulus, the cell membrane becomes more permeable to Na^+. As Na^+ enters the cell, the inside of the cell becomes positively charged (Phase 0, depolarization). Sodium channels become inactivated. K^+ leaves the cell and chloride (Cl^-) enters the cell, decreasing the positive charge (Phase 1, early repolarization). Calcium (Ca^{2+}) and Na^+ ions enter the cell while K^+ leaves the cell (Phase 2, plateau), allowing Ca^{2+} to initiate muscle contraction. K^+ leaves the cell (Phase 3, repolarization), returning the cell to its negative state. K^+ regains dominance over Na^+ diffusion and establishes equilibrium (Phase 4, resting membrane potential) before another stimulus is elicited.

PHASE 2

Phase 2, the plateau phase, is long, lasting more than 100 milliseconds (msec). Slow calcium channels allow the influx of calcium ions into the cells. Sodium may also diffuse into the cells via slow channels. These currents are balanced by the slow efflux of potassium ions out of the cells, thus maintaining a membrane potential of approximately 0 mV (i.e., the inside and outside environments of the cells are nearly equal electrically). The calcium influx into cells triggers the initiation of muscle contraction. This complex interrelationship of electrical stimulation leading to mechanical contraction is called excitation-contraction coupling. Phases 1 and 2 in ventricular myocardial and Purkinje cells are reflected by the ST segment on the ECG.

PHASE 3

Phase 3 is the phase of rapid repolarization. The cells regain their negative charge. This results from the efflux of potassium out of the cells while the other channels are inactivated, allowing the internal cellular environment to become negatively charged again. This process of repolarization, or electrical recovery of cells, is reflected by the T wave on the ECG.

PHASE 4

During the beginning of phase 4, a sodium-potassium pump is responsible for actively pumping sodium out of the cells and potassium back into the cells, against their concentration gradients, with the expenditure of energy from adenosine triphosphate (ATP). Electrolytes are returning to their area of greatest concentration, preparing for the next cardiac cycle. Cell negativity returns to normal (i.e., the resting membrane potential).

In phase 4, the charge of fast-response cells should remain stable at −90 mV until the next pacemaker-generated impulse arrives to excite the cells and start the process again. If cells become unstable owing to myocardial ischemia or hypokalemia, phase 4 may slope up and reach threshold; fast-response cells then fire an impulse, behaving as pacemaker cells. This is called altered automaticity; it causes a type of dysrhythmia called a premature beat.

PROCESSES OF DEPOLARIZATION AND REPOLARIZATION

As just discussed, depolarization is the process by which normally negatively charged (resting) cardiac cells become positively charged on the inside (electrically stimulated). This creates a wave of positive current. The current flows from endocardium to epicardium. Atrial depolarization proceeds first from right atrium to left atrium, generating a P wave. Ventricular depolarization proceeds from the interventricular septum in a left-to-right direction, continues to the ventricular apex and much of the right ventricle, and concludes with the basal (upper) portion of both ventricles and septum. This generates the QRS complex.

Repolarization, the electrical recovery of the cells,

proceeds from epicardium to endocardium, with all portions of both ventricles recovering relatively simultaneously. Ventricular repolarization is reflected by the ST segment and the T wave. Atrial repolarization also occurs but usually cannot be identified on the normal ECG.

REFRACTORY PERIODS

After depolarization of myocardial and Purkinje cells (phase 0), there is a period during which cells are unable to be re-excited or to respond to an electrical stimulus generated from pacemaker cells. An action potential cannot be initiated. This is known as the effective (or absolute) refractory period and extends from phase 0 through the middle of phase 3 (or from the beginning of the QRS complex to the top of the T wave).

During the last half of phase 3 repolarization (or the downslope of the T wave), an action potential can be initiated if the stimulus is of greater than normal strength. This is the relative refractory period. The full recovery time includes the time required for depolarization and complete repolarization (phase 0 to the end of phase 3). When cells have fully recovered, they are nonrefractory, responding to a stimulus of normal strength with a normal action potential.

SLOW-RESPONSE CELLS

The action potential of slow-response cells (nodal, or pacemaker, cells) differs from that of fast-response cells (Fig. 33–2). The resting membrane potential of pacemaker cells is less negative, at approximately −60 mV.

PHASE 4

Phase 4 is the phase of spontaneous diastolic depolarization. It is an unstable phase, providing automaticity in pacemaker cells. This is accomplished through a slow inward current, believed to be due largely to the slow influx of calcium and sodium, along with a decreased efflux of potassium. The influx of cations creates instability in the membrane potential. The cells decrease their negative charge and spontaneously reach their activation threshold, at approximately −40 mV; that is, phase 4 slopes up and reaches threshold. This initiates an action potential.

PHASE 0

Phase 0, or depolarization, occurs after the cells reach threshold. As calcium and sodium continue to enter the cells and potassium efflux is reduced, the electrical charge of the cells becomes less and less negative. They then generate or fire an electrical impulse, which is conducted to excitable myocardial and Purkinje cells as described earlier. The cells reach 0 mV.

PHASE 3

Pacemaker cells do not have a plateau phase, or phase 1 and 2. Slow repolarization begins, leading to phase 3, during which potassium efflux causes rapid repolarization and the return of negative charges to the cells. A sodium-potassium pump is then activated to return the electrolytes to their area of greatest concentration. This is preparation to begin the process again for the next cycle.

The sinoatrial (SA) node, which is the first structure in the heart's conduction system, is the primary pacemaker. It has the greatest number of nodal cells and consequently the fastest rate of automaticity. Secondary, or subsidiary, pacemakers have fewer nodal cells and therefore a slower rate of automaticity. Subsidiary pacemakers include atrioventricular (AV) junctional cells and ventricular Purkinje cells. They can serve as "escape," or latent, pacemakers when the primary pacemakers become dysfunctional.

CARDIAC CONDUCTION SYSTEM

The cardiac conduction system consists of specialized cells. It is responsible for the generation and conduction of electrical impulses that stimulate atrial and ventricular muscles to contract (Fig. 33–3). The conduction system consists of the sinoatrial node, internodal pathway and tracts, atrioventricular (AV) junctional area, and bundle branch system.

Sinoatrial Node

The conduction system begins with the sinoatrial (SA) node (also called the sinus node), located close

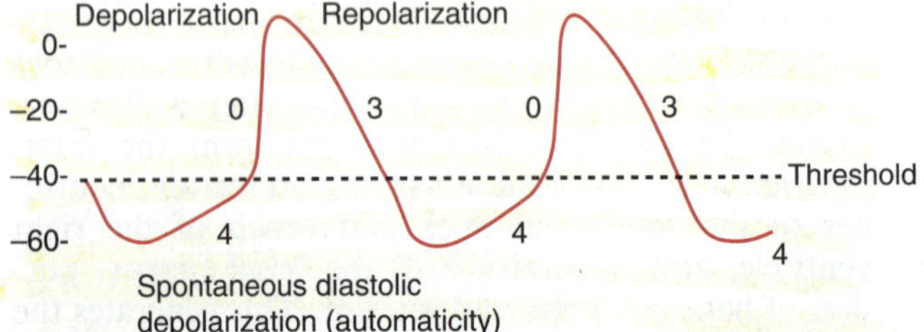

FIGURE 33–2 ◆ Action potential of a slow-response cell (pacemaker cell). At rest, the cell is less negative than the muscle cell. During Phase 4 (spontaneous diastolic depolarization), the pacemaker cell membrane is more permeable to Ca^{2+} and Na^{+} ions than to K^{+} ions. Ca^{2+} and Na^{+} enter the cell, decreasing the negative charge (the property of automaticity) until threshold is reached. Ca^{2+} and Na^{+} continue to enter the cell until the cell is no longer negatively charged (Phase 0, depolarization), and the cell fires an electrical stimulus. The cell is now more permeable to K^{+} and less permeable to Ca^{2+} and Na^{+}. K^{+} leaves the cell, returning the cell to its negative state (Phase 3, repolarization). The slow Ca^{2+} and Na^{+} channels regain dominance over K^{+}, creating instability in the resting state (Phase 4), allowing the process to begin again for another cycle.

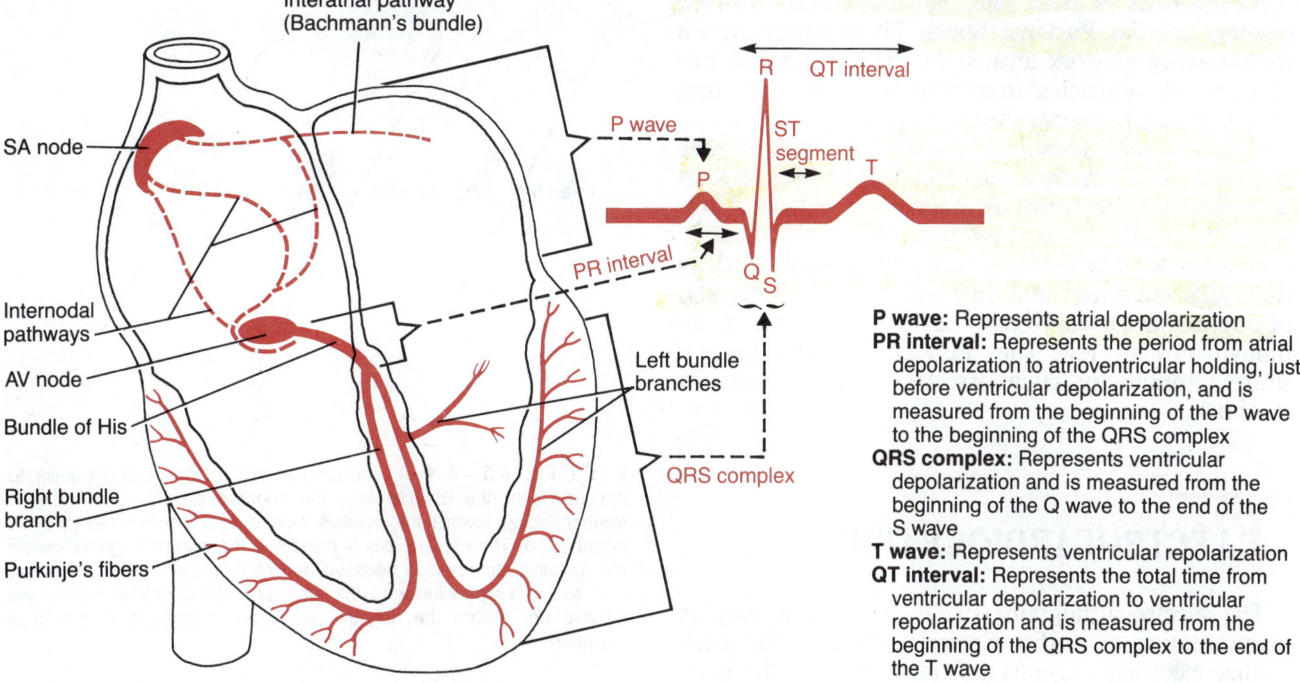

FIGURE 33-3 ◆ The cardiac conduction system.

to the epicardial surface of the right atrium near its junction with the superior vena cava. The SA node consists primarily of P (pacemaker) cells (nodal cells) and is the heart's primary pacemaker. It can spontaneously and rhythmically generate electrical impulses at a rate of 60 to 100/minute, possessing the property of automaticity.

The SA node is richly innervated by the sympathetic and parasympathetic nervous systems, which accelerate and decelerate the rate of discharge of the sinus node, respectively. This results in changes in the heart rate. In 55% to 60% of the population, the SA node is perfused by a branch of the right coronary artery (RCA) (Braunwald, 1992). In the remaining population, it is perfused by a branch from the left circumflex artery.

Internodal Pathway and Tracts

Anatomic evidence suggests that an anterior internodal pathway emerges from the SA node. This anterior internodal pathway also gives rise to an interatrial band called *Bachmann's bundle,* which sends fibers to the left atrium. In addition, there is a middle internodal tract and a posterior internodal tract. The anterior, middle, and posterior internodal tracts send fibers to the AV node. These tracts are thought to conduct impulses rapidly to both atria, leading to atrial depolarization. This is reflected by a P wave on the electrocardiographic (ECG) trace. Atrial muscle contraction follows. The function of these tracts remains controversial, because their existence has not been proven (Braunwald, 1992).

Atrioventricular Junctional Area

The AV junctional area consists of a transitional cell zone, the AV node itself, and the His bundle. The AV node lies just beneath the right atrial endocardium, between the tricuspid valve and the ostium of the coronary sinus. Here, T cells (transitional cells) cause impulses to slow down or be delayed in the AV node before proceeding to the ventricles. This delay is reflected by the PR segment on the ECG. This slow conduction provides a physiologic delay, allowing the atria to contract before ventricular stimulation and contraction. This contraction, known as the "atrial kick," contributes 15% to 30% of additional blood volume for a greater cardiac output. Nodal cells in the AV junctional area may occasionally demonstrate automaticity, giving rise to junctional beats or rhythms. In 85% to 90% of the population, the AV node is perfused by a branch of the right coronary artery (Braunwald, 1992). It is innervated by both the sympathetic and parasympathetic nervous systems.

Bundle Branch System

The bundle of His connects with the distal portion of the AV node and continues on to perforate the septum. It is perfused by branches from both the left anterior descending (LAD) and posterior descending coronary arteries. It extends as a right bundle branch down the right side of the interventricular septum to the apex of the right ventricle. On the left side, it extends as a left bundle branch, which further divides.

At the ends of both right and left bundle branch systems are the Purkinje fibers. These fibers are an interweaving network located on the endocardial surface of both ventricles, from apex to bases. The fibers then partially penetrate into the myocardium.

Purkinje cells make up the His bundle, bundle branches, and terminal Purkinje fibers. They are responsible for the rapid conduction of electrical impulses throughout the ventricles. This rapid conduction leads to ventricular depolarization, reflected by the QRS complex, and the subsequent ventricular muscle contraction. Nodal cells are also present, although they are few. They may occasionally demonstrate automaticity, giving rise to ventricular beats or rhythms.

ELECTROCARDIOGRAPHY

The electrocardiogram (ECG) provides a graphic representation of cardiac electrical activity. The weak cardiac electrical currents are transmitted to the body surface. The placement of electrodes on various sites on the body provides different leads, or views, of the heart's electrical activity. Electrode placement is the same for male and female clients. Electrodes consist of conductive medium on an adhesive pad. They attach to cables or wires connected to an ECG machine or to a monitor. The cardiac electrical current is transmitted via the electrodes and through the lead wires to the machine or monitor. The monitor provides one or more views of this electrical activity.

Lead systems are made up of a positive pole and a negative pole. An imaginary line joining these two poles is called the *lead axis.* The direction of electrical current flow in the heart is the *cardiac axis.* The relationship of the cardiac axis to the lead axis is responsible for the deflections seen on the ECG pattern:

- The baseline is the isoelectric line. It occurs when there is no current flow in the heart after complete depolarization and also after complete repolarization. Positive deflections occur above this line and negative deflections occur below this line. Deflections represent depolarization and repolarization of cells.
- If the direction of electrical current flow in the heart (cardiac axis) is parallel to the lead axis with the current moving toward the positive pole, a monophasic (single-component) positive deflection is inscribed (Fig. 33–4*A*).
- If the cardiac axis is parallel to the lead axis, but the current is moving away from the positive pole, toward the negative pole, a monophasic negative deflection is inscribed (see Fig. 33–4*B*).
- If the cardiac axis is exactly perpendicular to the lead axis, with the current going neither toward nor away from the positive pole but rather crossing the lead axis, a biphasic (two-component) deflection is inscribed. The deflection is equal in both positive and negative directions (see Fig. 33–4*C*).

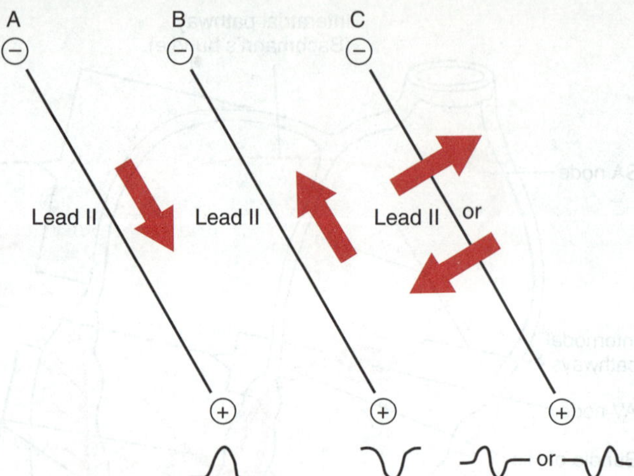

FIGURE 33–4 ◆ *A,* The cardiac axis *(bold arrow)* is parallel to the lead axis (the line between the negative and the positive electrodes), going toward the positive electrode; a positive deflection is inscribed. *B,* The cardiac axis is parallel to the lead axis, going toward the negative electrode; a negative deflection is inscribed. *C,* The cardiac axis is perpendicular to the lead axis, going neither toward the positive nor toward the negative electrode; a biphasic deflection is inscribed.

The strength, or magnitude, of the cardiac current determines the size or amplitude of the deflection: the greater the current magnitude, the larger the deflection. Cardiac disease can affect the current's magnitude. Myocardial infarction (MI) may decrease the amplitude, whereas ventricular hypertrophy increases the amplitude. In addition, the relationship of the lead axis to the cardiac axis affects the amplitude of deflections seen on the ECG. Leads parallel to the cardiac axis inscribe larger deflections than do perpendicular leads.

Lead Systems

The standard 12-lead ECG consists of 12 leads (or views) of the heart's electrical activity. Six of the leads are called limb leads because the electrodes are placed on the client's four limbs in the frontal plane. The remaining six leads are called chest (precordial) leads because the electrodes are placed on the client's chest in the horizontal plane (see Chap. 32).

LIMB LEADS

Standard bipolar limb leads consist of a positive and a negative electrode, which determine the lead axis, as well as a reference, or ground, electrode. Bipolar leads can be obtained by using a monitor with either three or five electrode cables or a 12-lead ECG machine. Leads I, II, and III are bipolar leads (Table 33–1).

TABLE 33–1 Electrode Placement for 12 Leads

Lead	Negative Electrode	Positive Electrode	Ground Electrode
I	• Right arm, or under the right clavicle	• Left arm, or under the left clavicle	• Right leg, or lowest rib, left mid-clavicular line
II	• Right arm, or under the right clavicle	• Left leg, or lowest rib, left mid-clavicular line	• Right leg, or under the left clavicle
III	• Left arm, or under the left clavicle	• Left leg, or lowest rib, left mid-clavicular line	• Right leg, or under the right clavicle
aVR	• Average potential of left arm (or under the left clavicle) and left leg (or lowest rib, left mid-clavicular line)	• Right arm, or under the right clavicle	• Right leg, or lowest rib, right mid-clavicular line
aVL	• Average potential of right arm (or under the right clavicle) and left leg (or lowest rib, left mid-clavicular line)	• Left arm, or under the left clavicle	• Same as for aVR
aVF	• Average potential of right arm (or under the right clavicle) and left arm (or under the left clavicle)	• Left leg, or lowest rib, left mid-clavicular line	• Same as for aVR
V_1	• Average potential of right arm, left arm, and left leg	• Fourth intercostal space (ICS), right sternal border	• Same as for aVR
V_2	• Same as for V_1	• Fourth ICS, left sternal border	• Same as for aVR
V_3	• Same as for V_1	• Midway between V_2 and V_4	• Same as for aVR
V_4	• Same as for V_1	• Fifth ICS, left mid-clavicular line	• Same as for aVR
V_5	• Same as for V_1	• Horizontal to V_4, left anterior axillary line	• Same as for aVR
V_6	• Same as for V_1	• Horizontal to V_4, left mid-axillary line	• Same as for aVR

- In lead I, the right arm electrode is negative and the left arm electrode is positive.
- In lead II, the right arm electrode is negative and the left leg electrode is positive.
- In lead III, the left arm electrode is negative and the left leg electrode is positive.

Unipolar limb leads consist of a positive electrode only. These leads can be obtained only by using a monitor with five electrode cables or a 12-lead ECG machine. The unipolar limb leads are leads aVR, aVL, and aVF, with "a" meaning augmented. "V" is a designation for a unipolar lead. The third letter denotes the positive electrode placement: "R" for right arm, "L" for left arm, and "F" for foot (left leg). The positive electrode is at one end of the lead axis. The other end is the center of the electrical field, at approximately the center of the heart.

CHEST LEADS

Chest (precordial) leads are also unipolar, or V, leads and therefore can be obtained only from a monitor with five electrode cables or a 12-lead ECG machine. There are six chest leads, determined by the placement of the chest electrode. The four limb electrodes are placed on the extremities, as designated on each electrode (right arm, left arm, right leg, and left leg). The fifth (chest) electrode is the positive, or exploring, electrode. It is placed in one of the following positions (see Table 33–1):

- V_1 on the fourth intercostal space (ICS), just to the right of the sternum
- V_2 on the fourth ICS, just to the left of the sternum
- V_3 midway between V_2 and V_4
- V_4 on the fifth ICS, on the left mid-clavicular line
- V_5 horizontal to (same level as) V_4, on the left anterior axillary line
- V_6 horizontal to V_4, on the left mid-axillary line

The nurse instructs the female client with large breasts to displace and hold the left breast so that electrode position can be accurate.

Continuous Electrocardiographic Monitoring

For continuous ECG monitoring, the electrodes are not placed on the client's limbs, because movement of the extremities causes "noise," or motion artifact, on the ECG signal. The nurse places the electrodes on the client's trunk, a more stable area, to minimize such artifact and to obtain a clearer signal. If the monitoring system provides five electrode cables, the nurse places the electrodes as follows:

- Right arm electrode just below the right clavicle
- Left arm electrode just below the left clavicle
- Right leg electrode on the lowest palpable rib, on the right mid-clavicular line
- Left leg electrode on the lowest palpable rib, on the left mid-clavicular line
- The fifth electrode is placed to obtain one of the six chest leads.

With this placement, the monitor lead select control may be changed to provide lead I, II, III, aVR, aVL, aVF, or one chest lead. The monitor automatically alters the polarity of the electrodes to provide the lead selected.

If the monitoring system provides only three electrode cables, the nurse places the right arm, the left arm, and the left leg electrodes as described above. In this case, the lead select provides only lead I, II, or III.

The popular MCL1 lead is a modified (M) bipolar chest (C) lead. It approximates the V_1 lead without requiring a five-electrode cable monitoring system because it is a bipolar lead system. To obtain MCL1, the nurse places the negative electrode just below the left (L) mid-clavicle, and the positive electrode in the V_1 position. The ground electrode may be placed anywhere but is usually placed under the right clavicle. The nurse uses this lead for bedside or telemetry monitoring to differentiate left from right electrical activity, such as left from right bundle branch block and left from right premature ventricular complexes (PVCs). It can also differentiate supraventricular beats that are aberrantly conducted from ventricular ectopic beats. Such differentiations are not addressed in this chapter. The MCL1 lead provides a right-sided view of cardiac electrical activity.

Another bipolar lead, MCL6, is frequently used. It can be achieved by placing the negative and ground electrodes as for MCL1 and moving the positive electrode to the V_6 position. This approximates the V_6 lead and provides a left-sided view of cardiac electrical activity. It is used for the same reasons as MCL1.

The clarity of continuous ECG monitor recordings is affected by skin preparation and electrode quality (Research Applications for Nursing). To optimize signal transmission, the nurse decreases skin impedance by cleaning the skin with soap and water. The nurse also shaves the area if it is hairy, wipes the electrode sites with an alcohol or other skin preparation pad, and dries the sites well. The gel applied to each electrode must be moist and fresh. The nurse attaches the lead electrode to the lead cable before applying the electrode to the skin. The nurse rubs the skin briskly with a gauze square or a washcloth (facecloth) until the skin is slightly reddened; the nurse then rolls the electrode onto the site for proper contact. Some electrode manufacturers provide a small black dot of fine sandpaper on the electrode backing to rub the skin. This action rubs off surface cells and increases capillary blood flow to the area. The nurse ensures that the contact site does not have any lotion, tincture, or other substance on it that increases skin impedance. Electrodes cannot be placed on abraded or irritated skin or over scar tissue.

ECG cables may be attached directly to a wall-mounted monitor (a hardwired system) if the client's activity is restricted to bed rest and sitting in a chair, as in a critical care unit. For an ambulatory client, the ECG cable is attached to a battery-operated transmitter (a telemetry system) held in a pouch worn by the client. The client's ECG is transmitted via antennae located in strategic places, usually in the ceiling, to a remote monitor. This allows the client freedom of movement within a certain radius without losing transmission of the ECG.

RESEARCH APPLICATIONS FOR NURSING

Effective Skin Preparation for Electrode Placement May Minimize Artifact

Clochesy, J. M., Cifani, L., & Howe, K. (1991). Electrode site preparation techniques: A follow-up study. *Heart & Lung, 20,* 27–30.

One of the problems with disposable skin electrodes has been the amount of artifact, or noise, that interferes with the transmission of electrical signals during cardiac monitoring. Proper skin preparation reduces skin resistance, which decreases artifact. The researchers replicated a study from 3 years earlier to determine the best way to prepare the skin to minimize artifact.

One hundred twenty healthy volunteers were randomly assigned to four groups: three treatment groups and one control group. Group 1 received the One Step Skin Prep, group 2 received the ECG Prep Pad for five strokes, group 3 received the ECG Prep Pad for one stroke, and group 4 received an alcohol pad. The results showed that the groups who received the One Step Skin Prep and the ECG Prep Pad for one stroke had significantly better results than did the other two groups. These findings were consistent with the earlier study that the researchers replicated.

Critique Studies that replicate previous reports help to validate their results. The researchers used a post-test–only control group design in which random assignment to four groups was used. This research method helps to control for intervening variables that could affect the results.

Possible nursing implications The method used to prepare the skin for electrode placement seems to affect the results. Artifact can be minimized by using one of the effective skin preparation techniques that reduce skin resistance.

Signal-Averaged Electrocardiography

Signal-averaged electrocardiography (SAECG) is a newer, noninvasive study that allows the physician to examine more closely the terminal portion of the QRS complex and the beginning of the ST segment for evidence of delayed potentials. These delays may trigger dysrhythmias such as ventricular tachycardia (Merva, 1993). Such small potentials are not visible on the surface ECG. They are obscured by noise in the ECG signals from muscle movement and electrical interference. Signal averaging minimizes such noise, achieving a smoother signal. Through computerization, 150 to 300 cycles of sinus rhythm are recorded, averaged together, and amplified. Because the quality of the ECG signal is critical to this data analysis, the nurse or the ECG technician must carefully prepare the electrode sites, ensure the quality of the electrodes, and apply the electrodes correctly. Lead placement is different from that with a 12-lead ECG and is indicated as leads X, Y, and Z.

The nurse explains the procedure to the client and instructs him or her to lie down, get comfortable, relax, and lie as still as possible during the procedure. This prevents excessive noise in the signal from muscle movement. The procedure lasts approximately 10 minutes. This test may help identify which post–myocardial infarction clients are at risk for ventricular tachycardia and sudden cardiac death and guide the selection of appropriate therapy.

Electrocardiographic Complexes, Segments, and Intervals

Complexes that make up a normal ECG consist of a P wave, a QRS complex, a T wave, and possibly a U wave. Segments include the PR segment, the ST segment, and the TP segment. Intervals include the PR interval, QRS duration, and the QT interval (Fig. 33–5).

THE P WAVE

The P wave is a deflection representing atrial depolarization. This is the electrical excitation of atrial myocardial cells after SA node (pacemaker) impulse formation and conduction to those cells. It results from phase 0 depolarization of atrial muscle cells. The impulse is conducted from cell to cell throughout the atria. The morphologic configuration (shape) of the P wave may be a positive, negative, or biphasic deflection, depending on the lead selected. When the electrical impulse is consistently generated from the SA node, the P waves have the same morphologic features in a given lead. If an impulse is then generated from a different (ectopic) focus, the morphologic features of the P wave change in that lead. This indicates that an ectopic focus has fired; that is, a focus other than the SA node has generated that impulse (e.g., atrial, junctional, or ventricular tissue).

THE PR SEGMENT

The PR segment is the isoelectric line from the end of the P wave to the beginning of the QRS complex, when the electrical impulse is traveling through the atrioventricular (AV) node. There it is delayed. It then travels through the ventricular conduction system to the Purkinje fibers, just before ventricular depolarization.

THE PR INTERVAL

The PR interval is measured from the beginning of the P wave to the end of the PR segment (beginning of the QRS complex). It represents the time required for atrial depolarization as well as the impulse delay in the AV node and the travel time to the Purkinje fibers. It normally measures from 0.12 to 0.2 second in duration.

THE QRS COMPLEX

The QRS complex represents ventricular depolarization, which is the electrical excitation of ventricular myocardial and Purkinje cells. It results from phase 0 depolarization of these ventricular cells. The impulse is conducted from cell to cell throughout the ventricles. The shape of the QRS complex, like that of the P wave, depends on the lead selected. The Q wave is the first negative deflection and is not present in all leads. When present, it is small and represents initial ventricular septal depolarization. The R wave is the first positive deflection. It may be small or large, depending on the lead. The S wave is a negative deflection following the R wave and is not present in all leads. If another positive deflection is present after the S wave, it is called an R′ (R prime) wave. A negative deflection following the R′ is an S′ (S prime) wave. R′ and S′ waves usually indicate ventricular conduction abnormalities.

THE QRS DURATION

The QRS duration represents the time required for depolarization of both ventricles. It is measured from the end of the PR segment (the beginning of the QRS complex) to the J-point (the junction where the QRS complex ends and the ST segment begins). It normally measures from 0.04 to 0.1 second.

THE ST SEGMENT

The ST segment is normally an isoelectric line and represents early ventricular repolarization, corresponding to phases 1 and 2 of the action potential when the membrane potential decreases to 0 mV. It occurs from the J-point to the beginning of the T wave. Its length varies with changes in the heart rate, the administration of medications, and electrolyte disturbances. It is normally not elevated more than 1 mm nor depressed more than 0.5 mm from the isoelectric line as seen in the TP segment. Its amplitude is measured at a point 2 mm after the J-point. It is affected by myocardial ischemia or infarction, conduction abnormalities, and the administration of medications.

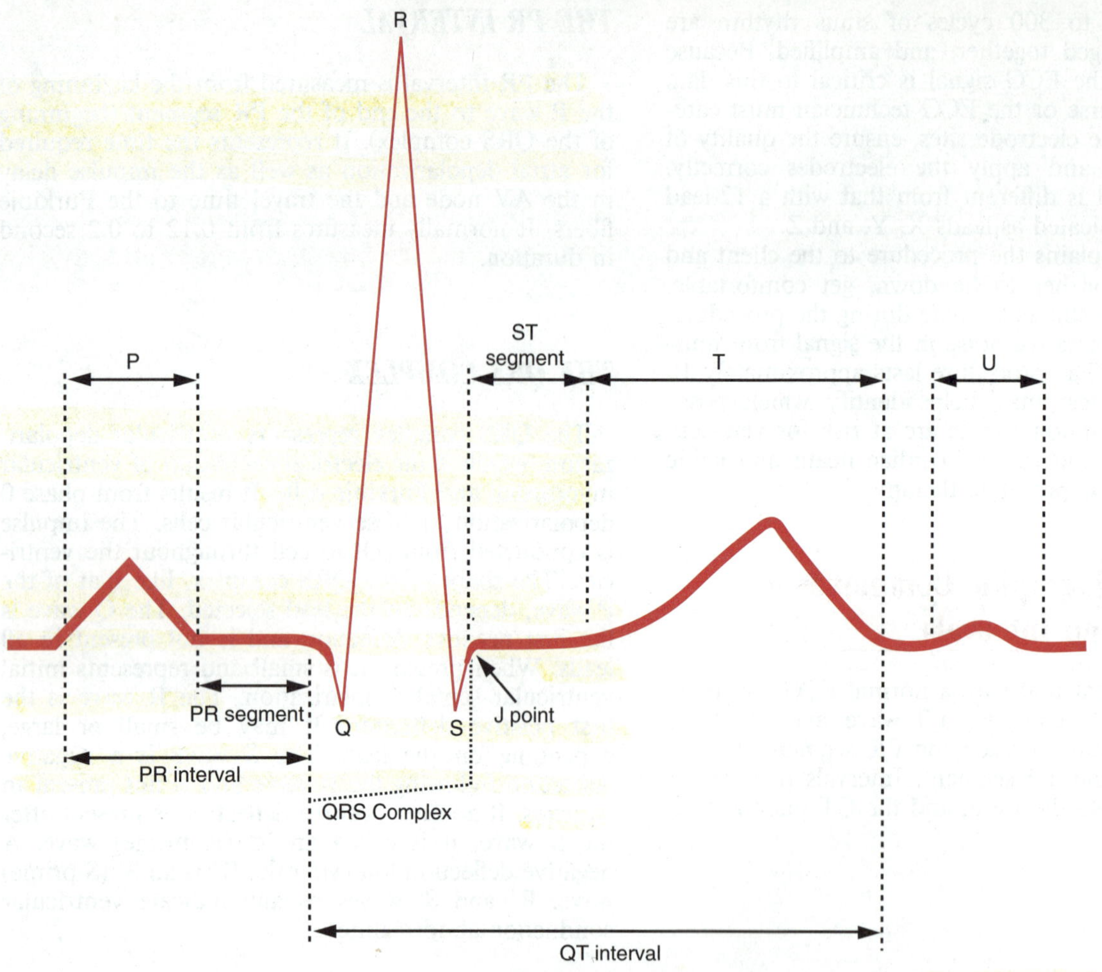

P wave:	Represents atrial depolarization.
PR segment:	Represents the time required for the impulse to travel through the AV node, where it is delayed, and through the Bundle of His, bundle branches, and Purkinje fiber network, just before ventricular depolarization.
PR interval:	Represents the time required for atrial depolarization as well as impulse travel through the conduction system and Purkinje fiber network, inclusive of the P wave and PR segment. It is measured from the beginning of the P wave to the end of the PR segment.
QRS complex:	Represents ventricular depolarization and is measured from the beginning of the Q (or R) wave to the end of the S wave.
J point:	Represents the junction where the QRS complex ends and the ST segment begins.
ST segment:	Represents early ventricular repolarization.
T wave:	Represents ventricular repolarization.
U wave:	Represents late ventricular repolarization.
QT interval:	Represents the total time required for ventricular depolarization and repolarization and is measured from the beginning of the QRS complex to the end of the T wave.

FIGURE 33–5 ◆ The components of a normal electrocardiogram.

THE T WAVE

The T wave follows the ST segment and represents ventricular repolarization. It corresponds to phase 3 of the action potential when the membrane potential decreases to its resting value. It is usually positive, rounded, and slightly asymmetric. If an ectopic stimulus excites the ventricles during this time, it may cause ventricular irritability and possible cardiac arrest in the vulnerable heart. This is known as the *R-on-T phenomenon.* T waves may become tall and peaked, inverted (negative), or flat as a result of myocardial ischemia, potassium or calcium imbalances, the administration of medications, or autonomic nervous system effects.

THE U WAVE

The U wave, when present, follows the T wave and may result from slow repolarization of ventricular Purkinje fibers. It is of the same polarity as T waves and is therefore usually positive, although generally smaller than the T wave. It is not normally seen in all leads and is more common in lead V_3. Abnormal prominence of the U wave suggests an electrolyte abnormality or other disturbance. It is important to identify it correctly so that it is not mistaken for a P wave.

THE QT INTERVAL

The QT interval represents the total time required for ventricular depolarization and repolarization. It is measured from the beginning of the QRS complex to the end of the T wave. This interval varies with the client's age and sex and changes in the heart rate. It lengthens with slower heart rates and shortens with faster heart rates. It is normally between 0.4 and 0.32 second for heart rates between 60 and 95 beats per minute, respectively. It may be prolonged by the administration of certain medications (e.g., type I-A antidysrhythmics and phenothiazines) or electrolyte disturbances, Prinzmetal's angina, or subarachnoid hemorrhage. A prolonged QT interval may lead to a unique type of ventricular tachycardia called torsades de pointes.

THE TP SEGMENT

The TP segment is the isoelectric line following the T (or U) wave and ending with the next P wave. During this time, the cells are at their resting membrane potential and there is no current flow. This segment lengthens as the heart rate decreases and shortens as the heart rate increases.

Electrocardiographic Paper

The ECG strip is printed on graph paper (Fig. 33–6), with each small block measuring 1 mm in height and width. ECG recorders and monitors are standardized at a speed of 25 mm/second. Time is measured on the horizontal axis. At this speed, each small block represents 0.04 second. Five small blocks make up one large block (5 mm), defined by darker bold lines and representing 0.2 second. Five large blocks (25 small blocks) represent 1 second, whereas 30 large blocks (150 small blocks) represent 6 seconds, and 300 large blocks (1500 small blocks) represent 60 seconds. Vertical lines in the top margin of the graph paper are usually 15 large blocks apart, representing 3-second segments (Fig. 33–7). If the recorder speed is changed to 50 mm/second, 1 small block represents 0.02 second and 1 large block stands for 0.1 second. This may be done during rapid heart rates to spread out complexes for easier identification.

The amplitude, or voltage, of complexes is measured on the vertical axis. One small block (1-mm amplitude) is equal to 0.1 mV. The ECG is calibrated to 1 mV (10 mm, or two vertical large blocks) for standardization. This allows comparison of complexes with a known electrical stimulus. The amplitude of a deflection is determined by the strength of the electrical force generating the current and its relationship to the lead axis.

Determination of Heart Rate

The heart rate may be estimated by counting the number of PP intervals (atrial rate) or RR intervals (ventricular rate) in 6 seconds and multiplying that number by ten to calculate the rate for a full minute (Fig. 33–8). For accuracy, timing should begin on the

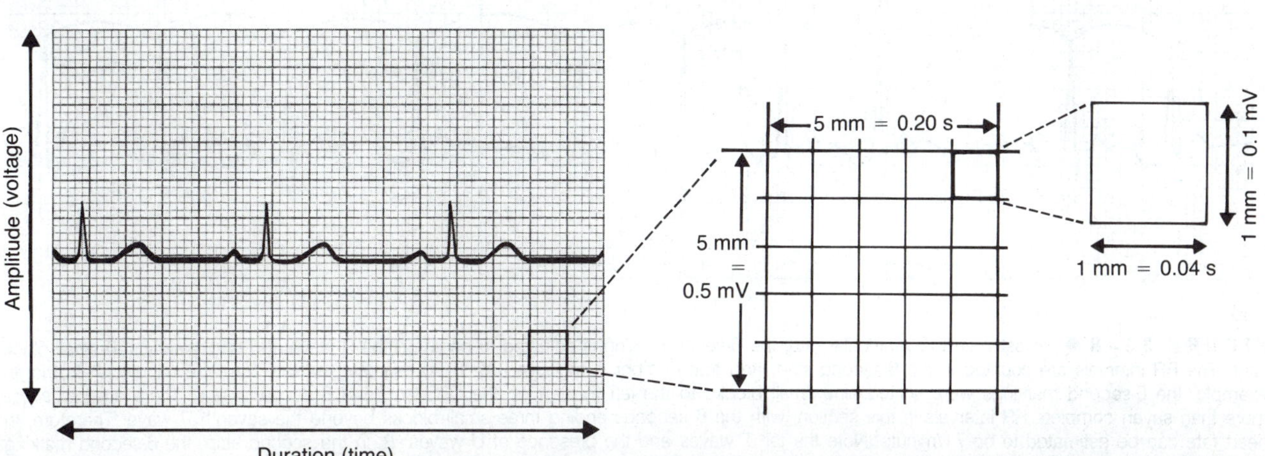

FIGURE 33–6 ◆ ECG waveforms are measured in amplitude (voltage) and duration (time).

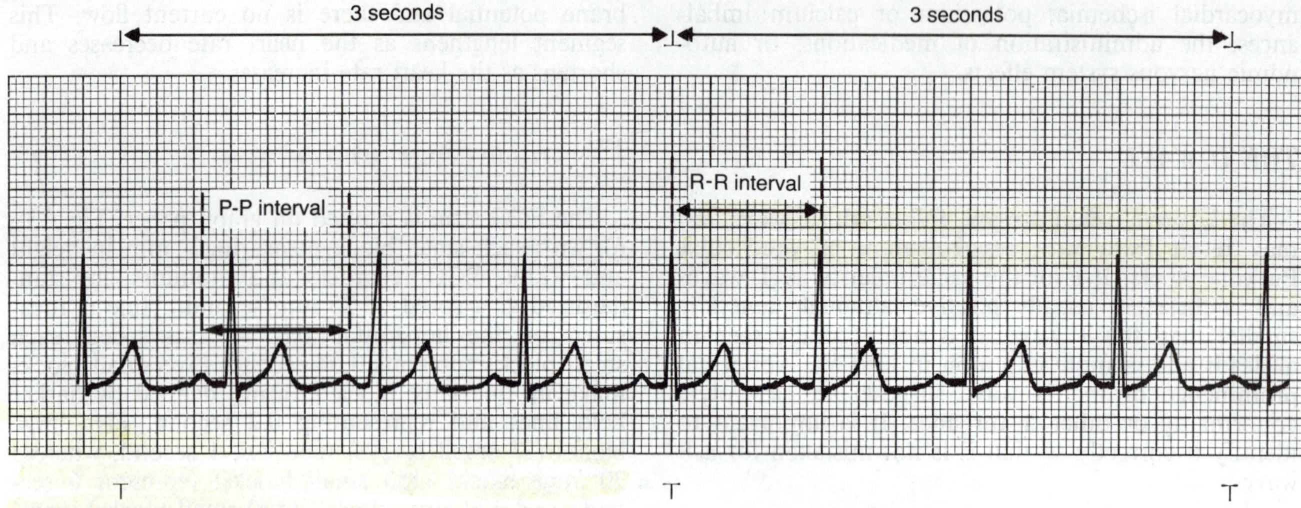

FIGURE 33-7 ◆ Each segment between the dark lines (above the monitor strip) represents 3 seconds, when the monitor is set at a speed of 25 mm/second.

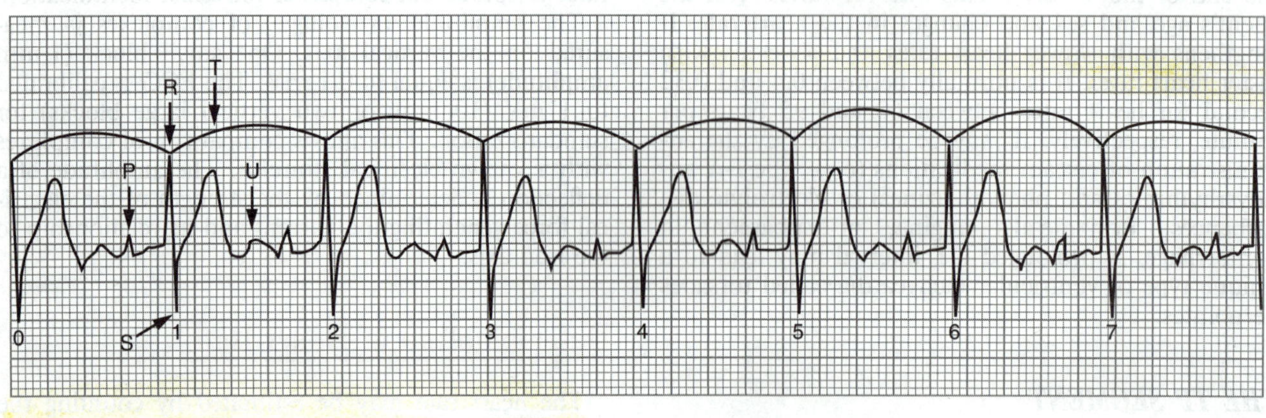

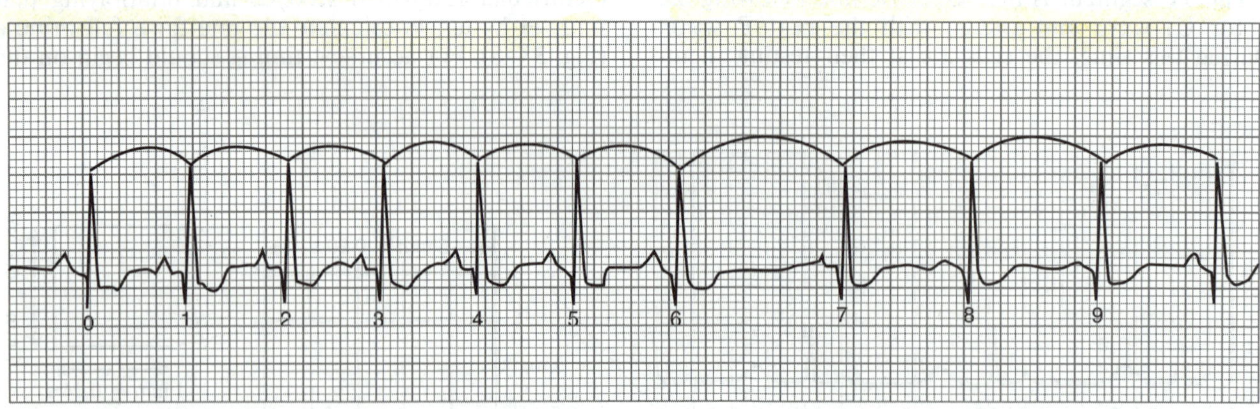

FIGURE 33-8 ◆ To estimate the ventricular rate, the 6-second timing is adjusted to begin on the R wave and end exactly 150 small blocks later. The RR intervals are counted in the 6-second strip, and that number is multiplied by 10 to estimate the rate for a full minute. *A*, In the first example, the 6-second markings were shifted nine small blocks to the left to start on the QRS and end 6 seconds later. There are just slightly more than seven complete RR intervals in this section, with the 6 seconds ending three small blocks beyond the seventh R wave. Therefore, the heart rate can be estimated to be 71/minute. Note the tall T waves and the presence of U waves. *B*, In the second strip, the 6-second markings were shifted seven small blocks to the right to start on the QRS and end 6 seconds later. There are approximately 9¾ RR intervals in this section, with the 6 seconds ending 13 small blocks beyond the ninth R wave. Therefore, the heart rate can be estimated to be 98/minute.

P wave or the QRS complex and end exactly 30 large blocks (150 small blocks) later. The initial complex is the reference point and counts as zero. Subsequent complexes are counted until the end of 6 seconds, to include a fraction of the last interval: for example, if there are exactly seven RR intervals, the heart rate is 70 beats per minute; if there are 9½ intervals, the heart rate is 95 beats per minute. This method may be used for both regular and irregular rhythms. It is called the 6-second strip method.

Another method, which may be used *only* if the rhythm is regular, relies on either of the following mathematic calculations:

- Count the number of small blocks in a PP or RR interval and divide 1500 (the number of small blocks in 1 minute) by that number. For example, 20 small blocks equals a heart rate of 75 beats per minute (1500/20 = 75).
- Count the number of large blocks in an interval and divide 300 (the number of large blocks in 1 minute) by that number. For example, three large blocks equals a heart rate of 100 beats per minute (300/3 = 100).

Commercially prepared ECG rate rulers are based on these calculations and may be used for regular rhythms.

Electrocardiographic Rhythm Analysis

Analysis of an ECG rhythm strip requires a systematic approach and is facilitated by the use of an ECG caliper. Although rhythm interpretation does not require an in-depth analysis of a 12-lead ECG, certain steps must be followed (Chart 33–1):

1. *Analyze the P waves.* The nurse checks that the P wave morphologic configuration (shape) is consistent throughout the strip. These uniform morphologic characteristics indicate that atrial depolarization is occurring from impulses originating from one focus, normally the sinoatrial (SA) node. The nurse determines whether there is one P wave occurring before each QRS complex. This establishes that a relationship exists between the P wave and the QRS complex. This indicates that impulses from one focus are responsible for both atrial and ventricular depolarization. The nurse may observe more than one P wave shape, or more P waves than QRS complexes, or absent P waves, or P waves coming after the QRS, each indicating that a dysrhythmia exists.
2. *Analyze the QRS complexes.* The nurse checks that the QRS complex morphologic configuration is consistent throughout the strip. The nurse may observe more than one QRS complex morphologic pattern or occasionally missing QRS complexes, indicating that a dysrhythmia exists.

CHART 33–1

Nursing Care Highlight

◆ Electrocardiographic Rhythm Analysis

1. Analyze the P waves.
2. Analyze the QRS complexes.
3. Determine the atrial rhythm or regularity.
4. Determine the ventricular rhythm or regularity.
5. Determine the heart rate.
6. Measure the PR interval.
7. Measure the QRS duration.
8. Interpret the rhythm.

3. *Determine the atrial rhythm or regularity.* The nurse checks the regularity of the atrial rhythm by assessing the PP intervals, placing one caliper point on a P wave and the other point on the next P wave. Then the caliper is moved from P wave to P wave along the entire strip ("walking out" the P waves) to determine the regularity of the rhythm. P waves of a different morphologic pattern (ectopic waves), if present, create an irregularity and do not walk out with the other P waves. A slight irregularity in the PP intervals, varying no more than three small blocks, is considered essentially regular if the P waves are all of the same morphologic pattern.
4. *Determine the ventricular rhythm or regularity.* The nurse checks the regularity of the ventricular rhythm by assessing the RR intervals, placing one caliper point on a portion of the QRS complex (usually the most prominent portion of the deflection) and the other point on the same portion of the next QRS complex. The caliper is then moved from QRS complex to QRS complex along the entire strip (walking out the QRS complexes) to determine the regularity of the rhythm. QRS complexes of a different morphologic pattern (ectopic QRS complexes), if present, create an irregularity and do not walk out with the other QRS complexes. A slight irregularity of no more than three small blocks between intervals is considered essentially regular if the QRS complexes are all of the same morphologic pattern.
5. *Determine the heart rate.* If the atrial and ventricular rhythms are regular, the nurse may use any of the methods previously described to calculate the heart rate. If the rhythms are irregular, the nurse must use the 6-second strip method for accuracy.
6. *Measure the PR interval.* The nurse places one caliper point at the end of the TP segment, where the P wave begins, and the other at the end of the PR segment, where the QRS complex begins. The PR interval normally measures between 0.12 and 0.2 second. The measurement should be constant throughout the strip. It cannot be measured if there are no P waves, or if P waves occur after the QRS complex.

7. *Measure the QRS duration.* The nurse places one caliper point at the beginning of the QRS complex and the other at the J-point, where the QRS complex ends. The QRS duration normally measures between 0.04 and 0.1 second. The measurement should be constant throughout the entire strip.
8. *Interpret the rhythm.* Using accepted rules, the nurse can now interpret the cardiac rhythm.

These steps can be reorganized and formatted as the basis for rules or criteria to differentiate normal and abnormal rhythms. The following format is used in this chapter:

Electrocardiographic Criteria

Rhythm: Atrial and ventricular rhythms
Rate: Atrial and ventricular rates
P waves: Presence, morphologic features (shape), relationship to QRS complexes
PR interval: Measurement and constancy
QRS duration: Measurement and constancy

NORMAL RHYTHMS

Normal Sinus Rhythm

Normal sinus rhythm (NSR) is the rhythm originating from the sinoatrial node (dominant pacemaker) that meets the following electrocardiographic (ECG) criteria (Fig. 33–9):

Electrocardiographic Criteria

Rhythm: Atrial and ventricular rhythms are regular.
Rate: Atrial and ventricular rates are 60 to 100 beats per minute.
P waves: Present; consistent morphologic configuration; one P wave before each QRS complex (1:1 relationship)
PR interval: 0.12 to 0.2 second and constant
QRS duration: 0.04 to 0.1 second and constant

Sinus Arrhythmia

Sinus arrhythmia is a variant of normal sinus rhythm. It results from changes in intrathoracic pressure during breathing and is therefore also considered normal. In this context, the term "arrhythmia" does not denote an absence of rhythm and is the accepted name of this rhythm. Negative intrathoracic pressure during inspiration causes venous pooling in the lungs and less venous return to the left ventricle. The heart rate increases because of reflex inhibition of vagal tone due to the reduced stroke volume. The positive intrathoracic pressure during expiration increases venous return to the left side of the heart from the lungs, increasing the stroke volume and allowing the heart rate to decrease again. This results in an irregular rhythm. Sinus arrhythmia has all the characteristics of normal sinus rhythm, except for rhythm. The PP and RR intervals vary, with the difference between the shortest and the longest intervals greater than 0.12 second (3 small blocks) (Fig. 33–10). Sinus arrhythmia may occasionally be due to nonrespiratory causes, such as the administration of digitalis or morphine. These drugs enhance vagal tone and cause decreased heart rate and irregularity unrelated to the respiratory cycle.

Electrocardiographic Criteria

Rhythm: Atrial and ventricular rhythms are irregular, with the shortest PP or RR interval varying at least 0.12 second from the longest PP or RR interval.
Rate: Atrial and ventricular rates may be normal or may be less than 60 beats per minute.
P waves: One P wave before each QRS complex; consistent morphologic configuration
PR interval: Normal, constant
QRS duration: Normal, constant

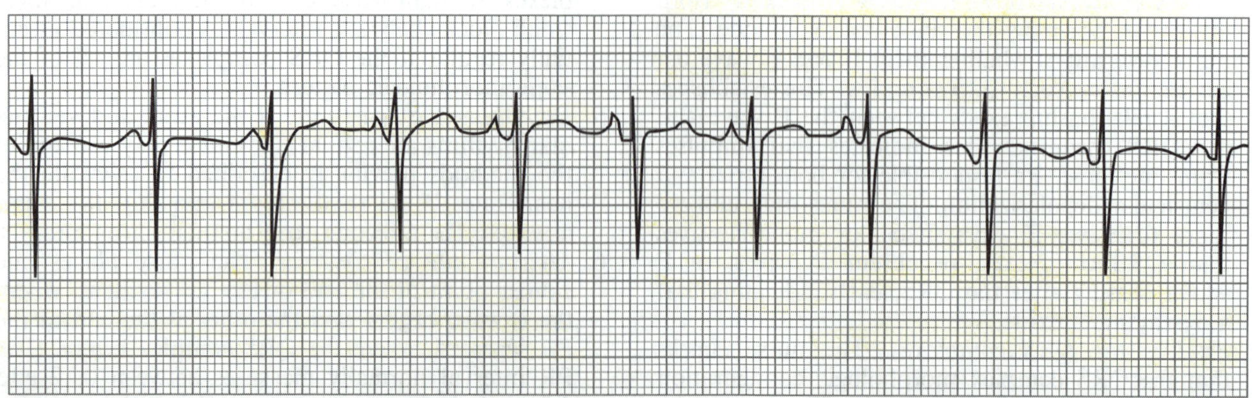

FIGURE 33–9 ◆ Normal sinus rhythm (NSR). Both atrial and ventricular rhythms are essentially regular (a slight variation in rhythm is normal). Atrial and ventricular rates are both 92/minute. There is one P wave before each QRS complex, and all the P waves are of a consistent morphology or shape. The PR interval measures 0.14 second and is constant; the QRS complex measures 0.08 second and is constant. The T waves vary in amplitude, from flat to positive, because of respirations (flat with inspiration, positive with expiration).

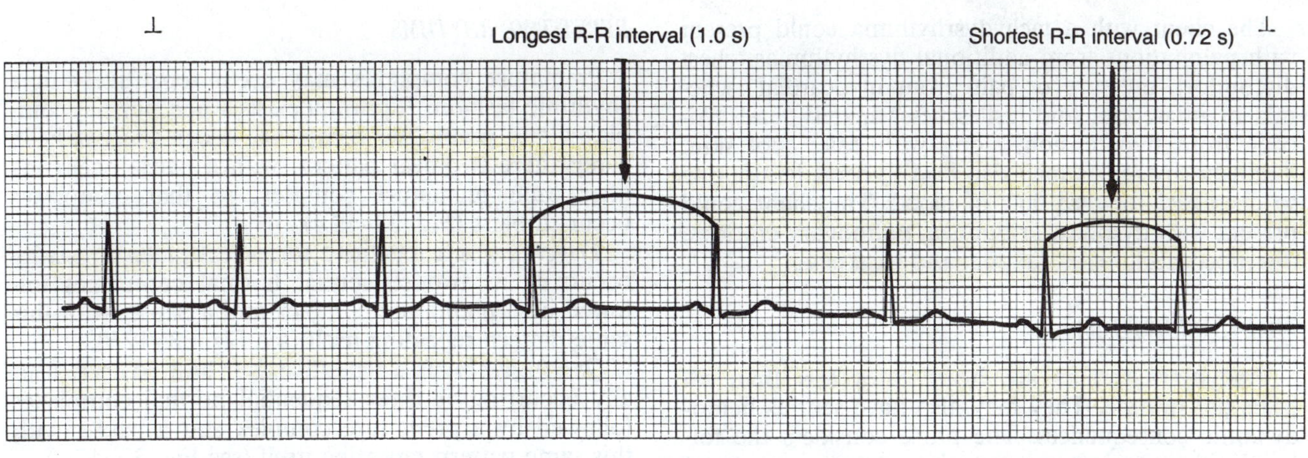

FIGURE 33–10 ◆ Sinus arrhythmia, considered normal. All the P waves have the same morphology, indicating that they are all from the sinus node. The rhythm is irregular, with the shortest RR interval (0.72 second) varying more than 0.12 second from the longest RR interval (1.0 second).

DYSRHYTHMIAS

OVERVIEW

Any disorder of the heartbeat is termed "dysrhythmia." Historically, the term arrhythmia has been used in the literature; however, it means an absence of cardiac rhythm. Although the terms are often used interchangeably, dysrhythmia, which means a disturbance in cardiac rhythm, is more accurate and is used here.

Dysrhythmias result from a disturbance in impulse formation (either from an abnormal rate or from an ectopic focus), from a disturbance in impulse conduction (delays and blocks), or from both mechanisms. Although many dysrhythmias have no clinical manifestations, many others have serious consequences. A summary is provided in Chart 33–2.

DYSRHYTHMIA TERMINOLOGY

TACHYDYSRHYTHMIAS

Tachydysrhythmias are heart rates greater than 100 beats per minute (BPM) and may have serious hemodynamic consequences in the client with coronary artery disease (CAD). Coronary artery blood flow occurs predominantly during diastole, when the aortic valve is closed, and is determined by diastolic time and blood pressure in the root of the aorta. The nurse must understand three important points to appreciate the seriousness of tachydysrhythmias.

- Tachydysrhythmias shorten the diastolic time and therefore the coronary perfusion time (the amount of time available for blood to flow through the coronary arteries to the myocardium)
- Tachydysrhythmias initially increase cardiac output and blood pressure. However, a continued rise in heart rate decreases the ventricular filling time because of a shortened diastole, decreasing the stroke volume. Consequently, at some point, cardiac output and blood pressure begin to decrease, reducing aortic pressure and therefore coronary perfusion pressure.
- Finally, tachydysrhythmias increase the work of the heart, increasing myocardial oxygen demand.

CHART 33–2

Key Features of Sustained Tachydysrhythmias and Bradydysrhythmias

- Chest discomfort, pressure, or pain, which may radiate to the jaw, the back, or the arm
- Restlessness, anxiety, nervousness, confusion
- Dizziness, syncope
- Palpitations (in tachydysrhythmias)
- Change in pulse strength, rate, and rhythm
- Pulse deficit
- Shortness of breath, dyspnea
- Tachypnea
- Pulmonary crackles
- Orthopnea
- S_3 or S_4 heart sounds
- Jugular venous distention
- Weakness, fatigue
- Pale, cool skin; diaphoresis
- Nausea, vomiting
- Decreased urinary output
- Delayed capillary refill
- Hypotension

The client with a tachydysrhythmia could present with palpitations from additional dysrhythmias, chest discomfort, pressure or pain from myocardial ischemia or infarction, and restlessness, anxiety, and syncope from hypotension, along with pale, cool skin. Tachydysrhythmias may also lead to heart failure due to decreased forward flow of blood. The client could present with dyspnea, orthopnea, pulmonary crackles, distended neck veins, fatigue, and weakness.

BRADYDYSRHYTHMIAS

Bradydysrhythmias are heart rates less than 60 beats per minute. They may also have serious hemodynamic consequences. The nurse considers the following three points to appreciate the seriousness of bradydysrhythmias:

- Coronary perfusion time is adequate because of a prolonged diastole. This is desirable.
- Coronary perfusion pressure may decrease if the heart rate is too slow to provide adequate cardiac output and blood pressure. This is a serious consequence.
- Myocardial oxygen demand is reduced from the slow heart rate. This is beneficial.

Therefore, the client may tolerate the bradydysrhythmia well if the blood pressure is adequate. If the blood pressure is not adequate, symptomatic bradydysrhythmias may lead to myocardial ischemia or infarction, dysrhythmias, hypotension, and heart failure.

PREMATURE COMPLEXES

Premature complexes are early complexes. They occur when a cardiac tissue, other than the sinoatrial (SA) node, becomes irritable and fires an impulse prematurely before the next sinus impulse is generated. This abnormal focus is called an *ectopic focus* and may be generated by atrial, junctional, or ventricular tissue.

After the premature complex, a slight pause occurs before the next sinus impulse fires. If it is determined that the sinus impulse after the pause comes exactly when it was due to occur, a complete compensatory pause exists, as is usually the case with premature ventricular complexes (PVCs) (Fig. 33–11*A*). This pattern indicates that the SA node was not affected by the ectopic impulse. If the sinus impulse after the pause comes earlier than it was due, a noncompensatory or incomplete compensatory pause exists with pacemaker resetting. This pattern indicates that the sinus node was depolarized by the ectopic impulse and consequently reset its timing to fire earlier than it was next scheduled to. This usually occurs with atrial and junctional premature complexes (see Fig. 33–11*B*). The client with premature beats may be unaware of them or may feel palpitations or a "skipping" of the heartbeat. If palpitations are frequent, the client may feel anxious or concerned.

REPETITIVE RHYTHMS

Premature complexes may occur repetitively in a rhythmic fashion. *Bigeminy* exists when normal complexes and premature complexes occur alternately in a repetitive two-beat pattern, with a pause occurring after each premature complex, so that complexes occur in pairs (Fig. 33–12*A*).

Trigeminy is a repetitive three-beat pattern, usually occurring as two sequential normal complexes followed by a premature complex and a pause, with this same pattern repeating itself (see Fig. 33–12*B*).

Quadrigeminy is a repetitive four-beat pattern, usually occurring as three sequential normal complexes followed by a premature complex and a pause, with this same pattern repeating itself (see Fig. 33–12*C*).

Such patterns may occur with atrial, junctional, or ventricular premature complexes. Clients may be unaware of the premature beats or may feel palpitations.

ESCAPE COMPLEXES AND RHYTHMS

Escape complexes or escape rhythms may occur when the sinoatrial (SA) node fails to discharge or is blocked, or a sinus impulse fails to depolarize the ventricles because of an atrioventricular (AV) nodal block. Escape complexes or rhythms come after a pause, serving as the subsidiary or escape pacemaker. Such impulses may originate from AV junctional or ventricular tissue. They cease when the SA node or the AV node regains the ability to function normally. If there are pauses followed by escape beats or rhythms, clients may feel lightheaded, dizzy, or faint during the pause.

CLASSIFICATION OF DYSRHYTHMIAS

Dysrhythmias are classified according to their site of origin. The sites include sinus, atrial, junctional, ventricular, and AV nodal tissue. Dysrhythmias may be caused by a disturbance in impulse formation or by conduction delays or blocks. The incidence and the prevalence of dysrhythmias are not precisely known because they usually result from an underlying condition, such as heart disease.

For each dysrhythmia presented here, the pathophysiology, etiology, physical assessment/clinical manifestations, and interventions are described. Information about specific drug therapy, pacing, cardioversion, cardiopulmonary resuscitation (CPR), and surgery is discussed later in the chapter. A summary of the common dysrhythmias and their treatment is provided in Table 33–2.

SINUS DYSRHYTHMIAS

The sinus node is the pacemaker in all sinus dysrhythmias. Sympathetic nerve fibers are distributed to the SA node, the atrial muscle, the AV node, and the ventricular muscle. Vagus nerve fibers from the parasympathetic system are distributed primarily to the

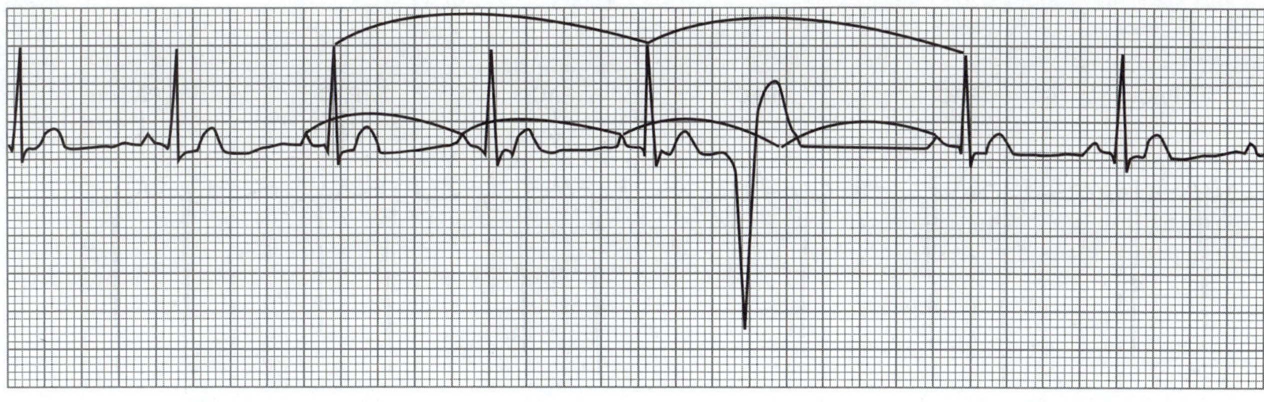

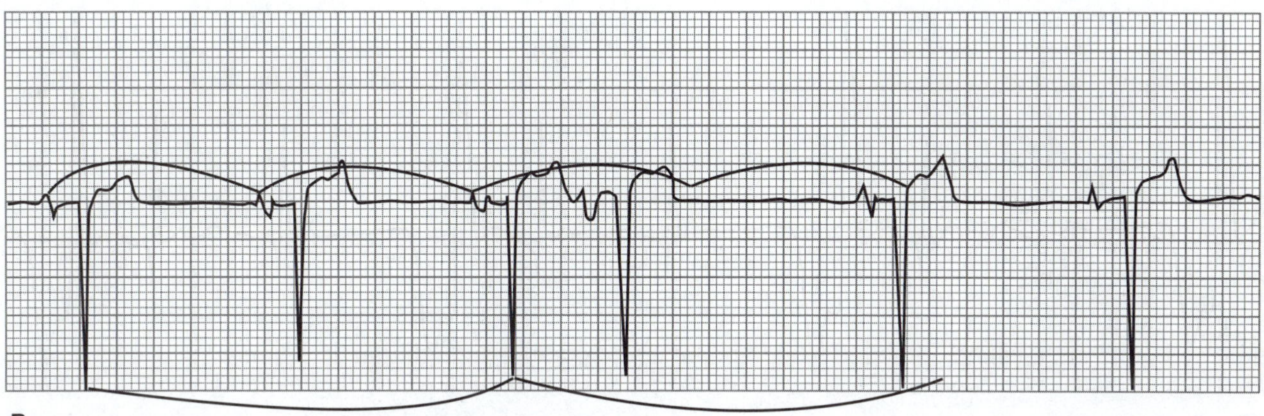

FIGURE 33-11 ◆ *A*, Normal sinus rhythm (NSR) with a premature ventricular contraction (PVC). There is a complete compensatory pause following the PVC, indicated by the fact that the sinus P wave following the pause comes exactly when it *was* due to occur. The P wave can also be determined by the RR intervals, measuring between two complete intervals, with the R wave following the pause coming exactly when it was due to occur. *B*, Normal sinus rhythm with a premature atrial *contraction* (PAC). There is an incomplete or noncompensatory pause following the PAC, indicated by the fact that the sinus P wave following the pause comes *before* it was originally due to occur. The QRS also comes before it would have been due.

SA and AV nodes, with little distribution to atrial and ventricular muscle. Innervation from these two systems is normally in balance to ensure a normal sinus rhythm. An imbalance increases or decreases the rate of SA node discharge, either as a normal response to activity or physiologic changes or as a pathologic response to illness. Types of sinus dysrhythmias include:

- Sinus tachycardia
- Sinus bradycardia
- Sinus pause

SINUS TACHYCARDIA

Pathophysiology Dominant sympathetic nervous system stimulation of the heart or vagal inhibition results in:

- An increased rate of SA node discharge, which increases the heart rate (positive chronotropic effect)
- An increased speed of conduction through the AV node and conduction system (positive dromotropic effect)
- An increased force of myocardial contraction (positive inotropic effect)

When the rate of SA node discharge exceeds 100 beats per minute, the rhythm is called sinus tachycardia (Fig. 33–13*A*). The rate rarely exceeds 160 beats per minute, but may reach 180 beats per minute. Sinus tachycardia initially enhances cardiac output and blood pressure. However, excessive increases in heart rate decrease coronary perfusion time and coronary perfusion pressure, while increasing myocardial oxygen demand.

ELECTROCARDIOGRAPHIC CRITERIA:

Rhythm: Atrial and ventricular rhythms are regular.

Rate: Atrial and ventricular rates are 100 to 180 beats per minute.

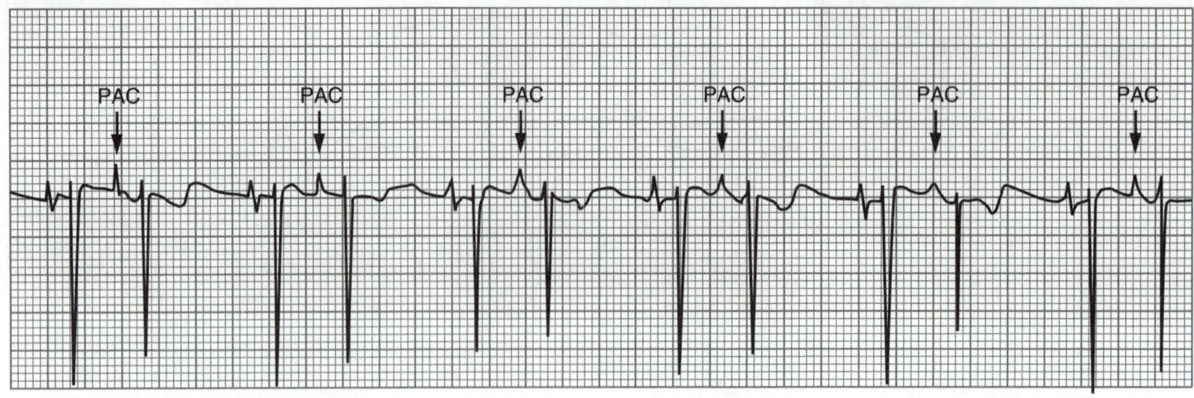

A

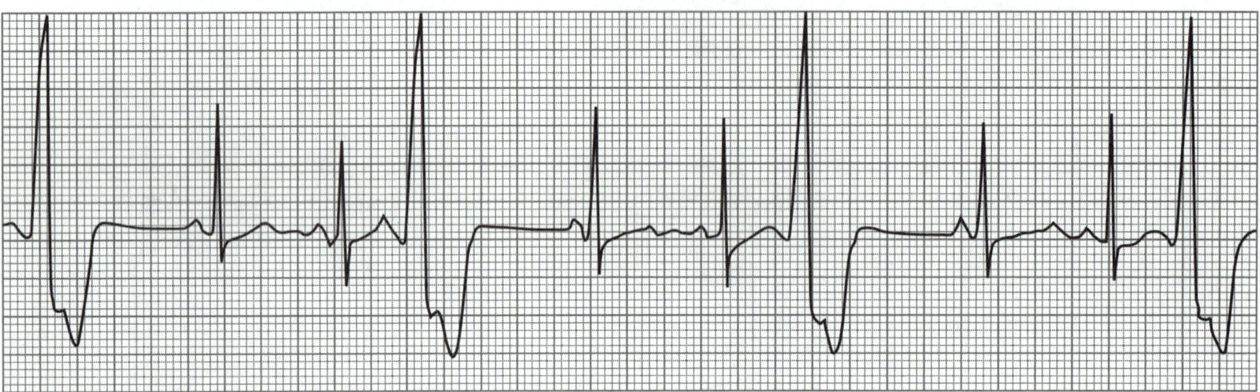

B

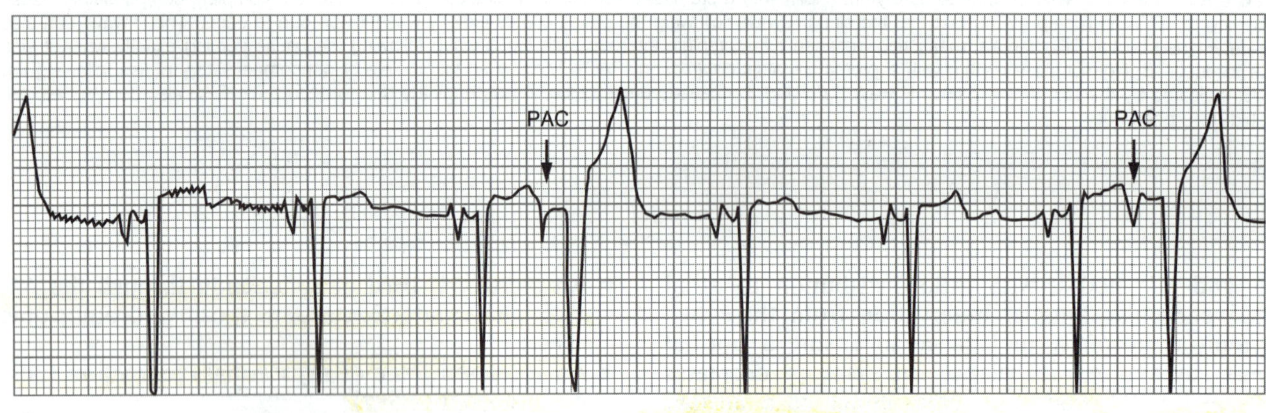

C

FIGURE 33–12 ◆ Repetitive rhythms. *A*, Atrial bigeminy. Every other complex is a premature atrial *complex* (PAC). *B*, Ventricular trigeminy. Every third complex is a premature ventricular contraction (PVC). *C*, Atrial quadrigeminy. Every fourth complex is an aberrant PAC.

P waves: One P wave before each QRS complex; consistent morphologic configuration. P waves may encroach on preceding T waves.

PR interval: Normal, constant

QRS duration: Normal, constant

Etiology Increased sympathetic stimulation is a normal response to physical activity but may also be caused by anxiety, pain, stress, fear, fever, anemia, hyperthyroidism, pulmonary embolus, and the administration of drugs such as catecholamines, atropine, caffeine, alcohol, nicotine, aminophylline, and thyroid drugs. It may also be a compensatory response to decreased cardiac output or blood pressure, as occurs in hypovolemia, shock, myocardial infarction, and heart failure.

Physical Assessment/Clinical Manifestations The client may be asymptomatic except for the increased pulse rate. However, if the rhythm is not well tolerated, the

TABLE 33–2 Common Dysrhythmias and Their Treatment

Dysrhythmia	Treatment*
Sinus tachycardia	• Correction of the underlying problem (e.g., fever, hypovolemia, pain, anxiety, and CHF) • Beta-adrenergic blockade if increased catecholamine secretion is the underlying problem

Sinus bradycardia	• Treatment necessary only if the client is symptomatic (has hypotension, diaphoresis, chest discomfort or pain, pulmonary congestion, or altered level of consciousness):
	  • Atropine
	  • Pacemaker
	  • Avoidance of parasympathetic stimulation, such as prolonged suctioning and stimulation of the gag reflex

Premature Beats and Ectopic Rhythms	

Supraventricular beats (PACs, PJCs)	• Correction of any underlying problem (e.g., anxiety, stress, caffeine and nicotine intake, CFH, effects of drugs, and CAL)
	• Medication administration
	  • Quinidine
	  • Procainamide
	  • Digitalis
	  • Propranolol
	  • Sedatives

Supraventricular rhythms	• Correction of any underlying problem (e.g., CHF, CAL, stress, and drugs)
	• Medication administration
	  • Verapamil
	  • Diltiazem
	  • Adenosine
	  • Digitalis
	  • Propranolol
	  • Esmolol
	  • Quinidine
	  • Procainamide
	• Vagal stimulation with carotid massage
	• Valsalva maneuvers
	• Overdrive atrial pacing
	• Synchronized cardioversion if the above measures are unsuccessful

Premature ventricular complexes and ventricular tachycardia (not sustained)	• Correction of any underlying problem (e.g., infection, electrolyte imbalance, effects of drugs, myocardial infarction, CHF, stress, fatigue, and nicotine)
	• Medication administration
	  • Lidocaine bolus and infusion
	  • Procainamide bolus and infusion
	  • Bretylium tosylate bolus and infusion
	  • Magnesium sulfate infusion
	  • Class I and II antidysrhythmics
	  • Amiodarone
	• Restoration of electrolyte balance

Atrial flutter	• Medication administration
	  • Diltiazem
	  • Verapamil
	  • Digitalis
	  • Propranolol
	  • Esmolol
	  • Quinidine
	  • Procainamide
	• Atrial overdrive pacing
	• Cardioversion
	• Catheter or surgical ablation

Atrial fibrillation	• Medication administration
	  • Digitalis
	  • Diltiazem
	  • Verapamil
	  • Quinidine
	  • Procainamide
	• Anticoagulation
	• Atrial overdrive pacing
	• Cardioversion
	• Surgery

Escape beats and rhythms	• Correction of the underlying cause if the client is symptomatic • Atropine administration • Pacemaker • Isoproterenol administration if pacemaker unavailable
Conduction Delays	
First-degree AV block	• Treatment necessary only if the client is symptomatic • Withhold digitalis (if the cause) • Atropine administration if block is associated with symptomatic bradycardia
Second-degree AV block type I	• Same as for first-degree AV block
Second-degree AV block type II	• Pacemaker • Isoproterenol administration if pacemaker unavailable
Third-degree AV block	• Pacemaker • Isoproterenol administration if pacemaker unavailable
Life-Threatening Dysrhythmias	

Sustained ventricular tachycardia	• Medication administration
	  • Lidocaine bolus and infusion
	  • Procainamide bolus and infusion
	  • Bretylium tosylate bolus and infusion
	  • Magnesium sulfate infusion
	• If unstable: synchronized cardioversion
	• If pulseless: defibrillation, CPR

Ventricular fibrillation	• Defibrillation
	• CPR
	• Medication administration
	  • Epinephrine
	  • Lidocaine
	  • Bretylium tosylate
	  • Procainamide
	  • Magnesium sulfate

Ventricular asystole	• CPR
	• Medication administration
	  • Epinephrine
	  • Atropine
	• Pacemaker

* CHF, congestive heart failure; CAL, chronic airway limitation.

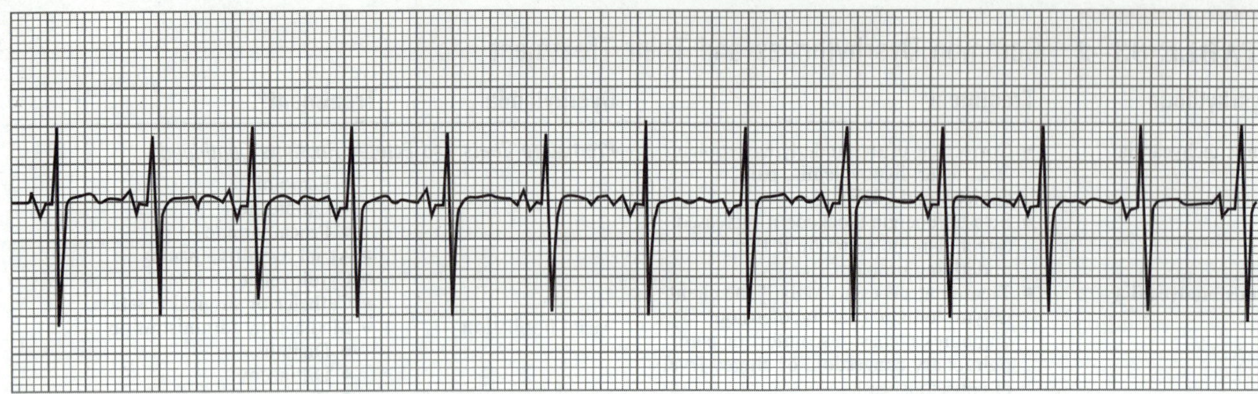

A

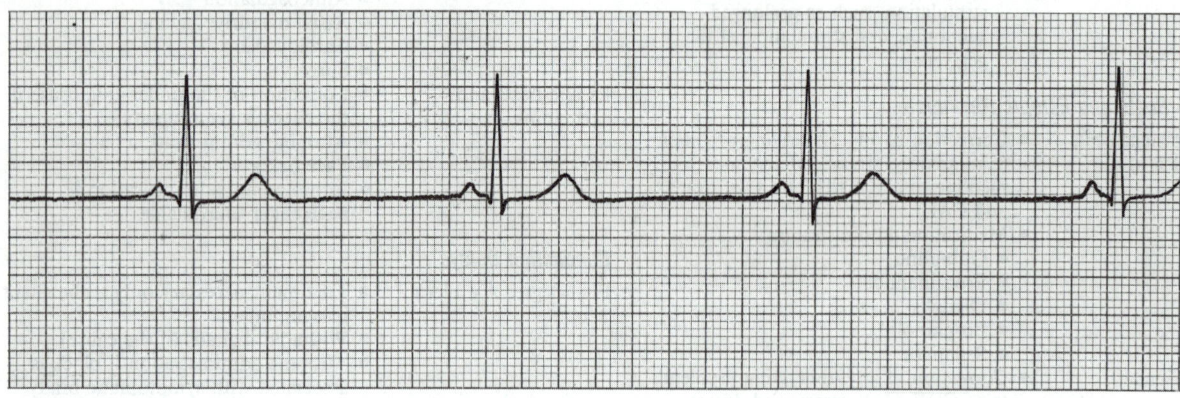

B

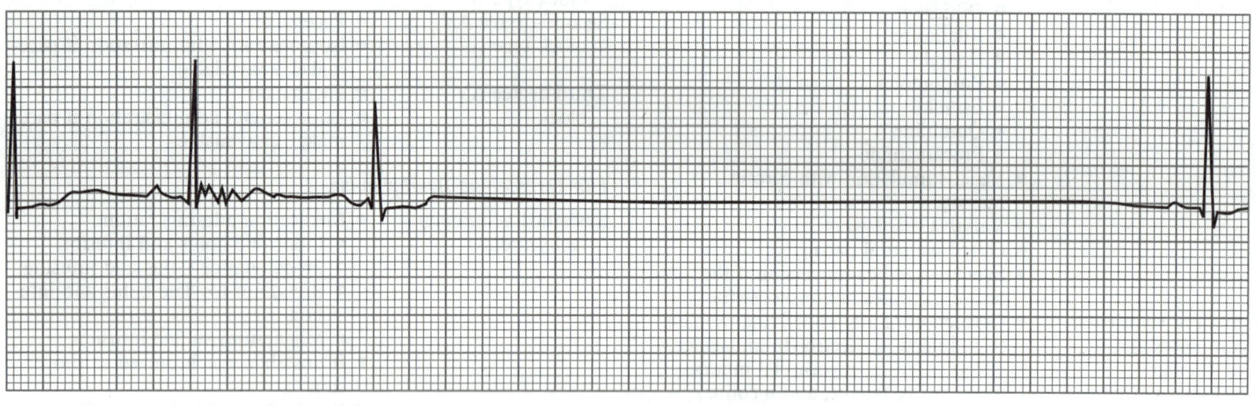

C

FIGURE 33–13 ◆ Sinus rhythms. *A*, Sinus tachycardia (HR = 110/minute, PR = 0.12 second, QRS = 0.08 second). *B*, Sinus bradycardia (HR = 35/minute, PR = 0.16 second, QRS = 0.10 second). *C*, Sinus pause (underlying HR = 60, PR = 0.20 second, QRS = 0.08 second, with just under a 5-second pause). PAC, premature atrial complex.

client is symptomatic. The nurse assesses the client for chest discomfort or pain, fatigue, weakness, shortness of breath, orthopnea, neck vein distention, and decreased blood pressure. The nurse also assesses for restlessness and anxiety from decreased cerebral perfusion and decreased urinary output from decreased renal perfusion. The electrocardiographic (ECG) pattern may show T wave inversion or ST segment elevation or depression in response to myocardial ischemia. The TP segment shortens.

Interventions The nurse and the physician collaborate to identify the cause of sinus tachycardia and select the appropriate treatment. The goal is to decrease the heart rate to normal levels by treating the underlying cause. For example, if the client has chest discomfort or pain, the nurse administers oxygen, assists the client to rest, and administers nitroglycerin or morphine and thrombolytic therapy as prescribed. The nurse administers diuretics and inotropic agents to the client in heart failure, initiates intravascular volume replacement for the hypovolemic client, administers antipyretics and antibiotics to the client with fever and infection, or provides comfort measures and administers analgesics or opioids to the client with noncardiac pain.

The nurse oxygenates and suctions the client with hypoxemia from excessive airway secretions, or administers beta-adrenergic blocking agents to the client with inappropriate sympathetic nervous system stimulation. The nurse provides emotional support, teaches the client, and administers antianxiety agents for clients who are anxious.

SINUS BRADYCARDIA

Pathophysiology Dominance of the parasympathetic nervous system, with excessive vagal stimulation to the heart, causes a decreased rate of sinus node discharge. This slows the heart rate and decreases the speed of conduction through the AV node and conduction system. When the rate of sinus node discharge is less than 60 beats per minute, the rhythm is called sinus bradycardia (see Fig. 33–13*B*). Sinus bradycardia increases coronary perfusion time but may decrease coronary perfusion pressure. However, myocardial oxygen demand is decreased.

Electrocardiographic Criteria

Rhythm: Atrial and ventricular rhythms are regular.

Rate: Atrial and ventricular rates are less than 60 beats per minute.

P waves: One P wave before each QRS complex; consistent morphologic pattern

PR interval: Normal, constant

QRS duration: Normal, constant

Etiology Increased parasympathetic stimulation of the heart by the vagus nerve is a normal response to decreased physical activity. It also often occurs in well-conditioned athletes because the strong heart muscle is extremely efficient in providing an adequate stroke volume, while not requiring a higher heart rate for a normal cardiac output. Excessive vagal stimulation may result from carotid sinus massage, vomiting, suctioning, Valsalva maneuvers such as bearing down for a bowel movement or gagging, inferior myocardial infarction, ocular pressure, pain, and hypothyroidism. Sinus bradycardia may also result from the administration of drugs such as beta-adrenergic blocking agents, calcium channel blockers, and digitalis. The TP segment is prolonged because of the slow heart rate.

Physical Assessment/Clinical Manifestations The client may be asymptomatic, except for the decreased pulse rate. However, the rhythm may not be well tolerated. The nurse assesses the client for dizziness, weakness, syncope, confusion, chest discomfort or pain, hypotension, diaphoresis, shortness of breath, and ventricular ectopy. T wave inversion or ST segment elevation or depression may occur in response to myocardial ischemia.

Interventions The treatment of choice for the client with a symptomatic sinus bradycardia is atropine administration. The nurse administers oxygen and atropine as prescribed to increase the client's heart rate to approximately 60 beats per minute. If the heart rate does not increase sufficiently, the nurse applies a noninvasive pacemaker (see later in this chapter) to increase the heart rate and notifies the physician. However, if atropine administration succeeds in achieving an adequate heart rate but the client remains hypotensive, the nurse initiates intravascular volume replacement as ordered, rather than administering another dose of atropine, because excessive atropine may induce tachycardia. If an offending drug is determined to be the cause, the nurse withholds the drug and notifies the physician for an order to temporarily or permanently discontinue use of the drug.

SINUS PAUSE

Pathophysiology Sinus pause is a general term for a sinus rhythm interrupted by a pause when an entire P-QRS-T sequence is absent (see Fig. 33–13*C*). Occasionally, more than one sequence is absent. Sinus pause occurs if a sinus impulse fails to emerge from the sinus node to depolarize atrial tissue (SA block) or if the SA node fails to generate an impulse (sinus arrest). The nurse does not usually need to differentiate between SA block and sinus arrest. Therefore, the broader term, sinus pause, is used in this chapter.

Electrocardiographic Criteria

Rhythm: Atrial and ventricular rhythms are irregular because of the pause; the underlying rhythm may be regular.

Rate: May be any rate; usually slow

P waves: One or more entire P-QRS-T sequences missing

PR interval: None during the pause because QRS complexes are missing

QRS duration: None, because the QRS complex is missing

Etiology Causes of sinus pause include excessive vagal stimulation, proximal right coronary artery occlusion, carotid sinus sensitivity, and the administration of digitalis, quinidine, beta-blockers, and calcium channel blockers. The duration of the pause is measured (in seconds) from the last P wave before the pause to the next P wave after the pause.

Physical Assessment/Clinical Manifestations Symptoms depend on the length of the pause, the overall heart rate, and the cardiac output. The client may be asymptomatic if pauses are short and infrequent. The nurse assesses the client for dizziness, shortness of breath, lightheadedness, pallor, hypotension, and syncope.

Interventions The physician identifies and treats the cause. For example, the administration of offending drugs is withheld. The nurse instructs the client to avoid activities causing vagal stimulation, such as straining for a bowel movement, rubbing the neck, raising the arms, and applying ocular pressure by rubbing the eyes. If the client is symptomatic, the nurse administers atropine as prescribed and, if necessary, initiates noninvasive pacemaker therapy (see later in this chapter). The nurse notifies the physician about the initiation of these interventions.

ATRIAL DYSRHYTHMIAS

With atrial dysrhythmias, the focus of impulse generation has shifted away from the sinus node to the atrial tissue, which now acts as an ectopic pacemaker, for one or more beats. This changes the axis (direction) of atrial depolarization, resulting in a P wave morphologic pattern (shape) that differs from that of sinus node origin. The types of atrial dysrhythmias include:

- Premature atrial complexes
- Wandering atrial pacemaker
- Atrial tachycardia
- Multifocal atrial tachycardia
- Atrial flutter
- Atrial fibrillation

PREMATURE ATRIAL COMPLEXES

Pathophysiology A premature atrial complex (PAC or APC) occurs when atrial tissue becomes irritable and this ectopic focus fires an impulse before the next sinus impulse is due, thus usurping the sinus pacemaker (Fig. 33–14*A*). The premature P wave from the atrial focus is early and has a different morphologic pattern from the P waves from the sinus focus. The premature P wave may not always be clearly visible, as it is often hidden in the preceding T wave. The T wave must be closely examined for any change in shape compared with that of other T waves, indicating a hidden P wave. PACs may appear as follows:

- Normally conducted PACs: The atrial impulse conducts normally through the AV node and through the ventricles, so that the abnormal P wave is followed by a normal QRS complex.
- Aberrantly conducted PACs: On occasion, the early atrial impulse may reach the ventricles when one of the bundle branches is still refractory from the preceding sinus impulse. One ventricle depolarizes first, followed by the other, after an aberrant conduction pathway and widening of the QRS complex. The abnormal P wave is followed by a wide QRS complex.

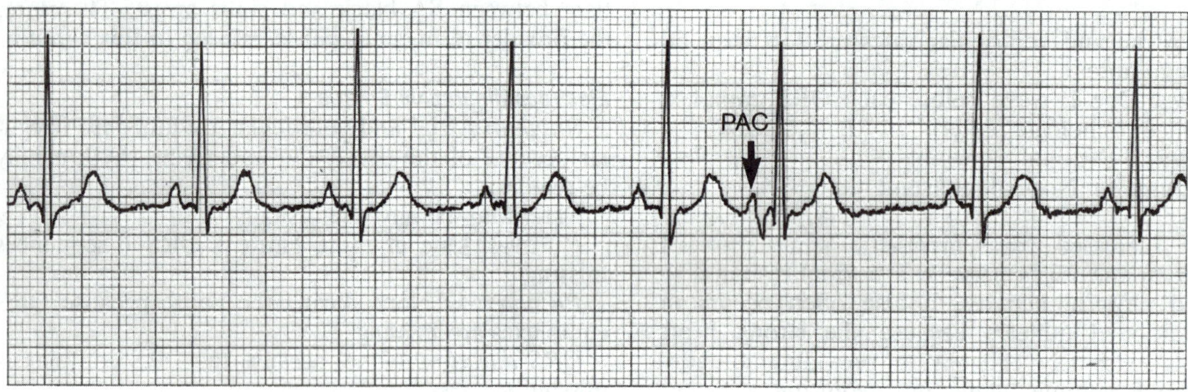

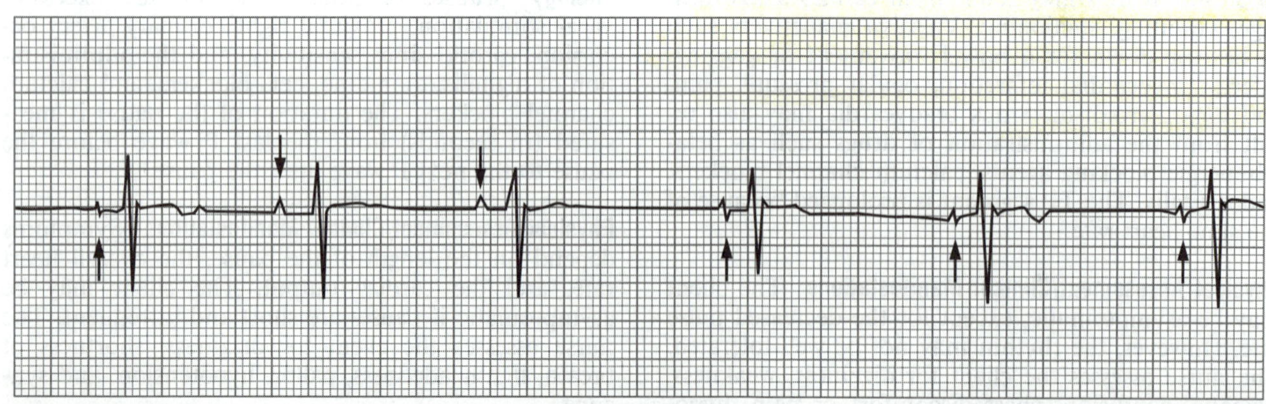

FIGURE 33–14 ◆ Atrial dysrhythmias. *A*, Normal sinus rhythm (NSR) with a premature atrial complex (PAC) at arrow. *B*, Wandering atrial pacemaker. The first, fourth, fifth, and sixth cycles have one P wave morphology; the second and third have a different P wave morphology.

- Nonconducted, or blocked, PACs: The atrial impulse may arrive too early and be unable to conduct to the ventricles at all, so that only the abnormal P wave is seen with no QRS complex following it.

Electrocardiographic Criteria

Rhythm: The underlying sinus rhythm is usually regular, unless sinus arrhythmia is present. Atrial and ventricular rhythms become irregular because of the early beat. The pause after a PAC is usually noncompensatory.

Rate: May be any rate, depending on underlying sinus rhythm. Atrial and ventricular rates are usually equal, unless there are nonconducted PACs.

P waves: One P wave occurs before each QRS complex if PACs are conducted. Sinus P waves have one consistent morphologic pattern. The premature atrial P wave is early with a different morphologic configuration.

PR interval: Normal and constant for sinus beats; normal for PAC, although may be different from sinus beats, or may be prolonged if PACs are early.

QRS duration: Usually normal and constant; may be wide if aberrantly conducted PACs are present; may be absent if nonconducted, or blocked, PACs occur.

Etiology The causes of atrial irritability include stress; fatigue; anxiety; inflammation; infection; intake of caffeine, nicotine, and alcohol; and the administration of drugs such as digitalis, catecholamines, sympathomimetics, amphetamines, and anesthetic agents. It may also result from myocardial ischemia, hypermetabolic states, electrolyte imbalance, or atrial stretch, as may occur with congestive heart failure, valvular disease, and pulmonary hypertension with cor pulmonale.

Physical Assessment/Clinical Manifestations The client is usually asymptomatic, except for possible heart palpitations, because there are no hemodynamic consequences.

Interventions No intervention is usually needed, except to treat the cause. If PACs occur frequently, they may herald the onset of more serious atrial tachydysrhythmias and therefore may warrant treatment. The nurse administers prescribed type IA antidysrhythmics, such as quinidine and procainamide, or other drugs such as digitalis and propranolol hydrochloride (Inderal, Apo-Propranolol✱). The nurse also initiates measures to reduce the client's stress and teaches the client to avoid substances known to increase atrial irritability as listed earlier.

WANDERING ATRIAL PACEMAKER

Pathophysiology With a wandering atrial pacemaker, the dominant sinus pacemaker gradually slows down. Latent pacemakers located in atrial and AV junctional tissue take over to control the heart rate, as escape rhythms, until the sinus rate gradually increases again. Consequently, the site of impulse origin shifts among sinus, atrial, and AV junctional sites, resulting in varying PP intervals, P wave morphologic features, and PR intervals (see Fig. 33–14*B*).

Electrocardiographic Criteria

Rhythm: Atrial and ventricular rhythms are somewhat irregular.

Rate: Atrial and ventricular rates are equal, often less than 60 beats per minute.

P waves: The morphologic pattern and position of P waves change.

PR interval: The PR interval varies with changes in P wave morphologic features and position.

QRS duration: Normal, constant

Etiology Wandering atrial pacemaker is usually caused by vagal slowing of the sinus pacemaker.

Physical Assessment/Clinical Manifestations The client is usually asymptomatic unless the overall heart rate is too slow. The nurse assesses the client for dizziness, weakness, syncope, confusion, chest discomfort or pain, hypotension, diaphoresis, and shortness of breath.

Interventions No intervention is usually needed unless a symptomatic bradycardia occurs. The nurse then administers atropine as prescribed or, if necessary, initiates noninvasive pacemaker therapy as ordered and notifies the physician.

ATRIAL TACHYCARDIA

Pathophysiology Atrial tachycardia involves the rapid stimulation of atrial tissue at a rate of 150 to 250 beats per minute. Atrial tachycardia may be due to the rapid, repetitive firing of an irritable ectopic atrial focus from atrial ischemia or the effects of drugs. More often, atrial tachycardia is due to a re-entry mechanism, in which one impulse circulates repeatedly in a circuitous atrial pathway, restimulating the atrial tissue repetitively at a rapid rate.

The term *paroxysmal atrial tachycardia* (PAT) is used when the rhythm is intermittent, initiated suddenly by a premature complex such as a PAC (Fig. 33–15*A*), and terminated suddenly with or without intervention. In some instances, the onset is more gradual (nonparoxysmal). During atrial tachycardia, the P waves have a different morphologic pattern than do sinus P waves but may not be seen if there is 1 : 1 conduction with rapid rates, because the P waves are obscured in the preceding T wave. Such a rhythm of sudden onset with obscured P waves and narrow QRS complexes may be called a *paroxysmal supraventricular tachycardia* (PSVT).

When the atrial rate is rapid, particularly if it is more than 200 beats per minute, the AV node cannot conduct each impulse to the ventricles. The AV node blocks some of the impulses, preventing them from reaching the ventricles. This block is a protec-

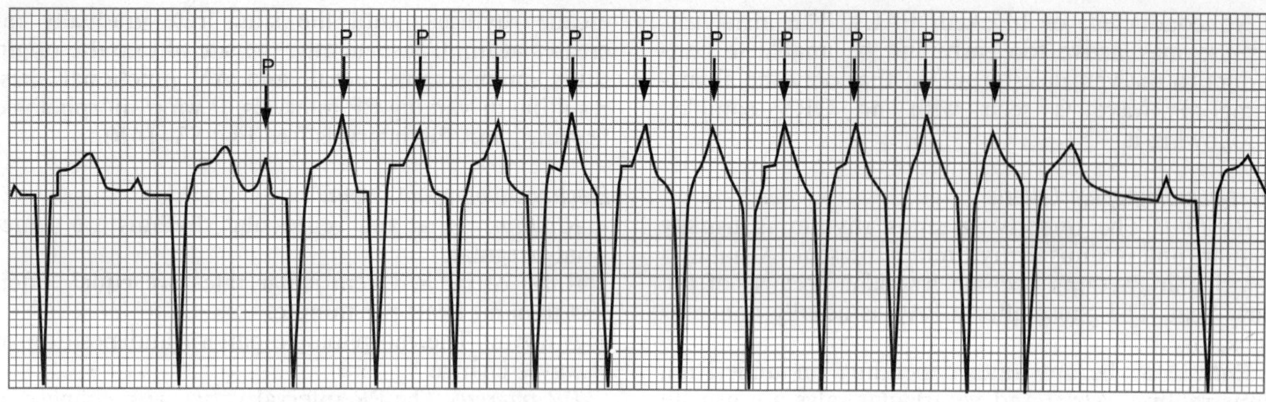

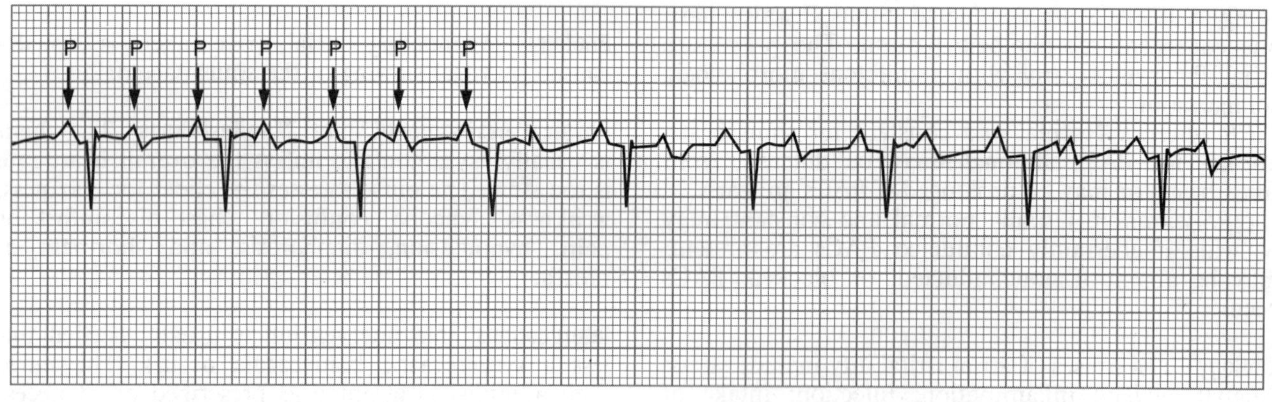

FIGURE 33–15 ◆ Atrial dysrhythmias. *A*, Normal sinus rhythm (NSR) with an 11-beat run of paroxysmal atrial tachycardia (PAT) with 1:1 conduction. *B*, Atrial tachycardia with 2:1 block. The atrial rate is 164/minute; the ventricular rate is 82/minute.

tive mechanism for the ventricles, which are stimulated at a slower rate than the atria. This is known as atrial tachycardia with 2:1 block (see Fig. 33–15*B*).

Electrocardiographic Criteria

Rhythm: The atrial rhythm is regular or nearly regular. The ventricular rhythm is regular if 1:1 conduction or a regular block is present. The ventricular rhythm is irregular if variable block occurs.

Rate: The atrial rate is 150 to 250 beats per minute. The ventricular rate is the same as the atrial rate if 1:1 conduction is present. The ventricular rate is less than the atrial rate if there is PAT with block, particularly if the atrial rate is greater than 200 beats per minute.

P waves: The morphologic pattern is different from that of sinus P waves. If 1:1 conduction is present, one P wave occurs before each QRS complex, but is seldom visible, being buried in preceding T waves. If there is PAT with block, more P waves than QRS complexes are present.

PR interval: The PR interval is usually not measurable with 1:1 conduction; it varies with tachycardia rate and degree of block.

QRS duration: Usually normal and constant. QRS complexes may be wide if aberrantly conducted.

Etiology The causes of atrial tachycardia are the same as those listed for PACs. PAT may occur in healthy young people without evidence of heart disease or in clients with rheumatic heart disease.

Physical Assessment/Clinical Manifestations The clinical manifestations depend on the rate of the ventricular response. In clients with a rapid ventricular response, the nurse assesses for palpitations, weakness, fatigue, shortness of breath, nervousness, anxiety, and syncope. Hemodynamic deterioration may occur in the client with cardiac disease, causing angina, heart failure, and shock. With a slower ventricular response, the client may be asymptomatic.

Interventions If PAT occurs in a healthy person and terminates spontaneously, no intervention is necessary other than eliminating causative factors. In sustained atrial tachycardia with a rapid ventricular response, the goals of treatment are to decrease the ventricular response, convert the dysrhythmia to a sinus rhythm, and treat the cause. Vagal stimulation may be successful, but often only transiently, and must be performed only by a physician. It may lead to excessive slowing of the heart or to vagal arrest.

The nurse assists the client to rest and administers oxygen and prescribed sedatives.

The nurse administers prescribed antidysrhythmic drugs, which slow the ventricular rate by increasing the AV block, such as adenosine (Adenocard), verapamil hydrochloride (Calan), diltiazem hydrochloride (Cardizem), digitalis, esmolol hydrochloride (Brevibloc), and propranolol hydrochloride (Inderal, Apo-Propranolol♣) (see Chart 33-4). Some of these drugs may also succeed in converting the dysrhythmia. If atrial tachycardia with block already exists, the nurse must suspect digitalis as the cause, withhold further doses, and notify the physician.

In the severely compromised client, the nurse assists the physician to attempt atrial overdrive pacing or to achieve cardioversion and regain hemodynamic stability. If atrial tachycardia is recurrent, the physician may prescribe digitalis alone or in combination with quinidine, procainamide, propranolol, diltiazem, or verapamil to prevent future recurrences.

MULTIFOCAL ATRIAL TACHYCARDIA

Pathophysiology Multifocal atrial tachycardia (MAT) is also known as chaotic atrial tachycardia. Several different ectopic atrial foci fire at a rate faster than 100 beats per minute. This results in varying PP intervals, changing P wave morphologic patterns, and varying PR intervals, with most, but not all, impulses conducted to the ventricles. Some P waves are not followed by a QRS complex (nonconducted P waves). The atrial and ventricular rhythms are both totally irregular (Fig. 33-16*A*).

Electrocardiographic Criteria

Rhythm: Atrial and ventricular rhythms are totally irregular.

Rate: The atrial rate is 100 to 130 beats per minute. The ventricular rate is greater than 100 beats per minute, although it is frequently less than the atrial rate.

P waves: At least three P wave morphologic patterns are seen. Some P waves may be hidden in T waves or blocked in the AV node.

PR interval: Variable

QRS duration: Usually normal, constant

Etiology MAT commonly occurs in clients with chronic pulmonary disease, as well as in older clients and diabetics. It may eventually develop into atrial fibrillation.

Physical Assessment/Clinical Manifestations Symptoms depend on the rate of ventricular response. The client may be asymptomatic or may present with manifestations similar to those of sinus or atrial tachycardia. The nurse assesses the client for shortness of breath, chest discomfort or pain, weakness, fatigue, anxiety, syncope, and hypotension.

Interventions The underlying disease process must be treated. The nurse administers oxygen and prescribed drugs, which decrease the atrial ectopy or slow the ventricular response, such as quinidine, digoxin (Lanoxin), propranolol hydrochloride (Inderal, Apo-Propranolol♣), and diltiazem hydrochloride (Cardizem). The physician does not order propranolol for clients with airway resistance disease, such as chronic asthma, because the drug may induce bronchospasm.

ATRIAL FLUTTER

Pathophysiology Atrial flutter is rapid atrial depolarization occurring at a rate of 250 to 350 times per minute. The most common rate is approximately 300 times per minute. An AV block limits the number of impulses that reach the ventricles as a protective mechanism (see Fig. 33-16*B*). When untreated, atrial flutter typically has a 2:1 block (Fig. 33-16*C*). In general, when a client's ventricular rate is 150 beats per minute, the nurse should suspect atrial flutter with 2:1 block and carefully scrutinize the ECG baseline for evidence of atrial flutter waves.

Electrocardiographic Criteria

Rhythm: The atrial rhythm is regular. The ventricular rhythm is regular if the block is consistent; the ventricular rhythm is irregular if the block is variable.

Rate: The atrial rate is 250 to 350 beats per minute. The ventricular rate is variable, depending on the block; it is usually rapid without treatment.

P waves: Flutter (F) waves are seen in a regular pattern, with a sawtooth or "picket fence" configuration and lack of an isoelectric segment between flutter waves. Some flutter waves may be partially hidden in QRS complexes.

PR interval: Actually FR interval, it may be constant or variable; it is usually not measured.

QRS duration: Usually normal and constant

Etiology Atrial flutter may be caused by rheumatic or ischemic heart disease, congestive heart failure, AV valve disease, septal defects, pulmonary emboli, thyrotoxicosis, alcoholism, or pericarditis and may occur after open heart surgery.

Physical Assessment/Clinical Manifestations The clinical manifestations depend on the rate of ventricular response. The client with a normal ventricular rate is usually asymptomatic. The nurse assesses the client for palpitations, weakness, fatigue, shortness of breath, nervousness, anxiety, syncope, and evidence of hemodynamic deterioration such as angina, heart failure, and shock. Carotid sinus massage transiently increases the AV block to facilitate rhythm interpretation but can be performed only by the physician.

Interventions The treatment goals are the same as those for atrial tachycardia. The nurse administers oxygen and prescribed drugs to slow the rapid ventricular response, such as diltiazem, verapamil, propranolol, and esmolol. Digoxin may convert the atrial flutter to atrial fibrillation, which is more responsive to treatment, or occasionally, it may convert atrial

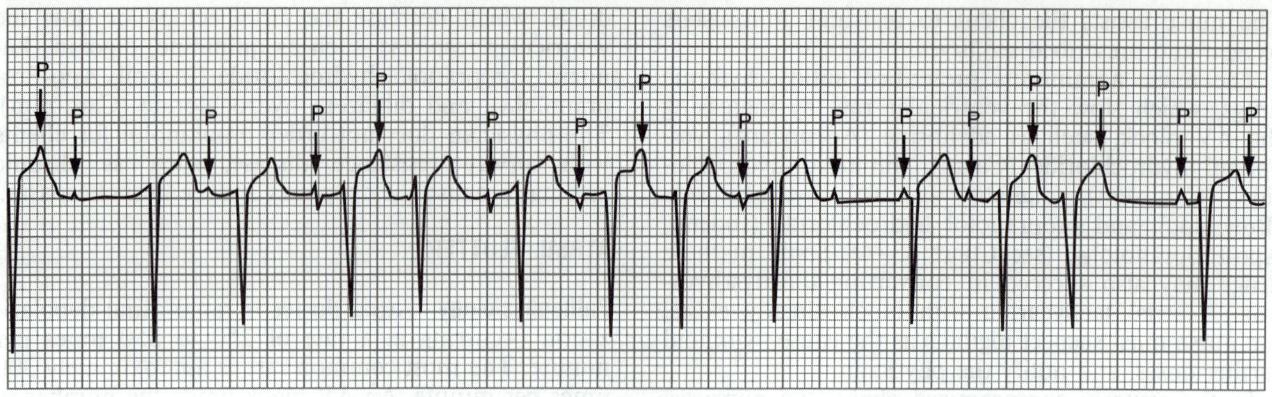

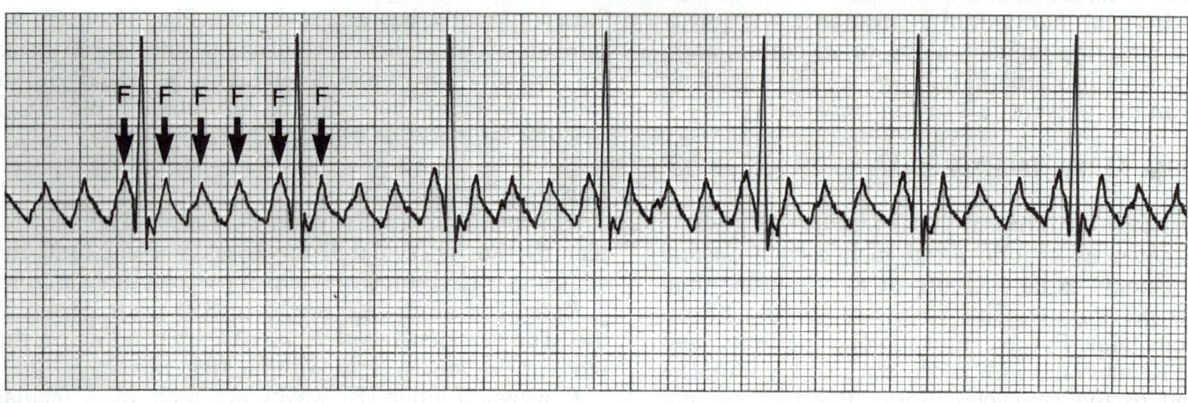

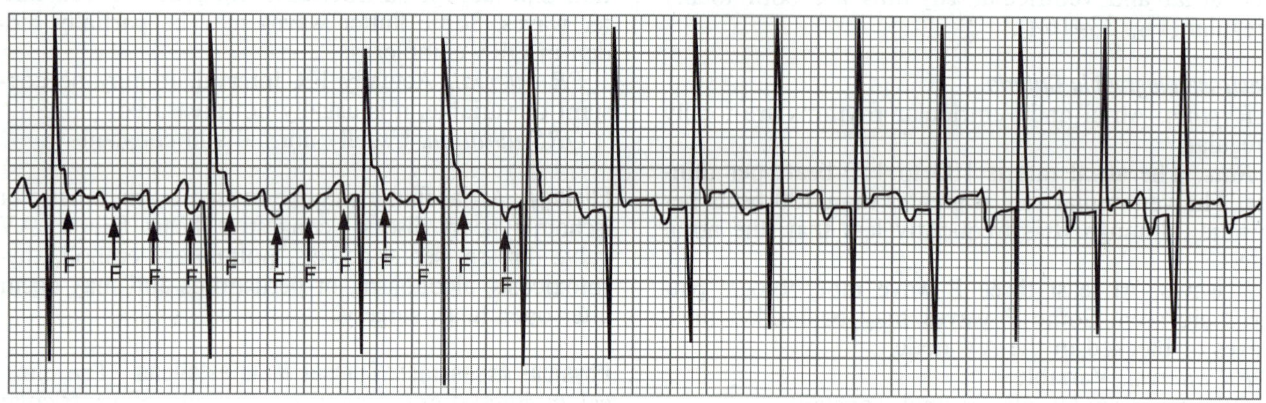

FIGURE 33–16 ◆ Atrial dysrhythmias. *A*, Multifocal atrial tachycardia (MAT) with an irregular rhythm; varying P wave morphologies and PR intervals. *B*, Atrial flutter (F) with 4:1 block. The atrial rate is 280/minute; the ventricular rate is 70/minute. *C*, Atrial flutter with 4:1 conduction, then an 11-beat run with 2:1 conduction, then back to 4:1.

flutter to sinus rhythm. Quinidine or procainamide must not be administered unless one of the above agents has slowed the ventricular response. Both drugs slow the atrial rate and increase AV conduction, which could cause a 1:1 conduction with an increase in ventricular rate and hemodynamic deterioration.

The nurse assists the physician to attempt rapid atrial overdrive pacing or to achieve cardioversion in the client who is hemodynamically compromised. If the client is medically refractory, the physician may recommend catheter ablation or surgical ablation to abolish the irritable focus. After undergoing such a procedure, the client is usually in a third-degree heart block and requires permanent pacemaker therapy (see later in this chapter).

ATRIAL FIBRILLATION

Pathophysiology Multiple, rapid impulses from many foci, at a rate of 350 to 600 times per minute, depolarize the atria in a totally disorganized manner. The result is chaos, with no P waves, no atrial contractions, loss of the atrial kick, and a totally irregular ventricular response (Fig. 33–17). The atria merely quiver in fibrillation (sometimes call "A fib"), which may lead to the formation of mural thrombi (within the cardiac wall) and potential embolic events.

Electrocardiographic Criteria

Rhythm: The atrial rhythm consists of an irregular undulating baseline. The ventricular rhythm is totally irregular.

Rate: The atrial rate cannot be counted because there are no P waves. The ventricular rate is usually 100 to 160 beats per minute or faster when untreated (uncontrolled A fib). The ventricular rate is 60 to 100 beats per minute when treated (controlled A fib). The ventricular rate is less than 60 beats per minute when excessive AV nodal block occurs with drug treatment, such as with digoxin (A fib with high-grade AV block).

P waves: P waves are absent; irregular fibrillatory (f) waves vary in amplitude and morphologic features in baseline.

PR interval: None

QRS duration: Usually normal and constant, although wide (aberrant) complexes are common

Etiology Atrial fibrillation occurs in clients with a history of rheumatic heart disease, particularly mitral stenosis, as well as in clients with:

- Myocardial infarction
- Atrial septal defect
- Congestive heart failure
- Cardiomyopathy
- Hypertensive cardiovascular disease
- Thyrotoxicosis
- Pulmonary emboli
- Wolff-Parkinson-White syndrome
- Congenital heart disease
- Chronic constrictive pericarditis
- Post–open heart surgery

Physical Assessment/Clinical Manifestations Atrial fibrillation may be intermittent or chronic. Symptoms depend on the ventricular rate. If the ventricular rate is rapid, the client may present as described for atrial tachycardia. However, the client in uncontrolled atrial fibrillation, with a ventricular rate greater than 100 beats per minute, is at greater risk for an inadequate cardiac output because of loss of the atrial kick. The nurse assesses the client for the presence of a pulse deficit, fatigue, weakness, shortness of breath, distended neck veins, dizziness, decreased exercise tolerance, anxiety, syncope, palpitations, chest discomfort or pain, and hypotension.

The client is at risk for systemic emboli, particularly an embolic stroke. Most emboli cause permanent severe neurologic impairment or death (Kater et al., 1992). Because approximately one third of clients with atrial fibrillation have thromboemboli, the nurse must be astute in assessing the client for evidence of embolic events. The nurse particularly notes changes in mentation, speech, sensory function, and motor function, reporting these to the physician immediately. Clients with atrial fibrillation who have valvular disease are particularly at risk for thromboemboli.

Interventions Treatment is the same as for atrial flutter. In addition, the nurse may administer anticoagulants, such as heparin (Hepalean✱) and sodium warfarin (Coumadin, Warfilone✱), as prescribed by the physician for clients considered to be at high risk for emboli. For elective cardioversion, the nurse must initiate anticoagulation therapy as prescribed to prevent a thromboembolic event. Atrial fibrillation of greater than 12 months' duration is not likely to respond to attempts at conversion to sinus rhythm by drug therapies.

Clients with recurring, symptomatic tachydysrhythmias resistant to medical therapies may benefit from the "maze" procedure, an open heart surgical technique (Kater et al., 1992). In this procedure, the nurse first prepares the client for electrophysiologic mapping studies for confirmation of the diagnosis of atrial fibrillation. The nurse then prepares the client for surgery. The surgeon places a maze of sutures in strategic places in the atrial myocardium to prevent electrical circuits from developing and perpetuating atrial fibrillation (Kater et al., 1992). Sinus impulses

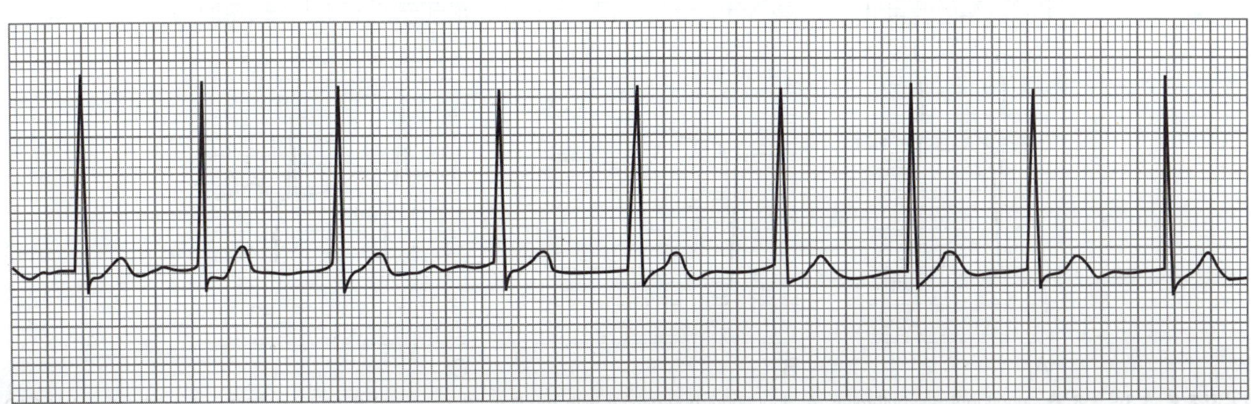

FIGURE 33–17 ◆ Atrial dysrhythmias. Atrial fibrillation, controlled, with a ventricular rate of approximately 80/minute.

can then depolarize the atria before reaching the AV node and preserve the atrial kick. The postoperative care of the client is similar to that after other open heart surgical procedures (see Chap. 37).

JUNCTIONAL DYSRHYTHMIAS

Nodal cells in the AV junctional area can generate electrical impulses and are therefore subsidiary or latent pacemaker cells. They have a slower rate of firing than do those of the sinus node and are usually suppressed. Occasionally, these cells do fire, with the wave of depolarization proceeding in two directions: retrograde (backward) into the atria and anterograde (forward) down the normal conduction system into the ventricles. The resultant ECG findings depend on the speed of conduction in each direction and may be manifested in one of three ways:

- If retrograde conduction into the atria is faster than anterograde conduction into the ventricles, the normal sequence of atrial depolarization preceding ventricular depolarization is preserved. The P wave is inscribed before the QRS complex, but with a short PR interval (less than 0.12 second) (Fig. 33–18*A*).
- If retrograde conduction depolarizes the atria at the same time as anterograde conduction depolarizes the ventricles, only the QRS complex is seen. The P wave is obscured by the QRS complex. There is no PR interval (see Fig. 33–18*B*).
- If anterograde conduction depolarizes the ventricles before retrograde conduction depolarizes the atria, the QRS complex is inscribed before the P wave, with a short RP interval (no PR interval) (see Fig. 33–18*C*).

Thus, the P wave may occur before, during, or after the QRS complex. In all three cases, there is a loss of the atrial kick because the atria cannot contract before the ventricles do. Retrograde depolarization of the atria causes the P wave to be inverted in leads II, III, and aVF. Several junctional rhythms are discussed:

- Junctional escape complexes
- Junctional escape rhythm
- Premature junctional complexes
- Accelerated junctional rhythm
- Junctional tachycardia

JUNCTIONAL ESCAPE COMPLEXES

Pathophysiology Junctional escape complexes occur when there is a pause in the underlying rhythm. The pause allows sufficient time for AV junctional cells to generate and to conduct an electrical impulse as a subsidiary pacemaker. The junctional complex occurs after the pause (Fig. 33–19*A*).

Electrocardiographic Criteria

Rhythm: Atrial and ventricular rhythms are irregular owing to a pause. The pause is followed by a late junctional complex. The underlying rhythm is usually sinus.

Rate: Any rate, but often slow

P waves: The underlying rhythm is one P wave before each QRS complex, sinus P waves, and then a pause. If blocked premature atrial contractions (PACs) occur, an early P wave of different morphologic pattern, not followed by a QRS complex, precedes the pause. In junctional escape beat, a P wave of different morphologic pattern may occur before, during, or after the QRS complex.

PR interval: The PR interval is constant for sinus beats; it may be normal or prolonged. Blocked PACs have no PR interval. In junctional escape beat, the P wave occurs before the QRS complex; the PR interval is less than 0.12 second in escape beat. If the P wave occurs during the QRS complex, there is no PR interval. If the P wave occurs after the QRS complex, there is an RP (not PR) interval.

QRS duration: Normal, constant

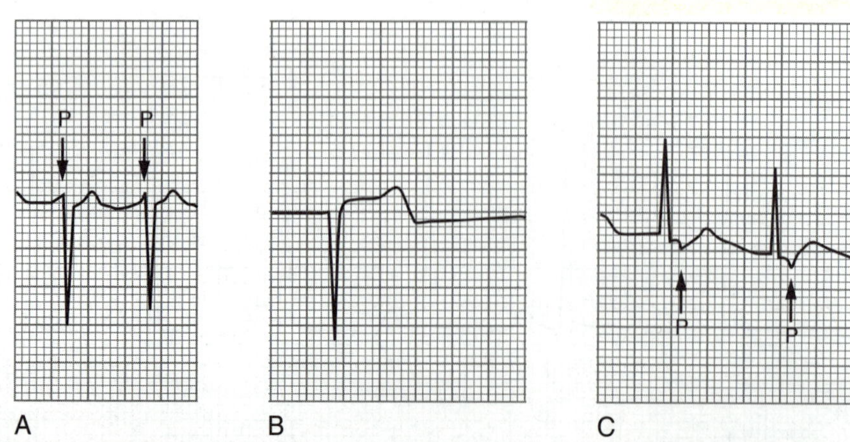

FIGURE 33–18 ◆ Junctional dysrhythmias. *A*, Junctional complexes with the P wave occurring *before* the QRS and a PR interval of 0.08 second. *B*, Junctional complex with no visible P wave, being buried in the QRS. *C*, Junctional complexes with the P wave occurring *after* the QRS.

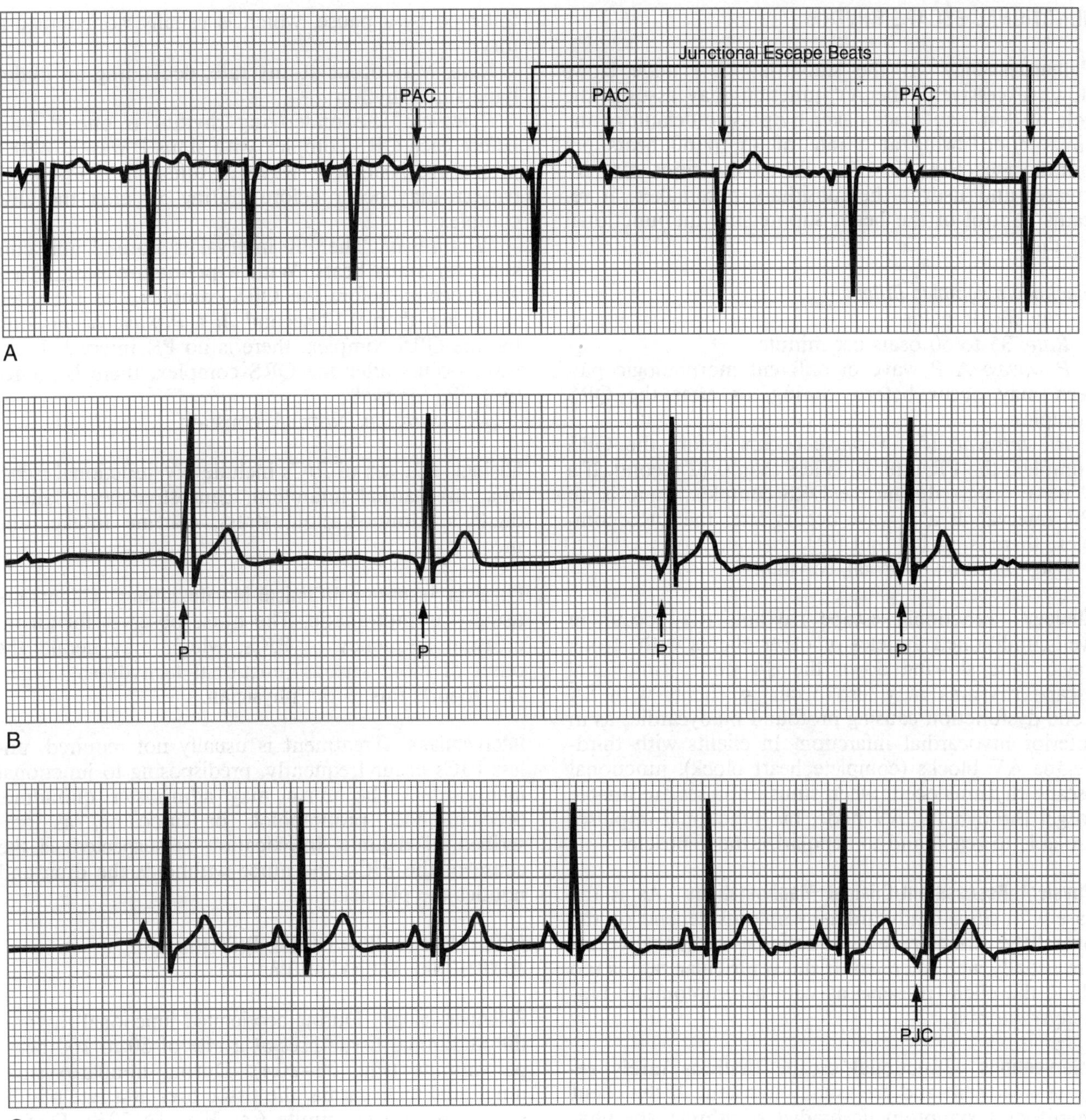

FIGURE 33-19 ◆ Junctional dysrhythmias. *A*, Normal sinus rhythm (NSR) with blocked premature atrial complexes (PACs) followed by junctional escape beats. *B*, Junctional escape rhythm with a rate of 40/minute. P waves occur before the QRS, and the PR interval is less than 0.12 second. *C*, Normal sinus rhythm with a premature junctional complex (PJC). The last beat has a premature inverted P before the QRS with a PR interval less than 0.12 second.

Etiology Pauses may occur in sinus bradycardia as the result of a sinus pause or may occur in normal sinus rhythm as the result of nonconducted PACs. The junctional escape complex fires as a latent pacemaker complex, interrupting the pause and providing an impulse to depolarize the ventricles and to improve the cardiac output.

Physical Assessment/Clinical Manifestations Clinical manifestations depend on the underlying rate and rhythm and the length and frequency of the pauses. The nurse assesses the client for symptoms of a bradydysrhythmia. If the ventricular rate is adequate, the client is usually asymptomatic.

Interventions Because junctional escape complexes are a normal response to a pause, the physician directs treatment at the cause of the pause. For example, symptomatic bradycardia is treated with atropine administration or noninvasive pacemaker therapy.

JUNCTIONAL ESCAPE RHYTHM

Pathophysiology If the sinoatrial (SA) node slows down excessively, the AV junction may assume the role of dominant pacemaker by passive default of the sinus node, firing at a rate of 35 to 60 beats per minute (see Fig. 33–19*B*). When the sinus rate increases and usurps the subsidiary pacemaker, it regains control of the heart, suppressing the junctional rhythm.

Electrocardiographic Criteria

Rhythm: Regular

Rate: 35 to 60 beats per minute

P waves: A P wave of different morphologic pattern may occur before, during, or after the QRS complex.

PR interval: If a P wave occurs before the QRS complex, the PR interval is less than 0.12 second. If a P wave occurs during the QRS complex, there is no PR interval. If a P wave occurs after the QRS complex, there is an RP (not PP) interval.

QRS duration: Normal, constant

Etiology Junctional escape rhythms may occur in well-conditioned athletes or other clients with strong vagal tone slowing down the SA node. Junctional escape rhythms may also occur in clients with SA node dysfunction causing profound bradycardia, as in inferior myocardial infarction. In clients with third-degree AV blocks (complete heart block), junctional escape rhythms occur when sinus impulses are unable to get through the AV node, but junctional impulses are able to reach and to depolarize the ventricles.

Physical Assessment/Clinical Manifestations As is the case with sinus bradycardia, symptoms depend on the overall ventricular rate. Junctional escape rhythms are usually well tolerated. If the ventricular rate is too slow, the client presents as with a symptomatic bradydysrhythmia.

Interventions Junctional escape rhythms rarely require treatment and are usually transient. If the client manifests a symptomatic bradydysrhythmia, the physician prescribes atropine or, if necessary, orders a noninvasive pacemaker.

PREMATURE JUNCTIONAL COMPLEXES

Pathophysiology Premature junctional complexes (PJCs), unlike escape beats, result from irritability in the AV junction. This irritability produces premature firing of an impulse from the ectopic junctional focus before the next sinus impulse is due. The complex is premature (early) and is followed by a pause, which is often noncompensatory (see Fig. 33–19*C*).

Electrocardiographic Criteria

Rhythm: The underlying rhythm is usually regular. The rhythm becomes irregular owing to an early beat followed by a pause, which is usually noncompensatory.

Rate: May occur at any rate, depending on underlying sinus rhythm

P waves: The underlying rhythm is one P wave before each QRS complex with sinus P waves. With a premature beat, a P wave of different morphologic pattern may occur before, during, or after the QRS complex.

PR interval: The PR interval is normal and constant for sinus beats. With a premature beat, if a P wave occurs before the QRS complex, the PR interval is less than 0.12 second. If a P wave occurs during the QRS complex, there is no PR interval. If a P wave occurs after the QRS complex, there is an RP (not PR) interval.

QRS duration: Normal, constant

Etiology Causes of PJCs include AV junctional ischemia, myocardial infarction, congestive heart failure, digitalis administration, stress, caffeine intake, and nicotine.

Physical Assessment/Clinical Manifestations Clients are usually asymptomatic. The nurse observes for an increasing frequency of PJCs, which may herald the onset of more serious junctional tachydysrhythmias, and reports this to the physician.

Interventions Treatment is usually not required, unless PJCs occur frequently, predisposing to junctional tachycardia. The nurse may administer quinidine, procainamide, propranolol, or lidocaine, as prescribed. If digitalis intoxication is suspected as the cause of the PJCs, the nurse withholds the drug and notifies the physician.

ACCELERATED JUNCTIONAL RHYTHM AND JUNCTIONAL TACHYCARDIA

Pathophysiology During accelerated junctional rhythm, the junctional tissue fires at a rate of 60 to 100 beats per minute (Fig. 33–20*A*). During nonparoxysmal junctional tachycardia, the tissue fires at a rate of 100 to 130 beats per minute (see Fig. 33–20*B*). During AV nodal tachycardia, formerly referred to as paroxysmal junctional tachycardia (PJT), there is a type of paroxysmal supraventricular tachycardia (PSVT). PSVT occurs suddenly at a rate of 150 to 250 beats per minute with 1:1 conduction. It is usually due to an AV nodal re-entry mechanism and may occur in people with no organic heart disease.

Electrocardiographic Criteria

Rhythm: Usually regular

Rate: Accelerated junctional rhythm: 60 to 100 beats per minute; nonparoxysmal junctional tachycardia: 100 to 130 beats per minute; PJT (actually AV nodal tachycardia or PSVT): 150 to 250 beats per minute.

P waves: A P wave of different morphologic pat-

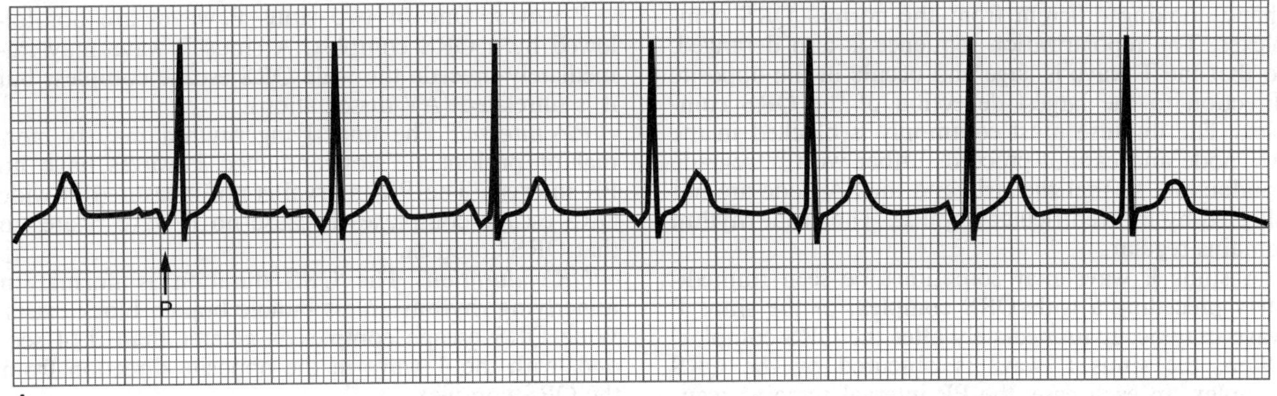

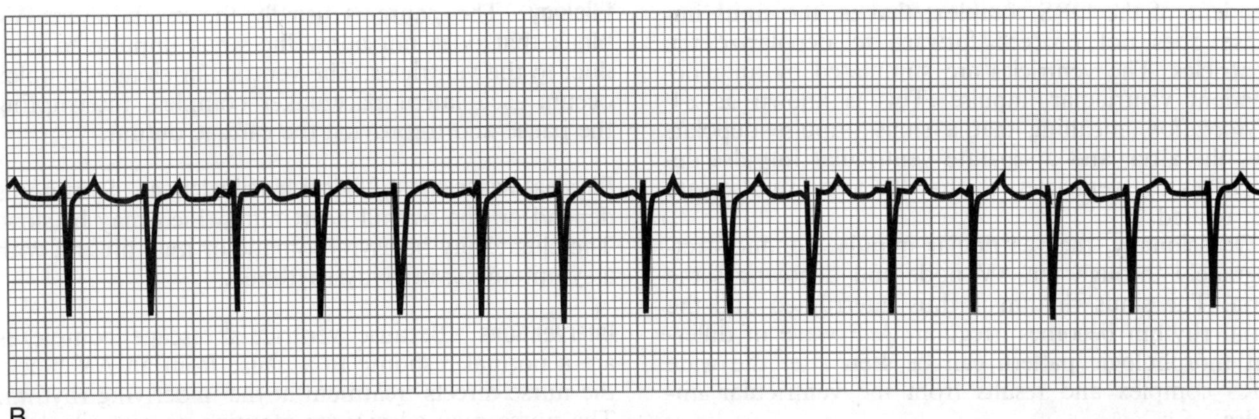

FIGURE 33-20 ◆ Junctional dysrhythmias. *A*, Accelerated junctional rhythm with a rate of 70/minute, inverted P waves before the QRS, and a PR interval less than 0.22 second. *B*, Junctional tachycardia with a rate of approximately 133/minute. P waves are before the QRS with a PR interval of 0.08 second.

tern may occur before, during, or after the QRS complex.

PR interval: If a P wave occurs before the QRS complex, the PR interval is less than 0.12 second. If a P wave occurs during the QRS complex, there is no PR interval. If a P wave occurs after the QRS complex, there is an RP (not PR) interval.

QRS duration: Normal, constant

Etiology These junctional rhythms are sometimes due to underlying heart disease, occurring with inferior myocardial infarction or myocarditis associated with acute rheumatic fever, or occur after cardiac surgery. However, they are most commonly the result of digitalis toxicity.

Physical Assessment/Clinical Manifestations Clients with accelerated junctional rhythms are usually asymptomatic. The client with nonparoxysmal junctional tachycardia may present with the same manifestations as those of sinus tachycardia. Clients with AV nodal tachycardia with a rapid ventricular response may become hemodynamically compromised, as with paroxysmal atrial tachycardia (PAT).

Interventions The underlying cause of the junctional rhythm must be treated. If digitalis toxicity is suspected as the cause, the nurse must withhold the drug and notify the physician. The physician orders ovine (Digibind) to bind with digoxin and reverse the toxicity. AV nodal tachycardia is treated in the same manner as PAT. If the client has recurrent re-entrant tachycardia, the physician may recommend catheter ablation or surgical ablation to abolish an irritable focus. After such a procedure, the client is usually in third-degree AV block and requires permanent pacemaker therapy (see later in this chapter).

VENTRICULAR DYSRHYTHMIAS

The ventricles have the fewest number of nodal cells and are the slowest subsidiary pacemaker, generally being usurped by faster, higher pacemakers. However, irritable ventricular cells may generate electrical impulses and fire prematurely. Because the impulse originates in and depolarizes one ventricle first, then spreads to depolarize the other, the resultant QRS complex is wide, usually measuring greater than 0.12 second. The QRS complex is bizarre or odd in shape, looking different from the normal QRS complexes. The repolarization sequence is also deranged, so that the T wave is large and occurs in the opposite direction to the largest deflection of the QRS complex. The impulse must commonly is blocked in the AV node and cannot proceed further with retrograde conduction, so that the atria and the SA node are not affected by the ventricular impulse. The atrial rhythm remains regular.

A sinus P wave may sometimes be seen immediately preceding a wide QRS complex, or the sinus P wave may occur immediately after the QRS complex. Often, the sinus P wave is obscured by the QRS complex. In each case, the PP interval remains regular. These P waves are not related to and are independent of the QRS complex; that is, the sinus impulse does not proceed forward to depolarize the ventricles. The ventricles are stimulated by an independent ventricular impulse. This is known as *AV dissociation,* meaning that a sinus impulse depolarizes the atria, and a separate ventricular impulse depolarizes the ventricles, so that the two impulses are not related.

Occasionally, the ventricular impulse conducts retrogradely through the AV node and depolarizes the atria. The sinus rhythm is thus interrupted and the atrial rhythm becomes irregular. A P wave of different morphologic pattern can be seen after the wide QRS complex and results from the ventricular impulse.

Several ventricular rhythms are discussed:

- Ventricular escape complexes
- Idioventricular rhythm
- Accelerated idioventricular rhythm
- Premature ventricular complexes
- Ventricular tachycardia
- Ventricular fibrillation
- Ventricular asystole

VENTRICULAR ESCAPE COMPLEXES

Pathophysiology If a sinus impulse is unable to be conducted to the ventricles because of an occasional AV block, ventricular nodal cells may fire as a subsidiary pacemaker. They provide an escape complex to depolarize the ventricles. The ventricular escape complex (wide QRS complex) comes after a pause. During the pause, one or two sinus P waves may be seen, not followed by normally conducted QRS complexes. The escape complex is a late complex and a normal mechanism in response to the AV block (Fig. 33–21*A*).

Electrocardiographic Criteria

Rhythm: The atrial rhythm is usually regular. The ventricular rhythm is irregular because of a pause followed by an escape beat.

Rate: The atrial rate may vary; it is usually normal. The ventricular rate is slower than the atrial rate; it is often slow.

P waves: One or two sinus P waves are not followed by a QRS complex. A sinus P wave may immediately precede the wide QRS escape complex, but it is unrelated (AV dissociation).

PR interval: The underlying rhythm may be normal or prolonged. Nonconducted P waves have no PR interval. The PR interval is not measured in wide QRS escape complexes because no P wave relates to that QRS complex.

QRS duration: The QRS duration is normal in underlying rhythm unless bundle branch block exists. Wide QRS escape complex is greater than 0.14 second, with the T wave in the opposite direction from the QRS complex.

Etiology The pause is usually the result of an AV block that does not allow the sinus impulse to conduct to the ventricles. The ventricular escape complex occurs as a latent pacemaker complex, interrupting the pause and improving the cardiac output.

Physical Assessment/Clinical Manifestations Symptoms depend on the overall heart rate, which may be slow. The client may be asymptomatic or may present with a symptomatic bradydysrhythmia.

Interventions Because ventricular escape complexes are a normal response to a pause from an AV block, the nurse directs treatment at the underlying rhythm. The nurse may administer atropine as prescribed for the AV block or, if necessary, initiate noninvasive pacemaker therapy and notify the physician.

IDIOVENTRICULAR RHYTHM (VENTRICULAR ESCAPE RHYTHM)

Pathophysiology During idioventricular rhythm (ventricular escape rhythm), the ventricular nodal cells pace the ventricles. Because their inherent rate of firing is slow, the rate–is usually less than 40 beats per minute (see Fig. 33–21*B*). If P waves are seen, they are independent of the QRS complexes and not related (AV dissociation).

Electrocardiographic Criteria

Rhythm: The atrial rhythm is usually absent because of downward displacement of the pacemaker with atrial standstill. The ventricular rhythm may be regular; it often becomes irregular.

Rate: There is no atrial rate. The ventricular rate is usually less than 40 beats per minute.

P waves: Usually absent

PR interval: None

QRS duration: Wide QRS complexes greater than 0.14 second may vary; T wave in opposite direction

Etiology Idioventricular rhythm is seen as a rhythm in the dying heart, where downward displacement of the pacemaker has occurred. It is also seen with third-degree AV block (complete heart block), when the block is subjunctional and sinus impulses are unable to reach and to depolarize the ventricles.

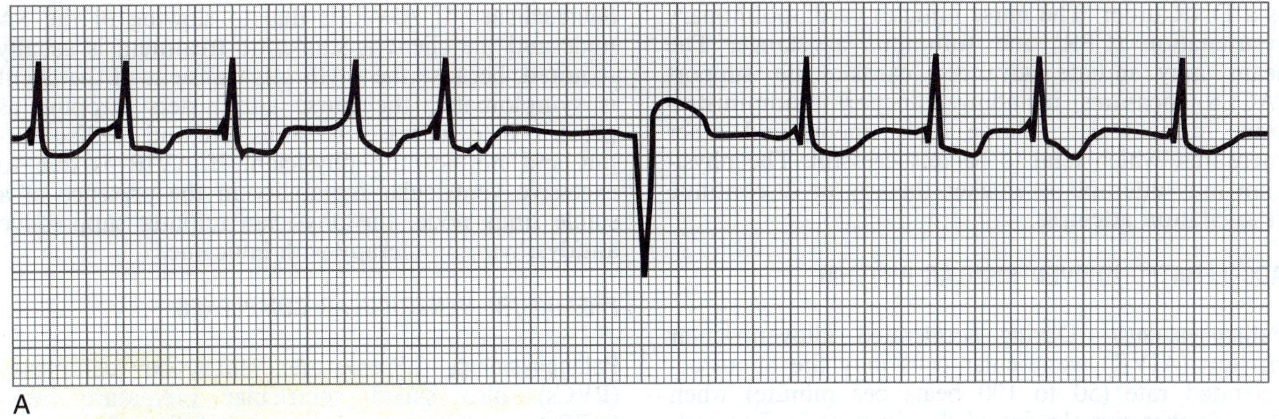

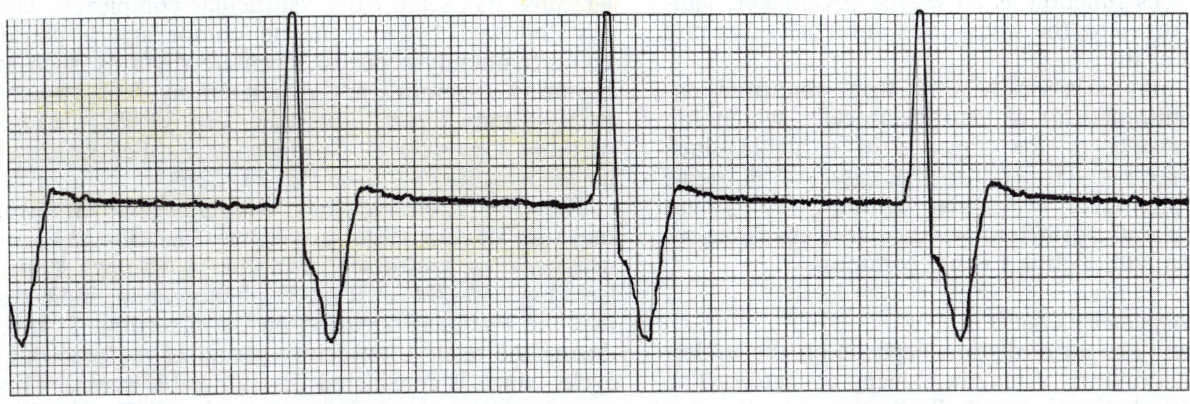

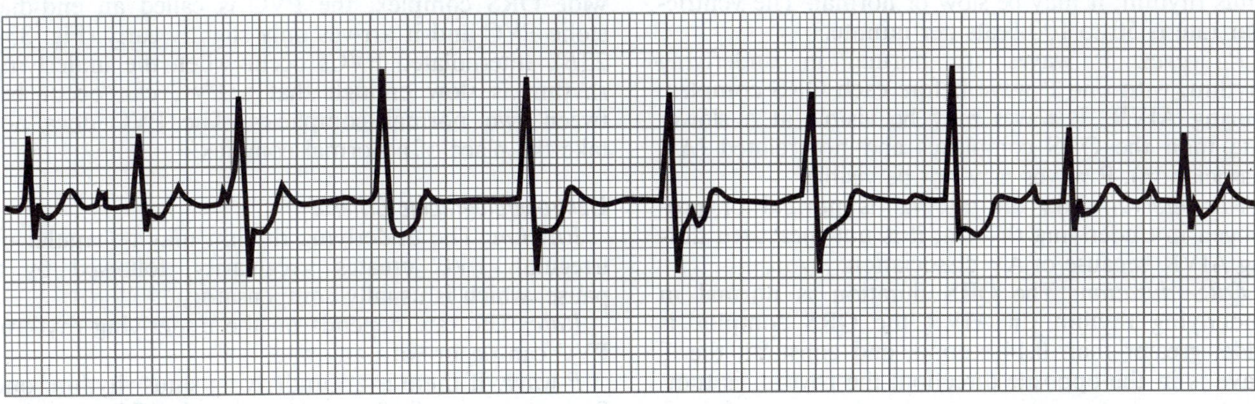

FIGURE 33-21 ◆ Ventricular dysrhythmias. *A*, Ventricular escape beat (sixth beat) with an underlying atrial fibrillation with wide QRS (bundle branch block). *B*, Idioventricular rhythm with a rate of 35/minute. *C*, Normal sinus rhythm (NSR) with first-degree AV block (PR interval greater than 0.20 second) at a rate of 100/minute, interrupted by a run of accelerated idioventricular rhythm (AIVR) initiated by a PVC and firing at a rate of 77/minute for six beats, then returning to NSR at a rate of 95/minute.

Physical Assessment/Clinical Manifestations Because idioventricular pacemakers are unstable and unreliable, the client is usually hypotensive, may be in shock, or may already be pulseless and therefore in cardiac arrest. The nurse assesses the client's pulse, blood pressure, level of consciousness, and pupil response. The nurse must know if the client is to be resuscitated or if there is a "do not resuscitate" (DNR) order.

Interventions Most often, idioventricular rhythms require immediate resuscitation measures, unless there is a DNR order. The nurse initiates cardiopulmonary resuscitation (CPR) and summons assistance. The team may initiate advanced cardiac life support (ACLS) measures, including epinephrine administration, intravascular volume replacement, and other measures, which tend to be unsuccessful. The physician may attempt pacemaker therapy or discontinue resuscitation attempts.

ACCELERATED IDIOVENTRICULAR RHYTHM

Pathophysiology During accelerated idioventricular rhythm (AIVR), ventricular cells may fire at an accelerated rate (50 to 100 beats per minute) when there is excessive slowing of the sinus node. The ventricular cells function as an escape pacemaker, temporarily usurping the sinus node until the sinus rate increases again.

AIVR may occasionally result from abnormal, enhanced automaticity of ventricular cells, which fire inappropriately in the presence of a stable sinus rhythm (see Fig. 33–21*C*). In that case, AIVR begins with a premature ventricular complex (PVC) and may accelerate further to ventricular tachycardia or fibrillation, although this is not common.

Electrocardiographic Criteria

Rhythm: The atrial rhythm depends on the underlying sinus rhythm; it may be slowing or regular. The ventricular rhythm is essentially regular.

Rate: The atrial rate depends on the underlying sinus rhythm; it may be slow or normal. The ventricular rate is 50 to 100 beats per minute.

P waves: P waves are normal in underlying rhythm, with one P wave before each QRS complex. During AIVR, P waves may be visible at a slower rate than the QRS complexes and not related (AV dissociation); P waves may not be visible.

PR interval: The PR interval is normal or prolonged in underlying rhythm; it is not measured during AIVR because of AV dissociation.

QRS duration: The QRS duration is normal in underlying rhythm. In AIVR the QRS complex is wide, greater than 0.14 second, and constant; the T wave is in the opposite direction; the rhythm is transient.

Etiology AIVR commonly occurs in inferior myocardial infarction as an escape pacemaker in response to excessive slowing of the sinus node. In such a case, it begins gradually, is usually considered benign, and is transient, lasting seconds to a minute and stopping with acceleration of the sinoatrial (SA) node (see Fig. 33–21*C*). When AIVR occurs because of enhanced automaticity of ventricular cells, it is usually caused by ischemia, acute myocardial infarction, hypokalemia, or digitalis toxicity.

Physical Assessment/Clinical Manifestations AIVR is usually well tolerated. Some clients may be symptomatic because of the loss of the atrial kick, resulting in a decreased cardiac output and blood pressure.

Interventions If AIVR is due to slowing of the SA node and the client is stable, no treatment is usually required, because the rhythm is transient. If the client is symptomatic, the nurse administers atropine as prescribed to increase the sinus rate and cardiac output and notifies the physician. If AVIR is due to excessive ventricular irritability in the presence of a stable sinus node, the physician initiates suppressive antidysrhythmic therapy with lidocaine.

PREMATURE VENTRICULAR COMPLEXES

Pathophysiology Premature ventricular complexes (PVCs), also called ventricular premature beats (VPBs), result from increased irritability of ventricular cells. PVCs are early ventricular complexes, usually followed by a complete compensatory pause. PVCs frequently occur in repetitive rhythms, such as bigeminy, trigeminy, and quadrigeminy. Two sequential PVCs are a pair, or couplet (Fig. 33–22*A*). Three or more successive PVCs are usually called ventricular tachycardia (VT) (see Fig. 33–22*B*).

The QRS complexes may be unifocal or uniform, meaning of the same shape (see Fig. 33–22*A*), or multifocal or multiform, meaning of different shapes (see Fig. 33–22*C*). R-on-T phenomenon indicates that the PVC has occurred on the preceding T wave during the relative refractory period of the preceding cycle, which is considered the vulnerable period. This may precipitate ventricular fibrillation (VF) (Fig. 33–23*A*). If a dissociated sinus P wave occurs before the wide QRS complex, the PVC is called an end-diastolic PVC and it arrives only slightly early (Fig. 33–23*B*). Interpolated PVCs occur when the underlying rhythm is slow enough that a PVC can occur between two normal complexes. The PVC does not take the place of a normal complex.

Electrocardiographic Criteria

Rhythm: The underlying rhythm may be regular or irregular. PVC creates irregularity, followed by a pause, which is usually compensatory.

Rate: The rate depends on the underlying rhythm; PVC can occur with any rate.

P wave: If there is an underlying sinus rhythm, one P wave occurs before each normal QRS complex. Sinus P waves are not related to PVC (AV dissociation); P waves may occur anywhere relative to PVCs.

PR interval: The PR interval is usually normal if the underlying rhythm is sinus; it is not measured with PVC because of AV dissociation.

QRS duration: The QRS duration is normal in sinus rhythm. In PVC, it is wider than 0.14 second and may vary; the T wave is in the opposite direction.

Etiology PVCs are common, and their frequency increases with age. PVCs may be insignificant or may occur with myocardial ischemia or infarction; congestive heart failure; hypokalemia; hypomagnesemia; the administration of catecholamines, sympathomimetic drugs, and digitalis; acidosis; anesthesia; stress; nico-

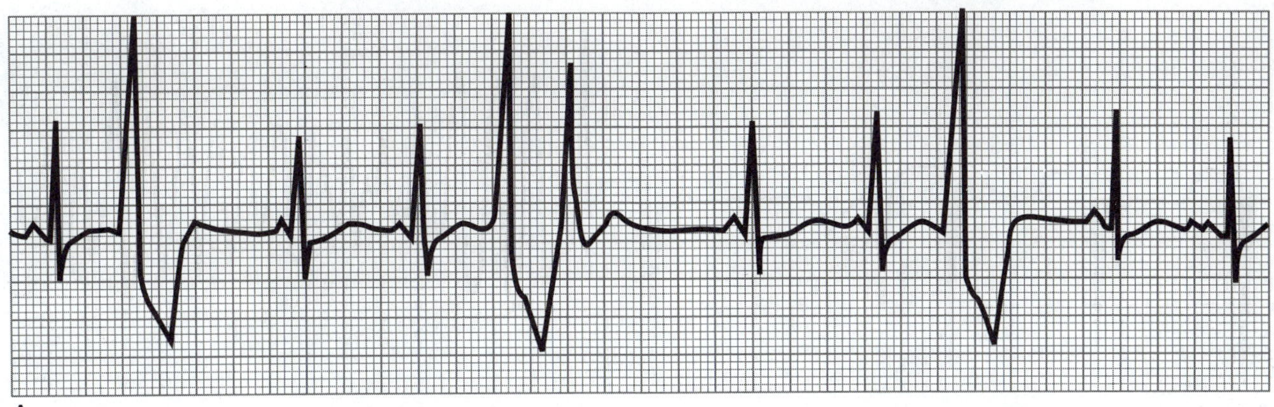
A

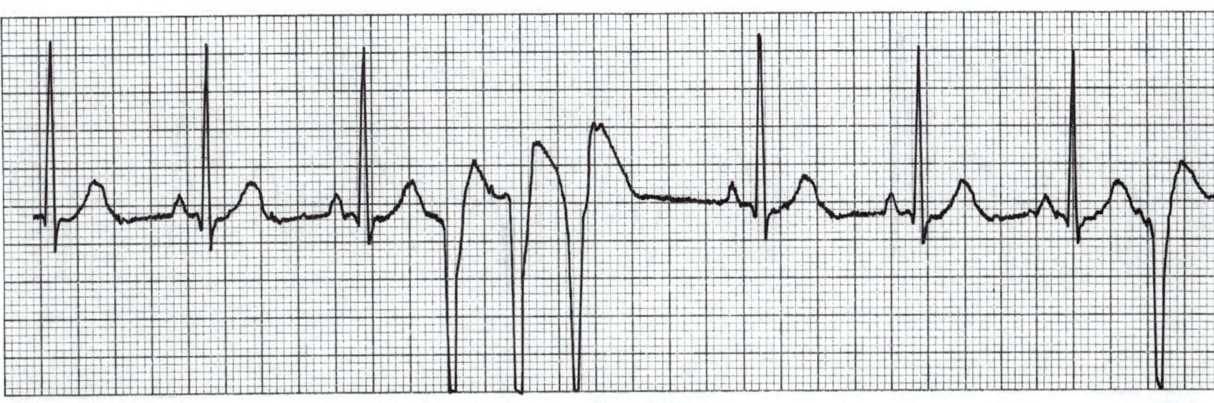
B

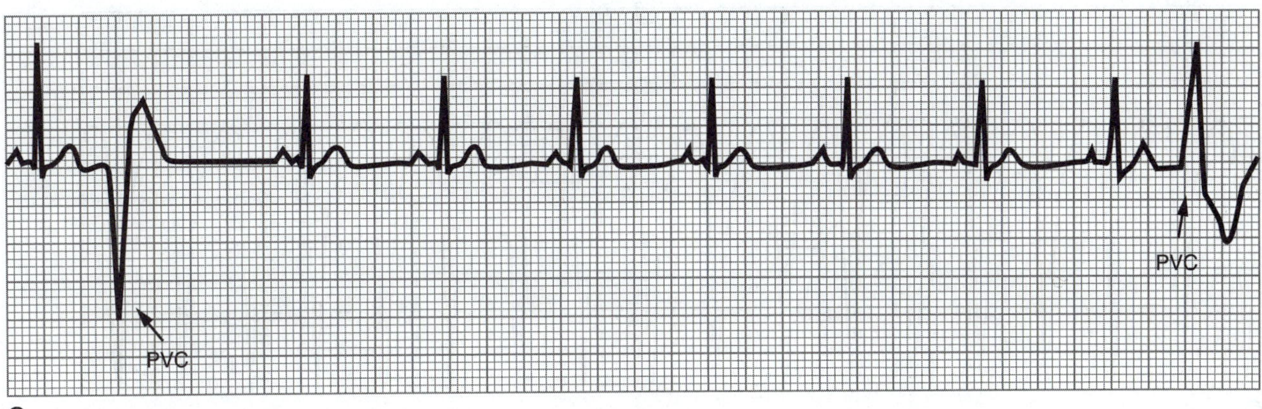

C

FIGURE 33–22 ◆ Ventricular dysrhythmias. *A*, Normal sinus rhythm (NSR) with unifocal premature ventricular complexes (PVCs); note the pair of PVCs. *B*, Normal sinus rhythm with a three-beat run of ventricular tachycardia (three consecutive PVCs) and another unifocal PVC. *C*, Normal sinus rhythm with multifocal PVCs (one negative and the other positive).

tine intake; ingestion of caffeine and alcohol; infection; trauma; or surgery.

Physical Assessment/Clinical Manifestations The client may be asymptomatic or may experience palpitations or chest discomfort owing to the increased stroke volume of the normal beat after the pause. Peripheral pulses may be diminished or absent with the PVCs themselves because the decreased stroke volume of the premature beats may decrease peripheral perfusion. In the setting of acute myocardial infarction, PVCs are considered warning dysrhythmias, possibly heralding the onset of VT or VF. For a client with chest discomfort or pain, the nurse reports to the physician whether PVCs increase in frequency, are multiform, are R-on-T, or occur in runs of VT.

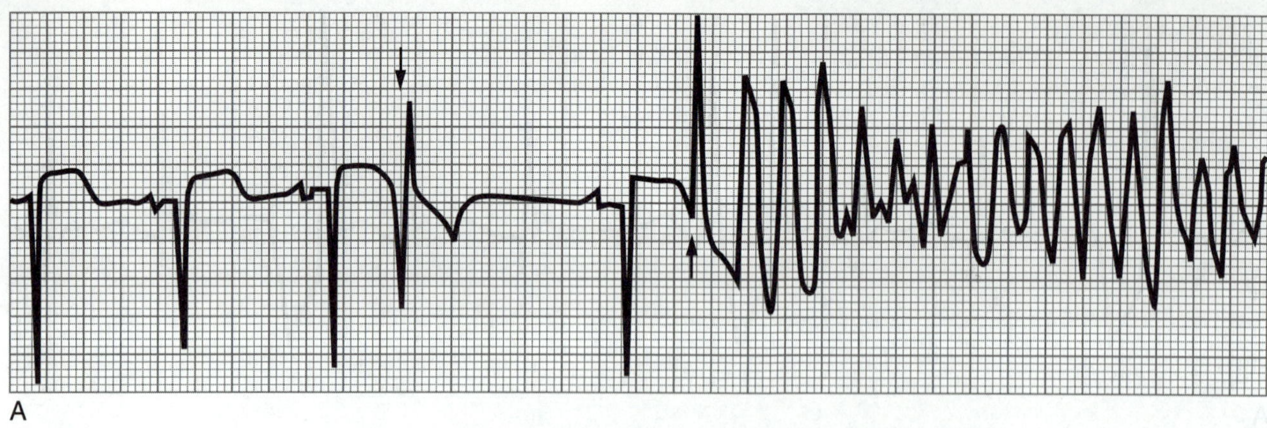

A

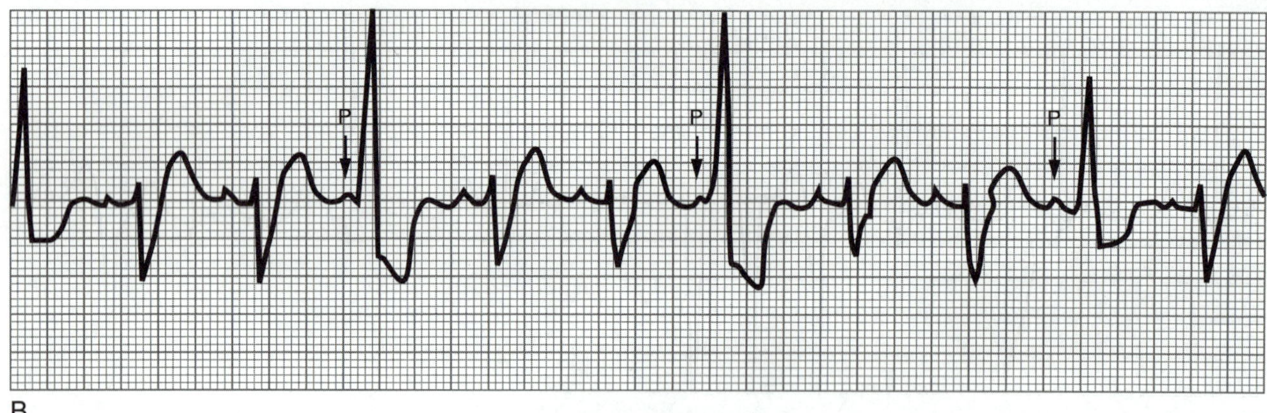

B

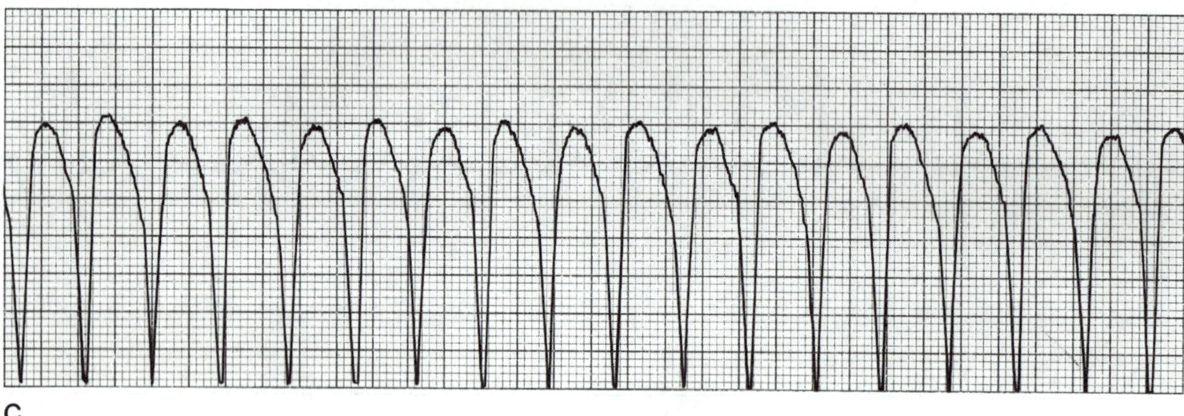

C

FIGURE 33-23 ◆ Ventricular dysrhythmias. *A*, Normal sinus rhythm (NSR) with R-on-T phenomenon. The first R-on-T had no consequence, but the second led to ventricular fibrillation. *B*, Normal sinus rhythm with a bundle branch block (wide QRS complexes) and trigeminal end-diastolic premature ventricular complexes (PVCs). Note the P waves before each PVC. The P waves are from the sinus node and are not related to the PVCs (AV dissociation). *C*, Sustained ventricular tachycardia at a rate of 166/minute.

Interventions If there is no underlying heart disease, PVCs are not usually treated, other than by eliminating any contributing cause (e.g., caffeine, stress). In the setting of acute myocardial ischemia or infarction, the nurse treats significant PVCs by administering oxygen and lidocaine as prescribed. Lidocaine is considered the drug of choice. The nurse may administer other drugs as ordered, including procainamide, bretylium tosylate, magnesium sulfate, propranolol, quinidine, mexiletine, tocainide, sotalol, and amiodarone (see Chart 33–4). The nurse administers potassium as ordered for replacement therapy if hypokalemia is the cause.

VENTRICULAR TACHYCARDIA

Pathophysiology Ventricular tachycardia (VT) (sometimes referred to as "V tach") occurs when there is repetitive firing of an irritable ventricular ectopic focus at a rate of 140 to 250 beats per minute or more (see Fig. 33–23*C*). VT may result from increased automaticity or a re-entry mechanism. VT may present as a paroxysm of three self-limiting beats or more, or it may be a sustained rhythm. The sinus node continues to discharge independently, depolarizing the atria but not the ventricles (AV dissociation), although P waves are seldom seen in sustained VT.

Electrocardiographic Criteria

Rhythm: It is usually not possible to determine the atrial rhythm. The ventricular rhythm is usually regular or nearly regular.

Rate: It is not possible to determine the atrial rate. The ventricular rate is 100 to 250 beats per minute but most commonly is 140 to 180 beats per minute.

P waves: P waves are usually not visible, being obscured in QRS complexes. There is AV dissociation.

PR interval: Not measured because of AV dissociation

QRS duration: Wide, greater than 0.14 second, may vary

Etiology VT is caused by ischemic heart disease, myocardial infarction, cardiomyopathy, hypokalemia, hypomagnesemia, valvular heart disease, heart failure, drug toxicity, or hypotension. In clients who go into cardiac arrest, 80% have VT as the initial rhythm before deteriorating into ventricular fibrillation as the terminal rhythm (Owen, 1991).

Physical Assessment/Clinical Manifestations Clinical manifestations of sustained VT partially depend on the ventricular rate. Slower rates are better tolerated. Clients may be hemodynamically compromised if the cardiac output decreases because of the shortened ventricular filling time or loss of the atrial kick. In some clients, VT causes cardiac arrest. The nurse assesses the client's pulse, respirations, blood pressure, level of consciousness, and pupil response.

Interventions For the stable client with sustained VT, the nurse administers oxygen and lidocaine as prescribed. If this is not successful, procainamide, bretylium tosylate, or magnesium sulfate may be given. The physician may prescribe an oral antidysrhythmic agent, such as sotalol hydrochloride (Betapace).

For the client with unstable VT, the nurse assists the physician immediately to attempt cardioversion followed by oxygen and antidysrhythmic therapy (Chart 33–3). The nurse may instruct the client to perform cough CPR if prescribed, telling the client to inhale deeply and cough hard every 1 to 3 seconds. Cough CPR is sometimes successful in either terminating the VT or at least briefly sustaining cerebral and coronary perfusion until other measures can be initiated (Eorgan & Greer, 1992). The physician may attempt rapid atrial or ventricular overdrive pacing if the VT is related to a significant bradydysrhythmia.

A precordial thump is sometimes successful in terminating VT, at least transiently. The physician or the ACLS-qualified nurse may only administer a precordial thump to a client with unstable VT if a defibrillator and pacemaker are immediately available (Emergency Cardiac Care Committee and Subcommittees [ECCC], American Heart Association, 1992).

For the client with pulseless VT, the physician or ACLS-qualified nurse must *immediately* defibrillate the client or administer a precordial thump and initiate CPR if a defibrillator is not immediately available. Full resuscitative measures are necessary if the rhythm does not quickly convert to a sinus rhythm. The nurse and resuscitation team initiate CPR and airway management and administer oxygen, epinephrine, and antidysrhythmic therapy with lidocaine, bretylium tosylate, procainamide, or magnesium sulfate.

After the rhythm has been successfully converted, attention is given to treating reversible causes, such as myocardial ischemia, hypokalemia, and hypomagnesemia. The nurse ensures that oxygen therapy and antidysrhythmic agent administration are continued and the client is closely monitored for PVCs and the recurrence of VT. The client with recurrent, medically refractory VT may require surgical intervention, such as coronary artery bypass graft (CABG) surgery,

CHART 33–3

Nursing Care Highlight ◆ The Client with Unstable Ventricular Tachycardia

- Assist the physician with cardioversion.
- Provide oxygen and antidysrhythmic drugs as ordered.
- Teach the client how to perform cough cardiopulmonary resuscitation (CPR), if ordered.
- Assist with or provide defibrillation (if you are qualified in advanced cardiac life support [ACLS]).
- Initiate CPR if the client does not respond to the above measures.
- Maintain a patent airway at all times.
- Monitor the client for premature ventricular complexes (PVCs) and the recurrence of VT.
- Assess for signs and symptoms of myocardial infarction, hypokalemia, or hypomagnesemia.

implantation of an automatic cardioverter/defibrillator, aneurysmectomy, encircling endocardial ventriculotomy, cryosurgery, and endocardial resection (see later in this chapter; also see Chap. 37.)

VENTRICULAR FIBRILLATION

Pathophysiology Ventricular fibrillation (VF) (sometimes called "V fib") is the result of electrical chaos in the ventricles. Impulses from many irritable foci fire in a totally disorganized manner, so that ventricular contraction cannot occur. There are no recognizable deflections. Instead, there are irregular undulations of varying amplitudes, from coarse to fine (Fig. 33–24*A*). The ventricles merely quiver, consuming a tremendous amount of oxygen. There is no cardiac output, therefore, no cerebral, myocardial, or systemic perfusion. This rhythm is *rapidly fatal* if not successfully terminated within 3 to 5 minutes.

Electrocardiographic Criteria

Rhythm: Irregular, chaotic undulations of varying amplitudes in baseline

Rate: Not measurable

P waves: Not visible

PR interval: Not measurable

QRS duration: None, fibrillatory waves may be coarse or fine.

Etiology VF may be the first manifestation of coronary artery disease. Clients with myocardial infarction are at great risk for VF. Other causes include myocardial ischemia, hypokalemia, hypomagnesemia, antidysrhythmic therapy, rapid supraventricular tachydysrhythmias, asynchronous pacing with competition, and severe metabolic derangements.

Physical Assessment/Clinical Manifestations On initiation of VF, the client becomes faint, immediately loses consciousness, and becomes pulseless and apneic. There is no blood pressure, and heart sounds are absent. Respiratory and metabolic acidosis develop. Seizures may occur. Within minutes, the pupils become fixed and dilated, and the skin becomes cold and mottled. Death ensues.

Interventions The goals of treatment are to terminate VF promptly and to convert it to an organized rhythm. The physician or the advanced cardiac life support (ACLS)–qualified nurse must immediately defibrillate the client because defibrillation is critical

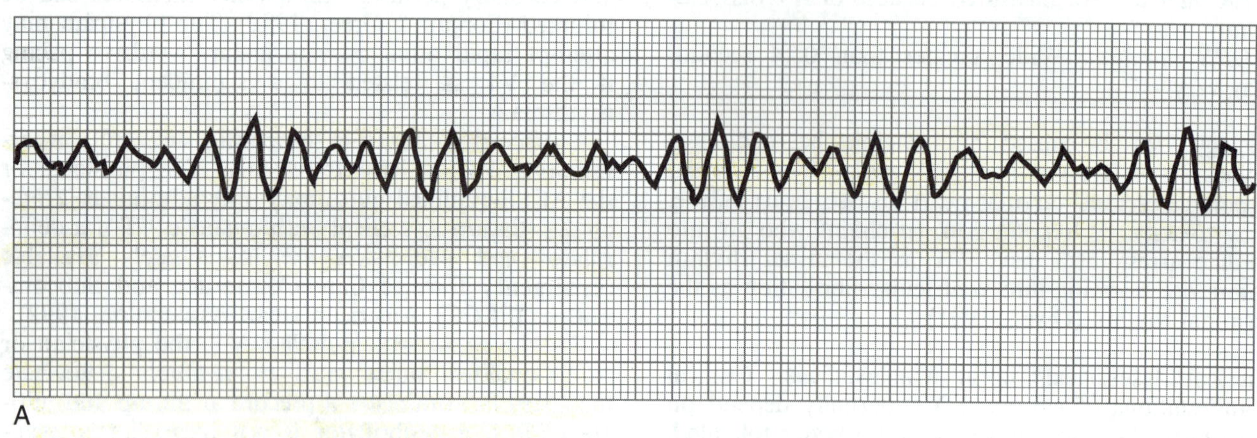

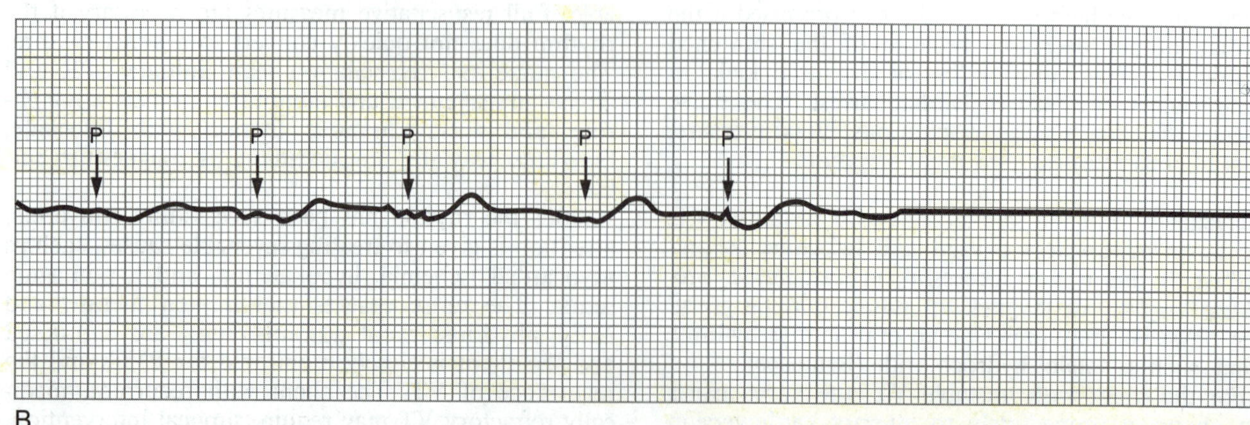

FIGURE 33–24 ◆ Ventricular dysrhythmias. *A*, Coarse ventricular fibrillation. *B*, Ventricular asystole, initially with 5 P waves, then no P waves (atrial and ventricular standstill).

to accomplish this goal and is the management priority. If a defibrillator is not readily available, the nurse may administer a precordial thump and initiate cardiopulmonary resuscitation (CPR) until the defibrillator arrives.

If the VF does not terminate after three rapid successive shocks of increasing energy, the nurse and resuscitation team resume CPR and provide airway management. They also administer oxygen, epinephrine, and antidysrhythmic therapy with lidocaine, bretylium tosylate, procainamide, or magnesium sulfate, along with attempting defibrillation frequently. Cough CPR may be successful in terminating the VF or at least briefly sustaining cerebral and coronary perfusion until definitive treatment can be initiated if the client coughs vigorously before losing consciousness (Eorgan & Greer, 1992). After successful conversion to a sinus rhythm, the nurse continues supportive therapy and assists the physician to treat potential causes of VF and to prevent its recurrence.

VENTRICULAR ASYSTOLE

Pathophysiology Ventricular asystole, sometimes called ventricular standstill, is the complete absence of any ventricular rhythm (see Fig. 33–24*B*). There are no electrical impulses in the ventricles, therefore *no* ventricular depolarization, no QRS complex, no contraction, no cardiac output, and no pulse, respirations, or blood pressure. The client is in full cardiac arrest. The sinoatrial (SA) node, in some cases, may continue to fire and depolarize the atria, with only P waves seen on the electrocardiogram (ECG); the sinus impulses do not conduct to the ventricles, and QRS complexes remain absent. In most cases, the entire conduction system is electrically silent, with no P waves seen on the ECG. There is only a mildly undulating line on the ECG. Fine VF may resemble asystole in some leads. Because treatment of these two rhythms differs significantly, the nurse must assess two ECG leads for an accurate rhythm interpretation.

Electrocardiographic Criteria

Rhythm: The atrial rhythm is usually absent. If P waves are present, atrial rhythm may be regular. The ventricular rhythm is absent.

Rate: No ventricular rate

P waves: P waves are usually absent. Occasionally, regular P waves may be seen if the SA node continues to function.

PR interval: None

QRS duration: QRS complexes are absent.

Etiology Ventricular asystole usually results from myocardial hypoxia, which may be a consequence of advanced heart failure. It may also be caused by severe hyperkalemia and acidosis. If P waves are seen, asystole is likely due to severe ventricular conduction blocks. Rarely, excessive vagal stimulation may cause asystole.

Physical Assessment/Clinical Manifestations Clients are in full cardiac arrest with loss of consciousness and absence of pulse, respirations, and blood pressure. Ventricular asystole is usually fatal.

Interventions The goal of treatment is to restore cardiac electrical activity. The nurse initiates CPR immediately and summons assistance. The nurse must assess another ECG lead to ensure that the rhythm is asystole and not fine VF, which warrants immediate defibrillation. When in doubt, the physician or the ACLS-qualified nurse should defibrillate. The nurse and resuscitation team manage the airway and administer oxygen, epinephrine, and atropine. The nurse assists the physician with the initiation of noninvasive pacing or invasive transvenous or epicardial pacing, although pacemaker therapy is generally not effective. An isoproterenol infusion may also be tried. The prognosis for clients with asystole is poor.

ATRIOVENTRICULAR BLOCKS

Atrioventricular blocks (AV blocks) exist when supraventricular impulses are excessively delayed or totally blocked in the AV node or intraventricular conduction system. Conduction may be transiently or permanently abnormal for a number of reasons. The nurse must remember that the SA node continues to function normally and that atrial depolarizations and P waves occur regularly. Because of the conduction dysfunction, ventricular depolarizations and QRS complexes are either delayed or blocked.

There are different degrees of AV block, as follows:

- In first-degree AV block, all sinus impulses eventually reach the ventricles.
- In second-degree AV block, some sinus impulses reach the ventricles, but others do not because they are blocked. Two types of second-degree block are discussed.
- In third-degree AV block, or complete heart block, none of the sinus impulses reaches the ventricles. The ventricles, therefore, are depolarized by a second, independent pacemaker.

AV blocks are differentiated by their PR intervals.

FIRST-DEGREE ATRIOVENTRICULAR BLOCK

Pathophysiology First-degree AV block is actually a conduction delay rather than a block. AV node conduction is slow, prolonging the PR interval to greater than 0.2 second. However, all sinus impulses eventually reach the ventricles. The underlying rhythm must still be identified (e.g., sinus tachycardia with first-degree AV block) (Fig. 33–25*A*).

Electrocardiographic Criteria

Rhythm: Atrial and ventricular rhythms are usually regular unless sinus arrhythmia is present.

Rate: The rate depends on the underlying rhythm; atrial and ventricular rates are equal.

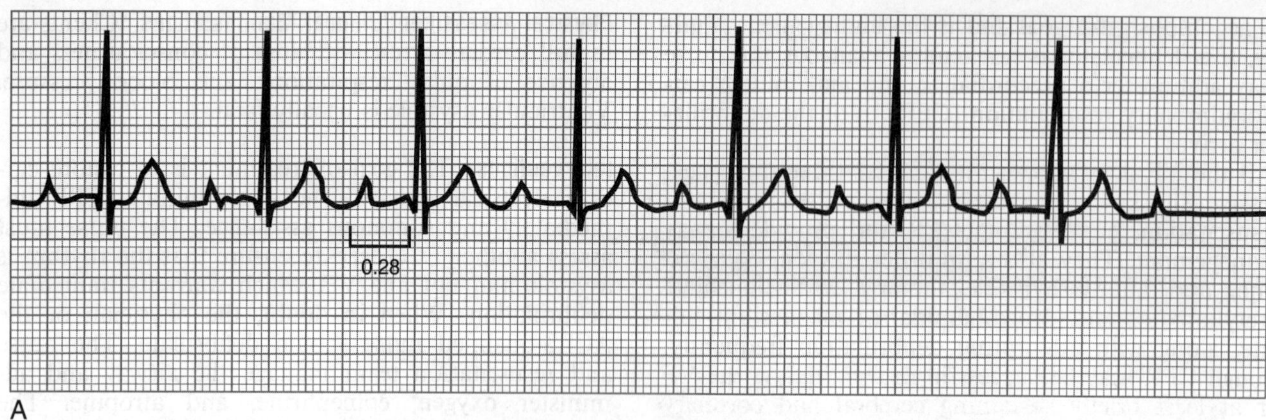

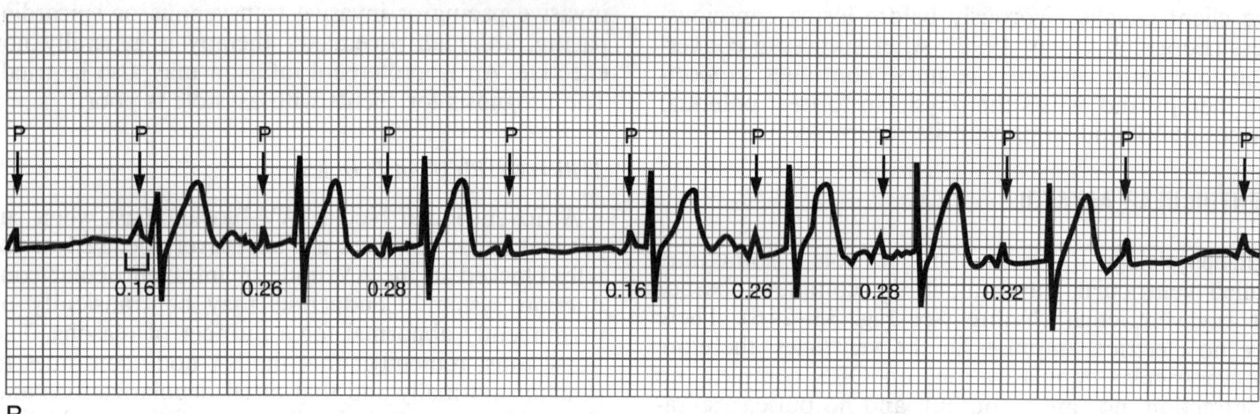

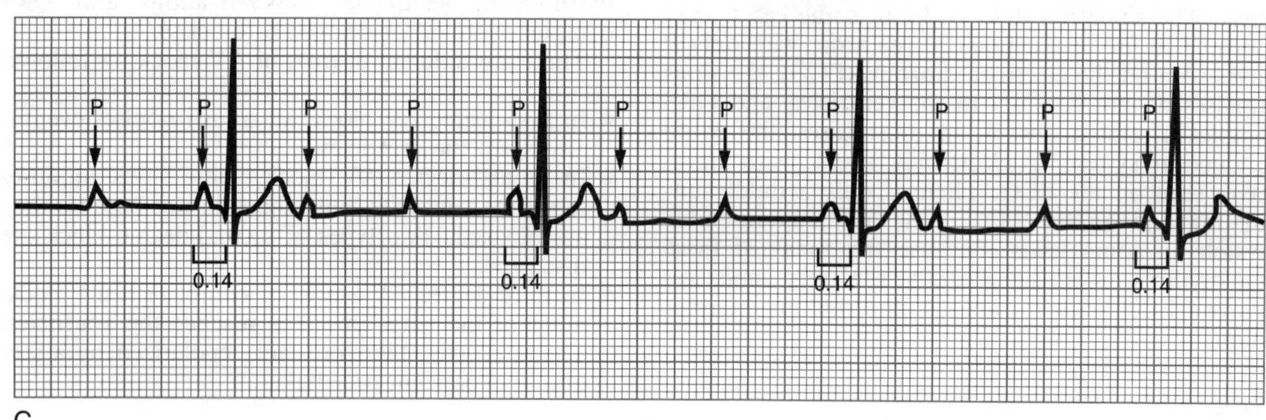

FIGURE 33–25 ◆ AV blocks. *A*, Normal sinus rhythm (NSR) with first-degree AV block (PR interval 0.28 second). *B*, Second-degree AV block type I (AV Wenckebach) with an irregular rhythm, grouped beating, and progressive prolongation of the PR interval until a P wave is completely blocked and not followed by a QRS complex. *C*, Second-degree AV block type II (Mobitz II) with 3:1 conduction and a constant PR interval.

P waves: One P wave precedes each QRS complex. A constant morphologic pattern is found.

PR interval: The PR interval is prolonged, greater than 0.2 second; it usually does not exceed 0.4 second.

QRS duration: Normal, constant

Etiology First-degree AV block may be due to AV nodal ischemia from occlusion of the right coronary artery, as with an inferior or posterior myocardial infarction. It may also result from hypokalemia; the administration of digitalis, beta-adrenergic blockers, and calcium channel blockers; excessive vagal stimulation; or degenerative AV nodal disease. First-degree AV block may be transiently seen during rapid supraventricular rates or early premature atrial complexes (PACs), in which case it is a physiologic rather than a pathologic delay in the AV node.

Physical Assessment/Clinical Manifestations First-degree AV block has no hemodynamic consequences and produces no symptoms. Any symptoms are the result of the underlying rhythm (e.g., sinus bradycardia). First-degree AV block may be insignificant and transient or may progress to more severe AV blocks, although this is uncommon.

Interventions In the stable client, no treatment is needed. If the first-degree AV block is due to drug therapy, the nurse must withhold the offending drug and notify the physician. If the PR interval is particularly long or is progressively getting longer, the nurse must notify the physician. When first-degree AV block is associated with symptomatic bradycardia, the nurse administers atropine as prescribed to accelerate AV conduction.

SECOND-DEGREE ATRIOVENTRICULAR BLOCK TYPE I (WENCKEBACH OR MOBITZ TYPE I)

Pathophysiology In second-degree AV block type I, each successive sinus impulse takes a little longer to conduct through the AV node. Each impulse arrives earlier and earlier in the relative refractory period of the impaired AV node, until one impulse is completely blocked and fails to depolarize the ventricles because the AV node has become completely refractory. This results in a nonconducted or dropped beat (missing QRS complex). There is progressive prolongation of the PR interval, followed by a dropped beat and a pause (the most characteristic feature of this rhythm). This pause allows sufficient time for the AV node to recover, so that the next beat is conducted with a shorter PR interval and the Wenckebach sequence is repeated. Although the atrial rhythm is regular, the ventricular rhythm is irregular, with an appearance of grouped beats, separated by pauses. Group size (conduction ratios) may be constant or may vary. In each group, there is normally one more P wave than there are QRS complexes, because of the dropped QRS complex (Fig. 33–25*B*). The QRS complexes are normal. A 2:1 Wenckebach block is sometimes seen, in which there are two P waves for every normal QRS complex, with PR intervals that do not vary.

Electrocardiographic Criteria

Rhythm: The atrial rhythm is regular. The ventricular rhythm is irregular, with grouped beating and shortening RR intervals in the group.

Rate: The atrial rate depends on the underlying sinus rhythm, which may be normal or slow. The ventricular rate is always less than the atrial rate because of dropped beats.

P waves: P waves are normal and constant. Some P waves are not conducted to ventricles and are not followed by a QRS complex.

PR interval: There is progressive lengthening of PR intervals until a dropped beat, which is followed by a pause, then a new sequence begins.

QRS duration: The QRS duration is usually normal and constant. One QRS complex is missing in each grouped sequence.

Etiology The causes of Wenckebach heart block are the same as for first-degree AV block. It is often a transient rhythm and may revert to first-degree AV block or even a normal sinus rhythm. It is frequently seen with inferior myocardial infarction, particularly if a right ventricular myocardial infarction coexists. It is also seen with rheumatic fever and digitalis administration.

Physical Assessment/Clinical Manifestations The client is usually asymptomatic if the frequency of dropped beats and the overall ventricular rate do not decrease the cardiac output. If the ventricular rate is too slow, decreasing the cardiac output, the client presents with symptoms of a symptomatic bradydysrhythmia. This rhythm is usually transient and terminates spontaneously.

Interventions No intervention is required in the stable client, because this rhythm rarely progresses to a more severe block. In the symptomatic client, the nurse administers atropine as prescribed. If atropine is not successful in speeding AV nodal conduction time and increasing the heart rate, the nurse initiates noninvasive pacemaker therapy as ordered and notifies the physician.

SECOND-DEGREE ATRIOVENTRICULAR BLOCK TYPE II (MOBITZ TYPE II)

Pathophysiology In Mobitz type II block, sinus impulses that conduct to the ventricles always do so with a constant PR interval. However, when the conduction system is suddenly and unexpectedly refractory and fails to conduct one or more sinus impulses, the result is dropped beats (P waves that are not followed by a QRS complex). Therefore, Mobitz type II block differs from Wenckebach block in that the PR intervals of conducted beats are constant (the most characteristic feature of this rhythm). Impulses may be blocked intermittently, making the ventricular rhythm irregular. Alternatively, the impulses may be blocked at regular intervals, such as in 2:1 block, in which case the ventricular rhythm is regular. The block is actually subjunctional, occurring below the bundle of His, involving a constant block in one of the bundle branches. The result is wide QRS complexes in conducted beats and an intermittent block in the other bundle branch. Thus, both branches are occasionally blocked and a QRS complex fails to occur (dropped beat) (see Fig. 33–25*C*).

Electrocardiographic Criteria

Rhythm: The atrial rhythm is regular. The ventricular rhythm may be regular or irregular, depending on the block.

Rate: The atrial rate depends on the underlying sinus rhythm; it may be normal or slightly fast. The ventricular rate is less than the atrial rate owing to dropped beats; this rate may be slow.

P waves: P waves are normal, with a constant morphologic pattern. One or more P waves are not conducted to ventricles.

PR interval: Constant in conducted beats

QRS duration: Usually wide, indicating that the block is subjunctional, with missing QRS complexes because of intermittent block of the other bundle

Etiology Second-degree AV block type II is less common than type I. It may occur with anterior myocardial infarctions and results from severe ischemic damage to the conduction system. It may also be caused by rheumatic heart disease or degenerative disease of the conduction system. It is a serious block that may progress suddenly to a third-degree AV block (complete heart block) and an ominous prognosis.

Physical Assessment/Clinical Manifestations Symptoms depend on the frequency of dropped beats and the overall ventricular rate. If the cardiac output is inadequate, the client presents with a symptomatic bradydysrhythmia. This rhythm may abruptly progress to a third-degree AV block.

Interventions In the asymptomatic client, the nurse assists the physician to initiate prophylactic pacing to avert the threat of sudden third-degree AV block. If slow ventricular rates are present, the nurse administers oxygen and atropine as prescribed. Atropine is usually ineffective because it does not reverse the subjunctional block. An isoproterenol (Isuprel) infusion may be administered with caution but may be dangerous. It is contraindicated in clients with myocardial infarction. Noninvasive or invasive pacing is preferred.

THIRD-DEGREE ATRIOVENTRICULAR BLOCK (COMPLETE HEART BLOCK)

Pathophysiology In third-degree AV block, none of the sinus impulses conduct to the ventricles. The SA node is usually the pacemaker for the atria, producing P waves at a normal or even accelerated rate. A separate, independent pacemaker paces the ventricles. Thus, AV dissociation exists. If the block is in the AV node, a junctional escape focus paces the ventricles, producing normal QRS complexes at a rate of 40 to 60 beats per minute (Fig. 33–26*A*). If the block is below the bundle of His (subjunctional), a ventricular escape focus paces the ventricles, producing wide QRS complexes at a rate less than 40 beats per minute (see Fig. 33–26*B*). In either case, the atrial and ventricular rhythms are both regular, but independent of each other, with more P waves than QRS complexes.

Because the P waves and the QRS complexes are totally independent of each other and bear no relationship to each other, the PR interval is inconstant, which is the most characteristic feature of this rhythm. The ventricular escape pacemaker is the least stable, least dependable pacemaker. It may abruptly fail, causing ventricular asystole, or it may predispose to irritability in the form of premature ventricular complexes (PVCs), ventricular tachycardia (VT), or ventricular fibrillation (VF).

Electrocardiographic Criteria

Rhythm: Atrial and ventricular rhythms are regular, but independent of each other owing to AV dissociation.

Rate: The atrial rate depends on the underlying sinus rhythm; it may be normal or slightly fast. If paced by a junctional escape rhythm, the ventricular rate is 40 to 60 beats per minute. If paced by a ventricular escape rhythm, the ventricular rate is usually less than 40 beats per minute.

P waves: Normal, constant morphologic pattern, but not related to QRS complexes (AV dissociation); more P waves than QRS complexes

PR interval: Inconstant, because of AV dissociation

QRS duration: With a junctional escape pacemaker, QRS complexes are normal and constant. With a ventricular escape pacemaker, the QRS complex is wide (greater than 0.14 second) and constant.

Etiology Third-degree AV block may be due to ischemic injury from coronary artery disease or myocardial infarction or to cardiac surgery, congenital heart disease, the effects of drugs, electrolyte disturbances, degenerative disease of the conduction system, digitalis toxicity, or calcific aortic stenosis.

Physical Assessment/Clinical Manifestations Clinical manifestations depend on the overall ventricular rate and cardiac output. Third-degree AV block may be well tolerated or may have serious hemodynamic consequences, particularly when the block is subjunctional. If cerebral perfusion is inadequate, clients may be confused and lightheaded or may experience episodes of syncope with or without seizures (Stokes-Adams attacks). Inadequate cardiac output may cause myocardial ischemia or infarction, heart failure, and hypotension. Third-degree AV block may predispose to cardiac arrest, causing VT, VF, or asystole. It is, therefore, regarded as a dangerous rhythm.

Interventions Third-degree AV block with a junctional escape pacemaker is often well tolerated and may require no treatment, particularly if it is transient. If the client is symptomatic, or in third-degree AV block with a ventricular escape pacemaker, the nurse assists the physician to initiate prophylactic pacing to avert the threat of cardiac arrest. Before pacemaker insertion, the nurse administers oxygen and atropine as prescribed, particularly if QRS complexes are narrow, to speed AV nodal conduction and heart rate. Atropine is usually not successful in subjunctional blocks with wide QRS complexes. Cautious use of isoproterenol (Isuprel) infusions may be necessary but is contraindicated in clients with acute myocardial infarction. Noninvasive or invasive pacing is preferred.

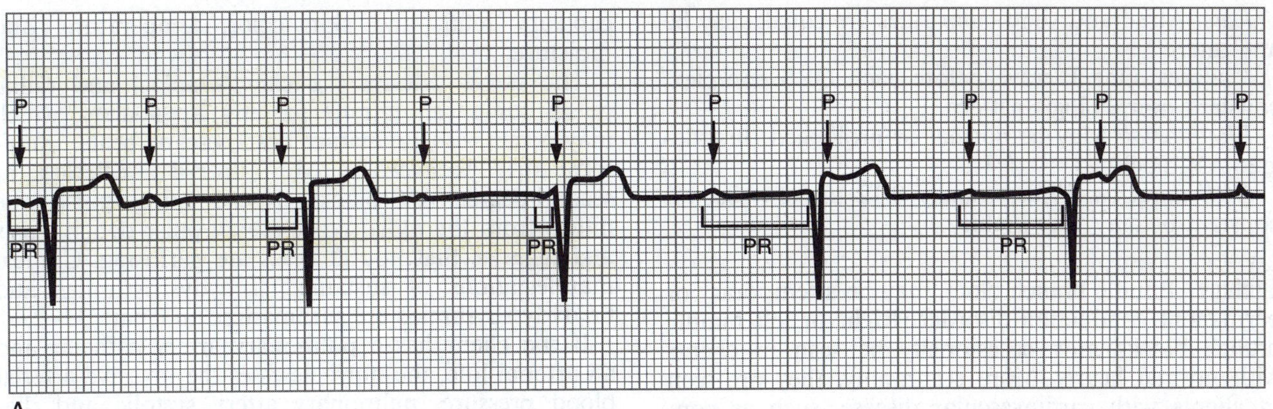

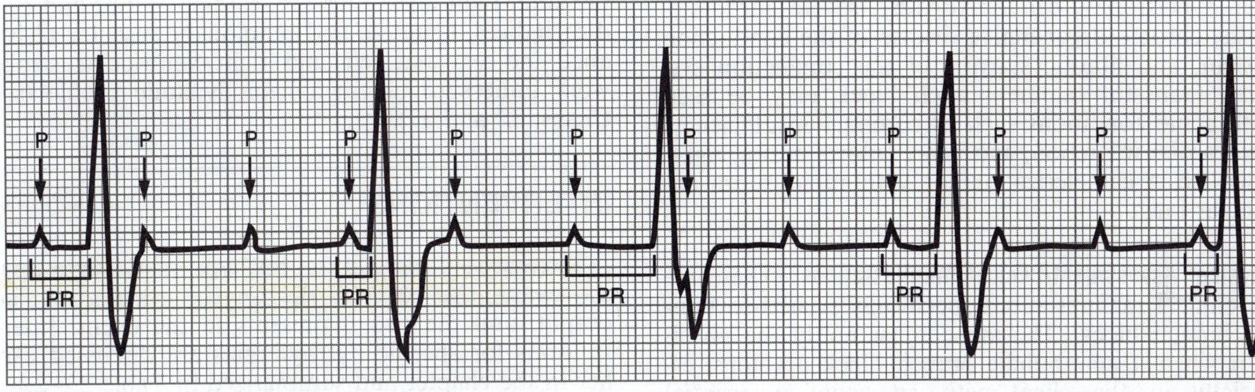

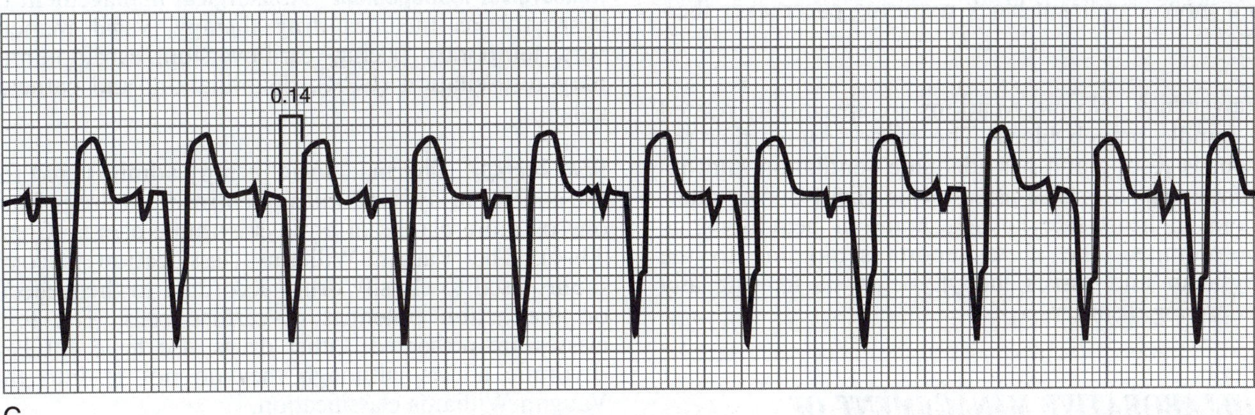

FIGURE 33–26 ◆ AV blocks. *A*, Third-degree AV block (complete heart block) with regular atrial and ventricular rhythms, inconstant PR intervals (AV dissociation), and a junctional escape focus (normal QRS complexes) pacing the ventricles at a rate of 38/minute. *B*, Third-degree AV block with regular atrial and ventricular rhythms, inconstant PR intervals (AV dissociation), and a ventricular escape focus pacing the ventricles at a rate of 35/minute, with wide QRS complexes. *C*, Normal sinus rhythm (NSR) with bundle branch block (wide QRS complexes measuring 0.14 second).

BUNDLE BRANCH BLOCKS

Pathophysiology Bundle branch block is a conduction delay or block within one of the two main bundle branches, below the bifurcation of the bundle of His. Because the block affects only one branch, it is called a monofascicular block. When one bundle branch is blocked, the supraventricular impulse is able to descend only down the normal bundle branch and to depolarize that ventricle. The other ventricle is depolarized afterward, as the wave of depolarization from the first ventricle proceeds from cell to cell to the other ventricle. Such slow depolarization prolongs the QRS duration to 0.12 second or longer. The underlying rhythm is usually sinus in origin (e.g., sinus rhythm with bundle branch block) (see Fig. 33–26*C*).

Electrocardiographic Criteria

Rhythm: Atrial and ventricular rhythms are usually regular.

Rate: Atrial and ventricular rates are equal; may be any rate.

P waves: One P wave before each QRS complex, constant morphologic pattern

PR interval: May be normal or prolonged (first-degree AV block)

QRS duration: Wide, usually 0.12 to 0.14 second, constant or may vary slightly

Etiology Bundle branch block may be a temporary or permanent conduction disorder. Right or left bundle branch blocks may occasionally be seen in clients with normal hearts. More commonly, they are seen in clients with cardiovascular disease, such as congenital heart disease, rheumatic heart disease, ventricular hypertrophy, cardiomyopathy, severe aortic stenosis, chronic degenerative disease of the conduction system, and fibrotic scarring of the conduction system. Transient bundle branch block may be seen with acute conditions such as coronary insufficiency, myocardial infarction, and heart failure; during right-sided heart catheterization; or with rapid supraventricular rates.

Physical Assessment/Clinical Manifestations There are no clinical manifestations specifically related to bundle branch block. The nurse must notify the physician when a new bundle branch block develops, especially in the client with an acute myocardial infarction. The conduction disorder may deteriorate to a more significant block requiring pacemaker therapy.

Interventions No interventions are specifically related to bundle branch block. The nurse ensures that the client is resting and has adequate ventilation and oxygenation. The nurse assesses the client during alterations in heart rate for symptoms of hemodynamic compromise. The nurse reports symptoms to the physician and assists the physician in treating any underlying disorder.

COLLABORATIVE MANAGEMENT OF DYSRHYTHMIAS

ASSESSMENT

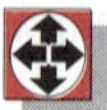

Dysrhythmias may be benign, serious, life-threatening, or lethal. The nurse must identify the client who is at risk for serious consequences from dysrhythmias.

Regardless of the type of dysrhythmia, the most important nursing assessment is the effect of the dysrhythmia on ventricular function and cardiac output. An adequate cardiac output is essential for perfusion of all body systems. The nurse assesses the client's heart rate and rhythm, blood pressure, level of consciousness, heart sounds, respiratory rate, work of breathing, breath sounds, neck veins, urinary output, capillary refill, and skin color, temperature, and moisture.

The nurse assesses the client's apical and radial pulses for a full minute for any irregularity, which may occur with premature beats, escape beats, multifocal atrial tachycardia (MAT), atrial fibrillation, or second-degree AV blocks. If the apical pulse rate differs from the radial pulse rate, a pulse deficit exists and suggests that not all beats are perfusing. Clinical manifestations of sustained tachydysrhythmias and bradydysrhythmias are summarized in Chart 33–2.

If the client has a pulmonary artery catheter and an arterial line, the nurse assesses the invasive arterial blood pressure, pulmonary artery systolic and diastolic pressures, pulmonary artery occlusive (wedge) pressure, right atrial pressure, cardiac output and cardiac indices, systemic and pulmonary vascular resistance indices, and left and right ventricular stroke work indices to obtain a hemodynamic profile (see Chaps. 32 and 37).

INTERVENTIONS

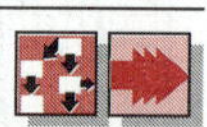

Treatment is specific to the type of dysrhythmia, the cause, the effect it has on the client's cardiac output, and the risk it presents to the client. Interventions for specific dysrhythmias are discussed earlier in the chapter and summarized in Table 33–2.

Nonsurgical Management Nonsurgical management of dysrhythmias includes drug therapy, vagal maneuvers, temporary pacing, cardioversion, cardiopulmonary resuscitation (CPR), defibrillation, and catheter ablation.

Drug Therapy Pharmacologic therapy administered for the control of dysrhythmias often includes drugs from one or more classes of antidysrhythmic agents (Chart 33–4). The Vaughn-Williams classification is commonly used to classify drugs according to their effects on the action potential of cardiac cells. The four classes are presented. Other drugs also have antidysrhythmic effects, although they do not fit into the Vaughn-Williams classification.

VAUGHN-WILLIAMS CLASSIFICATION Class I antidysrhythmics are membrane-stabilizing agents, stabilizing phase 4 to decrease automaticity. They depress the rate of depolarization by impeding the flow of sodium into the cell during phase 0. There are three subclassifications in this group. Type IA drugs moderately slow conduction and prolong repolarization, prolonging the QT interval. These drugs are used to treat or to prevent supraventricular and ventricular premature beats and tachydysrhythmias. Examples include quinidine sulfate and procainamide hydrochloride (Pronestyl). Type IB drugs shorten repolarization. These drugs are used to treat or prevent ventricular premature beats, ventricular tachycardia (VT), and ventricular fibrillation (VF). Examples include lidocaine and mexiletine hydrochloride (Mexi-

Text continued on page 864

CHART 33–4

Drug Therapy for Dysrhythmias

Drug	Usual Dosage	Nursing Interventions	Rationale
Class I Drugs			
Type IA			
Quinidine sulfate (Quinidine, Apo-Quinidine✱)	• 300–600 mg q8–12h PO • 6–10 mg/kg IV slowly, may be given IM	• Monitor blood pressure. • Watch for diarrhea, nausea, or vomiting and administer with food if these occur. • Monitor for widening QRS complex, prolonged QT interval, heart block, and onset or increase in number of PVCs.	• Hypotension is a common side effect. • Diarrhea is common during early therapy. Diarrhea and other gastrointestinal symptoms often decrease when quinidine is administered with food. • Toxic side effects necessitate stopping quinidine administration.
Procainamide hydrochloride (Pronestyl)	• 50 mg/kg/day PO in 4 divided doses • 20–30 mg IV, not to exceed 17 mg/kg, followed by infusion of 1–4 mg/min	• Monitor blood pressure. • Monitor for widening QRS complex, prolonged QT or PR interval, or heart block.	• Hypotension warrants drug discontinuation. • Toxic side effects necessitate stopping procainamide administration.
Disopyramide phosphate (Norpace)	• 100–200 mg q6h PO	• Monitor blood pressure. • Watch for shortness of breath and weight gain. • Monitor for widening QRS complex, prolonged QT or PR interval, or heart block	• Hypotension is a common side effect. • Disopyramide can cause heart failure in a client with CAD. • Toxic side effects necessitate stopping disopyramide administration.
Type IB			
Lidocaine (Xylocaine)	• 1–1.5 mg/kg IV bolus, then 0.5–0.75 mg/kg IV boluses q5–10min to a loading dose of 3 mg/kg, followed by 2–4 mg/min infusion • For VF or pulseless VT: 1–1.5 mg/kg IV bolus q3–5 min to a loading dose of 3 mg/kg, followed by 2–4 mg/min infusion	• Watch for confusion, paresthesias, slurring of speech, drowsiness, or seizure activity.	• CNS adverse effects predominate; they may require a decrease in dosage or discontinuation of the infusion.
Mexiletine hydrochloride (Mexitil)	• 200–300 mg q8h PO with food • 125–250 mg IV bolus for 5–10 min • 0.5–1.5 mg/min infusion	• Monitor blood pressure and heart rate. • Assess for tremors, blurred vision, dizziness, ataxia, or confusion.	• Hypotension and bradycardia may occur. • CNS adverse reactions predominate.
Tocainide hydrochloride (Tonocard)	• 400 mg q8h PO initially • 400–800 mg q8h PO • Maximum of 2.4 g/day • Take with food.	• Watch for tremors. • Monitor heart rate and blood pressure.	• Tremors indicate that the maximum dose is being approached. • Bradycardia and hypotension may occur.

Chart continued on following page

CHART 33–4

Drug Therapy for Dysrhythmias *Continued*

Drug	Usual Dosage	Nursing Interventions	Rationale
		• Teach the client to report shortness of breath, wheezing, chest pain, or cough, as well as dyspnea and distended neck veins or swelling of the extremities.	• Pulmonary fibrosis is a serious side effect, which necessitates discontinuation of the drug; the drug also may cause CHF.
Type IC			
Flecainide acetate (Tambocor)	• 100 mg bid PO • Maximum dose of 400 mg/day	• Monitor for an increase in frequency and severity of dysrhythmias. • Monitor heart rate and blood pressure. • Monitor for CHF, dizziness, visual disturbances, paresthesias, and tremors.	• Flecainide can induce dysrhythmias. • Bradycardia and hypotension may occur. • Side effects may require a decrease in dosage or discontinuation of the drug.
Propafenone hydrochloride (Rythmol)	• 150–300 mg q8h PO	• Monitor for an increase in dysrhythmias. • Monitor heart rate and blood pressure. • Monitor for CNS effects, dizziness, anxiety, ataxia, insomnia, confusion, and seizures, as well as CHF and gastrointestinal distress.	• Propafenone can induce dysrhythemias. • Bradycardia and hypotension may occur. • Side effects may require a decrease in dosage or discontinuation of the drug.
Moricizine hydrochloride (Ethmozine)	• 200–300 mg q8h PO	• Monitor for an increase in dysrhythmias. • Monitor heart rate and blood pressure. • Monitor for dizziness, hyperesthesias, anxiety, ataxia, insomnia, confusion, and seizures.	• Drug can induce dysrhythmias. • Bradycardia and hypotension may occur. • Side effects may require a decrease in dosage or discontinuation of the drug.
Class II Drugs			
Propranolol hydrochloride (Inderal, Apo-Propranolol✱)	• 10–80 mg qid PO before meals • 0.1 mg/kg slow IV bolus divided in 3 equal doses given at 2–3 min intervals, at rate of 1 mg/min	• Monitor heart rate and blood pressure. • Assess for shortness of breath or wheezing. • Assess for insomnia, fatigue, and dizziness.	• Bradycardia and decreased blood pressure are expected effects. • $Beta_2$-blocking effects on the lungs can cause bronchospasm. • Side effects may require decrease in dosage or discontinuation of the drug.
Acebutolol hydrochloride (Sectral)	• 600–1200 mg daily PO	• Monitor heart rate and blood pressure. • Assess for shortness of breath or wheezing. • Assess for insomnia, fatigue, and dizziness.	• Bradycardia and decreased blood pressure are expected effects. • $Beta_2$-blocking effects on the lungs can cause bronchospasm. • Side effects may require a decrease in dosage or discontinuation of the drug.
Esmolol hydrochloride (Brevibloc)	• Initially, 500 μg/kg/min for 1 min, then 50 μg/kg/min for 4 min IV	• Monitor heart rate and blood pressure.	• Bradycardia and decreased blood pressure are expected effects.

CHART 33-4

Drug Therapy for Dysrhythmia *Continued*

Drug	Usual Dosage	Nursing Interventions	Rationale
	• Titrate up, if necessary.	• Assess for shortness of breath or wheezing.	• $Beta_2$-blocking effects on the lungs can cause bronchospasm.
		• Assess for insomnia, fatigue, and seizures.	• Side effects may require a decrease in dosage or discontinuation of the drug.
Sotalol hydrochloride (Betapace)	• Initial dose of 80 mg PO bid • Dosage may be increased every 2–3 days to 240–320 mg/day in 2–3 divided doses, if necessary	• Assess ECG rhythm for torsades de pointes and other serious new ventricular dysrhythmias.	• Sotalol may have proarrhythmic effects.
		• Assess for fatigue, bradycardia, dyspnea, CHF, chest pain, hypotension, dizziness, hypoglycemia, nausea, and vomiting.	• Adverse reactions may warrant drug discontinuation.
		• Sotalol should not be administered to clients with hypokalemia or hypomagnesemia before correction of these imbalances.	• Hypokalemia or hypomagnesemia may prolong the QT interval and cause torsades de pointes.
		• Sotalol is contraindicated in clients with bronchial asthma, sinus bradycardia, or second- and third-degree AV block (unless a functioning pacemaker is present), prolonged QT syndrome, cardiogenic shock, and CHF.	• Sotalol has beta-blocking (class II) effects and class III effects.
Class III Drugs			
Bretylium tosylate (Bretylol, Bretylate✱)	• 5–10 mg/kg, diluted in 50 mL IV, for 8–10 min, may repeat in 1–2 hr; maximum of 30–35 mg/kg • 1–2 mg/min infusion • For VF or pulseless VT: 5 mg/kg IV undiluted, IV bolus, followed by defibrillation; may give 10 mg/kg IV bolus, followed by defibrillation, and repeat q5min to maximum of 30–35 mg/kg	• Observe cardiac monitor for PVCs, increased heart rate, and other dysrhythmias.	• PVCs and increased heart rate commonly occur within 30 min.
		• Monitor blood pressure.	• Hypertension may occur in the first hour, followed by significant hypotension.
		• Maintain the client in a supine position for up to 8 hr.	• Orthostatic hypotension is a significant problem until tolerance to the drug develops.
		• When the client begins to sit up or get out of bed, raise the head of the bed slowly and advise the client to make position changes slowly.	• The client could become dizzy and faint.
		• Anticipate vomiting during drug administration. Except in cardiac arrest, the drug must be diluted and given slowly.	• Vomiting is a common side effect.

Chart continued on following page

CHART 33-4

Drug Therapy for Dysrhythmias *Continued*

Drug	Usual Dosage	Nursing Interventions	Rationale
Amiodarone hydrochloride (Cordarone)	• 800–1600 mg qd PO in divided doses for 1–3 wk, then 600–800 mg qd for 1 mo, then 200–600 mg qd (average of 400 mg qd)	• Assess the client's knowledge of the treatment regimen and side effects.	• Drug has major side effects, which make noncompliance a problem; clients may take the drug for 1½–3 mo before full clinical effects are apparent.
		• Monitor heart rate, blood pressure, and cardiac rhythm when initiating therapy.	• Bradycardia, hypotension, and worsening dysrhythmia can occur.
		• Teach clients to report any muscle weakness, tremors, or difficulty with ambulation.	• Muscle-related side effects usually develop during the first week of treatment.
		• Teach clients to report shortness of breath, cough, pleuritic pain, or fever.	• Pulmonary side effects may indicate drug-induced pulmonary toxicity.
		• Teach clients to report any visual disturbances and to wear sunglasses outdoors in the daytime if they have photophobia.	• Corneal pigmentation occurs in most clients but generally does not interfere with vision; if it does, the dosage is decreased.
		• Teach clients to use barrier sunscreens.	• Photosensitivity reactions may occur.
		• Teach clients to report any signs of thyroid problems or hepatotoxicity.	• Thyroid problems or hepatotoxicity may occur, necessitating a decrease in dosage or discontinuation of the drug.
Class IV Drugs			
Verapamil hydrochloride (Calan, Isoptin✱)	• 2.5–5 mg IV, for 1–2 min for narrow-complex SVT or PSVT; after 15–30 min may give 5–10 mg IV for 1–2 min if necessary, and repeat to a maximum of 20 mg • 80–120 mg q6–8h PO	• Monitor heart rate and blood pressure.	• Bradycardia and hypotension are common side effects.
		• Teach clients to remain recumbent for at least 1 hr after IV administration.	• Hypotension may occur; may be reversed with calcium chloride ($CaCl_2$), 0.5–1 g slow IV.
		• Teach clients to change positions slowly when receiving oral therapy.	• Dizziness and orthostatic hypotension often occur until tolerance develops.
		• Teach clients to report dyspnea, orthopnea, distended neck veins, or swelling of the extremities.	• Heart failure may occur, necessitating a decrease in dosage or discontinuation of the drug.
Diltiazem hydrochloride (Cardizem)	• 0.25 mg/kg IV for 2 min • After 15 min, give 0.35 mg/kg IV for 2 min • 5–15 mg/hr IV infusion	• Monitor heart rate and blood pressure.	• Bradycardia and hypotension are common side effects.
		• Teach clients to remain recumbent for at least 1 hr after IV administration.	• Hypotension may occur.
		• Teach clients to report dyspnea, orthopnea, distended neck veins, or swelling of the extremities.	• Heart failure may occur, necessitating a decrease in dosage or discontinuation of the drug.

CHART 33-4

Drug Therapy for Dysrhythmias *Continued*

Drug	Usual Dosage	Nursing Interventions	Rationale
Other Drugs			
Digoxin (Lanoxin, Novodigoxin✱)	• Rapid digitalization: 0.5–1 mg PO or IV initially; 0.125–0.5 mg PO or IV q6h until a total of 1–1.5 mg is reached	• Assess apical heart rate for 1 min before each dose; withhold the dose if the heart rate is less than 60 beats per min.	• Decreased heart rate is an expected response, but bradycardia may indicate toxicity.
	• Maintenance: 0.125–0.25 mg qd or qod PO or IV (may be less for elderly)	• Assess for sudden increase of heart rate and change of rhythm from regular to irregular, or irregular to regular.	• Changes in heart rate or rhythm may indicate toxicity.
		• Teach clients to report anorexia, nausea, vomiting, diarrhea, paresthesias, confusion, or visual disturbances.	• Side effect can indicate toxicity.
		• Monitor serum potassium levels.	• Hypokalemia increases the risk of toxicity and ventricular dysrhythmias.
		• Monitor serum creatinine levels.	• Impaired renal function can cause toxicity; the dosage is altered if this occurs.
Atropine sulfate	• 0.5–1 mg IV bolus may be repeated q3–5min, if necessary, to a maximum of 0.04 mg/kg	• Monitor heart rate and rhythm after administration.	• Increased heart rate is expected.
	• For asystole, PEA, or EMD: 1 mg IV bolus q3–5min to a total of 0.04 mg/kg, if necessary	• Assess for chest pain after administration.	• Increased heart rate may cause ischemia in client with CAD.
		• Assess for urinary retention and dry mouth after administration.	• Atropine is an anticholinergic agent.
		• Avoid using in clients with angle-closure glaucoma.	• Atropine increases intraocular pressure.
Adenosine (Adenocard)	• 6 mg IV for 1–3 sec followed by 20-mL saline flush; may repeat in 1–2 min, if necessary, at 12 mg IV for 1–3 sec with 20-mL flush; may repeat 12 mg IV after 1–2 min, if necessary	• Monitor heart rate and rhythm after administration.	• A short period of asystole is common after administration; bradycardia and hypotension may occur.
		• Assess clients for facial flushing, shortness of breath, dyspnea, and chest pain.	• These side effects commonly occur.
		• Assess clients for recurrence of PSVT or ventricular ectopy.	• Recurrence of PSVT is common; PVCs may occur.
Magnesium sulfate	• 1–2 g diluted in 100 mL of D_5W administered for 1 to 2 min for VF or VT	• Assess ECG rhythm for conversion to sinus rhythm.	• Hypomagnesemia may precipitate refractory VF.
	• 1–2 g in 50–100 mL of D_5W for 5–60 min for loading dose; 0.5–1 g/hr for 24 hr for supplementation	• Assess clients for facial flushing, hypotension, and respiratory and CNS depression.	• Magnesium sulfate causes vasodilation and respiratory and CNS depression.

VF, ventricular fibrillation; VT, ventricular tachycardia; SVT, supraventricular tachycardia; PSVT, premature supraventricular tachycardia; PEA, pulseless electrical activity; EMD, electromechanical dissociation; PVC, premature ventricular contraction; CHF, congestive heart failure; CNS, central nervous system; CAD, coronary artery disease.

til). Type IC drugs markedly slow conduction and widen the QRS complex. These drugs are used primarily to treat or to prevent ventricular premature beats, VT, and VF. Examples include flecainide acetate (Tambocor) and propafenone hydrochloride (Rythmol).

Class II antidysrhythmics control dysrhythmias associated with excessive beta-adrenergic stimulation by competing for receptor sites and thereby decreasing heart rate and conduction velocity. Beta-adrenergic blocking agents, such as propranolol hydrochloride (Inderal) and esmolol hydrochloride (Brevibloc), are class II drugs. They are used to treat or to prevent supraventricular and ventricular premature beats and tachydysrhythmias. Sotalol hydrochloride (Betapace) is an antidysrhythmic agent with both noncardioselective beta-adrenergic blocking effects (class II) and action potential duration prolongation properties (class III). It is an oral agent recommended for the treatment of documented ventricular dysrhythmias, such as VT, that are life-threatening.

Class III antidysrhythmics lengthen the absolute refractory period and prolong repolarization and the action potential duration of ischemic cells. They decrease the disparity with normal cells to prevent a re-entry response. Class III drugs include bretylium tosylate (Bretylol, Bretylate✱) and amiodarone hydrochloride (Cordarone) and are used to treat or prevent ventricular premature beats, VT, and VF.

Class IV antidysrhythmics impede the flow of calcium into the cell during depolarization, thereby depressing automaticity of the sinoatrial (SA) and atrioventricular (AV) nodes, decreasing heart rate and prolonging AV nodal refractoriness and conduction. Calcium channel blockers, such as verapamil hydrochloride (Calan, Isoptin✱) and diltiazem hydrochloride (Cardizem), are class IV drugs. They are used to treat paroxysmal supraventricular tachycardia (PSVT) and AV nodal re-entry tachydysrhythmias, atrial flutter, and atrial fibrillation to slow down the ventricular response.

OTHER ANTIDYSRHYTHMIC DRUGS Other drugs, such as digoxin, atropine, adenosine, and magnesium sulfate, are frequently used to treat dysrhythmias. Digoxin increases vagal tone, slowing AV nodal conduction. It is useful in treating supraventricular tachydysrhythmias, particularly chronic atrial fibrillation, by controlling the rate of ventricular response. Atropine is a parasympatholytic or vagolytic agent. It is used to treat vagally induced symptomatic bradydysrhythmias. Adenosine is an endogenous nucleoside that slows AV nodal conduction to interrupt re-entry pathways. It is effective in terminating PSVT, a reentrant tachydysrhythmia. Magnesium sulfate is an electrolyte that is currently recommended to treat refractory VT or VF, because these clients may be hypomagnesemic, which causes ventricular irritability.

EMERGENCY CARDIAC DRUGS In addition to antidysrhythmics, several other drugs are used during cardiac arrest (Chart 33–5). Epinephrine (Adrenalin) is a first-line agent in all cardiac arrests. It is given predominantly for its alpha-adrenergic effects to increase vasomotor tone for myocardial and cerebral perfusion. Its beta-adrenergic effects may stimulate the heart and increase myocardial contractility to improve cardiac output. Dopamine hydrochloride (Intropin) is generally used for its beta-adrenergic effects after cardiac arrest but may be used for its alpha-adrenergic effects during resuscitation. Dobutamine hydrochloride (Dobutrex) is a beta-adrenergic agent used to improve myocardial contractility and increase cardiac output.

Norepinephrine may be used, if necessary, for its alpha-adrenergic effects to increase vasomotor tone and increase perfusion pressure. Sodium bicarbonate must be used only for treatment of metabolic acidosis, if necessary, based on arterial blood gas determinations. Improved chest compressions and hyperventilation with oxygen are preferred. Isoproterenol (Isuprel) is a beta-adrenergic agent that is rarely used to increase heart rate in an atropine-refractory, symptomatic bradydysrhythmia. Pacing is preferred. Calcium chloride, which increases myocardial contractility, is also rarely indicated. It is reserved for clients with hyperkalemia, hypocalcemia, or calcium channel–blocker toxicity, because it may cause cell damage and cerebrovascular vasospasm.

Vagal Maneuvers Vagal maneuvers induce vagal stimulation of the cardiac conduction system, specifically the SA and AV nodes. Vagal maneuvers are used to terminate supraventricular tachydysrhythmias. They include carotid sinus massage and Valsalva maneuvers.

CAROTID SINUS MASSAGE The physician massages over the carotid artery briefly, not to exceed 6 to 8 seconds, until there is a change in cardiac rhythm (Eagle et al., 1989). When stretch receptors within the carotid sinus are stimulated, the heart rate and blood pressure decrease via vagal stimulation. The nurse prepares the client for this procedure, instructs the client to turn the head slightly away from the side to be massaged, and observes the cardiac monitor for a change in rhythm. The nurse records an electrocardiographic (ECG) rhythm strip before, during, and after the procedure. After the procedure, the nurse assesses the client's vital signs and level of consciousness. Complications include bradydysrhythmias, asystole, ventricular fibrillation, and cerebral damage. This procedure is contraindicated in clients with cerebral arteriosclerosis and carotid bruits. A defibrillator and resuscitative equipment must be immediately available during the procedure.

VALSALVA MANEUVERS The physician instructs the client to bear down as if straining to have a bowel movement or induces the gag reflex in the client, both of which stimulate a vagal reflex (Eagle et al., 1989). The nurse prepares the client for the procedure; assesses the client's heart rate, heart rhythm, and blood pressure; observes the cardiac monitor;

CHART 33-5

Drug Therapy for Cardiac Arrest

Drug	Usual Dosage	Nursing Interventions	Rationale
Epinephrine (Adrenalin)	• 1-mg IV bolus followed by 20-mL saline flush q3–5min • If this fails, may consider: 2–5 mg IV bolus q3–5 min; 1-mg, 3-mg, and 5-mg IV bolus (3 min apart); or 0.1 mg/kg IV bolus q3–5 min • If necessary, may give endotracheally with dose at least 2–2½ times IV dose	• Monitor for return of rhythm and pulse when used for asystole or VF. • Assess for tachycardia, dysrhythmias, or hypertension. • Assess for the development of coarse VF when given during fine VF.	• Return of rhythm and pulse is the expected response. • Adverse reactions can occur with a dramatic response. • This may improve the response to defibrillation.
Dopamine hydrochloride (Intropin)	• 2.5–5 μg/kg/min IV infusion; titrate to desired clinical response • 1–2 μg/kg/min for renal and mesenteric vasodilation • 2–10 μg/kg/min for beta-adrenergic effects • 10–20 μg/kg/min for alpha-adrenergic effects	• Assess clients for increased blood pressure. • Monitor for tachycardia, dysrhythmias, or hypertension. • Monitor the IV site for infiltration. • Assess for urinary output <30 mL/hr, or pallor, cyanosis, pain, or numbness in the extremities.	• Increased blood pressure is the expected response. • Adverse reactions may occur. • Extravasation of drug can occur, causing necrosis. • Dosages >10 μg/kg/min cause vasoconstriction of renal and peripheral blood vessels; dosages of 2–5 μg/kg/min may improve urinary output by causing renal vasodilation and improving renal blood flow.
Dobutamine hydrochloride (Dobutrex)	• 2–20 μg/kg/min IV infusion	• Assess for increased blood pressure. • Assess for hypertension and dysrhythmias.	• Increased blood pressure is the expected response. • Adverse reactions may occur.
Norepinephrine (Levophed)	• 0.5–1 μg/min IV infusion, titrate to desired effect, up to 8–30 μg/min	• Assess for increased blood pressure. • Monitor for bradycardia. • Monitor for hypertension and dysrhythmias. • Monitor the IV site for infiltration. • Assess for urinary output <30 mL/hr or pallor, cyanosis, pain, or numbness in the extremities. • Assess for chest pain after resuscitation.	• Increased blood pressure is the expected response. • Reflex bradycardia may occur with a rise in blood pressure. • Adverse reactions may occur with a dramatic response. • Extravasation can occur, which necessitates immediate treatment with phentolamine injected at the site. • Norepinephrine is a powerful vasoconstrictor. • Norepinephrine increases myocardial oxygen demand.
Sodium bicarbonate	• 1 mEq/kg IV bolus given after the first 10 min of cardiac arrest if necessary • 0.5 mEq/kg IV bolus q10min thereafter, if necessary	• Assess arterial blood gas values for metabolic acidosis.	• Administration without evidence of metabolic acidosis can result in alkalosis, which can hinder resuscitation efforts.

Chart continued on following page

CHART 33–5

Drug Therapy for Cardiac Arrest *Continued*

Drug	Usual Dosage	Nursing Interventions	Rationale
Isoproterenol (Isuprel)	• 2–10 μg/min IV infusion; titrate to desired clinical response	• Assess for increased heart rate.	• Increased heart rate is the expected response.
		• Assess for tachycardia, hypotension, or hypertension.	• Adverse reactions may occur with a dramatic response.
		• Assess for chest pain after resuscitation.	• Isoproterenol increases myocardial oxygen demand.
		• Monitor for ventricular dysrhythmias.	• Isoproterenol increases ventricular irritability, especially in clients who are hypokalemic or who are receiving digitalis.
Calcium chloride ($CaCl_2$)	• 2–4 mg/kg IV slowly, may repeat, if necessary, q10min	• Calcium chloride is indicated only for cardiac arrest associated with hyperkalemia, hypocalcemia, or calcium channel blocker toxicity.	• Calcium chloride may cause cellular damage and cerebrovascular spasm.

VF, ventricular fibrillation.

and records an ECG rhythm strip before, during, and after the procedure to determine the effect of therapy. If gagging is induced, the nurse provides an emesis basin and oral hygiene if the client vomits and takes measures to prevent aspiration.

The nurse is cautious when performing procedures that may inadvertently cause vagal stimulation. For example, tracheal suctioning, enema administration, and rectal temperature checks can stimulate the vagus nerve and decrease the heart rate inappropriately. The nurse administers stool softeners, as prescribed. The nurse instructs the client not to strain to move bowels and to avoid constipation through proper diet and exercise. The client is also told to avoid inducing gagging during oral hygiene, which triggers a vagal response. The nurse assesses the heart rate and rhythm of a client who is vomiting, which may induce a vagal reflex. Some clients experience a vagal response when raising their arms above their head and must be instructed to avoid this movement.

Temporary Pacing Temporary pacing is a nonsurgical intervention that provides an electrical stimulus to the right atrial myocardium, right ventricular myocardium, or both when a stimulus does not exist, is blocked, or is firing too slowly to provide adequate cardiac output. The stimulus then spreads to the left side of the heart to complete depolarization, followed by contraction and cardiac output.

When a pacing stimulus is delivered to the heart, a spike is seen on the monitor or ECG strip. This is a straight vertical line of varying amplitude, depending on the type of pacemaker system used. The spike should be followed by evidence of depolarization. (i.e., a P wave indicating atrial depolarization or a QRS complex indicating ventricular depolarization). This is referred to as "capture," indicating that the pacemaker successfully depolarized, or captured, the chamber.

Temporary pacing is generally initiated in clients with symptomatic, atropine-refractory bradydysrhythmias, particularly second-degree AV block type II and third-degree AV block. It is also used with asystole, as may occur in clients with coronary artery disease, myocardial infarction, cardiac arrest, post–open heart surgery, vagal depression, carotid sinus syncope, cardioactive drug toxicity, sick sinus syndrome, and bradydysrhythmia induced by anesthesia or procedures using a radiopaque dye. Temporary pacing may also be initiated prophylactically in hemodynamically stable clients with left bundle branch block in certain situations:

- Before inserting a pulmonary artery catheter, which could cause a right bundle branch block, resulting in a complete heart block for the client
- Before performing other procedures that could cause bradydysrhythmias
- Before transporting a client who is at risk for a hemodynamically unstable bradydysrhythmia

A different type of pacing may be used to terminate symptomatic tachydysrhythmias. Occasionally, atrial overdrive pacing is attempted to terminate atrial tachydysrhythmias, such as atrial flutter. Overdrive pacing is accomplished by rapidly pacing the atrium to capture the heart and control depolarization, followed by no pacing, in the hope that the sinus node will regain control of the heart. Ventricular overdrive pacing may be done to terminate ventricular tachydysrhythmias in much the same way. Overdrive pacing is performed only by the physician. The nurse must have emergency equipment available in case the client becomes more unstable or goes into cardiac arrest.

MODES OF PACING There are two basic modes of pacing:

- Synchronous (demand) pacing
- Asynchronous (fixed-rate) pacing

Synchronous (Demand) Pacing. Temporary pacing is most commonly done in the demand mode. This means that the pacemaker's sensitivity is set to sense the client's own beats. When the client's intrinsic rate is above the rate set on the pulse generator, the pacemaker is inhibited from firing. When the client's rate is below that set on the generator, the pacemaker fires electrical impulses to stimulate depolarization (Fig. 33–27*A*).

Asynchronous (Fixed-Rate) Pacing. The asynchronous mode is used when the client is asystolic or profoundly bradycardiac, as may occur after open heart surgery. The pulse generator is set in an asynchronous mode, in which it does not sense any intrinsic beats of the client. The pacemaker continues to fire at a fixed rate as set on the generator, regardless of the client's intrinsic rhythm. This is not a problem as long as the client remains asystolic or has a rate slower than the pacemaker rate, because all beats come from the pacemaker and there is no competition from the client's beats (see Fig. 33–27*B*). If the client's rate increases and equals or exceeds the pacemaker rate, however, competition (undersensing) is noted. The danger is that a pacemaker stimulus may reach the heart during the vulnerable period during repolarization (such as an R-on-T phenomenon, with the pacer spike falling on the T wave) and possibly induce ventricular fibrillation. The nurse must observe for pacemaker competition and set the pacemaker to a synchronous mode to avert potential problems.

UNIVERSAL PACEMAKER CODE In 1974, the Intersociety Commission for Heart Disease established a three-position pacemaker code (ICHD code) to standardize the description of pacemaker systems (Underhill et al., 1989).

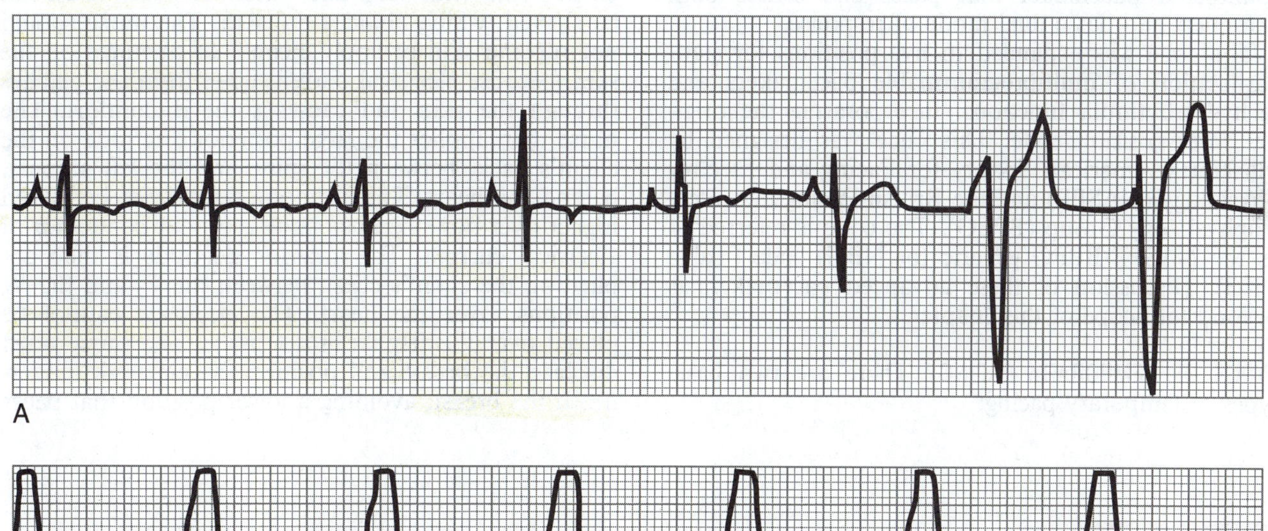

A

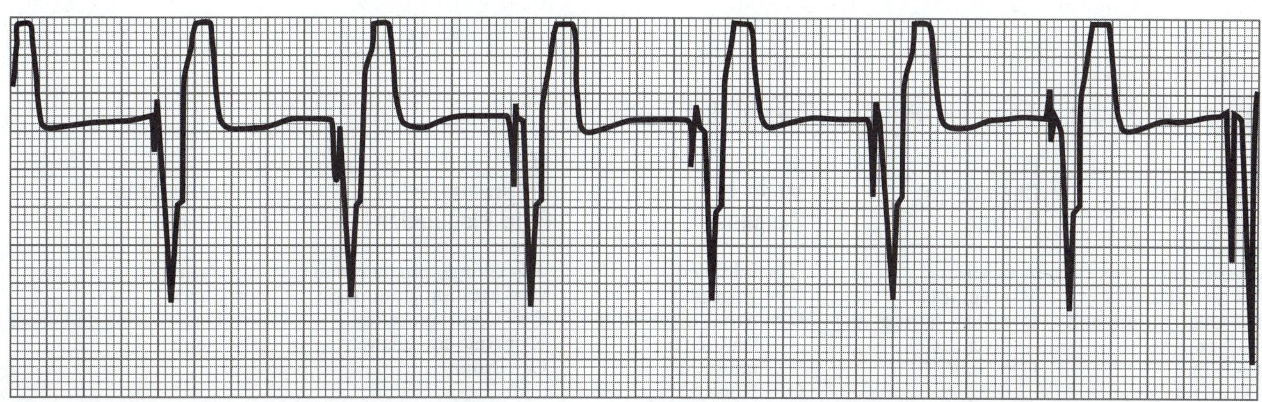

B

FIGURE 33–27 ◆ Modes of pacing. *A*, Synchronous (demand) ventricular pacing. *B*, Asynchronous (fixed-rate) ventricular pacing at a rate of 61 beats/minute.

- The first letter of the code represents the chamber being paced: "A" for atrium, "V" for ventricle, and "D" for dual (both atrium and ventricle).
- The second letter represents the chamber being sensed, using the same three letters. This indicates a demand pacing mode. If the pacemaker is asynchronous, the second letter is "O," because no chamber is sensed.
- The third letter represents the mode of response: "I" for inhibited, when the pacemaker senses an intrinsic beat and therefore does not fire; "T" for triggered, when the pacemaker senses an intrinsic beat and fires an impulse with the beat; "O" for no mode of response, when the pacemaker is asynchronous and therefore fires at a set rate; and "D" for dual mode of response, when the pacemaker can inhibit firing when it senses an impulse and can trigger when no impulse is sensed.

This code is used universally and makes it easier to identify quickly the primary functions of the pacemaker. AAI denotes an atrial demand pacemaker. AOO denotes an asynchronous atrial pacemaker. VVI denotes a ventricular demand pacemaker. VOO refers to an asynchronous ventricular pacemaker. DVI denotes a demand AV sequential pacemaker that can pace both chambers but senses only the ventricular chamber. DOO indicates an asynchronous AV sequential pacemaker. DDD denotes a demand dual-chambered pacemaker that paces and senses both chambers and has a dual mode of response.

The code was expanded to five positions for standardization of multiprogrammable pacemakers and tachydysrhythmia functions, incorporating the original three-position code. This code was designed by the North American Society for Pacing and Electrophysiology (NASPE) and the British Pacing and Electrophysiology Group (BPEG). The code is referred to as the NASPE/BPEG generic (or NBG) code (Table 33–3). Discussion of these advanced pacemakers is beyond the scope of this chapter.

TYPES OF TEMPORARY PACING There are two basic types of temporary pacing:

- Noninvasive temporary pacing
- Invasive temporary pacing

Noninvasive Temporary Pacing. Noninvasive temporary pacing (NTP) is accomplished through the application of two large patch electrodes. The electrodes are attached to an external pulse generator, which is attached to alternating current (AC) but may also be run on battery power (Fig. 33–28). The generator emits electrical pulses, which are transmitted through the cutaneous patches. It provides transcutaneous electrical current to stimulate ventricular depolarization when the client's heart rate is slower than the rate set on the pacemaker. Electrical currents of 60 milliamperes (mA) or more are usually required to achieve ventricular depolarization. The current is applied for 20 to 40 milliseconds (msec) (pulse width), producing a pacing stimulus or spike that occupies 0.02 to 0.04 second on the electrocardiographic (ECG) paper.

NTP is used as an emergency measure to provide demand ventricular pacing in a profoundly bradycardiac or asystolic client until invasive pacing can be instituted or the client's intrinsic rate returns to normal. It may be used prophylactically when performing procedures or transporting clients at risk for bradydysrhythmias.

Procedure. The nurse explains NTP to the client and prepares the equipment. The nurse washes the client's skin with soap and water. The skin must not be shaved, which abrades the skin. The nurse should not rub the skin or apply alcohol or tinctures on the skin, because electrical current flows from the patches through the skin and causes some discomfort. The nurse then applies the large posterior electrode on the client's back, between the spine and the left scapula, behind the heart. The electrode should not be placed higher over bone because bone is a poor conductor of electrical current. The anterior electrode is then applied on the client's chest, between the V_2 and the V_5 positions, over the heart. The electrode cannot be placed over the female breast tissue. The nurse must displace the breast and position the electrode underneath the breast, avoiding a lower position that paces

TABLE 33–3 The Five-Position Pacemaker Code*

I Chamber(s) Paced	II Chamber(s) Sensed	III Mode of Response	IV Programmability, Rate Modulation	V Antitachycardia Function(s)
A = Atrium	A = Atrium	I = Inhibited	P = Simple programmable	P = Pacing
V = Ventricle	V = Ventricle	T = Triggered	M = Multiprogrammable	S = Shock
D = Dual (atrium and ventricle)	D = Dual (atrium and ventricle)	D = Atrial triggered and ventricular inhibited	C = Communicating	D = Dual (pacing and shock)
O = None	O = None	O = None	R = Rate modulation	O = None
			O = None	

From Bernstein, A. D., et al. (1987). The NASPE/BPEG pacemaker code. *PACE, 10*(4), 794.

* The North American Society for Pacing and Electrophysiology (NASPE) and the British Pacing and Electrophysiology Group (BPEG) code (the NASPE/BPEG generic [NBG] code).

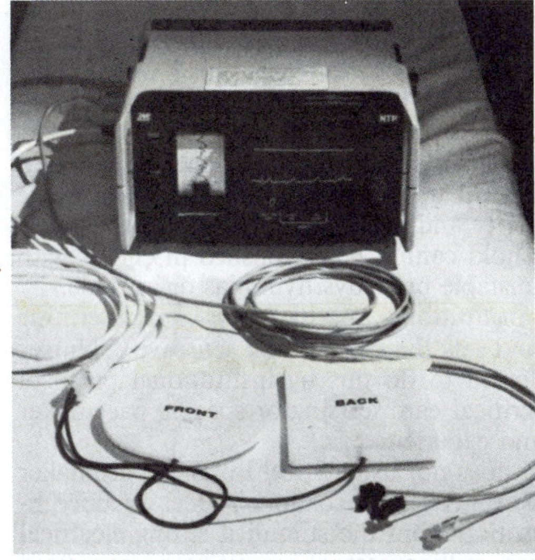

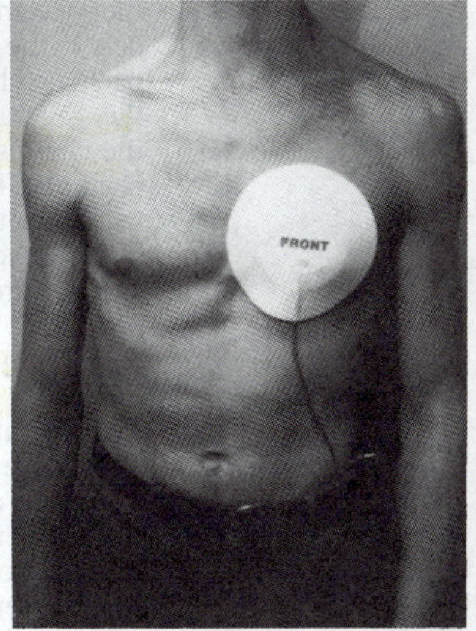

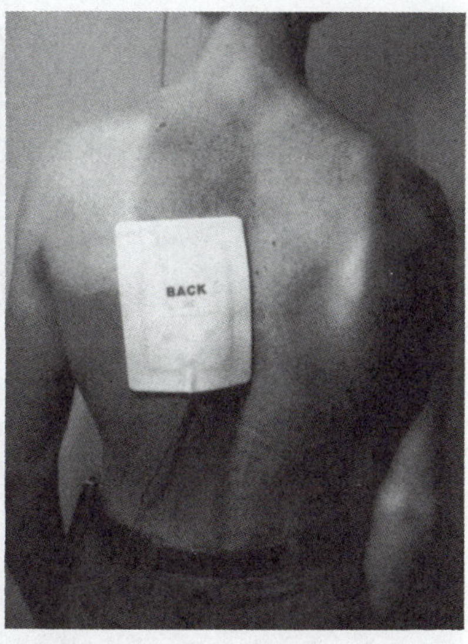

A

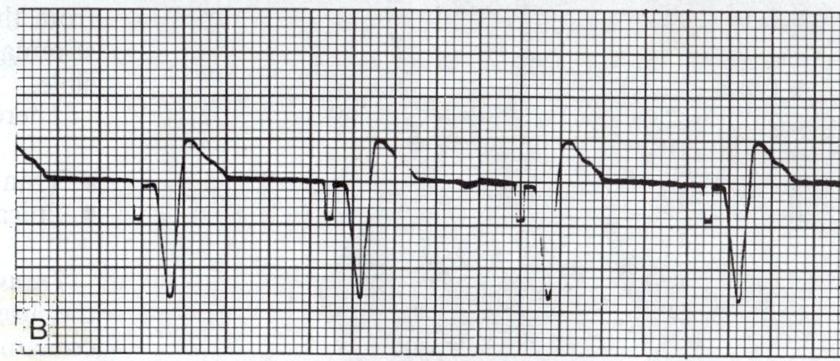

FIGURE 33-28 ◆ *A*, Equipment and electrode placement for transcutaneous external pacing. (From Schwartz, G. R., Bircher, N., Hanke, B. K., Mangelsen, M. A., Mayer, T., & Ungar, J. R. [1989]. *Emergency medicine: The essential update.* Philadelphia: W. B. Saunders.) *B*, ECG rhythm strip showing wide pacing spikes.

the diaphragm and causes discomfort and possible dyspnea.

The high electrical pacing current distorts the ECG signal transmission to the bedside monitor. The nurse must attach a filter cable from the back of the NTP unit to the bedside monitor to reduce interference and obtain a clear ECG signal on the bedside monitor and central console.

The nurse sets the pacing rate as ordered and establishes the stimulation threshold, which is the lowest current that achieves capture, with each pacing spike followed by a QRS complex. The QRS complex is wide because one ventricle depolarizes first, followed by the other. The nurse then sets the electrical current 10% above threshold levels. In some institutions, this is performed only by a physician.

The nurse palpates the client's right radial or carotid pulse and assesses the blood pressure using the client's right arm, ensuring that there is a mechanical response (ventricular contraction) to each pacing stimulus. Vital signs are not taken on the left side of the body because they may not be accurate, particularly if a high milliamperage is used. This large electrical current can cause muscle twitching, which may stimulate blood pressure sounds or simulate a pulse on the left side (Appel-Hardin, 1992).

Complications. Three complications may arise with NPT. The first includes discomfort from cutaneous and muscle stimulation and skin irritation and diaphoresis from the patch electrodes. The nurse must ensure that the electrodes are in good contact with the skin and that the milliamperage is set at the lowest level for effective capture. The electrode position may have to be changed. The nurse also administers prescribed analgesics or sedatives and provides comfort and support.

The second problem is loss of capture, when the pacing spike is not followed by a QRS complex. The nurse ensures that the electrodes are in good contact with the skin and, if necessary, increases the current until capture is regained; however, the greater the current is, the more discomfort is experienced by the client.

The third problem is inappropriate pacing, when the pacemaker does not sense the client's intrinsic QRS complex and therefore fires impulses at its preset rate, competing with the client's rhythm. The nurse must assess electrode contact and the effect of the client's position on pacemaker function. The client may have to avoid lying on his or her left side. If diaphoresis has caused poor contact and the electrodes must be replaced, the nurse must first turn the pacing function off. The nurse avoids electrical shocks when taking the electrodes off the client and possibly touching the pacing side of the electrodes.

Invasive Temporary Pacing. An invasive temporary pacemaker system consists of an external, battery-operated pulse generator and pacing electrodes or

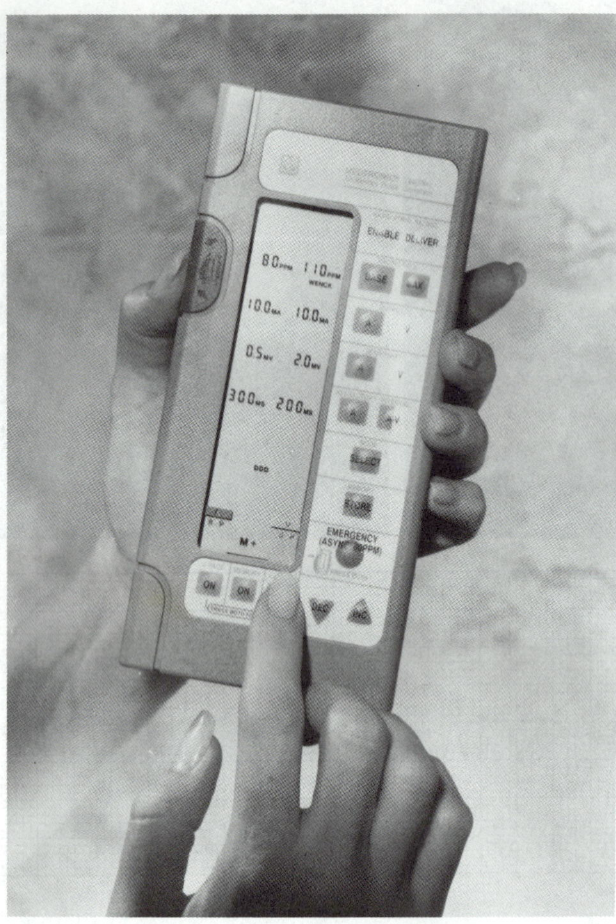

FIGURE 33–29 ◆ Temporary AV sequential pacemaker. (Courtesy of Medtronic, Inc.)

lead wires (Fig. 33–29). These wires attach to the generator on one end and are in contact with the heart on the other end. Electrical pulses, or stimuli, are emitted from the negative terminal of the generator, flow through a lead wire, and stimulate the myocardial cells to depolarize. The current seeks ground by returning through the other lead wire to the positive terminal of the generator, thus completing a circuitous route. The intensity of electrical current is set by selecting the appropriate current output, measured in milliamperes.

The nurse establishes the client's stimulation threshold, which is the lowest current (in milliamperes) that achieves capture, or depolarization. The nurse then sets the current two to three times higher, as determined by the physician, to allow for dynamic changes in the heart that may alter the threshold. Because the electrical stimulus is applied for only approximately 1 msec (pulse width), the spike is a straight vertical line on the ECG paper. The QRS complex is wide because the right ventricle depolarizes first, followed by the left ventricle.

The nurse also establishes the sensitivity threshold, which is the ability of the generator to sense the client's intrinsic cardiac electrical activity. To do this, the pacemaker rate must be decreased to 10 BPM below the client's intrinsic rate, so that there is no pacing. The nurse then decreases the sensitivity on the generator until the pacemaker no longer senses the client's complexes and begins firing impulses (i.e., pacing). The sensitivity is then set to be twice as great to ensure that the generator can detect low-amplitude intrinsic activity and inhibit firing appropriately. Sensitivity threshold cannot be established in clients with profound, unstable bradydysrhythmias or asystole.

In many institutions, only the physician determine thresholds and sets the current and sensitivity. Nurses who are allowed to do this by institutional protocol must have critical care nursing or specific pacemaker education and experience.

The client does not usually feel invasive pacemaker stimuli; however, clients occasionally feel an uncomfortable sensation from the stimuli if strong electrical currents (high milliamperage) are set to be generated from the pacemaker. The nurse should determine the stimulation threshold and decrease the current if possible.

There are two types of invasive temporary pacing:

- Transvenous pacing
- Epicardial pacing

Transvenous Pacing. Transvenous pacing involves the use of fluoroscopy to thread a sterile catheter, containing two lead wires, percutaneously through a vein to the right ventricle for temporary ventricular pacing. The catheter electrode tip (negative electrode) is in contact with the endocardial surface of the ventricle, where it fixates for stability (Fig. 33–30*A*). The positive electrode is located just proximal to the tip of the catheter. The bifurcated external end of the catheter is attached to the negative and positive terminals of a battery-operated pulse generator. The generator provides the electrical current to stimulate the myocardial cells to depolarize. The electrical current flows from endocardium to epicardium, and from the right side of the heart to the left, depolarizing all cells. The energy output required to achieve depolarization is usually less than 5 mA.

If the client needs the atrial kick from atrial contractions, a temporary AV sequential pacemaker is used, with one catheter tip in the right atrium and the other in the right ventricle (see Fig. 33–30*B*). This preserves the normal synchrony of atrial contraction preceding ventricular contraction. Some clients with a dysfunctional sinus node but intact AV node may require only temporary atrial pacing (see Fig. 33–30*C*).

Nursing management of the client after temporary transvenous pacemaker insertion includes continuous ECG monitoring, frequent assessment of vital signs and pacemaker insertion site, restriction of the client's movement to prevent lead wire displacement, and documentation of pacemaker settings.

Epicardial Pacing. Epicardial pacing is accomplished with separate lead wires loosely threaded on the epicardial surface of the heart after open heart

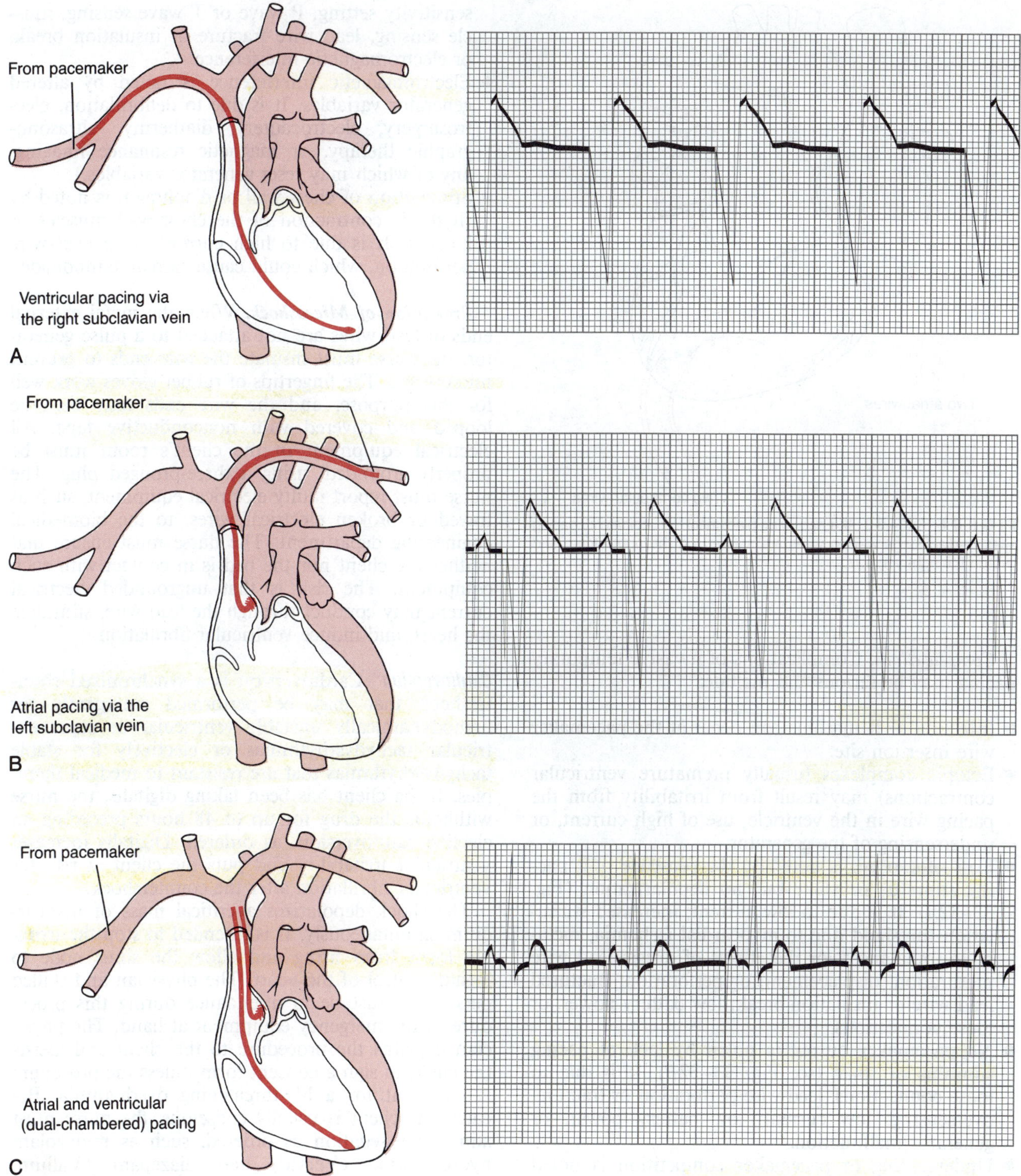

FIGURE 33–30 ◆ Pacemaker catheter electrode placement and corresponding ECG patterns in temporary transvenous pacing. *A*, Ventricular pacing at a rate of 75/minute. *B*, AV sequential pacing at a rate of 50/minute. *C*, Atrial pacing at a rate of 60/minute, with intrinsic QRS complexes.

surgery (Fig. 33–31). The other ends of the wires exit through the chest wall. They attach to the negative and positive terminals of a pulse generator. There are usually two wires on the atrium and two wires on the ventricle. The electrical current flows from epicardium to endocardium, from right to left. Epicardial pacing requires a higher energy output to achieve depolarization, with the current frequently set at 10 mA or higher. Nursing management of the client is detailed in Chapter 37.

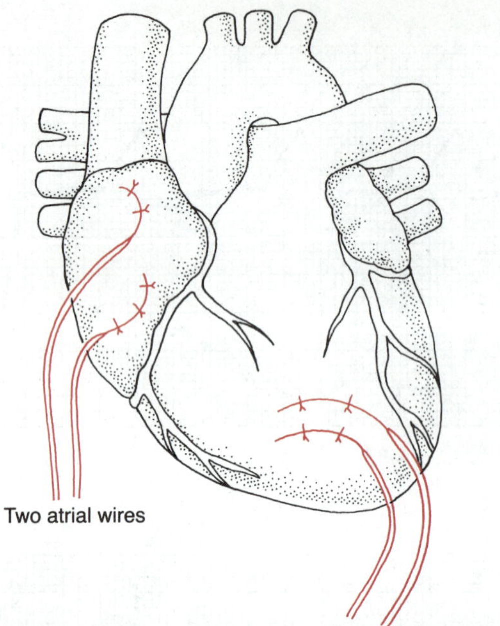

FIGURE 33-31 ◆ Lead wire placement for epicardial pacing after cardiac surgery. Two wires are sutured on the right atrium and two on the right ventricle.

Complications. Complications of invasive temporary pacing may be serious and include:

- Infection or hematoma can occur at the pacemaker wire insertion site.
- Ectopic complexes (usually premature ventricular contractions) may result from irritability from the pacing wire in the ventricle, use of high current, or undersensing of the generator.
- Loss of capture is noted by the presence of a pacing stimulus or spike but no depolarization (Fig. 33-32*A*). It is due to low current; increased stimulation threshold due to myocardial ischemia, metabolic imbalances, or the effects of drugs; lead wire maturation, displacement, or perforation; fractured lead wire or insulation break; low battery power; or loose connections.
- No pacemaker output is noted by lack of pacing stimulus or spike (see Fig. 33-32*B*). It is due to loose connections, lead wire perforation or fracture, oversensing, low current, low battery power, or generator malfunction.
- Undersensing or pacemaker competition is noted when pacing stimuli occur at a fixed rate in the presence of an adequate intrinsic rhythm (see Fig. 33-32*C*). It is due to decreased or asynchronous sensitivity setting, loose connections, lead wire maturation or displacement, the effects of myocardial ischemia or drugs causing inadequate cardiac signals, fractured lead wire or insulation break, low battery power, or faulty generator.
- Oversensing is noted when the pacemaker fails to fire in the presence of an inadequate intrinsic rhythm (see Fig. 33-32*D*). It is due to increased sensitivity setting, P wave or T wave sensing, muscle sensing, lead wire fracture or insulation break, or electromagnetic interference.
- Electromagnetic interference is noted by altered generator variables. It is due to defibrillation, electrosurgery, electrocautery, diathermy, ultrasonographic therapy, or magnetic resonance imaging, any of which may reset generator variables.
- Stimulation of chest wall or diaphragm is noted by rhythmic contraction of the chest wall muscles or hiccups. It is due to high current or to lead wire perforation, which could cause cardiac tamponade.

Prevention of Microshock. When the metal external ends of lead wires are not attached to a pulse generator, the nurse must insulate the wire ends to prevent microshock. The fingertips of rubber gloves work well for this purpose, and the wire ends may then be looped and covered with nonconductive tape. All electrical equipment in the client's room must be properly grounded, using a three-pronged plug. The nurse must report faulty electrical equipment, such as frayed or broken electrical wires, to the biomedical engineering department. The nurse must ensure that neither the client nor the bed is in contact with such equipment. The risk is that ungrounded electrical current may conduct through the lead wire, stimulate the heart, and induce ventricular fibrillation.

Cardioversion Cardioversion is a synchronized countershock that may be performed emergently for hemodynamically unstable ventricular or supraventricular tachydysrhythmias or electively for stable tachydysrhythmias that are resistant to medical therapies. If the client has been taking digitalis, the nurse withholds the drug for up to 48 hours preceding an elective cardioversion, as ordered. Digitalis increases ventricular irritability and puts the client at risk for ventricular fibrillation after the countershock.

The shock depolarizes a critical mass of myocardium simultaneously. It is intended to stop the irritable focus from firing and allow the sinus node to regain control of the heart. The physician and skilled personnel must be in attendance during this procedure, with emergency equipment at hand. The physician explains the procedure to the client and assists the client to sign a consent form unless the procedure is emergent for a life-threatening dysrhythmia. Because the client is usually conscious, the nurse must administer sedation as ordered, such as midazolam hydrochloride (Versed) and diazepam (Valium, E-Pam♣).

The nurse examines the client's skin to ensure that no electrocardiographic (ECG) electrodes and no topical nitroglycerin preparations are on the area where the paddles will be placed. If present, they must be removed and the skin quickly cleaned and dried. The physician or advanced cardiac life support (ACLS)–qualified nurse places conductive pads, one on the client's upper right chest below the clavicle and the other left of the nipple with the center in the mid-axillary line (ECCC, 1992). The nurse places the elec-

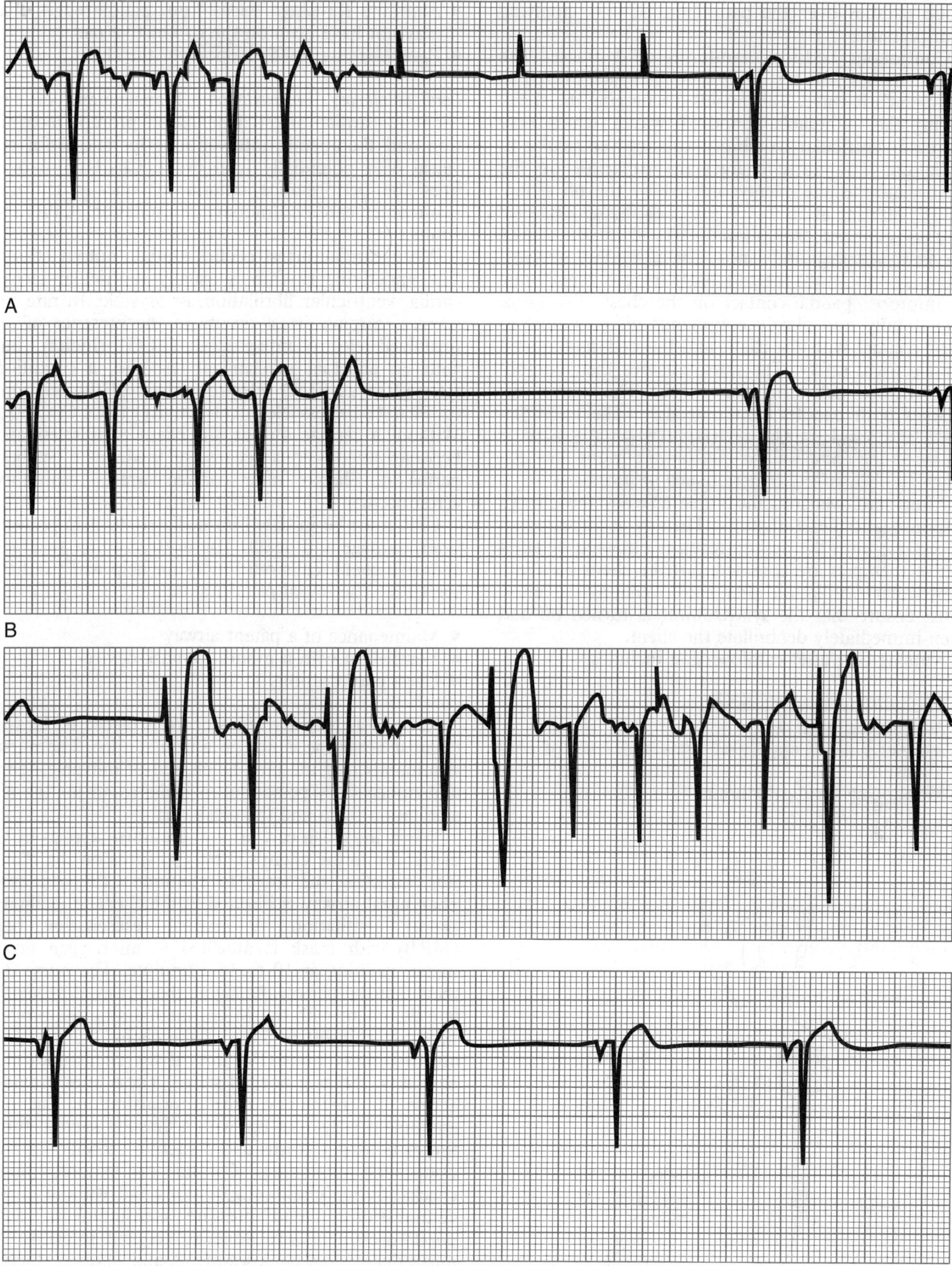

FIGURE 33–32 ◆ Complications of pacing. *A*, Loss of capture. Underlying rhythm is atrial fibrillation initially, followed by a 3.32-second pause, during which pacing spikes not followed by a QRS (capture) can be seen in a client with a *VVI* pacemaker. *B*, No pacemaker output. In the same client, note the lack of pacing spikes during another pause. *C*, Undersensing. Note the presence of inappropriate pacing spikes occurring at a fixed rate of 51 pulses per minute (PPM) throughout the atrial fibrillation. *D*, Oversensing. Sinus bradycardia at a rate of 45/minute in a client with a VVI pacemaker set at a rate of 50 pulses per minute.

trode paddles over the pads (Fig. 33–33), applying firm pressure.

Continuous bedside monitoring is desirable. The nurse ensures that the defibrillator is synchronized to the client's R wave. This avoids discharging the shock during the vulnerable period (T wave), which may increase ventricular irritability, causing ventricular fibrillation. The nurse charges the capacitor on the defibrillator to the energy ordered by the physician, usually starting at 50 to 100 joules. The nurse ensures that oxygen has been turned away from the client. Oxygen supports combustion, and a fire may result if there is arcing from the paddles. Arcing is usually due to improper paddle contact on the chest. The nurse then loudly and clearly commands all personnel to clear contact with the client and the bed, as required for electrical safety. The nurse ensures their compliance before delivering the shock. The nurse discharges both paddles simultaneously. The nurse delivers the shock at end-expiration when the heart is closer to the chest wall so that more current flow can reach the heart for a better chance of success.

After cardioversion, the nurse assesses the client's response and heart rhythm. Therapy is repeated, if necessary, until the desired result is obtained or alternative therapies are considered. If the client goes into ventricular fibrillation after cardioversion, the nurse must ensure that the synchronizer is turned off and then immediately defibrillate the client.

Nursing care after cardioversion includes:

- Maintaining a patent airway
- Administering oxygen
- Assessing the client's vital signs and level of consciousness
- Monitoring for dysrhythmias

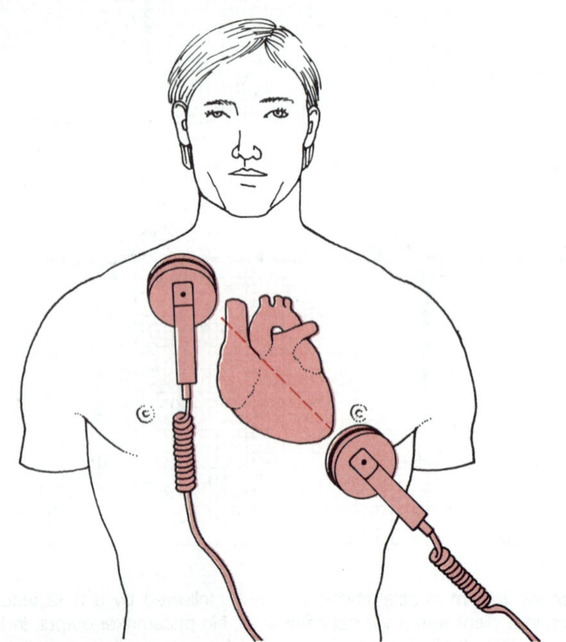

FIGURE 33–33 ◆ Standard electrode paddle placement for cardioversion or defibrillation.

- Assessing for chest burns from paddle edges that may not have been on the conductive pad
- Providing emotional support for the client

Cardiopulmonary Resuscitation Management of the client in cardiac arrest depends on prompt recognition and therapeutic interventions for successful reversal of a potentially fatal event. Chart 33–6 outlines the performance criteria for one-rescuer and two-rescuer cardiopulmonary resuscitation (CPR) for adults.

When cardiac arrest occurs, cardiac output ceases. The underlying rhythm is usually ventricular tachycardia, ventricular fibrillation, or asystole. In rare instances, cardiac arrest occurs in the presence of an organized electrocardiographic (ECG) rhythm, but with no effectual mechanical response, a condition referred to as EMD (electromechanical dissociation) or PEA (pulseless electrical activity) (ECCC, 1992). Without a cardiac output, the client is pulseless and becomes unconscious because of inadequate cerebral perfusion. Shortly after cardiac arrest, respiratory arrest occurs.

CPR must be initiated immediately to help prevent brain damage and death. The nurse, finding an unresponsive client, calls out loudly for help while initiating CPR. The initial priorities are:

- Maintenance of a patent airway
- Ventilation with a mouth-to-mask device
- Chest compressions

As soon as help arrives, a board is placed under the client if he or she is not on a firm surface. The nurse commands that the area be cleared of movable items and unnecessary personnel to make room for the resuscitation team and the crash cart.

When the crash cart arrives, the nurse applies ECG electrodes to the client's chest and turns on the monitor, directing the team to continue CPR. An oropharyngeal airway is inserted in the client to facilitate proper ventilation. A manual resuscitation bag (MRB) with mask is attached to an oxygen flowmeter, running at 10 to 15 L/minute. The nurse directs that the person managing the airway now ventilate the client with the MRB, maintaining the proper head-tilt, chin-lift position of the client. Nurses initiate two intravenous (IV) lines if the client does not have any, infusing normal saline. These lines provide access for emergency drug administration. Suction equipment is also set up, with a tonsillar suction tube for suctioning vomitus and a suction catheter for endotracheal suctioning. Carotid or femoral pulse checks, during chest compressions and without chest compressions; blood pressure measurements; and pupil assessments are done at frequent intervals. A nurse documents all assessments and findings, therapeutic measures, and the client's responses throughout the resuscitation.

The goal of resuscitation is the rapid return of a pulse, blood pressure, and consciousness in the client. This is rarely achieved by CPR and basic measures

CHART 33–6

Nursing Care Highlight ◆ Adult Cardiopulmonary Resuscitation

Interventions

One Rescuer

1. Determine unresponsiveness.

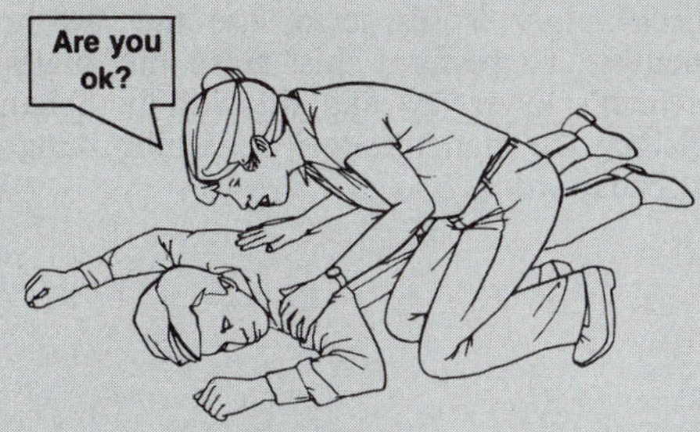

2. Call for help.

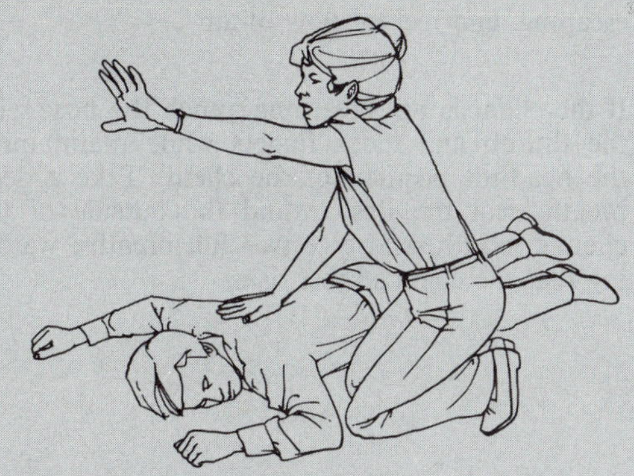

3. Position the client supine on a hard, flat surface. If the client is in bed, place a back board under the client as soon as help arrives.

4. Open the airway with a head-tilt, chin-lift maneuver. To perform this, place one hand on the client's forehead, applying firm backward pressure. Place the fingers of the other hand under the chin and lift it forward with teeth almost to occlusion.

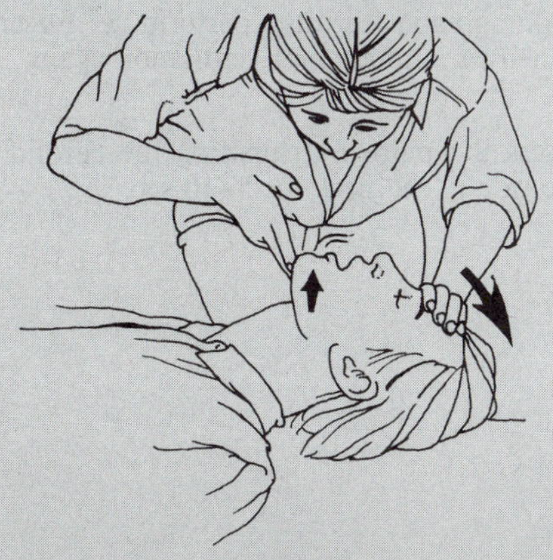

Chart continued on following page

CHART 33–6

Nursing Care Highlight ◆ Adult Cardiopulmonary Resuscitation *Continued*

Interventions

5. If neck injury is suspected, use the jaw-thrust maneuver. To perform this, grasp the angles of the client's lower jaw and lift with both hands, displacing the mandible forward while tilting the head backward.

6. Assess for breathlessness with the airway open. Look for the chest to rise and fall, listen for air escaping, and feel for flow of air.

7. If the client is not breathing, pinch the nose with the thumb and index fingers while maintaining the head-tilt position of the client. Take a deep breath, seal the lips around the outside of the client's mouth, and give two full breaths, watching that the client's chest rises.

8. If the chest does not rise, reposition the client's head and repeat ventilations.

9. If the chest still does not rise, perform 6–10 subdiaphragmatic thrusts, perform a finger-sweep maneuver, and attempt ventilation again.

10. Assess the pulse by palpating the carotid artery on one side of the neck for 5–10 sec.

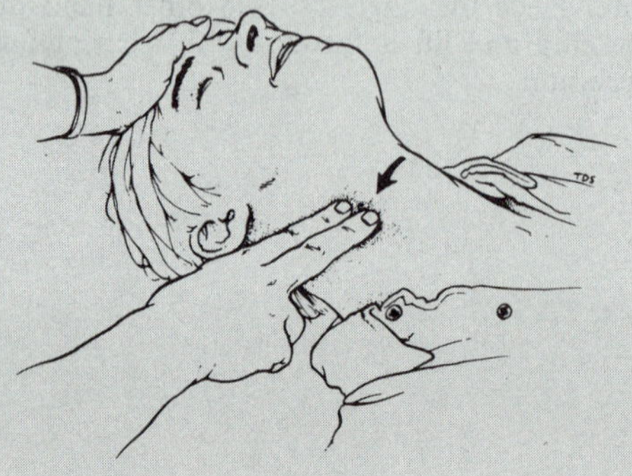

CHART 33–6

Nursing Care Highlight ◆ Adult Cardiopulmonary Resuscitation *Continued*

Interventions

11. If no pulse is palpated, determine proper hand position for chest compressions:
    a. Locate the notch where the rib margin meets the sternum and place the middle finger on this notch and the index finger next to it.

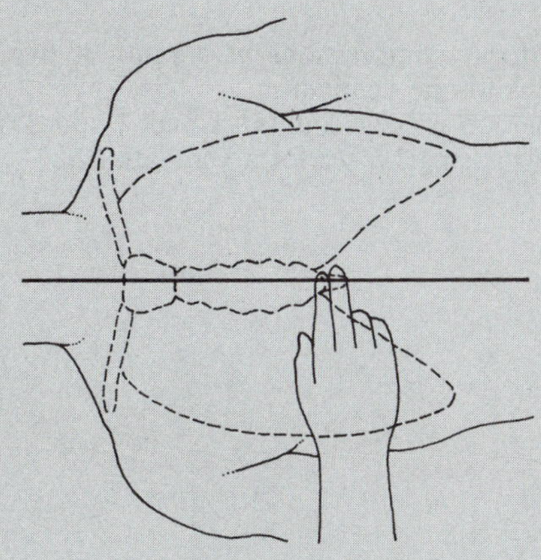

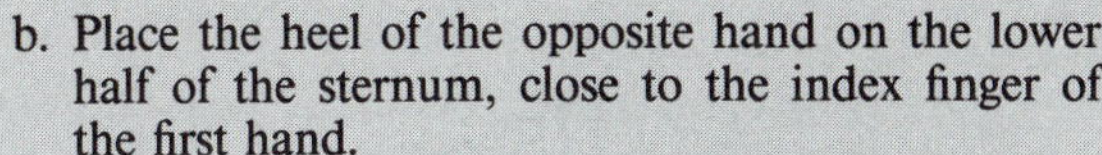

    b. Place the heel of the opposite hand on the lower half of the sternum, close to the index finger of the first hand.

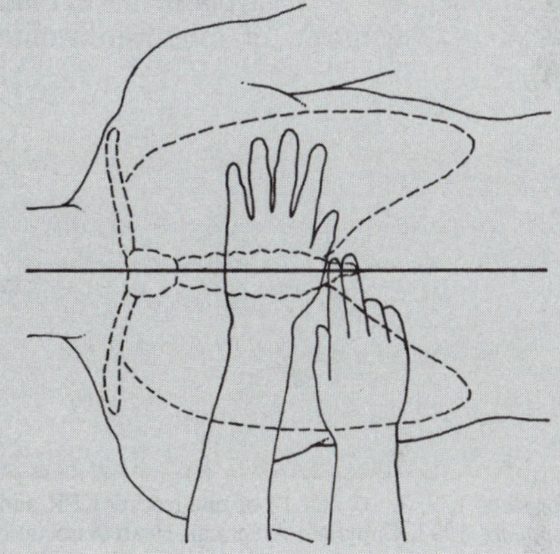

    c. Remove the first hand and place it on top of the hand on the sternum.

12. Begin chest compressions with elbows locked, arms straightened, and shoulders positioned directly over the hands. Depress sternum 1½–2 inches with each compression. Perform 15 compressions, counting "1 and 2 and 3 . . ." to 15. After 15 compressions, deliver two more ventilations.
13. Perform four complete cycles of 15 compressions with two ventilations.
14. Reassess the client's carotid pulse and breathing.

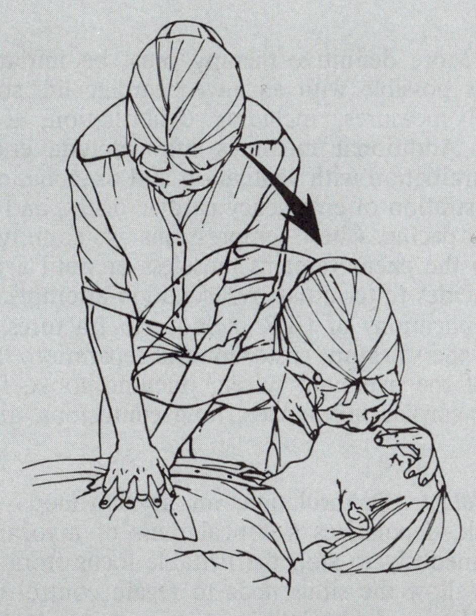

Chart continued on following page

CHART 33–6

Nursing Care Highlight ◆ Adult Cardiopulmonary Resuscitation *Continued*

Interventions

Two Rescuers

1. Perform compressions at a ratio of five compressions to one ventilation.
2. The compressor counts "1 and 2 and 3 and 4 and 5," pausing 1½ sec for a ventilation.
3. If available, use a clear plastic face mask with a one-way valve instead of mouth-to-mouth ventilation.

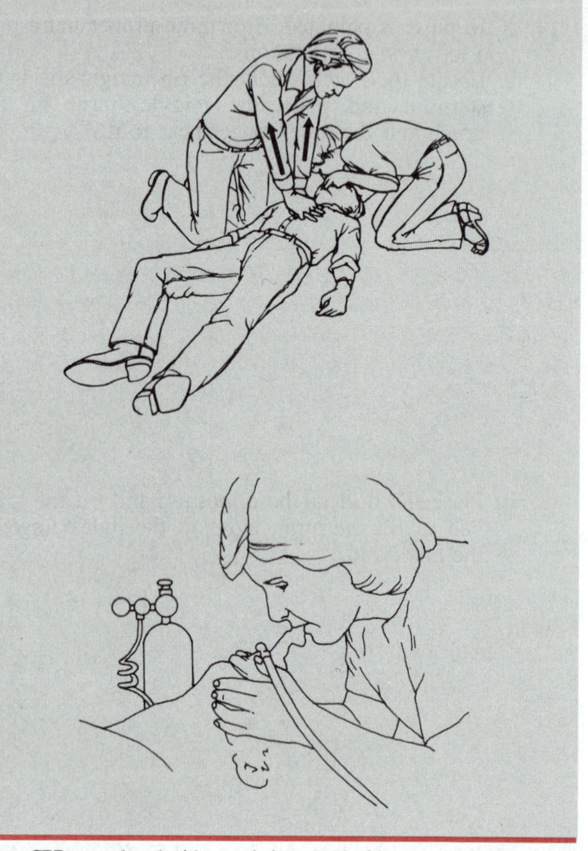

Illustrations for steps 1, 2, 7, 10, and 12 of one-rescuer CPR and for step 2 of two-rescuer CPR reproduced with permission. © *Healthcare provider's manual for basic life support,* 1993. Copyright American Heart Association.

alone. More definitive therapy must be initiated as soon as possible with advanced cardiac life support (ACLS) measures, including defibrillation, if warranted. Additional measures may include endotracheal intubation with ventilation and oxygenation, IV administration of emergency cardiac drugs, and occasionally pacing. Chest compressions are continued as long as the client remains pulseless or until a physician decides to terminate resuscitation attempts.

Complications of CPR include rib fractures, fracture of the sternum, costochondral separation, lacerations of the liver and spleen, pneumothorax, hemothorax, cardiac tamponade, lung contusions, and fat emboli.

Defibrillation Defibrillation, an asynchronous countershock, depolarizes a critical mass of myocardium simultaneously to stop the irritable focus from firing and to allow the sinus node to regain control of the heart. Early defibrillation is critical to terminate pulseless ventricular tachycardia (VT) or ventricular fibrillation (VF). It must not be delayed for any reason after the equipment and skilled personnel are present. The earlier that defibrillation is performed, the greater the chance of survival is.

If a defibrillator is not immediately available, an ACLS-qualified nurse may deliver a precordial thump to a pulseless client in VF. There is a slight chance that it may succeed in terminating the VF (ECCC, 1992). A precordial thump is performed by striking the lower half of the sternum with a closed fist from a height of 8 to 12 inches (12 to 30 cm) above the sternum. If the client remains in VF, CPR is resumed and the nurse prepares the client's chest for defibrillation.

The physician or the ACLS-qualified nurse places conductive gel pads, one on the client's upper right chest below the clavicle and the other to the left of the nipple with the center in the mid-axillary line (ECCC, 1992). The nurse places the electrode paddles over the pads (see Fig. 33–33), applies firm pressure, and charges the capacitor on the defibrillator to an initial energy of 200 joules. The nurse ensures that oxygen has been turned away from the client. The nurse loudly and clearly commands all personnel to clear contact with the client and the bed and ensures their compliance before delivering the shock.

After defibrillation, the nurse assesses the client's heart rhythm. If the first shock was unsuccessful, the nurse may deliver a second shock at 200 to 300 joules, followed by a third shock at 360 joules, if necessary. The shocks are given in rapid succession. Successive shocks decrease transthoracic impedance, allowing more current flow to reach the heart for a better chance of success. If defibrillation is successful, the nurse and team members maintain a patent airway, provide oxygen and ventilatory support, assess vital signs frequently, and continuously monitor the client for the recurrence of dysrhythmias. IV access, hemodynamic support, and antidysrhythmic medications are also essential.

AUTOMATIC EXTERNAL DEFIBRILLATION The American Heart Association promotes the use of automatic external defibrillators (AEDs) for use by laypersons and emergency medical technicians (EMTs) for prehospital cardiac arrests (ECCC, 1992). The client in cardiac arrest must be on a firm, dry surface. The rescuer places two large adhesive patch electrodes on the client's chest, in the same positions as for defibrillator paddles. The rescuer stops CPR and commands anyone present to move away so that no one is touching the client. This eliminates motion artifact when the machine analyzes the rhythm. The rescuer presses the analyze button on the machine. After rhythm analysis, which may take up to 30 seconds, the machine either advises that a shock is necessary or advises that a shock is not indicated. Shocks are recommended for pulseless VF only.

After issuing a command to clear all contact with the client, the rescuer charges the capacitor and presses both discharge buttons on the machine simultaneously, delivering the first shock at 200 joules. The shock is delivered through the patches, so it is hands-off defibrillation, which is safer for the rescuer. With sustained VF, two more shocks may be delivered, with the third at 360 joules. If the client remains in cardiac arrest, CPR is performed for 1 minute, and then another series of three shocks may be delivered, each at 360 joules. It is imperative that ACLS be provided as soon as possible. Use of AEDs results in earlier defibrillation of clients and therefore a greater chance of successful rhythm conversion and survival.

TRANSTELEPHONIC DEFIBRILLATION/MONITORING An innovation approved by the U. S. Food and Drug Administration in 1987 is the transtelephonic defibrillator/monitor (TTD) (Kuhrik et al., 1992). The rescuer places two large adhesive patch electrodes on the client in cardiac arrest or impending arrest, as for the AED. The TTD interacts with a base station via a telephone line. A clinician interprets the electrocardiographic (ECG) rhythm and maintains voice contact with the rescuer to obtain information and assessment findings. When the clinician deems a shock appropriate, the process is activated from the base station, with commands transmitted over the telephone line to the defibrillator. A voice synthesizer commands the rescuer to stand back and a shock is delivered. All decisions are made by a trained professional. This is reassuring to the lay rescuer. However, the client and the TTD must be near a telephone wall connection or a cellular phone for the system to work. TTD allows rapid defibrillation before the EMTs or paramedics arrive.

CURRENT-BASED DEFIBRILLATION Research is being conducted on the use of current-based defibrillation. Defibrillators in use deliver energy, measured in joules. It is not known what the optimal energy for defibrillation is, nor whether energy selected may be too low, which may be ineffective, or too high, which could result in myocardial damage. These problems would be avoided by the use of electrical current, measured in amperes, as it would take into account transthoracic impedance. Optimal defibrillation current has been found to be 30 to 40 mA (ECCC, 1992). Such defibrillators are under investigation.

Catheter Ablation Catheter ablation is an invasive procedure that may be used to abolish an irritable focus causing a supraventricular tachydysrhythmia. The client must undergo electrophysiologic studies and mapping procedures to locate the focus. Then, single or multiple synchronized electrical shocks are administered between one pole of the catheter and a metal paddle placed between the scapulae (Eagle et al., 1989). Newer ablation techniques have been developed that use radiofrequency waves to abolish the irritable focus. Although the irritable focus is abolished, damage may also occur to the normal conduction system, causing heart blocks. For this reason, the physician usually implants a permanent pacemaker.

Surgical Management Clients who experience life-threatening dysrhythmias may require surgical treatment for long-term management. The type of treatment depends on the nature of the dysrhythmia, but most often, the surgical intervention requires open heart surgery. (The preoperative and postoperative care of the client with open heart surgery is discussed in detail in Chapter 37.) Surgical management of dysrhythmias includes permanent pacing, coronary artery bypass grafting, aneurysmectomy, insertion of an automatic implantable cardioverter/defibrillator, and open chest cardiac massage.

Permanent Pacing Permanent pacemaker insertion is performed for the resolution of conduction disorders that are not temporary, including complete heart block and sick sinus syndrome. Permanent pacemakers are usually powered by a lithium battery and have an average life span of 10 years. After the battery power is depleted, the generator must be replaced, a procedure done under local anesthesia. Some pacemakers are nuclear powered and have a life span of 20 years or longer. Other pacemakers can be recharged externally.

TYPES OF PACEMAKERS Pacemakers may be single-chambered or dual-chambered. With single-chambered pacemakers, a lead wire is positioned in the chamber to be paced, most commonly the right ventricle. Occasionally, it is positioned in the right atrium for bradydysrhythmias originating from SA node disease with an intact atrioventricular (AV) conduction system.

Dual-chambered pacemakers have lead wires placed in the right atrium and the right ventricle (Fig. 33–34) for a more physiologic effect, preserving the atrial kick. A programmed AV interval, which closely relates to the PR interval, ensures a ventricular response shortly after atrial depolarization. One common type of dual-chambered pacemaker is the AV sequential pacemaker, which can sense only ventricular intrinsic activity. It paces both the atrium and the ventricle when the client's ventricular rate drops below that set on the generator.

Another dual-chambered pacemaker is the DDD (demand) pacemaker. It is able to sense both atrial and ventricular intrinsic activity and pace both the atrium and the ventricle. It allows sinus control of the ventricular rate to meet increased metabolic demands when the sinus node is functioning well. The DDD pacemaker has an upper rate limit, which prevents the ventricles from being paced too rapidly when the atrial rate goes above the upper rate set on the generator. If the client's sinus rate drops below the lower rate set, the generator paces both the atrium and the ventricle.

A newer type of dual-chambered pacemaker is the rate-responsive pacemaker. Various kinds are available, but each type senses some physiologic variable within the client with impaired sinus or atrial function to allow faster pacing rates to meet increased body demands. Many other types of pacing modes are available.

SURGICAL PROCEDURES For both single-chambered and dual-chambered pacemakers, the surgeon most commonly implants the pulse generator in a surgically made subcutaneous pocket at the shoulder in the right or left subclavicular area. The leads are introduced transvenously via the cephalic or the subclavian vein to the endocardium on the right side of the heart.

An alternative approach is to transthoracically introduce the leads and suture them to the epicardium, requiring a thoracotomy. In this procedure, the surgeon implants the pulse generator in a subcutaneous abdominal pocket. After the procedure, the nurse monitors the client's electrocardiographic (ECG) rhythm to ensure that the pacemaker is functioning correctly. The nurse also assesses the implantation site for evidence of bleeding, swelling, redness, tenderness, and infection. The dressing over the site should remain clean and dry, and the client should be afebrile and have stable vital signs. The physician may order activity restrictions to enhance lead fixa-

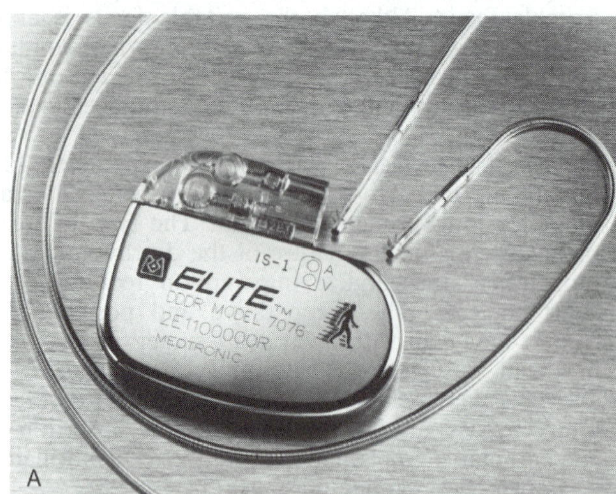

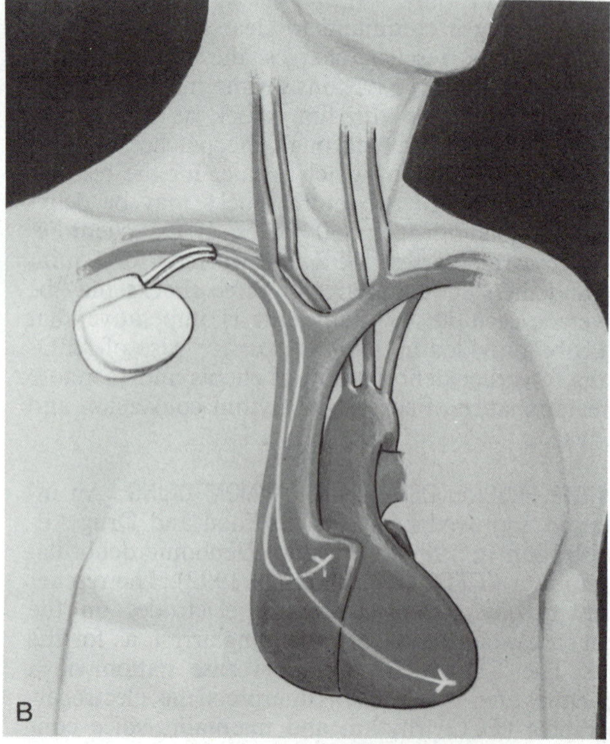

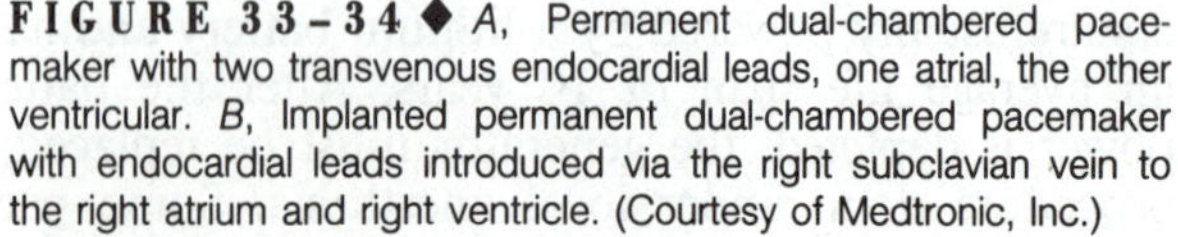
FIGURE 33–34 ◆ *A*, Permanent dual-chambered pacemaker with two transvenous endocardial leads, one atrial, the other ventricular. *B*, Implanted permanent dual-chambered pacemaker with endocardial leads introduced via the right subclavian vein to the right atrium and right ventricle. (Courtesy of Medtronic, Inc.)

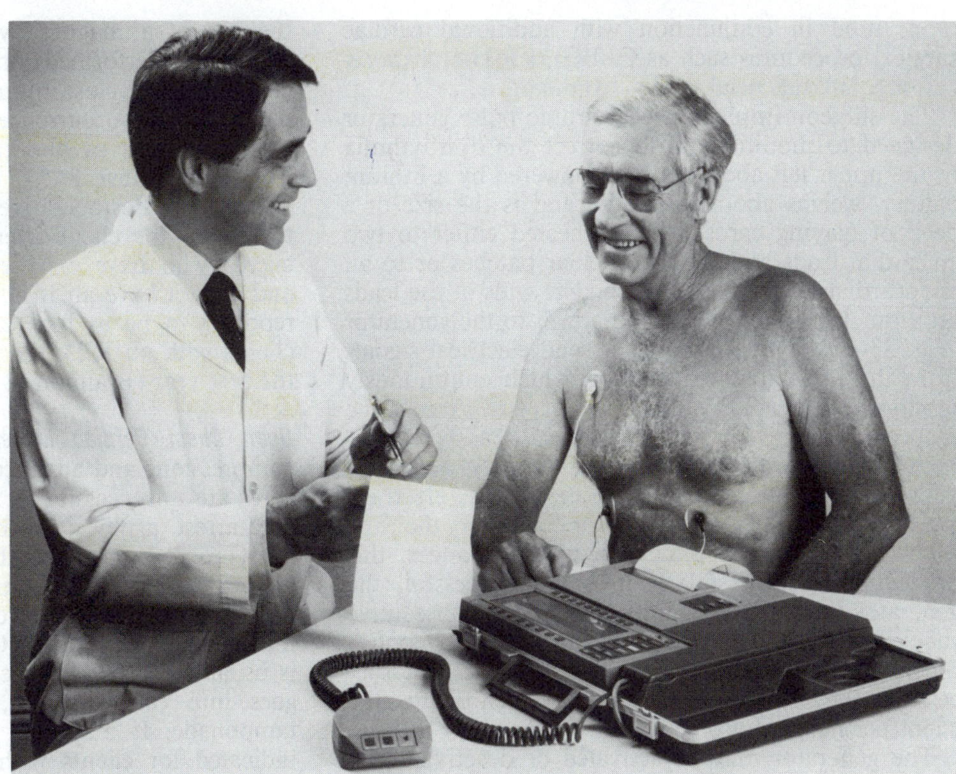

FIGURE 33-35 ◆ Permanent pacemaker check. The "head" of the device, at the end of the coiled line, is placed over the pulse generator to interrogate the pacemaker and reprogram it if necessary. (Courtesy of Hewlett-Packard Company.)

tion. After 24 hours, activity is gradually increased. Pacing complications of permanent pacemakers are identical to those for temporary invasive pacing.

Pacemaker checks are done on an outpatient basis at regular intervals. Reprogramming may be warranted if there are pacemaker problems. The pulse generator is interrogated using an electronic device to determine the pacemaker settings and battery life (Fig. 33-35). Reprogramming, if necessary, is accomplished by using a programming device, the "head" of which is placed on the client's skin over the pulse generator. With certain commands, the programming device can reprogram the mode in which the pacemaker is to function, the rate of firing, the sensitivity, and the amount of current it sends to the heart, as well as other variables in highly sophisticated pacemakers.

For clients who live too far from the pacemaker clinic or physician's office, pacemaker information can be sent via transtelephonic transmission of data. The client attaches ECG electrodes to the wrists and places the telephone receiver in a transmitting unit. The sound signals are relayed via telephone lines to the clinic or office, where they are converted and recorded as the client's ECG rhythm strip and information about the pacemaker variables. The nurse stresses the need to keep clinic appointments for more detailed pacemaker checks and reprogramming, if necessary, as well as assessment of the client.

Coronary Artery Bypass Grafting Coronary artery bypass grafting (CABG) is performed if the cause of the dysrhythmia is coronary artery insufficiency that is unresponsive to medical therapy. This procedure is described in Chapter 37.

Aneurysmectomy Ventricular aneurysms are a complication of myocardial infarction and may be the source of intractable ventricular tachydysrhythmias. The surgeon resects the aneurysm, a dyskinetic or ballooning portion of the ventricular wall. Resection of the area eliminates the dangerous irritable focus and therefore the cause of the dysrhythmias. Care of the client is similar to that for clients undergoing CABG, described in Chapter 37.

Insertion of an Implantable Cardioverter/Defibrillator The implantable cardioverter/defibrillator (ICD) is reserved for use in clients who have experienced at least one episode of sudden cardiac death unrelated to a myocardial infarction, clients who were successfully resuscitated, or clients in whom conventional medical attempts to control life-threatening dysrhythmias have not been successful. Clients undergo electrophysiologic studies to assess the inducibility of ventricular tachydysrhythmias and their response to medication. If the dysrhythmias can be induced despite medical therapy, the client may be considered a candidate for ICD implantation. A psychologic profile is done to determine whether the client will be able to cope with the discomfort and fear associated with internal defibrillation from the ICD.

One of four surgical approaches for implanting the device may be used: median sternotomy (most common, used in conjunction with additional cardiac surgical procedures such as CABG), left lateral thoracotomy, left subcostal, and subxiphoid.

The surgeon implants an electronic pulse generator designed to monitor and to correct the dysrhythmia in the upper left abdomen. It is powered by a lithium battery, weighs about ½ pound, and is the size of a deck of playing cards. It is connected either to two epicardial leads and two ventricular patches or to an endocardial lead and one patch. The ends of the leads are tunneled under the skin to attach to the generator (Fig. 33–36). The sensing leads send electrical signals from the heart to the generator, which continuously monitors the heart rhythm. If the rhythm exceeds the preprogrammed rate (rate cutoff), such as with ventricular tachycardia or fibrillation, the pulse generator takes 10 to 35 seconds to sense the cardiac electrical activity, charge its capacitor, and deliver the first shock, usually at 25 joules. In most instances, this procedure is successful. If it is not successful, the generator can deliver up to four more consecutive shocks to the heart, usually at 30 joules, to abolish the abnormal rhythm. If these shocks are not successful, the nurse must externally defibrillate the client per hospital protocol.

The generator may be activated or deactivated by the use of a magnet over the implantation site, a procedure performed only by the physician. The client requires close monitoring in the postoperative period for the occurrence of dysrhythmias and complications such as bleeding and cardiac tamponade. The nurse must know if the ICD is activated or deactivated. Postoperative care of the client is similar to that of the client after CABG (see Chap. 37). In clients who have experienced sudden cardiac death and do not have an ICD, the mortality rate has been reported to be as high as 73% in the first year. In clients with an ICD, the mortality reported is 3% in the first year (Brannon & Johnson, 1992).

Open Chest Cardiac Massage When external chest compressions and advanced cardiac life support measures are unsuccessful in resuscitating a client in cardiac arrest, a physician may decide to perform open chest cardiac massage through a thoracotomy approach or through the median sternotomy incision in post–cardiac surgery clients. Internal defibrillation may also be performed. Open chest cardiac massage is usually reserved for the cardiac surgical client who goes into cardiac arrest, often because of cardiac tamponade. It may also be beneficial but is rarely indicated for clients with hypothermia, crushing or

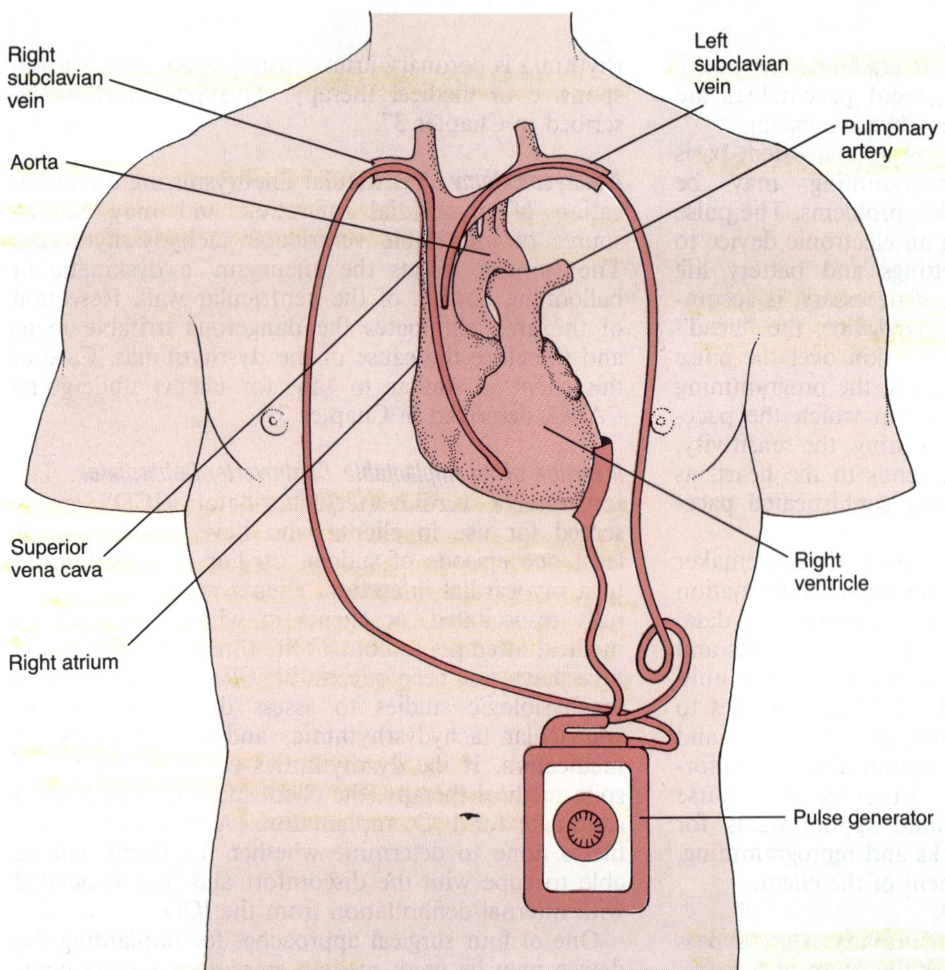

FIGURE 33–36 ◆ Automatic implantable cardioverter/defibrillator, with two epicardial sensing leads and two ventricular patches.

penetrating chest injuries, penetrating abdominal trauma, or chest deformities prohibiting external chest compressions.

DISCHARGE PLANNING

HOME CARE PREPARATION

The client may have been hospitalized because of an episode of dysrhythmic sudden cardiac death (cardiac arrest) or because of severe hemodynamic instability from a dysrhythmia. On the other hand, the client may have been hospitalized for a medical disorder, such as unstable angina, myocardial infarction, heart failure, diabetes, or chronic pulmonary disease, or for a surgical intervention or trauma and found to have dysrhythmias. Dysrhythmias may be benign, serious, or life-threatening.

Clients at risk for recurrence of dysrhythmias have considerable discharge planning needs. The nurse, in collaboration with members of the interdisciplinary health care team, must develop a comprehensive care plan to meet the client's needs. The care plan focuses on health teaching, psychosocial preparation, and health care resources.

HEALTH TEACHING

PREVENTION OF RECURRENCE Clients who have experienced a dysrhythmia that was associated with an acute disorder, such as electrolyte imbalance or ischemia related to a myocardial infarction, are instructed in the prevention, early recognition, and management of that disorder. The nurse teaches the client lifestyle modifications designed to prevent, decrease, or control the occurrence of dysrhythmias, as outlined in Chart 33-7.

CHART 33-7

Education Guide ◆ How to Prevent or Decrease Dysrhythmias

For Clients at Risk for Vasovagal Attacks Causing Bradydysrhythmias

- Avoid doing things that stimulate the vagus nerve, such as raising your arms above your head, applying pressure over your carotid artery, applying pressure on your eyes, bearing down or straining during a bowel movement, and stimulating a gag reflex when brushing your teeth or putting objects in your mouth.

For Clients with Premature Beats and Ectopic Rhythms

- Take the medications that have been prescribed for you, and report any adverse effects to your physician.
- Stop smoking, avoid caffeinated beverages as much as possible, and drink alcohol only in moderation.
- Learn ways to manage stress and avoid getting too tired.

For Clients with Ischemic Heart Disease

- If you have an angina attack, treat it promptly with rest and nitroglycerin administration as prescribed by your physician. This decreases your chances of experiencing a dysrhythmia.
- If chest pain is not relieved after taking the amount of nitroglycerin that has been prescribed for you, seek medical attention promptly. Also, seek prompt medical attention if the pain becomes more severe or you experience other symptoms, such as sweating, nausea, weakness, and palpitations.

For Clients at Risk for Potassium Imbalance

- Know the symptoms of decreased potassium levels, such as muscle weakness and cardiac irregularity.
- Eat foods high in potassium, such as tomatoes, beans, prunes, avocados, bananas, strawberries, and lettuce.
- Take the potassium supplements that have been prescribed for you.

DRUG THERAPY Clients receiving antidysrhythmic drugs after discharge from the hospital must have a thorough understanding of their medications. The nurse teaches clients the generic and trade names of their drugs, as well as their purposes, using basic terms that are easily understood. The nurse must provide clear instructions on dosage schedules and common side effects (see Chart 33-4). The nurse emphasizes the importance of reporting these side effects and any dizziness, nausea, vomiting, chest discomfort, or shortness of breath to the physician. Chart 33-8 highlights special considerations for elderly clients receiving antidysrhythmic therapy.

PULSE CHECK The nurse teaches all clients and their significant others or family members how to take the client's pulse. The nurse instructs them to report any signs of a change in heart rhythm, such as a significant decrease in pulse rate, a rate greater than 100 beats per minute, or increased irregularity.

PACEMAKER Clients who have a permanent pacemaker are given written and verbal information about the type and settings of their pacemaker. The nurse teaches them to report any pulse rate that is lower than that set on the pacemaker. The nurse also teaches clients with pacemakers to avoid strong electromagnetic fields, such as metal detectors. These may cause interference and could change the pacemaker settings, causing a malfunction. The nurse teaches the client the proper care of the pacemaker insertion site and the importance of reporting any fever or any redness, swelling, or drainage at the pacemaker insertion site. If the surgical incision is near either shoulder, the nurse teaches and demon-

CHART 33–8

Nursing Focus on the Elderly ◆ Dysrhythmias

Elderly clients are at increased risk for dysrhythmias because of changes in their cardiac conduction system. The sinoatrial node has fewer pacemaker cells. There is a loss of fibers in the bundle branch system. Therefore, elderly clients are at risk for sinus node dysfunction and may require pacemaker therapy. The most common dysrhythmias in the elderly are premature atrial contractions, premature ventricular contractions, and atrial fibrillation. Dysrhythmias tend to be more serious in elderly clients because of underlying heart disease, causing cardiac decompensation. Consequently, blood flow to organs, which may already be decreased because of the aging process, is further compromised, leading to multisystem organ dysfunction (Matteson & McConnell, 1988). The following are special nursing considerations for the elderly client with dysrhythmias:

- Evaluate the client with dysrhythmias immediately for the presence of a life-threatening dysrhythmia or hemodynamic deterioration.
- Assess the client with a dysrhythmia for angina, hypotension, heart failure, and decreased cerebral and renal perfusion.
- Consider the following causes of dysrhythmias when taking the client's history: hypoxia, drug toxicity, electrolyte imbalances, heart failure, and myocardial ischemia or infarction.
- Assess the client's level of education, hearing, learning style, and ability to understand and recall instructions to determine the best approaches for teaching.
- Assess the client's ability to read written instructions.
- Teach the client the generic and trade names of prescribed antidysrhythmic drugs, as well as their purposes, dosage, side effects, and special instructions for their use.
- Provide clear, written instructions in basic language and easy-to-read print.
- Provide a written drug dosage schedule for the client, taking into account all the medications the client is taking and possible drug interactions.
- Assess the client for possible side effects or adverse reactions to drugs, considering the client's age and health status.
- Teach the client to take his or her pulse and to report significant changes in heart rate or rhythm to the physician.
- Inform the client of available resources for blood pressure and pulse checks, such as blood pressure clinics, home health agencies, and cardiac rehabilitation programs.
- Instruct the client on the importance of keeping follow-up visit appointments with the physician and of reporting symptoms promptly.
- Include the client's family members or significant other in all teaching whenever possible.
- Instruct the client to avoid drinking caffeinated beverages, to stop smoking, to drink alcohol only in moderation, and to follow his or her prescribed diet.

strates range-of-motion exercises for the client to perform to prevent shoulder stiffness. The nurse instructs the client to carry a pacemaker identification card and to wear a medical alert (Medic-Alert) bracelet. Chart 33–9 outlines the major points for client and family teaching after the insertion of a permanent pacemaker.

IMPLANTABLE CARDIOVERTER/DEFIBRILLATOR Clients with an implantable cardioverter/defibrillator (ICD) usually continue to receive antidysrhythmic drugs after discharge from the hospital. The nurse stresses the importance of continuing to take these medications as prescribed. The nurse provides clear instructions about the purposes of the medications, the dosage schedules, special instructions for taking the medications, and side effects to report. The nurse teaches clients that if they experience an internal defibrillator shock, they must sit or lie down immediately and must notify the physician. Some clients describe the experience of a shock as a quick thud or kick in the chest, whereas other clients relate severe pain similar to that of external defibrillation. The nurse teaches family members that, although they may feel an electrical shock if they are touching the client during delivery of the shock, it is harmless. The nurse provides instructions to the client and family members on how to have access to the emergency medical services (EMS) system in their community. The nurse also recommends resources for the family to learn how to perform cardiopulmonary resuscitation (CPR).

The nurse also teaches clients with an ICD to avoid strong electromagnetic fields, such as large electrical generators, radio or television transmitters, airport metal detectors, and nuclear magnetic resonance imaging equipment. The nurse stresses that if the pulse generator emits a beeping sound, the client must move away from the area as quickly as possible to prevent deactivation of the device. The nurse instructs the client with an ICD to carry an ICD identification card and to wear a medical alert (Medic-

Alert) bracelet. Chart 33–10 highlights the important points for teaching clients and family members and significant others.

PSYCHOSOCIAL PREPARATION

Clients and families often fear recurrence of a life-threatening dysrhythmia. Clients with an ICD may dread or fear the activation of the ICD. The nurse provides the client and family members with the opportunity to verbalize their concerns and fears. The nurse provides emotional support, as well as information about support groups in the community, and makes appropriate referrals.

HEALTH CARE RESOURCES

The cardiac rehabilitation department nurse typically provides written and verbal information about dysrhythmias, antidysrhythmic drugs, pacemakers, and ICDs, as well as information about cardiac exercise programs, educational classes, and support groups. The nurse instructs the client on how to contact the local affiliate of the American Heart Association or the provincial affiliate of the Heart and Stroke Foundation in Canada for information about dysrhythmias, pacemakers, and CPR training. Clients with pacemakers may have transtelephonic systems for transmission of their rhythms to a clinic or health care provider's office. The nurse teaches clients how to use these systems.

The nurse instructs clients with an ICD to contact the local ambulance or paramedic services to inform them that they have these devices implanted. Depending on the surgical placement of the ICD patches, successful external defibrillation may be impeded if paddles are placed in the standard position. The nurse obtains information on the best external paddle placement from the physician and provides this information to the client. Paramedics must be

CHART 33–9

Education Guide ◆ Permanent Pacemakers

- Follow the instructions for pacemaker site skin care that have been specifically prepared for you. Report any fever or redness, swelling, or drainage from the incision site to your physician.
- Keep your pacemaker identification card in your wallet and wear a medical alert (Medic-Alert) bracelet.
- Take your pulse for one full minute at the same time each day and record the rate in your pacemaker diary. Take your pulse any time you feel symptoms of a possible pacemaker failure and report your heart rate and symptoms to your physician.
- Know the rate at which your pacemaker is set and the basic functioning of your pacemaker. Know what rate changes to report to your physician.
- Do not apply pressure over your generator. Avoid tight clothing or belts.
- You may take baths or showers without concern for your pacemaker.
- Inform other physicians and dentists that you have a pacemaker. Certain tests they may wish to perform (such as magnetic resonance imaging) could affect or damage your pacemaker.
- Know the indications of battery failure for your pacemaker as you were instructed, and report these findings to your physician if they occur.
- Do not operate electrical appliances directly over your pacemaker site, because this may cause your pacemaker to malfunction.
- Do not lean over electric or gasoline engines or motors. Be sure that electric appliances or motors are properly grounded.
- Avoid all transmitter towers for radio, television, and radar. Radio, television, other home appliances, and antennas do not pose a hazard.
- Be aware that antitheft devices in stores may cause temporary pacemaker malfunction. If symptoms develop, move away from the device.
- Inform airport personnel of your pacemaker before passing through a metal detector and show them your pacemaker identification card. The metal in your pacemaker will trigger the alarm in the metal detector device.
- Stay away from any arc welding equipment.
- Be aware that it is safe to operate a microwave oven unless it does not have proper shielding (old microwave ovens) or is defective.
- Report any of the following symptoms to your physician if you experience them: difficulty breathing, dizziness, fainting, prolonged weakness or fatigue, swelling of arms or legs, chest pain, weight gain, and prolonged hiccupping. If you have any of these symptoms, check your pulse rate and call your physician.
- If you feel symptoms when near any device, move 5 to 10 feet away from it and then check your pulse. Your pulse rate should return to normal.
- Keep all your physician and pacemaker clinic appointments.
- Take all medications prescribed for you as instructed.
- Follow your prescribed diet.
- Follow instructions on restrictions on physical activity, such as no sudden, jerky movement for 8 weeks to allow the pacemaker to settle in place.

CHART 33-10

Education Guide ♦ Implantable Cardioverter/Defibrillator (ICD)

- Follow the instructions for ICD site skin care that have been specifically prepared for you.
- Report to your physician any fever or redness, swelling, soreness, or drainage from your incision site.
- Do not wear tight clothing or belts that could cause irritation over the ICD generator.
- Avoid activities that involve rough contact with the ICD implantation site.
- Keep your ICD identification card in your wallet and consider wearing a medical alert (Medic-Alert) bracelet.
- Know the basic functioning of your ICD device and its rate cutoff, as well as the number of consecutive shocks it can deliver.
- Avoid magnets directly over your ICD because they can inactivate the device. If beeping tones are coming from the ICD, move away from the electromagnetic field immediately (within 30 sec) before the inactivation sequence is completed, and notify your physician.
- Inform all physicians and dentists caring for you that you have an ICD implanted, because certain diagnostic tests and procedures must be avoided to prevent ICD malfunction. These include diathermy, electrocautery, and nuclear magnetic resonance tests.
- Avoid other sources of electromagnetic interference, such as devices emitting microwaves (not microwave ovens); transformers; radio, television, and radar transmitters; large electrical generators; metal detectors, including hand-held security devices at airports; antitheft devices; arc welding equipment; and sources of 60-cycle (Hz) interference. Also avoid leaning directly over the alternator of a running motor of a car or boat.
- Report to your physician symptoms such as fainting, nausea, weakness, blackouts, and rapid pulse rates.
- Take all medications prescribed for you as instructed.
- Follow instructions on restrictions on physical activity, such as not swimming, driving motor vehicles, or operating dangerous equipment.
- Follow your prescribed diet.
- Keep all physician and ICD clinic appointments.
- Sit or lie down immediately if you feel dizzy or faint to avoid falling if the ICD discharges.
- Post emergency telephone numbers.
- Know how to contact the local emergency medical services (EMS) systems in your community. Inform them in advance that you have an ICD so that they can be prepared if they need to respond to an emergency call for you.
- Know how to perform cough CPR as instructed.
- Encourage family members to learn how to perform CPR. Family members should know that, if they are touching you when the device discharges, they may feel a slight shock but that this is not harmful to them.
- Follow instructions on what to do if the ICD successfully discharges, after which you feel well. This may include maintaining a diary of the date, the time, activity preceding the shock, symptoms, the number of shocks delivered, and how you feel after the shock. The physician may wish to be notified each time the device discharges.
- Avoid strenuous activities that may cause your heart rate to meet or exceed the rate cutoff of your ICD, because this causes the device to discharge inappropriately.
- Notify your physician if you are leaving town or are relocating for information regarding access to health care.

informed that, if the ICD fails to convert the rhythm, external defibrillation may be more successful if paddles are placed in the anterior/posterior position.

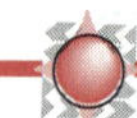

IMPLICATIONS FOR NURSING RESEARCH

Dysrhythmias can be frightening for most clients when they understand their significance. The treatment of dysrhythmias ranges from observation to open heart surgery. Possible questions for future nursing research include:

- ♦ How can the nurse best meet the needs of the elderly client for health teaching about medications?
- ♦ How can the nurse best alleviate the fear and anxiety that often accompany the diagnosis of dysrhythmia?
- ♦ What effects do specific nursing procedures have that may contribute to dysrhythmias?
- ♦ What nursing procedure modifications can be recommended to decrease the occurrence of dysrhythmias?

SELECTED BIBLIOGRAPHY

*American Heart Association. (1987). *Textbook of advanced cardiac life support.* Dallas: Author.

Appel-Hardin, S. (1992). The role of the critical care nurse in noninvasive temporary pacing. *Critical Care Nurse, 12*(3), 10–16, 18–19.

Barbiere, C. C., et al. (1992). Automated external defibrillators: An update of additions to the ACLS algorithms. *Critical Care Nurse, 12*(5), 17–20.

Barbiere, C. C., & Liberatore, K. (1993). From emergent transvenous pacemaker to permanent implant and follow-up. *Critical Care Nurse, 11*(3), 39–44.

Bashford, C. W. (1994). When a patient survives sudden cardiac death. *RN, 57*(4), 34–37.

Benz, M. R. (1991). Pharmacologic management of ventricular arrhythmias. *Critical Care Nursing Quarterly, 14*(3), 8–15.

*Bernstein, A. D., et al. (1987). The NASPE/BPEG generic pacemaker code for antibradyarrhythmia and adaptive-rate pacing and antitachyarrhythmia devices. *PACE, 10*(4), 794.

Berry, S. L., & Schleicher, C. A. (1992). Adjusting the beat: What to teach about antiarrhythmics. *American Journal of Nursing, 92*(6), 28–32.

Brannon, P., & Johnson, R. (1992). The internal cardioverter defibrillator: Patient-family teaching. *Focus on Critical Care, 19*(1), 41–42, 44–46.

Braunwald, E. (1992). *Heart disease: A textbook of cardiovascular medicine* (4th ed.). Philadelphia: W. B. Saunders.

Burke, L. J., et al. (1992). Living with recurrent ventricular dysrhythmias. *Focus on Critical Care, 19*(1), 60–62, 64–66, 68.

Campbell, C. D., et al. (1990). Detecting life-threatening arrhythmias. *Nursing 90, 20*(12), 34–40.

Canobbio, M. M., et al. (1991). Mechanism, diagnosis, and management of ventricular arrhythmias. *Critical Care Nursing Quarterly, 14*(2), 4–80.

Catalano, J. T. (1990). AV nodal arrhythmias. *Critical Care Nurse, 10*(6), 76, 78–80.

Clark, L., et al. (1992). The long and the short of sinus arrhythmias. *Heart & Lung, 21*(5), 507–508.

Clochesy, J. M., Cifani, L., & Howe, K. (1991). Electrode site preparation techniques: A follow-up study. *Heart & Lung, 20*, 27–30.

Coleman, S. (1992). Cardiac issues in CPR: What the future might hold. *Nursing 92, 22*(4), 54–57.

Collins, M. A. (1994). When your patient has an implantable defibrillator. *American Journal of Nursing, 94*(3), 34–39.

Connelly, A. G. (1992). An examination of stressors in the patient undergoing cardiac electrophysiologic studies. *Heart & Lung, 21*(4), 365–371.

*Conover, M. B. (1988). *Understanding electrocardiography, arrhythmias and the 12-lead ECG.* St. Louis: C. V. Mosby.

Cummins, R., et al. (1991). Improving survival from sudden cardiac arrest: The "chain of survival" concept. *Circulation, 83*, 1832–1847.

Deantonio, H. J., et al. (1992). Atrial fibrillation: Current therapeutic approaches. *American Family Physician, 45*(6), 2576–2584.

Doering, L. (1991). Psychosocial responses of patients with malignant ventricular arrhythmias: Assessment and treatment. *Critical Care Nursing Quarterly, 14*(2), 72–80.

Dolan, J. T., et al. (1991). *Critical care nursing: Clinical management through the nursing process.* Philadelphia: F. A. Davis.

Dougherty, A. H., et al. (1992). Acute conversion of paroxysmal supraventricular tachycardia with intravenous diltiazem. *American Journal of Cardiology, 70*(6), 587–592.

Drew, B. J. (1992). Using cardiac leads the right way. *Nursing 92, 22*(5), 50–54.

Drew, B. J., et al. (1991). Accuracy of bedside electrocardiographic monitoring: A report on current practices of critical care nurses. *Heart & Lung, 20*(6), 597–609.

*Eagle, K. A., et al. (1989). *The practice of cardiology: The medical and surgical cardiac units at the Massachusetts General Hospital* (2nd ed.). Boston: Little, Brown.

Emergency Cardiac Care Committee and Subcommittees, American Heart Association. (1992). Guidelines for cardiopulmonary resuscitation and emergency cardiac care—recommendations of the 1992 national conference. *JAMA, 268*(16), 2171–2302.

Eorgan, P. A., & Greer, J. L. (1992). Cough CPR: A consideration for high-risk cardiac patient discharge teaching. *Critical Care Nurse, 12*(6), 21–27.

Green, E., et al. (1992). Charting the future of emergency drug protocols. *Nursing 92, 22*(6), 55–57.

Gunderson, L. P., et al. (1991). Endotracheal suctioning-induced heart rate alterations. *Nursing Research, 40*(3), 139–143.

Guyton, A. C. (1991). *Textbook of medical physiology* (8th ed.). Philadelphia: W. B. Saunders.

Hanna, D. L. (1991). A primary care approach to cardiac arrhythmias. *Nurse Practitioner Forum, 2*(1), 48–54.

Harper, P., & VanRiper, S. (1993). Implantable cardioverter defibrillator: A patient education model for the illiterate patient. *Critical Care Nurse, 11*(3), 55–59.

Hessen, S. E. (1992). Clinical evaluation of the patient with ventricular arrhythmia. *Geriatrics, 47*(11), 63–68.

*Hurst, J. W., et al. (1986). *The heart, arteries and veins* (6th ed.). New York: McGraw-Hill.

Jacobson, C. (1991). Mechanisms of arrhythmia formation. *Critical Care Nursing Quarterly, 14*(2), 1–9.

Johnson, G. E., et al. (1992). *Pharmacology and the nursing process* (3rd ed.). Philadelphia: W. B. Saunders.

Kater, K. M., et al. (1992). Corralling atrial fibrillation with "maze" surgery. *American Journal of Nursing, 92*(7): 34–38.

Kelso, L. A. (1992). Dysrhythmias associated with digoxin toxicity. *AACN Clinical Issues in Critical Care Nursing, 3*(1), 220–225.

Kinney, M. R., et al. (1991). *Comprehensive cardiac care* (7th ed.). St. Louis: Mosby Year Book.

Klein, M. D. (1991). Atrial fibrillation: New findings about an old nemesis. *Hospital Practice, 26*(11), 75–76, 78, 81–82.

Kleinpell, R. M. (1992). The use of adenosine to treat paroxysmal supraventricular tachycardia: A case study. *Heart & Lung, 21*(2), 187–188.

Kopecky, S. L. (1992). Management decisions in lone atrial fibrillation. *Hospital Practice, 27*(6), 135–138, 143, 147–150.

Kopp, D. E., et al. (1992). Palpitations and arrhythmias: Separating the benign from the dangerous. *Postgraduate Medicine, 91*(1), 241–244, 247–248, 251.

Kuhrik, N., et al. (1992). Defibrillation over the phone. *American Journal of Nursing, 92*(11), 28–31.

Loebl, S., et al. (1991). *The nurse's drug handbook* (6th ed.). Albany: Delmar Publishers.

Lynn, L. A., et al. (1992). Coronary precautions: Should caffeine be restricted in patients after myocardial infarction? *Heart & Lung, 21*(4), 365–371.

Lynn-McHale, D. J., et al. (1991). Epicardial pacing after cardiac surgery. *Critical Care Nurse, 11*(8), 62–66, 68–74, 76–77.

Manion, P. A. (1993). Temporary epicardial pacing in the postoperative cardiac surgical patient. *Critical Care Nurse, 13*(2), 30–38.

*Marriott, H. J. L. (1988). *Practical electrocardiography* (8th ed.). Baltimore: Williams & Wilkins.

Mason, P., et al. (1992). Implantable cardioverter defibrillator: A review. *Heart & Lung, 21*(2), 141–147.

*Matteson, M. A., & McConnell, E. S. (1988). *Gerontological nursing: Concepts and practice.* Philadelphia: W. B. Saunders.

McKenry, L. M., & Salerno, E. (1992). *Mosby's pharmacology in nursing* (18th ed.). St. Louis: C. V. Mosby.

Merva, J. (1993). A closer look at the heart SAECG. *RN, 56*(5), 51–53.

Metzger, B., & Therrien, B. (1990). Effect of position on cardiovascular response during the Valsalva maneuver. *Nursing Research, 39*(4), 198–202.

Moser, S. A., et al. (1993). Updated care guidelines for patients with automatic implantable cardioverter defibrillators. *Critical Care Nurse, 11*(3), 62–71.

Niemann, J. T. (1992). Current concepts: Cardiopulmonary resuscitation. *New England Journal of Medicine, 327*(15), 1075–1080.

Owen, P. M. (1991). *Sudden cardiac death: Theory and practice.* Gaithersburg, MD: Aspen Systems.

Porterfield, L. M., et al. (1992). Automatic cardioverter-defibrillator. *Critical Care Nurse, 12*(1), 13–14.

Porterfield, L. M., & Porterfield, J. G. (1993). Radiofrequency ablation of a left-sided free-wall accessory pathway: A case study. *Critical Care Nurse, 11*(3), 46–49.

Repique, L. J., et al. (1992). Atrial fibrillation 1992: Management strategies in flux. *Chest, 101*(4), 1095–1103.

Sachter, J. J. (1992). Magnesium in the 1990s: Implications for acute care. *Topics in Emergency Medicine, 14*(1), 23–50.

Schoenbaum, M. P., et al. (1991). Proarrhythmia: Mechanisms, evaluation, and treatment. *Critical Care Nursing Quarterly, 14*(2), 10–18.

Sheehy, S. B. (1992). *Emergency nursing: Principles and practice* (3rd ed.). Philadelphia: Mosby Year Book.

Snowberger, P. (1991). Wandering atrial pacemaker. *RN, 54*(9), 36–37.

Snowberger, P. (1992). Sinus arrhythmia. *RN, 55*(1), 50–51.

Snowberger, P. (1993). Second-degree AV block. *RN, 56*(2), 43–45.

Snowberger, P. (1993). Third-degree heart block. *RN, 56*(6), 52–54.

Sorenson, L. M., et al. (1992). The maze procedure: A new treatment for atrial fibrillation. *AACN Clinical Issues in Critical Care Nursing, 3*(1), 209–219.

Strong, A. G. (1991). Nursing management of postoperative dysrhythmias. *Critical Care Nursing Clinics of North America, 3*(4), 709–715.

Teplitz, L. (1991). Nursing diagnoses for automatic implantable cardioverter defibrillator patients. *Dimensions in Critical Care Nursing, 10*(4), 188–201.

Teplitz, L. (1991). Surgical treatment of ventricular arrhythmias: Historical and current perspectives. *Critical Care Nursing Quarterly, 14*(2), 41–59.

Thelan, L. A., et al. (1990). *Textbook of critical care nursing: Diagnosis and management.* St. Louis: C. V. Mosby.

*Underhill, S. L., et al. (1989). *Cardiac nursing* (2nd ed.). Philadelphia: J. B. Lippincott.

Underhill, S. L., et al. (1990). *Cardiovascular medications for cardiac nursing.* Philadelphia: J. B. Lippincott.

Vaska, P. L. (1992). Sudden cardiac death in young athletes: A review for nurses. *AACN Clinical Issues in Critical Care Nursing, 3*(1), 243–254.

SUGGESTED READINGS

Berry, S. L., & Schleicher, C. A. (1992). Adjusting the beat: What to teach about antiarrhythmics. *American Journal of Nursing, 92*(6), 28–32.

This article discusses the mechanism of action of each class of antidysrhythmic agents. It provides a table reviewing five major antidysrhythmic agents, outlining their mechanism of action, dosage, serum drug level, possible side effects, client teaching, and nursing implications. The article includes useful explanations to incorporate when the nurse is teaching clients about their medications.

Collins, M. A. (1994). When your patient has an implantable cardioverter defibrillator. *American Journal of Nursing, 94*(3), 34–39.

This article provides an overview and update on implantable cardioverter defibrillators (ICDs). Types of ICDs and the nursing care and documentation involved are discussed. Special considerations during emergency treatment are also described.

Drew, B. J. (1992). Using cardiac leads the right way. *Nursing 92, 22*(5), 50–54.

This article stresses the need for correct electrocardiographic (ECG) electrode placement to obtain the most information for accurate interpretation of ECGs in dysrhythmia. It artistically demonstrates clearly the placement of electrodes for each lead. It summarizes the usefulness of certain leads, particularly MCL1.

Green, E., et al. (1992). Charting the future of emergency drug protocols. *Nursing 92, 22*(6), 55–57.

This article presents the advances that have been made in emergency drug administration as well as the controversies surrounding certain drugs. Drug dosages and methods of administration are discussed. It also includes precautions to consider when administering certain emergency drugs.

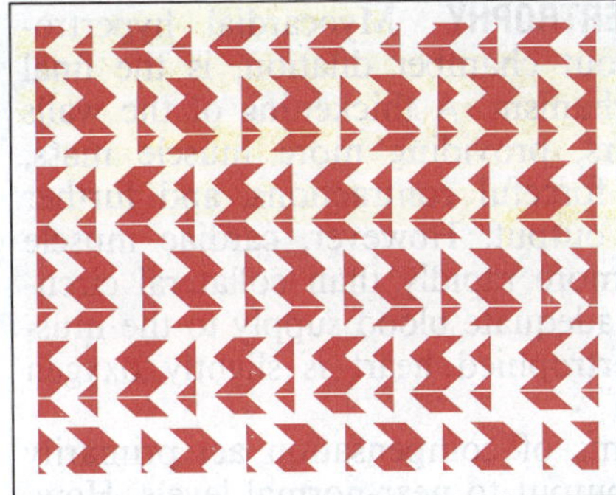

CHAPTER 34

Interventions for Clients with Cardiac Problems

CHAPTER HIGHLIGHTS

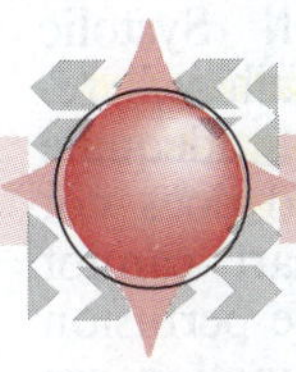

Primary cardiac dysfunction may have a number of causes, including impaired cardiac muscle function, structural cardiac defects, infections within the heart, and inflammatory conditions of the heart. Although most Americans do not consider heart disease an incurable illness, more people die of heart disease than of any other disorder. Moderately severe heart failure and dilated cardiomyopathy have 2-year survival rates of only 50%. Long-term survival of clients with heart disease depends on a coordinated interdisciplinary approach to ensure the best management of the illness and the highest possible quality of life.

Heart Failure

OVERVIEW

Heart failure, also called cardiac failure or pump failure, is the inability of the heart to pump sufficient blood to meet the demands of the body. Heart failure was once called "congestive heart failure" (CHF), but this term is not accurate because congestion, or fluid, is not always evident. Heart failure may be due to either increased cellular demands or, more commonly, impaired pumping of the heart. When the heart fails, cardiac output is diminished and peripheral tissue is not adequately perfused. Congestion of the lungs and periphery may also develop.

PATHOPHYSIOLOGY

COMPENSATORY MECHANISMS

When cardiac output is insufficient to meet the demands of the body, compensatory mechanisms operate to improve cardiac output. Although the compensatory mechanisms may initially increase cardiac output, they eventually have a damaging effect on pump function. Compensatory mechanisms include:

- Increased heart rate
- Improved stroke volume
- Arterial vasoconstriction
- Sodium and water retention
- Myocardial hypertrophy

In heart failure, stimulation of the sympathetic nervous system represents the most immediate compensatory mechanism. Stimulation of the adrenergic receptors causes an increase in heart rate and vasoconstriction.

INCREASED HEART RATE Because cardiac output equals heart rate times stroke volume, an increase in heart rate results in an immediate increase in cardiac output. The increase in heart rate is limited in its ability to compensate for decreased cardiac output. If the heart rate becomes too rapid, diastolic filling time is limited and cardiac output may start to fall.

IMPROVED STROKE VOLUME Stroke volume is also improved by sympathetic stimulation. With sympathetic stimulation, there is increased venous return to the heart, which stretches the myocardial fibers further. This increased stretch is referred to as *preload.* In accordance with Starling's law of the heart, increased myocardial stretch results in more forceful contraction, increasing stroke volume and cardiac output. However, after a critical point is reached, further volume and stretch reduce cardiac output.

ARTERIAL VASOCONSTRICTION Sympathetic stimulation also results in arterial vasoconstriction. Constriction of arteries has the beneficial effect of maintaining blood pressure and redistributing cardiac output in low-output states. However, constriction of arteries also increases *afterload,* the resistance against which the heart must pump. Afterload is the major determinant of myocardial oxygen requirements. As afterload increases, the left ventricle requires more energy to eject its contents and stroke volume may decline.

RETENTION OF SODIUM AND WATER Reduced blood flow to the kidneys, a common occurrence in low-output states, results in the activation of the renin-angiotensin-aldosterone mechanism. Vasoconstriction becomes more pronounced in response to angiotensin, whereas aldosterone secretion causes sodium and water retention. The volume of blood returning to the left ventricle is further increased by activation of this mechanism.

MYOCARDIAL HYPERTROPHY Myocardial hypertrophy, with or without chamber dilation, is the final compensatory mechanism. A thickening of the walls of the heart occurs, providing more muscle mass, resulting in more forceful contractions, and further increasing cardiac output. However, cardiac muscle may hypertrophy more rapidly than collateral circulation can provide adequate blood supply to the muscle. Often, a hypertrophied heart is slightly oxygen deprived.

These mechanisms of compensation act primarily to restore cardiac output to near-normal levels. However, during heart failure, these cardiac and peripheral circulatory adjustments may harm pump function. All of them contribute to an increase in myocardial oxygen consumption. When this occurs and myocardial reserve has been exhausted, clinical manifestations of heart failure develop.

CLASSIFICATION OF HEART FAILURE

Heart failure can be classified in many ways. Several important categories are discussed here.

SYSTOLIC VERSUS DIASTOLIC DYSFUNCTION Systolic dysfunction, sometimes called "forward failure," results when the heart is unable to eject adequate amounts of blood into the circulation and does not effectively empty itself. Because the heart cannot maintain an adequate cardiac output, tissue perfusion is diminished. Symptoms of systolic dysfunction are usually symptoms of decreased organ or system functioning. Diastolic failure, sometimes called "backward failure," represents a relaxation and filling abnormality of the ventricles. An increase in preload results in increased volume and pressure in the pulmonary vessels and pulmonary and/or systemic congestion.

LEFT VERSUS RIGHT VENTRICULAR FAILURE Because the two ventricles of the heart represent two separate pumping systems, it is possible for one to fail alone for a short period. Most heart failure begins with failure of the left ventricle and progresses to failure of both ventricles. Typical causes of left ventricular failure include:

- Hypertensive disease
- Coronary artery disease
- Valvular disease (involving the mitral or aortic valve)

Decreased tissue perfusion from poor cardiac output and pulmonary congestion from increased pressure in the pulmonary vessels indicate left ventricular failure.

Right ventricular failure may be caused by:

- Left ventricular failure
- Right ventricular myocardial infarction
- Pulmonary hypertension

In right ventricular failure, the right ventricle is unable to empty completely, increased volume and pressure develop in the systemic veins, and systemic venous congestion and peripheral edema develop. Figure 34–1 illustrates the pathophysiology of heart failure.

LOW-OUTPUT VERSUS HIGH-OUTPUT SYNDROME Low-output syndrome, the more common type of heart failure, occurs when the heart fails as a pump, resulting in impaired peripheral circulation and peripheral vasoconstriction. When cardiac output remains normal or above normal but the metabolic needs of the body are not met, high-output syndrome is present. It may be caused by:

- Increased metabolic needs (hyperthyroidism, fever, pregnancy)
- Hyperkinetic conditions (arteriovenous fistulas, Paget's disease)

FUNCTIONAL STATUS Heart failure may also be categorized by its effect on the client's functional status. Table 32–2 summarizes the New York Heart Association (NYHA) categories.

ETIOLOGY

The most common cause of heart failure is myocardial infarction (MI). The next most common causes are conditions such as systemic hypertension and pulmonary stenosis, which cause pressure or volume overload on the heart. Other direct causes of heart failure are myocardial dysfunction, filling disorders, and increased metabolic demand. Some of the

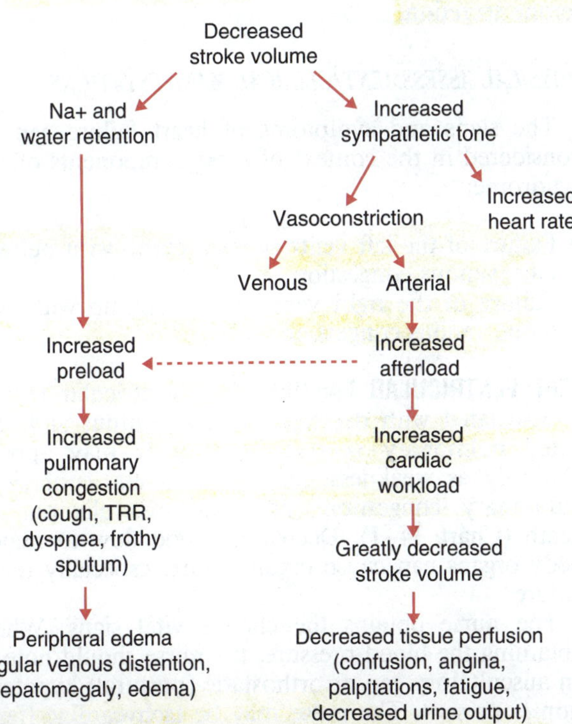

FIGURE 34–1 ◆ Pathophysiology of heart failure.

TABLE 34–1 Causes of Heart Failure

Pressure Overload
- Hypertension
- Aortic stenosis
- Hypertrophic cardiomyopathy

Volume Overload
- Aortic incompetence
- Mitral incompetence
- Tricuspid incompetence
- Overtransfusion
- Left-to-right shunts
- Hypervolemia

Myocardial Dysfunction
- Cardiomyopathy
- Myocarditis
- Coronary artery disease
- Ischemia
- Infarction
- Dysrhythmias
- Toxic disorders

Filling Disorders
- Mitral stenosis
- Tricuspid stenosis
- Cardiac tamponade
- Restrictive pericarditis

Increased Metabolic Demand
- Anemias
- Fever
- Beriberi
- Paget's disease
- Arteriovenous fistula

Reproduced by permission from Michaelson, C. R. (Ed.). (1983) *Congestive heart failure* (p. 45). St. Louis: C. V. Mosby.

conditions capable of causing heart failure are listed in Table 34–1.

INCIDENCE/PREVALENCE

Heart failure occurs most commonly in older adults, and its prevalence increases with age; 75% of clients with heart failure are older than 60 years. There are approximately 60 people with heart failure per 1000 population in the age group 65 years and older, but the prevalence increases to 100 per 1000 in people older than the age of 75 years (Wilson, 1992). Heart failure is more common in men than women at all ages. Approximately 50% of people with moderately severe heart failure survive 2 years.

COLLABORATIVE MANAGEMENT

ASSESSMENT

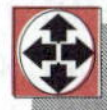

Manifestations of heart failure depend on the type of failure, the ventricle involved, and the underlying cause. Impaired tissue perfusion, pulmonary congestion, and edema dominate the picture of left ventricular failure. Systemic venous congestion and peripheral edema are associated with right ventricular failure.

HISTORY

When taking a history, the nurse should keep in mind the many conditions that can lead to heart failure. The nurse carefully questions the client about past medical history, including a history of high blood pressure, angina, myocardial infarction, rheumatic heart disease, valvular disorders, endocarditis, and pericarditis.

The nurse asks about the client's perception of his or her activity tolerance, breathing pattern, urinary pattern, and fluid volume status and the client's knowledge about heart failure.

LEFT VENTRICULAR FAILURE With left ventricular systolic dysfunction, the cardiac output is diminished, impaired tissue perfusion results, and the client often reports unusual fatigue. The nurse assesses the client's activity tolerance by asking if the client can perform normal activities of daily living (ADL) or climb flights of stairs without dyspnea (difficult breathing). Clients should be asked about their ability to perform simultaneous arm and leg work (e.g., walking while carrying a bag of groceries). Such activity may place an unacceptable demand on the failing heart. The client may describe weakness or fatigue as a feeling of heaviness in the arms and the legs. The nurse should ask clients to name their most strenuous activity in the past week. Many clients unconsciously limit their activities in response to fatigue or dyspnea and may not realize how limited they have become.

Cough may be the first manifestation because blood backs up behind the left ventricle into the pulmonary vessels. The client in early heart failure describes the cough as irritating, nocturnal, and usually nonproductive. As heart failure becomes more severe, the client may begin expectorating frothy pink-tinged sputum, a sign of pulmonary edema.

Decreased cerebral perfusion resulting from low cardiac output leads to changes in mental status. Confusion may occur with even mild or moderate heart failure in the older client. The nurse asks the client and his or her family members if any lapses in memory or periods of disorientation have occurred.

Perfusion to the myocardium is often impaired, especially if cardiac muscle has hypertrophied. The client may report chest discomfort or may describe palpitations, skipped beats, or a fast heartbeat.

Dyspnea, or abnormally uncomfortable breathing, is caused by a failing left ventricle, rising pulmonary venous pressure, and pulmonary congestion. The nurse carefully questions the client about the presence of dyspnea and when and how it developed. The client may refer to dyspnea as trouble in catching one's breath, breathlessness, or difficulty in breathing.

As exertional dyspnea develops, the client discontinues previously tolerated levels of activity owing to shortness of breath. Dyspnea at rest in the recumbent position is known as *orthopnea.* The nurse asks whether the client usually uses a number of pillows to sleep or sleeps in an upright position in a bed or a chair.

Clients who describe sudden awakening with a feeling of breathlessness 2 to 5 hours after falling asleep have paroxysmal nocturnal dyspnea. Sitting upright, dangling the feet, or walking usually relieves this condition.

RIGHT VENTRICULAR FAILURE Fluid volume changes result in peripheral edema. Edema develops in the lower legs and ascends to the thigh and the abdominal walls. Clients may note that shoes fit more tightly or indentations may develop on their swollen feet from shoes or socks. Clients may indicate that they have removed their rings because of swelling in their fingers and hands. The nurse asks the client about weight gain. An adult may retain 4 to 7 L of fluid (10 to 15 pounds [4.5 to 6.8 kg]) before pitting edema occurs.

Gastrointestinal complaints of nausea and anorexia may be a direct consequence of the liver engorgement due to fluid retention. Another finding related to fluid retention is diuresis at rest. The client describes frequent awakening at night to urinate. At rest, the body's metabolic requirements are decreased; cardiac function improves, decreasing systemic venous pressure. Edema fluid is thus mobilized and excreted.

The nurse takes a careful nutritional history, questioning the client about the use of salt and the types of food consumed. The nurse also questions the client concerning daily fluid intake. Clients in heart failure may experience increased thirst and take in excessive fluid (4000 to 5000 mL) because of aldosterone secretion.

PHYSICAL ASSESSMENT/CLINICAL MANIFESTATIONS

The signs and symptoms of heart failure can be considered in the context of these components of the syndrome:

- Failure of the left ventricle as a pump with pulmonary venous congestion
- Failure of the right ventricle as a pump with systemic venous congestion

LEFT VENTRICULAR FAILURE Left ventricular failure is associated with decreased cardiac output and elevated pulmonary venous pressure. It may appear clinically as weakness, fatigue, dizziness, confusion, pulmonary congestion, breathlessness, oliguria, or death (Chart 34–1). Decreased blood flow to major body organs can cause organ failure, especially renal failure.

The nurse obtains the client's vital signs. When obtaining the blood pressure, the nurse should note if an auscultatory gap or orthostatic (postural) hypotension is present. The pulse may be tachycardiac (fast) or may alternate in strength (pulsus alternans). The

CHART 34–1

Key Features of Left-Sided Heart Failure

Decreased Cardiac Output

- Fatigue
- Oliguria during the day
- Angina
- Confusion, restlessness
- Dizziness
- Tachycardia, palpitations

Pulmonary Congestion

- Hacking cough, worse at night
- Dyspnea
- Crackles in lungs
- Frothy pink-tinged sputum
- Tachypnea

nurse takes the apical pulse for a full minute, noting any irregularity in heart rhythm. An irregular heart rhythm resulting from premature atrial or ventricular contractions and atrial fibrillation is common in clients with heart failure. The nurse monitors the client's respiratory rate, rhythm, and character. The respiratory rate usually exceeds 20 breaths per minute.

The nurse also determines whether the client is oriented to person, place, and time. If there are concerns about orientation, a short mental status examination may be used (see Chapter 40). Objective data are important because many people are skillful at covering up memory losses in daily conversation.

The nurse palpates the precordium. Increased heart size is common, with a displacement of the apical impulse to the left. On auscultation, the nurse may hear a third heart sound (S_3) gallop, an early diastolic filling sound indicating an increase in left ventricular pressure. A fourth heart sound (S_4) can also occur, although it is not a sign of failure but a reflection of decreased ventricular compliance.

When the nurse assesses the lungs, crackles may be present. Late inspiratory crackles and fine profuse crackles that repeat themselves from breath to breath and do not diminish with coughing indicate heart failure. Crackles are produced by intra-alveolar fluid and are frequently noted first in the dependent areas of the lungs. Usually, crackles develop in the bases and spread upward as the condition worsens. The nurse identifies precisely the location of the crackles. Wheezes may also be auscultated.

RIGHT VENTRICULAR FAILURE Right ventricular failure is associated with increased systemic venous pressures. It gives rise to the clinical signs of jugular vein distention, hepatomegaly, dependent edema, and ascites (Chart 34–2).

On inspection, the nurse assesses the neck veins for distention (see Chap. 32). The nurse also measures the client's abdominal girth and assesses for the presence of hepatomegaly (liver engorgement), ascites, and jaundice. The collection of fluid in the abdomen (ascites) can reach volumes of more than 10 L.

In addition, the nurse examines the client for dependent edema. In the ambulatory client, edema is normally located in the ankles and legs. However, when the client is restricted to bed rest, the sacrum is dependent and edema accumulates there. Edema is an extremely unreliable sign of right ventricular failure so the nurse must weigh the client to document fluid retention.

PSYCHOSOCIAL ASSESSMENT

Acute episodes of heart failure may be precipitated in susceptible people by stressful life situations. Older adults may have acute exacerbations of heart failure in response to feelings of rejection, insecurity, frustration, or rage. The nurse needs to question clients sensitively about any recent stressors in their lives. The nurse asks clients to rate their current level of stress and describe any significant recent life changes.

Many clients with heart failure have symptoms that are not well controlled. These clients may have anxiety and frustrations related to dealing with a chronic illness. The nurse assesses clients and their families for fears, anxieties, and frustrations and also assesses their usual methods of coping (see Chapter 7).

Hope is a major determinant of well-being for clients in heart failure. Clients who are hopeful tend to feel better and to be more socially involved. Hopeful clients may be ignoring or suppressing certain realities of their illness, continuing with their lives despite their limitations. The nurse might ask clients what activities they engage in and who the significant people are in their life and how often they are able to interact with them.

LABORATORY ASSESSMENT

Electrolyte imbalance in heart failure reflects complications of failure as well as the use of diuretics and other drug therapies. Any impairment of renal function may be reflected by elevated blood urea nitro-

CHART 34–2

Key Features of Right-Sided Heart Failure

- Jugular venous distention
- Enlarged liver
- Anorexia and nausea
- Dependent edema (legs and sacrum)
- Polyuria at night

gen, serum creatinine, and creatinine clearance levels. Urinalysis may reveal proteinuria and high specific gravity.

Arterial blood gas values reveal hypoxia, because oxygen does not diffuse easily through fluid-filled alveoli. Respiratory alkalosis occurs because of hyperventilation; respiratory acidosis occurs because of carbon dioxide retention.

RADIOGRAPHIC ASSESSMENT

Chest x-rays can be helpful in diagnosing left ventricular failure. Typically, the cardiac silhouette is enlarged, representing hypertrophy or dilation. Pleural effusions develop less often and generally reflect biventricular failure.

OTHER DIAGNOSTIC ASSESSMENT

The electrocardiogram (ECG) demonstrates ventricular hypertrophy, dysrhythmias, and any degree of myocardial ischemia, injury, or infarction. It is not helpful in determining the presence or extent of heart failure.

Echocardiography is useful in diagnosing cardiac valvular changes, pericardial effusion, chamber enlargement, and ventricular hypertrophy. Radionuclide studies (thallium imaging or technetium pyrophosphate scanning) can also indicate the presence and cause of heart failure. Multigated angiographic (MUGA) scans provide information about left ventricular ejection fraction and velocity.

Pulmonary artery catheters allow direct measurement of cardiac pressures. These measurements are often necessary for the diagnosis and management of heart failure. The right atrial pressure may be normal in left ventricular failure and elevated in right ventricular failure. Pulmonary artery pressure and pulmonary artery wedge pressure (PAWP) are elevated in left-sided heart failure, because cardiac output is decreased. (See Chapter 32 for a more detailed description of the pulmonary artery catheter.)

ANALYSIS

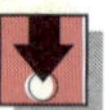

COMMON NURSING DIAGNOSES

The most common nursing diagnoses pertinent to the client with heart failure are:

1. Decreased Cardiac Output related to a reduction in stroke volume as a result of mechanical malfunctions
2. Impaired Gas Exchange related to altered oxygen supply
3. Activity Intolerance related to an imbalance between oxygen supply and demand, fatigue, or an electrolyte imbalance
4. High Risk for Inability to Sustain Spontaneous Ventilation related to pulmonary edema and respiratory muscle fatigue

ADDITIONAL NURSING DIAGNOSES

In addition to the common nursing diagnoses, some clients have one or more of the following diagnoses:

- Ineffective Individual Coping related to physical inactivity, major changes in lifestyle, loss of control over body function, or fear of death
- Altered Sexuality Patterns related to the effects of illness
- Hopelessness related to the effects of deteriorating physical status
- Altered Thought Processes related to impaired gas exchange or fear of the unknown
- Impaired Physical Mobility related to fatigue and activity intolerance

PLANNING AND IMPLEMENTATION

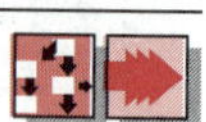

DECREASED CARDIAC OUTPUT

PLANNING: CLIENT GOALS The primary goal is that the client will resume and maintain an adequate cardiac output as evidenced by the following:

- A heart rate within the baseline value
- No signs of impaired tissue perfusion
- No dependent edema
- Clear lungs
- No neck vein distention
- Normal blood pressure

INTERVENTIONS Interventions are aimed at improving cardiac output. A clinical pathway for congestive heart failure is found on page 895. Therapy may be directed toward optimizing the two major components of cardiac output:

- Stroke volume (determined by preload, afterload, and contractility)
- Heart rate

Interventions to optimize stroke volume include:

- Reducing preload
- Reducing afterload
- Improving cardiac muscle contractility

Reducing Preload When ventricular fibers are overstretched, as in the failing heart, they contract less forcefully. Interventions aimed at preload reduction attempt to decrease volume and pressure in the left ventricle, optimizing ventricular muscle contraction.

DIET THERAPY In heart failure, diet therapy is aimed at reducing sodium and water retention.

Sodium Restriction. The physician may restrict sodium intake in an attempt to decrease fluid retention. Many clients with heart failure need to omit only

OUR LADY OF LOURDES MEDICAL CENTER
CRITICAL PATHWAY
CONGESTIVE HEART FAILURE DUE TO LEFT VENTRICULAR DYSFUNCTION NOT REQUIRING ADMISSION TO A CRITICAL CARE UNIT

	DAY #1 DATE____	DAY#2 DATE____	DAY#3 DATE____	DAY#4 DATE____
LOCATION OF PATIENT	CARDIOLOGY FLOOR (PREFERRED) OR MED SURG FLOOR	CARDIOLOGY FLOOR (PREFERRED) OR MED-SURG FLOOR	CARDIOLOGY FLOOR (PREFERRED) OR MED-SURG FLOOR	CARDIAC FLOOR (PREFERRED) OR MED SURG FLOOR
RESPONSIBLE SERVICE	INTERNAL MEDICINE OR CARDIOLOGY	INTERNAL MEDICINE OR CARDIOLOGY	INTERNAL MEDICINE OR CARDIOLOGY	INTERNAL MEDICINE OR CARDIOLOGY
CONSULTS	CARDIOLOGY, DIETARY AND PATIENT EDUCATION, AS NECESSARY. CARDIAC REHAB	CARDIOLOGY, DIETARY AND PATIENT EDUCATION, AS NECESSARY. CARDIAC REHAB	CARDIOLOGY, DIETARY AND PATIENT EDUCATION, AS NECESSARY. CARDIAC REHAB	CARDIOLOGY, DIETARY AND PATIENT EDUCATION, AS NECESSARY. CARDIAC REHAB
LAB	BUN, CREATININE, LYTES, BLOOD GLUCOSE, ALBUMIN, URIC ACID, CBC, URINALYSIS. IF ACUTE MI IS BEING EXCLUDED, CK ON ADMISSION AND Q8H X3. CK-MB IF TOTAL CK ELEVATED	BUN, CREATININE, LYTES	BUN, CREATININE, LYTES, DIGOXIN LEVEL.	NONE
RADIOLOGY	CHEST X-RAY, PA AND LATERAL	NONE	CHEST X-RAY, PA AND LATERAL	NONE
OTHER TESTS	EKG ON ADMISSION AND FOR ANGINA AS PER PROTOCOL - CHEST LEAD LOCATIONS MARKED WITH PEN. CARDIAC ECHO - DOPPLER ORDERED FOR DAY 1 OR DAY 2. PULSE OXIMETRY.	ECHO - DOPPLER HEART IF NOT DONE DAY 1	NONE	NONE
ACTIVITY	BED REST, DANGLE TID, OR OUT OF BED, AS TOLERATED	AMBULATE AS TOLERATED	AMBULATE AD LIB	AMBULATE AD LIB
NURSING CARE	CHECK AND RECORD BP, HEART RATE, AND RESPIRATORY RATE ON ADMISSION, 1 HR AFTER ADMISSION AND Q 2 HRS UNTIL STABLE. AFTER STABLE, RECORD BP HR, AND RR Q 4 H. CHECK AND RECORD TEMPERATURE ON ADMISSION AND Q 8 H THEREAFTER. WEIGH PATIENT ON ADMISSION (USE BED OR CHAIR SCALE IF NECESSARY: ESTIMATED WEIGHT NOT ALLOWED) I&O. ARRHYTHMIA AND ANGINA CARE PER PROTOCOLS.	RECORD I&O. MEASURE AND RECORD BP, HR, RR, AND TEMP EVERY 8 HOURS. RECORD AND EVALUATE RHYTHM STRIPS IF PATIENT ON TELEMETRY. WEIGH DAILY IN AM (POST-VOID, PRE-PRANDIAL). ARRHYTHMIA AND ANGINA CARE PER PROTOCOLS.	MEASURE AND RECORD BP, HEART RATE, RESP RATE Q 4 H. RECORD TEMP Q 8 H. WEIGH DAILY (POST-VOID), PRE-PRANDIAL).	ENCOURAGE AMBULATION
LINES, MONITORS, AND TUBES	TELEMETRIC MONITORING IF INDICATED. TEXAS OR FOLEY CATHETER AS INDICATED. PRN ADAPTER. SUPPLEMENTAL O2 PRN SOB, CHEST PAIN, OR O2 SAT<93%.	PRN ADAPTER. TELEMETRIC EKG MONITOR IF INDICATED. REMOVE TEXAS OR FOLEY CATHETER. O2, PRN SOB, CHEST PAIN, OR O2 SAT<93%.	DISCONTINUE TELEMETRIC MONITORING. REMOVE PRN ADAPTER AFTER TELEMETRY D/C'D. D/C O2 SUPPLEMENT.	NONE
MEDS	INTRAVENOUS DIURETICS. LOW DOSE ORAL ACE INHIBITOR. DIGOXIN LOAD, IF APPROPRIATE. ORAL OR CUTANEOUS NITRATES. MOM PRN. MAALOX, MYLANTA, PRN. TYLENOL PRN. DAYTIME SEDATIVE PRN. HS SEDATIVE PRN. HEPARIN 5000 U SC Q 12 H WHILE PATIENT IS NON-AMBULATORY. COLACE 100 MG BID.	IV DIURETIC; SWITCH TO ORAL DIURETIC IF DIURESIS ADEQUATE. CONTINUE ORAL OR CUTANEOUS NITRATE AS INDICATED. ACE INHIBITOR; INCREASE DOSE AS TOLERATED. DIGOXIN, MAINTENANCE DOSE. MOM PRN. MAALOX, MYLANTA PRN. TYLENOL PRN. DAYTIME SEDATIVE PRN. HS SEDATIVE PRN. D/C S.C. HEPARIN WHEN PATIENT AMBULATORY.	ORAL DIURETIC; ADJUST DOSAGE AS INDICATED. ORAL OR CUTANEOUS NITRATE. ACE INHIBITOR; INCREASE DOSE AS TOLERATED. DIGOXIN. MOM PRN. MAALOX, MYLANTA PRN. TYLENOL PRN. DAYTIME SEDATIVE PRN. HS SEDATIVE PRN.	ORAL DIURETIC. ORAL OR CUTANEOUS NITRATE. ACE INHIBITOR. DIGOXIN. MOM PRN. MAALOX, MYLANTA PRN. TYLENOL PRN.
DIET	CARDIAC DIET (3 GM SODIUM, LOW CHOLESTEROL) AS TOLERATED.	CARDIAC DIET	CARDIAC DIET	CARDIAC DIET
PATIENT AND FAMILY EDUCATION	UNIT AND ROOM ORIENTATION. EXPLANATION OF MEDS. INTRODUCTION TO CRITICAL PATHWAY. EXPLAIN ADVANCED DIRECTIVES.	EXPLANATION OF MEDS TO PATIENT AND FAMILY. REHAB TEACHING AS PER PROTOCOL.	EXPLANATION OF MEDS TO PATIENT AND FAMILY. REHAB TEACHING AS PER PROTOCOL. DIET INSTRUCTIONS.	FINAL REVIEW OF MEDICATIONS, DIET, AND DISCHARGE INSTRUCTIONS.
DISCHARGE PLANNING	SOCIAL SERVICES CONSULT AS INDICATED. HOME HEALTH SERVICES CONSULT AS INDICATED.		REMIND PATIENT THAT DISCHARGE IS PLANNED FOR AM OF DAY 4. NOTIFY FAMILY OF PLANNED DISCHARGE AND MAKE TRANSPORTATION ARRANGEMENTS. SOCIAL SERVICES RE-EVALUATION. CONFIRM ARRANGEMENTS FOR HOME HEALTH.	ASSIST PATIENT IN PREPARING TO LEAVE HOSPITAL AND WITH TRANSPORTATION ARRANGEMENTS. PATIENT DISCHARGED TO HOME.

THIS CRITICAL PATHWAY HAS BEEN DEVELOPED TO SERVE AS A GUIDELINE FOR THE "BEST CASE" MANAGEMENT OF PATIENTS HOSPITALIZED PRIMARILY FOR THE ABOVE NOTED DIAGNOSIS OR PROCEDURE WITHOUT COMPLICATING COMORBIDITIES.

ser:msw:weber\chf1

Clinical Pathway: Congestive heart failure. (Courtesy of Our Lady of Lourdes Medical Center, Camden, NJ.)

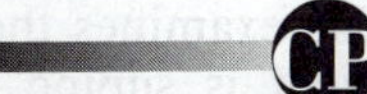

table salt (no added salt) from their diet, thus reducing the sodium intake to 1.5 g/day. If salt intake must be reduced further, the client may need to eliminate all salt in cooking, thus reducing sodium intake to 1.2 to 1.4 g/day. For clients with more severe heart failure, a strict low-sodium diet limits the salt intake to 0.2 to 1 g of sodium per day. The nurse collaborates with the dietitian to help the client select food that meets the prescribed therapeutic diet. Table 14–5 lists the sodium content of some common foods.

Fluid Volume Restriction. Few clients are placed on severe fluid restrictions. However, because clients with excessive aldosterone secretion may experience thirst and drink 3 to 5 L of fluid each day, their fluid intake may be limited to a more normal 2 L/day. Compliance with these simple strategies may be high, especially if the client experiences relief of any of the symptoms of volume excess. When a fluid restriction is imposed on the hospitalized client, the nurse adjusts oral and intravenous (IV) therapy accordingly.

The nurse weighs the client daily (1 kg of weight gain or loss equals 1 L of retained or lost fluid, respectively) and keeps accurate records of fluid intake and output. The same scale should be used every morning before breakfast for the most accurate assessment of weight.

DRUG THERAPY Common drugs prescribed to reduce preload are diuretics and venous vasodilators. Some of these drugs are described in Chart 34–3.

Diuretics. The physician adds diuretics to the regimen when diet and fluid restriction have not been effective in the management of heart failure. Diuretics are primarily effective for clients with pulmonary congestion and systemic vascular congestion. Diuretics enhance renal excretion of sodium and water by:

- Reducing the circulating blood volume
- Decreasing preload
- Reducing systemic and pulmonary congestion

The type and dosage of diuretic prescribed depend on the degree of heart failure and renal function. The high-ceiling (loop) diuretics, furosemide (Lasix, Furoside♣) and ethacrynic acid (Edecrin), are most effective for treating volume overload. However, the physician may initially use a thiazide diuretic, such as hydrochlorothiazide (Hydro-DiURIL, Urozide♣), for elderly clients. The action of the thiazide diuretic is self-limiting (i.e., diuresis decreases after edema fluid is lost). Thiazide diuretics may be preferred for older clients who are susceptible to dehydration and even vascular collapse from excessive diuresis with loop diuretics (Chart 34–4).

For many clients, loop diuretics are needed to ensure effective diuresis. The nurse must check orthostatic blood pressures in the elderly client receiving loop diuretics to detect volume depletion. The nurse also examines the client for flat neck veins when the client is supine, a loss of skin turgor, and a slow progressive weight loss despite an adequate diet. All of these signs, plus disorientation in the older client, may indicate excessive diuresis and volume depletion.

The nurse also needs to monitor for and prevent potassium deficiency (hypokalemia) from diuretic therapy, especially in the elderly. The signs of hypokalemia are nonspecific neurologic and muscular complaints, such as generalized weakness, depressed reflexes, and irregular heart rate. Therefore, to accurately identify hypokalemia, the physician and the nurse monitor serum potassium levels.

If the client's serum potassium levels are low, the physician has several alternatives:

- Adding a potassium-sparing diuretic to the regimen
- Requesting that clients increase their intake of potassium-rich foods diet
- Prescribing a potassium supplement

Venous Vasodilators. The physician may prescribe venous vasodilators for the client in heart failure. To compensate for the client's reduced cardiac output, significant constriction of venous and arterial blood vessels occurs, reducing the volume of fluid that the vascular bed can hold and increasing the preload. Venous vasodilators may benefit clients by:

- Return the venous vasculature to a more normal capacity
- Decreasing the volume of blood returning to the heart
- Improving left ventricular function

Nitrates may be administered intravenously, orally, or topically. These drugs cause primarily venous vasodilation but also a significant amount of arteriolar vasodilation. It is essential for the nurse to monitor the client's blood pressure when initiating nitrate therapy or increasing the dosage. Clients may initially report headache. The nurse should assure clients that they will develop a tolerance to this effect and the headache will cease or diminish. Unfortunately, when nitrates are uniformly administered during 24 hours, clients may also develop tolerance to the vascular effects, ceasing to respond to nitrates with vasodilation. Therefore, to prevent such tolerance, the physician may order the nitrate administration to be stopped for 8 to 12 hours of each day.

Reducing Afterload By relaxing arterioles, arterial vasodilators can reduce impedance to left ventricular ejection (afterload) and improve cardiac output. In the strictest sense, these drugs do not act as vasodilators but reverse some of the inappropriate or excessive vasoconstriction that is common in heart failure.

The use of angiotensin-converting enzyme (ACE) inhibitors, a group of arterial vasodilators, generally prolongs and improves the quality of life of clients in heart failure (see Chart 34–3). These medications suppress the renin-angiotensin-aldosterone system,

CHART 34–3

Therapy for Cardiac Failure

Drug	Usual Dosage	Nursing Interventions	Rationale
Drugs Used Primarily to Reduce Preload			
Diuretics Furosemide (Lasix, Furoside🍁)	• 40 mg qd or bid PO • 40 mg qd IV push • **Elderly:** Older adults may be more sensitive to the effects of the usual adult dose.	• Administer once daily when the client arises.	• The volume and frequency of urination increase for 6–8 hr after an oral dose.
		• Assess the client for adequate diuresis. Obtain daily weights (in the morning before breakfast). Note changes in breath sounds and edema.	• Weight is one of the most accurate noninvasive measurements of volume status.
		• Monitor the client's serum electrolytes (especially K^+, Na^+, and Cl^-). Provide K^+ supplementation if prescribed.	• Loop diuretics may produce excessive loss of these electrolytes.
		• Monitor the client for signs of dehydration. (Check for hypotension, dry mucous membranes, poor skin turgor, thirst, and oliguria.)	• Loop diuretics continue to cause diuresis even after the excessive fluid has been removed.
		• Note any report of ringing in the ears (tinnitus).	• Ringing in the ears may indicate toxicity.
Nitrates Isosorbide dinitrate (Isordil, Isonate, Coronex🍁, Novosorbide🍁)	• PO (tablet) 15–30 mg q6h • PO (sustained release) 40 mg q6–12h	• Observe the client for postural hypotension. Supervise ambulation until the dose response is determined.	• Relaxation of venous smooth muscle causes blood to pool in the veins when the client stands.
Nitroglycerin (Nitro-Dur)	• Transdermal ointment: starting dose of ½ inch q4–8h increasing to ½ inch q4–8h	• Identify whether the client is experiencing a headache. Inform the physician and provide relief.	• Headache diminishes with tolerance. Mild analgesics should provide relief until then.
Nitroglycerin (Nitrodisc)	• Transdermal patch: 2.5–15 mg/24 hr	• Administer PO dose 30 min before or 2 hr after meals. (If headache is a consistent problem, administering with meals may help.) Make sure the client does not chew.	• Oral nitrates are most rapidly absorbed from an empty stomach.
		• Administer the ointment on a hairless part of the body in a uniform layer using an applicator.	• Proper administration ensures consistent dose administration.
		• If so prescribed, allow a nitrate-free period at night.	• An 8- to 12-hr nitrate-free period prevents the development of tolerance to the vasodilating effect of nitrates.

Chart continued on following page

CHART 34-3

Therapy for Cardiac Failure *Continued*

Drug	Usual Dosage	Nursing Interventions	Rationale
		• Rotate the skin sites of transdermal nitrate administration.	• Nitrates cause skin irritation.
		• Remove transdermal nitrates before defibrillation.	• Skin burns have occurred, and explosion is possible.
Drugs Used Primarily to Reduce Afterload			
Angiotensin-Converting Enzyme Inhibitors Captopril (Capoten)	• To start: 6.25–12.5 mg PO tid • May increase to 50–100 mg PO tid	• Monitor the client's blood pressure closely for several hours after the first dose. Consult with the physician to determine the desired range for blood pressure.	• Hypotension may occur as a first-dose effect. It is most common in Na^+- or volume-depleted clients.
		• Monitor the serum potassium level carefully.	• Clients with impaired renal function may develop hyperkalemia.
		• Report fever and sore throat to the physician. Monitor the results of the complete blood count.	• Neutropenia, although rare, can be a hazardous complication.
Enalapril maleate (Vasotec)	• To start: 2.5–5 mg/day • May increase to 10–40 mg/day as a single dose or divided doses	• Administer 1 hr before or 2 hr after meals.	• Administration on an empty stomach enhances absorption.
		• Enalapril is similar to captopril but may be administered less frequently and with food.	• Enalapril has a longer half-life than captopril.
Cardiac glycosides Digoxin (Lanoxin, Novodigoxin✹)	• Loading dose of 1 mg divided over 24 hr • Then maintenance 0.125–5 mg PO qd • Usually 0.25–5 IV	• Ask the client about previous use of digitalis; provide the preparation previously taken. (Do not substitute one preparation for another.)	• Dosages, absorption rates, and duration of effects differ among drugs.
Digitoxin (Crystodigin) (infrequently used)	• Loading dose of 1.2–1.6 mg divided during 24 hr • Then 0.1 mg daily IV or PO	• Be alert for the following: • Myocardial infarction • Hypokalemia • Renal or hepatic disorders • Diuretic therapy • Diarrhea • Advanced age • Metabolic alkalosis	• Any of these factors may result in an increased sensitivity to digitalis and increase the risk of toxicity.
		• Monitor serum potassium levels and electrocardiograms.	• Hypokalemia is often associated with digitalis toxicity and dysrhythmias.
		• Take the apical pulse or check the cardiac monitor pattern before administering each dose of digitalis.	

CHART 34–3

Therapy for Cardiac Failure *Continued*

Drug	Usual Dosage	Nursing Interventions	Rationale
		• Monitor serum levels of digitalis. Therapeutic digoxin level is 0.9–2 ng/mL.	• There is a narrow margin between therapeutic and toxic doses of digitalis. Toxicity occurs in approximately 10% to 20% of clients receiving digitalis.
		• Observe for signs of digitalis toxicity and notify the physician if any occur: • Confusion • Dysrhythmias • Nausea or vomiting • Fatigue • Muscle weakness	

which was activated in response to decreased renal blood flow. ACE inhibitors benefit clients by:

- Reducing arterial resistance
- Decreasing pulmonary artery wedge pressure
- Increasing stroke volume and cardiac output

The physician usually starts ACE inhibitor doses slowly and cautiously. If the client is volume-depleted, administration of an ACE inhibitor may bring about a rapid drop in blood pressure. The nurse assesses the client's hydration status before beginning therapy with a prescribed ACE inhibitor (such as captopril). After the initial dose and each increased dose, the nurse monitors the client's blood pressure for several hours.

The nurse clarifies with the physician the guidelines for administering the vasodilator. For example, many physicians maintain clients in heart failure at systolic blood pressures ranging from 90 to 110 mmHg. When such a blood pressure is the client's maintenance level, the nurse assesses the client for orthostatic hypotension, confusion, poor peripheral perfusion, and reduced urinary output. Table 34–2 compares the effects of selected agents that reduce the preload and/or the afterload. (IV medications used to decrease preload and afterload are described in Chapter 37.)

Improving Contractility Traditionally, cardiac glycosides, such as digitalis derivatives, have been prescribed indefinitely to increase contractility and to decrease heart rate for clients in heart failure. Clients who benefit the most from digitalis may be those with systolic dysfunction, third heart sounds, and atrial fibrillation (Braunwald, 1992). Because cardiac glycosides have a narrow therapeutic range, they must be administered only when it is clear that they will benefit the client.

ACTION OF DIGITALIS The potential benefits of digitalis derivatives are:

- An increase in contractility
- A reduction in heart rate

CHART 34–4

Nursing Focus on the Elderly ◆ Heart Failure

- Assess older clients with confusion for indications of heart failure. People older than 80 years often present with restlessness or confusion as the initial manifestation of heart failure.
- Auscultate the lungs carefully, recognizing that dependent crackles may not be an indication of heart failure in the older adult.
- Do not expect crackles to clear rapidly after treatment. Crackles may persist in the lung bases of older adults for an extended period after pulmonary congestion has decreased.
- Be especially alert for the signs of digitalis toxicity in the elderly client because it occurs frequently.
- If loop diuretics are used for diuresis, monitor the client closely for signs of excessive diuresis, dehydration, and hypokalemia.
- In older clients receiving drug therapy for heart failure, monitor for orthostatic hypotension. Cardiovascular changes associated with aging make this likely to develop.

TABLE 34–2 Effects of Vasodilators*

Drug	Preload Reduction (Vasodilates Peripheral Veins)	Afterload Reduction (Vasodilates Arterioles)
Nitrates (nitroglycerin, isosorbide dinitrate)	+++	+
Hydralazine hydrochloride (Apresoline)	0	+++
Nifedipine (Procardia)	0	++
Sodium nitroprusside (Nipride)	+++	+++
Captopril (Capoten)	+	++
Prazosin (Minipress)	++	+

*0, no effect; +, mild effect; ++, moderate effect; +++, maximal effect.

- A slowing of conduction through the atrioventricular (AV) node

Digitalis also may have a mild diuretic effect. At toxic digitalis levels, increased automaticity occurs and ectopic beats (PVCs) may result.

DIGITALIS TOXICITY The most commonly prescribed cardiac glycoside is digoxin (Lanoxin, Novodigoxin✱). Digoxin is erratically absorbed from the gastrointestinal tract. Many medications, especially antacids, interfere with its absorption. It is eliminated primarily by renal excretion. The half-life in middle-aged adults is 36 hours: in older adults with diminished renal function, the half-life may be about 48 hours. Thus, elderly clients are particularly susceptible to digoxin toxicity.

Toxicity occurs in 10% to 20% of all clients taking digoxin, more commonly in older clients and clients with hypokalemia (low potassium levels). In older adults, mortality from digitalis toxicity may approach 40%. The presentation of digitalis toxicity may be nonspecific: anorexia, muscular weakness, fatigue, and confusion. Toxicity may cause nearly any dysrhythmia, but premature ventricular contractions (PVCs) are most commonly noted. The nurse monitors the apical pulse rate and heart rhythm of clients receiving digoxin. The nurse must identify when the heart rate is less than 60 beats per minute or greater then 100 beats per minute and when there is a significant change in rhythm or rate. It is equally important for the nurse to report the development of an irregular rhythm in a client with a previously regular rhythm and a regular rhythm in a client with a previously irregular one. The nurse also monitors serum digoxin and potassium levels to identify toxicity. Therapeutic digoxin levels range from 0.9 to 2 ng/mL. Chart 34–3 presents information about selected cardiac glycosides.

Any medication that increases the workload of the failing heart also increases its oxygen requirement. The nurse should be alert for the possibility that the client may experience angina (chest pain) in response to digoxin. IV medications that increase contractility are described in Chapter 37.

IMPAIRED GAS EXCHANGE

PLANNING: CLIENT GOALS The goals are that the client will:

- Have a normal rate, rhythm, and depth of respiration
- Have normal arterial blood gas values

INTERVENTIONS The nurse monitors the client's respiratory rate, rhythm, and character every 1 to 4 hours, at the same time auscultating breath sounds. The oxygen content of the blood in clients with heart failure is markedly reduced because of pulmonary congestion. The nurse administers supplemental oxygen as prescribed by the physician and determined by the client's arterial blood gas values.

The nurse also places the client in high-Fowler's position to maximize chest expansion and improve oxygenation. Repositioning the client and having the client perform coughing and deep breathing exercises every 2 hours help to improve oxygenation and to prevent atelectasis.

ACTIVITY INTOLERANCE

PLANNING: CLIENT GOALS The goals are that the client:

- Will not experience shortness of breath with exertion
- Will be able to perform activities of daily living

INTERVENTIONS Initially, the client in heart failure requires physical and emotional rest. Nursing care should be organized to allow periods of uninterrupted rest. The nurse observes and documents the client's physiologic response to activity.

As the client's condition improves, the nurse may need to identify the client's response to mild exercise.

The exercise might be walking a prescribed distance or merely moving from bed to chair. The nurse takes the client's blood pressure and pulse before, during, and after the activity. A blood pressure change of more than 20 mmHg or a pulse increase of more then 20 beats per minute may indicate that the activity is too stressful. Other indications that the client cannot tolerate the activity include dyspnea, fatigue, and chest pain.

HIGH RISK FOR INABILITY TO SUSTAIN SPONTANEOUS VENTILATION

PLANNING: CLIENT GOALS The goal is that the client will continue to maintain ventilation of adequate rhythm, rate, and depth.

INTERVENTIONS The nurse assesses clients for acute pulmonary edema, a life-threatening event that results from severe heart failure. The left ventricle fails to eject sufficient blood, and pressure increases in the lungs because of the accumulated blood. The increased pressure causes fluid to leak across the pulmonary capillaries and into the pulmonary interstitium. The client in pulmonary edema is usually extremely anxious, is tachycardiac, and has air hunger. He or she may have a moist cough productive of frothy, blood-tinged sputum, and the client's skin may be cold, clammy, or cyanotic. For the client who has acute pulmonary edema, the physician prescribes rapid-acting diuretics, such as furosemide (Lasix, Furoside♣). These diuretics are given intravenously over 1 to 2 minutes, usually at a starting dose of 40 mg and another 40 mg repeated if needed.

Oxygen is always ordered, and the client is placed in high-Fowler's position. IV morphine sulfate may be given, 1 to 2 mg at a time, to reduce venous return (preload), but the nurse should monitor respiratory rate and blood pressure closely. The physician may also order aminophylline (Aminophyllin, Corophyllin♣) to relieve bronchospasm. Vasodilators, such as nitroglycerin (Tridil) and sodium nitroprusside (Nipride), may be administered via continuous infusion pumps, but low dosages of these drugs must be given initially and increased slowly to avoid severe hypotension.

Once commonly used to decrease preload, rotating tourniquets and phlebotomy are now used rarely during the wait for medications to be effective. The nurse inserts a Foley catheter, if ordered, to assess the client's urinary output after diuretic administration and to minimize exertion related to voiding. Diuresis normally begins within 5 minutes of the administration of IV furosemide and peaks at 30 minutes. Chart 34–5 summarizes the care of the client with acute pulmonary edema.

Clients often respond dramatically and quickly to these interventions, but their condition can also deteriorate rapidly because of pulmonary congestion and severe hypoxemia. Clients frequently require intubation and ventilation to survive the acute episode. A skilled nurse is needed to assist with intubation. (Management of the client who is critically ill with heart failure is detailed in Chapter 37.)

DISCHARGE PLANNING

HOME CARE PREPARATION

For many clients, heart failure is a chronic disorder. Activity restrictions at home after hospital discharge range from minimal (New York Heart Association functional class I) to strict (functional class IV) for clients who have symptoms at rest (see Table 32–2).

The nurse, the occupational therapist, or the discharge planner evaluates the home environment, considering activity restrictions. The nurse determines whether the client needs to climb stairs and asks about the location of the bathroom and the bedroom. Clients with strict activity restrictions should avoid stair climbing, and alternative arrangements for toileting and sleeping may be required. For example, if a bathroom is not available on the same floor as the other rooms, clients may need to use a bedside commode and sponge bathe until they can climb stairs. The family or significant other may add a bathroom and/or a bedroom to the same floor if the client is not expected to get substantially stronger and the resources are available.

HEALTH TEACHING

The nurse assists clients in planning to reach an optimal level of functioning within the limits of their

CHART 34–5

Nursing Care Highlight ◆ Care of the Client with Pulmonary Edema

- Identify the client's chief complaint.
- If the client's blood pressure is adequate, place the client in high-Fowler's position.
- Auscultate the client's lungs briefly (posterior assessment).
- Ensure that vascular access is present and check for patency.
- Provide oxygen as ordered.
- Provide IV diuretic (usually furosemide) as prescribed.
- Anticipate urinary output in 5 to 15 minutes after diuretic administration; catheterize if ordered.
- Monitor blood pressure, respiratory rate, pulse, and cardiac rhythm, and the client's subjective feelings of ability to breathe.
- Provide additional medications as prescribed (usually morphine sulfate or nitroglycerin).
- Notify the physician if the client does not have a rapid improvement and diuresis.

cardiac function. The goal for clients who have experienced heart failure is to maximize rehabilitation gains and to prevent recurrent acute episodes. Activity schedules during all stages of heart failure are individualized to maintain the client without symptoms, or as symptom-free as possible. The nurse instructs the client to begin walking 200 to 400 feet/day and to increase the distance slowly during the first week. The client should try to walk at least three times/week but should discontinue this if symptoms such as dyspnea and chest pain occur.

The nurse and the client identify factors that might precipitate symptoms. The nurse instructs the client to watch for and report a weight gain of more than 2 pounds/day for 3 successive days, swelling of the ankles and feet, a persistent cough, or frequent urination during the night. Circumstances when the client should contact his or her health care provider include:

- Rapid weight gain (2 pounds/day for 2 or 3 days)
- Decrease in exercise tolerance lasting 2 to 3 days
- Cold symptoms lasting more than 3 to 5 days
- Excessive awakening at night to urinate
- Development of dyspnea or angina at rest

The nurse provides oral and written instructions about the medication regimen. If the client is taking digoxin, the family and the client are taught how to count a pulse rate. The nurse explains how to take the pulse daily and record it. Chart 34–6 lists instructions for the client taking digoxin at home. The nurse advises clients taking diuretics to take them in the morning to avoid waking during the night for voiding. The nurse reviews the signs and symptoms of hypokalemia with clients who are taking potassium-wasting diuretics (such as furosemide). The nurse instructs clients to report the occurrence of side effects to their physician or other health care provider. The nurse or the dietitian also supplies written information on high-potassium foods to clients and the people who will be managing or assisting with meal preparation (see Chap. 14).

Clients with chronic heart failure are advised to restrict their dietary sodium. The nurse or the dietitian provides written instructions on low- or restricted-sodium diets. Clients are also instructed to confer with their physician if they want to use commercial salt substitutes. Most salt substitutes contain potassium, and the renal status needs to be considered before one can recommend these products. To enhance the flavor of low-salt foods, the nurse suggests that clients use lemon, garlic, and herbs.

CHART 34–6

Education Guide ◆ Digoxin Therapy

- Noon is the best time of day to take this medication if you can remember to take it then.
- Continue administration of this medication unless you are told to stop it by your health care provider.
- Do not take digoxin at the same time as antacids or cathartics (laxatives).
- Take your pulse rate before taking each dose of digoxin. Notify your health care provider of a change in pulse rate (60 to 90 beats per minute is normal) or rhythm as well as increasing fatigue, muscle weakness, confusion, or loss of appetite (signs of digitalis toxicity).
- If you forget to take a dose, it may be delayed a few hours. However, if you do not remember it until the next day, you should take only your usual daily dose.
- Report for scheduled laboratory test (such as potassium and digoxin levels).
- If potassium supplements are prescribed, continue the dose until told to stop by your health care provider.

PSYCHOSOCIAL PREPARATION

Clients with chronic heart failure must make necessary adjustments in lifestyle. They must adhere to a medical regimen that includes dietary restrictions, activity restrictions, and drug therapy. Clients need careful, concise explanations of the treatment plan. Kison (1992) noted that education was a major factor in compliance with the follow-up regimen (Research Applications for Nursing).

The nurse encourages the client to verbalize fears and concerns about his or her illness and assists the client in exploring appropriate coping skills. Clients' participation in treatment can help alleviate and control symptoms.

HEALTH CARE RESOURCES

A home care nurse may be needed to assess the client's adherence to medication and diet therapy and to monitor for worsening heart failure. Clients with activity restrictions benefit from the services of a home care aide. A dietitian might be consulted to assist with menu planning and teaching. A physical therapist may be needed at home for the continuation of rehabilitation, including ambulation and exercise.

The American Heart Association is an excellent community resource for pamphlets, books, cookbooks, and videotapes related to heart failure and heart disease as well as a referral for various support groups in the community.

EVALUATION

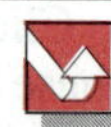

On the basis of the identified nursing diagnoses, the nurse evaluates the care of the client with heart failure.

RESEARCH APPLICATIONS FOR NURSING

Education Promotes Compliance Among Clients with Heart Disease

Kison, C. (1992). Health beliefs and compliance of cardiac patients. *Applied Nursing Research, 5,* 181–185.

This study examines the relationship between health beliefs and the compliance of clients with cardiac disease with their cardiac regimen, including checkups, drug therapy, and diet therapy. Thirty-one subjects, ranging from 41 to 70 years old, participated in the study. In general, the subjects reported the highest degree of compliance with their drug regimens. They were least compliant with interventions for stress reduction and management. College-educated subjects reported more benefits to physician checkups and were more compliant with the activity regimen than non–college-educated subjects. Some subjects admitted to smoking, even after heart surgery.

Critique This study examines an area that is essential in the rehabilitation of people with heart disease. It reaffirms that some people are more compliant than other people with secondary prevention in the management of their chronic illness. However, the sample was small and chosen from one cardiac rehabilitation program.

Possible nursing implications Nurses need to recognize that education is a major factor in compliance with cardiac follow-up care. More studies are needed to identify other factors and how nurses can be more effective in ensuring client compliance.

Expected outcomes may include that the client will:

- Demonstrate an adequate cardiac output as evidenced by blood pressure and pulse within desired levels, mental alertness, adequate urinary output, and strong peripheral pulses
- Demonstrate an acceptable fluid balance as evidenced by adequate urinary output, normal lung sounds, absence of edema, maintenance of weight, good skin turgor, and moist mucous membranes
- Tolerate gradual increases in activity without dyspnea, chest pain, fatigue, or changes in vital signs
- Demonstrate normal air exchange as evidenced by normal rate, rhythm, and depth of respiration and arterial blood gas values within acceptable limits
- Administer medications safely and recognize possible side and toxic effects
- Identify when he or she should contact the health care provider

Valvular Heart Disease

OVERVIEW

Valvular heart disease occurs when the heart valves cannot open fully (valvular stenosis) or close completely (valvular insufficiency or regurgitation). Acquired valvular dysfunctions most often involve the left side of the heart, especially the mitral valve. Acquired valvular dysfunctions in rank order of occurrence are:

- Mitral stenosis
- Mitral insufficiency
- Mitral valve prolapse
- Aortic stenosis
- Aortic insufficiency

The tricuspid valve is involved infrequently, and the pulmonic valve is affected rarely. Often, stenosis and regurgitation occur simultaneously in a defect called a mixed lesion. The following discussion covers the most common dysfunctions of the mitral and aortic valves.

MITRAL STENOSIS

PATHOPHYSIOLOGY

Mitral stenosis usually results from rheumatic carditis (see later). Rheumatic carditis can cause valve thickening by fibrosis and calcification. The valve leaflets fuse and become stiff, whereas the chordae tendineae contract and shorten. The valvular orifice narrows, preventing normal blood flow from the left atrium to the left ventricle. As a result of these changes:

- The left atrial pressure rises
- The left atrium dilates
- Pulmonary artery pressures increase
- The right ventricle hypertrophies

Pulmonary congestion and right-sided heart failure occur. The left ventricle receives insufficient end-diastolic blood volume, and thus the cardiac output is decreased.

Clients with mild mitral stenosis are usually asymptomatic. As the valvular orifice narrows, the client experiences dyspnea on exertion, orthopnea, paroxysmal nocturnal dyspnea (sudden dyspnea at night), and dry cough. As the pulmonary hypertension and congestion progress, hemoptysis and pulmonary edema appear. Right-sided heart failure can cause hepatomegaly, neck vein distention, and pitting edema late in the disorder.

The pulse may be normal on palpation, tachycardiac, or irregularly irregular, as in atrial fibrillation. Because the development of atrial fibrillation indicates that the client may decompensate, the physician should be notified immediately. On auscultation, the nurse notes a rumbling, apical diastolic murmur.

ETIOLOGY

Rheumatic fever is most often the cause of mitral stenosis. Nonrheumatic causes include atrial myxoma (tumor), calcium accumulation, and thrombus formation.

INCIDENCE/PREVALENCE

Two thirds to three fourths of all clients with mitral stenosis are women. About two thirds of the women with rheumatic mitral stenosis are younger than age 45.

MITRAL INSUFFICIENCY (REGURGITATION)

PATHOPHYSIOLOGY

The fibrotic and calcific changes occurring in mitral regurgitation cause the mitral valve to fail to close completely, allowing a backflow of blood. During the *systolic* phase, a great deal of pressure is generated within the left ventricle. Lack of closure of the mitral valve allows leakage of blood into the left atrium during ventricular systole. During the *diastolic* phase, regurgitant output is returned with the normal blood flow from the left atrium to the left ventricle, increasing the volume that must be ejected during systole. To compensate for the increased volume and pressure, the left atrium and ventricle dilate and hypertrophy.

Mitral insufficiency usually progresses slowly; clients may remain symptom-free for decades. Symptoms begin to occur when the left ventricle fails in response to increased blood volumes. The client most often reports fatigue and chronic weakness as a result of reduced cardiac output. Dyspnea on exertion and orthopnea develop later. Nursing assessment may reveal normal vital signs, atrial fibrillation, or changes in heart rate and respirations characteristic of left ventricular failure.

When right-sided heart failure results from left ventricular dysfunction, the neck veins become distended, the liver enlarges (hepatomegaly), and pitting edema is noted. On auscultation, the nurse hears a high-pitched systolic murmur at the apex, with radiation to the left axilla. Severe regurgitation often exhibits a third heart sound.

ETIOLOGY

Rheumatic heart disease is the predominant cause of mitral insufficiency. When mitral insufficiency results from rheumatic heart disease, it usually coexists with some degree of mitral stenosis. Nonrheumatic causes include papillary muscle dysfunction or rupture due to ischemic heart disease, infective endocarditis, and a congenital anomaly.

INCIDENCE/PREVALENCE

Mitral regurgitation resulting from rheumatic heart disease is more common in women than in men. Mitral regurgitation of a nonrheumatic etiology occurs more often in men.

MITRAL VALVE PROLAPSE

PATHOPHYSIOLOGY

Mitral valve prolapse occurs because the valvular leaflets enlarge and prolapse into the left atrium during systole. Usually, this is a benign abnormality, but it may progress to pronounced mitral regurgitation.

Most clients with mitral valve prolapse are asymptomatic. Clients may report chest pain, palpitations, or exercise intolerance. Atypical chest pain is a common complaint that clients describe as a sharp pain localized to the left side of the chest. Dizziness, syncope, and palpitations may be associated with atrial or ventricular dysrhythmias.

On physical examination, the nurse usually finds a normal heart rate and blood pressure. On auscultation, the first heart sound may be followed by a nonejection systolic click.

ETIOLOGY

The etiology of mitral valve prolapse is variable and is associated with a number of conditions, such as endocarditis, myocarditis, and acute or chronic rheumatic heart disease. Mitral valve prolapse is also present in otherwise apparently healthy people. A familial occurrence is well established.

INCIDENCE/PREVALENCE

Mitral valve prolapse affects 5% to 10% of people (Braunwald, 1992). Although it is present in all age groups, it is most common in women between the ages of 20 and 54.

AORTIC STENOSIS

PATHOPHYSIOLOGY

In people with aortic stenosis, the aortic valve orifice narrows, obstructing left ventricular outflow during systole. This increased resistance to ejection or afterload results in ventricular hypertrophy. As the stenosis progresses, the cardiac output becomes fixed. Increases in cardiac output are not possible with exertion. Because the left atrium may be unable to empty completely, the pulmonary system becomes congested. Eventually, right-sided heart failure can result.

The classic symptoms of aortic stenosis are dyspnea on exertion, angina, and syncope on exertion. When cardiac output falls in the late stages of the disease, the client has marked fatigue, debilitation, and peripheral cyanosis. A diamond-shaped systolic crescendo-decrescendo murmur is usually noted on auscultation.

ETIOLOGY

Congenital valvular disease or malformation is the predominant etiologic factor in aortic stenosis. Rheumatic aortic stenosis is always concomitant with rheumatic disease of the mitral valve. The client's age when the condition manifests itself usually suggests its cause. Congenital aortic stenosis with a bicuspid or a unicuspid valve occurs most frequently in persons younger than age 30. In clients between ages 30 and 70, it is attributed equally to congenital malformation and to rheumatic heart disease. Atherosclerosis and degenerative calcification of the aortic valve are the predominant factors in people older than age 70.

INCIDENCE/PREVALENCE

Aortic stenosis has become the most common valvular disorder in countries with aging populations. Of clients with aortic stenosis, 80% are men (Braunwald, 1992).

AORTIC INSUFFICIENCY (REGURGITATION)

PATHOPHYSIOLOGY

In clients with aortic insufficiency, the aortic valve leaflets do not close properly during diastole, and the annulus (the valve ring that attaches to the leaflets) may be dilated, loose, or deformed. This allows a regurgitation of blood from the aorta back into the left ventricle during diastole. The left ventricle, in compensation, dilates to accommodate the greater blood load and eventually hypertrophies.

Clients with aortic regurgitation remain asymptomatic for many years because of the compensatory mechanisms of the left ventricle. As the disease progresses and left ventricular failure occurs, the principal concerns of the client are exertional dyspnea, orthopnea, and paroxysmal nocturnal dyspnea. The client with severe disease may note palpitations, especially while lying on the left side. Many clients with aortic regurgitation experience nocturnal angina with diaphoresis (profuse sweating).

On palpation, the nurse notes a "bounding" arterial pulse. The pulse pressure is usually widened, with an elevated systolic pressure and diminished diastolic pressure. The classic auscultatory finding is a high-pitched, blowing, decrescendo diastolic murmur.

ETIOLOGY

Aortic insufficiency is less frequently caused by rheumatic heart disease. Nonrheumatic causes include infective endocarditis, congenital anatomic aortic valvular abnormalities, hypertension, and Marfan's syndrome (a rare, generalized, systemic disease of connective tissue).

INCIDENCE/PREVALENCE

Approximately 75% of clients with aortic regurgitation are men.

COLLABORATIVE MANAGEMENT

ASSESSMENT

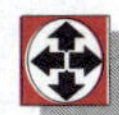

HISTORY

A client with valvular disease may have become ill at an early age or may have been disabled during the course of many years. The nurse collects information on the client's family health history, including valvular or other forms of heart disease to which the client may be genetically predisposed. The nurse questions the client about attacks of rheumatic fever, the specific dates when these occurred, and the use of antibiotic prophylaxis against recurrence of rheumatic fever. The nurse discusses the client's fatigue level, the level of activity that is tolerated, the presence of angina, and the occurrence of palpitations.

PHYSICAL ASSESSMENT/CLINICAL MANIFESTATIONS

The nurse obtains the client's vital signs, inspects the client for signs of edema, palpates and auscultates the client's heart and lungs, and palpates the client's peripheral pulses. Findings consistent with valvular malformation are summarized in Chart 34–7.

PSYCHOSOCIAL ASSESSMENT

Clients with valvular disorders often fear that symptoms will become worse and their disorders will progress to the point at which they may require surgery. Symptoms of shortness of breath or fatigue can interfere with activities of daily living. The nurse assesses for fears and frustrations related to these problems as well as coping skills of the client and the family.

LABORATORY ASSESSMENT

No laboratory tests are available to confirm a diagnosis of valvular heart disease.

RADIOGRAPHIC ASSESSMENT

In clients with mitral stenosis, the chest x-ray shows left atrial enlargement, prominent pulmonary arteries, and an enlarged right ventricle. In those with mitral regurgitation, the chest x-ray reveals an increased cardiac shadow, indicating left ventricular and left atrial enlargement.

In the later stages of aortic stenosis, the chest x-ray may show left ventricular enlargement and pulmonary congestion. In clients with aortic *insufficiency,* left atrial and left ventricular dilation appear on the

CHART 34–7

Key Features of Valvular Heart Disease

Mitral Stenosis	Mitral Insufficiency	Mitral Valve Prolapse	Aortic Stenosis	Aortic Insufficiency
• Fatigue • Dyspnea on exertion • Orthopnea • Paroxysmal nocturnal dyspnea • Hemoptysis • Hepatomegaly • Neck vein distention • Pitting edema • Atrial fibrillation • Rumbling, apical diastolic murmur	• Fatigue • Dyspnea on exertion • Orthopnea • Palpitations • Atrial fibrillation • Neck vein distention • Pitting edema • High-pitched holosystolic murmur	• Atypical chest pain • Dizziness, syncope • Palpitations • Atrial tachycardia • Ventricular tachycardia • Systolic click	• Dyspnea on exertion • Angina • Syncope on exertion • Fatigue • Orthopnea • Paroxysmal nocturnal dyspnea • Harsh, systolic crescendo-decrescendo murmur	• Palpitations • Dyspnea • Orthopnea • Paroxysmal nocturnal dyspnea • Fatigue • Angina • Sinus tachycardia • Blowing, decrescendo diastolic murmur
S_1 S_2 S_1 S_2 S_1	S_1 S_2 S_3 S_1 S_2 S_3	click click S_1 S_2 S_1 S_2	S_1 S_2 S_1 S_2	S_1 S_2 S_1 S_2 S_1

chest x-ray. If heart failure is present, pulmonary venous congestion is also evident.

OTHER DIAGNOSTIC ASSESSMENT

For clients with valvular heart disease, echocardiography is usually indicated because it is an excellent tool for defining abnormal movement of the valve leaflets. Exercise tolerance testing (ETT) is sometimes performed to evaluate symptomatic response, to assess functional capacity, and to enhance auscultatory findings.

In clients with either mitral or aortic stenosis, cardiac catheterization is frequently indicated to assess the severity of the stenosis and its other effects on the heart.

The physician also orders an electrocardiogram (ECG) to assess abnormalities such as left ventricular hypertrophy, as seen with mitral regurgitation and aortic regurgitation, or right ventricular hypertrophy, as seen in severe mitral stenosis. Atrial fibrillation is a common finding in both mitral stenosis and mitral regurgitation.

ANALYSIS

COMMON NURSING DIAGNOSIS

Clients with valvular disorders commonly have a diagnosis of Decreased Cardiac Output related to structural problems (narrow valves with decreased forward flow of blood or incompetent valves with backflow of blood).

ADDITIONAL NURSING DIAGNOSES

In addition to the common diagnosis, some clients may experience one or more of the following:

- Impaired Gas Exchange related to altered blood flow
- Activity Intolerance related to an imbalance between oxygen supply and demand
- Anxiety related to a threat to or a change in health status
- Altered (Cardiopulmonary) Tissue Perfusion related to interruption of blood flow

PLANNING AND IMPLEMENTATION

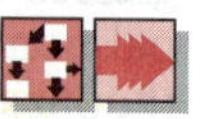

DECREASED CARDIAC OUTPUT

PLANNING: CLIENT GOALS The major goal is that the client will experience restoration and maintenance of hemodynamic status as evidenced by:

- A stable blood pressure and pulse rate
- Clear lung fields
- Mental alertness and orientation
- Adequate urinary output
- Improved activity tolerance

INTERVENTIONS Management of valvular heart disease depends on which valve is affected and the degree of valve impairment. Some clients can be managed without surgery, but other clients require open heart surgery and careful monitoring.

Nonsurgical Management Nonsurgical management includes drug therapy and rest.

Drug Therapy A major concern in valvular heart disease is maintaining cardiac output despite the development of atrial fibrillation. Atrial fibrillation occurs frequently in both mitral stenosis and mitral regurgitation because of distention of the atria. With mitral valvular disease, left ventricular filling is especially dependent on atrial contraction. When atrial fibrillation develops, atrial contraction is no longer effective. Cardiac output can decrease by 25% to 30%, and heart failure may occur. Ineffective atrial contraction may also lead to stasis of blood and thrombosis in the left atrium. For these reasons, therapy is instituted to restore normal sinus rhythm or, if that is unsuccessful, to slow the ventricular rate.

If medical therapy is instituted, digitalis is the drug of choice and is usually given intravenously. If digitalization slows the ventricular rate but atrial fibrillation does not resolve, quinidine gluconate (Quinaglute, Quinate✱) or procainamide hydrochloride (Pronestyl hydrochloride, Procan-SR) may be added to the regimen. A beta-blocking agent, such as propranolol hydrochloride (Inderal, Apo-Propranolol✱), or a calcium channel blocker, such as verapamil hydrochloride (Calan), may also be considered. If atrial fibrillation is rapid and the client is unresponsive to medical treatment, synchronized countershock (cardioversion) may be attempted.

When a client has valvular heart disease and chronic atrial fibrillation, anticoagulation with sodium warfarin (Coumadin, Warfilone✱) is usually a part of the medical treatment plan to prevent thrombus formation. Thrombi may form in the atria or on defective valve segments, resulting in systemic emboli. As a result, clients may experience one or more cerebrovascular accidents (CVAs). Therefore, the nurse assesses the client's baseline neurologic status and regularly reassesses the client for neurologic changes. Prophylactic antibiotic therapy is required for all clients with valve disease before any invasive procedure. Procedures for which clients require antibiotic coverage include bronchoscopy, endoscopy, sigmoidoscopy, colonoscopy, genitourinary instrumentations, surgery, and dental procedures of any type. Table 34–3 outlines appropriate antibiotic prophylaxis for clients with heart disease.

If left ventricular failure and pulmonary congestion are present in clients with valve disorders, digoxin, diuretics, vasodilating agents, and oxygen are also administered (see earlier).

Rest Rest is often an important part of treatment. Activity may be limited because the client's cardiac output cannot meet the increased metabolic demands, and angina or heart failure can result.

Surgical Management Surgical repair or replacement of heart valves has a major effect on the prognosis of valvular heart disease. Correct timing is crucial. Repair or replacement of the valve is usually performed before irreversible dysfunction occurs. Surgical therapy is the only definitive treatment of aortic stenosis and is recommended when left ventricular failure, angina, or syncope develops.

Reparative Procedures Reparative procedures are becoming popular because of continuing problems with thrombi, endocarditis, and left ventricular dysfunction after valvular replacement. Reparative procedures do not result in a normal valve, but they usually "turn back the clock," resulting in a more functional valve and an improvement in cardiac output. Turbulent blood flow through the valve often persists, and degeneration of the repaired valve is possible.

BALLOON VALVULOPLASTY Balloon valvuloplasty, an invasive nonsurgical procedure, is possible for stenotic mitral and aortic valves. Careful selection of clients is necessary; most clients selected for balloon valvuloplasty are older and are at high risk for surgical complications or have refused operative treatment. However, some young adults with noncalcified congenital aortic stenosis may also benefit.

The physician passes a balloon catheter from the femoral vein through the atrial septum and to the mitral valve. The balloon is then inflated, enlarging the mitral orifice. The physician inserts the catheter for aortic valvuloplasty through the femoral artery and advances it to the aortic valve, where it is inflated, enlarging the orifice.

After the procedure, the nurse observes the client closely for bleeding from the catheter insertion site and institutes precautions for arterial puncture if appropriate. Bleeding is likely after valvuloplasty because of the large size of the catheter. The nurse also observes the client for signs of a regurgitant valve by closely monitoring the client's heart sounds, cardiac output, and pattern on the monitor. Because vegetations (thrombi) may have been dislodged from the valve, the nurse observes for any indication of systemic emboli (see Endocarditis later in this chapter).

DIRECT, OR OPEN, COMMISSUROTOMY Direct commissurotomy, the reparative procedure of choice for those with pure mitral stenosis, is accomplished with cardiopulmonary bypass during open heart surgery. The surgeon visualizes the valve, removes thrombi from the atria, incises the fused commissures (leaflets), and debrides calcium from the leaflets widening the orifice.

MITRAL ANNULOPLASTY Mitral annuloplasty is the reparative procedure for mitral insufficiency in clients with a mobile, noncalcified valve. The annulus is the valve ring that attaches to and supports the leaflets. The physician may suture the leaflets to an annuloplasty ring or take tucks in the client's annulus. Leaflet repair is frequently performed at the same time. Elongated leaflets may be tucked over and shortened; shortened leaflets may be repaired by lengthening the chordae that bind them in place.

TABLE 34–3 Antibiotic Prophylaxis for Clients with Heart Disease

Procedure	Standard Regimen	For Clients Allergic to Penicillin
Dental procedures and surgery of the upper respiratory tract	• Penicillin alone • Parenteral-oral combined: aqueous crystalline penicillin G (1,000,000 U IM) mixed with procaine penicillin G (600,000 U IM). Give 30 min to 1 hr before the procedure and then give penicillin V (formerly called phenoxymethyl penicillin) 500 mg q6h PO for 8 doses. • Oral: penicillin V (2 g orally 30 min to 1 hr before the procedure PO and then 500 mg q6h for 8 doses PO)	• Erythromycin (1 g orally 1½–2 hr before the procedure)
Clients with prosthetic heart valves	• Penicillin plus streptomycin: aqueous crystalline penicillin G (1,000,000 U IM) mixed with procaine penicillin G (600,000 U IM) plus streptomycin (1 g IM). Give 30 min to 1 hr before the procedure; then penicillin V 500 mg q6h for 8 doses PO.	• Vancomycin (1 g IV over 30 min to 1 hr). Start initial vancomycin infusion ½–1 hr before the procedure; then erythromycin 500 mg q6h PO for 8 doses.
Genitourinary tract and gastrointestinal tract surgery or instrumentation*	• Aqueous crystalline penicillin G (2,000,000 U IM or IV) or ampicillin (1 g IM or IV) plus gentamicin (1.5 mg/kg—not to exceed 80 mg—IM or IV) or streptomycin (1 g IM). Give initial doses 30 min to 1 hr before the procedure. If gentamicin is used, give a similar dose of gentamicin and penicillin (or ampicillin) q8h for 2 additional doses.† If streptomycin is used, then give a similar dose of streptomycin and penicillin (or ampicillin) q12h for 2 additional doses.†	• Vancomycin (1 g IV given over 30 min to 1 hr) plus streptomycin (1 g IM). A single dose of these antibiotics begun 30 min to 1 hr before the procedure is probably sufficient, but the same dose may be repeated in 12 hr.†

* In clients with significantly compromised renal function, it may be necessary to modify the dosage of antibiotics used. Some of these dosages may exceed the manufacturer's recommendations for a 24-hr period. Because they are recommended only for a 24-hr period in most cases, however, it is unlikely that toxicity will occur.

† During prolonged procedures, or in case of delayed healing, it may be necessary to provide additional doses of antibiotics. For brief outpatient procedures such as uncomplicated catheterization of the bladder, one dose may be sufficient.

Annuloplasty and leaflet repair result in an annulus of the appropriate size and leaflets that can close completely. Thus, regurgitation is eliminated or markedly reduced. (Care of the client undergoing open heart surgery is discussed in more detail in Chapter 37.)

Replacement Procedures The development of prosthetic (synthetic) and biologic (tissue) valves has improved the surgical therapy and prognosis of valvular heart disease. Prosthetic valves come in a wide variety (Fig. 34–2). Although prosthetic valves are very durable, all clients must receive oral anticoagulation over a lifetime because of the possibility of clot formation.

Biologic valves are usually xenografts (valves from other species), such as porcine valve (from a pig) (Fig. 34–3) or a bovine valve (from a cow). However, homografts, valves donated from human cadavers, are also possible. Since tissue valves are associated with little risk of clot formation, long-term anticoagulation is not indicated. However, xenografts are not as durable as prosthetic valves and usually they must be replaced every 7 to 10 years.

The mitral valve should be replaced if the leaflets are calcified and immobile. The surgeon excises the valve during cardiopulmonary bypass surgery, and the new valve, either biologic or prosthetic, is sutured into place.

An aortic valve is replaced for most symptomatic adults with aortic stenosis and aortic insufficiency. As with mitral valve replacement, the surgeon excises the aortic valve during cardiopulmonary bypass surgery and sutures the new valve into place.

PREOPERATIVE CARE Clients undergoing valve surgery have open heart surgery similar to the procedure for clients undergoing a coronary artery bypass graft (CABG) (see Chap. 37). Ideally, surgery is an elective, planned procedure. Therefore, the nurse can assist in preparing the client by instructing the client and family members or a significant other about the

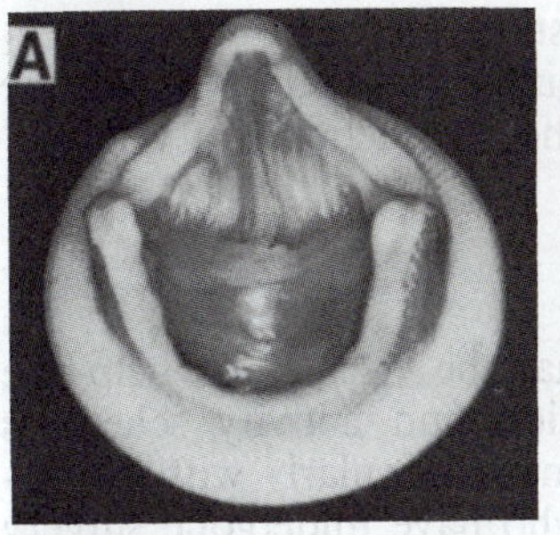

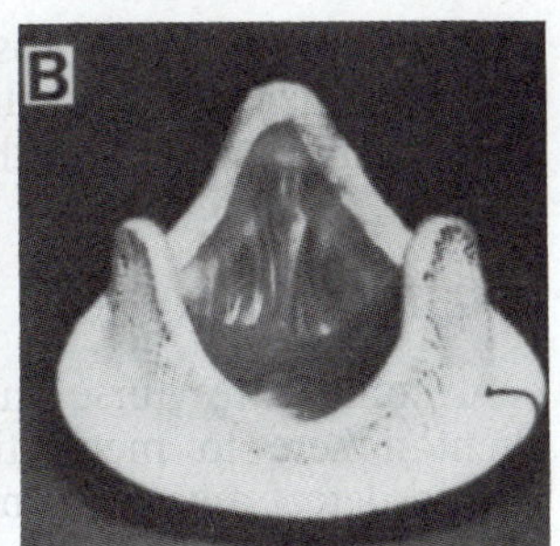

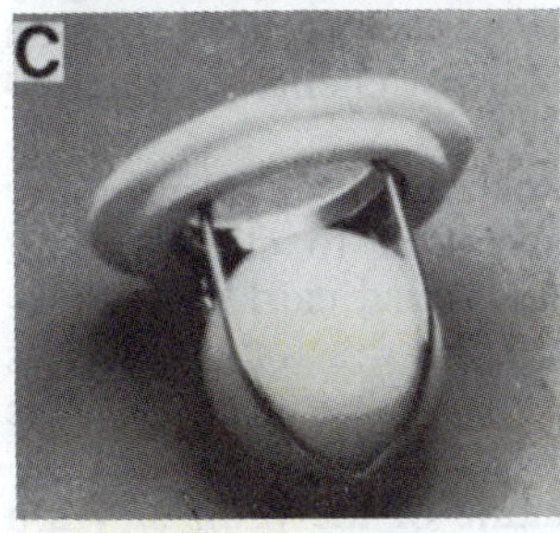

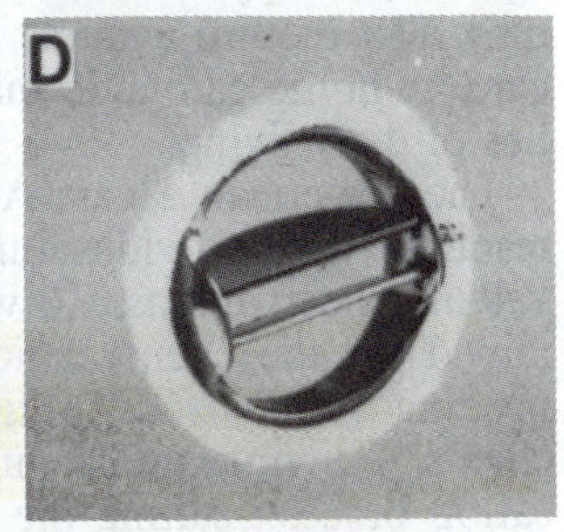

FIGURE 34–2 ◆ Prosthetic heart valves. *A*, Starr-Edwards. *B*, Björk-Shiley. *C*, Medtronic Hill. *D*, St. Jude Medical. (From Sabiston, D. C., Jr. [1991]. *Textbook of surgery: The biological basis of modern surgical practice* [14th ed.]. Philadelphia: W. B. Saunders.)

management of postoperative pain, incision care, and strategies to prevent respiratory complications (see Chaps. 19 and 21).

The nurse may also introduce the client and the family or the significant other to the staff and the environment of the surgical critical care unit, where the client will be transferred after surgery. Clients receiving oral anticoagulants stop taking these medications at least 72 hours before the procedure.

POSTOPERATIVE CARE Nursing interventions for clients undergoing open heart surgery for valve disorders are similar to those for clients undergoing a CABG (see Chap. 37). However, there are a few significant differences, First, because clients undergoing aortic valve replacements may be at a higher risk for postoperative hemorrhage than those undergoing CABG, the nurse is especially vigilant for indications of bleeding.

Clients with valve replacements are also more likely to have significant reductions in cardiac output postoperatively, especially those with aortic stenosis or left ventricular failure from mitral valve disease. The nurse is particularly attentive to monitoring the client's cardiac output and identifying any indications of pump failure. High filling pressures (pulmonary artery wedge pressure greater than 18 mmHg) may be required to maintain an acceptable cardiac output in the immediate postoperative period. The physician may prescribe digoxin (Lanoxin, Novodigoxin✽) for 3 to 6 months postoperatively to maintain cardiac output and to prevent atrial fibrillation. Clients who have had valve replacements with prosthetic valves require lifetime prophylactic anticoagulation therapy to prevent thrombus formation.

DISCHARGE PLANNING

HOME CARE PREPARATION

The client with valvular heart disease may be discharged home on medical therapy or postoperatively after valve repair or replacement. Because fatigue is a common problem for clients with valve disorders, the nurse helps the client and family ensure that the home environment is conducive to providing rest. If stair climbing overexerts the client and if access to the client's bedroom or bathroom is up or down stairs, alternative arrangements for sleeping and toileting need to be made. The client may benefit from the use of a bedside commode, a reclining chair, or a wheelchair to conserve energy.

HEALTH TEACHING

The teaching plan for the client with valvular heart disease includes:

- The disease process
- Medications, including diuretics, vasodilators, cardiac glycosides, antibiotics, and anticoagulants
- Prophylactic use of antibiotics
- Good oral hygiene
- A plan of work, activity, and rest to conserve energy
- The purpose and nature of surgical intervention, if appropriate

Because these clients are at risk for infective endocarditis, the nurse teaches them to brush their teeth twice a day with a soft manual toothbrush, followed by oral rinses. Clients are instructed to avoid irrigation devices, electric toothbrushes, and flossing, because these activities may cause gums to bleed, allowing bacteria to enter mucous membranes and the bloodstream. The nurse advises frequent checkups by a dentist who is aware of the client's valve disorder.

The nurse instructs clients to inform all health care providers of the valvular heart disease history before any treatment; the clients are also told that they require antibiotic administration before all invasive

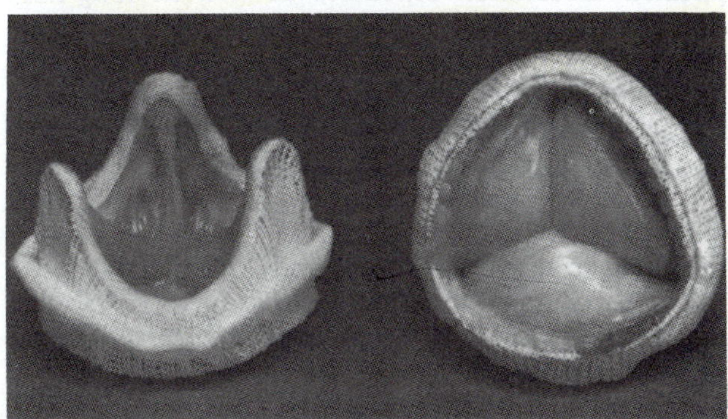

FIGURE 34–3 ◆ Biologic heart valve: The Carpentier-Edwards porcine xenograft. (From Sabiston, D. C., Jr., & Spencer, F. C. [1989]. *Gibbon's surgery of the chest* [5th ed.]. Philadelphia: W. B. Saunders.)

CHART 34-8

Education Guide ♦ Valvular Heart Disease

- Notify all of your health care providers that you have a defective heart valve.
- Remind the health care provider of your valvular problem when you have any dental work (cleaning, filling, or extraction) or any examination by instrument (cystoscopy, endoscopy, or sigmoidoscopy).
- Request antibiotic prophylaxis before and after these procedures if the health care provider does not offer it.
- Clean all wounds and apply antibiotic ointment to prevent infection.
- Notify your health care provider immediately if you experience fever, petechiae (pinpoint red dots on your skin), or shortness of breath.

procedures and tests. Instructions for the client are described in Chart 34-8.

The nurse teaches clients taking anticoagulants how to manage their drug therapy successfully and to prevent bleeding. For example, the client should use an electric razor to avoid skin cuts. The client should report any bleeding or excessive bruising to the health care provider. (For more information on anticoagulants, see Chapter 35.)

The nurse teaches clients who have undergone valve surgery how to care for the sternal incision. The nurse instructs clients to watch for and report any fever or drainage or redness at the site. Clients should not lift heavy objects (over 10 pounds [4.5 kg]) and should exercise caution when driving to allow for optimal healing of the sternotomy incision. Clients who have had valvular surgery should also avoid any dental procedures for 6 months.

PSYCHOSOCIAL PREPARATION

Clients with valvular heart disease may have complicated medication schedules as well as long-term antibiotic or anticoagulant therapy. These circumstances may potentially lead to noncompliance. The nurse ensures that the client is an active participant in care decisions. The nurse also provides clear, concise instructions about medication schedules.

Limitations on physical activity can be depressing and frustrating for the client. The nurse encourages the client to discuss any fears and anxieties.

The psychologic response to valve surgery is similar to that after coronary artery bypass surgery. Clients may experience an altered self-image as a result of the changes required in lifestyle or the visible medial sternotomy incision. In addition, clients with prosthetic valves may have to adjust to a soft but audible clicking sound of the prosthetic valve. The nurse encourages clients to verbalize their feelings about the sternotomy incision and the prosthetic heart valve.

HEALTH CARE RESOURCES

A home care nurse may be needed to help the client adhere to medication and activity schedules and to detect any problems, particularly with anticoagulant therapy. Clients who have undergone surgery may also require a nurse for assistance with incision care. A home care aide may assist clients with activities of daily living.

The American Heart Association is a community resource that provides information to clients about valvular heart disease. A wallet-sized card can be obtained for the client, which identifies him or her as needing prophylactic antibiotics. The nurse advises clients receiving anticoagulants to obtain an identification bracelet stating the name of the drug they are taking.

EVALUATION

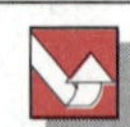

The nurse evaluates the care of the client with valvular disease with reference to the expected outcomes of treatment. Expected outcomes include that the client will:

- Demonstrate restoration and maintenance of cardiac output, including vital signs within normal limits, mental alertness, adequate urinary output, and strong peripheral pulses
- Demonstrate activity tolerance within his or her level of cardiac reserve as evidenced by the ability to perform activities of daily living without dyspnea, chest pain, fatigue, or changes in vital signs
- Remain normovolemic as evidenced by adequate urinary output, normal lung sounds, absence of edema, and maintenance of weight
- Comply with the prescribed medication regimen
- State the importance of the prophylactic use of antibiotics

INFLAMMATIONS AND INFECTIONS

Inflammations and infections of the heart frequently follow systemic infections. Recovery from these infections is often prolonged, and such clients are at great risk for future heart problems. Inflammation and infection may involve the endocardium (endocarditis), the pericardium (pericarditis), or the entire heart (rheumatic carditis).

Infective Endocarditis

OVERVIEW

PATHOPHYSIOLOGY

Infective endocarditis (previously called bacterial endocarditis) refers to a bacterial or fungal infection involving the endocardium, which includes the valves. Infective endocarditis was formerly classified as acute and subacute bacterial endocarditis (SBE). Acute endocarditis represented the infection of a normal valve by a virulent organism, such as *Staphylococcus aureus*. It usually resulted in rapid destruction of the heart valve and the client's death. SBE represented the infection of an existing defect by a less virulent organism, such as *Streptococcus viridans*. Such classic presentations of infective endocarditis are now used less frequently (Korzeniowski & Kaye, 1992).

ETIOLOGY

Infective endocarditis occurs primarily in clients who:

- Are intravenous drug abusers
- Have had valve replacements
- Have mitral valve prolapse or other structural cardiac defects.

Conditions predisposing a client to endocarditis are listed in Table 34–4.

In a client with a cardiac defect, a stream of blood often flows rapidly from a high-pressure area to a low-pressure zone. A sterile platelet fibrin thrombus (vegetative lesion) forms on a section of endocardium eroded by the rapid flow. During a bacteremia, bacteria become trapped in the low-pressure "sinkhole" and are deposited in the vegetation. The vegetative lesion grows, and the endocardium and valve are destroyed. After the infectious process begins, valvular insufficiency may result, or the vegetations may become so large that blood flow through the valve is obstructed and the valve appears to be stenotic.

Possible ports of entry for infecting organisms include:

- The oral cavity (especially if dental procedures have been performed within the previous 3 to 6 months)
- Rashes, lesions, or abscesses of the skin
- Infections (cutaneous, genitourinary, or gastrointestinal)
- Surgery or invasive procedures, such as tonsillectomy, endoscopy, bronchoscopy, cystoscopy, and prosthetic valve replacement, and IV drug abuse

TABLE 34–4 Conditions Predisposing to Endocarditis

Cardiac surgery
Cardiac defects
- Rheumatic heart disease
- Congenital heart disease
- Mitral valve prolapse

Intravenous drug abuse
Intravenous foreign bodies or devices, such as
- Intravenous catheters
- Pacemaker electrodes
- Dialysis shunts
- Hyperalimentation catheters

Immunosuppression related to
- Diabetes
- Burns
- Cancer
- Hepatitis
- Human immunodeficiency virus (HIV)

INCIDENCE/PREVALENCE

The incidence of infective endocarditis is much lower today because of the use of antibiotics. Fewer than 1% of all clients with cardiac dysfunction have infective endocarditis. Rheumatic fever, once the primary cause of infective endocarditis, now accounts for only about 30% of cases. Most clients with infective endocarditis have an identifiable predisposing cardiac defect (Korzeniowski & Kaye, 1992).

COLLABORATIVE MANAGEMENT

ASSESSMENT

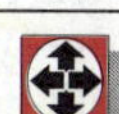

Clinical manifestations of infective endocarditis include fever, anorexia, fatigue, weight loss, cardiac murmurs, heart failure, embolic complications, and classic peripheral manifestations. The severity of the symptoms may depend on the virulence of the infecting organism.

Assessment consistently reveals fever. Clients may have high-grade fevers, with temperatures ranging from 39.4° to 40° C (103° to 104° F). However, clients with less virulent infections usually have temperatures from 37.2° to 38.8° C (99° to 102° F). Other symptoms of infection include chills, malaise, night sweats, anorexia, weight loss, and fatigue (Chart 34–9).

CARDIOVASCULAR MANIFESTATIONS

The nurse assesses the client's cardiovascular status. Most clients with infective endocarditis have murmurs, although some clients with acute infective endocarditis may not have them in the early stages of the disease. The nurse carefully auscultates the precordium, noting and documenting any new murmurs (usually regurgitant in nature) or any changes in the

CHART 34–9

Key Features of Infective Endocarditis

- Fever associated with chills, night sweats, and fatigue
- Cardiac murmur (newly developed or change in existing)
- Development of heart failure
- Evidence of systemic embolization
- Petechiae
- Splinter hemorrhages
- Osler's nodes
- Janeway's lesions

intensity or quality of an old murmur. An S_3 or S_4 heart sound may also be heard.

Heart failure is the most common complication of infective endocarditis. The nurse assesses for right-sided heart failure (as evidenced by peripheral edema, weight gain, and anorexia) as well as left-sided heart failure (as evidenced by fatigue, shortness of breath, and crackles on auscultation of breath sounds).

EMBOLIC COMPLICATIONS

Arterial embolization is a major complication in up to 50% of clients with infective endocarditis. Fragments of vegetation break loose and travel randomly through the circulation. When the left side of the heart is involved, vegetation fragments are carried to the spleen, the kidneys, the gastrointestinal (GI) tract, the brain, and the extremities. When the right side of the heart is involved, emboli enter the pulmonary circulation.

Clients with splenic infarction describe sudden abdominal pain with radiation to the left shoulder. When performing an abdominal assessment, the nurse notes rebound tenderness on palpation. The classic pain described by the client with renal infarction is flank pain with radiation to the groin, accompanied by hematuria or pyuria.

Emboli to the central nervous system cause either transient ischemic attacks (TIAs) or a cerebrovascular accident (CVA). The client may appear confused, have reduced concentration and aphasia, or have dysphagia. Pleuritic chest pain, dyspnea, and cough are often described by the client who is experiencing pulmonary infarction related to embolization.

PERIPHERAL MANIFESTATIONS

There are a number of classic peripheral manifestations of endocarditis. For instance, petechiae (pinpoint red spots) occur in up to 40% of these clients. The nurse examines the mucous membranes, the palate, the conjunctivae, and the skin above the clavicles for small red, flat lesions. The nurse also examines the distal third of the nail bed for the black longitudinal lines or small red streaks called "splinter hemorrhages" (Fig. 34–4).

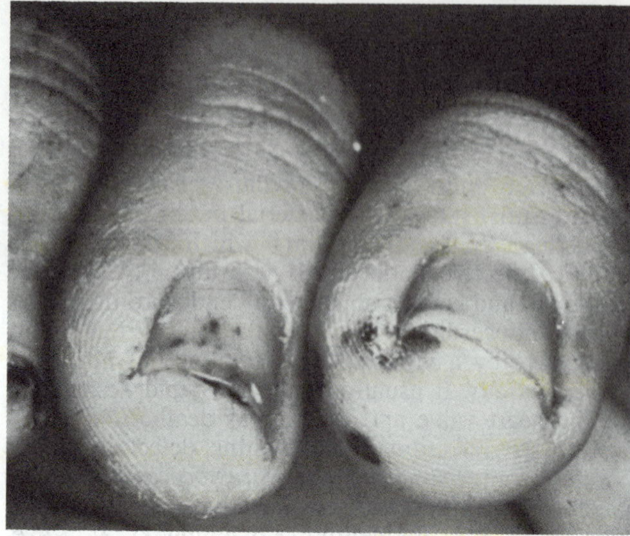

FIGURE 34–4 ◆ Splinter hemorrhage lesions in endocarditis. (From Braunwald, E. [1992]. *Heart disease* [4th ed.]. Philadelphia: W. B. Saunders.)

Osler's nodes and Janeway's lesions are also considered classic manifestations of endocarditis, although they may occur with other conditions. The nurse inspects the pads of the fingers, hands, and toes for Osler's nodes, which are reddish tender lesions with a white center. Janeway's lesions (Fig. 34–5) are nontender hemorrhagic lesions found on the fingers, toes, nose, or earlobes. Splenomegaly and clubbing of

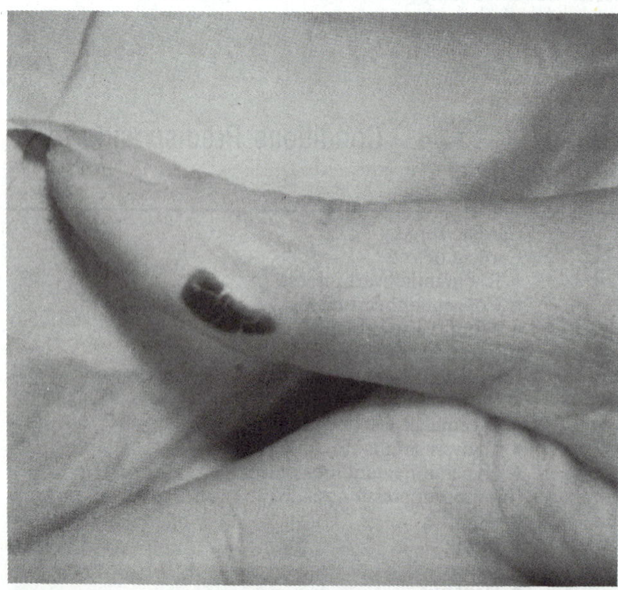

FIGURE 34–5 ◆ Janeway's lesions in endocarditis. (From Braunwald, E. [1992]. *Heart disease* [4th ed.]. Philadelphia: W. B. Saunders.)

the fingers may occur in clients who have had infective endocarditis for longer than 6 weeks.

LABORATORY ASSESSMENT

A positive blood culture is of prime diagnostic and therapeutic importance. Both aerobic and anaerobic specimens are obtained for culture. Low hemoglobin and hematocrit levels may also be found.

INTERVENTIONS

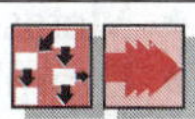

Interventions for endocarditis usually do not include surgery, although in some cases surgery is required to correct or eliminate one or more factors contributing to the disease process.

Nonsurgical Management The major component of treatment for endocarditis is drug therapy. Other interventions help to prevent the life-threatening complications associated with endocarditis.

Drug Therapy Antibiotics are the mainstay of treatment, with the choice of antibiotics depending on the specific organism involved. Antibiotics are given in sufficiently high dosages, most often intravenously, with the course of treatment lasting 4 to 6 weeks. In most cases, the ideal antibiotic is one of the penicillins.

Until recently, clients with endocarditis were hospitalized for up to 6 weeks for IV antibiotic therapy. Now clients are hospitalized for 5 to 7 days to institute IV therapy and then are discharged for continued IV therapy at home. During hospitalization, the nurse assesses the client's response to therapy. Clients are responding to antimicrobial therapy and may be considered for home therapy when they:

- Are afebrile
- Have negative blood cultures
- Have no signs of heart failure or embolization
- Show decreased clubbing

Anticoagulants are of no value in preventing embolization from vegetations. They are avoided unless they are required to retard thrombus formation on a prosthetic valve because they may result in bleeding.

Other Interventions Complete bed rest need not be enforced unless clients have fever or signs of heart failure. However, the nurse carefully monitors activities to allow adequate rest. The nurse assists clients in range-of-motion exercises and frequent position changes to decrease the risk of thrombus formation. The client wears antiembolism stockings to promote venous return. The nurse also explains proper oral and general body hygiene and consistently uses appropriate medical and surgical aseptic technique when caring for the client to protect the client from contact with potentially infective organisms. Nursing assessment for rapid pulse, fatigue, dyspnea, signs of heart failure, new heart murmurs, and early signs of embolization continues during the client's hospitalization.

Surgical Management If the client begins to show signs of hemodynamic compromise, the physician may consider surgery. Current surgical interventions for infective endocarditis include:

- Removing the infected valve (either biologic or prosthetic)
- Removing congenital shunts
- Repairing injured valves and chordae tendineae
- Draining abscesses in the heart or elsewhere

Preoperative and postoperative care of clients having surgery involving the valves is similar to that described earlier for clients undergoing a valve replacement.

DISCHARGE PLANNING

HOME CARE PREPARATION

Discharge planning for clients with infective endocarditis is essential to resolve infective endocarditis and to avoid complications. Clients and families involved in the treatment need to be motivated and have the knowledge, physical ability, and resources to administer IV antibiotics.

The nurse arranges for appropriate supplies to go home with the client. Supplies include IV tubing, alcohol wipes, needles, normal saline solution, and heparin or saline lock flush solution drawn up in syringes. A heparin or saline lock or central catheter is positioned at a new venous site that is easily accessible to the client or a family member.

The nurse contacts the pharmacist who will be preparing the antibiotics and arranges for ordering of related supplies for the client.

HEALTH TEACHING

The teaching plan for the client with infective endocarditis includes:

- Instruction in the cause of the disease and its course
- Medication regimens
- The technique for administering IV antibiotics
- Practices that help avoid and identify future infections

The nurse teaches the client, family members, or a significant other how to administer the antibiotic and care for the infusion site and how to maintain aseptic technique. The client or a family member demonstrates this technique before the client is discharged from the hospital.

The nurse encourages the client to maintain proper hygiene, particularly oral hygiene. Clients are advised to use a soft toothbrush to brush their teeth at least twice a day and to rinse the mouth with water after brushing. Clients should not use irrigation devices or floss the teeth because bacteremia may result.

Clients must inform their health care providers, including their dentists, of their endocarditis history. The nurse should teach clients to remind health care providers of their endocarditis and to request prophylactic antibiotic coverage each time they visit a health care provider who performs an invasive procedure. This is essential because studies have documented low compliance with prophylaxis regimens by health care providers (Guzzetta, 1992).

The nurse teaches the client self-monitoring for the manifestations of endocarditis, including the complications of heart failure and embolic phenomena. The client is instructed to monitor his or her temperature daily and record it for up to 6 weeks. Clients are also taught to report fever, chills, malaise, weight loss, or increase in fatigue to their primary care provider.

PSYCHOSOCIAL PREPARATION

Many clients find it difficult to cope with the chronic nature of infective endocarditis, the lengthy intervention needed, and the potential financial drain of antibiotic prophylaxis. Clear, concise explanations about the disease process and the reasons for lengthy intervention promote compliance with the intervention program. Consistent encouragement from a supportive spouse, a family member, or a significant other can help facilitate recovery.

HEALTH CARE RESOURCES

A home care nurse may be needed for follow-up care, especially for clients who self-administer IV antibiotics. The home care nurse can be contacted to monitor the client's progress and detect any complications.

The American Heart Association is a community resource that provides information about infective endocarditis to clients and health care professionals. A wallet-sized card can be obtained for the client, which identifies him or her as needing prophylactic antibiotics and lists the recommended uses of prophylactic antibiotic therapy as well as the specific antibiotics, dosage, and route of administration.

Pericarditis

OVERVIEW

Pericarditis is an inflammation or alteration of the pericardium, the membranous sac that encloses the heart. There are two general types of pericarditis:

- Acute pericarditis
- Chronic constrictive pericarditis

Acute pericarditis can be caused by:

- Viruses
- Bacteria (*Streptococcus, S. aureus,* meningococcus, or *Mycobacterium tuberculosis*)
- Trauma
- Uremia
- Post-myocardial infarction (MI) syndrome (Dressler's syndrome)
- Postpericardiotomy syndrome
- Metastatic tumors
- Lymphomas
- Radiation therapy
- Rheumatoid arthritis or other systemic connective tissue disease

Acute pericarditis can also be idiopathic. Acute viral pericarditis commonly follows a respiratory infection and is more common in men aged 20 to 50 years. Dressler's syndrome occurs in less than 5% of clients who experience an MI, from 1 to 12 weeks after infarction.

Chronic constrictive pericarditis is caused by

- Tuberculosis
- Radiation therapy
- Trauma
- Renal failure
- Metastatic cancer

In chronic constrictive pericarditis, the pericardium becomes rigid, preventing adequate filling of the ventricles and eventually resulting in cardiac failure.

COLLABORATIVE MANAGEMENT

ASSESSMENT

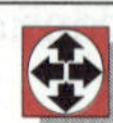

Assessment findings include substernal precordial pain that radiates to the left side of the neck, the shoulder, or the back. Pain is classically pleuritic and is aggravated by breathing (mainly on inspiration), coughing, and swallowing. The pain is worse when the client is in the supine position and can be relieved by the client's sitting up and leaning forward. Differentiation must be made between the pain of pericarditis and that of acute myocardial infarction.

The nurse may hear a pericardial friction rub with the diaphragm of the stethoscope positioned at the left lower sternal border. This is a scratchy, high-pitched sound; it is produced when the inflamed, roughened pericardial layers create friction as their surfaces rub together.

Clients with acute pericarditis may have an elevated white blood cell count and ECG changes consisting of ST-T wave elevation in all leads, with a T wave inversion occurring after ST segments return to baseline. Clients with infectious pericarditis always have fever. Blood specimens for culture may be obtained to assess for possible bacterial infection.

Clients with chronic constrictive pericarditis show signs of right-sided heart failure, including dyspnea, exertional fatigue, hepatomegaly, and orthopnea. These clients may have thickening of the pericardium on echocardiography or computed tomography (CT) scan. ECG changes include inverted or flat T waves. Atrial fibrillation is common.

INTERVENTIONS

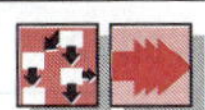

Drug Therapy The physician prescribes analgesics or nonsteroidal anti-inflammatory drugs (NSAIDs) for the relief of pain in clients with acute pericarditis. Clients who do not respond to these methods of pain relief within 48 hours may receive corticosteroid therapy. The physician prescribes antibiotics if the cause is a bacterial infection. Clients should rest and maintain a comfortable position, usually sitting up and leaning forward. The usual clinical course of acute pericarditis is short-term, from 2 to 6 weeks; however, episodes may recur (Client Care Plan).

Drug therapy for clients with chronic constrictive pericarditis includes digoxin (Lanoxin, Novodigoxin✱) and diuretics for symptoms of right-sided heart failure.

Assessing for Complications of Pericarditis A significant complication of pericarditis is pericardial effusion, which occurs when the space between the parietal and visceral layers of the pericardium fills with fluid. Pericardial effusion puts the client at risk for cardiac tamponade, an accumulation of fluid in the pericardial cavity. Tamponade restricts diastolic ventricular filling, and cardiac output drops. Findings of cardiac tamponade include:

- Decreased cardiac output
- Jugular venous distention with clear lungs
- Muffled heart sounds
- Pulsus paradoxus, a systolic blood pressure 10 mmHg or more higher on expiration than on inspiration (Chart 34–10)

Management of Acute Cardiac Tamponade Acute tamponade may occur when small volumes (20 to 50 mL) of fluid accumulate in the pericardium. The nurse reports any suspicion of this complication to the physician immediately. The physician may initially manage the decreased cardiac output with increased fluid volume administration. The physician may also order a chest x-ray or echocardiogram to confirm the diagnosis. However, these tests may not be helpful because the fluid volume around the heart may be small. Hemodynamic monitoring in a specialized critical care unit usually demonstrates compression of the heart, with all pressures (right atrial, pulmonary artery, and wedge) being similar and elevated (plateau pressures).

The physician may elect to perform a pericardiocentesis to relieve the pressure on the heart. Under echocardiographic or fluoroscopic and hemodynamic monitoring, the cardiologist inserts an 8-inch (20.3-cm) long 16- or 18-gauge pericardial needle into the pericardial space. The physician and the nurse monitor the needle's position, recognizing that ST and T wave changes indicate myocardial injury and misplacement of the needle. When the needle is properly positioned, a catheter is inserted and all available pericardial fluid is withdrawn. The nurse monitors the pulmonary artery, wedge, and right atrial pressures during the procedure. The pressures should return to normal as the fluid compressing the heart is removed.

After the pericardiocentesis, the nurse closely monitors the client for the recurrence of tamponade. Often, pericardiocentesis alone does not resolve acute tamponade. The nurse should be prepared to provide adequate fluid volumes to increase cardiac output and to prepare the client for emergency sternotomy if tamponade recurs.

If the client experiences a recurrence of tamponade or recurrent effusions or adhesions from chronic pericarditis, a portion or all of the pericardium may need to be removed to allow adequate ventricular filling and contraction. The surgeon may perform a

CHART 34–10

Nursing Care Highlight ◆ Care of the Client with Pericarditis

- Assess the nature of the client's chest discomfort. (Pericardial pain is typically substernal: it is worse on inspiration and decreases when the client leans forward.)
- Auscultate for a pericardial friction rub.
- Assist the client to a position of comfort.
- Provide anti-inflammatory agents as prescribed.
- Explain that anti-inflammatory agents usually decrease the pain within 48 hr.
- Avoid the administration of aspirin and anticoagulants because these may increase the possibility of tamponade.
- Auscultate the blood pressure carefully to detect paradoxical blood pressure (pulsus paradoxus), a sign of tamponade:
  - Palpate the blood pressure and inflate the cuff above the systolic pressure.
  - Deflate the cuff gradually, and note when sounds are first audible on expiration.
  - Identify when sounds are also audible on inspiration.
  - Subtract the inspiratory pressure from the expiratory pressure to determine the amount of pulsus paradoxus (>10 mmHg is an indication of tamponade).
- Inspect for other indications of tamponade, including jugular venous distention with clear lungs, muffled heart sounds, and decreased cardiac output.
- Notify the physician if tamponade is suspected.

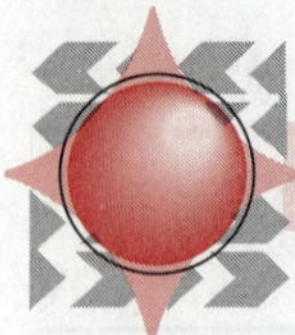

CLIENT CARE PLAN

The Client with Pericarditis

Nursing Diagnosis No. 1: Pain related to inflammation process

Expected Outcomes	Nursing Interventions	Rationale
Clients will state that pain is absent or markedly diminished.	◆ Ask the client to describe the pain. • Note the location and the intensity of the pain. • Determine whether breathing, coughing, or lying down aggravates the pain. • Assess for pericardial friction rub and ST and T wave changes.	◆ Accurate description of the pain is essential to confirm that the pain is pericardial. Friction rubs and ST and T wave changes often occur concurrently with pericardial pain.
	◆ Provide NSAIDs, steroids, or antibiotics as directed.	◆ These medications reduce inflammation and relieve pain in pericarditis when the cause is immunologic or infectious.
	◆ Assist the client to a position of comfort, usually a side-lying position, high-Fowler's position, or sitting up and leaning forward.	◆ These positions usually enhance the client's comfort.
	◆ Continue the client reassessment q2h including: vital signs, pain, and the presence of a friction rub. Notify the physician if the pain has not resolved by 48 hr.	◆ Pericarditis pain that has not resolved after 48 hr of therapy usually requires a change in medication (e.g., steroids instead of NSAIDs).

Nursing Diagnosis No. 2: Anxiety related to pain, lack of knowledge, or concern that pain is due to coronary artery disease

Expected Outcomes	Nursing Interventions	Rationale
The client will state that anxiety is diminished.	◆ Assess the client's knowledge of pericarditis. ◆ If appropriate, describe the inflammatory process occurring in pericarditis and explain why it causes chest pain. ◆ Reassure the client that pericarditis is not a "heart attack."	◆ The client may assume that the chest pain is from the angina or a heart attack.
	◆ Explain that pericardial pain often takes 48 hr to resolve.	◆ Pain that persists may be frightening to the client.
	◆ Explain all procedures and tests simply and completely. ◆ Assist the client with relaxation techniques.	◆ Unfamiliarity with the environment may increase anxiety.

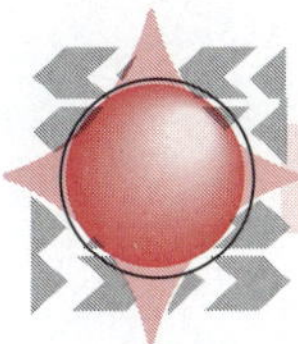

CLIENT CARE PLAN

The Client with Pericarditis *Continued*

Nursing Diagnosis No. 3: High risk for decreased cardiac output related to cardiac tamponade

Expected Outcomes	Nursing Interventions	Rationale
The client's cardiac output will remain adequate as evidenced by blood pressure and pulse within the client's acceptable range, mental alertness, adequate urinary output, and clear lungs.	◆ Assess the client's vital signs, chest pain, breath sounds, and the presence of a friction rub q2h. ◆ Note any indications of tamponade (decreased cardiac output, distended neck veins, clear lungs, or paradoxical pulse). ◆ Notify the physician, prepare emergency equipment, and prepare for rapid volume infusion if tamponade is suspected.	◆ Tamponade is a serious complication of pericarditis with pleural effusion. Monitoring for its occurrence and preparing for emergency treatment are important nursing responsibilities.

pericardial window, the removal of a portion of the pericardium permitting the excessive pericardial fluid to drain into the pleural space. In more severe cases, pericardiectomy, removal of the toughened encasing pericardium, may be necessary.

Rheumatic Carditis

OVERVIEW

Rheumatic carditis, occurring in about 40% of clients with rheumatic fever, is a sensitivity response. It develops after an upper respiratory tract infection with group A beta-hemolytic streptococci. The precise mechanism by which the infection causes inflammatory lesions in the heart is not established. However, inflammation is evident in all layers of the heart. The inflammation results in impaired contractile function of the myocardium, thickening of the pericardium, and valvular damage.

Rheumatic myocarditis is characterized by the formation of Aschoff's bodies, small nodules in the myocardium that are replaced by scar tissue. A diffuse cellular infiltrate also develops and appears to be responsible for the heart failure. The pericardium becomes thickened and covered with exudate, and a serosanguineous pleural effusion may develop. However, the most serious damage occurs to the endocardium, with inflammation of the valve leaflets developing. Hemorrhagic and fibrous lesions form along the inflamed surfaces of the valves, resulting in stenosis or regurgitation primarily of the mitral and aortic valves.

Rheumatic fever may be a complication of 3% of group A beta-hemolytic throat infections. Although the primary attacks occur most often in childhood, rheumatic fever may occur in adulthood. It develops more frequently than was previously thought (Kupper & Duke, 1992). The incidence of rheumatic carditis had been decreasing consistently until the mid-1980s. At that time, a strain of organisms emerged that was capable of triggering the rheumatic immune response but not causing a sore throat severe enough for the client to seek medical attention.

COLLABORATIVE MANAGEMENT

Rheumatic carditis is one of the major indicators of rheumatic fever. Clinical manifestations are:

- Tachycardia
- Cardiomegaly
- Development of a new murmur or a change in an existing murmur
- A pericardial friction rub
- Precordial pain
- Changes in the ECG (prolonged PR interval)
- Indications of heart failure
- Evidence of an existing streptococcal infection

Primary prevention is extremely important. The nurse teaches all clients with indications of streptococcal pharyngitis to consult their health care providers and receive appropriate antibiotic therapy. Indications of streptococcal pharyngitis include:

- Moderate-to-high fever
- Abrupt onset of a sore throat
- A reddened throat with exudate
- Enlarged tender lymph nodes

Penicillin is the antibiotic of choice for treatment. Erythromycin (ERYC, Erythromid✱) is the alternative for penicillin-sensitive clients.

The signs of rheumatic carditis must be recognized promptly, and antibiotic therapy must be instituted immediately for secondary prevention. The client is urged to continue the antibiotic administration for the full 10 days to prevent reinfection. The nurse suggests ways to manage the fever, such as maintaining hydration and administering antipyretics. The nurse encourages the client to obtain adequate rest.

The nurse emphasizes tertiary prevention in client education, explaining that a recurrence of rheumatic carditis is probable with reinfection by a streptococcal organism. Thus, antibiotic therapy is essential for streptococcal infection. The nurse also informs the client that antibiotic prophylaxis is necessary for the rest of the client's life to prevent infective endocarditis (see earlier).

OTHER DISORDERS OF THE HEART

Cardiomyopathy

OVERVIEW

Cardiomyopathy is a subacute or chronic disorder of cardiac muscle. It is not common, occurring in only 10 to 20 per 100,000 population. The cause is usually unknown.

Treatment is usually palliative, not curative; approximately 50% of clients die within 2 years of symptom onset. Clients have to deal with a shortened life span along with numerous changes in lifestyle.

Cardiomyopathies can be broadly divided into two etiologic categories:

- Primary (disease of the heart muscle without a known cause)
- Secondary (disease of the heart muscle with a known or suspected cause)

Secondary causes may include:

- Infectious processes (e.g., viral and bacterial infection)
- Metabolic disorders (e.g., thiamine deficiency and scurvy)
- Immunologic disorders (e.g., leukemia)
- Pregnancy and postpartum disorders
- Toxic processes (e.g., alcohol use and chemotherapy)
- Infiltrative processes (e.g., amyloidosis and cancer)

Cardiomyopathies are also classified into three categories on the basis of abnormalities in structure and function (Table 34–5):

- Dilated cardiomyopathy
- Hypertrophic cardiomyopathy
- Restrictive cardiomyopathy

DILATED CARDIOMYOPATHY

In the most common type of cardiomyopathy, dilated cardiomyopathy (DCM), there is extensive damage to the myofibrils and interference with myocardial metabolism. There is normal ventricular wall thickness but dilation of both ventricles and impairment of systolic function. Because of an inefficient contractile state, the heart ejects less than 40% of the blood in the left ventricle (normal is about 70%). This reduced cardiac output results in heart failure. DCM is twice as common in men as in women and occurs most often in middle age.

HYPERTROPHIC CARDIOMYOPATHY

The cardinal feature of hypertrophic cardiomyopathy (HCM), once called idiopathic hypertrophic subaortic stenosis (IHSS), is massive symmetric ventricular hypertrophy with small ventricular cavities. The left ventricular hypertrophy leads to a hypercontractile left ventricle with rigid ventricular walls. Obstruction in the left ventricular outflow tract is seen in 75% to 80% of clients with HCM. The abnormal stiffness of the ventricle in HCM results in diastolic filling abnormalities. In approximately 50% of clients, HCM is transmitted as a single-gene autosomal dominant trait.

RESTRICTIVE CARDIOMYOPATHY

Restrictive cardiomyopathy, the least common of the three cardiomyopathies, denotes restriction of filling of the ventricles. It is caused by endocardial and/or myocardial disease and produces a clinical picture similar to that with constrictive pericarditis.

COLLABORATIVE MANAGEMENT

ASSESSMENT

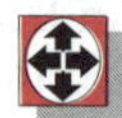

Findings in cardiomyopathy depend on the variations in the pathophysiology. Left ventricular or biventricular failure is the outcome of the characteristic changes in *dilated* cardiomyopathy. Clients may be asymptomatic for months to years and have left ventricular dilation that is identified on x-ray. Symptoms of left ventricular failure, as described by the client, are fatigue, weakness, and activity intolerance. About 25% of clients initially report chest pain, possibly due to associated myocardial ischemia. Right ventricular failure occurs late in the disease and is associated with a poor prognosis.

The clinical picture of *hypertrophic* cardiomyopathy (HCM) results from the hypertrophied septum, which in 80% of cases causes a mechanical obstruc-

TABLE 34–5 Pathophysiology, Signs and Symptoms, and Treatment of Cardiomyopathies

Dilated Cardiomyopathy	Hypertrophic Cardiomyopathy: *Nonobstructed*	Hypertrophic Cardiomyopathy: *Obstructed*	Restrictive Cardiomyopathy
Pathophysiology			
Fibrosis of myocardium and endocardium Dilated chambers Mural wall thrombi prevalent	Hypertrophy of all walls Hypertrophied septum Relatively small chamber size	Same as for nonobstructed, except for obstruction of left ventricular outflow tract associated with the hypertrophied septum and mitral valve incompetence	Mimics constrictive pericarditis Fibrosed walls cannot expand or contract Chambers narrowed; emboli common
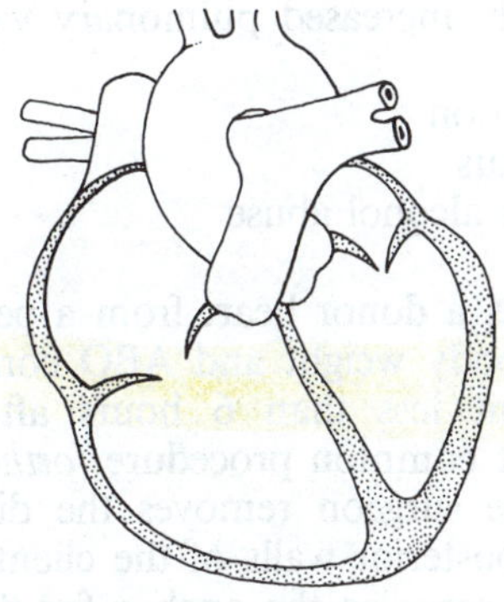	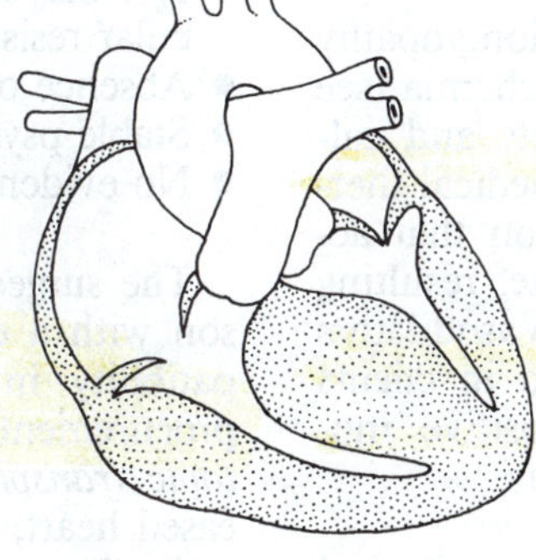		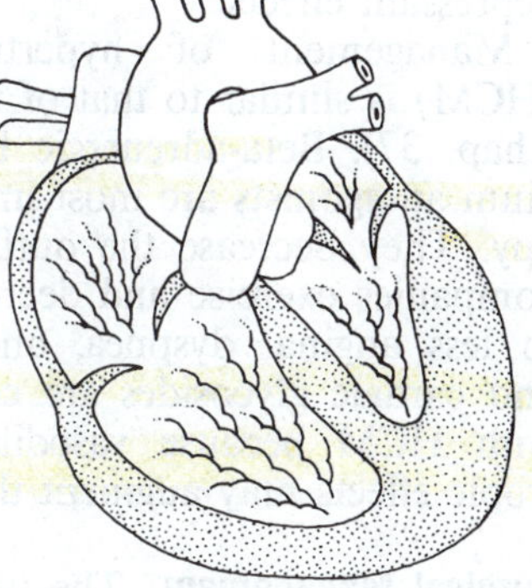
Signs and Symptoms			
Fatigue and weakness Heart failure (left sided) Dysrhythmias or heart block Systemic or pulmonary emboli S_3 and S_4 gallops Moderate-to-severe cardiomegaly	Dyspnea Angina Fatigue, syncope, palpitations Mild cardiomegaly S_4 gallop Ventricular dysrhythmias Sudden death common Heart failure	Same as for nonobstructed except with mitral regurgitation murmur Atrial fibrillation	Dyspnea and fatigue Heart failure (right sided) Mild-to-moderate cardiomegaly S_3 and S_4 gallops Heart block Emboli
Treatment			
Symptomatic treatment of heart failure Vasodilators Control of dysrhythmias Surgery: heart transplant	For both: Symptomatic treatment Beta-blockers Conversion of atrial fibrillation Surgery: ventriculomyotomy or muscle resection with mitral valve replacement Digitalis, nitrates, and other vasodilators contraindicated with the obstructed form		Supportive treatment of symptoms Treatment of hypertension Conversion from dysrhythmias Exercise restrictions Emergency treatment of acute pulmonary edema

Data from Wynne, J., & Braunwald, E. (1988). The cardiomyopathies and myocarditis. In E. Braunwald (Ed.), *Heart disease: A textbook of cardiovascular medicine* (3rd ed.). Philadelphia: W. B. Saunders.

tion and thereby reduces stroke volume and cardiac output. Most clients are asymptomatic until late adolescence or early adulthood. The primary symptoms of HCM are exertional dyspnea (90% of clients), angina (75% of clients), and syncope. The chest pain is atypical in that it usually occurs at rest, is prolonged, has no relation to exertion, and is not relieved by the administration of nitrates. A high incidence of ventricular dysrhythmias is associated with HCM. Sudden death occurs and may be the first manifestation of the disease.

The earliest clinical finding in *restrictive* cardiomyopathy is exertional dyspnea. Cardiac output cannot increase during periods of exertion because of the fixed ventricular volume. The client also reports weakness and dyspnea.

Echocardiography, radionuclide imaging, and angiocardiography during cardiac catheterization are performed to diagnose and to differentiate cardiomyopathies.

INTERVENTIONS

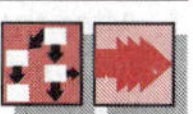

The care of clients with dilated or restrictive cardiomyopathy is the same as that for clients with heart failure (see earlier).

Nonsurgical Management Drug therapy includes the use of diuretics, vasodilating agents, and cardiac glycosides to increase cardiac output. Combined arterial and venous vasodilators are useful in clients with symptoms of biventricular failure. Because clients are at risk for sudden death, the nurse urges them to report any dizziness or fainting, which might indicate a dysrhythmia. Antidysrhythmic drugs are used to control dysrhythmias, including tachycardia. If cardiomyopathy has developed in response to a toxin, clients are instructed to avoid further exposure. The nurse teaches all clients with cardiomyopathy to abstain from alcohol ingestion because of its cardiac depressant effects.

Management of hypertrophic cardiomyopathy (HCM) is similar to that of myocardial ischemia (see Chap. 37). Beta-adrenergic blocking agents and calcium antagonists are most important in medical therapy. They decrease the outflow obstruction that accompanies exercise and decrease heart rate, resulting in less angina, dyspnea, and syncope. Vasodilators and cardiac glycosides are contraindicated in clients with HCM because vasodilating and positive inotropic effects may augment the obstruction.

Surgical Management The type of surgery performed depends on the type of cardiomyopathy.

Excision of Hypertrophied Septum The most commonly used surgical treatment includes excising a portion of the hypertrophied ventricular septum. Surgery results in long-term improvement in exercise tolerance in about 70% of clients with HCM (Braunwald, 1992).

Heart Transplantation Heart transplantation is the treatment of choice for clients with severe dilated cardiomyopathy (DCM). Each year, about 2000 clients in the United States receive cardiac transplants for cardiomyopathy or end-stage heart failure. Most clients who have a heart transplant have DCM. Criteria for candidate selection (Braunwald, 1992) include:

- Life expectancy less than 1 year
- Age younger than 65 years (variable)
- New York Heart Association (NYHA) class III or IV
- Normal or only slightly increased pulmonary vascular resistance
- Absence of active infection
- Stable psychosocial status
- No evidence of drug or alcohol abuse

The surgeon transplants a donor heart from a person with a comparable body weight and ABO compatibility into a recipient less than 6 hours after procurement. In the most common procedure *(orthotopic transplantation),* the surgeon removes the diseased heart, leaving the posterior walls of the client's atria. The remnant atria serve as the anchor for the donor heart; anastomoses are made between the recipient and donor atria, aorta, and pulmonary arteries (Fig. 34–6). Because a remnant of the client's atria remains, two unrelated P waves are visible on electrocardiography.

The transplanted heart is denervated, unresponsive to vagal stimulation. The client's heart rate approxi-

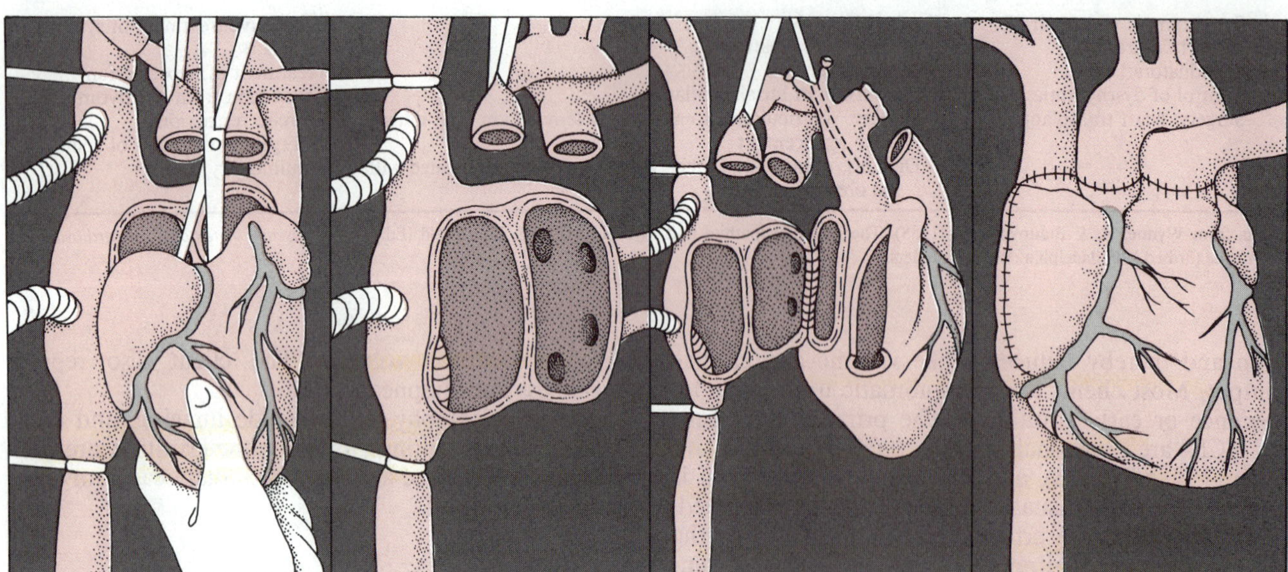

FIGURE 34–6 ◆ Heart transplantation.

mates 100 beats per minute, responding slowly with increases in heart rate, contractility, and cardiac output to exercise or stress. In the early postoperative phase, isoproterenol (Isuprel) is often required to support the heart rate and maintain cardiac output. Atropine, digitalis, and carotid sinus pressure do not have their usual effects on the heart because of denervation.

Many clients experience at least one episode of acute rejection of the transplanted heart in the first 3 months after transplantation and then approximately one episode a year. Symptoms of rejection of the heart are nonspecific, occurring late in the rejection process. They include:

- Hypotension
- Cardiac dysrhythmias
- Weakness
- Fatigue
- Dizziness

To detect rejection, the surgeon performs endomyocardial biopsies at regularly scheduled intervals and whenever symptoms occur.

To suppress natural defense mechanisms and prevent transplant rejection, clients require immunosuppressant therapy for the rest of their lives. Most commonly, the physician prescribes triple drug therapy with cyclosporine (Sandimmune), azathioprine (Imuran), and prednisone (Deltasone, Winpred✱).

Eighty percent to 90% of clients survive 1 year after transplantation; most return to NYHA class I or II status. Five years after transplantation, many of the surviving clients (20% to 40%) have evidence of coronary artery disease (CAD). Because the heart is denervated, clients do not experience angina and regularly scheduled exercise tolerance tests and angiography are required to identify CAD.

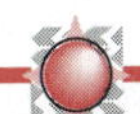

IMPLICATIONS FOR NURSING RESEARCH

Nursing research is concerned with ways to improve the clients' compliance with therapy and enhance the quality of life for clients with cardiac disorders. Questions for future nursing research include:

- ◆ What interventions most enhance the quality of life for clients in heart failure?
- ◆ How can nurses best address quality-of-life issues for women, meeting their functional and psychosocial needs?
- ◆ What influences clients with severe heart failure or cardiomyopathy to make advance directives concerning their care?
- ◆ What is the economic impact of the care of the client with heart failure?

SELECTED BIBLIOGRAPHY

American Heart Association. (1992). *Heart and stroke facts.* Dallas: Author.

Barden, C., & Burgman, V. (1990). Balloon angioplasty: Nursing care implications. *Critical Care Nurse, 10*(6), 22–30.

Braunwald, E. (1992). *Heart disease: A textbook of cardiovascular medicine* (4th ed.). Philadelphia: W. B. Saunders.

Brown, K. K. (1993). Boosting the failing heart with inotropic drugs. *Nursing93, 23*(4), 34–43.

*Fardy, P. S., Yanowitz, F. G., & Wilson, P. K. (1988). *Cardiac rehabilitation, adult fitness, and exercise testing* (2nd ed.). Philadelphia: Lea & Febiger.

Galvao, M. (1990). Role of angiotensin-converting enzyme inhibitors in congestive heart failure. *Heart & Lung, 5,* 505–511.

Gawlinski, A., & Jensen, G. (1991). The complications of cardiovascular aging. *American Journal of Nursing, 91*(11), 26–30.

Govoni, L. E., & Hayes, J. E. (1992). *Drugs and nursing implications.* Norwalk, CT: Appleton & Lange.

Guzzetta, C. E. (1992). Infective endocarditis. In B. M. Dossey, C. E. Guzzetta, & C. V. Kenner (Eds.), *Critical care nursing* (3rd ed., pp. 515–536). Philadelphia: J. B. Lippincott.

Havens, L. L., & Weaver, J. W. (1992). Cardiovascular system. In M. O. Hogstel (Ed.), *Clinical manual of gerontologic nursing* (pp. 70–90). St. Louis: Mosby Year Book.

Holden, T. (1992). Seeing Joan through. *American Journal of Nursing. 92*(12), 26–30.

Kison, C. (1992). Health beliefs and compliance of cardiac patients. *Applied Nursing Research, 5,* 181–185.

Korzeniowski, O., & Kaye, D. (1992). Infective endocarditis. In E. Braunwald (Ed.), *Heart disease: A textbook of cardiovascular medicine* (4th ed., pp. 1078–1105). Philadelphia: W. B. Saunders.

Kupper, N. S., & Duke, E. S. (1992). Inflammatory and valvular heart disease. In S. M. Lewis & I. C. Collier (Eds.), *Medical-surgical nursing* (3rd ed., pp. 888–917). St. Louis: Mosby Year Book.

*Laurent-Bopp, D. (1989). Heart failure. In S. L. Underhill, S. L. Woods, E. S. Froelicher, & C. J. Halpenny (Eds.), *Cardiac nursing* (2nd ed.). Philadelphia: J. B. Lippincott.

Letterer, R. A., Carew, B., Reid, M., & Woods, P. (1992). Learning to live with congestive heart failure. *Nursing92, 22*(5), 34–41.

McGraw, J. P. (1992). Perfusion. In P. S. Kidd & K. D. Wagner (Eds.), *High acuity nursing* (pp. 107–118). Norwalk, CT: Appleton & Lange.

Murphy, T. G., & Bennett, E. J. (1992). Low tech, high touch perfusion assessment. *American Journal of Nursing, 92*(5), 36–46.

Palarski, V., & Washburn, S. (1992). Overcoming LVD in cardiac rehab. *American Journal of Nursing, 92*(9), 52–57.

Purcell, J. A. (1990). Advances in the treatment of dilated cardiomyopathy. *AACN Clinical Issues in Critical Care Nursing, 1*(1), 31–45.

Recker, D. (1994). Patient perception of preoperative cardiac surgical teaching—done pre- and postadmission. *Critical Care Nurse, 14*(1), 52–58.

*Schroeder, S. A., & Chatton, M. J. (1988). General care symptoms and disease prevention. In S. A. Schroeder, M. A. Krupp, & L. M. Tierrey (Eds.), *Current medical diagnosis and treatment* (pp. 1–16). Norwalk, CT: Appleton & Lange.

Schwertz, D. W., & Piano, M. R. (1990). New inotropic drugs for treatment of heart failure. *Cardiovascular Nursing, 26*(2), 7–12.

Scordo, K. A. (1992). Helping your patient cope with mitral valve prolapse syndrome. *Nursing92, 22*(10), 34–39.

Smith, D. F., & Bumann, R. (1993). Assessing and treating decreased cardiac output. *MEDSURG Nursing, 2,* 351–357.

Sulzbach, L. M., & Dossey, B. M. (1992). Acute pericarditis. In B. M. Dossey, C. E. Guzzetta, & C. V. Kenner (Eds.), *Critical care nursing* (3rd ed., pp. 501–514). Philadelphia: J. B. Lippincott.

Swearubgen, P. L., & Keen, J. H. (Eds.). (1992). *Manual of critical care* (2nd ed.). St. Louis: Mosby Year Book.

Urban, N. (1990). Hemodynamic clinical profiles. *AACN Clinical Issues in Critical Care Nursing. 1*(1), 119–130.

U.S. Department of Health and Human Services, Agency for Health Care Policy and Research. (1994). *Heart failure: Evaluation and care of patients with left-ventricular systolic dysfunction.* Rockville, MD: Author.

*Wassertheil-Smoller, S., Alderman, M. H., & Wylie-Rosell, J. (1989). *Cardiovascular health and risk management: The role of nutrition and medication in clinical practice.* Littleton, MA: PSG Publishing.

Wenger, N. K., & Hellerstein, H. K. (Eds.). (1992). *Rehabilitation of the coronary patient.* New York: Churchill Livingstone.

Wilson, R. F. (1992). *Critical care manual: Applied physiology and principles of practice* (2nd ed.). Philadelphia: F. A. Davis.

Wynne, J., & Braunwald, E. (1992). The cardiomyopathies and myocarditides: Toxic chemical and physical damage to the heart. In E. Braunwald (Ed.), *Heart disease: A textbook of cardiovascular medicine* (4th ed., pp. 1394–1450). Philadelphia: W. B. Saunders.

Yakabowich, M. (1992). What you should know about administering nitrates. *Nursing92, 22*(9), 53–55.

SUGGESTED READINGS

Palarski, V., & Washburn, S. (1992). Overcoming LVD in cardiac rehab. *American Journal of Nursing, 92*(9), 52–57.

This article discusses the special cardiac rehabilitation considerations that are needed for people with left ventricular dysfunction (LVD). Specific exercises and ambulation techniques are described to help the client slowly regain strength.

Scordo, K. A. (1992). Helping your patient cope with mitral valve prolapse syndrome. *Nursing92, 22*(10), 34–39.

This comprehensive article on mitral valve prolapse includes a discussion of pathophysiology, assessment findings, and interventions, including drug therapy. A symptom checklist that clients can use to monitor this health problem is also included.

Yakabowich, M. (1992). What you should know about administering nitrates. *Nursing92, 22*(9), 53–55.

This article describes the drug actions, administration tips, and adverse reactions associated with nitrate administration. A table compares the four major nitrates, differentiating clinical indications, onset of action, and duration of action for each drug.

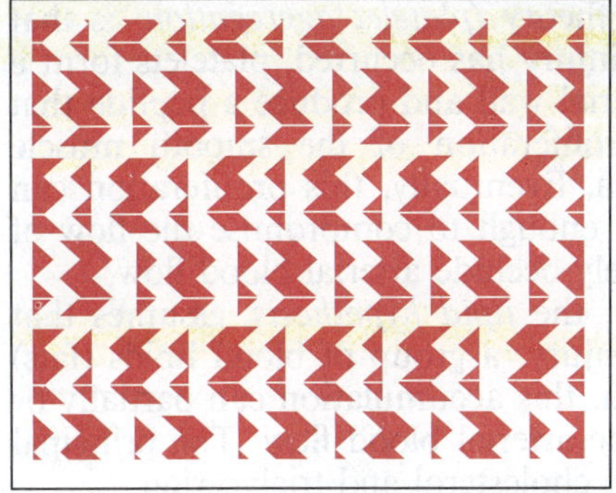

CHAPTER 35

Interventions for Clients with Vascular Problems

CHAPTER HIGHLIGHTS

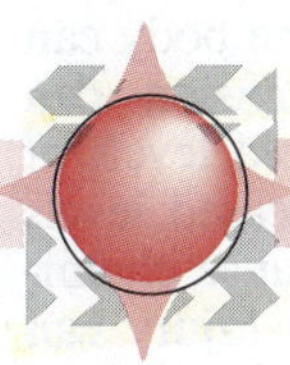

Disorders of the vascular (blood vessel) system cause many problems for people and may lead to complete shutdown of all body organs or eventually death. Each year, vascular disorders leave millions of people limbless, disabled, or dead, and the economic considerations are overwhelming.

Although vascular disease can affect any portion of the human body, such as the heart, brain, and kidneys, the peripheral vascular system and its associated diseases are described here.

Arteriosclerosis and Atherosclerosis

OVERVIEW

Arteriosclerosis is a thickening, or hardening, of the arterial wall. Atherosclerosis, a type of arteriosclerosis, involves the formation of plaque within the arterial wall. Atherosclerosis is the most common cause of arterial obstruction. The process of atherosclerosis can lead to cardiovascular diseases, such as coronary artery disease (CAD); cerebrovascular disease; and peripheral vascular disease (PVD). Cardiovascular disease is the primary cause of death in the United States. Nearly one million people died of heart and blood vessel disease in 1989 (American Heart Association, 1992).

PATHOPHYSIOLOGY

The exact pathophysiology of atherosclerosis is not known, but it is thought to occur in the following way (Fig. 35–1). A fatty streak appears on the intimal surface (inner lining) of the artery. At this stage, the fatty streak may appear flattened or elevated, but it generally does not affect the integrity of the arterial wall.

Next, a fibrous plaque develops. This plaque is described as a white, glistening, fibrous elevation that covers a lipid core. At this stage, the plaque is elevated enough to partially or completely occlude the blood flow of an artery.

In the final stage, the fibrous lesions become calcified, hemorrhagic, ulcerated, or thrombosed. The rate of progression of this process may be influenced by:

- Genetic factors
- Certain diseases (e.g., diabetes mellitus)
- Lifestyle habits, including smoking, eating habits, and level of exercise

ETIOLOGY

THEORIES

The exact etiology of atherosclerosis is unknown, but several theories attempt to explain its cause. It is believed that an injury to the intimal layer of the artery may initiate the development of atherosclerosis. One popular theory *(platelet aggregation)* is that after the intimal injury has occurred, platelets form a cluster at the arterial wall and produce a peptide that stimulates the proliferation of the smooth muscle cells of the intima. Eventually, this proliferation can narrow the artery enough to compromise the flow of blood or completely occlude arterial blood flow.

Another theory, the *lipid hypothesis,* assumes that after an intimal injury, a group of blood lipids (fats) accumulate. Again, this accumulation can partially or completely occlude arterial blood flow. The principal lipids involved are cholesterol and triglyceride.

Many theorists believe that a combination of these two events is the most appropriate view of the atherosclerotic process and that this can occur in any arterial wall of the body. Usually, the disease affects the larger arteries, such as the coronary arterial beds, the major branches of the aorta, the visceral branches of the aorta, the terminal abdominal aorta, the carotid and vertebral arteries, or any combination of these.

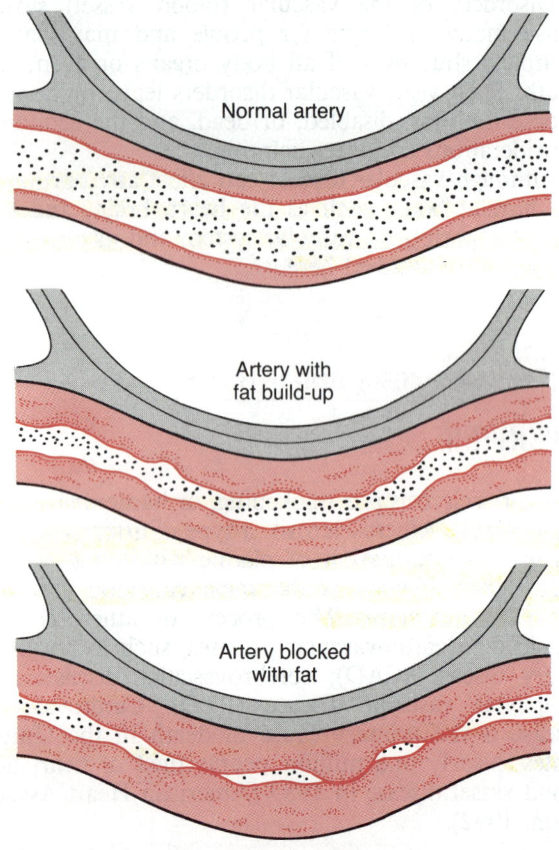

FIGURE 35–1 ◆ Pathophysiology of atherosclerosis.

FACTORS CAUSING ARTERIAL INJURY

Intimal injury of the major arteries of the body can be attributed to many factors. Hypertension can cause a mechanical injury, whereas elevated levels of low-density lipoproteins (LDLs) and decreased levels of high-density lipoproteins (HDLs) can cause chemical injuries to the intimal wall. Chemical injury can also be caused by elevated levels of toxins in the bloodstream, which may occur with renal failure, or by circulating carbon monoxide in the bloodstream from cigarette smoking. The intimal wall can be weakened by the natural process of aging or by physiologic disorders, such as diabetes.

Genetic predisposition and diabetes have a fairly direct effect on the development of atherosclerosis. Some families demonstrate inherited hyperlipidemia, an elevation in levels of blood lipids. In these people, the liver makes excessive cholesterol, which accounts for the development of atherosclerosis. In some people with hereditary atherosclerosis, however, the blood cholesterol level is normal. The reason for the development and progression of plaque in these people is not understood.

People with severe diabetes mellitus frequently have premature and severe atherosclerosis, often involving the microvasculature. This occurs because diabetes promotes an increase in LDL in plasma. In addition, intimal arterial damage may result from the effect of hyperglycemia.

Factors indirectly related to atherosclerosis include obesity, a sedentary lifestyle, and stress. Clients who are obese are at greater risk, most often because of concomitant elevations in cholesterol levels. Long-term physical activity is important in maintaining ideal body weight; it is also thought to help in maintaining optimal blood pressure and cholesterol levels and improved glucose tolerance. The effect of stress may be due to its effect on the sympathetic and parasympathetic release of catecholamines and an acute rise in blood pressure.

INCIDENCE/PREVALENCE

It is not known exactly how many people have atherosclerosis, but small plaques are almost always present in the arteries of young adults. The incidence can be better quantified by assessing diseases that result from this process. Although the process of atherosclerosis does not appear to differ between men and women, coronary artery disease (CAD) is much less common in premenopausal women than in age-matched men because of the lipid-lowering effect of estrogen. Postmenopausal women have similar rates of CAD as men in their same age group. People in the United States have a higher incidence of CAD related to atherosclerosis than in other industrialized nations (American Heart Association, 1992).

COLLABORATIVE MANAGEMENT

ASSESSMENT

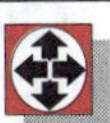

A client with early atherosclerosis may not have symptoms of disease. However, the nurse inspects the client for typical changes related to decreased oxygen supply, such as pallor around the lips and nail beds, rubor (red hue) of the skin, thickened or clubbed nails, dry skin, or loss of hair in the extremities.

VITAL SIGN ASSESSMENT

Because of the high incidence of hypertension in clients with atherosclerosis, the nurse assesses the blood pressure in both arms. The heart is also thoroughly assessed because concomitant cardiac disease is often present.

The nurse palpates pulses at all of the major sites on the body and notes any differences. The nurse should palpate the carotid arteries separately because of the risk of inadequate cerebral perfusion. The nurse also palpates for temperature differences in the lower extremities and checks capillary filling. Prolonged capillary filling (>3 seconds) generally indicates poor circulation. An extremity with significant atherosclerotic disease may be cool or cold, with a diminished or absent pulse.

ASSESSMENT FOR BRUITS

After palpating the pulses, the nurse auscultates each large artery from the carotid to the dorsalis pedis with a stethoscope or a Doppler probe. Many clients with vascular disease have a bruit in the larger arteries. A bruit is described as a turbulent, swishing sound, which can be soft or loud in pitch. The mere existence of a bruit is considered abnormal, but the role it plays in indicating the severity of vascular disease is not understood. Bruits often occur in the carotid, aortic, femoral, and popliteal arteries and usually indicate some degree of narrowing of the arterial wall. The nurse should document the location of a bruit and its pitch. The nurse also notes the rate and intensity of the pulse in each artery during auscultation. A decrease in intensity and audibility or a complete loss of a pulse, as the nurse progresses distally with auscultation, may indicate an arterial occlusion. The nurse notes at which point the pulse intensity changes and reports these findings immediately to the physician.

LABORATORY ASSESSMENT

Serum cholesterol levels are often elevated in clients with atherosclerosis. It is recommended that clients keep their cholesterol levels below 200 milligrams per deciliter (mg/dL). The National Cholesterol Education Program has recommended screening guidelines based on three classifications of cholesterol levels (Table 35–1).

Elevated cholesterol levels must be validated by low-density lipoprotein (LDL) and high-density-lipoprotein (HDL) determinations. Elevated LDL levels indicate that a person is at an increased risk for atherosclerosis. Low or normal levels of HDL also indicate an increased risk. In some people, particularly women, an elevated cholesterol level may be due to an elevated HDL level, which is not considered a risk. Although not routinely measured, *Apo B* is a major component of LDL and is a more sensitive predictor of coronary artery disease (CAD) in men than are standard cholesterol measures. *Apo A*, a major component of HDL, is a much more sensitive predictor of CAD in women (Penckofer & Holm, 1993).

TABLE 35–1 Classification of Serum Cholesterol Levels

Serum Cholesterol Level (mg/dL)	Classification	Intervention
< 200	• Optimal level	• Provide dietary information • Determine cholesterol levels again within 5 years
200–239 with *no* CAD or risks for CAD	• Borderline high blood cholesterol	• Provide dietary information • Determine cholesterol level again within 1 year
200–239 *with* CAD or risks for CAD 240 or higher, with or without CAD or risks for CAD	• High blood cholesterol	• Obtain serum LDL and HDL cholesterol levels • If LDL is 130–159, advise client to follow fat-modified diet, and repeat LDL annually • If LDL is 160 or higher, provide dietary therapy and frequent monitoring

CAD, coronary artery disease; LDL, low-density lipoprotein; HDL, high-density lipoprotein.

Triglyceride levels may also be elevated with atherosclerosis. A level of 150 mg/dL is indicative of hyperlipidemia.

INTERVENTIONS

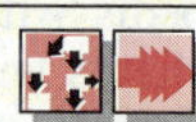

Atherosclerosis is a disease that progresses for years before clinical manifestations are evident. Clients with or at risk for atherosclerosis can often be identified by cholesterol screening. Because of the high incidence of atherosclerosis in the United States, all people 20 years of age and older are advised to have their serum cholesterol level evaluated.

Diet Therapy Clients with LDL values of 130–159 mg/dL are advised to follow a fat-modified diet. The nurse or dietitian instructs clients with LDLs of 160 or greater to follow a more structured diet aimed at decreasing saturated fat and cholesterol and, if appropriate, promoting weight loss. A decrease in fat, particularly saturated fat, is considered more important than simply decreasing the cholesterol number because saturated fat is one of the main determinants of cholesterol synthesis in the body.

In the United States, 37% of the total caloric intake in the diets of many people is made up of fat and this overconsumption of fat and cholesterol leads to hypercholesterolemia—an elevated total blood cholesterol level (Whitney et al., 1991). Elevated cholesterol levels, however, can often be decreased if fat in the diet is limited to no more than 30% of the caloric intake.

To assess what 30% of the caloric intake is, clients first need to determine their ideal daily caloric intake. Then they can calculate their fat limit in grams (see Table 35–3). In addition to tracking fat in grams, people need to assess the fatty acid content of foods.

STEP ONE DIET The Step One American Heart Association diet, which is often recommended to decrease serum cholesterol, calls for a total fat intake of less than 30%, with less than 10% of total caloric intake coming from saturated fat, up to 10% of total calories coming from polyunsaturated fat, and 10%–15% coming from monounsaturated fat. Cholesterol intake with this diet is limited to less than 300 mg daily.

In collaboration with the dietitian, the nurse educates the client about the fat content of foods in terms of the total degree of fat (Table 35–2) and saturation. Meats and eggs contain mostly saturated fats. Because canola (rapeseed) oil is rich in monounsaturated fat and safflower and sunflower oil are rich in polyunsaturated oils, they are recommended over highly saturated oils, such as palm or coconut oil. Cholesterol is found only in animal sources, such as meat and eggs, which are also high in saturated fats.

STEP TWO DIET The client's serum cholesterol levels are retested 6 and 12 weeks after the initial dietary intervention. If the cholesterol level has not significantly decreased, the client may be referred to a registered dietitian for instruction on a more restricted diet, such as the Step Two Diet. The Step Two Diet limits saturated fat to less than 7% of total calories and cholesterol to less than 200 mg/day.

In addition to elevated LDLs, other variations of hyperlipidemias put clients at risk for atherosclerosis. A low-fat, low-cholesterol diet, however, can play a significant role in improving a lipid profile, regardless of the lipid alteration.

Smoking Cessation Cigarette smoking lowers levels of HDL cholesterol and dramatically increases the rate of progression of atherosclerosis. The nurse advises all clients who smoke and are at risk for atherosclerosis to stop smoking. The nurse describes the relationship of smoking to atherosclerosis and assesses the client's willingness to change this behavior. A smoking cessation group, such as the American Cancer Society's "Fresh Start," may help the client with this difficult process.

Clients may also consider using the nicotine patch, which helps relieve nicotine withdrawal symptoms. The patch is about 50% effective in helping clients to stop smoking and is prescribed by a physician or nurse practitioner. The dose is determined by the client's weight and the extent to which he or she smokes. Clients are urged to completely stop smoking when the nicotine patch is initiated. The nurse informs clients that if they continue to smoke while using the patch, their risks for adverse effects are increased because the peak levels of nicotine are higher than those experienced from smoking alone. Serious cardiovascular effects, such as angina and/or dysrhythmias, may result from the patch, although the most common side effect is skin irritation. Patches cost approximately $100 a month, or a total of $300 over 3 months.

Exercise Regular exercise is recommended to promote optimal lipid levels, and it can actually prevent atherosclerosis. Exercise can also lead to regression of atherosclerotic plaque and the building of collateral circulation in people with atherosclerosis. The level of exercise required to provide protection from atherosclerotic disease has not been established. The nurse instructs clients at risk for or with atherosclerosis—when it results from hyperlipidemia, hypertension, or diabetes—to undergo an exercise tolerance (treadmill or stress) test before undertaking a strenuous exercise program, such as aerobics or running.

Drug Therapy Clients with elevated total and LDL cholesterol levels that do not respond adequately to dietary intervention are started on lipid-lowering agents (Chart 35–1). Because most of these drugs produce major side effects, they are generally given only when nonpharmacologic management has been unsuccessful. Bile acid sequestrants, such as cholestyramine (Questran) or Nicotinic acid (Nicobid), may be recommended initially as long as there is no contraindication for the client. Because the lipid-lowering agent Clofibrate (Atromid-S, Claripex) may be asso-

TABLE 35–2 Fat Content of Selected Foods

Food	Fat (g)	Calories
Beef (3 oz with removable fat trimmed)		
Corned beef	16	213
Eye of round (roasted)	5	151
London broil, braised (choice)	12	208
T-bone steak, broiled (choice)	9	182
Luncheon Meats (1 slice)		
Louis Rich 96% fat-free turkey pastrami	0	25
Oscar Mayer bologna	4	50
Weaver Chicken Frank with cheese	12	140
Seafood (3 oz cooked unless otherwise indicated)		
Haddock	1	95
Lobster	1	83
Swordfish	4	132
Tuna, canned in oil and drained	7	158
Tuna, canned in water and drained	0	111
Shrimp	1	84
Shrimp, breaded and fried	10	206
Poultry (3 oz roasted unless otherwise indicated)		
Chicken breast, meat with skin	7	165
Chicken breast, meat only	3	142
Chicken drumstick, meat with skin, batter dipped and fried, 1 average	11	193
Chicken drumstick, meat only, 1 average	2	76
Turkey, light meat with skin	7	168
Turkey, light meat only	3	133
Turkey, dark meat with skin	10	188
Turkey, dark meat only	6	160
Eggs		
1 large	5	75
Fleischmann's Egg Beaters, ¼ c	0	25
Morningstar Scramblers, ¼ c	3	60
Milk and Other Dairy Products		
Milk (1 c)		
Whole	8	150
2% fat	5	120
1% fat	3	100
Skim	0	90
Cream (1 tbsp)		
Half and half	2	20
Heavy whipping cream	6	52
Sour cream	3	26
Cheese		
American, 1 oz	9	106
Cheddar, 1 oz	9	114
Cottage cheese, creamed, 1 c	9	217
Cottage cheese, 1% fat, 1 c	2	164
Cream cheese, 1 oz	10	99
Ricotta, ½ c	16	216
Ricotta, part-skim, ½ c	10	171
Swiss, 1 oz	8	107
Weight Watchers American Pasteurized Process Cheese Product, 1 slice	2	45
Yogurt		
Colombo, plain, 8 oz	7	150
Colombo, plain, nonfat lite, 8 oz	0	110
Breads		
Bagel, 1	1	163
English muffin, 1	1	135
Whole-wheat bread, 1 slice	1	61
Other Grains		
Pasta, 1 c cooked	1	159
White rice, 1 c cooked	1	223
Pancakes, 4-in plain	2	62
Waffles, 7-in plain	8	206
French toast, 1 slice	7	153
Fruits and Vegetables		
Apple, 1 medium	1	81
Banana, 1 medium	1	105
Orange, 1 medium	1	65
Raisins, ⅓ c	1	150
Avocado, ½ medium	15	153
Broccoli, ½ c cooked	0	23
Carrot, raw, 1 medium	0	31
Corn, canned, ½ c	1	66
Green beans, ½ c cooked	0	22
Peas, ½ c cooked	0	67
Spreads and Oils		
Butter, 1 tsp	4	36
Margarine, 1 tsp	4	34
Diet margarine, 1 tsp	2	17
Vegetable oil (corn, safflower, olive, peanut, soybean, sunflower, and sesame), 1 tbsp	14	120
Vegetable oil, spray, 2.5-s spray	1	6
Salad Dressings		
Blue cheese, 1 tbsp	8	77
French, 1 tbsp	6	67
Italian, 1 tbsp	7	69
Russian, 1 tbsp	8	76
Thousand Island, 1 tbsp	6	59
Sweets		
Apple pie, ⅛	12	282
Cheesecake, ⅛	13	278
Chocolate pudding, 1 c	12	385
Chocolate syrup, 2 tbsp	1	92
Fudge topping, 2 tbsp	5	124
Ice cream, Sealtest, vanilla, chocolate, or strawberry, ½ c	6	140
Orange sherbet, ½ c	3	92
Popsicle ice pop	0	50
Snack Foods		
Lay's Bar-B-Q Flavored Potato Chips, 1 oz	9	150
Orville Redenbacher's Natural Microwave Popping Corn, 4 c popped	7	110
Popcorn, air-popped, 1 c	0	23
Pringle's Light Potato Chips, 1 oz	8	150

From Tufts University (1989). What is a gram of fat . . . and how many should you eat? *Tufts University Diet and Nutrition Letter, 7,* 4–5.

CHART 35-1

Drug Therapy for Hyperlipidemia

Drug	Usual Dosage	Nursing Interventions	Rationale
Bile acid sequestrants, e.g., cholestyramine (Questran, Cholybar)	• 12–24 g	• Encourage clients to increase fluid intake and consider stool softeners if needed	• Chloestyramine is constipating
Nicotinic Acid (Nicobid, Nicolar, Nia-Bid [niacin])	• 3–6 g	• Encourage clients to take with meals	• Flushing of skin and pruritus are common side effects, which can be minimized when drug is taken with meals
Fibric acid, usually derivatives, e.g., Gemfibrozil (Lopid) and clofibrate (Atromid-S)	• 120 mg • 1–2 mg	• Instruct clients to take with meals if nausea or gastrointestinal discomfort occurs	• Although well tolerated, nausea and gastrointestinal discomfort may occur and can be prevented if taken with meals.
HMG-CoA reductase inhibitors, e.g., Lovastatin (Mevacor)	• Starting dose 20 mg; increased to 40–80 mg	• Instruct clients to report muscle tenderness	• Although rare, myositis has occurred as a side effect

ciated with reduced life expectancy, it is given only to those clients who are at risk for pancreatitis or when another extenuating circumstance warrants its use. It often takes 4 to 6 weeks before total cholesterol and LDL levels respond.

Hypertension

OVERVIEW

Hypertension is generally defined as a systolic blood pressure greater than or equal to 140 mmHg and/or a diastolic blood pressure greater than or equal to 90 mmHg. Generally, the presence of hypertension is determined by three separate readings unless the systolic pressure is 210 mmHg or higher and the diastolic is 120 mmHg or more.

Hypertension has been classified into four stages (Table 35–3). The significance of this disease is that it is a major risk factor for coronary, cerebral, renal, and peripheral vascular disease. However, control of hypertension has resulted in significant decreases in cardiovascular morbidity and mortality.

TABLE 35–3 Stages of Hypertension

Stage 1	Systolic, 140–159 mmHg Diastolic, 90–99 mmHg
Stage 2	Systolic, 160–179 mmHg Diastolic, 100–109 mmHg
Stage 3	Systolic, 180–209 mmHg Diastolic, 110–119 mmHg
Stage 4	Systolic, ≥ 210 mmHg Diastolic, ≥ 120 mmHg

From U.S. Department of Health and Human Services (1993). *The Fifth Report of the Joint National Committee on Detection, Evaluation, and Treatment of High Blood Pressure* (NIH Publication). Washington, D.C.: U.S. Government Printing Office.

PATHOPHYSIOLOGY

The systemic arterial pressure is a product of the cardiac output and the total peripheral resistance (Fig. 35–2). Cardiac output is determined by stroke volume and heart rate. Control of peripheral resistance is maintained by the autonomic nervous system and circulating hormones, such as norepinephrine and epinephrine. Consequently, any factor producing an alteration in peripheral resistance, heart rate, or stroke volume affects the systemic arterial pressure.

REGULATION OF BLOOD PRESSURE

Stabilizing mechanisms exist in the body to exert an overall regulation of systemic arterial pressure and to prevent circulatory collapse. Four control systems

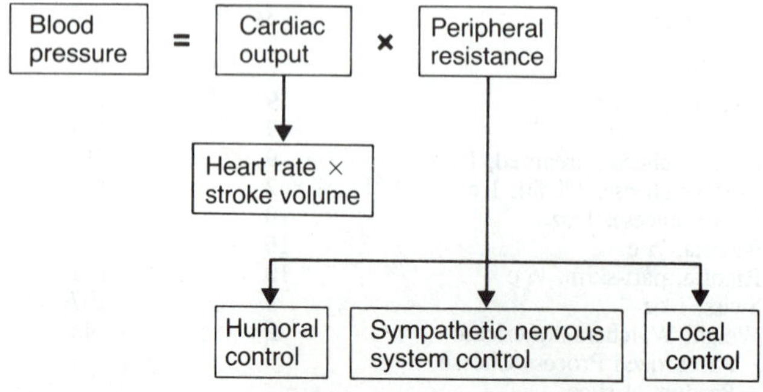

FIGURE 35–2 ◆ The components of blood pressure.

play a major role in maintaining blood pressure:

- The arterial baroreceptor system
- The regulation of body fluid volume
- The renin-angiotensin-aldosterone system
- Vascular autoregulation

ARTERIAL BARORECEPTORS The arterial baroreceptors are found primarily in the carotid sinus but also in the aorta and the wall of the left ventricle. These baroreceptors monitor the level of arterial pressure. The baroreceptor system counteracts a rise in arterial pressure through vagally mediated cardiac slowing and vasodilation with decreased sympathetic tone. Therefore, reflex control of circulation elevates the systemic arterial pressure when it falls and lowers it when it rises. Why this control fails in hypertension is unknown. There is evidence for upward resetting of baroreceptor sensitivity, so that pressure rises are inadequately sensed even though pressure decreases are not.

REGULATION OF BODY FLUID VOLUME Changes in fluid volume also affect the systemic arterial pressure. If there is an excess of salt and water in a person's body, the blood pressure rises through complex physiologic mechanisms that change the venous return to the heart, producing a rise in cardiac output. If the kidneys are functioning adequately, a rise in systemic arterial pressure produces diuresis and a fall in pressure. Pathologic conditions that change the pressure threshold at which the kidneys excrete salt and water alter the systemic arterial pressure.

RENIN-ANGIOTENSIN-ALDOSTERONE SYSTEM Renin, angiotensin, and aldosterone also regulate blood pressure (Fig. 35–3) (see also Chap. 15). The kidney produces renin, an enzyme that acts on a plasma protein substrate to split off angiotensin I, which is removed by a converting enzyme in the lung to form angiotensin II, then angiotensin III. Angiotensin II and III have strong vasoconstrictor action on blood vessels and are the controlling mechanism for aldosterone release. The significance of aldosterone in hypertension is most evident in primary aldosteronism. By increasing the activity of the sympathetic nervous system, angiotensin II and III also appear to inhibit sodium excretion, resulting in an elevation in blood pressure.

Inappropriate secretion of renin may cause increased peripheral vascular resistance in essential (primary) hypertension. In high blood pressure, renin levels should be expected to fall because the increased renal arteriolar pressure should inhibit renin secretion. In most people with essential hypertension, however, renin levels are normal.

VASCULAR AUTOREGULATION The process of vascular autoregulation, which keeps perfusion of tissues in the body relatively constant, appears to be important in causing hypertension accompanying salt and water overload. This mechanism is poorly understood.

COMPLICATIONS OF HYPERTENSION

Sustained blood pressure elevation in clients with essential (primary) hypertension results in damage to blood vessels in vital organs. Essential hypertension produces medial hyperplasia (thickening) of the arterioles. As the blood vessels thicken and perfusion decreases, body organs are damaged; these changes can result in myocardial infarctions, cerebrovascular accidents, peripheral vascular disease, or renal failure.

Malignant hypertension is a severe type of elevated blood pressure that is rapidly progressive. A person with malignant hypertension usually has symptoms such as morning headaches, blurred vision, and dyspnea, and/or symptoms of uremia (accumulation in the blood of substances ordinarily eliminated in the urine). Clients are often in their 30s, 40s, or 50s. The diastolic blood pressure is greater than 110 mmHg and frequently much higher, ranging from 130 to 170 mmHg. Unless intervention occurs promptly, a client with malignant hypertension may experience renal failure, left ventricular failure, or stroke.

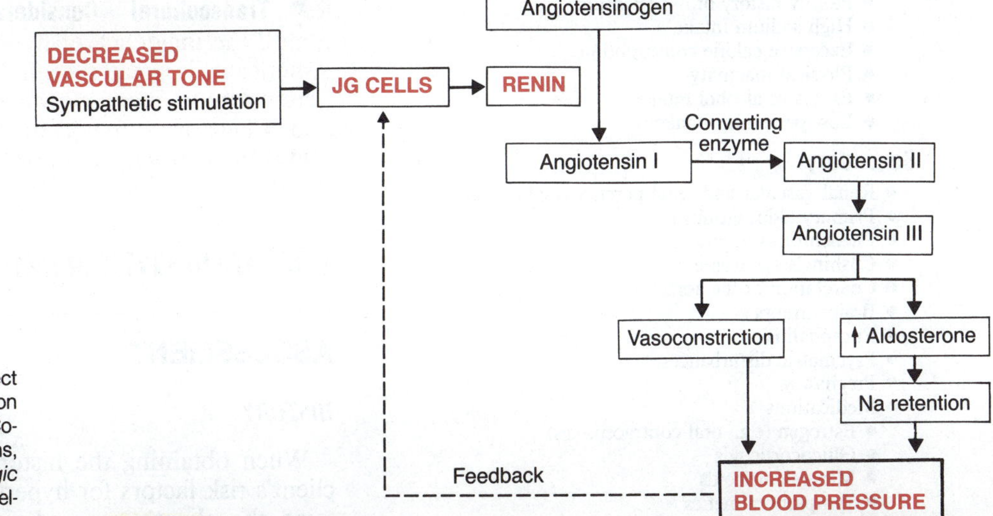

FIGURE 35–3 ◆ The effect of the renin-angiogensin system on blood pressure control (From Cotran, R. S., Kumar, V., & Robbins, S. L. [1989]. *Robbins pathologic basis of disease* [4th ed.]. Philadelphia: W. B. Saunders.)

ETIOLOGY

Hypertension can be essential (primary) or secondary (Table 35–4). Essential hypertension accounts for 95% of all cases (Kaplan, 1991).

ESSENTIAL HYPERTENSION

Although there is no known cause for essential hypertension, several associated risk factors have been derived on the basis of common characteristics of people with this disease:

- A family history of hypertension
- High sodium intake
- Excessive calorie consumption
- Physical inactivity
- Excessive alcohol intake
- Low potassium intake

A family history of hypertension is a major risk factor. In families with hypertension, there may be a defect in renal secretion of sodium or a heightened sympathetic nervous response to stress.

SECONDARY HYPERTENSION

Specific disease states and medications can increase a person's susceptibility to hypertension; a person with this type of elevation in blood pressure has secondary hypertension.

DISEASES Renal vascular and renal parenchymal diseases are two of the most common causes of secondary hypertension. Hypertension can develop when there is any sudden damage to the kidneys. Renovascular hypertension is associated with narrowing of one or more of the main arteries carrying blood directly to the kidneys. Renal parenchymal diseases are related to infection, inflammation, and changes in kidney structure and function.

Dysfunction of the adrenal medulla or the adrenal cortex can cause secondary hypertension. Adrenal-mediated hypertension is due to primary excesses of aldosterone, cortisol, and catecholamines. In *primary aldosteronism*, excessive aldosterone causes hypertension and hypokalemia (low potassium levels). Primary aldosteronism usually arises from benign adenomas of the adrenal cortex. *Pheochromocytomas* originate most commonly in the adrenal medulla and result in excessive secretion of catecholamines. In *Cushing's syndrome*, excessive glucocorticoids are excreted from the adrenal cortex. The cause of Cushing's syndrome may be either adrenocortical hyperplasia or adrenocortical adenoma (see Chap. 63).

Coarctation of the aorta is a congenital narrowing of the aorta that may cause hypertension. Occurring at any level of the thoracic or abdominal aorta, the narrowing restricts blood flow through the aortic arch, resulting in an elevated blood pressure above the constriction. After surgical repair, the elevation in blood pressure eventually subsides.

Secondary hypertension is also associated with other neurogenic disturbances, such as brain tumors, encephalitis, and psychiatric disturbances.

MEDICATIONS Medications that can cause secondary hypertension include estrogen, glucocorticoids, mineralocorticoids, sympathomimetics, cyclosporine, and erythropoietin. The use of estrogen-containing oral contraceptives is probably the most common cause of secondary hypertension in women. Discontinuation of medications capable of causing hypertension often reverses this problem.

TABLE 35–4 Etiology of Hypertension

Essential (Primary)
- No known cause
- Associated risk factors
  - Family history of hypertension
  - High sodium intake
  - Excessive calorie consumption
  - Physical inactivity
  - Excessive alcohol intake
  - Low potassium intake

Secondary
- Renal vascular and renal parenchymal disease
- Primary aldosteronism
- Pheochromocytoma
- Cushing's syndrome
- Coarctation of the aorta
- Brain tumors
- Encephalitis
- Psychiatric disturbances
- Pregnancy
- Medications
  - Estrogen (e.g., oral contraceptives)
  - Glucocorticoids
  - Mineralcorticoids
  - Sympathomimetics

INCIDENCE/PREVALENCE

It is estimated that 62,770,000 people 6 years of age and older in the United States have high blood pressure, and the incidence increases with age.

Transcultural Considerations In the United States, the incidence of hypertension among African-Americans is greater than that for Caucasians. Hypertension is more prevalent in African-Americans and Caucasians living in the southeastern United States than in African-Americans and Caucasians living in other parts of the country (U.S. DHHS, 1993).

COLLABORATIVE MANAGEMENT

ASSESSMENT

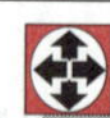

HISTORY

When obtaining the history, the nurse considers a client's risk factors for hypertension. The nurse ascertains the client's age, ethnic origin or race, family history of hypertension, average dietary intake of calories, sodium- and potassium-containing foods, alcohol intake, and exercise habits.

The nurse assesses past and present history of renal or cardiovascular disease as well as current use of medications.

PHYSICAL ASSESSMENT/CLINICAL MANIFESTATIONS

When a diagnosis of hypertension is made, most clients have no symptoms; however, they may experience headaches, dizziness, or fainting as a result of the elevated blood pressure. The nurse obtains blood pressure readings in both of the client's arms. Two or more readings are taken at each visit, with the average reading obtained used as the value for the visit. To detect postural (orthostatic) changes, the nurse should also take readings with the client in the supine (lying) or sitting position and at least 2 minutes later with the client standing.

Funduscopic examination of the eyes is done by a skilled practitioner to observe vascular changes in the retina. The appearance of the retina can be a reliable index of the severity and prognosis of hypertension. The Keith-Wagener (KW) classification of retinal changes in hypertension is commonly used to stage changes:

- Stage I is characterized by minimal arteriolar narrowing.
- Stage II involves more marked narrowing of arterioles, and arteriovenous nicking (changes at the arteriovenous crossings).
- Stage III shows circular or flame-shaped hemorrhages fluffy "cotton wool" exudates.
- Stage IV, the most severe, is the same as stage III but with the addition of papilledema (malignant hypertension is always associated with papilledema).

Physical assessment is helpful in diagnosing several conditions that produce secondary hypertension. The presence of abdominal bruits is typical of clients with renovascular disease. Tachycardia, sweating, and pallor suggest pheochromocytoma or adrenal medulla tumor. Coarctation of the aorta is often characterized by elevation of blood pressure in the arms, with normal or low blood pressure in the lower extremities. Femoral pulses are also delayed or absent.

PSYCHOSOCIAL ASSESSMENT

The nurse assesses for psychosocial stressors that can worsen the client's hypertension and that may affect the client's ability to collaborate in a treatment. The nurse also assesses the client for job-related, economic, or other life stressors as well as the client's response to these stressors.

Some clients may have difficulty coping with the lifestyle changes needed to control hypertension. The nurse assesses the coping strategies that the client has used in the past (see Chap. 7).

LABORATORY ASSESSMENT

Although no laboratory tests are diagnostic of essential hypertension, several laboratory tests can assess possible causes of secondary hypertension. The presence of protein, red blood cells, pus cells, and casts in the urine; elevated levels of blood urea nitrogen (BUN); and elevated serum creatinine levels indicate renal disease. In clients with a pheochromocytoma, a urinary test for the presence of catecholamines is positive. An elevation of levels of serum corticoids and 17-ketosteroids in the urine is diagnostic of Cushing's syndrome.

RADIOGRAPHIC ASSESSMENT

There are no specific x-rays that can result in a diagnosis of hypertension. Routine chest radiography may be of assistance in recognizing left ventricular hypertrophy that results from hypertension.

Intravenous pyelography (IVP) is performed when clinical findings suggest renovascular hypertension. Renal arteriography is undertaken to establish the exact location and the extent of any lesions, the degree of obstruction, and the basic pathologic change in the renal arteries.

OTHER DIAGNOSTIC ASSESSMENT

An electrocardiogram (ECG) is of value in determining the degree of cardiac involvement. Left atrial abnormality is the first electrocardiographic sign of cardiac involvement resulting from hypertension.

ANALYSIS

COMMON NURSING DIAGNOSES

The common nursing diagnoses for a client with hypertension are:

1. Knowledge Deficit related to information misinterpretation or unfamiliarity with information resources.
2. Noncompliance related to side effects of medications and/or lack of support system or economic resources (e.g., money, transportation).

ADDITIONAL NURSING DIAGNOSES

The client may also have one or more of the following diagnoses:

- Altered Tissue Perfusion (renal, cerebral, cardiopulmonary, and peripheral) related to decreased blood flow
- Altered Nutrition: High Risk for More than Body Requirements related to learned eating behaviors, ethnic and cultural values, lack of social support for weight loss, and/or imbalance between activity level and caloric intake

- Fatigue related to altered body chemistry (medications)
- Altered Sexuality Patterns related to effects of medical treatment (drugs)
- Ineffective Individual Coping related to effects of chronic illness and major changes in lifestyle

PLANNING AND IMPLEMENTATION

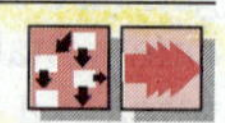

KNOWLEDGE DEFICIT

PLANNING: CLIENT GOALS The goal is that the client will verbalize an understanding of the management of hypertension.

INTERVENTIONS For the client with essential hypertension, the nurse initially recommends the following lifestyle modifications:

- Sodium restriction
- Weight reduction
- Moderation of alcohol intake
- Exercise
- Relaxation techniques
- Tobacco avoidance

These modifications are considered the foundation of hypertension control. If these modifications are unsuccessful, the physician considers the use of antihypertensive drugs.

There is no surgical treatment for essential hypertension. However, surgery may be indicated for certain causes of secondary hypertension, such as renal vascular disease, coarctation of the aorta, and pheochromocytoma.

Sodium Restriction The nurse advises all clients with hypertension to decrease their sodium chloride intake from the average of 150 mmol/L (150 mEq/L) to less than 100 mmol/L (100 mEq/L) each day (less than 2.3 g of sodium). To accomplish this goal, the nurse advises clients to:

- Avoid adding salt at the table
- Avoid cooking with salt
- Avoid adding seasonings that contain sodium
- Limit eating canned, frozen, or other processed foods

The nurse reviews a 3-day dietary recall with the client to identify whether sodium intake has been excessive. The nurse suggests spices, herbs, fruits, and other non–salt-containing substances, such as powdered garlic and onion, to enhance the flavor of meat, chicken, seafood, and snacks. The nurse instructs clients to read the labels on processed foods and to avoid those that are high in sodium. Salt substitutes are an alternative to salt, but the client needs a physician's order to use them. The order is necessary because salt substitutes are high in potassium, and the client may have hyperkalemia (high potassium levels) associated with a concomitant problem, such as renal impairment. Although hyperkalemia is unusual, it can also occur in clients who are taking potassium-sparing diuretics.

Although salt is restricted, the client should include recommended daily allowances of potassium, calcium, and magnesium in the diet. Studies are not conclusive, but data suggest that low levels of these electrolytes are associated with high blood pressure (U.S. DHHS, 1993).

Weight Reduction If a client's weight is more than 10% above ideal, the nurse encourages the client to lose weight. The nurse discusses the rationale for reducing or maintaining weight and plans a weight-reducing diet with the dietitian and client. The nurse may then refer the client to a group or organization for weight reduction.

Diets varying in total fat have little or no effect on blood pressure (Sacks, 1989). However, because of the relationship of saturated fat and cholesterol to weight, a weight-reduction plan is formulated with the following limits:

- Total fat, less than 30% of daily caloric intake
- Saturated fat, less than 10%
- Cholesterol, less than 300 mg/day

Table 35–5 describes how to calculate grams of fat.

Moderation of Alcohol Intake The nurse instructs clients to limit alcohol intake to no more than 1 ounce of ethanol (2 ounces of liquor, 8 ounces of wine, 24 ounces of beer) daily. The client is taught that alcohol consumption may elevate arterial blood pressure and can add "empty" calories.

TABLE 35–5 How to Determine Dietary Fat Limits

Procedure	Example
1. Begin with the number of calories consumed in a day.	• 1800 kcal
2. Multiply the number of calories by 0.30 (30% of total calories) to determine the maximal number of calories that should be obtained from fat.	• 1800 × 0.30 = 540 kcal/day from fat
3. Divide by 9 (1 g of fat contains 9 kcal) to determine the maximal number of grams of fat in the diet per day.	• 540 ÷ 9 = 60 g/day of fat. To limit fat intake to no more than 30% of calories, the client must take in no more than 60 g of fat daily.

Adapted from Tufts University (1989). What is a gram of fat . . . and how many should you eat? *Tufts University Diet and Nutrition Letter, 7,* 6.

Exercise With the physician's approval, the nurse can help the client develop a regular exercise program. It is recommended that the client perform regular aerobic exercise, such as brisk walking, running, cycling, swimming, or stair climbing, 30 to 45 minutes three to five times a week. The client should initiate exercise gradually and should stop and notify the physician if severe shortness of breath, fainting, or chest pain occurs. Clients should avoid muscle-building isometric exercise (weight lifting, wrestling, rowing) because it may raise blood pressure to dangerous levels.

Tobacco Avoidance Although cigarette smoking is unrelated to hypertension, it is a major risk factor for cardiovascular disease. Therefore, the client who smokes is strongly urged to stop. With input from the nurse and physician, the client plans a smoking cessation program that best fits into his or her lifestyle. The nurse explains the nicotine patch and smoking cessation programs and implements follow-up to assess the client's plans for quitting (see earlier).

Drug Therapy Drug therapy is individualized for each client, with consideration given to the client's culture, age, concomitant illness, severity of blood pressure elevation, and cost of drugs and follow-up. Therapy may not be instituted for clients with diastolic readings between 90 and 94 mmHg because there is controversy about the advantage of treatment in this group.

Treatment of hypertension generally begins with a single drug. Once-a-day drug therapy is best, because the more doses required each day, the higher the risk that a client will not follow the treatment regimen. Several classifications of medications are available to control hypertension. Examples of commonly used drugs are listed in Chart 35–2.

DIURETICS There are three basic types of diuretics used to decrease blood volume and lower blood pressure:

- Thiazide diuretics, such as hydrochlorothiazide (HydroDIURIL, Urozide✱), prevent sodium and water reabsorption in the distal tubules while promoting potassium excretion.
- Loop (high-ceiling) diuretics, such as furosemide (Lasix, Furoside✱), depress sodium reabsorption in the ascending loop of Henle and promote potassium excretion.
- Potassium-sparing diuretics, such as spironolactone (Aldactone, Novospiroton✱), act on the distal tubule to inhibit reabsorption of sodium ions in exchange for potassium, thereby retaining potassium.

Diuretics are the drugs of choice in clients who have asthma, chronic airway limitation, chronic renal disease, and selected clients with congestive heart failure. They are particularly effective in African-American clients.

Diuretics are relatively inexpensive, and adherence to the medication regimen is enhanced because the drug can usually be prescribed on a once-a-day or, at most, a twice-a-day schedule. However, the frequent voiding that occurs after a person takes a diuretic may interfere with one's daily activities. The most frequent side effect associated with diuretics is hypokalemia (low potassium levels). The nurse monitors the client's serum potassium level and assesses for signs and symptoms of irregular pulse and muscle weakness, which may indicate hypokalemia. The nurse advises clients receiving potassium-depleting diuretics to eat foods high in potassium, such as bananas and orange juice. However, the client may need a potassium supplement to maintain adequate serum potassium levels (see Chap. 16). The nurse assesses clients taking potassium-sparing diuretics for hypokalemia and hyperkalemia. Both of these electrolyte disturbances are characterized by weakness and irregular pulse.

BETA-ADRENERGIC BLOCKING AGENTS Beta-blockers lower blood pressure by blocking beta-receptors in the heart and peripheral vessels, reducing cardiac rate and output. By blocking beta-adrenergic receptors in the heart, beta-blockers cause a decrease in heart rate and decreased contractility. Bradycardia (slow heart rate) and heart failure may result. Beta-blockers can also prohibit bronchodilation by blocking beta-receptors in the lungs. Therefore, clients with a history of asthma or bronchospasm are generally not given these drugs and all clients taking these drugs must be monitored for shortness of breath and wheezing.

Common side effects of beta-blockers include fatigue, weakness, depression, and sexual dysfunction, although the potential for side effects depends on the "selective" blocking effects of the drug. A variety of beta-blockers are available, and they differ from each other in terms of their cardioselectivity (primarily $beta_1$ effects, with less $beta_2$ effects), lipid solubility, and sympathomimetic activity throughout the body.

Diabetic clients who take beta-blockers may not have the usual signs and symptoms of hypoglycemia because the sympathetic nervous system is blocked. Counterregulatory responses to hypoglycemia, such as gluconeogenesis, may also be inhibited by certain beta-blockers.

CALCIUM CHANNEL BLOCKING AGENTS Calcium channel blockers, such as verapamil hydrochloride (Calan), nifedipine (Procardia, Adalat), and diltiazem (Cardizem) lower blood pressure by interfering with the transmembrane flux of calcium ions, resulting in reduced vasoconstriction. These medications are thought to be particularly effective for elderly and African-American clients. Verapamil and diltiazem can affect atrial-ventricular conduction and often lower the heart rate. Oral nifedipine can reduce blood pressure quickly, often decreasing blood pressure by 25% within 30 minutes. Sublingual administration of nifedipine, given by puncturing the capsule and placing the liquid contents under the tongue, acts within 10 to 15 minutes.

CHART 35–2

Drug Therapy for Hypertension

Drug	Usual Dosage	Nursing Interventions	Rationale
Diuretics			
Thiazides			
Chlorothiazide (Diuril) Hydrochlorothiazide (Esidrix, HydroDIURIL)	• 125–500 mg/day • 12.5–50 mg/day	• Monitor potassium levels and watch for muscle weakness or irregular pulse. • Encourage intake of foods high in potassium (e.g., bananas and orange juice).	• Hypokalemia is a common occurrence. • Depleted potassium needs to be replaced.
Loop Diuretics			
Furosemide (Lasix, Furoside✱) Ethacrynic acid (Edecrin)	• 20–40 mg/day • 25–100 mg/day	• Same as for thiazide diuretics.	• Same as for chlorothiazide
Potassium-Sparing Diuretics			
Spironolactone (Aldactone)	• 25–100 mg/day	• Monitor potassium levels and watch for muscle weakness or irregular pulse.	• Hypokalemia or hyperkalemia may occur.
Beta-Blocking Agents			
Propranolol (Inderal, Apo-Propranolol✱) Atenolol (Tenormin) Nadolol (Corgard)	• 40–240 mg/day • 25–100 mg once a day • 20–240 mg/day	• Monitor pulse rate. • Watch for shortness of breath or cough. • Instruct client to report any difficulty in sexual function, fatigue, weakness, or depression. • Instruct clients with diabetes to monitor blood glucose levels.	• A drop in pulse is expected, and bradycardia may occur. • Bronchospasm caused by blockage of beta-receptors in the lungs may occur. • Although these are common side effects, newer beta-blocking agents may be more "selective" in terms of side effects. • Hypoglycemic symptoms may be blocked in clients taking beta-blocking agents.
Calcium Channel Blockers			
Nifedipine (Procardia, Adalat)	• 10–30 mg tid	• Monitor blood pressure. • Assess for dizziness. • Assess lower lower extremities.	• A drop in blood pressure occurs within 30 minutes after oral administration. • Pedal edema can occur as a result of peripheral vasodilation.
Verapamil (Calan, Isoptin)	• 40–80 mg q 8 h, 240 mg SR once a day	• Monitor blood pressure and pulse. • Encourage intake of foods high in fiber.	• Hypotension and decreased heart rate may occur. • Constipation is a common side effect.
Diltiazem hydrochloride (Cardizem)	• 30–60 mg q 8 h	• Monitor blood pressure and pulse.	• Hypotension and decreased heart rate may occur.
Angiotensin-Converting-Enzyme Inhibitors			
Captopril (Capoten)	• 6.25 mg tid initially, increased to 50 mg tid	• Instruct client to stay in bed for 3 h after the first dose.	• Severe hypotension may follow the first dose.

CHART 35-2

Drug Therapy for Hypertension *Continued*

Drug	Usual Dosage	Nursing Interventions	Rationale
Enalapril (Vasotec)	• 2.5 mg/d initially increased to 10–40 mg/day	• Monitor blood pressure.	• Hypotension needs to be detected promptly.
Central Alpha Agonists			
Clonidine hydrochloride (Catapres)	• 0.1–1.2 mg h.s. or 0.1–0.3 mg once a week transdermally	• Administer at bedtime.	• Sedation is a common side effect.
		• Instruct client to report rash associated with transdermal route.	• Bothersome skin rashes occur in about 25% of clients using transdermal patch.
Methyldopa (Aldomet)	• 250–500 mg qid	• Instruct client to sit on the side of the bed for several minutes before arising and to avoid changing position suddenly.	• Postural hypotension is a common complication.
		• Warn clients that sedation can occur when drug is initiated and dose is increased.	• This information can assist clients in planning activity and rest periods.
		• Instruct male clients to report any difficulty in sexual function.	• Impotence is a common side effect.
Vasodilators			
Hydralazine (Apresoline)	• 10–50 mg qid	• Monitor pulse rate.	• Tachycardia may occur as a result of reflex increase in sympathetic activity.

ANGIOTENSIN-CONVERTING ENZYME (ACE) INHIBITORS ACE inhibitors are also used as single or combination agents in the treatment of hypertension. The angiotensin-converting enzyme converts angiotensin I to angiotensin II, one of the most powerful vasoconstrictors in the body. ACE inhibitors include captopril (Capoten), enalapril (Vasotec), and lisinopril (Prinivil). These drugs are most effective in young Caucasian adults but are not as effective in African-American clients or older adults.

The client receiving an ACE inhibitor for the first time is instructed to stay in bed for 3 to 4 hours to avoid the severe hypotensive effect that can occur with initial use. The nurse monitors the client's blood pressure every 15 minutes after this first dose. *Postural (orthostatic) hypotension* may occur with subsequent doses, but it is less severe. The nurse checks for postural hypotension by taking the blood pressure when the client is lying, sitting, and standing. If there is a significant decrease in the systolic blood pressure (>20 mmHg), the nurse notifies the physician. The elderly client is at the greatest risk for postural hypotension because of the cardiovascular changes associated with aging (Chart 35-3) (also see Chap. 32).

CENTRAL ALPHA AGONISTS Central alpha agonists act on the central nervous system, preventing reuptake of norepinephrine, resulting in a lowering of peripheral vascular resistance and blood pressure. Common central alpha agonists include clonidine (Catapres) and methyldopa (Aldomet, Apo-Methyldopa♣). Methyldopa can cause unique side effects, such as hemolytic anemia and inflammatory disorders of the liver, although they happen rarely. Because of this potential, clonidine is the more commonly used central alpha agonist. Clonidine can also be given as a transdermal patch, providing control of blood pressure for as long as 7 days. Side effects common to clonidine and methyldopa include sedation, postural hypotension, and impotence.

VASODILATORS Vasodilators lower blood pressure by relaxing vascular smooth muscle tone, thus reducing total peripheral resistance. Vasodilators include minoxidil (Loniten), nitroglycerin (Nitro-Bid), and nitroprusside (Nipride).

ALPHA-ADRENERGIC RECEPTOR AGONISTS Alpha-adrenergic agonists, such as prazosin (Minipress), dilate

CHART 35-3

Nursing Focus on the Elderly ◆ Hypertension

- Before initiating drug therapy, obtain blood pressure measurements with the client lying, sitting, and standing to assess for postural changes.
- Monitor the client's standing blood pressure during treatment.
- Instruct the client to avoid caffeine and nicotine for 1 hour before blood pressure measurements to obtain accurate readings.
- Teach the client that dizziness is a symptom of hypotension that should be reported.
- Instruct clients how to avoid orthostatic (postural) hypotension by avoiding sudden changes in position. Clients should arise from bed in three stages: sit in bed for 1 minute; sit on the side of the bed with legs dangling for 1 minute; stand, holding onto a nonmovable object for 1 minute before walking. Clients should also be cautious about heat exposure (hot tub), alcohol intake, and exercise, which can lead to orthostatic hypotension.

the arterioles and veins. These drugs can lower blood pressure quickly, but their use is limited because of frequent and bothersome side effects.

The Joint National Committee on Detection, Evaluation, and Treatment of High Blood Pressure (1993) has recommended that initial therapy for hypertension include either a thiazide diuretic or a beta-blocker unless these drugs are contraindicated or ineffective or there are special indications for agents such as calcium antagonists or ACE inhibitors. If after 1 to 3 months a client's blood pressure does not decrease adequately in response to initial therapy, the physician may increase the dose of the drug, substitute a drug from another class of antihypertensives, or add a second drug from another class. Because of changes in recommendations and the availability of more drug options and more information on drug tolerance, the nurse sees a variety of drug protocols used by the physician to meet the individual needs of clients with hypertension.

NONCOMPLIANCE

PLANNING: CLIENT GOALS The goal is that the client will adhere to the therapeutic regimen, thus minimizing the risk of target organ damage.

INTERVENTIONS Clients who require pharmacologic treatment to control essential hypertension usually need to take medication for the rest of their lives. Frequently, clients stop taking antihypertensive medications, assuming that because they have no symptoms the hypertension is under control. Clients may also assume that if their blood pressure returns to normal levels with antihypertensives, they no longer need them. Clients may also stop taking antihypertensives because of adverse side effects or cost.

The nurse and the client discuss the goals of therapy, including potential side effects of the client's individualized treatment, to help the client identify potential problems. The nurse then assists the client in tailoring the therapeutic regimen to the client's activities of daily living.

Clients who do not comply with antihypertensive treatment are at great risk for target organ damage and hypertensive crisis (malignant hypertension). Clients in hypertensive crisis are admitted to critical care units, where they receive intravenous antihypertensive therapy such as nitroprusside (Nipride), nitroglycerin (Nitro-Bid, Tridil IV), labetalol (Normodyne), diazoxide (Hyperstat), or sublingual nifedipine (Procardia, Adalat).

DISCHARGE PLANNING

HOME CARE PREPARATION

If possible, the client should obtain a blood pressure monitor for use at home so that the pressure can be checked periodically. The nurse evaluates the client's ability to learn how to check his or her blood pressure. If the client cannot monitor blood pressure, a family member or significant other may be taught how to perform this procedure.

If weight reduction is a goal, the nurse suggests that the client have a scale in the home.

HEALTH TEACHING

The nurse instructs the client about sodium restriction, weight maintenance or reduction, alcohol restriction, stress management, and exercise (see earlier). If necessary, the nurse also explains about the need to stop smoking.

For clients taking medication for hypertension, the nurse provides oral and written information about the indications, dosage, times of administration, side effects, and drug interactions (see Chart 35-2). The nurse stresses that the medication must be taken as prescribed and that when all of it has been consumed, the prescription must be renewed on a continual basis. Abrupt discontinuation of medications, such as beta-blockers, can result in angina (chest pain) or myocardial infarction.

The nurse urges clients to report unpleasant side effects, such as sexual dysfunction. In many instances, an alternative medication can be prescribed to minimize certain side effects.

If the client has access to equipment to measure blood pressure, the nurse instructs the client or a family member or significant other, or both, in the proper technique for measuring blood pressure. The nurse shows the client how to record all readings in a diary and to bring the diary to all medical appointments so that progress can be followed. Regardless of the therapy to be used, the nurse plans follow-up for all clients.

PSYCHOSOCIAL PREPARATION

Hypertension is a chronic illness, and clients may not be prepared to accept this fact. The nurse allows clients to verbalize feelings about this disease and its treatment. Clients are advised that their involvement in the treatment can lead to control of this disease and can prevent complications.

HEALTH CARE RESOURCES

A home health nurse may be needed for follow-up to monitor blood pressure. The nurse evaluates the ability of the client or the family to obtain accurate blood pressure measurements and assesses their compliance with treatment. If clients cannot purchase equipment to monitor blood pressure, the nurse may suggest the American Heart Association, the Red Cross, or a local pharmacy for free blood pressure checks.

EVALUATION

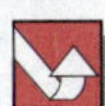

On the basis of the identified nursing diagnoses, the nurse evaluates the care of the hypertensive client. The expected outcomes are that the client will:

- Explain the rationale for treatment of hypertension
- Maintain blood pressure of less than 140/90 mmHg
- Demonstrate no signs or symptoms of target organ damage, such as renal or heart disease

ARTERIAL DISORDERS

Peripheral Arterial Disease

OVERVIEW

Peripheral vascular disease (PVD) includes disorders that alter the natural flow of blood through the arteries and veins of the peripheral circulation. PVD affects the lower extremities much more frequently than the upper extremities. Generally, a client with a diagnosis of PVD has arterial disease (peripheral arterial disease) rather than venous involvement. Some clients have both arterial and venous disease.

PATHOPHYSIOLOGY

Peripheral arterial disease (PAD) is a chronic condition in which partial or total arterial occlusion deprives the lower extremities of oxygen and nutrients. Body tissues cannot live without an adequate oxygen and nutrient supply, and tissue eventually dies. Atherosclerosis is the most common cause of chronic altered blood flow. Fatty substances accumulate at the site of vessel wall injury and alter or totally occlude blood flow within the arteries. Tissue damage generally occurs below the arterial obstruction.

Obstructions are classified as inflow or outflow, according to the arteries involved and their relationship to the inguinal ligament (Fig. 35–4). *Inflow* obstructions involve the distal end of the aorta and the com-

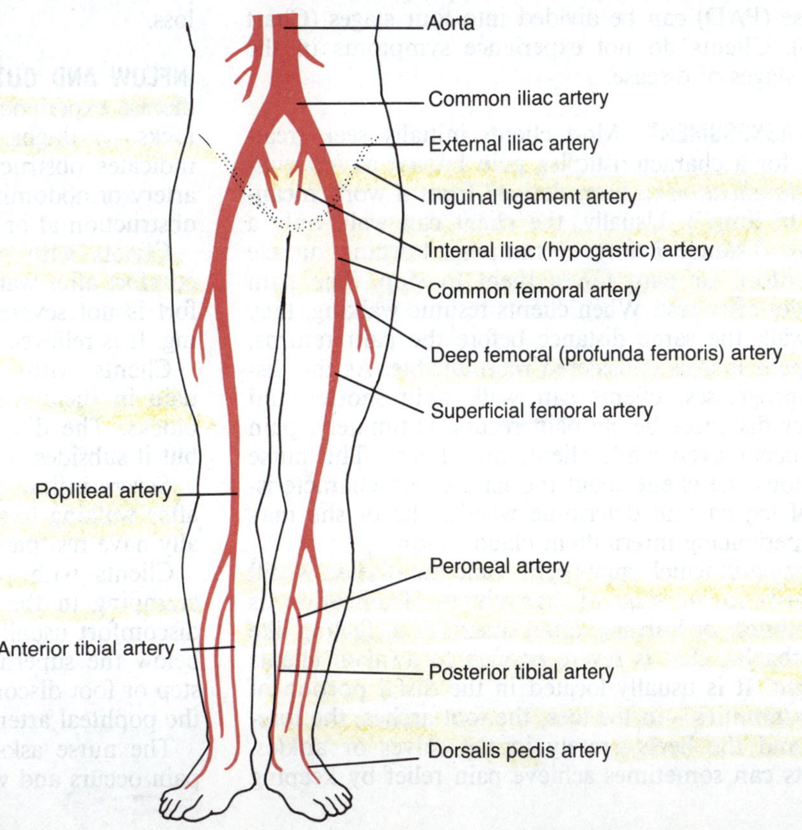

FIGURE 35–4 ◆ Common locations of inflow and outflow lesions.

mon, internal, and external iliac arteries. They are located above the inguinal ligament. *Outflow* obstructions involve infrainguinal arterial segments (the femoral, popliteal, and tibial arteries) and are below the superficial femoral artery (SFA). Gradual inflow occlusions may not cause significant tissue damage; gradual outflow occlusions typically do.

ETIOLOGY

Because atherosclerosis is the most common cause of chronic arterial obstruction, the risk factors for atherosclerosis apply to peripheral arterial disease as well. These include hypertension, hyperlipidemia, diabetes mellitus, cigarette smoking, obesity, and familial predisposition. Advancing age also increases the risk of disease related to atherosclerosis.

INCIDENCE/PREVALENCE

In the United States, at least 10% of people over age 70 and 1% to 2% of people aged 37 to 69 have symptomatic, chronic peripheral arterial disease (Porter et al., 1991). PAD generally occurs in men older than age 45 and in postmenopausal women.

COLLABORATIVE MANAGEMENT

ASSESSMENT

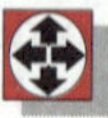

HISTORY

The clinical course of chronic peripheral arterial disease (PAD) can be divided into four stages (Chart 35-4). Clients do not experience symptoms in the early stages of disease.

PAIN ASSESSMENT Most clients initially seek treatment for a characteristic leg pain known as *intermittent claudication* (a term derived from a word meaning "to limp"). Usually, the client can walk only a certain distance before a cramping, burning muscle discomfort, or pain forces them to stop. The pain subsides after rest. When clients resume walking, they can walk the same distance before the pain returns. The pain is thus considered reproducible. As the disease progresses, clients can walk only shorter and shorter distances before pain recurs. Ultimately, pain may occur even while clients are at rest. The nurse questions the client about the nature and characteristics of leg pain to determine whether he or she may be experiencing intermittent claudication.

Rest pain, which may begin while the disease is still primarily in the stage of intermittent claudication, is a numbness or burning, often described as feeling like a toothache, that is severe enough to awaken clients at night. It is usually located in the distal portion of the extremities—in the toes, the foot arches, the forefeet, and the heels—rarely in the calves or ankles. Clients can sometimes achieve pain relief by keeping the limb in a dependent position. Clients with rest pain have advanced disease that may result in limb loss.

CHART 35-4

Key Features of Chronic Peripheral Arterial Disease

Stage I: Asymptomatic
- No claudication is present.
- Bruit or aneurysm may be present.
- Pedal pulses are decreased or absent.

Stage II: Claudication
- Muscle pain, cramping, or burining occurs with exercise and is relieved with rest.
- Symptoms are reproducible with exercise.

Stage III. Rest Pain
- Pain while resting commonly awakes the client at night.
- Pain is described as numbness, burning, toothache-type pain.
- Pain usually occurs in the distal portion of the extremity—toes, arch, forefoot, or heel—rarely in the calf or the ankle.
- Pain is relieved by placing the extremity in a dependent position.

Stage IV: Necrosis/Gangrene
- Ulcers and blackened tissue occur on the toes, the forefoot, and the heel.
- Distinctive gangrenous odor is present.

INFLOW AND OUTFLOW DISEASE Clients with *inflow* disease experience discomfort in the lower back, buttocks, or thighs. Lower back or buttock discomfort indicates obstruction at or above the common iliac artery or abdominal aorta. Thigh discomfort indicates obstruction at or above the profunda femoris artery.

Clients with *mild* inflow disease experience discomfort after walking about two blocks. This discomfort is not severe but causes the client to stop walking. It is relieved with rest.

Clients with *moderate* inflow disease experience pain in these areas after walking about one or two blocks. The discomfort is described more like pain, but it subsides with rest most of the time.

Severe inflow disease causes the client severe pain after walking less than one block. These clients usually have rest pain.

Clients with *outflow* disease describe burning or cramping in the calves, ankles, feet, and toes. Calf discomfort usually indicates arterial obstruction at or below the superficial femoral or popliteal artery. Instep or foot discomfort indicates an obstruction below the popliteal artery.

The nurse asks specific questions about when the pain occurs and whether or not it occurs at rest.

Clients with *mild* outflow disease experience discomfort after walking about five blocks. This discomfort is relieved by rest.

Clients with *moderate* outflow disease have pain after walking about two blocks, and intermittent rest pain may be present.

Clients with *severe* outflow disease are usually unable to walk more than one-half block and usually experience rest pain. They may hang their feet off the bed at night for comfort.

Clients with outflow disease complain more frequently of rest pain than do clients with inflow disease.

PHYSICAL ASSESSMENT/CLINICAL MANIFESTATIONS

Specific findings for peripheral arterial disease (PAD) depend on the severity of the disease. The nurse may observe loss of hair on the lower calf, ankle, and foot; dry, scaly skin; and thickened toenails. With severe arterial disease, the extremity is cold and gray-blue or darkened. The nurse may also note elevational pallor and dependent rubor.

The nurse palpates all pulses in both legs. With chronic PAD, the pulses below the level of obstruction may be decreased or absent. The affected extremity is cool to cold when compared with the nonaffected extremity. If both extremities are cool, the causative factor may be room temperature.

The nurse may also note early signs of ulcer formation or complete ulcer formation. The nurse must differentiate arterial and venous stasis ulcers from diabetic ulcers, which may have a different cause (Chart 35-5).

Arterial ulcers usually are painful and develop on the toes, between the toes, or on the upper aspect of the foot.

Diabetic ulcers develop on the plantar surface of the foot, over the metatarsal heads, and on the heel —anywhere that pressure is exerted. Diabetic ulcers may not be painful because of diabetic neuropathy.

Venous stasis ulcers cause minimal pain and occur in the ankle area. The foot is warm, and distal pulses are palpable. The nurse notes discoloration of the lower extremity at the ulcer site.

PSYCHOSOCIAL ASSESSMENT

In clients with chronic arterial disease, disabling pain can cause depression and anxiety. Pain becomes a part of the client's life. Mobility is limited, and some people may need to change or relinquish their jobs.

Many clients experience fear. The fear of losing a limb or life can cause anxiety, grief, and depression. The nurse assesses each client's coping mechanisms, noting symptoms of maladjusted coping, such as severe anxiety or depression. If limb loss occurs, the client must deal with disfigurement. Assessing the client's feelings about prosthetics and other assistive devices can be important when the nurse is developing interventions for future care.

LABORATORY ASSESSMENT

The laboratory findings in arterial disease are the same as those for atherosclerosis (see earlier).

RADIOGRAPHIC ASSESSMENT

The most common x-ray for peripheral arterial disease is arteriography of the lower extremities. Because arteriography involves injecting contrast medium into the arterial system, the risks, which include hemorrhage, thrombosis, embolus, and death, are serious. Arteriography is often performed before surgery to pinpoint the exact location of the occlusion. The nurse prepares the client for the procedure and carefully implements follow-up care (see Chap. 32).

OTHER DIAGNOSTIC ASSESSMENT

The advent of noninvasive evaluation of arterial disease has become a popular method of diagnosis. Noninvasive testing provides information about the arterial system with minimal risk to the client.

SEGMENTAL SYSTOLIC BLOOD PRESSURE MEASUREMENTS Segmental systolic blood pressure measurements of the lower extremities at the thigh, calf, and ankle are a noninvasive method of assessing peripheral arterial disease (PAD). Normally, blood pressure readings in the thigh and calf are higher than those in the upper extremities. With the presence of arterial disease, these pressures are lower than the brachial pressure.

With *inflow* disease, pressures taken at the thigh level indicate the severity of disease. Mild inflow disease may cause a difference of only 10 to 30 mmHg in pressure on the affected side compared with the brachial pressure.

Severe inflow disease can cause a pressure difference of greater than 40 to 50 mmHg. The ankle pressure is normally equal to or greater than the brachial pressure.

To evaluate *outflow* disease, the nurse compares ankle pressure with the brachial pressure, which provides a ratio known as the ankle/arm (or ankle/brachial) index (ABI). This value can be derived by dividing the ankle blood pressure by the brachial blood pressure.

With mild outflow disease, the client has an ankle/arm index of 0.8 to 1.0; pressures are decreased by about 10 to 30 mmHg.

The client with moderate outflow disease has an ankle/arm index of 0.5 to 0.8, with pressure differences of 20 to 40 mmHg.

An ankle/arm index less than 0.5 indicates severe outflow disease.

EXERCISE TOLERANCE TESTING Exercise tolerance testing (by stress test or treadmill) may give valuable information about clients who are experiencing claudication (muscle pain) without rest pain. The nurse

CHART 35–5

Key Features of Lower Extremity Ulcers

Feature	Arterial Ulcers	Venous Ulcers	Diabetic Ulcers
History	Client complaints of claudication after walking approximately 1–2 blocks Rest pain usually present Pain at ulcer site Two or three risk factors present	Chronic nonhealing ulcer No claudication or rest pain Moderate ulcer discomfort Client complaints about ankle or leg swelling	Diabetes Peripheral neuropathy No complaints of claudication
Ulcer location and appearance	End of the toes Between the toes Deep Ulcer bed pale, with even edges Little granulation tissue	Ankle area Brown pigmentation Ulcer bed pink Usually superficial, with uneven edges Granulation tissue present	Plantar area of foot Metatarsal heads Pressure points on feet Deep Pale, with even edges Little granulation tissue
	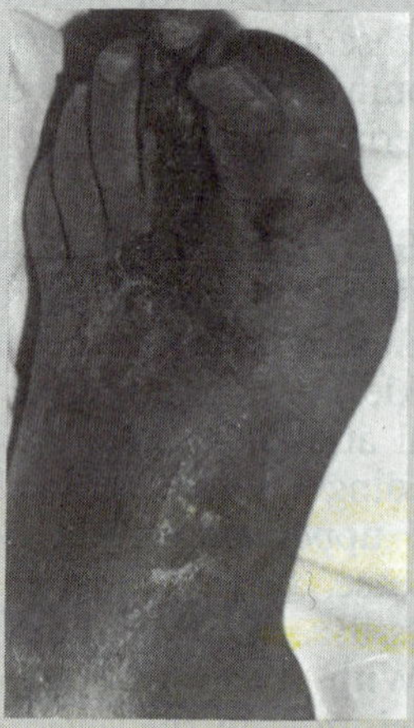	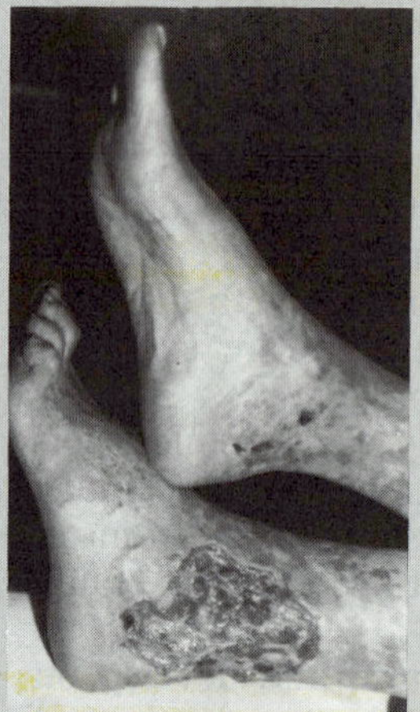	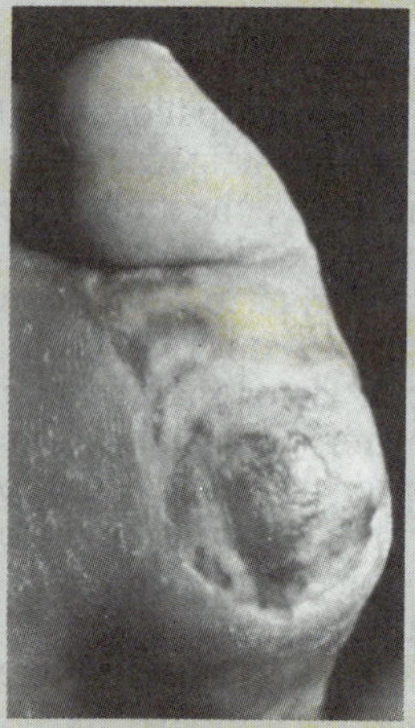
Other assessment findings	Cool or cold foot Decreased or absent pulses Atrophy of skin Hair loss Pallor with elevation Dependent rubor Possible gangrene When acute, neurologic deficits noted	Ankle discoloration and edema Full veins when legs slightly dependent No neurologic deficit Pulses present May have scarring from previous ulcers	Pulses usually present Cool or warm foot Painless
Treatment	Treat underlying cause (surgical revascularization) Prevent trauma and infection Client education, stressing foot care	Long-term wound care (Unna's boot, damp-to-dry dressings) Elevate extremity Client education Prevent infection	Rule out major arterial disease Control diabetes Client education regarding foot care Prevent infection

Photograph of diabetic ulcer from Kozak, G. P., Hoar, C. S., Jr., Rowbotham, J. L., Wheelock F. C., Jr., Gibbons, G. W., & Campbell D. (1984). *Management of diabetic foot problems.* Philadelphia: W. B. Saunders.

or technician obtains resting pulse volume recordings and has the client walk on a treadmill until the symptoms are reproduced. At the time of symptom onset or after approximately 5 minutes, the nurse or technician obtains another pulse volume recording. Normally, there may be an increased waveform with minimal, if any, drop in the ankle pressures. In clients with arterial disease, the waveforms are decreased (dampened) and there is a decrease in the ankle pressure of the affected limb of 40 to 60 mmHg for 20 to 30 seconds. If the return to normal pressure is delayed (longer than 10 minutes), the results suggest abnormal arterial flow in the affected limb.

PLETHYSMOGRAPHY Plethysmography can also be performed to evaluate arterial flow in the lower extremities. This measurement provides graph or tracing readings of arterial flow in the limb. If an occlusion is present, the waveforms are dampened to flattened, depending on the degree of occlusion.

ANALYSIS

COMMON NURSING DIAGNOSES

The common nursing diagnoses found in clients with peripheral arterial disease are:

1. Altered Tissue Perfusion (peripheral) related to decreased blood flow
2. Impaired Skin Integrity related to decreased circulation

ADDITIONAL NURSING DIAGNOSES

Additional nursing diagnoses related to arterial disease include:

- Pain related to obstructive process
- Fear related to effects of possible limb loss
- Impaired Physical Mobility related to pain and intolerance to activity
- Activity Intolerance related to pain

PLANNING AND IMPLEMENTATION

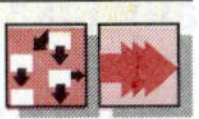

ALTERED TISSUE PERFUSION (PERIPHERAL)

PLANNING: CLIENT GOALS The major goal is that the client will show an increased arterial blood flow to the extremities, as evidenced by the presence of pulses bilaterally and warm skin.

INTERVENTIONS The nurse first determines whether the altered tissue perfusion is of arterial or venous origin. An accurate assessment often provides this information, but in some people both conditions may exist. In this case, each disease must be considered separately when appropriate interventions are planned.

Nonsurgical Management The interventions of exercise, position changes, promotion of vasodilation, drug therapy, and invasive nonsurgical procedures are used to increase arterial flow to the affected limb.

Exercise Exercise may improve arterial blood flow to the affected limb through build-up of the *collateral* circulation. (Collateral circulation provides blood to the affected area through smaller vessels that develop and compensate for the occluded vessels.) Exercise is individualized for each client, but people with severe rest pain, venous ulcers, or gangrene should not participate. Other clients with peripheral arterial disease (PAD) can benefit from exercise that is initiated gradually and is slowly increased; an excellent exercise for these clients is walking. The nurse instructs the client to walk until the point of claudication, stop and rest, then walk a little farther. Eventually, clients are able to walk longer distances as collateral circulation develops. The nurse collaborates with the physician and physical therapist in determining an appropriate exercise program.

Positioning Positioning of the client to promote circulation has been somewhat controversial. Some clients have swelling in their extremities. Because swelling prevents arterial flow, these clients should elevate their feet at rest, but the nurse teaches clients to refrain from raising their legs above the heart level. Extreme elevation *slows* arterial blood flow to the feet.

In severe cases, clients with PAD and swelling may sleep with the affected limb hanging from the bed or they may sit upright in a chair for comfort. The nurse instructs all clients with PAD to avoid crossing their legs, which may interfere with blood flow.

Promoting Vasodilation Vasodilation can be achieved by providing warmth to the affected extremity and preventing long periods of exposure to cold. The nurse encourages the client to maintain a warm environment at home and to wear socks or insulated shoes at all times. The client is cautioned *never* to apply direct heat to the limb, such as with the use of heating pads or extremely hot water. Sensitivity is decreased in the affected limb, and the client may get burned without feeling it.

The nurse encourages clients to prevent exposure of the affected limb to the cold because cold temperatures cause vasoconstriction (decreasing of the diameter of the blood vessels) and therefore decrease arterial blood flow. Emotional stress, caffeine, and nicotine also can cause vasoconstriction. The nurse emphasizes that complete abstinence from smoking or chewing tobacco is the most effective method of preventing vasoconstriction. The vasoconstrictive effects of each cigarette may last up to 1 hour after the cigarette is smoked.

DRUG THERAPY For clients with chronic peripheral arterial disease (PAD), prescribed drugs include hemorrheologic and antiplatelet agents. Pentoxifylline (Trental) is a hemorrheologic agent that increases the flexibility of red blood cells; it decreases blood viscosity by inhibiting platelet aggregation and decreasing fibrinogen and thus increases blood flow in the extremities. Many clients report limited improvement in their daily lives after taking pentoxifylline. Moreover, clients with extremely limited endurance for walking have reported improvement to the point that they can perform some activities (e.g., walk to the mailbox or dining room) that were previously impossible.

The most commonly used drugs for clients with

PAD are the antiplatelet agents, such as aspirin (acetylsalicylic acid, Ancasal✱) and dipyridamole (Persantine, Apo-Dipyridamole✱). Aspirin, 325 mg/day, is typically recommended for life for all clients with chronic PAD.

Controlling hypertension can improve tissue perfusion by maintaining pressures that are adequate to perfuse the periphery but not vasoconstrict the vessels. Nurses should make clients aware of the effect of blood pressure on the circulation and should instruct clients in methods of control. For example, clients taking beta-blockers may experience drug-related claudication or an exacerbation of their symptoms. The physician, nurse practitioner, and/or nurse closely monitor clients with PAD who are receiving beta-blockers.

PERCUTANEOUS TRANSLUMINAL ANGIOPLASTY Another nonsurgical but invasive method of improving arterial flow is percutaneous transluminal angioplasty (PTA) (Fig. 35–5). One or more arteries are dilated with a balloon catheter advanced through a cannula, which is inserted into or above an occluded or stenosed artery. When the procedure is successful, it opens the vessel lumen and improves arterial blood flow, creating a smooth inner vessel surface. Clients who are candidates for PTA must have occlusions or stenoses that are accessible to the catheter. The physician often uses PTA for clients who are poor surgical candidates who cannot withstand general anesthesia or for whom amputation may be inevitable. Clients can experience reocclusion after this procedure, and the procedure may be repeated. Some clients have been occlusion-free for up to 3 to 5 years, whereas others experience reocclusion within a year of PTA.

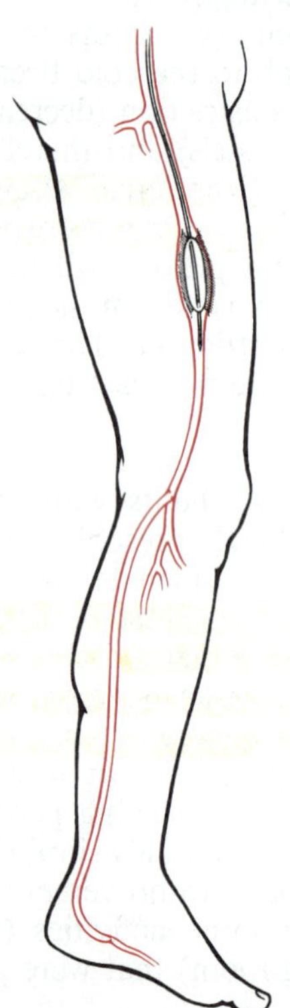

FIGURE 35–5 ◆ Percutaneous transluminal angioplasty.

LASER-ASSISTED ANGIOPLASTY Another invasive procedure is laser-assisted angioplasty. A laser probe is advanced through a cannula similar to that used for percutaneous transluminal angioplasty (PTA). Laser-assisted angioplasty is usually reserved for clients with smaller occlusions in the distal superficial femoral, proximal popliteal, and common iliac arteries. Heat from the laser vaporizes the arteriosclerotic plaque to open the occluded or stenosed artery. If significant stenosis remains after the artery is opened, a PTA balloon catheter may be inserted to further dilate the artery.

Preparation of the client for PTA or laser-assisted angioplasty is similar to that for diagnostic angiography. The nurse keeps the client on nothing by mouth (NPO) after midnight and scrubs the groin area with an antiseptic soap according to hospital policy. Some clients are shaved. Post-procedure nursing care involves observing for bleeding at the puncture site. The nurse closely observes vital signs and frequently checks the distal pulses in both limbs. These clients are typically restricted to bed rest, with the limb straight for approximately 6 to 8 hours before ambulation. Many of these clients receive anticoagulant therapy, such as heparin (Heplean✱), for approximately 3 days and then dipyridamole (Persantine, Apo-Dipyridamole✱) for 3 to 6 months. Clients usually take aspirin on a permanent basis.

ATHERECTOMY The technique of mechanical rotational abrasive atherectomy is used to improve blood flow to ischemic limbs in people with peripheral arterial disease. The rotational atherectomy device (Rotablator) is a high-speed rotary, metal bur ranging in sizes from 1.25 to 4.5 mm in diameter. The distal half of the bur is embedded with fine abrasive bits, which at rotational speeds of 100,000 to 120,000 rotations per minute result in fine-particle destruction of tissue. The Rotablator is designed to preferentially scrape "hard" surfaces (such as plaque) while minimizing damage to the vessel surface.

Surgical Management Clients with severe rest pain or claudication that interferes with the ability to work or threatens loss of a limb become surgical candidates. Arterial revascularization is the surgical procedure most commonly used to increase arterial blood flow in an affected limb.

Surgical procedures are classified as inflow or outflow. Inflow procedures involve bypassing arterial occlusions above the superficial femoral arteries (SFAs). Outflow procedures involve surgical bypassing of arterial occlusions at or below the superficial femoral arteries. For clients who have both inflow and outflow problems, the inflow procedure (for larger arteries) is done before the outflow repair.

Inflow procedures include aortoiliac, aortofemoral, and axillofemoral bypasses. Outflow procedures include femoropopliteal and femorotibial bypasses. Inflow procedures are more successful, with less chance of reocclusion or postoperative ischemia. Outflow procedures are less successful in relieving ischemic pain and are associated with a higher incidence of reocclusion.

Graft materials for the bypasses are selected on an individual basis. For outflow procedures, the preferred graft material is an autogenous saphenous vein. However, these clients can experience systemic vascular disease and may need this vein for coronary artery bypass. When the saphenous vein is not usable, the client's cephalic or basilic arm veins may be used.

Grafts made of synthetic materials, such as polytetrafluoroethylene, Gore-Tex, and Dacron, have also been used when autogenous veins were not available. Although synthetic grafts have achieved adequate patency in arteries above the knee, they have failed to achieve satisfactory results in infrapopliteal outflow vessels. In addition, autogenous veins are often not long enough for use in these vessels. Composite grafts constructed from multiple vein segments offer even better patency to arteries below the knee.

Preoperative Care Preparing the client for surgery is similar to that described for the client having general or epidural anesthesia (see Chap. 19). Documentation of vital signs and peripheral pulses provides a baseline of information for comparison during the postoperative phase. Depending on the surgical procedure, the client may have an intravenous (IV) line, urinary catheter, central venous catheter, and/or arterial line. To prevent postoperative infection, clients typically receive antibiotic therapy for about 48 hours before the procedure.

Operative Procedures The anesthesiologist or nurse anesthetist places the client under general, epidural, or spinal anesthesia. Epidural or spinal induction is preferred for older adults to decrease the risk of cardiopulmonary complications in this group. If arterial bypass is to be accomplished by autogenous grafts, the surgeon excises the appropriate veins through an incision. The occluded artery is then exposed through an incision, and the conduit veins or synthetic graft material is sutured above and below the occlusion to facilitate blood flow around the occlusion.

For *aortoiliac* and *aortofemoral* bypass surgery, the surgeon makes a midline incision into the abdominal cavity to expose the abdominal aorta, with additional incisions into each groin (Fig. 35–6). Graft material is tunneled from the aorta to the groin incisions, where it is sutured in place.

In an *axillofemoral* bypass (Fig. 35–7) the surgeon makes an incision beneath the clavicle and tunnels graft material subcutaneously with a catheter from the chest to the iliac crest, into a groin incision, where it is sutured in place. Neither the thoracic nor abdominal cavity is entered. For this reason, the axillofemoral bypass is used for high-risk clients who cannot tolerate a procedure requiring abdominal surgery.

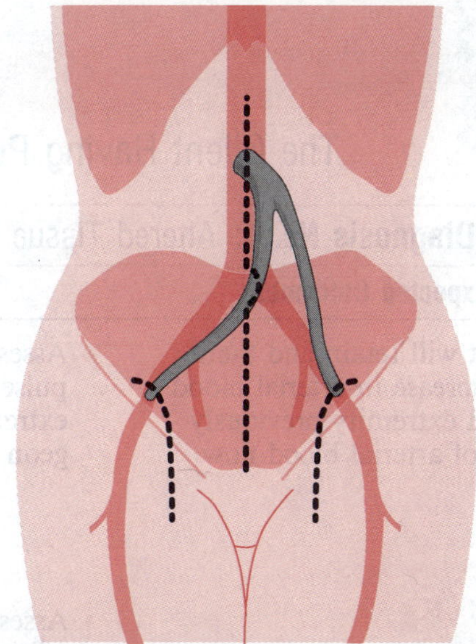

FIGURE 35–6 ◆ In aortoiliac and aortofemoral bypass surgery, a midline incision into the abdominal cavity is required, with an additional incision in each groin.

Postoperative Care Graft occlusion often occurs within the first 24 hours. Therefore, astute nursing care is crucial. The Client Care Plan highlights the most important aspects of postoperative care.

ASSESSMENT FOR GRAFT OCCLUSION The nurse monitors the patency of the graft by checking the extremity every 15 minutes for the first hour, then hourly for changes in color, temperature, and pulse intensity.

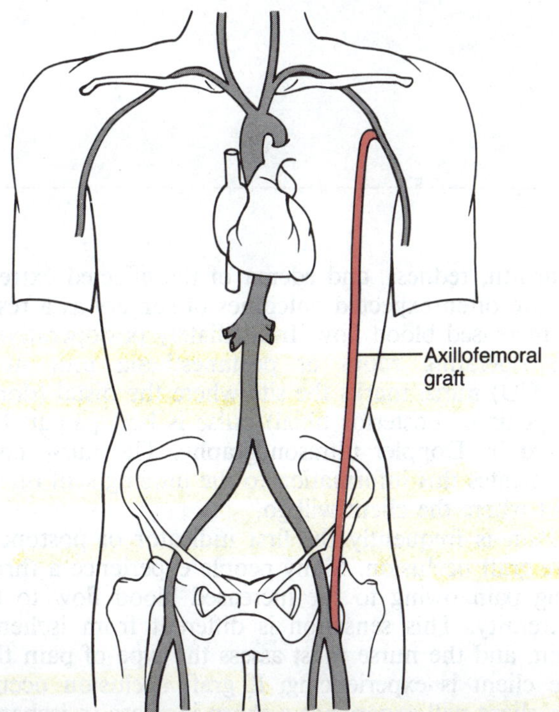

FIGURE 35–7 ◆ An axillofemoral bypass graft.

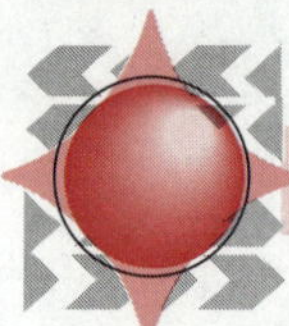

CLIENT CARE PLAN

The Client Having Peripheral Arterial Revascularization (Bypass) Surgery

Nursing Diagnosis No. 1: Altered Tissue Perfusion (Peripheral)

Expected Outcomes	Nursing Interventions	Rationale
The client will retain and maintain an increase in arterial blood flow to an extremity previously deprived of arterial blood flow.	◆ Assess color, temperature, and pulse intensity of the affected extremity hourly. Notify the surgeon of a significant change.	◆ Color, temperature, and pulse intensity immediately postoperatively indicate optimal arterial flow achieved with revascularization. Any increase in pallor or cyanosis or decrease in temperature or pulse intensity indicates postoperative graft occlusion.
	◆ Assess the client for pain in the affected extremity, and report, if described, as "severe, similar to the pain before surgery."	◆ Severe pain, similar to the pain felt before surgery, is frequently the first indicator of postoperative graft occlusion.
	◆ Monitor the client's blood pressure, and report if it is increased or decreased beyond the client's normal limits.	◆ Hypotension may indicate hypovolemia, which can increase the risk of clotting. Hypertension may put stress on the graft.
	◆ Instruct the client to keep the affected extremity straight, limit movement, and avoid flexion of the knee and hip. Consult with the surgeon about turning the client.	◆ Pressure on the graft can facilitate clot formation.
	◆ Assess the incision for drainage, edema, and temperature.	◆ Edema of the affected extremity is an expected outcome, but excessive edema should be reported. ◆ A small amount of bloody drainage is expected, but excessive bleeding is abnormal. ◆ Warmth, erythema, or a hard, tender area around the incision may indicate infection.

Warmth, redness, and edema of the affected extremity are often expected outcomes of surgery as a result of increased blood flow. Immediately postoperatively, the operating room or postanesthesia unit nurse (PACU) nurse marks the site where the distal (dorsalis pedis or posterior tibial) pulse is best palpated or heard by Doppler ultrasonography. The nurse communicates this information to the nursing staff on the unit where the client will go.

Pain is frequently the first indicator of postoperative graft occlusion. Many people experience a throbbing pain owing to the increased blood flow to the extremity. This sensation is different from ischemic pain, and the nurse must assess the type of pain that the client is experiencing. If graft occlusion occurs, the client will experience a sharp increase in ischemic pain, described as similar to the pain felt before surgery. The nurse reports severe pain to the surgeon immediately.

PROMOTION OF GRAFT PATENCY To promote graft patency, the nurse monitors the client's blood pressure and notifies the surgeon if the pressure increases or decreases beyond normal limits. Hypotension may indicate hypovolemia, which can increase the risk of clotting. Range of motion of the affected limb is usually limited, with bending of the hip and knee contraindicated. The nurse consults with the surgeon on a case-by-case basis regarding limitations of movement, including turning. Clients are restricted to bed rest for at least 24 hours postoperatively.

The nurse instructs all clients to cough and deep breathe every 1 to 2 hours and to use an incentive spirometer. Clients who have had aortoiliac or aortofemoral bypass are allowed nothing by mouth (NPO) for at least 1 day postoperatively. Clients who have undergone bypass surgery of the lower extremities not involving the aorta or abdominal wall (femoropopliteal or femorotibial bypass) may be on NPO status the night of surgery but are often allowed clear liquids the morning after surgery.

TREATMENT OF GRAFT OCCLUSION If manifestations of graft occlusion occur, the nurse notifies the surgeon immediately. Perfusion through the graft must be resolved promptly to avoid ischemic injury to the limb. Emergency *thrombectomy* (removal of the clot), which the surgeon may perform at the bedside, is the most common treatment for acute graft occlusion. Thrombectomy is associated with excellent results in prosthetic grafts but variable results in autogenous vein grafts, which often necessitate graft revision and even replacement.

Local intra-arterial *thrombolytic therapy* with urokinase (Abbokinase) may be used for acute graft occlusions in selected clients, in settings where health providers are experts on its use. The physician considers thrombolytic therapy when the surgical alternative (e.g., thrombectomy with or without graft revision or replacement) carries high morbidity or mortality or when surgery for this type of occlusion has traditionally yielded poor results. When the physician uses urokinase, the nurse closely assesses the client for signs and symptoms of bleeding.

ASSESSMENT OF INFECTION Graft or wound infections can be life-threatening and can endanger the client's limb. The nurse uses sterile technique when in contact with the incision and observes for symptoms of infection at or around the graft and incision sites. If the area over the graft becomes hard, tender, red, or warm, the client may have an infection. The nurse notifies the surgeon if any of these symptoms occurs.

IMPAIRED SKIN INTEGRITY

PLANNING: CLIENT GOALS The primary goal is that the client will not experience an ulcer. If an ulcer develops, the goal is that the ulcer will heal.

INTERVENTIONS Prevention is the most important intervention associated with impairment of skin integrity or ulcer formation. The nurse explains how ulcers occur. Arterial ulcers can occur because of minor trauma or inadequate foot care. The nurse instructs clients about proper foot care and preventive measures. An ulcer may develop despite preventive measures, necessitating wound interventions.

Nonsurgical Management Management of arterial ulcers can be difficult. Some ulcers are chronic in nature, but many are acute. The underlying cause of arterial obstruction must first be determined. Arterial ulcers do not respond well to treatment if the arterial blood flow to the affected limb is not improved.

Nonsurgical treatment of the ulcer can vary. Because all ulcers are fertile ground for infection, the nurse uses sterile technique for wound care. The physician prescribes intravenous antibiotic therapy if the ulcer is accompanied by cellulitis (a reddened, inflamed area). For arterial ulcers, the physician may order damp-to-dry saline dressings. The nurse secures the dressing with a roll bandage (such as Kling or Kerlix), applying tape only on the bandage. Because Kling has elastic properties, the nurse applies this bandage loosely to prevent further impairment of arterial circulation. The nurse *never* uses tape directly on the skin because of the risk of causing further tissue damage. In some facilities, the use of Kling is not permitted for leg or foot ulcers.

Arterial ulcers are often odorous. The nurse notes any change in odor, secretions, or redness extending up the foot or leg and notifies the physician immediately if any of these manifestations are present. Close observation by the nurse can enable prompt treatment to prevent further complications.

Surgical Management The surgeon performs a surgical *debridement* early in the management of leg ulcers. This procedure may be necessary several times before healing can occur. *Arterial bypass grafting* (described earlier) may be performed to improve perfusion to the ulcerated area and to facilitate healing. If infected and gangrenous ulcers do not improve with antibiotics and debridement, *amputation* may be necessary to avoid septicemia and possible death, and to decrease disabling pain. The trend is toward limited, distal amputations such as amputation of an affected toe or toes, but the extent depends on the level of the ulceration. (For a discussion of the care of clients with an amputation, see Chapter 51.)

Preoperative Care If the wound is superficial, the physician may debride it with local anesthesia. The client needs reassurance and education about the procedure and its indications. The physician may prescribe a preoperative medication to relax the client before the procedure.

Operative Procedure Surgical debridement involves removing the dense eschar (outer) tissue so that the wound can granulate, form healthier tissue, and heal.

Postoperative Care After surgical debridement, the nurse observes for any bleeding at the ulcer site. The nurse administers pain medication as prescribed. Aseptic dressing changes are necessary to prevent infection. The nurse continues to observe for signs of infection, such as elevated temperature or purulent wound drainage.

DISCHARGE PLANNING

HOME CARE PREPARATION

Clients with arterial compromise may need assistance with activities of daily living (ADL) if activity is limited by pain. The client may need to limit or avoid stair climbing depending on the severity of disease. Clients who have undergone surgery usually need temporary help with activities of daily living.

HEALTH TEACHING

The nurse instructs all clients on methods to promote vasodilation (see Planning and Implementation). Clients receive individualized instruction about positioning and exercise. The nurse teaches clients to avoid raising their legs above the level of the heart unless they also have venous stasis. The nurse provides written and oral instructions on foot care and methods to prevent injury and ulcer development for all clients (Chart 35–6).

The nurse teaches clients receiving pentoxifylline (Trental) to take the drug as prescribed, whether or not they notice improvement. It often takes 6 to 8 weeks for the drug to be effective, and the effect may not be apparent. The nurse instructs the client to take pentoxifylline with meals to prevent side effects of nausea and vomiting.

Clients receiving dipyridamole (Persantine) are instructed to take the medication 1 hour before meals to promote optimal absorption. The nurse advises clients taking aspirin to take the drug with meals or milk and crackers and to report any nausea or vomiting.

Clients who have had surgery require additional instruction on incision care (see Chap. 21). The nurse encourages all clients to avoid smoking and to limit dietary fat intake to less than 30% of the total daily calories.

CHART 35–6

Education Guide ◆ Foot Care for the Client with Peripheral Vascular Disease

- Keep your feet clean by washing them with a mild soap in room-temperature water.
- Keep your feet dry, especially between the toes and ankles.
- Avoid injury to your feet and ankles. Wear comfortable, well-fitting shoes. Never go without shoes.
- Keep your toenails clean and filed. Have someone cut them if you cannot see them clearly. Cut your toenails straight across.
- To prevent dry, cracked skin, apply a lubricating lotion to your feet.
- Prevent exposure to extreme heat or cold. Never use a heating pad on your feet.
- Avoid constricting garments.
- If a problem develops, see a podiatrist or physician.
- Avoid extended pressure on your feet or ankles, such as occurs when you lean against something.

PSYCHOSOCIAL PREPARATION

The client who is hospitalized with chronic arterial obstruction may fear recurrent occlusion or further narrowing of the artery. Clients often fear that they might lose a limb or become debilitated in other ways. Indeed, chronic peripheral arterial disease (PAD) may worsen, especially in clients with diabetes mellitus. The nurse, however, reassures clients that their participation in prescribed exercise, diet, and pharmacologic therapy, along with cessation of smoking, can limit further atherosclerotic plaque formation.

The client who undergoes amputation of a limb requires significant support to assist in coping with changes in gait and disturbance in body image. (see Chap. 51).

HEALTH CARE RESOURCES

Clients who must limit activity because of peripheral arterial disease may benefit from the assistance of a home health aide. The client who has undergone surgery may require a home health nurse to assist with incision care. Clients who have had amputations usually need physical therapy to assist with ambulation as well. The nurse or discharge planner arranges for home care resources before the client is discharged.

EVALUATION

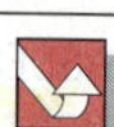

Evaluation of the client with arterial occlusive disease is based on outcome criteria for each nursing diagnosis. The expected outcomes are that the client will:

- Demonstrate improved peripheral tissue perfusion, manifested by palpable or audible pedal pulses and the absence of claudication (muscle pain)
- Remain free of arterial ulcers
- Demonstrate improved activity tolerance as evidenced by performance of activities of daily living and exercise
- Verbalize an understanding of interventions that can help prevent complications of arterial disease

Acute Peripheral Arterial Occlusion

OVERVIEW

Although chronic peripheral arterial disease (PAD) progresses slowly, the onset of acute arterial occlusions may be sudden and dramatic. An embolus is the most common cause of peripheral occlusions, although a local thrombus may be the cause. Occlusion may affect the upper extremities, but it is more common in the lower extremities. Emboli originating from the heart are the most common cause of acute arterial occlusions. Most clients with an embolic occlusion have had an acute myocardial infarction and/or atrial fibrillation within the preceding weeks.

COLLABORATIVE MANAGEMENT

ASSESSMENT

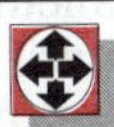

Clients with acute arterial occlusion describe severe pain below the level of the occlusion that occurs even at rest. The affected extremity is cool or cold, pulseless, and mottled. Minute areas on the toes may be blackened or gangrenous.

INTERVENTIONS

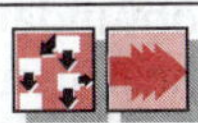

The physician must initiate treatment promptly to avoid permanent damage or loss of an extremity. Anticoagulant therapy with heparin (Hepalean✱) is usually the first intervention to prevent further clot formation. The physician may order a bolus up to 10,000 units. The client may also undergo angiography.

A surgical thrombectomy or embolectomy with local anesthesia may be performed to remove the occlusion. The physician makes an incision, followed by an arteriotomy (a surgical opening into an artery). The physician then inserts a Fogarty catheter into the artery and retrieves the embolus. It may be necessary to close the artery with a patch graft.

Postoperatively, the nurse monitors the affected extremity for improvement in color, temperature, and pulse as well as other extremities for signs and symptoms of new thrombi or emboli. Pain should significantly diminish after the surgical procedure, although mild incisional pain remains. The nurse watches closely for complications caused by reperfusing the artery after thrombectomy or embolectomy, which include spasms and swelling of the skeletal muscle. Swelling of the skeletal muscles is characterized by edema, pain on passive movement, poor capillary refill, numbness, and muscle tenseness. Fasciotomy (surgical opening into the tissues) may be necessary to prevent further injury and save the limb.

The use of systemic thrombolytic therapy for acute arterial occlusions has been disappointing because bleeding complications have outweighed the benefits obtained. However, local intra-arterial thrombolytic therapy with urokinase (Abbokinase) has emerged as an occasional alternative to surgical treatment in selected clients in settings where health providers are familiar with its use and its complications. When urokinase is given, the nurse monitors the client for signs and symptoms of bleeding.

Aneurysms

OVERVIEW

An aneurysm is a permanent localized dilation of an artery, which enlarges the artery to at least 1½ times its normal diameter.

TYPES OF ANEURYSMS

An aneurysm may be described as *fusiform* (a diffuse dilation affecting the entire circumference of the artery) or *saccular* (an outpouching affecting only a distinct portion of the artery). *Dissecting hematomas,* traditionally called "dissecting aneurysms," are more accurately described as "aortic dissections" (see later). Aortic dissections differ from aneurysms, in that they are formed when blood accumulates in the wall of an artery.

Aneurysms tend to occur at specific anatomic sites (Fig. 35–8), most commonly, the abdominal aorta. Aneurysms often occur at a point where the artery is not supported by skeletal muscles or on the lines of curves or flexion in the arterial tree.

PATHOPHYSIOLOGIC PROCESS

An aneurysm forms when the middle layer (media) of the artery is weakened, producing a stretching effect in the inner layer (intima) and outer layers (adventitia) of the artery. As the artery widens, tension in the wall increases and further widening occurs, thus enlarging the aneurysm. Hypertension (high

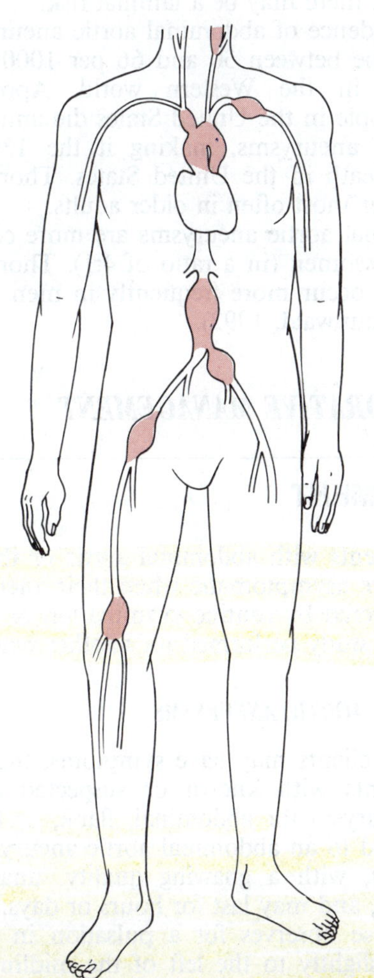

FIGURE 35–8 ◆ Common anatomic sites of arterial aneurysms.

blood pressure) produces more tension and enlargement within the artery. As the aneurysm grows, the risk of arterial rupture increases.

Abdominal aortic aneurysms account for approximately 75% of all aneurysms. Most of these aneurysms are located between the renal arteries and the aortic bifurcation. Of all abdominal aortic aneurysms greater than 6 cm in diameter, 50% rupture within 1 year; of those aneurysms smaller than 6 cm in diameter, 15% to 20% rupture.

Thoracic aneurysms account for approximately 25% of all aneurysms. They commonly develop between the origin of the left subclavian artery and the diaphragm. They are located in the descending, ascending, and transverse sections of the aorta.

Aneurysms can cause symptoms by exerting pressure on surrounding structures or by rupturing. Rupture of an aneurysm is the most frequent complication and is life-threatening because abrupt and massive hemorrhagic shock occurs with the rupture. Thrombi within the wall of an aneurysm can also be the source of emboli in distal arteries below the aneurysm.

Atherosclerosis is the most common cause of all aneurysms, with hypertension and cigarette smoking being contributing factors. Syphilis and Ehlers-Danlos syndrome are other causes of abdominal aortic aneurysms, and there may be a familial risk.

The incidence of abdominal aortic aneurysms, estimated to be between 30 and 66 per 1000 people, is increasing in the Western world. Approximately 15,000 people in the United States die annually from abdominal aneurysms, making it the 13th leading cause of death in the United States. Thoracic aneurysms occur most often in older adults.

Abdominal aortic aneurysms are more common in men than women (in a ratio of 4:1). Thoracic aneurysms also occur more frequently in men (in a ratio of 3:1) (Braunwald, 1992).

COLLABORATIVE MANAGEMENT

ASSESSMENT

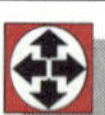

Most clients with abdominal aortic or thoracic aneurysms are asymptomatic when their aneurysms are first discovered by routine examination or during radiographic study performed for another reason.

ABDOMINAL AORTIC ANEURYSMS

Because clients may have symptoms, the nurse assesses clients with known or suspected abdominal aortic aneurysm for abdominal, flank, or back pain. Pain related to an abdominal aortic aneurysm is usually steady, with a gnawing quality, unaffected by movement, and may last for hours or days.

The nurse observes for a pulsation in the upper abdomen slightly to the left of the midline between the xiphoid process and the umbilicus. A detectable aneurysm is at least 5 cm in size. The nurse then auscultates for a bruit over the mass but avoids palpating the mass because it may be tender and there is a risk of rupture.

Although some clients have symptoms when the aneurysm is intact, many clients are asymptomatic until the time of rupture. If expansion and impending rupture of an abdominal aortic aneurysm is suspected, the nurse assesses for severe pain of sudden onset in the back or lower abdomen, which may radiate to the groin, buttocks, or legs.

Clients with a rupturing abdominal aortic aneurysm are critically ill in hemorrhagic (hypovolemic) shock. Signs include hypotension, diaphoresis, mental obtundation, oliguria, and dysrhythmias. Retroperitoneal hemorrhage is manifested by hematomas in the flanks. Rupture into the abdominal cavity causes abdominal distention.

THORACIC ANEURYSMS

When a thoracic aneurysm is suspected, the nurse assesses the client for back pain and manifestations of compression of the aneurysm on adjacent structures. Signs include shortness of breath, hoarseness, and difficulty swallowing.

Thoracic aneurysms are not often detected by physical assessment, but occasionally a mass may be visible above the suprasternal notch.

The client with suspected rupture of a thoracic aneurysm is assessed for sudden and excruciating back or chest pain. Rupture of a thoracic aneurysm is also indicated by hemorrhagic shock (see Chap. 36).

RADIOGRAPHIC ASSESSMENT

An abdominal x-ray or lateral film of the spine often shows an abdominal aortic aneurysm. The "eggshell" appearance of the aneurysm is essentially diagnostic (Fig. 35–9).

Computed tomographic (CT) scanning is the standard tool for assessing the size and location of an aortic aneurysm. A thoracic aneurysm can be diagnosed by chest x-ray. A CT scan is used to assess size and location. Aortic arteriography is performed for all clients who are to undergo surgical repair of a thoracic aneurysm.

OTHER DIAGNOSTIC ASSESSMENT

Ultrasonography is a noninvasive technique that provides an accurate diagnosis as well as information about the size and location of an abdominal aortic aneurysm.

INTERVENTIONS

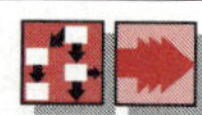

The size of the aneurysm and the presence of symptoms are the most important parameters in the determination of treatment.

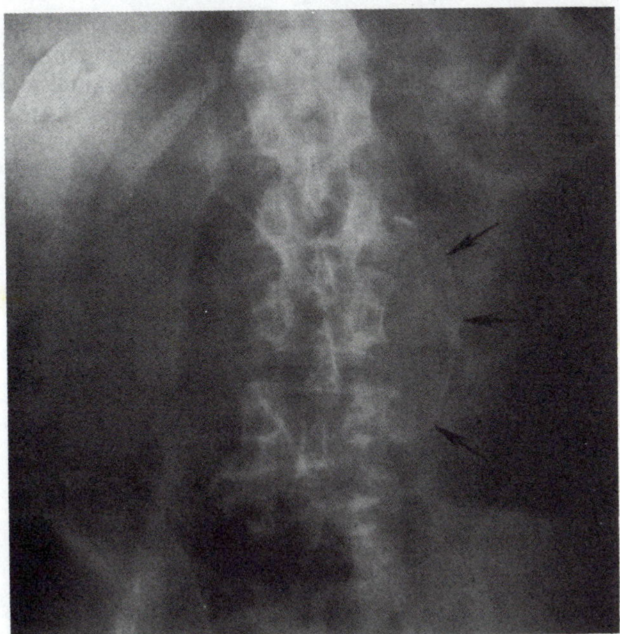

FIGURE 35-9 ◆ X-ray of the abdomen of a client with an abdominal aortic aneurysm *(arrows).* Note the "eggshell" appearance of the border of the aneurysm, caused by calcification. (From Sabiston, D. C. [1991]. *Textbook of surgery: The biological basis of modern surgical practice* [14th ed.]. Philadelphia: W. B. Saunders.)

Nonsurgical Management The goal of nonsurgical management is to maintain the blood pressure at a normal level in order to decrease the risk of rupture and monitor the growth of the aneurysm.

Because elevated blood pressure can increase the rate of aneurysmal enlargement, hypertension is an important risk factor for rupture. Clients with hypertension are treated with antihypertensives to decrease the rate of enlargement and the risk for early rupture (see hypertension management earlier).

For clients with small or asymptomatic aneurysms, frequent CT scans are necessary to monitor the growth of the aneurysm. The nurse emphasizes the importance of following through with scheduled tests to monitor the growth. The nurse also explains the clinical manifestations of aneurysms that need to be promptly reported.

Surgical Management Surgical management of an aneurysm may be an elective or an emergency procedure.

Clients with an abdominal aortic aneurysm 6 cm in diameter or wider undergo elective surgery. Some surgeons favor surgical treatment for clients with aneurysms 4 to 6 cm in diameter if the client is in good health. Clients in good health with aneurysms smaller than 4 cm and clients in poor health with aneurysms 4 to 6 cm in diameter undergo nonsurgical treatment until the aneurysm reaches 6 cm.

Clients with thoracic aneurysms measuring 7 cm or more in diameter and clients with smaller aneurysms that are producing symptoms are advised to have elective surgery. Clients with aneurysms smaller than 7 cm in diameter that are not causing symptoms are treated nonsurgically until symptoms occur or the aneurysm enlarges to 7 cm.

For all clients with either a rupturing abdominal aortic or a thoracic aneurysm, emergency surgery is performed.

The most common procedure performed for clients with an abdominal aortic aneurysm is an abdominal aortic aneurysm (AAA) resection or repair (aneurysmectomy). The mortality rate for elective AAA resection is 2% to 5%. The mortality rate for emergency surgery for expanding abdominal aortic aneurysms is 5% to 15% and 50% for those that have ruptured.

The major surgery for clients with a thoracic aneurysm is a thoracic aneurysm repair. Elective resection of these aneurysms is associated with a 10% mortality rate.

Abdominal Aortic Aneurysm Resection In an abdominal aortic aneurysm (AAA) resection, the physician excises the aneurysm from the abdominal aorta to prevent or repair its rupture. The goal is to secure stable aortic integrity and tissue perfusion throughout the body.

PREOPERATIVE CARE Interventions are similar to those for clients undergoing surgery with general anesthesia (see Chap. 19). A bowel preparation and emphasis on coughing and deep breathing are very important. Because a significant blood loss often occurs during AAA resection, clients planning elective surgery may be advised to bank their blood for autologous (self) transfusions postoperatively.

The nurse assesses all peripheral pulses to serve as a baseline for comparison postoperatively. The nurse may mark where the pulse is palpated or heard by Doppler ultrasonography to facilitate locating the pulse postoperatively.

Clients with ruptured aneurysms are brought to the operating suite directly from the emergency department. Preoperative care of clients with ruptured aneurysms involves administration of large volumes of intravenous (IV) fluids to maintain tissue perfusion.

OPERATIVE PROCEDURE The surgeon makes a midline abdominal incision from the xiphoid process to the symphysis pubis, or a wide transverse incision from flank to flank, to expose the aneurysm. Clamps are applied just above the aneurysm and below it, the aneurysm is excised, and a preclotted Dacron graft is sutured in an end-to-end fashion (Fig. 35-10).

POSTOPERATIVE CARE Immediately postoperatively, the client is admitted to a critical care unit for 24 to 48 hours. In addition to providing the routine postoperative care discussed in Chapter 21, the nurse assesses for and assists in the prevention of the postoperative complications that can occur after an AAA repair. These complications include:

- Graft occlusion or rupture causing hemorrhage
- Hypovolemia and/or renal failure

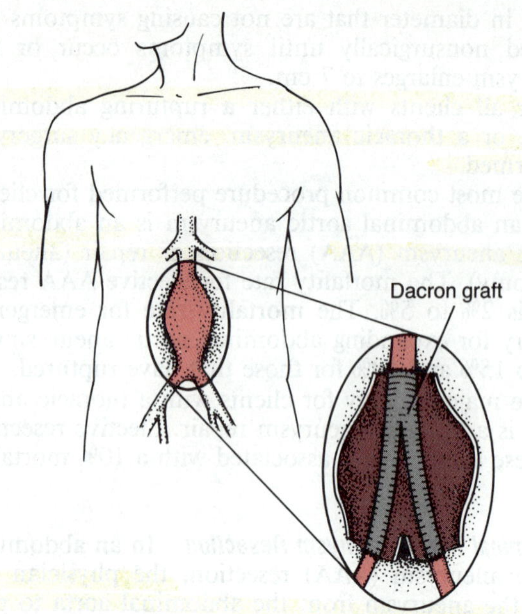

FIGURE 35–10 ◆ Surgical repair of abdominal aortic aneurysm with a woven Dacron graft.

- Respiratory distress
- Paralytic ileus

Graft Occlusion or Rupture. The nurse assesses vital signs and circulation every 15 minutes for the first hour, then hourly with assessment of pulses distal to the graft site (including posterior tibial and dorsalis pedis). The nurse reports any signs of graft occlusion or rupture, including:

- Changes in pulses
- Cool to cold extremities below the graft
- White or blue extremities or flanks
- Severe pain
- Abdominal distention

The nurse limits elevation of the head of the bed to 45 degrees to avoid flexion of the graft.

Hypovolemia or Renal Failure. Hypovolemia and renal failure occur because there is often a large blood loss during surgery or before if rupture occurred. The nurse assesses urine output via Foley catheter hourly. If urine output is less than 50 mL/hour, the nurse notifies the surgeon. Although advances in surgical technique have decreased the risk of renal failure after clamping during surgery, renal failure may occur. Renal failure caused by acute tubular necrosis is more common after emergency surgery. In addition to monitoring urine output, the nurse and physician monitor serum creatinine and blood urea nitrogen levels daily.

Respiratory Distress. The nurse assesses the client's respiratory rate and depth every hour and auscultates breath sounds every 4 hours to monitor for respiratory complications. Often, the client is maintained on a ventilator at least overnight to facilitate respiratory exchange. The nurse administers opioids for pain, as ordered, and turns and suctions the client according to protocol. The nurse ensures firm abdominal support of the incision with a pillow or bath blanket, while the client is coughing, to prevent the incision from separating. After the client is extubated, the nurse assesses that the client turns, coughs, and deep breathes every 1 to 2 hours and increases his or her mobility as ordered.

Paralytic Ileus. Paralytic ileus after AAA repair is expected for 3 to 4 days. Clients have a nasogastric tube to low suction until bowel sounds return. The nurse listens for bowel sounds every 8 hours and reports their return to the physician. The nurse assesses for prolonged absence of bowel sounds and distention, which may indicate a prolonged ileus or a bowel infarction.

Thoracic Aneurysm Repair Repair of thoracic aneurysms is tailored to each client; the procedure depends on the type and location of the aneurysm. Total cardiopulmonary bypass (CPB) is necessary for excision of aneurysms in the ascending aorta, and partial bypass is often used during excision of aneurysms in the descending aorta.

PREOPERATIVE CARE The care of the client undergoing thoracic aneurysm resection is similar to that provided for the client having thoracic surgery (see Chap. 31). Clients undergoing cardiopulmonary bypass receive care similar to that described in Chapter 37.

OPERATIVE PROCEDURE The surgeon uses either a thoracotomy or a median sternotomy approach to enter the thoracic cavity. The surgeon exposes the aneurysm and excises it. After excising the aneurysm, the surgeon usually sews a Dacron graft or prosthesis onto the aorta. Saccular aneurysms, which have an outpouching from a distinct portion of the arterial wall, can sometimes be removed without resection of the aorta.

POSTOPERATIVE CARE The care of a client who has undergone thoracic aneurysm repair is similar to that after other chest surgery. Clients undergoing cardiopulmonary bypass receive care similar to that described in Chapter 37. The nurse assesses for and assists in the prevention of postoperative complications that can occur after a thoracic aneurysm repair. These complications include:

- Hemorrhage
- Paraplegia
- Respiratory distress
- Cardiac dysrhythmias

Hemorrhage. The nurse assesses vital signs at least hourly, reporting any signs of hemorrhage (a drop in blood pressure, an increase in pulse rate, rapid respirations, diaphoresis), to the physician immediately. The nurse assesses for bleeding or separation at the graft site by noting significant increases in chest drainage from the chest tubes.

Paraplegia. Inadvertent interruption of the blood

supply to the spinal cord during thoracic aneurysm repair can result in paraplegia. The nurse assesses the client hourly for sensation and motion in all extremities and reports deficits immediately.

Respiratory Distress. After thoracic aneurysm repair, clients are especially susceptible to respiratory distress from atelectasis or pneumonia. This problem occurs as a result of both cardiopulmonary bypass and incisional discomfort. Both atelectasis and pneumonia may cause shallow breathing and poor cough effort. These clients are often maintained on a ventilator, at least overnight after surgery. For clients with a median sternotomy, the surgeon firmly splints the incision to prevent separation of the sternum.

Cardiac Dysrhythmias. The nurse assesses all clients recovering from thoracic aneurysm repair for cardiac dysrhythmias. The stress of the thoracic surgery, added to the increased incidence of arteriosclerosis in this group, may predispose these clients to a myocardial infarction, cardiac dysrhythmias, or heart failure.

DISCHARGE PLANNING

HOME CARE PREPARATION

Most clients after aneurysm repair are discharged home. In rare instances, the postoperative client may be discharged to an extended (long-term) care facility for rehabilitation in the absence of family or other support systems.

HEALTH TEACHING

For clients who have not undergone surgical aneurysm repair, the teaching plan emphasizes the importance of compliance with the schedule of computed tomography (CT) scanning to monitor the size of the aneurysm. The nurse educates the client receiving treatment for hypertension about the importance of continuing to take prescribed medication. The client and family or significant other are instructed about signs and symptoms that they must promptly report to their health care provider:

- Clients with abdominal aortic aneurysms must report abdominal fullness or pain or back pain.
- Clients with thoracic aneurysms must report chest or back pain, shortness of breath, difficulty swallowing, or hoarseness.

The nurse teaches the client who has undergone repair of the aneurysm about activity restrictions, wound care, and pain management. Clients may not engage in activities that involve lifting heavy objects (usually more than 15 to 20 pounds, or 6.8 to 9.1 kg) for 6 to 12 weeks postoperatively. The nurse advises the client to use discretion in activities that involve pulling, pushing, or straining, such as vacuuming, changing bed linens, moving furniture, mopping or sweeping, raking leaves, mowing grass, and chopping wood. Clients should temporarily avoid such hobbies as tennis, swimming, horseback riding, and golf, although putting practice is allowed. Because of postoperative weakness, the client is usually restricted from driving a car for several weeks after discharge.

PSYCHOSOCIAL PREPARATION

Clients who have not undergone aneurysm repair may fear rupture and subsequent death. The nurse assesses for the client's and family's perceptions of this potential situation. The nurse reinforces the rationales for CT monitoring of aneurysmal size and for controlling hypertension, and encourages clients to verbalize their fears.

HEALTH CARE RESOURCES

The nurse assesses the availability of transportation to and from appointments for clients needing CT monitoring. If transportation is a problem, the nurse consults the social worker to assist in arranging this service.

Clients who have undergone surgery may require the services of a home health nurse for assistance with dressing changes. A home health aide may be needed to assist with activities of daily living.

Aneurysms of the Peripheral Arteries

OVERVIEW

Although femoral and popliteal aneurysms are relatively uncommon, they are often associated with an aneurysm in another location of the arterial tree. To detect a popliteal aneurysm, the nurse palpates a pulsating mass in the popliteal space. To detect a femoral aneurysm, the nurse palpates a pulsatile mass over the femoral artery. The nurse evaluates both extremities because more than one femoral or popliteal aneurysm may be present.

COLLABORATIVE MANAGEMENT

The client may exhibit symptoms of limb ischemia, and the nurse assesses for diminished or absent pulses, cool to cold skin, and pain. Pain may also be present if an adjacent nerve is compressed. The recommended treatment for either type of aneurysm, regardless of the size, is surgery because of the risk of thromboembolic complications associated with their presence.

To treat a femoral aneurysm, the physician excises the aneurysm and restores circulation using a Dacron graft or an autogenous saphenous vein graft. Most surgeons prefer to bypass rather than resect a popliteal aneurysm.

Postoperatively, the nurse monitors for lower limb ischemia. The nurse palpates pulses below the graft to assess graft patency. Often, Doppler ultrasonography is necessary to assess blood flow when pulses are not palpable. Sudden development of pain or discoloration of the extremity is reported immediately to the physician because it may indicate graft occlusion.

Aortic Dissection

OVERVIEW

Aortic dissection has traditionally been referred to as a "dissecting aneurysm." However, because this condition is more accurately described as a dissecting hematoma, the term aortic dissection has gained favor.

Aortic dissection is thought to be caused by a sudden tear in the aortic intima, opening the way for blood to enter the aortic wall. Degeneration of the aortic media might be a prerequisite for this condition, with hypertension an important contributing factor.

Aortic dissection is a relatively common event, occurring in at least 2000 people in the United States annually. It is frequently associated with connective tissue disorders such as Marfan's syndrome. It also occurs in older people, peaking in adults in their 50s and 60s and in women in their third trimester of pregnancy.

Because the circulation of any major artery arising from the aorta can be impaired in clients with aortic dissection, this condition is highly lethal and represents an emergency situation.

Dissections are classified in various ways. Debakey et al.'s classification contains three groups:

- Type 1: Is characterized by an intimal tear in the ascending (proximal) aorta, with extension of the dissection into the descending (distal) aorta
- Type 2: Originates in and is limited to the ascending (proximal) aorta
- Type 3: Arises within the descending (distal) thoracic aorta and often progresses distally

Proximal dissections occur almost twice as often as distal dissections. Although the ascending aorta and descending thoracic aorta are the most common sites, dissection can also occur in the abdominal aorta and other arteries.

COLLABORATIVE MANAGEMENT

The most common presenting symptom of aortic aneurysm is pain, with painless dissection occurring rarely. The pain is described as "tearing," "ripping," and "stabbing" and tends to move from its point of origin. Depending on the site of dissection, the client may feel pain in the anterior chest, back, neck, throat, jaw, or teeth.

Diaphoresis, nausea, vomiting, faintness, and apprehension are also common. Blood pressure is usually elevated, unless complications, such as cardiac tamponade or rupture, have occurred. A decrease or absence of peripheral pulses is common, as is aortic regurgitation, characterized by a musical murmur heard better along the right sternal border. Neurologic deficits, such as altered level of consciousness, paraparesis, and cerebrovascular accidents, can also occur.

Chest x-ray, Doppler echocardiogram, computed tomography (CT), and aortic angiography are commonly used to confirm the diagnosis.

The goals of emergency treatment include:

- The elimination of pain
- A reduction of blood pressure to 100 to 120 mmHg
- A decrease in the velocity of left ventricular ejection

The physician prescribes intravenous (IV) sodium nitroprusside (Nipride) by continuous drip initially to lower the blood pressure. If this regimen is ineffective, trimethaphan (Arfonad) may be used. Propranolol (Inderal, Apo-Propranolol♣) is given in increments of 1 mg IV to decrease left ventricular ejection.

Subsequent treatment depends on the location of the dissection. Generally, clients receive continued medical treatment for uncomplicated distal dissections and surgical treatment for proximal dissections.

For clients receiving long-term medical treatment, the systolic blood pressure must be maintained at or below 130 to 140 mmHg. Beta-blockers (propranolol) and calcium channel antagonists are indicated.

Clients receiving surgical intervention for a proximal dissection always require total cardiopulmonary bypass (see Chap. 37). The surgeon excises the intimal tear and obliterates entry in the false opening by suturing edges of the dissected aorta. Usually, a prosthetic graft is used.

Buerger's Disease

OVERVIEW

Buerger's disease (thromboangiitis obliterans) is a relatively uncommon occlusive disease limited to the medium and small arteries and veins. The distal upper and lower limbs are the most frequently affected. Typically, Buerger's disease is identified in young adult males who smoke. Larger arteries, such as the femoral and brachial, become involved in the late stages of the disease. The veins are less commonly involved.

The disease often extends into the perivascular tissues, resulting in fibrosis and scarring that binds the artery, vein, and nerve firmly together. For people who have this disease, cessation of cigarette smoking usually arrests the disease process but persistence in smoking causes occlusion in the more proximal vessels.

The cause of Buerger's disease is unknown, although there is a strong association with tobacco smoking. A familial or genetic predisposition and autoimmune etiologic factors are also possible.

COLLABORATIVE MANAGEMENT

ASSESSMENT

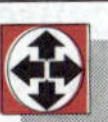

The first clinical manifestation of Buerger's disease is usually claudication (pain in the muscles resulting from an inadequate blood supply) of the arch of the foot. Intermittent claudication may occur in the lower extremities. The pain may be ischemic, occurring in the digits while the client is at rest. Often, there is an aching pain that is more severe at night. Paroxysmal shock-like pain can be the result of ischemic neuropathy. Clients often experience increased sensitivity to cold and complain of coldness and numbness. On physical examination, the nurse notes that the pulses are often diminished in the distal extremities and the extremities are cool and red or cyanotic in the dependent position.

A diagnosis of Buerger's disease is commonly based on a physical finding of peripheral ischemia, often in association with migratory superficial phlebitis. Ulcerations and gangrene may be seen in the digits. The ulcerations are usually sharply demarcated. The gangrenous lesion can be small or can affect the entire digit.

Arteriograms can be useful in delineating the degree of disease present in the arteries. Commonly, arteriography reveals multiple segmental occlusions in the smaller arteries of the forearm, hand, leg, and foot. Plethysmographic studies of the fingers or toes may be diagnostic of the disease in the early stages. These studies can also be useful in following the progression of the disease in more proximal arteries.

INTERVENTIONS

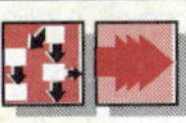

Nursing interventions are directed at:

- Preventing the progression of the disease
- Avoiding vasoconstriction
- Promoting vasodilation
- Relieving pain
- Treating ulceration and gangrene

To prevent progression of Buerger's disease, complete abstinence from tobacco in all forms is essential. The client is instructed to prevent extreme or prolonged exposure to cold to prevent vasoconstriction. The nurse instructs the client about medications that are prescribed for vasodilation, such as nifedipine (Procardia, Adalat). (See Chapter 8 for interventions and nursing management for pain relief.)

The treatment of clients with Buerger's disease is similar to that of clients with peripheral arterial disease (see earlier).

Subclavian Steal

OVERVIEW

Subclavian steal occurs in the upper extremities from a subclavian artery occlusion or stenosis. The result is altered blood flow and ischemia in the arm. Subclavian steal can occur in people at any age but is more common in those with risk factors for atherosclerosis. Symptoms include:

- Tiredness in the arm with exertion
- Paresthesias
- Lightheadedness
- Dizziness
- Exercise-induced pain in the forearm when the arms are elevated

COLLABORATIVE MANAGEMENT

Physical examination usually reveals a significant difference in the blood pressures between the arms. A difference greater than 20 mmHg is considered significant. Another important finding is a subclavian bruit, which can occur on the affected side. The subclavian pulse may be decreased on the occluded side when compared with the opposite side. The client's arm may also be discolored or cyanotic; however, this finding generally occurs only in severe cases.

Surgery is the recommended intervention when a client has cyanosis or pain. One of three procedures may be used:

- Endarterectomy of the subclavian artery
- Carotid-subclavian bypass
- Dilation of the subclavian artery

Nursing care encompasses postoperative care of the client and monitoring the arterial flow in the affected arm. The nurse should check brachial and radial pulses frequently and observe for ischemic changes. The nurse also observes the arm for edema, redness, or any other signs.

Thoracic Outlet Syndrome

OVERVIEW

Thoracic outlet syndrome is a compression of the subclavian artery at the thoracic outlet by anatomic structures, such as a rib or muscle. The arterial wall may be damaged, producing thrombosis or embolization to distal arteries of the arms. The three common sites of compression in the thoracic outlet are:

- The interscalene triangle
- Between the coracoid process of the scapula and the pectoralis minor tendon
- Most commonly, the costoclavicular space

COLLABORATIVE MANAGEMENT

Thoracic outlet syndrome is more common in females and in people whose occupations require holding their arms up or leaning over, such as baseball players, golfers, or swimmers. It is also seen in clients who have had trauma such as whiplash or after clavicular fracture. Clients generally complain of neck, shoulder, and arm pain that may be intermittent. The client may also have numbness and moderate edema of the extremity. The pain and numbness are worse when the arm is placed in certain positions, such as over the client's head or out to the side. The client may have overdeveloped neck and shoulder muscles, and the affected arm may appear cyanotic.

Treatment includes physical therapy, exercises, and avoiding aggravating positions, such as elevating the arms. Surgical treatment involves resection of the anatomic structure that is compressing the artery. Surgery is performed only if a client has severe pain, has lost hand function, or is responding poorly to conservative treatment.

Raynaud's Phenomenon

OVERVIEW

Raynaud's phenomenon is caused by vasospasm of the arterioles and arteries of the upper and lower extremities, usually unilaterally. *Raynaud's disease* occurs bilaterally. The two terms are sometimes used interchangeably and, although they are related, there are some differences. Raynaud's phenomenon usually occurs in people older than 30 years; Raynaud's disease can occur between the ages of 17 and 50 years. Raynaud's phenomenon can occur in either sex, but Raynaud's disease is more common in women.

The pathophysiology is the same for both. The etiology is unknown. Clients often have an associated systemic connective tissue disease, such as systemic lupus erythematosus or progressive systemic sclerosis (see Chap. 23).

As a result of vasospasm, the cutaneous vessels are constricted and blanching of the extremity occurs, followed by cyanosis. When the vasospasm is relieved, the tissue becomes reddened or hyperemic. The client's extremities are numb and cold, and the client may complain of pain and swelling. Ulcers may also be present. These attacks are intermittent and can be aggravated by cold or stress. In severe cases, the attack lasts longer and gangrene of the digits can occur.

COLLABORATIVE MANAGEMENT

Treatment involves relieving or preventing the vasoconstriction by drug therapy. Commonly prescribed drugs are reserpine (Serpasil, Novoreserpine♣), nifedipine (Procardia), cyclandelate (Cyclospasmol), and phenoxybenzamine (Dibenzyline). These agents may help to relieve the symptoms, but they can cause uncomfortable side effects, such as facial flushing, headaches, hypotension, and dizziness.

For severe symptoms that cannot be alleviated by drugs, a lumbar sympathectomy can be performed. The physician cuts the sympathetic nerve fibers that cause vasoconstriction of blood vessels in the lower extremities. This method is effective when clients are experiencing foot symptoms. For the upper extremities, a similar procedure—sympathetic ganglionectomy—may provide symptom relief. The long-term effectiveness of these treatments is questionable.

Education of the client is important in prevention of complications. The nurse explains methods to prevent vasoconstriction, such as minimizing exposure to cold and decreasing stress. The client is instructed to wear warm clothes, socks, or gloves when exposed to cool or cold temperatures. Clients should keep their homes at a comfortably warm temperature. The nurse helps the client to identify stressors and provides suggestions for reducing them.

Popliteal Entrapment

Popliteal entrapment causes ischemic symptoms in the affected leg or foot because of anatomic compression of the popliteal artery. Popliteal entrapment occurs in young people, most often in men complaining of intermittent claudication of one or both extremities.

Physical examination may reveal ischemic changes of the affected extremity, with normal function of the unaffected limb. When the client is at rest, the nurse may note diminished distal pulses, although this is a rare finding.

Diagnosis of popliteal entrapment is possible only after an accurate client history, physical examination, and arteriography.

The recommended treatment is surgical repair of the anatomic compression. Reconstruction of the popliteal artery may be necessary to restore arterial blood flow to the limb.

Nursing care involves preventing general postoperative complications and evaluating the patency of the graft or artery postoperatively. The nurse observes for ischemic changes and evaluates distal pulses frequently postoperatively.

VENOUS DISORDERS

Peripheral Venous Disease

To function properly, veins must be patent (unobstructed) with competent valves. Vein function also necessitates the assistance of the surrounding muscle beds to help pump blood toward the heart. If one or more veins are not operating efficiently, they become distended and clinical manifestations occur.

Two distinct phenomena alter the blood flow in veins:

- Thrombus formation (*venous thrombosis)* can lead to pulmonary embolism, a life-threatening complication (see Chap. 31).
- Defective valves lead to *venous insufficiency* and *varicose veins,* which are not life-threatening but are problematic.

Venous Thrombosis

OVERVIEW

Thrombus formation constitutes one of health care's greatest challenges. A thrombus (also called a thrombosis) is a blood clot believed to result from an endothelial injury, venous stasis, and/or hypercoagulability. However, the thrombosis may not be specifically attributable to one element, or it may involve all three elements. Thrombosis is often associated with an inflammatory process. When a thrombus develops, inflammation can occur around the thrombus, thickening the vein wall and consequently leading to embolization (the formation of an embolus).

Thrombophlebitis refers to a thrombus that is associated with inflammation; *phlebothrombosis* is a thrombus without inflammation. Thrombophlebitis can occur in superficial veins; however, it most frequently occurs in the deep veins of the lower extremities.

Deep venous (vein) thrombophlebitis, commonly referred to as deep venous thrombosis (DVT), not only is more common but also is more serious than superficial thrombophlebitis because it presents a greater risk for *pulmonary embolism,* in which a dislodged blood clot travels to the pulmonary artery.

Thrombus formation has been associated with stasis of blood flow, endothelial injury, and/or hypercoagulability, or Virchow's triad (Carroll, 1993). The precise cause of these events remains unknown; however, a few predisposing factors have been identified. Thrombosis has commonly occurred in people undergoing certain surgical procedures. The highest incidence of clot formation occurs in clients who have undergone hip surgery or open prostate surgery. Other conditions that seem to promote thrombus formation are pregnancy, ulcerative colitis, and heart failure.

Immobility can predispose a person to thrombosis. This can occur during prolonged bed rest, such as when a client is confined to bed during the perioperative period. *Phlebitis* (vein inflammation) associated with invasive procedures, such as intravenous therapy, can predispose clients to thrombosis. Severe infections, systemic lupus erythematosus, polycythemia vera, oral contraceptives, and trauma have also been linked to thrombosis.

COLLABORATIVE MANAGEMENT

ASSESSMENT

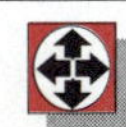

The classic signs and symptoms of deep vein thrombosis (DVT) are calf or groin tenderness and pain, with or without leg swelling. Pain in the calf on dorsiflexion of the foot (Homan's sign) is another possible indicator of DVT, although the reliability of this assessment finding is controversial. The nurse examines the area that the client describes as painful, comparing this site with the contralateral limb. The nurse gently palpates the site, observing for warmth and edema. Signs and symptoms, however, may be absent with thrombophlebitis. Because there are often silent clinical findings, the nurse must have a high index of suspicion for this disorder when caring for clients at high risk.

Localized edema in one extremity may suggest thrombophlebitis. The nurse may measure and compare right and left calf and thigh circumferences for changes over time as an indicator of DVT or venous insufficiency. However, serial leg measurements may not be the most reliable indicator of DVT. Swarczinski and Dijkers (1991) found that serial leg measurements were not useful or reliable in determining the presence of DVT in clients with spinal cord injury (Research Applications for Nursing).

Although diagnostic tests for DVT are available, physical examination findings are often adequate for diagnosis. If a definitive diagnosis is lacking from physical examination alone, other diagnostic tests may be performed, such as: venography, doppler studies, and impedance phlebography.

Venography with contrast medium visualizes clot formation in approximately 95% of people with DVT. However, this study is generally not performed because it may precipitate thrombosis and is very painful.

Doppler ultrasonography is a noninvasive test frequently used as the initial diagnostic test for DVT if a definitive diagnosis cannot be made by physical examination. Normal venous circulation is characterized by audible signals, whereas thrombosed veins produce little or no flow.

Impedance phlebography (IPG), another noninvasive test, has its limitations, although it has become more accurate in diagnosing clots.

INTERVENTIONS

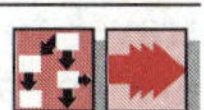

The focus of treatment for thrombophlebitis is to prevent complications, such as pulmonary emboli, and to prevent an increase in size of the thrombus. Deep venous thrombophlebitis (thrombosis) is the

RESEARCH APPLICATIONS FOR NURSING

Serial Leg Measurements May Not Help to Identify Deep Vein Thrombosis

Swarczinski, C., & Dijkers, M. (1991). The value of serial leg measurements for monitoring deep vein thrombosis in spinal cord injury. *Journal of Neuroscience Nursing, 23,* 306–314.

This study examined the effectiveness of using serial leg measurements to detect or monitor the progress of deep vein thrombosis (DVT). Each of 30 clients hospitalized in an acute care setting with spinal cord injury was evaluated for DVT using serial leg measurements every day and a diagnostic procedure, the radiofibrinogen uptake test (RFUT), every 3 days.

There was no significant correlation between the findings on the RFUT and leg measurements. Because spinal cord injury clients demonstrate leg atrophy soon after experiencing trauma, the effects of atrophy could have obscured an increase in leg circumference from DVT.

Critique The researchers attempted to validate a traditional nursing intervention of measuring leg circumference as a part of nursing assessment for clients who have or are at risk for DVT. The sample was limited to 30 clients with the same medical diagnosis in one acute care setting.

Possible nursing implications This study shows the need to question and validate some of the interventions that nurses have routinely been doing without a scientific basis. It clearly raises questions about the need for the nurse to take the time to measure leg circumferences if it is not helpful.

most common type of thrombophlebitis. All clients with DVT are hospitalized for treatment.

Nonsurgical Management Deep vein thrombosis (DVT) is most often treated medically, using a combination of rest, drug therapy, and preventive measures.

Rest Supportive therapy for DVT includes bed rest and elevation of the extremity. Some physicians order intermittent or continuous warm, moist soaks to the affected area. All clients are evaluated for signs and symptoms of pulmonary embolus (PE), which include shortness of breath and chest pain. Emboli may also travel to the brain or heart, but these complications are not as common as PE (see Chap. 31).

Drug Therapy Anticoagulants are the drugs of choice for a client with DVT and for clients at risk for DVT. Heparin is used for an existing clot, but other agents, such as aspirin and dextran, may be used for clot prevention.

HEPARIN THERAPY Most clients with a confirmed diagnosis of an existing blood clot are started on a regimen of intravenous (IV) heparin (Hepalean✱) therapy. Heparin is an anticoagulant agent that, at low doses, interacts with antithrombin III to produce selective inhibition of clotting factor X. At higher doses, heparin inhibits practically all clotting factors. The ultimate result is inhibition of fibrin formation (Lehne et al., 1994). Heparin does nothing to the existing clot. The physician prescribes heparin to prevent the formation of other clots, which often develop in the presence of an existing clot, and to prevent enlargement of the existing clot. Over a long period of time, the existing clot is slowly absorbed by the body.

Heparin is initially given by a bolus IV dose of approximately 100 units/kg, followed by constant infusion. The infusion is regulated by a reliable electronic infusion device that protects against accidental free flow of solution. The physician or clinical pharmacist orders concentrations of heparin (in 5% dextrose in water) and the number of units or milliliters per hour to maintain a therapeutic activated partial thromboplastin time (APTT). APTTs are obtained daily, or more frequently, and are reported to the physician as soon as the results are available, to allow adjustment of heparin dosage. Therapeutic levels of APTTs are usually 1½ to 2 times normal control levels. The nurse assesses clients for signs and symptoms of bleeding, which include hematuria, frank or occult blood in the stool, ecchymosis, petechiae, an altered level of consciousness, or pain.

Heparin can also decrease platelet counts. Mild reductions are common. Severe platelet reductions, although rare, result from the development of antiplatelet bodies. The physician discontinues heparin administration if severe *heparin-induced* thrombocytopenia (<100,000 mm³) occurs. An oral anticoagulant may be substituted for heparin, if necessary (Lehne et al., 1994).

The nurse also ensures that protamine sulfate, the antidote for heparin, is available, if needed, for excessive bleeding. Chart 35–7 highlights important nursing care and client education associated with anticoagulant therapy.

To prevent DVT, heparin may be given in low doses subcutaneously. The physician usually orders a dose of 5000 units every 8 to 12 hours for high-risk clients, especially after orthopedic surgery (Carroll, 1993). Other pharmacologic agents that may be used for prophylaxis are:

- Low-molecular-weight heparin (e.g., enoxaparin)
- Dextran, an intravenous plasma expander
- Dihydroergotamine (DHE)
- Warfarin (Coumadin, Warfilone✱)
- Aspirin

WARFARIN THERAPY After treatment for deep vein thrombosis (DVT) with heparin therapy, and after the signs and symptoms of DVT have greatly resolved, the client is usually started on oral warfarin

CHART 35–7

Nursing Care Highlight ◆ The Client Receiving Anticoagulant Therapy

- Carefully check the dosage of anticoagulant to be administered, even if the pharmacy prepared the medication.
- Monitor the client for signs and symptoms of bleeding, including hematuria, frank or occult blood in the stool, ecchymosis, petechiae, altered mental status (indicating possible cranial bleeding), or pain (especially abdominal pain, which could indicate abdominal bleeding).
- Monitor vital signs frequently for decreased blood pressure and increased pulse (indicating possible internal bleeding).
- Have antidotes available as needed, e.g., protamine sulfate for heparin and vitamin K for warfarin (Coumadin, Warfilone✱).
- Monitor activated partial thromboplastin time (APTT) for clients receiving heparin; monitor prothrombin time (PT) or International Normalized Ratio (INR) for clients receiving warfarin.
- Apply prolonged pressure over venipuncture sites and injection sites.
- When administering *subcutaneous* heparin, apply pressure over the site and do not massage.
- Teach the client going home on an anticoagulant to:
  - Use only an electric razor.
  - Take precautions to avoid injury, for example, do not use tools like hammers or saws, where accidents commonly occur.
  - Report signs and symptoms of bleeding, such as blood in the urine or stool, nosebleeds, ecchymosis, or altered mental status.
  - Take the prescribed dosage of medication at the precise time that it was ordered to be given.
  - Not stop taking the medication abruptly; the physician usually tapers the anticoagulant gradually.

sodium. Warfarin works in the liver to inhibit synthesis of the four vitamin K–dependent clotting factors. It takes 3 to 4 days before warfarin can exert therapeutic anticoagulation. For this reason, warfarin administration is started while the intravenous (IV) heparin is being infused. The heparin continues to provide therapeutic anticoagulation until this effect is achieved with warfarin. IV heparin is discontinued at that time. Therapeutic levels of warfarin are monitored by measuring prothrombin time (PT). A therapeutic prothrombin time with warfarin administration is often 1½ to 2 times normal control levels (International Normalized Ratio [INR] of 1.5 to 2.0). The initial dosage of warfarin is usually 10 to 15 mg daily for 1 to 2 days. Maintenance therapy ranges from 2.5 to 7.5 mg given once a day in the evening. Clients usually receive warfarin for up to 6 months after an episode of DVT.

Nursing assessment for bleeding is similar to that described for clients receiving heparin. The nurse ensures that vitamin K, the antidote for warfarin, is available in case of excessive bleeding (see Chart 35–7).

THROMBOLYTIC THERAPY The use of systemic thrombolytic therapy for deep vein thrombosis (DVT) is effective in dissolving thrombi quickly and completely. The greatest advantage is thought to be the prevention of valvular damage and consequential venous insufficiency, or "post-phlebitic syndrome." However, thrombolytic therapy is contraindicated postoperatively, during pregnancy, and after childbirth, trauma, cerebrovascular accidents, or spinal injuries.

To be most effective, thrombolytic therapy must be initiated within 5 days after the onset of symptoms.

Tissue plasminogen activator (t-PA) is the thrombolytic that has been studied for DVT. It should be used for at least 3 days but not more than 5. The nurse caring for clients receiving t-PA must monitor closely for signs and symptoms of bleeding (see also Chap. 37).

Prevention and Treatment of Peripheral Edema The client's legs should be elevated when in bed and when in the chair. To help prevent chronic venous insufficiency, clients with active and resolving deep vein thrombosis are often instructed to wear knee or thigh-high compression or elastic stockings.

Surgical Management A deep venous thrombus is rarely removed surgically unless there is a massive occlusion that does not respond to medical treatment and the thrombus is of recent (1 to 2 days) onset. *Thrombectomy* is the most common surgical procedure for removing the thrombus. Preoperative and postoperative care of clients undergoing thrombectomy are similar to that for clients undergoing arterial surgery (see earlier).

Inferior Vena Caval Interruption For clients with recurrent deep vein thrombosis and/or pulmonary emboli that do not respond to medical treatment and for clients who cannot tolerate anticoagulation, inferior vena caval (IVC) interruption may be indicated to prevent pulmonary emboli.

Preoperative care is similar to that provided for clients receiving local anesthesia (see Chap. 19). If clients have recently been taking anticoagulants, such as warfarin (Coumadin, Warfilone✱) or heparin (Hepalean✱), the nurse consults with the physician about interrupting this therapy in the preoperative period to avoid hemorrhage.

The surgeon inserts a filter device, or "umbrella," percutaneously into the inferior vena cava (Fig. 35–11). The device is meant to trap emboli in the inferior vena cava before they progress to the lungs. Holes in the device allow blood to pass through, thus not significantly interfering with the return of blood to the heart. Popular IVC filters include the bird's-nest filter and the Greenfield filter.

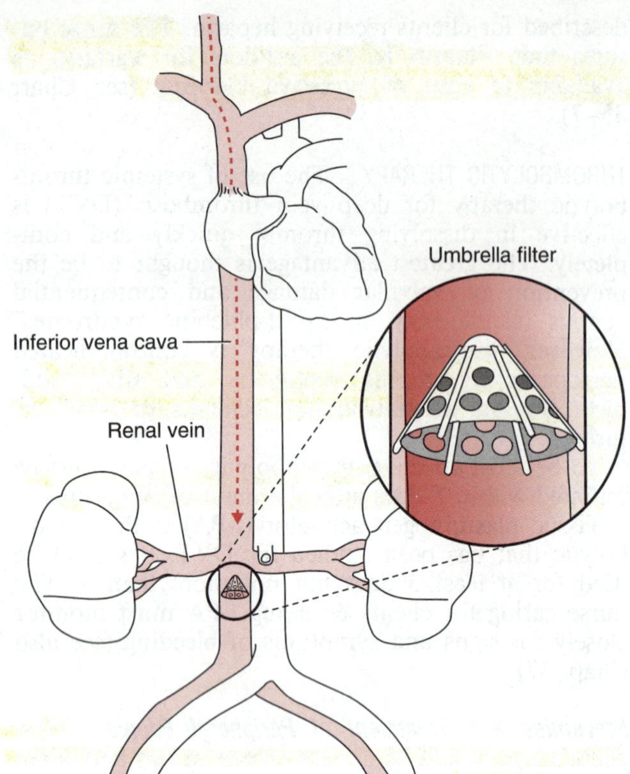

FIGURE 35–11 ◆ An inferior vena caval (IVC) filter.

Postoperatively, the nurse inspects the incision on the right side of the chest for bleeding and signs or symptoms of infection. Other postoperative nursing care is similar to that for any client having surgery (see Chap. 21).

Ligation or External Clips If an inferior vena cava (IVC) filter is not successful in preventing pulmonary emboli or if the filter becomes blocked with thrombi, the surgeon may perform ligation or insert external clips on the inferior vena cava to prevent pulmonary emboli.

Preoperative care for clients undergoing ligation of the vena cava or placement of an external clip is similar to that for clients undergoing abdominal laparotomy. If the client is receiving anticoagulation therapy, the nurse consults with the surgeon about temporary interruption of therapy.

Ligation and insertion of external clips in the inferior vena cava are often performed by means of an abdominal laparotomy. In a ligation, the surgeon ties off the inferior vena cava to block emboli. Application of an external clip, such as the Adams-DeWeese, narrows the inferior vena cava to four serrated transverse slits, 3 to 5 mm in diameter. If laparotomy is performed, the external clip procedure is preferred because there are fewer hemodynamic and venous complications and a low frequency of recurrent pulmonary emboli associated with its use.

Postoperative care for the client with IVC ligation or external clip placement is similar to that for the client after an abdominal laparotomy.

DISCHARGE PLANNING

HOME CARE PREPARATION

Clients recovering from thrombophlebitis or deep vein thrombosis are usually ambulatory when they are discharged from the hospital. The primary focus of planning for discharge is to educate the client about the hazards of anticoagulation therapy (see Chart 35–7). The nurse helps the client identify situations and equipment that might cause trauma, such as the use of a straight-edged razor. The nurse helps the client and family or significant others make arrangements to avoid hazardous situations and to procure alternative types of equipment, if needed, such as an electric razor.

HEALTH TEACHING

The nurse teaches clients recovering from deep vein thrombosis to stop or avoid smoking and to avoid the use of oral contraceptives to decrease the risk of recurrence. Most clients are discharged on a regimen of warfarin (Coumadin, Warfilone✱). The nurse instructs clients and their families to avoid potentially traumatic situations, such as participation in contact sports. The nurse provides all clients with written and oral information about the signs and symptoms of bleeding (see earlier). The client must report any of these manifestations to the health care provider immediately.

The anticoagulant effect of warfarin may be reversed by the omission of one or two doses of the drug or by the administration of vitamin K. In case of injury, clients are directed to apply pressure to bleeding wounds and to seek medical assistance immediately. The nurse encourages clients to carry an identification card or wear a medical alert (Medic-Alert) bracelet that states that they are taking warfarin.

The nurse also instructs clients to inform their dentist and other health care providers that they are taking warfarin before receiving treatment or prescriptions. Prothrombin times are affected by many prescription and over-the-counter medications, such as antacids, antihistamines, aspirin, mineral oil, oral contraceptives, and large doses of vitamin C. The action of warfarin is also affected by high-fat and vitamin K–rich foods, such as cabbage, cauliflower, broccoli, asparagus, lettuce, turnip, spinach, kale, fish, liver, and coffee. Clients are therefore instructed to eat a well-balanced diet and to avoid taking additional medications without consulting a physician. The nurse arranges for clients to have determinations of prothrombin time 1 to 2 weeks after discharge.

If the physician prescribes antiembolism stockings, the nurse teaches clients how and when to apply them (see Venous Insufficiency).

PSYCHOSOCIAL PREPARATION

Clients who have experienced deep vein thrombosis (DVT) may fear recurrence of a thrombus and may also be concerned about treatment with coumadin and the risk for bleeding. The nurse assures such clients that participation in the prescribed treatment frequently helps in resolving this problem and that ongoing assessment of prothrombin levels should minimize the risks of bleeding.

HEALTH CARE RESOURCES

Clients discharged on warfarin need access to a pharmacy to renew prescriptions and, if feasible, to obtain a Medic-Alert bracelet. Clients also need access to a laboratory for frequent monitoring of prothrombin times.

Venous Insufficiency

OVERVIEW

Venous insufficiency occurs as a result of prolonged venous hypertension, which stretches the veins and damages the valves. This can lead to a back-up of blood and further venous hypertension, resulting in edema. Edema occurs as the by-products of red blood cells break down and infiltrate the surrounding tissues. Because the client cannot eliminate waste products, they accumulate within the tissues. With time, this stasis (stoppage) results in venous stasis ulcers, swelling, and cellulitis.

Venous efficiency is altered when thrombosis occurs or when valves are not functioning correctly. Defective valves can result from prolonged venous hypertension, which stretches the veins and damages valves. This can occur in people who stand or sit in one position for long periods, such as teachers and office personnel. Pregnancy and obesity can also cause chronically distended veins, which lead to damaged valves. Thrombus formation can contribute to valve destruction.

Chronic venous insufficiency often occurs in clients who have had thrombophlebitis, although a history of this problem is not obtainable in 25% of these clients (Tierney & Erskine, 1988).

COLLABORATIVE MANAGEMENT

ASSESSMENT

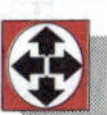

Clients with venous insufficiency may have edema in both extremities. There may be *stasis dermatitis* or discoloration along the ankles, extending up to the calf. In people with long-term venous insufficiency or stasis, *ulcers* often form. Ulcer formation can result from the edema or from minor injury to the limb. Venous ulcers typically occur over the malleolus, more often medially than laterally. The ulcer usually has irregular borders. Generally, these ulcers are chronic and difficult to heal (see Chart 35-5). Many clients live with ulcers for years, and recurrence is common. Some clients may lose one or both limbs if ulcers are not controlled.

INTERVENTIONS

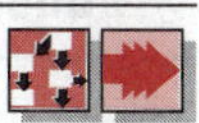

The focus of treating venous insufficiency is to decrease edema and promote venous return from the affected extremity. Clients are not usually hospitalized for venous insufficiency alone unless it is complicated by an ulcer or another disorder is occurring simultaneously.

Nonsurgical Management Treatment of chronic venous insufficiency is primarily nonsurgical, unless it is complicated by a venous stasis ulcer that requires surgical debridement. The goal of managing venous stasis ulcers is twofold:

- To heal the ulcer
- To prevent stasis with recurrence of ulcer formation

Treatment of Edema Clients with chronic venous insufficiency wear elastic or compression stockings, which fit from the middle of the foot to just below the knee or to the thigh. Clients should wear the stockings during the day and evening. The nurse instructs clients to elevate their legs for at least 20 minutes four or five times per day but to avoid long periods of sitting or standing in place. When the client is in bed, the legs should be elevated above the level of the heart (Chart 35-8).

The nurse and physician should also confer about the use of intermittent sequential pneumatic compression of the lower extremities for clients with past or present venous stasis ulcers. A sequential gradient compression device, such as the Home Rx Vascular Compression System, is used. If the client is being treated for an open venous ulcer, the device is applied over a dressing such as an Unna boot (see Dressings). The nurse instructs the client to apply the pump twice a day—1 hour in the morning and 2 hours at night—during the period of healing. Because of the high incidence of venous ulcer recurrence, clients with chronic venous insufficiency whose ulcers have healed are encouraged to continue compression therapy for life.

Treatment of Venous Stasis Ulcers Venous stasis ulcers are slightly more manageable than ulcers resulting from arterial disease. They are chronic in nature, with some clients manifesting the same ulcer for years. Ulcers often heal, only to reoccur later in the same area. The client may have simultaneous ulcers for several years.

DRESSINGS Two types of occlusive dressings are used for venous stasis ulcers: oxygen-permeable and oxygen-impermeable. Because the role of atmospheric oxygen in wound healing is controversial, opinions

CHART 35–8

Education Guide ◆ Venous Insufficiency

Elastic Stockings

- Wear elastic stockings as prescribed, usually during the day and evening.
- Put the stockings on upon awakening and before getting out of bed.
- When applying the stockings, do not "bunch up" and apply like socks. Instead, place your hand inside the stocking and pull out the heel. Then place the foot of the stocking over your foot and slide the rest of the stocking up. Be sure that rough seams on the stocking are on the outside, not next to your skin.
- Do not push stockings down for comfort because they may function like a tourniquet and further impair venous return.
- Put on a clean pair of stockings each day. Wash them by hand (not in a washing machine) in a gentle detergent and warm water.
- If the stockings seem to be "stretched out," replace them with a new pair.

Do's and Don'ts

- Elevate your legs for at least 20 minutes four or five times a day. When in bed, elevate your legs above the level of your heart.
- Avoid prolonged sitting or standing.
- Do not cross your legs; crossing at the ankles is acceptable for short periods of time.
- Do not wear tight, restrictive pants; avoid girdles and garters.

vary with regard to which type of dressing is preferred. The oxygen-permeable polyethylene film (e.g., Op Site) and an oxygen-impermeable hydrocolloid dressing (e.g., DuoDerm) are common. Hydrocolloid dressings are left in place for a minimum of 3 to 5 days for best effect.

A potential problem is that some occlusive dressings stick to the skin and can cause more damage to friable skin. Newer dressings have calcium alginate (e.g., Sorbsan), which prevents maceration of healthy tissue.

If the client is ambulatory, an Unna boot may be used. This dressing is constructed of gauze that has been moistened with zinc oxide. The physician applies the boot to the affected limb, from the toes to the knee, after the ulcer has been cleaned with normal saline solution. Povidone-iodine (Betadine) and hydrogen peroxide are not used because they destroy granulation tissue. The Unna boot is then covered with an elastic wrap and hardens like a cast; this promotes venous return and prevents stasis. The Unna boot also forms a sterile environment for the ulcer. The physician should change the boot approximately once a week. The nurse instructs the client about what to look for if arterial occlusion should occur from an Unna boot that is too tight.

DRUG THERAPY The physician may prescribe topical agents to chemically debride the ulcer, eliminating necrotic tissue and promoting healing. The proteolytic enzyme Sutilains (Travase) is most effective for superficial limb ulcers. Fibrinolysin and deoxyribonuclease (Elase) are most effective after dry eschar (outer) tissue has been surgically removed. Because these agents can injure healthy tissue, the nurse protects the surrounding skin with an oil-based agent such as petroleum jelly (Vaseline). Injury to healthy tissue can prolong healing time.

If an infection occurs or cellulitis develops, systemic antibiotics are more effective than local ointments. Ointments are not well absorbed in the presence of edema. They may also inhibit the ulcer's healing by occluding the ulcer and prohibiting the needed interactions with air.

Surgical Management Surgery for chronic venous insufficiency is not usually performed because historically it has not been successful. Attempts at transplanting vein valves have had limited success. Surgical debridement of venous ulcers is similar to that performed for arterial ulcers (see earlier).

DISCHARGE PLANNING

HOME CARE PREPARATION

The nurse helps clients with chronic venous insufficiency to plan for opportunities and facilities that allow for elevation of the lower extremities in and outside the home. In addition, clients with venous stasis ulcers need to plan for care of the ulcers.

HEALTH TEACHING

The nurse instructs clients with chronic venous stasis to:

- Avoid standing still if possible
- Elevate their legs when sitting
- Avoid crossing their legs
- Avoid wearing tight girdles, tight pants, and narrow-banded knee-high socks

The physician prescribes support hose or antiembolism stockings. The nurse teaches clients to apply these stockings before they get out of bed in the morning and to remove them just before going to bed at night (see Chart 35–8). The nurse also advises clients that they will probably need to wear these stockings for the rest of their lives.

To improve circulation and aid in weight reduction, the nurse prescribes an exercise program on an individual basis with the physician's input. The nurse encourages all clients to maintain an optimal weight and may consult with the dietitian to plan a weight-reducing diet. The nurse instructs clients with venous stasis ulcers how to care for the ulcers at home (see earlier).

PSYCHOSOCIAL PREPARATION

Clients with venous stasis disease, especially those with venous stasis ulcers, may require long-term emotional support to assist them in meeting chronic needs. They may also need assistance in coping with necessary lifestyle adjustments, such as changes in occupation.

HEALTH CARE RESOURCES

Clients with venous stasis ulcers may need the assistance of a home health nurse to perform dressing changes. Clients with Unna boots will need weekly transportation to their health provider for dressing changes. The nurse will need to arrange for a sequential compression device in the home if the physician prescribes one.

Varicose Veins

OVERVIEW

Varicose veins are distended, protruding veins that appear darkened and tortuous. They can occur in anyone, but they are common in clients older than 30 years whose occupations require prolonged standing. Varicose veins are also frequently seen in:

- Pregnant women
- Clients with systemic problems, such as heart disease
- Obese clients
- Clients with a family history of varicose veins

As the vein wall weakens and dilates, venous pressure increases and the valves become incompetent (defective). The incompetent valves enhance the vessel dilation, and the veins become tortuous and distended. The client may complain of pain, especially after standing and may experience a fullness in the legs. Nursing assessment reveals distended protruding veins.

The Trendelenburg test assists with the diagnosis. The client is placed in a supine position with elevated legs. As the client sits up, the veins would normally fill from the distal end; however, if there are varicosities, the veins fill from the proximal end.

COLLABORATIVE MANAGEMENT

Conservative measures are the treatment of choice. These involve wearing elastic stockings and elevating the extremities as much as possible. Clients who continue to have pain or unsightly veins, despite this treatment, may opt for either sclerotherapy or surgical removal of the vein.

Sclerotherapy is performed on small or a limited number of varicosities. The physician injects a solution, such as sodium tetradecyl, directly into the vein. A pressure dressing is applied over the sclerosed vein to keep vessels free of blood for 24 to 72 hours. The surgeon performs an incision and drainage of trapped blood in the sclerosed vein 14 to 21 days after injection, followed by application of a second pressure dressing for 12 to 18 hours.

Varicose veins are surgically removed when they are larger than 4 mm in diameter or are in clusters. The surgeon may use the stab avulsion technique if the saphenous veins are competent. The surgeon exposes varices through 2- to 3-mm stab incisions, grasping the veins with hooks, and dividing and avulsing each vein.

The surgeon may need to strip (remove) affected veins if the saphenous vein is incompetent. The surgeon threads a long wire through an incision above an affected vein, pulling it down through the vein and out through an incision below the vein. After this procedure, the client's legs are bandaged with firm elastic (Ace) bandages.

Postoperatively, the nurse assesses the groin and entire leg for bleeding through the elastic bandage. The nurse instructs the client to keep the legs elevated and to perform range-of-motion exercises of the legs at least hourly. Clients are ambulatory and are often discharged from the hospital by the first postoperative day. At this time, the nurse instructs clients to:

- continue to wear elastic stockings
- walk
- limit sitting
- avoid standing in one place
- elevate their legs when sitting

Phlebitis

Phlebitis is an inflammation of the superficial veins caused by an irritation, such as intravenous therapy (also see Chap. 15). The client has a reddened, warm area radiating up an extremity, commonly an arm. The client may also experience pain, soreness, and swelling of the extremity.

Treatment involves application of warm, moist soaks, which dilate the vein and promote circulation. Sometimes a heating unit is used to keep the soaks warm. Rarely, ice packs are used. The nurse applies the soaks, making sure that the temperature is not warm enough to burn the client, and assesses for complications, such as tissue necrosis, infection, or pulmonary embolus. After a few days of conservative therapy, the inflammation usually subsides.

Vascular Trauma

OVERVIEW

Many types of trauma can result in vascular injury. Injuries to the blood vessels in the upper and lower extremities account for approximately 70% of all vascular injuries to the human body. Vascular injuries to the blood vessels include punctures, lacerations, and transections. Acute blunt or penetrating trauma may result in a false aneurysm or hematoma. Arteriovenous fistulas may be seen after penetrating injuries. The more common causes of penetrating injuries to the blood vessels are gunshot and knife wounds.

Blunt trauma, which is less common, can result from high-speed automobile accidents as a result of the shearing force of rapid deceleration. Vascular trauma can also occur during arterial puncture for arteriographic or hemodynamic studies in which a dissection, hematoma, or occlusive lesion occurs.

COLLABORATIVE MANAGEMENT

The history and physical examination aid in establishing the diagnosis in the client with vascular injury. The nurse questions the client or family about the following:

- The mechanism of injury
- The site of injury
- The amount of blood loss
- Symptoms present after the injury

The nurse assesses for circulatory, sensory, or motor impairment but is aware that despite significant trauma, impairment may not be apparent, especially if deep vessels have been injured. Arteriography provides essential information about the vascular injury. Emergency or urgent surgical intervention is warranted for clients with ischemia to maximize successful revascularization.

Management of vascular injuries is often initiated in a hospital emergency department. Careful triage by the nurse is crucial. Snyder and associates (1989) suggest three types of vascular injuries, with variations in the time at which definitive treatment is essential:

- *Category I:* These injuries expose clients to immediate threats of survival and must be treated immediately (e.g., tension pneumothorax, cardiac tamponade, exsanguinating hemorrhage).
- *Category II:* These injuries are serious but not quite as severe, allowing time for more extensive evaluation before treatment is initiated. (e.g., major fractures, abdominal trauma in the presence of stable vital signs, genitourinary trauma).
- *Category III:* These injuries permit management of the injury at a more leisurely pace (e.g., lacerations, simple lacerations, contusions).

The most important principles in the management of vascular trauma are:

- Establishment of a patent airway
- Control of bleeding
- Restoration of blood flow.

The method of repair varies with the type of vascular injury. Techniques include vein bypass grafting, lateral suture repair, thrombectomy (excision of blood clot), resection with end-to-end anastomosis, and vein patch grafting.

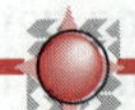

IMPLICATIONS FOR NURSING RESEARCH

Nursing research is aimed at promoting wellness through education of clients. Specific questions that nursing research should address include:

- ♦ What methods can be used to identify individuals at risk for vascular disease?
- ♦ How can nurses promote wellness and prevention of vascular disease?
- ♦ What can nurses do to identify clients with undetected hypertension?
- ♦ How do the risk factors for coronary artery disease apply to clients with vascular disease?
- ♦ Can reliable and simple screening tests be developed to detect vascular disease in the early stages?

SELECTED BIBLIOGRAPHY

Aaronson, L., Carlon-Wolfe, W., & Schoener, S. (1991, March/April). Pressures that fall on rising. *Geriatric Nursing*, 67.

American Heart Association (1992). *1992 Heart and stroke facts.* Dallas, TX: Author.

Bergan, J. J. (1991). Varicose veins: Chronic venous insufficiency. In W. S. Moore (Ed.), *Vascular surgery* (3rd ed., pp. 680–687). Philadelphia: W. B. Saunders.

*Bickerstaff, L. K., Hollier, L. H., Van Peenen, H. J., et al. (1984). Abdominal aortic aneurysm: The changing natural history. *Journal of Vascular Surgery, 1,* 6–12.

Bright, L. D., & Georgi, S. (1993). Peripheral vascular disease: Is it arterial or venous? *American Journal of Nursing, 92*(9), 34–47.

Capasso, V. C., & Coté, K. (1993). The management of patients undergoing arterial reconstructive surgery. *MEDSURG Nursing, 2*(1), 11–20.

Carroll, P. (1993). Deep venous thrombosis: Implication for orthopaedic nursing. *Orthopaedic Nursing, 12*(3), 33–43.

Dennis, K. E., Morrison, A. S., & Howes, D. G. (1991). Beta-blocker therapy: Identification and management of side effects. *Heart & Lung, 20,* 459–463.

DeWeese, J. A. (1990). Surgery for aortoiliac occlusion. In J. Bergan & J. Yao (Eds.), *Techiques in arterial surgery* (pp. 17–26). Phildelphia: W. B. Saunders.

Dickinson, R. (1990). Our way, VI ulcers heal. *RN, 53*(7), 32–36.

*Fahey, V. A. (1988). *Vascular nursing.* Philadelphia: W. B. Saunders.

Farmer, J. A., & Gotto, A. M. (1991). Risk factors for coronary artery disease. In E. Braunwald (Ed.), *Heart disease: A textbook of cardiovascular medicine* (4th ed., pp. 1125–1160). Philadelphia: W. B. Saunders.

Flanagan, D. P. (1991). Aneurysms of the peripheral arteries. In W. S. Moore (Ed.), *Vascular surgery* (3rd ed., pp. 325–349). Philadelphia: W. B. Saunders.

Fogelman, A. M., Edwards, P. A., & Haberland, M. E. (1991). Atherosclerosis: Pathology, pathogenesis, and medical management. In W. S. Moore (Ed.), *Vascular surgery* (3rd ed., pp. 80–85). Philadelphia: W. B. Saunders.

Goldstone, J. (1991). Aneurysms of the aorta and iliac arteries. In W. S. Moore (Ed.), *Vascular surgery* (3rd ed., pp. 304–324). Philadelphia: W. B. Saunders.

Jarvis, C. (1992). *Physical examination and health assessment.* Philadelphia: W. B. Saunders.

Johannsen, J. M. (1993). Update: Guidelines for treating hypertension. *American Journal of Nursing, 93*(3), 42–53.

*Kannel, W. B., Doyle, J. T., Ostfeld, A. M., Jenkins, C. D., Kuller, L., Podell, R. N., & Stamler, J. S. (1984). Optimal resources for primary prevention of atherosclerotic diseases. *Circulation, 70,* 157A–195A.

Kaplan, N. M. (1991). Systemic hypertension: Mechanisms and diagnosis. In E. Braunwald (Ed.), *Heart disease: A textbook of cardiovascular medicine* (4th ed., pp. 817–851). Philadelphia: W. B. Saunders.

Kaplan, N. M. (1991). Systemic hypertension: Therapy. In E. Braunwald (Ed.), *Heart disease: A textbook of cardiovascular medicine* (4th ed., pp. 852–874). Philadelphia: W. B. Saunders.

Lehne, R. A., et al. (1994). *Pharmacology for nursing care* (2nd ed.). Philadelphia: W. B. Saunders.

*Lim, L. T. (1987). Extremity arterial penetrating injury. In C. B. Ernst & J. C. Stanley (Eds.), *Current therapy in vascular surgery.* Toronto: B. C. Decker.

Mannick, J. A., & Whittemore, A. D. (1991). Aortoiliac occlusive disease. In W. S. Moore (Ed.), *Vascular surgery* (3rd ed., pp. 350–363). Philadelphia: W. B. Saunders.

Murdaugh, C. L. (1991). The person with coronary artery disease risk factors. In C. E. Guzzetta & B. M. Dossey (Eds.), *Cardiovascular nursing holistic practice* (pp. 197–219). St. Louis: Mosby Year Book.

*National Cholesterol Education Program. (1988). *Report of the Expert Panel on Detection, Evaluation, and Treatment of High Blood Cholesterol in Adults.* Bethesda, MD: National Heart, Lung, and Blood Institute.

Perry, M. (1991). Vascular trauma. In W. S. Moore (Ed.), *Vascular surgery* (3rd ed., pp. 560–577). Philadelphia: W. B. Saunders.

Porter, J. M., Taylor, L. M., & Harris, E. J. (1991). Nonatherosclerotic vascular disease. In W. S. Moore (Ed.), *Vascular surgery* (3rd ed., pp. 97–130). Philadelphia: W. B. Saunders.

Quinones-Baldrich, W. J. (1991). Thrombolytic therapy for vascular disease. In W. S. Moore (Ed.), *Vascular surgery* (3rd ed., pp. 237–261). Philadelphia: W. B. Saunders.

Ross, R. (1991). The pathogenesis of atherosclerosis. In E. Braunwald (Ed.), *Heart disease: A textbook of cardiovascular medicine* (4th ed., pp. 1106–1124). Philadelphia: W. B. Saunders.

Sacks, F. M. (1989). Dietary fats and blood pressure: A critical review of the evidence. *Nutrition Review, 47:*291–300.

Schell, M. (1990). Cholesterol, lipoproteins, lipid profiles: A challenge in patient education. *Focus on Critical Care, 17*(3), 203–211.

Seeley, J. (1992). A comprehensive method of management for patients with chronic venous insufficiency and venous ulcers. *Ostomy/Wound Management, 38*(8), 45–48.

Snyder, W. H., Thal, E. R., & Perry, M. O. (1989). Vascular injuries of the extremities. In R. B. Rutherford (Ed.), *Vascular surgery* (3rd ed., pp. 613–637). Philadelphia: W. B. Saunders.

Swarczinski, C., & Dijkers, M. (1991). The value of serial leg measurements for monitoring deep vein thrombosis in spinal cord injury. *Journal of Neuroscience Nursing, 23,* 306–314.

*Tierney, L. M., & Erskine, J. M. (1988). Blood vessels & lymphatics. In S. Schroeder, M. A. Krupp, & L. M. Tierney (Eds.), *Current medical diagnosis & treatment 1988* (pp. 266–293). Norwalk, CT: Appleton & Lange.

Trottier, D. J., & Kochar, M. C. (1992). Hypertension & high cholesterol. *American Journal of Nursing, 92*(11), 40–43.

U.S. Department of Health and Human Services (1993). *The Fifth Report of the Joint National Committee on Detection, Evaluation, and Treatment of High Blood Pressure* (NIH Publication). Washington, D. C.: U.S. Government Printing Office.

Veith, F. J., Gupta, S. K., Wengerter, K. R., & Rivers, S. P. (1991). Femoral-popliteal-tibial occlusive disease. In W. S. Moore (Ed.), *Vascular surgery* (3rd ed., pp. 364–389). Philadelphia: W. B. Saunders.

Whitney, E. N., Cataldo, C. B., & Rolfes, S. R. (1991). *Understanding normal and clinical nutrition* (3rd ed.). St. Paul: West Publishing Co.

Workman, M. L. (1994). Anticoagulants and thrombolytics: What's the difference? *AACN Clinical Issues in Critical Care Nursing,* 5(1), 26–35.

SUGGESTED READINGS

Dennis, K. E., Morrison, A. S., & Howes, D. G. (1991). Beta-blocker therapy: Identification and management of side effects. *Heart & Lung, 20,* 459–463.

This article reports on a study testing a scale to identify and quantify side effects of beta-blocker therapy. Seventy clients receiving beta-blockers for hypertension participated in the study. The most problematic side effects related to lack of sleep, dreams, lack of energy, diminished interest in sexual activity, and changes in vision.

Dickinson, R. (1990). Our way, VI ulcers heal. *RN, 53*(7), 32–36.

This article describes successful interventions for ulcers related to chronic venous insufficiency with a case study approach. The author provides a detailed description and photographs of Unna boots and Jobst pneumatic boots, with nursing implications for each. In addition to being informative, this article offers Continuing Education Credit.

Schell, M. (1990). Cholesterol, lipoproteins, lipid profiles: A challenge in patient education. *Focus on Critical Care, 17*(3), 203–211.

This article explains lipid metabolism, alterations in lipid profiles, and treatment for clients with hyperlipidemia. Tables describing different types of hyperlipidemia and drugs for this disorder, as well as common questions asked by clients, are particularly helpful for the nurse planning client education to reduce the risk of atherosclerosis.

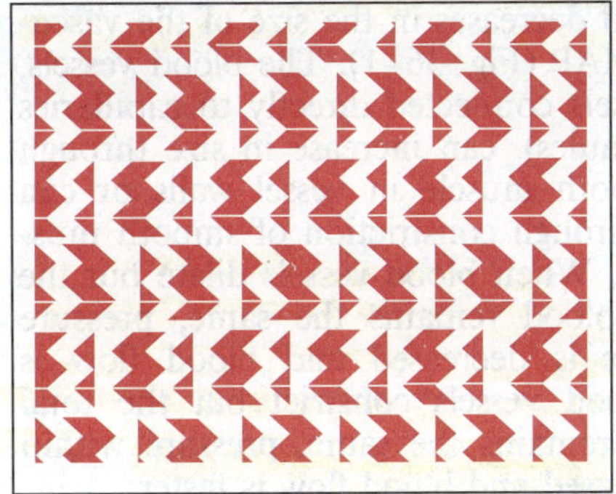

CHAPTER 36

Interventions for Clients in Shock

CHAPTER HIGHLIGHTS

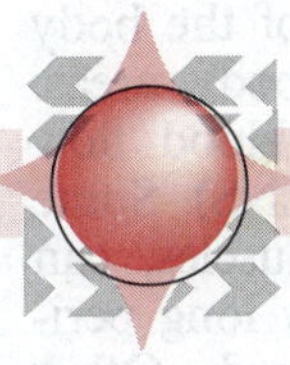

Shock can result from many different situations and can lead to death. Hospitalized clients are most frequently at risk for shock, although shock can occur any place at any time. Because the consequences of shock may be devastating and because shock can be prevented or halted, all nurses should be able to anticipate who is likely to develop shock, to recognize the clinical manifestations of shock, and to know how to intervene appropriately for all types of shock. Table 36-1 lists important concepts related to shock.

OVERVIEW

Tissues and cells within the human body need a continuous supply of oxygen for proper metabolism and function. The cardiovascular system delivers oxygen to all tissues and removes wastes that develop from normal cellular metabolism. The important components of the cardiovascular system for this homeostatic function are the blood, the blood vessels, and the heart. When even one component of the cardiovascular system does not function properly for any reason, the syndrome of shock can result.

Shock is a pathologic condition rather than a disease state. It is initiated by abnormal cellular metabolism that occurs when insufficient oxygen is delivered to the tissues (Guyton, 1991; Houston, 1990). Shock was previously classified by the site of origin of the problem causing shock as hypovolemic, cardio-

TABLE 36–1 Key Concepts Related to Shock

- Shock results when too little oxygen reaches cells and tissues.
- Anyone is susceptible to shock.
- Shock progresses in a predictable, orderly fashion.
- Shock is reversible when the compensatory mechanisms are supported and the underlying causes are eliminated.
- Most clinical manifestations of shock are related to the body's compensatory responses to shock and not the cause of shock.
- The nurse always considers the possibility and probability of shock development.
- Subtle changes in heart rate, level of consciousness, and behavior may herald the onset of shock.
- Clients experiencing the early phase of sepsis-induced distributive shock may be warm and pink with a high cardiac output.
- Oxygen administration is an appropriate therapy for any type of shock.
- Changes in systolic blood pressure are *not* reliable indicators of initial and nonprogressive stages of shock.

genic, vasogenic, and septic. Shock is now classified by the specific functional impairment manifested. The current classification system (Effron & Chernow, 1992) includes:

- Hypovolemic shock
- Cardiogenic shock
- Distributive shock
- Obstructive shock

Table 36–2 categorizes specific conditions causing shock. Because this functional classification is used by researchers and guides clinicians, it is used in this chapter.

Many clinical manifestations of shock are similar, regardless of the cause or the resulting functional impairment. These common findings are due to physiologic compensatory mechanisms. Manifestations unique to any one type of shock are due to specific tissue dysfunction. The common clinical features of shock are listed in Chart 36–1.

Oxygenation of any organ or tissue depends on how much oxygenated arterial blood perfuses (moves into and through) the organ or tissue. Organ perfusion is related to mean arterial pressure (MAP). Because the cardiovascular system is a closed but continuous circuit, the factors that influence MAP include:

- Total blood volume
- Cardiac output
- Size of the vascular bed

Total blood volume and cardiac output are directly related to MAP, so that increases in either total blood volume or cardiac output usually increase MAP. Decreases in either total blood volume or cardiac output usually decrease MAP.

The size of the vascular bed is inversely related to MAP, so that increases in the size of the vascular bed decrease MAP and decreases in the size of the vascular bed increase MAP (Fig. 36–1). The blood vessels, especially the vessels connected directly to capillaries (arterioles and venules), can increase in size through relaxation of smooth muscle in vessel walls or can decrease in size through constriction of smooth muscle in vessel walls. When blood vessels dilate but the total volume of blood remains the same, pressure within the vessels is decreased and blood flow is slower. When blood vessels constrict but the total volume of blood remains the same, pressure within the vessels is increased and blood flow is faster.

Blood vessels contain nerves from the sympathetic division of the autonomic nervous system. Some of these nerves continuously stimulate vascular smooth muscle, so that blood vessels are normally partially contracted. This state of partial contraction is called *sympathetic tone.* An increase in sympathetic stimulation causes the vascular smooth muscle to constrict further, increasing MAP; a decrease in sympathetic stimulation causes the vascular smooth muscle to dilate, decreasing MAP.

Blood flow to body organs varies to adjust to changes in tissue oxygen needs. The body can selectively increase blood flow to some areas of the body while diminishing blood flow to other body areas. The most powerful control of regional blood flow comes from the central nervous system (CNS). Some organs, such as the skin and skeletal muscles, can tolerate low levels of oxygen for relatively long periods without dying or becoming damaged. Other organs, such as the heart, the brain, and the liver, tolerate hypoxic conditions (low levels of tissue oxygenation) poorly, and even just a few minutes without adequate oxygen results in serious or permanent damage.

PATHOPHYSIOLOGY

The underlying problem common to all types of shock, regardless of cause, is the effects of anaerobic cellular metabolism (metabolism without oxygen), which result from inadequate tissue oxygenation (Shoemaker, 1987). These effects cause adverse changes in physiologic function. Because these changes can profoundly disturb physiologic function, the body initiates compensatory mechanisms in an attempt to maintain or to restore tissue perfusion and oxygenation even while the triggering events of shock are still present.

When the conditions that cause shock remain uncorrected, shock progresses in a predictable sequence consisting of:

1. Initial stage
2. Nonprogressive stage
3. Progressive stage
4. Refractory stage

The stages of shock can be identified on the basis of:

- How well the client's compensatory mechanisms are working

TABLE 36–2 Types and Causes of Shock

Shock Type	Overall Cause	Specific Cause or Risk Factors

Hypovolemic shock	• Body fluid depletion	• Hemorrhage
		  • Trauma
		  • Gastrointestinal ulcer
		  • Surgery
		  • Inadequate clotting
		    • Hemophilia
		    • Liver disease
		    • Malnutrition
		    • Bone marrow suppression
		    • Cancer
		    • Anticoagulation therapy
		• Dehydration
		  • Vomiting
		  • Diarrhea
		  • Heavy diaphoresis
		  • Diuretic therapy
		  • Nasogastric suction
		  • Diabetes insipidus
		  • Hyperglycemia

Cardiogenic shock	• Direct pump failure	• Myocardial infarction
		• Cardiac arrest
		• Ventricular dysrhythmias
		  • Fibrillation
		  • Tachycardia
		• Cardiac amyloidosis
		• Cardiomyopathies
		  • Viral
		  • Toxic
		• Myocardial degeneration

Distributive shock	• Decreased vascular volume or tone	• Neural-induced
		  • Pain
		  • Anesthesia
		  • Stress
		  • Spinal cord injury
		  • Head trauma
		• Chemical induced
		  • Anaphylaxis
		  • Sepsis
		  • Capillary leak
		    • Burns
		    • Extensive trauma
		    • Hepatic dysfunction
		    • Hypoproteinemia

Obstructive shock	• Indirect pump failure	• Cardiac tamponade • Arterial stenosis • Pulmonary embolus • Pulmonary hypertension • Constrictive pericarditis • Thoracic tumors

- The severity of the clinical manifestations
- The reversibility of tissue damage

The primary triggering event leading to the recognizable picture of shock is a sustained decrease in mean arterial pressure (MAP) that results from decreased cardiac output, decreased circulating blood volume, or expansion of the vascular bed. A decrease in MAP of 5 to 10 mmHg from the client's baseline value is immediately detected by pressure-sensitive, afferent nerve receptors (baroreceptors) located in the aortic arch and the carotid sinus (Guyton, 1991). This information is transmitted to an integration center in the brain, which then stimulates compensatory mechanisms to ensure continued perfusion and oxygenation of vital organs while limiting blood flow to less vital body areas. This selective shunting of blood (moving blood into selected areas while bypassing other areas) leads to the physiologic changes and clinical manifestations of various stages of shock.

If the events that caused the initial decrease in MAP are halted at this point, the compensatory mechanisms can return the body to a normal perfused and oxygenated state, even without outside intervention. If the initiating events continue and MAP decreases further, some tissues perform metabolic ac-

CHART 36-1

Key Features of Shock

Cardiovascular

- Decreased cardiac output
- Increased pulse rate
- Thready pulse quality
- Decreased blood pressure
- Narrowed pulse pressure
- Postural hypotension
- Low central venous pressure
- Flat neck and hand veins in dependent positions
- Slow capillary refill in nail beds
- Diminished peripheral pulses

Respiratory

- Increased respiratory rate
- Shallow depth of respirations
- Decreased arterial PCO_2
- Decreased arterial PO_2
- Cyanosis, especially around lips and nail beds

Neuromuscular

- Early
  - Anxiety
  - Restlessness
- Late
  - Decreased central nervous system activity (lethargy to coma)
  - Generalized muscle weakness
  - Diminished or absent deep tendon reflexes
  - Sluggish pupillary response to light

Renal

- Decreased urinary output
- Increased specific gravity
- Sugar and acetone present in urine

Integumentary

- Cool to cold
- Pale to mottled to cyanotic
- Moist, clammy
- Mouth dry, paste-like coating present

Gastrointestinal

- Decreased motility
- Diminished or absent bowel sounds
- Nausea and vomiting
- Constipation
- Increased thirst

tivities under anaerobic conditions, creating an increase in lactic acid and other harmful metabolites (such as kinins, degradative enzymes, and oxygen radicals). These substances cause electrolyte and acid-base imbalances that can exert generalized, tissue-damaging effects and depress myocardial activity. Such effects are temporary and reversible if the cause of shock is corrected within 1 to 2 hours after onset of shock. When causal conditions continue for longer periods without supportive interventions, the resulting acid-base imbalance, electrolyte imbalances, and increased levels of toxic metabolites damage the cells within vital organs so much that full recovery from shock is no longer possible. Table 36-3 summarizes the progression of shock.

INITIAL STAGE OF SHOCK

The initial, or early, stage of shock is present when the initiating factors cause MAP to decrease from the client's baseline level by less than 10 mmHg. During this stage of shock, adaptive and compensatory mechanisms are activated and are so effective at returning MAP to normal levels that oxygenated blood flow to all vital organs is maintained. Cellular changes observed in this stage are a decrease in aerobic metabolism and an increase in anaerobic metabolism with increased production of lactic acid (although overall cellular metabolism is still aerobic). Compensation, occurring through vascular constriction and heart rate increase, is relatively complete, and both cardiac output and MAP are maintained within the normal range. Because vital organ function is not disrupted during the initial stage, the signs and symptoms of this stage of shock are subtle and difficult to detect. A heart rate increase from the client's baseline level may be the only manifestation of this stage of shock.

NONPROGRESSIVE STAGE OF SHOCK

The nonprogressive, or compensatory, stage of shock is observed when initiating conditions have caused a 10- to 15-mmHg drop in MAP. Renal and chemical compensatory mechanisms are activated because cardiovascular compensation alone is not enough to maintain MAP and to supply needed oxygen to vital organs.

Sustained decreased MAP is sensed by the kidneys and the baroreceptors, resulting in the release of renin, antidiuretic hormone (ADH), aldosterone, and the catecholamines epinephrine and norepinephrine (Lancaster, 1990). Renal compensation is regulated through the actions of renin, aldosterone, and ADH (see Chap. 14). Renin is secreted by the kidney and initiates the angiotensinogen reactions (see Chap. 14, Fig. 14-6), which eventually cause decreased urinary output, increased reabsorption of sodium, and systemic vasoconstriction. ADH is secreted by the posterior pituitary gland. The activity of ADH both increases renal reabsorption of water and causes peripheral vasoconstriction. These actions together attempt to compensate for shock by increasing central vascular volume (Guyton, 1991; Lancaster, 1990).

Tissue hypoxia is present in nonvital organs and in the kidney but is not great enough to cause severe symptoms or permanent damage (Rice, 1991b). Because some metabolism is anaerobic, acid-base and electrolyte changes occur in response to the buildup of metabolites. These changes include acidosis and hyperkalemia (see Chaps. 16 and 18).

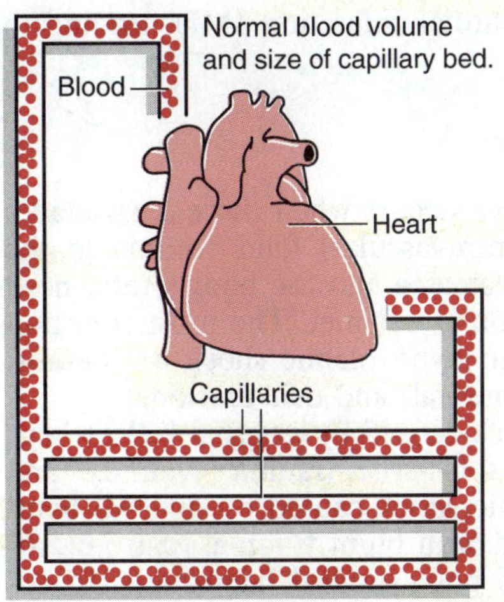

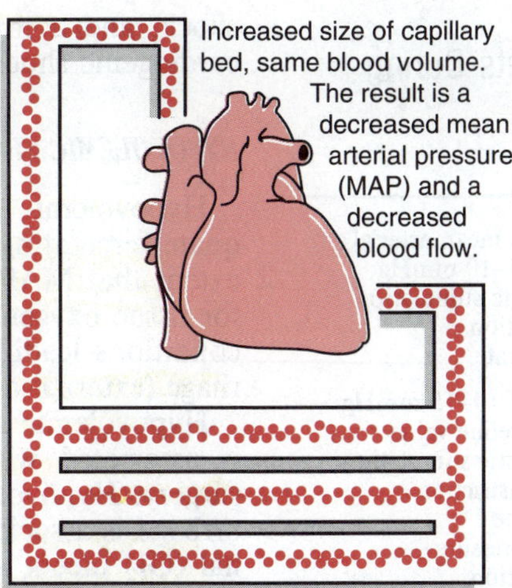

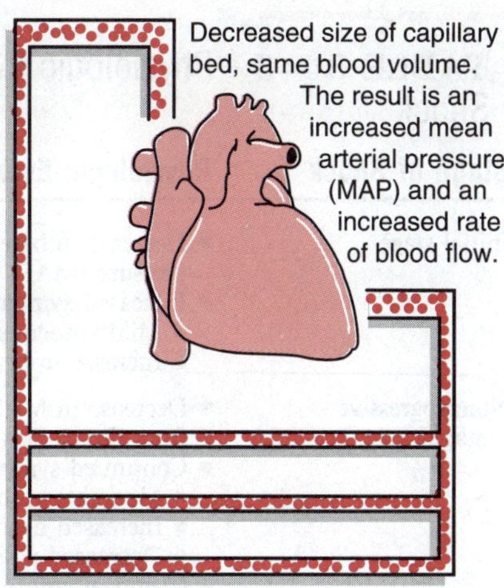

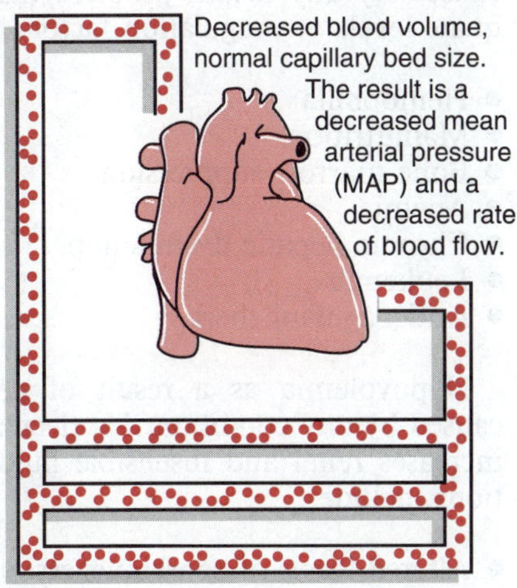

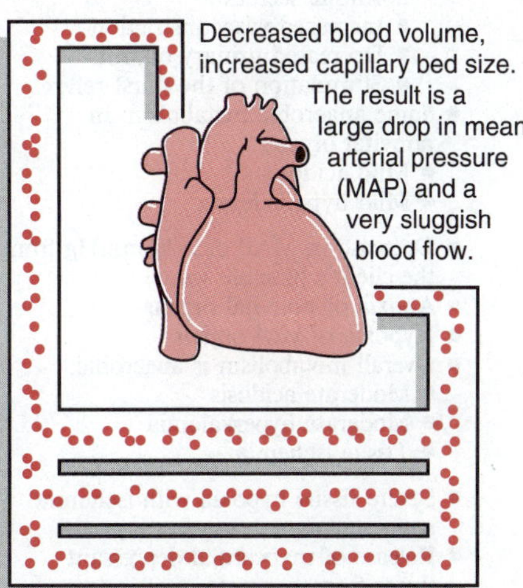

FIGURE 36-1 ◆ Interaction of blood volume and the size of the capillary bed affecting mean arterial pressure.

If the client's condition is stable and compensatory mechanisms are supported by medical and nursing interventions, the client can remain in this stage for hours without sustaining permanent damage. Halting the conditions that initiated shock and providing supportive interventions are necessary to prevent the progression of shock. When appropriate interventions are carried out, the effects of the nonprogressive stage of shock are reversible.

PROGRESSIVE STAGE OF SHOCK

The progressive stage of shock, sometimes called the intermediate stage, is characterized by a sustained decrease in MAP of greater than 20 mmHg from the client's baseline level. Compensatory mechanisms are functioning but are no longer able to maintain sufficient oxygen supply, even to vital organs. The heavy use of oxygen in tissues participating in compensatory mechanisms makes the problem of general inadequate oxygenation even worse. Hypoxia is present in vital organs, whereas less vital organs experience anoxia and ischemia. As a result of inadequate oxygenation and a buildup of toxic metabolites, some tissues have extensive cell damage and cell death (Klein, 1990).

The progressive stage of shock is a life-threatening emergency. Cells of vital organs can tolerate this situation for only a short time before being permanently damaged. Immediate interventions are required to reverse the effects of this stage of shock. Tolerance of this stage is highly individual and depends greatly on the client's pre-existing state of health. In general, the client's life can be saved if conditions causing the progressive stage of shock are corrected within an hour after the onset of this stage.

REFRACTORY STAGE OF SHOCK

The refractory stage of shock is sometimes called the irreversible stage. It is reached when so much cell death and tissue damage have occurred because of too little oxygen getting to the tissues that overwhelming functional changes are present in vital organs. This stage is termed refractory because the body is unable to respond appropriately to any therapeutic interventions and the syndrome of shock continues (Rice, 1991b; Summers, 1990). The remaining

TABLE 36–3 Physiologic Events During Shock

Stage of Shock	Physiologic Event

Initial stage	• Decrease in baseline mean arterial pressure (MAP) of 5–10 mmHg
	• Increased sympathetic stimulation
	  • Mild vasoconstriction
	  • Increase in heart rate

Nonprogressive stage	• Decrease in MAP of 10–15 mmHg from the client's baseline value
	• Continued sympathetic stimulation
	  • Moderate vasoconstriction
	  • Increased heart rate
	  • Decreased pulse pressure
	• Chemical compensation
	  • Renin, aldosterone, and antidiuretic hormone secretion
	    • Increased vasoconstriction
	    • Decreased urinary output
	    • Stimulation of the thirst reflex
	• Some anaerobic metabolism in nonvital organs
	  • Mild acidosis
	  • Mild hyperkalemia

Progressive stage	• Decrease in MAP of >20 mmHg from the client's baseline value
	• Anoxia of nonvital organs
	• Hypoxia of vital organs
	• Overall metabolism is anaerobic.
	  • Moderate acidosis
	  • Moderate hyperkalemia
	  • Tissue ischemia

Refractory stage	• Severe tissue hypoxia with ischemia and necrosis • Release of myocardial depressant factor from pancreas • Buildup of toxic metabolites

cells perform metabolic functions anaerobically. Therapy is ineffective in saving the life of the client, even if the underlying cause of the shock is corrected and MAP temporarily returns to normal. So much tissue damage has occurred and has resulted in the systemic release of toxic metabolites and destructive enzymes that cellular deterioration of vital organs continues. The most profound change that continues to occur is deterioration of the myocardium. One factor contributing to the deterioration of the myocardium is the release of myocardial depressant factor (MDF) from the ischemic pancreas (Wilson, 1992).

ETIOLOGY

Because shock is a manifestation of a pathologic condition rather than a separate disease state, the causes of shock vary. Specific conditions leading to hypovolemic, cardiogenic, distributive, and obstructive shock are listed in Table 36–2. More than one type of shock can be present at the same time. For example, trauma caused by an automobile accident may trigger both hemorrhage, leading to hypovolemic shock, and a myocardial infarction (MI), leading to cardiogenic shock.

HYPOVOLEMIC SHOCK

Hypovolemic shock occurs when there is an inadequate circulating (intravascular) fluid volume to the extent that MAP decreases and the body's total need for tissue oxygenation is not met. The most common conditions leading to hypovolemic shock are hemorrhage (external or internal) and dehydration.

Hypovolemic shock caused by external hemorrhage is associated with soft-tissue trauma, wounds, and surgery. Hypovolemic shock caused by internal hemorrhage is associated with blunt trauma, gastrointestinal (GI) ulcers, and poor surgical hemostasis. In addition, external and internal hemorrhage can be caused by any health problem that results in inadequate levels of coagulation factors. These include:

- Hemophilia
- Malnutrition
- Bone marrow suppression
- Anemia
- Chronic hepatic dysfunction
- Leukemia
- Anticoagulant therapy

Hypovolemia as a result of dehydration can be caused by any condition that decreases fluid intake or increases renal and insensible fluid loss. Such conditions include:

- Altered levels of consciousness
- Musculoskeletal immobility
- Heavy exercise
- Excessive wound drainage
- Nasogastric suction
- Vomiting
- Diarrhea
- Hyperglycemia
- Diuretic therapy
- Diabetes insipidus

CARDIOGENIC SHOCK

Cardiogenic shock occurs when the actual heart muscle is unhealthy and contractility is directly impaired. Direct pump failure can result from:

- Cardiac arrest
- Serious dysrhythmias (ventricular fibrillation or tachycardia)
- Valvular pathologic changes
- Toxic or viral cardiomyopathies
- Cardiac amyloidosis
- Myocardial degeneration

Such conditions decrease cardiac output and afterload, thus reducing MAP. (Chapter 37 provides an in-depth discussion of specific conditions leading to cardiogenic shock.)

DISTRIBUTIVE SHOCK

Distributive shock is characterized by a loss of sympathetic tone, vasodilation, pooling of blood in venous and capillary beds, and increased vascular permeability, which all contribute to decreased mean arterial pressure (MAP). The origin of these reactions is neural or chemical. Neurogenically induced loss of MAP occurs when sympathetic stimulation of nerves regulating the vascular smooth muscle is inhibited and the smooth muscle relaxes, causing vasodilation. Chemically induced distributive shock has three common origins:

- Anaphylaxis
- Sepsis
- Capillary leak syndrome

NEURAL-INDUCED DISTRIBUTIVE SHOCK Neural-induced vasodilation can be a normal local response to injury, but shock results when the vasodilation is systemic. Common conditions that can cause a systemic loss of sympathetic tone include:

- Severe pain
- Prolonged exposure to heat
- Psychologic stress
- Neurologic damage
- Spinal cord injury
- Injection of nerve block anesthetics over a large area (spinal, epidural, and caudal anesthesia)

CHEMICAL-INDUCED DISTRIBUTIVE SHOCK Chemical-induced distributive shock occurs when specific types of chemicals or foreign substances within the blood and blood vessels stimulate widespread changes in blood vessel walls. Usually, the chemicals are exogenous (come from outside the body), but this type of shock can be induced by substances normally found in the body.

Anaphylaxis Anaphylaxis is associated with the type I (delayed hypersensitivity) immune reaction (see Chap. 24). Although it usually begins within seconds to minutes after exposure to a specific allergen, this reaction is termed delayed because the person rarely has this type of reaction the first time the allergen is encountered. Rather, this reaction occurs on subsequent exposure to the same allergen (Guyton, 1991). Table 24–8 lists some common allergens associated with anaphylaxis.

Anaphylaxis is due to an antigen-antibody reaction occurring systemically in response to contact with a substance to which the individual has a severe hypersensitivity (allergy). The widespread antigen-antibody reaction involves the interaction of the allergen, immunoglobulin E (IgE), basophils, and mast cells. It occurs within the walls of blood vessels, myocardial cells, and bronchial epithelium (see Chaps. 22 and 24). This reaction damages cells and causes the release of massive amounts of histamine and other vasoactive amines. These substances are distributed rapidly throughout the circulatory system, causing massive vasodilation and increased capillary permeability, which result in profound hypovolemia and vascular collapse. Decreased myocardial contractility and dysrhythmias can be seen during anaphylaxis, but it is not known whether these symptoms are direct results of myocardial changes induced by the antigen-antibody reaction or are due to the profound hypovolemia. Antigen-antibody reactions in bronchial tissues cause severe edema and pulmonary obstruction, which greatly reduce pulmonary gas exchange. These pulmonary problems in combination with inadequate circulation cause the person to experience extreme hypoxia. Without intervention, this condition results in death.

Sepsis Sepsis leading to distributive shock occurs when microorganisms are present in the blood and other normally sterile areas of the body. Often, sepsis is associated with disseminated intravascular coagulation (DIC). Although distributive shock has been reported among clients with viral and yeast sepsis, it is more commonly associated with bacteremia. Organisms implicated in sepsis include gram-negative bacteria (*Pseudomonas aeruginosa, Escherichia coli,* and *Klebsiella pneumoniae*) and gram-positive bacteria (*Staphylococcus* and *Streptococcus*) (Bell, 1990; Epstein & Bakanauskas, 1991; Houston, 1990; Littleton, 1988; McMorrow & Cooney-Daniello, 1991; Mostow, 1990). Table 36–4 lists some of the conditions that predispose the client to sepsis-induced distributive shock.

The initiation of the syndrome of sepsis-induced distributive shock results from the large amounts of metabolites and toxins (including endotoxin) that are produced by the bacteria and secreted into the client's blood. These bacteria-produced toxins react with blood vessels and cell membranes. The resulting reactions, through leukocyte recognition, stimulate a variety of inflammatory and immune responses (see Chap. 22). These toxin-host interactions stimulate systemic complement activation, altered microcirculation within vascular organs (including selective coagulation and thrombus formation), increased capillary permeability, cell injury, and increased cellular metabolism (in combination with an inability of some cells to take up necessary oxygen). Metabolism

TABLE 36–4 Conditions That Predispose the Client to Sepsis-Induced Distributive Shock

- Malnutrition
- Immunosuppression
- Large open wounds
- Mucous membrane fissures in prolonged contact with bloody or drainage-soaked packing
- Gastrointestinal ischemia
- Loss of gastrointestinal integrity
- Exposure to invasive procedures

becomes anaerobic because of decreased MAP, thrombus formation in capillaries, and poor cellular uptake of oxygen. Although bacterial toxins are generally implicated in initiating these events, some evidence indicates that the bacteria in the extracellular fluid, as well as the toxins, can directly initiate septic shock.

Capillary Leak Syndrome Capillary leak syndrome leading to distributive shock occurs when there is a shift of fluid from the vascular space to the interstitial space. Such shifts are caused by increased capillary permeability, loss of plasma osmolarity, and increased vascular hydrostatic pressure. Specific conditions associated with fluid shifts include:

- Severe burns
- Bullous dermatologic disease
- Hepatic dysfunction or enlargement
- Abdominal ascites
- Acute peritonitis
- Paralytic ileus
- Severe malnutrition
- Surgical wounds
- Hyperglycemia
- Sodium-wasting renal disease
- Hypoproteinemia
- Trauma

OBSTRUCTIVE SHOCK

Obstructive shock results from conditions that affect the ability of the normal heart muscle to pump effectively. Some of the causes of obstructive shock (Houston, 1990) include:

- Cardiac tamponade
- Pulmonary embolism
- Pulmonary hypertension
- Arterial stenosis
- Constrictive pericarditis
- Thoracic tumors interfering with blood flow or mechanically preventing adequate myocardial contraction
- Aortic aneurysm

The heart itself is normal, but conditions outside the heart prevent either adequate filling of the heart or adequate contraction of the healthy heart muscle.

INCIDENCE/PREVALENCE

The exact incidence of shock is not known, because shock is a manifestation of a pathologic condition rather than a separate disease entity. However, some degree of shock is a common complication among hospitalized clients and frequently is the reason why clients seek health care assistance initially. Hypovolemic shock is the most common type of shock experienced by clients in emergency departments and after surgery or procedures that involve invasion of a major artery. Cardiogenic shock is the most frequent complication of myocardial infarction and is present in an estimated 15% of clients who experience damage to 40% or more of the myocardium (Houston, 1990; Rubenstein & Federman, 1992). The frequency of distributive shock as a result of sepsis, which ranges in mortality from 40% to 85%, is increasing among clients who are immunocompromised or who have infections (Littleton, 1988; Mostow, 1990).

COLLABORATIVE MANAGEMENT OF HYPOVOLEMIC SHOCK

This chapter presents the collaborative management of clients experiencing hypovolemic shock caused by hemorrhage and distributive shock caused by sepsis. The collaborative management of clients experiencing conditions leading to cardiogenic shock is presented in Chapters 34. The collaborative management of clients experiencing obstructive shock caused by pulmonary embolism is presented in Chapter 31.

ASSESSMENT

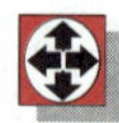

HISTORY

The nurse collects data on risk factors, as well as causative factors, related to hypovolemic shock. Age is important because hypovolemic shock associated with trauma is more frequently seen in young adults. Clients are asked specific questions about recent illness, trauma, or procedures or chronic conditions that may lead to the development of shock. Such conditions include:

- Gastrointestinal ulcers
- General surgery
- Hemophilia
- Liver disease or dysfunction
- Prolonged vomiting or diarrhea

The use of some medications may directly cause changes leading to hypovolemic shock or may indicate the presence of a disease or a problem that can contribute to hypovolemic shock. Such medications include aspirin and aspirin-containing drugs, diuretics, and antacids.

The nurse inquires about the client's fluid intake and output during the previous 24 hours. Information about urinary output is especially critical because the initial and nonprogressive stages of shock are characterized by a diminished urinary output, even when fluid intake is normal.

The nurse assesses the client and the immediate environment for obvious evidence of factors leading to shock. Areas to examine for possible hemorrhage include the gums, wounds, and sites of dressings, drains, and vascular access. The client is observed for the presence of any swelling, skin discoloration, or visible manifestations of pain that may indicate the presence of significant internal hemorrhage.

PHYSICAL ASSESSMENT/CLINICAL MANIFESTATIONS

Most of the observable manifestations of hypovolemic shock result from the physiologic changes associated with accompanying compensatory efforts. Manifestations of shock are first evident as changes in cardiovascular function. As shock progresses, functional changes in the renal, pulmonary, integumentary, musculoskeletal, and central nervous systems become evident.

CARDIOVASCULAR MANIFESTATIONS Because the pathologic changes of shock involve a decrease of mean arterial pressure (MAP) and the resulting early compensatory mechanisms are cardiovascular, the earliest clinical findings in hypovolemic shock are associated with the cardiovascular system.

Pulse The nurse assesses the central and peripheral pulses for rate and quality. In the initial stage of hypovolemic shock, the pulse rate increases to maintain cardiac output and MAP at normal levels, although the actual stroke volume per beat is usually decreased. Because the cardiac output is decreased, the distal peripheral pulses are more difficult to palpate and are easily blocked with minimal pressure. As hypovolemic shock progresses, superficial peripheral pulses may be absent.

Blood Pressure Indirect blood pressure reading using a pneumatic cuff, sphygmomanometer, and a stethoscope is the most common method of blood pressure measurement used on medical-surgical units. Research Applications for Nursing discusses the accuracy of different methods of indirect blood pressure measurement compared with that of the more invasive direct measurement of blood pressure.

Changes in blood pressure are not always present in the initial stages of hypovolemic shock. An important concept to consider when assessing the blood pressure of a client at risk for shock is the normal baseline blood pressure level for the client. Although a blood pressure measurement of 90/50 may indicate the presence of severe shock in one person, it may represent the normal blood pressure value for another healthy, but slightly built, adult.

When compensatory efforts include vasoconstriction, the result is an increased diastolic pressure level, while the systolic pressure level remains the same. As a result, the pulse pressure, or the difference between the systolic and diastolic pressure measurements, is diminished. The nurse monitors the client's blood pressure for changes from baseline levels and changes from the previous measurement. For accuracy, the nurse uses the same equipment on the same extremity. When the client's condition permits, the nurse measures the blood pressure with the client in the lying, sitting, and standing positions.

RESEARCH APPLICATIONS FOR NURSING

Blood Pressure Readings at Different Sites May Vary for the Same Client

Byra-Cook, C., Dracup, K., & Lazik, A. (1990). Direct and indirect blood pressure in critical care patients. *Nursing Research, 39*(5), 285–288.

This clinical study, using 50 critical care unit clients as subjects, compares the accuracy of four different indirect blood pressure measurement techniques against the standard of direct arterial pressure measured by an intra-arterial catheter in the radial artery. The four techniques consisted of a standard pneumatic cuff with sphygmomanometer reading taken at two sites using the bell and the diaphragm of a stethoscope. The two sites were the antecubital fossa and the brachial artery of the upper arm. All indirect measurements correlated well with the direct intra-arterial measurements. The most accurate measurements were obtained using the diaphragm over the upper arm site and the least accurate measurements were obtained using the bell over the upper arm site.

Critique The investigators used a sound scientific approach in comparing the sensitivity of different techniques for indirect blood pressure measurement. Although differences in techniques reached statistical significance, the clinical effect of the differences remains to be demonstrated.

Possible nursing implications Because decisions about treatment during episodes of shock are based on the changes in blood pressure, each hospital unit should establish guidelines for the most accurate indirect blood pressure measurement technique. By providing consistency in measurement techniques, documented changes in blood pressure are more likely to be actual rather than an artifact of different techniques.

As hypovolemic shock progresses and cardiac output changes, the systolic pressure level decreases, diminishing the pulse pressure even further. When hypovolemic shock continues and interventions are not adequate, compensatory mechanisms fail and both the systolic and diastolic pressures decrease. At this stage, indirect blood pressure is difficult to auscultate. The nurse may need to use palpation or a Doppler device to ascertain the systolic blood pressure.

INTEGUMENTARY MANIFESTATIONS In hypovolemic shock, the skin is affected indirectly by altered perfusion and not by pathologic changes in the skin. Because the skin can tolerate low oxygen levels and other vital organs cannot, early compensatory mechanisms for hypovolemic shock involve profound vasoconstriction in the skin and superficial tissues to the extent that perfusion of these tissues is minimal or absent.

The nurse assesses the skin for temperature, color, and degree of moisture. The skin feels cool or cold to the touch, and the color is pale to cyanotic. Color changes are first evident in mucous membranes and in the skin around the mouth. Because pallor or cyanosis may be difficult to observe on many areas of a client who has dark skin, the nurse particularly assesses color changes in oral mucous membranes. As hypovolemic shock progresses, color changes in clients who have lighter skin are noted in the extremities and then in the central trunk area. The skin also feels clammy or moist to the touch. This manifestation is not due to increased perspiration but occurs because the normal fluid lost through the skin does not evaporate quickly on cold skin.

The nurse evaluates capillary refill time by pressing on the client's fingernail until it blanches and then observing how fast the nail bed resumes color when pressure is released. Normally, the nail bed capillaries resume color as soon as pressure is released. Capillary refill in clients experiencing hypovolemic shock is usually slow and sometimes absent.

RESPIRATORY MANIFESTATIONS The nurse assesses the rate, depth, and ease of respiration and auscultates the lungs for the presence of any abnormal breath sounds. The clinical manifestations of hypovolemic shock include an increased respiratory rate. This finding is a compensatory mechanism to assist in providing adequate oxygenation to critical tissues. When shock has progressed to the stage at which lactic acidosis is present, the depth of respirations increases with the rate.

RENAL/URINARY MANIFESTATIONS The renal system compensates for the decreased MAP associated with hypovolemic shock by conserving body water through decreasing glomerular filtration and increasing the reabsorption of filtrate. The nurse measures the urinary output every hour. The nurse assesses the urine for such variables as color, specific gravity, and the presence of blood or protein. Urinary output is diminished (compared with fluid intake) or even absent in severe shock. When hypovolemic shock is severe and pressure in the renal artery is low, nephron perfusion does not occur. Of the four vital organs (heart, brain, liver, and kidney), only the kidney can tolerate hypoxia and anoxia for up to an hour without permanent damage to tubular epithelial cells. When hypoxic or anoxic conditions persist beyond this time, the client is at grave risk for ischemic acute tubular necrosis and subsequent renal failure (Lancaster, 1990).

CENTRAL NERVOUS SYSTEM MANIFESTATIONS The nurse assesses the client's level of consciousness and orientation to person, time, and place. Most causes of hypovolemic shock do not interfere with the generation and maintenance of nerve impulse transmission. Rather, central nervous system manifestations of hypovolemic shock are associated with cerebral hypoxia. In the initial and nonprogressive stages of hypovolemic shock, the client may be restless or agitated and may experience anxiety or a feeling of impending doom that has no obvious cause. As hypoxia progresses, the client becomes confused and lethargic. Lethargy progresses to somnolence and loss of consciousness as cerebral hypoxia intensifies.

MUSCULOSKELETAL MANIFESTATIONS Although musculoskeletal manifestations are not an early or a cardinal symptom of shock, they may be present and cause discomfort for the client. Tissue hypoxia, anaerobic metabolism, and lactic acidosis cause skeletal muscle weakness and pain. This weakness is generalized, with no specific pattern of presentation. The accompanying electrolyte disturbances in progressive and refractory stages of shock compound this muscle weakness by interfering with the generation and transmission of action potentials. In this situation, deep tendon reflexes are diminished or absent.

The nurse assesses the client's muscle strength by having the client squeeze the nurse's hand and try to keep the arms flexed while the nurse pulls downward on the lower arms. The nurse assesses deep tendon reflexes by lightly tapping the patellar tendons and Achilles tendons with a reflex hammer and observing the degree of reflexive movement.

PSYCHOSOCIAL ASSESSMENT

Changes in mental status and behavior may be early indicators of hypovolemic shock. The nurse observes the client closely and documents the client's behavior. The nurse assesses the client's current mental status by evaluating the level of consciousness (LOC). The nurse notes whether the client is asleep or awake. If the client is asleep, the nurse attempts to awaken the client and documents the ease with which the client is aroused. If the client is awake, the nurse establishes whether the client is oriented to person, time, and place. The nurse avoids asking questions that can be answered with a "yes" or a "no" response. The nurse documents the manner in which the client responds to the questions. The following points are considered during evaluation:

- Is it necessary to repeat questions to obtain a response?
- Does the response answer the question asked?
- Does the client have difficulty with word choices during the responses?
- Is the client irritated or upset by the questions?
- Can the client concentrate on a question long enough to provide an appropriate response, or is his or her attention span limited?

If possible, the nurse questions family members or a significant other to determine whether the behavior and mental status are typical of this client.

CHART 36–2

Lab Profile ♦ Hypovolemic Shock

Test	Normal Range for Adults	Significance of Abnormal Findings
pH	• 7.35–7.45	• *Decreased* • Insufficient tissue oxygen causing anaerobic metabolism and acidosis
PaO_2 (arterial)	• 80–100 mmHg	• *Decreased* • Anaerobic metabolism
$PaCO_2$ (arterial)	• 35–45 mmHg	• *Increased* • Anaerobic metabolism
Lactic acid	• 0.6–1.8 mEq/L	• *Increased* • Anaerobic metabolism with buildup of metabolites
Hematocrit	• Males: 42%–52% • Females: 37%–47%	• *Decreased* • Hemorrhage • *Increased* • Dehydration
Hemoglobin	• Males: 14–18 g/dL • Females: 12–16 g/dL	• *Decreased* • Hemorrhage • *Increased* • Dehydration
Potassium	• 3.5–5.0 mEq/L	• *Increased* • Acidosis

LABORATORY ASSESSMENT

No single laboratory finding confirms or rules out the presence of shock, although changes in laboratory data may support the diagnosis of hypovolemic shock. Chart 36–2 lists the common laboratory assessment findings associated with hypovolemic shock. As shock progresses, the combination of an increase in anaerobic metabolism, cell damage, and the presence of specific compensatory mechanisms causes physiologic changes that are reflected as abnormal arterial blood gas values. Most commonly, the pH decreases, the arterial partial pressure of oxygen (PaO_2) decreases, and the arterial partial pressure of carbon dioxide ($PaCO_2$) increases. Changes in other laboratory values may be associated with specific causes of hypovolemic shock.

Hematocrit and hemoglobin concentrations decrease with hypovolemic shock caused by hemorrhage. When hypovolemic shock is the result of dehydration, the hematocrit and hemoglobin values are elevated.

INTERVENTIONS

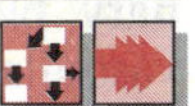

Interventions for clients who are experiencing hypovolemic shock are focused on reversal of hypovolemic shock, restoration of fluid volume, and prevention of ischemic complications. Some of these actions may be accomplished through supportive and drug therapies. Surgery may be necessary to correct the underlying problem leading to hypovolemic shock. Chart 36–3 summarizes nursing care priorities for clients experiencing hypovolemic shock.

Nonsurgical Management Interventions are aimed at increasing the body fluid compartment volumes to within normal ranges and supporting the client's operating compensatory mechanisms. Intravenous (IV) therapy, fluid replacement therapy, and drug therapies are the management choices for this problem.

Intravenous Therapy The two categories of substances commonly used for fluid volume replacement during hemorrhagic hypovolemia are colloids and crystalloids. Colloids contain large molecules (usually composed of proteins or starches); IV colloid solutions are

CHART 36–3

Nursing Care Highlight ♦ The Client in Hypovolemic Shock

- Ensure a patent airway.
- Start an IV line or maintain an established line.
- Increase the rate of IV fluid delivery.
- Administer oxygen.
- Elevate the client's feet, keeping his or her head flat or elevated to a 30-degree angle.
- Examine the client for overt bleeding.
- If overt bleeding is present, apply direct pressure to the site.
- Take the client's vital signs every 5 min until stable.
- Administer medications as ordered.
- Do not leave the client.

used to restore plasma volume and colloidal osmotic pressure (see Chap. 14). IV crystalloid solutions are administered for fluid and electrolyte replacement; they contain nonprotein substances, such as minerals, salts, and sugars. These fluids may be used individually or in combination as therapy for hypovolemic shock.

COLLOID FLUID REPLACEMENT Protein-containing colloid fluids are good for restoring vascular osmotic pressure as well as fluid volume. Blood and blood products are frequently used for this purpose and are the treatment of choice when hypovolemia is caused by blood loss. These products include whole blood, packed red blood cells, and plasma.

Whole blood and packed red blood cells increase the hematocrit and hemoglobin concentrations as well as the vascular fluid volume. Whole blood is used to replace large volumes of blood loss because it provides increased intravascular volume while improving the oxygen-carrying capacity of the blood. Packed red blood cells are given for moderate blood loss because they replenish the red blood cell deficit and improve the oxygen-carrying capacity without giving excessive fluid volume. (Chapter 39 discusses nursing care issues in blood and blood product administration.)

Human plasma, an acellular blood product containing some clotting factors, is administered to correct plasma deficits and restore osmotic pressure when the hematocrit and hemoglobin levels are within normal ranges. Plasma protein fractions (such as Plasmanate) and synthetic plasma expanders, such as hetastarch (hydroxyethyl starch, Hespan), effectively increase plasma volume and are frequently used as an early treatment of hypovolemic shock before a cause is established.

CRYSTALLOID FLUID REPLACEMENT Crystalloid solutions are commonly administered to help establish and maintain an adequate fluid and electrolyte balance. Two common crystalloid solutions are Ringer's lactate and normal saline. Ringer's lactate contains physiologic concentrations of sodium, chloride, calcium, potassium, and lactate in water (see Chap. 15). This isotonic solution is an effective volume expander, and the lactate is an effective buffer in the presence of acidosis. Normal saline (0.9% sodium chloride in water) is a fluid replacement that can increase the plasma volume; it is most frequently used when there has been no loss of red blood cells.

Drug Therapy If the volume deficit is severe and the client does not respond sufficiently to the replacement of fluid volume and blood products, the administration of medications that increase venous return, improve myocardial contractility, or ensure adequate myocardial perfusion through dilation of coronary vessels may be necessary. Chart 36–4 presents the drugs commonly used to treat hypovolemic shock.

VASOCONSTRICTING AGENTS A variety of drugs stimulate venous return by causing vasoconstriction and decreasing venous pooling of blood. These actions increase cardiac output and mean arterial pressure (MAP), helping to improve tissue perfusion and oxygenation. Most of these drugs produce serious side effects, and their dosages must be carefully calculated (sometimes titrated) on the basis of the client's size and degree of response. Drugs with systemic peripheral vasoconstricting activity include:

- Dopamine hydrochloride (Intropin, Revimine✱)
- Epinephrine (Adrenalin)
- Mephentermine (Wyamine)
- Methoxamine (Vasoxyl) hydrochloride
- Norepinephrine (Levophed)
- Phenylephrine (Neo-Synephrine) hydrochloride

AGENTS ENHANCING MYOCARDIAL CONTRACTILITY Some drugs directly stimulate adrenergic receptor sites on the myocardium (especially $beta_1$-receptors) and increase the contractile response of the cardiac muscle cells. Such agents include:

- Dobutamine hydrochloride (Dobutrex)
- Amrinone (Inocor)
- Epinephrine (Adrenalin)
- Isoproterenol (Isuprel)

Other agents enhance myocardial contractility by slowing the heart rate through altering electrical conduction and allowing the left ventricle a longer filling time. When the filling time is increased, more blood enters the left ventricle and stretches the myocardial fibers. Thus, greater recoil is achieved and more blood leaves the left ventricle during contraction. Some of these drugs also stimulate the ventricles at the same time. Agents with these types of actions include digoxin (Lanoxin) and deslanoside (Cedilanid-D).

AGENTS ENHANCING MYOCARDIAL PERFUSION The treatment of shock includes the administration of agents that produce systemic vasoconstriction to help enhance venous return and increase MAP. However, it is important to ensure that the myocardium is adequately perfused so that aerobic metabolism is maintained in the heart and maximum contractility can be achieved. Agents that selectively dilate coronary blood vessels while causing minimal systemic vasodilation are used for this purpose. Care is taken, because higher dosages can cause some systemic vasodilation and increase shock. Such agents include nitroglycerin (Nitroject, Nitrol, Nitrostat, Tridil), isosorbide dinitrate (Isordil), and nitroprusside (Nipride✱, Nitropress).

Oxygen Therapy Oxygen therapy is useful whenever shock is present. Oxygen can be administered by:

- Mask
- Hood

CHART 36–4

Drug Therapy for Hypovolemic Shock

Drug	Usual Dosage	Nursing Interventions	Rationale
Vasoconstrictors			
Dopamine hydrochloride (Intropin, Revimine✱)	• 5–30 μg/kg/min IV (for hypotension) • 2–5 μg/kg/min IV (for renal perfusion)	• Assess the client for chest pain. • Monitor urinary output hourly. • Assess blood pressure every 15 min. • Assess the client for headache.	• Dopamine increases myocardial oxygen consumption. • Higher doses decrease renal perfusion and urinary output. • Hypertension is a symptom of overdose. • Headache is an early symptom of drug excess.
Epinephrine (Adrenalin)	• 0.5–1 mg IV initially, followed by 0.5 mg every 5 min • May also be given by intracardiac injection	• Monitor the client for dysrhythmias. • Assess the client for chest pain.	• Epinephrine may cause ventricular tachyarrhythmias. • Vasoconstriction may impair cardiac oxygenation.
Norepinephrine (Levophed)	• 0.1–0.2 μg/kg/min continuous IV infusion to maintain blood pressure at 90–100 mmHg	• Assess for extravasation. • Observe the client's extremities for color and perfusion.	• Norepinephrine can cause severe tissue damage and necrosis. • Norepinephrine can cause such vasoconstriction that peripheral ischemia may result.
Agents Enhancing Contractility			
Amrinone (Inocor)	• 0.75–1.5 mg/kg bolus • 5–20 μg/kg/min continuous IV infusion	• Assess blood pressure every 15 min. • Do not administer through the same tubing as furosemide.	• Hypertension is a symptom of overdose. • Amrinone and furosemide form a precipitate.
Atropine sulfate	• 0.5–1 mg IV every 5 min, up to a total of 2 mg	• Take pulse every 5 min. • Monitor urinary output every 30 min. • Administer cautiously to clients with glaucoma.	• Atropine sulfate may cause a rebound tachycardia. • Atropine sulfate may cause urinary retention. • Atropine sulfate may precipitate an episode of acute angle-closure glaucoma.
Dobutamine hydrochloride (Dobutrex)	• 2.5–20 μg/kg/min continuous IV infusion	• Assess the client for chest pain. • Assess blood pressure every 15 min.	• Dobutamine increases myocardial oxygen consumption. • Hypertension is a symptom of overdose.
Agents Enhancing Myocardial Perfusion			
Sodium nitroprusside (Nitropress, Nipride✱)	• 0.5–10 μg/kg/min continuous IV infusion	• Assess blood pressure every 15 min.	• Hypotension may result from the systemic dilation of veins and arteries.

- Nasal cannula
- Nasopharyngeal tube
- Endotracheal tube
- Tracheostomy tube

Most commonly, masks and nasal cannulas are used to provide oxygen to clients experiencing shock. The nurse administers oxygen to the client in the amount of liters per minute (for administration via cannula) or concentration by percentage (for administration by mask) specified by the physician's order.

Monitoring A major nursing responsibility in caring for the client in hypovolemic shock is monitoring vital signs and level of consciousness (LOC). On the standard medical-surgical nursing unit, the nurse monitors the client's:

- Pulse
- Blood pressure
- Pulse pressure
- Central venous pressure
- Respiratory rate

- Skin and mucous membrane color
- Pulse oximetry values

The nurse performs these assessments at least every 15 minutes until the shock is under control and the client's condition improves. More extensive monitoring of cardiac output (hemodynamic monitoring), including intra-arterial monitoring, SVO_2 (mixed venous oxygen saturation), and pulmonary artery wedge pressures, is done in critical care settings.

Clients with shock who require more invasive monitoring, such as central venous pressure (CVP), pulmonary artery (PA) pressure, and pulmonary artery wedge pressure (PAWPs), should be transported to a critical care unit. Chapter 37 provides in-depth discussion of the uses and nursing responsibilities associated with various types of hemodynamic monitoring.

Insertion of a CVP catheter allows monitoring of the client's right atrial or superior vena cava pressure as well as providing venous access for volume replacement or infusion of pharmacologic agents. Changes in CVP accurately reflect the syndrome of hypovolemic shock. As the circulating volume decreases, the amount of blood returning to the right atrium also decreases, causing the CVP to decrease from baseline levels.

Intra-arterial catheter placement provides a means to monitor blood pressure continuously and serves as an access for arterial blood sampling. Intra-arterial catheters are inserted into an artery (radial, brachial, femoral, or dorsalis pedis artery). The arterial catheter is attached to pressure tubing and a transducer. The transducer converts the pressure in the artery (mechanical energy) into an electrical signal that is expressed as a visible waveform on an oscilloscope and a digital numeric value is displayed.

Surgical Management The nurse monitors the client's fluid loss and uses the nonsurgical interventions described earlier to stabilize the client's hemodynamic status. After a definitive diagnosis is established, surgical intervention may be necessary to correct the underlying cause of shock. Such interventions include:

- Vascular repair or revision
- Surgical hemostasis of major wounds
- Oversewing of bleeding ulcers
- Chemical scarring (chemosclerosis) of varicosities

COLLABORATIVE MANAGEMENT OF SEPSIS-INDUCED DISTRIBUTIVE SHOCK

ASSESSMENT

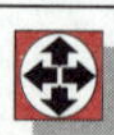

Distributive shock caused by sepsis does not resemble other types of shock, in that it has two distinctive phases (Fig. 36–2). The first phase is relatively long, frequently lasting from hours to days. The clinical manifestations during this phase are subtle. However, when the client is recognized to be in the first phase of sepsis-induced distributive shock and

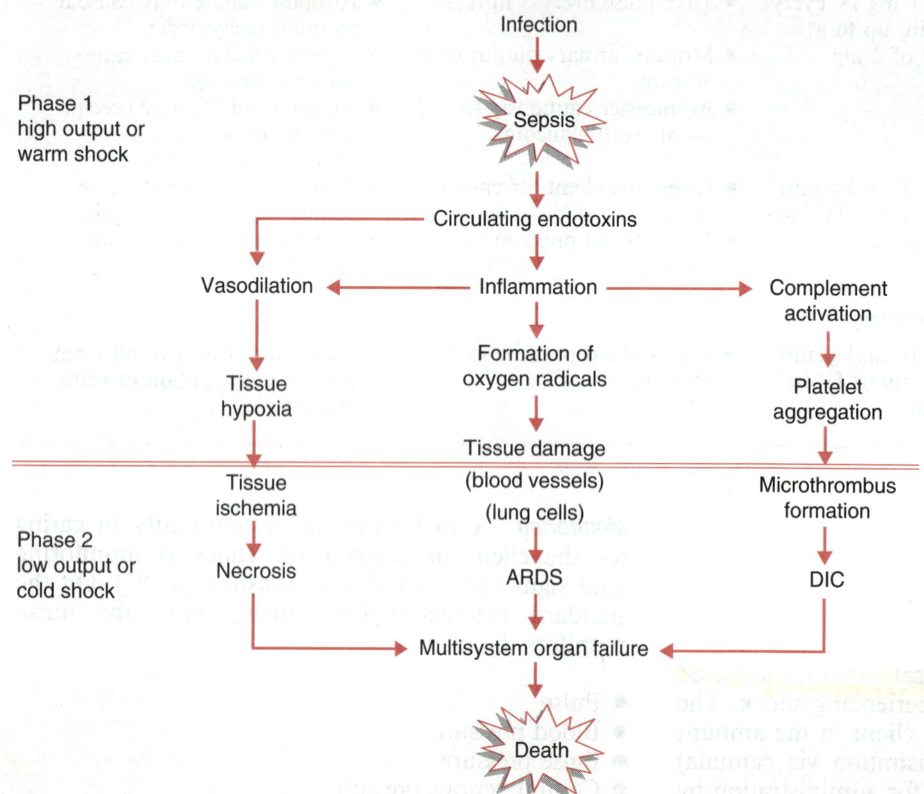

FIGURE 36–2 ◆ The sequence of sepsis-induced distributive shock.

the appropriate interventions are made, the client has a good chance for recovery. The second phase of sepsis-induced distributive shock has a sudden onset and a rapid downhill course. If sepsis-induced distributive shock progresses without intervention to the second phase, chances for the client's recovery are slim. The identification of the first phase of sepsis-induced distributive shock can make the biggest difference in survival among affected clients.

HISTORY

The nurse collects data about risk factors, as well as causative factors, related to sepsis-induced distributive shock. Age is important because sepsis-induced distributive shock can develop more easily among elderly, debilitated people with any degree of immunosuppression. Chart 36–5 lists some of the factors that increase the elderly person's risk of shock. Clients are asked specific questions about recent illness, trauma, or procedures or chronic conditions that may lead to sepsis and distributive shock. Such conditions include:

- Gastrointestinal surgery
- Surgery involving the nasal mucosa
- Any immunodeficient condition
- Malignancies
- Urinary tract or other infections

The use of some medications may directly cause changes leading to shock. A medication regimen may also indicate the presence of a disease or a problem that can contribute to sepsis-induced distributive shock. Such medications include aspirin and aspirin-containing drugs, antibiotics, and chemotherapeutic agents.

CHART 36–5

Nursing Focus on the Elderly ◆ Risk Factors for Shock

Type of Shock	Specific Risk Factor
Hypovolemic shock	• Diuretic therapy • Diminished thirst reflex • Immobility
Cardiogenic shock	• Diabetes mellitus • Presence of cardiomyopathies
Distributive shock	• Diminished immune response • Reduced skin integrity • Presence of cancer • Peripheral neuropathy • Cerebrovascular accidents • Institutionalization (hospital or extended-care facility) • Malnutrition • Anemia
Obstructive shock	• Pulmonary hypertension • Presence of cancer

PHYSICAL ASSESSMENT/CLINICAL MANIFESTATIONS

Many of the clinical manifestations of the first phase are unique to sepsis-induced distributive shock and, frequently, opposite from those associated with all other types of shock. Chart 36–6 summarizes the clinical manifestations of the first phase of sepsis-induced distributive shock. These findings, affecting the cardiovascular, integumentary, and pulmonary systems, result from the body's reaction to the presence of endotoxins.

CARDIOVASCULAR MANIFESTATIONS Endotoxins in the client's blood and other extracellular fluids interact with leukocytes, as well as with blood vessel walls, and trigger an inflammatory reaction. In addition, some endotoxins appear to stimulate myocardial tissue directly. As a result, cardiac output is actually *increased* during the first phase of sepsis-induced distributive shock. This phase may be termed the high-output phase. The increased cardiac output is reflected by tachycardia, increased stroke volume, a normal-to-elevated systolic blood pressure, and a normal central venous pressure. In addition, the increased cardiac output causes good perfusion of the skin so that the client may appear to have normal skin color with pink mucous membranes and feel warm to the touch. In some institutions, the high-output phase of sepsis-induced distributive shock is called warm shock. This situation is temporary, and eventually the cardiac output greatly diminishes in clients experiencing sepsis-induced distributive shock.

As sepsis-induced distributive shock progresses, disseminated intravascular coagulation (DIC) may accompany it. The presence of the endotoxins and the inflammatory reactions stimulate complement activation (see Chap. 22). These actions cause thousands of small clots to form in the tiny capillaries of vascular organs (e.g., liver, kidney, brain, spleen, and heart). These small clots interfere with the oxygenation in those organs, causing hypoxia and ischemia and making overall metabolism anaerobic. In addition, the enormous number of small clots use up clotting factors and fibrinogen faster than they can be regenerated by the liver, making the client much more susceptible to hemorrhage. These occurrences mark the beginning of the second phase of sepsis-induced distributive shock. Because some of the blood has already clotted, most of the clotting factors are gone, and blood vessels are dilated, the client is hypovolemic in this phase of distributive shock. The cardiac output now decreases dramatically, as does systolic blood pressure and pulse pressure. This phase is called the low-output phase of sepsis-induced distributive shock or cold shock, and the clinical manifestations strongly resemble those of the later stages of all forms of shock.

CHART 36-6

Key Features of Phase 1 Sepsis-Induced Distributive Shock

Assessment	Findings
General	
Assess the mental status and level of consciousness.	• Irritability, restlessness, lethargy, disorientation, and inappropriate euphoria
Check the oral temperature.	• Normal, subnormal, or elevated temperature
Cardiovascular System	
Check the pulse and blood pressure. Document the pulse pressure with each blood pressure reading.	• Tachycardia: normal mean arterial blood pressure; widening pulse pressure
Check peripheral pulses.	• "Bounding" peripheral pulses
Auscultate heart sounds at four valvular sites and record the onset of murmur or gallop	• No murmur or gallop
Respiratory System	
Observe the rate, rhythm, and effort of breathing. Observe the symmetry of chest expansion.	• Tachypnea, hyperventilation
Percuss and auscultate the lungs. Note the onset of adventitious sounds.	• Crackles and decreased breath sounds
Check blood gas levels.	• Respiratory alkalosis
Integumentary System	
Inspect and palpate the skin. Note color, vascularity, moisture, temperature, texture, thickness, mobility, and turgor. Assess the oral mucosa.	• Warm flushed skin and peripheral edema

PULMONARY MANIFESTATIONS In the high-output phase of sepsis-induced distributive shock, respiratory rate and depth are increased. Often, the client actually experiences a respiratory alkalosis (see Chap. 18).

When sepsis-induced distributive shock progresses to the low-output phase, the possible life-threatening pulmonary complication of adult respiratory distress syndrome (ARDS) may occur. Although this complication has many causes, its association with sepsis is thought to be related to the formation of oxygen free radicals, which exert destructive actions on the type I and type II pulmonary epithelial cells (Wilson, 1992). Oxygen free radicals can form as a result of oxygen therapy and in response to cellular destruction and the subsequent release of oxidizing enzymes. The presence of ARDS in a client who has sepsis-induced distributive shock is an ominous clinical sign and is usually associated with a high mortality rate.

INTEGUMENTARY MANIFESTATIONS Often, clients in the early phase of sepsis-induced distributive shock are not recognized as having a problem because the appearance of the skin and mucous membranes leads health care professionals to believe that circulation is unimpaired. Clients feel warm to the touch and their lips and mucous membranes appear well oxygenated.

When distributive shock progresses so that circulation is compromised, the client's skin is cool and clammy with pallor or cyanosis present. In clients with disseminated intravascular coagulation, petechiae and ecchymoses occur anywhere and everywhere. Blood may ooze from gums, other mucous membranes, venipúncture sites, and around IV lines.

PSYCHOSOCIAL ASSESSMENT

Often, the indicator that all is not well with a client at the beginning of sepsis-induced distributive shock is a change in affect or behavior. The nurse compares the client's presenting behavior, verbal responses, and general affect with those assessed earlier in the day or the day before and notes changes. Clients may seem just slightly different in their reactions to greetings, comments, or jokes. They may be less patient than usual or act restless or fidgety. Clients may verbalize statements such as, "I feel as if something is wrong but I don't know what." If this behavior represents a change for the client, the nurse always considers the possibility and probability of shock.

LABORATORY ASSESSMENT

The presence of bacteria in blood and other extracellular fluids supports the diagnosis of sepsis. The nurse obtains specimens of urine, blood, sputum, and any drainage for culture to identify the causative organisms for both diagnostic and therapeutic purposes. Other abnormal laboratory findings associated with sepsis-induced distributive shock include changes in the white blood cell count; the differential leukocyte count may demonstrate a left shift (see Chap. 22). Changes in the hematocrit and hemoglobin levels usually are not evident until late in septic shock when the client is hemorrhaging. At that point, the hematocrit and hemoglobin concentrations are low, as are the fibrinogen levels and the platelet count (Epstein & Bakanauskas, 1991).

INTERVENTIONS

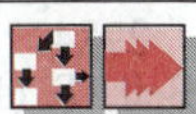

Interventions for the client experiencing sepsis-induced distributive shock focus on correcting the conditions contributing to shock and on preventing complications. Chart 36–7 summarizes the nursing care priorities for clients experiencing sepsis-induced distributive shock.

Control of fluid volume deficit associated with septic shock is accomplished through supportive and drug therapies. IV therapy is the same as that described for hypovolemic shock.

Drug Therapy The same agents used to enhance cardiac output and restore vascular volume in hypovolemic shock are appropriate for sepsis-induced distributive shock. A major focus is the administration of antibiotics to combat sepsis. In addition, agents to counteract disseminated intravascular coagulation (DIC) may be required. Sepsis-induced distributive shock and DIC have two distinctly different phases, and drug therapies for each phase of sepsis-induced distributive shocks are different. Drug therapy in the first phase is aimed at preventing coagulation. Drug therapy in the second, late phase of sepsis-induced distributive shock is aimed at increasing the blood's ability to clot.

ANTIBIOTICS Although sepsis and distributive shock can be caused by any microorganism, the most common agents are gram-negative bacteria. When blood cultures have identified the presence of specific bacteria, IV antibiotics with known activity against the bacteria are administered. When the causative agent is not known, multiple agents with wide activity are prescribed. These agents include vancomycin (Vancocin, Diatracin♣), one of the aminoglycosides (amikacin, gentamicin, kanamycin, tobramycin), and a systemic penicillin derivative (ampicillin, cloxacillin, ticarcillin).

ANTIBODIES Endotoxin antibodies are being tested for efficacy against sepsis-induced distributive shock. Monoclonal antibodies have been developed against different components of the actual bacteria producing the endotoxin and against part of the endotoxin itself. This therapy shows promise in reducing the extensive mortality associated with sepsis-induced distributive shock (Allen & Clochesy, 1993; Klein & Witek-Janusek, 1992).

ANTICOAGULANTS When clients are identified as being in the early phase of sepsis-induced distributive shock and are beginning to form numerous small clots, heparin is given to limit the unnecessary clotting and to prevent the consumption of clotting factors.

CHART 36–7

Nursing Care Highlight ♦ The Client in Sepsis-Induced Distributive Shock

- Ensure a patent airway.
- Start or maintain an established IV line.
- Administer oxygen.
- Administer antibiotics.
- Obtain specimens of blood, urine, wound drainage, and sputum for culture.
- Increase the rate of IV fluid delivery.
- Use aseptic technique for any invasive procedure.
- Handle the client gently.
- Examine the client for overt bleeding, especially of gums, injection sites, and IV sites.
- Elevate the client's feet, keeping his or her head flat or elevated to a 30-degree angle.
- Take the client's vital signs every 5 min until they are stable.
- Administer medications as ordered:
  - Heparin during phase 1
  - Clotting factors during phase 2
- Do not leave the client.

CLOTTING FACTORS When sepsis-induced distributive shock progresses to the point at which microthrombi have formed to such an extent that the client no longer has sufficient clotting factors to prevent hemorrhage, clotting factors are administered intravenously. These factors are obtained as a precipitate from pooled human serum. Individual clotting factors may be given separately, although most clients in sepsis-induced distributive shock are generally deficient in all factors. Administration of fresh frozen plasma also helps to replace clotting factors.

Providing a Safe Environment Primary prevention is possible for some types of shock by identifying clients at risk for conditions and complications leading to sepsis and preventing those complications. Strict adherence to aseptic technique during invasive procedures and during the manipulation of nonintact skin and mucous membranes of clients who are immunocompromised to any degree can help to prevent or to limit sepsis and sepsis-induced distributive shock.

Secondary prevention (early detection) of the clinical manifestations of shock is a major nursing responsibility. Because shock is a common complication of many conditions found in hospitalized clients, the nurse always considers the possibility of sepsis-induced distributive shock. For early detection, the nurse continuously assesses measurements indicative of impending shock for specific changes from normal values or from baseline levels. After distributive shock is recognized, the nurse rapidly takes actions to halt or to change the conditions contributing to shock, to support the client's physiologic compensatory mechanisms, and to prevent life-threatening complications.

Oxygen Therapy Oxygen therapy is useful whenever inadequate tissue perfusion and inadequate oxygenation are present, such as during distributive shock. Oxygen can be administered by:

- Mask
- Hood
- Nasal cannula
- Nasopharyngeal tube
- Endotracheal tube
- Tracheostomy tube

Most commonly, masks and nasal cannulas are used to administer oxygen to clients experiencing shock. The nurse administers oxygen to the client in the amount of liters per minute (for administration via cannula) or concentration by percentage (for administration by mask) specified by the physician's prescription.

IMPLICATIONS FOR NURSING RESEARCH

A review of current nursing literature reveals the need for nursing research on the effectiveness of specific interventions for the hospitalized client who is in the early stage of shock, especially sepsis-induced distributive shock. In addition, the development of assessment tools to enhance early detection of shock in the client at risk is clearly needed. Nursing research is needed to answer the following questions related to the care of clients experiencing shock:

- ◆ How effective are nursing measures in preventing sepsis-induced distributive shock?
- ◆ What effect does early recognition of signs and symptoms have on preventing the progression and complications of hypovolemic shock?
- ◆ What are the effects of nursing measures on perfusion in the presence of shock?
- ◆ Which noninvasive delivery method of oxygen therapy (nasal cannula or mask) is more effective in maintaining adequate PO_2 levels?
- ◆ How do hospital infection control reports influence the incidence of nosocomial infections?
- ◆ Which specific nursing care procedures are most closely associated with the development of sepsis-induced distributive shock?
- ◆ How effective are urgent care outpatient centers in the early detection of shock?

SELECTED BIBLIOGRAPHY

Allen, C., & Clochesy, J. (1993). Patients with sepsis. In J. Clochesy, C. Breu, S. Cardin, E. Rudy, & A. Whittaker (Eds.), *Critical care nursing* (pp. 1245–1257). Philadelphia: W. B. Saunders.

* American Heart Association. (1986). Standards and guidelines for cardiopulmonary resuscitation (CPR) and emergency cardiac care (ECC). *JAMA, 255*(21), 2841–2984.

Bell, T. (1990). Disseminated intravascular coagulation and shock. *Critical Care Nursing Clinics of North America, 2*(2), 255–262.

Burns, K. (1990). Vasoactive drug therapy in shock. *Critical Care Nursing Clinics of North America, 2*(2), 167–178.

Byra-Cook, C., Dracup, K., & Lazik, A. (1990). Direct and indirect blood pressure in critical care patients. *Nursing Research, 39*(5), 285–288.

Clochesy, J., Breu, C., Cardin, S., Rudy, E., & Whittaker, A. (1993). *Critical care nursing.* Philadelphia: W. B. Saunders.

Colletti, R., Dew, R., & Goulart, A. (1993). Antiendotoxin therapy in sepsis. *Critical Care Nursing Clinics of North America, 5*(2), 345–354.

Daleiden, A. (1993). Physiology and treatment of hemorrhagic shock during the early postoperative period. *Critical Care Nursing Quarterly, 16*(1), 45–59.

Effron, M., & Chernow, B. (1992). Shock. In E. Rubenstein & D. Federman (Eds.), *Scientific American: Medicine* (pp. I card III Shock 1–12). New York: Scientific American.

Epstein, C., & Bakanauskas, A. (1991). Clinical management of DIC: Early nursing interventions. *Critical Care Nurse, 11*(10), 42–53.

Guyton, A. (1991). *Textbook of medical physiology* (8th ed.). Philadelphia: W. B. Saunders.

Houston, M. (1990). Pathophysiology of shock. *Critical Care Clinics of North America, 2*(2), 143–149.

Kadota, L. (1993). Hemodynamic monitoring. In J. Clochesy, C. Breu, S. Cardin, E. Rudy, & A. Whittaker (Eds.), *Critical care nursing* (pp. 155–182). Philadelphia: W. B. Saunders.

Klein, D. (1990). Physiologic response to traumatic shock. *American Association of Critical Care Nurses Clinical Issues, 1*(3), 505–521.

Klein, D. (1991). Shock: Physiology, signs, symptoms. *Nursing 91, 21*(11), 74–76.

Klein, D., & Witek-Janusek, L. (1992). Advances in immunotherapy of sepsis. *Dimensions in Critical Care Nursing, 11*(2), 75–89.

Lancaster, L. (1990). Renal response to shock. *Critical Care Nursing Clinics of North America, 2*(2), 221–228.

* Littleton, M. (1988). Pathophysiology and assessment of sepsis and septic shock. *Critical Care Nursing Quarterly, 11*(1), 30–47.

McCormac, M. (1990). Managing hemorrhagic shock. *American Journal of Nursing, 90*(12), 22–27.

McMorrow, M., & Cooney-Daniello, M. (1991). When to suspect septic shock. *RN, 54*(10), 32–37.

Mostow, S. (1990). Management of gram-negative septic shock. *Hospital Practice, 25*(10), 121–130.

O'Neal, P. (1994). How to spot early signs of cardiogenic shock. *American Journal of Nursing, 94*(5), 36–40.

Rice, V. (1991a). Shock, a clinical syndrome: An update part 1: An overview of shock. *Critical Care Nurse, 11*(4), 20–24.

Rice, V. (1991b). Shock, a clinical syndrome: An update

part 2: The stages of shock. *Critical Care Nurse, 11*(5), 74–82.

Rice, V. (1991c). Shock, a clinical syndrome: An update part 3: Therapeutic management. *Critical Care Nurse, 11*(6), 34–39.

Rice, V. (1991d). Shock, a clinical syndrome: An update part 4: Nursing care of the shock patient. *Critical Care Nurse, 11*(7), 28–42.

Roach, A. (1990). Antibiotic therapy in septic shock. *Critical Care Nursing Clinics of North America, 2*(2), 179–191.

Russell, S. (1994). Hypovolemic shock: Is your patient at risk? *Nursing94, 24*(4), 34–39.

Russell, S. (1994). Septic shock: Can you recognize the clues? *Nursing94, 24*(4), 40–48.

Shelton, B. (1994). Disorders of hemostasis in sepsis. *Critical Care Nursing Clinics of North America, 6*(2), 373–387.

* Shoemaker, W. (1987). Circulatory mechanisms of shock and their mediators. *Critical Care Medicine, 15,* 787–794.

Stengle, J., & Dries, D. (1994). Sepsis in the elderly. *Critical Care Nursing Clinics of North America, 6*(2), 421–427.

Stroud, M., Swindell, B., & Bernard, G. (1990). Cellular and humoral mediators of sepsis syndrome. *Critical Care Nursing Clinics of North America, 2*(2), 151–160.

Suhl, J. (1993). Patients with shock. In J. Clochesy, C. Breu, S. Cardin, E. Rudy, & A. Whittaker (Eds.), *Critical care nursing* (pp. 1258–1270). Philadelphia: W. B. Saunders.

Summers, G. (1990). The clinical and hemodynamic presentation of the shock patient. *Critical Care Nursing Clinics of North America, 2*(2), 161–166.

Truett, L. (1991). The septic syndrome: An oncologic treatment challenge. *Cancer Nursing, 14*(4), 175–180.

Wilson, R. (1992). *Critical care manual: Applied physiology and principles and therapy* (2nd ed.). Philadelphia: F. A. Davis.

Young, L. (1990). DIC: The insidious killer. *Critical Care Nurse, 10*(9), 26–33.

Zeigler, E., & Smith, C. (1992). Anti-endotoxin monoclonal antibodies. *New England Journal of Medicine, 326,* 1165.

SUGGESTED READINGS

Burns, K. (1990). Vasoactive drug therapy in shock. *Critical Care Nursing Clinics of North America, 2*(2), 167–178.

This article reviews the types and actions of various fluid replacement and pharmacologic agents used in the general treatment of hemorrhagic, cardiogenic, neurogenic, anaphylactic, and septic shock. Drug dosages and administration tips are provided. Some specific nursing actions associated with drug administration or complications of shock are addressed.

Epstein, C., & Bakanauskas, A. (1991). Clinical management of DIC: Early nursing interventions. *Critical Care Nurse, 11*(10), 42–53.

This excellent article provides a detailed description of the sequence of events and pathophysiology associated with the development of disseminated intravascular coagulation (DIC) and septic shock. A system-by-system assessment guide for overt and covert changes associated with DIC enhances the usefulness of this article. The authors present a care plan with interventions for preventing as well as for addressing actual problems. Interventions are listed with complete rationales and expected outcomes.

Klein, D. (1991). Shock: Physiology, signs, symptoms. *Nursing 91, 21*(11), 74–76.

The outstanding features of this article are the in-depth assessment guide for identifying clients with or at risk for septic shock and the complete explanations of the physiology and pathophysiology of septic shock. The assessment guide includes rationales for the clinical manifestations observed during early, intermediate, and late stages of septic shock. A description of specific nursing measures is a foundation for the plan of care appropriate for most clients with septic shock.

Littleton, M. (1988). Pathophysiology and assessment of sepsis and septic shock. *Critical Care Nursing Quarterly, 11*(1), 30–47.

This article briefly reviews the major physiologic events associated with shock. Color pictures enhance the textual descriptions of such concepts as sympathetic nervous system regulation of cardiac output, anaerobic metabolism, DIC, and progression of shock. The article visually depicts the interrelatedness of different types of shock and summarizes the most common manifestations of each type.

Stengle, J., & Dries, D. (1994). Sepsis in the elderly. *Critical Care Nursing Clinics of North America, 6*(2), 421–427.

This excellent article compares the clinical manifestations of sepsis in elderly people with those considered "classic for the adult population," emphasizing the subtle changes that can be easily overlooked in an elderly client. In addition, the authors describe risk factors, usual clinical course, and treatment.

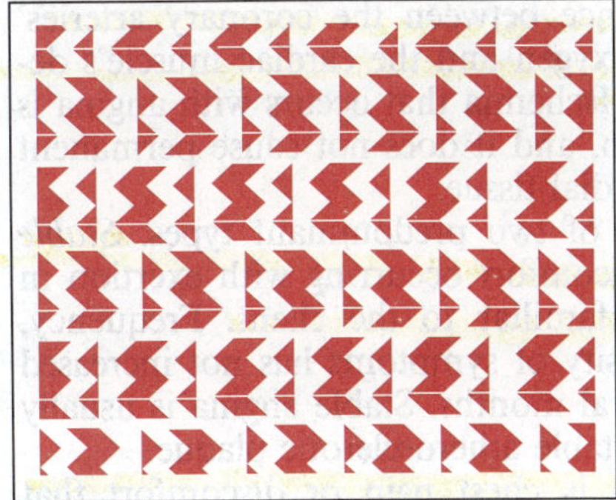

CHAPTER 37

CHAPTER HIGHLIGHTS

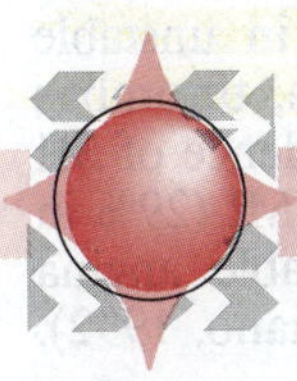

Interventions for Critically Ill Clients with Coronary Artery Disease

Coronary care units started in the 1960s as a means of limiting client death after myocardial infarctions (MIs), or heart attacks. Since that time, deaths from myocardial infarction have been reduced approximately 30% (American Heart Association [AHA], 1992). This reduction is partly due to better health promotion, but management of the client with coronary artery disease also changed dramatically during this time.

Most deaths today from myocardial infarction happen before the client reaches the hospital because of dysrhythmias. During the past 5 years, in-hospital mortality from myocardial infarction has dropped from 15% to 5%. Advances in cardiac care, especially new strategies for opening and maintaining the patency of obstructed coronary vessels, contributed to this decline.

OVERVIEW

Since 1940, coronary artery disease (CAD) has been the leading cause of death in the United States. This disease affects the arteries that provide blood, oxygen, and nutrients to the myocardium. When blood flow through the coronary arteries is partially or completely blocked, ischemia and infarction (necrosis) of the myocardium may result. Ischemia occurs when insufficient oxygen is supplied to meet the requirements of the myocardium. Infarction occurs when severe ischemia is prolonged and irreversible damage to tissue results.

PATHOPHYSIOLOGY

Atherosclerosis is the leading contributor to coronary artery disease and death in Western civilizations (see Chap. 35).

Three basic processes occur in atherosclerosis:

- Overgrowth of intimal smooth muscle cells with accumulation of macrophages and T cells
- Formation of a connective tissue matrix in the vessel intima
- Accumulation of lipids, especially cholesterol, in the connective tissue

These processes narrow the vessel lumen (Fig. 37–1). Blood flow through the restricted lumen may be adequate to perfuse myocardial tissue when the client is at rest.

At rest, the heart extracts a larger amount of oxygen (75%) from its blood flow than does any other major organ in the body. When additional oxygen is needed to meet increased tissue demands, an increase in coronary artery blood flow is required. Once the lumen of a coronary artery is obstructed by more than 70%, blood flow may not be able to increase in response to tissue demands. Increases in myocardial oxygen requirements (e.g., exercise or aortic stenosis) or transient reductions in blood flow (e.g., hypotension or coronary spasm) may result in inadequate oxygen supply to and ischemia of the myocardium. Ischemic myocardium is oxygen-deprived myocardium, and the client normally experiences angina.

ANGINA PECTORIS

Angina pectoris, a name derived from a Latin phrase, means "strangling of the chest." Angina is a temporary imbalance between the coronary arteries' ability to supply oxygen and the cardiac muscle's demand for oxygen. Ischemia that occurs with angina is limited in duration, and it does not cause permanent damage of myocardial tissue.

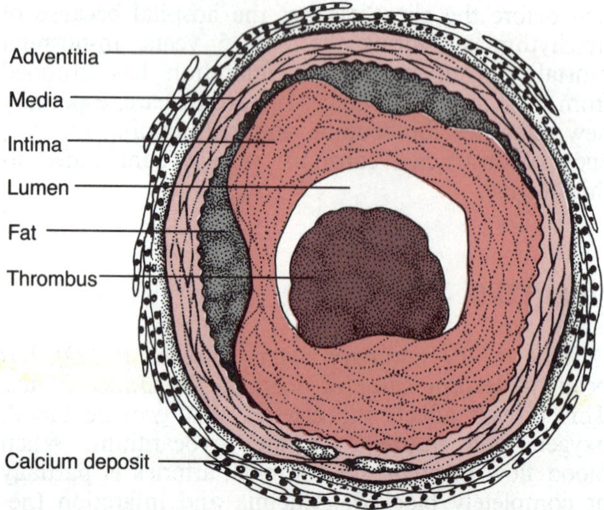

FIGURE 37–1 ◆ A cross-section of an atherosclerotic coronary artery.

Angina may be of two predominant types. *Stable* angina is chest discomfort occurring with exertion in a pattern that is familiar to the client. Frequency, duration, or intensity of symptoms has not increased over the past several months. Stable angina is usually associated with a stable atherosclerotic plaque.

Unstable angina is chest pain or discomfort that occurs at rest or with minimal exertion. An increase in the number of attacks and an increase in the intensity of the pain characterize unstable angina. The pain may last longer than 15 minutes or be poorly relieved by rest or nitroglycerin. Unstable angina describes a broad spectrum of disorders, including:

- New-onset angina
- Variant angina (Prinzmetal's)
- Preinfarction angina
- Crescendo angina

The atherosclerotic plaque may rupture in unstable angina, with resultant platelet aggregation, thrombus formation, and vasoconstriction. The incidence of MI (10% to 30% per year) and of death from MI (29% in 5 years) is higher for clients with unstable angina than for those with stable angina (Matrisciano, 1992).

MYOCARDIAL INFARCTION

Myocardial infarction (MI) occurs when myocardial tissue is abruptly and severely deprived of oxygen. When blood flow is acutely reduced by 80% to 90%, ischemia develops. Ischemia can lead to necrosis of myocardial tissue if blood flow is not restored. Most MIs are the result of atherosclerosis of a coronary artery, subsequent thrombosis, and occlusion of blood flow. However, other factors may be implicated, such as coronary artery spasm, platelet aggregation, and emboli from mural thrombi (within the cardiac wall).

MIs often begin with infarction (necrosis) of the subendocardial layer of cardiac muscle. This layer has the longest myofibrils in the heart, the greatest oxygen demand, and the poorest oxygen supply.

Around the initial area of infarction in the subendocardium are two zones:

- The zone of injury, tissue that is injured but not necrotic
- The zone of ischemia, tissue that is oxygen-deprived

This pattern is illustrated in Figure 37–2.

THE PROCESS OF INFARCTION Infarction is a dynamic process. It does not occur instantly but evolves over several hours. Hypoxia from ischemia may lead to local vasodilation of blood vessels and acidosis.

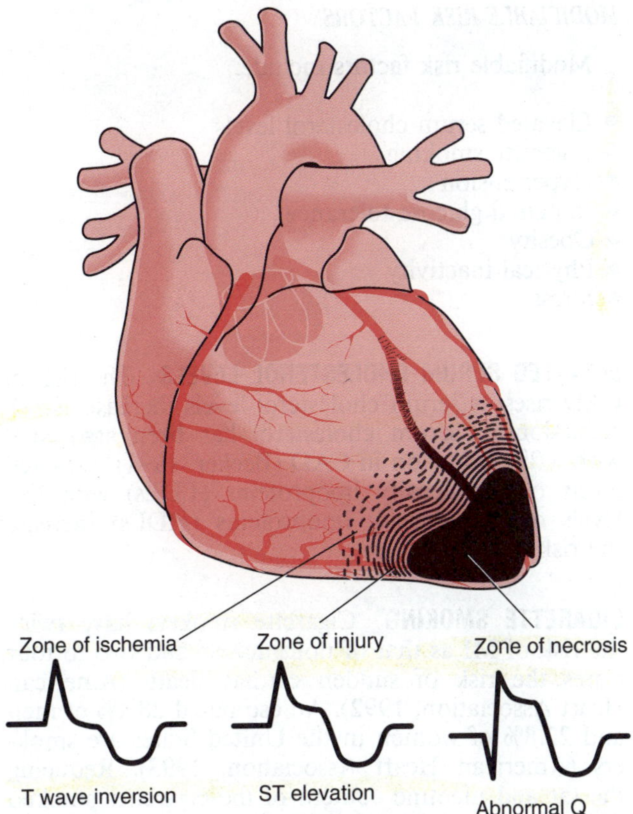

FIGURE 37–2 ◆ The ECG changes seen in myocardial infarction.

Imbalances of potassium, calcium, and magnesium as well as acidosis may lead to suppression of normal pacemaker and contractile functions. Automaticity and ectopy are enhanced. Catecholamines released in response to hypoxia and pain may increase the heart's rate and force of contraction. These factors increase oxygen requirements in tissue already oxygen-deprived. The area of infarction may extend into the zones of injury and ischemia.

The actual extent of the zone of infarction depends on three factors:

- Collateral circulation
- Anaerobic metabolism
- Workload demands on the myocardium

The infarction may involve only the subendocardium (called a subendocardial or non–Q wave MI), or it may spread to the epicardium or to all three layers of cardiac muscle. When all three layers are involved, the MI is termed transmural. Subendocardial MIs have less effect on wall motion and cardiac output then transmural infarctions do.

PHYSIOLOGIC RESPONSE TO INFARCTION Obvious physical changes do not occur in the heart until 6 hours after the infarction, when the infarcted region appears blue and swollen. After 48 hours, the infarct turns gray with yellow streaks as neutrophils invade the tissue and begin to remove the necrotic cells. By 8 to 10 days after infarction, granulation tissue forms at the edges of the necrotic tissue. Over 2 to 3 months, the necrotic area eventually develops into a shrunken, thin, firm scar (Pasternak et al., 1992). Scar tissue permanently changes the size and shape of the entire left ventricle (ventricular remodeling). Remodeling may decrease left ventricular function and increase morbidity and mortality.

CLASSIFICATION OF MYOCARDIAL INFARCTION BY LOCATION The client's response to an MI also depends on which coronary artery or arteries were obstructed and which part of the left ventricle wall was damaged: anterior, lateral, septal, inferior, or posterior. Figure 37–3 details the major coronary arteries, and Table 37–1 describes the structures they perfuse.

Clients with obstruction of the left anterior descending (LAD) artery usually have anterior and/or septal MIs because the LAD artery perfuses the anterior wall and most of the septal wall of the left ventricle. Anterior wall MIs account for 25% of all MIs and, at 25%, have the highest mortality rate. Clients with anterior MIs are most likely to experience left ventricular heart failure and ventricular dysrhythmias, because a large segment of the left ventricle wall may have been damaged.

The circumflex artery supplies the lateral wall of the left ventricle and possibly portions of the posterior wall or the sinoatrial (SA) and atrioventricular (AV) nodes. Clients with obstruction of the circumflex artery may experience posterior wall MI (2% of MIs) or lateral wall MI (3% of MIs), and sinus dysrhythmias.

The right coronary artery perfuses the SA and AV nodes in most people as well as the diaphragmatic portion of the left ventricle. Clients with obstruction

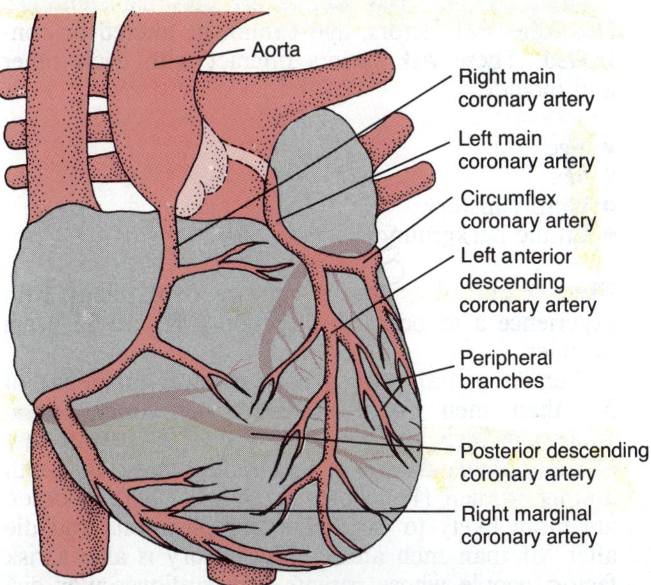

FIGURE 37–3 ◆ The coronary arterial system.

TABLE 37–1 Major Coronary Vessels and the Structures They Perfuse

Left Anterior Descending Coronary Artery

- Most of the left ventricular muscle mass and septum

Left Circumflex Coronary Artery

- The posterior wall of the left ventricle
- The SA node in 39% of clients
- The AV node in 12% of clients
- The left ventricular muscle in 10% of clients

Right Coronary Artery

- The right ventricle
- The inferior portion of the left ventricle
- The SA node in 59% of clients
- The AV node in 88% of clients

SA, sinoatrial; AV, atrioventricular.

of the right coronary artery often have inferior MIs. Inferior wall MIs account for approximately 17% of all MIs and have a mortality rate of about 10%. Clients are most likely to experience bradydysrhythmias or AV conduction defects, especially transient second-degree heart blocks. About one-third of clients with inferior MIs have right ventricular MI and right ventricular failure (Braunwald, 1992).

ETIOLOGY

Atherosclerosis is the primary factor in the development of coronary artery disease (CAD). Numerous risk factors contribute to atherosclerosis (see Chap. 35). Risk factors are classified as nonmodifiable and modifiable.

NONMODIFIABLE RISK FACTORS

Nonmodifiable risk factors are personal elements, also called set factors, that cannot be altered or controlled. These risk factors interact with each other and include:

- Age
- Sex
- Family history
- Ethnic background

The risk of CAD increases with age. Most clients who experience a myocardial infarction (MI) are 65 years or older.

Premenopausal women have a lower incidence of MI than men do. However, for postmenopausal women in their 70s, the incidence of MI equals that of men. Heart disease is the leading cause of death among women (Penckofer & Holm, 1993). Women are more likely to experience complications and die after MI than men are. Family history is also a risk factor; people whose parents had cardiovascular disease are more susceptible.

MODIFIABLE RISK FACTORS

Modifiable risk factors include:

- Elevated serum cholesterol levels
- Cigarette smoking
- Hypertension
- Impaired glucose tolerance
- Obesity
- Physical inactivity
- Stress

ELEVATED SERUM CHOLESTEROL LEVELS The risk of CAD rises as serum cholesterol levels increase. A 1% reduction in serum cholesterol has been associated with a 2% reduction in CAD (Becker, 1991). Elevated levels of low-density lipoproteins (LDLs) with low levels of high-density lipoproteins (HDLs) increase the risk further.

CIGARETTE SMOKING Cigarette smokers have twice the risk of MI as that of nonsmokers and two to four times the risk of sudden cardiac death (American Heart Association, 1992). An estimated 28.4% of men and 22.8% of women in the United States are smokers (American Heart Association, 1993). Reducing the tar and nicotine content of the cigarettes smoked does not reduce the risk of CAD.

OTHER FACTORS *Hypertension* increases the workload of the heart, which increases the risk of MI. *Impaired glucose tolerance* (e.g., in diabetes) seriously increases the risks.

Obesity is associated with increased serum cholesterol, elevated blood pressure, and abnormal glucose tolerance. It may also have an independent effect on risk of CAD. The distribution of adipose tissue seems to be important; clients with fat deposited about the waist are at greater risk than are clients with fat distributed about the hips.

Physical inactivity is a major risk factor for people in Western countries because such a large number are inactive. Regular physical activity helps maintain body weight and muscle mass while optimizing blood pressure and lipid values.

The effect of *stress* on the development of CAD is controversial. Some evidence indicates that job stress may be associated with left ventricular hypertrophy. The role of *type A behavior* in the development of CAD is also controversial. Type A people are aware of time constraints, are highly ambitious, and are occasionally hostile. Type A behavior has been associated with a twofold increase in angina.

Clients with several risk factors (hypertension, obesity, smoking, high cholesterol levels, and diabetes) have several times the risk of CAD as do those without these characteristics.

Although many factors place a client at risk for heart disease, there are well-documented, effective ways of promoting cardiovascular health. Some of these methods are described in Chart 37–1.

CHART 37–1

Health Promotion ◆ Prevention of Coronary Artery Disease

Smoking
- If you smoke, quit.
- If you don't smoke, don't start.

Diet
- Follow a prudent daily diet:
  - Consume sufficient calories for your body:
    - Obtain 50%–55% of your calories from carbohydrates.
      - Obtain 30%–35% of your calories from complex carbohydrates.
      - Obtain 10% of your calories from simple sugars.
    - Obtain 30%–35% of your calories from fat.
      - Obtain 15% of your calories from monounsaturated fat.
      - Obtain 10% of your calories from polyunsaturated fat.
      - Obtain the remainder of your calories (5%–10%) from saturated fat.
    - Obtain 12%–20% of your calories from protein.
  - Limit your cholesterol intake to 300 mg daily.
  - Limit your sodium intake to 130 mEq daily.

Cholesterol
- Have your cholesterol and low-density lipoprotein (LDL) levels checked regularly.
- If they are elevated, follow your health care provider's advice.

Physical Activity
- If you are middle-aged or older or have a history of medical problems, check with your health care provider before starting an exercise program.
- Appropriate exercise should be enjoyable, burn 400 calories/session, and sustain a heart rate of 120–150 beats per minute, depending on your age.
- Exercise moderately at least three times each week, preferably five. If you are unable to exercise moderately three to five times each week, walk daily for 30 minutes at a comfortable pace.
- Exercise periods should be at least 20–30 minutes long with 10-minute warm-up and 5-minute cool-down periods.

Diabetes
- Manage your diabetes with your health care provider.

Blood Pressure
- Have your blood pressure checked regularly.
- If it is elevated, follow your health care provider's advice.
- Continue to monitor your blood pressure at regular intervals.

Obesity
- Avoid severely restricted or fad diets.
- Consider a restriction in intake of saturated fats, simple sugars, and cholesterol-rich foods.
- Increase your physical activity.

Transcultural Considerations Modifiable risk factors vary for people of differing race and ethnic backgrounds. African-Americans do not have significantly higher overall heart disease rates than other groups. However, the incidence of diabetes is 33% higher in African-Americans, and hypertension is four times more common in African-American men. Obesity is significantly more common in African-American women than in the corresponding Caucasian-American populations (U.S. Department of Health and Human Services [DHHS], 1992).

Hispanics have lower death rates from heart disease than non–Hispanics. However, smoking continues in 43% of Hispanic men (higher than in other American populations) (DHHS, 1992). Overweight is more of a problem for Hispanic women, especially Mexican-American women (Jarvis, 1992), and may be associated with lower-than-average physical activity.

Tremendous diversity among the Asian and Pacific Island American populations makes generalizations about the population difficult. However, Filipino-Americans seem to have an increased incidence of hypertension.

The major modifiable cardiovascular risk factors for Native Americans seem to be obesity and diabetes. The increase in obesity in Native Americans has paralleled the increase in diabetes (DHHS, 1992). In many tribes, more than 20% of the members have diabetes.

INCIDENCE/PREVALENCE

Approximately 1,500,000 myocardial infarctions (MIs) occur each year in the United States, and about a third of these people die (American Heart Association, 1992). Approximately 240,000 women die each year from MI (Penckofer & Holm, 1993).

It is not clear how many people experience angina each year. However, 750,000 people are hospitalized each year with the diagnosis of unstable angina (Matrisciano, 1992). It is estimated that more than 6 million people who have experienced angina or MI are still living (American Heart Association, 1992). The estimated cost of caring for people with CAD is in excess of $100 billion yearly.

COLLABORATIVE MANAGEMENT

ASSESSMENT

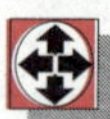

HISTORY

If chest discomfort is present at the time of the interview, the nurse delays collection of historical data until interventions for pain and dysrhythmias are initiated and the discomfort resolves. The nurse obtains information about how the client has managed the current episode of chest discomfort and which medications the client is taking. When the client is *pain-free,* the nurse obtains information about family history and modifiable risk factors, including eating habits, lifestyle, and physical activity levels.

PHYSICAL ASSESSMENT/CLINICAL MANIFESTATIONS

The nurse asks the client to describe his or her immediate concern. The nurse notes the presence of chest, epigastric, jaw, back, or arm discomfort and asks the client to rate the discomfort on a scale of 1 to 10, with 10 being the highest level of discomfort. Clients often describe the discomfort as tightness, a burning sensation, pressure, or indigestion. The nurse asks the client what he or she has already done to try to relieve the pain.

PAIN ASSESSMENT The nurse should rapidly yet completely assess the client with ongoing chest pain. Chest discomfort may occur from a variety of causes (see Table 32–1). It is important to differentiate between the types of chest pain and to identify the source. Both the physician and nurse may question the client to determine the characteristics of the discomfort. Appropriate questions for the nurse to ask concerning the discomfort include:

- Location
- Radiation
- Intensity
- Duration
- Precipitating and relieving factors

Chart 37–2 compares and contrasts anginal and infarction pain. Because anginal pain is ischemic pain, it usually improves when the disparity between oxygen supply and demand is resolved. For example, rest reduces tissue demands, and nitroglycerine improves oxygen supply. Discomfort from an MI does not usually resolve with such simple measures.

The nurse also notes the presence of any additional symptoms, including:

- Nausea
- Vomiting
- Diaphoresis
- Dizziness
- Weakness
- Palpitations
- Shortness of breath

CHART 37–2

Key Features of Angina and Myocardial Infarction

Angina	Myocardial Infarction
Substernal chest discomfort	Substernal chest pressure
• Radiating to the left arm	• Radiating to the left arm, back, or jaw
• Precipitated by exertion or stress	• Occurring without cause, primarily early in the morning
• Relieved by nitroglycerin or rest	• Relieved only by opioids
• Lasting <15 min	• Lasting 30 min or more
• Few associated symptoms	• Frequent associated symptoms: • Nausea • Diaphoresis • Dyspnea • Feelings of fear and anxiety • Dysrhythmias

The presence of these symptoms without chest discomfort is also significant. In 15% to 25% of clients with MI, chest pain or discomfort may be mild or absent. About 25% of older adults experiencing MI may present with a primary complaint of shortness of breath. Many elderly clients do not typically experience chest discomfort but develop disorientation or confusion as the primary clinical manifestation of MI.

CARDIOVASCULAR ASSESSMENT The nurse immediately obtains a blood pressure measurement, determines the heart rate, and interprets the cardiac monitor pattern to assess for dysrhythmias. Sinus tachycardia with premature ventricular contractions (PVCs) frequently occurs in the first few hours after MI. If an intravenous access is available, the nurse ensures that it is patent because the client will most likely receive intravenous fluids and medications. If an access is not available, the nurse initiates one or contacts the appropriate person to establish an intravenous route as quickly as possible. The nurse may administer oxygen according to protocols or the physician's order.

Next, the nurse assesses distal peripheral pulses and skin temperature. The skin should be warm, with all pulses palpable. In clients with unstable angina or myocardial infarction, poor cardiac output may be manifested by cool, diaphoretic skin and diminished or absent pulses.

The nurse auscultates for an S_3 gallop, which often indicates heart failure, a serious and common complication of MI. The nurse also assesses respiratory rate and breath sounds for signs of heart failure. An increased respiratory rate is common because of anxiety and pain, but the presence of crackles or wheezes may indicate heart failure. Auscultation of an S_4 heart sound is a common finding in clients who have had a previous MI or hypertension.

Clients with MI may experience a temperature elevation for several days after infarction. Temperatures as high as 102° F (38.9° C) may occur in response to myocardial necrosis.

PSYCHOSOCIAL ASSESSMENT

Denial is a common early reaction to chest discomfort associated with angina or myocardial infarction (MI). On average, the client with acute MI waits more than 2 hours before seeking medical attention. Clients often rationalize that their symptoms are due to indigestion or overexertion. In some situations, denial is a normal part of adapting to a stressful event. However, denial that interferes with identification of a symptom, such as chest discomfort, can be harmful to the client. The nurse explains the significance of reporting any discomfort, emphasizing that he or she will attempt to relieve the discomfort immediately.

Fear, anxiety, and anger are other common reactions of clients and families. Nursing assessment focuses on assisting clients and their families in identifying these feelings. The nurse allows the client and family time to explain their understanding of the event and clarifies any misconceptions.

LABORATORY ASSESSMENT

CARDIAC ENZYMES A myocardial infarction can be confirmed by abnormally high blood levels of cardiac enzymes and isoenzymes. Of all the cardiac enzymes, creatine kinase (CK) is considered the most sensitive and reliable indicator for diagnosis of MI. Total CK levels rise within 3 hours after the onset of chest pain and peak within 24 hours after damage and death of cardiac tissue. Because total CK also rises with brain or muscle injury, an elevation is not specific for myocardial damage.

When cardiac muscle tissue dies, the CK specific to myocardial cells—CK-MB isoenzyme—enters the bloodstream (serum does not normally contain CK-MB isoenzymes). Peak elevation occurs approximately 12 to 24 hours after the onset of chest pain, with levels returning to normal 48 to 72 hours later. Elevated CK-MB levels are the best laboratory confirmation of the diagnosis of a transmural MI. However, CK-MB rises with any event that causes myocardial damage, such as CPR, coronary artery bypass grafting, and thrombolytic therapy.

The physician may also use serum measurement of lactate dehydrogenase (LDH) to confirm MI. However, identification of LDH is not as reliable as that of CK-MB. LDH levels start to rise within 12 to 24 hours after MI, peak between 48 and 72 hours, and fall to normal in 7 days. Serum levels of LDH_1 isoenzyme rise higher than do serum levels of LDH_2 in the presence of MI. (See Chapter 32 for a more detailed discussion of cardiac enzymes.)

OTHER LABORATORY TESTS The finding of an elevated white blood cell count (10,000 to 20,000 cells/mm^3) helps in the diagnosis of MI. It typically appears on the second day and lasts up to a week.

No laboratory test can confirm the diagnosis of angina. Serum enzyme determinations are not useful in assessing the presence of angina. However, serum enzymes remaining within normal limits are an indication that the client has not had an acute MI.

RADIOGRAPHIC ASSESSMENT

Unless there is associated cardiac dysfunction (e.g., valvular disease) or heart failure, the chest x-ray is not diagnostic for angina or for MI.

OTHER DIAGNOSTIC ASSESSMENT

ELECTROCARDIOGRAPHY Twelve-lead electrocardiograms (ECGs) allow the health care provider to examine the heart from varying perspectives and note both the occurrence and location of ischemia (angina) or necrosis (infarction).

Ischemic myocardium does not repolarize normally. Thus, 12-lead ECGs obtained during an anginal episode reveal ST depression, T wave inversion, or both. *Variant angina,* due to coronary spasm, usually causes elevation of the ST segment during anginal attacks. These ST and T wave changes usually subside when the ischemia is resolved and the pain is relieved. If the client is not experiencing angina at the moment of the test, the ECG for the client with angina is normal.

When infarction occurs, three ECG changes are usually observed:

- ST segment elevation
- T wave inversion
- Abnormal Q wave (wider than 0.04 seconds or more than one-third the height of the QRS complex)

The Q wave develops because necrotic cells do not conduct electrical stimuli. Hours to days after the MI, the ST and T wave changes will return to normal, but the Q wave usually remains permanently.

By identifying in which of the 12 leads the ECG changes are occurring, the physician can identify the extent and location of the infarction.

OTHER DIAGNOSTIC TESTS The physician often orders an *exercise tolerance test* (stress test) after the acute stages of an anginal episode or MI to:

- Assess for ECG changes consistent with ischemia
- Evaluate medical therapy
- Identify clients who might benefit from referral for invasive therapy

Thallium scans use radioisotope imaging to assess for ischemia or necrotic muscle tissue related to angina or MI. Areas of decreased or absent perfusion, referred to as cold spots, identify ischemia or infarction. *Multigated acquisition* (MUGA) scans may be used to evaluate left ventricular function.

Cardiac catheterization may be performed to determine the extent and location of obstructions of the coronary arteries. Cardiac catheterization, the "gatekeeper" to invasive management, allows the cardiologist and cardiac surgeon to identify clients who might benefit from percutaneous transluminal angioplasty (PCTA) or coronary artery bypass grafting (CABG). (Chapter 32 describes each of these tests in detail.)

ANALYSIS

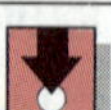

COMMON NURSING DIAGNOSES

The client with coronary artery disease (CAD) may have either angina or myocardial infarction (MI). If MI is suspected or cannot be completely ruled out, the client is admitted to a coronary or critical care unit for continuous monitoring.

On the basis of the assessment data, the nurse often identifies the following common diagnoses for the client with CAD:

1. Pain related to imbalance between myocardial oxygen supply and demand
2. Altered Tissue Perfusion (cardiopulmonary) related to interruption of blood flow
3. Activity intolerance related to imbalance between oxygen supply and demand
4. Ineffective Individual Coping related to effects of acute illness, major changes in lifestyle, and/or loss of control over a body part
5. Decreased Cardiac Output related to dysrhythmias
6. Decreased Cardiac Output related to left or right ventricular dysfunction

ADDITIONAL NURSING DIAGNOSES

In addition to the common nursing diagnoses, some clients may also experience one or more of the following diagnoses:

- Fear related to threat of death
- Altered Sexuality Patterns related to pain and effects of illness
- Impaired Physical Mobility related to pain and/or fear of movement

PLANNING AND IMPLEMENTATION

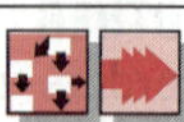

PAIN

PLANNING: CLIENT GOALS The major goal is that the client will state that chest pain is alleviated.

INTERVENTIONS The objective of management is to eliminate chest discomfort by:

- Providing pain relief
- Decreasing myocardial oxygen demand
- Increasing myocardial oxygen supply

Chart 37-3 summarizes appropriate interventions for the client with chest discomfort.

Drug Therapy After the nurse has evaluated the chest pain, obtained the client's vital signs, ensured the patency of an intravenous (IV) access, and notified the physician, if appropriate, the nurse may administer the prescribed pain medication. The initial medication prescribed is usually sublingual nitroglycerin (Chart 37-4).

NITROGLYCERIN Nitroglycerin, a nitrate often referred to as "nitro," increases collateral blood flow, redistributes blood flow toward the subendocardium, and causes dilation of the coronary arteries. The nurse instructs the client to hold the tablet under the tongue and provides 5 mL of water, if necessary, to allow the tablet to dissolve. Pain relief should begin within 1 or 2 minutes and be clearly evident in 3 to 5 minutes. After 5 minutes, the nurse rechecks the client's pain intensity and vital signs. If the client's blood pressure is less than 100 systolic or 25 mmHg lower than the previous reading, the nurse lowers the head of the client's bed and notifies the physician. If the client is experiencing some but not complete relief and vital signs remain stable, another nitroglycerin tablet may be used. A total of three tablets may be needed to relieve anginal pain.

Angina usually responds to nitroglycerin. The client typically states that the pain is relieved or

CHART 37-3

Nursing Care Highlight ◆ The Client with Chest Discomfort

- Obtain the client's description of the chest discomfort.
- Obtain the client's vital signs (blood pressure, pulse, respiration).
- Assess the client's vascular access.
- Consult standing orders or notify the physician for specific intervention.
- Obtain a 12-lead ECG, if indicated.
- Provide pain relief medication as ordered.
- Administer oxygen therapy as prescribed.
- Remain calm; stay with the client if possible.
- Assess the client's vital signs and intensity of pain 5 min after administration of medication.
- Remedicate (if vital signs remain stable), and check the client every 5 min.
- Notify the physician if vital signs deteriorate or pain is not relieved after three doses of nitroglycerin.

CHART 37-4

Drug Therapy for Coronary Artery Disease

Drug	Usual Dosage	Nursing Interventions	Rationale
Nitrates			
Nitroglycerin (Nitrostat, Tridil)	• 0.3–0.4 mg q5min sublingually, up to three tablets	• Instruct the client to lie down with the head of the bed at a level of comfort when taking the sublingual form.	• Hypotension can be dramatic, immediate, and intensified by the upright position.
		• Monitor blood pressure. Pay attention to orthostatic changes.	• A decrease in blood pressure occurs with vasodilation.
		• Instruct the client to allow the sublingual tablet to dissolve and to avoid swallowing the tablet.	• The sublingual dose is absorbed through the sublingual mucous membranes.
		• Check the expiration date on sublingual tablets. Tablets should be replaced every 3–5 mo.	• The efficacy of the tablets decreases with time.
		• Determine whether pain is relieved.	• Additional medication may be required to relieve pain.
		• Monitor for headache.	• Vasodilation is generalized.
Isosorbide dinitrate (Isordil, Iso-Bid)	• 2.5 mg q4–6h sublingually • 5–30 mg qid PO	• Instruct the client taking sublingual forms to lie down before administration.	• The hypotensive effect can be dramatic and immediate with sublingual administration.
	• 40-mg sustained-release tablet 2–3 times daily	• Monitor blood pressure and assess for dizziness.	• A decrease in blood pressure occurs with vasodilation.
		• Schedule sustained-release form with an 8–12 hr dose-free interval.	• Tolerance may develop.
Nitroglycerin patch (Nitro-bid Patch)	• Transdermally started at 5 mg/24 hr (10 cm^2 system)	• Remove the patch from the client before defibrillation.	• The client may develop a burn.
		• Rotate application sites.	• Rotation prevents skin irritation.
		• Apply the patch to a clean, dry, hairless area.	• The drug is better absorbed when the skin is clean, dry, and hairless.
Beta-Blockers			
Propranolol (Inderal)	• 10–80 mg bid–qid to 240 mg/day PO	• Assess heart rate before administration.	• Beta-blocking effects cause a decrease in heart rate.
	• 1–3 mg at rate not to exceed 1 mg/min IV	• Monitor blood pressure.	• The hypotensive effect is due to a decrease in cardiac output, suppressed renin activity, and beta-blocking effects.
		• Observe for signs of heart failure.	• Heart failure may occur as a result of a decrease in cardiac output.
		• Assess for shortness of breath and wheezing.	• $Beta_2$-blocking effects in the lungs can cause bronchoconstriction.
Metoprolol (Lopressor, Betaloc✱), a cardioselective beta-adrenergic blocker	• 100–450 mg/day PO • 5 mg IV over 2 min may be repeated twice for a total of 15 mg	• Assess heart rate prior to administration; do not administer if heart rate <50.	• Beta-blockers may cause further decreases in heart rate.
		• Monitor BP and hold for systolic <90.	• Decreased blood pressure is an anticipated effect.
		• Assess client for cough, shortness of breath, edema, and weight gain.	• These are indications of heart failure.

Chart continued on following page

CHART 37–4

Drug Therapy for Coronary Artery Disease *Continued*

Drug	Usual Dosage	Nursing Interventions	Rationale
Calcium Channel Blockers			
Nifedipine (Procardia, Adalat)	• 10–30 mg tid PO or sublingually	• Monitor blood pressure and assess for dizziness.	• Vasodilation can cause dramatic hypotension, which occurs within minutes, especially after sublingual administration.
		• Assess for headache and edema of the lower extremities.	• These are common side effects.
Verapamil hydrochloride (Calan, Isoptin)	• 40–80 mg qid PO or 240-mg sustained-release tablet once a day • 5–10 mg over 2 min IV	• Monitor heart rate.	• This agent slows SA and AV node conduction.
		• Monitor blood pressure and assess for dizziness.	• Vasodilation decreases blood pressure.
		• Assess for constipation.	• This is a common side effect.
Diltiazem hydrochloride (Cardizem)	• 30–60 mg qid PO or 180–240 mg sustained-release tablet once a day	• Monitor blood pressure and assess for dizziness.	• Vasodilation decreases blood pressure.
		• Monitor heart rate.	• This drug slows SA and AV node conduction, but the decrease is not as great as that which occurs with verapamil.
Antiplatelet Agents			
Aspirin (Empirin, Apo-asa✱)	• 80–325 mg PO	• Suggest that the client take the daily dose with food.	• Gastric irritation may occur.
		• Question the client about ringing in the ears.	• Tinnitus may occur with aspirin toxicity.
		• Emphasize to the client that aspirin is an important cardiac medication and should be continued unless the client is told to stop.	• Studies document significantly better survival rates for clients with coronary artery disease receiving aspirin.

markedly diminished. When simple measures, such as three repeated sublingual nitroglycerin tablets, do not relieve chest discomfort, the client may be experiencing MI. The nurse should inform the physician immediately and prepare the client for transfer to a specialized unit where the client can be closely monitored and appropriately managed.

In a specialized unit, the physician may prescribe IV nitroglycerin for management of the chest pain. The nurse begins the nitroglycerin infusion slowly, checking the client's blood pressure and pain level every 3 to 5 minutes. The nitroglycerin dose is increased until the pain is relieved, the blood pressure falls excessively, or the maximal prescribed dose is reached. The nurse continues to monitor the blood pressure frequently (Chart 37–5).

MORPHINE SULFATE The physician may prescribe morphine sulfate (MS) to relieve chest discomfort that is unresponsive to nitroglycerin. Morphine relieves pain, decreases myocardial oxygen demand, and reduces circulating catecholamines. It is administered in 2- to 5-mg increments intravenously every 5 to 15 minutes until the maximal prescribed dose is reached or until the client experiences relief or signs of toxicity.

Signs of morphine toxicity include:

- Respiratory depression
- Hypotension
- Severe vomiting

The nurse monitors the client's vital signs and cardiac rhythm every few minutes. These strategies are often enough to relieve the client's pain. If these methods are not adequate, additional interventions, identified later under Altered Tissue Perfusion (Cardiopulmonary), may be attempted.

Other Interventions Several interventions may assist in

CHART 37–5

Drug Therapy with Intravenous Vasodilators and Inotropes

Drug	Usual Dosage	Nursing Interventions	Rationale
Sodium nitroprusside (Nipride)	• IV only by infusion device • Begin with 0.2 μg/kg/min • May increase gradually to 3 μg/kg/min	• Monitor BP q2–5 min when initiating therapy. If BP drops excessively, elevate the legs, decrease the dose, and increase fluids per unit policies.	• This agent is a potent, rapidly reversible vasodilator acting on both peripheral venous and arterial musculature. BP may drop in 2 min.
		• Monitor PAWP, SVR, BP, heart rate, and urine output frequently.	
		• Titrate medication to obtain the desired effect.	
		• Protect from light.	• This agent is light-sensitive.
		• Maintain dose at less than 3 μg/kg/min if possible.	• Doses >3 μg/kg/min are associated with thiocyanate or cyanide toxicity.
		• In clients requiring doses >3 μg/kg/min for >24–36 hr, monitor for metabolic acidosis, confusion, or hyperreflexia. Examine blood thiocyanate level.	• These are indications of the toxic effects of cyanide.
Nitroglycerin (Tridil)	• IV only by infusion device started at 0.3 μg/kg/min and gradually increased to 3 μg/kg/min	• Monitor BP q1–3 min when initiating therapy. If BP drops excessively, elevate the legs and decrease the dose according to unit policies.	• This agent dilates coronary arteries. It is a more potent systemic venous vasodilator than an arterial vasodilator. BP may drop in 1 min.
		• Monitor RAP, PAWP, SVR, BP, heart rate, and urine output frequently.	
		• Titrate medication to obtain the desired effect.	
		• Intermittent administration of IV nitroglycerin should be considered.	• Tolerance may develop rapidly to nitroglycerin administered by continuous IV.
		• Monitor the client for headache.	• Headache is a frequent side effect of initial nitroglycerin therapy.
Sympathomimetics			
Dopamine (Intropin)	• IV only by infusion device • Starting dose 2–5 μg/kg/min • Titrate up to 20 μg/kg/min	• Determine the reason for use and the expected result.	• This agent is a dose-dependent activator of alpha, beta, and dopaminergic receptors.
		• Observe the client's heart rate, ECG, BP, PAWP, SVR, CO, and urine output q5min to q1h.	• 2–5 μg/kg/min stimulates dopaminergic receptors, which promotes renal and mesenteric blood flow.

Chart continued on following page

CHART 37–5

Drug Therapy with Intravenous Vasodilators and Inotropes *Continued*

Drug	Usual Dosage	Nursing Interventions	Rationale
		• Titrate the dose carefully to maintain the dose range and obtain the desired effect.	• 5 μg/kg/min stimulates beta-receptors. This increases heart rate and contractility. • >10–15 μg/kg/min, alpha effects predominate. This causes peripheral constriction.
		• Infuse through a central line.	• Extravasation can cause tissue necrosis and sloughing.
		• Monitor the client for ectopy and angina.	• These are adverse effects.
Dobutamine (Dobutrex)	• IV only by infusion device, 2–5 μg/kg/min	• Observe the client continuously during administration. • Titrate the drug on the basis of heart rate, ECG findings, BP, PAWP, CO, SVR, and urine output.	• This agent is a very strong $beta_1$-receptor activator and a moderately strong $beta_2$-activator.
		• Monitor for atrial and ventricular ectopy.	• Dysrhythmias are an adverse effect.

relieving chest pain. Supplemental oxygen may increase the amount of oxygen available to myocardial tissue. Therefore, oxygen is often prescribed and administered at 2 to 4 L by nasal cannula. If the client's blood pressure is stable, the nurse may assist the client in assuming any position of comfort. Placing the client in semi-Fowler's position often enhances the client's comfort and tissue oxygenation. A quiet, calm environment and explanations of interventions often reduces the client's anxiety and assist in relief of chest pain.

When the pain has subsided and the client is stabilized, the physician may change the client's medication to an oral or topical nitrate. Before administration of long-term oral and topical nitrates, a 12-hour nitrate-free period may be instituted to prevent tolerance. Clients may complain initially of headache. The physician may prescribe acetaminophen (Tylenol, Exdol✱) before the nitrate to prevent some of this discomfort.

ALTERED TISSUE PERFUSION (CARDIOPULMONARY)

PLANNING: CLIENT GOALS The major goal is that the client will demonstrate improved myocardial perfusion as evidenced by a reduction in chest discomfort and a resolution of ST and T wave changes.

INTERVENTIONS Because myocardial infarction (MI) is a dynamic process, restoration of perfusion to the injured area often reduces infarct size, improves left ventricular function, and decreases morbidity and mortality.

Thrombolytic Therapy Thrombolytic agents are used to dissolve thrombi in the coronary arteries and restore myocardial blood flow. Examples include streptokinase (Kabikinase), tissue plasminogen activator (t-PA, Activase), and anisoylated plasminogen-streptokinase activator complex (APSAC). The physician can administer thrombolytics intravenously or by the intracoronary route during cardiac catheterization. Thrombolytic agents are most effective when administered within the first 6 hours of the coronary event.

Thrombolytic therapy should be given in a unit where the client can be continuously monitored. It is indicated for clients who have chest pain of greater than 30 minutes' duration unrelieved by nitroglycerin with indications of transmural ischemia and injury as shown by the electrocardiogram. Contraindications include recent abdominal surgery or cerebrovascular accident (CVA). Bleeding may occur more readily if these conditions are present. Table 37–2 lists the current contraindications to thrombolytic therapy.

ASSESSMENT OF BLEEDING All thrombolytics lyse existing clots, and bleeding may develop anywhere in the body. Therefore, the nurse must monitor the client for signs of obvious or occult bleeding by:

- Documenting hemoglobin and hematocrit values
- Checking blood pressure and pulse
- Assessing for abdominal and back pain
- Noting changes in the color of urine and stool
- Assessing neurologic signs

The nurse may need to apply pressure dressings to puncture sites or wounds to limit bleeding. Bleeding

TABLE 37–2 Contraindications to Thrombolytic Therapy

Absolute
• Active internal bleeding
• Cerebrovascular processes
• Recent cerebrovascular accident
• Recent spinal surgery
• Cerebral surgery
• Prolonged cardiopulmonary resuscitation (CPR)
Relative
• Chronic renal failure
• Liver dysfunction
• Severe uncontrolled hypertension
• Pregnancy or recent delivery
• Trauma within last 10 days
• Surgery within last 10 days

occurs more frequently in women who receive this therapy than in men. The nurse immediately reports any indications of bleeding to the physician.

Some concerns in administration are associated with the thrombolytics. *Streptokinase* is a first-generation thrombolytic agent. It is not fibrin-specific; thus, it may create systemic bleeding problems. Streptokinase may also induce an antigenic response, because it is a bacteria protein. It can cause a hypersensitivity reaction in clients who have had previous exposure. Therefore, the nurse questions the client about previous streptococcal infections or doses of streptokinase. To prevent an allergic reaction, the physician may prescribe steroids or antihistamines before the administration of streptokinase. During administration, the nurse observes the client closely for evidence of an allergic or anaphylactic response (see Chap. 24). The half-life of the drug is 16 minutes.

Second-generation thrombolytics include tissue plasminogen activator (t-PA, Activase) and anisoylated plasminogen-streptokinase activator complex (APSAC, Eminase). *t-PA* is fibrin-specific, has a short half-life (3 to 5 minutes), and lacks antigenicity. Because some studies have associated t-PA with a more frequent occurrence of cerebrovascular bleeding, the nurse carefully documents neurologic findings. t-PA is much more expensive than streptokinase.

APSAC is a streptokinase derivative; it has a longer half-life (90 to 105 minutes) than that of streptokinase but the same antigenic properties.

NURSING CARE FOR CLIENTS RECEIVING THROMBOLYTICS

The nurse monitors the client for indications that the clot has been lysed and the artery has been reperfused. These indications include:

- Abrupt cessation of chest pain
- Sudden onset of ventricular dysrhythmias
- Resolution of ST segment depression
- A peak at 12 hours of CK-MB

To maintain the patency of the coronary artery after thrombolytic therapy, the physician usually prescribes IV nitroglycerin and heparin. The nurse monitors the partial thromboplastin time (PTT; the usual appropriate range is 1½ to 2 times control) and maintains the heparin infusion for 1 to 3 days, as prescribed. Later, most clients receive aspirin (Ancasal✱) daily (80 to 325 mg) to prevent platelet aggregation at the site of the obstruction.

Other Drug Therapy Beta-adrenergic blocking agents (e.g., propranolol [Inderal, Apo-Propranolol✱]) decrease infarction size, ventricular dysrhythmias, and mortality rates in clients with myocardial infarction (MI). The physician usually prescribes a beta-blocking agent within the first 24 hours after MI. Beta-blockers seem to work by slowing the heart rate. Thus, these agents prolong the period of diastole and increase myocardial perfusion while reducing the force of myocardial contraction. With beta-blockade, the heart is capable of performing 25% to 30% more work without ischemia.

During beta-blocker therapy, the nurse:

- Monitors the heart rate (heart rates are often slowed to 60)
- Checks the BP
- Measures the PR interval
- Checks the client's level of consciousness
- Monitors for any chest discomfort

The nurse assesses the client's lungs for crackles (indicative of heart failure) and wheezes (indicative of bronchospasm). Hypoglycemia, depression, and forgetfulness are also problems with beta-blockade, especially in older clients (see Chart 37–4).

The physician may prescribe calcium channel blockers to enhance myocardial perfusion in clients with angina. Calcium channel blockers are indicated primarily for clients with angina because they have been associated with higher mortality rates in MI clients. The primary effect of calcium channel blockers is coronary artery vasodilation and vasospasm. The nurse monitors the client receiving calcium channel blockers for hypotension and headache.

ACTIVITY INTOLERANCE

PLANNING: CLIENT GOALS The long-term goal is that the client will resume activities of daily living (ADL) and return to usual role functioning without experiencing chest discomfort, dyspnea, or fatigue.

INTERVENTIONS Activity intolerance is reduced by a planned program of cardiac rehabilitation implemented primarily by the nurse and physical therapist. Cardiac rehabilitation is a process of actively assisting the client with cardiac disease to achieve and maintain a vital and productive life while remaining within the heart's ability to respond to increases in activity and stress. Cardiac rehabilitation can be divided into three phases:

- Phase 1 begins with the acute illness and ends up with discharge from the hospital.
- Phase 2 begins after discharge and continues through convalescence at home.
- Phase 3 refers to long-term conditioning.

In the acute phase (phase 1), the nurse promotes rest yet ensures some limited mobility. The nurse assists with some activities of daily living, such as bathing and toileting. Clients progress at their own rate to increasing activity levels, depending on their clinical status, age, and physical capabilities. For example, for the first 24 to 36 hours, the client may be maintained on bed rest but allowed to stand to void or to use the bedside commode. The second day, the client may dangle at the side of the bed or be out of bed sitting in a chair as tolerated, usually for 30 minutes three times a day. When the client is restricted to bed or chair, range-of-motion exercises can help prevent thrombus formation and maintain muscle strength and tone.

The next step in phase 1 is ambulation of the client in the room and to the bathroom. Finally, the nurse encourages progressive ambulation in the hallway—usually 50, 100, then 200 feet three times a day. In addition, the client may begin showering for 5 or 10 minutes with warm water; a stool should be available for the client to sit on if necessary.

The nurse assesses the client's heart rate, blood pressure, respiratory rate, and level of fatigue with each level of activity. Decreases in systolic blood pressure greater than 20 mmHg, changes in pulse rate of 20 beats/minute, and complaints of dyspnea or chest pain indicate intolerance of activity. When such signs and symptoms develop, the nurse notifies the physician and does not advance the client to the next level. Older adults with coronary artery disease often have needs and concerns different from those of younger adults (Chart 37–6).

CHART 37–6

Nursing Focus on the Elderly ◆ Coronary Artery Disease

- Recognize that chest pain may not be evident in the older client; associated symptoms, such as dyspnea and confusion, may prevail.
- Although older adults have a greater reduction in mortality from myocardial infarction (MI) with the use of thrombolytics, they also have the most severe side effects. Monitor older clients receiving thrombolytics extremely carefully.
- Dysrhythmia may be a normal age-related change rather than a complication of MI. Determine whether the dysrhythmia is causing significant symptoms, then notify the physician.
- Monitor antidysrhythmic doses carefully; overdoses of lidocaine can occur in older adults at normal dose ranges.
- If beta-blockers are used, assess the client carefully for the development of side effects. Exacerbation of the depression already present in older adults is a significant problem with beta-blockade.
- Plan slow, steady increases in activity. Older adults with minimal previous exercise show particular benefit from a gradual increase in activity.
- Older adults should plan longer warm-up and cool-down periods when participating in an exercise program. Their pulse rates may not return to baseline until 30 minutes or longer after exercise.

INEFFECTIVE INDIVIDUAL COPING

PLANNING: CLIENT GOALS The major goal is that the client will:

- Indicate a reduction in anxiety
- Verbalize his or her feelings
- State that he or she is beginning to experience some control over his or her life

INTERVENTIONS The nurse assesses the client's level of anxiety while allowing the client to express any anxiety and attempt to define its origin. Simple, repeated explanations of therapies, expectations, and surroundings may help the client. During the acute phase of illness, the physician may prescribe anxiolytic (antianxiety) medications, such as alprazolam (Xanax). The nurse identifies the client's current coping mechanisms; the most common are:

- Denial
- Anger
- Depression

Denial is a defense mechanism that allows the client to minimize a threat and use problem-focused coping mechanisms. The client may avoid discussing what has happened yet comply with treatment regimens. This type of denial decreases the client's anxiety, and the nurse should not discourage it. However, denial that results in a client's "acting out" and refusing to follow treatment regimens can be harmful. Because this behavior is usually due to extreme anxiety or fear, threats only worsen the behavior. The nurse remains calm and avoids confronting the client but clearly indicates when a behavior is not acceptable and is potentially harmful.

Anger may represent an attempt by the client to regain control of his or her life. The nurse encourages the client to verbalize the source of frustration and provides the client with opportunities for decision-making and control.

Depression may be a client's response to grief and loss of function. The nurse listens as the client verbalizes feelings of loss, being careful not to offer false or general reassurances. The nurse acknowledges that the client is depressed but expects the client to perform activities of daily living and other activities within restrictions. The nurse identifies all improvements in the client's condition and shares them with the client. (Chapter 7 describes interventions and positive coping strategies.)

DECREASED CARDIAC OUTPUT RELATED TO DYSRHYTHMIAS

PLANNING: CLIENT GOALS The major goals are that the client will:

- Resume a normal sinus or baseline rhythm
- Be hemodynamically stable

INTERVENTIONS Dysrhythmias are the cause of death in most clients with myocardial infarction (MI) who die before they can be hospitalized. Even in the early hospitalization period, 70% to 90% of MI clients experience some abnormality of cardiac rhythm. Whenever a dysrhythmia develops in a client with coronary artery disease (CAD), the nurse:

- Identifies the dysrhythmia
- Assesses the client's hemodynamic status
- Evaluates the client for chest discomfort

Dysrhythmias are treated (Pasternak et al., 1992) when:

- They are causing hemodynamic compromise
- They are increasing myocardial oxygen requirements
- They predispose to lethal ventricular dysrhythmias

Inferior MI Typical dysrhythmias for a client with an inferior MI are bradycardias and second-degree AV blocks resulting from ischemia of the AV node. These rhythms tend to be transient. The nurse monitors the client's cardiac rhythm and rate and hemodynamic status. If the client becomes hemodynamically unstable, a temporary pacemaker may be necessary.

Anterior MI Clients with *anterior* MIs are likely to exhibit ventricular irritability (premature ventricular contractions, PVCs). Third-degree or bundle branch block in the client with an anterior MI indicates that a large portion of the left ventricle is involved. The physician may insert a pacemaker. The nurse should observe the client closely to detect the development of heart failure. (Appropriate interventions for dysrhythmias are described in Chapter 33.)

DECREASED CARDIAC OUTPUT RELATED TO LEFT OR RIGHT VENTRICULAR DYSFUNCTION

PLANNING: CLIENT GOALS The goal is that the client will resume hemodynamic stability as evidenced by:

- Blood pressure within the client's acceptable range
- Adequate urine output
- Mental alertness
- Absence of pulmonary edema
- Palpable peripheral pulses

INTERVENTIONS Decreased cardiac output related to heart failure is a relatively common complication after MI. The most severe form of heart failure, *cardiogenic shock,* accounts for most in-hospital deaths after MI.

Nonsurgical Management The type of nonsurgical management used to increase cardiac output depends on the location of the MI and the type of heart failure that resulted from the infarction.

Managing Left Ventricular Failure When a client with MI experiences damage to the left ventricle, rupture of the intraventricular septum, or tear of a papillary muscle, a reduction occurs in the amount of blood that the heart can eject. This reduction in ejection fraction results in a decreased cardiac output and greater left ventricular residual volumes. Volume and pressure increase first in the left ventricle but eventually in the pulmonary vasculature. When volume and pressure are markedly increased in the pulmonary vasculature, pulmonary complications develop.

NURSING ASSESSMENT AND MONITORING The nurse assesses for the development of left ventricular failure and pulmonary edema by auscultating for crackles and identifying their location in the lung fields. Wheezing, tachypnea, and frothy sputum may also occur with pulmonary edema. The nurse auscultates the heart, paying particular attention to the presence of an S_3 heart sound. The nurse monitors for the following signs of poor organ perfusion that may result from decreased cardiac output:

- A change in the client's orientation or mental status
- Urine output less than 30 mL/hr
- Cool, clammy extremities with decreased or absent pulses
- Unusual fatigue
- Recurrent chest pain

In specialized units, hemodynamic monitoring may be instituted to assess the client's preload, afterload, and cardiac output. Hemodynamic monitoring requires the insertion of a pulmonary artery catheter (see Chap. 32). The nurse obtains and records hemodynamic measurements, which include:

- Right atrial (RA) pressure
- Pulmonary artery (PA) systolic and diastolic pressures
- Pulmonary artery wedge pressure (PAWP; a measure of preload)
- Systemic vascular resistance (SVR; a measure of afterload)
- Cardiac output (CO)
- Cardiac index (CI)

Single values of these measurements are less significant than is the trend of values combined with the client's clinical manifestations. These measurements help both the nurse and the physician to identify heart failure and guide the administration of fluids and vasoactive drugs.

CLASSIFICATION OF HEART FAILURE AFTER MYOCARDIAL INFARCTION Killip categorized heart failure after myocardial infarction (MI) into four classes, according to prognosis (Table 37–3). Clients with class I heart failure often respond well to reduction in preload with IV diuretics. The nurse:

- Monitors the urine output hourly
- Checks the client's vital signs frequently
- Continues to assess for signs of heart failure
- Reviews laboratory data to identify the serum potassium level

Clients with class II and class III failure may require diuresis and more aggressive medical intervention, such as reduction of afterload or enhancement of contractility. Intravenous nitroprusside or nitroglycerin may be used to decrease both preload and afterload. These drugs are administered as continuous infusions in specialized units where the pulmonary artery wedge pressure and blood pressure can be closely monitored. The client's blood pressure can drop in response to excessive vasodilation (see Chart 37–5).

Positive inotropes, such as dopamine (Intropin), dobutamine (Dobutrex), and amrinone (Inocor), increase the force of cardiac contraction. They are administered by continuous IV infusion. The effects of these drugs on the vasculature and heart rate vary and may be dose-dependent. The nurse must understand the anticipated effect of the drug and the desired dose range. The nurse titrates the infusions to optimize cardiac output. The nurse must use caution when administering these drugs because of the potential risk of increasing myocardial oxygen consumption and further decreasing cardiac output. The nurse continues to assess the client, paying particular attention to the development of chest pain.

CARDIOGENIC SHOCK Killip class IV is cardiogenic shock. In cardiogenic shock, necrosis of more than 40% of the left ventricle has occurred, usually as a result of occlusions of all three major coronary vessels. Most clients have a stuttering pattern of chest pain resulting in piecemeal extension of the MI. Manifestations of cardiogenic shock include:

- Tachycardia
- Hypotension
- Blood pressure less than 90 or 30 mmHg less than the client's baseline
- Urine output less than 30 mL/hr
- Cold, clammy skin with poor peripheral pulses
- Agitation, restlessness, or confusion
- Pulmonary congestion
- Tachypnea
- Continuing chest discomfort

Early detection is essential because established cardiogenic shock has a mortality rate of 65% to 100%.

Medical Management. Medical interventions aim to relieve pain and decrease myocardial oxygen requirements through preload and possibly afterload reduction (see Chart 37–5). The physician orders intravenous morphine, which is used to decrease pulmonary congestion and relieve pain. Oxygen is administered; intubation and ventilation may be necessary. The nurse uses the information gained from hemodynamic monitoring to titrate drug therapy. Preload reduction may be cautiously attempted with diuretics, nitroglycerin, or nitroprusside, as described with Killip class III clients. Because vasodilation may result in a further decline in blood pressure, the nurse monitors systolic pressure constantly. Vasopressors and positive inotropes may be used to maintain organ perfusion, but such drugs increase myocardial oxygen consumption and can worsen ischemia.

Use of an Intra-aortic Balloon Pump. When clients do not respond to drug therapy with improved tissue perfusion, decreased workload of the heart, and increased cardiac contractility, an intra-aortic balloon pump (IABP) may be inserted. Insertion of an intra-aortic counterpulsation device, such as the IABP, is an invasive intervention that is used to:

- Improve myocardial perfusion during an acute MI
- Reduce afterload
- Facilitate left ventricular emptying

The physician can insert an IABP percutaneously or through surgical cutdown. Inflation of the IABP during diastole increases the client's diastolic pressure and improves coronary perfusion. Deflation of the balloon just before systole reduces afterload at the time of systolic contraction. This facilitates emptying of the left ventricle and improves cardiac output. The balloon catheter is attached to a pump console, which is triggered by an ECG tracing and arterial waveform (Fig. 37–4).

Immediate Reperfusion. Immediate reperfusion is an invasive intervention that is showing some promise for clients with cardiogenic shock (Pasternak et al., 1992). The client is taken to the cardiac catheterization laboratory and an emergency left-sided heart

TABLE 37–3 The Killip Classification of Heart Failure

Class	Findings
• Class I	Absent crackles and S_3
• Class II	Crackles in the lower half of the lung fields and possible S_3
• Class III	Crackles more than halfway up the lung fields and frequent pulmonary edema
• Class IV	Cardiogenic shock

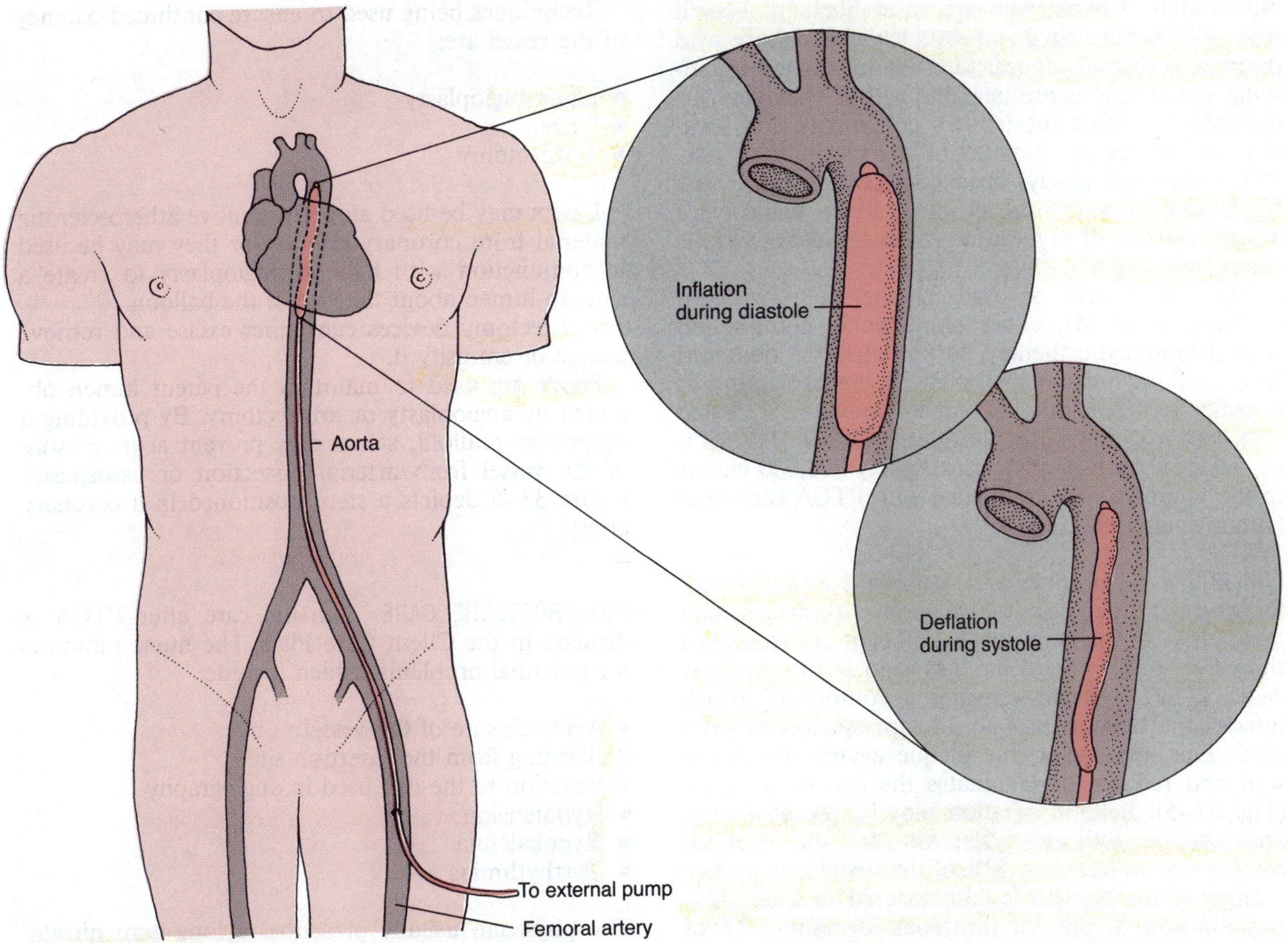

FIGURE 37–4 ◆ Intra-aortic balloon pumping. An intra-aortic balloon catheter is inserted into the femoral artery and advanced into the descending aorta. The polyethylene balloon lies just distal to the left subclavian artery. Immediately after it is inserted, the catheter is connected to the external pump.

catheterization is performed. If the client has a treatable lesion or lesions, the surgeon performs an immediate percutaneous transluminal coronary angioplasty (PTCA) in the catheterization laboratory or the client is transferred to the operating suite for coronary artery bypass graft (CABG). (Surgical management is discussed later.)

Managing Right Ventricular Failure Conditions other than left ventricular failure may result in decreased cardiac output after MI. In approximately 30% of clients with inferior MIs, right ventricular infarction and failure develop. In this instance, the right ventricle fails independently of the left. Decreased cardiac output with a paradoxical pulse, clear lungs, and jugular venous distention result when the client is in semi-Fowler's position.

A right ventricular MI may be documented by an ECG using right-sided precordial leads and by echocardiography. The goal of medical management is to improve right ventricular stroke volume by increasing right ventricular fiber stretch or preload. To enhance right ventricular preload, the nurse administers sufficient fluids (as much as 200 mL/hr) to increase right atrial (RA) pressure to 20 mmHg, as ordered. The nurse monitors the pulmonary artery wedge pressure (PAWP) (attempting to maintain it below 15 to 20) and auscultates the lungs to ensure that left-sided failure is not developing. The nurse monitors the client's cardiac output to ensure that fluid administration is having the desired effect.

Surgical Management Clients who continue to have chest discomfort despite medical therapy may require invasive correction by percutaneous transluminal angioplasty or coronary artery bypass graft to resolve angina or prevent MI. Before invasive treatment, a left-sided cardiac catheterization with coronary angiogram (see Chap. 32) is performed to document that the client's lesions are correctable and that left ventricular pump function is adequate.

Percutaneous Transluminal Coronary Angioplasty Percutaneous transluminal coronary angioplasty (PTCA) is an invasive but technically a nonsurgical technique. It is performed to reduce the frequency and severity of chest discomfort for clients with angina. The risk of complications is not significant.

INDICATIONS Clients who are most likely to benefit from PTCA have single- or double-vessel disease with discrete, proximal, noncalcified lesions. When identifying which lesions are treatable with PTCA, the cardiologist considers the lesion's complexity and location as well as the amount of myocardium at risk. PTCA does not always open complex lesions. Treating lesions located in the left main artery would place a large amount of myocardial tissue at risk should the vessel close acutely.

PTCA may also be used for the client with an evolving acute MI, either alone or in conjunction with thrombolytic therapy, to reperfuse the damaged myocardium. Indications for PTCA are expanding. It is estimated that 50% of clients previously treated with coronary artery bypass graft (CABG) will soon be treated with PTCA. Approximately 300,000 clients in the United States are treated with PTCA each year (Braunwald, 1992).

PROCEDURE The physician performs PTCA under fluoroscopic guidance in the cardiac catheterization laboratory. A balloon-tipped catheter is introduced through a guide wire to the occlusion in the coronary vessel. The physician activates a compressor which inflates the balloon at 4 to 14 atmospheres of pressure. This compresses the plaque against the vessel wall and reduces or eliminates the occluding lesion (Fig. 37–5). Balloon inflation may be repeated until angiography indicates decrease of the stenosis (narrowing) to less than 50% of the vessel's diameter.

Intravenous heparin is administered in a continuous infusion to prevent thrombus formation; IV or intracoronary nitroglycerin or sublingual nifedipine is given to prevent coronary spasm. PTCA initially reopens the vessel in more than 90% of appropriately selected clients. However, restenosis occurs in 20% to 40% of these clients (Halfman-Franey & Coburn, 1990).

Techniques being used to ensure continued patency of the vessel are:

- Laser angioplasty
- Stents
- Arthrectomy

Lasers may be used alone to remove atherosclerotic material from coronary arteries, or they may be used in conjunction with balloon angioplasty to create a smooth lumen about the size of the balloon.

Arthrectomy devices can either excise and retrieve plaque or emulsify it.

Stents are used to maintain the patent lumen obtained by angioplasty or arthrectomy. By providing a supportive scaffold, stents may prevent acute closure of the vessel from arterial dissection or vasospasm. Figure 37–6 depicts a stent positioned in a coronary artery.

POSTPROCEDURE CARE Nursing care after PTCA is detailed in the Client Care Plan. The nurse monitors for potential problems, which include:

- Acute closure of the vessel
- Bleeding from the insertion site
- Reaction to the dye used in angiography
- Hypotension
- Hypokalemia
- Dysrhythmias

The physician usually prescribes a long-term nitrate, calcium channel blocker, and aspirin therapy for clients after PTCA. The nursing interventions for clients receiving these medications are described in Chart 37–4. The nurse provides the client with careful explanations of drug therapy and any recommended lifestyle changes.

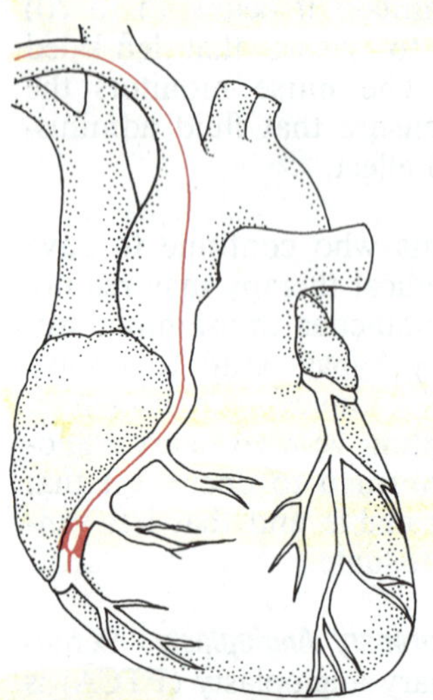

1. The balloon-tipped catheter is positioned in the artery.

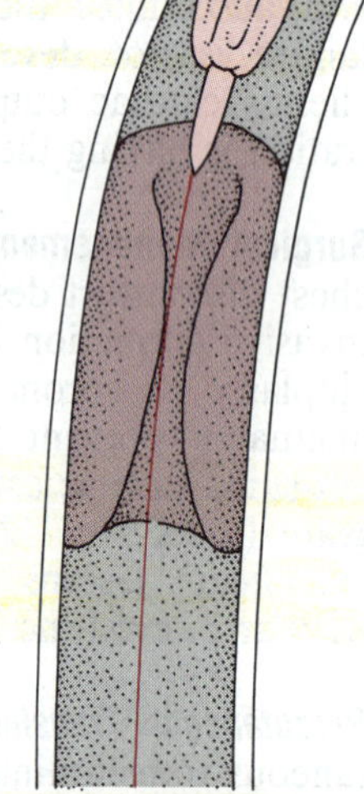

2. The uninflated balloon is centered in the obstruction.

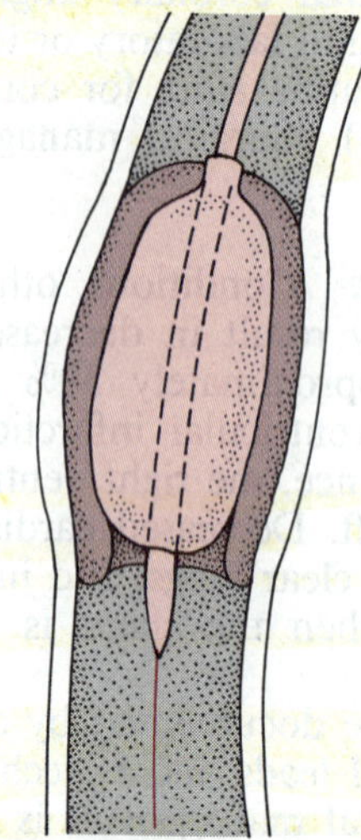

3. The balloon is inflated, which flattens plaque against the artery wall.

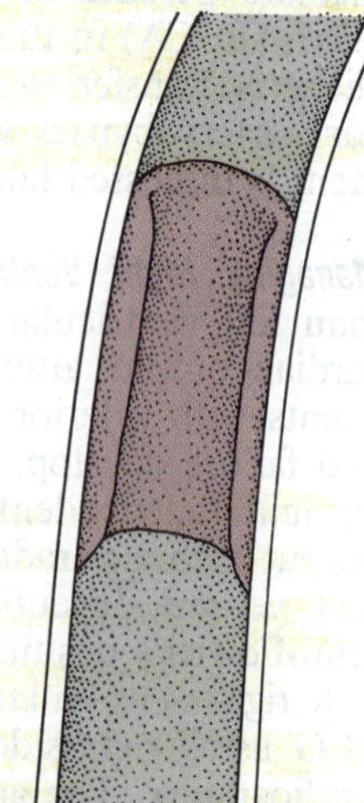

4. The balloon is removed, and the artery is left unoccluded.

FIGURE 37–5 ◆ Percutaneous transluminal angioplasty.

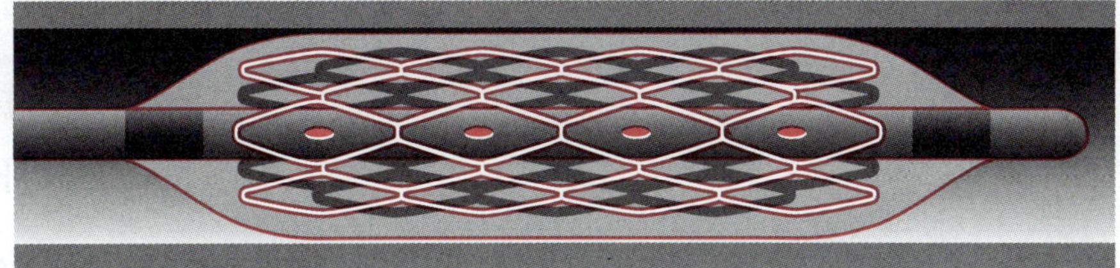

FIGURE 37-6 ◆ A coronary stent open after balloon inflation.

Coronary Artery Bypass Graft Surgery Coronary artery bypass graft (CABG), performed in approximately 400,000 people in the United States each year, is the most common type of cardiac surgery. It is a common procedure for older adults; more than 50% of all CABGs are performed on clients older than 65 years. The occluded coronary arteries are bypassed with the client's own venous or arterial blood vessels or synthetic grafts. CABG is indicated when clients do not respond to medical management of coronary artery disease (CAD) or when disease progression is evident. The decision for surgery is based on the client's symptoms and the results of cardiac catheterization.

Candidates for surgery (Swearingen & Keen, 1992) are clients who have:

- Angina with greater than 60% occlusion of the left main coronary artery
- Unstable angina with severe two-vessel or moderate three-vessel disease
- Ischemia with heart failure
- Acute myocardial infarction (MI)
- Signs of ischemia or impending MI after angiography or percutaneous transluminal coronary angioplasty (PTCA)

The vessels to be bypassed should have proximal lesions occluding more than 70% of the vessel's diameter but good distal run-off. Bypass of less occluded vessels may result in poor perfusion through the graft and early obstruction. CABG is most effective when good ventricular function remains and the ejection fraction is more than 40% to 50%. Clients with lower ejection fractions are poorer risks.

For most clients, the risk is low and the benefits of bypass surgery are clear. Surgical treatment of CAD does not appear to affect the client's life span. Early mortality rates are 1% to 2%. Left ventricular function is the most important long-term indicator of survival after CABG. CABG does improve quality of life for most clients. Eighty percent to 90% of clients are pain-free 1 year after CABG, and 70% remain pain-free at 5 years. The percentage of clients experiencing some pain increases sharply after 5 years (Whitman & Guzzetta, 1992).

PREOPERATIVE CARE CABG surgery may be planned as an elective procedure or as an emergency procedure. Clients for elective surgery are often admitted the morning of surgery. Preoperative preparations and teaching are completed during pre-hospitalization interviews. Clients must understand that some medication will need to be adjusted because of the surgery. The nurse ensures that appropriate medications have been discontinued preoperatively and that the necessary ones have been administered (Table 37-4).

Pre-hospitalization Preparation. The nurse familiarizes the client and family with the cardiac surgical critical care environment and prepares the client for postoperative care. The nurse demonstrates and has the client return a demonstration of how to splint the chest incision, cough, deep breathe, and perform arm and leg exercises (see Chap. 19). The nurse stresses the following:

- The client should identify any pain that he or she is experiencing to the nursing staff
- Most of the pain will be in the sternal incision
- Pain medication will be available

The nurse explains that the client should expect to have a sternal incision, possibly a leg incision, one or two chest tubes, a Foley catheter, and several IV fluid catheters postoperatively. An endotracheal tube will be connected to a ventilator for 6 to 24 hours postoperatively. The client and family must understand that the client will not be able to talk while the endotracheal tube is in place. The client should breathe with the ventilator and not fight it (see Chap. 31). When describing the postoperative course, the nurse emphasizes that close monitoring and the use of sophisticated equipment are standard treatment.

Psychosocial Preparation. Preoperative anxiety is common. Clients often wait 1 to 6 weeks for CABG surgery to be scheduled and performed. As the length

TABLE 37-4 Medication Administration Before Coronary Artery Bypass Graft Surgery

Medications Often Discontinued

- Digitalis 12 hr before surgery
- Diuretics 2-3 days before surgery
- Aspirin and anticoagulants 1 wk before surgery

Medications Often Administered

- Potassium chloride to maintain K between 3.5 and 4.0
- Scheduled beta-blockers
- Scheduled calcium channel blockers
- Scheduled antidysrhythmics
- Scheduled antihypertensives
- Prophylactic antibiotic 20-30 min before surgery

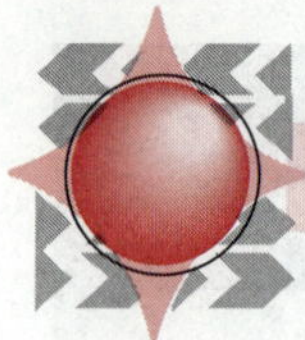

CLIENT CARE PLAN

The Client Recovering from Angioplasty

Nursing Diagnosis No. 1: High Risk for Altered Cardiopulmonary Tissue Perfusion related to vessel reocclusion

Expected Outcomes	Nursing Interventions	Rationale
The client will have no evidence of cardiac injury or ischemia. ◆ No complaints of chest discomfort. ◆ BP >100 mmHg. ◆ CK-MB within normal limits. ◆ ECG within the client's normal parameters. ◆ Heart rate <120. ◆ No ST and T wave changes. ◆ Rhythm normal for the client.	◆ Monitor VS q15min × 4, q30min × 4, then q1–4h. Observe the client closely for development of hypotension. For systolic BP <100 or 20 mmHg below the client's baseline, place the client supine, notify the physician, and prepare for volume administration.	◆ Reocclusion is the primary cause of morbidity and mortality after angioplasty. Reocclusion occurs in 8.3% of clients (40% have MIs, and 4% die). ◆ Hypotension may be a response to antianginal or vasodilatory medications. However, it may also be an indication of reocclusion.
	◆ Instruct the client to report the development of chest pain immediately. ◆ Note duration, location, quality, and radiation of the chest pain. ◆ Monitor the ECG continuously for the development of dysrhythmias, tachycardia, and ST or T wave changes. ◆ Note the presence of diaphoresis.	◆ Reocclusion can be detected by ECG changes, diaphoresis, and the client's complaints of chest pain.
	◆ If the chest pain recurs or reocclusion is suspected, notify the physician and prepare an emergency 12-lead ECG or respond according to protocol.	◆ Prompt assessment and intervention are necessary to prevent infarction after reocclusion.

Nursing Diagnosis No. 2: High Risk for Injury at cannulation site related to mechanical irritation, bleeding, thrombus, or infection

Expected Outcomes	Nursing Interventions	Rationale
The client will maintain adequate perfusion in the cannulated extremity. ◆ Peripheral pulse palpable. ◆ Extremity warm and pink. ◆ Sensation and movement in digits intact. ◆ No evidence of hematoma formation at site.	◆ Leave the sheaths in place until they are removed by trained personnel and the PTT is within parameters. ◆ Monitor circulation to the affected limb q15min × 4, q30min × 4, then q1–4h after sheath removal.	◆ Sheaths used for angioplasty are larger than those used for cardiac catheterization alone and are more likely to result in damage to the vessel in which they have been introduced.
	◆ Notify the physician if the client experiences: weak or thready pulses; coolness, paleness or numbness; and tingling of the extremity. ◆ Monitor the sheath site for signs of external and subcutaneous	◆ Detection of vessel injury is a high priority in nursing care after angioplasty.

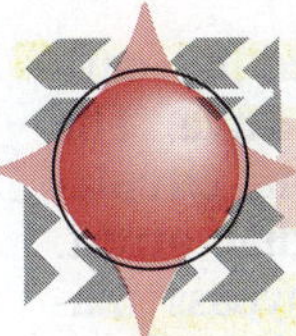

CLIENT CARE PLAN

The Client Recovering from Angioplasty *Continued*

Nursing Diagnosis No. 2: High Risk for Injury at cannulation site related to mechanical irritation, bleeding, thrombus, or infection

Expected Outcomes	Nursing Interventions	Rationale
	bleeding. (If bleeding occurs, apply manual pressure and notify the physician.) ♦ Instruct the client to notify the nurse and place manual pressure on the site should a sensation of warmth or wetness be felt at the site.	
	♦ Maintain immobilization of the site for at least 6 hr or until discontinued by protocol or the physician. ♦ Elevate the head of the bed slowly per protocol. ♦ Maintain a pressure dressing and sandbag at the site.	♦ Simple strategies may decrease the risk of injury to the insertion vessel.

Nursing Diagnosis No. 3: Altered Health Maintenance related to cannulation procedure and coronary artery vascular changes

Expected Outcomes	Nursing Interventions	Rationale
The client will recall and follow instructions for self-care after angioplasty. The client will follow recommendations for lifestyle revision.	♦ Instruct the client: ♦ To wait 1–2 wk and to check with the physician before returning to normal activities (including work) ♦ To avoid heavy lifting for several weeks ♦ To apply manual pressure if there is bleeding from the insertion site. If the bleeding is a large amount or oozing persists for >15 min, the client should notify the health care provider.	♦ Clients are returned home while they are still recuperating, usually after 1 or 2 days. They must be prepared to continue care and return to a productive lifestyle.
	♦ Review AHA recommendations for healthy lifestyle and refer to cardiac rehabilitation: ♦ Prudent (low-cholesterol, low-fat) diet ♦ Exercise ♦ Smoking cessation ♦ Control of BP and diabetes (see Chart 37–1)	♦ Initial evidence suggests that angioplasty clients are less adherent to suggested lifestyle modifications than CABG clients are. Nurses must emphasize the appropriate lifestyle changes in their teaching and refer clients to appropriate community support sites for continued rehabilitation.

of time a client waits increases, the client's anxiety may increase. An appropriate nursing assessment should identify the level of a client's anxiety and the coping methods the client has used successfully in the past.

Some clients may find it helpful to define their fears. Common sources of fear include:

- Fear of the unknown
- Fear of bodily harm
- Fear of death

Clients may benefit from detailed information about the surgery, or they may feel overwhelmed by so much material. Some clients need to discuss their feelings in detail or describe the experiences of people they know who have undergone CABG. The nurse assesses the client's anxiety level and helps the client to cope. Preoperative anxiety has been positively associated with postpericardiotomy delirium (Dolan, 1991).

OPERATIVE PROCEDURE Coronary artery bypass surgery is performed with the client under general anesthesia and undergoing cardiopulmonary bypass (CPB). The anesthesiologist or nurse anesthetist administers anesthesia and intubates the client. Once the client is anesthetized, one surgical team may begin harvesting the saphenous vein if it is to be used for the graft. The cardiac surgical team begins the procedure with a median sternotomy incision and visualization of the heart and great vessels.

Cardiopulmonary bypass is accomplished by cannulation of the inferior and superior vena cava. The purpose of CPB is to provide oxygenation, circulation, and hypothermia during induced cardiac arrest. Blood is diverted from the heart to the bypass machine, where it is heparinized, oxygenated, and returned to the circulation through a cannula placed in the ascending aortic arch or femoral artery (Fig. 37–7). During bypass, the client's core temperature is cooled to 82.6° to 89.6° F (28° to 32° C). Cooling decreases the rate of metabolism and demand for oxygen. The heart is perfused with a cold cardioplegia solution, which decreases myocardial oxygen consumption and causes the heart to stop during diastole. This ensures a still operative field and prevents myocardial ischemia.

Once the heart is arrested, the grafting procedure can begin. The surgeon uses the saphenous vein or the internal mammary artery to bypass lesions in the coronary arteries (Fig. 37–8). The graft is anastomosed (sutured) proximally to the aorta and distally to the coronary artery just beyond the occlusion. Thus, myocardial perfusion is improved. After flow rates through the grafts are measured, the heart is rewarmed slowly. The cardioplegia solution is flushed from the heart. The heart regains its rate and rhythm, or it may be defibrillated to return it to a normal rhythm. When the procedure is completed, the client is rewarmed by CPB and weaned from the bypass machine while the grafts are observed for patency and leakage. The surgeon then places atrial and ventricular pacemaker wires and mediastinal chest tubes.

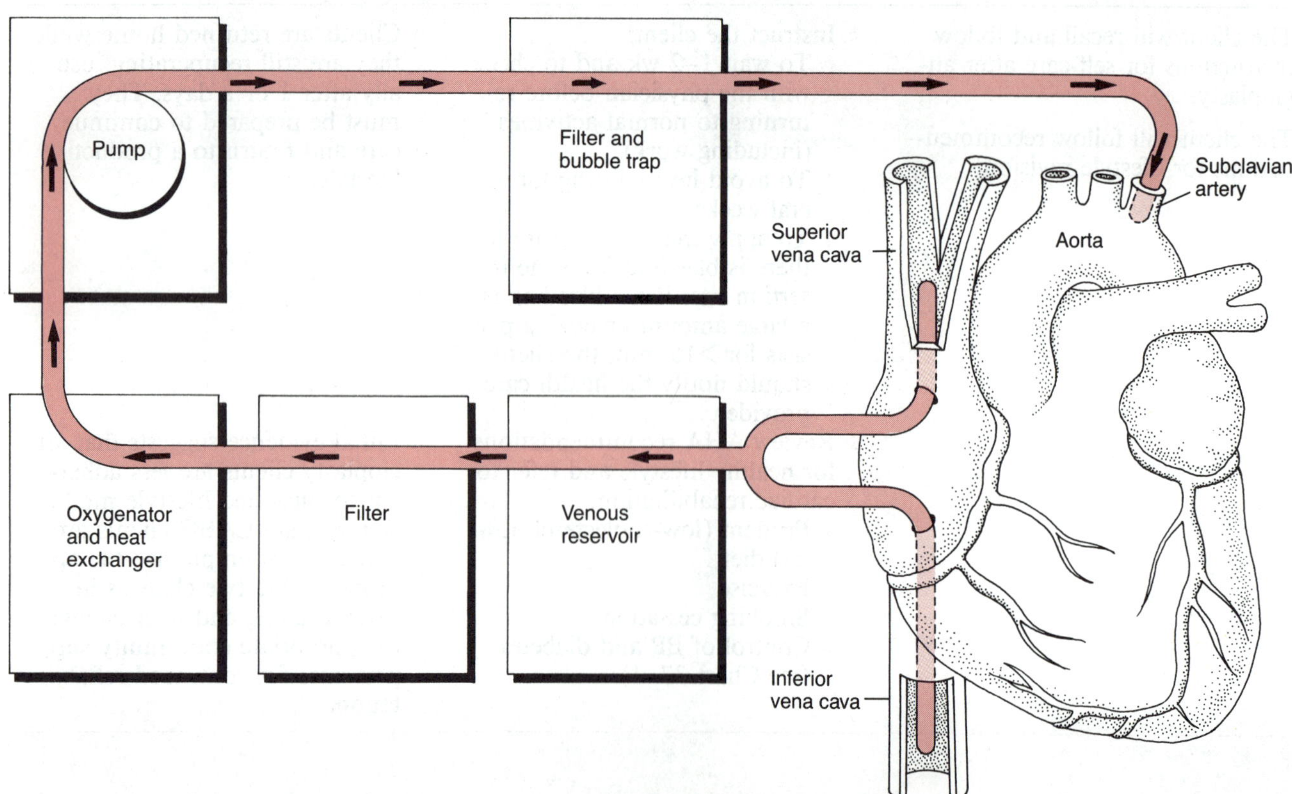

FIGURE 37–7 ◆ The heart-lung bypass circuitry used during cardiopulmonary bypass.

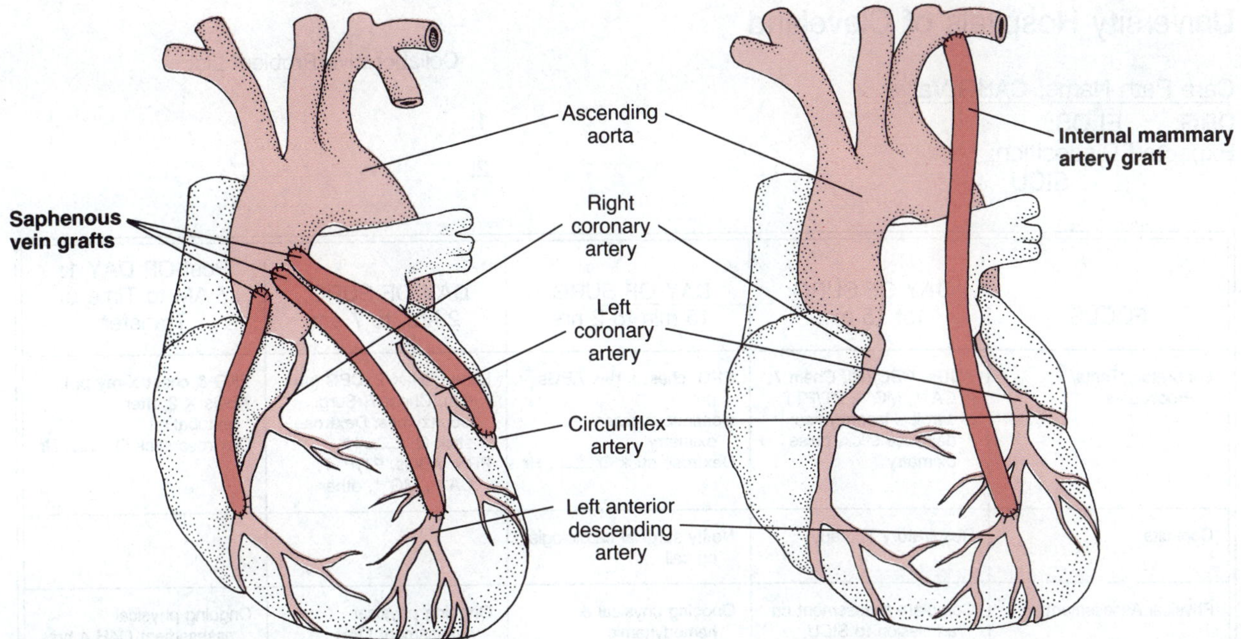

FIGURE 37–8 ◆ Two methods of coronary artery bypass grafting. Saphenous vein revascularization is more common, but results appear to be longer lasting with internal mammary artery revascularization. The procedure used depends on the nature of the coronary artery disease and the condition of the vessels available for grafting.

Finally, the surgeon closes the sternum with wire sutures.

POSTOPERATIVE CARE After surgery, the client is transported to a post–open heart surgery unit. There, the client undergoes mechanical ventilation for 6 to 24 hours. The client requires highly skilled nursing care from a nurse qualified to care for post–cardiac surgery clients. The nurse connects mediastinal tubes to water seal drainage systems and grounds the epicardial pacer wires and tapes them to the client. The nurse monitors pulmonary artery and arterial pressures and the client's heart rate and rhythm, which are displayed on a monitor. A sample clinical pathway for postoperative clients having CABG surgery is found on page 1008.

The nurse closely assesses the client for dysrhythmias, such as ventricular ectopic rhythms, bradydysrhythmias, or heart block. The nurse treats symptomatic dysrhythmias according to unit protocols or the physician's order. If the client has symptomatic bradydysrhythmias or heart block, the nurse connects the pacer wires to a pacemaker box and sets the appropriate rate as ordered (see Chap. 33). The nurse also monitors for other complications of CABG surgery, including:

- Fluid and electrolyte imbalance
- Hypotension
- Hypothermia
- Hypertension
- Bleeding
- Cardiac tamponade
- Altered cerebral perfusion

Table 37–5 lists some of the possible postoperative complications of CABG.

TABLE 37–5 Some Possible Postoperative Complications of Coronary Artery Bypass Graft Surgery

Decreased Cardiac Output

- Reduced preload
  - Hypovolemia
  - Hemorrhage
- Increased preload
  - Heart failure
  - Cardiogenic shock
- Increased afterload
  - Hypothermia
  - Increased sympathetic activity
- Dysrhythmias
  - Bradydysrhythmias
  - Conduction defects
  - Tachydysrhythmias
- Myocardial infarction

Pulmonary Dysfunction

- Atelectasis
- Pneumonia
- Pulmonary edema
- Hemothorax/pneumothorax

Neurologic Dysfunction

- Transient neurologic deficits
- Postpericardiotomy delirium
- Cerebrovascular accident

Acute Renal Failure

Gastrointestinal Dysfunction

- Stress ulcer
- Paralytic ileus

Infection

University Hospitals of Cleveland

Collaborative Problem List

Care Path Name: CABG/Valve

DRG: ELOS:

Expected Disposition:
SICU

1.

2.

FOCUS	DAY OF SURG: 1st 15 min.	DAY OF SURG: 15 min to 2 hrs.	DAY OF SURG: 2 hrs. to 7 am	Post-OP DAY 1: 7 AM to Time of Transfer
Laboratory/Tests/ Procedures	ABGs, CBC/diff, Chem 7, CA^{++}, MG^{++}, PT/PTT, surgical isoenzymes; dextrose stick, pulse oximetry	EKG, chest x-ray, ABGs prn Continuous pulse oximetry Dextrose stick Q ___ Hr	Labs q8H × 2: CBC (no diff), Chem 7, Surg, isoenzymes, Dextrose stick Q ___ Hr PRN: ABGs, PT/PTT, CA^{++}, MG^{++}, other	EKG & chest X-ray prn ABGs × 2 after extubation Dextrose stick Q ___ Hr
Consults	Respiratory Therapy	Notify surgical cardiologist on call		
Physical Assessment	Complete assessment on admission to SICU, continuous EKG & hemodynamics Q15 min. & prn I & O	Ongoing physical & hemodynamic assessment & Vital signs Q15 min. I & O Wean vent as tolerated	Ongoing physical assessment Q4H Evaluate for extubation, 8–10 Hrs post-op; extubate if ABGs adequate, weaning parameters WNL, and awake. OR Evaluate weaning parameters at 0500; plan extubation, if ready as above, between 0600-0700. VS/Hemodynamic eval Q 1–2 Hrs I & O Wt in AM Assess bowel sounds	Ongoing physical assessment Q4H 4 hrs post-extubation assess for transfer to HH2 in collaboration with ICU team and surgical attending, and cardiologist when necessary VS/Hemodynamic eval Q 2–4 H I & O
Activity	Bedrest	Bedrest: turn Q2H	Bedrest: turn Q2 Hrs	Chair in AM/OOB TID
Treatments	Connect to Vent/mode IMV Insert NG tube to ___ Chest tube: autotransfusion-30 cm suction or H_2O seal Document initial CT output Blood repl: autotransfuse Q4H or when 500cc, up to 1L Blood products as ordered IAPB/Pacer: stand by Foley: sp gr Q6H	Warming lights or Bair hugger for temp less than 36 degrees C NG tube to ___ Isolate epicardial wires (using 3cc syringe with syringe cannula) Chest tube: utotransfusion-30 cm suction or H_2O seal CT/MSCT output Q15 min. Blood repl: autotransfuse Q4H or when 500cc, up to 1L Blood products as ordered Foley: sp gr Q6H	NG tube to ___ D/C NG tube at time of extubation if bowel sounds present Chest tube: autotransfusion-30 cm suction or H_2O seal CT/MSCT output Q1H Blood repl: autotransfuse Q4H or when 500cc, up to 1L Blood products as ordered Foley: sp gr Q6H	Evaluate for NG tube removal D/C chest tube(s) per protocol: cannot be transferred if mediastinal CT remains in pt. Portable chest x-ray post CT removal Change epicardial wire dsg when MSCT D/C D/C Swan Ganz cath if hemodynamically stable D/C foley if urine output adequate Evaluate to D/C A-line after post extubation ABGs done & patient to be transferred Incentive spiro Q1H WA Encourage C & DB O_2 at ___ L/min, NC Blood products as ordered

FOCUS	DAY OF SURG: 1st 15 min.	DAY OF SURG: 15 min to 2 hrs.	DAY OF SURG: 2 hrs. to 7 am	Post-OP DAY 1: 7 AM to Time of Transfer
Diet	NPO	NPO	NPO	Clear liquid post extubation; advanced as tolerated to low chol/low salt
Medications	IV: D5 1/4 NS (___ KCL/L) or ___ Antibiotics ___ Pain: MS 2–12 mg IV/IM Q1H prn Other: Meperidine Digoxin Nitroglycerin Nitroprusside Dopamine Epinephrine Norepinephrine Lidocaine Amrinone Insulin Coverage Dobutamine Esmolol Procainamide PRN: KCL bolus	IV: D5 1/4 NS (___ KCL/L) or ___ Antibiotics ___ Pain: MS 2–12 mg IV/IM Q1H prn Other: Meperidine Digoxin Nitroglycerin Nitroprusside Dopamine Epinephrine Norepinephrine Lidocaine Amrinone Insulin Coverage Dobutamine Esmolol Procainamide PRN: KCL bolus	IV: D5 1/4 NS (___ KCL/L) or ___ Antibiotics ___ Pain: MS 2–12 mg IV/IM Q1H prn Other: Meperidine Digoxin Nitroglycerin Nitroprusside Dopamine Epinephrine Norepinephrine Lidocaine Amrinone Insulin Coverage Dobutamine Esmolol Procainamide PRN: KCL bolus	Enteric ASA Dipyridamole Pain: MS 2–12 mg IV/IM Q1H prn Other: Digoxin Dopamine Lidocaine Insulin Coverage Procainamide PRN: KCL bolus
Discharge Planning				
Teaching/Learning				
Intermediate Outcomes		Adequate ABGs Hemodynamically stable	Extubate by 7 AM Hemodynamically stable without pharmacologic support Chest tube output ≤ 75 cc/H	Hemodynamically stable without pharmacologic support Neurologically intact Mediastinal chest tubes D/C Arterial line D/C
Date Intermediate Outcome Met/Not Met				
Reviewed by: RN Signature Days				
Reviewed by: RN Signature Evenings				
Reviewed by: RN Signature Nights				

Outcomes:	Met	Not Met	Comments	Date/Initials
Hemodynamically stable; respiratory parameters adequate for patient				

Clinical Pathway: Coronary artery bypass graft or valve replacement. (Courtesy of University Hospitals of Cleveland, Cleveland, OH.)

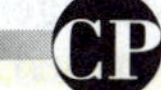

Management of Fluid and Electrolyte Imbalance. Assessing fluid and electrolyte balance is a high priority in the early postoperative period. Clients usually have edema, and fluids may be limited to 1500 to 2000 mL. However, decisions concerning fluid administration are made on the basis of the client's:

- Blood pressure
- Pulmonary artery wedge pressure (PAWP)
- Right atrial pressure
- Cardiac output
- Cardiac index
- Systemic vascular resistance
- Urine output

An experienced nurse interprets assessment findings and adjusts fluid administration on the basis of standing unit policies or specific orders from the physician.

Management of Hypotension. Hypotension (systolic blood pressure less than 90) is a significant problem because it may result in the collapse of a vein graft. The nurse reviews the assessment parameters to identify what might be causing the hypotension. Decreased preload (decreased PAWP) can result from hypovolemia or vasodilation. If the client is hypovolemic, it might be appropriate to increase fluid administration or administer blood. The physician may treat the client with a low PAWP, decreased systemic vascular resistance, and vasodilation with vasopressor therapy to increase the blood pressure. However, if hypotension is the result of left ventricular failure (increased PAWP), intravenous inotropes might be necessary (see earlier discussion of decreased cardiac output).

Serum electrolytes (especially calcium, magnesium, and phosphorus) may be reduced postoperatively and are monitored carefully by both the physician and the nurse. Because the serum potassium level can fluctuate dramatically, electrolyte levels are checked frequently. Potassium depletion is common and may result from hemodilution, diuretic therapy, and nasogastric suction. To prevent dysrhythmias, potassium concentrations are maintained between 4 and 5.

If the serum potassium level is severely depleted, the physician may order IV potassium replacement. The dose of potassium administered exceeds the usual recommended level of no more than 10 mEq of potassium per hour. For a potassium bolus, 40 to 80 mEq is mixed in 100 mL of IV solution and given at a rate as high as 40 mEq/hr. The drug must be given through a central line, and the rate of administration should be controlled by an infusion pump. The client must be on a cardiac monitor for extremely careful observation.

Management of Hypothermia. Although the client is rewarmed to 98.6° F (37° C) before being removed from bypass, it is not uncommon for the temperature to drift downward after the client leaves the surgical suite. The nurse monitors the client's body temperature and institutes rewarming procedures should the temperature drop below 96.8° F (36° C). Rewarming might be accomplished by warm blankets, rewarming lights, or thermal blankets. The danger of rewarming a client too quickly is that the client may begin shivering, resulting in metabolic acidosis and hypoxia. To prevent shivering, rewarming should proceed no faster than 1.8° F (1° C) per hour. The nurse discontinues rewarming when the client's temperature approaches 98.6° F (37° C) and the client's extremities feel warm.

Management of Hypertension. Hypothermia is a significant risk for the client undergoing coronary artery bypass graft (CABG) surgery because it promotes vasoconstriction and hypertension. Other factors contributing to hypertension in the CABG client include:

- Cardiopulmonary bypass
- Medications
- The client's own sympathetic activity

When hypertension is defined as a systolic blood pressure greater than 140 to 150, most CABG clients experience hypertension (Antman, 1992). Hypertension is dangerous because increased pressure promotes leakage from suture lines and may cause bleeding. The nurse titrates intravenous nitroprusside or nitroglycerin to return the blood pressure to acceptable limits (see Chart 37–5).

Management of Bleeding. Bleeding occurs to a limited extent in all clients postoperatively. The nurse measures the mediastinal and chest tube drainage at least hourly and reports drainage exceeding 100 to 150 mL/hr to the surgeon. The nurse must maintain the patency of the mediastinal and chest tubes. One effective way of promoting chest tube drainage is to prevent a dependent loop from forming in the tubing. Gentle milking or stripping of the chest tubes may be permitted, but nurses should observe unit policies because these procedures are controversial.

Management of Cardiac Tamponade. If the client is bleeding and the mediastinal tubes are not kept patent, blood may accumulate around the heart. The myocardium is compressed, and cardiac tamponade results. The fluid accumulating around the heart compresses the atria and ventricles, prevents them from filling adequately, and reduces cardiac output. Hallmarks of cardiac tamponade include:

- Sudden cessation of previously heavily draining mediastinal drainage
- Jugular venous distention but clear lung sounds
- Pulsus paradoxus (blood pressure greater than 10 mmHg higher on expiration than on inspiration)
- An equalizing of PAWP and right atrial pressure

Tamponade can be confirmed by echocardiogram or chest x-ray. Pericardiocentesis (see Chap. 34) may not be appropriate for tamponade after CABG because the blood in the pericardium may have clotted. Volume expansion and emergency sternotomy with drainage are then the treatments of choice.

Management of Altered Levels of Consciousness. The client may demonstrate changes in the level of consciousness, which may be permanent or transient. Transient changes related to anesthesia, cardiopulmonary bypass, or hypothermia occur in approximately 25% of clients. Transient neurologic deficits may include:

- Slowness to arouse
- Memory loss
- Confusion

Clients with transient neurologic deficits usually return to baseline neurologic status over 4 to 8 hours. Permanent deficits may be associated with a cerebrovascular accident (CVA) during surgery. The client may demonstrate:

- Abnormal pupillary response
- Failure to awaken from anesthesia
- Seizures
- Absence of sensory or motor function

The nurse checks the client's neurologic status every 30 to 60 minutes until the client has awakened from anesthesia, then every 2 to 4 hours.

Pain Management. The nurse must differentiate between sternotomy pain, which is expected after CABG, and anginal pain, which might indicate graft failure. Typical sternotomy pain is localized, does not radiate, and often becomes worse when the client coughs or breathes deeply. The client may describe the pain as sharp, aching, or burning. Pain may stimulate the client's sympathetic nervous system, which increases the client's heart rate and vascular resistance while decreasing cardiac output. The nurse administers the prescribed medication, in adequate doses, frequently enough to limit pain. However, during the process of weaning the client from mechanical ventilation, it may be necessary to limit pain medication because of the respiratory depressant effects of analgesia.

TRANSFER FROM THE SPECIAL CARE UNIT Ventilation is usually provided for 6 to 24 hours postoperatively, until the client is breathing adequately and is hemodynamically stable. During the first 24 to 48 hours, the client usually is weaned from the ventilator; has pacer wires, hemodynamic monitoring lines, and mediastinal tubes removed; and is transferred to an intermediate care unit. For the remaining 4 to 5 days of hospitalization, the nurse encourages the client to splint, cough, turn, and deep breathe to raise secretions and prevent atelectasis. The nurse guides the client in a gradual resumption of activity (Client Care Plan). The nurse continues to monitor the client for decreased cardiac output, pain, dysrhythmias, and infection.

Approximately one third of clients with CABG and two thirds of clients with valve replacements develop supraventricular dysrhythmias (especially atrial fibrillation) during the postoperative period, most commonly on the second or third postoperative day. The nurse examines the monitor pattern for atrial fibrillation. When auscultating the heart, the nurse listens for an irregularly irregular rhythm. (See Chap. 33 for interventions for atrial fibrillation.)

Sternal wound infections develop between 5 days and several weeks postoperatively in about 2% of clients and represent a significant complication. The nurse is alerted to the presence of *mediastinitis* by:

- Fever continuing beyond the first 4 days after CABG
- Instability or redness of the sternum
- Purulent drainage from suture sites
- An increased white blood cell count

The physician may perform a needle biopsy to confirm a sternal infection. Surgical debridement, antibiotic wound irrigation, and intravenous antibiotics are usually indicated. Four to 6 weeks of intravenous antibiotics are required if sternal osteomyelitis has developed.

Postpericardiotomy syndrome is a source of chest discomfort in 10% to 40% of post–cardiac surgery clients. The syndrome is characterized by:

- Pericardial and pleural pain
- Pericarditis
- A friction rub
- An elevated temperature and white blood cell count
- Dysrhythmias

Postpericardiotomy syndrome may occur days to weeks after surgery and seems to be associated with blood remaining in the pericardial sac. The nurse observes the client for the development of pericardial or pleural pain. For most clients, the syndrome is mild and self-limiting. However, the client may require treatment similar to that for pericarditis. The nurse should be prepared to detect pericardial tamponade (see Chap. 34).

Older adults may have different needs and experience slightly different problems after CABG. Nursing concerns related to the older CABG client are detailed in Chart 37–7.

DISCHARGE PLANNING

HOME CARE PREPARATION

Clients who have experienced myocardial infarction (MI), angina, or coronary artery bypass graft (CABG) surgery are usually discharged home with pharmacologic therapy and specific activity prescriptions. Hospital stays are approximately 5 to 7 days for MI and CABG clients and only 2 days for percutaneous transluminal coronary angioplasty (PTCA) clients, so clients are still recovering when they are discharged. Continuing recovery depends on effective discharge planning.

Clients who recover from anginal episodes or MI may need assistance with activities of daily living (ADL) on a temporary basis to allow rest. Clients

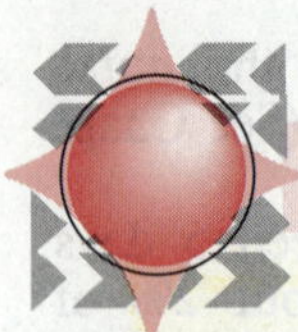

CLIENT CARE PLAN

The Cardiac Surgery Client After Transfer from the Special Care Unit

Nursing Diagnosis No. 1: Ineffective Airway Clearance related to pain from sternal incision

Expected Outcomes	Nursing Interventions	Rationale
The client will have a respiratory rate <20 and clear breath sounds.	◆ Auscultate the client's lungs and check respiratory rate, rhythm, and depth q4–8h. ◆ Examine the most recent analysis of blood gases.	◆ Continuous assessment of the client's respiratory status detects abnormalities early.
	◆ Have the client place his or her palms in the midaxillary line at the level of the 8th rib. Have the client inhale deeply so the hands move outward. ◆ Instruct the client to hold inspiration 1–2 sec. ◆ Repeat several times/hour. ◆ Encourage the client to use an incentive spirometer.	◆ This technique encourages bilateral chest expansion and deep inspiration, which is painful but necessary for a client with a sternal incision.
	◆ Have the client splint the incision, sit in a forward flexed position, and cough strongly from the chest with a double cough several times each hour.	◆ An effective cough is necessary to raise secretions and prevent atelectasis.
	◆ Encourage the client to sit, get out of bed, and walk.	◆ Early and repeated mobilization decreases the likelihood of atelectasis and pneumonia.
	◆ Provide adequate fluids and hydration.	◆ Adequate hydration helps liquefy secretions.

Nursing Diagnosis No. 2: Decreased Cardiac Output related to dysrhythmia

Expected Outcomes	Nursing Interventions	Rationale
The client will not experience dysrhythmias. Blood pressure will be within the client's acceptable range.	◆ Assess the client's cardiac rhythm.	◆ Atrial dysrhythmias occur in about one third of clients after CABG and in two thirds of clients after valve surgery.
	◆ If the client is monitored, observe for the development of dysrhythmias (especially atrial fibrillation and supraventricular tachycardia).	◆ Atrial fibrillation is irregular; new-onset atrial dysrhythmia is usually rapid.
	◆ If the client is not monitored, note whether the client has an increase in rate and a change from a regular to an irregular rhythm.	◆ Atrial dysrhythmias may be associated with reduced ventricular filling and decreased cardiac output because of the rapid rate or the absence of an atrial kick.
	◆ If the client develops an atrial dysrhythmia, check the client's BP, level of consciousness, and peripheral perfusion and notify the physician.	

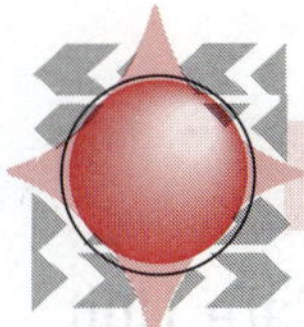

CLIENT CARE PLAN

The Cardiac Surgery Client After Transfer from the Special Care Unit *Continued*

Nursing Diagnosis No. 2: Decreased Cardiac Output related to dysrhythmia

Expected Outcomes	Nursing Interventions	Rationale
	♦ Prepare the client for conversion as directed by the physician.	♦ The physician might choose to use medications or cardioversion to return the client to a sinus rhythm.

Nursing Diagnosis No. 3: High Risk for Infection related to surgical incisions, invasive lines, and altered nutrition

Expected Outcomes	Nursing Interventions	Rationale
The client will not experience infection.	♦ Monitor temperature q4–8h and WBC qd.	♦ After cardiac surgery, the client will commonly have an elevated temperature for several days. An elevated WBC and temperature after 3–4 days usually indicate infection.
	♦ Assess suture lines and chest tube insertion sites daily for redness, induration, and purulent discharge.	♦ Wound infections may occur in the median sternotomy or leg incision sites or the chest tube insertion sites.
	♦ If active infection is present, limit the client's activities to activities of daily living and short periods of sitting.	
	♦ Assess the sternal suture line for "bogginess" or "stepping."	♦ Instability of the sternum is an indication of infection.
	♦ If the sternum is unstable, avoid upper body or trunk exercises.	
	♦ Notify the physician if any signs of infection occur.	♦ Infection, especially of the sternal incision, requires immediate medical and probably surgical intervention.

Nursing Diagnosis No. 4: Activity Intolerance related to surgery, possible heart failure, and fear of pain

Expected Outcomes	Nursing Interventions	Rationale
Vital signs will remain stable during activity.	♦ Assess the client for tachycardia, orthostatic hypotension, and fatigue before, during, and after each activity.	♦ Inactivity and blood loss during surgery may cause these.
The client will not experience lightheadedness, dizziness, or extreme fatigue with activity.	♦ Report the development of dizziness, lightheadedness, extreme fatigue, or angina.	♦ Activities should cease if these problems develop or if BP drops more than 10–20 mmHg or pulse increases more than 10 beats/min.
The client will increase the amount of time she or he is active each day.	♦ Once the client is hemodynamically stable, begin activity and advance daily as tolerated.	

Continued on following page

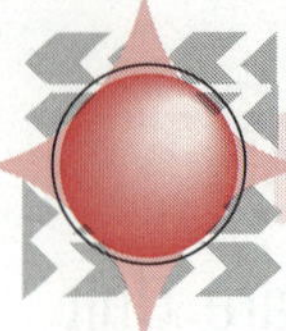

CLIENT CARE PLAN

The Cardiac Surgery Client After Transfer from the Special Care Unit *Continued*

Nursing Diagnosis No. 4: Activity Intolerance related to surgery, possible heart failure, and fear of pain

Expected Outcomes	Nursing Interventions	Rationale
The client will climb one flight of stairs and walk without difficulty before discharge. The client will plan to exercise regularly at home.	◆ Post-CABG:	
	◆ *Day 1:* ROM in bed 4×/day. ◆ *Day 1 or 2:* Sit at bedside 3×/day; ROM (e.g., foot circles and leg lifts).	◆ ROM exercises are essential for restoring flexibility and maintaining muscle tone.
	◆ *Day 2 or 3:* Walk 50–75 ft 3×/day for the remainder of hospitalization. Increase distance, pace, and time of walk daily. Before discharge, supervise stair climbing.	◆ Steadily increasing the amount of walking will increase the client's tolerance of activity.
	◆ If client becomes fatigued on longer walks, encourage short, frequent walks.	◆ Short, frequent walks of low intensity raise a client's tolerance for activity more effectively than one long walk does.
	◆ Advise the client to limit pushing or pulling and avoid lifting for 6 weeks after discharge.	◆ This is a common postoperative restriction if the client has sternal incisions to prevent damage to the suture line.
	◆ Encourage clients to continue to progress activity at home.	

who have undergone CABG or are recovering from MI complicated by heart failure or shock often require more assistance with ADL because of their limited activity tolerance. Many clients benefit from involvement in a structured cardiac rehabilitation program, which allows them to increase their activity level while being monitored at home.

HEALTH TEACHING

After the nurse has identified the needs of the client and family as well as their readiness to learn, a teaching plan is developed. The plan usually includes:

- Teaching about the normal anatomy and physiology of the heart
- The pathophysiology of angina and myocardial infarction (MI)
- Risk factor modification
- Cardiac medications
- Activity and exercise protocols
- Stress management

The nurse informs the client about the normal function of the heart and coronary arteries and explains angina and MI. Clients are taught that after MI, myocardial healing begins early and is usually complete in 6 to 8 weeks. Clients who have undergone CABG are told that the sternotomy heals in about 6 to 8 weeks.

Clients who have undergone CABG require instruction on incisional care for the sternum and the donor site (most often the leg). The client should inspect the incisions daily for any redness, swelling, or drainage. The leg of the donor site is often edematous. The nurse instructs the client to:

- Avoid crossing legs
- Wear elastic hose until the edema subsides
- Elevate the surgical limb when sitting in a chair

RISK FACTOR MODIFICATION Modification of risk factors is a necessary part of a client's management and involves changing the client's health maintenance patterns. Such modifications may include:

- Smoking cessation
- Altered dietary habits
- Regular exercise
- Blood pressure control
- Blood glucose control

CHART 37-7

Nursing Focus on the Elderly ◆ Coronary Artery Bypass Graft Surgery

- Be aware that perioperative mortality rates are higher for the older client (4%–9%) than for the client younger than 60 years (1%–2%).
- Monitor neurologic and mental status carefully because older adults are more likely to have transient neurologic deficits after coronary artery bypass graft (CABG) surgery than younger adults are.
- Observe for side effects of cardiac drugs because elders are more likely to develop toxic effects from positive inotropes (dobutamine) and potent antihypertensives (nitroglycerin or nitroprusside).
- Monitor the client closely for dysrhythmias because older adults are more likely to have dysrhythmias, such as atrial fibrillation or supraventricular tachycardia, after CABG surgery.
- Be aware that recuperation after CABG surgery is slower for older clients. The average length of stay for clients older than 70 years is 10.5 days, compared with 7 days for clients younger than 70 years.
- Teach the client and family that during the first 2 to 5 weeks after discharge, fatigue, chest discomfort, and lack of appetite may be particularly bothersome for older clients.

Smoking Cessation For clients who smoke, the nurse explains the detrimental effects on the cardiovascular system of smoking tobacco, especially cigarettes. The nurse encourages the client to attempt to quit even if he or she has been unsuccessful in the past. Although cessation of smoking is difficult and many clients are not successful the first or even second time they attempt it, continued efforts to quit eventually result in success.

Diet Therapy The nurse also encourages the client to follow a prudent diet. Only 30% to 35% of the calories in the diet should be from fat, and the fat consumed should be primarily monounsaturated or polyunsaturated. Clients should avoid saturated fats and other foods rich in cholesterol. The nurse instructs the client not to add salt at the table and to use spices other than salt when cooking. Booklets and cookbooks that can assist the client in learning to cook with reduction of fats, oils, and salt are available from the American Heart Association. In addition, the client can be instructed to read labels with greater care, looking particularly for saturated fats (such as palm and coconut oils) in many processed foods. The nurse collaborates with the dietitian when teaching the client about the diet.

Physical Activity The nurse collaborates with the physical therapist as part of cardiac rehabilitation. A program of physical activity has beneficial effects on cardiac performance and is encouraged by the nurse during preparation for discharge. The nurse instructs the client to remain at home during the first week after discharge and to continue a walking program there. The client may engage in normal daily activities that do not precipitate angina but should avoid lifting or pulling heavy objects for the first 6 to 8 weeks. Chart 37-8 lists suggested instructions for exercise.

The client may begin a simple walking program by walking 400 feet twice a day the first week after discharge and increasing the distance as tolerated, usually weekly, until he or she can walk 2 miles. The nurse instructs the client to take his or her pulse before, halfway through, and after exercise. The client should stop exercising if the target pulse rate is exceeded or the client experiences dyspnea or angina.

After a limited exercise tolerance test, the nurse encourages the client to join a formal exercise program, ideally one that assists the client in monitoring cardiovascular progress. The program should include 5- to 7-minute warm-up and cool-down periods as well as 30 minutes of aerobic exercise. The client should engage in aerobic exercise a minimum of three, but preferably five, times a week.

Sexual Activity Sexual activity is often of great concern to clients and their sexual partners. The nurse informs the client and partner that engaging in their usual sexual activity is unlikely to cause any damage to the client's heart. Clients can resume sexual intercourse on the advice of the physician, usually after exercise tolerance is assessed. If the client can walk one block or climb two flights of stairs without symptoms, usually he or she can safely resume sexual activity.

CHART 37-8

Education Guide ◆ Activity for the Client with Coronary Artery Disease

- Begin by walking the same distance at home as in the hospital (usually 400 feet) three times each day.
- Carry nitroglycerin with you.
- Check your pulse before, during, and after the exercise.
- Stop the activity for a pulse increase of more than 20 beats per minute, shortness of breath, angina, or dizziness.
- Exercise outdoors when the weather is good.
- Gradually increase the walking until the distance is ¼ mile twice daily (usually the end of the second week).
- After an exercise tolerance test and with your physician's approval, walk at least three times each week, increasing the distance by ½ mile every other week, until the total distance is 2 miles.
- Avoid straining (lifting, pushups, pull-ups, and straining at bowel movements).

The nurse suggests that initially the client time intercourse after a period of rest. Clients might try having intercourse in the morning when they are well rested or wait 1½ hours after exercise or a heavy meal. The client may take nitroglycerin before intercourse as a prophylactic measure. The position selected should be comfortable for both the client and the partner (e.g., side-lying) so that no undue stress is placed on the client's heart or suture line.

Blood Pressure Control Control of high blood pressure involves teaching the hypertensive client and the family or significant other to take the client's blood pressure. Clients are instructed to take their blood pressure on a daily basis initially and to keep a record. The nurse teaches the client to report a blood pressure of 140/90 or higher to the primary health care provider.

Blood Glucose Control Clients with diabetes mellitus are assessed for their participation in efforts to control hyperglycemia. The nurse reviews the prescribed dosage of insulin or oral hypoglycemic agents with the client and family. The client should demonstrate accurate testing of blood for glucose levels.

CARDIAC MEDICATIONS The nurse assists the client in understanding:

- The type of cardiac medications prescribed
- The benefit of each drug
- The potential side effects to watch for
- The correct dosage and time of day to take each drug

Medication regimens vary considerably from client to client. However, many clients with angina are discharged taking aspirin, a calcium channel blocker, and a nitrate. Clients who have experienced a myocardial infarction (MI) may require aspirin, a beta-blocker, a nitrate, and possibly an angiotensin-converting enzyme (ACE) inhibitor or an antidysrhythmic. The regimen can be complex. The nurse must determine that the client can comply with the instructions.

Use of sublingual nitroglycerin deserves special attention. The nurse instructs the client to carry nitroglycerin tablets at all times and to keep the tablets in a light-resistant container. Nitroglycerin tablets should be replaced every 3 to 5 months before they lose their potency and stop tingling when the client places one under the tongue. Chart 37–9 gives instructions for clients about management of chest discomfort at home.

OCCUPATION/VOCATION Two thirds of clients who experience a first MI can return to their former occupations, yet only about half of clients who have undergone coronary artery bypass grafts (CABG) surgery usually do. With the client and the family, the nurse explores the type of occupation the client is engaged in. The nurse refers the client for vocational counseling if adjustments are necessary.

CHART 37–9

Education Guide ◆ Management of Chest Pain at Home

- Keep fresh nitroglycerin available for immediate use.
- At the first indication of chest discomfort, cease activity and sit down.
- Place one nitroglycerin tablet under your tongue and allow it to dissolve.
- Wait 5 minutes for relief.
- If no relief results, repeat the nitroglycerin and wait 5 more minutes.
- If there is no relief, repeat and wait 5 more minutes.
- If there is still no relief, call for transportation to a health care facility.

PSYCHOSOCIAL PREPARATION

Having angina, experiencing an acute MI, or undergoing CABG may be the most frightening experience in a client's life. Any of these experiences may also cause an altered self-image. Common coping mechanisms are:

- Anxiety
- Denial
- Anger
- Depression

Clients need reassurance and an opportunity to express grief, fears, and anxieties about their acute illness or future recovery. Teaching and counseling sessions with family members and significant others about the illness and preventive measures reduce anxiety and tension. A nursing study by Artinian (1993) found that the spouse is the most important support system for the client who has had CABG surgery (Research Applications for Nursing).

A cardiac rehabilitation program can benefit clients. They can identify with others who have experienced the same illness and receive emotional support. The goal of cardiac rehabilitation is to return the client to his or her normal or higher-than-normal level of physical and psychosocial wellness. If needed, the nurse teaches methods of stress reduction, such as relaxation techniques or the use of biofeedback response (see Chap. 7).

HEALTH CARE RESOURCES

The American Heart Association is an excellent source for booklets, films, video cassettes, cookbooks, and professional service referrals for the client with coronary artery disease. Many local affiliates have their own cardiac rehabilitation programs for clients to join.

Within the community, cardiac rehabilitation programs may be affiliated with local hospitals, commu-

RESEARCH APPLICATIONS FOR NURSING

Discharge of the Cardiac Surgical Client May Be More Successful When Spouses Feel Prepared to Handle Home Care

Artinian, N. T. (1993). Spouses' perceptions of readiness for discharge after cardiac surgery. *Applied Nursing Research, 6,* 80–88.

This study examines the perception of 67 women about their readiness for their husbands' discharge after cardiac surgery. Data were obtained by use of a written questionnaire 6 weeks after the client's discharge. Of the spouse sample, 62% thought they were ready for the discharge. Four key people were identified as being the most helpful in preparation for discharge: the nurse, the physician, immediate family members (especially children), and friends who had the same experience. The factors that influenced readiness for discharge were the availability of social support, coping strategies, personal resources (like religious faith), and knowing what to expect in advance.

Critique In view of early discharges to lower hospital costs, discharge planning and teaching are critical for successful client outcomes. This study examines how well the spouses of cardiac surgical clients are prepared to handle home care. More studies of this nature are needed to help nurses with discharge planning.

Possible nursing implications Only 62% of the sample thought they were ready for the client's discharge; more than one third were *not* prepared. Nurses need to ensure that clients and their families are thoroughly prepared for discharge. Knowledge of what to expect is particularly helpful so that the caregiver spouse can anticipate changes in care, if needed.

nity centers, or other facilities, such as clinics. Many shopping malls open before shopping hours to allow a measured walking program indoors; this is particularly popular with the elderly client and also provides a good support group.

Mended Hearts is a nationwide program with local chapters that provides education and support to CABG clients and their families. Smoking cessation programs and clinics as well as weight reduction programs are found within the community. Many hospitals sponsor health fairs, blood pressure screening, and risk factor modification programs as well.

EVALUATION

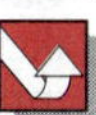

The expected outcomes may include that the client will:

- State that the chest discomfort is markedly diminished or absent. (Absence of chest pain is evidenced by resolution of ST and T wave changes and absence of facial grimacing, moaning, or guarded posture.)
- Maintain a normal sinus rhythm or a normal rhythm for the client
- Maintain blood pressure, respiratory rate and pattern, breath sounds, and peripheral pulses within acceptable parameters
- Identify concerns about living with coronary artery disease (CAD)
- State the risk factors for CAD and plan appropriate lifestyle changes
- Explain safe administration of all medications, including nitroglycerin
- Describe how he or she will respond should chest pain recur
- Increase exercise gradually and resume activities of daily living without chest pain, dyspnea, or fatigue.

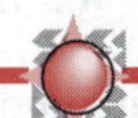

IMPLICATIONS FOR NURSING RESEARCH

All levels of health promotion and illness prevention are areas for research, including:

- ◆ Primary prevention: What are the most effective strategies for encouraging appropriate exercise?
- ◆ Secondary prevention: What are effective ways of encouraging clients to recognize chest discomfort and to proceed immediately for health care?
- ◆ Tertiary prevention: What are the most effective strategies for discouraging invalidism and encouraging clients to return to work?

Other areas for nursing research in regard to the client with coronary artery disease (CAD) include the following questions:

- ◆ What intervention strategies work most successfully to encourage coping in the spouses of clients with CAD?
- ◆ What are the differences between men and women in manifestations of CAD?
- ◆ Why do women bleed more after thrombolytic therapy?
- ◆ Why do women have a poorer survival rate after myocardial infarction (MI) and coronary artery bypass graft (CABG)?
- ◆ What interventions are most successful in enhancing quality of life after MI in women?
- ◆ What is the effect of angioplasty on quality of life?
- ◆ What is the economic impact of the treatment of CAD on the person, community, and nation?

SELECTED BIBLIOGRAPHY

American Heart Association. (1992). *1992 Heart and Stroke Facts.* Dallas, TX: Author.

American Heart Association. (1993). *1993 Heart and Stroke Statistics.* Dallas, TX: Author.

Antman, E. (1992). Medical management of the client undergoing cardiovascular surgery. In E. Braunwald (Ed.), *Heart disease: A textbook of cardiovascular medicine* (4th ed., pp. 1670–1693). Philadelphia: W. B. Saunders.

Aragon, D., & Martin, M. (1993). What you should know about thrombolytic therapy for acute MI. *American Journal of Nursing, 93*(9), 24–31.

Artinian, N. T. (1991). Stress experience of spouses of coronary artery bypass patients during hospitalization and 6 weeks after discharge. *Heart & Lung, 20,* 52–59.

Artinian, N. T. (1993). Spouses' perceptions of readiness for discharge after cardiac surgery. *Applied Nursing Research, 6,* 80–88.

Beach, E. K., Plocica, A. R., Weaver, M., & Utz, S. (1992). The spouse—a factor in recovery after acute myocardial infarction. *Heart & Lung, 21,* 30–38.

Beattie, S. (1993). CABG surgery: The second time around. *American Journal of Nursing, 93*(8), 42–45.

Becker, D. (1991). Debunking the cholesterol myth. *Journal of Cardiovascular Nursing, 5*(2), 5–8.

Braunwald, E. (Ed.). (1992). *Heart disease: A textbook of cardiovascular medicine* (4th ed.). Philadelphia: W. B. Saunders.

Brown, K. K. (1993). Boosting the failing heart with inotropic drugs. *Nursing, 23*(4), 34–43.

Bruce, S. L., & Grove, S. K. (1994). The effect of a coronary artery risk evaluation program on serum lipid values and cardiovascular risk levels. *Applied Nursing Research, 7*(2), 67–74.

Clark, S. (1990). Nursing interventions for the depressed cardiovascular patient. *Journal of Cardiovascular Nursing, 5*(1), 54–64.

Cronin, L. A. (1993). Saving the heart with thrombolytic drugs. *Nursing, 23*(8), 34–42.

Dault, L. H., Groene, J., & Herick, R. (1992). Helping your patient through cardiac catheterization. *Nursing, 22*(2), 52–55.

Dolan, J. (1991). *Critical care nursing: Clinical management through nursing process.* Philadelphia: F. A. Davis.

Finesilver, C., & Metzler, D. (1991). Right ventricular infarction: The critically different MI. *American Journal of Nursing, 91*(4), 32–39.

Gallo, J. A., & Todd, B. A. (1990). Mediastinitis after cardiac surgery. *Critical Care Nurse, 10*(6), 64–66.

Gawlinski, A., & Jensen, G. A. (1991). The complications of cardiovascular aging. *American Journal of Nursing, 91*(11), 26–30.

Gerber, R. M., (1990). Coronary artery disease in the elderly. *Journal of Cardiovascular Nursing, 4*(4), 23–34.

Gortner, S. R., Dirks, J., & Wolfe, M. M. (1992). The road to recovery for elders after CABG. *American Journal of Nursing, 92*(8), 44–49.

Grayboys, T. B., Biegelsen, B., Lampert, S., et al. (1992). Results of a second opinion among patients recommended for coronary angiography. *Journal of the American Medical Association, 268,* 2537–2540.

Green, E. (1992). Solving the puzzle of chest pain. *American Journal of Nursing, 92*(1), 32–37.

Halfman-Franey, M., & Coburn, C. (1990). Techniques in cardiac care: Lasers, stents, and arthrectomy devices. *AACN Clinical Issues in Critical Care Nursing, 1*(1), 87–109.

Halfman-Franey, M., Tukan, T., Bergstrom, D., & Hoffman, M. (1991). Using stents in the coronary circulation: Nursing perspectives. *Focus on Critical Care, 18*(2), 132–140.

Hanisch, P. J. (1991). Identification and treatment of acute myocardial infarction by electrocardiographic site classification. *Focus on Critical Care, 18*(6), 480–488.

Harrell, J., Welty, P., Jackson, M., & Jarr, S. (1992). Bedmaking in the coronary care unit. *Heart & Lung, 21,* 297 (Abstract).

Hawthorne, M. H. (1994). Gender differences in recovery after coronary artery surgery. IMAGE: Journal of Nursing Scholarship, *26*(1), 75–80.

Jarvis, C. (1992). *Physical examination and health assessment.* Philadelphia: W. B. Saunders.

Kleven, M. (1990). The critical care nurse's role in the noninvasive assessment of myocardial reperfusion. *AACN Clinical Issues in Critical Care Nursing, 1*(1), 110–118.

Kline, E. (1990). Clinical controversies surrounding thrombolytic therapies in acute myocardial infarction. *Heart & Lung, 19,* 596–601.

Matrisciano, L. (1992). Unstable angina: An overview. *Critical Care Nurse, 12*(8), 30–38.

McMillan, J. Y., & Little, C. D. (1991). Right ventricular infarction. *Focus on Critical Care, 18*(2), 158–163.

Murdaugh, C. (1990). Coronary artery disease in women. *Journal of Cardiovascular Nursing, 4*(4), 35–40.

Palarski, V., & Washburn, S. (1992). Overcoming LVD in cardiac rehab. *American Journal of Nursing, 92*(9), 52–57.

Pasternak, R., Braunwald, E., & Sobel B. (1992). Acute myocardial infarction. In E. Braunwald (Ed.), *Heart disease: A textbook of cardiovascular medicine* (4th ed., pp. 1200–1291). Philadelphia: W. B. Saunders.

Peberdy, M., & Ornato, J. (1992). Coronary artery disease in women: A review. *Heart Disease & Stroke, 1,* 315–319.

Penckofer, S., & Holm, K. (1993). What you should know about women and heart disease. *Nursing, 23*(6), 42–46.

Reigel, B., & Dossey, B. M. (1992). Acute myocardial infarction. In B. M. Dossey, C. E. Guzzetta, & C. V. Kenner (Eds.), *Critical care nursing: Body, mind, and spirit* (3rd ed., pp. 413–442). Philadelphia: J. B. Lippincott.

Reigel, B., & Dracup, K. (1992). Does overprotection produce cardiac invalidism after myocardial infarction? *Heart & Lung, 21,* 529–539.

Swearingen, P. L., & Keen, J. H. (1992). *Manual of critical care: Applying nursing diagnoses to adult critical illness* (2nd ed.). St. Louis: Mosby Year Book.

U.S. Department of Health and Human Services (DHHS). (1990). *Healthy people 2000: National health promotion and disease prevention objectives.* Washington, DC: U.S. Government Printing Office.

Weigle, D. S. (1992). The pathophysiology of obesity: Implications for treatment. *Clinician Reviews, 2*(5), 81–102.

Whitman, G. R., & Guzzetta, C. E. (1992). Cardiac surgery. In B. M. Dossey, C. E. Guzzetta, & C. V. Kenner (Eds.), *Critical care nursing: Body, mind, and spirit* (3rd ed., pp. 443–500). Philadelphia: J. B. Lippincott.

Wilson, R. F. (1992). *Critical care manual: Application physiology and principles of therapy* (2nd ed.). Philadelphia: F. A. Davis.

Wingate, S. (1991). Women and coronary heart disease: Implications for the critical care setting. *Focus on Critical Care, 18*(3), 212–228.

Workman, M. L. (1994). Anticoagulants and thrombolytics: What's the difference? *AACN Clinical Issues in Critical Care Nursing, 5*(1), 26–34.

Yakabowich, M. (1992). What you should know about administering nitrates. *Nursing, 22*(9), 52–55.

SUGGESTED READINGS

Brown, K. K. (1993). Boosting the failing heart with inotropic drugs. *Nursing, 23*(4), 34–43.

This comprehensive article describes the indications for, actions of, and adverse effects associated with inotropic drugs. The author provides an excellent quick reference table and several charts to highlight the most important information for the nurse.

Penckofer, S., & Holm, K. (1993). What you should know about women and heart disease. *Nursing, 23*(6), 42–46.

This article discusses the differences and similarities between men and women who have heart disease. The authors identify several risk factors that women have, such as iron retention, and point out that smoking among women is a major problem. They also describe concerns about misdiagnosis and undertreatment of women with heart disease.

Workman, M. L. (1994). Anticoagulants and thrombolytics: What's the difference? *AACN Clinical Issues in Critical Care Nursing, 5*(1), 26–34.

This article reviews the essential features that stimulate and limit the action of blood coagulation. The differences between anticoagulants and thrombolytic agents in terms of mechanisms of action, clinical uses, duration of therapy, cost, and complications are highlighted.

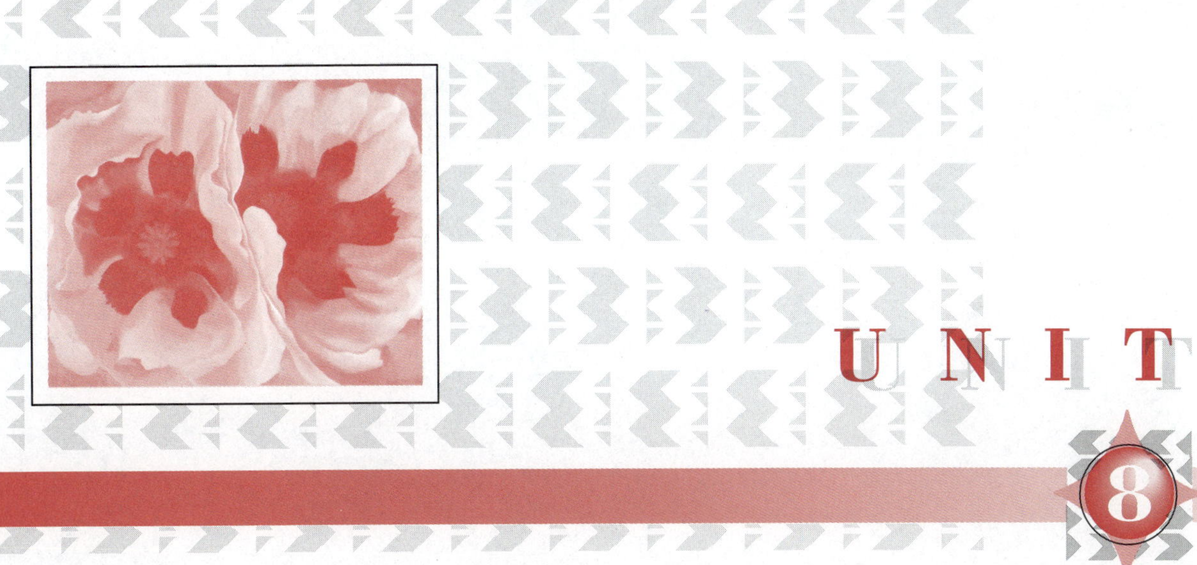

UNIT 8

Problems of Tissue Perfusion: Management of Clients with Problems of the Hematologic System

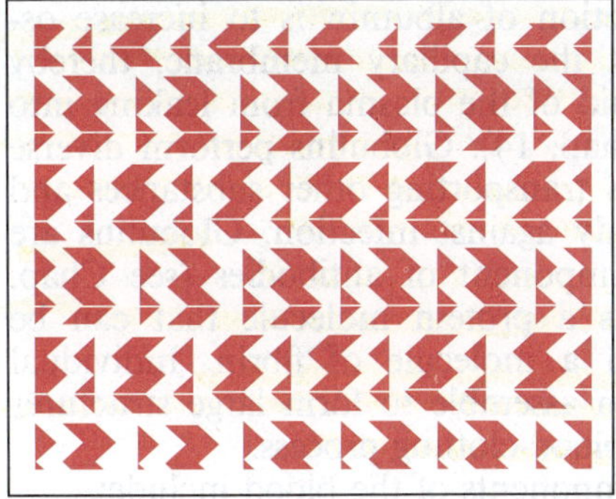

CHAPTER 38

Assessment of the Hematologic System

CHAPTER HIGHLIGHTS

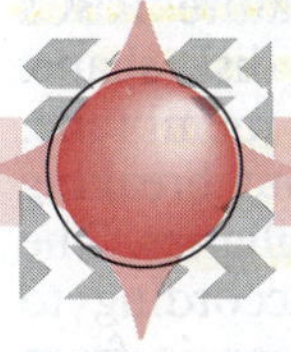

The hematologic system has many essential functions. In addition, the blood and lymph fluids are not confined to any one space in the body but circulate into all body tissues and organs. As a result, the functions of the hematologic system influence the health and well-being of all body systems. Therefore, hematologic assessment is an important skill for the nurse. This chapter together with Chapter 22 (Inflammation and the Immune Response) reviews the normal physiology of the hematologic system and assessment skills necessary to assess accurately the client's hematologic status.

ANATOMY AND PHYSIOLOGY REVIEW

Bone Marrow

The bone marrow is a blood-forming (hematopoietic) organ. It produces most of the cellular elements of the blood, including:

- Red blood cells (RBC)
- White blood cells (WBC)
- Platelets

The bone marrow is directly involved in some aspects of the immune response, including antibody-mediated and cell-mediated immunity (see Chap. 22).

Each day, the bone marrow in a healthy adult produces and releases about 2.5 billion red blood cells, 2.5 billion platelets, and 1 billion granulocytes per kilogram of body weight (Williams et al., 1990).

In the fetus, blood components are formed in the liver, the spleen, and, by the last trimester, the bone marrow. At birth, blood-producing marrow is present in every bone (Hays, 1990). The flat bones (sternum, skull, pelvic and shoulder girdles) contain active blood-producing marrow throughout life. In small, irregularly shaped bones and in the long bones, the amount of functional bone marrow decreases as a person ages until, by age 18 years, blood production is limited to the ends of the long bones. During adulthood, fatty tissue replaces inactive bone marrow. In elderly people, the proportion of fatty marrow increases to about one half of the marrow that is found in the sternum and the ribs, and only a relatively small portion of the remaining marrow continues active blood production. When a persistent increased demand for blood cells is present, however, some inactive marrow sites can again become functional and produce blood cells (Rapaport, 1987).

As described in Chapter 22, the bone marrow produces all blood cells, initially producing stem cells. The bone marrow contains pluripotent stem cells, immature and undifferentiated cells capable of maturing into any of several lines of blood cells. A pluripotent stem cell can differentiate into a red blood cell, a white blood cell, or a platelet line, depending on the needs of the body (see Fig. 22–3).

The next stage in cell development is the committed stem cell (also called the precursor cell or the unipotent stem cell). A committed stem cell has one specific maturational pathway and matures or differentiates into only one cell type. Committed stem cells are in the active phase of growth but require the presence of a specific growth factor (poietin) for further development and maturation (Metcalf, 1992). For example, erythropoietin is a growth factor made in the kidneys that is specific for the red blood cell line. A variety of other growth factors influence white blood cell and platelet maturation (see Chaps. 22, 26, and 39).

Blood Components

Blood is composed of plasma and cellular elements. Plasma is part of the extracellular fluid of the body. It is similar to the interstitial fluid that is found between tissue cells; however, plasma contains about 7% protein, whereas interstitial fluid normally contains less than 2% protein. There are three major types of plasma proteins:

- Albumin
- Globulins
- Fibrinogen

The primary function of albumin is to increase osmotic pressure at the capillary membrane, thereby preventing the fluid of the plasma from leaking into the tissues (see Chap. 14). Globulins perform diverse functions, such as transporting other substances and protecting the body against infection. Globulins are also the main component of antibodies (see Chap. 22). Fibrinogen is a protein molecule that can be activated to form a molecule of fibrin. Individual molecules of fibrin assemble to form large structures important in the blood-clotting process.

The cellular components of the blood include:

- Red blood cells
- White blood cells
- Platelets

These blood components differ in anatomic features, sites of maturation, and functions.

RED BLOOD CELLS (ERYTHROCYTES)

Red blood cells (RBCs), or erythrocytes, make up the largest proportion of blood cells. Mature RBCs have no nucleus; they have a biconcave disk shape. This feature, together with a pliable membrane, allows RBCs to change their shape without breaking as they pass through narrow, winding capillaries. The number of RBCs a person has varies according to sex, age, and general health, but the range is from 4,400,000 to 5,500,000/mm^3.

As shown in Figures 38–1 and 38–2, RBCs originate from the pluripotent stem cell, enter the myeloid pathway, and progress in stages to the mature RBC, the erythrocyte. Healthy mature RBCs have a life span of approximately 120 days after being released into circulation from the bone marrow. As RBCs age, their membranes become more fragile. These old cells are trapped and destroyed by fixed macrophages in the tissues, the spleen, and the liver. Some intracellular parts of destroyed RBCs, such as iron, are recycled and used in the formation of new RBCs.

RBCs are responsible for the formation of hemoglobin (Hgb). Each normal mature RBC contains many thousands of hemoglobin molecules (Guyton, 1991). The heme portion of each hemoglobin molecule requires the presence of a molecule of iron. Only when the heme molecule is complete with iron can it transport up to four molecules of oxygen. Therefore, iron is a critical component of hemoglobin (Fairbanks & Beutler, 1990). The globin portion of the hemoglobin molecule carries carbon dioxide. In addition, because RBCs contain the enzyme carbonic anhydrase and because hemoglobin is an excellent buffer, RBCs greatly assist in maintaining acid-base balance (see Chaps. 17 and 18).

The most important feature of the hemoglobin molecule is its ability to combine loosely and reversibly with oxygen. With only a small drop in oxygen tension at the tissue level, there is a considerable increase in the transfer of oxygen from hemoglobin to tissues. This transfer is also known as *oxygen dis-*

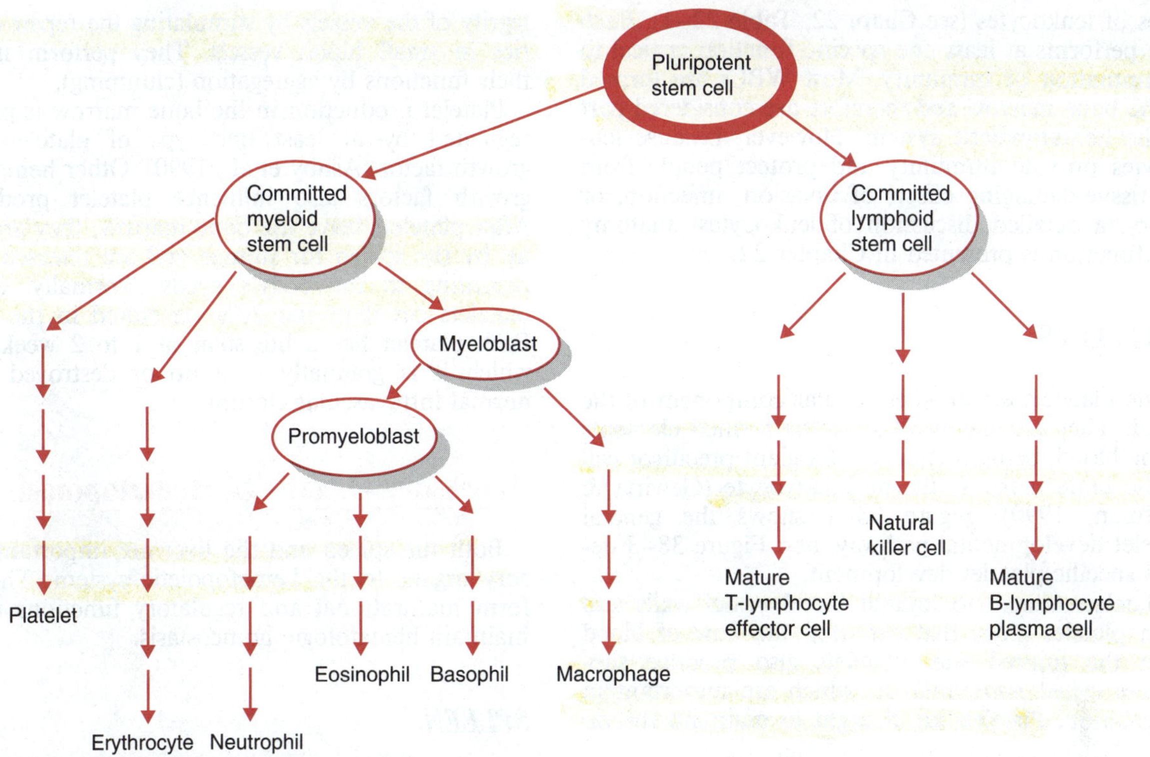

FIGURE 38–1 ◆ Bone marrow cell differentiation and maturational pathways. (© 1992 by M. Linda Workman. All rights reserved.)

sociation. Some pathologic conditions can alter the speed and quantity of oxygen release to the tissues.

The total number of RBCs a person has is precisely regulated. Regulation occurs through the process of erythropoiesis (selective maturation of pluripotent stem cells into mature erythrocytes) to prevent overconcentration of RBCs. The trigger for control of erythropoiesis is tissue oxygenation. The kidney produces the RBC growth factor (erythropoietin) at a rate consistent with RBC destruction to maintain a constant normal level of circulating RBCs. When tissue oxygenation is less than normal, a condition known as *hypoxia,* the kidney increases the production and release of erythropoietin (Hays, 1990). This growth factor then stimulates the bone marrow to increase the rate and total amount of RBC production (Pollin & DeLuca, 1992). When tissue oxygenation is excessive, the kidney decreases the production of erythropoietin, resulting in an inhibition of RBC production.

A number of substances are essential for the formation of hemoglobin and RBCs. These critical substances include iron, vitamin B_{12}, folic acid, copper, pyridoxine, cobalt, and nickel (Williams et al., 1990). A lack of any of these substances can lead to anemia. Anemia is a feature of any of a variety of conditions in which either the function or the number of erythrocytes is insufficient to meet tissue oxygen demands (see Chap. 39).

WHITE BLOOD CELLS (LEUKOCYTES)

The white blood cells (WBCs), or leukocytes, are the second category of blood cells. There are multiple

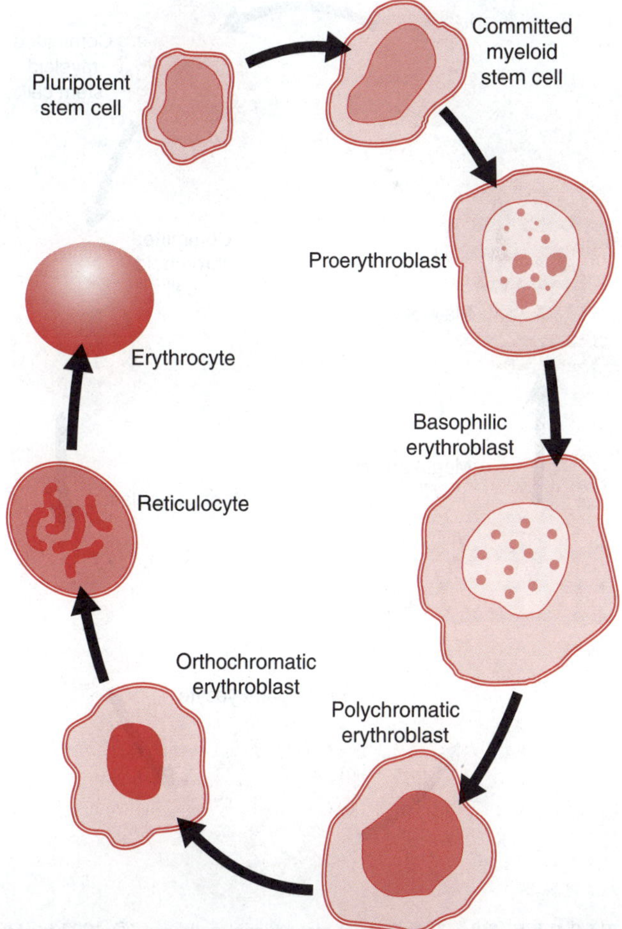

FIGURE 38–2 ◆ Erythrocyte maturational pathway. (© 1992 by M. Linda Workman. All rights reserved.)

types of leukocytes (see Chap. 22, Table 22–1). Each type performs at least one specific function critical to inflammation or immunity. Most WBCs are formed in the bone marrow and therefore are considered part of the hematopoietic system. However, because leukocytes provide immunity and protect people from the tissue-damaging effects of invasion, infection, or injury, a detailed discussion of leukocytes' anatomy and function is presented in Chapter 22.

PLATELETS

The platelets are another cellular component of the blood. They are the smallest of the formed elements of the blood, being fragments of a giant precursor cell in the bone marrow, the megakaryocyte (Gewirtz & Hoffman, 1990). Figure 38–1 shows the general platelet developmental pathway, and Figure 38–3 depicts specific platelet development.

Platelets adhere to injured blood vessel walls and form platelet plugs that can stop the flow of blood from the injured site. Platelets also produce substances called *phospholipids,* which are important in coagulation. Platelets are thought to maintain the integrity of the vessels by stimulating the repair of injuries in small blood vessels. They perform most of their functions by aggregation (clumping).

Platelet production in the bone marrow is precisely regulated by at least one type of platelet-specific growth factor (Ashby et al., 1990). Other hematologic growth factors also influence platelet production. After platelets leave the bone marrow, they are taken up by the spleen for storage and are released slowly according to the body's needs. Normally, 80% of platelets circulate and 20% are stored in the spleen. Each platelet has a life span of 1 to 2 weeks, after which it is gradually used up or destroyed during normal intravascular clotting.

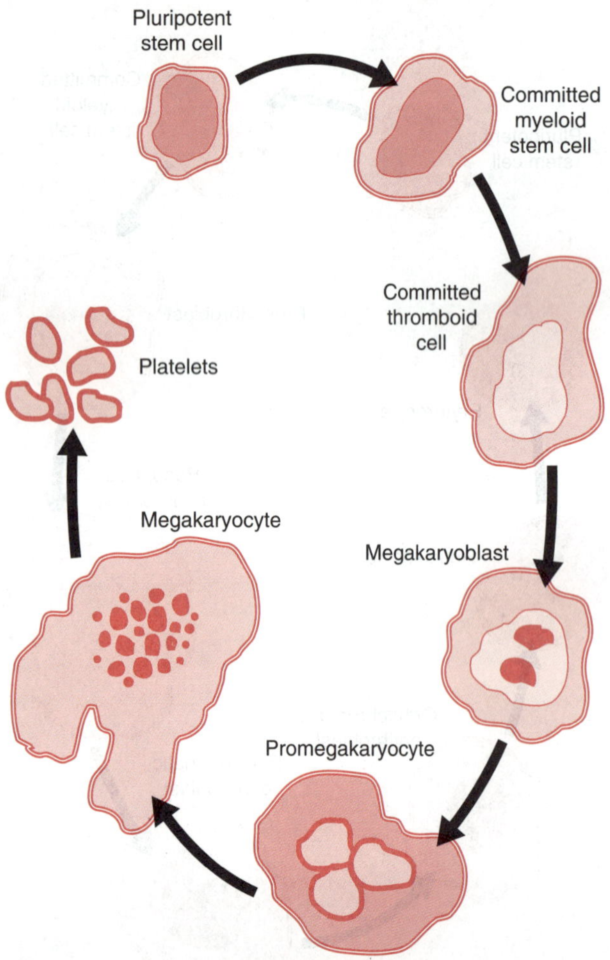

FIGURE 38–3 ◆ Platelet maturational pathway. (© 1992 by M. Linda Workman. All rights reserved.)

Accessory Organs of Hematopoiesis

Both the spleen and the liver are important accessory organs to the hematopoietic system. They perform maturational and regulatory functions to help maintain hematologic homeostasis.

SPLEEN

The spleen is located beneath the diaphragm to the left of the stomach. It contains three types of tissue:

- White pulp
- Red pulp
- Marginal pulp

These three tissues maintain an equilibrium between blood cell synthesis and blood cell destruction and assist with immunologic defensive mechanisms. White pulp is filled with lymphocytes and macrophages. This area filters the circulating blood to some degree and removes unwanted cells (such as bacteria and old RBCs). Red pulp is composed of vascular sinuses that are storage sites for erythrocytes and platelets. Marginal pulp contains the termination sites of many arteries and other blood vessels.

During hematopoiesis, the spleen destroys aged or imperfect RBCs through phagocytosis and mechanical deformation, assists in iron metabolism by breaking down the hemoglobin released from these destroyed cells, stores platelets, and filters antigens. Clients who have had splenectomies have impairment of some immune functions. As a result, splenectomized clients are not efficient at ridding the body of many blood-borne pathogenic microorganisms and are at a greatly increased risk for infection and sepsis (Workman et al., 1993).

LIVER

The liver is important for normal erythropoiesis. Its functions become even more important if red blood cell production in the marrow is abnormal. The liver is the primary site of production for most of the blood-clotting factors and prothrombin. In addition, proper liver function, including bile production, is critical to the formation of vitamin K in the intestinal tract. (Vitamin K is essential in the formation of blood-clotting factors VII, IX, and X and prothrombin.) Large quantities of whole blood and blood cells can be stored in the liver. The liver also converts bilirubin (one end-product of hemoglobin breakdown) to bile and stores extra iron within a storage protein called ferritin. Small amounts of erythropoietin are synthesized in the liver.

In some people, when marrow production of blood cells is impaired for prolonged periods, the liver can resume its blood-producing capacities that ceased after fetal life. This activity is called extramedullary hematopoiesis and is not considered a normal function of the adult liver (Rapaport, 1987).

Hemostasis

Hemostasis is the process in which selective localized blood clotting occurs in the lumens of damaged blood vessels while blood circulation to all areas is maintained. It is a complex process that balances the production of clotting factors against the production of factors that dissolve clots. The foundations of hemostasis are first the formation of a platelet plug and then a series of events that eventually cause the formation of a fibrin clot. Intrinsic and extrinsic factors are involved in fibrin clot formation and blood coagulation.

PLATELET AGGREGATION

Platelets normally circulate as individual cell-like structures. They are not attracted to each other until they are activated or until the presence of other substances causes the membranes of the platelets to change (actually become sticky) and allows aggregation to occur. When platelets become activated and aggregate, they can form large, semisolid plugs within the lumens of blood vessels (as well as in holes in blood vessel walls) and disrupt blood flow. Some of the substances capable of causing or allowing platelets to aggregate include adenosine diphosphate (ADP), calcium, thromboxane A_2, and collagen (Ashby et al., 1990). Platelets themselves can be stimulated to secrete some of these substances, whereas other substances enabling platelet aggregation are exogenous. Formation of a platelet plug can result in the stimulation of a cascade reaction that ultimately causes blood coagulation to occur through the formation of a fibrin clot.

THE BLOOD-CLOTTING CASCADE

In the blood-clotting cascade, the beginning of the sequence is rapidly amplified or enhanced to the extent that the final result is much larger than might be predicted by the size of the triggering event. Cascades work almost like a landslide, in which a few small pebbles rolling down a steep hillside can unbalance large rocks and dislodge pieces of soil, causing a final enormous movement of earth. Just like landslides, physiologic cascade reactions are hard to stop after they have been set into motion. Platelet plug formation stimulating the clotting cascade can result from intrinsic factors or extrinsic factors.

INTRINSIC FACTORS

Platelet plugs can begin to form when events inside blood vessels change. Trauma to the blood itself, especially to the blood cells, or exposure of the blood to collagen in the linings of blood vessels can stimulate platelet aggregation, the formation of a platelet plug, and the beginning of the clotting cascade (Fig. 38–4; see also Fig. 39–2). Other intrinsic events stimulating platelet aggregation include:

- Antigen-antibody reactions
- The presence of circulating debris
- Prolonged venous stasis
- The presence of bacterial endotoxins

Having the cascade continue to the point of fibrin clot formation depends on the presence of sufficient amounts of all the various clotting factors and cofactors. These factors are presented in Table 38–1.

EXTRINSIC FACTORS

Platelet plugs can begin to form when events external to the blood vessels change. The most common extrinsic events stimulating the clotting cascade are trauma to tissues and damage to blood vessels. The platelet plug is formed within seconds of the trauma. The platelet plug causes the blood-clotting cascade to be initiated sooner than by the intrinsic pathway because some of the steps of the intrinsic pathway are bypassed.

The result of initiation of the clotting cascade by intrinsic factors or extrinsic factors is the same—the formation of a fibrin clot resulting in coagulation.

FIBRIN CLOT FORMATION

Fibrinogen is a large, inactive protein molecule made in the liver and secreted into the blood. An enzyme, thrombin, removes the end portions of fibrinogen, converting it to the active molecule fibrin. Individual fibrin molecules can associate or be linked in a special way to form fibrin threads. The fibrin threads come together in a lattice-like meshwork, forming a net-like structure that is a scaffold for a blood clot (Fig. 38–5).

After the fibrin scaffold is formed, a stabilizing factor (clotting factor XIII) tightens up the scaffold, making it more dense. Platelets stick to the threads of the scaffold and attract other blood cells and proteins

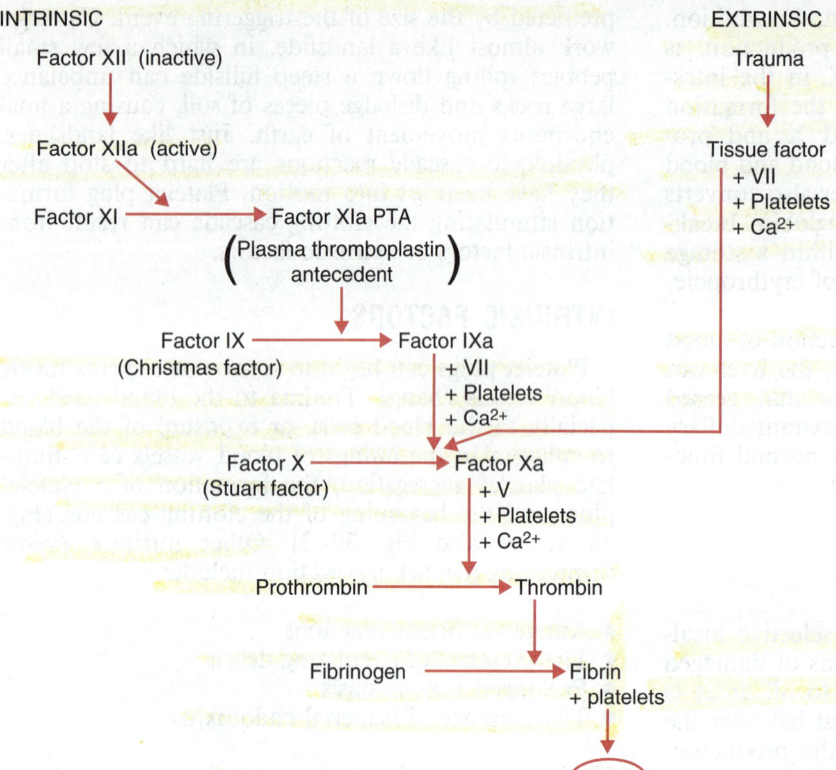

FIGURE 38-4 ◆ Summary of blood-clotting cascade. (© 1992 by M. Linda Workman. All rights reserved.)

to form an actual blood clot. As this clot retracts, the serum (plasma without the clotting factors) is extruded, and clot formation is complete.

FIBRINOLYSIS

Because blood coagulation occurs through a rapid cascade-type process, in theory whenever the cascade is set into motion, it keeps forming fibrin clots until all blood, throughout the entire body, has coagulated. Such widespread coagulation is not compatible with life. Therefore, whenever the blood-clotting cascade is initiated, counterclotting or anticoagulant forces are also initiated to limit clot formation to necessary areas and to maintain a normal flow of blood within the vascular space. When blood-clotting actions are appropriately balanced with anticlotting actions, coagulation occurs only where it is needed and normal circulation is maintained.

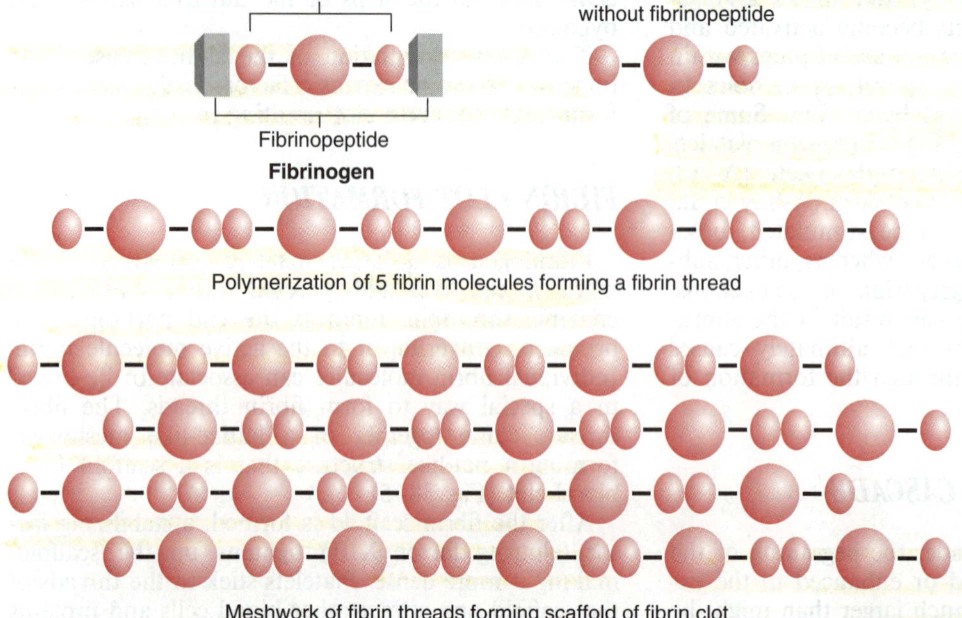

FIGURE 38-5 ◆ Activation and polymerization of fibrin to form fibrin clot. (© 1992 by M. Linda Workman. All rights reserved.)

TABLE 38–1 The Coagulation Factors

Factor	Action
I: fibrinogen	• Factor I is converted to fibrin by the enzyme thrombin. Individual fibrin molecules form fibrin threads, which are the scaffold for clot formation and wound healing.
II: prothrombin	• Factor II is the inactive precursor of thrombin. Prothrombin is activated to thrombin by coagulation factor X (Stuart-Prower factor). After it is activated, thrombin converts fibrinogen (coagulation factor I) into fibrin and activates factors V and VIII. • Synthesis is vitamin K dependent.
III: tissue thromboplastin	• Factor III interacts with factor VII to initiate the extrinsic clotting cascade.
IV: calcium	• Calcium (Ca^{2+}), a divalent cation, is a cofactor for most of the enzyme-activated processes required in blood coagulation. • Calcium also enhances platelet aggregation and makes red blood cells clump together.
V: proaccelerin	• Factor V is a cofactor for activated factor X, which is essential for converting prothrombin to thrombin.
VI: discovered to be an artifact	• No factor VI is involved in blood coagulation.
VII: proconvertin	• Factor VII activates factors IX and X, which are essential in converting prothrombin to thrombin. • Synthesis is vitamin K dependent.
VIII: antihemophilic factor	• Factor VIII together with activated factor IX enzymatically activates factor X. In addition, factor VIII combines with another protein (von Willebrand's factor) to help platelets adhere to capillary walls in areas of tissue injury. • A lack of factor VIII is the basis for classic hemophilia (hemophilia A).
IX: plasma thromboplastin component (Christmas factor)	• Factor IX, when activated, activates factor X to convert prothrombin to thrombin. • This factor is essential in the common pathway between the intrinsic and extrinsic clotting cascades. • A lack of factor IX is the basis for hemophilia B. • Synthesis is vitamin K dependent.
X: Stuart-Prower factor	• Factor X, when activated, converts prothrombin into thrombin. • Synthesis is vitamin K dependent.
XI: plasma thromboplastin antecedent	• Factor XI, when activated, assists in the activation of factor IX. However, a similar factor must exist in tissues. People who are deficient in factor XI have mild bleeding problems after surgery but do not bleed excessively as a result of trauma.
XII: Hageman factor	• Factor XII is critically important in the intrinsic pathway for the activation of factor XI.
XIII: fibrin-stabilizing factor	• Factor XIII assists in forming cross-links among the fibrin threads to form a strong fibrin clot.

The fibrinolytic system dissolves the fibrin clot with special enzymes (Fig. 38–6). The central event of fibrinolysis is the conversion of plasminogen to plasmin. Plasmin, an active enzyme, then digests fibrin, fibrinogen, prothrombin, and factors V, VIII, and XII, thus breaking down the fibrin clot (Colman et al., 1994).

Hematologic Changes Associated with Aging

Changes in the cellular and plasma components of the blood occur with aging and make accurate assessment of the hematologic system in elderly people more difficult. Chart 38–1 provides techniques to assess the hematologic system in this population. Total body water is decreased among elderly clients. This change is a consequence of an age-related reduction of the thirst reflex and a simultaneous decrease in the ability of the older kidney to concentrate urine. In addition, elderly people tend to have a lower concentration of plasma proteins (possibly related to a decreased dietary intake of proteins), which also causes some loss of vascular fluid into the interstitial space by decreasing the plasma oncotic/osmotic pressure (Chap. 15).

As the bone marrow ages, it produces fewer blood cells. Total red blood cell counts and white blood cell counts (especially lymphocytes) are lower among elderly people, although platelet counts do not appear to change with age. Lymphocytes from elderly clients are less reactive to antigens and have a loss of immune function. Antibody levels and responses are lower in older adults. The leukocyte count does not rise as high in response to infection in elderly people as in young people (Workman et al., 1993).

Another hematologic parameter that changes with age is hemoglobin level. Hemoglobin levels in men and women fall after middle age. Iron-deficient diets may play a role in this phenomenon.

HISTORY

Demographic Data

Age and sex are important variables to obtain in assessments of the client's hematologic status. Bone marrow and lymphoid activity diminish with age. At all ages, women have lower blood cell counts compared with men, but this difference is more profound during the years of menstruation. This sex difference may be related to a dilutional effect of female hormones, which cause an increased volume of vascular fluid, or differences in bone marrow activity. It is also important for the nurse to collect information on occupation, hobbies, and the geographic location of

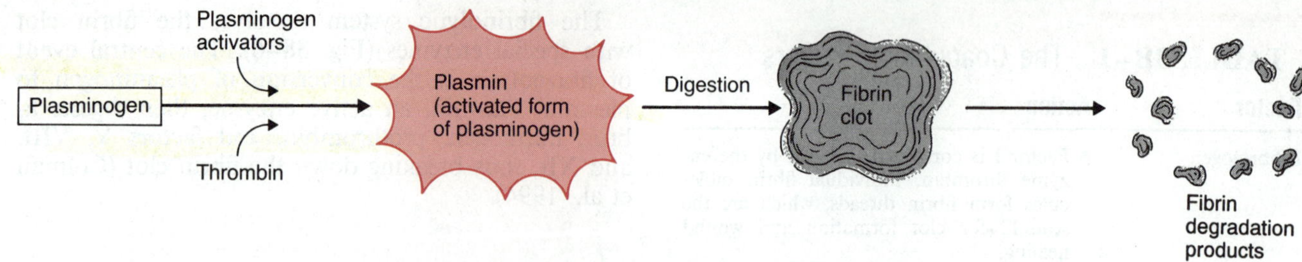

FIGURE 38-6 ◆ The process of fibrinolysis.

housing. These data may reveal exposure to specific agents or chemicals that affect bone marrow proliferation and hematologic function.

Personal and Family History

Because many types of bleeding disorders are inherited, the nurse must obtain an accurate family history. The nurse asks whether anyone in the family has had hemophilia, frequent nosebleeds, postpartum hemorrhages, excessive bleeding after dental extractions, or continuous heavy bruising in response to relatively mild trauma. Of particular importance is whether anyone in the family has sickle cell disease or sickle cell trait. Although sickle cell disease is seen primarily among African-Americans, anyone may have the trait. Research Applications for Nursing discusses social implications in the assessment of sickle cell disease or trait.

Personal factors to be included in the hematologic assessment are:

- Liver function
- The presence of known immunologic or hematologic disorders
- Current medication use

Because liver function is important in the synthesis of clotting factors, the nurse asks about jaundice, anemia, and gallstones.

The nurse questions the client about use of blood "thinners" such as sodium warfarin (Coumadin, Warfilone✱) and aspirin. A person who consumes large quantities of aspirin may have bleeding problems, and many over-the-counter medications contain

CHART 38-1

Nursing Focus on the Elderly ◆ Hematologic Assessment

Assessment Area	Findings in Hematologic Disorders	Normal Changes in the Elderly	Significance/Alternatives
Nail beds (for capillary refill)	• Pallor or cyanosis may indicate a hematologic disorder.	• Thickened or discolored nails make visualization of skin color beneath the nails impossible.	• Use another body area, such as the lip, to assess central capillary refill.
Hair distribution	• Thin or absent hair on the trunk or extremities may indicate poor circulation to a particular area.	• Progressive loss of body hair is a normal facet of aging.	• A relatively even pattern of hair loss that has occurred over an extended period is not significant.
Skin moisture	• Skin dryness may indicate any of a number of hematologic disorders.	• Skin dryness is a normal facet of aging.	• Skin moisture is not usually a reliable indicator of an underlying pathologic condition in the elderly.
Skin color	• Skin color changes, especially pallor and jaundice, are associated with some hematologic disorders.	• Pigment loss and skin yellowing are common changes associated with aging.	• Pallor in an elderly person may not be a reliable indicator of anemia; laboratory testing is required. Yellow-tinged skin in an elderly person may not be a reliable indicator of increased serum bilirubin levels; laboratory testing is required.

RESEARCH APPLICATIONS FOR NURSING

Health Care Professionals Are Not Always the Most Effective Health Educators for the Public

Holmes, A., Hatch, J., & Robinson, G. (1992). A lay education approach to sickle cell disease education. *Journal of the National Black Nurses Association, 5*(2), 26–36.

This study examined the feasibility of using lay African-American volunteers in a community outreach program to teach the public about sickle cell trait or disease and the resources available to people at risk. The reasons for conducting this study are related to (1) a historical lack of trust on the part of many African-Americans in Caucasian health care professionals and (2) lack of progress in the area of sickle cell trait or disease screening and counseling.

A total of 48 lay volunteers from the African-American community were recruited and trained as educators and counselors. Preliminary results indicate that these lay educators remained committed to the task, were well accepted by the community, and were recognized as being sensitive to the social, genetic, and sexual issues associated with sickle cell trait or disease screening and counseling.

Critique Although this study publishes only preliminary findings, it is an excellent resource on the concepts of community-based health assessment. In addition, it points out how important the interpretation of the social significance of a health problem can be in encouraging people to use available resources.

Possible nursing implications Nurses may have the latest accurate information to disseminate to the public about a specific health problem. However, if the nurse is not accepted by a group at risk because of perceived cultural differences or socioeconomic barriers, the information is not helpful. A more effective role of the nurse may be that of helping to train lay educators to bridge the gap between the health care community and a population at risk.

aspirin or other salicylates that disrupt platelet aggregation. The nurse determines all medications that the client is using or has used in the past 3 weeks. The nurse notes the use of antibiotics because prolonged antibiotic therapy can lead to coagulopathies or bone marrow depression. Table 38–2 lists drugs known to alter hematologic function. Previous radiation therapy, especially if marrow-forming bones were in the radiation path, may result in some permanent impairment of hematologic function.

Diet History

Specific dietary patterns can alter cell quality and blood coagulation. The nurse asks clients to record

TABLE 38–2 Drugs Impairing the Hematologic System

Generic Name	Common Trade Names
Drugs Causing Bone Marrow Suppression	
Altretamine	Hexalen, Hexastat♣
Amphotericin B	Fungizone
Azathioprine	Imuran
Chemotherapeutic agents*	
Chloramphenicol	Chloromycetin, Novochlorocap♣
Chromic phosphate	Phosphocol
Colchicine	(generic only)
Didanosine	Videx
Eflornithine	Ornidyl
Foscarnet sodium	Foscavir
Ganciclovir	Cytovene
Interferon alfa	Actimmune, Alferon, Intron-A, Roferon-A, Wellferon-A♣
Pentamidine	Pentam 300, NebuPent, Pentacarinat♣
Sodium iodide	Iodopen
Zalcitabine	Hivid
Zidovudine	AZT, Retrovir, Novo-AZT♣
Drugs Causing Hemolysis	
Acetohydroxamic acid	Lithostat
Chlorpropamide	Diabinese, Glucamide, Novopropamide♣
Doxapram	Dopram
Glyburide	Diabeta, Micronase, Euglucon♣
Mefenamic acid	Ponstel, Ponstan♣
Menadiol diphosphate	Synkayvite
Methyldopa	Aldomet, Dopamet♣
Nitrofurantoin	Macrodantin, Novofuran♣
Amoxicillin	Amoxil, Augmentin, Apo-Amoxi♣
Penicillin G benzathine	Bicillin, Crystapen
Penicillin V	Pen Vee K, Pen Vee, Nu-Pen-VK♣
Primaquine	(generic only)
Procainamide hydrochloride	Procan-SR, Promide, Pronestyl hydrochloride
Quinidine polygalacturonate	Cardioquin, Quinalan, Novoquinidin♣
Quinine	Legatrin, Quindan
Sulfonamides	Sulfamethoxazole (Gantanol), sulfisoxazole (Gantrisin, Novosoxazole♣)
Tolbutamide	Oramide, Orinase, Apo-Tolbutamide♣, Mobenol♣
Vitamin K	AquaMEPHYTON, Konakion
Drugs Disrupting Platelet Action	
Aspirin	Anacin, Ascriptin, Bufferin, Ecotrin, Entrophen♣, Riphen♣, Triaphen♣
Carbenicillin	Geopen, Pyopen♣
Carindacillin	Geocillin
Dipyridamole	Persantine, Apo-dipyridamole♣, Novodipiradol♣
Moxalactam	Moxam
Pentoxifylline	Trental
Sulfinpyrazone	Anturane, Antazone♣, Novopyrazone♣
Ticarcillin	Ticar
Ticlopidine	Ticlid
Valproic acid	Dalpro, Depakene, Epival♣

Data from United States Pharmacopeial Convention, Inc. (1993). *Volume I: Drug information for the health care professional* (13th ed.). Taunton, MA: Rand McNally.

*General categories of chemotherapeutic agents include alkylating agents, antimitotics, antitumor antibiotics, and antimetabolites.

everything they have eaten during the previous week. This information is helpful in determining the causes of anemias, hypocalcemia, and protein-deficient immunosuppression. Diets high in fat and carbohydrates and low in protein, iron, and vitamins can cause many types of anemia as well as a decrease in the energy-requiring functions of all blood cells.

The nurse also questions the client about alcohol consumption. Chronic alcoholism is associated with nutritional deficiencies and liver impairment, both of which can adversely affect the hematologic system.

Some dietary habits can enhance blood clotting. Diets high in vitamin K may increase the rate of blood coagulation (Furie, 1990). The nurse assesses the amount of raw, green leafy vegetables that the client consumes and whether the client routinely takes supplemental vitamins. The nurse also assesses the amount of calcium consumed, either within the diet or in supplements.

Socioeconomic Status

The nurse assesses the client's ability to understand and follow instructions related to proper diet, specific procedures and tests, and therapeutic regimens. The nurse also determines the client's personal resources, such as finances and social support. A person with a marginal income may have a diet low in iron and protein. The nurse determines which community resources are available to the client. The nurse notes the client's occupation. The nurse asks whether the work involves exposure to noxious or toxic agents.

Current Health Problem

The nurse determines whether the client has noted swelling of lymph nodes or excessive bruising or bleeding and whether the bleeding was spontaneous or induced by trauma. The nurse also inquires about the amount and duration of bleeding after routine dental work. The nurse assesses whether the client has menorrhagia, excessive menstrual flow. Clients are asked to estimate the number of pads or tampons used during the most recent menstrual cycle and whether this amount represents a change from the client's usual pattern of menstrual flow. The nurse asks whether clots are present in the menstrual blood. If clots are present, the client is asked to estimate clot size using coins or fruit for comparison ("clots are dime-sized" or "clots are the size of lemons").

The nurse determines whether the client experiences dyspnea (difficulty breathing) on exertion, palpitations, frequent infections, fevers, recent weight loss, headaches, or paresthesias. Any or all of these symptoms may accompany hematologic disease.

The single most common symptom of anemia is fatigue. The nurse questions the client about feeling tired, needing more rest, or losing endurance during normal activities. Clients are asked to compare the extent and intensity of their activities during the past month with those of the same month a year ago. The nurse asks about other symptoms associated with anemia such as vertigo, tinnitus, anorexia, dysphagia, and a sore tongue.

PHYSICAL ASSESSMENT

The nurse performs a comprehensive physical assessment, inclusive of all body systems. A comprehensive assessment is particularly necessary for the hematologic system because its dysfunction affects the whole body. Certain problems are specific for hematologic assessment in elderly clients, as noted in Chart 38-1.

Assessment of the Integumentary System

The nurse inspects the color of the skin for pallor or jaundice. Mucous membranes and nail beds are observed for pallor or cyanosis. Pallor of the gums, conjunctivae, and palmar creases indicates decreased hemoglobin levels. The gums also are assessed for actively bleeding areas in response to applying light pressure or brushing the teeth with a soft-bristled brush. Any lesions or draining areas are noted. The nurse assesses for signs of bleeding in the form of petechiae and large bruises (ecchymoses). Petechiae are pinpoint hemorrhagic lesions in the skin. Bruises may be confluent or clustered. For hospitalized clients, the nurse determines whether the client is bleeding from obvious sites or from covert sites, such as nasogastric tubes, endotracheal tubes, central lines, peripheral intravenous sites, or Foley catheters. The nurse also notes skin turgor and itching because dry skin or intense itching can indicate hematologic disease.

Transcultural Considerations The nurse may have difficulty in assessing people with darker skin for pallor, jaundice, or the presence of petechiae and bruising. The oral mucous membranes and the conjunctiva of the eye are areas where pallor and cyanosis are more easily detected. The roof of the mouth can be assessed for jaundice. Petechiae may be visible only on the palms of the hands or the soles of the feet. Bruises can be seen as darker areas of skin. In addition, bruises may be palpated as slight swellings or irregular skin surfaces. The nurse asks the client whether pain is present when skin surfaces are touched lightly or palpated. (Chapter 66 provides additional information on techniques for the accurate assessment of darker skin.)

Assessment of the Head and Neck

The nurse notes pallor or ulceration of the oral mucosa. The tongue may be completely smooth in pernicious anemia and iron deficiency anemia. The tongue may be smooth and red in clients with nutritional deficiencies, and these manifestations may be accompanied by fissuring at the corners of the mouth. The nurse observes for jaundice of the sclera.

All lymph node areas are inspected and palpated. The nurse documents any lymph node enlargement, noting whether palpation of the enlarged node causes pain. In addition, the nurse determines whether the enlarged node moves with palpation or remains fixed in position.

Assessment of the Respiratory System

The nurse measures the rate and depth of respiration while the client is at rest as well as during and after mild physical activity (such as walking 20 steps in 10 seconds). The nurse notes whether the client can complete a ten-word sentence without stopping for a breath. The nurse determines whether the client is fatigued easily, whether the client experiences shortness of breath at rest or on exertion, and whether the client requires additional pillows to sleep comfortably at night. Many anemias cause these symptoms.

Assessment of the Cardiovascular System

The nurse observes for the presence of heaves, distended neck veins, edema, or signs of phlebitis. The nurse auscultates for murmurs, gallops, irregular rhythms, and abnormal blood pressure. For clients with anemia, blood pressure tends to be lower than normal. In conditions of hypercellularity, blood pressure is greater than normal. Severe anemias can precipitate right ventricular hypertrophy and subsequent heart disease.

Assessment of the Renal/Urinary System

Because the kidneys are extremely vascular, bleeding problems may manifest as hematuria (blood in the urine). Hematuria may be overt or occult. The nurse inspects a voided sample of urine for color. Hematuria may present as grossly bloody red or dark brownish gold urine. Because blood contains significant amounts of proteins, the nurse tests the urine for the presence of protein with a urine test dipstick. In addition, the nurse tests the urine sample for the presence of occult blood (Hemoccult test).

Assessment of the Musculoskeletal System

Increased rib or sternal tenderness is an important sign that may indicate the presence of hematologic malignancy. The nurse examines the superficial surfaces of all bones by applying intermittent firm pressure with the fingertips. The nurse also assesses the client's range of joint motion and notes whether swelling or joint pain is present.

Assessment of the Abdomen

The normal adult spleen is usually not palpable. Enlarged spleens may be detected by percussion, although palpation is more reliable. The spleen lies just beneath the abdominal wall and is identified by its movement during respiration. During palpation, the client lies in a relaxed, supine position while the nurse, standing on the client's right, palpates the left upper quadrant. The nurse palpates for the spleen gently and cautiously because an enlarged spleen may be tender and easily ruptured.

Palpation of the edge of the liver in the right upper quadrant of the abdomen is commonly used to detect hepatic enlargement. The normal liver may be palpable as much as 4 to 5 cm below the right costal margin but is usually not palpable in the epigastrium. Both the liver and the spleen may be enlarged in hematologic disease.

A common cause of anemia among older adults is a gastrointestinal lesion that bleeds chronically. If the lesion is located in the stomach or the small intestine, obvious blood may not be visible in the stool or such a small amount is passed each day that the client is not aware of it. Therefore, the nurse obtains and tests a stool specimen for the presence of occult blood.

Assessment of the Central Nervous System

A thorough examination of cranial nerves and neurologic function is necessary in many clients with hematologic disease. Vitamin B_{12} deficiency impairs cerebral, olfactory, spinal cord, and peripheral nerve function, and severe chronic deficiency may lead to irreversible neurologic degeneration. A variety of neurologic abnormalities may develop in clients who have hematologic malignancies as a consequence of bleeding, infection, or tumor spread. When the client has a known or suspected bleeding disorder and has experienced any head trauma, the nurse expands the physical assessment to include frequent neurologic checks and mental status examinations (see Chap. 40).

Other important signs and symptoms associated with impaired hematologic function include fever, chills, and night sweats.

PSYCHOSOCIAL ASSESSMENT

The person with hematologic abnormalities may have a chronic illness, such as hemophilia or cancer, or an acute exacerbation of a chronic disease, such as pernicious anemia. In either instance, each person brings his or her own coping style to the illness. After developing a rapport with the client, the nurse can ascertain what coping mechanisms the client has used in the past during illness or other crises.

The nurse also asks the client and family members about social support networks, community resources, and financial health. A problem in any of these areas can interfere with the client's compliance with therapy and, ultimately, recovery.

DIAGNOSTIC ASSESSMENT

Laboratory Tests

In hematologic disease, the most definitive signs are often the laboratory test results. Chart 38–2 lists pertinent laboratory data associated with hematologic function.

TESTS OF CELL NUMBER AND FUNCTION

COMPLETE BLOOD COUNT

A complete blood count (CBC) includes a number of studies:

- Red blood cell (RBC) count
- White blood cell (WBC) count
- Hematocrit
- Hemoglobin level

The RBC count is a count of circulating red blood cells in 1 mm^3 of venous blood. The WBC count is a count of the number of all leukocytes present in 1 mm^3 of venous blood. To ascertain the percentages of different kinds of leukocytes circulating in the blood, a WBC count with differential leukocyte count is performed (Chap. 22). The hemoglobin (Hgb) level represents the total amount of hemoglobin in peripheral blood. The hematocrit (Hct) is calculated as the percentage of red blood cells in the total blood volume.

CHART 38–2

Lab Profile ◆ Hematologic Assessment

Test	Normal Values	Significance of Abnormal Findings
Tests of the Hematologic System		
Red blood cell (RBC) count	• Females: 4.2–5.4 million/mm^3 • Males: 4.7–6.1 million/mm^3	• *Decreased levels* indicate possible anemia or hemorrhage. • *Elevations* indicate possible chronic anoxia or polycythemia vera.
Hemoglobin (Hgb)	• Females: 12–16 g/dL • Males: 14–18 g/dL **Canada:** • Females: 120–150 g/L • Males:140–165 g/L	• Same as for RBC
Hematocrit (Hct)	• Females: 37%–47% • Males: 42%–52%	• Same as for RBC
Mean corpuscular volume (MCV)	• 80–95 μm^3	• *Elevations* indicate possible macrocytic RBCs. • *Decreased levels* indicate possible microcytic RBCs.
Mean corpuscular hemoglobin (MCH)	• 27–31 pg	• *Elevations* are associated with macrocytic anemia. • *Decreased levels* are associated with microcytic anemia.
Mean corpuscular hemoglobin concentration (MCHC)	• 32–36 g/dL (32%–36%)	• *Decreased levels* indicate possible hypochromic cells. • *Elevations* are associated with spherocytosis.
White blood cell (WBC) count	• 5000–10,000/mm^3	• *Elevations* indicate possible infection or leukemia. • *Decreased levels* indicate possible bone marrow failure.
Reticulocyte count	• 0.5%–2% of total RBC	• *Decreased levels* indicate possible inadequate RBC production. • *Elevations* indicate possible polycythemia vera.
Total iron-binding capacity (TIBC)	• 250–420 μg/dL	• *Decreased levels* indicate possible iron deficiency anemia, hemorrhage, or hemolysis. • *Elevations* indicate possible iron deficiency.

CHART 38-2

Lab Profile ◆ Hematologic Assessment *Continued*

Test	Normal Values	Significance of Abnormal Findings
Serum haptoglobin	• 100–150 mg/dL	• *Decreased levels* indicate possible hemolytic liver disease. • *Elevations* indicate possible inflammatory disease.
Iron (Fe)	• 60–190 μg/dL	• *Decreased levels* indicate possible iron deficiency anemia, hemorrhage. • *Elevations* indicate iron excess: hemochromatosis, megaloblastic anemia, certain liver disorders.
Serum ferritin	• Females: 12–300 ng/ml • Males: 10–150 ng/ml	• Same as for iron.
Platelet count	• 150,000–400,000/mm^3	• *Decreased levels* indicate possible bone marrow failure, hypersplenism, or accelerated consumption of platelets. • *Elevations* indicate possible hemorrhage, polycythemia vera, or malignancy.
Hemoglobin electrophoresis	• Hgb A_1: 95%–98% • Hgb A_2: 2%–3% • Hgb F: 0.8%–2% • Hgb S: 0% • Hgb C: 0%	• *Variations* indicate hemoglobinopathies.
Direct Coombs' and indirect Coombs' tests	• Negative	• *Positive findings* indicate antibodies to RBCs.
Coagulation Tests		
Prothrombin time (PT)	• 11–12.5 sec (85%–100%)	• *Elevations* indicate possible deficiency of factors V and VII.
Partial thromboplastin time (PTT)	• 30–40 sec	• *Elevations* indicate possible deficiency of factors II, V, VIII, IX, XI, or XII.
Bleeding time	• 1–9 min	• *Elevations* indicate possible thrombocytopenia, marrow infiltration, or inadequate platelet function.
Euglobulin lysis time	• 90 min–6 hr	• *Decreased levels* indicate possible fibrinolysis.
Fibrin split products (FSPs)	• < 10 μg/mL	• *Elevations* indicate possible disseminated intravascular coagulation or fibrinolysis.

Data from Pagana, K., & Pagana, T. (1990). *Diagnostic testing and nursing implications* (3rd ed.). St. Louis: C. V. Mosby.

In addition to determining the total amounts of any particular blood cell type, CBC studies can measure other variables of the circulating cells. These measurements include the mean corpuscular volume (MCV), the mean corpuscular hemoglobin (MCH), and the mean corpuscular hemoglobin concentration (MCHC). The MCV measures the average volume or size of a single red blood cell. The MCV is useful for classifying anemias. When the MCV is elevated, the cell is said to be macrocytic, or abnormally large, as seen in megaloblastic anemias. When the MCV is decreased, the cell is abnormally small, or microcytic, as seen in iron deficiency anemia. The MCH is the average amount of hemoglobin in a single red blood cell. The MCHC measures the average concentration of hemoglobin in a single red blood cell. When the MCHC is decreased, the cell has a hemoglobin deficiency and is hypochromic, as in iron deficiency anemia.

RETICULOCYTE COUNT

Another hematologic test that is often helpful is the reticulocyte count, which determines bone marrow function. A reticulocyte is an immature red blood cell, and an elevated reticulocyte count indicates increased red blood cell (RBC) production by the bone marrow. Normally, about 2% of circulating RBCs are reticulocytes. An elevated reticulocyte count is desirable in an anemic client or after hemorrhage. Such an elevation indicates that the bone marrow is responding appropriately to a decrease in the total red blood cell mass. An elevated reticulocyte count without a precipitating cause may indicate pathologic conditions, such as polycythemia vera.

HEMOGLOBIN ELECTROPHORESIS

Hemoglobin electrophoresis detects abnormal forms of hemoglobin, such as hemoglobin S in sickle cell disease. Hemoglobin A is the major component of hemoglobin in the normal red blood cell.

LEUKOCYTE ALKALINE PHOSPHATASE

Leukocyte alkaline phosphatase (LAP) is an enzyme produced by normal mature neutrophils. Elevated LAP levels occur during episodes of infection or stress. An elevated neutrophil count without an accompanying elevation in LAP level is associated with chronic myelogenous leukemia.

COOMBS' TEST

The Coombs' test is an important hematologic test used for blood typing. It exists in two forms:

- Direct Coombs' test
- Indirect Coombs' test

The direct test detects the presence of antibodies against red blood cells (RBCs) (also called antiglobulins) that may be attached to a person's RBCs. Although healthy people can make these antibodies, certain diseases, such as systemic lupus erythematosus, mononucleosis, and lymphomas, are associated with the production of antibodies directed against the client's own RBCs. The presence of these antibodies usually causes a hemolytic anemia.

The indirect Coombs' test detects the presence of circulating antibodies against RBCs. The test is used to determine whether the client has serum antibodies to the type of RBCs that he or she is about to receive by blood transfusion.

SERUM FERRITIN, TRANSFERRIN, AND TOTAL IRON-BINDING CAPACITY

Serum ferritin, transferrin, and the total iron-binding capacity (TIBC) test are measures of iron levels. Abnormal levels of iron and TIBC are characteristic of many diseases, including iron deficiency anemia.

The serum ferritin test measures the quantity of iron present as free iron in the plasma. Because the amount of serum ferritin is proportionally related to the amount of intracellular iron, representing 1% of the total body iron stores, the serum ferritin level provides a means to assess a person's total iron stores. People who have serum ferritin levels within 10 g of the normal range for their sex have adequate iron stores. People whose serum ferritin levels are more than 10 g lower than the normal range for their sex have inadequate iron stores and have difficulty recovering from any hemorrhagic event.

Transferrin is a protein that transports iron from the gastrointestinal tract to the intracellular storage sites. Because the amount of transferrin cannot be easily measured, measuring the amount of iron that can be bound to serum transferrin provides an indirect way to determine whether an adequate amount of transferrin is present. This test is the total iron-binding capacity test. In healthy people, only about 30% of the transferrin is bound to iron in the blood. One can measure the TIBC by taking a sample of blood and adding measured amounts of iron to it. When the blood no longer binds the iron but allows it to precipitate, the TIBC can be calculated. TIBC increases when a person is deficient in serum iron and stored iron levels. Such a value indicates that an adequate amount of transferrin is present but less than 30% of it is bound to serum iron.

TESTS MEASURING BLEEDING AND COAGULATION

CAPILLARY FRAGILITY TEST

The capillary fragility test, or Rumpel-Leede test, measures vascular hemostatic function. The test is done by increasing intracapillary pressure in the arm by occluding venous outflow or by applying controlled negative pressure to a skin area. Usually, a blood pressure cuff is inflated to a pressure halfway between the systolic and diastolic pressures; inflation is maintained for 5 minutes. The petechiae that appear distal to the cuff are counted. Normally, five to ten petechiae appear. The capillary fragility test can help determine whether excessive bleeding or bruising results from increased capillary fragility rather than impaired platelet action.

BLEEDING TIME TEST

The bleeding time test evaluates vascular and platelet activity during hemostasis. A small incision (using a special spring-loaded lancet that ensures uniform wound depth) is made in the forearm while a blood pressure cuff remains inflated at 40 mmHg. Blood is blotted from the site at 30-second intervals, and the time required for the bleeding to stop is recorded. Normal bleeding time ranges from 1 to 9 minutes.

PROTHROMBIN TIME

The prothrombin time (PT) evaluates the adequacy of the extrinsic coagulation cascade. PT is prolonged when factors II, V, VII, and X are deficient or when liver disease is present. Sodium warfarin (Coumadin, Warfilone✱) therapy is monitored by the use of PT levels. Appropriate warfarin therapy prolongs the PT by 1½ to 2 times the client's normal PT value. The PT test results are given in seconds, along with a control value. A normal PT is nearly equal to the control value.

PARTIAL THROMBOPLASTIN TIME

The partial thromboplastin time (PTT) assesses the intrinsic coagulation cascade. It evaluates the presence of factors II, V, VIII, IX, XI, and XII. When any of these factors is deficient, as in hemophilia or disseminated intravascular coagulation (DIC), the

PTT is prolonged. Because factors II, IX, and X are vitamin K–dependent and are produced in the liver, liver disease can decrease their concentration and prolong the PTT. Heparin (Calciparin, Liquémin, Hepalean✱) therapy is monitored by PTT. Desired ranges for therapeutic anticoagulation are 1½ to 2½ times normal values.

PLATELET AGGLUTINATION/AGGREGATION

Platelet aggregation, or the ability to clump, can be tested by mixing the client's plasma with a substance called ristocetin. The degree of aggregation is noted. Aggregation can be impaired in von Willebrand's disease and during the use of a variety of drugs such as aspirin, anti-inflammatory agents, and psychotropic agents.

Radiographic Examinations

Assessment of the client with a suspected hematologic abnormality can include radioisotopic imaging. Isotopes are used to evaluate the bone marrow for sites of active erythropoiesis and sites of iron storage. Radioactive colloids are routinely used to determine organ size and liver and spleen function.

The client is given a radioactive isotope intravenously about 3 hours before the procedure. The client is then taken to the nuclear medicine department for the scan, where he or she must lie still for about an hour. There are no special client preparations or follow-up care for these tests.

Standard x-rays may be used in the diagnosis of some hematologic disorders. For example, multiple myeloma causes a characteristic destruction of bone with a "Swiss cheese" appearance on x-ray.

Other Diagnostic Tests

BONE MARROW ASPIRATION AND BIOPSY

Bone marrow aspiration or biopsy is frequently done to evaluate the client's hematologic status when other tests show persistent abnormal findings. Results can provide important information about bone marrow function, including red blood cell, white blood cell, and platelet production. Bone marrow aspiration and biopsy are similar procedures. In a bone marrow aspiration, cells and fluids from the bone marrow are obtained by suction. In a bone marrow biopsy, solid tissue and cells are obtained by coring out an area of bone marrow with a large-bore needle.

A physician's order and a signed, informed consent are obtained from the client before a bone marrow aspiration or biopsy is done. Bone marrow aspiration may be performed by a physician, a sanctioned clinical nurse specialist, or a physician assistant, depending on the agency's policy and regional law. The procedure may be performed at the client's bedside, in an examination room, in a laboratory, or in a physician's office.

On learning what specific tests will be performed on the marrow, the nurse consults the procedure manual and the hematology laboratory to determine how to handle the specimen. Some tests necessitate the addition of heparin or other special solutions to the specimen.

CLIENT PREPARATION Most clients experience anxiety or fear before a bone marrow aspiration. Clients who have experienced a bone marrow aspiration previously may have less or more anxiety, depending on how the previous experience was perceived. The nurse can help reduce anxiety and allay fears by providing accurate information and continuous emotional support. Some clients like to have their hands held during the procedure; other clients may want the nurse to hug or hold their entire upper body during the procedure.

The nurse explains the procedure to the client and tells the client that the nurse will be present during the entire procedure. Occasionally, a friend or family member is permitted to be present to hold the client's hand and provide additional emotional support. If a local anesthetic is to be used, the nurse tells the client that the injection will be felt as a stinging or burning sensation. The nurse tells the client to expect a heavy sensation of pressure and pushing while the needle is being inserted. Some clients also can hear a crunching sound or feel a scraping sensation as the needle punctures the bone. The nurse explains that as the marrow is being aspirated by mild suction in the syringe, a sensation of pulling will be experienced. This sensation, although brief, is painful. If a biopsy is performed, the client may feel more pressure and discomfort as the needle is rotated into the bone.

The client is assisted onto an examining table, and the site is exposed. The most common site for bone marrow aspiration or biopsy is the iliac crest. If this site is not available or if more marrow is needed, the sternum can be used. If the iliac crest is the site, the client is usually placed in the prone position, although the client can be in the side-lying position. Depending on the tests to be performed on the specimen, a laboratory technician may also be present to ensure appropriate handling of the specimen.

PROCEDURE The procedure usually lasts from 5 to 15 minutes. Clients may be uncomfortable and may experience pain. The type and the amount of anesthesia or sedation depend on:

- The physician's preference
- The client's preference and previous experience with bone marrow aspiration and biopsy
- The setting

A local anesthetic solution might be injected into the skin around the site. The client may receive a mild tranquilizer or a rapid-acting agent for conscious sedation, such as midazolam hydrochloride (Versed) or lorazepam (Ativan, Apo-Lorazepam✱, Novolorazem✱). Some clients do well with guided imagery or techniques for autohypnosis.

The procedure for either aspiration or biopsy is invasive, and sterile precautions are observed. The skin over the site is cleaned with a disinfectant solution. For an aspiration, the needle is inserted with a twisting motion and the marrow is aspirated by pulling back on the plunger of the syringe. When sufficient marrow has been aspirated to ensure accurate analysis, the needle is carefully and rapidly withdrawn while the tissues are supported at the site. For a biopsy, a small skin incision is made and the biopsy needle is inserted through the skin opening. Pressure and several twisting motions are performed to ensure coring and loosening of an adequate amount of marrow tissue. External pressure is applied to the site until hemostasis is ensured. A pressure dressing or sandbags may be applied to minimize bleeding at the site.

FOLLOW-UP CARE The site is covered with a dressing after hemostasis is achieved. The site of the aspiration is observed closely for 24 hours for signs of bleeding and infection. A mild analgesic (aspirin free) is prescribed for the discomfort. Ice packs are applied over the aspiration sites to limit bruising. The nurse instructs the client to inspect the sites every 2 hours for the first 24 hours and to note the presence of active bleeding or bruising. The nurse advises clients not to engage in contact sports or any other activity that might result in trauma to the site for 48 hours.

Information obtained from bone marrow aspiration or biopsy reflects the degree and quality of bone marrow activity present. The counts made on a marrow specimen can indicate whether stem cells, blast cells, committed cells, and more mature cell forms are present in the expected quantities and proportions. In addition, bone marrow aspiration or biopsy can confirm the presence of cancer cells that have spread from other tumor sites.

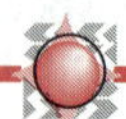

IMPLICATIONS FOR NURSING RESEARCH

Nursing research relevant to the hematologic system has focused on characterizing the manifestations of fatigue. Other questions to be answered include:

- ◆ What physical assessment findings accurately reflect anemia in people with dark skin?
- ◆ What nonpharmacologic nursing interventions are effective for reducing the discomfort of clients undergoing bone marrow aspiration or bone marrow biopsy?
- ◆ Is there a difference in iron stores and total iron-binding capacity among people older than 65 years who take daily vitamin supplements with iron compared with those of people older than 65 years who do not take daily vitamin supplements?
- ◆ Is there a role for erythropoietin therapy in the treatment of anemia caused by blood loss?

SELECTED BIBLIOGRAPHY

Ashby, B., Daniel, J., & Smith, J. (1990). Mechanisms of platelet activation and inhibition. *Hematology/Oncology Clinics of North America, 4*(1), 1–26.

Colman, R., Hirsch, J., Marder, V., & Salzman, E. (1994). *Hemostasis and thrombosis: Basic principles and clinical practice* (3rd ed.). Philadelphia: J. B. Lippincott.

Erslev, A., & Lichtman, M. (1990). Structure and function of the marrow. In W. Williams, E. Beutler, A. Erslev, & M. Lichtman (Eds.), *Hematology* (4th ed., pp. 37–47). New York: McGraw-Hill.

Fairbanks, V., & Beutler, E. (1990). Iron metabolism. In W. Williams, E. Beutler, A. Erslev, & M. Lichtman (Eds.), *Hematology* (4th ed., pp. 329–339). New York: McGraw-Hill.

Furie, B. (1990). Disorders of the vitamin K–dependent coagulation factors. In W. Williams, E. Beutler, A. Erslev, & M. Lichtman (Eds.), *Hematology* (4th ed., pp. 1510–1513). New York: McGraw-Hill.

Gewirtz, A., & Hoffman, R. (1990). Human megakaryocyte production: Cell biology and clinical considerations. *Hematology/Oncology Clinics of North America, 4*(1), 43–64.

Guyton, A. (1991). *Textbook of medical physiology* (8th ed.). Philadelphia: W. B. Saunders.

*Haeuber, D., & DiJulio, J. (1989). Hemopoietic colony stimulating factors: An overview. *Oncology Nursing Forum, 16*(2), 247–255.

Hays, K. (1990). Physiology of normal bone marrow. *Seminars in Oncology Nursing, 6*(1), 3–8.

Holmes, A., Hatch, J., & Robinson, G. (1992). A lay education approach to sickle cell disease education. *Journal of the National Black Nurses Association, 5*(2), 26–36.

Metcalf, D. (1992). Hemopoietic regulators. *Trends in Biochemical Sciences, 17*(8), 286–289.

Pagana, K., & Pagana, T. (1990). *Diagnostic testing and nursing implications* (3rd ed.). St. Louis: C. V. Mosby.

Pollin, S., & DeLuca, E. (1992). How to use the new weapon against anemia. *RN, 55*(1), 36–38.

*Rapaport, S. (1987). *Introduction to hematology* (2nd ed.). Philadelphia: J. B. Lippincott.

*Simmons, A. (1989). *Hematology: A combined theoretical and technical approach.* Philadelphia: W. B. Saunders.

United States Pharmacopeial Convention, Inc. (1993). *Volume I: Drug information for the health care professional* (13th ed.). Taunton, MA: Rand McNally.

Williams, W., Beutler, E., Erslev, A., & Lichtman, M. (1990). *Hematology* (4th ed.). New York: McGraw-Hill.

Williams, W., & Nelson, D. (1992). Examination of the marrow. In W. Williams, E. Beutler, A. Erslev, & M. Lichtman (Eds.), *Hematology* (4th ed., pp. 24–34). New York: McGraw-Hill.

Workman, M., Ellerhorst-Ryan, J., & Koertge, V. (1993). *Nursing care of the immunocompromised patient.* Philadelphia: W. B. Saunders.

SUGGESTED READINGS

Haeuber, D., & DiJulio, J. (1989). Hemopoietic colony stimulating factors: An overview. *Oncology Nursing Forum, 16*(2), 247–255.

This clinically focused article explains the physiologic actions and clinical uses of the currently approved colony-stimulating factors. Side effects and nursing implications are addressed.

Hays, K. (1990). Physiology of normal bone marrow. *Seminars in Oncology Nursing, 6*(1), 3–8.

This excellent article describes the blood-forming functions of bone marrow. Terms are explained simply and concisely. The reference list contains both informational and research-based sources.

Pollin, S., & DeLuca, E. (1992). How to use the new weapon against anemia. *RN, 55*(1), 36–38.

This article provides a simple description of the uses of erythropoietin to combat anemia. The clinical situation presented focuses on clients who have anemia due to chronic renal failure. Nursing issues such as complications of erythropoietin use and contraindications are discussed.

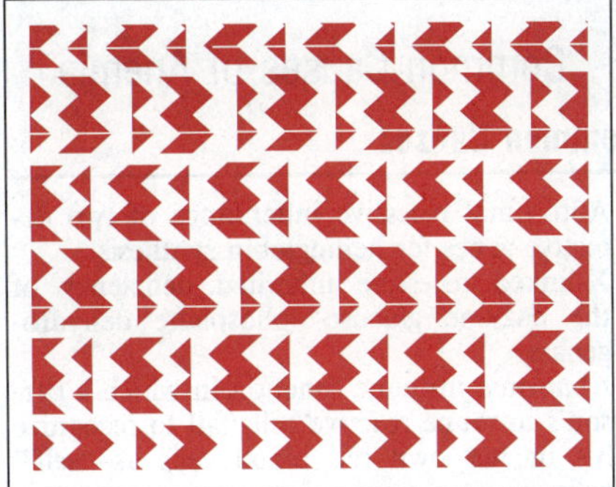

CHAPTER 39

Interventions for Clients with Hematologic Problems

CHAPTER HIGHLIGHTS

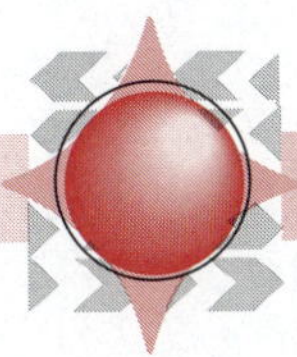

Disorders of the hematologic system can involve problems in the synthesis, function, or normal destruction of any cellular component of the blood. Depending on the type, degree, and rate of onset of the specific disorder, clients may experience minimal disruption of their activities of daily living (ADL) or devastating, life-threatening crises. Because all body tissues and organs use blood components to maintain normal physiologic function, disorders of the hematologic system may manifest as altered function in many unrelated organs.

RED BLOOD CELL DISORDERS

As discussed in Chapter 38, the major cellular component of the blood is the population of red blood cells (RBCs), or erythrocytes. Physiologic function depends on maintaining the circulating volume of erythrocytes within the normal range for the person's age and gender and ensuring that the erythrocytes can perform their normal functions. Disorders of RBCs include problems in RBC production, function, and destruction. These problems may result in an insufficient number or function of RBCs (anemia) or an excess of RBCs (polycythemia).

ANEMIA

Anemia is defined as a reduction in either the number of red blood cells (RBCs), the quantity of hemoglobin, or the hematocrit (the volume of packed RBCs per deciliter, of blood). Anemia is a clinical sign, rather than a diagnosis, because it is a manifestation of a number of abnormal conditions. Anemia can result from:

- Dietary deficiency states
- Hereditary disorders
- Bone marrow disease
- Bleeding states

There are many types and causes of anemia. Some anemias arise from a deficiency in one or more of the components needed to make fully functional RBCs. Such anemias can be caused by deficiencies of iron, vitamin B_{12}, folic acid, or intrinsic factor. Additional causes include decreased development of the RBC line precursors, decreased rate of erythrocyte production, or increased destruction of RBCs. Table 39–1 lists common causes of various types of anemia.

Despite the many causes of anemia, the effects of anemia on the client (Chart 39–1) and the corresponding nursing care are similar for all types of anemia. Many organ system disorders can result in an anemic condition through chronic blood loss. Any client who has anemia requires a detailed assessment to determine the cause. This part of the chapter covers the most common types of anemia and their interventions, followed by a collaborative management plan focusing on nursing diagnoses common to all clients with anemia.

TABLE 39–1 Common Causes of Anemia

Type of Anemia	Common Causes
Sickle cell anemia	• Autosomal recessive inheritance of two defective genes for hemoglobin synthesis.
G6PD deficiency anemia	• X-linked recessive inherited deficiency of the enzyme glucose-6-phosphate dehydrogenase.
Autoimmune hemolytic anemia	• Abnormal immune function in which a person's immune reactive cells fail to recognize his or her own red blood cells as "self" cells.
Iron deficiency anemia	• Inadequate iron intake due to: • Iron-deficient diet • Chronic alcoholism • Malabsorption syndromes • Partial gastrectomy • Rapid metabolic (anabolic) activity due to: • Pregnancy • Adolescence • Infection
Vitamin B_{12} deficiency anemia	• Dietary deficiency • Failure to absorb vitamin B_{12} from intestinal tract due to: • Partial gastrectomy • Pernicious anemia
Folic acid deficiency anemia	• Dietary deficiency • Malabsorption syndromes • Drugs: • Oral contraceptives • Anticonvulsants • Methotrexate
Aplastic anemia	• Exposure to myelotoxic agents • Radiation • Benzene • Chloromycetin • Alkylating agents • Antimetabolites • Sulfonamides • Insecticides • Viral infection (unproven) • Epstein-Barr virus • Hepatitis B • Cytomegalovirus

Anemias Resulting from Increased Destruction of Red Blood Cells

Sickle Cell Disease

OVERVIEW

Sickle cell disease is an autosomal codominant hereditary disorder that causes a single amino acid change in the beta chain of the hemoglobin molecule, creating an abnormal type of hemoglobin. This abnormal hemoglobin is *hemoglobin S (Hb S)* instead of hemoglobin A (Hb A). Hb S is sensitive to changes in the oxygen content of the red blood cell (RBC). Insufficient oxygen causes the abnormal beta chains to contract and pile together within the cell, distorting the overall shape of the RBC. These cells assume a sickle shape (Fig. 39–1). When this happens, the cells become rigid, clump together, and form clusters that obstruct capillary blood flow. This condition leads to further tissue hypoxia (reduced oxygen supply) and more sickling, causing blood vessel obstructions and infarctions in the locally affected tissues. Situations that precipitate sickling include:

- Hypoxia
- Vascular stasis
- Low environmental and/or body temperatures
- Acidosis
- Strenuous exercise
- Anesthesia
- Dehydration
- Infections

Usually, sickled cells resume a normal shape when the precipitating condition is removed and proper oxygenation occurs. However, membranes of the cells can become damaged over time, with irreversibly sickled cells the end result. Additionally, the altered membranes of cells with Hb S make them more fragile and more easily destroyed in the spleen and in other organs that have long, twisted capillary pathways. The average life span of a sickle cell is approximately 20 days, considerably less than the 120-day life span of normal RBCs (Williams et al., 1990). This reduced life span is responsible for hemolytic anemia in clients with sickle cell disease.

When the client inherits one abnormal gene of the pair regulating hemoglobin structure, the condition is

CHART 39–1

Key Features of Anemia

Integumentary Manifestations

- Pallor, especially of the ears, the nail beds, the palmar creases, the conjunctiva, and around the mouth
- Cool to the touch
- Intolerance of cold temperatures

Cardiovascular Manifestations

- Tachycardia at basal activity levels, increasing with activity and during and immediately after meals
- Murmurs and gallops heard on auscultation when anemia is severe
- Orthostatic hypotension

Respiratory Manifestations

- Dyspnea on exertion

Neurologic Manifestations

- Increased somnolence and fatigue
- Headache

called *sickle cell trait.* The client can pass on the condition to offspring but has only mild manifestations of the disease under severe precipitating conditions because only about 50% of the person's hemoglobin is abnormal.

Transcultural Considerations Sickle cell disease occurs frequently in African-Americans as well as in African, Mediterranean, Asian, Caribbean, Middle Eastern, and Central American populations (Wethers et al., 1989). Approximately one of every ten African-Americans has the sickle cell trait. One of every 400 African-American infants born has inherited two abnormal genes (one from each parent) and has overt sickle cell disease. People who have sickle cell disease have easily induced clinical manifestations and chronic anemia as a result of increased RBC destruction.

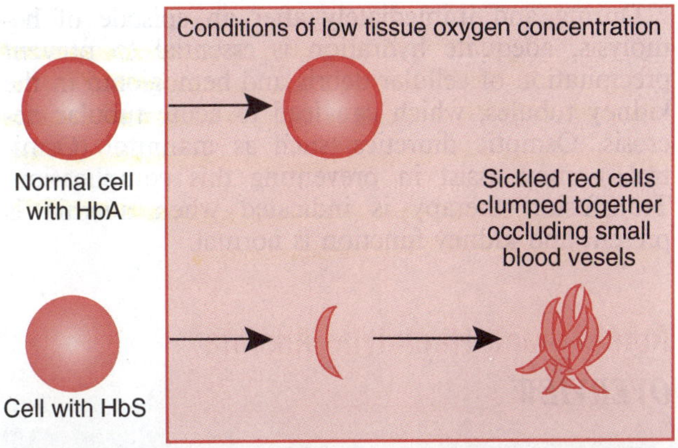

FIGURE 39–1 ♦ Red blood cell actions under conditions of low tissue oxygenation. (© M. Linda Workman, 1992. All rights reserved.)

The client with sickle cell disease experiences periodic episodes of extensive cellular sickling called *crises.* Many clients are in good health much of the time, with crises occurring sporadically in response to precipitating conditions that stimulate local or systemic hypoxemia (deficient oxygen in the blood). The crises have a sudden onset and can be as frequent as weekly or as seldom as once a year.

Pain is the most common symptom clients experience during sickle cell crisis (Bojanowski, 1989). Jaundice may also be present as a result of increased RBC destruction and release of bilirubin. Tissue damage and scarring as a result of infarcts are common complications of sickle cell disease. Infarcts may occur in any tissue but are most common in organs of the chest and abdomen, especially the spleen. Other clinical manifestations vary with the site of tissue damage (Chart 39–2).

CHART 39–2

Key Features of Sickle Cell Disease

Hematologic Manifestations

- Fragile red blood cells that sickle and clump under conditions of low tissue oxygenation, venous stasis, lower environmental or body temperature
  - Anemia
- Tissue hypoxia and ischemia
  - Pain
  - Hardened, enlarged spleen

Respiratory Manifestations

- Pulmonary infarcts
  - Chest pain
  - Pneumonia

Genitourinary Manifestations

- Renal ischemia
  - Decreased urine concentration
- Priapism

Cardiovascular Manifestations

- Cardiac ischemia
  - Myocardial infarctions
  - Chest pain
  - Congestive heart failure
- Cerebral vascular accidents

Musculoskeletal Manifestations

- Necrosis of femur head
- Pain in extremities with moderate physical exercise

COLLABORATIVE MANAGEMENT

The management of sickle cell disease focuses on prevention and treatment of crises. Clients are taught to avoid the specific activities that lead to hypoxia and hypoxemia. In addition, clients are taught to recognize the early signs and symptoms of crisis so that appropriate treatment can be initiated early to prevent undue pain, complications, and permanent tissue damage. Additionally, clients are counseled about the hereditary aspects of this problem, and information concerning prenatal diagnosis and options is offered.

The treatment of crises includes:

- Pain management
- Fluid replacement to ensure adequate hydration and maintenance of blood flow
- Oxygen therapy
- Correction of the specific condition causing or contributing to hypoxia

Chart 39–3 lists specific priorities for the nurse caring for clients with sickle cell crisis. Transfusions usually are not administered unless profound anemia (aplastic crisis) is present without an accompanying vascular occlusion. In some treatment centers, bone marrow transplantation is being performed in an attempt to permanently correct the problem of abnormal hemoglobin. Because bone marrow transplantation is expensive and may result in chronic and life-threatening complications, its risks and benefits need to be seriously considered for each client.

CHART 39–3

Nursing Care Highlight ◆ The Client in Sickle Cell Crisis

- Administer oxygen.
- Administer pain medication as ordered.
- Hydrate the client with normal saline intravenously and with beverages of choice (without caffeine) orally.
- Remove any constrictive clothing.
- Encourage the client to keep extremities extended to promote venous return.
- Do not raise the knee gatch of the bed.
- Elevate the head of the bed no more than 30 degrees.
- Keep room temperature at or above 72° F.
- Avoid taking blood pressure with external cuff.
- Check circulation in extremities every hour:
  - Pulse oximetry of fingers and toes
  - Capillary refill
  - Peripheral pulses
  - Toe temperature

Glucose-6-Phosphate Dehydrogenase Deficiency Anemia

OVERVIEW

Many forms of congenital hemolytic anemia result from defects or deficiencies of one or more enzymes within the red blood cell (RBC). Most of these enzymes are needed to complete some critical step in intracellular energy production. More than 200 such disorders have been identified. The most common type of congenital hemolytic anemia is associated with a deficiency of the enzyme glucose-6-phosphate dehydrogenase (G6PD). This disease is inherited as an X-linked recessive disorder and affects about 15% of all African-American males (Cotran et al., 1989).

G6PD stimulates critical reactions in the glycolytic pathway. Because RBCs contain no mitochondria (sites of high-efficiency production of the energy compound adenosine triphosphate [ATP] through the Krebs cycle), active glycolysis is essential for energy metabolism. Cells that have reduced amounts of G6PD are more susceptible to hemolysis during exposure to specific drugs (e.g., phenacetin, sulfonamides, aspirin [acetylsalicylic acid], quinine derivatives, thiazide diuretics, and vitamin K derivatives) and toxins (Williams et al., 1990). Newly produced RBCs from clients with G6PD deficiency have relatively sufficient quantities of G6PD; however, as the cells age, the concentration of this enzyme diminishes drastically.

After exposure to any of the above-mentioned agents, the client experiences acute intravascular hemolysis lasting from 7 to 12 days. During this acute phase, the client has anemia and jaundice. The hemolytic reaction is self-limited because only older erythrocytes, containing less G6PD, are destroyed.

COLLABORATIVE MANAGEMENT

It is imperative that the precipitating drug or the agent responsible for the hemolytic reaction be identified and totally removed. People should be screened for this deficiency before donating blood because administration of cells deficient in G6PD can be hazardous for the recipient.

During and immediately after an episode of hemolysis, adequate hydration is essential to prevent precipitation of cellular debris and hemoglobin in the kidney tubules, which can lead to acute tubular necrosis. Osmotic diuretics, such as mannitol (Osmitrol✱), may assist in preventing this complication. Transfusion therapy is indicated when anemia is present and kidney function is normal.

Autoimmune Hemolytic Anemia

OVERVIEW

Increased red blood cell (RBC) destruction through the process of hemolysis can occur in response to many situations, including:

- Mechanical trauma
- Microbial infection (especially malarial infections)
- Autoimmune reactions directed against self blood components

All of these situations increase the rate at which RBCs are destroyed by causing lysis (disintegration) of the RBC membrane. The most common types of hemolytic anemias in industrialized countries are the autoimmune hemolytic anemias (Packman & Leddy, 1990).

In clients with autoimmune hemolytic anemia, RBC destruction occurs because the immune system components attack their own RBCs. The exact mechanism that causes immune components to no longer recognize the client's own blood cells as self and to initiate destructive processes against the RBCs is not known. Some hemolytic anemias are present with other autoimmune disorders (such as systemic lupus erythematosus) or lymphoproliferative disorders. Regardless of the cause, the RBC is viewed as nonself by the immune system and is destroyed.

There are two types of autoimmune hemolytic anemia: warm and cold antibody.

The *warm antibody* type is usually associated with IgG antibody excess. These antibodies are most active at 37°C (98° F) and may be stimulated by drugs, chemicals, or other autoimmune problems.

The *cold antibody* type is associated with fixation of complement proteins on IgM. This action occurs best at 30° C (86° F) and is commonly associated with a Raynaud-like response in which the arteries in the distal extremities constrict profoundly in response to cold temperatures or stress.

COLLABORATIVE MANAGEMENT

Treatment depends on clinical severity. Steroid therapy for mild to moderate immunosuppression is the first line of treatment and is temporarily effective in most clients. Splenectomy and more intensive immunosuppressive therapy with cyclophosphamide (Cytoxan, Procytox✱) and azathioprine (Imuran) may be instituted if steroid therapy fails. Plasma exchange therapy to remove attacking antibodies is effective for clients who do not respond to immunosuppressive therapy (Packman & Leddy, 1990).

Anemias Resulting from Decreased Production of Red Blood Cells

Anemias associated with decreased production of red blood cells (RBCs) can result from pathologic alterations in any of a variety of physiologic mechanisms. Some anemias arise from failure or inability of the bone marrow to properly synthesize RBCs. Other anemias occur because the body cannot synthesize or absorb a specific component necessary for RBC production.

Iron Deficiency Anemia

OVERVIEW

The adult body contains between 2 and 6 g of iron, depending on the size of the person and the amount of hemoglobin in the cells. Approximately two thirds of this iron is contained in hemoglobin; the other third is stored in the bone marrow, spleen, liver, and muscle (see Chap. 38). If a person has an iron deficiency, the iron stores are depleted first, then hemoglobin is reduced. As a result, RBCs are small (microcytic) and the client has relatively mild manifestations of anemia, including weakness and pallor.

Iron deficiency anemia is the most common type of anemia and can result from:

- Blood loss
- Increased metabolic energy demands
- Syndromes of gastrointestinal malabsorption
- Dietary inadequacy

The basic problem of iron deficiency anemia is a decreased supply of iron for the developing RBC. Iron deficiency anemia can occur at any age but is more frequently noted in women, the elderly, and people with poor diets.

COLLABORATIVE MANAGEMENT

The primary treatment of clients with iron deficiency anemia is to increase the oral intake of iron. Iron is obtained from food. Common food sources of iron are listed in Table 39–2. An adequate diet supplies a person with about 12 to 15 mg of iron per day, of which only 5% to 10% is absorbed. The amount of iron normally absorbed daily from the diet is sufficient to meet the needs of healthy men and healthy women after the childbearing age, but it is not sufficient to supply the greater needs of menstruating women and adolescents during growth spurts. Fortunately, if iron intake is inadequate or if bleeding or pregnancy occurs, the gastrointestinal (GI) tract is capable of increasing the absorption of iron to about 20% to 30% of the total daily intake (Fairbanks & Beutler, 1990).

Vitamin B_{12} Deficiency Anemia

OVERVIEW

Proper production of red blood cells (RBCs) depends on adequate deoxyribonucleic acid (DNA) synthesis in the precursor cells so that mitosis and further maturation into functional erythrocytes occur. All DNA synthesis requires adequate amounts of folic acid (folate) to ensure the availability of the nucleotide thymidine to stimulate DNA synthesis. One function of vitamin B_{12} is to serve as an essential cofactor to activate the enzyme system responsible for

TABLE 39–2 Common Food Sources of Iron, Vitamin B_{12}, and Folic Acid

Essential Element	Common Food Source
Iron	• Liver (especially pork and lamb) • Red meat • Organ meats • Kidney beans • Whole wheat breads and cereals • Green leafy vegetables • Carrots • Egg yolks • Raisins
Vitamin B_{12}	• Liver • Organ meats • Dried beans • Nuts • Green leafy vegetables • Citrus fruit • Brewer's yeast
Folid acid	• Liver • Organ meats • Eggs • Cabbage • Broccoli • Brussels sprouts

Data from Pennington, J. (1992). *Bowe's and Church's food values of portions commonly used* (16th ed.). Philadelphia: Lippincott.

transporting folic acid from the extracellular fluid into the cell, where DNA synthesis occurs. Thus, a deficiency of vitamin B_{12} indirectly causes anemia by inhibiting folic acid transportation and limiting DNA synthesis in RBC precursor cells. As a result, these precursor cells undergo improper DNA synthesis and mitosis. Instead, the immature precursor cells increase in size and only a few are released from the bone marrow. This type of anemia is called *megaloblastic* (macrocytic) because of the large size of these abnormal cells.

A deficiency of vitamin B_{12} can result from either inadequate intake of this substance (dietary deficiency) or lack of absorption of ingested vitamin B_{12} from the intestinal tract. Anemia caused by failure to absorb vitamin B_{12} (*pernicious* anemia) results from a deficiency of intrinsic factor (normally secreted by the gastric mucosa), which is necessary for intestinal absorption of vitamin B_{12}.

Anemia that results from vitamin B_{12} deficiency may be mild or severe, usually develops slowly, and produces few symptoms. Clients usually have severe pallor and slight jaundice. Clients also have glossitis (a smooth, beefy-red tongue), fatigue, and weight loss. Because vitamin B_{12} also is necessary for normal nervous system functioning, especially of the peripheral nerves, clients with pernicious may also have neurologic abnormalities, such as paresthesias (abnormal sensations) in the feet and the hands and disturbances of balance and gait (Chart 39–4).

CHART 39–4

Key Features of Vitamin B_{12} Deficiency Anemia

- Severe pallor
- Slight jaundice
- Smooth, beefy red tongue
- Fatigue
- Weight loss
- Paresthesias of the hands and feet
- Difficulty with gait

COLLABORATIVE MANAGEMENT

When anemia is the result of a dietary deficiency of vitamin B_{12}, clients must increase their intake of foods rich in vitamin B_{12} (animal proteins, eggs, dairy products). Vitamin supplements may be prescribed when anemia is severe. For clients who have anemia as a result of a deficiency of intrinsic factor, vitamin B_{12} must be administered parenterally on a regular schedule (usually weekly for initial treatment, then monthly for maintenance).

Folic Acid Deficiency Anemia

OVERVIEW

In addition to folic acid deficiencies produced by vitamin B_{12} deficiency, primary folic acid deficiency can also cause a megaloblastic anemia. Clinical manifestations are similar to those of vitamin B_{12} deficiency without the accompanying nervous system manifestations because folic acid does not appear to affect neuronal function. The absence of neurologic problems is an important diagnostic finding because it differentiates folic acid deficiency from vitamin B_{12} deficiency. The disease develops slowly, and symptoms may be attributed to other coexisting diseases. Gastrointestinal disturbances include dyspepsia and glossitis.

There are three common causes of folic acid deficiency:

- Poor nutrition
- Malabsorption
- Drugs

Poor nutrition, especially a diet lacking in leafy green vegetables, liver, yeast, citrus fruits, dried beans, nuts, and greens, is the most common cause. A diet that is low in folic acid is seen in chronic alcohol abusers and in people receiving parenteral alimentation without folic acid supplement.

Malabsorption syndromes, such as Crohn's disease, are the second most common cause of folic acid deficiency.

Additionally, the ingestion of specific drugs impedes the absorption and conversion of folic acid to its active form (tetrahydrofolate) and can also lead to folic acid deficiency and anemia. Such drugs include methotrexate, some anticonvulsants, and oral contraceptives.

COLLABORATIVE MANAGEMENT

Folic acid deficiency anemia is largely preventable. Prevention is aimed at identifying high-risk clients, such as the older, debilitated alcoholic; others prone to malnutrition; and those with increased folic acid requirements. A diet high in folic acid and vitamin B_{12} also prevents a deficiency (see Table 39–2). By routinely incorporating questions about dietary habits in a health history, the nurse can determine which clients are at risk for diet-induced anemias and can provide appropriate follow-up.

Aplastic Anemia

OVERVIEW

Aplastic anemia is a deficiency of circulating erythrocytes resulting from arrested development of red blood cells (RBCs) within the bone marrow. It is caused by an injury to the hematopoietic precursor cell, the pluripotent stem cell. Although aplastic anemia sometimes occurs alone, it is usually accompanied by agranulocytosis (a reduction in leukocytes) and thrombocytopenia (a reduction in platelets). These three problems occur simultaneously because the bone marrow produces not only RBCs but also white blood cells (WBCs) and platelets. Consequently, if the bone marrow is abnormal for any reason or if it has been exposed to a myelotoxin (any substance that is toxic and damaging to bone marrow), production of erythrocytes, leukocytes, and thrombocytes slows greatly. *Pancytopenia* (a deficiency of all three cell types), is common in aplastic anemia. The onset of aplastic anemia may be insidious or rapid.

The development of aplastic anemia, although relatively rare, is associated with chronic exposure to several myelotoxic agents (Table 38–2).

In about 50% of cases, the etiology of aplastic anemia is unknown. Aplastic anemia may occur as a sequela of viral infection (Cotran et al., 1989). The mechanism by which the damage to the bone marrow occurs is unknown.

COLLABORATIVE MANAGEMENT

Blood transfusions are the mainstay of treatment for clients with aplastic anemia. Transfusions are discontinued as soon as the bone marrow begins to produce RBCs. Transfusion for anemia is indicated only when the anemia causes real disability or when bleeding is life-threatening because of thrombocytopenia. Unnecessary transfusion, however:

- Increases the opportunity for the development of immune reactions to platelets
- Shortens the life span of the transfused cell
- Possibly increases the rate of rejection of transplanted marrow cells

Because clients with some types of aplastic anemia have a disease course consistent with that of clients with autoimmune problems, immunosuppressive therapy may be helpful. Agents that selectively suppress lymphocyte activity, such as antilymphocyte globulin (ALG), antithymocyte globulin (ATG), and cyclosporine (Sandimmune) have brought about partial or complete remissions (Adamson & Erslev, 1990). In more severe cases, general immunosuppressive agents, such as prednisone and cyclophosphamide (Cytoxan, Procytox♣), have been effective.

When the client has an enlarged spleen that is either destroying normal RBCs or suppressing their development, splenectomy is considered. Bone marrow transplantation has resulted in a cure for some clients, although cost, availability, and complications limit this technique for treatment of aplastic anemia (Loughran & Storb, 1990).

COLLABORATIVE MANAGEMENT FOR THE CLIENT WITH ANEMIA

ASSESSMENT

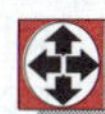

HISTORY

The nurse collects demographic data because gender and age are key risk factors for some types of anemia. The nurse should ask about occupation and hobbies, which may yield important clues about chronic exposure to substances that are linked to some types of anemia.

The nurse determines whether the client is aware of how long he or she has been anemic. Additionally, the nurse asks whether anyone else in the family is anemic or if there is a positive family history of specific types of anemia. Clients are asked if obvious conditions of blood loss, such as trauma, melena (blood in the stool), hematemesis, hematuria, and menorrhagia (excessive menstrual flow), have occurred recently. The client is asked to try to quantify any known blood loss. The nurse asks women how many pads or tampons they use per day during the menstrual cycle.

The nurse should determine the presence of any underlying alcohol or drug abuse because substance abuse is often associated with malnutrition, a possible cause of anemia. The nurse reviews exposure to medications and potentially harmful industrial or household toxins. Causative agents include:

- Thiazide diuretics
- Chloramphenicol
- Aspirin
- Quinine derivatives
- Anticonvulsants
- Sulfonamides
- Alkylating agents
- Benzene
- Insecticides

The nurse obtains a thorough diet history to determine daily caloric, protein, and vitamin intake. The nurse asks the client to list everything consumed during the previous week to determine possible dietary deficiency of iron, folate, or vitamin B_{12}.

The client is asked about the presence of any associated symptoms, such as:

- Chronic fatigue and shortness of breath
- Increased susceptibility to infection
- Anorexia
- Weight loss
- Indigestion
- Sore mouth and tongue
- Bone pain and deformity
- Chronic depression

The nurse also asks whether the client has experienced:

- Headaches
- Behavior changes
- Increased somnolence
- Decreased alertness
- Decreased attention span
- Lethargy
- Muscle weakness
- Increased fatigue

Having the client relate the previous 24 hours' activities may disclose additional information about activity intolerance, changes in behavior, and the presence of unexplained fatigue. The nurse asks about changes in sleep/rest patterns, ability to climb stairs, and activities that induce shortness of breath. Obtaining a subjective baseline assessment of the client's perceived energy level using a scale of 1 to 10 (1 represents not tired and plenty of energy, and 10 represents total exhaustion) can be useful to the nurse in evaluating the effectiveness of later treatments (Blesch et al., 1991).

PHYSICAL ASSESSMENT/CLINICAL MANIFESTATIONS

When a person becomes anemic, several compensatory mechanisms develop. Many of the physical findings seen in an anemic client are a result of these mechanisms.

CARDIOVASCULAR MANIFESTATIONS Cardiovascular manifestations of anemia include:

- Bounding arterial pulses
- Vascular bruits
- Cardiac enlargement
- Murmurs
- Dependent edema
- Pallor
- Spider angiomas

The client's cardiac output increases to increase tissue oxygenation. Signs of compensatory cardiac activity include tachycardia, a systolic flow murmur, and orthostatic hypotension. The client may have angina (chest pain) if there is pre-existing heart disease.

RESPIRATORY MANIFESTATIONS The client's respiratory rate may increase in an attempt to increase oxygenation. This accounts for the symptoms orthopnea and dyspnea (difficulty breathing) upon exertion.

INTEGUMENTARY MANIFESTATIONS Vasoconstriction occurs in the skin, producing the characteristic pallor. The client may have jaundice if the anemia is associated with a rapid destruction of erythrocytes.

MISCELLANEOUS MANIFESTATIONS An increase in the rate of RBC production may result in client complaints of bone pain and sternal tenderness. Other symptoms often seen in the anemic client include:

- Chronic fatigue
- Shortness of breath
- Increased susceptibility to infection
- Anorexia
- Weight loss
- Indigestion
- Sore mouth and tongue
- Headaches
- Vertigo
- Loss of consciousness

A shift of blood flow away from the kidneys may also occur in anemia, causing diminished urinary output.

PSYCHOSOCIAL ASSESSMENT

The nurse caring for the client with anemia continually assesses for the psychologic impact of the illness and hospital environment on the client, the family, and social and sexual roles. Anemia is often a chronic disease, which can lead to psychosocial problems. Self-concept, including such aspects as body image and role perception, serves as a frame of reference for reality. Illness, especially when it is chronic, alters the self-concept by interfering with perceptions of self. Clients may experience a feeling of loss over changes in their lives as a result of chronic illness; chronic depression is also common in anemic clients.

LABORATORY ASSESSMENT

Laboratory studies useful in the diagnosis and monitoring of anemia include:

- Complete blood count (CBC)
- Mean corpuscular hemoglobin
- Mean corpuscular volume
- Mean corpuscular hemoglobin concentration
- Iron levels and total iron-binding capacity test
- Bone marrow examination
- Hemoglobin electrophoresis
- Peripheral blood smears

Anemic clients usually have decreased erythrocyte counts, hematocrit values, and hemoglobin levels. Other findings may be abnormal, depending on the cause of the anemia.

ANALYSIS

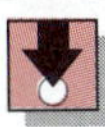

COMMON NURSING DIAGNOSES

Common nursing diagnoses for the client with anemia are:

1. Fatigue related to decreased oxygen-carrying capacity of the blood
2. Altered Nutrition: Less than Body Requirements related to inadequate dietary intake

ADDITIONAL NURSING DIAGNOSES

Clients may also have one or more of the following diagnoses:

- High Risk for Impaired Skin Integrity related to decreased tissue perfusion
- Altered Oral Mucous Membrane related to decreased tissue perfusion
- Anxiety related to chronic illness
- Pain related to hypoxia

PLANNING AND IMPLEMENTATION

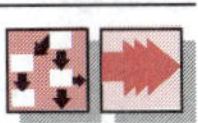

The plan of care for the client with anemia focuses on the common nursing diagnoses and is aimed at supporting the physiologic compensatory mechanisms.

FATIGUE

PLANNING: CLIENT GOALS The major goal is that the client will not become excessively fatigued while carrying out activities of daily living.

INTERVENTIONS Interventions are aimed at reducing distressing symptoms and restoring hematologic homeostasis.

Rest Rest is essential. The nurse encourages the client to rest frequently throughout the day to lower oxygen requirements and to reduce the strain on the client's heart and the lungs. If possible, the client should try to shorten the working day. Clients with severe anemia are usually hospitalized and restricted to bed rest until they improve. The nurse helps extremely weak clients in bathing, turning, eating, and providing self-care. The nurse protects the client from frequent visitors, continuous telephone interruptions, and excessive noise.

Blood Replacement Therapy Blood transfusions are indicated for some types of anemia. Transfusions increase the oxygen-carrying capacity of blood and replace missing red blood cells and some coagulation factors. Indications for treatment with blood components are summarized in Table 39–3. Also see Transfusion Therapy later in this chapter.

ALTERED NUTRITION: LESS THAN BODY REQUIREMENTS

PLANNING: CLIENT GOALS The major goals are that the client will:

- Receive optimal protein, calories, vitamins, and minerals
- Avoid iron deficiency anemia, folic acid deficiency anemia, or vitamin B_{12} deficiency anemia

INTERVENTIONS For anemias caused by deficiencies of vitamin B_{12}, folic acid, or iron, increased intake of these substances is therapeutic. The client can accomplish this with drug and diet therapy.

Drug Therapy Drug therapy for vitamin B_{12} and folic acid deficiency anemias consists of vitamin supplements, which can be given parenterally or orally until symptoms abate. Both of these vitamins are added routinely to total parenteral nutrition (TPN) and tube feeding solutions. Medicinal iron can be administered orally or parenterally; however, the preferred route is oral.

The drugs of choice for oral administration are ferrous sulfate and ferrous gluconate. Iron preparations must be administered correctly. Because iron is a gastric irritant, it is always given with meals. The nurse dilutes liquid oral iron preparations and administers them through a straw to avoid staining the client's teeth.

The nurse explains that iron preparations often change the color of stools to black and that the change in color is due to iron supplementation, not insidious gastrointestinal bleeding.

Parenteral iron therapy is indicated for clients who have an intolerance to oral iron preparations or who continue to experience blood loss. Iron dextran is the drug of choice. Iron dextran causes darkening and discoloration of the skin around the injection site and is administered intramuscularly by Z-track injection technique (Chart 39–5). The Z-track method pre-

TABLE 39–3 Indications for Treatment with Blood Components

Component	Volume	Infusion Time	Indications
Packed red blood cells (PRBCs)	• 200–250 ml	• 2–4 hr	• Anemia, hemoglobin <8
Washed red blood cells (WBC-poor PRBCs)	• 200 ml	• 2–4 hr	• History of allergic transfusion reactions • Bone marrow transplant clients
Platelets Pooled	• Approx. 300 ml	• 15–30 minutes	• Thrombocytopenia platelet count <20,000 • Clients who are actively bleeding with a platelet count <80,000
Platelets Single donor	• 200 mL	• 30 minutes	• History of febrile or allergic reactions
Fresh frozen (FFP)	• 200 mL	• 15–30 minutes	• Deficiency in plasma coagulation factors
Cryoprecipitate	• 10–20 mL/U	• 15–30 minutes	• Hemophilia VIII or von Willebrand's disease
White blood cells (WBCs)	• 400 mL	• 1 hr	• Sepsis, neutropenic infection not responding to antibiotic therapy

CHART 39–5

Nursing Care Highlight ◆ Administering Intramuscular Medications by the Z-Track Method

- Draw medication up into the syringe using aseptic technique.
- Add 0.25 mL of air to the syringe.
- Discard the needle used to draw up the medication.
- Place a new needle (22-gauge, 2–3 inches long) on syringe.
- Make certain that the injection site is in a bright light.
- *Select the dorsal gluteal site only.*
- Identify appropriate landmarks for administration into the upper, outer quadrant.
- Once the site is selected, pull the skin and subcutaneous tissues sideways away from the muscle.
- Clean the site while holding the skin and subcutaneous tissues off to the side.
- Insert the needle deeply into the muscle tissue.
- Aspirate to determine needle placement.
- When iron dextran is being administered, the medication is black; look very closely to determine whether or not blood is being aspirated into the syringe.
- If blood is aspirated, withdraw needle and begin procedure again from the first step.
- If no blood is aspirated, inject medication slowly, followed by injection of the air bubble.
- Quickly withdraw the needle.
- Release the skin and subcutaneous tissue.
- *Do not massage the injection site.*

vents the irritating and staining medications from leaking back through the path made by the needle during administration.

Diet Therapy The nurse explains which foods are high in vitamin B_{12}, folic acid, and iron (see Table 39–2).

Prevention of Complications For clients with vitamin B_{12} deficiency anemia, injury as a result of neurologic alterations is possible. The nurse advises the client to use caution when climbing stairs and using the bathroom. A hazard-free environment is necessary to meet this goal, and the nurse emphasizes its importance. If the client is experiencing paresthesias of the feet, he or she should test the bath water before stepping into the bathtub to avoid burns. For clients with any type of anemia, fainting can occur and lead to injury. The nurse advises the client to rise slowly from a seated position.

DISCHARGE PLANNING

The anemic client can usually be treated at home. Clients with severe cases of aplastic anemia, sickle cell disease, and other anemias may be treated in the hospital.

HOME CARE PREPARATION

Depending on the diagnosis, the nurse considers various factors in regard to the client's home environment. The nurse assesses the environment for potential hazards before the hospitalized client is discharged if the client is susceptible to falls. If the client is experiencing excessive fatigue and shortness of breath as a result of anemia, stair climbing may be a problem. The nurse works with the social services department to identify adaptations in home life.

HEALTH TEACHING

For any of the hereditary anemias, such as sickle cell disease, nurses educate clients and their families about these issues:

- Genetic transmission of the disease
- Signs and symptoms of crises
- Management of crises on an outpatient basis
- Indications on when to seek medical attention

Clients with sickle cell disease are often given opioid analgesics for self-management of sickle cell crises at home. The nurse teaches the client and family about correct administration of the drugs. The nurse specifically instructs clients and family members to keep iron supplements out of the reach of children because an overdose can be lethal. For diet-induced anemias, the nurse includes nutritional counseling as a part of nursing care from the time of diagnosis. The nurse explains to clients and family members that the client will need assistance with activities of daily living.

PSYCHOSOCIAL PREPARATION

Explaining the importance of proper diet and sufficient rest to the client and the family increases the likelihood of compliance. Clients who are anemic need to plan frequent visits to health care personnel for monitoring and therapy. Involvement of the family may increase the client's motivation and ensure a complete recovery. Most clients can work while they are anemic, although they may need frequent rest periods. Allowing the client to ventilate his or her feelings regarding restrictions in activities of daily living can increase coping abilities.

HEALTH CARE RESOURCES

Before the nurse can expect a client to comply with a healthy diet, health care resources must be evaluated. A healthy diet is more expensive than a high-calorie, high-carbohydrate diet. The client may need financial assistance, and the nurse can provide the necessary referrals to social services. For many anemic clients who are extremely weak, a home care nurse or aide may be necessary to assist with activities of daily living and ambulation. The hospital nurse documents the client's needs on the transfer chart and communicates these needs to the home care agency.

EVALUATION

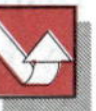

On the basis of the identified nursing diagnoses, the nurse evaluates the care of the anemic client. The expected outcomes may include that the client will:

- State that he or she is not fatigued after performing activities of daily living
- Select correctly from a list those foods that contain significant quantities of iron and vitamin B_{12}
- Describe and comply with drug therapy as needed
- State correctly the signs and symptoms of anemia
- State which health care resource person should be notified when symptoms of anemia occur

POLYCYTHEMIA

Polycythemia is a condition in which the number of red blood cells (RBCs) in whole blood is above normal levels. There is hyperviscosity, or increased blood "thickness." Polycythemia may be transitory, subsequent to other conditions, or chronic. One type of polycythemia that is fatal if left untreated is polycythemia vera.

Polycythemia Vera

OVERVIEW

Polycythemia vera (PV) is characterized by one of these findings:

- A sustained increase in blood hemoglobin concentration to 18 g/dL
- A red blood cell (RBC) count of 6 million/mm
- A hematocrit increase to 55% or greater

PV is a red blood cell malignancy. There are three major hallmarks of this condition:

- A relentless, unrestrained production of massive numbers of erythrocytes
- Production of an excessive number of leukocytes
- An overproduction of thrombocytes

As described in Chart 39–6, at first there is extreme hypercellularity of the peripheral blood in peo-

CHART 39–6

Key Features of Polycythemia Vera

- Persistently elevated hematocrit value (>55%)
- Hypertention
- Dark, flushed appearance of the hands and face
- Distention of superficial veins
- Weight loss
- Fatigue
- Intense itching
- Enlarged hemorrhoids
- Swollen, painful joints
- Enlarged, firm spleen
- Infarctions of the heart
  - Chest pain
  - Congestive heart failure
- Cerebral vascular accidents
- Bleeding tendency

ple with PV (Workman et al., 1993). The skin, especially of the face, and mucous membranes have a dark, flushed (plethoric) appearance. These areas may appear purplish or cyanotic because the blood in these tissues is incompletely oxygenated. Most clients experience intense itching sensations related to vasodilation and variation in tissue oxygenation. The viscosity ("thickness") of the blood is greatly increased, causing a corresponding increase in vascular friction and peripheral resistance. Superficial veins are visibly distended. Blood moves more slowly through all tissues and places increased demands on the pumping action of the heart, resulting in hypertension. In some highly vascular areas, blood flow may become so slow that vascular stasis occurs. Vascular stasis causes thrombosis within the smaller vessels to the extent that the vessels are occluded and the surrounding tissues experience hypoxia, progressing to anoxia, further progressing to infarction and necrosis. Tissues most prone to this complication are the heart, spleen, and kidneys, although infarction with loss of tissue/organ function can occur in any organ or tissue.

Because the actual number of cells in the blood is greatly increased and the cells are not completely normal, individual cell life spans are shorter. The shorter life spans, coupled with increased cell production, result in a rapid turnover of peripheral blood cells. This rapid turnover increases the amount of intracellular products (released when cells die) in the blood, adding to the general "sludging" of the blood. These products include uric acid and potassium, which can cause the associated symptoms of gout and hyperkalemia.

In addition to hypercellularity and hypermetabolism, later clinical manifestations of polycythemia vera are related to abnormal blood cells. Even though the numbers of circulating erythrocytes is greatly increased, their oxygen-binding capacity is impaired and the client experiences severe generalized hypoxia. In spite of the RBC excess, most clients with polycythemia vera are susceptible to bleeding problems because of an apparent associated platelet dysfunction (Williams et al., 1990).

COLLABORATIVE MANAGEMENT

Polycythemia vera is a malignant disease that progresses in severity over time. If left untreated, few people with polycythemia vera live longer than 2 years. Conservative management with repeated phlebotomies (two to five times per week) can prolong life for 5 to 10 years. (Phlebotomy is the routine collection of the client's red blood cells to decrease the number of RBCs and to diminish blood viscosity.) Maintaining adequate hydration and promoting venous return are essential to prevent thrombus formation. Therapies are prescribed to prevent the formation of clots and include anticoagulant drugs. Chart 39–7 lists information for the client with polycythemia vera.

CHART 39–7

Education Guide ◆ Polycythemia Vera

- Drink at least 3000 mL of liquids each day.
- Avoid tight or constrictive clothing, especially garters or girdles.
- Wear gloves when outdoors in temperatures lower than 50° F.
- Keep all health care related appointments.
- Contact your physician at the first sign of infection.
- Take anticoagulants as ordered.
- Wear support hose or stockings while you are awake and up.
- Elevate your feet whenever you are seated.
- Exercise slowly and only on the advice of your physician.
- Stop activity at the first sign of chest pain.
- Use an electric razor, not a manual one.
- Use a soft-bristled toothbrush to brush your teeth.
- Do not floss between your teeth.

As the disease progresses, the client needs more intensive therapies that suppress bone marrow activity, including oral alkylating agents and/or irradiation with injections of radioactive phosphorus. An experimental treatment aimed at cure, allogeneic bone marrow transplantation, is promising, but the results are too limited to determine its application to polycythemia vera.

WHITE BLOOD CELL DISORDERS

As discussed in Chapter 22, white blood cells (WBCs or leukocytes) provide protection from invading nonself cells and cancer cells in several ways. These protective functions depend on maintaining normal numbers and ratios of many specific mature circulating leukocytes. When any one type of WBC is present in either abnormally high or abnormally low amounts, hematopoietic function and immune function may be altered to some degree, causing the client to be at risk for specific complications. This part of the chapter covers the pathologic changes and nursing care requirements for clients with disorders characterized by overgrowth of specific types of WBCs. (See Chapter 24 for the pathologic alterations and care requirements for clients with leukocyte-related problems of immunodeficiency, allergy, and autoimmune disorders.)

Leukemia

OVERVIEW

The leukemias are a group of malignant disorders involving abnormal overproduction of a specific white blood cell type, usually at an immature stage, in the bone marrow. Leukemia may be acute, with a sudden onset and short duration, or chronic, with a slow onset and persistent symptoms over a period of years.

The types of leukemia are categorized by the specific maturational pathway from which the abnormal cells arose (Maguire-Eisen, 1990). Leukemias in which the abnormal cells arise from within the committed lymphoid maturational pathways (see Fig. 22–3) are lymphocytic or lymphoblastic. Leukemias in which the abnormal cells arise within the committed myeloid maturational pathways are myelocytic or myelogenous. Several subtypes exist for each of these diseases and are classified by the degree of maturity of the abnormal cell and the specific cell type involved (Table 39–4).

PATHOPHYSIOLOGY

The basic pathologic defect in leukemia is a malignant transformation of the stem cells or early committed precursor leukocyte cells, causing an abnormal proliferation of a specific type of leukocyte. The immature leukocytes, which are functionally and structurally abnormal, are produced in excessive quantities in the bone marrow, essentially shutting down normal bone marrow production of erythrocytes, platelets, and other functionally mature leukocytes. This situation leads to anemia, thrombocytopenia, and leukopenia of the unaffected white blood cell types, even though the number of immature, abnormal WBCs in the circulation is greatly elevated. Unless treatment is instituted, clients usually die from infection or hemorrhage. For clients with acute leukemias, these pathologic changes occur rapidly and progress quickly to death without intervention. Chronic leukemia may be present for many years before overt pathologic changes related to the illness occur.

ETIOLOGY

Epidemiologic studies suggest that many different genetic and environmental factors may be involved in the development of leukemia. Although only a few of these factors have been identified as having a definite role, the basic mechanism appears to involve gene damage of cells, leading to transformation of those cells from a normal state to a malignant state. The following constitute possible risk factors (Maguire-Eisen, 1990):

- Ionizing radiation
- Chemicals and drugs
- Marrow hypoplasia
- Environmental interactions
- Genetic factors
- Viral factors
- Immunologic factors
- Interactive factors

Exposure to large quantities of ionizing radiation appears to be a major risk factor. Exposures ranging from therapeutic irradiation (for such diseases as ankylosing spondylitis and Hodgkin's lymphoma) to environmental irradiation (such as the atomic bomb at

TABLE 39–4 Differentiating Characteristics of the Four Types of Leukemia

Leukemia Type	Age at Onset (yr)	Sex	Race	Cell of Origin	Specific Markers	Comments
Acute lymphocytic (ALL)	• <15	• M	• Caucasian	• B cell	• CALLA+ • Hyperdiploidy • TDT+	• Prognosis poorer for adults than for children • Prognosis better than in AML • Curable in children
Acute myelogenous (AML)	• 15–39	• Equal incidence		• Myeloblast • Myelocyte • Promyelocyte • Myelomonocyte	• TDT– • t(9;22) • t(15;17)	• Prognosis generally poor • Heterogeneous tumor cell populations • Best prognosis with bone marrow transplant
Chronic myelogenous (CML)	• >50	• M		• Myeloid cell	• Ph[1] chromosome	• Prognosis generally poor; worse if no Ph[1] chromosome • No blockage of maturation of nonmalignant leukocytes • Blastic crisis indicative of more acute disease
Chronic lymphocytic (CLL)	• >50	• M	• Caucasian	• B cell	• Trisomy 12	• Prognosis poor • Long (4–10 yr) course with rare conversion to acute form • Only leukemia with a possible genetic predisposition

Hiroshima or the accident at Chernobyl) are associated with leukemia.

Many chemicals and drugs have been linked to the development of leukemia (see Table 38–2).

Marrow hypoplasia can increase the risk of leukemia. A reduction or alteration in the production of hematopoietic cells may be responsible. Examples of conditions associated with the later development of leukemia include Fanconi's anemia, paroxysmal nocturnal hemoglobinuria during its aplastic phase, and myelodysplastic syndromes (Carson & Callaghan, 1991).

An increase in the frequency of leukemia in the following populations suggests a possible genetic involvement: identical twins of clients with leukemia and people with Down syndrome, Bloom's syndrome, Fanconi's anemia, and Klinefelter's syndrome. Chromosomal aberration may be an important factor in these syndromes.

Deficiency in the immune system may favor the development of leukemia. It has not been determined whether leukemia among immunodeficient people is a result of immunosurveillance failure or if the pathologic mechanisms that cause the immune deficiency also trigger malignant transformation of leukopoietic cells.

The interaction of multiple host and environmental factors may result in leukemia. Because each person tolerates the interaction of these factors differently, it is difficult to determine the origin of any specific leukemia.

INCIDENCE/PREVALENCE

The leukemias account for 3% of all newly diagnosed cases of cancer and 4% of all cancer deaths (American Cancer Society, 1994). The incidence and frequency of leukemia depend on many factors, including:

- The morphologic type of white blood cell affected
- Age
- Sex
- Race
- Geographic locale

An estimated 28,200 new cases of leukemia were projected in the United States for 1994 (American Cancer Society, 1994). In the United States, leukemia is categorized into any one of four basic types. These types differ in the cell type affected and the rate of progression of the leukemia.

Acute myelogenous leukemia (AML) occurs with a similar frequency in all ages and is the most common form of leukemia in adults.

Acute lymphocytic leukemia (ALL) constitutes about 10% of adult leukemias.

Chronic myelogenous leukemia (CML) constitutes about 20% of adult leukemias and occurs more frequently in people above age 50.

Chronic lymphocytic leukemia (CLL) is the rarest type of leukemia and occurs primarily in people older than 50 years of age.

Characteristics and risk factors associated with four types of leukemia are presented in Table 39–4.

COLLABORATIVE MANAGEMENT

ASSESSMENT

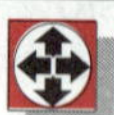

HISTORY

The nurse asks the client about risk factors and causative factors. Age is important because the incidence of leukemia increases with age. The client's occupation and hobbies may reveal specific environmental exposures that increase the risk of leukemia. Previous illnesses and medical history may indicate exposure to ionizing radiation or medications that also increase risk.

Because of leukemia-related alterations of immune function, the risk for infection is increased in clients with leukemia. The nurse asks clients about the frequency and severity of infectious processes (such as colds, influenza, pneumonia, bronchitis, and unexplained episodes of fever) during the preceding 6 months.

Because platelet function may be diminished in people with leukemia, the nurse questions the client about any overt or hidden excessive bleeding episodes, such as:

- A tendency to bruise easily
- Nosebleeds
- Increased menstrual flow
- Bleeding from the gums
- Rectal bleeding
- Hematuria (blood in the urine)
- Prolonged bleeding after minor abrasions or lacerations

If the client has experienced such an episode, the nurse asks whether this type and extent of bleeding constitute the client's usual response to injury or represent a change in injury pattern.

Clients with leukemia frequently experience weakness and fatigue resulting from anemia and increased metabolic and energy demands of the leukemic cells. The nurse asks the client whether he or she has experienced any of the following:

- Headaches
- Behavior changes
- Increased somnolence
- Decreased alertness
- Decreased attention span
- Lethargy, muscle weakness
- Diminished appetite
- Weight loss
- Increased fatigue

Having the client relate the previous 24 hours' activities may disclose additional information about activity intolerance, changes in behavior, and the presence of unexplained fatigue. The nurse determines how long the client has had any of these debilitating symptoms.

PHYSICAL ASSESSMENT/CLINICAL MANIFESTATIONS

Leukemia involves one or more pathologic mechanisms in the bone marrow that influence the composition and activity of various blood components. Because blood influences the health and functional capacity of all organs and systems, many areas remote from the actual site of origin of malignant cells may be affected (Chart 39–8). The following clinical manifestations are associated with the acute leukemias (Cotran et al., 1989). Some of these findings may also be present in clients with chronic leukemia in the blast phase.

CARDIOVASCULAR MANIFESTATIONS Cardiovascular manifestations of leukemia are usually related to anemia. The client's heart rate may be increased and blood pressure decreased. Murmurs and bruits may be present. Capillary filling time is increased.

RESPIRATORY MANIFESTATIONS Respiratory manifestations of leukemia are primarily associated with anemia and infectious complications. The client's respiratory rate increases as the degree of anemia becomes greater. If respiratory tract infections are present, the client may experience signs and symptoms of pneumonia, including cough and shortness of breath. Abnormal breath sounds are present on auscultation.

INTEGUMENTARY MANIFESTATIONS The client's skin and mucous membranes may manifest abnormalities associated with leukemia. The skin may be pale and cool to the touch as a result of the accompanying anemia. Pallor is especially evident on the face, around the mouth, and in the nail beds. The conjunctiva of the eye also is pale, as are the creases on the palmar surface of the hand (most evident when the skin over the palm of the hand is stretched). Petechiae (raised red spots) may be present on any area of skin surface, especially the lower extremities. The petechiae may be unrelated to any obvious trauma. The nurse carefully inspects the skin for the presence of any skin infections or traumatized areas that have failed to heal. The nurse inspects the client's mouth for evidence of bleeding from the gums and the presence of any sore or lesion of the oral cavity indicating infection.

GASTROINTESTINAL MANIFESTATIONS Gastrointestinal manifestations may be related to the increased bleeding tendency and to the fatigue. Weight loss, nausea, and anorexia are common. The nurse examines the rectal area for fissures and tests the stool for the presence of occult blood. Many clients with leukemia have diminished bowel sounds and constipation.

CHART 39–8

Key Features of Acute Leukemia

Integumentary Manifestations
- Ecchymoses
- Petechiae
- Open infected lesions
- Pallor of the conjunctiva, the nail beds, and the palmar creases and around the mouth

Gastrointestinal Manifestations
- Bleeding gums
- Anorexia
- Weight loss
- Enlarged liver and spleen

Renal Manifestations
- Hematuria

Cardiovascular Manifestations
- Tachycardia at basal activity levels
- Orthostatic hypotension
- Palpitations

Respiratory Manifestations
- Dyspnea on exertion

Neurologic Manifestations
- Fatigue
- Headache
- Fever

Musculoskeletal Manifestations
- Bone pain
- Joint swelling and pain

Hepatosplenomegaly and abdominal tenderness also may be present from leukemic infiltration of abdominal viscera.

CENTRAL NERVOUS SYSTEM MANIFESTATIONS Cranial nerve disturbances, headache, and papilledema as a result of leukemic infiltration of the meninges or central nervous system (CNS) may be present. In advanced cases, seizure activity and coma may occur. Although clients often have fever, this manifestation may be more a response to the presence of infection than to malignancy-related changes in the CNS.

MISCELLANEOUS MANIFESTATIONS Other manifestations include bone and joint tenderness as a result of marrow involvement and bone resorption. Leukemic cell growth or infiltration may produce enlarged lymph nodes or masses.

PSYCHOSOCIAL ASSESSMENT

The client with newly diagnosed leukemia is extremely anxious. The average layperson equates a diagnosis of any cancer with a death sentence.

Current therapies have greatly improved the prognoses of most cancers, yet the public is largely unaware of these advances. The nurse spends time with the client and family to ascertain what the diagnosis means to them and what they expect from the future. Without knowing the client's expectations and feelings, the nurse cannot educate and support clients and family members in an individualized manner. The nurse must determine areas of concern before developing a meaningful plan of care.

A diagnosis of leukemia has dramatic implications for a client's lifestyle. Hospitalization for initial treatment often lasts several weeks. Clients become bored and experience feelings of loneliness and isolation. The nurse assesses the client's coping patterns, including activities that the client finds enjoyable and methods that help the client to relax. A care plan to prevent diversional activity deficit is particularly beneficial for such clients (Radziewicz & Schneider, 1992). After initial therapy, clients may be able to resume work, depending on their occupation. However, clients often must make adjustments to accommodate changes in their functional status. In addition, repeated hospitalizations may be necessary.

LABORATORY ASSESSMENT

The client with acute leukemia usually has:

- Decreased hemoglobin and hematocrit levels
- A decreased platelet count
- An altered white blood cell (WBC) count

The WBC count may be low, normal, or elevated, but usually it is quite elevated, with counts of 20,000 to 100,000 common. Clients with higher WBC counts on diagnosis have a poorer prognosis (Carson & Callaghan, 1991).

The definitive test for leukemia includes various examinations of cells obtained as a result of bone marrow aspiration and biopsy. The bone marrow is full of leukemic blast phase cells. The composition of various cell surface proteins (antigens) on the leukemic cells assists in the diagnosis of the type of leukemia. Such markers include the presence or absence of:

- The T-11 protein
- The enzyme terminal deoxynucleotidyl transferase (TDT)
- The common acute lymphoblastic leukemia antigen (CALLA)

These markers also indicate prognosis.

Coagulation variables are usually abnormal for clients with acute leukemia. Reduced levels of fibrinogen and other coagulation factors are typical. Whole blood clotting time (Lee-White clotting test) is increased, as is the activated partial thromboplastin time (PTT).

Chromosomal analysis of the malignant bone marrow cells may be performed to determine the presence of specific marker chromosomes, which can be used:

- To assist in the diagnosis of leukemia type
- To predict prognosis
- To determine the effectiveness of therapy

RADIOGRAPHIC ASSESSMENT

Specific symptoms determine the feasibility of specific tests. For instance, a client with dyspnea needs chest radiography to determine whether leukemic infiltrates are present in the lung. Skeletal x-ray films may help to determine the degree of bone reabsorption present with subperiosteal involvement.

ANALYSIS

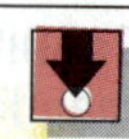

COMMON NURSING DIAGNOSES

The following nursing diagnoses are commonly seen in adult clients with acute myelogenous leukemia (AML), the most common type of adult leukemia:

1. High Risk for Infection related to decreased immune response
2. High Risk for Injury related to thrombocytopenia
3. Fatigue related to decreased tissue oxygenation and increased energy demands

ADDITIONAL NURSING DIAGNOSES

In addition, many clients with AML have one or more of the following nursing diagnoses:

- Impaired Skin Integrity related to prolonged immobility
- Altered Oral Mucous Membrane related to effects of chemotherapy and pancytopenia
- Total Self Care Deficit related to progressive debilitation and weakness
- Altered Nutrition: Less than Body Requirements related to anorexia, nausea, and vomiting
- Anxiety related to fear of death
- Powerlessness related to an inability to control the progression of the disease
- Altered Family Processes related to acute, life threatening illness of an individual family member
- Altered Role Performance related to perceived inability to fulfill parental and other family roles and prolonged hospitalization
- Diversional Activity Deficit related to prolonged hospitalizations.

PLANNING AND IMPLEMENTATION

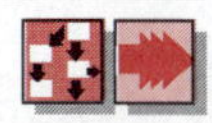

HIGH RISK FOR INFECTION

PLANNING: CLIENT GOALS The major goals are that the client will:

- Remain free from cross-contamination–induced infection
- Remain free of autocontamination-induced infection
- Not experience sepsis

INTERVENTIONS Infection is a major cause of death in the immunosuppressed client, and septicemia is a common sequela. Infection of clients with leukemia occurs through:

- Autocontamination (the client's normal flora overgrows and penetrates the internal environment)
- Cross-contamination (microorganisms from another person or the environment are transmitted to the client)

The three most common sites of infection are:

- The skin
- The respiratory tract
- The gastrointestinal tract

Gram-negative bacteria are frequently the cause of infection, although gram-positive and fungal infections do occur (Oniboni, 1990). Interventions are aimed at:

- Interrupting or halting the infection processes
- Controlling infection
- Initiating early, effective treatment regimens for specific infections

The accompanying client care plan outlines specific interventions for the client with acute myelogenous leukemia (AML).

Drug Therapy for Leukemia Drug therapy for clients with acute myelogenous leukemia (AML), the most common type occurring in adults, is divided into three distinctive phases:

- Induction
- Consolidation
- Maintenance

INDUCTION THERAPY Induction therapy is intensive and consists of combination chemotherapy initiated at the time of diagnosis. This therapy is aimed at achieving a rapid, complete remission of all manifestations of disease (Maguire-Eisen, 1990). Different institutions and different physicians vary the agents used and the treatment schedule. A typical course of aggressive chemotherapy for the induction of remission in clients with acute myelogenous leukemia (AML) includes intravenous (IV) administration of cytosine arabinoside (at 200 mg/m^2 of body surface area per day) for 7 days with concomitant administration of daunorubicin (30 to 45 mg/m^2/per day) for the first 3 days.

A major problem is that one side effect of these agents is severe bone marrow suppression. As a result, the client becomes even more vulnerable to infection than before the treatment started. Prolonged hospitalizations are common while the client is immunosuppressed. Recovery of hematopoiesis requires at least 2 to 3 weeks, during which time the client must be protected from life-threatening infections. Other adverse reactions include:

- Nausea
- Vomiting
- Diarrhea
- Alopecia (hair loss)
- Stomatitis
- Renal toxicity
- Hepatic toxicity
- Cardiac toxicity

CONSOLIDATION THERAPY Consolidation therapy usually consists of another course of either the same agents as used for induction at a different dosage level or a different combination of chemotherapeutic agents. This treatment occurs early in remission, and its intent is to cure (Wujcik, 1990). At some institutions, consolidation therapy is a single course of chemotherapy; at other institutions, consolidation therapy consists of regularly scheduled repeated courses of chemotherapy over a period of 1 to 2 years.

MAINTENANCE THERAPY Maintenance therapy may be prescribed for months to years after successful induction and consolidation therapies. The purpose is to maintain the remission achieved through induction and consolidation. Agents used for maintenance are milder, are often given orally, and may be taken for 2 to 5 years.

Drug Therapy for Infection Drug therapy is a primary defense against infections that tend to develop in clients undergoing therapy for acute myelogenous leukemia. Agents used depend on the sensitivity of the specific organism causing the infection and the extent of the infection. Agents are categorized by specificity as antibacterial, antiviral, or antifungal.

ANTIBIOTIC AND ANTIBACTERIAL AGENTS Antibiotic and antibacterial agents used for prophylaxis or treatment of infection in clients with acute myelogenous leukemia usually include at least one of the aminoglycosides (amikacin, gentamicin, and tobramycin) and a systemic penicillin. Additional powerful antibiotics

Text continued on page 1062

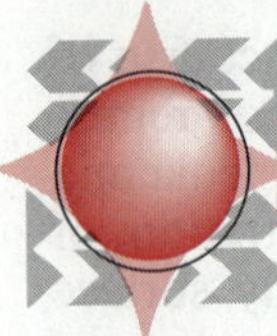

CLIENT CARE PLAN

The Client with Acute Myelogenous Leukemia

Nursing Diagnosis No. 1: High Risk for Infection related to decreased immune response

Expected Outcomes	Nursing Interventions	Rationale
The client will remain free from cross-contamination–induced infection. ◆ Limits close contact with other people. ◆ Maintains a core body temperature of < 100° F (38° C). ◆ Does not have pathogenic organisms in cultures of blood, urine, or wound drainage.	◆ Initiate protective isolation procedures according to institutional policy (e.g., thorough hand washing between clients, reverse isolation, private room, wear masks, etc.).	◆ These procedures reduce the number of vector-transmissible microorganisms.
	◆ Keep supplies for the client (e.g., paper cups, straws, dressing materials, gloves) separate from supplies for other clients.	◆ Separation of these supplies limits the potential for cross-contamination infection.
	◆ Limit the number of care personnel entering the client's room.	◆ This precaution decreases the client's exposure to nonself microorganisms.
	◆ Have the client maintained in a private room.	◆ Isolation reduces traffic and exposure to nonself microorganisms.
	◆ Limit visitors to healthy adults.	◆ This precaution prevents transmission of microorganisms by small children who may incubate microorganisms and inadvertently transmit them to the client by not adhering to infection control procedures.
	◆ Reduce exposure to environmental microorganisms by eliminating raw fruits and vegetables in the client's diet and by not having standing water in the client's room (e.g., remove vases, humidifiers, and water games).	◆ These measures prevent contact with potentially harmful microorganisms.
	◆ Clean the client's room at least once per day.	◆ A clean environment inhibits proliferation of environmental microorganisms.
The client will remain free from auto-contamination–induced infection. ◆ Complies with prescribed hygiene measures. ◆ Maintains a core body temperature of < 100° F (38° C). ◆ Does not have pathogenic organisms in cultures of blood, urine, or wound drainage.	◆ Instruct or assist the client with daily bathing using antimicrobial soap.	◆ Antisepsis reduces microorganisms on skin surfaces.
	◆ Touch the client gently to avoid injuring the skin.	◆ Keeping the skin intact prevents new portals of entry for microorganisms.
	◆ Instruct and assist the client to perform oral hygiene every 4 hours, including the use of antimicrobial rinses, mouth swabs, and moisturizing rinses.	◆ Proper hygiene reduces the number of oral tract microorganisms.
	◆ Change IV tubing every 48 hours.	◆ Fresh tubing reduces the risk for contamination.
	◆ Prevent rectal trauma by initiating a bowel program including stool softeners and laxatives and sitz baths.	◆ Preventing constipation reduces intestinal stasis and bacterial overgrowth.

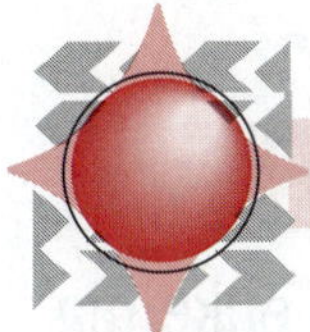

CLIENT CARE PLAN

The Client with Acute Myelogenous Leukemia *Continued*

Nursing Diagnosis No. 1: High Risk for Infection related to decreased immune response

Expected Outcomes	Nursing Interventions	Rationale
	♦ Change wound dressings daily, teaching the client or performing central venous catheter site care per institutional protocol.	♦ Fresh dressings reduce the number of colony-forming microorganisms at the site of a portal of entry and allows inspection of the site for signs and symptoms of infection.
	♦ Teach clients to identify signs and symptoms of infections and instruct them to inform a health care professional should any new symptom occur.	♦ Often clients are more in touch with subtle changes that occur to their own person. Involving the client can help with early detection of infection.
	♦ Avoid invasive procedures, such as injections, rectal temperatures, and urinary catheterization.	♦ Invasive procedures and trauma can disrupt mucosal linings and skin, resulting in a portal of entry for infectious organisms.
	♦ Encourage the client to cough and deep breathe; counsel regarding smoking cessation.	♦ These measures help to prevent respiratory infection.
The client will not experience septicemia ♦ Does not experience a "left shift" in white blood cell (WBC) populations. ♦ Maintains a core body temperature of <100° F (38° C). ♦ Does not have pathogenic organisms in cultures of blood, urine or wound drainage. ♦ Maintains a pulse rate and blood pressure (BP) within normal limits.	♦ Assess the client for signs and symptoms of infection. ♦ Measure oral temperature q 4 h. ♦ Inspect wound areas for redness, swelling or drainage q 8 h. ♦ Auscultate lungs q 8 h. ♦ Check urine for odor and cloudiness. ♦ Monitor pulse and BP q 4 h.	♦ These assessments identify the infectious process early so that appropriate interventions can be initiated.
	♦ Monitor the differential WBC, especially the absolute neutrophil count (ANC).	♦ These values determine the client's risk for infection and indicate a return of immune function.
	♦ If symptoms of infection are present, notify the physician immediately and be prepared to:	♦ Appropriate treatment can be instituted:
	♦ Obtain blood specimens through the venous access device and the peripheral vein before antibiotic therapy is initiated.	♦ It is important to determine whether microorganisms are present in the blood and whether the venous access device is the source of contamination.
	♦ Obtain specimens for culture of open lesions, urine, and sputum.	♦ It is important to determine the origin of the infection and to identify the infecting organism.
	♦ Administer prescribed antibiotic, antifungal, and/or antiviral therapy.	♦ These therapeutic measures limit proliferation of microorganisms within the client and prevent progression to sepsis.

Continued on following page

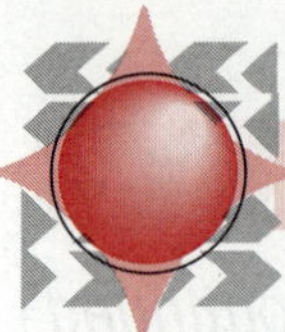

CLIENT CARE PLAN

The Client with Acute Myelogenous Leukemia

Nursing Diagnosis No. 2: High Risk for Injury related to excessive bleeding secondary to thrombocytopenia

Expected Outcomes	Nursing Interventions	Rationale
The client will not experience injury. ♦ Has intact skin and mucous membranes. ♦ Manifests no bruising or petechiae. ♦ Does not participate in activities that increase the risk for falls and other injuries.	♦ Handle the client gently.	♦ Gentle handling prevents trauma to sensitive tissues.
	♦ Use soft-bristle toothbrush or sponge tooth cleaners. Avoid dental floss.	♦ It is important to prevent damage to oral mucous membranes.
	♦ Avoid intravenous, intramuscular, and subcutaneous injections.	♦ Avoiding injections prevents trauma to the skin and bleeding.
	♦ Apply firm but gentle pressure to a needlestick site for at least 10 minutes after removal of the needle.	♦ Gentle pressure prevents excessive capillary blood loss.
	♦ Offer mechanically soft foods that are cool to warm in temperature.	♦ These dietary measures avoid mucous membrane injury.
	♦ Permit the client to use only an electric razor for shaving.	♦ Electric razors reduce the risk for abrasions or lacerations.
	♦ Pad side rails and sharp corners of bed.	♦ Padding reduces the risk of contusion injuries.
	♦ Remove extra furniture from the client's room.	♦ Removing extra furniture increases the client's space and reduces the risk of bumping into environmental objects and becoming injured.
	♦ Discourage the client from engaging in activities involving the use of sharp objects (e.g., hand sewing, whittling.	♦ Eliminating sharp objects in hobbies reduces the risk of injury.
	♦ Use soft cloths, mild soap, and a light touch when bathing the client.	♦ These measures prevent abrasion injury.
	♦ Avoid dressing the client in clothing that is tight or rubs.	♦ Loose clothing reduces risk for abrasion injury.
	♦ Avoid taking blood pressures with a standard, external, inflatable cuff.	♦ It is important to prevent skin injury from cuff pressure.
	♦ Instruct the client to avoid blowing or picking the nose.	♦ It is important to minimize the risk of trauma to nasal mucous membranes.
	♦ Avoid rectal suppositories, enemas, and rectal thermometers.	♦ Rectal mucosa bleeds easily; avoiding these items prevents rectal trauma.
The client will not experience significant blood loss. ♦ Has normal hematocrit and hemoglobin values. ♦ Has no manifestation of overt bleeding from wounds or body orifices.	♦ Examine the client q 4 h for signs and symptoms of bleeding, including: ♦ Increase in abdominal girth ♦ Presence of petechiae ♦ Oozing from mucous membranes	♦ These measures help determine sites and extent of bleeding.

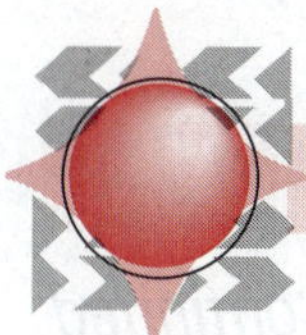

CLIENT CARE PLAN

The Client with Acute Myelogenous Leukemia *Continued*

Nursing Diagnosis No. 2: High Risk for Injury related to excessive bleeding secondary to thrombocytopenia

Expected Outcomes	Nursing Interventions	Rationale
♦ Maintains pulse rate and BP within normal limits.	♦ Increase in bruise size ♦ Drainage on dressings and around IV sites ♦ Scleral hemorrhage ♦ Persistent headaches ♦ Vaginal or rectal bleeding ♦ Epistaxis	
	♦ Examine all body fluids and excrement for the presence of overt or occult blood. ♦ Vomitus ♦ Urine ♦ Stool	
	♦ Administer ice and topical agents (e.g., Gelfoam, thrombin) to wound sites.	♦ Ice and topical agents promote blood clotting at the wound site.
	♦ When the client is menstruating, count the number of pads or tampons used and weigh each before and after use.	♦ Noting the number of pads and tampons used during menstruation can help determine the rate and amount of blood loss.
	♦ Administer oral medications to stop menses.	♦ Interrupting menstruation prevents excessive blood loss.
	♦ Instruct the client in the signs and symptoms of overt and occult hemorrhage.	♦ If clients know the signs and symptoms of overt hemorrhage, they can participate in self-care and accept responsibility in health maintenance.
	♦ Instruct the client to avoid drug products that contain aspirin and non-steroidal anti-inflammatory agents.	♦ Aspirin and NSAIDs may trigger bleeding episodes. Limiting their use can prevent excess bleeding.
	♦ Monitor laboratory values (e.g., platelet count, hematocrit, coagulation studies).	♦ Laboratory findings can pinpoint potential and actual blood loss and help to determine the need for blood product replacement therapy.
	♦ Administer blood products as ordered.	♦ To provide cells necessary for coagulation and tissue oxygenation.

Nursing Diagnosis No. 3: Fatigue related to anemia and increased energy demands

Expected Outcomes	Nursing Interventions	Rationale
The client will be able to participate in some self-care activities without becoming excessively fatigued.	♦ Assist the client in selecting food items high in protein and calories.	♦ High-protein and high-calorie foods restore nutritional balance and increase available energy substrates.

Continued on following page

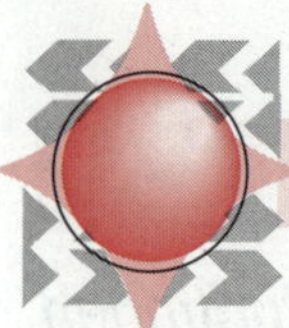

CLIENT CARE PLAN

The Client with Acute Myelogenous Leukemia *Continued*

Nursing Diagnosis No. 3: Fatigue related to anemia and increased energy demands

Expected Outcomes	Nursing Interventions	Rationale
♦ Verbalizes symptoms of mild fatigue. ♦ Performs self-care activities within limitations. ♦ Identifies alternative means of performing daily activities that require less energy than normal.	♦ Provide small meals that require little chewing.	♦ Small meals prevent the client from becoming fatigued while eating.
	♦ Administer blood products as ordered.	♦ Blood products replace red blood cells and hemoglobin, ameliorating anemia and decreasing fatigue.
	♦ Assist the client in turning and self-care activities.	♦ These measures conserve the client's energy.
	♦ Allow the client to rest between nursing interventions.	♦ Rest conserves the client's energy.
	♦ Cancel activities not essential to the client's immediate well-being.	♦ Eliminating nonessential activities conserves the client's energy.

may include vancomycin and drugs from the tetracycline and third-generation cephalosporin classes.

ANTIFUNGAL AGENTS Antifungal agents are used when a fungal infection has been diagnosed or is strongly suggested. The major systemic antifungal agents are amphotericin B, ketoconazole (Nizoral), and nystatin (Mycostatin, Nadostine♣, Nilstat).

ANTIVIRAL AGENTS Antiviral agents may be prescribed prophylactically but not until a viral infection is diagnosed. The most common systemic antiviral agent in use today is acyclovir (Oniboni, 1990).

These drugs, although helpful in combating severe infections, are associated with a wide range of serious adverse effects, especially ototoxicity and nephrotoxicity. The nurse carefully monitors clients treated with such drugs for signs of hearing impairment and renal insufficiency.

Infection Control For the nurse who is caring for leukemic clients, a major objective is to protect them from infection. Nurses must use extreme care during all nursing procedures. Frequent, thorough hand washing is of the utmost importance. Anyone with an upper respiratory infection who must enter the client's room must wear a mask. Nurses must observe strict procedures when performing dressing changes or when assisting a physician with the insertion of a central venous catheter. The nurse maintains strict aseptic technique in the care of these catheters at all times. A focus of nursing research is to determine which types of dressings are most effective in protecting the client from infection (Research Applications in Nursing).

If possible, the nurse ensures that a client is in a private room to minimize cross-contamination. Because infection in immunosuppressed people is most commonly caused by organisms that are normal inhabitants of the body, protective (reverse) isolation has been eliminated from the Centers for Disease Control and Prevention (CDC) guidelines for infection control. However, other environmental precautions still exist for clients with leukemia. For instance, no standing collections of water, such as in vases, denture cups, or humidifiers, are allowed in the client's room because they are excellent breeding grounds for microorganisms.

Some institutions prescribe a "minimal bacteria diet" for the client during the neutropenic period. Any uncooked foods, such as raw fruit and vegetables, and pepper are eliminated from the diet because they contain large numbers of microorganisms. Whether clients benefit from this diet is controversial.

In some institutions, the immunosuppressed client is in a room with a high-efficiency particulate air (HEPA) filtration or laminar air flow system. These systems decrease the number of airborne pathogens. Whether these restrictions benefit clients is also debatable (Oniboni, 1990).

The nurse constantly assesses the client for the presence of infection. This task is difficult because manifestations of infection may not be obvious in clients with leukopenia. The development of fever and the formation of pus (both indicators of infection) depend on the presence of leukocytes. Therefore, leukopenic clients may have severe infections without the presence of pus and with relatively low fevers.

The nurse monitors the client's daily complete

RESEARCH APPLICATIONS FOR NURSING

Transparent Adherent Dressings May Be a Viable Alternative for Clients Undergoing Bone Marrow Transplantation

Shivanam, J. C., McGuire, D., Freedman, S., Sharkazy, E., Bosserman, G., Larson, E., & Grouleff, P. (1991). A comparison of transparent adherent and dry gauze dressings for long-term central catheters in patients undergoing bone marrow transplant. *Oncology Nursing Forum, 18*(8), 1349–1356.

This clinical study compared the use of dry sterile gauze dressings (DSGDs) and transparent adherent dressings (TADs) at the sites of central venous catheters for incidence of infection, cost effectiveness, client comfort, and the time involved for nursing care. The study population were clients undergoing bone marrow transplantation as treatment for leukemia or lymphoma. The transparent adherent dressings were changed every 4 days, and the dry sterile gauze dressings were changed daily. Skin specimens were obtained for culture on the first day of the study, followed by five periodic cultures. No significant differences between the two dressings were found for the incidence of infection or local complications. The transparent adherent dressings were preferred by clients, caused less skin irritation, and were more cost-effective than the dry sterile gauze dressings.

Critique This randomized prospective study was well controlled. The investigators stratified the sample to examine the factors of type of transplant, client age, and length of time the central venous catheter was in place. Limitations of this study were the small size of sample subgroups and a high number of incidents in which the dressings needed to be modified because of pain, exudate, or skin irritation.

Possible nursing implications The transparent adherent dressing causes less skin irritation, is preferred by clients, costs less, and requires less nursing time to maintain. Although larger studies are needed to confirm these results, nurses should consider this dressing as a viable alternative for dressing care.

blood count (CBC) with differential white blood cell (WBC) count. The nurse inspects the oral mucosa during every nursing shift for the presence of lesions indicating fungal or viral infection. The nurse auscultates the client's lung sounds every 8 hours for the presence of crackles, wheezes, or diminished breath sounds. Each time the client voids, the nurse inspects the urine for odor and cloudiness. The nurse asks the client whether any sensation of urgency, burning, or pain is present during urination.

The nurse takes the client's vital signs at least every 4 hours to assess for the presence of fever. A temperature elevation of even 0.5° (°F or °C) above the baseline is significant for a leukopenic client and indicates the presence of an infection until proven otherwise.

Many hospital units that specialize in the care of neutropenic clients have specific protocols for antibiotic therapy if infection is suspected. Physicians are notified immediately, and specific specimens are obtained for culture. Blood for bacterial and fungal cultures is obtained from peripheral sites and from the central venous line. Urine and sputum specimens are also obtained. Specimens from open lesions are taken for culture, and chest x-ray films are made. After the specimens are obtained, the client begins a regimen of intravenous antibiotics.

SKIN CARE Skin care is important for preventing infection in the leukemic client. The skin may be the client's only intact defense. The nurse teaches ambulatory clients thorough hygiene care and encourages them to bathe daily. If the client is immobile, turning is necessary every hour and skin lubricants are applied.

RESPIRATORY CARE Respiratory care, including pulmonary hygiene, is performed every 2 to 4 hours. The nurse auscultates the lungs for the presence of crackles, wheezes, or diminished breath sounds. The nurse encourages the client to cough and deep breathe or to perform sustained maximal inhalations every hour while awake.

Bone Marrow Transplantation Bone marrow transplantation (BMT) is a relatively new technique; it has had a successful 20-year history and is now considered a standard treatment option for clients with leukemia. Even as recently as the late 1980s, clients undergoing BMT would have been seen only in major medical centers. Today, BMT units are becoming commonplace, even in community hospital settings. With long-term survival after transplantation increasing, nurses can expect to be caring for these people, if not during the actual transplantation or BMT recovery period, then during the post-transplant period in a variety of health care settings.

Bone marrow transplantation is the treatment of choice for clients with leukemia who have closely matched donors and who are experiencing temporary remission with induction therapy. Because of the successful history of BMT in clients with leukemia, this therapy is now being used for clients with lymphoma, aplastic anemia, inborn errors of metabolism, and many solid tumors (Ford & Eisenberg, 1990).

For many malignant disorders, the dose-limiting toxicity of treatments is bone marrow suppression. The aim of BMT is to rid the client of all leukemic or other malignant cells through administering high doses of chemotherapy, often in conjunction with whole body irradiation. These treatments are lethal to the bone marrow, and, without replacement of bone marrow function through transplantation, the client would die of infection or hemorrhage.

The transplanted bone marrow can be from another person (allogeneic transplantation) or from the client during a period of complete remission (autologous transplantation). Because the bone marrow is the actual site of production of leukemic cells, and because it can be difficult to ensure that all leukemic cells have been eradicated during induction therapy, the goal is that the extremely high doses of chemotherapy will destroy all of the affected marrow. The new, healthy marrow then begins the process of hematopoiesis, which results in normal, properly functioning cells and, it is hoped, a permanent cure.

Although marrow donated from a person whose human leukocyte antigens (HLA) match the client's is assumed to be disease-free, autologous marrow, even if harvested during remission, may contain abnormal cells. In some centers, the harvested autologous marrow is "purged" with chemotherapy or monoclonal antibody treatments in an effort to remove any residual leukemia cells. It is not known whether clients who receive purged marrow have better long-term responses than those who receive untreated marrow (Whedon, 1991).

Bone marrow transplantation procedures have several phases:

- Harvest
- Conditioning regimen
- Transplantation
- Engraftment
- Post-transplantation recovery

HARVEST PROCEDURE Bone marrow is harvested either from the client directly (autologous marrow) or from an HLA-matched person (allogeneic marrow). For allogeneic marrow a suitable donor is selected after family members are tested for HLA types. The most preferred transplantations are those between HLA-identical siblings, but transplantation can also be successful between those with closely matched HLA types. The chance of matching with any given sibling is 25%. Several donor registries have been formed that keep records of people who are willing to donate marrow. The goal is to provide marrow for clients who do not have a family member HLA match.

After a suitable donor is identified by tissue typing, the donor is taken to the operating room, where marrow is harvested through multiple aspirations from the iliac crests to retrieve sufficient bone marrow for the transplant. About 500 to 1000 mL of marrow is aspirated, which is approximately 3% to 5% of the donor's marrow supply (Whedon, 1991). The marrow is then filtered and may be further processed in an attempt to purge the autologous marrow of any residual cancer cells or to deplete the allogeneic marrow of T cells, which may later cause graft-versus-host disease (described later). Allogeneic marrow is transfused into the recipient immediately; autologous marrow is frozen for later use.

The nurse monitors the donor for signs and symptoms of fluid loss, assessing for complications of anesthesia and managing postoperative pain. During surgery, donors may lose a significant amount of fluid in addition to the volume of marrow donated. Donors are often hydrated with saline infusions before and immediately after surgery. Occasionally, the donor may require an infusion of packed red blood cells.

The nurse assesses the harvest sites to ensure that the dressings are dry and intact and that the donor is not bleeding excessively. Donors often experience pain in the hip region at the harvest sites. Usually this pain is managed effectively by medications with oral non–aspirin-containing analgesics, but individual differences do occur. Some donors refuse pain medication, but others require opioid analgesics for relief.

CONDITIONING REGIMEN Figure 39–2 outlines the timing and steps typically involved during bone marrow transplantation. The day the client actually receives the bone marrow is considered day T-0. Pretransplantation conditioning days are counted in reverse chronologic order relative to the transplantation day (just like the countdown to a launch of a satellite or rocket). Post-transplantation days are counted in chronologic order from day of transplantation to discharge.

Clients who are to receive the donated marrow must first undergo a conditioning regimen before transplantation. The conditioning depends on the client's diagnosis and type of transplant to be received. The conditioning regimen can serve two purposes:

- To obliterate, or "wipe out," the client's own bone marrow, thus preparing the client for optimal graft take
- To give higher than normal doses of chemotherapy and/or radiotherapy to obliterate, or wipe out, a malignancy, such as breast cancer

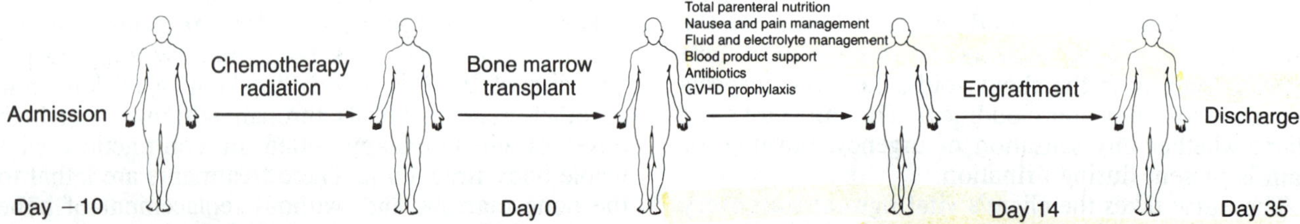

FIGURE 39–2 ◆ Timing and steps of allogeneic bone marrow transplantation. (Modified from Ford, R. [1991]. Bone marrow transplantation. In S. Baird, R. McCorkle, & M. Grant [Eds.], *Cancer nursing: A comprehensive textbook* [pp. 385–406]. Philadelphia: W. B. Saunders.)

Usually, anywhere from 5 to 10 days is required. The conditioning regimen always includes intensive chemotherapy and sometimes includes radiotherapy, usually total body irradiation (TBI). Each conditioning regimen is tailored to each client, with the client's specific disease, overall health, and previous treatment for the condition taken into account.

A typical conditioning regimen for an adult client receiving an allogenic bone marrow transplant for treatment of acute myelogenous leukemia is as follows (Workman et al., 1993):

1. Days T-7 through T-5: high-dose chemotherapy to obliterate the client's own bone marrow cells and to eradicate any leukemic cells still present in the client. Specific agents include busulfan, carmustine, cyclophosphamide, cytosine arabinoside, etoposide, and melphalan (Ford, 1991). Usually only one agent is used, and the dose is many times that used for normal chemotherapy.
2. Days T-4 through T-2: delivery of fractionated total body irradiation (smaller doses of radiation given over a period of time instead of one larger dose). The typical radiation dose for total body irradiation is 1200 rad. The client usually receives no cell-killing treatment on day T-1.

During conditioning, bone marrow and normal tissues begin to respond immediately to the chemotherapy and radiotherapy. The client experiences all the expected side effects associated with both therapies. Because the chemotherapy is administered in such high doses, the side effects are much more intense than those seen with either normal chemotherapy or radiation. These side effects include:

- Severe nausea and vomiting
- Stomatitis
- Diarrhea
- Bone marrow suppression

TRANSPLANTATION Day T-0 is bone marrow transplantation day. This day is separated from the chemotherapy conditioning days by at least 2 days to ensure that the chemotherapeutic agent has been cleared from the client and will not exert any cytotoxic effects on the transplanted bone marrow. The client should have few, if any, circulating white blood cells at this point, indicating successful conditioning.

The transplantation itself is very simple. The bone marrow is administered through the client's central line in a fashion similar to that in an ordinary blood transfusion, although blood administration tubing is not used. Usually, the marrow is infused over a 30-minute period, although it may also be administered by intravenous push directly into the central line with syringes.

ENGRAFTMENT The transfused bone marrow cells circulate only briefly in the peripheral blood. Most of the cells, especially the stems cells, find their way to the marrow-forming sites of the recipient's bones and establish residency there. The mechanism by which the donated marrow cells "home in" on the appropriate sites is not understood.

Engraftment is the key to the whole process. In order for the donated marrow to "rescue" clients after large doses of chemotherapy and/or radiotherapy wipe out their own bone marrow, the donated marrow must survive and grow in the clients' bone marrow sites. When successful, the engraftment process can take 2 to 5 weeks. Engraftment has occurred when the client's white blood cell, erythrocyte, and platelet counts begin to rise.

PREVENTION OF COMPLICATIONS The post-transplantation period is difficult. Because the client remains without any natural immunity until the donor marrow begins to proliferate and engraftment occurs, infection is a major problem. The client also has severe thrombocytopenia during this period. The nursing care requirements for these clients are virtually identical to those for clients undergoing aggressive induction therapy for acute myelogenous leukemia (AML). Helping the client to maintain hope through this long recovery period is difficult. Complications are often severe and life-threatening. The nurse should try to provide realistic hope (Research Applications for Nursing).

In addition to the problems related to the period of pancytopenia (too few circulating blood cells), other immediate hazards associated with bone marrow transplantation include:

- Failure to engraft
- Development of graft-versus-host disease (GVHD)
- Veno-occlusive disease (VOD)

Failure to Engraft. Sometimes the donated marrow fails to engraft. This possibility is discussed in advance with the client and the donor. Failure to engraft occurs more frequently among allogeneic transplant recipients than among autologous transplant recipients. The causes may be related to:

- Insufficient numbers of cells transplanted
- Attack or rejection of donor cells by residual immunologically competent recipient cells
- Infection of transplanted cells
- Biologic factors

If the transplanted bone marrow fails to engraft, the client will die unless another transplantation is attempted and is successful.

Graft-versus-Host Disease. Graft-versus-host disease (GVHD) is an immunologic event that occurs if:

- The recipient is *not* immunocompetent.
- Donor tissue has active leukocytes, especially effector T cells and T-cell precursors.

Because the recipient is totally immunosuppressed, the recipient cannot recognize the donated bone marrow cells as foreign or nonself. Instead, the im-

RESEARCH APPLICATIONS FOR NURSING

Helping Clients to Control Their Responses to Leukemia and Bone Marrow Transplantation May Help Sustain Hope

Ersek, M. (1992). The process of maintaining hope in adults undergoing bone marrow transplant for leukemia. *Oncology Nursing Forum, 19*(6), 883–889.

This qualitative study explored how leukemic clients maintain hope while undergoing bone marrow transplantation. Ten men and women were interviewed three times, once before and twice after bone marrow transplantation. Two major themes emerged. The first theme was "dealing with it," or how clients confronted the negative possibilities of their illness. The second theme was "keeping it in its place," or how the clients controlled their responses to the therapy and the illness. Clients who believed themselves to be hopeful spent more time detailing the process of keeping it in its place than with the process of dealing with it. Successful strategies used by clients in the second theme included viewing the situation as a challenge, keeping distracted, focusing on loved ones, joking about the illness, and setting long-term goals.

Critique The sample size was small, and the composition of the sample population was homogeneous, limiting the generalizability of the results to clients of other races and educational levels. Only clients who viewed themselves as "hopeful" participated in the study.

Possible nursing implications Nurses may be able to foster hope in clients who are facing life-threatening illnesses by helping them focus on strategies that allow them to keep it in its place rather than deal with it. Although the strategies revealed by this study may be appropriate, nurses should encourage clients to develop personal strategies that work for them.

munocompetent cells of the donated marrow recognize the client's (recipient) cells, tissues, and organs as foreign and mount an immune offense against them; the graft is actually trying to attack the host.

Although all host tissues can be attacked and harmed, the tissues that most commonly manifest symptoms of this damage are the skin, the gastrointestinal tract, and the liver. Approximately 30% to 70% of all allogeneic bone marrow transplant recipients experience some degree of GVHD, and more than 15% of the clients who experience GVHD die from its complications (Whedon, 1991). The presence of GVHD indicates that the transplanted cells are competent and have successfully engrafted.

Clients with GVHD are managed with immunosuppressive agents and support of the systems sustaining the heaviest damage. Care is taken to avoid suppressing the new immune system to the extent that either the client becomes more susceptible to infection or the transplanted cells stop engrafting (Vogelsand & Wagner, 1990).

Veno-occlusive Disease. Veno-occlusive disease (VOD) involves occlusion of the hepatic venules by thrombosis and phlebitis. This condition occurs in up to 20% of the clients who receive a bone marrow transplant, and symptoms usually occur within the first 30 days after transplantation. Clients who have received high doses of chemotherapy, especially alkylating agents, are at risk for life-threatening hepatic complications. Clinical signs include:

- Jaundice
- Pain in the right upper quadrant
- Ascites (fluid accumulating in the abdomen)
- Weight gain
- Hepatomegaly

Because there is no known way of opening the hepatic vessels, treatment is supportive. Fluid management is crucial. Early detection enhances the chances of client survival. The nurse assesses the client daily for weight gain, fluid accumulation, increases in abdominal girth, and hepatomegaly (Grandt, 1989).

HIGH RISK FOR INJURY

Because normal bone marrow production is severely limited in clients with acute myelogenous leukemia (AML), the number of circulating platelets is severely diminished, creating a condition of thrombocytopenia. This condition puts the client with AML at a greatly increased risk for excessive bleeding in response to minimal trauma.

PLANNING: CLIENT GOALS The goal is that the client will remain free from bleeding.

INTERVENTIONS As a result of chemotherapy-induced pancytopenia, the client's platelet count is decreased. During the period of greatest bone marrow suppression (the nadir), the platelet count may be extremely low ($<10,000/mm^3$). The client is at great risk for bleeding once the platelet count falls below $50,000/mm^3$, and spontaneous bleeding frequently occurs when the platelet count is lower than 20,000 (Erickson, 1990). The nurse's major objectives are to protect the client from situations that could lead to bleeding and to closely monitor the amount of bleeding that is occurring.

The nurse assesses the client frequently for evidence of bleeding, in the form of oozing, confluent ecchymoses, petechiae, or purpura. All stools, urine, nasogastric drainage, and vomitus are examined visually for the appearance of blood and are tested for occult blood. The nurse measures any blood loss as accurately as possible. The nurse measures the client's abdominal girth during every nursing shift. Increases in abdominal girth can indicate internal hemorrhage. Bleeding precautions are instituted (Chart 39–9).

The nurse monitors laboratory values daily. The complete blood count (CBC) results are reviewed daily to determine the client's risk for bleeding as well as to determine whether actual blood loss has occurred. Clients with a platelet count below 20,000/mm^3 may need a platelet transfusion. For clients with severe blood loss, packed red blood cells may be ordered (see Transfusion Therapy later).

FATIGUE

Because normal bone marrow production is severely limited in clients with acute myelogenous leukemia (AML), the number of circulating erythrocytes is severely diminished, creating a condition of anemia, leading to fatigue. Because leukemic cells tend to have higher rates of metabolism and greater utilization of oxygen, the anemic client with leukemia is at risk for severe fatigue.

CHART 39–9

Nursing Care Highlight ◆ Bleeding Precautions

- Handle the client gently.
- Use a lift sheet when moving and positioning in bed.
- Avoid intramuscular injections and venipunctures.
- When injections or venipunctures are necessary, use the smallest-gauge needle for the task.
- Apply firm pressure to the needle stick site for 10 minutes or until the site no longer oozes blood.
- Apply ice to areas of trauma.
- Test all urine and stool for the presence of occult blood.
- Observe IV sites every 2 hours for bleeding.
- Avoid trauma to rectal tissues:
  - Do not take temperatures rectally.
  - Do not give enemas.
  - Administer well-lubricated suppositories with caution.
  - Advise client not to have anal intercourse.
- Measure abdominal girth daily.
- Teach the client to use an electric razor.
- Teach the client to avoid mouth trauma:
  - Use soft-bristled toothbrush or toothsponges.
  - Do not floss between teeth.
  - Avoid dental work, especially extractions.
  - Avoid hard foods.
  - Make sure that dentures fit and do not rub.
- Encourage the client not to blow the nose or insert objects into the nose.
- Teach the client to avoid contact sports.
- Teach clients to wear shoes with firm soles whenever they are ambulating.

PLANNING: CLIENT GOALS The major goals are that the client will:

- Not experience an increase in fatigue
- Show an increase in activity above baseline activity

INTERVENTIONS Interventions are aimed at the following:

- Decreasing the effects of anemia
- Conserving the client's energy expenditure

Diet Therapy Diet therapy is indirectly related to fatigue and subsequent activity intolerance. The client must ingest enough calories to meet at least basal energy requirements. Increasing the dietary intake can be difficult when the client is extremely fatigued. The nurse provides small, frequent meals that are high in protein and carbohydrates. Food items that are liquid or easy to chew require less effort to eat.

Blood Replacement Therapy Blood transfusions are sometimes indicated for clients with fatigue. Transfusions increase the blood's oxygen-carrying capacity and replace missing red blood cells (RBCs) and some coagulation factors (see Table 39–3). For the leukemic client experiencing fatigue related to anemia, packed RBCs are usually the blood component of choice. (See Transfusion Therapy for a discussion of nursing care during transfusions.)

Conservation of Energy The nurse examines the hospitalized client's schedule of prescribed and routine activities. Those activities that do not have a direct positive effect on the client's condition are assessed in terms of their usefulness to the client. If the actual or potential benefit of the activity does not outweigh its actual or potential worsening of the client's fatigue, the nurse consults with other members of the health care team about eliminating or postponing the activity. Activities that are candidates for cancellation or postponement include hair washing, physical therapy, and certain invasive diagnostic tests not required for the assessment or the treatment of current problems.

DISCHARGE PLANNING

The leukemic client is discharged to the home setting after induction chemotherapy or bone marrow transplantation. Follow-up care is provided on an outpatient basis.

HOME CARE PREPARATION

Planning for home care for the client with leukemia begins as soon as a client achieves remission. Clients may need assistance at home until their condition improves. The nurse assesses the available support mechanisms. Many clients require the services of a visiting nurse to assist with dressing changes for central venous catheters, to assist with hyperalimentation infusions, and to answer questions. Occasionally, the client may require home transfusion therapy for one or more blood components.

HEALTH TEACHING

The client and the family need to be educated about the importance of continuing therapy and appropriate medical follow-up, despite the unpleasant side effects of therapy. Many clients go home with a central venous catheter in place and require instructions about its care and maintenance. Chart 39–10 lists general guidelines for central venous catheter care at home. These guidelines may be altered depending on the home setting, assistance available, and agency policy.

Protecting the client from infection after discharge from the hospital is just as important as when the client was hospitalized. The nurse urges the client to use proper hygiene and avoid crowds or others with infections. Neither clients nor their household contacts should receive immunization with a live virus for diseases such as poliomyelitis, measles, or rubella for 1 year after transplantation. The client should continue mouth care regimens at home. The nurse emphasizes that the client should immediately notify the physician if he or she experiences any fever or other sign of infection.

Because recovery of platelets is usually slower than recovery of white blood cells, many clients return home still at risk for bleeding. The nurse reinforces the safety and bleeding precautions that were initiated in the hospital. The client should follow these precautions until the platelet count is above 50,000. The nurse instructs the client and family:

- To assess for petechiae
- To avoid trauma and sharp objects
- To apply pressure to wounds for 10 minutes
- To report any unusual symptoms, including blood in the stool or urine, or headache that does not respond to acetaminophen

CHART 39–10

Education Guide ◆ Home Care of the Central Venous Catheter

- To maintain patency, flush the catheter briskly with heparinized saline (10 U/mL) once a day and after completing infusions.
- Change the Luer lock cap on each catheter lumen weekly.
- Change the dressing every other day:
  - Use clean technique with thorough hand washing.
  - Clean the exit site with alcohol and povidone-iodine (Betadine).
  - Apply antibacterial ointment to the site.
  - Cover the site with dry sterile gauze dressing, taped securely, or with transparent adherent dressing.
- To prevent tension, always tape the catheter to yourself.
- Look for and report any signs of infection (redness, swelling, or drainage at the exit site).
- In case of a break or puncture in the catheter lumen, immediately clamp the catheter between yourself and the opening. *Notify your physician immediately.*

PSYCHOSOCIAL PREPARATION

The nurse's responsibility in psychosocial preparation of the client for discharge from the hospital is very important. A diagnosis of leukemia is a threat to the client's self-esteem and role within the family. Clients are confronted with the reality of death, and treatment causes major adjustments in the way they view themselves. The client and family experience changes in the client's body image, level of independence, and lifestyle. Some clients feel threatened by the environment, seeing everything as potentially infectious. The nurse helps the client and the family redefine priorities, understand the illness and its treatment, and find hope. The nurse makes referrals to support groups sponsored by organizations such as the American Cancer Society ("I Can Cope," "Make Today Count"), which can be enormously beneficial to both the client and the family.

HEALTH CARE RESOURCES

Clients with limited social support may need assistance at home until their strength and energy return. A home care aide may suffice for some clients, whereas a visiting nurse may be needed for other clients to reinforce teaching. The client may need equipment to facilitate activities of daily living and ambulation. In addition, financial resources are assessed by the nurse. Treatment of cancer is very expensive, and the nurse works closely with the social services department to ensure that insurance is adequate. If the client is without insurance, other sources are explored.

Because prolonged outpatient contact and follow-up will be necessary, clients will need transportation to the outpatient facility. Many local divisions of the American Cancer Society offer free transportation to clients with any form of cancer, including leukemia. The Leukemia Society of America, Inc., offers limited financial assistance for clients with leukemia, sponsors support groups, and provides several publications for clients and health care providers.

EVALUATION

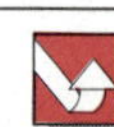

On the basis of the identified nursing diagnoses, the nurse evaluates the care of the client with leukemia. The expected outcomes may include that the client will:

- State the signs and symptoms of infection

- Know whom to contact if signs and symptoms of infection are present
- Describe the mouth care regimen
- Have minimal or no disruption in the oral mucous membranes
- Remain free from episodes of bleeding
- Maintain appropriate weight for height and body build
- Be able to participate in activities of daily living
- Recognize symptoms of fatigue and alter activity before fatigue becomes excessive
- Have no evidence of skin breakdown
- Verbalize decreased feelings of fear
- Identify role change within the family
- Verbalize increasing feelings of control of the response to the disease process and treatment regimens

Malignant Lymphoma

Although malignant lymphomas reflect abnormal proliferation of one type of leukocyte (lymphocytes), they differ from the leukemias in the degree of differentiation of the affected cells and the location of the production of these cells. Lymphomas are malignancies characterized by a proliferation of committed lymphocytes rather than the stem cell precursors (as in leukemia). This proliferation occurs not in the bone marrow but in the other lymphoid tissues scattered throughout the body, especially the lymph nodes and spleen. As such, lymphomas are actually solid tumors rather than cellular suspensions within the blood and bone marrow.

There are two major categories of lymphomas: Hodgkin's and non-Hodgkin's.

Hodgkin's Lymphoma

OVERVIEW

Hodgkin's lymphoma is a cancer that can affect any age group, although the incidence peaks first in people in their mid to late 20s with another peak in people over 50 years. Men and women are affected equally in the first group, but the disease is more prevalent in men in the older group (Carson & Callaghan, 1991).

Factors implicated as possible causes of Hodgkin's lymphoma include viral infections and previous exposure to alkylating chemical agents. This cancer usually originates in a single lymph node or a single chain of nodes. The lymphoid tissues within the node undergo malignant transformation and usually initiate some inflammatory processes at the same time. These nodes contain a specific transformed cell type, the Reed-Sternberg cell, a characteristic marker of Hodgkin's lymphoma. The initially localized disease first metastasizes (spreads) to other adjacent lymphoid structures and eventually invades nonlymphoid tissues.

Assessment most often reveals a greatly enlarged but painless lymph node or nodes, usually the earliest manifestation of Hodgkin's lymphoma. Clients often experience fever, malaise, and night sweats (Table 39–5). More specific clinical manifestations depend on the site (or sites) of malignancy and the extent of the disease.

COLLABORATIVE MANAGEMENT

Diagnosis and grade are established when biopsy of a node or a mass reveals the presence of Reed-Sternberg cells. After diagnosis, the client undergoes extensive staging procedures to determine the exact extent of disease (see Table 39–5). Staging has to be detailed and accurate because the treatment regimen is determined by the extent of disease. Staging procedures for Hodgkin's lymphoma include the following:

- Biopsies of distant lymph nodes
- Lymphangiography
- Computed tomography (CT) of the thorax and the abdomen
- Complete blood count
- Liver function studies
- Bilateral bone marrow biopsies

TABLE 39–5 Manifestations and Staging Criteria for Hodgkin's Lymphoma

Stage	Manifestations
Stage Ia	• Disease is confined to a single lymph node region or only one extranodal site.
Stage Ib	• Disease is confined to a single lymph node region or only one extranodal site. The client also experiences some or all of the following systemic symptoms: persistent fever, night sweats, and significant weight loss (>10%).
Stage IIa	• Disease is confined to either two or more lymph node regions on the same side of the diaphragm or contiguous extranodal sites on the same side of the diaphragm.
Stage IIb	• Disease is confined to either two or more lymph node regions on the same side of the diaphragm or contiguous extranodal sites on the same side of the diaphragm. Client also experiences some or all of the following systemic symptoms: persistent fever, night sweats, and significant weight loss (>10%).
Stage IIIa	• Disease extends to lymph node regions on both sides of the diaphragm.
Stage IIIb	• Disease extends to lymph node regions on both sides of the diaphragm. The client also experiences some or all of the following systemic symptoms: persistent fever, night sweats, and significant weight loss (>10%).
Stage IIIs	• Disease extends to lymph node regions on both sides of the diaphragm. The client also experiences some or all of the following systemic symptoms: persistent fever, night sweats, and significant weight loss (>10%). The spleen is also involved in disease.
Stage IV	• Disease has widely disseminated foci of involvement, including one or more extranodal tissues and organs.

Such great progress has been made with the treatment regimens that Hodgkin's lymphoma is now one of the most curable types of cancer. Generally, for stages I and II disease without mediastinal node involvement, the treatment of choice is extensive external radiation of involved lymph node regions. With more extensive disease, radiation coupled with an aggressive multiagent chemotherapy regimen is the most effective means of achieving a complete response. (See Chapter 26 on general care for clients receiving radiation and/or chemotherapy.)

Specific nursing management of the client undergoing treatment for Hodgkin's lymphoma focuses on the side effects of therapy, especially:

- Drug-induced pancytopenia, which results in increased risk for infection, bleeding, and anemia
- Severe nausea and vomiting
- Skin irritation and breakdown at the site of radiation
- Impaired hepatic function either by disease extension to the liver or by the multiagent chemotherapy
- Permanent sterility for male clients receiving radiation in an inverted Y pattern to the abdominopelvic region along with specific chemotherapeutic agents (clients should be informed of this side effect and given the option of storage of sperm in a sperm bank before treatment)

Non-Hodgkin's Lymphoma

OVERVIEW

Non-Hodgkin's lymphoma is the classification for all cancers originating from lymphoid tissues that are not diagnosed as Hodgkin's lymphoma. There are more than 12 subtypes of non-Hodgkin's lymphoma, including low-grade, intermediate, and high-grade.

The low-grade lymphomas usually arise from B-cell lymphocytes and generally progress slowly. Although clients with low-grade lymphomas have a longer survival, the diseases are less responsive to treatment; consequently, cures are rare.

At the other end of the spectrum are the high-grade lymphomas. These aggressive tumors are usually of mixed cellularity and have rapid doubling times. Clients with high-grade lymphomas are more responsive to chemotherapy, and the chances for long-term cure are greater.

Most non-Hodgkin's lymphomas arise from lymph nodes, but these lymphomas can originate in virtually any tissue or organ. A low-grade lymphoma can convert to a higher-grade lymphoma. Most non-Hodgkin's lymphomas occur among older adults. Definitive causes are unknown, but the following factors have been implicated:

- Viral infection
- Exposure to ionizing radiation
- Exposure to toxic chemicals

COLLABORATIVE MANAGEMENT

Because lymphomas may arise from lymphoid cells in any tissue and because the malignancy can spread to any organ, assessment reveals no specific clinical manifestations, other than lymphadenopathy, that are common to all types of lymphoma. Diagnosis is made from the histologic features apparent on biopsy specimens of any suspicious node or mass. Classification of specific lymphoma subtype is based on a complex grading of the presence or absence of surface markers, cytogenetic features, cell size, and expression of viral antigens. Staging is similar to that for Hodgkin's lymphoma (see Table 39–5).

Depending on the cell type, prognosis ranges from excellent to poor. Overall, however, clients with non-Hodgkin's lymphomas have a poorer prognosis than those with Hodgkin's lymphoma. Some types of non-Hodgkin's lymphoma run a protracted course, extending over many years, and are not treated in the early phases. However, for most types of non-Hodgkin's lymphoma, death ensues rapidly if the client is not treated. Treatment consists of radiation therapy and multiagent chemotherapy. Nursing care needs are similar to those of clients with Hodgkin's lymphoma, with additional organ-specific problems taken into account when disease is widely disseminated.

COAGULATION DISORDERS

Coagulation disorders are synonymous with bleeding disorders. Such disorders are characterized by abnormal or increased bleeding as a result of defects in one or more components regulating hemostasis. Bleeding disorders may be spontaneous or traumatic, localized or generalized, and lifelong or acquired. Bleeding disorders can originate from a defect in the hemostatic processes at the vascular level, the platelet level, or the clotting factor level. Figure 39–3 outlines the blood clotting cascades and sites where specific defects and drugs disrupt the hemostatic processes.

PLATELET DISORDERS

Platelets play a very important role in hemostasis. For both the intrinsic and extrinsic pathways, coagulation starts with platelet adhesion and formation of a platelet plug. Any condition that either diminishes the number of platelets or interferes with the ability of platelets to adhere (to one another, blood vessel walls, collagen, or fibrin threads) can be manifested as increased bleeding. Platelet disorders can be inherited, acquired, or temporarily induced by the ingestion of substances that limit platelet production or inhibit aggregation.

When the actual number of platelets is below that which is needed for normal coagulation, the condition is called *thrombocytopenia*. Thrombocytopenia may occur as a result of other conditions or treat-

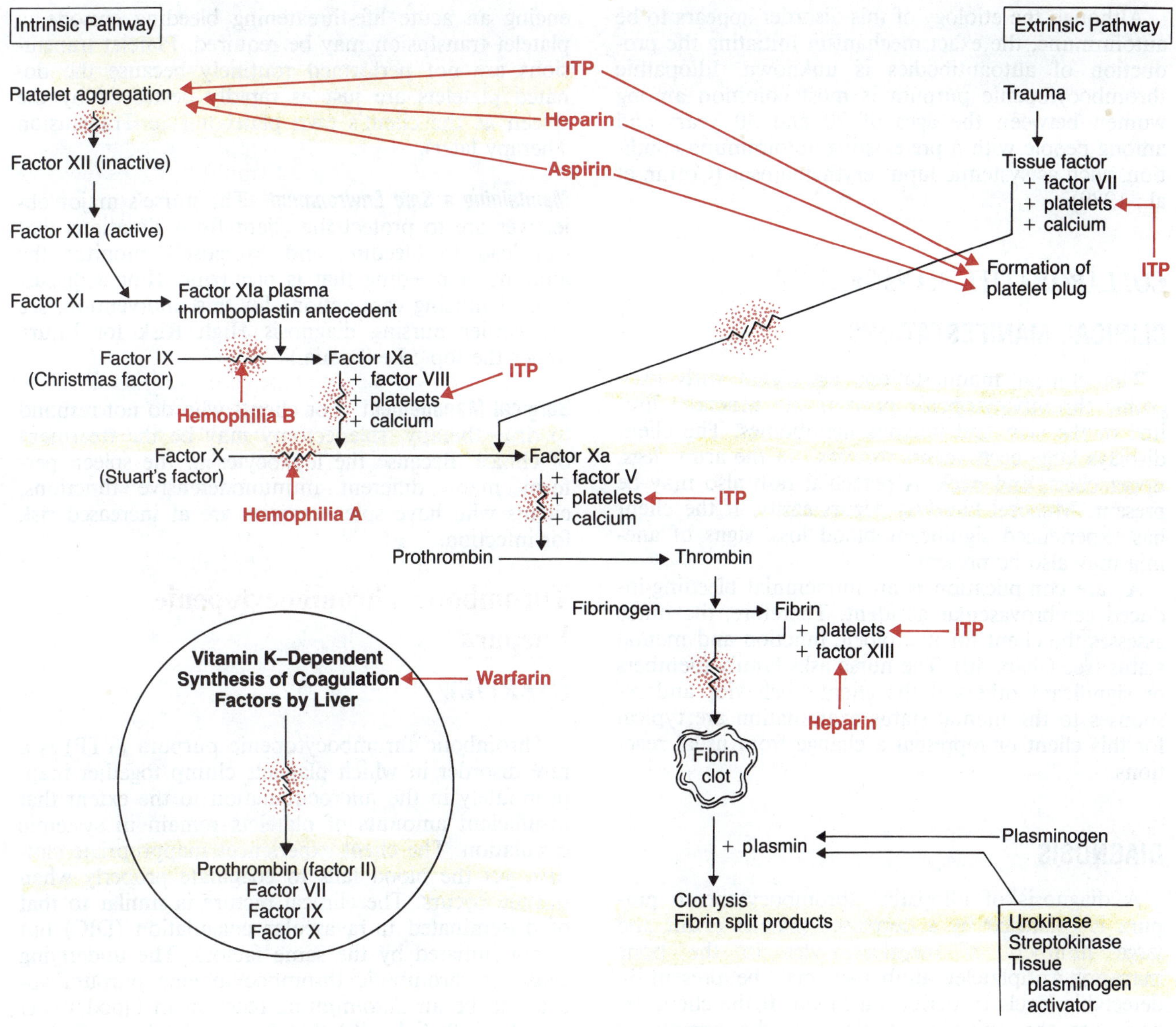

FIGURE 39-3 ◆ Sites of disruption of the coagulation mechanisms by drugs and disease.

ments that suppress general bone marrow activity. Additionally, thrombocytopenia can occur by processes that specifically limit platelet formation or increase the rate of platelet destruction. The two thrombocytopenic conditions affecting adults are autoimmune thrombocytopenic purpura and thrombotic thrombocytopenic purpura.

Autoimmune Thrombocytopenic Purpura

OVERVIEW

Before the underlying cause of autoimmune thrombocytopenic purpura was identified, this condition was known as idiopathic thrombocytopenic purpura (ITP). Although the cause is now thought to be an autoimmune reaction, the condition is still commonly known as ITP. In this condition, the total number of circulating platelets is greatly diminished, even though platelet production in the bone marrow is normal.

Clients with idiopathic thrombocytopenic purpura make an antibody directed against the surface of their own platelets (an antiplatelet antibody). This antibody coats the surface of the platelets, making them more susceptible to attraction and destruction by phagocytic leukocytes, especially macrophages (see the discussion of opsonization in Chapter 22). Because the spleen contains a large concentration of fixed macrophages and because the blood vessels of the spleen are long and tortuous, antibody-coated platelets are destroyed primarily in the spleen. When the rate of platelet destruction exceeds the rate of platelet production, the number of circulating platelets decreases and blood clotting slows.

Although the etiology of this disorder appears to be autoimmune, the exact mechanism initiating the production of autoantibodies is unknown. Idiopathic thrombocytopenic purpura is most common among women between the ages of 20 and 40 years and among people with a pre-existing autoimmune condition, such as systemic lupus erythematosus (Cotran et al., 1989).

COLLABORATIVE MANAGEMENT

CLINICAL MANIFESTATIONS

The clinical manifestations associated with idiopathic thrombocytopenic purpura are generally limited to the skin and mucous membranes. The client displays large ecchymoses (bruises) on the arms, legs, upper chest, and neck. A petechial rash also may be present. Mucosal bleeding occurs easily. If the client has experienced significant blood loss, signs of anemia may also be present.

A rare complication is an intracranial bleeding-induced cerebrovascular accident. Therefore, the nurse assesses the client for neurologic function and mental status (see Chap. 40). The nurse asks family members or significant others if the client's behavior and responses to the mental status examination are typical for this client or represent a change from usual reactions.

DIAGNOSIS

A diagnosis of idiopathic thrombocytopenic purpura is indicated by a decreased platelet count and large numbers of megakaryocytes in the bone marrow. Antiplatelet antibodies may be present in detectable levels in peripheral blood. If the client experiences any episodes of bleeding, the hematocrit and hemoglobin levels are low.

INTERVENTIONS

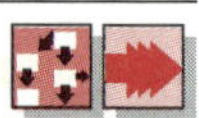

Nonsurgical Management As a result of the decreased platelet count, the client is at great risk for bleeding. Interventions include therapy for the underlying condition as well as protection of the client from trauma-induced bleeding episodes.

Drug Therapy Agents that have assisted in controlling idiopathic thrombocytopenic purpura include drugs that suppress immune function to some degree. The premise for the use of these agents is to inhibit immune system synthesis of autoantibodies directed against platelets. Such agents include corticosteroids and azathioprine. More aggressive therapy can include low doses of chemotherapeutic agents, such as the antimitotic agents and cyclophosphamide.

Blood Replacement Therapy For the client with a platelet count of less than 20,000/mm³ who is experiencing an acute life-threatening bleeding episode, a platelet transfusion may be required. Platelet transfusions are not performed routinely because the donated platelets are just as rapidly destroyed by the spleen as the client's own platelets (see Transfusion Therapy later).

Maintaining a Safe Environment The nurse's major objectives are to protect the client from situations that can lead to bleeding and to closely monitor the amount of bleeding that is occurring. (For a discussion of nursing care actions for this intervention, see the earlier nursing diagnosis High Risk for Injury under the topic Leukemia.)

Surgical Management For clients who do not respond to drug therapy, splenectomy may be the treatment of choice. Because the leukocytes in the spleen perform many different immunodefensive functions, clients who have splenectomies are at increased risk for infection.

Thrombotic Thrombocytopenic Purpura

OVERVIEW

Thrombotic thrombocytopenic purpura (TTP) is a rare disorder in which platelets clump together inappropriately in the microcirculation to the extent that insufficient amounts of platelets remain in systemic circulation. The client experiences inappropriate clotting, yet the blood fails to coagulate properly when trauma occurs. The clinical picture is similar to that of disseminated intravascular coagulation (DIC) but is not initiated by the same factors. The underlying cause of thrombotic thrombocytopenic purpura appears to be an autoimmune reaction in blood vessel cells (endothelial cells) that makes platelets aggregate in the microcirculation.

COLLABORATIVE MANAGEMENT

The focus of treatment for clients with thrombotic thrombocytopenic purpura rests with inhibiting the inappropriate platelet aggregation and with disrupting the underlying autoimmune process. Immunosuppressive therapy reduces the intensity of this disorder. Interventions to inhibit platelet aggregation include plasma exchange therapy and the administration of platelet aggregation inhibitors, such as aspirin, alprostadil (Prostin), and plicamycin.

CLOTTING FACTOR DISORDERS

Bleeding disorders can result from a clotting factor defect. Defects may include:

- The inability to synthesize a specific clotting factor
- Synthesis of insufficient quantities of a clotting factor
- Synthesis of a less active form of a clotting factor

Most clotting factor disorders are congenitally transmitted gene abnormalities of one clotting factor. The few acquired clotting factor disorders are related to the inability to synthesize many of the clotting factors at the same time as a result of liver damage or an insufficiency of clotting cofactors and precursor products. Common congenital disorders that result in defects at the clotting factor level include the hemophilias and von Willebrand's disease. Disseminated intravascular coagulation (DIC) may be considered an acquired clotting disorder, but it is more closely associated with the clinical presentation of sepsis-induced distributive shock (see Chap. 36).

Hemophilia

OVERVIEW

Hemophilia comprises several hereditary bleeding disorders resulting from deficiencies of specific clotting factors. Hemophilia A (classic hemophilia) results from a deficiency of factor VIII. It accounts for 80% of the cases of hemophilia. Hemophilia B (Christmas disease) is a deficiency of factor IX and accounts for 20% of the cases.

The incidence is 1 in 10,000 (Cotran et al., 1989). Hemophilia is an X-linked recessive trait. Female carriers risk transmitting the gene for hemophilia to half of their daughters (who then are carriers) and to half of their sons (who will have overt hemophilia). Hemophilia A is, with rare exceptions, a disease of men, none of whose sons will have the gene for hemophilia and all of whose daughters will be obligatory carriers of the trait (Gobel, 1990).

The bleeding disorder associated with hemophilia A is so severe that before blood transfusions were available, hemophiliacs rarely survived past the age of 3 years. With the availability of blood transfusion and factor VIII therapy, mean survival time has increased so greatly that hemophilia now is commonly seen among adult clients as well as children.

The clinical pictures of hemophilia A and B are identical. The client has abnormal bleeding in response to any trauma because of an absence or deficiency in the specific clotting factor. Hemophiliacs form platelet plugs at the bleeding site, but the clotting factor deficiency impairs the hemostatic response and the capacity to form a stable fibrin clot. This produces abnormal bleeding, which may be mild, moderate, or severe, depending on the degree of factor deficiency.

COLLABORATIVE MANAGEMENT

Assessment of the client with hemophilia reveals the following:

- Excessive hemorrhage from minor cuts or abrasions caused by the abnormal platelet function
- Joint and muscle hemorrhages that lead to disabling long-term sequelae
- A tendency to bruise easily
- Prolonged and potentially fatal postoperative hemorrhage

The laboratory test results for a true hemophiliac demonstrate a prolonged prothrombin time, a normal bleeding time, and a normal prothrombin time (Rapaport, 1987). The most common health problem associated with hemophilia is degenerating joint function resulting from chronic bleeding into the joints, especially at the hip and knee.

The bleeding problems of hemophilia A can be well managed by either regularly scheduled intravenous (IV) administration of factor VIII cryoprecipitate or intermittent administration as needed, depending on activity level and injury probability (see Transfusion Therapy). However, the cost of the cryoprecipitate is high and prohibitive for many people with hemophilia. In addition, because the precipitated clotting factors are currently derived from pooled human serum, the risk of viral contamination is present, even with the use of heat-inactivated serum. Major complications of therapy for hemophilia during the 1980s were infection with hepatitis B virus, cytomegalovirus, and the human immunodeficiency virus (HIV). Although the use of heat-inactivated serum and the elimination of HIV-positive donor serum from the pool have reduced these risks, they have not yet been eliminated. New techniques for mass producing factor VIII may lead to uncontaminated and less expensive sources of this vital substance.

TRANSFUSION THERAPY

Any component of the blood may be removed from one person and transfused into another person for the benefit of the recipient. Components may be transfused individually or collectively with varying degrees of benefit to the recipient.

Nursing actions during transfusions are aimed largely at prevention or early recognition of adverse transfusion reactions. Preparation of the client for transfusion therapy is imperative, and the blood product administration procedure for the institution should be carefully followed. Before administering any blood product to a client, the nurse reads the agency's policies and procedures governing this activity. The information contained in Chart 39–11 is a general guideline.

Legally, a physician's order is needed to administer blood or its components. The order specifies the type of component to be delivered, the volume to be transfused, and any special conditions the physician judges to be important. The nurse verifies the order for accuracy and completeness. The nurse also evaluates the need for transfusion, considering both the client's clinical condition and the laboratory values. In many hospitals, a separate consent form must be obtained for the administration of blood products before a transfusion is performed.

CHART 39–11

Nursing Care Highlight ◆ Guidelines for Transfusion Therapy

Nursing Actions	Rationale
Prior to Infusion	
1. Assess laboratory values.	• Many institutions have specific guidelines for blood product transfusions (i.e., platelet count <20,000 or hemoglobin <8.0).
2. Verify the medical order.	• Legally, a physician's order is required for transfusions. The order should state the type of product, dose, and transfusion time.
3. Assess the client's vital signs, urine output, skin color, and history of transfusion reactions.	• Determine whether the client can tolerate infusion. Baseline information may be needed to help identify transfusion reactions.
4. Obtain venous access. Use a central line or 19-gauge needle if possible.	• The larger-bore needle allows cells to flow more easily without occluding the lumen of the catheter.
5. Obtain blood products from a blood bank. Transfuse immediately.	• Once a blood product has been released from the blood bank, the product should be transfused as soon as possible. (For example, red blood cell transfusions should be completed within 4 hours of removal from refrigeration.)
6. With another registered nurse, verify the client by name and number, check blood compatibility, and note expiration time.	• Human error is the most common cause of ABO incompatibility reactions.
7. Administer the blood product using the appropriate filtered tubing.	• Filters are needed to remove aggregates and possible contaminants.
8. If the blood product needs to be diluted, use *only* normal saline solution.	• Hemolysis occurs if any other intravenous solution is used.
9. Remain with the client during the first 15 to 30 minutes of the infusion.	• Hemolytic reactions occur most often within the first 50 mL of the infusion.
10. Infuse the blood product at the ordered rate.	• Fluid overload is a potential complication of rapid infusion.
11. Monitor vital signs.	• Vital sign changes often indicate transfusion reactions.
12. When the transfusion is completed, discontinue infusion and dispose of the bag and tubing properly.	• Blood-borne pathogens may be spread inadvertently through improper disposal.
13. Document.	• The client record should indicate type of product infused, product number, volume infused, time of infusion, and any adverse reactions.

A blood specimen is obtained for cross-matching (the testing of the donor's blood and the recipient's blood for compatibility). The procedure and responsibility for obtaining this specimen are specified by hospital policy. In most hospitals, a new cross-matching specimen is required at least every 48 hours.

Because of the viscosity of blood components, a 19-gauge needle or larger is used, whenever possible, for venous access. Both Y tubes and straight tubing sets are available for blood component administration. A blood filter (approximately 170 μ) is included with component administration equipment and must be used for the transfusion of all blood products. This filter removes aggregates from the stored blood products. If the client is receiving a massive transfusion, a microaggregate filter (20 to 40 μ) may be used (Jassak & Godwin, 1991).

Normal saline is the solution of choice for administration with blood component therapy. Ringer's lactate and dextrose in water are contraindicated for administration with blood or blood products because these solutions cause either clotting or hemolysis of the blood cells. *Medications are never added to blood products.*

Before the transfusion is initiated, it is essential to determine that the blood component delivered is the correct one for the client. Two registered nurses simultaneously check the physician's order, the client's identity, and whether the hospital identification band name and number are identical to those on the blood component tag. The blood bag label, the attached tag, and the requisition slip are examined to ensure that the ABO and Rh types are compatible.

The nurse takes the client's vital signs, including temperature, immediately before initiating the transfusion. Infusion begins slowly. If a severe client reaction is to occur, it usually happens with administration of the first 50 ml of blood. A nurse remains with the client for the first 15 to 30 minutes. The nurse assesses vital signs 15 minutes after initiation of the transfusion to detect signs of a transfusion reaction. If there are no signs of a reaction, the infusion rate can be increased to transfuse 1 unit in about 2 hours (depending on the client's cardiovascular status). The nurse takes the client's vital signs every ½ hour throughout the transfusion or as specified by agency policy.

Blood components without large amounts of red blood cells (RBCs) can be infused more quickly. The identification checks are the same as for RBC transfusions. Physiologic changes in elderly clients may necessitate that blood products be transfused at a slower rate. See Chart 39–12 for other nursing care needs of older clients undergoing transfusion therapy.

Types of Transfusions

RED BLOOD CELL TRANSFUSIONS

Red blood cells (RBCs) are administered to replace erythrocytes lost as a result of trauma or surgical interventions. Clients with clinical conditions that result in the destruction or abnormal maturation of RBCs may also benefit from RBC transfusions. Packed RBCs, supplied in 250-mL bags, are a concentrated source of RBCs and are the most common component administered to clients deficient in RBCs.

Blood transfusions are actually transplantations of tissue from one person to another. The donor and recipient blood must be carefully checked for compatibility in order to prevent potentially lethal reactions (Table 39–6). Compatibility is determined by two different types of antigen systems (cell surface proteins): the ABO system antigens and the Rh antigen, present on the membrane surface of red blood cells.

Red blood cell antigens are inherited from parents. For the ABO antigen system, a person inherits one of the following:

- A antigen (type A blood)
- B antigen (type B blood)
- Both A and B antigens (type AB blood)
- No antigens (type O blood)

Within the first few years of a child's life, circulating antibodies develop against the blood type antigens that were not inherited (Pavel, 1990). For example, a child with type A blood will form antigens against type B blood. A child with type O blood has not inherited either A or B antigens and will form antibodies against RBCs that contain either A or B antigens. If erythrocytes that contain a foreign antigen are infused into a recipient, the donated tissue can be recognized by the immune system of the recipient as nonself, and the client may have a reaction to the transfused products.

The mechanism of the Rh antigen system is slightly different. A person who is Rh-negative is born without the antigen and does not form antibodies unless he or she is specifically sensitized to the antigen. Sensitization can occur with RBC transfusions from an Rh-positive person or from exposure during pregnancy and birth. Once an Rh-negative person has been sensitized and antibody development has occurred, any exposure to Rh positive blood can result in a transfusion reaction. Antibody development can be prevented by administration of Rh immune globulin as soon as exposure to the Rh antigen is suspected (Pavel, 1990). People who have Rh-posi-

CHART 39–12

Nursing Focus on the Elderly ◆ Transfusion Therapy

- Assess the client's circulatory, renal, and fluid status before initiating the transfusion.
- Use no larger than a 19-gauge needle.
- Try to use blood that is less than 1 week old. (Older blood cell membranes are more fragile, break easily, and release potassium into the circulation.)
- Take vital signs (especially pulse, blood pressure, and respiratory rate) every 15 minutes throughout the transfusion. Changes in these parameters can indicate fluid overload and may also be the only indicators of adverse transfusion reactions.

Overload:

- Rapid bounding pulse
- Hypertension
- Swollen superficial veins

Transfusion reaction:

- Rapid thready pulse
- Hypotension
- Increased pallor, cyanosis
- Administer blood slowly, taking 3–4 hours for each unit of whole blood, packed red blood cells, or plasma.
- Avoid concurrent fluid administration into any other intravenous site.
- If possible, allow 2 full hours after the administration of 1 unit of blood before administering the next unit.

TABLE 39–6 Compatibility Chart for Red Blood Cell Transfusions

	Recipient			
Donor	**A**	**B**	**AB**	**O**
A	x		x	
B		x	x	
AB			x	
O	x	x	x	x

tive blood can receive an RBC transfusion from an Rh-negative donor, but Rh-negative people must not receive Rh-positive blood.

PLATELET TRANSFUSIONS

Platelets are administered to clients who have a platelet count below 20,000 mm³ and to thrombocytopenic clients who are actively bleeding or scheduled for an invasive procedure. Platelet transfusions are usually pooled from as many as ten donors. The platelet does not have to be of the same blood type as the client's. For clients who are candidates for bone marrow transplant or who require multiple platelet transfusions, single-donor platelets may be ordered. Single-donor platelets are obtained from one person. This type of donation decreases the amount of antigen exposure to the recipient and helps to prevent the formation of platelet antibodies, thus reducing the chances of allergic transfusion reactions to future platelet transfusions.

Platelet infusion bags usually have a volume of 300 mL for pooled platelets and 200 mL for single-donor platelets. Because the platelet is an easily destroyed cell, platelet transfusions are given immediately after being brought to the client's room. They are administered rapidly, usually over 15 to 30 minutes. A special transfusion set with a smaller filter and shorter tubing is used.

Standard transfusion sets are not used with platelets because the filter traps the platelets and the longer tubing increases platelet adherence to the lumen.

Additional platelet filters are available for removal of white blood cells in the platelet concentrate. These filters are connected directly to the platelet transfusion set and are used for clients who have a history of febrile reactions or who will require multiple platelet transfusions.

The nurse takes the client's vital signs before the infusion, 15 minutes after infusion is initiated, and at the completion of the infusion. The client may be premedicated with meperidine or hydrocortisone to minimize the possibility of a reaction. Clients can become febrile and experience rigors (severe chills) during transfusion of platelets, but these symptoms are not considered a true transfusion reaction. Intravenous administration of amphotericin B, an antifungal agent given to many leukemic clients, is discontinued during platelet transfusion and is not be resumed for at least 1 hour after platelet transfusion.

PLASMA TRANSFUSIONS

Historically, plasma infusions have been administered to replace blood volume. Occasionally, plasma is still used for this purpose. It is more common for plasma to be immediately frozen after donation. Freezing preserves the clotting factors, and the plasma can then be used for clients with clotting disorders. Fresh frozen plasma (FFP) is infused immediately after thawing while the clotting factors are still viable.

ABO compatibility is required for transfusion of plasma products.

The volume of the infusion bag is approximately 200 mL. The infusion takes place as rapidly as the client can tolerate, generally over 30 to 60 minutes, through a regular Y-set or straight filtered tubing (Gobel, 1990).

CRYOPRECIPITATE

Cryoprecipitate is a product derived from plasma. Clotting factors VIII and XIII, von Willebrand factor, fibronectin, and fibrinogen are precipitated from pooled plasma to produce cryoprecipitate. This highly concentrated blood product is administered to clients with clotting factor disorders. The volume is 10 to 20 mL/unit. Although cryoprecipitate can be administered as an infusion, it usually is given by IV push within 3 minutes. Dosages are individualized, and it is best if the cryoprecipitate is ABO-compatible (Gobel, 1990).

GRANULOCYTE TRANSFUSIONS

At some centers, neutropenic clients with infections receive granulocyte transfusions for replacement of white blood cells. However, this practice is highly controversial because the potential benefit to the client must be weighed against the potential severe reactions that often accompany granulocyte transfusions. The surface of granulocytes contains numerous antigens that can cause severe antibody/antigen reactions when infused into a recipient whose immune system recognizes these antigens as nonself. In addition, transfused granulocytes have a very short life span and are probably of minimal benefit to the client (see Chap. 22). There is some evidence that treatment with antibiotics alone for the infected neutropenic population results in better survival rates (Anderson & Braine, 1990).

Transcultural Consideration Although transfusion with blood products is a relatively common occurrence in acute care settings, the nurse remains sensitive to the needs of those people who view receiving the blood or blood products of others as repugnant or sinful. Approximately 800,000 Jehovah's Witnesses live in the United States (Marelli, 1994). The tenets of this religion include that receiving blood from other people or animals is the same as "consuming" blood—an action specifically denounced in the Old Testament. Devout Jehovah's Witnesses believe that to receive blood condemns them to eternal damnation. When possible, transfusion therapy with human blood products is avoided for this group. When clients are transfused with blood products against their will, the nurse shows respect for the client's distress and religious beliefs.

Some of the newer therapies for clients with anemia or hypovolemia may reduce the need for transfusion of human or animal blood products. One such therapy is the increasing use of hemoglobin substitutes, also known as "artificial blood." These agents increase the oxygen-carrying and oxygen-releasing power of the client's own blood.

Transfusion Reactions

Clients can experience four types of transfusion reactions:

- Hemolytic
- Allergic
- Febrile
- Bacterial

The nurse is vigilant to prevent serious complications through early detection and initiation of appropriate treatment.

HEMOLYTIC TRANSFUSION REACTIONS

Hemolytic transfusion reactions are caused by blood type or Rh incompatibility. When blood containing antibodies against the recipient's blood is infused, antigen-antibody complexes are formed and released into the circulation. These complexes can destroy the transfused cells and can initiate inflammatory responses in the blood vessel walls and organs of the recipient. The ensuing reaction may be mild, with fever and chills, or severe, with disseminated intravascular coagulation (DIC) and circulatory collapse. Other clinical signs include:

- Apprehension
- Headache
- Chest pain
- Low back pain
- Tachycardia
- Tachypnea
- Hypotension
- Hemoglobinuria
- A sense of impending doom

The onset of this type of reaction may be immediate or may not occur until subsequent units have been transfused.

ALLERGIC TRANSFUSION REACTIONS

Allergic transfusion reactions are most often seen in clients with a history of allergy. The client may have urticaria, itching, bronchospasm, or, occasionally, anaphylaxis. Onset of this type of reaction is usually during the transfusion or up to 24 hours after the transfusion. Clients with histories of allergy can be given buffy coat–poor or washed red blood cells in which the white blood cells and plasma are removed from the blood. This procedure minimizes the possibility of an allergic reaction.

FEBRILE TRANSFUSION REACTIONS

Febrile transfusion reactions occur most commonly in clients with antibodies directed against the transfused white blood cells, a situation seen after multiple transfusions. The recipient experiences:

- Sensations of cold
- Tachycardia
- Fever
- Hypotension
- Tachypnea

Again, the physician can order buffy coat–poor red blood cells or single-donor human leukocyte antigen (HLA)–matched platelets. Leukocyte filters may also be used to trap white blood cells and prevent their transfusion into the client.

BACTERIAL TRANSFUSION REACTIONS

Bacterial transfusion reactions are seen after transfusion of contaminated blood products. Usually, a gram-negative organism is the source because these bacteria grow rapidly in blood stored under refrigeration. Symptoms include:

- Tachycardia
- Hypotension
- Fever
- Chills
- Shock

Onset is rapid. (See Chapter 36 for care of the client experiencing sepsis-induced distributive shock.)

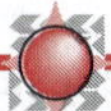

IMPLICATIONS FOR NURSING RESEARCH

The gaps in knowledge in caring for the hematologically impaired client are immense. It is a challenge to examine nursing care practices for relevance and effectiveness and creatively modify and test new and different intervention strategies. A few questions to stimulate nursing research in the area of caring for clients with hematologic disorders include:

- Does the normal skin flora of clients with neutropenia differ from the normal skin flora of clients with normal granulocyte function?
- Which cleaning techniques are effective in reducing

the colony count of the skin over the site of an implanted venous access device?
- What assessment criteria are essential for early identification of oral infections in neutropenic clients?
- Which mouth care regimens most effectively reduce pain in clients with stomatitis?
- Which mouth care regimens effectively reduce oral infections in clients with stomatitis and neutropenia?
- Is relaxation therapy more effective than guided imagery in controlling the nausea from chemotherapy?
- Does a regular exercise regimen influence immune activity in clients receiving immunosuppressive agents?
- What role does hope play in the client's coping with a potentially fatal disease?
- Which analgesics are most effective in controlling the bone pain from lymphoma?
- Which types of isolation and environmental control practices are most effective in preventing infection in neutropenic clients?

SELECTED BIBLIOGRAPHY

Adamson, T., & Erslev, A. (1990). Aplastic anemia. In W. Williams, E. Beutler, A. Erslev, & M. Lichtman (Eds.), *Hematology* (4th ed., pp. 158–172). New York: McGraw-Hill.

American Cancer Society. (1994). *Cancer facts and figures 1994.* Atlanta: Author.

Anderson, K. C., & Braine, H. G. (1990). Specialized cell component therapy. *Seminars in Oncology Nursing, 6*(2), 140–149.

Baranowski, L. (1992). Current trends in blood component therapy: The evolution of a safer, more effective product. *Journal of Intravenous Nursing, 15*(3), 136–149.

Blesch, K. S., Paice, J. A., Wickham, R., et al. (1991). Correlates of fatigue in people with breast or lung cancer. *Oncology Nursing Forum, 18*(1), 81–87.

*Bojanowski, C. (1989). Use of protocols for emergency department patients with sickle cell anemia. *Journal of Emergency Nursing, 15*(2), 83–87.

Carson, C., & Callaghan, M. (1991). Hematopoietic and immunologic cancers. In S. Baird, R. McCorkle, & M. Grant (Eds.), *Cancer nursing: A comprehensive textbook* (pp. 536–566). Philadelphia: W. B. Saunders.

Clark, J. C., & McGee, R. F. (Eds.) (1992). *Core curriculum for oncology nursing* (2nd ed.). Philadelphia: W. B. Saunders.

*Cotran, R., Kumar, V., & Robbins, S. (1989). *Robbins pathologic basis of disease* (4th ed.). Philadelphia: W. B. Saunders.

Erickson, J. (1990). Blood support for the myelosuppressed patient. *Seminars in Oncology Nursing, 6*(1), 61–66.

Ersek, M. (1992). The process of maintaining hope in adults undergoing bone marrow transplant for leukemia. *Oncology Nursing Forum, 19*(6), 883–889.

Fairbanks, V., & Beutler, E. (1990). Iron metabolism. In W. Williams, E. Beutler, A. Erslev, & M. Lichtman (Eds.), *Hematology* (4th ed., pp. 329–339). New York: McGraw-Hill.

Ford, R. (1991). Bone marrow transplantation. In S. Baird, R. McCorkle, & M. Grant (Eds.). *Cancer nursing: A comprehensive textbook.* (pp. 385–406). Philadelphia: W. B. Saunders.

Ford, R., & Eisenberg, S. (1990). Bone marrow transplant: Recent advances and nursing implications. *Nursing Clinics of North America, 25*(2), 405–422.

Gobel, B. H. (1990). Plasma and plasma derivative therapy for coagulation disorders. *Seminars in Oncology Nursing, 6*(2), 129–135.

*Grandt, N. C. (1989). Hepatic veno-occlusive disease following bone marrow transplantation. *Oncology Nursing Forum, 16*(6), 813–817.

Jassak, P. F., & Godwin, J. (1991). Blood component therapy. In S. Baird, R. McCorkle, & M. Grant (Eds). *Cancer nursing: A comprehensive textbook.* (pp. 370–384). Philadelphia: W. B. Saunders.

Jassak, P., & Riley, M. B. (1994). Autologous stem cell transplant: An overview. *Cancer Practice, 2*(2), 141–145.

Loughran, T. P., & Storb, R. (1990). Treatment of aplastic anemia. *Hematology/Oncology Clinics of North America, 4*(3), 559–575.

Maguire-Eisen, M. (1990). Diagnosis and treatment of adult acute leukemia. *Seminars in Oncology Nursing, 6*(1), 17–24.

Marelli, T. (1994). Use of a hemoglobin substitute in the anemic Jehovah's Witness patient. *Critical Care Nurse, 14*(1), 31–38.

National Blood Resource Education Program's Nursing Education Working Group. (1991). Transfusion nursing: Trends and practices for the '90s. *American Journal of Nursing, 91*(6), 42–56.

Oniboni, A. C. (1990). Infection in the neutropenic patient. *Seminars in Oncology Nursing, 6*(1), 50–60.

Packman, C., & Leddy, J. (1990). Acquired hemolytic anemia due to warm-reacting autoantibodies. In W. Williams, E. Beutler, A. Erslev, & M. Lichtman (Eds.), *Hematology* (4th ed., pp. 666–675). New York: McGraw-Hill.

Pavel, J. N. (1990). Red blood cell transfusions for anemia. *Seminars in Oncology Nursing, 6*(2), 117–122.

Peterson, K. (1992). Nursing management of autologous blood transfusion. *Journal of Intravenous Nursing, 13*(3), 128–134.

Radziewicz, R., and Schneider, S. M. (1992). Using diversional activity to enhance coping. *Cancer Nursing, 15*(4), 293–298.

*Rapaport, S. (1987). *Introduction to hematology* (2nd ed.). Philadelphia: J. B. Lippincott.

Shivanam, J. C., McGuire, D., Freedman, S., Sharkazy, E., Bosserman, G., Larson, E., & Grouleff, P. (1991). A comparison of transparent adherent and dry gauze dressings for long-term central catheters in patients undergoing bone marrow transplant. *Oncology Nursing Forum, 18*(8), 1349–1356.

United States Department of Health and Human Services (1993). *Sickle cell disease: Screening, diagnosis, management, and counseling in newborns and infants.* Rockville, MD: Agency for Health Care Policy and Research.

United States Pharmacopeial Convention, Inc. (1993). *Volume I: Drug information for the health care professional* (13th ed.). Taunton, MA: Rand McNally.

Vogelsang, G. B., & Wagner, J. E. (1990). Acute graft-versus-host disease. *Hematology/Oncology Clinics of North America, 4*(3), 625–639.

*Wethers, D., Pearson, H., & Gaston, M. (1989). Newborn screening for sickle cell disease and other hemoglobinopathies. *Pediatrics, 83*(5), 813–814.

Whedon, M. B. (1991). *Bone marrow transplantation prin-*

ciples, practice and nursing insights. Boston: Jones and Bartlett.

Williams, W., Beutler, E., Erslev, A., & Lichtman, M. (1990). *Hematology* (4th ed.). New York: McGraw-Hill.

Workman, M., Ellerhorst-Ryan, J., & Koertge, V. (1993). *Nursing care of the immunocompromised patient.* Philadelphia: W. B. Saunders.

Wujcik, D. (1990). Options for postremission therapy in acute leukemia. *Seminars in Oncology Nursing, 6*(1), 25-30.

SUGGESTED READINGS

Erickson, J. (1990). Blood support for the myelosuppressed patient. *Seminars in Oncology Nursing, 6*(1), 61-66.

This article is a good overview of the types of blood products commonly administered to immunosuppressed clients. Red blood cell transfusions and platelet transfusions are discussed in detail. The author also reviews nursing care regarding proper infusion and potential adverse reactions.

Ford, R., & Eisenberg, S. (1990). Bone marrow transplant: Recent advances and nursing implications. *Nursing Clinics of North America, 25*(2), 405-422.

The authors present an excellent discussion of bone marrow transplant therapy (BMT). Information includes indications for BMT, the different types of BMT, phases of transplantation, and potential complications of this intensive therapy. Nursing care for management of infections is outlined.

Jassak, P., & Riley, M. B. (1994). Autologous stem cell transplant: An overview. *Cancer Practice, 2*(2), 141-145.

This informational article helps the reader to understand the rationale for bone marrow transplantation. A complete description of the transplantation process is provided. The authors highlight supportive care issues, particularly those required after the client goes home.

Maguire-Eisen, M. (1990). Diagnosis and treatment of adult acute leukemia. *Seminars in Oncology Nursing, 6*(1), 17-24.

The pathophysiology of acute lymphoblastic and acute myelogenous leukemia is the focus of this article. Epidemiologic factors, diagnostic parameters, and common chemotherapeutic treatment regimens are discussed. This is a valuable article for students who have clinical experience caring for acute leukemia clients or who are considering this setting for employment.

Marelli, T. (1994). Use of a hemoglobin substitute in the anemic Jehovah's Witness patient. *Critical Care Nurse, 14*(1), 31-38.

The author uses a case report approach to present the clinical applications and limitations of Fluosol DA, a hemoglobin substitute, used to treat anemia. Jehovah's Witness views on blood transfusion are presented along with historical and physiologic information about Fluosol DA. Specific nursing needs for clients receiving hemoglobin substitutes are addressed.

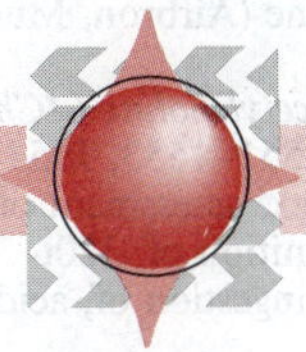

Index

Note: Page numbers in *italics* indicate illustrations; page numbers followed by t, b, and c indicate tables, boxed material, and charts, respectively.

NANDA-Approved Nursing Diagnoses

This list represents the NANDA-approved nursing diagnoses for clinical use and testing (1994).

Activity Intolerance
* Activity Intolerance, Risk for
\# Adaptive Capacity: Intracranial, Decreased
Adjustment, Impaired
Airway Clearance, Ineffective
Anxiety
* Aspiration, Risk for
Body Image Disturbance
* Body Temperature, Risk for Altered
Breastfeeding, Effective
Breastfeeding, Ineffective
Breastfeeding, Interrupted
Breathing Pattern, Ineffective
Caregiver Role Strain
* Caregiver Role Strain, Risk for
Communication, Impaired Verbal
\# Community Coping, Ineffective
\# Community Coping, Potential for Enhanced
\# Confusion, Acute
\# Confusion, Chronic
Constipation
Constipation, Colonic
Constipation, Perceived
Decisional Conflict (Specify)
Decreased Cardiac Output
Defensive Coping
Denial, Ineffective
Diarrhea
\# Disorganized Infant Behavior
\# Disorganized Infant Behavior, Risk for
Disuse Syndrome, Risk for
Diversional Activity Deficit
* Dysfunctional Ventilatory Weaning Response (DVWR)
Dysreflexia
\# Energy Field Disturbance
\# Environmental Interpretation Syndrome, Impaired
Family Coping; Compromised, Ineffective
Family Coping: Disabling, Ineffective
Family Coping: Potential for Growth
Family Processes, Altered
\# Family Processes: Alcoholism, Altered
Fatigue
Fear
Fluid Volume Deficit
* Fluid Volume Deficit, Risk for
Fluid Volume Excess
Gas Exchange, Impaired
Grieving, Anticipatory
Grieving, Dysfunctional
Growth and Development, Altered
Health Maintenance, Altered
Health Seeking Behaviors (Specify)
Home Maintenance Management, Impaired
Hopelessness
Hyperthermia
Hypothermia
Incontinence, Bowel
Incontinence, Functional
Incontinence, Reflex
Incontinence, Stress
Incontinence, Total
Incontinence, Urge
Individual Coping, Ineffective
Infant Feeding Pattern, Ineffective
* Infection, Risk for
* Injury, Risk for
Knowledge Deficit (Specify)
\# Loneliness, Risk for
\# Management of Therapeutic Regimen: Community, Ineffective
\# Management of Therapeutic Regimen: Families, Ineffective
\# Management of Therapeutic Regimen: Individual, Effective
Management of Therapeutic Regimen (Individuals), Ineffective
\# Memory, Impaired
Noncompliance (Specify)
Nutrition: Less than Body Requirements, Altered
Nutrition: More than Body Requirements, Altered
Nutrition: Potential for More than Body Requirements, Altered
Oral Mucous Membrane, Altered
\# Organized Infant Behavior, Potential for Enhanced
Pain
Pain, Chronic
Parental Role Conflict
\# Parent/Infant/Child Attachment, Risk for Altered
Parenting, Altered
* Parenting, Risk for Altered
\# Perioperative Positioning Injury, Risk for
* Peripheral Neurovascular Dysfunction, Risk for
Personal Identity Disturbance
Physical Mobility, Impaired
* Poisoning, Risk for
Post-Trauma Response
Powerlessness
Protection, Altered
Rape-Trauma Syndrome
Rape-Trauma Syndrome: Compound Reaction
Rape-Trauma Syndrome: Silent Reaction
Relocation Stress Syndrome
Role Performance, Altered
Self Care Deficit
  Bathing/Hygiene
  Dressing/Grooming
  Feeding
  Toileting
Self Esteem, Chronic Low
Self Esteem Disturbance
Self Esteem, Situational Low
* Self-Mutilation, Risk for
Sensory/Perceptual Alterations (Specify)(Visual, Auditory, Kinesthetic, Gustatory, Tactile, Olfactory)
Sexual Dysfunction
Sexuality Patterns, Altered
Skin Integrity, Impaired
* Skin Integrity, Risk for Impaired
Sleep Pattern Disturbance
Social Interaction, Impaired
Social Isolation
Spiritual Distress (distress of the human spirit)
\# Spiritual Well-Being, Potential for Enhanced
* Suffocation, Risk for
Sustain Spontaneous Ventilation, Inability to
Swallowing, Impaired
Thermoregulation, Ineffective
Thought Processes, Altered
Tissue Integrity, Impaired
Tissue Perfusion, Altered (Specify Type)(Renal, Cerebral, Cardiopulmonary, Gastrointestinal, Peripheral)
* Trauma, Risk for
Unilateral Neglect
Urinary Elimination, Altered
Urinary Retention
Violence, Risk for: Self-Directed or Directed at Others, Risk for

---

\# New diagnoses added in 1994 classified at level 1.4 using new criteria for staging.
* Diagnoses with modified label terminology in 1994. (This change was recommended by the NANDA Taxonomy Committee and adopted to remain consistent with the ICD.)